Disorders Quick Look Up

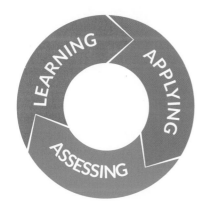
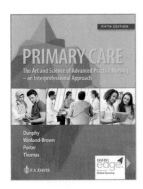
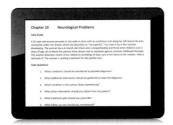
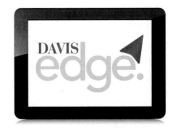

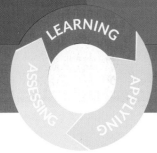
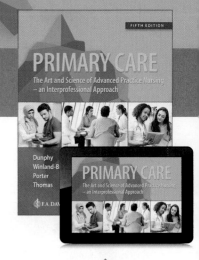

STEP #1 Build a solid foundation.

New color-coded icons help to categorize and emphasize three major areas for Advanced Practice Nurses.

An integrated eBook version of your text lets you study anytime, anywhere.

Nursing Assessment

Nursing Therapies

Nursing Perspectives

Differential Diagnosis 12.2: Pediculosis

Rash present	Atopic dermatitis (eczema)
	Bullous pemphigoid
	Burrowing insects/larvae (scabies)
	Contact dermatitis
	Dandruff
	Dermatitis herpetiformis
	Dermatographism (Darier's disease)
	Drug eruptions
	Ecthyma
	Erythroderma
	Folliculitis
	Impetigo
	Insect bites
	Lichen planus
	Malignancy (cutaneous T-cell lymphoma)
	Miliaria (heat rash)
	Neurotic excoriation
	Pityriasis rosea
	Pregnancy induced
	Prurigo nodularis
	Pyoderma (impetigo)
	Psoriasis
	Scabies
	Seborrheic dermatitis
	Tinea (capitis, corporis, pedis, cruris)
No rash pre	

Drugs Commonly Prescribed 12.2: Pediculosis

DRUG	INDICATION	ADVERSE REACTIONS AND PRESCRIBING CONSIDERATIONS
Topical		
Permethrin 1% lotion or 5% cream OTC (Nix)	Presence of lice/nits; may use on children older than 2 months	May need to reapply in 7–14 days. Use nit-remover products before application of permethrin. Apply to towel-dried, affected area; leave on 10 minutes, then wash off.
Pyrethrin 0.3% with piperonyl butoxide shampoo or gel OTC (RID, R&C shampoo)	Presence of lice/nits	May need to reapply in 7–14 days. Use shampoo for head or pubic lice, gel for body lice. Contraindicated in persons sensitive to ragweed. Apply to dry hair until wet; leave on 10 minutes, then wash off.

Differential Diagnosis boxes help you reach the specific diagnosis to determine the best treatment.

Drugs Commonly Prescribed charts summarize the key drugs used to treat a particular condition.

The Patient's Voice 10.1: Postherpetic Neuralgia

My mother died of postherpetic neuralgia (PHN).

My mother was 80 years old and had recently won the golf championship at her club. She had been a widow for 25 years and decided that she wanted to move in with me, her daughter, and her only granddaughter (age 3). We lived 4 hours away. At first she was very independent, driving around by herself and going shopping while I worked. That only lasted a few months. Then the decline began. First, she broke a wrist, which incapacitated her, and then she got pneumonia, which weakened her. Then she got "shingles" (herpes zoster), which did her in. She was diagnosed at the earliest onset of pain, yet treatment wasn't started until the vesicles erupted. She had ophthalmic herpes, so her vision was affected. She developed PHN very early, and due to the persistent pain, she became reclusive. She stopped going out, retreating to her room, and eventually wouldn't get out of bed. Nothing helped the pain. I'm convinced it was because preventive treatment wasn't started early. As she became more depressed and stayed in bed, she got weaker and weaker and just gave up. She complained of shooting pain over half of her head that was worse at night, so she'd be awake all night, and sleep all day. Nobody could help—not her primary-care provider, neurologist, ophthalmologist, psychologist, or me. She died in her sleep, and I'm convinced it was the result of PHN.

I've learned three things from this experience. First, if older persons are optimally functioning, don't move them out of their familiar supportive environment. Second, treat all cases of herpes aggressively, as you don't know who is going to develop PHN. As my mom used to say, "An ounce of prevention is worth a pound of cure." This leads to the third, probably most important lesson: get every older adult vaccinated!

The Patient's Voice highlights the important role of the Advanced Practice Nurse as a holistic practitioner through stories that illustrate how a disorder can affect patients and their families.

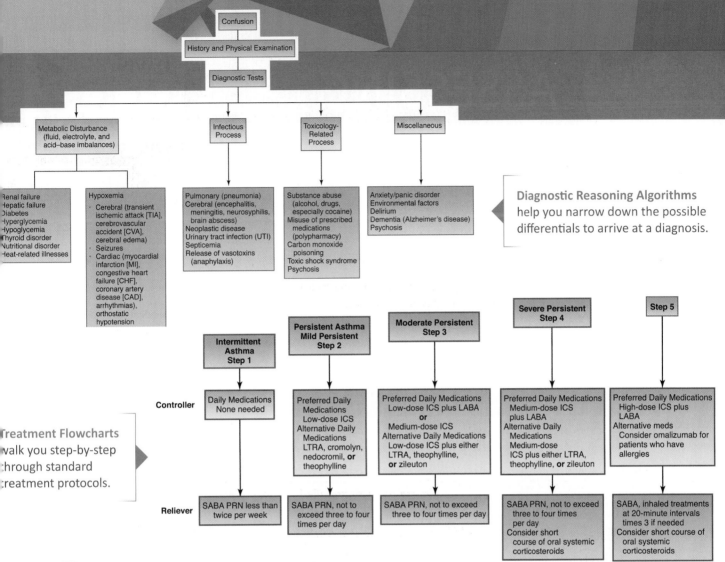

Diagnostic Reasoning Algorithms help you narrow down the possible differentials to arrive at a diagnosis.

Treatment Flowcharts walk you step-by-step through standard treatment protocols.

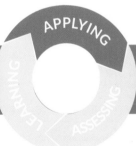

APPLYING

STEP #2

Practice in a safe environment.

Online Case Studies hone your clinical decision-making skills with real-world scenarios that challenge you to diagnose and treat patients successfully.

Chapter 10   Neurological Problems

Case Study

A 35-year-old woman presents to the walk-in clinic with an erythemic rash along her left lateral rib area, somewhat under her breast, which she describes as "very painful." You note it has a few vesicles developing. The woman has a 6-month-old infant who is breastfeeding and three other children over 3 years of age, all of whom the parents have chosen not to vaccinate against common childhood illnesses. The woman describes recent stress related to providing 24-hour care in her home to her mother, who is seriously ill. The woman is seeking treatment for the painful rash.

Case Questions

1. Which conditions should be considered as possible diagnoses?

2. What additional information should be gathered to make the diagnosis?

3. Which condition is the woman likely experiencing?

4. What other information should you obtain from the patient?

Topics include...

- Ears, Eyes, Nose & Throat Problems
- Cardiovascular Problems
- Neurological Problems
- Respiratory Problems
- Endocrine and Metabolic Problems
- Skin Problems
- Health Promotion
- Care of Older Adults
- Palliative/Chronic Pain
- Sports Assessment
- Human Trafficking
- Genetic and Genomic Assessments
- Suicide Risk Assessment
- Opioid Addiction

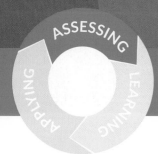

ASSESSING

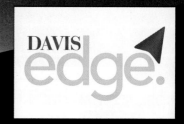

STEP #3

Study smarter, not harder.

Davis Edge is the interactive, online Q&A review platform that provides the practice you need to master Primary Care content and to improve your scores on classroom exams. Access it from a laptop, tablet, or mobile device for review and study on the go.

Quiz

Assignment 1

Questions 1. A 21-year-old man who has ingested "herbal ecstasy" containing ephedrine is agitated and tremulous. Blood pressure 230/128 mm Hg; pulse 152/min; and respirations 24/min. Sinus tachycardia is noted on cardiac monitoring. Intravenous administration of which of the following is the preferred initial therapy to reduce the blood pressure?

- ○ Acetazolamide
- ○ Adenosine
- ◉ Nifedipine
- ○ Phentolamine

Assignments are made by your instructor. Or, create your own practice quizzes as a study tool to review before an exam.

Comprehensive rationales explain why your responses are correct or incorrect. Page-specific references direct you to the relevant content in *Primary Care*.

Question 4. A 21-year-old man who has ingested "herbal ecstasy" containing ephedrine is agitated and tremulous. Blood pressure 230/128 mm Hg; pulse 152/min; and respirations 24/min. Sinus tachycardia is noted on cardiac monitoring. Intravenous administration of which of the following is the preferred initial therapy to reduce the blood pressure?

- 1. Acetazolamide
- 2. Adenosine
- ✗ • 3. Nifedipine
- ✓ 4. Phentolamine

Rationales

Option 1:	Acetazolamide is a carbonic anhydrase inhibitor diuretic that is used to prevent and treat acute high mountain sickness. It has no sympatholytic effect.
Option 2:	Adenosine is administered to patients who have paroxysmal supraventricular tachycardia. However, this agent should not be given to patients who have asthma or chronic obstructive lung disease because adenosine can precipitate acute bronchospasm.
Option 3:	Nifedipine is a dihydropyridine calcium channel blocker. It has no anti-arrhythmic effect. It is a potent vasodilator that elicits a strong reflex beta adrenergic response resulting in tachycardia. This limits its efficacy in treatment of angina pectoris unless the patient is also taking a beta adrenergic blocker. Long-acting nifedipine is commonly used to treat the patient who has isolated systolic hypertension.
Option 4:	Ephedrine and cocaine cause stimulation of the sympathetic nervous system in the brain and peripherally. Patients have hypertension, tachycardia, agitation, psychosis, and seizures. Intravenous administration of phentolamine (an alpha-adrenergic blocker) is indicated to lower blood pressure.

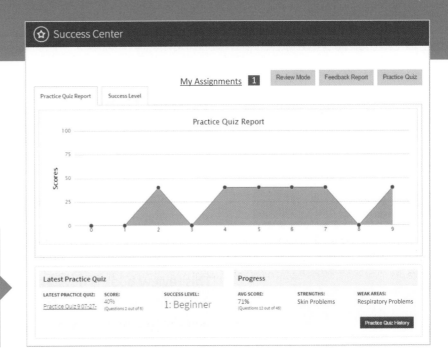

The Success Center is where you can access your quizzing assignments from your instructor, as well as receive a snapshot of your progress to identify your strengths and weaknesses.

Feedback Report

Feedback Report

Create Practice Quiz On Weak Areas | Course Topic ▾

Strengths and Weaknesses will appear for a specific course topic or concept once you have answered a minimum of 10 questions in that area. Select to view by Course Topic or Concept from the drop down box above. Choose 'Create quiz on weak areas' above to begin creating a new quiz based on all weak areas.

Course Topic	Strength / Weakness	Number of Questions Answered	Success Level	Create Quiz
Neurological Problems	● Needs More Practice	10	1: Beginner	Create Practice Quiz
Cardiovascular Problems	● Needs More Practice	25	1: Beginner	Create Practice Quiz
Gender-Related Health Problems	Strengths and Weaknesses will appear for a specific course topic or concept once you have answered a minimum of 10 questions in that area	6	1: Beginner	Create Practice Quiz

The Feedback Report drills down to show your performance in individual content areas. It's easy to create new practice quizzes that focus on your areas of weakness or to select the topics or areas of practice where you want to focus your studies.

★ ★ ★ ★ ★

"My experience with Davis Edge not only helped my scores, but my confidence as a test taker and a student. Without this powerful tool, I don't think I would be where I am today."

– Rachel O.

95%

of students surveyed received a B or higher in their class using Davis Edge.

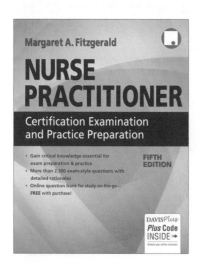
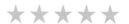
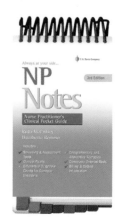
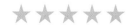

PRIMARY CARE

The Art and Science of Advanced Practice Nursing
—An Interprofessional Approach

FIFTH EDITION

PRIMARY CARE
The Art and Science of Advanced Practice Nursing
—An Interprofessional Approach

FIFTH EDITION

Lynne M. Dunphy, PhD, APRN, FNP-BC, FAAN, FAANP
Research Professor
Christine E. Lynn College of Nursing
Florida Atlantic University
Boca Raton, Florida

Jill E. Winland-Brown, EdD, APRN, FNP-BC
Professor Emeritus
Christine E. Lynn College of Nursing
Florida Atlantic University
Boca Raton, Florida
Family Nurse Practitioner
VIM/Hands Clinic
Ft. Pierce, Florida

Brian Oscar Porter, MD, PhD, MPH, MBA
Clinical Drug Development Physician-Scientist
Private Biopharmaceutical Industry
and
Medical House Officer
Veterans Affairs New Jersey Health Care System–Lyons Campus
Lyons, New Jersey

Debera J. Thomas, DNS, RN, FNP/ANP
Dean and Professor
Orvis School of Nursing
University of Nevada–Reno
Professor Emeritus
Northern Arizona University
Flagstaff, Arizona

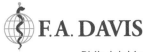

F.A. DAVIS

Philadelphia

F. A. Davis Company
1915 Arch Street
Philadelphia, PA 19103
www.fadavis.com

Copyright © 2019 by F. A. Davis Company

Printed in the United States of America

Last digit indicates print number: 10 9 8 7 6 5 4 3 2 1

Publisher: Susan Rhyner
Developmental Editor: Kathleen Scogna
Manager of Project and eProject Management: Catherine Carroll
Content Project Manager: Amanda Minutola
Design & Illustration Manager: Carolyn O'Brien

As new scientific information becomes available through basic and clinical research, recommended treatments and drug therapies undergo changes. The author(s) and publisher have done everything possible to make this book accurate, up-to-date, and in accord with accepted standards at the time of publication. The author(s), editors, and publisher are not responsible for errors or omissions or for consequences from application of the book, and make no warranty, expressed or implied, in regard to the contents of the book. Any practice described in this book should be applied by the reader in accordance with professional standards of care used in regard to the unique circumstances that may apply in each situation. The reader is advised always to check product information (package inserts) for changes and new information regarding dose and contraindications before administering any drug. Caution is especially urged when using new or infrequently ordered drugs.

Library of Congress Cataloging-in-Publication Data

Names: Dunphy, Lynne M. Hektor, editor. | Winland-Brown, Jill E., 1948-
  editor. | Porter, Brian Oscar, editor. | Thomas, Debera J., editor.
Title: Primary care : the art and science of advanced practice nursing /
  [edited by] Lynne M. Dunphy, Jill E. Winland-Brown, Brian Oscar Porter,
  Debera J. Thomas.
Other titles: Primary care (Dunphy)
Description: Fifth edition. | Philadelphia, PA : F.A. Davis Company, [2019] |
  Includes bibliographical references and index.
Identifiers: LCCN 2018039369 (print) | LCCN 2018039940 (ebook) | ISBN
  9780803695290 | ISBN 9780803667181 (hard cover)
Subjects: | MESH: Advanced Practice Nursing | Primary Care Nursing
Classification: LCC RT82.8 (ebook) | LCC RT82.8 (print) | NLM WY 128 | DDC
  610.73—dc23

LC record available at https://lccn.loc.gov/2018039369

The contents of this textbook and the independent contributions of Dr. Porter do not represent official views of Novartis, the VA, the FDA, the NIH, or any other U.S. federal government agency.

To Our Families:

To my husband, Jim, for his patience, support, and affection, which have been
ENDLESS . . .
To my parents, Joan and Arthur, for their immense love, and to my brother,
Jim, for his good humor, steadfastness, and vacation planning!

Lynne M. Dunphy

To my husband, Harvey, who is my soulmate.
To my parents, who instilled a sense of purpose in me and never let me give up on myself.
To my children: my sons, who have grown into wonderful friends—Ken, Nathan, Eddie,
and Mason—and my daughter, Cydney, for all that we've shared in the past
and look forward to in the future.

Jill E. Winland-Brown

As with all my professional endeavors, this work is ultimately for my family—my beauti-
ful and endlessly supportive wife, Carolyn; our gifted and talented sons, Mitchel and MJ;
our creative and loving daughter, Cheyanne; and our brilliant yet goofy youngest son,
Brennan. I also dedicate this work to my mother and professional inspiration,
Dr. Luz Sobong Porter, and my dear aunt, Dr. Loreto Calibo Sobong, both pioneers in
their fields, as well as the physician role models in my family—Uncle Boy, Auntie Espie,
Uncle En, and Auntie Esther.

Brian Oscar Porter

To my husband, Bob Coan, who is learning to be a rancher on our new
property outside of Reno and who keeps me grounded.
To my parents, who inspired me to believe that I could do anything.
To my dog, Miller, who makes sure I get my exercise, and my cat, Neffer Kitty,
for never failing to wake me up at 4:00 a.m. for breakfast
and start the day early!

Debera J. Thomas

Preface

We are very excited and proud to present this fifth edition of our primary care textbook, *Primary Care: The Art and Science of Advanced Practice Nursing.* Maintaining the commitment to a holistic, caring-based approach to primary care practice, our *Circle of Caring* model keeps the patient and family—and in some cases, the community—at the center of care, surrounded by a team of care providers.

Unit I, *Caring-Based Nursing: The Art,* contains five chapters that continue to provide a caring-based interprofessional approach to primary care, conceptualized by a *Circle of Caring,* presented in Chapter 1, which is further operationalized in the remainder of the text. Chapter 2 in Unit I lays out an ontological base for caring-in-practice and extends this across disciplines, Chapter 3 grounds caring-based primary care in the context of community and health promotion, and Chapter 4 reviews the basis for a caring-based, interprofessional approach to diagnosis and treatment that includes precision medicine. Chapter 5 discusses evidence-based practice, critical to providing value-based care.

Unit II, *Caring-Based Nursing: The Science,* uses the traditional system-based approach to provide the essential information necessary to provide safe and effective primary care to patients. Each body system section has chapters that begin with "Common Complaints," a symptom-based approach to clinical phenomena that lays out the associated differential diagnoses of each complaint with which a patient may present, as well as emphasizing the correct questions that a new practitioner needs to ask.

Following "Common Complaints," each section then provides chapters on the most frequently encountered of these differential diagnoses under "Common Problems." Each problem is defined, and the associated epidemiology and causes are outlined, as well as the pathophysiological processes. Dr. Brian Porter has again provided a thoughtful and in-depth update on the pathophysiology of the disorders developed within these chapters, as well as a thorough review of diagnostic processes and management plans. The addition of more of our medical and physician assistant colleagues as content experts and authors has provided a true team-based approach, new insights, and depth to the information provided.

Within each disorders-based chapter, the subjective and objective manifestations of each problem are elaborated, as well as the associated diagnostic testing that might typically be used in a comprehensive work-up. A review of potential differential diagnoses for the disorder is provided, including the underlying reasoning and critical thinking involved in reaching a specific diagnosis. This helps shape team-based treatment decisions, made in concert with patient and family preferences. Consistent with our caring model, a holistic database is established and built on the patient's voice and experience. Management strategies, including pharmacological therapy and surgical interventions, when indicated, are described, as well as complementary therapies and behavioral health interventions to provide a holistic plan of care. Follow-up and referral practices are included, along with patient education—the all-important teaching–learning component of caring-based primary care practice.

Unit III, *Caring-Based Nursing: The Practice,* includes content on palliative care and the management of chronic pain, ethical and legal issues affecting advanced practice nursing, and a substantive chapter on the business of practice. We include an update of a practical approach to psychotherapy for primary care, known as the "15-minute hour." This is especially important in an age of rising behavioral health issues and the need for integrated mind–body approaches. Finally, we include an important message for all advanced practice nurses: a chapter on caring for self.

Expanded Contributorship and Team-Based Practice

In this fifth edition, we have expanded our contributorship to include physician and physician assistant colleagues in addition to nurse practitioners, and we are pleased to embrace a truly interprofessional approach to primary care, which leads to sound, team-based practice. We have never believed that caring is the domain of any one discipline; rather we embrace caring as a mode of relating, accessible to all, and lived out between the care provider and the person seeking care.

Organizational Changes and Design Enhancements

Importantly, we made major organizational changes to both the structure and content of the text in this edition, to increase ease of readability as well as to optimize learning. Body systems in Unit II are now denoted by sections, with smaller chapters devoted to common complaints and conditions, making it easier for students to read and digest information.

Wanting to enhance the pedagogical value of all key features, color-coding has also been introduced in three major box categories: Nursing Assessments (red), Advanced Practice Nursing Therapies (yellow), and Advanced Practice Nursing Perspectives (blue), which should aid students in making connections and retaining information. As in past editions, tables, figures, and recurring displays are provided throughout the text, including drugs commonly prescribed, therapeutic procedures that a primary care clinician might be called on to perform, screening guidelines, diagnostic reasoning algorithms, treatment standards and guidelines, advanced assessment techniques, as well as sidebars for history and risk factors. Also included are "Nursing Situations" (essential case studies), along with abstracts of current nursing-based research, and anecdotes from patients drawn directly from practice experience in "The Patient's Voice." This variety of information will assist any primary care provider, regardless of discipline or training background, in establishing and implementing a holistic, caring practice base. These changes were made based on reader feedback and our own assessments, with much encouragement and concrete support from the FA Davis team.

NEW FACULTY AND STUDENT RESOURCES

With each edition of this text, we have added numerous resources to enhance student learning and provide faculty and preceptor support. We are particularly excited about the addition of the Davis Edge online quizzing system to this edition's resource package. Davis Edge is an adaptive platform that affords faculty and students access to more than 1,000 board-style questions, with complete and detailed rationales for all correct answers and incorrect distractors. Davis Edge provides faculty with a powerful assessment tool that seamlessly integrates with learning management systems and gradebooks. As students take quizzes in Davis Edge, the system provides data back to faculty as well, tracking student progress and reporting on areas of student strength and weakness (as individuals and at the cohort level) to assist with remediation. All questions in Davis Edge are completely different from those in the faculty test bank, so that quizzing and exams are separate experiences.

For students, the Davis Edge platform offers nearly endless opportunities to ensure that they comprehend and retain the information presented in chapters. The program also provides integrated access to the e-book version of the text, so students can quickly look up and refresh their knowledge base as a part of their quizzing experience.

In addition to Davis Edge, faculty resources in this edition include 48 new case studies with rationales, updated PowerPoints to support faculty lectures and course packs, and an expanded and updated test bank for faculty.

Conclusion

As long-time nurse practitioner faculty and practicing clinicians, we remain committed to providing an in-depth book with a comprehensive and holistic approach that can be used across the nurse practitioner curriculum, as well as in a variety of other primary care curricula—and that includes participation by practitioners from other disciplines, such as medicine, pharmacy, and social work. This text provides a high-level pathophysiological foundation, evidence-based diagnostic and management strategies, and a holistic plan of care that is consistent with this advanced level of practice. Although we realize that health professional students will always need supplementary information to provide the currency and occasionally depth of information required for clinical practice, the reader will be able to find a large amount of information in this comprehensive and complete text, complemented by an ever-expanding collection of ancillaries.

It is a most exciting time for primary care and advanced practice nursing. The professional nursing doctorate—the Doctor of Nursing Practice or DNP—is providing primary care practitioners of nursing with a well-grounded base of pathophysiology, diagnosis, management, and follow-up, situated in a caring-based model. With the advent of readily accessible health information—both accurate and inaccurate—within arm's reach of a smart phone, an app, or a personal computer, consumers are more informed and empowered than ever. In turn, now it is time for primary care practitioners to provide consumers with healthcare driven by an equally powerful framework—primary care practice within a *Circle of Caring*. Caring-based relationships—and the team-based, patient-centered care encapsulated in this model—are the necessary foundation to create healing environments so essential for effective primary care practice today.

Acknowledgments

There are numerous people to thank for helping this book become a reality: Susan Rhyner, Publisher—our wonderful, *patient*, always supportive, always optimistic editor, whom we have come to know well, and who is, most of all, our friend.

Amanda Minutola, our new Content Project Manager, who has had to work *very* hard to keep us all in line—and always managed to do this with professionalism and humor.

Kathleen Scogna, our Developmental Editor from afar, who was efficient, enthusiastic, and patient. Kathleen worked tirelessly to "pull it all together" and maintained her composure at all times, even the most trying!

The entire F. A. Davis production team—*all* of whom were always patient, flexible, and terrific!

All of our students, past and present, who continue to teach us as much, if not more, than we teach them!

We also acknowledge the following chapter authors of the fourth edition of this book, without whom this new edition would not have been possible:

Susan K. Chase, EdD, APRN, FNP-BC

Lauren Gallagher, MS, APRN, FNP-BC

Bette K. Idemoto, PhD, RN, ACNS-BC, CCRN

Ruth McCaffrey, DNP, APRN, FNP-BC, GNP, FAAN, FAANP

Jacqueline Rhoads, PhD, RN, CCRN, ACNP-CS

Edwin W. Schaefer, ND, APRN, FNP-BC

Terry South, MSN, APRN, NP-C

Michael Zycowicz, DNP, APRN, FNP-BC, FAANP, FAAN

And most of all, we acknowledge all our patients over the years, who taught us to "hear" their voices.

About the Authors

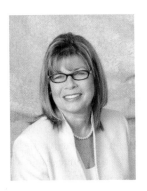

Lynne M. Dunphy, PhD, APRN, FNP-BC, FAAN, FAANP Dr. Lynne Dunphy is Research Professor at the Christine E. Lynn College of Nursing, Florida Atlantic University, Boca Raton, Florida. Dr. Dunphy was the Inaugural Routhier Chair for Practice from 2006–2016 at the College of Nursing at the University of Rhode Island, Kingston, Rhode Island. She also served as Associate Dean for External Affairs during 2012–2014. She was a Robert Wood Johnson Executive Nurse Fellow and was the founding nursing lead of the Rhode Island Action Coalition, dedicated to the implementation of the Institute of Medicine's recommendations for the Future of Nursing. Dr. Dunphy served for 4 years on the Board of the National Organization of Nurse Practitioner Faculties (NONPF) and as Co-Chair and Lead Co-chair of the American Academy of Nursing's Primary Care Expert Panel.

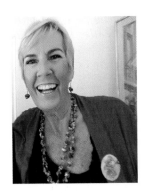

Jill E. Winland-Brown, EdD, APRN, FNP-BC Dr. Winland-Brown was born in Boston but raised in Pennsylvania. After high school, she went to Newport Hospital School of Nursing, Salve Regina College, Newport, Rhode Island, for her BSN; Boston College for her MS; and Florida Atlantic University for her EdD and post master's FNP. Her first teaching position was at the University of Rhode Island, after which she moved to Florida. She taught in the undergraduate and graduate programs at FAU and was Assistant Dean and then moved to the Northern Campus as Director. Children include his, mine, and ours, although after 37 years, all five are ours. In whatever little free time is left, her loves are the beach and tennis. Dr. Winland-Brown was also on the ANA Center for Ethics and Human Rights Advisory Board. She currently volunteers 8 hours per week as a nurse practitioner at a Volunteers in Medicine Clinic and precepts NP students.

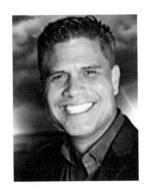

Brian Oscar Porter, MD, PhD, MPH, MBA Dr. Porter is a triple board–certified and licensed immunologist/allergist, internist, and pediatrician. After completing both his MD and PhD in immunology and microbiology at the University of Miami School of Medicine (Miami, Florida), as well as his MPH at the Harvard School of Public Health (Boston, Massachusetts), Dr. Porter completed combined residency training in Internal Medicine and Pediatrics at the Virginia Commonwealth University Medical Center (Richmond, Virginia), followed by fellowship training in Allergy and Immunology at the National Institutes of Health (Bethesda, Maryland), where he also served as an Adjunct Intramural Investigator in the Laboratory of Immunoregulation and Principal Investigator on two National Institutes of Health–based clinical and translational research protocols in primary and acquired immunodeficiency. Dr. Porter then joined the U.S. Food and Drug Administration's Center for Drug Evaluation and Research (Silver Spring, Maryland) as a Primary Reviewer and Medical Officer, before transitioning into the private pharmaceutical industry as a clinical drug development physician-scientist focusing on biological immunotherapies and global product development strategy. To complement this work, most recently Dr. Porter earned an MBA from the Northwestern University–Kellogg School of Management (Miami, Florida). Dr. Porter has held leadership roles in several biopharmaceutical companies, including Human Genome Sciences, GlaxoSmithKline, and most recently Novartis Pharmaceuticals, where he currently serves as Vice-President and Therapeutic Area Head for Autoimmunity and Skeletal Diseases* (East Hanover, New Jersey). He also continues to work actively as a clinician in the Veterans Affairs New Jersey Health Care System as a Medical House Officer* (Lyons, New Jersey). Dr. Porter credits his multidisciplinary approach to human health largely to the influence and encouragement of his mother, Dr. Luz Sobong Porter, a nurse clinician, educator, and researcher, who always involved him in her work and was one of his primary research collaborators.

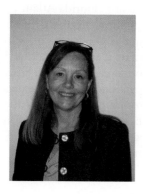

Debera J. Thomas, DNS, RN, FNP/ANP Dr. Thomas is Professor and Dean of Nursing at the Orvis School of Nursing at the University of Nevada, Reno, and a Professor Emeritus at Northern Arizona University in Flagstaff, Arizona. Her teaching career began in 1978 at Augustana Hospital School of Nursing in Chicago, Illinois. She has held numerous faculty and administrative positions at institutions including Kent State University, Case Western Reserve University, Florida Atlantic University, University of Connecticut, and Northern Arizona University. In her free time, Debera is a potter. She prefers wheel throwing and functional ceramics and works in high fire clay. On most weekends, you can find her caring for her 10 acres of gardens, vineyard, and house outside of Reno, NV.

The contents of this textbook and the independent contributions of Dr. Porter fall outside of his current employment and do not represent official views of Novartis Pharmaceuticals, the U.S. Department of Veterans Affairs, or any other U.S. federal government agency.

Contributors

Rehan Aziz, MD
Associate Professor of Psychiatry and Neurology
Rutgers University–Robert Wood Johnson Medical School
New Brunswick, New Jersey
>*Chapter 67 Mood Disorders; Chapter 69 Obsessive-Compulsive Disorders*

Ronke Babalola, MD, MPH
Assistant Professor of PsychiatryRutgers University-Robert Wood Johnson Medical School
New Brunswick, New Jersey
>*Chapter 71 Neurodevelopmental Disorders*

Barbara Beausejour, APRN, FNP-BC
The Joseph C. & Ann S. Day Medical Center
Stuart, Florida
>*Chapter 31 Inflammatory Respiratory Disorders*

Anne Boykin, PhD, RN
Founding Dean and Professor Emeritus
Florida Atlantic University
Christine E. Lynn College of Nursing
Boca Raton, Florida
>*Chapter 2 Caring and the Advanced Practice Nurse*

Susan J. Bulfin, DNP, APRN, FNP-BC
Associate Professor of Practice and DNP Program Director
Christine E. Lynn College of Nursing
Florida Atlantic University
Boca Raton, Florida
>*Chapter 1 Primary Care in the Twenty-First Century: A Circle of Caring; Chapter 46 Common Reproductive System Complaints; Chapter 67 Mood Disorders*

Rebecca Carley, MS, DNP, APRN, Adult NP
Associate Clinical Professor
University of Rhode Island
Kingston, Rhode Island
>*Chapter 82 Putting Caring Into Practice: Caring for Self*

Katherine Chadwell, DNP, MBMSc, APRN, GNP-BC
Assistant Professor
Christine E. Lynn College of Nursing Boca Raton, Florida
>*Chapter 4: The Art of Diagnosis and Treatment*

Margaret Colyar, DSN, APRN, FNP-BC, PNP-BC
Nurse Practitioner
Hannibal Clinic
Hannibal, Missouri
>*Chapter 76 Sports Physicals*

Debbie Nogueras Conner, PhD, ANP/FNP-BC, FAANP
Associate Professor and Director of Campus Health and Wellness
Chair Family Nurse Practitioner Program
Franklin University
Columbus, Ohio
>*Chapter 43 Common Urinary Complaints; Chapter 44 Urinary Tract Disorders; Chapter 45 Kidney and Bladder Disorders; Chapter 49 Prostate Disorders; Chapter 50 Penile and Testicular Disorders*

Brandi Cotton-Parker, PhD, APRN, PMHNP-BC
Psychiatric Nurse Practitioner
Gateway Healthcare, Inc.
Pawtucket, Rhode Island
>*Chapter 81 The 15-Minute Hour: Practical Approaches to Behavioral Health for Primary Care*

Mae De La Calzada-Jeanlouie, DO, MS
Attending Physician
Emergency Medicine/Medical Toxicology
Trinitas Regional Medical Center
Elizabeth, New Jersey
and
Veterans Affairs New Jersey Health Care System–East Orange Campus
East Orange, New Jersey
>*Chapter 73 Common Injuries; Chapter 74 Toxic Exposures; Chapter 75 Environmental Exposures*

Ilene Decker, PhD, RN
Retired Professor
Northern Arizona University
Flagstaff, Arizona
>*Chapter 5 Evidence-Based Practice*

Sally Doshier, EdD, MS, RN
Associate Professor
Northern Arizona University
Flagstaff, Arizona
>*Chapter 5 Evidence-Based Practice*

Dorothy J. Dunn, PhD, APRN, FNP-BC, AHN-BC
Associate Professor
Northern Arizona University
Flagstaff, Arizona
>*Chapter 3 Health Promotion; Chapter 5 Evidence-Based Practice*

Lynne M. Dunphy, PhD, APRN, FNP-BC, FAAN, FAANP
Research Professor
Christine E. Lynn College of Nursing
Florida Atlantic University
Boca Raton, Florida
> *Chapter 1 Primary Care in the Twenty-First Century: A Circle of Caring; Chapter 4 The Art and Diagnosis of Treatment; Chapter 18 Common Eye Complaints; Chapter 19 Lid and Conjunctival Pathology; Chapter 20 Visual Disturbances and Impaired Vision; Chapter 21 Common Ear, Nose, and Throat Complaints; Chapter 22 Hearing and Balance Disorders; Chapter 23 Inflammatory and Infectious Disorders of the Ear; Chapter 24 Inflammatory and Infectious Disorders of the Nose, Sinuses, Mouth, and Throat; Chapter 25 Epistaxis; Chapter 26 Temporomandibular Disorders; Chapter 27 Dysphonia; Chapter 52 Common Musculoskeletal Complaints; Chapter 53 Spinal Disorders; Chapter 54 Soft-Tissue Disorders; Chapter 55 Osteoarthritis and Osteoporosis; Chapter 64 Common Psychosocial Complaints; Chapter 65 Substance Use Disorders; Chapter 66 Schizophrenia Spectrum Disorders; Chapter 67 Mood Disorders; Chapter 68 Anxiety, Stress, and Trauma-Related Disorders; Chapter 69 Obsessive-Compulsive Disorders; Chapter 70 Behavioral Disorders Related to Physical/Physiological Disturbances; Chapter 71 Neurodevelopmental Disorders; Chapter 76 Sports Physicals; Chapter 77 Primary Care of Older Adults; Chapter 81 The 15-Minute Hour: Practical Approaches to Behavioral Health for Primary Care*

Jacinta D. Elder, MD, MSc
Staff Physician
Internal Medicine, Functional, and Integrative Medicine
JenCare Senior Medical Centers
Louisville, Kentucky
> *Chapter 60 Common Hematological and Immunological Complaints; Chapter 61 Hematological Disorders*

Susan Garnett, MSN, APRN, FNP-BC
> *Chapter 11 Common Skin Complaints; Chapter 13 Fungal Skin Infections; Chapter 14 Bacterial Skin Infections; Chapter 15 Viral Skin Infections*

Angela K. Golden, DNP, APRN, FNP-C, FAANP
Former President
American Association of Nurse Practitioners
Owner
NP from Home, LLC
Munds Park, Arizona
> *Chapter 58 Diabetes Mellitus*

Kimberly Rae Gould, DNP, RN, FNP-BC
Assistant Clinical Professor
Northern Arizona University
Flagstaff, Arizona
> *Chapter 48 Vaginal, Uterine, and Ovarian Disorders; Chapter 51 Sexually Transmitted Infections*

Kim S. Griswold, MD, MPH, AS, RN
Department of Family Medicine
State University of New York (SUNY) at Buffalo
Buffalo, New York
> *Chapter 65 Substance Use Disorders*

Joseph Holbrook, BS, BSN, MS, APRN
Nurse Practitioner
VIM/Hands Clinic
Ft. Pierce, Florida
xPress Urgent Care
Port St. Lucie, Florida
> *Chapter 72 Common Urgent Care Complaints; Chapter 73 Common Injuries; Chapter 75 Environmental Exposures*

Mary Hooshmand, MSN, PhD, RN
Associate Dean and Assistant Professor
School of Nursing
University of Miami
Coral Gables, Florida
> *Chapter 4 The Art of Diagnosis and Treatment*

Sarah Horn, MD
Neurologist
Philadelphia, Pennsylvania
> *Chapter 6 Common Neurologic Complaints; Chapter 7 Seizure Disorders; Chapter 8 Degenerative Disorders; Chapter 9 Cerebrovascular Accident (Stroke); Chapter 10 Infectious and Inflammatory Neurological Disorders*

Kathryn B. Keller, PhD, RN, CNE
Professor
Christine E. Lynn College of Nursing
Boca Raton, Florida
> *Chapter 34 Common Cardiovascular Complaints; Chapter 35 Cardiac and Associated Risk Disorders; Chapter 36 Dysrhythmias and Valvular Disorders; Chapter 37 Disorders of the Vascular System*

Michael B. Keller, MD
Department of Medicine
Johns Hopkins Hospital and School of Medicine
Baltimore, Maryland
> *Chapter 6 Common Neurologic Complaints; Chapter 36 Dysrhythmias and Valvular Disorders; Chapter 37 Disorders of the Vascular System*

Beth M. King, PhD, APRN, PMHCNS-BC, PMHNP-BC
Associate Professor
Christine E. Lynn College of Nursing
Florida Atlantic University Boca Raton, Florida
> *Chapter 64 Common Psychosocial Complaints*

Jason V. Lambrese, MD
Child and Adolescent Psychiatrist
Cleveland Clinic
Cleveland, Ohio
> *Chapter 70 Behavioral Disorders Related to Physical/Physiological Disturbances; Chapter 71 Neurodevelopmental Disorders*

Mary Lavin, DNP, APRN, FNP-BC
Associate Clinical Professor
University of Rhode Island
Kingston, Rhode Island
> *Chapter 82 Putting Caring Into Practice: Caring for Self*

Dianne Loomis, DNP, APRN, FNP-BC
Associate Clinical Professor
State University of New York (SUNY) at Buffalo
Buffalo, New York
    Chapter 65 Substance Use Disorders

Conor Luskin, PA-C
Physician Assistant
Rothman Institute
Sewel, New Jersey
    *Chapter 52 Common Musculoskeletal Complaints; Chapter 53
Spinal Disorders; Chapter 54 Soft-Tissue Disorders; Chapter 55
Osteoarthritis and Osteoporosis*

Donna Maheady, APRN, CPNP, EdD
Adjunct Faculty
Utica College
St. Petersburg, Florida
    Chapter 16 Dermatitis

Lori Martin-Plank, PhD, APRN, FNP-BC, GNP-BC, FAANP
Clinical Assistant Professor, College of Nursing
University of Arizona
Tucson, Arizona
    *Chapter 52 Common Musculoskeletal Complaints; Chapter 55
Osteoarthritis and Osteoporosis; Chapter 77 Primary Care of
Older Adults*

Ruth McCaffrey, DNP, APRN, FNP-BC, GNP, FAAN, FAANP
    *Chapter 18 Common Eye Complaints; Chapter 21 Common
Ear, Nose, and Throat Complaints; Chapter 22 Hearing and
Balance Disorders; Chapter 25 Epistaxis; Chapter 26 Temporo-
mandibular Disorders; Chapter 27 Dysphonia; Chapter 77
Primary Care of Older Adults; Chapter 78 Palliative Care
and Pain Management*

Eugenia Millender, PhD, RN, MS, PMHNP-BC, CDE
Associate Professor
College of Nursing
Florida State University
Tallahassee, Florida
    Chapter 68 Anxiety, Stress, and Trauma-Related Disorders

Patricia A. Pastore, MS, APRN, FNP-BC
Retired-Women's Wellness Primary Care
Veterans Administration, Western New York Health Care
System
Buffalo, New York
    Chapter 65 Substance Use Disorders

Brian Oscar Porter, MD, PhD, MPH, MBA
Clinical Drug Development Physician-Scientist
Private Biopharmaceutical Industry
and
Medical House Officer
Veterans Affairs New Jersey Health Care System–Lyons Campus
Lyons, New Jersey
    *Chapter 1 Primary Care in the Twenty-First Century: A Circle
of Caring; Chapter 11 Common Skin Complaints; Chapter 12
Parasitic Infestations; Chapter 13 Fungal Skin Infections; Chapter
14 Bacterial Skin Infections; Chapter 15 Viral Skin Infections;
Chapter 16 Dermatitis; Chapter 17 Skin Lesions; Chapter 18*
*Common Eye Complaints; Chapter 19 Lid and Conjunctival
Pathology; Chapter 20 Visual Disturbances and Impaired Vision;
Chapter 21 Common Ear, Nose, and Throat Complaints;
Chapter 22 Hearing and Balance Disorders; Chapter 23 Inflam-
matory and Infectious Disorders of the Ear; Chapter 24 Inflam-
matory and Infectious Disorders of the Nose, Sinuses, Mouth, and
Throat; Chapter 25 Epistaxis; Chapter 26 Temporomandibular
Disorders; Chapter 27 Dysphonia; Chapter 28 Common Respira-
tory Complaints; Chapter 30 Infectious Respiratory Disorders;
Chapter 31 Inflammatory Respiratory Disorders; Chapter 32
Lung Cancer; Chapter 33 Smoking Addiction; Chapter 34
Common Cardiovascular Complaints; Chapter 35 Cardiac
and Associated Risk Disorders; Chapter 36 Dysrhythmias and
Valvular Disorders; Chapter 37 Disorders of the Vascular System;
Chapter 43 Common Urinary Complaints; Chapter 44 Urinary
Tract Disorders; Chapter 45 Kidney and Bladder Disorders;
Chapter 46 Common Reproductive System Complaints;
Chapter 47 Breast Disorders; Chapter 48 Vaginal, Uterine, and
Ovarian Disorders; Chapter 49 Prostate Disorders; Chapter 50
Penile and Testicular Disorders; Chapter 51 Sexually Transmitted
Infections; Chapter 52 Common Musculoskeletal Complaints;
Chapter 53 Spinal Disorders; Chapter 56 Common Endocrine
and Metabolic Complaints; Chapter 57 Glandular Disorders;
Chapter 58 Diabetes Mellitus; Chapter 59 Metabolic Disorders;
Chapter 60 Common Hematological and Immunological
Complaints; Chapter 61 Hematological Disorders; Chapter 62
Immunological Disorders; Chapter 63 Infectious Disorders;
Chapter 72 Common Urgent Care Complaints; Chapter 73
Common Injuries; Chapter 74 Toxic Exposures; Chapter 75
Environmental Exposures*

Cathleen Provins, RN, MSN, PhD, CCRN-K, NE-BC,
ACNP-BC
Assistant Professor
Mercer University
Atlanta, Georgia
    Chapter 20 Visual Disturbances and Impaired Vision

Humberto Reinoso, PhD, FNP-BC, ENP-BC
Clinical Assistant Professor and Graduate Clinical Coordinator
Georgia Baptist College of Nursing
Mercer University
Atlanta, Georgia
    *Chapter 19 Lid and Conjunctival Pathology; Chapter 23
Inflammatory and Infectious Disorders of the Ear; Chapter 24
Inflammatory and Infectious Disorders of the Nose, Sinuses,
Mouth, and Throat; Chapter 77 Primary Care of Older Adults*

Marcella M. Rutherford, PhD, MSN, MBA, RN
Dean, College of Nursing
Nova Southeastern University
Ft. Lauderdale, Florida
    Chapter 80 The Business of Advanced Practice Nursing

Denese Sabatino, MSN, APRN, NP-C, CCRN
Advanced Registered Nurse Practitioner
Cleveland Clinic
Weston, Florida
    *Chapter 35 Cardiac and Associated Risk Disorders; Chapter 36
Dysrhythmias and Valvular Disorders; Chapter 37 Disorders of
the Vascular System*

Savina O. Schoenhofer, PhD, RN
Professor Emeritus
Alcorn State University
School of Nursing
Natchez, Mississippi
    Chapter 2 Caring and the Advanced Practice Nurse

Virginia Sheikh, MD, MHS
Medical Officer
U.S. Food and Drug Administration
Silver Spring, Maryland
    Chapter 63 Infectious Disorders

Martin T. Strassnig, MD
Associate Professor of Integrated Medical Sciences
Charles E. Schmidt College of Medicine
Florida Atlantic University
Boca Raton, Florida
    Chapter 66 Schizophrenia Spectrum Disorders

John Suen, MD
Clinical Assistant Professor
College of Medicine
Florida State University
Vero Beach, Florida
    Chapter 29 Sleep Apnea

Michael E. Thase, MD
Professor of Psychiatry
Perelman School of Medicine
University of Pennsylvania
Philadelphia, Pennsylvania
    Chapter 66 Schizophrenia Spectrum Disorders

Debera J. Thomas, DNS, RN, FNP/ANP
Family and Adult Nurse Practitioner
Dean and Professor
Orvis School of Nursing
University of Nevada Reno
Reno, Nevada
and
Professor Emeritus
Northern Arizona University
Flagstaff, Arizona
    Chapter 1 Primary Care in the Twenty-First Century: A Circle
    of Caring; Chapter 3 Health Promotion; Chapter 5 Evidence-
    Based Practice; Chapter 38 Common Abdominal Complaints;
    Chapter 39 Infectious Gastrointestinal Disorders; Chapter 40
    Gastric and Intestinal Disorders; Chapter 41 Gallbladder and
    Pancreatic Disorders; Chapter 42 Cirrhosis and Liver Failure;
    Chapter 43 Common Urinary Complaints; Chapter 44 Urinary
    Tract Disorders; Chapter 45 Kidney and Bladder Disorders;
    Chapter 46 Common Reproductive System Complaints; Chapter
    47 Breast Disorders; Chapter 48 Vaginal, Uterine, and Ovarian
    Disorders; Chapter 49 Prostate Disorders; Chapter 50 Penile and
    Testicular Disorders; Chapter 51 Sexually Transmitted Infec-
    tions; Chapter 56 Common Endocrine and Metabolic Complaints;
    Chapter 57 Glandular Disorders; Chapter 58 Diabetes Mellitus;
    Chapter 59 Metabolic Disorders

Denise Vanacore, PhD, APRN, ANP-BC, FNP, PMHNP-BC
Director of Primary & Behavioral Health Services
Frances M. Maguire School of Nursing & Health Professions
Gwynedd Mercy University
Gwynedd Valley, Pennsylvania
    Chapter 70 Behavioral Disorders Related to Physical/
    Physiological Disturbances

Patricia Vanhook, PhD, MSN, APRN, FNP-BC, FAAN,
FAANP
Associate Professor and Associate Dean
College of Nursing
East Tennessee State University
Johnson City, Tennessee
    Chapter 52 Common Musculoskeletal Complaints; Chapter 53
    Spinal Disorders; Chapter 54 Soft-Tissue Disorders; Chapter 55
    Osteoarthritis and Osteoporosis

Josie Weiss, PhD, FNP-BC, PNP-BC, FAANP
Associate Professor
College of Nursing
University of Central Florida
Orlando, Florida
    Chapter 79 Ethical and Legal Issues of a Caring-Based Practice

Timothy Wilson, DNP, APRN, FNP, PMHNP
Private Practice
Delray, Florida
    Chapter 64 Common Psychosocial Complaints

Jill E. Winland-Brown, EdD, APRN, FNP-BC
Professor and Family Nurse Practitioner
Christine E. Lynn College of Nursing
Florida Atlantic University
Boca Raton, Florida
    Chapter 1 Primary Care in the Twenty-First Century: A Circle
    of Caring; Chapter 6 Neurological Complaints; Chapter 7
    Seizure Disorders; Chapter 8 Degenerative Disorders; Chapter
    9 Cerebrovascular Accident (Stroke); Chapter 10 Infectious and
    Inflammatory Neurological Disorders; Chapter 11 Common Skin
    Complaints; Chapter 12 Parasitic Infestations; Chapter 13
    Fungal Skin Infections; Chapter 14 Bacterial Skin Infections;
    Chapter 15 Viral Skin Infections; Chapter 16 Dermatitis;
    Chapter 17 Skin Lesions; Chapter 28 Common Respiratory
    Complaints; Chapter 29 Sleep Apnea; Chapter 30 Infectious
    Respiratory Disorders; Chapter 31 Inflammatory Respiratory
    Disorders; Chapter 32 Lung Cancer; Chapter 33 Smoking
    Addiction; Chapter 34 Common Cardiovascular Complaints;
    Chapter 35 Cardiac and Associated Risk Disorders; Chapter 36
    Dysrhythmias and Valvular Disorders; Chapter 37 Disorders of
    the Vascular System; Chapter 60 Common Hematological and
    Immunological Complaints; Chapter 61 Hematological Disorders;
    Chapter 62 Immunological Disorders; Chapter 63 Infectious
    Disorders; Chapter 72 Common Urgent Care Complaints;
    Chapter 73 Common Injuries; Chapter 74 Toxic Exposures;
    Chapter 75 Environmental Exposures; Chapter 79 Ethical and
    Legal Issues of a Caring-Based Practice

Reviewers

Margaret Ackerman, DNP, AGPCNP-C
Coordinator, Adult-Gero NP program
Salem State University
Salem, Massachusetts

Debra K. Bailey, RN, FNP-BC, PhD, CDE
Associate Professor of Nursing
Colorado Mesa University
Grand Junction, Colorado

Amber A. Barnes, DNP, AARN, DP-C
Adjunct Faculty, Adult Nurse Practitioner
Rocky Mountain University of Health Professions
Provo, Utah

Teri Berry, DNP, FNP-C
Adjunct Graduate Nursing Faculty
Maryville University
St. Louis, Missouri

Cathleen Crowley-Koschnitzki, DNP, CNM, WHNP-BC, FNP-C
Associate Professor
Chamberlain College of Nursing
Downers Grove, Illinois

Mykale Elbe, DNP, FNP-BC
Assistant Professor, Coordinator of FNP program
Maryville University
St. Louis, Missouri

Lindsey Hobson, MSN, APRN, FNP-BC
Nurse Practitioner/Adjunct Faculty/Interim FNP Director
Indiana University East
Richmond, Indiana

Patricia Krauskopf, PhD, FNP-BC, FAANP
Professor & Helen Zebarth Chair in Nursing
Shenandoah University
Winchester, Virginia

Roberta McCauley, DNP, FNP-BC, NEA-BC
DNP Program Director, Graduate Nursing Department Chair
Shenandoah University, School of Nursing
Winchester, Virginia

Christina L. Nordick, DNP, FNP-BC
Assistant Professor
University of St Francis
Joliet, Illinois

Marilyn Perkowski, RN, MED, MSN, APRN, CNP
Professor of Instruction
University of Akron
Akron, Ohio

Maria Rosen, PhD, APRN-BC
Associate Dean Graduate Nursing Studies
MCPHS University
Worcester, Massachusetts

Dawn M. Specht, MSN, PhD, RN, APN, CEN, CPEN, CCRN, CCNS, AGACNP-BC
Assistant Professor
American Sentinel University
Aurora, Colorado

Felicia Stewart, DNP, FNP-C, RN-BC
Assistant Professor, Family Nurse Practitioner
Indiana State University, Wellness for Life
Terre Haute, Indiana

Contents

Special Features

Complementary Therapies

Drugs Commonly Prescribed

Treatment Standards/Guidelines

ADVANCED PRACTICE NURSING PERSPECTIVE FEATURES

The Patient's Voice

Evidence-Based Nursing Practice

DIAGNOSTIC REASONING ALGORITHMS

TREATMENT FLOWCHARTS

Nursing—The Seasons of My Life

Nursing is the spring of my life—
Each experience is fresh and new.
There's wonderment
Like flowers washed with morning dew.

Nursing is the summer of my life—
A time to perfect all I know.
There's confidence
A world where I can grow.

Nursing is the autumn of my life—
Ablaze with experience rich and glowing.
There's compassion
From richness of caring and knowing.

Nursing is the winter of my life—
A tapestry, a mosaic of all I am.
There's challenge
To find the spring again.

—Charlotte Dison, RN

Caring-Based Nursing
The Art

Advanced practice nursing is not filling the gap with medical care where it does not exist; it is filling the existing gap in health care with the core of nursing practice… The core of advanced practice nursing lies within nursing's disciplinary perspective on human–environment and caring relationships that facilitate health and healing. This core is delineated specifically in the theoretic foundations of nursing. True advanced nursing practice is theory-based [and] fully integrated into the nurse's way of being and practicing.

–Marlaine Smith. The core of advanced practice nursing. *Nurs Sci Q.* 1995;8(1):2–3.

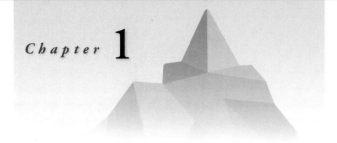

Chapter **1**

Primary Care in the Twenty-First Century
A Circle of Caring

Lynne M. Dunphy, PhD, APRN, FNP-BC, FAAN, FAANP

Brian Oscar Porter, MD, PhD, MPH, MBA

Jill E. Winland-Brown, EdD, APRN, FNP-BC

Debera J. Thomas, DNS, RN, FNP/ANP

Susan J. Bulfin, DNP, APRN, FNP-BC

WHERE WE HAVE BEEN AND WHERE WE ARE GOING

Our health-care system is in flux. It is constantly being remade as political battles over health-care funding shift rapidly. Educational models are also in the process of being reformed; interprofessional education and team-based care are required norms. It "takes a village" to provide quality, cost-effective, population-based, and person-centered care. Advanced practice registered nurses (APRNs), specifically Primary care nurse practitioners, are ideal care providers to take a leadership role in the evolving health-care system. They are especially critical as care providers in safety-net settings, such as community health centers (CHCs).

Heeding the recommendations of the Institute of Medicine's report *The Future of Nursing: Leading Change, Advancing Health* (2011) that all nurses practice to their full scope of education, many states have implemented important changes in the APRN scope of practice regulations. However, the scope of practice for APRNs remains inconsistent across states and APRN autonomy faces persistent threats (Livanos, 2017). This chapter reviews the disciplines of nursing and medicine from a historical perspective, highlighting the different strengths that each brings to the care of patients. The *Circle of Caring* practice model on which this text is based is presented as a way of making primary-care practice, which must incorporate aspects of what has been traditionally defined as medical practice, richer by integrating nursing-based understanding of the lived experience of patients and families.

The American health-care system continues to struggle with fiscal realities, as well as questions of quality and access to care. Technological advancements, an aging population, chronic illnesses, and alarming increases in behavioral health issues, such as those manifested in the opioid epidemic, are additional themes that color the ongoing political debate over the American health-care system, as politicians and the public alike ask, "Is health care a right or a privilege?" The Affordable Care Act (2010), despite ongoing efforts to dismantle it, has nevertheless achieved major reforms. Regardless of legislative changes, payment reform will most likely continue to evolve from a fee-for-service payment system to payment for quality, cost, and satisfaction with care. Currently, however, more often than not illness continues to be treated episodically, outside the context of home, family, community, and people's day-to-day lives, in isolation from the trajectory of the life of the individual. The major goals of *Healthy People 2020* (U.S. Department of Health and Human Services, 2010) of increasing quality and years of healthy life and the elimination of health disparities are far from being met. In fact, after decades of improvement, reversals are being seen in these areas.

Despite increasing evidence of the need for strengthening health-promotion and disease prevention strategies, including principles of behavioral change and the need for caring and relationship-building interactions in the clinician–patient relationship, these shifts are not easily accomplished. Health-care disciplines are in the throes of change, and change is never easy. Disciplinary and professional turf battles abound as health-care reimbursement shrinks. Some physician groups oppose an expansion of nurse practitioners' scope of practice, citing concerns over patient safety. Much of the controversy plays out in state capitals, where medical boards and legislators determine the scope of practice for non-physician providers, including nurse practitioners. Recent skirmishes have even included care coordination services, traditionally a nursing domain, but since reimbursement for care coordination was established by the Centers for Medicare and Medicaid Services in 2015 medical boards in some states attempted to legislate that these payments must go through the physician, not a nurse practitioner (NP). There are also considerations at the federal level that impact nurse practitioners' ability to be reimbursed for the care they provide.

Increased access to primary care for more of the population, although morally essential, may become more difficult. Health inequities have proven intractable and indeed are worsening: African Americans are 7 times as likely to die from HIV/AIDS as non-Hispanic whites (American Public Health Association, 2015); additionally, they are 3 times as likely to be admitted to the hospital for asthma exacerbations as non-Hispanic whites (AHRQ, 2015). Moreover, the gap in life expectancy between the wealthiest and poorest areas in the United States continues to widen to more than 20 years (Chetty et al., 2016).

One of the fundamental ways scientists measure the well-being of a nation is tracking the rate at which its citizens die and how long they can be expected to live. For the first time in more than 100 years, life expectancy in the United States has *fallen*. In 2015, the overall death rate for Americans rose because mortality from heart disease and stroke increased after declining for years. Deaths were also up from Alzheimer's disease, respiratory disease, kidney disease, and diabetes. More Americans also died from unintentional injuries and suicide. Overall, the rise was driven by increases in deaths from 8 of the top 10 leading causes of death in the United States. Some researchers speculate that the rise in opioid addiction and overdose could be due to economic factors causing despair, and wide availability in the United States of guns account for the rise in unintentional injuries and suicide. This trend was further exaggerated in 2016 (CDC Life Expectancy, 2016) and is concerning, especially when the death rate is decreasing and life expectancy is still on the rise in most other industrialized countries.

In the past, the burden of chronic-illness care was provided in hospitals and specialty practices, whereas today a substantial portion of that care must be provided in primary-care settings and communities. In turn, there is a rising demand for primary-care services and a decreasing supply of professionals providing these services (Health Resources & Services Administration, 2013). As the population ages and the number of older Americans rises, so will the burden of chronic illness. Increasing numbers of older adults live with multiple chronic illnesses; currently, 87% of Americans aged 65 to 79 years live with one chronic condition, and more than 45% have three or more chronic comorbidities (Bodenheimer et al., 2016). By 2020, a projected 157 million patients will have a chronic disease. Cancer, cognitive disorders, and diabetes will increase by 50% by 2023 (Bodenheimer et al., 2016). The number of individuals with disabilities is projected to grow from about 5.1 million in 1986 to 22.6 million in 2040, or nearly 350%, even as the elderly population overall will grow by only 175% (Administration on Aging, 2012).

Healthy People 2020 highlighted the importance of addressing the social determinants of health by including "Create social and physical environments that promote good health for all" as one of the four overarching goals for the decade (Secretary's Advisory Committee on Health Promotion and Disease Prevention Objectives for 2020, 2010). This emphasis was also highlighted by a 2008 report from the World Health Organization called *Closing the gap in a generation: Health equity through action on the social determinants of health*. The emphasis is also shared by other U.S. health initiatives such as the National Partnership for Action to End Health Disparities (National Partnership for Action, 2011) and the National Prevention and Health Promotion Strategy: America's Plan for Better Health and Wellness (2011) from the Surgeon General. In 2008, Berwick and colleagues identified "improving the health of populations" as one element in the Institute

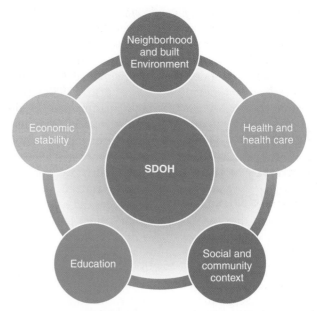

Figure 1.1 Social determinants of health (SDOH). The five key social determinants of health as defined by *Healthy People 2020* are shown in this diagram. From *U.S. Department of Health and Human Services/Office of Disease Prevention and Health Promotion.* Healthy People 2020. *www.healthpeople.gov/2020/ topics-objectives/topic/ social-determinants-of-health. Accessed November 24, 2017.*

for Healthcare Improvement's Triple Aim for improving the U.S. health-care system. Empowerment of individuals, families, and communities is critical, and both primary-care practice and community-based services must be cojoined in a meaningful way to ensure a seamless journey through a system of care across the life span. See Figure 1.1 for a visual representation of the social determinants of health (from *Healthy People 2020*).

In this milieu, APRN care providers will be needed more than ever, specifically nurse practitioners who provide primary care. This chapter makes the case that historically nurses have always cared for community (Dunphy, 2018), and have since the time of Florence Nightingale, focused explicitly on health (Nightingale, 1860). Nurses excel in coordination of community-care services, and their nursing background is situated in person and community, as well as health promotion and disease prevention, and support of patient and family empowerment. Nurses know that health starts in homes, schools, workplaces, neighborhoods, and communities. Health means self-care, eating well, staying active, not smoking, getting the recommended immunizations and screening tests, and seeing a health-care provider when sick. Health is determined in part by access to social and economic opportunities; the resources and supports available in homes, neighborhoods, and communities; the quality of schooling; the safety of workplaces; the cleanliness of water, food, and air; and the nature of social interactions and relationships. This is what the *social determinants of health* are all about. The conditions in which people live explain in part why some Americans are healthier than others and why Americans more generally are not as healthy as they could be (Kolata, 2015, 2016).

In a keynote address at the Centennial Conference of the National League for Nursing in 1993, Donna Shalala, former Secretary of the Department of Health and Human Services, stated that patients, families, groups, and communities are calling for the appearance of the "good fairy" in health care—someone who really hears them and their concerns, the nitty-gritty of their day-to-day experiences and struggles. Patients and their families need someone to hear why they did not take the medication that their health-care provider prescribed— that they could not tolerate, could not afford, could not get to the pharmacy to pick-up, or that had directions for administration that they could not understand or even read. Patients and their families need us to hear why they did not undergo the mammogram that was ordered— because they were afraid; or to hear why their baby was not immunized—because putting food on the table was more important. ARNPs are ideally suited to be this caring ear, even when providing expert clinical care.

THE TIP OF THE ICEBERG

The health problems encountered in day-to-day practice are merely the tip of the iceberg on which our health-care system has traditionally focused. Reimbursement streams pay for the "tip" of this iceberg: a visit to a primary-care provider to place a diagnostic label, for billing purposes, onto the symptomatology of the patient and a "treatment"—typically a pharmaceutical product— aimed at treating that symptom or underlying disease. Whether health-care reform will be able to continue to effect meaningful change within a value-based system of reimbursement rooted in quality outcomes, cost containment, and patient satisfaction remains to be seen.

The true causality of what brought the patient into the primary-care setting is the much larger part of the iceberg that lies under the surface and has often been invisible in health care. This hidden "under-structure" is composed of the *social determinants of health* built of various lifestyle and health equity issues, such as environmental challenges, the overall health and safety of communities, socioeconomic status, spiritual issues, family concerns, psychological stressors, and biological–genetic factors that have an impact on health. The nursing perspective—Donna Shalala's "good fairy"—is even more critical in today's world than it was in 1993. Nurses have always understood social determinants of health (Thurman & Pftziner, 2017; Wald, 2015). Nurses understand the *whole* of the "patient's iceberg" (Fig. 1.2). They are educated to see both above *and* below the water and to intervene accordingly. In turn, social determinants of health are inextricably bound up with the lower part of the iceberg—often unseen, invisible, and unidentified.

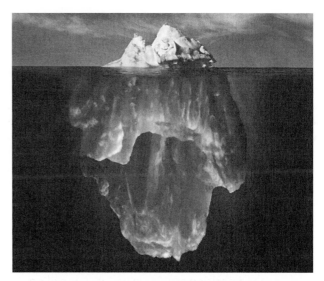

Figure 1.2 Nurses understand the *whole* of the patient's "iceberg"; they are educated to see both above *and* below the water and to intervene accordingly.

This point was recently made by Judge-Ellis and Wilson (2017) who issued a call-to-action for each NP to "…name a personal philosophy, claim the nursing identity and time needed to practice advanced practice nursing and explain the value of this practice to all" (p 588). In short, NPs need to "own" their individual practice.

The classical medical model, on the other hand, focuses on disease, an abnormality in the structure and function of bodily organs and systems, and is concerned with the malfunction or maladaptation of biological or psychophysiological processes in the individual. In his textbook of family practice, Robert Rakel makes a distinction between the terms *disease* and *illness* (Rakel, 2011). *Illness* is "all the sensations of a patient and all the ramifications of a disorder." *Disease,* however, "is a theoretical and taxonomic concept, a useful tool that enables the health-care provider to make inferences and predictions concerning phenomena." As such, the two concepts of illness and disease belong to two different universes of discourse: *disease* in the world of theory and *illness* in the lived experience of the patient. Benner and Wrubel (1989) also distinguish between disease and the experience of disease, or illness. *Illness* is defined as the way the sick person and his or her social network perceive and respond to disease. Illness is inextricable from the context of the patient's life, including the intersections of social, political, economic, spiritual, and cultural factors—in other words, the whole of the iceberg, which includes all of the community-based determinants of health.

Historically, nursing has been concerned with the whole person and the promotion of health across the life span— what Florence Nightingale referred to as "the Laws of Health." Nurses also have traditionally focused on people's responses to the illness experience in the context of their day-to-day lives. Much of the challenge in the role of the

APRN is the negotiation of seemingly disparate worlds: the reconciliation of an essentially holistic nursing model with a health-care system still focused predominantly on disease-oriented care. It is precisely this nexus between more discrete diagnostic categories of disease and a more holistic view of the continuum between health and illness—the iceberg—that gives nursing its identity, richness, diversity, and usefulness. Today's primary-care practitioners dwell in this nexus and must bridge these two realities—the world of disease and the world of illness, including the context of the patient's life in all its complexity. The increasing and necessary placement of APRNs into primary-care settings and teams across the health-care continuum provides nursing with the opportunity to effect change on both the micro and macro levels—in the lives of individual patients and families, as well as in the well-being of communities, including the global community.

A recent Hastings Center Report discussed the difficulty in making prevention a meaningful part of health-care reform because it involves changing behavior. The author notes that changing health behaviors involves changing habits that have "complex developmental, psychological, cultural, and socioeconomic roots" (Blacksher, 2009). In addition, health promotion and disease prevention require comprehensive policy changes that support the often tedious, unglamorous work of behavioral change, as well as community-based services. In addition to care of the sick, the real-life, day-to-day health needs of people (such as those in the grip of the opioid crisis), their social and economic circumstances, and their communities are all part of the traditional domain of nursing practice, as stated by Florence Nightingale. Nightingale understood these links and discussed them, as well as care of the sick, in her prophetic *Notes on Nursing* (1860). More recently, nurse theorist Margaret Newman and colleagues asserted that the NP–patient relationship has become the central focus of the nursing discipline. They state:

It is the nature of the nurse-patient relationship that unites the practice if nursing …. nursing actions occur within the context of a unified commitment. That commitment is to a caring relationship focused on understanding the meaning of the current situation for the people involved and appreciating the pattern of evolving forces shaping health, so that appropriate actions can be realized (Newman et al., 2008, p 17).

Nurse historian Ellen Baer notes that the services demanded of primary-care providers today are broader in scope than those within the domain of medicine before the 1960s. Supportive functions, previously the domain of the clergy or multigenerational families, began falling within the purview of the primary-care provider. Likewise, the conceptual shift to health promotion, coupled with increased knowledge about healthy lifestyles, requires that primary-care providers be well grounded in their patients' community context. In making her case for the role of the nurse in primary care, Baer concludes: "The best reason for nurses to provide primary care is because they are nurses. Nursing's focus on people; its blend of medical, behavioral, and social science expertise; and its commitment to caring, teaching, counseling, and supporting patients are the characteristics of nursing that make nurses so uniquely qualified to provide primary health care services" (Baer, 1993). In another history of advanced practice nursing, Dunphy (2018) asserts that "nurses have always cared for community."

This text provides a nursing-based approach to primary care and includes content on health promotion and disease prevention, as well as the diagnosis, management, and treatment of disease in the primary-care setting. The essentials of disease pathology and management necessary for safe and satisfactory functioning in the clinical area are integrated into a view of the wholeness of persons, an understanding of human responses, and a repertoire of therapeutic options. This information will enable the primary-care provider, regardless of disciplinary background, to become an orchestrator of health and wellness, as well as a skilled negotiator and mediator in the space that exists between health and illness, between disease and the "lived experience of the patient" in the context of his or her community. APRNs must understand the discipline of nursing to effectively fill the gap between health and illness with true nursing care. Nurses on teams and in interprofessional educational settings must be confident and secure about their knowledge base and its intrinsic value, as well as the critical nature of their contributions to the care of the patient and the subsequent outcomes of that care.

The American Association of Colleges of Nursing (AACN) has called for all APRN preparation to take place in practice-based programs at the doctoral level—the Doctor of Nursing Practice (DNP). In 2006, the AACN *Essentials of Doctoral Education for Advanced Nursing Practice* was approved (AACN, 2009). Essential VIII, Advanced Nursing Practice, was further defined as a set of advanced nursing practice competencies (Box 1.1).

The DNP is a catalyst, allowing nursing to develop and expand nursing knowledge and practice through health promotion and disease prevention practices, essential for disciplinary distinction and growth (Burman et al., 2009). As noted by Burman et al., "Ultimately our vision for NP care to be consistently 'different,' yet just as essential as physician care, leading to positive outcomes in health promotion and disease management" (2009). The American Association of Nurse Practitioners (AANP) statement on the uniqueness of NP practice echoes the statements above.

"What sets NPs apart from other health-care providers is their unique emphasis on the health and well-being of the whole person. With a focus on health promotion, disease prevention, and health education and counseling, NPs guide patients in making smarter health and lifestyle choices, which in turn can lower patient's out-of-pocket-costs" (AANP, 2017).

Box 1.1   Essential VIII: Advanced Nursing Practice Competencies

1. Conduct a comprehensive and systematic assessment of health and illness parameters in complex situations, incorporating diverse and culturally sensitive approaches.
2. Design, implement, and evaluate therapeutic interventions based on nursing science and other sciences.
3. Develop and sustain therapeutic relationships and partnerships with patients (individuals, family, or group) and other professionals to facilitate optimal care and patient outcomes.
4. Demonstrate advanced levels of clinical judgment, systems thinking, and accountability in designing, delivering, and evaluating evidence-based care to improve patient outcomes.
5. Guide, mentor, and support other nurses to achieve excellence in nursing practice.
6. Educate and guide individuals and groups through complex health and situational transitions.
7. Use conceptual and analytic skills in evaluating links among practice, organizational, population, fiscal, and policy issues.

Source: American Association of Colleges of Nursing. *Essentials of doctoral education for advanced nursing practice.* http://www.aacnnursing.org/DNP/DNP-Essentials. Published 2006. Accessed November 22, 2017.

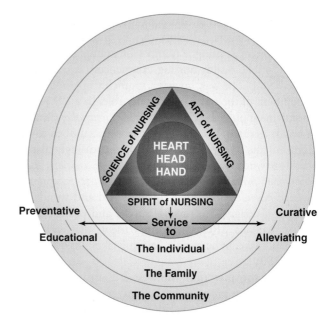

Figure 1.3 The professional equipment of the modern nurse and the scope of her responsibilities. Source: *Dock LL, Stewart IM.* A short history of nursing: From the earliest times to the present day. *3rd ed. New York, NY: G.P. Putnam's Sons; 1931: 337.*

HISTORICAL PERSPECTIVES ON ADVANCED PRACTICE NURSING

Nursing as a discipline and a profession with a theoretical base can be traced to Florence Nightingale. As long ago as 1860, Nightingale in *Notes on Nursing* proclaimed that there were laws of sickness and laws of health. There was not enough known, she wrote, about the laws of health. Nursing the "room," meaning the environment surrounding the patient, was as important as nursing the patient. Somewhat controversially, she also wrote that nursing and medicine were like "cats and dogs" and should not be mixed.

The early public health nurses of Lillian Wald's Henry Street Settlement House at the turn of the 20th century created their own vision of health and illness, and lived and worked in the community they served. Lavinia Dock, one of the first Henry Street nurses, evolved a model (Fig. 1.3) that has implications for the current health-care system. New and emerging primary-care models are attempting to recapture population-based care, health promotion, and disease prevention in more meaningful and reimbursable ways, such as through team approaches and the ideas of patient-centered medical homes (PCMHs) and affordable care organizations, in which health-care systems are integrated across the continuum of care.

Nurses' functions have always been rooted in population-based, public health approaches, and nursing has always

claimed domains that were educational and preventive as well as curative. Nurses alleviated illness and actualized self and "other" through service to the individual, family, and community. As noted by Blacksher in an editorial in the *Hastings Center Report on Prevention,* "Health happens where people live, learn, love, work, and play" (2009). These activities flow from the spirit, science, and art of nursing or the "heart, head, and hand" of nursing (a phrase popularized by Virginia Henderson [1966]). The first instances of standardized protocols, for example, evolved from the work of the early school nurses and the New York City Public Health Department. These early public health nurses enjoyed an autonomy of practice similar to that exercised by today's primary-care providers. Dock and Stewart (1920) likened the relationship between nursing and medicine to workers on a team who complement and supplement each other; the relationship is based on neither independence nor subordination but on interdependence and cooperation.

Henderson's 1966 book *The Nature of Nursing* was an attempt to provide nursing with its own explanatory model for practice. Building on her own experiences in nursing (Henderson also spent time as a public health nurse at the Henry Street Settlement) and on her understanding of physiology, she tried to place nursing on a continuum with medical care. Henderson argued that nurses had to place themselves (figuratively) "inside" patients in order to become their "counterpart, alter ego, or helper" (1966).

Martha Rogers, another foundational nurse-theoretician, argued for the necessity of an independent basis of nursing science out of which autonomous nursing practice grows. According to Rogers, "Primary care by nurses is as old as modern nursing," citing a number of examples rooted in her early public health nursing experiences (as quoted by Hektor, 1989). She was, however, staunchly opposed to the development of the nurse practitioner role. In a 1975 position statement published in the *American Journal of Nursing*, she boldly asserted, "Not all nurses have succumbed to the blandishments of euphemisms and the increasingly blatant perfidy spawned by such terms as *pediatric associate, nurse practitioner, primary-care practitioner, geriatric practitioner, physician extender,* and other equally weird and wonderful cover-ups—designed to provide succor and profit for the nation's shamans" (Rogers). Those patients that ended up in hospitals were, in her words, "our mistakes" (as quoted by Hektor, 1989).

Despite the fact that the first NP program was a graduate nursing program at the University of Colorado, overall the early nurse practitioner "movement" evolved with little connection to academia and the flurry of nursing conceptual models and theories that proliferated throughout the 1970s and 1980s. These pioneering nurse practitioners, rooted in practice, usually in a primary-care setting, and often "trained" in certificate programs, had little patience with the abstractions of nursing theory that provided little meaning for their day-to-day practice. They needed and valued the medical model to care for their patients. Yet most remained nurses at heart, devoted to health promotion, disease prevention, and providing holistic care to their patients. Nurses in today's DNP programs bring 4 years of a nursing baccalaureate base with them, as well as their practice as *nurses*. Thus, the DNP is a strong base on which to build advanced nursing practice.

Very few nursing models have addressed or attempted to make sense of the dichotomy of nurse practitioner practice and medical care. Some argue that no dichotomy exists. A number of others, however, identify the relationship between advanced nursing practice and medical practice as an issue requiring ongoing attention. Cody (1994) views medicine as still dominating nursing politically, and he states that many nurses "actually value having medical tasks delegated to them." On a more ominous note, he points out that nursing must realize what is merely delegated from another (more powerful) discipline can also be taken away. He concludes, "Only when nurses everywhere are guided by a theory base specific to nursing will nursing have achieved parity with other scholarly disciplines." In a coauthored article, Barbara Bates, MD, and Joan Lynaugh, NP, venture some thoughts on the relationship between nursing and medicine: medicine, they speculate, is concerned with structure; nursing is focused on function (Lynaugh & Bates, 1973).

In an unpublished paper, Lynaugh discusses the respective roles of nurses and physicians in greater depth. She notes that the biomedical model of disease and cure, which swept across the Western world, seemed far more compelling and promising than nursing's holism, environmentalism, and "watchful waiting" approach to illness (Lynaugh & Bates, 1973). Nurses, she elaborates, seem to be both inarticulate in explaining their work and "touchingly confident" that altruism will eventually be rewarded. Years of medical dominance have drawn a veil over the work of nursing. This invisibility is serious because it compromises the public's access to good nursing care in an era in which reimbursement for care is restricted to payment based exclusively on the phenomena of interest to physicians. The power relationships among patient, nurse, and physician are complicated by economic issues, professional territoriality on all sides, and profound questions of disciplinary identity; therefore, adjustments in these relationships will come slowly, step by step, but inevitably. An essential component of this process is making the "invisible" work of nurses more visible. It is the part of the iceberg that is below the water that takes up so much of nursing's time and energy and is so unnamed and unseen. Demonstration of nursing's contribution to patient care is vital. This is accomplished, in part, through the clear articulation of nursing's theoretical base.

In the day-today realities of practice and needs of patients and families, these issues are often obscured. There are, after all, the needs of patients that unite APRNs and physicians. Fairman and D'Antonio (2008) argue that as providers of care, APRNs and MDs work well together more often than not, and will engage in collaborative relationships when caring for patients. The real rub between nursing and medicine lies in the politicized agendas of each as advanced by their respective professional organizations

As nursing theory embraces the mode of midrange theory development and testing, with real-life clinical applications for practice, the applicability to advanced practice nursing and the utilization of theory-based practice should increase. This still begs the question, however, of an underlying theoretical basis for advanced practice nursing. It can be argued, as Burman et al. (2009) do in an article titled "Reconceptualizing the Core of Nurse Practitioner Education and Practice," that "the heart and soul of nursing is health promotion both in healthy persons and those dealing with chronic illness." Nursing practice as a DNP should focus more explicitly on health promotion, changing health behaviors, and chronic disease management, thus advancing a unique nursing science. These are traditional nursing domains and strengths. These authors state that advanced practice nurses "can fill the growing societal need for expert clinicians to assume major leadership roles in clinical management and evaluation of outcomes research arenas. DNP programs include extensive clinical practicum and have a strong focus on scholarly and evidence-based practice."

The AACN (2015) encourages DNP nursing faculty to consider a broad range of community-based academic–practice partnerships. Collaborating with clinical partners, particularly in underserved areas, will provide students with rich and varied opportunities to impact health outcomes in meaningful ways. Academic–practice partnerships are forming with the expectation that DNP students not only prepare for the highest level of nursing practice, but also develop a DNP scholarly project focused on adding value to the practice site. The AACN Task Force (2015) also encourages innovation in the design and dissemination of the final DNP project.

In a recent survey by Dols, Hernández, and Miles (2017), 90 DNP program directors identified the overwhelming majority of DNP projects as quality improvement or evidence-based practice. To fully engage with partner site leaders, nursing faculty and students need a strong background in improvement science methods to identify areas where improvement is feasible and measurable. Improvement models such as Lean (Toyota Production System) and Institute for Health Care Improvement-Quality Improvement can provide frameworks for developing projects that focus on maximizing quality while minimizing waste or inefficiency.

Both approaches emphasize the "design and continual refinement of processes as the way to reduce variation and increase value in outcomes" (Scoville & Little, 2014, p 16).

By providing the education and support necessary for nurse leaders to develop the skills in improvement science methodology, we can create meaningful impact throughout our country with DNP projects. As DNP students and practice partners mutually identify population needs, innovative evidence-based processes can be codesigned. DNP projects aimed at better quality, availability, and more cost-effective care will continually drive system transformation. Dissemination of DNP projects will ensure the advanced practice nurse becomes increasingly visible by highlighting local, regional, and national impact.

CHANGING MODELS OF ADVANCED NURSING PRACTICE AND RESEARCH

Expert practice domains of the clinical nurse specialist and nurse practitioner (both delineated as APRNs by the AACN 2008 White Paper) were originally identified by Fenton and Brykczynski in 1993 and evolved from domains identified in Patricia Benner's 1984 book *From Novice to Expert*. In 1990, these identified domains were used by the National Organization of Nurse Practitioner Faculties, the long-time leader in education of nurse practitioners (Zimmer et al., 1990), to create a framework for primary-care NP curricula.

In a study by Lewis and Brykczynski (1994), the authors elaborated on the *practical* knowledge as well as the *healing* role of nurse practitioners. In the discussion of their findings, the authors state that to bring about healing, nurse practitioners fight for patient's rights and access to care—going beyond the call of duty by, visiting schools and other diverse settings such as jails, prisons, homeless shelters, residential housing communities, federally qualified health centers, and CHCs; making phone calls; driving patients to appointments; and attending funerals. The practitioners in the study describe both the professional and personal satisfaction derived from their caring practices, even when the rewards of such actions were limited. Lewis and Brykczynski (1994) situate the work of these practitioners within a caring paradigm, citing Sally Gadow, Jean Watson, and Madeline Leininger. They also cite the 1991 work of Benner, who, in studying the effectiveness of expert nurses, found that mere technique and knowledge were not enough, and that caring, or a certain level of human involvement, was required for expert "human practice." Indeed, expert "human practice" should be a goal of all primary-care providers.

Johnson (1993) cites clear evidence of a nursing perspective in NP primary-care practice. According to Johnson, nurse practitioner–patient dialogue incorporates the voice of medicine and the voice of the "lifeworld" (of the patient). The skilled practitioner "knows self" and how to share his or her own personal experience to either enhance the patient's progress or strengthen the provider–patient bond. An element of camaraderie was viewed as positive and not in opposition to maintaining a professional stance. *Coordination, continuity*, and *advocacy* were the major functions the NPs in this study believed that they contributed to the practice. All primary-care practice needs these functions, which constitute some of the foundational ideas of a patient-centered medical home.

Swanson (1995) proposed "A Spirit-Focused Conceptual Model of Nursing for the Advanced Practice Nurse" in which she identified the core of every person, both patient and nurse, as the spirit. She describes the act of nursing as a goal-directed interpersonal relationship between the patient and nurse, based on traditional nursing process components such as assessing, planning, intervening, and evaluating. Interventions are broad based, ranging from play, music, and stories to utilization of counseling principles such as active listening and anticipatory guidance. The use of this approach in primary-care practice could be adapted by any primary-care practitioner.

The Shuler Nurse Practitioner Practice Model (Shuler & Davis, 1993) is an ambitious attempt to describe the nurse practitioner's integrated role. Building on a holistic nursing assessment, the next step is the mutual identification of unmet patient health needs to identify health problems. The treatment plan must be mutually agreeable and oriented toward self-care; disease prevention and health-promotion activities are incorporated into the treatment plan. Nonpharmacological treatments, including alternative and complementary healing practices, are also integrated into the plan. These approaches are framed within the concept of functioning within a multidisciplinary team and could be seen as particularly relevant in today's team-based clinical care settings.

In addition, this model is seen as enhancing both the patient's and the nurse practitioner's personal movement toward wellness. Patients are encouraged to examine their lives honestly and to identify areas that are not "balanced." The patient's physical and psychological ability to participate in wellness activities is assessed. Creative, uninhibited problem-solving and identification of appropriate wellness activities are pursued. The model emphasizes that the primary-care practitioner's personal commitment to health and wellness can have a direct impact on her or his ability to influence positive patient outcomes.

Another interesting approach to nursing phenomena, not elaborated as unique for APRNs but with wide applicability for the autonomy of the advanced practice nursing role, is "symptom management." This approach evolved from the University of California, San Francisco, School of Nursing Symptom Management Faculty Group (1994) and has since been revised based on research studies testing the model (Dodd et al., 2001). Proponents of this approach note that when the underlying cause of the patient's problem and the presenting symptoms are managed concurrently, patients are more likely to benefit and remain in treatment.

The Symptom Management group proposes that symptoms be viewed as subjective experiences reflecting changes in a person's biopsychosocial function, sensation, or cognition. They contrast this view of the word *symptom*, a subjective phenomenon, with the word *sign*, which is used to mean an abnormality indicative of disease, which can be observed by another person and sometimes by the patient, and is thus identified as objective. The model they propose to address symptoms has three dimensions:

1. The symptom experience (subjective)
2. Symptom management strategies
3. Symptom outcomes

Snyder and Mirr (1995) conceptualize advanced practice within a nursing paradigm built around human responses as a focus for nursing interventions. They identify the following foci for advanced practice nursing:

1. Self-care limitations
2. Impaired functioning in areas of rest, sleep, ventilation, circulation, nutrition, and the like
3. Pain and discomfort
4. Emotional problems related to illness and treatment, life-threatening events, or daily experiences, such as anxiety, loss, or loneliness
5. Distortion of symbolic functions reflected in interpersonal and intellectual processes such as hallucinations
6. Deficiencies in decision-making ability to make personal choices
7. Self-image changes required by health status
8. Dysfunctional perceptual orientations to health
9. Strains related to life processes such as birth, development, and death
10. Problematic affiliative relationships

Patient problems, conceptualized in this manner, are amenable to uniquely nursing-based interventions. Attention to human responses, as such, provides the missing link to much that is absent within today's contemporary health-care system. Many of these responses are tied to *social determinants of health*—such as where one lives and works. Our current health-care system, however, is not structured in such a way to make many of these practices sustainable, as such interventions are not typically coded for reimbursement.

Ryan's (2009) integrated theory of health behavior change (ITHBC) is based on the belief that health-promotion activities are an integral part of the long-term health and well-being of both healthy people and those with chronic illnesses. For health promotion to be successful, people must take responsibility for initiating and maintaining both health behavior changes and prevention behaviors. APRNs are in a position to facilitate and support health behavior changes in their patients, and therefore APRNs require knowledge of what drives people to make these changes. This is especially true in today's health-care system, which requires patients and their families to take responsibility for increasingly complex conditions in the home. This trend will continue to escalate as hospital care will be increasingly reserved only for acutely ill patients.

The ITHBC can be used by APRNs to tailor interventions for individual patients in such a way that positively affects their long-term health status. Health behavior change is directly influenced by "fostering knowledge and beliefs, increasing self-regulation skill and ability, and enhancing social facilitation" (Ryan, 2009). Social facilitation involves both social influence and support, which is of particular importance to APRNs, who are in a unique position to be a source of both for their patients. New research demonstrates that a patient's health behaviors are strongly influenced by the health behaviors of those in the patient's social network. Thus, models such as ITHBC have great relevance for APRNs in primary-care settings today.

Cumbie et al. (2004) Model of Promoting Process Engagement is a patient-centered theory developed to assist APRNs to manage the care of chronically ill patients. In this model, the APRN chooses interventions based on each patient's needs and expectations of his or her care, and are developed in collaboration with the patient. "Interventions focus on motivational strategies designed to facilitate and support individuals as they make sense of health information, engage in health promoting activities, and sustain health-related behavioral change" (Cumbie et al., 2004). People are influenced by a number of internal and external variables that cause them to either resist or engage in beneficial health behaviors (Cumbie et al., 2004). To promote engagement, the APRN must help patients make sense of health information, so that this information becomes meaningful to them.

APRNs can use the intervention structure of the model to help their patients become actively involved in managing chronic illness. Engagement strategies include patient-centered assessment followed by therapeutic interview and communication techniques (Cumbie et al., 2004). When the patient's health–illness situation is understood, the APRN works with patients to determine their health priorities and to develop mutually agreed upon health goals and a plan of action to meet these goals (Cumbie et al., 2004). Case management, advocacy, and referral are activities of the ongoing collaborative process, which is the part of the intervention that is used to "sustain health process engagement" (Cumbie et al., 2004).

Another promising direction is Nurse Coaching, which promotes integrative approaches for health and well-being (Dossey et al., 2015), and can be used by APRNs to promote behavioral change. It supports the need for clinicians to help their patients develop a plan for healthy living and to support them in making the stepwise journey to health. This builds on the theoretical model of health and health promotion that embraces the integration of body, mind, and spirit. Utilizing motivational interviewing, nonjudgmental acceptance of the patient, the transtheoretical model of behavioral change, appreciative inquiry, cultural perspectives, and "rituals of healing"; this largely nursing-based model extends nursing practice.

CHANGING MODELS OF MEDICAL PRACTICE AND RESEARCH

Changes are taking place in traditional medical practice as well. Given its lack of fiscal sustainability, the American health-care system has gone through significant change over the past 10 years. Cost-consciousness by governments and third-party payers, the availability of medical information (and misinformation) to patients via the Internet, the move from hospital-based to community-based provision of health care, multiculturalism, a growing interest in holistic care and alternative therapies, an increasingly litigious environment, and the ever-expanding use of technology—all of these factors continue to force re-examination of traditional professional roles.

Advances in therapeutics over the course of the 20th century, which are often taken for granted today, were far more impactful than therapeutic advances that had been developed prior to this period. Medicine was now able to intervene—specifically, powerfully, and radically—in the course of previously fatal diseases. Today, no disorder, however complex, seems beyond the possibility of understanding and cure, provided the health-care system is willing to invest in research and development. As a result, the impact of medicine is felt far beyond the immediacies of the patient–provider encounter. Alcoholism, for example, viewed as a moral disorder in earlier times, is now a phenomenon conceptualized as a disease, with an array of psychological and pharmacological interventions available to practitioners.

A review of the progress of medicine in combating disease is a journey from an integrated view of illness and therapeutics to one of discrete diseases with distinct causes and an armamentarium of ever-expanding and specific therapeutics. From the time of the ancient Greeks and Romans until well into the 19th century, illness was seen as an imbalance in the economy of the entire body, which could be expressed in the relationships between input or output of food, sweat, secretions, urine, phlegm, and the like. Treatment was focused on restoring harmony and balance between body and environment (a view promulgated by Nightingale, 1860/1969). Specific symptoms were not treated; instead, a systemic physiological effect was sought through such methods as inducing or facilitating sweating, fever, diuresis, and/or vomiting. These interventions, it was theorized, would assist the body to recover its balance.

Throughout the course of the 19th century, however, this integrated view of disease and therapeutics was increasingly challenged by notions of discrete disease states with specific causes. Illnesses seemed less amenable to purges, bleeding, and diuretics (the so-called holistic approaches) than was previously thought. Quite late in the modern era, the first active principles of some of the oldest and most useful botanicals were isolated, and later some were even synthesized. A new dimension was added to the emerging concept of specificity of therapeutics by the discovery of sulfonamides in the late 1930s and penicillin in the early 1940s. Not only could therapy be directed at particular symptoms, but for the first time, therapeutics could become "radical," matching the power of the surgeon's knife—that is, they could eradicate the primary cause of an illness, in this case, specific microorganisms.

Increasingly specific therapeutic measures, such as the use of antisera, the isolation of blood fractions, and the synthesis of polypeptide hormones and biologic immunotherapies, are developments seen over the last several decades. Advances in laboratory analysis and diagnostic techniques confer on therapeutics the capability of effecting cure at the molecular loci of disease. The era of specific and radical therapeutics has only just begun. Thus, what seems certain is the continued trend toward even greater specificity in the diagnosis and treatment of disease, extending to the genetic level. This will continue to have profound effects on the medical profession, on society, and on inherent power imbalances among patients, nurses, and physicians, as new diagnostic and therapeutic technologies will surely raise questions of access to care and equitable distribution among all patients.

Medicine's successes have led to a generation of physician-specialists with an increasingly narrow focus on human disease and technologically advanced medical interventions that are often far removed from the day-to-day lives of patients. The effectiveness of modern therapeutics adds a powerful strain of reductionism and positivism to the 20th-century medical ethos. Although this has been a useful stance for the creation of highly effective medical interventions, when universalized to all realms of medical practice, this stance may be antithetical to the fulfillment of the more sensitive moral and social responsibilities of medicine. Care—when defined as helping the patient and family to cope, offering reassurance, educating, and relieving worry—does not require a high level of scientific sophistication, but it does require human understanding.

In the past when physician remuneration was less driven by technological advances and he or she was a highly integrated member of the community, these issues could be negotiated more successfully between doctor and patient, with more dedicated time for two-way physician–patient interaction. The doctor of today, however, is at risk of being seen more often as an unfamiliar interventionist, with multiple competing priorities and limited time for direct patient interaction. This raises a fearful dilemma for patients who must trust the physician because of his or her specialized knowledge and power to heal, while that trust may be undermined by a fear of the physician's self-interest. Additionally, social responsibilities in a broader sense—in a public health sense—have become neglected, as population-based health indicators in the United States continue to lag behind those of other developed nations.

Despite the emphasis on medical advancements purported by many sectors of the health-care industry, including for-profit medical therapeutics and pharmaceutical companies, as well as large health-care delivery systems—there has nonetheless been a dawning recognition of the *limits* of medical progress and its partner, technological innovation. Beginning with the AIDS epidemic in the early 1980s through the current struggle with multidrug-resistant organisms, it has become increasingly clear that not all aspects of human health and wellness can be controlled solely through medical technology and the development of newer therapeutics, particularly given the persistence of chronic diseases and cancer as the leading causes of death in developed, resource-rich societies. Moreover, overwhelming evidence exists that technological innovations are drivers of health-care costs. In numerous studies over time, 60% of the improvement in population-based health status is tied to improved socioeconomic factors, particularly education and income. With the notable exception of the health care of the elderly, this means that only approximately 40% of improvements in health status result from medical care.

Thus, there has been an increasing call for a better balance between cure-oriented and care-oriented medicine. Chronic disease continues to be the most difficult and expensive type of health problem to manage, as demonstrated in the failure of cure-oriented medicine to completely eradicate the most common causes of morbidity, such as heart disease and cancer. People are living longer with these conditions, but in the face of persistent morbidity; in fact, much of medicine is focused on the long-term management, rather than cure, of chronic disease. Care-oriented medicine, on the other hand, reflects well-coordinated medical assistance to enable patients to manage disease, combined with the marshaling of critical family-based and social supports—again, traditional nursing strengths and domains.

Prevention as an approach to health and wellness can only go so far, however, as sickness and death can be forestalled, but not eradicated, and the costs of illness deferred or minimized, but not eliminated entirely. According to Callahan (2009), "Serious progress would mean turning back the clock: learning to take care of ourselves, to tolerate some degree of discomfort, to accept the reality of aging and death, and to see our personal doctor as someone as likely to talk to as to have us scanned."

Modern medicine is not unaware of this quandary; indeed, these issues are widely discussed in medical circles and among policy makers. A loss of 60% of the nation's hospital beds has been predicted in some reports. There is a converging agreement among health-care delivery and health-care policy experts that allopathic medicine, as it has developed across the 20th century, does not make a population healthy in and of itself. Much of the health status of a community stems from habits, lifestyle choices, environmental factors, and both patient- and population-level genetics. All too often, allopathic medicine as utilized in the modern health-care system only operates at the margins of these health determinants, yet the American health-care system has been structured on this mode of care in terms of both the delivery and reimbursement of health care by professionals (Commonwealth Fund Commission on a High Performance Health Care System, 2008).

A TRANSFORMATIVE TEMPLATE: THE CIRCLE OF CARING

Both the traditional medical and nursing models are predicated on a subjective and objective database, a labeling of the patient's problems and responses, a therapeutic plan, and an evaluation of the outcome. The *Circle of Caring* model builds on these features and expands them to include the following:

- A broadened and contextualized database, more typical of a holistic nursing assessment that gives the health-care provider a more in-depth understanding of the patient's situation, life, strengths, and weaknesses, including social determinants of health.
- A labeling of the patient's concern that more actively incorporates the patient's responses to the meaning of illness in his or her day-to-day life, as well as standard medical diagnostic language.
- A holistic and creative approach to an individualized therapeutic plan that includes nursing interventions based on evidence, including complementary therapies as appropriate, incorporated with standardized pharmacological, surgical, and other nonpharmacological interventions.
- A view of outcomes based on the patient, family, social group, and community perceptions of improvement, as

well as the more traditional, quantified outcome measures such as mortality and morbidity, with emerging primary-care quality indicators and costs of care also built into these outcomes. This integrates the health of populations into the outcomes of care.

The *Circle of Caring* model is a synthesized view of the problem-solving methodology that may be used in a variety of settings—primary care, acute care, and community-based settings. The model is diagrammed in Figure 1.4. The basic problem-solving process used by nurses is represented by the boxes in the middle of the diagram. This process is encircled by a visual representation of caring—the interpersonal process that occurs among the caregiver and the patient, which also reflects the family, social group, and community of the patient.

The ability to provide effective and meaningful care for the patient is based on of caring; qualities of authentic presence, patience, courage, advocacy, commitment, and knowing. These qualities of caring enable the nurse to hear the patient's "call" and to fashion creative nursing responses. It is this authenticity in the nurse–patient encounter that allows the nurse to enter the lifeworld of that person and be truly compassionate in their care.

A Broadened, Contextualized Database

A contextualized approach—the lived experience of the patient in the context of his or her community—is central to this model and is one that most nurses have learned in their undergraduate nursing programs. Although the patient's subjective perception of this experience is captured in the history portion of the assessment database, the *Circle of Caring* is based on hearing the patient's story in all its complexity, as well as eliciting the patient's own unique meaning of *health*. In addition, increased attention is focused on the interplay among perceptual, psychodynamic, socioeconomic, cultural, and environmental factors that have an impact on the patient's health status—in other words, increased awareness and attention to *social determinants of health*.

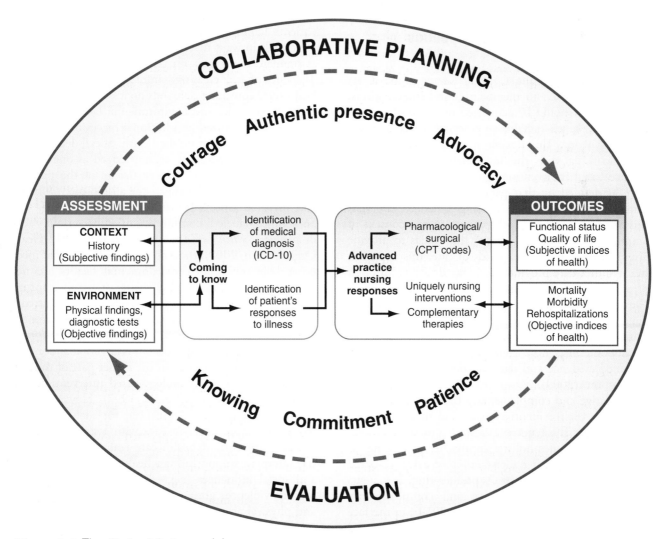

Figure 1.4 The *Circle of Caring* model.

The Nature of Patient Responses

The 2010 American Nurses Association's Social Policy Statement defined nursing as the "diagnosis and treatment of human responses to actual and potential health problems." The *Circle of Caring* model may be used effectively with the traditional tools of nursing diagnosis. Boykin and Schoenhofer (2001) conceptualized the phenomenon of human responses as "calls for nursing." As such, these calls remain unique, interactional, and contextualized, and thus not amenable to any form of generic labeling. It is through coming to know people as caring persons that the nurse is able to fully hear each patient's call.

Labeling the patient's problem (i.e., the "call for nursing"), be it in medical or nursing diagnostic terminology or in a more generic format, helps to address patient responses more effectively. Labeling, thus, involves the acknowledgment and knowledge of the complex interplay of perceptual, psychodynamic, socioeconomic, cultural, and environmental factors that contribute to health. APRNs are especially skilled at eliciting and understanding this complexity and at fashioning nursing-based responses that are uniquely suited to the individual.

A Creative Approach to Therapeutics and Interventions

Another hallmark of the *Circle of Caring* model is its broadened approach to therapeutics and interventions. This approach should be actualized in day-to-day practice by APRNs, yet remains an especially invisible piece of nursing work. This flexible nursing-based approach entails working with the individual patient to tailor evidence-based interventions geared to the meaning of *health* as defined by that patient. Building on current standards of medical and nursing practice, interventions are fine-tuned for each patient, in the context of community. Although a focus of this text is to provide current evidence-based standards of care, this approach often requires care providers to make decisions through narrowly prescribed filters. As noted by Payne, "there is an art to clinical practice that extends beyond hard science and numbers and often requires swift, sound, decision-making in an environment of incomplete evidence. Sometimes no formula or calculation based on quantified evidence and data can determine the appropriate action" (2009).

Alternative and complementary therapies are considered within their evidentiary basis and meaningfulness for the patient. This requires a creative approach to therapeutics that includes holistic approaches to healing, as well as a sophisticated understanding of evidence-based practice. Research in this area is proliferating, as patients increasingly call for alternative and complementary approaches to their treatment (Riffle, 2010), in the face of rapid growth of this multibillion dollar industry and largely unregulated direct-to-consumer marketing.

In the practice of nursing as caring (see Chapter 2), the nurse is described as "an artist who responds creatively to calls for nursing with unique nursing responses." Any taxonomy of nursing must, of necessity, have universal applicability. What distinguishes so many of nursing's interventions, however, is precisely their uniqueness and the tailoring of an individual response to each patient. A broadened approach to therapeutics and interventions based on a contextualized database implies attention to the context of the patient's life, the *social determinants of health* for the patient, and his or her family and community.

POPULATION-BASED APPROACHES

Current outcomes-based research demonstrates the need to incorporate patients' perceptions as measured both objectively (by functional assessments and similar methods) and subjectively. Quality-of-life measures and, most important, the various and individualistic meanings of health and illness must be taken more fully into consideration. The *patient experience* is a frequently used measure of quality care in both the acute and primary-care settings. Plans must be assessed according to their potential to assist patients, families, social groups, and communities to meet their goals in ways that are meaningful to them, not just as standard items on a checklist of preventive measures. The voice of an increasingly informed, information-savvy health-care consumer demands no less.

Multiple social and environmental factors impacting health are recognized as additional pieces of the health-care puzzle—those of public health. Social determinants of health are increasingly acknowledged as one component of the enormous understructure of the primary-care iceberg discussed earlier—the all-too-often "unseen" and invisible aspects beneath the water (see Fig. 1.2). Sometimes labeled community-oriented primary care or *primary health care* (according to the World Health Organization, 2008), these approaches to care that incorporate the social and environmental factors are now understood to be essential elements of a truly reformed health-care system, and in some cases are also referred to as population-based care or preventive care, and in other contexts referred to as *social determinants of health* (see Fig. 1.1). This holistic approach was largely abandoned by allopathic medical science in the earlier part of the 20th century in favor of technology-based interventions and medical specialization (Brandt, 1997). However, modern medicine recognizes the need for such approaches to provide more effective care with lasting effects and to deal with current health-care realities that highlight the interplay among human health and environmental and social influences (e.g., the health effects of community violence, gun violence, teen pregnancy, sexual and physical abuse, and HIV infection). As with medicine, nursing has renewed its emphasis on population-based approaches, reaffirming its historic roots. There is now a shared understanding of the importance of these approaches. This is an ideal climate in which to build interprofessional education—shared *core* understandings of care, but with variations in ways to implement or practice these understandings.

The PCMH is anticipated to be one of the main drivers in providing a more responsive, more effective, and less expensive health-care delivery system. This concept is "a philosophical transformation of the way that care is delivered" (Nutting et al., 2009). Patient care within a PCMH should have a whole-person orientation and be coordinated across the health-care system, replacing a fragmented, episodic health-care delivery system. New reimbursement models should reflect the added value of the PCMH to the patient by providing for continuous coordinated care and expanded access to services that fall outside of the fee-for-service system. The process of transition into a PCMH model is a lengthy and complicated one and will require a champion who can allocate resources to this effort and both support and coordinate the process of change. This requires strong leadership and excellent organizational skills—additional areas in which APRNs excel.

Additionally, leaders are needed to guide teams of health-care providers and support staff who work with specific patient populations (e.g., diabetic patients or those with congestive heart failure). This leader might be the same person who advocates for the process of change, or it might be someone different who is focused solely on the provision of care to individual patients. Effective implementation of the PCMH model requires someone to delegate duties among the team of providers and to make decisions, along with the patient, about aspects of care such as referral to specialists.

Regardless of who assumes this role, the PCMH leader must be able to move the organization forward to meet the accreditation requirements and to receive enhanced reimbursement as a PCMH practice. Similar to Joint Commission: Accreditation, Health Care, Certification (JCAHO) or Magnet recognition programs, a PCMH practice must meet specific criteria and inspection requirements by one of four current accrediting agencies: the National Committee for Quality Assurance (NCQA), JCAHO, the Utilization Review Accreditation Committee, and/or the Accreditation Association for Ambulatory Health Care. For example, receiving recognition as a PCMH practice by the NCQA depends on meeting specific elements in six standard categories (Table 1.1).

Widescale adoption of this model is fundamentally changing the primary-care landscape. At present, the physician's skill set is not geared toward care coordination or managing transitions in care, because these functions have been historically performed by nurses. However, the challenges in our health-care system call for creative thinking and innovative improvements in care. Various technologies will continue to emerge, and health care will continue to evolve, but the interpersonal caring base on which nursing has always been grounded will continue to be widely needed and a driving force.

TABLE 1.1 National Committee for Quality Assurance Patient-Centered Medical Home: Structure of Concepts, Criteria, and Competencies

Concepts. The overarching themes of the PCMH. To earn recognition, your practice must complete criteria in each of six concept areas.
Criteria. Specific activities in which a practice engages to demonstrate that it meets recognition requirements. The practice must pass all 40 core criteria and at least 25 credits of elective criteria across concept areas.
Competencies. Competencies categorize the criteria. Competencies do not offer credit.

Concept Areas

CONCEPT	DESCRIPTION
Team-Based Care and Practice Organization	Helps structure a practice's leadership, care team responsibilities, and how the practice partners with patients, families, and caregivers
Knowing and Managing Your Patients	Sets standards for data collection, medication reconciliation, evidence-based clinical decision support, and other activities
Patient-Centered Access and Continuity	Guides practices to provide patients with convenient access to clinical advice and helps ensure continuity of care
Care Management and Support	Helps clinicians set up care management protocols to identify patients who need more closely managed care.
Care Coordination and Care Transitions	Ensures that primary and specialty care clinicians are effectively sharing information and managing patient referrals to minimize cost, confusion, and inappropriate care
Performance Measurement and Quality Improvement	Helps practices develop ways to measure performance, set goals, and develop activities that will improve performance

FURTHER UNDERSTANDING THE CIRCLE OF CARING

The *Circle of Caring* model (see Fig. 1.3) has grown out of, and is rooted in, the assumption that caring is the central concept of nursing and is uniquely known and expressed in nursing. Boykin and Schoenhofer (2001) contend that the special contributions of nursing to nurturing the wholeness of persons and environment through caring. Additionally, they affirm all nursing takes place within nursing situations, as "shared lived experiences in which caring between the persons of nurse and nursed enhances the process of living and growing in caring" (see Chapter 2 of this text). Watson (1988) viewed caring as an intersubjective human process based on the belief that "persons learn from one another how to be human by identifying ourselves with others or finding their dilemmas in ourselves." Boykin and Schoenhofer (2001) extended this concept and defined caring in nursing as "the intentional and authentic presence of the nurse with another who is recognized as a person living caring and growing in caring."

Mayeroff (1971) discussed the primacy of caring as a process in contrast to caring as a product, with caring viewed as an end in and of itself. Mayeroff also identified "ingredients" of caring: knowing, alternating rhythms, patience, honesty, courage, humility, trust, and hope. Boykin and Schoenhofer (2001) viewed caring in nursing "as a mutual human process in which the nurse responds with authentic presence to a call from another." The caring attributes of the *Circle of Caring* are based on these—knowing, patience, authentic presence, commitment, courage, and advocacy—and are elaborated by Boykin and Schoenhofer in Chapter 2 of this text. It is the caring attributes that characterize the nurse–patient relationship, enabling healing. Healing is meant in the broadest sense of the word: it might imply a good death, for example.

This chapter has focused on the professions of nursing and medicine. Today, interprofessional practice includes many other disciplines, such dentistry, social work, pharmacy, and physical and occupational therapy. Seemingly disparate partners may also play a role in health care, such as lawyers and advocates working for social equity, local and global businesses creating healthier communities, and local, state, and federal governments developing healthier housing and safer community environments.

- No single discipline, perspective, or role can heal the current problems ailing the U.S. health-care system. All are needed more than ever to shape a healthful future, and all must rethink their roles, functions, and professional cultures. Moving away from the hierarchical role structures of the hospital setting creates an opportunity to redefine the content and processes of clinical practice and negotiate a new and as yet undefined space. The boundaries of practice continue to expand and contract for all stakeholders during this transformative

period. The larger questions for all health-care professions include the following: How will all health-care professionals be accountable to their patients?

- Are physicians and APRNs willing to share accountability in a responsible manner?
- Is the Institute of Medicine's *Bridge to Quality* becoming a reality?
- How can disciplines work together in a meaningful way to achieve the goals and objectives of *Healthy People 2020*?
- How can medicine and nursing, as well as other disciplines, work together to achieve the triple aim of health-care reform: improving the patient experience of care (including quality and satisfaction), improving the health of populations, and reducing the per capita cost of health care?
- How do we integrate the proposed fourth aim—healthier (and happier) work environments?

Lynaugh, in an unpublished paper from 1989, specifically discussing medicine and nursing, suggests that both disciplines can occupy the same territory to the benefit of patient care; however, she notes that tension is created by proximity, stating that "physicians and nurses quarrel occasionally when they jostle each other in the narrow passageway of patient care." This can be further extrapolated to other health-care professions. However, Lynaugh makes the case that tension is preferable to the distrust and ignorance that stem from silence and distance between disciplines. She advocates a "productive tension" and social parity between health-care professions that will benefit the care of all patients. Health-care professionals are *all* natural allies, with the best interests of the patient at their core. In turn, all perspectives are needed, working together, for effective change to occur in the health-care system.

In daily practice, primary-care providers hear the frustration of patients and families in dealing with today's health-care system. Although the technology of medical care continues to improve, the interactional and collaborative aspects of care are often underdeveloped. A *Circle of Caring* model is needed for patients, families, social groups, and communities. This model is also a way to document and describe the practice of primary-care providers, who respond to calls from patients and who imaginatively, creatively, and powerfully foster meaningful responses in the context of the situation. These responses may be fashioned on the micro level in the one-to-one clinician–patient relationship in primary or acute care or on the macro level, as nursing-based knowledge unites with traditional public health approaches and is applied to the care of communities and populations (see Chapter 3).

This transformative model, the *Circle of Caring,* incorporates the strengths of nursing, public health, and medicine, and reformulates them in a new model of care. Primary-care practitioners are the appropriate providers to demonstrate the efficacy of an integrated model of caregiving, rooted in the lived experience of the patient as experienced in the context of the larger community. This text offers you the necessary tools to provide care in ways that will be meaningful for patients, their families, their social groups, and the larger communities in which they live.

 For additional resources please visit https://davisedge.fadavis.com/

REFERENCES

AACN. (2015) Current Issues and Clarifying DNP Recommendations – I sent this document yesterday

Administration on Aging. Aging into the 21st century. U.S. Department of Health & Human Services. www.aoa.gov/AoARoot/Aging.Statistics/future_growth/aging21/health.aspx. Accessed September 16, 2017.

Agency for Healthcare Research and Quality. National healthcare quality and disparities report. http://nhqrnet.ahrg.gov/inhqrdr/data/query. Published 2015. Accessed August 15, 2017.

American Association of Colleges of Nursing (AACN). Essentials of doctoral education for advanced nursing practice. www.aacn.nche.edu/dnp/PDF/essentials. Published 2009.

American Association of Nurse Practitioners. AANP statement on unique perspective of the nurse practitioner. htpp://www.aanp/org/all-about-nps/what-is-an-np/. Published 2017. Accessed November 18, 2017.

American Nurses Association (ANA). *Nursing: A social policy statement.* Kansas City, MO: ANA; 2010.

American Public Health Association. Health disparities: the basics. http://www.apha.org/media/files/pdf/factsheets/healthdisparity_primer_final.ashx. Accessed August 15, 2017

APRN Consensus Work Group & the National Council of State Boards of Nursing APRN Advisory Committee. Consensus model for APRN regulation: Licensure, accreditation, certification & education. APRN joint dialogue group report. http://c.ymcdn.com/sites/www.nonpf.org/resource/resmgr/consensus_model/aprnconsensusmodelfinal09.pdf. Published July 2008. Accessed November 24, 2017.

Arias E, Heron M, Xu JQ. United States life tables, 2013. National vital statistics reports; vol. 66 no 3. Hyattsville, MD: National Center for Health Statistics; 2017.

Atlas SJ. Patient-physician connectedness may affect quality of care. *Ann Intern Med.* 2009;150:325–335.

Baer E. Philosophical and historical bases of primary care nursing. In: Mezey MD, McGivern DO, eds. *Nurses, nurse practitioners: Evolution to advanced practice.* 2nd ed. New York, NY: Springer; 1993:114.

Benner P. *From novice to expert.* Menlo Park, CA: Addison-Wesley; 1984.

Benner P, Wrubel J. *The primacy of caring.* Menlo Park, CA: Addison-Wesley; 1989.

Blacksher E. Health reform: What's prevention got to do with it? *Hastings Cent Rep.* 2009;39(6):49.

Bodenheimer T, Chen E, Bennett HD. Confronting the growing burden of chronic disease: Can the U.S. health care workforce do the job? *Health Aff.* 2009;28:64–74.

Bodenheimer T, Grumbach K. *Understanding health policy: A clinical approach.* 7th ed. New York, NY: Appleton & Lange; 2016.

Boykin A, Schoenhofer S. *Nursing as caring: A model for transforming practice.* Sudbury, MA: Jones and Bartlett and National League for Nursing Press; 2001.

Boykin A, et al. Aesthetic knowing grounded in an explicit conception of nursing. *Nurs Sci Q.* 1994;7(4):158–161.

Brandt AM. Just say no: Risk, behavior, and disease in twentieth-century America. In: Walters R, ed. *Scientific authority and twentieth century America.* Baltimore, MD: Johns Hopkins University Press; 1997:82–98.

Burman ME, et al. Reconceptualizing the core of nurse practitioner education and practice. *Am Acad Nurse Pract.* 2009;21:11–17.

Callahan D. Medical progress: Unintended consequences. In: Callahan D, ed. *Connecting American values with health reform.* Garrison, NY: Hastings Center; 2009:12–14.

Central Intelligence Agency. The world factbook. https://www.cia.gov/library/publications/resources/the-world-factbook/rankorder/2091rankhtml. Published 2014. Accessed August 15, 2017.

Chetty R, Stepner M, Abraham S, Lin S, Scuderi B, Turner N, Bergeron A, Cutler D. The association between income and life expectancy in the United States, 2001–2014. *JAMA.* 2016;315(16):1750–1766.

Cody WK. Nursing theory-guided practice: What it is and what it is not. *Nurs Sci Q.* 1994;7(3):144–145.

Committee on Facilitating Interdisciplinary Research. *Facilitating interdisciplinary research.* Washington, DC: National Academy of Sciences, National Academy of Engineering, National Academy of Medicine; 2005.

Cooke M, et al. American medical education 100 years after the Flexner Report. *N Engl J Med.* 2006;355(13):1339–1344.

Cumbie SA, et al. Advanced practice nursing model for comprehensive care with chronic illness: Model for promoting engagement. *Adv Nurs Sci.* 2004;27(1):70–80.

Dacher E. Reinventing primary care. *J Altern Ther Health Med.* 1995;1(5):29–34.

Decker J, et al. Use of medical care for chronic conditions. *Health Aff.* 2009;28(1):26–35.

Department of Health and Human Services. *Report to Congress: National strategy for quality improvement in health care.* Washington, DC: Department of Health and Human Services; 2011.

Dock LL, Stewart IB. *A short history of nursing.* New York, NY: G.P. Putnam's Sons; 1920.

Dodd M, et al. Advancing the science of symptom management. *J Adv Nurs.* 2001;33(5):668–676.

Dols J, Hernández C, Miles H. The DNP project: Quandaries for nursing scholars. *Nurs Outlook.* 2017;65(1):84–93.

Dunphy LM. Doing what had to be done. In: Joel L, ed. *Advanced practice nursing: Essentials for role development.* 4th ed. Philadelphia, PA: F.A. Davis; 2018:2–15.

Eisenberg L. Disease and illness: Distinctions between professional and popular ideas of sickness. *Cult Med Psychiatry.* 1977;1:9.

Fairman J, D'Antonio P. Reimagining nursing's place in the history of clinical practice. *J Hist Med Allied Sci.* 2008;63(4):435–446.

Fenton MV, Brykczynski, KA. Qualitative distinctions and similarities in the practice of the clinical nurse specialists and nurse practitioners. *J Prof Nurs.* 1993;9:313.

Gordon M. *Nursing diagnosis: Process and application.* 2nd ed. New York, NY: McGraw-Hill; 1987.

Health Resources and Services Administration, Bureau of Health Professions, National Center for Health Workforce Analysis. *Projecting the supply and demand for primary care practitioners through 2020.* Washington, DC: U.S. Department of Health & Human Services; 2013.

Hektor LM. Martha E. Rogers: A life history. *Nurs Sci Q.* 1989;2: 63–73.

Henderson V. *The nature of nursing.* New York, NY: Macmillan; 1966.

Howie JGR. A new look at illness in general practice: A reclassification of illness based on antibiotic prescribing. In: Rakel R, ed. *Textbook of family practice.* 4th ed. Philadelphia, PA: WB Saunders; 2011.

Institute of Medicine. Health care quality initiative. *Crossing the quality chasm: A new health care system for the 21st century.* Washington, DC: National Academy Press; 2001.

Institute of Medicine. *Health professions education: A bridge to quality.* Washington, DC: National Academy Press; 2003.

Institute of Medicine. *The future of nursing: Leading change, advancing health.* Washington, DC: National Academy Press; 2011.

Johnson R. Nurse practitioner–patient discourse: Uncovering the voice of nursing in primary care practice. *Schol Inq Nurs Pract Int J.* 1993;7(3):143.

Judge-Ellis T, Wilson TR. Time and NP practice: Naming, claiming, and explaining the role of nurse practitioners. *Nurse Pract.* 2017;13(9):583–589.

Kochanek KD, Murphy SL, Xu JQ, Arias E. Mortality in the United States, 2016. NCHS Data Brief, no 293. Hyattsville, MD: National Center for Health Statistics. 2017.

Kolata G. Death rates rising for middle-aged white Americans, study finds. *New York Times.* November 2, 2015. https://nyti. ms/1KUrGdg. Accessed November 24, 2017.

Kolata G, Cohen S. Drug overdoses propel rise in mortality rates for young whites. *New York Times.* January 16, 2016. https://nytim. ms/1OWwoOR. Accessed November 24, 2017.

Lewis PH, Brykczynski KA. Practical knowledge and competencies of the healing role of the nurse practitioner. *J Am Acad Nurse Pract.* 1994;6(5):207–213.

Livanos N. Physicians look to disrupt longtime regulatory tradition for APRNs. *J Nurs Regul.* 2017;9(3):59–62.

Lynaugh J, Bates B. The two languages of nursing and medicine. *Am J Nurs.* 1973;73(1):66.

Madden M. Conceptualizations of advanced nursing practice. In: Hamric AB, Spross JA, Hanson CM, eds. *Advanced practice nursing: An integrative approach.* 1st ed. Philadelphia, PA: WB Saunders; 1996:25–41.

Massachusetts: Institute for Healthcare Improvement. http://ihi.org. Published 2014. Accessed November 30, 2017.

Mayeroff M. *On caring.* New York, NY: Harper & Row; 1971.

Mishler EG. *The discourse of medicine: Dialectics of medical interviews.* Norwood, NJ: Ablex; 1984.

Mitchell G. Nursing diagnosis: An obstacle to caring ways. In: Boykin A, ed. *Power, politics, and public policy.* New York, NY: National League for Nursing Press; 1995.

National Organization of Nurse Practitioner Faculties. National Organization of Nurse Practitioner Faculties Domains and Core Competencies of Nurse Practitioner Practice. www.nonpf.com/ associations/10789/files/DomainsandCoreComps2006.pdf. Published March 2006.

National Partnership for Action. HHS action plan to reduce racial and ethnic health disparities and the national stakeholder strategy for achieving health equity. http://minorityhealth.hhs.gov/npa. Published 2011.

National Prevention and Health Promotion Strategy. The National prevention strategy: America's plan for better health and wellness, June 2011. https://www.surgeongeneral.gov/priorities/prevention/ strategy/index.html.

Newman MA, Smith MC, Pharris MD, Jones D. The focus of the discipline revisited. *Adv Nurs Sci.* 2008;31(1):16–27.

Nightingale F. *Notes on nursing: What it is and what it is not.* Dover, New York; 1860/1969.

Nutting P, Miller W, Crabtree B, Jaen CT, Steward E, Strange K. Initial lessons from the First National Demonstration project on practice transformation to a patient-centered medical home. *Ann Fam Med.* 2009;7(3):254–260.

Parker M. Exploring the aesthetic meaning of presence in nursing practice. In: Gaut D, ed. *The presence of caring in nursing.* New York, NY: National League for Nursing Press; 1992.

Payne R. The quality mantra: Proceed carefully. *Hastings Cent Rep.* 2009;39(6):14.

Rakel R, ed. *Textbook of family practice.* 4th ed. Philadelphia, PA: WB Saunders; 2011.

Reed PG. A treatise on nursing knowledge development for the 21st century: Beyond postmodernism. *Adv Nurs Sci.* 1995;17(3):70.

Riffle K. CAM therapies for nurse practitioners. *Adv Nurse Pract.* http://nurse-practitioners.advanceweb.com/Editorial/content. Accessed December 17, 2017.

Rogers ME. Nursing: To be or not to be? *Nurs Outlook.* 1972;20: 42–46.

Rogers ME. The nurse practitioner movement: Pro and con. *Am J Nurs.* 1975;75(10):1834–1843.

Ryan P. Integrated theory of health behavior change: Background and intervention development. *Clin Nurse Spec.* 2009;23(4):161–170.

San Francisco School of Nursing Management Faculty Group. A model for symptom management. *Image J Nurs Sch.* 1994; 26(4):272–276.

Scoville R, Little K. Comparing lean and quality improvement. IHI white paper. Cambridge, MA: Institute for Healthcare Improvement; 2014.

Secretary's Advisory Committee on Health Promotion and Disease Prevention Objectives for 2020. *Healthy People 2020: An opportunity to address the societal determinants of health in the united states.* http://www.healthypeople.gov/2010/hp2020/advisory/ SocietalDeterminantsHealth.htm. Published July 26, 2010. Accessed October 10, 2017,

Shalala DE. Nursing and society: The unfinished agenda for the 21st century. *Nurs Health Care.* 1993;14(6):4–7.

Shuler PA, Davis JE. The Shuler Nurse Practitioner Practice Model. *J Am Acad Nurse Pract.* 1993;5(1):11–17.

Shuler PA, et al. Providing holistic health care for the elderly: Utilization of the Shuler Nurse Practitioner Model. *J Am Acad Nurse Pract.* 2001;13(7):297–303.

Snyder M. Defining nursing interventions. *Image J Nurs Sch.* 1996; 28(2):137.

Snyder M, Mirr S. Independent nursing intervention. 2nd ed. Albany, NY: Delmar; 1995.

Spross JA, Lawson MT. Conceptualizations of advanced practice nursing. In: Hamric AB, Spross JA, Hanson CM, eds. *Advanced practice nursing: An integrative approach.* 4th ed. St. Louis, MO: Saunders Elsevier; 2008:33–74.

St. Anthony's: *ICD-10-CM: Code book for physician payment.* Vols 1 and 2. Cincinnati, OH: St. Anthony Publishing; 2005.

Stewart M, et al. *Patient-centered medicine: Transforming the clinical method.* Thousand Oaks, CA: Sage; 1995.

Swanson C. A spirit-focused conceptual model of nursing for the advanced practice nurse. *Issues Comp Pediatr Nurs.* 1995;18:267–275.

Thurman W, Pfitzinger-Lippe M. Returning to the profession's roots: Social justice in nursing education for the 21st century. *Adv Nurs Sci.* 2017;40(2):184–193.

U.S. Department of Health and Human Services. *Healthy people 2020.* McLean, VA: International Medical Publishing; 2010.

University of California, San Francisco School of Nursing Symptom Management Faculty Group. A model for symptom management. *Image J Nurs Sch.* 1994;26:272–276.

Watson J. *Nursing: Human science and human care.* Norwalk, CT: Appleton-Century-Crofts; 1988.

Whitcomb M, Nutter D. *Learning medicine in the 21st century: The general professional education of the physician.* Carnegie Institute study: Educating doctors to provide high quality care: A vision for medical education in the United States. Washington, DC: Association of Medical Colleges; 2004.

World Health Organization, Commission on Social Determinants of Health. Closing the gap in a generation: Health equity through action on the social determinants of health. http://www.who.int/social_determinants/enExternal Accessed August 2018.

Zimmer P, et al. *Advanced practice nursing: Nurse practitioner curriculum guidelines.* Seattle, WA: National Organization of Nurse Practitioner Faculty; 1990.

RESOURCES

Centers for Disease Control and Prevention. United States life tables, 2013
https://www.cdc.gov/nchs/data/nvsr/nvsr66/nvsr66_03.pdf

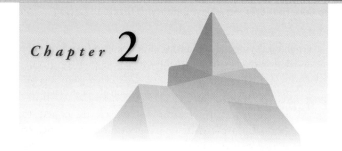

Chapter **2**

Caring and the Advanced Practice Nurse

Anne Boykin, PhD, RN

Savina O. Schoenhofer, PhD, RN

Advanced practice registered nursing (APRN) is a special way of nursing. Although the APRN role blends elements of medical practice and generic primary care, it is based on the traditional nursing approach of caring as a way of being, knowing, and doing. The emphasis on the learning of medical and scientific knowledge and skills in advanced nursing science programs sometimes obscures the fact that these programs are aimed at the development of advanced practice nurses, not physicians.

The advanced practice of nursing must be firmly grounded in the knowledge and skills of caring. The framework presented in this text is intended to help students, faculty, and providers retain a caring-based nursing focus while addressing advanced practice nursing in an interdisciplinary environment.

Dunphy's advanced practice nursing model, the *Circle of Caring* (see Chapter 1), introduces the term "caring process" as a pivotal element. In familiar usage, the term "process" (e.g., "nursing process" or "problem-solving process") means a series of cognitive or psychomotor steps or things to do. In the *Circle of Caring* model, "process" means "unfolding." Caring processes are ways to express a way of being and living as a caring person in the profession of advanced nursing. There is no defined set or list of caring processes; rather, there are as many caring processes as there are persons and situations.

CARING

Caring is the essence of being human, and nursing is a deeply human relationship; thus, caring is the essence of nursing. The meaning of caring as the essential nature of humanness cannot be condensed within a single limiting definition; rather, caring can be understood, recognized, and developed both philosophically and practically. Caring expressed in nursing is the intentional and authentic presence of the nurse with another person who is living, caring, and growing in caring (Boykin & Schoenhofer, 2001).

All human service disciplines are based on caring. Nursing is unique, however, in that caring directly characterizes a nurse's knowledge base and service. In contrast, in the discipline of medicine, the fundamental commitment to caring is directly reflected in the diagnosis and treatment of human structural and functional problems manifested primarily in physical terms. The nature of the APRN role permits a direct focus on care and caring that also incorporates the focus of medicine. An APRN does not practice medicine but rather draws on and transforms characteristic medical methods of practice for nursing purposes, just as the practice of holistic medicine draws on and transforms characteristic nursing ways of practice for medical purposes.

Caring is the matrix, the medium, the "stuff" within which the APRN–patient relationship is brought to life. In this relationship, the APRN lives his or her commitment to caring by facilitating a personal connection that communicates "I acknowledge you as a caring person, one who is worthwhile and deserving of my respect, my attention, my commitment, my care." That effort to create a personal connection also communicates the practitioner's acceptance of the trust being placed in him or her as a caring person, as one who is available and able to participate effectively in the life of the other. Within the caring relationship, each participant has the opportunity for enhancing personhood, that is, for living life grounded in caring and for growing in one's capacity to express caring in meaningful and satisfying ways. Knowing another as a caring person requires a commitment to entering the world of the nursed with the explicit intention of knowing the person individually and uniquely. Entering into the world of another with caring intention requires that the practitioner know himself or herself as caring and be open to growing in the relationship. A truly collaborative relationship (in contrast to one in which the collaboration is taken at face value or in some way limited) emerges in the context of this caring intention.

All APRNs, including nurse practitioners (NPs) in primary care, practice a specialized form of nursing. In APRN practice, specialized opportunities for creating situations of care call forth unique patterns of caring. Although a person seeking care may present with an issue that is characterized as typically medical, the APRN is cocreating a relationship with the person in which care is experienced and possibilities for personally meaningful ways of living unfold.

Specialized patterns of caring in the role of APRN blend knowledgeable perspectives of the health situation and recommendations for characteristically medical ways of ameliorating presenting issues (treatment) with generalized patterns of nursing care. Generalized patterns of nursing care are represented in the *Circle of Caring* model as follows:

- Courage
- Authentic presence

- Advocacy
- Knowing
- Commitment
- Patience

Specialized patterns of care are incorporated in the uniqueness of caring processes. Knowledge of general patterns of care is important; however, that knowledge must be creatively used in actual, unfolding processes of care if the situation is to be considered nursing. These themes of caring can serve as a conceptual structure or framework to assist the practitioner in examining, recognizing, and understanding the fullness of caring in practice. Though interconnected, each individual theme is addressed theoretically and then in action in a practice situation to illustrate caring processes.

Courage

Courage is a human act (Tillich, 1952). Courage comes to light in making deliberate choices resulting in acts that express who we are and what is important to us. Courage is the daily application of values, the living out of one's beliefs in spite of obstacles and challenging situations. Expressions of courage affirm our being.

This understanding of courage offers an ethical grounding for the practice of advanced nursing. It requires that, in each nursing situation, the nurse live the values held dear. The nurse risks entering each situation with the fullness of his or her being, willing to be rejected or not understood, or, perhaps equally risky, being accepted and known.

As part of courage, the nurse also understands and acts on the obligation to come to know that which matters to those seeking care. What shapes the moments the nurse has with people is the intention to know them as caring, to hear their stories, and to create nurturing responses reflective of the uniqueness of the situation. Courage manifests itself because of the nurse's deliberate choices to carry out, in a particular time and place, the beliefs that serve as the core of advanced nursing practice. Courage manifests itself in making one's nursing vocation a commitment to these values and beliefs that undergird caring.

Authentic Presence

Nursing is communicated through authentic presence. Authentic presence is a unique way of being with others, unique in that it is a way of ordering and balancing self so as to grow in one's beauty and spirit. Such presence with self requires trust, courage, and the desire to know. One who is authentic with self and others is able to see things from the inside that others see only from the outside. There is an inner genuine awareness that is congruent with feelings, attitudes, and actions lived moment to moment. The commitment to truly know oneself frees one to be with others in authentic presence.

Authentic presence may be understood as intentionally being with another in the fullness of one's personhood. The caring that is communicated through authentic presence is the initiating and sustaining medium of nursing within the nursing situation. Nurses are called to be authentically present in nursing situations. Stories of nursing practice portray the depth of such experiences. The degree to which one knows oneself influences one's presence with others and thus the degree of commitment possible in the situation.

Advocacy

Advocacy is a way in which nurses have traditionally expressed caring. There are many opportunities for advocacy, that is, many situations in which "speaking up for" another is an important aspect of the role. From a depth of knowledge and understanding, the practitioner speaks up for the person as unique and worthwhile, as having personal hopes, dreams, intentions, and preferences that are honorable. Gadow's (1990) formulation of existential advocacy calls for the nurse to advocate for alternative interpretations of the situations that arise from experience and specialized knowledge. Existential advocacy is contrasted with advocacy that is either paternalistic or consumer oriented. Paternalistic advocacy is characterized by a sense of "as the expert, I know what is best for you and your life." Consumer-oriented advocacy takes the approach that "I'll just give you the facts and options; you sort them out by yourself."

In existential advocacy, self is brought into the situation as a full partner, sharing alternative perspectives for consideration, although not insisting on them or imposing them. The patient enters into the relationship seeking to connect with the practitioner as a whole person, not just as a set of facts. When the practitioner takes the paternalistic stance (dismissive and overbearing, offering an all-or-none option) or the consumer-oriented stance (withdrawn to an objective distance, offering an essentially value-free set of options), the patient experiences the loss of an opportunity to connect with another assumed to be truly concerned, knowledgeable, and giving. When the nurse offers existential advocacy, the nursed feels truly known, respected, and connected in a way that affirms humanity and being.

Knowing

Knowing as an aspect of caring encompasses "knowing that," "knowing about," "knowing directly," and "unknowing." "Knowing that" and "knowing about" refer to descriptions and analyses of the patient's situation in the context of facts and information. Caring competence requires knowledge of facts and data points that are empirically and objectively derived. "Knowing directly" involves being deeply attuned to the person-as-person and comes through intentionality and authentic presence. "Unknowing" refers to an openness to unfolding, a humble sense that all is not yet known. The practitioner who truly embraces unknowing recognizes that what might be right or timely in general terms may be neither right nor timely for the particular person seeking care in a particular moment.

Carper (1978) described patterns of knowing fundamental to nursing: personal, empiric, ethical, and aesthetic knowing. The practitioner draws on the personal way of knowing as essential intuitive knowing. Empiric knowing is an avenue for drawing on science and skilled observation. Ethical knowing prompts the practitioner to ask, "What are the personal and professional values that enter into this situation?" And thus, "What is right for this situation?" Esthetic knowing develops as the practitioner incorporates knowing gained from the other patterns in the context of fully living the situation as she or he cocreates with the nursed an integrated understanding of the unfolding whole picture.

The *Circle of Caring* is developed and strengthened as the practitioner and patient communicate their unfolding knowing of self, of each other, and of the situation. Knowing, as described briefly here, contributes to enhanced personhood, to the affirmation and growth of self and other as caring persons.

Commitment

Is there any greater act of courage than the commitment to another? Commitment is a sign of that which we value. Choosing to be a member of the discipline and profession of nursing speaks to the deep valuing and lifelong commitment of service to humankind. Commitment directs obligations or what "ought to be" in particular situations. Because these commitments are so internalized as values, however, one's obligation is not experienced as a burden but as a response that is right, deliberate, conscious, and caring (Roach, 2002).

Nurses in advanced practice roles frequently face challenges to commitment. Choices made in practice reflect one's devotion to particular commitments. Often the values of an economically based health-care system, of which nursing is such an integral part, do not support or seem to be in line with the substantive nature of caring and its essential relation to practice. A struggle to preserve nursing's values often results. The APRN has the unique opportunity to demonstrate how a commitment to the values of nursing influences the outcomes of care.

The practice of advanced nursing must be firmly rooted in the values of the nurse. In addition to many essential types of knowledge and skills, he or she must be able to draw on the knowledge of nursing, especially knowledge of caring, to create environments for care that honor person-as-person and that humanize care.

Nursing always occurs in a relational context. As a human science, nursing calls for the continued commitment to understand better the lived experience of the nursed, to truly hear their stories, and to respond in ways that matter, ways that nurture and sustain persons as they live and grow in caring. Central to advanced practice is the commitment to know self and others as caring.

Patience

Patience as a key theme in caring refers to trusting people to grow in their own time and in their own way (Mayeroff, 1971). Patience is not passive but rather an active openness to "the moment alive with possibilities." Humility and courage are intimately connected to patience. The ability to remain actively engaged with the person while honoring individual circumstances and freedom of choice is an act of courage and leads to the kind of patience that communicates caring.

CARING PROCESSES

The two Nursing Situations below illustrate ways in which advanced nursing practice is truly an expression of caring processes. The first story was shared by a family nurse practitioner (FNP) in practice in a family clinic in a small rural southern town.

Nursing Situation: Like a Pebble in a Pond—The Circle of Caring

The incident that I am describing involved an 18-year-old female college student—I'll call her Lucy—and her mother, Mrs. K. Lucy presented at my clinic with a history of shortness of breath and flu-like symptoms for several months. She and her mother had been to multiple health-care providers seeking a diagnosis and resolution of Lucy's problem. I had never seen this patient, so I went through the usual process of taking a history of the present illness, past medical history, social history, and a thorough physical examination. I then ordered what I determined to be the necessary tests. The outcome was a referral to a pulmonologist in a nearby city with the eventual successful resolution of her illness.

The interesting part of this story is what happened years later regarding this clinical incident. My husband and I went into a newly opened used bookstore in our community. On entering, there was no one but the owner and the two of us in the store. When the owner saw me, she came over and hugged me like a long-lost friend—it was Mrs. K! I did not even remotely recognize her and was sure she had mistaken me for someone else. She looked at my husband and stated, "She saved my daughter's life." She then began to cry as she related her feelings about the event and what had transpired. Mrs. K was embarrassed by her emotions (so was I), but she was determined to tell her story.

Mrs. K said that she had taken her daughter to multiple health-care providers seeking help for her child. She felt they did not take the case seriously and "blew her off" even as her daughter worsened. When Mrs. K and Lucy came to me, Mrs. K was desperate for help for her daughter. Mrs. K described her feelings regarding the clinical visit, grateful that I had listened and believed what she was saying. She then quoted something I had said to her that she said had given her hope and comfort. I told her that "I will do everything possible to find out what is wrong in order to help Lucy get better. We will not give up until we knew what is going on with Lucy." Mrs. K said a burden was lifted from her because at last she felt that "someone cared." Mrs. K told us that with the referral, the problem was diagnosed and resolved. It was her profound belief that I had literally saved her daughter's life. I do not remember Lucy's final diagnosis at this point in time, and I don't know how much actual assistance I gave in the final resolution of her illness; but I will always remember Mrs. K's gratitude for a caring response to her feelings of helplessness while dealing with the health-care system. Mrs. K's belated description of her heartfelt feelings regarding her daughter's illness and my interventional actions made a profound impression on me as a provider. The need for a caring response to each of our patients is evident; yet, we may never know how much such caring can impact a life.

As shared by Carolyn B. Dollar, PhD, APRN-BC, FNP

In this story, the most prominent caring processes are authentic presence and commitment, as the FNP offered self in a way that truly communicated caring to this beleaguered family. The FNP's commitment to caring for the family and her courage and patience in tackling an issue that obviously had been given a "pass" by previous health-care providers illustrate the importance of opportunities to hear and respond effectively to calls for caring in advanced nursing practice. Referral is an act of advocacy that is frequently an element of NP practice, and when it is recognized as an opportunity for caring through advocacy, it becomes an even more integral expression of advanced nursing. The fact that the FNP offered this particular story as an exemplar of caring in advanced nursing practice makes evident the merging of knowing in past–present–future: the FNP continues to be open to knowing self and others through appreciating the mother's report of the impact of an act of caring initiated in the rather distant past.

A second story from an APRN practicing in a specialty clinic in an urban health sciences center showcases the centrality of the nurse–patient caring relationship in the midst of treatment situations involving complicated biomedical technology.

Nursing Situation: Spirited Caring

My APRN role has been a rewarding challenge. The story that I am going to share was pivotal to my development as an APRN. The story focuses on a pleasant, jolly, gem of a patient, with a warm smile—I'll call her Mrs. J. Her energy lit up the room. This independent free spirit also worked as a volunteer at the clinic. She served cookies and other baked goods to the patients undergoing chemotherapy. Her strong faith and compassion for others impressed me as a busy provider. To the nursing staff, she stood out as a patient and volunteer. Her faith helped her in aiding the sicker patients to maintain hope. Her genuine concern for others encouraged nursing staff and family members to have compassion for others. Mrs. J was always the first to ask, "How are you doing?" This unique patient was a beacon of light in a dark, sobering environment.

My favorite patient and I developed a good rapport as I saw her weekly in the Coumadin clinic. She was my first patient on my very first day. When she stepped into my office and noted my frazzled appearance, she grabbed my hands and prayed with me. Because we are in the Bible belt, I considered that to be normal. She later apologized because she did not know my religious beliefs. I assured her that her actions had calmed me and made my day go a little better. Mrs. J had been doing exceptionally well although she had been diagnosed with cancer. She had a history of stage II breast cancer but had been in complete remission for 2 years.

One Friday, she presented to the clinic at four o'clock in the afternoon. She had been complaining of vision changes and had her son bring her to the clinic. I knew something was wrong because this independent woman always presented to visits alone. Mrs. J's primary care provider was not available by phone, and her oncologist was out of town. She reported a headache with vision changes, which seemed strange for a woman who had undergone chemotherapy with adjuvant radiation therapy without difficulties. She explained that 4 days before this clinic visit, she experienced the worst headache she had ever had. Her clinical presentation led me to order a computed tomography (CT) scan of the head with contrast. After reading her CT, the radiologist called me immediately. He had identified a large mass that was pressing against her sulcus. At this point, I had to find her hematologist, start her on high-dose steroids, find the neurosurgeon on call, and prepare her for everything that was about to take place. I was so consumed by my actions that I nearly forgot to care for the patient.

Mrs. J demonstrated sincere compassion when I had to give her the hard news. She grabbed my hands and prayed for me and the other health-care providers. She prayed that we would make the right decisions regarding her health care. Just as we had started our relationship, we were ending it. Her demonstration of faith was a unique testament to her life. Her strength in a time of weakness showed the vigor of her faith. Though she was a devout Catholic and I am a Methodist, we had to rely on our genuine concern for each other and our beliefs in a higher being to get us through this difficult time. Compassion and faith were integral components in our provider–patient relationship.

The experience taught us that compassion and faith coupled with therapeutic communication can get you through the toughest of situations. In revisiting this story, I am reminded of the need to foster a sense of caring and respect for patients' beliefs as I mature and develop as a nurse. The patient's actions were surprising. I had been taught about putting my compassion and faith into action. However, I had never seen it done. It was affirming as an APRN to recall how we cried and laughed and came to the sobering realization that this disease might beat her. However, we had given it our best effort. This experience was beneficial to me because it was my first time being the bearer of bad news to a patient. Consumed as we are with time management, compassion and faith are not always exhibited, shared, or utilized in my daily practice. However, by revisiting this story, I am challenged to treat others as I treated my special patient. The core values that guided my practice in the past have been rekindled while reflecting on my nursing experience. Nursing is a rewarding challenge if you allow it to be.

As shared by C'Sara Strong, MSN, CFNP

This story needs no interpretation; it can be easily recognized as an exquisite example of creating a holistic fabric of caring integrating a multitude of harmonious patterns: interpersonal, clinical, and technological.

These stories illustrate the use of caring processes. As situations are studied and relived, students, faculty, and providers discover the limitless ways caring is expressed. As nurses, we live out our personhood—our living grounded in caring—in unique and special ways. We bring to our practice our humanness, our expertise in caring, and our intention to participate fully in the life experiences of those we are privileged to nurse, and thus to bring the benefits of nursing to those seeking care.

  For additional resources please visit
https://davisedge.fadavis.com/

REFERENCES

Boykin A, Schoenhofer SO. *Nursing as caring: A model for transforming practice.* Sudbury, MA: Jones & Bartlett; 2001.

Carper B. Fundamental patterns of knowing in nursing. *Adv Nurs Sci.* 1978;1(1):13–23.

Gadow S. A model for ethical decision making. In: Pence T, et al., eds. *Ethics in nursing: An anthology.* New York, NY: National League for Nursing; 1990:52–55.

Johns C. *Becoming a reflective practitioner.* 4th ed. Hoboken, NJ: Wiley-Blackwell; 2013.

Leininger M, McFarlane MR. *Transcultural nursing: Concepts, theories, research, and practice.* New York, NY: McGraw-Hill, Medical Publishing Division; 2002.

Locsin RC. *Technological competency as caring in nursing: A model for practice.* Indianapolis, IN: Sigma Theta Tau International Honor Society of Nursing; 2005.

Mayeroff M. *On caring.* New York, NY: HarperPerennial; 1971.

Paterson J, Zderad LT. *Humanistic nursing.* New York, NY: National League for Nursing; 1988.

Roach MS. *The human act of caring: A blueprint for the health professions.* Ottawa, ON: Canadian Hospital Association; 1987.

Roach S. *Caring: The human mode of being. A blueprint for the health professions.* Ottawa, ON: CHA Press; 2002.

Smith MC, Turkel MC, Wolf ZR. *Caring in nursing classics: An essential resource.* New York, NY: Springer Publishing Co; 2012.

Tillich P. *The courage to be.* New Haven, CT: Yale University Press; 1952.

Watson J. *The philosophy and science of caring.* Revised edition. Boulder, CO: University Press of Colorado; 2008.

Watson J. *Assessing and measuring caring in nursing and health sciences.* New York, NY: Springer Publishing Co; 2009.

Wolf Z, King B, France N. Antecedent context and structure of communication during a caring moment: Scoping review and analysis. *Int J Hum Caring.* 2015;19(2):7–21.

RESOURCES

Anne Boykin Institute (ABI) for Advancement of Caring in Nursing
http://nursing.fau.edu/outreach/anne-boykin-institute/resources.php

Archives of Caring of the Christine E. Lynn College of Nursing
http://nursing.fau.edu/archives/

Boykin and Schoenhofer on Nursing as Caring
https://www.youtube.com/watch?v=AZbrs5iOGaQ

International Association for Human Caring (IAHC)
http://www.humancaring.org/

International Journal for Human Caring (IJHC)
www.humancaring.org

Journal of Art and Aesthetics in Nursing and Health Sciences
www.JAANHS.org.

Nursing as Caring Theory into Practice
https://www.youtube.com/watch?v=d8DDWYMO1Fk

Nursing Situations: Teaching, Learning, Living Caring
https://www.youtube.com/watch?v=9_AEmRFAPo&feature=youtu.be

Watson Caring Science Institute
http://watsoncaringscience.org/

Chapter 3

Health Promotion

Dorothy J. Dunn, PhD, APRN, FNP-BC, AHN-BC
Debera J. Thomas, DNS, RN, FNP/ANP

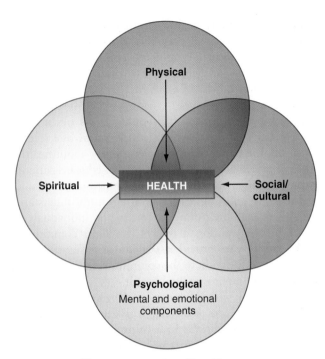

Figure 3.1 The components of health.

HEALTH

The goal of all health-care providers and their patients is to promote health and prevent disease. Engaging in health-promoting activities helps individuals live longer and healthier lives. To put this goal in perspective, the basic tenets of health must first be explored.

What is health? Several disciplines and organizations have tried to define health, and the definition continues to evolve. Some view health as the absence of disease, but this definition does not consider other important human characteristics that include physical, social, spiritual, cultural, and emotional dimensions. In 1948, the World Health Organization (1948) defined health as a "state of complete physical, mental and social well-being"; this definition provides a more holistic view of health because it incorporates the social and mental aspects of a human being, as well as the physical dimension. In fact, this definition has not been amended since its inception in 1948. However, this definition fails to recognize the spiritual and cultural dimensions of a person. According to the American Holistic Nurses' Association (Mariano, 2013), health can be described as a state or process in which an individual experiences a sense of well-being, harmony, and unity of one's body-mind-spirit within an ever-changing environment. Health is, therefore, a state in which the physical, psychological, social, spiritual, and cultural attributes of a person are in balance, creating harmony within the body (Fig. 3.1).

The balance of each of these dimensions is an important parameter when considering health. A patient may be physically healthy, but his or her spiritual, cultural, social, and psychological dimensions may not be balanced, and therefore the patient is not experiencing optimal health. If we believe that the whole is greater than the sum of its parts, then we cannot accurately determine someone's health status without evaluating these attributes.

Historically, the medical evaluation of a patient was based only on physical signs and symptoms of a disease. If the patient lacked symptoms, we considered him or her healthy. We now know that this type of assessment is incomplete and does not consider how the other attributes

of a person either contribute to or subtract from health status. We also know that many patients have medical problems that have not yet presented as signs and symptoms of a disease.

When assessing a patient, it is imperative to also evaluate his or her social, psychological, spiritual, and cultural well-being, as well as the physical state. In performing a complete health assessment, the provider should ask questions related to the person's social and dietary habits; current living and work situation environment; and feelings, beliefs, values, and life satisfaction, as well as questions about his or her philosophical and spiritual beliefs.

Along with physical signs and symptoms, all these parts of a patient's history inform diagnosis and treatment plans. The focus on all component parts of a person helps to provide a more holistic view that can assist in making a comprehensive assessment of the current health status of the patient. The determination of health is based on the synthesis of all the parameters of health and should be incorporated into all patient assessments.

HEALTH PROMOTION

Health promotion can be defined as activities and preventive measures that contribute to an individual's state of optimal health. Such activities and preventive measures include immunizations, fitness/exercise programs, breast self-awareness, appropriate nutrition, relaxation, stress management, social support, prayer, meditation, healing rituals, cultural practices, and promoting environmental health and safety. Health and well-being are created by a balance of physical, psychological, spiritual, cultural, and social components of health. Health promotion requires a commitment on the part of the individual patient, the health-care provider, and the community. Health-promotion efforts are achieved only when everyone works in partnership to achieve goals that will enhance health and well-being.

Health-promotion efforts should always begin with the clinician because the clinician plays a pivotal role in educating the patient and the community about health-promoting behaviors. The clinician can educate patients about how their environment can contribute to health or disease. In addition, the community must understand the impact that environment can have on individuals so that health-promotion activities can be a community effort. Health-care providers play an important role by providing consultation to the community and the legislature regarding environmental health.

Consultation with influential members of the community can assist efforts to develop legislation that supports healthy living conditions in a community. In addition, legislative efforts can help provide funding to maintain or improve environmental health. When patients commit to their own health, living conditions in the community must also be healthy to sustain and support their efforts. Basic community resources, such as water and sanitation, must be monitored for potential threats to health and well-being, and these resources are the responsibility of community and local government agencies. Health-care providers and patients need to work in collaboration with these agencies to ensure that resources essential to health, are maintained or improved. To be successful, health promotion must be a group effort.

Historically, health promotion has been viewed as an effort to prevent disease and illness. Most sources cite three levels of prevention: primary prevention is the prevention of disease; secondary prevention consists of early screening and detection of disease; and tertiary prevention is the restoration of health after illness or disease has occurred. Focusing health-care efforts on all three levels of prevention is important to promoting health, but during the last two decades, primary prevention has become the focus of health promotion.

During the first half of the 20th century, health-care efforts were directed at patients who were already ill. The prevailing belief at the time was that patients should seek health care when they were ill. During this time, most health-care practitioners cared for patients at the tertiary level by (1) preventing further insult or injury after the disease or illness had occurred by stabilizing the patient's condition to prevent deterioration; (2) helping patients recover from the current illness or disease through treatment; and (3) whenever possible, to help restore patients to their previous state of health.

Advancements in technology during the second half of the 20th century contributed to better diagnostic testing, helping to shift the focus of health care to secondary prevention. Providers began to emphasize the importance

of screening "at risk" patients at appropriate intervals for known diseases and illnesses. A focus on secondary levels of prevention has led health-care providers to encourage early detection and treatment.

With the focus on screening and early detection, treatment can be instituted before overt signs and symptoms appeared, thereby preventing some of the long-term sequelae associated with disease. For example, blood pressure is checked in a patient with no symptoms of hypertension, and if elevated, a plan of treatment is initiated. The goal is to maintain the patient's blood pressure within normal limits and minimizing the development of catastrophic complications such as stroke or myocardial infarction. Box 3.1 summarizes questions the clinician should consider in consultation with the patient before routinely screening for any condition.

In determining whether screening is appropriate, health-care providers should keep in mind that early signs of chronic disease often surface in midlife, that is, in persons aged 40 to 65 years. In general, the earlier disease is identified, the easier it is to treat, and the more likely it is to have a successful outcome. In addition, individuals in midlife tend to focus more on behaviors to extend life and prevent disability than do younger people. Adults aged 20 to 40 years focus more on relationships, family, self-image, and career development, whereas those older than age 65 spend more time responding to and coping with overt, established illness. As life expectancy increases and older adults anticipate living longer, more attention is focused on health enhancement, adding quality years to the life span of older persons.

Focusing on primary prevention enables providers to assess patients' potential risk factors, including lifestyle and family history, and to help them make lifestyle changes that will foster health and prevent disease and disability. Health-care providers are aware that health or wellness is best achieved through primary prevention strategies. However, when this is not possible, secondary and tertiary levels

---

Box 3.1   Questions to Consider Before Ordering Screening Tests

1. Does the condition must have a significant affect on the quality and quantity of life?
2. Are there acceptable treatment options available?
3. Does detection of the condition while it is asymptomatic significantly reduce morbidity and mortality if treated?
4. Does treatment in the asymptomatic phase yield a therapeutic result superior to that obtained by delaying treatment until symptoms appear?
5. Are there tests available that are acceptable to patients and at a reasonable cost that detect the condition in the asymptomatic period?
6. Is evidence of the condition sufficient to justify the cost of the screening?

of prevention are employed. Each health-care interaction between a patient and clinician is an opportunity to promote health at the primary, secondary, and tertiary levels. Optimal wellness or health for all patients is the goal.

Health-care providers can use the levels of prevention in several ways: on an individual level, with small groups (families), and with larger groups such as a community. Individual encounters provide an opportunity to educate patients about their individual risk factors and changes they can make to prevent, or at least delay, the onset of disease(s) and the potential sequelae of disease (implementing primary and secondary prevention strategies). Incorporating family members into the educational process of health promotion can provide support and reinforcement for patients during the early phase of risk reduction. This incorporation of family may also serve the individual family members by educating them regarding their own risk for disease. Family members can also serve as advocates for patients by helping to synthesize the information given and providing the patient with a support system to make healthy lifestyle changes.

Health-care providers can be instrumental in developing health-promotion strategies in a community. This can be accomplished by developing interventions that include identifying community groups at risk for certain diseases and developing community-wide educational programs that will educate this group about their potential risks. Community-based educational programs reach a broad audience with the potential to have a significant impact on the health status of a community (Fig. 3.2).

Expanding knowledge has increased our awareness that many diseases today can be minimized or potentially avoided with early assessment and management. The effects from diseases such as hypertension, cardiovascular disease, and diabetes on patients' lives can be minimized or avoided with early interventions. For example, most patients diagnosed with diabetes have had the disease for at least 5 years. Diabetes has serious consequences in many organ systems if it is not diagnosed early and treated aggressively. The development of a community-wide diabetes education and screening program can help identify patients who are at high risk for the disease. With

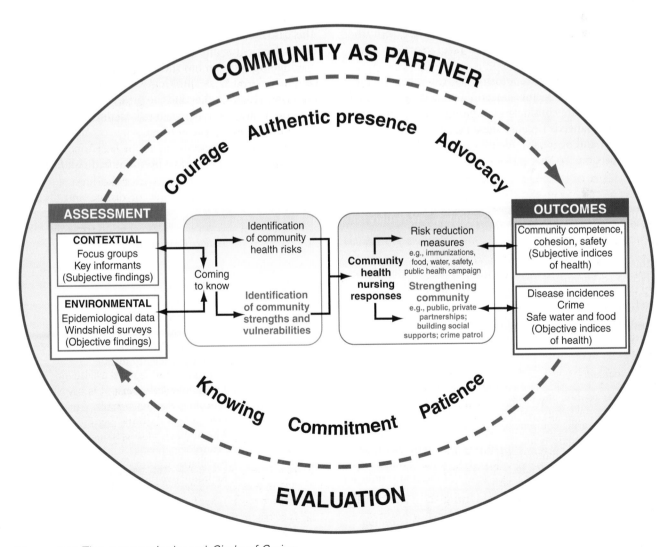

Figure 3.2 The community-based *Circle of Caring*.

early diagnosis and treatment, long-term complications associated with diabetes such as peripheral neuropathy, cardiovascular complications, and retinopathies can be minimized.

Clinicians can take a leadership position within a community by developing targeted programs for early identification and treatment. This type of widescale intervention can reduce morbidity and mortality rates. Early diagnosis, before signs/symptoms of a disease are present, can have a significant impact on the outcomes of disease. If patients are identified early, educated about the importance of healthy nutrition and lifestyle, and treated aggressively, the outcome may be a long and healthy life. Table 3.1 provides examples of primary, secondary, and tertiary prevention.

RISK FACTORS IN HEALTH PROMOTION

The identification of risk factors is an essential component of health promotion. Some patients have no known risk factors, whereas others have many. The key component of effective health promotion is to screen patients for potential known risk factors and intervene. Not all diseases can be prevented, and not every person with unhealthy lifestyle choices will get a disease, but the elimination or alteration of certain risk factors can affect disease outcomes.

Some risk factors are modifiable, whereas others are not. Nonmodifiable risk factors, including sex, age, and genetic/family history, are considered nonmodifiable because they cannot be changed. Because these factors are nonmodifiable, early, and aggressive identification of all risk factors should be done so that patients with nonmodifiable risk

factors can make any possible changes in the modifiable risk factors and affect a more favorable outcome.

Modifiable risk factors include weight, diet, social habits, lifestyle choices, and stress. For example, 38-year-old Mr. Hart is being seen for a physical examination. He has not had a physical in 20 years. His past medical history is negative for any diseases, surgeries, or illnesses. His social history includes the use of alcohol and cigarettes; he works an average of 60 hours per week as an emergency medical technician and does not exercise. His family history reveals that his father, paternal uncle, and grandfather had all had a myocardial infarction before age 50. Mr. Hart's physical examination reveals the following: height, 69 inches; weight, 230 pounds; and a body mass index (BMI) of 34. Mr. Hart's laboratory results include a cholesterol level of 250 mg/dL, a high-density lipoprotein (HDL) of 30 mg/dL, and a low-density lipoprotein (LDL) of 160 mg/dL. Box 3.2 reviews the risk factors for heart disease for Mr. Hart.

Although Mr. Hart cannot change his age, sex, or family history, there are several factors that he can change. With improvements in his diet, regular exercise, stress reduction, moderation of alcohol intake, and smoking cessation, Mr. Hart can reduce his risk for heart disease. This case illustrates the importance of early identification of risk factors for intervention.

Ongoing research has shown the relationship between certain risks such as smoking, consuming alcohol, and ingesting a high-fat diet and the presence of disease. However, the relationship between risk factors and disease can be confounding, because often a person may develop a disease without experiencing any risk factors. For example, some patients will have no identified risk factors for

TABLE 3.1   Examples of Primary, Secondary, and Tertiary Prevention

Primary Prevention	*Secondary Prevention*	*Tertiary Prevention*
Immunizations	*Screening for:*	*Treatment to prevent further sequelae of:*
Health education		
Skin cancer prevention measures	Skin cancer	Cardiovascular disease
Weight control	Oral cancer	Respiratory disease
Seatbelt use	Lung cancer	Gastroenterology disease
Violence prevention	Breast cancer	Genitourinary disease
Substance abuse	Testicular cancer	Endocrine diseases
	Prostate cancer	Immunodeficiency disease
Education on:	Diabetes	Infectious disease
	Hypertension	Dermatological disease
Smoking, alcohol, and drugs	Cardiovascular disease	Oncology disease
Environmental hazards avoidance	Ovarian cancer	Gynecological disease
Protective hearing equipment	Cervical cancer	Musculoskeletal disease
Protective eye equipment	Fecal occult blood	Neurologic disease
Safety helmets for motorcycles,	Sexually transmitted infections	Psychiatric disease
skateboards, and bicycles	Tuberculosis infection	Reproductive disease
Nutrition counseling	Pediatric developmental screening	
Exercise	Lead screening	
Stress reduction	Anemia screening	
Eliminating allergen exposure	Height, weight, and BMI screening	

Box 3.2 Risk Factors for Mr. Hart

Nonmodifiable Risk Factors

- Male sex
- Age
- Family history

Modifiable Risk Factors

- Weight
- Sedentary lifestyle
- Elevated cholesterol
- Elevated LDL and suboptimal HDL
- Alcohol consumption
- Smoking
- Stress level

---

a disease, yet will still develop the disease. Conversely, some patients may have several identified risk factors and yet never go on to develop the disease. Evidence-based research will continue to focus on efforts to identify as yet unknown risk factors or health-promoting determinants that could influence the outcomes for disease.

INFLUENCES ON HEALTH PROMOTION

Many factors influence health-promotion activities today. Government initiatives, community health programs, and media attention all focus attention on the importance of health literacy, health promotion, and disease prevention.

Health Literacy

Most persons will encounter health information when they seek health care, and most persons will encounter health information that they cannot understand. More than a measurement of reading skills, health literacy also includes writing, listening, speaking, arithmetic, and conceptual knowledge. *Health literacy* is commonly defined as the degree to which individuals have the capacity to obtain, process, and understand basic information and services needed to make appropriate decisions regarding their health (Affordable Care Act, 2010).

Health literacy is required when acute illness, injury, or chronic-disease management necessitates that a person seek health care. Consider that nurses are charged with "the protection, promotion, and optimization of health and abilities, prevention of illness and injury, alleviation of suffering through diagnosis and treatment of human response, and advocacy in the care of individuals, families, communities, and populations" (American Nurses Association, 2010, p 10). Therefore, nurses must accept the challenge to screen and assess for health literacy levels at each health-care encounter. Many instruments

are available to assess a person's level of health literacy. For example, the Newest Vital Scale (NVS) instrument can be used to quickly assess health literacy within 3 minutes. The NVS can provide results comparable to more time-consuming literacy tests such as the Test of Functional Health literacy in Adults or Rapid Estimate of Adult Literacy in Medicine-Short Form. Other instruments have been developed for other languages (AHRQ, 2016).

By identifying those at risk for misunderstanding instructions and the ability to adhere to recommendations in all aspects of care, health-care providers will have a positive impact on health promotion, prevention strategies, and treatment adherence successes for individuals who seek health care.

Government Initiatives

Three major government initiatives that have had great impact on health promotion in the United States are the National Prevention Strategy (NPS), *Healthy People 2020*, and the U.S. Preventive Services Task Force (USPSTF).

National Prevention Strategy

The Affordable Care Act (ACA), passed in 2010, created the National Prevention Council, which in turn developed the NPS. In 2011, the National Prevention Council released *National Prevention Strategy: America's Plan for Better Health and Wellness*, a comprehensive plan that describes evidence-based and achievable means for improving health and well-being for all Americans at every stage of life. These efforts are designed to stop disease before it starts and to create strategies for a healthy and fit nation, recognizing that prevention must be part of daily life. The goal of the NPS is to transform us from a system of sick care to one based on wellness and prevention. In addition, an Advisory Group on Prevention, Health Promotion, and Integrative and Public Health has made final recommendations to the Surgeon General and National Prevention Council that reaffirm the value of and their commitment to the following four strategic directions of the NPS (Surgeon General, 2016):

- Health and safe community environments
- Clinical and community preventive services
- Empowered people
- Elimination of health disparities

Within this framework, seven priorities are identified to reduce the burden of the leading causes of preventable death and major illness:

- Tobacco-free living
- Preventing drug abuse and excessive alcohol use
- Healthy eating
- Active living
- Injury and violence-free living

- Reproductive and sexual health
- Mental and emotional well-being

Healthy People 2020

Healthy People 2020 is a foundational resource for the NPS four strategic directions and seven priorities and is based on the accomplishments of four previous *Healthy People* initiatives: (1) the 1979 Surgeon General's Report, *Healthy People: The Surgeon General's Report on Health Promotion and Disease Prevention*; (2) *Healthy People 1990: Promoting Health/Preventing Disease: Objective for the Nation*; (3) *Healthy People 2000: National Health Promotion and Disease Prevention Objectives*; and (4) *Healthy People 2010: Objectives for Improving Health*. *Healthy People 2020* is the result of a multiyear process that reflects input from a diverse group of individuals and organizations.

Over the course of the decade, the four foundation health measures will be used to monitor progress toward promoting health, preventing disease and disability, eliminating disparities, and improving quality of life (Box 3.3). There are nearly 600 objectives in *Healthy People 2020* with more than 1,300 measures. The topic areas were developed by experts from numerous following federal agencies, including the Administration on Aging, Agency for Healthcare Research and Quality, Centers for Disease Control and Prevention (CDC), and the U.S. Food and Drug Administration.

Healthy People 2020 focuses on identifying, measuring, tracking, and reducing health disparities through a determinants-of-health approach. Over the past two decades, *Healthy People's* overarching goals have focused on disparities. In *Healthy People 2000*, the goal was to reduce health disparities among Americans; in *Healthy People 2010*, it was to eliminate, not just reduce, health disparities. In *Healthy People 2020*, the goal is expanded further to achieve health equity, eliminate disparities, and improve health for all groups. Currently, *Healthy People 2020* is

assessing health disparities in the U.S. population by tracking rates of illness, death, chronic conditions, behaviors, and other types of outcomes in relation to demographic factors, including race and ethnicity, gender, sexual identity and orientation, disability status and special healthcare needs, and geographic location (Box 3.4).

Thirteen new topic areas have been added for 2020 (Box 3.5). Each of the *Healthy People 2020* topic areas includes related evidence-based interventions and resources

---

Box 3.3   *Healthy People 2020* Foundation Health Measures

1. General health-status measures such as life expectancy at birth and at age 65, healthy life expectancy, years of potential life lost, physically and mentally unhealthy days, self-assessed health status, limitation of activity, and chronic disease prevalence.
2. Health-related quality of life and well-being such as physical, mental, and social health–related quality of life, well-being/satisfaction, and participation in common activities.
3. Determinants of health, a range of personal, social, economic, and environmental factors that include biology, genetics, behavior, access to care, and environment in which people are born, live, learn, play, work, and age.
4. Disparities that include race/ethnicity, gender, physical and mental ability, and geography.

Box 3.4   Topic Areas for *Healthy People*

- Access to Health Services
- Adolescent Health*
- Arthritis, Osteoporosis, and Chronic Back Conditions
- Blood Disorders and Blood Safety*
- Cancer
- Chronic Kidney Disease
- Dementias, Including Alzheimer's Disease*
- Diabetes
- Disability and Health
- Early and Middle Childhood*
- Educational and Community-Based Programs
- Environmental Health
- Family Planning
- Food Safety
- Genomics*
- Global Health*
- Health Communication and Health Information Technology
- Health-Care–Associated Infections*
- Health-Related Quality of Life and Well-being*
- Hearing and Other Sensory or Communication Disorders
- Heart Disease and Stroke
- HIV
- Immunization and Infectious Diseases
- Injury and Violence Prevention
- Maternal, Infant, and Child Health
- Lesbian, Gay, Bisexual, and Transgender Health*
- Medical Product Safety
- Mental Health and Mental Disorders
- Nutrition and Weight Status
- Occupational Safety and Health
- Older Adults*
- Oral Health
- Physical Activity
- Preparedness*
- Public Health Infrastructure
- Respiratory Diseases
- Sexually Transmitted Diseases
- Sleep Health*
- Social Determinants of Health*
- Substance Abuse
- Tobacco Use
- Vision

*New for *Healthy People 2020*.

from the USPSTF Clinical Preventive Services, Guide to Community Preventive Services, and Healthfinder.gov's Quick Guide to Healthy Living Information for Consumers. *Healthy People 2020* also hosts an online community using Twitter, LinkedIn, and webinars. Leading health indicators reflect high-priority health issues and communicate actions that can be taken to address them. These indicators will be used to assess the health of the nation over the decade, to facilitate collaboration across sectors, and to motivate action at the national, state, and community levels to improve the health of the U.S. population.

According to the *Healthy People* initiative, *health promotion* is defined as any strategy that helps individuals make personal choices in a social context about lifestyle that will have a positive influence on the individual's health prospects. *Health protection* is defined as those interventions that are related to the environment made by regulatory bodies to protect a large population group. *Preventive services* include screening for disease, counseling, medication to prevent disease, or immunization interventions for individuals in the clinical setting. The last priority area of surveillance and data systems was essential to track all of the changes that would occur with programs focusing on meeting the goals of *Healthy People 2020*.

The *Healthy People 2020* initiatives continue to have a significant impact on primary health care in the United States. The incorporation of health-promoting and disease prevention strategies has become the foundation for primary care. It is believed that all of the goals of *Healthy People 2020* are achievable with support from individual health-care providers, local and national government agencies, and, most important, the active participation of individual patients.

Healthy People 2020 stresses the importance of each individual taking personal responsibility for his or her own health, in partnership with his or her health-care professional. For the public to have an effective role in illness prevention, individuals must work in partnership with clinicians who have been educated in health promotion and disease prevention strategies.

Healthy People 2030 is the next step in the *Healthy People* initiative. The Secretary's Advisory Committee on National Health Promotion and Disease Prevention Objectives for 2030 is a federal advisory committee composed of nonfederal, independent, subject-matter experts who will be responsible for making recommendations to the Secretary of the U.S. Department of Health and Human Services for developing and implementing the national health promotion and disease prevention objectives for 2030. This committee has been charged with developing the components of *Healthy People 2030*, which include a mission and vision statement, framework, organizational structure, and selection criteria for developing measurable, nationally representative objectives. It is expected to make recommendations to ensure that selection criteria address public health issues shown to be high-impact priorities from national data, limit the number of objectives, identify leading health indicators, and implement *Healthy People 2030* (U.S. Department of Health and Human Services, Office of Disease Prevention and Health Promotion, 2017).

U.S. Preventive Services Task Force

The USPSTF is composed of private sector experts who make recommendations to the health-care community regarding clinical prevention strategies. This group was first convened by the U.S. Public Health Service in 1984 and since 1998 has come under the umbrella of the Agency for Healthcare Research and Quality. Their mission, as mandated by Public Law Section 915, is to conduct scientific evidence reviews of a broad array of clinical preventive services; develop recommendations for the health-care community; and provide ongoing administrative, research, and technical support to disseminate the findings.

The USPSTF meets and systematically reviews scientific evidence for each of the current health-care screening guidelines, as well as preventive medications, immunizations, and counseling, and makes recommendations based on these reviews. Through consensus, the task force assigns a grade to each recommendation based on net benefits for patients and the strength of evidence for each of the current recommendations.

The result of the task force's efforts is an online *Procedure Manual* that can be used by clinicians who provide preventive services. The *Procedure Manual* provides recommendations for screening, including the following: cancer screening and chemoprevention strategies; screening for heart and valvular disease, infectious disease, injury and violence, mental health issues, and substance abuse; metabolic, nutritional, and endocrine screening; and pediatric screening guidelines. Nurse practitioners can use its evidence-based recommendations for clinical preventive services. The USPSTF *Procedure Manual* (2015) is available for distribution from several sources and has its own Web site. An evidence-based prevention resource for nurse practitioners is available through the USPSTF web site.

The USPSTF not only makes recommendations for screening select populations but also prioritizes services. All of the recommendations issued by the USPSTF are optional; providers and patients may decide not to implement certain recommendations based on shared decision making. For example, patients who have a significant family history for a particular type of cancer may need to be screened earlier than recommended for the general population but only after careful discussion with the patient weighing the pros and cons and the possibility of false-positive results.

The work of this task force continues. Some of the current recommendations, such as lead poisoning and iron-deficiency anemia screenings, have been included as part of the well-child visits in pediatrics for many years. It is important that screening programs be continued or eliminated based on the strength of scientific evidence available and not just on tradition (see Box 3.1).

With the rapid evolution of technology in health care, it is important to be knowledgeable about current health-care information. Resources such as the NPS, *Healthy People 2020*, and the USPSTF recommendations are essential tools to help clinicians keep up to date with current best practices. These initiatives have Web sites that provide updates to the current printed reports. The NPS encourages partnerships among federal, state, tribal, local, and territorial governments; business, industry, and other private sector partners; philanthropic organizations; community-and faith-based organizations; and everyday Americans to improve health through prevention. Initiatives such as *Healthy People 2020* and the USPSTF recommendations are excellent examples of well-researched tools that can help to enhance health promotion and disease prevention. The result will be comprehensive care to patients with the goal of optimal health for all.

Immunization Practices

Immunization administration is one of the best examples of primary health promotion. Immunizations provide the patient's body with the ability to build up antibodies to a potential life-threatening illness before exposure to the offending agent. The guidelines for immunization continue to evolve and change over time. Currently, immunizations begin at birth and are continued throughout life. During early childhood, infants and children (birth through 6 years old) are immunized with a wide variety of vaccines, including hepatitis B (Hep B); hepatitis A (Hep A); diphtheria, tetanus, and acellular pertussis; inactivated polio vaccine; *Haemophilus influenzae* type B; measles, mumps, and rubella; varicella-zoster virus (VZV); pneumococcal conjugate vaccine; influenza (flu); pneumococcal vaccine; and rotavirus. The 2017 Advisory Committee on Immunization Practices (ACIP, 2017) recommends immunizations for children aged 7 to 18 years to protect against tetanus, diphtheria, and pertussis; meningococcal conjugate vaccine (MCV) is recommended at this age as well. At age 11 to 12, boys and girls should receive the human papillomavirus vaccine, but as new evidence emerges the practice may change. Teens who received MCV for the first time between ages 13 and 15 should receive a one-time booster between ages 16 and 18. All children should receive approximately 25 vaccines by the time they reach 5 years of age. After this point, they should continue to receive one Tdap and then tetanus booster every 10 years.

Recommendations for adults include annual flu immunizations, as well as pneumococcal, meningococcal, Hep A, and Hep B immunizations for those with certain risk factors related to their health, job, or lifestyle. Older adults should receive a VZV immunization at age 60 to prevent shingles and a pneumococcal polysaccharide vaccine at age 65 to protect them from pneumonia. Immunization schedules change rapidly; the most current information can be obtained at the CDC's web site, which offers current immunization guidelines for children and adults.

Immunizations are an effective form of primary health promotion, but they are not without controversy. Over the past several years, some consumers have argued that immunizations are not safe and in fact cause diseases such as autism and attention-deficit hyperactivity disorder. To date, the etiology of these diseases has not been found to be a result of immunization administration. However, there is always the potential for vaccines to cause side effects; therefore, patient education is paramount.

Each clinician must provide patients and their families with accurate information regarding immunization administration, including potential side effects and known contraindications to immunization, and keep a copy of a written consent for each immunization on file. This consent must be obtained for each immunization before it is administered. If, after administration of a vaccine, a patient develops a significant reaction (such as very high fever, uncontrollable crying for more than 2 hours, lethargy, coma, etc.), the patient should be evaluated in a timely manner, and the potential adverse reaction to the vaccine should be reported. In 1986, the National Childhood Vaccine Injury Act required that all health-care providers report any severe adverse reactions to the Vaccine Adverse Event Reporting System and CDC. The length of time from administration to the appearance of an adverse reaction that is a reportable event is between 7 and 30 days and is dependent on whether the vaccine contains a live virus. When in doubt, it is best to report the event.

Information regarding potential reactions for each vaccine is available in the *Red Book* developed by the American Academy of Pediatrics or on the CDC Web site's Morbidity and Mortality Weekly Report (MMWR). Immunization is still one of the best methods for preventing illness and disease or the serious sequelae that can develop from specific diseases such as polio, diphtheria, *H. influenzae*, and others.

Individual Influences

The key to successful health promotion is the motivation and commitment of the patient. To obtain a successful outcome, the patient must be willing to make lifestyle changes. The clinician should provide patients with health education that informs them of their current risk factors, the possibility of reducing or eliminating risk factors by lifestyle changes, and the potential benefits of implementing these changes. Once the clinician has provided the information to the patient, the decision to act rests with the patient. An ideal scenario for health promotion would involve both patient and clinician working in partnership toward mutually agreed on health goals. However, the choice to engage in this partnership is the patient's decision. For example, 36-year-old K.J. is being seen for a routine physical examination and reveals a smoking history of a pack a day of cigarettes for 20 years. She is counselled about her smoking habit and the associated risk for cardiac, respiratory, and peripheral vascular disease. She states that she understands that smoking is not good for her health but currently is not willing to quit. This scenario illustrates that despite the best efforts of the clinician, the patient still has the right to not engage in health-promoting behaviors.

Many factors can influence a patient's motivation to engage in health-promotion activities, such as willingness to alter lifestyle practices, belief that making the changes will affect health, and belief that promoting health can prevent disease. These factors influence whether a patient decides to make lifestyle changes. Several health models have been developed to identify factors that influence a patient's willingness to act and make changes. Nola Pender's 1997 health-belief model provides a framework for health-care providers to use in assessing patients' readiness to make lifestyle changes to promote their own health (Pender, 2010). Pender's model describes and defines several factors that affect a patient's decision to act (Fig. 3.3). She divides these factors into two types: cognitive-perceptual factors and modifying factors. Cognitive-perceptual factors include items such as importance of health, perceived control of health, and perceived barriers to health-promoting behaviors. Modifying factors include biological characteristics, situational factors, and demographic characteristics.

Pender states that these factors will affect a patient's willingness to act (which she terms "cues to take action"). For example, 17-year-old Jonathan had not been consistently wearing a seat belt while riding in or driving a car until 2 months ago. His friend Kyle was involved in a motor vehicle collision (MVC) in which Kyle was seriously injured. Kyle's parents informed Jonathan that Kyle's injury could have been prevented if Kyle had been wearing a seat belt. In this situation, Jonathan has changed his perception (cognitive-perceptual factors) about the importance of wearing a seat belt (health-promoting behavior) based on interpersonal influences (his friend's involvement in an MVC). His "cue to action" was hearing that the injuries incurred by Kyle could have been avoided had Kyle been wearing his seat belt.

This scenario illustrates that although various factors can influence positive health changes, the "cues to action" for patients may vary. In this scenario, it would be interesting to find out if the MVC caused Kyle to change his behavior regarding seat belt use. It is important that clinicians strive to offer patients a variety of scenarios to promote health.

Today's focus on primary disease prevention is empowering for patients, in contrast to the situation 20 years ago, when most patients were not given the option of actively participating in their health care. Health care today provides many opportunities for patients and clinicians to optimize health through health promotion and disease prevention.

Community Influences

Community efforts can also substantially enhance health-promotion efforts. As described previously, the burden of responsibility regarding sanitation, hygiene, and clean water supplies rests with the local community government. A person who lives in a community that lacks appropriate waste disposal, air pollution controls, or law enforcement is exposed to greater health risks than is an individual who lives in a community in which each of these environmental issues has been effectively addressed.

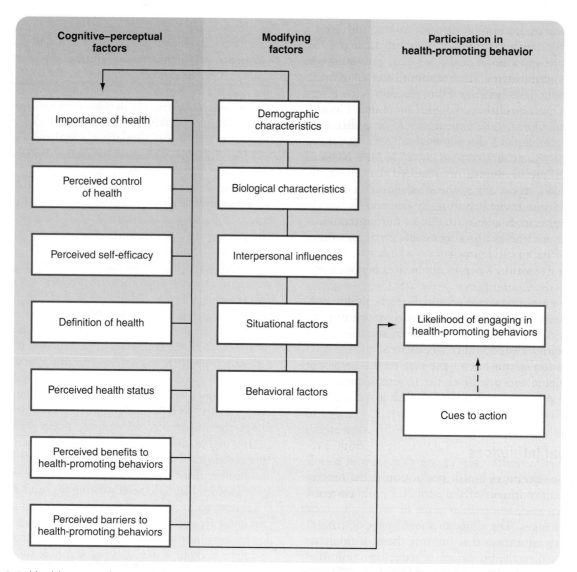

Figure 3.3 Health promotion model. *(Source: Pender N. Health promotion in nursing practice. 5th ed. Upper Saddle River, NJ: Prentice-Hall; 2006.)*

Health-care providers need to work in partnership with local government agencies to ensure that healthy living conditions are a right for each citizen and not dependent on an individual's race or ethnicity, geography, or socioeconomic status. Clinicians can provide education and expertise to local government agencies for understanding the connection between effective sanitation measures and health. Each health-care provider can also alert the local community to possible outbreaks of illness and disease that can affect the greater community at large.

One of the major transitions that occurred from the earlier initiatives of *Healthy People* to *Healthy People 2000/2010/2020* was the shift from a largely federal government initiative to more involvement from local and community agencies. It was believed that this shift in responsibility would result in a significant improvement in meeting the goals of the initiative.

Community programs aimed at providing health information are one way that local communities can assist with this initiative. Offering forums for dialogue between health-care providers and local citizens is an excellent way to educate a broader audience. If these types of efforts are supported by community leaders, there will be a larger impact in the community. The development of health-promoting legislation is another way that local communities can help affect change. For example, the passage of smoking restrictions in public areas is an excellent example of how local efforts can improve the health of the communities they serve. Legislative policies and interventions that affect the health of individuals and communities, such as housing, labor, energy, transportation, education, justice, and so forth, can be initiated by local and regional agencies. *Healthy People 2020* encourages the active participation of all civic and community agencies to help meet the goals for 2020.

Communities can also respond to the "call for action" from *Healthy People 2020* by ensuring that their citizens have equal access to health care, which is a priority for the *Healthy People* initiatives. For example, it is often difficult for indigenous populations to access health-care services in their communities because of the rural nature of Indian Reservations. The Navajo Nation is the largest Indian Reservation in the United States, covering 27,000 square miles and spanning parts of Utah, Arizona, and New Mexico. The nearest health-care facility can be a 3-hour drive away.

In addition, many communities do not have systems in place to support the efforts of patients who have language or financial barriers to seek care in their community. Often, a disadvantaged patient's only access to care is through the hospital emergency department. At that time, tertiary measures of prevention are employed and are very costly. Community hospitals can work together with local government agencies to develop health programs/settings that will provide access to health care for all citizens, not just those who have health insurance or whose primary language is English.

The long-range goals of establishing these types of health programs are a reduction in direct hospital costs and an improvement in the quality of life for all citizens. Saving money is a major concern for both hospitals and local communities, and improving access to nonemergent health care can provide significant savings to both. Providing access to health-care services to groups of people who lack the means to access care in traditional settings will do much to improve the health disparities currently affecting our nation.

The ACA was signed into law on March 23, 2010, and the Supreme Court rendered a final decision on June 28, 2012, to uphold the heath-care law. The ACA puts consumers in charge of their health care, allowing for improved access to care, stability and flexibility of care, and information needed to make informed choices about their health.

Other Influences

Health-promotion strategies can be effective only when we have adequate knowledge of diseases affecting any given population. With this knowledge, individuals, families, health-care providers, community partners, and governmental agencies can work together to alleviate or minimize the impact of disease on patients. The evaluation of current health indicators is important to change the course of illness and disease. Evaluating and reviewing the current leading causes of death in the United States is one way to evaluate past trends. Once this evaluation is made, it can be determined whether these diseases can be prevented or reversed with lifestyle changes.

The leading causes of death in this country are published by the National Center for Health Statistics. The top 10 causes of death in the United States for 2014 are listed in Table 3.2. Our current knowledge regarding

TABLE 3.2 Top 10 Causes of Death (National Vital Statistics Report for 2014)		
Cause of Death	**Statistics**	**Amendable to Intervention**
Heart disease	614,348	Yes
Cancer	591,699	Some
Chronic lower respiratory disease	147,101	Yes
Accidents (unintentional injuries)	136,053	Yes
Stroke (cerebrovascular disease)	133,103	Yes
Alzheimer's disease	93,541	Early diagnosis to slow progression
Diabetes mellitus	76,488	Yes
Influenza and pneumonia	55,227	Yes
Nephritis, nephrotic syndrome, and nephrosis	48,146	Yes
Intentional self-harm (suicide)	42,773	Yes

Source: Kochanek KD, Murphy SL, Xu JQ, Tejada-Vera B. *Deaths: Final data for 2014*. National vital statistics reports; vol 65 no 4. Hyattsville, MD: National Center for Health Statistics; 2016.

these diseases indicates that healthy lifestyles can indeed positively affect their outcomes. For example, heart disease has been the leading cause of death in the United States for many years. A healthy lifestyle can prevent or at least ameliorate heart disease in most individuals. The previously discussed health scenario of Mr. Hart is an excellent example of risk factors for heart disease. Mr. Hart had several lifestyle factors that put him at risk for heart disease: smoking, alcohol consumption, being overweight, and elevated cholesterol and LDL levels. Making different lifestyle choices could potentially help Mr. Hart to control his heart disease to live a long and healthy life, without the devastation of a myocardial infarction or possibly even death from heart disease.

Most of the current top 10 causes of death could be avoided or delayed with healthy lifestyle choices, providing hope for the future health status for patients. With early health assessment and screenings, clinicians can intervene by helping patients to make healthier life choices and lowering their risk for devastating health consequences.

PRACTICAL EPIDEMIOLOGY

It is essential for clinicians to monitor trends in health and disease that may affect patients' health. In the role of health promoters for both their patients and the larger community, clinicians gather and contribute raw epidemiological data to various health organizations. Clinicians then consume the analyses of these data in the research reports and journals produced by these organizations.

Epidemiology is the evaluation of distribution patterns and determinants of health and disease in populations. The focus of epidemiology is to study the trends of disease occurrences in groups rather than in individuals. The goal of epidemiologic studies is to discover and evaluate the trends of illness or disease in groups of people in order to determine cause and effect and thereby prevent further disease. For example, a single case of swine flu (H1N1) is a concern, but it is not the focus of epidemiology. Instead, increasing numbers of cases of the H1N1 virus become an epidemiologic issue when they occur at the same time and in the same place. When susceptible populations are studied for the presence of a particular infection or disease, distribution patterns and symptoms may begin to emerge.

When disease statistics are given, reports often refer to the prevalence and incidence rates of a certain disease. The terms prevalence and incidence are commonly used to describe disease trends (Table 3.3). The *prevalence* rate refers to the number of cases of a particular disease at a particular point in time divided by the percentage of the population at a point in time. Prevalence does not distinguish between *new* and *old* cases. For example, if the current prevalence rate for a disease was 1 million, it indicates the number of new and old cases of the disease in the current population. The *incidence rate* is the number of *new* cases of a disease diagnosed at a point in time (e.g., 1 year).

Additional common terms used to study trends include *morbidity, mortality, sporadic, endemic, pandemic,* and *epidemic.* Morbidity and mortality rates are often described together. *Morbidity* is the number of people who have been diagnosed with a disease divided by the number of total population at risk. The number of people

TABLE 3.3 Prevalence and Incidence Rates	
Prevalence Rate	**Incidence Rate**
New and old cases of "B" disease at a specific point in time	New cases of "C" disease at a specific point in time
Number of cases divided by total population at specific point in time	Number of cases divided by total population at a specific point in time

who have died from a particular disease divided by the total population is the *mortality* (Table 3.4).

To understand the difference between morbidity and mortality, consider HIV. During 2003, the estimate for the number of persons living with HIV/AIDS in the United States was 1,185,000 (morbidity rate). During the same year, the total number of deaths from AIDS was 17,934 (mortality rate). The current rates for HIV infection indicate that significant strides have been made in prevention of HIV, which has in turn influenced the incidence, prevalence, morbidity, and mortality associated with the disease. More people are living longer with HIV as a result of significant advances in treatment and management.

Certain illnesses affect the population during annual predictable cycles. Terminology regarding these cycles includes *epidemic, endemic, sporadic,* and *pandemic* (Table 3.5). For example, the influenza (flu) virus is known to be prevalent during the winter season and can

TABLE 3.4 Morbidity and Mortality Formulas	
Morbidity Formula	**Mortality Formula**
Number of new cases of "D" disease divided by total population at risk	Number of deaths from "E" disease divided by total population at risk

TABLE 3.5 Epidemiologic Terms	
Term	**Definition**
Sporadic	Outbreaks of an illness/disease that occur occasionally and are unrelated in space and time
Epidemic	Presence of an event (illness or disease) at a much higher rate than expected based on past history
Endemic	Presence of an illness/disease constantly present or present at a rate that is expected based on history
Pandemic	Presence of an event in epidemic proportions affecting many communities and countries in a short period of time

 The Patient's Voice 3.1

DELIA

Delia, a 41-year-old woman, comes in for a complete physical examination and completes a primary health-promotion questionnaire. "This is the first time any primary-care provider has asked me so many in-depth questions about my own health and well-being. After doing this, I realize that there are many things in my life that impact my health. It made me take a personal inventory of everything from emotional, social, cultural, and psychological aspects of my life." She indicates that she is willing to work with her primary-care provider to begin to change some of her current health and lifestyle patterns to enhance her own health and well-being. "This has been a very enlightening exercise for me and I can't wait to begin the journey to balance my life to be healthier."

cause significant morbidity and mortality. The ability to predict the active cycle of this virus helps health-care practitioners to educate and immunize patients before predicted outbreaks. These health-promotion efforts are effective means of decreasing the prevalence and incidence of the influenza virus. Each year, predictions are made regarding the number of patients who, without health-promotion efforts, will experience the flu. In the past, there have been years in which the number of patients experiencing the flu was significantly higher than expected. This is called an *epidemic* and is defined as the presence of an event (illness or disease) at a much higher rate than expected based on past history.

Although there is some seasonal variation in the incidence of the common cold, it is known to be present throughout the year. *Endemic* is the term used when the presence of an event is constant at or about the same frequency as expected based on past history. A *sporadic* outbreak occurs when there are occasional cases of an event unrelated in space or time. For example, a gastrointestinal virus may be present in 3 patients this month, 20 patients 2 months from now, and 100 patients in 6 months. The virus is present but is not causing illness at a specific time and place. It is rare to hear of a patient having the flu during the summer season. A *pandemic* is defined as the presence of an event in epidemic proportions affecting many communities and countries in a short period of time. For example, in 2005 to 2006, there was widespread concern regarding avian or "bird" flu. It was found in several countries in a short period of time, and there was concern that it would reach pandemic proportions by affecting many people in many countries.

The CDC generally monitors and reports the incidence, prevalence, morbidity, and mortality rates of diseases and specifically monitors the rates of infectious diseases. This information is distributed in the weekly MMWR report. The report contains useful information about current infectious diseases that are a threat to local and global communities and provides the latest guidelines for treatment of infectious diseases. It is a helpful tool to investigate current infectious disease trends and potential health-promotion practices that may minimize or eliminate the threat of infectious disease.

CONCLUSION

Health promotion is one of the most powerful tools available today to prevent disease and disability. Clinicians should use health-promotion strategies at the primary, secondary, and tertiary levels of prevention. Each level of prevention is important, but the ultimate goal is primary prevention because it has the most significant impact on disease. Actively engaging in primary prevention strategies, such as health promotion, creates a wonderful opportunity for patients and health-care providers to work together as a team with the common goal of wellness and the prevention of disease. When primary prevention strategies are not feasible, *Healthy People 2020* and the USPSTF provide clinicians with guidelines to initiate secondary prevention strategies, such as early screening and detection of illness and disease. The utilization of these guidelines and health-focused initiatives will help to improve the health of the nation. With all of the current health-promotion strategies in place and a focus on disease prevention, it may be possible to eliminate or minimize the most expensive level of health-promotion: tertiary prevention. As we embrace the second decade of the 21st century, we continue to build momentum on primary health-promotion strategies with the goal of ensuring optimal health and wellness for all citizens.

 For additional resources please visit **https://davisedge.fadavis.com/**

REFERENCES

Advisory Committee on Immunization Practices (ACIP). Recommended immunization schedule United States. https://www.cdc.gov/vaccines/schedules/hcp/index.html. Published 2017.

Agency for Healthcare Research and Quality (AHRQ). *Health literacy measurement tools.* https://healthit.ahrq.gov/health-it-tools-and-resources/consumer-engagement-and-human-factors/health-it-literacy-guide. Published 2016. Accessed August 2018.

American Nurses Association. *Nursing's social policy statement: The essence of the profession.* 3rd ed. Silver Spring, MD: American Nurses Association; 2010.

Dossey B, Keegan L. *Holistic nursing: A handbook for practice.* 6th ed. Burlington, MA: Jones & Bartlett Learning; 2013.

Mariano C. *Holistic nursing: scope and standards of practice.* In: Dossey B, Keegan L, eds. *Holistic nursing: A handbook for practice.* 6th ed. Burlington, MA: Jones & Bartlett Learning; 2013:60.

National Center for Health Statistics. Healthy people 2010 final review. Hyattsville, MD; 2012.

Pender N. *Health promotion in nursing practice.* 6th ed. Upper Saddle River, NJ: Prentice-Hall; 2010.

U.S. Department of Health & Human Services. Final recommendations of the advisory group on prevention, health promotion, and integrative and public health to the Surgeon General and the National Prevention Council. https://www.surgeongeneral.gov/priorties/advisorygrp/advisory-group-prevention.html. Published 2016.

U.S. Department of Health and Human Services. *Healthy people 2000.* Washington, DC: U.S. Government Printing Office; 1996.

U.S. Department of Health and Human Services. *Healthy people 2010.* Washington, DC: U.S. Government Printing Office; 2000.

U.S. Department of Health and Human Services. *Healthy people 2020.* www.healthypeople.gov/2020/topicsobjectives2020/default.aspx. Accessed August 2018.

U.S. Department of Health and Human Services. Office of Disease Prevention and Health Promotion. Secretary's advisory committee on national health promotion and disease objectives for 2030. https://www.healthypeople.gov/2020/About-Health-People/Development-Healthy-People-2030/AdvisoryBoard. Published 2017.

U.S. Department of Health, Education and Welfare, Public Health Service. The Surgeon General's report on health promotion and disease prevention. Washington, DC: U.S. Department of Health and Human Services; U.S. Government Printing Office; 1979.

U.S. Preventive Services Task Force. Recommendations for primary care practice. https://www.uspreventiveservicestaskforce.org. Published 2017.

World Health Organization. Constitution of the World Health Organization. http://www.who.int/about/definition/en/print.html. Published 1948.

RESOURCES

Agency for Healthcare Research and Quality
    www.ahrq.gov
American College of Nurse Practitioners
    www.nurse.org/acnp
American Academy of Family Physicians
    www.aafp.org
American Academy of Nurse Practitioners
    www.aanp.org
American College of Sports Medicine
    www.acsm.org
    www.physsportsmed.com
Centers for Disease Control and Prevention
    www.cdc.gov/cdc.html
National Institutes of Health
    www.nih.gov
National Institute of Nursing Research
    www.nih.gov/ninr
National Library of Medicine
    www.nlm.nih.gov
Occupational Safety and Health Administration
    www.osha.gov
U.S. Department of Health and Human Services
    www.hhs.gov
U.S. Food and Drug Administration
    www.fda.gov
U.S. Preventive Services Task Force
    https://www.uspreventiveservicestaskforce.org/Page/Name/home

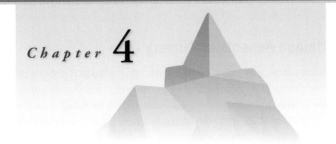

Chapter 4

The Art of Diagnosis and Treatment

Mary Hooshmand, MSN, PhD, RN

Katherine Chadwell, DNP, MBMSc, APRN, GNP-BC

Lynne M. Dunphy, PhD, APRN, FNP-BC, FAAN, FAANP

Health-care policy reform continues to drive critical changes in the health-care system. But regardless of how the system evolves, nurse practitioners (NPs) will be central in delivering much of primary care. NPs are able to offer unique services in primary care for several reasons. All health-care providers provide care by making treatment and screening choices based on current research findings. Evidence-based care works best when systems of care are established so that local protocols and tracking systems support the diagnosis and treatment decisions of providers and adhere to a standard of care.

NPs are able to enact evidence-based care particularly well because they bring a nursing perspective of whole-person care to patient encounters in settings that in some cases have been traditionally more disease centered than person centered. Instead of focusing solely on the patient's diagnosis, clinicians can work with patients to improve overall health by considering the individual's life situation. A care plan may include medications as well as recommendations for diet, activity, rest, stress management, and health promotion. Evidence-based practice requires more than a "diagnose and treat" mentality. There is more to do in a primary-care visit than set up a treatment plan. Treatment decisions are made based on patient values, preferences, and resources while also considering guidelines and research-based recommendations. Learning to practice primary care is an art, and it requires a certain kind of thinking.

CLINICAL JUDGMENT IN PRIMARY CARE

Clinical Judgment and the Circle of Caring

The *Circle of Caring* model, introduced in Chapter 1, provides a framework for advanced practice nursing. It includes aspects of the more traditional medical model approach within a model that has nursing as its origin. The *Circle of Caring* incorporates elements of the patient's experience, including the context of that experience in the patient's life and the environment in which care is delivered. It includes traditional modes of assessment, such as history taking, that are similar to those of the medical model, as well as a basis in the nursing perspective, functional health patterns, and other holistic measures. Objective findings include physical assessment data, laboratory test data, and functional measures. The *Circle of Caring* demonstrates that the clinician uses these data as part of a data-collection process that leads to the identification of both medical diagnoses as listed in the International Classification of Diseases, 10th Revision and the human responses to those specific diagnoses or nursing diagnoses as listed in taxonomies such as the North American Nursing Diagnosis Association International (NANDA-I). The NANDA-I list includes consideration of problem prevention and wellness promotion and goes beyond a narrow problem-solving framework. A full understanding of the patient situation provides a basis for planning interventions based on best available evidence. Patient preferences are considered as the patient and provider together design a treatment plan that may include pharmacologic measures but will also include lifestyle choices and complementary modalities to approach healing and wellness. The *Circle of Caring* reflects that outcomes of NP practice include improved mortality and morbidity statistics for aggregates of patients; optimized use of the health-care system that provides early, relatively inexpensive treatments to prevent more expensive problems later; and improved functional status and quality of life, as judged by the patient. All of this occurs in an environment consistent with the Institute of Medicine's recommendations that all patients have access to care based on best available evidence, as well as care that takes into account the patient's preferences and values.

Not only is the *Circle of Caring* an expanded way of thinking about both the nursing and the medical clinical process, but it also denotes the way in which the NP and patient relate to each other within this model. The NP is able to make appropriate diagnosis and intervention selections on the basis of knowing the patient, being committed to using appropriate clinical guidelines, and having patience when working with the patient, who may be required to make substantial lifestyle change as a result of illness or risk factors. In addition, both patient and nurse exhibit courage in that they engage in this most human of endeavors, that of caring. Throughout assessment, diagnosis, and treatment, the NP brings an authentic presence, which is in itself humanizing and healing, and is willing to be an advocate for the patient in personal or professional realms. The *Circle of Caring* requires a balance. The nurse and patient working together need to create a meaningful treatment plan and a plan for follow-up support. The *Circle of Caring* depicts a complex yet rewarding practice that enriches both patient and nurse.

The *Circle of Caring* model includes the medical model perspective that nurses with baccalaureate degrees may not have learned in an academic setting or practiced in hospital or community settings. It also includes a broader sense of nursing than practice at the baccalaureate level allows. Therefore, the NP role includes elements from the medical realm and from an expanded nursing base.

Essential to high-quality clinical judgment is the ability of the nurse to form a link between the patient's experience of his or her health concerns and the range of diagnostic and therapeutic choices available to achieve a range of possible outcome states. The nurse must be expert at eliciting the true story of the patient and recognizing patterns that are presented in the data in order to arrive at an appropriate diagnosis and therapeutic plan. This chapter focuses on merging the results of research with diagnostic reasoning and clinical judgment to facilitate their application by the NP.

Purpose and Goal of Diagnostic Reasoning

From the patient's point of view, the purpose of a visit to a clinician may be to solve a physical problem. Beyond problem-solving, the practitioner must always keep in mind that every visit is an opportunity for disease prevention, for screening for high-risk problems, and for health promotion based on appropriate guidelines. The patient must know that his or her initial concerns are taken seriously and are not ignored. The NP can establish a tone that attends to body, mind, and spirit in every visit. Diagnostic reasoning to solve problems, promote health, and screen for disease or illness all require a sensitivity to complex stories, contextual factors, and a sense of probability and uncertainty. At times, the patient will schedule a visit stating one concern, but during the visit other issues arise that become more important. Headache might be caused by a stressful job or family situation, or the patient might not want to tell the scheduler that domestic violence or a sexual concern is really what is bothering the patient. Clinicians learn to pay attention to the "By the way, I was wondering about…" lead-ins to real concerns. Chapter 81 details "The 15 Minute Hour: Practical Approaches to Behavioral Health for Primary Care" that provides strategies for getting to the heart of the patient's true concerns, as well as introducing motivational interviewing techniques to assist the patient and family in making needed behavioral changes.

The mental tasks of eliciting and sorting through large amounts of data, clustering data elements into meaningful patterns, connecting patterns to reasonable diagnostic statements, considering risk factors, and selecting appropriate interventions require the highest order of cognitive processes. It is these analytical functions that distinguish advanced practice nursing and are the reason patients seek our services. The human element of caring helps elicit rich data and establish the trust necessary to encourage patients to adjust their living patterns in the short or long range.

Unique Aspects of Primary Care

Many students come to advanced practice programs with extensive experience in acute- or critical-care nursing. They are committed to learning an expanded mode of practice but may be overwhelmed by the amount of new material that must be mastered. Even students with community health experience find that the issues faced in primary care are different from those encountered in their previous practice and require new knowledge and skills. Primary care is a new world with a different set of problems to be solved, different kinds of constraints on choices, and a different culture of care. Entering this world with sensitivity to its differences can help reduce anxiety for new NP students and can explain other reactions to this new nursing setting that might arise.

The types of problems addressed in primary care are different from those encountered in acute- or critical-care settings. Upper respiratory infections, common abdominal complaints, skin rashes, and vaginal discharges are problems not often encountered in acute-care settings. Even chronic conditions present differently in primary care. Hypertension, congestive heart failure, arthritis, or diabetes present with day-to-day management problems that are different from the crises that acute-care nurses must respond to in tertiary-care settings. Patients with psychosocial problems, such as anxiety and depression, frequently present with vague, nonspecific somatic complaints.

The pace of care is different in primary care. Nurses who are seeking refuge from busy acute-care duties will be surprised by the mental fatigue that comes from diagnosing and treating up to 30 different patients or families in a day. The sheer variety of possible problems faced in a day's time is exciting and interesting, but it is also challenging. Primary care includes more than problem-solving and symptom management. It involves screening for problems as yet undetected and supporting health promotion and disease and injury prevention at every opportunity. It also involves dealing with patients with chronic diseases who need to make behavioral changes, which can present a challenge. Teaching patients of all ages about how their bodies work, risk reduction, and treatment options helps patients assume more responsibility for their own wellness. These activities support patients in increasing their health literacy so that they can be active participants in their own care. Researchers from Canada are exploring how NPs help patients participate in their own care more actively through a concern for their comfort and for a sense of coherence in their lives (Sangster-Gormley & Frisch, 2013). Establishing trust and believing that the NP cares about the whole person promote true patient-centered care.

Uncertainty

Primary care and the increased autonomy that NPs enjoy also bring an increase in uncertainty. Patient problems are not already labeled when the NP sees the patient. Many different conditions present in similar ways. Even the "hard numbers" of laboratory tests must be evaluated for their reliability. Once a diagnosis is made, multiple treatment approaches are available even for simple problems. Further, patients do not always carry out recommended treatment plans (Michaels et al., 2008). Many problems require lifelong lifestyle adjustment. At the end of the day, the clinician may have nagging doubts about the decisions that were made on many levels. New practitioners especially need support to develop confidence in their diagnostic and treatment-planning capabilities, but even experienced practitioners describe learning to live with the uncertainties involved in primary care. Intellectual honesty and humility are important aspects of thoughtful practice and can be cultivated, but they must be balanced with confidence that is based on experience; this serves to increase the effectiveness of the provider.

Nursing and the Medical Model

NPs perform in both the nursing and the medical domains. The nursing domain contains consideration of individual and family responses to actual or potential threats to health. It involves helping patients cope with disease processes that may be occurring, and it anticipates human distress and works on the level of what an illness experience means to the patient. By becoming an NP, nurses do not leave their nursing model of practice. As NPs gain skill in the medical domain of practice, they learn new diagnostic reasoning possibilities and new treatment options for

specific medical problems. These new skills are built on the nursing framework, but they do not replace the nursing basis for practice. NPs have been proven to be effective and efficient care providers for patients with acute and chronic health problems. The process of clinical judgment is unique in primary care because patients and their families will actually carry out the care (Elliott, 2010). Patients are actively involved in their own care, and the clinician must take that into account in designing a treatment or health-promotion plan. Although much of this textbook is designed to provide a background for managing medical problems, all that the nurse has learned in caring for patients still applies. A NP's approach to patient problems is invariably very individualized and, therefore, less easy to summarize in a textbook. Nevertheless, the nursing model supports and nurtures the NP's practice. It provides the basis for the *Circle of Caring.*

Patient–Advanced Practice Nurse Linkages

A model for how the provider and patient work together in a clinical encounter is presented in Figure 4.1. Clinical judgment is not a process that happens in the mind of the practitioner alone: it happens in a dialogue that occurs between patient and provider. The quality of communication and the agreement about what the encounter is meant to accomplish will improve both effectiveness and satisfaction with the patient encounter for both parties. The model includes patient factors, provider factors, and environmental factors, all of which have an influence on the clinical judgment process (Chase, 2004).

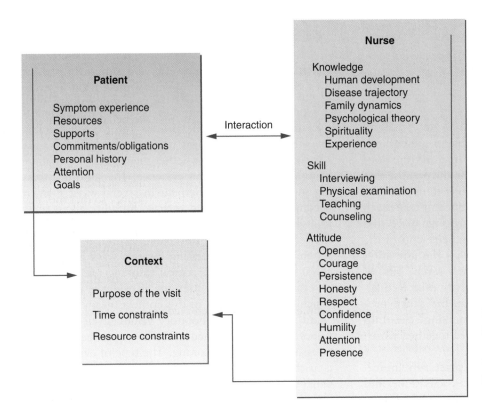

Figure 4.1 Patient–advanced practice nursing linkages. *Source: Chase SK. Clinical judgment and communication in nurse practitioner practice. Philadelphia, PA: F.A. Davis; 2004.*

The Patient–advanced practice nurse linkage model is based on research in diagnostic reasoning in general and the particulars of the primary-care encounter. Johnson (1993) described the discourse between patient and nurse as having several phases: establishing the agenda for the encounter; eliciting information from the patient, including being alert to cues and helping to problem solve; and conducting the physical examination, including attending to comfort level, preparing and informing, and developing a plan of care and using a teachable moment. Teaching in this case is not content centered but patient centered, based on understanding the perspective of the patient. Finally, the NP personalizes solutions based on knowing the patient. A large quantitative study investigating overall satisfaction with care has shown that patients are equally satisfied with care access and overall care experience when care is provided by a NP or physician assistant compared with a visit to a physician in both adult and pediatric settings. Patients were more satisfied, however, with NP and physician assistant care when rating the quality of practitioner interaction (Roblin et al., 2004). A review of the literature on NPs' communication style (Charlton et al., 2008) characterized NP communication style as either biomedical or biopsychosocial. The biopsychosocial style was associated with higher patient satisfaction and better adherence to treatment plans. A qualitative study of health outcomes achieved in a home visiting model for young disadvantaged mothers showed that the nature of the relationship between carer and recipient goes beyond protocols with a result of enhanced personhood and new possibilities developed by these young women (SmithBattle, 2009). The personal relationship between NP and patient within which this work is done is unique.

THE CLINICAL PROCESS AND ITS LIMITATIONS

Human Memory Limitations

One of the most useful models available to understanding diagnostic reasoning is that of the information-processing model. This model is built on the premise that the human brain has both short- and long-term memory, and that these forms of memory are different from each other. Short-term memory is the processing space that can hold new pieces of information and elements of the patient history and physical data. It has the limitation of being able to hold only approximately seven "bits" of information. Much of the mental activity used in diagnostic reasoning is done to maximize the active processing space and to clustering or "chunking" cues into collections of data that can be managed together, which helps to maximize processing capacity.

In contrast, long-term memory is practically unlimited. It can hold vast quantities of facts, sensations, and experiences. To bring these facts or experiences to bear

on a given situation, long-term memories must be accessible. Research has shown that the ability to retrieve a fact depends on the frequency with which the fact is brought forward for use. This is why in some cases repetitive exercises assist in cementing long-term memory. Another factor that affects retrievability of facts from long-term memory is the organizational structure with which the fact is associated. Body systems and functional health patterns are systems of data organization that help busy clinicians retrieve relevant bits of information as needed.

Although the information-processing model is a useful starting point, it leaves out many of the complexities of the human experience. The human brain is able to sense patterns of data and include emotional responses to interactions with human beings. The ability to empathize with a patient, to be available personally, and to be invested with the patient in maximizing health make the human decision maker much more valuable than any computer or protocol system could ever be. Patients come to a health-care provider for more than a diagnosis; they come for a human connection. The human aspect of the nurse–patient relationship adds to, rather than detracts from, diagnostic accuracy. One researcher called this "getting alongside" (Elliott, 2010) when describing the ways that NPs listen to the patient's perspective on his or her problem.

Technology does play a role in assisting clinicians by prompting routines and offering diagnostic and therapeutic options that might have been missed (Lee et al., 2009; Topol, 2012). Technology should not be viewed as a threat, but rather as an adjunct to human judgment, and should not become a barrier to provider–patient communication; in fact, there is increasing evidence that it can actually enhance this communication (Hooshmand & Yao, 2017).

Critical Thinking

Diagnostic reasoning can be seen as a kind of critical thinking. *Critical thinking* has been defined as reflective thinking because the process involves questioning one's thinking to determine whether all possible avenues have been explored and whether the conclusions that are being drawn are based on evidence. This kind of thinking supports clinical judgment in several ways. First, it becomes a habit of mind to have humility about one's thought processes and to know that even the most experienced thinker can be mistaken. Second, it becomes a systematic way of generating creative ways of thinking about problems. Third, critical thinking returns one to an examination of the strength of evidence for a given conclusion. "Evidence" in this context means more than "hard" data such as laboratory values. Even laboratory values must be examined critically when they are used to assist diagnostic reasoning. The type of evidence that is useful includes subjective impressions of the ways patients present themselves. The patient's initial complaint may be fatigue, but any patient who describes a bone-chilling inability to generate energy for daily living (compared with a fulfilled fatigue that comes after a challenging situation is completed) is providing data the NP can use to investigate potentially serious health problems.

Critical thinking can include creative thinking—in this sense, the NP is creative in developing potential problem lists. A patient may complain of abdominal pain. The pattern is unclear or may indicate irritable bowel syndrome. The creative NP will explore stress management issues as a way of generating diagnostic and therapeutic choices that could include a diet and symptom log, increased fiber in the diet, a walking program, or a quick follow-up visit to check on symptoms. Creativity may also be required in developing goals with patients for their short- or long-term problems. In addition to creative processing, critical thinking includes systematic thinking that evaluates each new piece of data as it either supports some diagnostic hypotheses or reduces the likelihood of others.

Intuition

Another kind of thinking that develops with experience is that of intuition. Research on intuition shows that it develops after long experience in the particular setting and that it is based on unconscious thought that is probably an exquisite pattern matching. The experienced clinician is reminded of a situation that occurred in the past when presented with a certain new situation. Past experience provides a picture of what will likely happen. The experienced clinician often could not list the specific data points that led to the conclusion. In fact, in some studies of computerized "artificial intelligence," experienced clinicians were asked to "think aloud" as a research device aimed at identifying the steps involved in reaching a diagnosis. Experienced clinicians reported that being asked to do that kind of thinking changed their thought process and slowed them down. Although intuition characterizes expert practice, it is not a goal in itself. Being able to reflect on one's thinking processes opens the process to analysis, sharing, and improvement (Thompson & Yang, 2009).

Developing Expertise

Benner et al. (1996) have done extensive work describing differences in clinical judgment based on experience. NP students, even those who are experts in hospital or specialty care, find it disconcerting to enter a world where they feel like novices again. Even skills that were a part of their old practice feel awkward. Their minds often do not generate ideas smoothly, and they focus on their own performance of skills more than on the patient's situation. With the experience of the clinical practicum, however, the student gains skill and by graduation is probably functioning at the advanced beginner level. Features of diagnostic reasoning used in the various stages of expertise are summarized in Table 4.1.

TABLE 4.1 Skill Acquisition in Advanced Practice Nursing Practice

Skill Level	*Features of Clinical Judgment*
Novice	Rule-based actions, unaware of context
Advanced beginner	Sensitive to aspects of the situation, able to formulate principles, needs help setting priorities
Competent	Goal-directed actions, feeling of mastery based on experience, deliberate planning
Proficient	Sees situation as a whole, immediate grasp of meaning, recognizes patterns of normalcy or aberrance, uses maxims to guide action
Expert	Transcends rules, intuitive grasp of the wholeness of situation, creative response to particularities of situation, flexible response to situations

DIAGNOSTIC PROCESS OVERVIEW

In general, the diagnostic process involves collecting data from a variety of sources (e.g., the history, physical examination, and diagnostic test results) and then generating a working hypothesis about the cause of the patient's signs and symptoms. In collecting data and generating a hypothesis, the clinician uses probabilistic reasoning, pattern matching, planning, problem-solving, and critical reflection. These processes are commonly summarized by describing the steps in the nursing process or the clinical reasoning process. Research has shown that many clinicians, physicians, nurses, occupational and physical therapists, dentists, and others use a similar method. Although research that uses simulated case studies to examine methods of clinician reasoning tends to oversimplify what happens in real life, it is helpful to review a simplified description of the diagnostic process as outlined here.

Research indicates that expert clinicians generate a list of possible diagnoses or diagnostic hypotheses early in the clinical encounter. Further, the likelihood that the diagnostic choice will be correct is higher if the correct diagnosis is included in the initial hypothesis list. In generating hypotheses, the NP considers a number of labels that could be associated with the initial complaint and considers potential problems for each patient based on the patient's age and demographics and the setting of the practice.

For experienced clinicians, data acquisition during history taking and physical examination is most effective if it is hypothesis driven—that is, when the information selected and gathered is related to the list of possible diagnoses. For common problems, the data collection approach becomes routine and, therefore, takes less active-processing space in short-term memory. In contrast, novices tend to use a "shotgun" approach and ask a little bit about everything that might be possible, not considering which diagnoses are most likely. Hypothesis-driven data collection means that data that would confirm or disprove a specific hypothesis is specifically sought and recorded. It is not enough to note only those data that fit with one possible problem. Competing hypotheses must be ruled out by seeking nonconfirmatory data. In doing this, the clinician must be open to changing the priority list of hypotheses based on new information. For example, rhinitis may present similar to a viral infection, but if, when asked whether the symptoms have occurred before, the patient says, "Yes, I had the same thing 2 weeks ago." This decreases the likelihood of viral illness and increases the likelihood of allergy.

An approach to data collection that is completely symptom driven, however, can result in leaving out important concepts. The agenda for the visit includes not only the patient's agenda but also expands the visit to provide health promotion.

Data are clustered together into meaningful "chunks" of information that explain and account for the different elements of the history. Clinicians are alert to any data bits that do not fit the pattern of what is expected. They are alert to the feeling in themselves that "something is just not right here." This can indicate that the problem is more serious than initially appeared or that there are data bits that are not yet accounted for. Diagnosticians are persistent in trying to fit the pieces of data into a coherent picture. One must be on guard not to ignore discrepant data. Research has shown that "we see what we expect to see" in many cases, so an openness to the patient situation must be maintained in order to continue "seeing" all the data present.

A maxim of practice is that "common things occur commonly." Students are frequently excited to make a diagnosis for the rare or exotic condition. This can be the result of a rich experience in acute- or critical-care settings where the most serious cases were seen. In primary care, common problems predominate. The adage that "when you hear hoof beats, think horses, not zebras" applies. In real life, "zebra" diagnoses are rare. Rare conditions can be considered with the differential list, but their lower probability must be taken into consideration.

Experienced clinicians keep their antennae raised for the most serious conditions. Abdominal pain could be from gas, but if it is from a ruptured ectopic pregnancy, a dissecting abdominal aortic aneurysm, or a ruptured appendix, immediate surgical consultation is necessary. The clinician must make it a point to collect and document data that rule out any potentially life-threatening condition.

Diagnoses are frequently interrelated. Obesity, hypertension, hyperlipidemia, and type 2 diabetes mellitus (DM) frequently occur together. When evaluating competing hypotheses, the NP can cluster related problems together. The lifestyle recommendations for all these conditions are the same. The medication approach might differ. For nursing diagnoses, many occur together. Clinicians should try

to approach the core diagnosis, which, if managed appropriately, will ameliorate all the others. For instance, ineffective coping with stress can result in an array of symptoms including altered sleep patterns, constipation, difficulty concentrating, and interpersonal tension. By dealing with the underlying problem, the other problems might not need direct intervention. If the NP focuses only on the superficial problem level, the problems may still remain. Table 4.2 summarizes habits that promote effective clinical judgment. Table 4.3 describes common errors in diagnostic thinking that are made even by experts.

Clustering history data into a likely problem list helps to focus the physical examination, laboratory test evaluation, and initial management plan. Physical examination for a problem-focused visit serves to rule in or rule out competing diagnostic hypotheses. A new hypothesis rarely emerges during a physical examination, but this

TABLE 4.2 Habits That Support Clinical Judgment	
Phase of Diagnostic Reasoning	*Habits That Support Clinical Judgment*
Data acquisition	Use systematic or hierarchically organized approach (general to specific). Review multiple systems.
Hypothesis formulation	Generate hypotheses early in encounter. Develop competing hypotheses. Consider life- or function-threatening problems. Consider "zebras" but recognize them as such.
Hypothesis evaluation	Recognize interrelation of diagnoses. Consider probabilities in context. Consider likelihood of altering course of problem with treatment. Rule out life- or function-threatening problems.
Problem naming	Choose most fundamental problem. Include multiple perspectives (biopsychosocial, spiritual, medical, nursing). Include illness prevention and health promotion.
Goal setting	Include patient in goal setting. Make goals explicit and realistic.
Therapeutic option consideration	Include modalities from multiple paradigms. Consider patient preferences. Consider context and cost in economic and human terms.
Evaluation	Plan for follow-up visit or phone call. Consider symptom or treatment logs or diaries. Measure and document the outcome of your practice for the individual. Report the effectiveness of your practice in the aggregate.

Source: Chase SK. *Clinical judgment and communication in nurse practitioner practice.* Philadelphia, PA: F.A. Davis; 2004:43. Used with permission.

TABLE 4.3 **Errors in Diagnostic Reasoning**	
Phase of Clinical Judgment	*Diagnostic Errors*
Data collection	Not obtaining all relevant clues Misjudging importance of clues Overemphasizing clues that favor top hypotheses Ignoring data that disconfirm working hypothesis Forgetting that some data are unreliable Ignoring pertinent negative findings
Hypothesis	Not generating enough competing hypotheses Oversimplifying Not generating hypotheses early Not including correct diagnosis on hypothesis list Failing to revise hypothesis list (premature closure) Selecting "favorite" hypotheses Generating too many hypotheses and getting lost Overestimating low-probability situations Underestimating high-probability situations

Source: Chase SK. *Clinical judgment and communication in nurse practitioner practice.* Philadelphia, PA: F.A. Davis; 2004. Used with permission.

might occur for a problem that the patient cannot see or that causes no symptoms, such as a skin lesion. Laboratory tests also provide information that is not available any other way.

Finally, a working diagnosis is reached, even though there might still be some uncertainty. A management plan is discussed with the patient in light of mutually shared goals and guidelines for practice based on published research. Honest conversation about the patient's ability and willingness to follow treatment recommendations will result in more realistic plans. Written instructions often help patients implement complicated treatment directions. Part of the treatment plan always includes a plan for follow-up. Patients need to know when to return for a visit and under what circumstances they should telephone. Documenting these plans in the patient record reduces the possibility of misunderstanding and places appropriate responsibility with the patient. Some patients need support in learning how to engage the health-care system in an effective way. This is one aspect of health literacy that the NP can support.

A simple encounter for a self-limiting acute illness might proceed like this: a patient requests an appointment for a "sore throat." The patient is known by the NP as a resourceful, independent young adult. Before even entering the room, the clinician draws from experience with other patients who have complained of sore throat and begins to generate a list of hypotheses. Contextual

factors enter into the reasoning: it may be allergy season in that particular area, or the clinician may have seen a large number of other patients with similar complaints who have tested positive for *Streptococcus* infection. The clinician enters the room and notes the general appearance of the patient. Is the patient ill-appearing, flushed, fatigued, or mildly irritated? These observations may serve to adjust the hypothesis list. The patient's story is elicited, beginning with HPI, along with a review of data already present in the record regarding past medical history and medications. Further questions regarding current life stresses and exposures may also serve to adjust the hypothesis list. The history narrows the hypothesis list to a short one, although experienced clinicians have ways of preventing the common diagnostic error of premature closure and work to consider alternative conditions that could also be represented by the same cluster of symptoms.

The physical examination serves to verify hypotheses and to screen out unlikely, though troubling, alternative diagnoses. The hypothesis list is narrowed further as data are weighed to see whether they fit the pattern of the highest-favored hypothesis; disconfirming data are also elicited to avoid leaping to conclusions too early. Finally, diagnostic tests may be chosen to firm up the diagnosis if the findings of the tests will have a bearing on how the patient's care is to be managed. Once findings of relevant tests have been obtained, treatment decisions are considered, including patient factors such as resources, reliability, and the risk of the patient not following through on instructions. For example, insufficiently treated strep throat could result in rheumatic heart disease. Besides prescribing medication, consider comfort measures that are likely to assist the patient and judge the appropriateness of health promotion and educational opportunities at the moment. For example, is this a good time to give the patient smoking cessation materials? Finally, a plan to evaluate the treatment plan is made. Is a follow-up appointment necessary? Would a telephone call be useful? For which date should the next "well" visit be scheduled? The list of decisions made in this rather simple example is long. Given a few data or situational changes, the management of the patient's care could be quite different, and a new-patient visit requires even deeper background data collection. Patients who present with more complex, long-term problems require even more complex decision making by the clinician. In observing the experienced clinician, many of these mental processes may not be apparent. Many of these processes occur as a kind of internal dialogue, but they occur nonetheless.

ELEMENTS OF THE DIAGNOSTIC PROCESS

A more detailed examination of each step in the diagnostic reasoning process is presented in the following sections.

History

History of Present Illness

Taking a history is the first step in the diagnostic reasoning process. Problems cannot be found, strengths identified, or appropriate direction known without a real grounding in the life experience of the individual patient. If the patient's visit is for "episodic" care or one in which a new complaint is being addressed, the history begins with a history of present illness (HPI). There are a number of mnemonics that can help the clinician remember the essential data elements; the "OLD CART" mnemonic is presented in Box 4.1.

Immediately on hearing the chief complaint, the clinician begins to sort out diagnostic possibilities. The list of possibilities helps to generate questions to follow-up on the HPI and in other areas of the history. Specific questions are asked that help distinguish between competing diagnostic hypotheses. For example, the question, "Do you feel the pain more often on an empty stomach or several hours after eating?" helps distinguish between ulcer and gallbladder disease. In general, asking open-ended questions helps the patient give his or her perspective and provides a richer database. An open-ended question is one that cannot be answered by a "Yes" or "No" response. Eliciting the patient's story will assist the clinician in understanding the illness experience from the patient's point of view. Frequently interrupting the patient's story distracts and places the story in the context of the examiner and not in the context of the patient's own life.

The clinician continues to clarify the patient's story until a clear picture of the illness appears. This can require patience because patients do not know which facts "fit together" to support diagnostic hypotheses. Patients may get the chronological order confused or not recall the exact onset of their problems. They may also have more than one problem and may not be able to distinguish which symptoms cluster together. The picture may not be completely clear at this point of history taking, but other areas of history can fill in some gaps. Periodically, the clinician can restate the emerging understanding of the story to clarify and summarize it. This summary allows the patient to clarify any misunderstandings. One important issue to address as part of the HPI is what the *patient* thinks may be wrong. Patients know their own bodies, and parents know their own children better than anyone and may have important insights to share. On the other hand, if a patient shares his or her fear of a serious diagnosis, the clinician can also explain reasons why many of those fears may be unfounded. A recurring headache does not necessarily indicate a brain tumor.

Visits for periodic health screening, to establish a new patient–provider relationship, or to follow-up on an existing problem do not use the HPI in the same sense unless a new problem is also identified. The clinician can ask, "What do you want to accomplish today?" or "What is the most important issue for us to deal with today?" This is particularly useful for the patient with a long list of problems or complaints. A plan for follow-up for other problems may need to be addressed.

Past Medical History

Past medical history helps to refine the hypothesis list by offering new explanations for symptoms or by ruling out others. The history also gives suggestions of risk factors for other problems that are being considered. If a patient reports that his or her gallbladder was removed 10 years ago, cholecystitis is now off the hypothesis list, but abdominal adhesions might go onto the list. Past medical history is frequently divided into childhood and other illnesses, surgical history, other hospital admissions, history of trauma, pregnancies, and psychiatric diagnoses. Travel outside the United States and any possible exposure to infectious or toxic agents can be explored. Treatment for cancer in the distant past is important in that the treatments may have increased the risk of other conditions. For example, some chemotherapy agents can lead to heart failure in later years.

The history includes information regarding all medications that patients take, including prescription and over-the-counter medications, as well as vitamins and

Box 4.1	**OLD CART Mnemonic**			
Onset	When did this problem start? How did it start? Has it changed over time? For an injury, exactly how did the injury occur (the mechanism of injury)?	**D**uration	Are the symptoms constant, fluctuating, getting better or worse?	
		Characteristics	How are the symptoms experienced? Dull ache, sharp pain, heat, or electrical?	
Location	Where exactly are the symptoms experienced? Can a specific location be identified, or is the problem more generalized? Has the symptom moved?	**A**ggravating factors	What makes the symptoms worse?	
		Relieving factors	What makes the symptoms better?	
		Treatment	What have you done so far to try to help the problem?	

herbal remedies. Patients also need to be asked whether they take any medications that have been prescribed for other members of the family. Even for patients who are well known to the practice and whose medications are listed on the chart, asking the patient what medications he or she is currently taking allows the clinician to learn what the patient remembers about the medication regimen. For patients with multiple prescriptions, it sometimes helps to use the "brown bag" method: ask the patient to bring in all the medications he or she is taking, then go over them one by one. This helps to determine whether the medications that have been ordered are really being taken. This review of medications also gives the clinician information about the patient's understanding of his or her medications and helps to determine any difficulties he or she is having with the prescribed regimen. Immunization status is part of the history. Many parents bring their child's immunization cards with them to office visits. This allows any additional immunization series to be documented. Adults often forget that they need immunizations for things such as tetanus or pneumonia.

Allergies can be discussed at this time and reviewed. The kind of reaction the medications or food caused can help to distinguish an adverse effect from a true allergy. By noting the adverse effect, one can avoid confusing it with an allergy, which is characterized by rash, hives, wheezing, or other hypersensitivity reactions.

Health maintenance practices can be questioned, as well as risk reduction techniques such as seat-belt use and exercise habits.

Family History

Family history provides information for a part of the risk factor pattern for this patient. The most efficient way to represent the family history is to draw a genogram (Fig. 4.2). This method of representation can be used to record family patterns of births, ages at death, and causes of death. The genogram can also record family members with whom the patient currently lives. Try to include information for at least two generations back, as well as for any children and their health status. The genogram can be used to map difficulties, such as alcoholism or the quality of relationships in the family, by drawing slashes across the relationship lines that are troubled or by using thick lines to represent relationships that are strongly supportive. Judgment is required to determine whether this level of information is useful. If there is no room in the patient's record for a genogram, list the major diseases that have familiar patterns, such as diabetes, heart disease, arthritis, psychiatric problems, alcoholism, and cancer.

Social History

Social history in a medical model interview includes such things as work patterns. Even if the patient is retired, the

Genogram of Family History

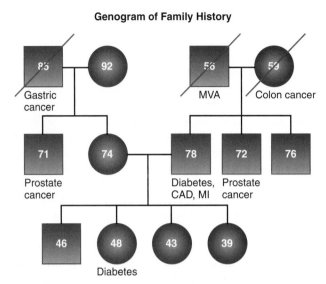

Figure 4.2 Genogram of family history. *Source: Chase SK.* Clinical judgment and communication in nurse practitioner practice. *Philadelphia, PA: F.A. Davis; 2004.*

type of work in which the patient had engaged is important because worksite exposures can be risk factors for many potential problems. Work background also gives the clinician a sense of how the person might handle new information and what kind of resources he or she might have at his or her disposal. Medical model histories also include the use of alcohol, tobacco, and illegal drugs. Nursing histories are more expanded in this area. Include such information as leisure time activities, risk factors and exposures, and the patient's resources and activity level. If a full functional health pattern is collected, much of this information can be recorded there. If the documentation system in use in a particular setting does not accommodate functional health patterns, expand the social history section to reflect nursing issues.

Review of Systems

This section of the history is often completed by the patient immediately before the physical examination. It is organized by body systems. Whenever the review is completed, it can include problems and symptoms that are current or related to past medical history and prompt the patient to report any past difficulties. This also helps remind patients of conditions they may have forgotten and can help to refine the hypothesis list further or to screen out potential new problems. When introducing a body system, start questions in general terms and then proceed to more specific items. When documenting this section, students frequently forget that these data are appropriately recorded as subjective data because they are reported from the patient's point of view. Please see the Review of Systems table under the Reference Resources section in DavisPlus for sample questions that can be used during the review of systems.

Functional Health Patterns

Functional health patterns, developed by Marjory Gordon, serve as a database for determining nursing diagnoses. NPs engage in some activities that require making medical diagnoses, but their practice base is always nursing. The value that NPs bring to a practice is an enhanced ability to assist patients with lifestyle changes and an ability to support patients as they cope with illness. The openness and thoroughness that patients report when cared for by an NP are dependent on the NP practicing from a database that is broader and more personal than that of the traditional medical model. Even in practice settings using a medically dominated model, the nurse has an obligation to represent nursing's contribution to care. The type of data recorded in the functional health pattern in the medical record can reflect a nursing approach.

For episodic visits, some patterns are more important than others, and the list can be prioritized accordingly. For example, for a patient with a sore throat, important data are nutrition (Is he or she able to eat and drink sufficiently?), sleep and rest (Is sleep interrupted?), activity and exercise (Does he or she feel fatigued?), and role relationship (Is he or she able to work? Are there children in the home?). Inability of the patient to carry out any normal, day-to-day function is often a "red flag"—an indicator for the NP that a potentially serious disease process may be developing.

The purpose of the functional health pattern is to determine the extent to which illness is affecting the person's ability to live his or her "normal" life. What accommodations must be made, even for a self-limiting condition? This is nursing's central question. What is the human response to the health problem? Advanced Assessment 4.1 presents the 11 functional health patterns and sample questions that can be used to elicit data for each functional pattern area.

At this phase of history taking, the hypothesis list is taking shape. The initial diagnostic possibilities generated are weighed as each new piece of information is gathered. Some data serve to support one hypothesis in favor of another; some data are noncontributory. Some data serve to rule out specific hypotheses. The problem list may contain physical disorders with signs or symptoms that are visible, along with other physical disorders that are presumed to be

Advanced Assessment 4.1: Functional Health Patterns: Questions to Elicit Data

Pattern	Sample Questions	Pattern	Sample Questions
Health perception	Do you have a regular health-care provider?	Cognitive/perceptual concept	Any hearing or vision problems? Any memory changes? How do you like to learn new things? Any pain or discomfort?
Health management	How often do you go to your health-care provider? What do you do to stay healthy?	Self-perception/ self-concept	How would you describe yourself? Do you feel good about yourself? Any changes in how you feel about your body? Do you get angry or down at times?
Nutrition/ metabolic	What did you eat yesterday or on a typical day? What do you drink? How is your appetite? Any skin problems?	Role relationship self-perception/ self-concept	Who lives with you? Do you have friends? What kind of work do you do? Do you have other responsibilities?
Elimination	What are your bowel and bladder elimination patterns? Do you have unexpected loss of control?	Sexuality/ reproductive Role relationship	Any problems with your sexuality? Any changes? If sexually active, do you practice safe sex? Do you use birth control? What mode of birth control do you use?
Activity/ exercise	How far can you walk before feeling tired? Do you have energy to do the things you want? Do you need any assistance with feeding, bathing, toileting, dressing, getting around (activities of daily living)? Do you need any help with cooking, shopping, or cleaning (instrumental activities of daily living)?	Coping/stress tolerance	How do you cope with stress? Any use of alcohol, drugs? Do you have someone to talk things over with?
Sleep/rest	How many hours do you sleep? Any trouble falling asleep or with early wakening? Do you feel rested?	Value/belief	What is most important to you in your life? Are you religious? Any values about life that health-care providers should know? Do you have a health-care proxy (medical power of attorney) or living will (advance directive)?

present based on the patient's story, emotional distress related to specific disorders, general emotional disorders, family or social disorders, or even spiritual distress. The patient's problem list may contain more than one diagnosis from any of the biological, psychosocial, or spiritual realms. It may also include health risks. Further data are available to help refine the hypothesis list by performing the physical examination and ordering diagnostic tests.

Physical Examination

The physical examination serves to clarify diagnostic hypotheses and to detect unanticipated problems of which the patient is unaware. In primary care, there is a wide range of ways of performing the physical examination. Textbooks of physical assessment outline a general head-to-toe model that is useful for an initial visit with a full physical examination or a periodic reassessment. In most practices, an initial patient visit is scheduled for more time, and in coding schemes the visit may be reimbursed at a higher level because of its comprehensiveness. Students in nursing or medical school learn to perform the head-to-toe examination in an organized way. In actual practice, however, clinicians must learn to focus their physical assessment skills and make the physical examination appropriate to the patient's complaint and history. If the patient complains of headache, a review of head, eyes, ears, nose, and throat and a neurologic examination are indicated, as well as a skin survey. For joint pain, a review of musculoskeletal tenderness, range of motion, and strength might be indicated. The body systems that are examined depend on the working hypothesis list that the clinician has generated. Examination skills need to be organized at a general screening level, with subroutines of examination techniques that can be adapted to specific findings and complaints. Positive or negative findings that serve to refine the hypothesis list must be noted and recorded in the documentation system that is in use. At times, a condition is in evolution, and the symptoms may not be clear when the patient comes for a visit. Nonetheless, the rich data reporting from that visit—even though the diagnosis is not clear—can serve to make the diagnosis more accurate later, when the condition evolves further. Full documentation serves to protect both patient and provider. The physical examination can also be a time to provide feedback and teaching about findings and about self-care. There is some evidence that thorough physical examinations are becoming rarer in medicine. An over-reliance on blood, radiological, and other tests to confirm diagnoses increases costs of care and reduces contact with the patient (Sanders, 2009). The ritual of the physical examination is evidence of person-to-person attention and may be perceived as the kind of professional caring expected in a health-care visit.

Diagnostic Tests

Diagnostic tests can be used to confirm or to rule out diagnostic hypotheses or as screening devices for conditions with subtle presentations that need to be picked up early, such as lead poisoning in children. Diagnostic tests vary in their usefulness based on their sensitivity, specificity, and predictive value. When considering or evaluating a test, consider that there are patient, test, and disease factors that affect the interpretation of the tests. The prevalence of a condition is the number of cases present in a given population at a particular point in time. The incidence of a condition reflects the total number of cases during a specified time period. For example, the number of cases of flu in a year (incidence) is greater than the number of people who have the flu on a given day (prevalence). Both incidence and prevalence rates are important considerations in making accurate diagnoses. Laboratory tests and radiographic or other imaging can assist in screening for conditions and in making diagnoses. For chronic conditions, tests are used to monitor progress in managing the condition.

No test is perfect, and test results can be inaccurate. When a patient who does not have a condition has a positive test result, it is called a "false-positive result." When a patient does have a condition but has a negative test result, it is called a "false-negative result." The sensitivity of a test is greater when it has few false negatives. Sensitivity equals the number of true positives for a test divided by the number of tested individuals who truly have the disease. The specificity of a test is greater when it has few false positives. The specificity of a test is equal to the number of true negatives divided by the number of all tested individuals who do not have the disease. Table 4.4 represents the relationship between test results and actual conditions.

In clinical practice, the predictive value of a test is the important consideration. Given a positive test result, what is the likelihood that the patient actually has the condition? Positive predictive value is equal to true positives divided by all positives. Negative predictive value is equal

TABLE 4.4 Tests: Characteristics and Diseases			
Test Reading	*Disease Present*	*Disease Absent*	*Total*
Positive	True positive (TP) A	False-positive (FP) B	All positives A + B
Negative	False-negative (FN) C	True negative (TN) D	All negatives C + D
Totals	All diseased A + C	All healthy B + D	Grand Total

Source: Chase SK. *Clinical judgment and communication in nurse practitioner practice.* Philadelphia, PA: F.A. Davis; 2004. Used with permission.

to true negatives divided by all negatives. Predictive value is in part dependent on the prevalence of the condition. If a condition is highly likely, a positive test result is more likely to be accurate. If a condition is very unlikely, a positive test result needs to be questioned, perhaps with different tests.

When deciding whether to order a test, cost, convenience, sensitivity and specificity, and risk of missing a condition are considered. One can ask whether the test result would affect the potential treatment plan. If not, the test might not be necessary. It is not appropriate to order a test merely to increase the clinician's confidence and comfort. Appropriate screening for life-threatening or life-altering conditions must be considered. Clinicians can use the U.S. Preventive Services Task Force guidelines or other research-based guidelines for deciding on screening tests for specific patients. It is important to always consider the individual patient's situation. For example, the age for first mammogram has changed over the years based on research data and is dependent, in part, on a strong family history or other risk factors for breast cancer.

Differential Diagnosis

A differential diagnosis list is the list of possible diagnoses, usually in priority order. When clinicians discuss a case, the list of differential diagnoses is usually considered. Supports for developing a rich differential diagnosis list include several guides. One approach suggests considering the problem from the "skin in." This means that if the patient complains of chest pain, the clinician can consider all the possible causes of chest pain, beginning at the skin, and visualize all the structures in the area that could possibly be affected. For example, chest pain at skin level could indicate early herpes zoster sensitivity and pain. Below the skin, the musculoskeletal system (including the rib cage) could be causing pain, from costochondritis or from muscle strain. The clinician can consider pain below the rib cage as a source of pain. Could the patient have pneumonia, pneumothorax, or pulmonary embolus? Next is the esophagus. Could the pain be from esophagitis, gastroesophageal reflux, or hiatal hernia? Next consider the pericardium as a possible source of pain, as with pericarditis. Finally, consider cardiac pain. This "skin in" approach keeps the student from jumping to early conclusions without considering a wide range of problems. It, thus, avoids the common diagnostic error of premature closure.

An evolving problem list can become quite long, even on an initial visit. The Nursing Situation below describes one approach to differential diagnosis.

Nursing Situation: A Nurse Practitioner's Approach to Differential Diagnosis

An NP describes her approach to a new patient.

My initial diagnosis at that time, just by speaking with him, without any laboratory test results and examining him physically,

was this: his diabetes was in poor control. His hypertension was in poor control. He had some rhinitis, probably allergic, but he was not having a problem. He has known unequal pupils since he had surgery and had damage to the pupillary musculature, but it does not affect his vision; if you did not happen to know that, you might be very concerned about it, you know? It is real important to put that in the problem list. He had a transurethral resection for benign prostatic hyperplasia. He had a real bad pars plana with secondary hip pain, and he kept going to people with back pain, and nobody ever stood him up and looked at his feet. He also had seborrheic dermatitis. The guy is an Irishman with pale skin and washed-out blue eyes, and he never used sunscreen. He had lots of skin cancers. The doctor kept calling him back to cut out the skin cancers but never told him to use sunscreen.

For this patient, the NP goes on to describe her approach to ordering diagnostic tests. Note that the hypotheses precede the test consideration. She describes her initial treatment plan:

OK, first thing you need is your laboratory parameters to check the problems that you have just defined. I would do blood counts, chemistries, thyroid function, glycohemoglobin, urines, prostate-specific antigen. The first time I see a patient, I always do the whole gamut. This guy also had had a bilateral total hip replacement, so I reviewed the subacute bacterial endocarditis prophylaxis because he had never been told about it. I started him on Prinivil, an angiotensin-converting enzyme inhibitor because he has diabetes and had previously been on Hytrin, but it was not doing the trick, and it was not protecting his kidneys. I started him on Glucotrol. He had not been on anything other than Micronase, which he quit using because he really did not know how to use the stuff. I also talked to him about his seborrhea and sunscreen.

The NP sees the wholeness of the patient's situation. This is a different approach than treating discrete problems as they come up. The NP's description of her approach to this patient continues:

He had had previous health care, and he thought he was doing fine. He just had never had it all put together. As far as he was concerned, he happened to have some elevated blood pressure and some elevated blood glucose, but nobody had ever put it all together in terms of the effects on the whole body. He went to someone for his glucose, and he went to somebody for his blood pressure. The guy was not a train wreck, but he had a number of problems that had been overlooked until he saw me and somebody (me) made a list. For example, he had not had a recent eye examination. For any patients with diabetes, I make sure they get an eye examination every single year. And that is how I started. His wife is also a patient of mine—a great cook, which is a tragedy for a diabetic—and he, like most husbands, will eat what he is given. So she needed some education as to what is the proper thing to eat and when and how they could cheat.

The NP is able to pull all of this patient's concerns and problems together in a way that honors his wholeness and his family dynamics. Her concern is for preventing future problems that are likely to develop, given his pattern of risk factors. Her method of collecting data and clustering it together to form a comprehensive picture of his life results in an effective, personal plan.

The differential diagnosis list should always include any conditions that are life, organ, or function threatening. An NP describing a different patient situation stated:

I always think in terms of the most dangerous or the most serious thing first—not necessarily the most catastrophic, but the most serious problem. If I know somebody has an abdominal aortic aneurysm (AAA) and he comes in with abdominal pain and it's sensitive, well, he probably has diverticulitis, but if I blow the diagnosis and go that way and it turns out that his aneurysm is dissecting, then he is dead. So I will treat his diverticulitis, but I will get the abdominal ultrasound right away. I consider the most urgent, deadly thing first. Cancer can be deadly, but it usually is not an emergency. It will kill you, but it is not going to kill you tomorrow. But an AAA can blow at any time. I had someone with an aneurysm blow in here once while I had the surgeon and the OR team waiting for him in the ER. We knew we had an aneurysm that was about to blow because I put my hand on his belly and it was throbbing and the patient was hypotensive and he was sweating. He had come in to the hospital because he was ready to go on vacation and just wanted to check this out before he left. So, you think of the most life-threatening situation first.

The following Nursing Situation illustrates how the diagnosis often involves more than medical problems.

Nursing Situation: An Advanced Practice Nurse's View of Nursing Versus Medical Problems

One pediatric NP described her interaction with an immigrant father who brought in a 3-year-old girl with a runny nose. The father was not disciplining the child, even though she was being difficult, because he had been reported to Human Services for hitting this child previously at 8 months of age.

I see myself making a dual diagnosis—a nursing diagnosis as well as a medical diagnosis. If the father does not discipline his child at the appropriate time in an appropriate way, that is a knowledge deficit. So I made a nursing decision there, and I intervened on the basis of that nursing decision, but I also made a medical decision, in that the child had an upper respiratory infection and I prescribed what I thought to be the appropriate medication for that. So, I see myself making nursing diagnoses as well as medical diagnoses and trying to somehow mesh these two to care for the family holistically because there is no way you can care for a child without caring for the family. That is my belief.

When asked if her full response was documented in the treatment plan, she responded:

Yeah, well, it sure does not fall under "upper respiratory infection." In this case, I did not know when the family was going to apply for insurance, so I certainly did not want to put "behavior disorder" down. Instead, I put down under my diagnosis, "knowledge deficit, re: discipline." In my treatment plan, I noted that I discussed discipline and that I gave the father "time out" guidelines and how to reward good behavior. I also noted that the father is coming back to me in 2 weeks to report differences in his approach to discipline and how it worked out. Nobody ever leaves my office without knowing when he or she needs to come back, and I document when I tell them to come back in my treatment plan.

Developing a Management Plan

Once the problem list has been clarified, the clinician needs to use his or her clinical judgment about how to best manage those problems. Although NPs bill for services in the medical realm, meaning selecting an ICD code for billing that designates a medical diagnosis and CPT code for treatment (see Chapter 80, The Business of Advanced Practice Nursing), they also operate in the nursing domain. NP students learn by "presenting the patient" to their preceptors. This skill involves presenting the data collected in history and physical assessment, organizing the content, along with major findings, in a coherent way to the preceptor and then reviewing treatment options. The preceptor then confirms and clarifies the data collection with the patient and proceeds to treatment planning. Initially, students may need to use a template to ensure that they are organized as they begin this process. With experience, the organization of patient data will become more obvious. This same skill of organizing patient data is useful when communicating with consulting providers. They need a clear summary of the case for efficient consultation.

NPs should consider a broad range of interventions for patients in addition to prescription medications. The discussion in Chapter 1 of Engebretson's (1997) *A Multiparadigm Approach to Nursing* is useful to consider here. In addition, Eisenhauer (1994) has argued that different levels of nursing interventions are useful when addressing patient problems. At the most basic level, interventions deal with symptom relief, such as ice for acute muscle pain, followed by heat application for strained muscles or a prescription for pain medication. At a higher level of complexity, interventions address functional patterns, such as stress and coping. The provider could schedule a follow-up visit to determine whether a stressful condition is being managed more successfully after a brief teaching or counseling session. At the next highest level, an intervention could be concerned with life patterns, such as recommending a course of rehabilitation to help a patient to regain confidence in exercising after a cardiac event. Finally, at the highest level, interventions such as spiritual support could be chosen to help patients and their families cope with life processes such as a terminal condition. This typology of intervention is useful to consider when selecting an approach to a problem. If, for example, a patient has been unable to lose weight using simple diet instruction, a higher-order intervention, such as counseling, may be required to address the source of the problem at a deeper level.

The Diagnostic Process in Action

A simple encounter for a self-limiting acute illness might proceed as follows:

A patient requests an appointment for a "sore throat." The patient is known by the NP as a resourceful, independent young adult. Before even entering the room, the clinician draws from experience with other patients who have complained of sore throat and begins to generate a list of hypotheses. Contextual factors enter into the reasoning: it may be allergy season in that particular area, or the clinician may have seen a large number of other patients with similar complaints who have tested positive for *Streptococcus* infection. The clinician enters the room and notes the general appearance of the patient. Is the patient ill-appearing, flushed, fatigued, or mildly irritated? These observations may serve to adjust the hypothesis list. The patient's story is elicited, beginning with HPI, along with a review of data already present in the record regarding past medical history and medications. Further questions regarding current life stresses and exposures may also serve to adjust the hypothesis list. The history narrows the hypothesis list to a short one, although experienced clinicians have ways of preventing the common diagnostic error of premature closure and work to consider alternative conditions that could also be represented by the same cluster of symptoms.

The physical examination serves to verify hypotheses and to screen out unlikely, though troubling, alternative diagnoses. The hypothesis list is narrowed further as data are weighed to see whether they fit the pattern of the highest-favored hypothesis; disconfirming data are also elicited to avoid leaping to conclusions too early. Finally, diagnostic tests may be chosen to firm up the diagnosis if the findings of the tests will have a bearing on how the patient's care is to be managed.

Once findings of relevant tests have been obtained, treatment decisions are considered, including patient factors such as resources, reliability, and the risk of the patient not following through on instructions. For example, insufficiently treated strep throat could result in rheumatic heart disease. Besides prescribing medication, the clinician should also consider comfort measures that are likely to assist the patient as well as judge the appropriateness of health promotion and educational opportunities at the moment. For example, is this a good time to give the patient smoking cessation materials? Finally, a plan to evaluate the treatment plan is made. Is a follow-up appointment necessary? Would a telephone call be useful? For which date should the next "well" visit be scheduled? The list of decisions made in this rather simple example is long. Given few data or situational changes,

the management of the patient's care could be quite different, and a new-patient visit requires even deeper background data collection. Patients who present with more complex, long-term problems require even more complex decision making by the clinician. In observing the experienced clinician, many of these mental processes may not be apparent. Many of these processes occur as a kind of internal dialogue, but they occur nonetheless.

CURRENT DIAGNOSTIC PROCESS TRENDS

Evidence-Based Practice

There is an emphasis in health care today to promote evidence-based practice (EBP). In a just society, patients have equal access to the most up-to-date treatment approaches and are also able to make informed choices about their treatment. To justify a treatment approach, proponents of EBP argue that there must be evidence, either from clinical trials or from case studies, that the approach is likely to benefit the patient. Obviously, it is easier to demonstrate the benefit of a certain drug that has been tested on a large number of individuals than it is to demonstrate the effectiveness of individual counseling. However, it is important for clinicians not to limit their practice to medicine based on clinical trials alone. This may require clinical research to demonstrate case studies of creative nursing intervention success. A research study that investigated how clinicians used guidelines in day-to-day practice showed that practitioners seldom referred directly to guidelines when planning care. They did, however, use internalized guidelines and could discuss what they were and how they were formed. Their own and colleagues' experience were also part of forming this knowledge in practice (Gabbay and LeMay, 2004). Guidelines for practice are available from government agencies or from specialty or disease-related groups such as the American Heart Association or the American Academy of Pediatrics. These guidelines can form the basis for protocol development and for peer evaluation.

Shared Decision Making

With the increased availability of health-care choices and treatment options, providers as well as families are faced with multiple treatments and care options, including choice of medications, laboratory tests, procedures, surgeries, home versus inpatient care, to name a few. In the past, these choices were driven primarily by provider preferences, affiliations, and insurance plans. As health-care providers strive to incorporate evidence into practice, providers must balance the choices with the needs and desires of the individual patient and family.

Shared decision making is a patient-centered care model that encourages the patient and family to be involved, fully informed, and engaged in all decisions related to their care with the premise that they can ask questions and express personal values and opinions related to their care. The process incudes the use of evidence-based decision aids providing patients and families with updated clinical information and decision tools based on current standards. Additionally, this process presumes the providers will respect the patient preferences, values, and opinions incorporating them into the recommendations and treatments (Agency for Health Care Quality and Research, 2015). This type of shared decision making has been linked to improved patient satisfaction, increased compliance, improved health outcomes, and reduced costs (Lee & Emanuel, 2013; Stacey et al., 2011). With NPs historically at the forefront of patient-centered care, they are in a pivotal position to promote shared decision making for all recipients of health care.

Outcome Considerations

In many instances, the patient's and provider's chosen outcomes for an encounter are clear. The simple, acute health problem is to be resolved. The screening measures recommended for the person's age-group are ordered to rule out the presence of nascent disease. When dealing with more chronic problems or problems that provide the patient with what may be reduced quality of life, the NP must be more sensitive to outcome determination.

DOCUMENTATION

Preparing concise, comprehensive, and meaningful documentation of one's thoughts and activities as a provider of primary care is a skill that takes time to develop. The purposes of documentation are to record the patient's report of symptoms, past medical history, lifestyle and family factors, positive and negative findings on physical examination, and the clinician's decisions and actions. An accurate record is essential to remind the clinician of findings and actions for the next follow-up visit. In a large practice, other providers will be seeing the patient and will need the benefit of the clinician's observations and actions during previous visits. The effectiveness of a treatment plan can be judged only if the plan has been adequately described. For example, if teaching about diet was provided at one visit but not recorded, the same teaching might be repeated at the next visit, to the frustration of the patient who was looking for more new information. This frustration might be misunderstood by the next provider as a lack of cooperation with the treatment plan. Finally, documentation can serve as protection for the provider or the practice in the rare case in which litigation is brought by the patient or family. In addition, third-party payers may be auditing the patient's record to determine whether the level of the visit that was billed was justified and whether the interventions billed were actually delivered. Additional details on billing and coding are provided in Chapter 80. In the student situation, the depth and comprehensiveness

of documentation can assist the preceptor or faculty in determining the student's progress in learning judgment.

SOAP Format

General principles for documentation are commonly applied using the SOAP (subjective, objective, assessment, and plan) format of charting. If other systems of charting are used, the principles still apply.

Subjective

The subjective portion of the record includes all data from the patient's report: the HPI, past medical history, family history, social history, functional health patterns data, and review of systems. The clinician can include here, in an easily visible way, current medications, immunization status, allergies to foods or medications, past hospitalizations (if appropriate), and, for women, the last menstrual period and menstrual cycle information. Even when a woman is being treated for simple problems, her pregnancy status must be known before certain medications are prescribed. It is an error to confuse physical findings noticed during the examination with subjective data from the patient. If the patient's particular way of describing a problem seems important, use the patient's exact words and include quotes. This is not necessary if the description is simple and without nuance.

It is helpful to develop an outline form for documentation that includes all essential data elements in a way that is retrievable. Writing in full sentences and paragraphs does not allow for easy retrieval of data by other providers. An outline template also serves as a memory tool for the new clinician. This template is useful in organizing patient presentation for the preceptor.

Objective

The objective section of the record includes all data obtained through objective means. This is not limited to numerical data. The objective portion of the record should begin with a brief description of the overall impression of the patient. Such phrases as "tired looking," "energetic," or "worried" can convey much of the patient impression that is useful in diagnostic reasoning. Vital signs and pertinent findings from the physical examination, as well as laboratory data, should also be included. Diagnostic judgments should not be included in this section; this part of the record should consist of "just the facts."

At first, students may not be able to focus on which pieces of data are significant to a problem and tend to include every piece of data available. All data need not be recorded, but "pertinent negatives" need to be recorded. These include data that by being normal tend to rule out a possible diagnosis. Recording pertinent negatives helps to show that a diagnosis was considered and why it was ruled out. It does not take long, however, for both the subjective and objective sections to be recorded with reasonable skill, even for advanced beginner students. When following patients over time, flow sheets can be useful for tracking data. For example, a flow sheet can show the effect of a change in medication management of hyperlipidemia or blood pressure or track a patient's weight over months or years.

Assessment

The assessment portion is an area of documentation in which much variability can be found. The assessment must include active problems that are being managed during the current visit. It can also include chronic problems that may have an impact on the treatment plan. Often, practices include a health-promotion line on the problem list to remind each clinician that the visit should reflect the preventive focus of that practice. For the list to serve both patient and practitioner well, a simple diagnostic label may not be enough. For example, if the patient has hypertension that is being managed by lifestyle change and medication, the effectiveness of control of the problem can be recorded in the assessment section. Assessment is ongoing in the management of health problems. For example, a patient's problem list might read as follows: (1) hypertension (HTN) stage 1, well controlled; (2) type 2 DM, poorly controlled; (3) obesity, unchanged. This documentation directs evaluation and intervention adjustment much more clearly than a simple list of "HTN, DM, obesity." It is helpful for practices to maintain an active problem list near the front of the patient record or in a part of the electronic record; this is particularly useful when dealing with chronic conditions and is recommended. The clinician can initiate such a tool in any practice, even if a blank progress note sheet is filed at the beginning of that section of the patient's record.

When reviewing the assessment part of the record, students can evaluate their own thinking by asking themselves if all data that were used to justify the naming of a problem are included in the subjective and objective section of the note. Further, one can ask whether all data were accounted for in the assessment section. In some cases, a clear problem cannot be identified. Abdominal pain that does not fit a clear diagnostic pattern can be reported in the problem list by simply naming the complaint. The clinician can reflect diagnostic hypotheses by writing "abdominal pain, rule out (R/O) irritable bowel syndrome." Or "cough, viral bronchitis versus allergy." Students are often reluctant to admit that they cannot name the problem. It is a mistake, however, to name a problem in error, simply to have a problem on the list. The patient will not be well served if the record fails to reveal competing diagnostic hypotheses. In primary care, uncertainty is reasonable and expected. Even if the problem is not completely specified, the problem list is the basis for the intervention schedule in the treatment plan.

Plan

The plan for treatment is most effective if it is described in detail, including specific directions for each intervention.

Three general sections are included in planning. First, any diagnostic testing that is to be conducted should be listed. The results of these diagnostic tests will help to clarify the assessment but, of course, are not yet available to the provider. Second, educational approaches are to be laid out. Every visit is a teaching opportunity. Patient education might include specifics of the problems being managed, such as symptom control for upper respiratory infections, medication teaching, diet and activity recommendations, and risk reduction, such as smoking cessation information or a discussion of seat-belt usage. The documentation of the plan includes details regarding any therapeutic plan that is to be carried out—including prescriptions, various therapies, counseling, activity promotion or restriction, dietary changes, or any of the therapeutics discussed earlier. When recording prescriptions, be sure to include all the data that were written on the prescription list, including number or volume of doses to be dispensed and number of refills allowed. This is important because patients may call for refills before they are due, and if a different provider takes the call, he or she may have an unclear idea of how the patient's condition had been managed. This is especially important when prescribing drugs that are prone to abuse.

Finally, the treatment plan is not complete without clear plans for follow up. When will the patient be seen again, and under what circumstances is the patient instructed to call back? For example, when treating a viral infection, remind the patient to call back if not better in 2 days or if a fever develops. By documenting your instructions for follow up, you allow other providers to manage the patient's care better if the patient calls when you are not available.

Plans are most effective when they include a sense of the goal of treatment. If the condition is simple and self-limiting, the goal of treatment may be obvious and need not be stated. For chronic or complex problems, however, the short- and long-term goals of therapy need to be discussed and recorded. By engaging the patient in this discussion, the choices that the patient makes in altering lifestyle and following a treatment plan may be clearer. For example, the patient with hypertension, diabetes, and obesity might have as a goal to lose 4 pounds in a month. The planned intervention to help the patient achieve this goal might be walking three times a week and one less restaurant meal a week. The feedback on the short-term goal at the next visit can help to keep the patient motivated to sustain lifelong change.

Finally, when reviewing the documentation for personal or peer evaluation, the clinician must consider whether the note conveys the scope and tone of the visit. Does it reflect the type of visit that occurred? If the patient were to ask to see the record, would the information be clear? The NP should write the note in such a way that the patient could agree with what has been stated. Discussions of sensitive issues such as family problems can be left in general terms. This is a useful approach when one considers that others, such as third-party payers or lawyers, might have access to the record in the future. If the provider and the patient disagree on a treatment plan—for example, on the use of medications—the record can reflect the disagreement in nonjudgmental terms, such as "Patient requested prescription for muscle relaxants, which was discussed as being unlikely to benefit the shoulder pain described." This kind of note can assist in determining patterns of behavior or documenting difficulties over time.

Documentation is an opportunity for clinicians at all levels to review the level of their thought. In general, NPs document visits more completely and less often have charts refused for payment by third-party payers than other clinicians do. It is best to develop a system for maintaining current, accurate records. Saving up quick scratches of notes and writing all formal patient notes at the end of a busy day is not the recommended approach. Dictation and computer systems allow for complete record-keeping and help to keep time spent on the task more manageable.

Documentation Systems

Documentation systems are usually "invented" by each practice. This gives NPs in practice the opportunity to rectify problems in the records that they use, such as omissions due to restrictive coding or limited space. Most systems in which NPs work are dominated by the medical model. NPs can ensure that contributions from a nursing perspective are not invisible by claiming credit and billing for the care actually provided. They should not agree to a system of billing "incident to" the physician, except where truly warranted. Unless NPs "own" their practice through their own, independent billing for services, nursing-based care is lost and outcomes related to NP practice are not captured. NPs educated at the Doctor of Nursing Practice (DNP) level should have the opportunity to shape the practice environment that they manage or share with other providers (Flanagan et al., 2009). This includes active participation of the DNP in the implementation of electronic health record (EHR) systems in the practice setting to assure the advanced practice nursing components are integrated into the EHR.

REDUCTION OF MEDICAL ERRORS

The reduction of medical errors and the support of patient safety are important in the health-care arena. The Institute of Medicine has called for attention to the processes and systems of care in order to reduce error and enhance safety (Kohn et al., 2000). A study of reported medical errors in primary care showed that most errors were considered administrative, such as information filed in the wrong place or at the wrong time, charts not being available at the time of the visit, and lack of documentation. Errors also occurred in obtaining or processing a laboratory specimen. Some errors were reportedly due to lack of clinical knowledge or skills, such as a wrong or missed diagnosis or wrong treatment choices (Dovey et al., 2005). Attention to decision making and follow-through is important to all primary-care providers. NPs can contribute to shaping the practice in their setting by, for example, developing systems to ensure that important laboratory results are addressed in a timely manner. All of these efforts are part of quality-oriented guidelines developed for the patient-centered medical homes (PCMHs) discussed in Chapter 1. These are the health-care systems of the future, and they are still emerging. NPs have an opportunity and an obligation to participate in and influence that emergence with their own unique knowledge base, to translate their knowledge into systems that support patient engagement.

THE DIGITAL FUTURE

The Affordable Care Act now requires all health-care providers to adopt EHRs and demonstrate "meaningful use" of clinical data. Providers must meet specific objectives in their charting, which include lists of patient drugs, computerized order entry, maintaining an active allergy list and an active problem list, and implementing decision support systems. NPs, along with physicians, are eligible for incentive payments if a certain percentage of their patient load is in the Medicare or Medicaid system and if objectives are met.

The use of electronic media in all facets of health care is a reality. Patients now have access to information about health promotion and about specific health-care concerns from the Internet; they can also communicate with health-care providers through e-mail, telehealth visits, and/or sensors to transfer physiologic data, and in some cases, continually. It is all about connectivity. General and individualized health information is now available to both consumers and providers of health care in "real time" through smartphones and tablets. Health records are maintained electronically and made accessible to providers and patients throughout a care delivery system. The U.S. Veterans Administration (VA) has been a leader in the use of technology and have been early adopters of electronic medical records. The VA Blue Button Program now provides veterans with access to their personal health records that allows them to manage all their health information in a single electronic health file. In addition, some practices send a weekly e-mail to their patients with health-related information. This has multiple benefits including education regarding preventive services and health practices, personalized messaging, and reminders, and as a marketing tool providing health information while promoting health services available in the community. The EHRs of the future have the potential to move beyond being a medical record in one setting to being the patient health record across practices managed by the patient, a self-managed patient navigation system for scheduling and coordinating care, and a source of health information for both preventive and disease management tailored to the individual patient.

Telehealth, sometimes referred to as telemedicine, has the capacity to open access to health care for people at remote sites. Telehealth is increasingly used to provide care to vulnerable populations residing in rural, remote, and medically underserved communities. According to a recent study by Harvard Medical School and the RAND Corporation, between 2004 and 2014, the number of telehealth visits for mental health services grew 45.1% annually (Mehrotra et al., 2016). The VA operates one of the country's largest telehealth programs, with some 700,000 veterans receiving medical care and advice via their computers and mobile devices in 2016. In August 2017, the VA announced a major expansion of this program with the launch of a tool called VA Video Connect, which will be available to every VA hospital across the country. VA Video Connect links veteran's access to doctors from more than 50 specialties, from dermatology to dentistry, with a special focus on mental health services, particularly in rural areas where such services are not readily accessible in-person.

Laws and policies are currently inconsistent from state to state and across health plans regarding telemedicine. Health insurance companies now reimburse practices for telehealth services. As of 2016, 48 states have enacted laws providing limited Medicaid coverage, whereas 32 states now have a private-payer reimbursement policy (National Conference of State Legislatures, 2016). Soon, lack of access to a computer may not be a barrier to participating in telemedicine as technology evolves and consumers of health care seek connectivity to providers. Business leaders predict that the next phase of medical innovation will incorporate smartphones and a variety of mobile apps to monitor patients' health and transmit the data to health-care providers on a regular basis or in advance of an office visit (Topol, 2012). It is only a matter of time until "body scanners" will be used to transmit a wide variety of physiological data to a distant location where a team of health-care providers is located. Just as in the debate over online education, some speculate that telemedicine can never achieve the same benefits as "hands-on" medical care; others feel that with adept use of technology, in some instances, clinician–patient communication may be enhanced. A recent study with parents of children with special health care needs comparing telehealth to traditional face-to-face care indicated no differences in parent perceptions of providers as caring. In addition, families receiving specialty care via telemedicine reported the system of care as significantly more family centered (Hooshmand, 2010). Although more research is indicated regarding the human connection as we introduce new technologies, this debate will dominate future conversation about the value of "human touch" and the benefits of the remote practice of

the NP. Systems of care and providers need to ensure that caring, family-centered care, and the human connection are addressed as they integrate new technologies into practice settings (Hooshmand & Yao, 2017).

Personalized, predictive, and precision are all similar terms that address health care, which considers individual genetic variations, lifestyle, and environmental factors in the treatment and prevention of disease (U.S. National Library of Medicine, 2016). The completion of the Human Genome Project, advances in molecular biology, particularly related to "omic" science (genome, epigenome, metabolome, proteome, transcriptome, etc.), considerable advances in biotechnology, and improved ability to address analyses of large data sets are driving the perfect storm that has the propensity to transform health care (National Institute of Health, 2016; Chen & Snyder, 2013). These advances in genomics and technology have given rise to the exciting field of precision medicine. This term is not to be confused with personalized medicine, inferring treatments prescribed uniquely for each individual person. Precision medicine refers to a prevention and treatment approach targeted currently to groups of individuals based on genes, environment, and lifestyle. For example, various forms of cancers, such as breast cancer, may be treated differently based on a person's genetics using specific targeted medications. Consumers and providers alike are seeking patient-specific solutions to address health-care concerns. As precision medicine advances, the goal would be to advance to targeted treatments specifically for the individual patient, truly personalized medicine at the individual level. NPs in primary-care settings can anticipate rapid growth of precision medicine and increased consumer knowledge. It is anticipated that precision medicine will open the door for more targeted and effective treatment plans for multiple disease conditions to further improve patient outcomes. DNPs will be challenged to translate this evidence as it evolves into practice solutions and ultimately individual patient treatment plans.

Caring stands as a cornerstone of nursing practice, and over the last 40 years a substantial body of work has emerged in nursing supporting the science of caring both from a research and practice perspective (Smith, 2013). According to Watson and Smith (2002), caring in nursing is relational, steeped in deep moral and ethical foundations, and examined through deliberation and expressed through moral actions. Nursing theories on caring are well suited to addressing precision health concerns and challenges as we come to know the wholeness of a person in the moment.

Health care approached from a personalized health perspective creates a different paradigm of care that calls for a more holistic approach that will require person engagement to be successful (Mirnezami et al., 2012). However, it is often easier to push an agenda forward than it is to reflect on the wholeness of the person behind the science. The very nature of precision health itself is person centered. Persons are interested in precision health and want to know more about their health in this way. Nursing has a unique view and the very act of nursing engagement in precision health is creating a caring environment. The successful navigation of precision health challenges through the lens of caring offers an opportunity to illuminate persons and create an enduring spirit of what matters most. Perhaps the call is for "precision caring" in the midst of precision health.

ETHICS

Every clinical judgment is an ethical judgment. Clinical judgment begins with respect for persons and supports each individual's autonomy. Some decisions call for balancing such principles as beneficence against autonomy; for example, as when a patient chooses not to follow a treatment plan. Truth telling by the clinician can do much to establish trust and to develop a plan the patient can accept. Ethical judgments are involved as well in the allocation of scarce resources, the most prominent for NPs being their own time. If one patient constantly requires more time than is allotted, other patients are made to wait or are given less time for their visits. Being a patient advocate means ascertaining that the health-care system provides for each patient everything that is reasonable to which the patient is entitled; such advocacy is a role of the NP. A survey of NPs in one mid-Atlantic state showed that 61% agreed that they sometimes weighed the needs of the patient against the interests of the managed care organization (Ulrich et al., 2003). Fidelity to the patient until the problem has been solved or resolved is another aspect of NP practice that is based on ethical principles. One could make the case that NPs have an ethical and professional responsibility to help design and implement systems to collaborate in the establishment of PCMHs that truly reflect the intent of that model that "hear" the voice of the patient.

Additionally, as technology advances, the NP is in a prime position to assure that ethical considerations are integrated into the decision-making, planning, and integration phases assuring balance between technology and the four pillars of bioethics: (1) respect for autonomy (informed and voluntary decisions), (2) nonmaleficence (do no harm), (3) beneficence (benefits), and (4) justice (fairness) (Beuchamp & Childress, 2013).

The privilege of being an NP and entering as a partner into patients' lives to support their health and wholeness requires true human presence, clear clinical judgment, and a commitment to do one's best. The *Circle of Caring* includes patient and nurse together as they enter a relationship that has the potential to enhance the humanity of both.

REFERENCES

Agency for Healthcare Research and Quality. Shared decision-making. https://www.ahrq.gov/cahps/quality-improvement/improvement-guide/6-strategies-for-improving/communication/strategy6i-shared-decisionmaking.htm. Accessed June 2017.

Beauchamp TL, Childress JF. *Principles of biomedical ethics.* 7th ed. New York, NY: Oxford University Press; 2013.

Benner P. *From novice to expert: Excellence and power in clinical nursing practice.* Menlo Park, CA: Addison-Wesley; 1984.

Benner PE, Tanner C, Chesla C. *Expertise in nursing practice: Caring clinical judgment and ethics.* New York, NY: Springer; 1996.

Billings JA, Stoeckle JD. *The clinical encounter: A guide to the medical interview and case presentation.* 2nd ed. St. Louis: Mosby; 1999.

Charlton CR, et al. Nurse practitioners' communication styles and their impact on patient outcomes: An integrated literature review. *J Am Acad Nurs Pract.* 2008;20:382–388.

Chase SK. *Clinical judgment and communication in nurse practitioner practice.* Philadelphia, PA: F.A. Davis; 2004.

Chen R, Snyder M. Promise of personalized omics to precision medicine. *Wiley Interdiscip Rev Syst Biol Med* 2013;5(1):73-82.

Dovey SM, et al. A preliminary taxonomy of medical errors in family practice. *Qual Safe Health Care.* 2005;11:233.

Eisenhauer LA. A typology of nursing therapeutics. *Image J Nurs Sch.* 1994;26:261.

Elliott N. "Mutual intacting": A grounded theory study of clinical judgment practice issues. *J Adv Nurs.* 2010;66:2711–2721.

Elstein A, et al. *Medical problem solving.* Cambridge, MA: Harvard University Press; 1979.

Engebretson J. A multiparadigm approach to nursing. *Adv Nurs Sci.* 1997;20:21.

Flanagan ME, et al. The effect of provider- and workflow-focused strategies for guideline implementation on provider acceptance. *Implement Sci.* 2009;4:71.

Gabbay J, LeMay A. Evidence based guidelines or collectively constructed "mindlines?" Ethnographic study of knowledge management in primary care. *Br Med J.* 2004;329(7473):1013.

Genetics Home Reference, U.S. National Library of Medicine, National Institute of Health. What is the difference between precision medicine and personalized medicine? What about pharmacogenomics? https://ghr.nlm.nih.gov/primer/precisionmedicine/precisionvspersonalized. Published 2016.

Gordon M, et al. Clinical judgment: An integrated model. *Adv Nurs Sci.* 1994;16(4):55.

Guadagnoli E, Ward P. Patient participation in decision-making. *Soc Sci Med.* 1998;47(3):329–39.

Hooshmand M. Comparison of telemedicine to traditional face-to-face care for children with special needs: An analysis of cost, caring, and family-centered care. [PhD dissertation]. University of Miami; 2010.

Hooshmand M, Yao K. Challenges facing children with special health-care needs and their families: Telemedicine as a bridge to care. *Telemed J E Health* 2017;23(1):18–24.

Johnson R. Nurse practitioner–patient discourse: Uncovering the voice of nursing in primary care practice. *Sch Inq Nurs Pract.* 1993;7:143.

Kohn LT, et al., eds. *To err is human: Building a safer health system.* Washington, DC: National Academy Press; 2000.

Lee EO, Emanuel EJ. Shared decision making to improve care and reduce costs. *N Engl J Med.* 2013;368:6–8.

Lee NJ, et al. The effect of a mobile clinical decision support system on the diagnosis of obesity and overweight in acute and primary care encounters. *Adv Nurs Sci.* 2009;32:211–221.

Lewis PH, Brykczynski KA. Practical knowledge and competencies of the healing role of the nurse practitioner. *J Am Acad Nurse Pract.* 1994;6:207.

Mehrotra A, Huskamp HA, Souza J, Uscher-Pines L, Rose S, Landon BE, Jena AB, Busch AB. Rapid growth in mental health telemedicine use among rural medicare beneficiaries, wide variation across states. *Health Aff (Millwood)* 1. 2017;36(5):909–917.

Michaels C, et al. Saying "no" to professional recommendations: Client values, beliefs, and evidence-based practice. *J Am Acad Nurse Pract.* 2008;20:585–589.

Mirnezami R, Nicholson J, Darzi A. Preparing for precision medicine. *N Engl J Med* 2012;366(6):489–491.

National Conference of State Legislatures. State coverage for telehealth services [Internet]. http://www.ncsl.org/research/health/state-coverage-for-telehealth-services.aspx. Published 2016 [cited 2017].

National Institute of Health. Precision medicine initiative. https://www.nih.gov/precision-medicine-initiative-cohort-program. Published 2016.

North American Nursing Diagnosis Association. *NANDA nursing diagnoses: Definitions and classification, 1997–1998.* Philadelphia, PA: NANDA; 1996.

Radwin LE. Research on diagnostic reasoning in nursing. *Nurs Diag.* 1990;1(2):70.

Reed K. Telemedicine: Benefits to advanced practice nursing and the communities they serve. *J Am Acad Nurse Pract.* 2005;17:176.

Roblin DW, et al. Patient satisfaction with primary care: Does type of practitioner matter? *Med Care.* 2004;42:579.

Rubin RH. *Primary care.* Philadelphia, PA: WB Saunders; 1995.

Sanders L. *Every patient tells a story.* New York, NY: Broadway Books; 2009.

Sangster-Gormley E, Frisch N. Articulating new outcomes of nurse practitioner practice. *J Am Acad Nurs Pract.* 2013;25:653–658.

Smith M. Caring and the discipline of nursing. In: Smith M, Turkel M, Wolf Z, eds. *Caring classics in nursing.* New York, NY: Springer Publishing Company; 2013:309–320.

SmithBattle L. Pregnant with possibilities: Drawing on hermeneutic thought to reframe home-visiting programs for young mothers. *Nurs Inq.* 2009;16:191–200.

Stacey D, Bennett CL, Barry MJ. Decision aids for people facing health treatment or screening decisions. *Cochrane Database Syst Rev.* 2011;10:CD001431.

Thompson C, Yang H. Nurses' decisions, irreducible uncertainty and maximizing nurses' contribution to patient safety. *Healthc Q.* 2009;12(Spec No Patient):e178–e185.

Topol E. *The creative destruction of medicine: How the digital revolution will create better health care.* New York, NY: Basic Books; 2012.

Ulrich CM, et al. Ethical conflict associated with managed care: Views of nurse practitioners. *Nurs Res.* 2003;52:168.

Watson J, Smith MC. Caring science and the science of unitary human beings: A trans_theoretical discourse for nursing knowledge development. *J Adv Nurs,* 2002;37(5):452–461.

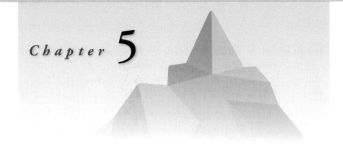

Chapter 5

Evidence-Based Practice

Ilene Decker, PhD, RN

Dorothy J. Dunn, PhD, APRN, FNP-BC, AHN-BC

Sally Doshier, EdD, MS, RN

Debera J. Thomas, DNS, RN, FNP/ANP

In health care, research findings are used to generate evidence to guide clinical practice, such as decisions regarding which diagnostic tests or treatment approaches are effective. This decision-making process is commonly known as evidence-based practice (EBP). EBP refers to using findings from the systematic review and appraisal of the most reliable studies to provide the best evidence for making decisions about health care in combination with the practitioner's clinical expertise and practice-based knowledge, as well as the patient's preferences. Therefore, the purpose of EBP is to incorporate evidence into practice using a systematic approach that integrates the review and appraisal of best evidence, the practitioner's clinical expertise, and patient or population values, concerns, and socioeconomic factors to guide care delivery (Melnyk & Fineout-Overhold, 2015; Sackett et al., 1996). The key steps involved in implementing EBP are summarized in Box 5.1. Understanding the process of EBP allows practitioners to compose succinct clinical questions to find the best evidence to improve patient outcomes.

Box 5.1 Key Steps in Implementing Evidence-Based Practice

1. Ask the burning clinical question.
2. Collect the most relevant and best evidence from a review of the literature, including published literature reviews, meta-analyses, and clinical practice guidelines.
3. Critically evaluate the evidence.
4. Integrate the best evidence with personal clinical expertise, patient preferences and values, and when making a practice decision or change.
5. Evaluate the change in outcomes after implementing into practice.
6. Disseminate findings.

Source: Melnyk BM, Fineout-Overholt E. *Evidence-based practice in nursing & healthcare: A guide to best practice.* 3rd ed. Philadelphia, PA: Wolters Kluwer; 2015.

EBP is an interdisciplinary approach that began in medicine as evidence-based medicine and spread to other disciplines, such as nursing, social work, and psychology. This chapter focuses on the predominant methods used to establish evidence for practice across disciplines.

THE AIMS OF NURSING RESEARCH FOR CLINICAL APPLICATION

Although there are differences in perspectives among health disciplines, the research conducted in each field has a common thread: the systematic pursuit of knowledge to answer important questions relevant to each profession, to translate research findings into practice, and to promote the use of research findings by healthcare providers at all levels of practice to improve patient outcomes. Nursing research uses the scientific process to generate new understandings and to validate existing knowledge about persons, the environment, health, and nursing practice. In particular, nursing research focuses on human responses to health and illness situations. Therefore, the goal of nursing research is to conduct studies to develop a body of nursing knowledge. EBP, on the other hand, involves gathering information from the published literature to make decisions about its application to clinical practice. Both approaches begin with a question. The difference is that in nursing research, the question is tested using an appropriate research methodology. In EBP, the question is used to search the literature for already completed studies that you can critically appraise to answer your clinical question.

Findings from research studies provide evidence for practice. Evidence does not fall into simple categories such as "evidence based" or "not evidence based." Conclusions from research studies are limited by study design and methods. This probabilistic nature of research studies has led to the classification of evidence along a continuum to describe the strength of the results measured in a study. Sackett (1989) first described five hierarchical levels of evidence with randomized controlled trials (RCTs) at the highest level, which can generate strong recommendations, and case series or expert opinions at the lowest level, which can yield weak recommendations. Over the past two decades, there have been several variations of the classification system by professional organizations and journals (Burns et al., 2011).

Clinicians are encouraged to use the highest level of evidence to inform their practice. However, many of the questions that arise in nursing practice are not easily answered using only one type of evidence or the highest level of evidence such as highly controlled, experimental methods. Important questions to be asked when using research for EBP are "What findings constitute evidence?" and "How will the findings be used?" This approach assumes that it is better to use the type of evidence that best answers the clinical question rather than applying the same level of evidence to all questions. If the clinical situation requires a better understanding of what the experience of emergent cardiac catheterization is for postmenopausal women with acute myocardial ischemia, providers need to look for the form of evidence (or findings) that best suits the situation. This evidence will not be found in the results of RCTs; it will be found in studies specifically designed for understanding human experiences of health in a personal and meaningful way (such as phenomenological studies or those using grounded theory). Critical appraisal of evidence and knowledge to improve health care can be found by using not only systematic reviews and meta-analyses but also qualitative research that connects evidence to elements of patient preferences and values (Stevens, 2015).

A BRIEF HISTORY OF EVIDENCE-BASED PRACTICE

The origins of EBP have been traced back to Archie Cochrane, a Scottish epidemiologist, who published the *Effectiveness and Efficiency: Random Reflections on Health Services* in 1972. Cochrane encouraged the medical profession to establish a collection of RCTs based on quality appraisal criteria to validate the rigor of the published research. He further advocated for RCTs in a key note address to the Royal College of Physicians Symposium held in London in September 1978 by the Office of Health Economics in which he stated, "It is surely a great criticism of our profession that we have not organised a critical summary by speciality or sub-speciality, updated periodically, of all relevant RCTs" (Teeling Smith & Wells, 1978, p 9). The first group to heed his call was the National Perinatal Epidemiology Unit (NPEU) established in 1978 at Oxford University. The NPEU was a leader in conducting RCTs to assess the effects of perinatal health services, as well as in the retrieval of information and the development and use of systematic reviews and meta-analyses to synthesize research results. This work laid the foundation for the development of the Cochrane Collaboration, inaugurated in October 1993. Hence, the term "evidence-based medicine" was coined and appeared in the literature in the early 1990s. The Cochrane Library was launched in 1996 (Starr & Chalmers, 2003).

EBP was first conceptualized by nursing as research utilization (RU). RU dates to Florence Nightingale, who used data to improve sanitary conditions during her work in military hospitals during the Crimean War. The term "research utilization" first appeared in the literature in the 1970s, and in 1976, Stetler and Marram developed an RU model (currently known as the Stetler Model) as a method to address the need to use nursing research findings in practice. The Stetler Model

"formulated a series of critical-thinking and decision-making steps designed to facilitate safe and effective use of research findings" (Stetler, 2001, p 273). The model also contained criteria for critically appraising research from single studies and determining the feasibility of using research findings in practice. Feasibility, as defined in the model, "involves ... assessment of the degree of risk, as compared to the expected benefit of research-based change and ... determination of the availability of needed resources and, if applicable, the cooperation, support, or readiness of stakeholders" (p 273).

RU has evolved into the broader concept of EBP. Although RU and EBP have commonalities, EBP is patient centered and takes into consideration the experiential knowledge and preferences of the provider and patient in a way that RU does not. Some authors argue that "research utilization can tend to focus on the implementation of exceptionally reliable research studies before determining their merit or value in a clinical practice area" and ... "the importance of patient preferences, and values have the potential to become lost to what is believed to be the best evidence" (Mackey & Bassendowsky, 2016, p 53).

DEVELOPMENT OF BEST PRACTICE GUIDELINES

In the past, clinical practice was guided by the premise that "common" practice is "correct" practice, despite the scientific evidence available either to support or refute the outcomes of such practice. Under this premise, "common practice" is sufficient evidence that the practice is appropriate. This approach may have been useful in the past, when practice decisions were less complicated and fewer diagnostic tests or interventions were available. Today, with the complexities involved in clinical decision making, research-based evidence is required. Although elements of the traditional approach remain, the majority of guidelines are now developed from available scientific evidence. One method to enhance patient outcomes is the use of EBP clinical practice guidelines.

The Agency for Health Care Policy and Research was instrumental in leading the way toward EBP, improving outcomes, and publishing national guidelines on a variety of health-care problems, such as smoking cessation, early detection and treatment of Alzheimer's disease, and caring for HIV-infected patients. The Healthcare Research and Quality Act of 1999 reauthorized this agency and renamed it the Agency for Healthcare Research and Quality (AHRQ). The mission of the AHRQ is to improve the quality, safety, efficiency, and effectiveness of health care for all Americans.

AHRQ clinical practice guidelines are used not only as references for health-care providers but also as the framework for insurance utilization review, quality assurance, and reimbursement. In addition, adherence or nonadherence to established guidelines (such as those published by the AHRQ) has played an increasing role in influencing medical malpractice litigation outcomes.

The implementation of AHRQ guidelines in clinical practice has not been without significant challenges. Originally, the AHRQ believed that providers would modify their practices to improve care if they were provided with clinically credible and useful information and that practitioner involvement in developing the guidelines would facilitate the use of guidelines in practice. Neither of these assumptions proved accurate: studies indicated wide variation between a practitioner's knowledge of the recommended management of a particular health problem based on the guidelines and the practitioner's actions. Additional research has identified several barriers to implementing guidelines in practice, and the AHRQ's role in supporting EBP has been redefined to include keeping relevant information in the public domain, serving as an impartial, neutral broker of the information; encouraging multidisciplinary input in all projects; advocating for patients' perspectives and needs; and protecting special populations.

Structurally, the AHRQ's role includes promoting initiatives focused on developing effective methods for implementing guidelines and analyzing the outcomes of care when clinical guidelines are widely disseminated and used. There are three parts to this initiative: (1) institution of EBP centers (EPCs), (2) development of the online National Guideline Clearinghouse (NGC), and (3) product research and evaluation.

EPCs constitute the first part of the AHRQ initiative. EPCs involve a private–public partnership between the AHRQ and a variety of health-care organizations to produce evidence reports and technology assessments on several priority health-care topics. Topics for EPC assessments are nominated by providers or others in the health-care industry and are chosen on the basis of the selection criteria provided in Box 5.2. Final evidence reports are intended for use in practice guidelines, quality improvement programs, and the formation of policy at the state or federal level.

The second part of the AHRQ's initiative is the development of the online NGC. The creation of the clearinghouse is a result of a private–public partnership among AHRQ, the American Association of Health Plans, and the American Medical Association. This electronic repository for clinical practice guidelines provides widespread access to a number of guidelines from various professional groups. Box 5.3 lists examples of organizations that have supported or published EBP guidelines. Guidelines published in the NGC are required to meet established AHRQ criteria and can be accessed through the Internet. Consistent reference to these guidelines has been used throughout this text.

A final aspect of the AHRQ's initiative involves product research and evaluation. This includes an array of research and evaluation activities aimed at the development of evidence for use in guidelines, implementation strategies, and the quality of practice when clinical practice guidelines are used (e.g., outcome-based research). These initiatives reflect the new role the AHRQ has with respect to supporting EBP and are intended to improve the scientific basis of guidelines, decrease duplication of efforts, distribute evidence on a national level, enhance uniformity, and reinforce public and private partnerships within the health-care sector.

Box 5.2   Criteria for Inclusion of Clinical Practice Guidelines in National Guideline Clearinghouse (NGC)

A clinical practice guideline must meet all of the following criteria to be included in the NGC:

1. The clinical practice guideline contains systematically developed statements that include recommendations, strategies, or information that assists physicians and/or other health-care practitioners and patients make decisions about appropriate health care for specific clinical circumstances.

2. The clinical practice guideline was produced under the auspices of medical specialty associations; relevant professional societies, public or private organizations, government agencies at the federal, state, or local level; or health-care organizations or plans. A clinical practice guideline developed and issued by an individual not officially sponsored or supported by one of the above types of organizations does not meet the inclusion criteria for NGC.

3. Corroborating documentation can be produced and verified that a systematic literature search and review of existing scientific evidence published in peer-reviewed journals was performed during the guideline development. A guideline is not excluded from NGC if corroborating documentation can be produced and verified detailing specific gaps in scientific evidence for some of the guideline's recommendations.

4. The full-text guideline is available on request in print or electronic format (for free or for a fee) in the English language. The guideline is current and the most recent version produced. Documented evidence can be produced or verified that the guideline was developed, reviewed, or revised within the last 5 years.

Source: Agency for Healthcare Research and Quality, 2017.

Box 5.3   Examples of Clinical Practice Guidelines and Evidence-Based Guidelines Developed/ Published by Organizations and Agencies

Alzheimer's Association
    Guideline for Alzheimer's disease management
    www.alz.org
American Academy of Allergy, Asthma and Immunology
    Allergen immunotherapy: a practice parameter second update
    www.aaaai.org
American College of Physicians
    Guidelines follow a rigorous development process and are based on the highest-quality scientific evidence
    www.acponline.org/clinical_information/guidelines
Faculty of Sexual and Reproductive Healthcare
    Contraception for women aged over 40 years
    www.fsrh.org
Society for Acupuncture Research
    Acupuncture evidence-based treatment guidelines
    www.acupunctureresearch.org

Global Initiative for Asthma
    Global strategy for asthma management and prevention
    http://ginasthma.org
National Association of Pediatric Nurse Practitioners
    Identifying and preventing overweight in childhood (clinical practice guideline)
    www.napnap.org
National Health Care for the Homeless Council, Inc.
    Adapting your practice: general recommendations for the care of homeless patients.
    www.nhchc.org
World Health Organization (WHO)
    WHO recommendations for the prevention of postpartum hemorrhage
    www.who.int/reproductivehealth/publications/maternal_perinatal_health/9789241548502/en

---

APPLYING CLINICAL PRACTICE GUIDELINES TO CLINICAL PRACTICE

Wide variation in practice patterns within and across provider type, specialty practice, and geographic region has been a major impetus for establishing both federal and organization-specific guidelines. This realization has led to efforts to form a broad consensus about how to diagnose and treat a number of common health conditions at national and local levels in the form of clinical practice guidelines, practice policies, and recommendations. Although some providers perceive these attempts to standardize aspects of clinical practice as stripping them of their decision making, the intent is to improve the provider's ability to make informed decisions that lead to better, more reliable outcomes for patients.

Practice Standards and Guidelines

The terms "clinical practice standards" and "practice guidelines" are often used interchangeably. However, they tend to originate from distinct processes, and the purpose of each is somewhat different. Standards relate to a framework for practice. Guidelines focus more on individual patient-care decisions. Academic researchers, professional practice organizations, private entities, and other groups may develop both practice standards and guidelines.

Practice standards are intended to be used under all circumstances and define correct overall practice. They are generally considered to be inflexible and should not be interpreted as adaptable to fit different contexts. The American Nurses Association (ANA) has issued practice standards for nurses, which includes broad requirements for nursing practice in any setting and at any level of practice. Practice standards are designed to provide direction to nurses on which to guide and evaluate their practice (ANA, 2015).

Two types of standards are delineated by the ANA: standards of care for clinical practice and standards of professional performance. Standard 13 (ANA, 2015) describes the nurses obligation to utilize research findings in practice. This expectation indirectly refers to the use of clinical guidelines and other resources. The American Association of Nurse Practitioners (AANP) establishes the standards of practice for nurse practitioners. The standards encompass many aspects of practice, including qualifications, process of care, care priorities, and research as a basis for practice (AANP, 2013).

Practice guidelines are not cookbooks that take the decision making away from providers; instead, they allow for flexibility when making individual patient-care decisions. Guidelines are intended to provide a reference point and general direction for decision making and are not meant to be interpreted as rigid criteria that must be followed regardless of the context in which they are being used. Nonetheless, guidelines should be followed in the majority of cases unless there is a clear rationale for deviating from them to serve the particular needs of individuals. Tailoring care to the needs of a particular patient is a cornerstone of EBP. The usefulness of applying guidelines in clinical decision making has become increasingly recognized over the past decade and is now an expectation in the delivery of health care.

DEVELOPMENT OF EVIDENCE-BASED PRACTICE GUIDELINES AND GRADING OF EVIDENCE

The essential components of guideline development are as follows: (1) identification/clarification of the topic, (2) establishment of an expert panel, (3) a systematic review of the literature, (4) development of evidence-based tables, (5) writing draft recommendations based on the evidence, (6) external review of the recommendations, and (7) final acceptance of the revised recommendations by the panel. Panel members are chosen according to the focus and intent of the guidelines and may include physicians, nurse practitioners, clinical nurse specialists, ethicists, pharmacists, therapists, and health-care consumers.

One of the most important aspects of developing guidelines is appraising the quality of the evidence used to make each recommendation and then grading the recommendation based on the level of evidence. Various grading systems are currently in use. For example, the U.S. Preventive Services Task Force's (USPSTF) uses a three-tiered system to rate evidence and a five-point rating scale (A through E ratings) to grade recommendations (USPSTF, 2016). Another system, known as GRADE, is a relatively new methodology that is becoming more popular among medical organizations (Grade Working Group, 2017). It is important to keep in mind the lack of standardization for defining the level of evidence. This must be considered when selecting criteria and the appropriate rating scale based on the clinical question.

Table 5.1 describes various databases and scales that are used to rate evidence.

The following discussion explains a common hierarchy used to evaluate evidence based on research design. This hierarchy was modified by Melnyk and Fineout-Overholt (2015) from Guyatt and Rennie (2002). It rates evidence on a scale of I to VII based on the type of research design, as follows.

Level I evidence—systematic review or meta-analysis of RCTs: Systematic reviews are considered among the highest level of evidence on which to base a change in practice. Some systematic reviews are also called meta-analyses, which involve a specific type of statistical analysis that is applied to a group of studies. The systematic review includes all RCT studies and similar research that address a similar clinical question. A review of the literature allows

TABLE 5.1	Sources of Evidence and Level of Evidence		
Sources of Evidence	*Different Types of Evidence*	*Specific Use*	*Examples of Types/Levels of Evidence*
Cochrane Library[1] SR and meta-analyses attempt to identify, appraise, and synthesize empirical evidence to inform decision making.	Five types: • Intervention reviews • Diagnostic test accuracy reviews • Methodology reviews • Qualitative reviews • Prognosis reviews	Findings are based on results that meet certain criteria; reliable studies provide the best evidence, reducing impact of bias. • Identification of relevant studies from different sources • Selection for inclusion and evaluation of strengths and limitations based on predefined criteria • Systematic collection of data • Appropriate synthesis of data	• Database of SRs • DARE: Database of Abstracts of REviews • Cochrane Central Register of Controlled (Clinical) Trials • National Health Service Economic Evaluation Data Base • Gold standard for developing SRs. Flow chart created from preappraised studies and clinical trials
Preferred Reporting Items for Systematic Reviews and Meta-Analyses (PRISMA)[2] Starting point for developing clinical practice guidelines. Addresses several conceptual and practical advances in the science of SRs.	Reporting reviews of evaluating randomized trials, reviews of interventions (meta-analyses).	Adopts the definitions of SR and meta-analysis used by Cochrane Collaboration.	• Identification: Records identified through databased searching, then records duplicates removed. • Screening: Records screened, records excluded • Eligibility: Full-text articles assessed for eligibility, full-text articles excluded with reasons • Included: Studies included in qualitative synthesis, studies included in quantitative syntheses

Continued

TABLE 5.1   Sources of Evidence and Level of Evidence—cont'd

Sources of Evidence	Different Types of Evidence	Specific Use	Examples of Types/Levels of Evidence
Joanna Briggs Institute Levels of Evidence[3]	Levels of evidence for effectiveness (RCT, quasi-experimental, pretest, post-test, descriptive) Levels of evidence for diagnosis (test accuracy among patients, diagnostic case studies) Level of evidence for prognosis (cohort studies, case series) Level of evidence for economic evaluations (decision makers, costs, health outcomes) Level of evidence for meaningfulness (qualitative)	Considers evidence-based health care as decision making that considers the feasibility, appropriateness, mean-ingfulness, and effec-tiveness of health-care practices.	Level 1: experimental design Level 2: quasiexperimental designs Level 3: observational-analytic designs Level 4: observational-descriptive studies/case studies Level 5: expert opinion and bench research
Johns Hopkins Nursing[4] Evidence Levels and Quality Guide	Level I: experimental, RCT, SR of RCTs Level II: quasiexperimental Level III: nonexperimental, qualitative Level IV: opinion of expert(s), consensus panels Level V: literature reviews, quality improvement, case reports, experi-ential opinions of experts	PET framework P: practice question E: evidence T: translation Problem-solving approach to clinical decision making within a health-care organiza-tion	Levels I–III A: High quality—consistent generalizable results, thor-ough reference to scientific evidence B: Good quality—reasonable consistent results, some ref-erence to scientific evidence C: Low quality/major flaws—inconsistent results, insuf-ficient sample size, conclu-sions cannot be drawn Levels IV–V A: High quality—consistent results, sponsored by pro-fessional, public, private, or government agencies developed or revised with-in 5 years B: Good quality—reasonably consistent results C: Low quality/major flaws—not sponsored by an official organization, limited literature search, not revised in 5 years
Melnyk & Fineout-Overholt (2015)[5] Rating system for the hierarchy of evidence for intervention/treatment questions	Level I: SR or meta-analysis of RCTs Level II: at least one RCT Level III: controlled trial without randomization Level IV: case–control or cohort studies Level V: SR of descriptive and qual-itative studies (meta-synthesis) Level VI: single descriptive or quali-tative study Level VII: opinion of authorities or reports of expert committees	PICOT question for-mat to determine key search parameters in databases Quick critical appraisal guides for evaluat-ing specific evidence depending on level	

Abbreviations: PICOT, patient or population/intervention/comparison/outcome/time; RCT, randomized clinical trial; SR, systematic review.

1. Cochrane Review-Cochrane Library. About Cochrane reviews. http://www.cochranelibrary.com/about/about-cochrane- systematic-reviews.html. Published 1999–2017.
2. Moher D, Liberati A, Tetzlaff J, Altman DG. Preferred Reporting Items for Systematic Reviews and Meta-Analyses: The PRISMA statement. *PLoS Med.* 2009;6(7): e1000097.
3. Joanna Briggs Institute. New JBI levels of evidence. https://joannabriggs.org/assets/docs/approach/JBI-Levels-of-evidence-2014.pdf. Published 2013.
4. The Institute for Johns Hopkins Nursing. *Nursing evidence-based practice: Model and guidelines.* 2nd ed. Indianapolis, IN: Sigma Theta Tau International; 2012.
5. Melnyk BM, Fineout-Overholt E. *Evidence-based practice in nursing & healthcare: A guide to best practice.* 3rd ed. Philadelphia, PA: Wolters Kluwer; 2015.

for a compilation of all the studies to give strength to outcomes. This review is a rigorous approach and provides a high level of evidence due to the minimization of bias. The Cochrane Library has an extensive compilation of systematic reviews.

Level II evidence—single well-designed RCTs: RCTs are increasingly considered the most respected method for establishing the cause of disease or the efficacy of a treatment/intervention. For example, the U.S. Food and Drug Administration requires evidence of a drug's efficacy from two independently conducted randomized trials before approving the drug's use in the United States. The National Institutes of Health is increasingly funding RCTs, and agencies or organizations developing clinical guidelines now consider the evidence from RCTs to supersede findings from case–control or cohort studies.

The strength of RCTs to establish cause or efficacy lies in the ability of this design to maintain a high degree of control within experimental conditions. If there are different effects between the groups (e.g., blood pressure, the development of pressure ulcers, the prevention of pregnancy), the differences can generally be attributed to the intervention, exposure, or treatment rather than "extraneous" factors. Moreover, the random assignment of subjects into the treatment or control group allows for a high degree of confidence in making causal inferences about the effects of an exposure, intervention, or treatment.

RCTs also frequently employ the use of double-blinding to further strengthen support for identifying a cause-and-effect relationship. When RCTs are double-blind, neither the principal investigators nor the participants know who is in the control or experimental group until either significant differences are noted in a (blind) analysis of the data or the study is complete. The purpose of double-blinding is to eliminate the potential for participants in the experimental or control group to treat themselves differently or to be treated differently by investigators.

Level III evidence—well-designed controlled trials without randomization: Quasiexperimental research designs evaluate the effectiveness of an intervention/treatment, but subjects are not randomly assigned to either the treatment or control group. In these designs, many of the other same methods to ascertain the internal validity of the study instituted in RCTs, such as control of extraneous variables and standardization of treatment, are implemented. For example, De Cunto Taets and de Figueiredo (2016) conducted a study to verify whether comatose patients experience pain during a bed bath. They collected saliva from patient before and during a bed bath and measured substance P levels in the saliva samples. This study evaluated the effective of a common nursing intervention but did not randomize the patients to a treatment or control group.

Level IV evidence—well-designed case–control or cohort studies: These types of studies are especially useful in answering clinical questions that address prognosis or causation. With this design, the study is generally initiated after the disease has developed. A group of individuals who have the disease (cases) and those who do not (controls) are selected and compared in terms of their prior exposures that are thought to be associated with the development of a particular type of disease. Case–control studies are also considered observational studies because they do not manipulate the exposure (what may also be referred to as the intervention). The course of the disease is observed without interference. The lack of control over the exposure in case–control studies (along with other observational studies) risks introducing selection bias into the study, which may confound the results. These potential shortcomings have some researchers arguing that case–control studies are essentially worthless because of the inherent potential for bias.

Despite the arguments against the value of the case–control design, it is the most commonly used epidemiological design in the medical literature today. For example, the association between unopposed estrogen use in postmenopausal women and the development of endometrial cancer was established through several case–control studies.

The Nurses' Health Study is an example of a well-known prospective cohort study. It is a large, ongoing cohort study that enrolled more than 120,000 married female nurses who were aged 30 to 55 years in 1976. The nurses completed a baseline questionnaire about a number of demographic and health characteristics. Follow-up questionnaires at 2-year intervals asked about the development of disease and any new exposures. By comparing the exposed and unexposed groups on a number of variables (e.g., those who took hormone replacement and those who did not; those who ate high-fat foods and those who did not) and the onset of disease within each group, the study has provided important information about the relationships of these variables with the development of cancer and cardiovascular disease in women.

Another example of a prospective cohort study is the Framingham Heart Study. In this study, investigators identified and examined 5,127 men and women from Framingham, Massachusetts, who were 30 to 59 years old in the 1950s. When the study was initiated, all 5,127 participants were determined to be free from coronary heart disease. Participants in the study have provided ongoing lifestyle and health status information and have been re-examined at regular intervals since 1952 for the development of coronary events. Prospective data from this study have been pivotal in identifying several major risk factors associated with coronary artery disease (CAD) and have been one of the sources of evidence for recommending lifestyle modifications to prevent CAD.

Level V evidence—systematic reviews of descriptive and qualitative studies: The purpose of descriptive research is to accurately portray the characteristics of a population or a clinical situation. Descriptive research can be quantitative or qualitative in design. In quantitative designs, the findings address the incidence, prevalence, or measurable characteristics of the population using descriptive statistics (frequencies, means, mode, etc.).

In qualitative designs, the population or clinical situation is displayed in a narrative format for the purpose of increasing the understanding of the various dimensions of the phenomena of interest. Common qualitative designs used in nursing research include phenomenology, ethnography, grounded theory, and historical analysis.

Level VI evidence—single descriptive or qualitative studies: Case studies fall into this category. They are ranked lower because of their likelihood of decreased objectivity. These studies describe the history of one individual or a small group of patients. Case studies are generally told in story form. The value of this study type is to alert a provider to an adverse event or a rare disease or to add to a provider's knowledge base. It is important to recognize that no inferences can be made from a case study to the general population.

Level VII evidence—opinion of authorities and/ or reports of expert committees: This level of evidence is just as it states: it is someone's opinion. This type of evidence follows the traditional approach for "correct" or "common" practice and may or may not be based on strong evidence. This level of evidence should not be a sole determination of changing practice or determining the proper course of treatment. However, there are times when this is the only evidence, and it is utilized to begin treatment in rare situations that do not have higher levels of evidence.

It is important to note that there is an increasing trend toward regarding evidence from RCTs as the only valid type of evidence appropriate for use in the practice setting. The danger in this perspective is disregarding what we have learned and can continue to learn from observational studies such as case–control and cohort studies.

The most sobering outcome of reliance on RCTs is the failure to teach providers to think and critically evaluate information. There are many circumstances in which randomization is impossible and where observational methods have provided invaluable information. For example, how did we come to understand the relationship between alcohol use in pregnancy and fetal alcohol syndrome; smoking and cardiopulmonary disease; birth defects and thalidomide; the transmission of HIV and viral hepatitis; and the development of endocarditis in intravenous drug use? Knowledge of these associations came from observational studies. Randomizing pregnant women into experimental or control group to either drink alcoholic beverages or not or designing an experimental trial to determine how the transmission of HIV in humans occurs is not ethically possible (or desirable). How we know what we know in practice must be determined through a critical appraisal of the information available.

APPLICATION OF CLINICAL PRACTICE GUIDELINES

Providers who use clinical guidelines must learn techniques and skills that focus on finding and evaluating relevant practice guidelines. They must also develop a systematic method with which to evaluate EBP guidelines at the point of patient care.

Evaluation of Clinical Practice Guidelines

Clinicians who use clinical guidelines should evaluate their usefulness by examining the following major characteristics:

- **Who created the guideline, and what is the date of revision or origination?** Authorship and funding of the guideline may be important if there is the potential for bias. In addition, the best guideline will be created using multidisciplinary groups and follow a systematic approach as recommended by AHRQ. The guideline must be current, meaning it was created or revised in the past 2 to 3 years and used the most current evidence.
- **Are the guidelines clinically important?** To establish clinical importance, guidelines should convince you that following them will provide more benefits for your patients than their potential associated harms or costs.
- **How strong are the recommendations?** As discussed previously, the strength of a recommendation is largely determined by the strength of available evidence used to make the recommendations (see "Development of Evidence-Based Practice Guidelines and Grading of Evidence" earlier in the chapter).
- **Are the guideline recommendations applicable to your patients?** Guidelines are developed for a variety of settings and for different practitioners. First, it is necessary to determine the group for which the guidelines were written (e.g., primary-care providers, specialists,

or quality assurance reviewers) and whether they suit the intended purpose. Second, a determination is made on whether the individual patient has the characteristics of patients for whom the guidelines were intended. For example, if the patients you care for have a higher or lower prevalence of a disease or different set of risk factors for disease than those in the guidelines, the recommendations may not apply. The patient population for whom the guidelines are intended will likely be dictated by the sample characteristics of the studies used to develop them as evidence. Before applying recommendations to any one patient, first determine whether this patient's characteristics are consistent with those for which the guideline was intended and modify the guidelines when required (remember, they are meant to be flexible and adapted to individual needs when necessary).

Application of Clinical Guidelines

The following example serves as a brief case study in applying clinical guidelines: a 52-year-old male patient with hypertension is in the office. The patient is on a diuretic and a beta blocker with well-controlled blood pressure. The provider is trying to determine whether the patient should be tested for causes of secondary hypertension. Using the Eighth Report of the Joint National Committee on Prevention, Detection, Evaluation, and Treatment of High Blood Pressure (JNC 8), the evidence demonstrates that the improved clinical outcomes associated with treating underlying causes of secondary hypertension are based on several well-designed studies; however, the costs and risks of adverse outcomes associated with diagnostic tests to rule out a cause such as renal artery stenosis may be greater than the benefits when applied to the entire population. Thus, guidelines do not recommend that every person who develops hypertension undergo extensive testing. Rather, specific characteristics of patients presenting with hypertension assist us in narrowing the population to those individuals who would reap the benefits of screening beyond any potential harm of the tests. A second patient presents with new-onset elevated blood pressure. He is 28 years old with no family history of hypertension. This patient would meet the criteria in the JNC 7 for investigation of possible renal stenosis.

EVALUATING THE EVIDENCE TO CHANGE PRACTICE

Distinguishing between intermediate and clinical outcomes is also critical before applying research findings to practice. Outcome research has been increasingly funded in recent years. An outcome is generally considered the dependent variable of the study. Intermediate outcomes include measurements such as bone mineral density, hemoglobin levels, and eosinophil level. Clinical outcomes include measures such as the number of hip fractures, a person's functional status, peak flow values, or the number of acute asthma exacerbations experienced.

Improvement in intermediate outcomes does not necessarily lead to improvements in clinical outcomes. For example, in early studies of using fluoride to treat osteoporosis, bone mineral density values improved greatly when given to osteoporotic women, but the number of fractures over time did not differ from those in women who were given placebos. Thus, intermediate outcomes, although important to study to gain an understanding of disease processes and treatment, should not be substituted for clinical outcome data.

An example of evaluating evidence to change practice is the use of angiotensin-converting enzyme (ACE) inhibitors in patients with congestive heart failure (CHF). In the early 1990s, several clinical trials demonstrated that the use of ACE inhibitors improved clinical outcomes in patients with CHF, not only with regard to mortality but also in exercise tolerance, symptom severity, progression to left ventricular dysfunction, and fewer hospitalization rates. The consistency of the findings and the fact that they came from well-designed RCTs provided unequivocal evidence that ACE inhibitor use was beneficial for the majority of patients with CHF. As a result, the American College of Cardiology, the American Heart Association, and the AHRQ developed clinical guidelines for the treatment of CHF that strongly encourage ACE inhibitors as standard therapy. The use of ACE inhibitors is now considered a standard of care and should be incorporated into the care of persons with CHF. For the provider at the point of care, the clinical guideline produced by these organizations provides point-of-care evidence to utilize with a patient.

DEVELOPING A POINT-OF-CARE STRATEGY

One aspect of providing evidence-based care is the ability to access summaries of large amounts of information using mobile technologies. During a busy clinical day, it is unlikely that providers will implement the full EBP process. For example, it is not practical for a busy clinician to collect the most relevant and best evidence from a review of the literature including published literature reviews, meta-analyses, and clinical practice guidelines and to critically evaluate the evidence. Providers need key answers to their questions at the point of care.

Ely et al. (1999) reported that providers generally have less than 2 minutes or less to spend searching for answers to clinical questions. Therefore, it is more feasible for clinicians to use preappraised summaries of evidence to assist them in making clinical decisions.

A point-of-care strategy involves the following tasks: (1) asking a clinical question, (2) having evidence resources readily available, (3) completing the search using those resources, (4) examining the results of the search, and finally (5) applying the findings to the individual patient. See Box 5.4 for a framework for point-of-care search strategy for EBP. Education of practitioners in developing point-of-care use of EBP should become an essential part of nursing degree programs.

The first step in the process of sorting through information relevant to any given clinical situation is to formulate the clinical issue into a searchable, answerable question. To do this, the clinician asks two types of questions. The first is a clinical question such as, "What is the best method for X?" The second is a question essential to find evidence to answer the clinical question. For example, "Between the

---

Box 5.4   A Framework for Point-of-Care Search Strategy

1. Ask the clinical question.
2. Select the evidence resource. The following lists suggested resources:
   - National Guideline Clearinghouse: www.guideline.gov
   - Cochrane Collaboration: www.cochrane.org
   - Essential Evidence Plus: www.essentialevidenceplus.com
   - UpToDate: www.uptodate.com/home/index.html
   - DynaMed: https://dynamed.ebscohost.com
   - Smartphone or tablet options:
     - Skyscape constellation: www.skyscape.com/estore/ProductDetail.aspx?ProductId=1180
     - Pepid primary care: www.pepid.com
3. Search.
4. Examine the evidence found in the search. Consider the level of evidence the search provided (meta-analysis, systematic reviews).
5. Apply the evidence to your patient.

Case scenario 1: A 72-year-old man is in the office for recent onset and worsening difficulty breathing. Pulse oximetry reading is 84 (sea level), and he is complaining of difficulty in completing activities of daily living due to the shortness of breath even while at rest. His wife states that he is more lethargic, and this is confirmed on examination. Examination also finds peripheral cyanosis and nonpitting pedal edema that the patient did not have on his last office visit.

1. The question: What are the criteria for admission for chronic obstructive pulmonary disease (COPD) exacerbation?
2. Selected resource: National Guideline Clearinghouse
3. Search term: "COPD acute exacerbation admission"
4. Examine the evidence: This 2016 guideline ("Care of the hospitalized patient with acute exacerbation of COPD") lists the following indications for hospital admission: marked increase in intensity of symptoms, such as sudden development of resting dyspnea; severe underlying COPD; onset of new physical signs; new or increased oxygen requirements (e.g., cyanosis, peripheral edema); failure of exacerbation to respond to initial medical management; presence of serious comorbidities such as pneumonia, congestive heart failure, arrhythmia, renal or liver failure; frequent exacerbations; older age; insufficient home support.

5. Explain the guideline recommendations to the patient and discuss his preferences. The clinician explained that he is experiencing increasing shortness of breath and his oxygen saturation was dangerously low. Because he is not responding to current plan of care, hospitalization is recommended to protect him from serious complications. The patient states that he is willing to go to the hospital. Call for advanced life support transport.

Case scenario 2: A 3-year-old child is diagnosed in the clinic with acute otitis media (AOM). He appears mildly ill and has an axillary temperature of 100.6°F. Child has no known allergy to medication and is otherwise a healthy 3-year-old. Child is in day care during the day at a camp; parents are migrant workers.

1. The question: What is the recommended antibiotic for AOM in a 3-year-old child?
2. Selected search places: UpToDate (www.uptodate.com)
3. Search term: "AOM children"
4. Examine the evidence: azithromycin (systemic): pediatric drug information. For children older than 24 months to provide a wait-and-see approach if nonsevere illness, mild otalgia, temperature less than 102.2°F (child is not severely ill and has a temperature less than 102.2°F), a follow-up can be ensured to start antibiotics if symptoms persist or worsen (this child's parents are about to move on to the next migrant camp with unknown available health care). The nurse practitioner (NP), who has experience working in this migrant camp, decides that the wait-and-see approach is probably not appropriate. The recommended antibiotic is amoxicillin 90 mg/kg per day divided in two doses, for 5 to 7 days for a maximum of 3 grams per day.
5. Explain to the patient (family) the results found and discuss the family preferences. The mother states that the child had amoxicillin for one other ear infection and had "pretty bad" diarrhea; she is asking if another antibiotic could be used instead because it is often difficult to have bathroom facilities while traveling to new camps. She also wonders if there is a medication that can be given just once or twice a day, because she is often in the fields for very long days. With this mother's request in mind, the NP gives the child azithromycin 10 mg/kg once daily for 3 days with a maximum dose of 500 mg.

Sources: National Guideline Clearinghouse. Care of the hospitalized patient with acute exacerbation of COPD. https://www.guideline.gov/summaries/summary/50686/care-of-the-hospitalized-patient-with-acute-exacerbation-of-copd. Published 2017. Accessed September 26, 2017; UpToDate. Acute otitis media in children: Treatment. http://www.uptodate.com/contents/acute-otitis-media-in-children-treatment. Accessed September 26, 2017; UpToDate. Azithromycin (systematic). Pediatric drug information. https://www.uptodate.com/contents/azithromycin-systemic-pediatric-drug-information?source=see_link. Accessed October 25, 2017.

two best methods for X, which one will work the best in my clinical situation and population?" Evidence for clinical questions is best found when the question is posed in a searchable format. In the foregoing example, the clinical question asks, "In X population, how does X compared with Y affect Z?"

There is an abundance of readily available resources that provide access to summaries of the best evidence on specific clinical issues. These resources facilitate the retrieval and use of preappraised information for use at the point of care. Campbell, et al. (2015), building on the work of Banzi et al. (2010), identifies available EBP point-of-care resources as "web-based medical compendia specifically designed to deliver predigested, rapidly accessible, comprehensive, periodically updated, and evidence-based information (and possibly also guidance) to clinicians" (p 313). The authors present a comprehensive evaluation of 20 point-of-care resources. These resources were evaluated for general characteristics, content presentation, and editorial quality. The top resources identified were UpToDate, Nursing Reference Centre, Mosby's Nursing Consult, BMJ Best Practice, and JBI COnNECT+. Many point-of-care resources are downloadable databases for PDAs and smartphones that are periodically updated. Decisions about which resources to use depends on the specific needs of the provider.

Applying evidence to care can be a complicated process. Research is establishing a number of moderating factors for applying evidence in practice. Often, it is difficult for providers to trust the information and balance the findings with their personal clinical knowledge and expertise. In addition, patient preference may conflict with EBP recommendations and preclude their implementation.

NURSING SCIENCE: BUILDING THE EVIDENCE FOR PRACTICE

Historically, nurses have been involved in conducting research. The establishment of the National Institute for Nursing Research marked a new era by aligning nursing science with other respected institutes within the National Institutes of Health. This development increased both federal funding for nursing research and the visibility of nursing science on a national level. Investment in nursing research continues to grow in terms of resources, funding, training, and the expectation for using research as the basis, or evidence, for practice. Many methods of knowing contribute to our knowledge or understanding of the world, and a combination of methods (or various ways of triangulating) will provide a clearer, more encompassing answer to questions asked within the discipline to provide the best individualized care for patients. The example (Box 5.5) of using multiple types of research to care for the family with a child diagnosed with diabetes demonstrates the value of multiple methods of evidence.

Box 5.5   A Framework for Evaluating Health Science Literature

Learning to evaluate health science literature is critical. It can be a time-consuming process, but it is necessary to reading an article for use in practice.

1. Look at the title to determine whether it reflects your specific interest.
2. Validate that the content is relevant to your original interest and the title by reading the abstract.
3. Evaluate and determine what is being studied:
   - What are the study questions or hypotheses?
   - What are the specific variables under study?
   - How are the variables defined and measured?
4. Evaluate and determine who is being studied:
   - What are the characteristics of the study sample or subjects?
   - How were subjects selected for the study?
   - Is there an adequate sample size?
5. Evaluate and determine the type of study design and assess its validity:
   - Do the designs of the studies support the statements made?
   - Have other studies in similar (or different) samples found consistent results?
6. Evaluate and determine how data have been analyzed:
   - What are the descriptive statistics used to describe the sample characteristics?
   - Could the degree or pattern of missing data influence the results?
   - Were the inferential statistics used appropriate for the study question and design?
   - Remember that statistical tests of significance do not determine causation or clinical significance.
7. Evaluate what you have determined thus far:
   - Have you been skeptical?
   - Have you judged the quality of the literature based on the journal in which it was published?
   - Do you realize that there is no such thing as a "perfect" study?
   - How have you judged the author's treatment of contradictory results?
   - Remember that validity and reliability are crucial aspects of the study.
8. Discuss your evaluation with colleagues and seek other opinions (such as in a journal club):
   - Do your colleagues agree with your evaluation?
   - Do the results or recommendations suggest a change in your clinical practice? If so, what change is suggested and how will it be implemented?

There are numerous examples of nursing research that have contributed to the knowledge base of nursing. Critically appraising studies regarding the appropriate use of results is one of the most important skills clinicians will need to use in practice. Using a framework for guidance can assist clinicians in taking the appropriate steps toward meeting this obligation. Some of the steps in applying the framework presented here are similar to those used for

evaluating clinical practice guidelines. Two of the many sources to find literature are PubMed and the Cumulative Index of Nursing and Allied Health Literature. A framework for evaluating journal articles in the health science literature is presented in Box 5.6. This framework provides an organized approach to interpreting the information found in a variety of articles, be it a review of the current knowledge in an area or original research findings.

Box 5.6   Example: Integration of Evidence-Based Practice and Nursing Research–Based Practice

The management of an 8-year-old child with type 1 diabetes requires a multidisciplinary approach of which the family is an integral part. Following are two resources available to the advanced practice registered nurse to assist in the management of the child with diabetes.

Evidence-Based Practice Guidelines

The American Diabetes Association (ADA) Professional Association supports the development of clinical guidelines for the management of diabetes. The ADA uses an evidence-grading system for standards of medical care in diabetes (level of evidence are graded A to E). The foundation of the guideline for the management of diabetes is the recommendations made as to glycemic control. These include the following:

1. Lowering A1C has been associated with a reduction of microvascular and neuropathic complications of diabetes (A).
2. Developing or adjusting the management plan to achieve normal or near-normal glycemia with an A1C goal of <7% is reasonable if it can be achieved without excessive hypoglycemia (B).
3. A lower A1C is associated with a lower risk of myocardial infarction and cardiovascular death (B).
4. Aggressive glycemic management with insulin may reduce morbidity in patients with severe acute illness, preoperatively, after myocardial infarction, and in pregnancy (B).
5. Less stringent treatment goals may be appropriate for patients with a history of severe hypoglycemia, patients with limited life expectancies, very young children or older adults, and individuals with comorbid conditions (E).

The panel rated the strength of the evidence supporting the first recommendation as "A." An "A" indicated that there was clear evidence from well-conducted, generalizable, randomized clinical trials that were adequately powered, or at the least supportive evidence from well-conducted randomized controlled trials that were adequately powered, including evidence from a well-conducted trial at one or more institutions. Evidence supporting the second through fifth recommendations were rated as "B." An evidence rating of "B" indicated that there was supportive evidence from well-conducted cohort studies. The final recommendation was given an evidence rating of "E." Evidence rated as E indicated that support for the recommendation was from expert consensus or clinical experience.

The guidelines also addressed nutrition and psychosocial assessment and care. The recommendations listed under psychosocial assessment and care are as follows:

1. Preliminary assessment of psychological and social status should be included as part of the medical management of diabetes (E).
2. Psychosocial screening should include but is not limited to attitudes about the illness, expectations for medical management and outcomes, affect/mood, general and diabetes-related quality of life, resources (financial, social, and emotional), and psychiatric history (E).
3. It is preferable to incorporate psychological treatment into routine care rather than to wait for identification of a specific problem or deterioration in psychological status (E).

Nursing Research

Sullivan-Bolyai and colleagues (2004) conducted a study to describe the experiences of parents managing their child's type 1 diabetes with the use of continuous subcutaneous insulin infusions (CSII), commonly referred to as the insulin pump. In this qualitative study, 14 mothers and 7 fathers were interviewed and asked to describe the day-to-day experience of managing their child's diabetes. The children ranged in age from 2 to 11 years, and their mean age was 7.2 years of age. Parents in this study agreed that the pump was very effective in managing their child's diabetes and believed that their child's glucose was under much better control with the pump compared with using multiple daily injections (MDIs). The results of Sullivan-Bolyai et al.'s research indicated that some parents are reluctant to change to an alternative method of achieving glycemic control for their child. But all of the parents in their study, once familiar with the device, were very satisfied with the results and reported a better quality of life after they changed methods. Another important finding was that parents reported more freedom and flexibility in their lives once their child was switched from MDIs to the insulin pump. Some parents reported that once the child was placed on the insulin pump, they often were tempted to impose stricter controls on their child's glucose levels.

Impact on Advanced Practice Nursing

The ADA guidelines indicate that there is strong, reliable evidence to support interventions that assist the child with diabetes

Box 5.6   Example: Integration of Evidence-Based Practice and Nursing Research–Based Practice—cont'd

to maintain normal to near-normal glycemic levels, with less convincing evidence given to support less stringent control in very young children. Two methods currently used to achieve control are MDI and CSII, commonly called the insulin pump.

These guidelines also include a mandate for the primary-care provider to provide psychosocial assessment and care. One assessment needed is the parents' comfort with technology and resources. Technology once limited to secondary and tertiary health-care settings is now available in the community and is often managed by laypersons and caregivers.

The method used to achieve glycemic control of the child is ultimately the parents' decision. However, advanced practice registered nurses (APRNs) who care for these children and families will be influential in the education and support of these families as they make complex health-care decisions for their child. Using the guidelines as the goals for management, APRNs can provide parents with evidence-based rationales for

glycemic management of their child and assist them in their choices.

Relaying information to parents based on nursing research, such as the research conducted by Sullivan-Bolyai et al., may relieve some initial hesitancy in parents about switching from MDI to SCII to manage their child's diabetes. One important consideration in using this research in practice is that the sample for the above research was described as Caucasian and well-educated. Will these same experiences be similar in other samples? However, perceptions of parents that their child's diabetes is under better control with the insulin pump and that this method has improved their quality of life can be useful to APRNs in their care of families managing this complex health condition.

This brings the evidence to the point of care, and using the providers' confidence in the evidence, their own experience with MDI or CSII, and the parents' comfort with technology demonstrate the essence of evidence-based practice.

Sources: American Diabetes Association Professional Association. *Standards of medical care in diabetes. Diabetes Care* 2017;40:S4–S5; Sullivan-Bolyai S, et al. Parents' reflections on managing their children's diabetes with insulin pumps. *J Nurs Scholarsh.* 2004;36:316–323.

CLINICAL DECISION MAKING AND THE PATIENT'S HEALTH-CARE DECISIONS

The decisions advanced practice registered nurses make in practice are fundamental to the quality of care given. Although collecting and evaluating evidence is critical to providing safe care, the importance of taking into consideration the patient's beliefs and desired outcomes is basic to making any health-care decision. There are two main steps of decision making in clinical practice: (1) collecting and analyzing evidence (or data) on the benefits, potential harms, and costs of various options and (2) making a judgment about how to use the available evidence to achieve the health outcome desired. This step includes the provider's experience with the population of patients served and his or her knowledge of available resources in the community.

Applying analytical procedures for determining the credibility or reliability of data to be employed as evidence is only one aspect of the decision-making process. An equal challenge in making practice decisions involves making a judgment about how to use the evidence. This second step is not a question of facts but of patient values or preferences. One of the most substantial qualities of advanced practice nursing is establishing a relationship with patients, providing them with the most current information, and allowing them to make health-care decisions they determine are best for them. In this respect, it is not entirely important to integrate the clinicians practice knowledge with the patient's perspective. Figure 5.1 illustrates this interaction of evidence, patient preferences, and clinician expertise.

To clarify this point, consider Ms. Jones, a 47-year-old woman with type 2 diabetes. She is in the office for a quarterly visit. She has not met her A1C goal through metformin and lifestyle changes. Because of the patient's history and laboratory values, the provider finds evidence supporting the addition of insulin. However, the patient absolutely refuses, despite significant explanations of the benefits. With this patient's refusal, the clinician revisits the current guidelines and selects an oral medication to add to the patient's regimen. The patient agrees to add another oral medication.

There will be times, however, that what the patient desires is not appropriate. Ms. Smith, who is 22 years old, comes to the office asking for Synthroid. The patient

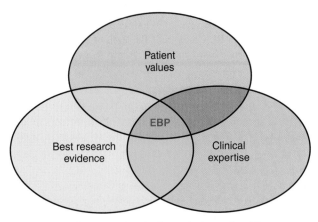

Figure 5.1 Schematic of triangulation of evidence-based practice. Source: *Sackett DL, Rosenberg W, McGray JA, Haynes RB, Richardson WS. Evidence-based medicine: What it is and what it isn't.* BMJ. *1996;312:71-72.*

explains that she has tried everything to lose weight and has a friend who was started on Synthroid and lost 30 pounds. The clinician performs a review of systems and a physical examination and orders the appropriate diagnostics. When the patient's laboratory results do not confirm a need for thyroid replacement, she educates the patient about the results and explains why she is not prescribing the medication simply because she is asking for it. Clearly, these cases identify the use of patients' preferences when the evidence will support a change in the "best" options, while not prescribing based solely on patient preferences.

 For additional resources please visit
https://davisedge.fadavis.com/

REFERENCES

Ackley, BJ, Swan, BA, Ladwig, G, Tucker S. *Evidence-based nursing care guidelines: Medical-surgical interventions.* St. Louis, MO: Mosby Elsevier; 2008.

Agency for Healthcare Research and Quality. Reauthorization fact sheet. http://archive.ahrq.gov/about/ahrqfact.htm. Published 1999.

Agency for Healthcare Research and Quality. Clinical guidelines and recommendations. https://www.ahrq.gov/professionals/clinicians-providers/guidelines-recommendations/index.html. Published 2017.

Agency for Healthcare Research and Quality. National Clearinghouse Guidelines. https://www.ahrq.gov/research/findings/factsheets/errors-safety/ngc/national-guideline-clearinghouse.html.

Amend R, Golden A. Practice at the point of care. *J Nurse Pract.* 2011; 7(4): 303–308.

American Associate of Nurse Practitioners. Standards of practice for nurse practitioners. https://www.aanp.org/images/documents/publications/standardsofpractice.pdf. Published 2013.

American Diabetes Association. *Standards of medical care in diabetes. Diabetes Care.* 2017;40:S4–S5. https://professional.diabetes.org/sites/professional.diabetes.org/files/media/dc_40_s1_final.pdf.

Banzi R, Liberati A, Moschetti I, Tagliabue L, Moja L. A review of online evidence-based practice point-of-care information summary providers. *J Med Internet Res.* 2010;12(3):e26.

Branham S, DelloSritto R, Hilliard T. Lost in translation: The acute care nurse practitioners' use of evidence based practice. A qualitative study. *J Nurs Educ Pract.* 2014;4(6):53–59.

Burns PB, Rohrich RJ, Chung KC. The levels of evidence and their role in evidence-based medicine. *Plastic Reconstr Surg.* 2011; 128(1):305–310.

Campbell JM, Umapathysivam K, Xue Y, Lockwood C. Evidence-based practice point of care resources: A quantitative evaluation of quality, rigor, and content. *Worldviews Evid Based Nurs.* 2015;12(6):313–327.

De Cunto Taets GG, de Figueiredo NMA. A quasi-experimental nursing study on pain in comatose patients. *Rev Bras Enferm.* 2016;69(5). http://www.scielo.br/scielo.php?pid=S0034-1672016000500927&script=sci_arttext&tlng=en.

Ely JW, Osheroff JA, Ebell MH, et al. Analysis of questions asked by family doctors regarding patient care. *Br Med J.* 1999; 319(7206):358–361.

Grade Working Group. What is GRADE? http://www.gradeworkinggroup.org/#. Published 2016.

Guyatt G, Rennie D, eds. *Users' guides to the medical literature: A manual for evidence-based clinical practice.* Chicago, IL: American Medical Association; 2002.

Mackey A, Bassendowski S. The history of evidence-based practice in nursing education and practice. *J Prof Nurs.* 2017;33(1): 51–55.

Melnyk BM, Fineout-Overholt E. *Evidence-based practice in nursing & healthcare: A guide to best practice.* 3rd ed. Philadelphia, PA: Wolters Kluwer; 2015.

Sackett DL. Rules of evidence and clinical recommendations on the use of antithrombotic agents. *Chest.* 1989;95:2S–4S.

Sackett DL, Rosenberg W, McGray JA, Haynes RB, Richardson WS. Evidence-based medicine: What it is and what it isn't. *BMJ.* 1996;312:71–72.

Spring, S. American Nurses Association (2015). Nursing: Scope and Standards of Practice, (3rd edition).

Starr M, Chalmers I. The evolution of the Cochrane Library, 1988–2003. http://siivola.org/markku/krit/jarkytyksen_jalkipuinti_Cochrane_history.pdf. Published 2003. Accessed October 25, 2017.

Stetler CB. Updating the Stetler Model of research utilization to facilitate evidence-based practice. *Nurs Outlook.* 2001;49(6): 272–279.

Stevens KR. Critically appraising knowledge for clinical decision making. In Melnyk BM, Fineout E, eds. *Evidence-based practice in nursing & healthcare: A guide to best practice.* 3rd ed. Philadelphia, PA: Wolters Kluwer; 2015.

Sullivan-Bolyai S, Knafl K, Tamborlane, W, Grey M. Parents' reflections on managing their children's diabetes with insulin pumps. *J Nurs Scholarsh.* 2004;36(4):316–323.

Teeling Smith G, Wells N, eds. *Medicines for the year 2000.* A symposium held at the Royal College of Physicians, September 1978, by the Office of Health Economics. London: Office of Health Economics. https://www.ohe.org/publications/medicines-year-2000.

Caring-Based Nursing
The Science

The march of professionally educated nurses onto the panoramic scene in the nation's health services re-defines the boundaries of nursing practice.... Inter-professional collaboration is imbued with the essence of conjoined learning to provide a higher degree of service than could be offered by one profession.

–Martha E. Rogers: *Reveille in Nursing.* Philadelphia, PA: F.A. Davis: 1964: 77.

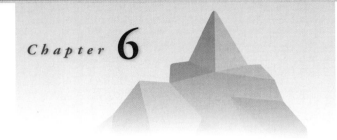

Chapter **6**

Common Neurological Complaints

Jill E. Winland-Brown, EdD, APRN, FNP-BC

Sarah Horn, MD

Michael B. Keller, MD

CONFUSION

Confusion is not a disease process or disease state but rather a symptom. *Confusion* is an inability to think quickly or coherently. A confused patient may be disoriented to time, place, or person and usually demonstrates impairment of cognitive functioning. It is usually demonstrated by inappropriate reactions to environmental stimuli, may arise suddenly or gradually, and may be either temporary or irreversible. Stressful events, lack of sleep or food, or sensory deprivation may precipitate confusion. Age is not a reliable predictor; however, older adults are most at risk because of polypharmacy (multiple prescription drugs), the aging process, preexisting dementia, and the presence of chronic disease.

DIFFERENTIAL DIAGNOSIS

Confusion is a key sign of neurologic disorders. The clinician must be diligent in determining its cause. The physical examination will provide clues. One major difficulty lies in differentiating symptoms of delirium from dementia. The clinician must establish whether the patient has delirium, a delirium superimposed on another condition such as Alzheimer's disease (AD), or another neurocognitive disorder apart from delirium, such as dementia. Once the disease has been identified and treatment started, the symptom of confusion may disappear. Differential diagnoses for confusion involve almost all body systems (Fig. 6.1).

Dementia

Dementia is a decline in mental functioning, affecting memory, cognition, language, and personality. An acute transient disturbance in thought process is a result of delirium, whereas persistent or more severe confusion, with or without psychomotor hyperactivity characterized by a significant time span between symptom appearance and death, defines dementia. Clinically significant confusion states in older patients may lead the practitioner to suspect dementias such as AD; multi-infarct dementia as a result of cerebrovascular accident (CVA)—vascular dementia; depression, which can cause dementia; or excessive consumption of alcohol or drugs, which can also cause dementia. (AD and CVA are discussed in Chapters 8 and 9.) Estimates from the *Healthy People 2020* report state that the prevalence of dementia among people older than 70 years of age is almost 15%. In individuals older than age 90, this number rises to almost 40%. The direct and indirect costs of dementia are an estimated $159 to $15 billion (Office of Disease Prevention and Health Promotion, 2017).

The Diagnostic and Statistical Manual of Mental Disorders (fifth edition; American Psychiatric Association, 2013) defines dementia as significant cognitive impairment that represents a significant decline from a previous level of functioning. Cognitive impairment refers to a decline in at least one of the following cognitive domains: language, executive function, attention, perceptual-motor function, social cognition, learning, and memory. The disturbance must interfere with independence in everyday activities and not be better accounted for by another neurocognitive disorder.

The history and physical examination, along with diagnostic studies, may reveal the presence of a medical condition or drug toxicity. Screening with the tools listed in Table 6.1 should be followed by a comprehensive neurologic examination along with laboratory and diagnostic tests to rule out any reversible causes of dementia.

Treatment for dementia is disease specific. Treatment of AD consists of both pharmacologic and nonpharmacologic measures. Pharmacologic therapy consists primarily of *N*-methyl-D-aspartate (NMDA).

NMDA receptor antagonists (memantine) and cholinesterase inhibitors (such as donepezil and rivastigmine) are both used to treat dementia. These agents appear to be most useful for moderate to severe AD;

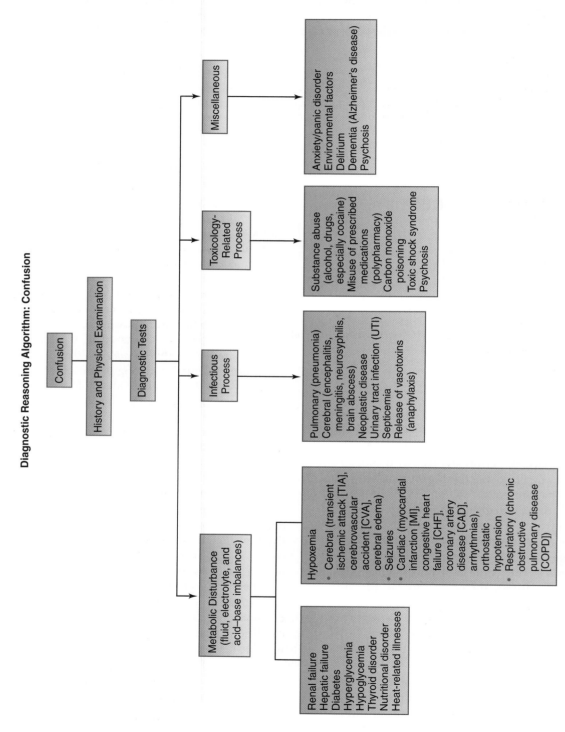

Figure 6.1 Diagnostic reasoning algorithm: confusion.

TABLE 6.1	**Delirium Versus Dementia**	
	Delirium (Acute Delusional State)	*Dementia (Chronic)*
Onset	Abrupt onset over a short period of time—days to weeks	Slowly evident over months or years
Timing	Confusion fluctuates throughout the day	Subtle decline
Duration	Hours to weeks	Months to years
Causes	Cerebral event Organic brain syndrome Distended bladder, constipation Sensory deprivation (poor eyesight/poor hearing) Fever, infection—sepsis, glomerulonephritis, chronic kidney disease Actively dying Polypharmacy Adverse reaction/abrupt withdrawal of a medication, serotonin syndrome Alcohol withdrawal delirium Hypoxemia Metabolic (thyroid function or organ failure) Stroke	Alzheimer's disease Lewy body dementia Parkinson's disease Vascular dementia Motor neuron disease Potentially reversible conditions: Medications Metabolic/endocrine disorders Trauma Infections Nutritional deficiencies Poisoning
Symptoms	Hallmark—inattention (73%) Sleep–wake cycle disturbance (73%) Memory problems Psychomotor retardation (37%) Agitation (27%) Perceptual disturbances and hallucinations (26%) Language disturbance (25%)	Subtle short-term memory changes Moderate: Multicognitive deficits—aphasia, apraxia, agnosia, impairment of occupational and social functioning A failing sense of direction Being repetitive Struggling to adapt to change *Severe:* Incontinence, inability to perform ADLs, inability to speak more than six intelligible words in a day, progressive weight loss of 10% of body weight in the past 6 months
Screening tools	MMSE MOTYB screening tool CAM	SLUMS MoCA AD8 informant interview MC-FAQ MMSE: 24 early dementia 12–24 intermediate dementia <12 severe dementia FAST: score of 7—admit to hospice Clock-drawing test
Treatment	Stabilize the environment; glasses or hearing aids if sensory deprivation; antipsychotics (haloperidol, chlorpromazine) if sedation is desired; for long-term prescription—risperidone, olanzapine for sedation	*Nonpharmacologic interventions:* Behavior management Caregiver intervention programs Cognitive stimulation Reality orientation therapy Recreational activities *Pharmacologic interventions:* Cholinesterase inhibitors Antidepressants Antipsychotics

Continued

TABLE 6.1	**Delirium Versus Dementia—cont'd**	
	Delirium (Acute Delusional State)	*Dementia (Chronic)*
Prevention/ help	Avoid illness—health-promotion efforts Avoid alcohol Decrease number of medications Normalize environment Check eyeglass prescription Use hearing aids if needed	No sure way to prevent dementia; support families in ways to assist the client's brain to stay healthy longer (e.g., being physically and socially active, mind exercises) Reduce blood pressure; reduce homocysteine and cholesterol levels; control diabetes mellitus; healthy diet; cease smoking; being current on vaccines

Abbreviations: ADLs, activities of daily living; CAM, confusion assessment method; FAST, FAST Functional Assessment Staging; MC-FAQ, Mini-Cog with Functional Assessment Questionnaire; MMSE, Mini-Mental State Examination; MoCA, Montreal Cognitive Assessment; MOTB, months of the year backwards; SLUMS, St. Louis University.

Sources: Alzheimer's Association. Delirium or dementia—do you know the difference? http://www.alz.org/norcal/in_my_community_17590.asp. Accessed May 5, 2014); Blazer DG, van Nieuwenhuizen AO. Evidence for the diagnostic criteria of delirium. *Curr Opin Psychiatry.* 2012;25(3):239–243; Medscape. Delirium and dementia at the end of life. http://www.medscape.org/viewarticle/499458. Accessed May 5, 2014.

the combination of both memantine and donepezil may be more effective than either alone. Nonpharmacologic measures include cognitive rehabilitation, exercise, and occupational therapy. Antipsychotic drugs such as haloperidol (Haldol), quetiapine (Seroquel), risperidone (Risperdal), olanzapine (Zyprexa), and aripiprazole (Abilify) continue to be used to treat agitation and aggression, but there is limited evidence of clinical benefit. Caution must be taken as to the risks of increased cerebrovascular events. Risperidone is the only recommended antipsychotic and should only be used for 3 months. Carbamazepine (Tegretol) is an anticonvulsant that may control impulsivity and aggression. Patients with panic disorders may respond to lorazepam (Ativan) or oxazepam (Serax). Referral to a specialist may help in treatment of agitation and confusion. Management goals for the family and caregivers should be supportive, specific, and consistent.

Delirium

Delirium is sometimes called an acute confusional state. The clinician must distinguish between delirium and dementia when evaluating confusion in the older adult. Patients with a history of dementia have a higher incidence of delirium, whereas delirium may also exist as a state by itself without any evidence of dementia. See Table 6.1 for the differences between delirium and dementia. They do, however, share common characteristics and causes. Once the cause of the delirium is corrected, the patient should return to his or her previous state of cognitive functioning.

There are many screening tools with varying degrees of sensitivity and specificity to detect cognitive changes that may be used to aid the clinician in the first step toward an accurate diagnosis (see Table 6.1). It is helpful to use the same tool at each visit for consistency in monitoring the patient's mental functioning.

Metabolic Disturbances

Fluid, electrolyte, and acid–base imbalances may be the result of metabolic problems, which can alter a patient's level of consciousness, producing confusion. The extent of the imbalance determines the severity of the patient's confusion. Typically, the patient is dehydrated and has poor skin turgor, dry skin, and a low-grade fever. Additional signs and symptoms such as dizziness, confusion, altered level of consciousness, hypotension, and coma, along with an extensive history and physical examination, will usually lead the clinician to a diagnosis. Routine laboratory tests, including electrolytes, urinalysis, chest x-ray examination, and electrocardiogram (ECG), may be performed. Treatment should be focused on restoration of appropriate fluid and electrolyte balance by specific correction of the primary metabolic disorder.

Infectious Process

Confusion may also be the result of an infectious process that can cause extensive tissue and organ impairment through the release of toxins. If the infectious process is allowed to continue, ischemia often occurs, producing cell injury and death. Severe generalized infections (such as septicemia or bacteremia) can produce symptoms suggestive of delirium, whereas infections that affect the nervous system (such as meningitis) cause confusion, headache, and nuchal rigidity. Specific signs and symptoms of infections include fever, tachycardia, tachypnea, decreased blood pressure, confusion, and irritability. Diagnostic studies should include routine tests and those associated with the suspected infectious agent. Treatment should focus on managing the primary cause of the infection.

Tissue Hypoxia and Ischemia

Cardiovascular disorders can cause confusion as a result of tissue hypoxia and ischemia. Confusion may be insidious and may come and go. The patient typically appears ill and has significant changes in vital signs (decreased blood pressure, elevated and/or irregular pulse, and tachypnea), edema, cyanosis, reduced level of consciousness, confusion, severe headache, agitation, vomiting, and motor deficits. Diagnostic examinations should include routine laboratory testing, arterial blood gases, chest x-ray, and ECG. Treatment depends on the problem or disease identified.

Neoplastic diseases that cause confusion include systemic cancers and intracranial lesions to the brain, secondary to the extensive tissue and organ destruction caused by the invading cancer. Signs and symptoms depend on the areas of the body where the cancer is located. Extensive cerebral edema, compression, and cell injury produce ischemic states and result in cell and tissue death. This destruction impairs the circulation, increases intracranial pressure, and results in confusion, headaches, disorientation, tremors, seizures, memory loss, gait disturbances, dehydration, changes in levels of consciousness, vomiting, and sensory and motor deficits. Diagnostic studies should include basic routine tests. Additional studies and treatment measures will vary depending on the type of cancer.

DIZZINESS AND VERTIGO

Dizziness and vertigo are often used synonymously, but they do not have the same meaning. *Dizziness* is the sensation of unsteadiness or feeling off balance, faintness, light-headedness, and a feeling of movement within the head. Loss of consciousness rarely occurs, but the feeling of faintness encourages the patient to lie down, which may cause the feelings to disappear. *Vertigo* is the false sensation of rotation or movement of the patient or the patient's surroundings. Vertigo may result from an inner ear disease or a disturbance of the vestibular center or pathway in the central nervous system (CNS).

It is important to distinguish between vertigo and dizziness. Episodes of dizziness are brief and may be mild or severe, with an abrupt or gradual onset. Both dizziness and vertigo may be accompanied by nausea, vomiting, nystagmus, and unsteady gait. Dizziness occurs as a result of inadequate blood flow and oxygen supply to the brain and spinal cord. If other neurologic symptoms occur, such as numbness or facial, arm, or leg weakness, it is more suggestive of a brainstem problem.

DIFFERENTIAL DIAGNOSIS

Differential diagnoses of dizziness are classified into four categories: peripheral vestibular disease, systemic disorders, CNS disorders, and anxiety states. The history and physical examination are essential to pinpoint a diagnosis (Fig. 6.2). Key questions to ask a patient regarding dizziness include duration, severity, and nature of the episodes and any associated symptoms such as hearing loss and weakness. Key points to assess include physical examination of the ear to rule out cerumen impaction or otitis media; hearing tests, including whisper, Weber, and Rinne; a thorough neurologic assessment; and the Hallpike maneuver to distinguish between benign vertigo and vertigo resulting from a CNS

lesion. The Hallpike maneuver is performed by rotating the patient's head to one side and then lowering it slowly to 30 degrees below the bodyline. The patient should be observed for nystagmus during head rotation and vertical positioning. In patients with benign vertigo, there may be rotational nystagmus and possible severe vertigo, which usually occurs in one direction. This resolves quickly and cannot be reproduced after two to three repetitions. The clinician should suspect a central lesion when the vertical nystagmus is of a longer duration and continues with each repetition.

Peripheral Vestibular Disease

Peripheral vestibular disease accounts for up to 44% of all cases of dizziness and vertigo. Many patients who experience dizziness may have a diseased vestibular nerve. Most often the problem is located in the labyrinth of the middle ear. The problem may be caused by otoliths precipitated in the labyrinth. Signs and symptoms of vestibular disease include dizziness, nausea and vomiting, diaphoresis, difficulty with balance, vertigo, tinnitus, fluctuating hearing loss, feelings of pressure in the ear, and diplopia. Diagnostic studies include audiological evaluation, electronystagmography, magnetic resonance imaging, magnetic resonance angiography, brainstem-evoked responses, and basic laboratory screening as guided by history and physical examination. Antihistamine/anticholinergic medications, such as meclizine (Antivert) or promethazine, are the most commonly prescribed medications for vertigo. These agents suppress the vestibular end-organ receptors and inhibit activation of vagal responses. Patients are instructed to take the medication for a week, then to try to taper the drug slowly. Diamox is used to decrease edema in the labyrinth. Antiemetics should be considered when nausea and vomiting are severe. These agents suppress central vestibular pathways, which activate the vagal stimulus. Prochlorperazine (Compazine) orally (PO) or by suppository or trimethobenzamide (Tigan) PO or by suppository will usually bring relief to the patient. Vestibular exercises can help the patient with the symptoms of vertigo. Exercises are helpful in dislodging the otoliths. They may also help the patient acclimate to the symptoms. Exercises have been shown to decrease the duration of vertigo or produce longer symptom-free periods. The patient is instructed to reproduce the feelings of vertigo by placing the affected ear down, then assume a supine position and hold that position until the vertigo disappears. The vertigo may return when the patient sits up. The patient should repeat these maneuvers at least five times a day or until the vertigo no longer returns. Patients with persistent symptoms should be referred for assessment of nerve function. Surgery may be indicated when conservative measures fail to relieve the vertigo.

Systemic Disorders

Systemic disorders may cause dizziness or light-headedness. Patients typically complain of light-headedness or feelings

Diagnostic Reasoning Algorithm: Dizziness and Vertigo

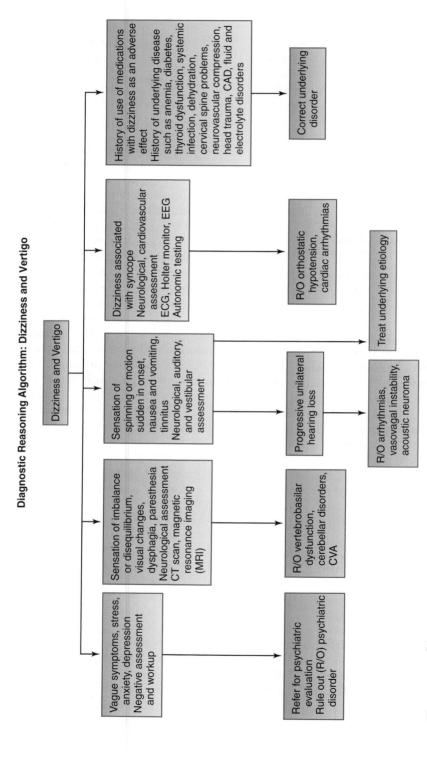

Figure 6.2 Diagnostic reasoning algorithm: dizziness and vertigo.

that they are about to faint or pass out. Dizziness may be aggravated by postural changes or exertion. Pallor, dyspnea, tachycardia, bounding pulse, weakness, hypotension, blurred vision, decreased breath sounds, headache, diaphoresis, and agitation suggest systemic problems. These symptoms should prompt the practitioner to look for signs of anemia, cardiovascular disease, hyperventilation, drug reactions, endocrine disorders, fluid and electrolyte imbalances, and psychiatric problems. Systemic diseases require diagnostic examination and treatment that is specific for the cause of the dizziness.

Central Nervous System Disorders

CNS disorders that disrupt the pathway between the vestibular apparatus and the brain may cause dizziness. Facial numbness, hemiparesis, diplopia, dysarthria, headache, nausea, and vomiting are some common signs and symptoms suggesting CNS dysfunction. Diagnostic examination and treatment depend on the underlying disorder.

HEADACHE

One of the most common of all human ailments is thought to be the headache. A headache is a pain or ache in the head that sometimes restricts activity, reduces the level of functioning, and decreases work performance. The prevalence of headaches has a great impact on society because of lost or reduced effectiveness at home, work, or school. Individual burdens result from pain and the disabling effects of various headache syndromes. About 90% of all headaches are without pathologic cause. Practitioners need to avoid underestimating the significance of headache as an early manifestation of serious neurologic disease.

Headaches may be classified into two general categories: primary and secondary headaches. Primary headaches include tension-type headaches, migraines, and cluster headaches. Table 6.2 presents a comparison of these three categories of headaches. Secondary headaches are a symptom of an injury or an underlying illness. Types of headaches are as follows:

- *Tension-type headache*, also referred to as a muscle contraction headache, presents as a mild to moderate bilateral, nonpulsating, tightening pain that is not aggravated by routine physical activity. It is usually not accompanied by nausea and vomiting or photophobia.
- *Migraine headache* may last for 4 to 72 hours and may or may not be precipitated by an aura. It is usually unilateral, of moderate to severe intensity with a pulsating quality, aggravated by routine physical activity, and accompanied by nausea, vomiting, and photophobia.
- *Cluster headache* usually occurs at night and may last from 15 to 180 minutes. There is usually severe

TABLE 6.2 **Primary Headaches: A Comparison of the Different Types**			
Type	*Tension-Type Headache*	*Migraine*	*Cluster*
Signs and symptoms	Nausea and vomiting Bilateral pressure or bandlike pain	Unilateral pulsating episodic pain Nausea and vomiting Photophobia and phonophobia	Periorbital nighttime unilateral nonpulsatile pain Photophobia Tearing Nasal stuffiness
History and physical examination findings	Sleep cycle disturbances Social stressors Neck arthritis Neck muscle spasm	May be similar	May be similar
Diagnostic tests	MRI: rule out lesions, hemorrhage, cerebral venous sinus thrombosis, etc. CT: rule out hemorrhage LP: measure opening pressure, rule out meningitis	Same	Same
Treatment	Support Biofeedback Stress management Massage Drugs: aspirin, acetaminophen (Tylenol), NSAIDs, muscle relaxants Preventive treatment	Avoidance education Drugs: Abortive: triptans, NSAIDs, antiemetics Prophylactic: propranolol, nortriptyline, topiramate	100% oxygen by mask, sumatriptan, indomethacin

Abbreviations: CT, computed tomography; LP, lumbar puncture MRI, magnetic resonance imaging.

unilateral orbital, supraorbital, and/or temporal pain that is accompanied on the same side of the face with sweating, lacrimation, nasal congestion, ptosis, rhinorrhea, eyelid edema, and/or conjunctival injection.

The Headache Classification Committee of the International Headache Society has a headache classification system and operational diagnostic criteria for the different headache syndromes. This system was designed to describe and identify headaches to allow for more accurate diagnosis and research. For primary headaches other than migraine, there are four subgoups: exertional headache, headaches associated with direct physical stimuli, epicranial headaches, and other hypnic (a sleep-related headache that occurs in the elderly) headaches.

Migraine has two major subtypes: migraine with aura and migraine without aura. The diagnosis of migraine with aura must include the presence of one or more of the following fully reversible neurologic symptoms: visual, motor, sensory, speech, brainstem, or retinal. The symptoms of an aura typically develop gradually and are usually followed by a headache. Auras are fully reversible and last 5 to 60 minutes. For migraine without aura, two of the following characteristics are required: unilateral location, pulsating quality, moderate to severe intensity, and exacerbation by physical activity. In addition, at least one of the following must be present: nausea or vomiting, photophobia, or phonophobia. Chronic migraines are classified as those that occur on at least 15 days of the month for more than 3 months.

EPIDEMIOLOGY AND CAUSES

More individuals complain about headaches than any other condition experienced, and they affect anyone of any age. Each year, approximately 45 million individuals complain of headaches, and more than 8 million individuals of all ages visit a health-care provider with this complaint annually, with the incidence decreasing with age. In the United States, some researchers estimate the annual cost of headaches, including costs of direct medical care and lost productivity, to exceed $17 billion. Women are two to three times more likely to be affected than men across all age-groups, with the incidence in women increasing during adolescence and peaking at menopause.

Tension-type headache is a highly prevalent condition that can be disabling. It is the most common type of headache, with an estimated 80% to 90% of the population experiencing tension headaches at some period in their lives. It occurs more often in women (86%) than in men (65%). Its prevalence peaks at about age 30 to 38. Tension headache occurs more frequently in whites (40%), especially with increasing educational levels (48%). Although few people with tension-type headaches lose time from work, more than 40% of people affected reported decreased effectiveness at work, home,

or school because of this type of headache. These muscle contraction headaches may either be primary (without underlying pathology) or secondary (the result of pathology such as trauma, infection, arthritis, or tumor).

Migraine headaches are the second most common type of headache with high prevalence and socioeconomic impacts. The *Global Burden of Disease Survey 2010* (Martelletti et al., 2013) ranks migraine as the third most prevalent disorder with the seventh highest specific cause of disability in the world. Racial differences in migraine prevalence are striking: African Americans and nonwhites of Hispanic or other nonspecified ethnic origin are at least twice as likely as whites or Asians to be migraine sufferers. An inverse relationship exists between migraine and age. Prevalence of migraine is highest in adults younger than age 40 and lowest in those older than age 60. Migraine headaches occur in 4% to 5% of school-age children. It is not unusual for migraine headaches to begin during childhood between ages 5 and 8 years. Migraine syndromes are painful and often disabling, accounting for a loss of more than 157 million workdays to headache pain each year. About 5 million persons in the United States have at least one migraine attack per month. Moderate to severe disability is claimed by more than 11 million persons with migraines. In one study of patients who met the International Headache Society criteria for migraine, fewer than half had actually received a diagnosis of migraine.

Migraine headaches are often hereditary and in women, often can be traced to hormonal shifts. In familial migraine headaches, the cause is associated with mutations in calcium-channel genes. The causes of menstrual migraine are explained by hormonal fluctuations and typically occur around the time of menstruation. Decreasing estrogen levels can trigger a migraine that is either endogenously or exogenously induced (e.g., by a week-off [21-day] oral contraceptive pill or by hormonal replacement therapy).

There are multiple and varied precipitating factors or "triggers" of migraine headaches. A migraine headache may occur shortly after or just before a period of stress. One type of migraine, sometimes known as an exertional migraine, is associated with strenuous physical activity, but in general, women who exercise regularly are less likely to get migraines or at least experience them with less severity. Some sports, however, may precipitate a headache, resulting in common phrases such as "swimmer's migraine" or "runner's headache." Weight lifting, cycling, and hockey have been identified as other possible culprits. Researchers believe that the relationship between exercise and sports activities and migraine is associated with increased pressure on the head or a strained neck muscle. Physical activity at high altitudes is another factor that may trigger a migraine between 6 hours and 4 days after arrival. Other factors associated with exercise may be an inadequate warm-up or dehydration. Certain foods containing tyramine or phenylethylamine are known triggers of migraine. These vasoactive substances cause both vasodilation and vasoconstriction of the cerebral vessels. Examples of vasodilator agents include alcohol and sodium nitrate. Sodium nitrate is used as a preservative and is present in processed meats and food coloring. Vasoconstrictor agents, on the other hand, stimulate the release of noradrenalin and adrenalin, causing vascular constriction of the cerebral vessels. Caffeine—either consumption or withdrawal—can trigger migraines. Although consuming smaller amounts of coffee may protect a person from a headache, sudden caffeine withdrawal may trigger a migraine because of rebound vasodilation. Monosodium glutamate can also produce a migraine. Eighty-five percent of individuals report some sort of trigger that will kick off their headache. Box 6.1 presents common triggers of migraine headaches.

Cluster headaches fall under the category of trigeminal autonomic cephalalgias, which are a group of primary headache disorders associated with severe, unilateral head pain accompanied by ipsilateral autonomic symptoms. Cluster headaches are named for their pattern of occurrence: they usually come in groups (clusters) over the span of several weeks or months, then disappear for months or even years. Cluster headaches are one of the most painful types of headaches. They typically occur in middle-aged men, with the first onset between ages 20 and 30, and typically cluster on a seasonal basis, with anywhere from 3 to 18 months between headaches. Approximately 69 out of 100,000 individuals have cluster headaches. A dysfunction of the hypothalamus may account for the periodicity and clocklike regularity of cluster headaches.

Older adults have fewer headaches overall. However, when an older adult presents with a new-onset headache, suspicion should be high for an underlying systemic disease such as temporal arteritis or intracranial lesion. These headaches require immediate medical evaluation.

Temporal arteritis or giant cell arteritis (GCA) affects men and women equally and occurs predominantly in adults older than age 60. Its incidence increases with age and is rare in the young. Associated symptoms include scalp allodynia, jaw claudication, and concurrent polymyalgia rheumatica. Other symptoms are local swelling; tenderness and pulselessness of the temporal artery; and systemic symptoms of fever, anorexia, weight loss, and chills. Systemic markers of inflammation also are present. Prompt diagnosis is important since temporal arteritis can cause permanent vision loss if left untreated.

A "thunderclap headache" is an abrupt and severe, sudden onset headache that reaches maximal intensity in under 1 minute. This type of headache requires emergent evaluation since it is often caused by a subarachnoid hemorrhage. The headache from subarachnoid hemorrhage commonly occurs from a ruptured intracranial aneurysm, such as a "berry" aneurysm or dissecting arterial aneurysm of the carotid or vertebral vessels. A berry aneurysm, or berry-shaped aneurysm, results from a congenital abnormality of intracranial vessels, primarily at the circle of Willis. Ruptured intracranial aneurysms are the primary cause of subarachnoid hemorrhage. Less often, a subarachnoid hemorrhage is caused by an atrioventricular malformation (AVM) or bleeding disorder. An AVM is a congenital disorder that results in the formation of a tangled collection of dilated arteries and veins. Symptoms are usually seen in persons aged 20 to 40 years. Two-thirds of people affected by a subarachnoid hemorrhage are aged 40 to 60 years; women are affected slightly more frequently. In the United States, 10 to 15 cases occur per 100,000 population per year. Activities such as lifting, straining, sexual intercourse, or emotional excitement can precipitate a hemorrhage.

The headache from a subdural hematoma is of venous origin, typically resulting from a head injury that is usually mild and easily forgotten by the patient. It occurs predominantly in persons older than age 50 and is more common in men. Alcohol abuse and use of anticoagulants

---

Box 6.1 Common Triggers of Migraine Headaches

Hormonal

- Low estrogen level, increased prostaglandin level

Environmental

- High-pitched noises, excessive sun, bright lights, weather changes, strong odors, video display terminals

Diet

- Vasodilating agents: alcohol, sodium nitrate
- Vasoconstricting agents: caffeine, tyramine (bananas, ripe cheese, nuts, pods of broad beans [Italian pole, lima, or butter beans]), chicken livers, yogurt, avocado, sour cream

Phenylethylamine

- Some cheeses, red wine, chocolate

Monosodium glutamate

- Chinese food, canned soups, frozen dinners

Artificial sweeteners
Lifestyle

- Stress, sports, swimming, cycling, hockey, weight lifting, running, inadequate warm-ups

Physical activity at high altitudes

- Cycling, climbing, skiing

Fatigue
Changes in sleep schedule

- Excessive sleep, too little sleep

Cigarette smoking
Dehydration

contribute to its occurrence. It rarely is associated with a fractured skull.

Arterial dissection, although occurring infrequently in young adults, is characterized by cephalic pain or headache of sudden onset, often preceding transient ischemic attack (TIA) or stroke symptoms. Carotid or vertebral artery dissection causes acute unilateral neck pain that is sudden and often radiates to the ipsilateral face or eye. The headache is related to cervical manipulation, sustained exertion, or trauma. Recognition and proper treatment are important since arterial dissections can lead to stroke.

Increased intracranial pressure causes headaches that worsen with lying flat, bending over, or with the Valsalva maneuver. There may be an associated cranial nerve VI palsy, pulsatile tinnitus, or transient visual obscuration, including a graying out of vision, typically with position changes. Funduscopic examination reveals papilledema. Idiopathic intracranial hypertension (pseudotumor) is a common cause, although it is a diagnosis of exclusion after mass lesion, cerebral venous sinus thrombosis, and meningitis are ruled out. Proper diagnosis of cerebral venous sinus thrombosis is important since it can lead to life-threatening infarcts and brain hemorrhage. Common causes associated with this type of thrombosis are pregnancy and oral contraceptive use. In meningeal irritation, headache is often the most prominent feature, along with photophobia, pain with eye movement, neck stiffness, and positive Brudzinski and Kernig signs. Encephalitis is associated with a new-onset generalized headache, accompanied by confusion, altered level of consciousness, focal neurologic signs, or seizures. Signs of infection and meningismus may be present. Changes associated with these conditions can be detected with lumbar puncture (LP) and brain imaging.

PATHOPHYSIOLOGY

Inside the skull, only certain structures are sensitive to pain; these include the meninges, arteries, and skull. The brain parenchyma itself is not pain sensitive. Increased pressure on and inflammation of the meninges, as well as distention of or traction on the arteries, will cause pain. Head trauma usually causes headaches through all these pain-inducing mechanisms.

Besides head trauma, many other medical problems can initiate a headache secondarily—strokes (ischemic and hemorrhagic); intracranial infections; tumors; metabolic disorders (hypercapnia, hypoglycemia, and hypoxia); sudden hypertension; changes in intracranial pressure; drugs and drug withdrawal syndrome; cranial nerve pain; and eye, ear, nose, sinus, teeth, and jaw disorders. The primary headache syndromes—chronic tension-type headaches, migraine headaches, and cluster headaches—are those in which the headache is the primary problem.

Pain signals are transmitted from most structures in the head by branches of the trigeminal nerve (Fig. 6.3), although pain from the back of the head and the posterior fossa of the skull are transmitted by branches of the first three cervical spinal nerves. First-order pain fibers from these nerves synapse in the brainstem and upper spinal cord, and from there, the second-order pain fibers project to sensory nuclei in the thalamus. Regardless of its cause, headache pain is the result of activating these trigeminothalamic and cervicothalamic pain circuits.

Primary headache syndromes, however, are not caused only by the normal activation of trigeminal or cervical pain receptors inside the skull. In addition, primary headache syndromes require hypersensitization of the trigeminothalamic or cervicothalamic circuitry at one or

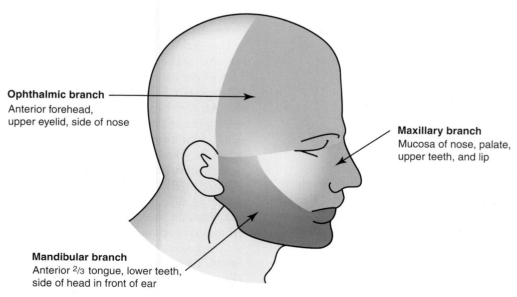

Ophthalmic branch
Anterior forehead,
upper eyelid, side of nose

Maxillary branch
Mucosa of nose, palate,
upper teeth, and lip

Mandibular branch
Anterior 2/3 tongue, lower teeth,
side of head in front of ear

Figure 6.3 The three branches of the trigeminal nerve.

more points along their route from the primary afferent axons to the thalamic sensory nuclei.

One part of this circuitry on which many headache studies have focused is the thalamus. When pain stimuli pass through the thalamus, the signals are modulated by serotonergic axons coming from the dorsal raphe nuclei in the midbrain. It is thought that an abnormal reduction in serotonergic activity in the thalamus is a part of the hypersensitization in primary headache syndromes. Among the observations consistent with this idea are the following:

- Serotonin agonists (ergotamine, dihydroergotamine, and triptans) can reduce the pain and frequency of migraines and can reduce the duration and frequency of cluster headaches.
- Increasing the effectiveness of serotonergic synapses with a selective serotonin reuptake inhibitor can reduce the frequency of tension-type headaches.
- Reserpine, a drug that depletes CNS synapses of serotonin, can precipitate migraine headaches.

Chronic Tension-Type Headaches

Chronic tension-type headaches produce mild to moderate pain that feels like a constant, bilateral head tightness and that lasts from a half hour to a week. These headaches do not pulsate, do not cause nausea, and usually are not made worse by physical activity. Chronic tension-type headaches occur repeatedly (typically many times a month), have a gradual onset during the day, and are more common in people with depression.

Although patients with chronic tension-type headaches have muscle tenderness, their headaches do not appear to be caused by unusual muscle tension or contraction. Instead, in patients with this type of primary headache, the head and neck pain circuitry is hypersensitized so that normal stimuli and typical muscle strains lead to headaches. The basic cause of the hypersensitization is not known, although it is thought that chronic tension-type headaches result from abnormalities in the serotonin, norepinephrine, or dopamine pathways that originate in the brainstem and that modulate the trigeminothalamic or cervicothalamic pain circuits.

Migraine Headaches

Migraine headaches produce moderate to severe unilateral pain lasting from 4 hours to 3 days. These headaches throb, cause nausea, and are made worse by activity. Migraine headaches happen repeatedly (typically one to three times per month) and can be triggered by certain stimuli, most commonly alcohol, stress, menstruation, or diet.

Migraine headaches occur as a set of events that unfold in a predictable pattern. First, there is a prodrome, which begins hours or days before the headache. The prodrome is often a psychological change—it can be drowsiness, depression, euphoria, hyperactivity, difficulty concentrating, irritability, or increased sensitivity to noises, lights, or smells. The prodrome is thought to reflect disturbances in the hypothalamic-limbic system.

Following the prodrome, patients with migraine experience a unilateral throbbing headache, which is accompanied by anorexia and nausea (with vomiting in one-third of cases) and by a heightened sensitivity to noises, lights, and smells. The basis for the pain is a hypersensitized trigeminothalamic circuit, which makes the normally innocuous pulsing of cerebral blood flow feel painful. The hypersensitivity can affect all trigeminal nerve stimuli on the same side of the head, so that normal pressures (caused by, e.g., combing, shaving, taking a shower, or wearing glasses or earrings) on the skin of the face and scalp also feel painful.

In an experimental model, migraine-like headaches can be initiated by electrical stimulation of areas in the midbrain. In this region, focal stimuli set off a cascade of specific reactions including an increase in local blood flow and a hypersensitization of the trigeminothalamic pain circuits.

In the less common type of migraine (migraine with aura), the headache is preceded by sensory phenomena called an aura. An aura is usually either a set of patterns in the visual fields or a sequence of strange feelings moving from the hand, up the arm, and onto the face. The aura coincides with a slowly spreading wave of chemical and metabolic changes that moves across the cerebral cortex from initial foci in the occipital lobe(s). As the wave reaches a region, it briefly activates the local neurons and increases the local blood flow. After the wave passes, the neurons are refractory and the local blood flow decreased. It is thought that this wave contributes to the hypersensitization of the trigeminothalamic circuits and that the wave also elicits the headache pain that follows the aura. Experimentally, it has been found that agents that reduce migraine headaches (specifically, the adrenergic agonist norepinephrine, the alpha$_2$-agonist clonidine, and the beta blocker propranolol) also stop or slow this wave of cortical depression.

Like individuals with epilepsy, patients with migraine headaches have cortical neurons that are permanently hyperexcitable. Between migraine attacks, migraine patients experience other headaches with unusual frequency, and they can get headaches and perceptual distortions from minor visual stresses such as patterns of glare. The neuronal hyperexcitability underlying this continuous sensitivity can be inherited, and there are indications that it is due to abnormalities in certain ion channels in nerve cell membranes.

Cluster Headaches

Cluster headaches cause severe unilateral pain behind the eye or temple lasting from 30 minutes to longer than 1 hour. The pain is constant, deep, and piercing and can radiate to the forehead, neck, or shoulder. These headaches do not pulsate and do not cause nausea, and they usually do now worsen with physical activity. The pain may be accompanied by eye or nose symptoms, such as tearing, swollen conjunctivae, runny nose, nasal congestion, eyelid droop, eyelid edema, facial sweating, or pupillary constriction. Cluster headaches come in groups that last 2 to 3 months. During one of these periods, headaches can occur as often as eight per day or as few as one every other day. Typically, a patient has one or two clusters of headaches per year.

Cluster headaches appear to be triggered by an abnormality in the ipsilateral circadian pacemaker, which is located in the ventral hypothalamus. The headache pain is caused by a hypersensitized ophthalmic nerve (the ophthalmic branch of the trigeminal nerve). The autonomic symptoms are caused by concurrent excitation of parasympathetic fibers running with the ophthalmic nerve. It is not known what causes these nerve problems.

CLINICAL PRESENTATION

Subjective

Patients with episodic tension headaches rarely seek health care. Patients with chronic tension headaches who present with symptoms of anxiety and depression often do not attribute their headaches to these symptoms. The astute clinician can relate patients' subjective comments to the stress and anxiety that they are experiencing in their lives and help each patient to attribute his or her headache to that cause, thereby encouraging patients to seek treatment for the underlying stress, anxiety, and/or depression.

Forty percent of all patients with muscle contraction headaches have a positive family history of headaches. Any headache that is abrupt, explosive, severe, and described as the worst headache of the patient's life is suggestive of a traction or inflammatory headache and is most often due to intracranial hemorrhage, a medical emergency.

Two basic types of migraine headaches occur: those with aura and those without. A typical migraine without aura (previously called "common migraine") is often unilateral (60%) but may become generalized. The headache lasts 2 to 72 hours or longer and is of pulsating quality. Most patients describe the pain as intense, throbbing, or pulsating. It is moderate to severe in intensity, inhibiting or prohibiting daily activities. It can be aggravated by routine physical activity and is often relieved by sleep. During the attack, nausea and vomiting, photophobia, and phonophobia are common. Adults often experience both photophobia and phonophobia, whereas children are more likely to have one or the other.

In migraine with aura (previously called "classic migraine"), the aura develops over minutes and usually lasts less than an hour. It is typically followed by a headache, although the headache may also start before or at the same time as the aura. Patients typically have one or more symptoms associated with the aura that are characteristically cortical in nature. Visual symptoms are the most common and include scotoma (blind spots), photopsia (flashing lights), and fortification spectra (zigzag pattern). Complex auras can cause focal neurologic signs such has hemiplegia, paresthesias, or aphasia. The aura phase may include additional symptoms of euphoria or depression, fatigue, hunger, and hyperosmia.

Migraine attacks may occur sporadically, with just a few headaches per year, or may be more frequent, with eight or more occurrences each month. Other symptoms may be associated with migraines, such as anorexia, constipation, pallor, dizziness, tremors, or diaphoresis. Some patients complain of cold hands or feet or experience polyuria, hunger, diarrhea, or body aches following the migraine.

The patient with a headache from a subarachnoid hemorrhage presents with a sudden, abrupt, and unrelenting headache. Associated symptoms include nausea and vomiting, photophobia, and decreased level of consciousness. With small "warning leak" hemorrhages, the patient may complain of severe hemifacial pain spreading to the neck or back. The headache may have begun after exercise or intercourse.

Objective

Careful attention to the patient's history is essential, including the headache's onset, location, character, and severity; frequency and duration; associated signs and symptoms; prodromal symptoms; precipitating factors; an association with sleep patterns; emotional factors and the patient's family and social history. Information should be sought regarding other family members who suffer from headaches, the type of headache, and the age at occurrence (Fig. 6.4). This information is essential to delineate the diagnosis and rule out other problems.

Patients with migraines usually have a parent who also has from migraines. Information regarding the age at onset with migraines is also important because migraine frequently starts before age 20. A social history may elicit stressors or precipitating factors for the headache. Identifying the possible precipitating factors for the migraine can assist the practitioner in developing an individual prescription plan to decrease the severity or frequency of the attacks. The patient's lifestyle, dietary habits, possible job-related stress, and environmental factors should be explored. Practitioners may consider postponing a complete medical history to a pain-free period for the patient once serious disorders have been ruled out. The final step of the medical history is obtaining a record of all previous work-ups and past treatments performed, including their effectiveness.

In women, information should be sought regarding the relationship of the migraine to the menstrual cycle. Headaches usually occur after ovulation and before and during menstruation. Migraines that occur before menses are considered premenstrual and associated with premenstrual syndrome. Women are more likely to have their first migraine in the year of menarche and often cease to have

Diagnostic Reasoning Algorithm: Headache

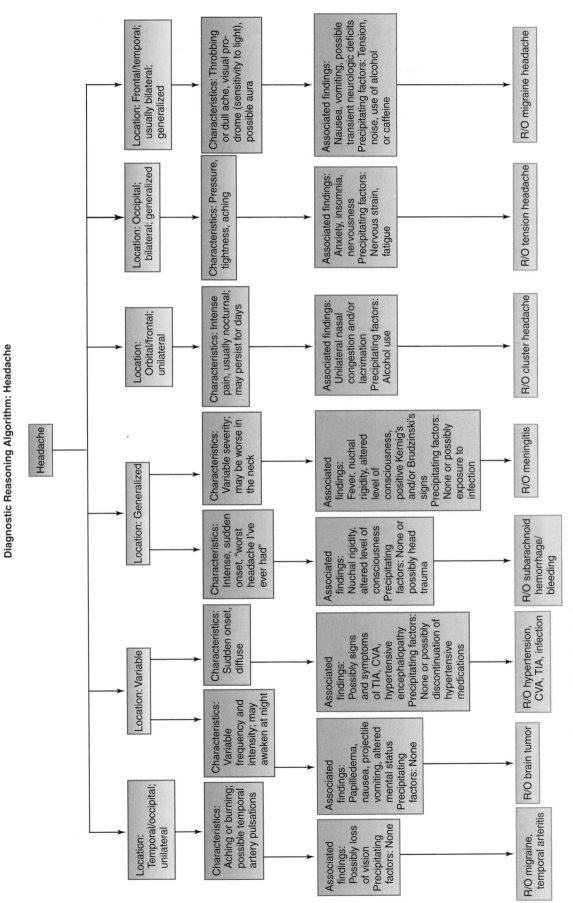

Figure 6.4 Diagnostic reasoning algorithm: headache.

migraine headaches during pregnancy. The use of oral contraceptive pills or hormonal replacement therapy should be explored. Initial menstrual cycles in patients starting hormonal medications are characterized by unstable blood estrogen concentrations. The use of hormonal medications for the first time may precipitate a migraine or cause migraines to increase in frequency or to be preceded by auras. Most women with migraines do not experience an aura. For women who do experience an aura, the use of any combined hormonal contraceptive is contraindicated due to a threefold increase in the risk of ischemic stroke (Curtis et al., 2016).

In contrast to migraine, the patient with a cluster headache experiences severe, unilateral, orbital, supraorbital, or temporal pain lasting 15 minutes to 3 hours. The pain is most commonly sharp and burning in quality. Frequently, the headache occurs at night, awakening the patient. No aura is present, and nausea and vomiting are rare. Attacks commonly occur in "clusters" or groups and can last up to several weeks or even months. Often, one of the following signs can be demonstrated on the affected side: conjunctival injection, miosis, ptosis and eyelid edema, nasal congestion, rhinorrhea, and forehead and/or facial sweating.

Physical findings associated with a headache resulting from a subarachnoid hemorrhage are visual blurring, diplopia, fever, alteration of consciousness, nuchal rigidity, and focal neurologic signs.

A headache is frequently seen in patients with GCA. The intensity of headache in GCA can be severe with the quality of the pain described as deep, burning, and throbbing. A symptom specific to temporal arteritis is "claudication" of the muscles of mastication. Because of ischemia of the muscles, the patient complains of pain in the jaw on prolonged chewing. Localized tenderness of the affected artery is often found. The practitioner should be alert to the potential complication of blindness. Diplopia is a common sign preceding visual impairment. Once visual impairment occurs, however, it can progress quickly to blindness in several hours. On physical examination, few abnormalities are revealed. A low-grade fever may appear. The temporal arteries may be tender and more visible or pronounced on palpation but have absent or decreased palpations.

The single most commonly occurring symptom with a subdural hematoma is headache. It is subacute and usually progresses. Characteristically, this secondary headache is generalized and worsens with changes in posture. It can occur during the night and may cause the patient to awaken in the morning earlier than usual. Associated symptoms are nausea, vomiting, confusion, seizures, or weakness. The practitioner should be alert to changes in personality, decreasing level of consciousness, excessive sleepiness, or sensory changes. Less common findings are focal neurologic signs, such as hemiparesis or pathological reflexes. Papilledema rarely occurs because of the large volume of cerebrospinal fluid.

DIAGNOSTIC REASONING

Diagnostic Tests

A computed tomography (CT) scan or an magnetic resonance imaging (MRI) study is recommended if the patient's headache pattern is atypical, has changed in pattern or character, or is accompanied by seizures, personality changes, or an abnormal neurologic finding. Patients with migraines commonly have normal physical findings between attacks. Extensive diagnostic testing for a patient with a migraine is not warranted. A complete blood count (CBC), chemistry profile, and urinalysis may be obtained to rule out systemic illness in the patient with typical migraine with no change in pattern and a normal physical examination. Nonspecific electroencephalogram (EEG) abnormalities can occur; however, some of these findings are normal and others often do not require treatment. An EEG is not useful in the routine evaluation of a patient with a headache and is not recommended to exclude a structural cause for headache. Neither a CT scan nor an MRI is warranted in adult patients whose headaches fit within the broad definition of tension or migraine headache and who have not demonstrated any recent substantial change in headache pattern, occurrence of seizures, or presence of focal neurologic signs or symptoms.

In an older adult patient with late-onset migraines, brain imaging is recommended to exclude secondary causes of migraine, or "symptomatic migraine." In older adults, a good indication of the need for imaging studies is an unusual presentation or change in symptoms from the patient's typical headaches.

Physical examination of patients with cluster headaches usually reveals normal physical findings. If there has been no change in the pattern or pain of the cluster headache and a normal physical examination is found, a CBC, chemical profile, and urinalysis may be completed to rule out a systemic illness.

Headaches from a subarachnoid hemorrhage should be identified quickly and an immediate CT scan performed. In some patients with a small hemorrhage, the result may be negative. The benefit from the CT scan diminishes with time; that is, there is less sensitivity if the scan is obtained more than 7 days after headache onset. If the results are positive, an immediate neurosurgical referral is initiated. If the CT scan is negative and suspicion remains high, an LP may be performed.

With GCA, the erythrocyte sedimentation rate (ESR) may be strongly elevated, from 50 mm to more than 100 mm. C-reactive protein (CRP) may also be elevated. Levels of both ESR and CRP may be normal and should not be used alone to rule out GCA. In this case, referral is essential, and a biopsy of the temporal artery (the gold standard) is recommended. Other laboratory findings may include anemia and an elevated alkaline phosphatase level.

A subdural hemorrhage is best evaluated by CT, which has a greater sensitivity to early hemorrhage. The CT reveals the bleeding as hyperdense, isodense, or hypodense depending on the chronicity. If bleeding is isodense, there may be a shift of midline structures without any further evidence of abnormalities on CT, in which case MRI may be used to determine if a hematoma is present.

Differential Diagnosis

A complete history is paramount to distinguish and diagnose headaches and to rule out life-threatening events, such as subarachnoid hemorrhage or meningitis. Patients may have more than one type of headache, so each event must be identified. A thorough history should be taken, including family, social, and medical history. A family history may reveal migraine headaches in other family members. A social history may identify stress or other precipitating factors for the headache. A general medical history, including a review of systems, may lead to a diagnosis other than migraine headache. The clinician should explore any recent or past history of head or neck traumas and previous medical procedures contributing to a headache, such as LP, spinal anesthesia, or surgeries. After an LP, for example, a bilateral headache may develop over the next few days. It typically worsens upon standing and is relieved when the patient is recumbent. Possible causes of headache might be related to current medical conditions, especially hypothyroidism, hypertension, and asthma. Identifying current medications, both prescription and over-the-counter (OTC) agents, help in distinguishing the headache. Chronic daily headaches are frequently associated with the daily use of nonprescription pain relievers, including NSAIDs, acetaminophen, and compounds containing caffeine.

Sudden onset of pain may suggest serious pathology such as subarachnoid hemorrhage, meningitis, or brain tumor. A headache that has been present over a period of years is more likely to be from a primary headache disorder such as migraine, cluster, or tension-type headaches. The character of pain in migraines also is helpful in distinguishing a migraine headache from a tension-type headache. A tension-type headache is dull and nonpulsating; it changes in intensity. Its duration may be 30 minutes to 7 days, and it is not associated with nausea or vomiting. Although tension-type headaches may limit some activities, they are generally not aggravated by physical activity and do not incapacitate the individual.

Testing should include motor and sensory function testing to detect serious organic disease. A diagnosis of migraines with aura requires the presence of one or more fully recoverable neurologic symptoms (visual, motor, or sensory). This finding helps the practitioner distinguish migraine from a progressive, organic disorder that requires further assessment. Migraine aura must be differentiated from a TIA, which causes neurologic symptoms that are rapid in onset as opposed to the slowly evolving symptoms of migraine aura. Differentiating a migraine with aura from a TIA may be difficult. Age, for instance, may play a role in the differential diagnosis because a TIA is rare in the young. Migraine aura also tends to cause "positive" symptoms (e.g., extra sensations) such as flashing lights or tingling, in contrast to a TIA, which tends to cause "negative" symptoms (e.g., loss of sensation), such as numbness or visual field cut.

Red flags indicative of secondary problems include the following:

- Progressive or fundamental change in headache that worsens over time
- Patient states, "This is the worst headache of my life!"
- New-onset headaches before the age of 5 or after age 50
- Persistent headache precipitated by a Valsalva maneuver, exertion, or sex
- Fever, acute glaucoma, hypertension, myalgias, weight loss, or scalp tenderness
- Neurologic signs and symptoms: confusion, altered level of consciousness, changes in memory, papilledema, sensory deficits, reflex asymmetry, or gait disturbances
- Headache with syncope or seizures

MANAGEMENT

Immediate hospitalization is required for the person with a severe (secondary) headache occurring suddenly or with signs of meningeal irritation. A patient who states that he or she is having "the worst headache of my life" is a red flag. Possible causes are intracranial hemorrhage or meningeal infection. If examination reveals evidence of symptoms or signs of increased intracranial pressure or severe intractable migraine, urgent hospitalization is indicated.

Because the majority of headaches (tension-type and migraines) can be recurrent and chronic, the principle of management is to design an individual treatment plan that identifies therapeutic goals for the patient. Goals should include strategies to avoid possible triggers and the ability to abort an attack, to obtain relief from pain and associated symptoms, and to decrease the frequency and severity of attacks.

Management for a tension-type headache is focused on the use of NSAIDs, cool compresses, and stress-reduction techniques. NSAIDs and acetaminophen are recommended for acute treatment in patients with tension-type headache. Drug therapy for acute headache should generally not exceed more than 2 days per week on a regular basis. More frequent treatment may result in medication-overuse chronic daily headaches.

Migraine treatment can be divided into abortive, prophylactic, and nonpharmacologic treatment. Nonpharmacologic measures are useful for minor migraines or as an adjunct to pharmacologic treatment to prevent or decrease the severity of a headache. These methods include identifying and eliminating known triggers. Maintaining a strict schedule for sleep and meals can prevent a headache related to fatigue and hunger. If exercise precipitates an attack, an adequate warm-up before working out is recommended. Biofeedback, relaxation techniques, and regular aerobic exercise are encouraged. Deep breathing, massage, and hot or cold therapy sometimes ease the pain, but excessive cold (e.g., ice packs) or caffeine can backfire.

Most migraine attacks vary in the effect on the patient's ability to function. In mild attacks, the effect is minimal. In moderate attacks, visual activities are moderately impaired. In severe attacks, however, the patient is unable to continue normal activities or can continue them only with severe discomfort. In some severe attacks, the patient is incapacitated, often requiring treatment in the provider's office, urgent care setting, or emergency department.

Drug therapy should be added when these measures are not completely effective. Early abortive treatment of migraines with effective medications improves a variety of outcomes, including duration, severity, and associated disability. It is appropriate for the clinician to take

a trial-and-error approach to identify medications most successful in the relief of headaches and associated symptoms with the fewest adverse effects and minimal costs and a return to normal functioning for each patient. Some patients may require a combination of medications, such as a triptan as an abortive medication and a daily preventive medication. NSAIDs are a common first-line abortive treatment for patients with migraine. Triptans are also a commonly prescribed abortive migraine treatment. Drugs Commonly Prescribed 6.1 and Complementary Therapies 6.1 present a list of medications commonly used to treat migraines and complementary therapies that may to help treat headaches.

First-line treatment for the relief of acute attacks of cluster headaches includes subcutaneous injection of sumatriptan or intranasal zolmitriptan is recommended. Oxygen inhalation is highly effective for cluster headaches when administered at the beginning of an attack

Drugs Commonly Prescribed 6.1: Migraine Headache: Adults

DRUG	ADVERSE REACTIONS AND PRESCRIBING CONSIDERATIONS
Abortive	
Triptans (serotonin receptor agonists)	
Almotriptan (Axert) Eletriptan (Relpax) Frovatriptan (Frova) Naratriptan (Amerge) Rizatriptan (Maxalt) Sumatriptan (Imitrex, Alsuma) Naratriptan (Amerge) Zolmitriptan (Zomig)	Side effects: paresthesias, asthenia, nausea, dizziness, chest or neck tightness, heaviness, somnolence. Contraindicated in ischemic heart disease or other significant cardiovascular disease or cerebrovascular disease. There is a risk of rebound headache if triptans are used more than twice a week. Imitrex is also available as an injection and nasal spray.
Ergot derivatives	
Ergotamine 1 mg/caffeine 100 mg (Cafergot) Ergotamine 2 mg/caffeine 100 mg (Cafergot supp) Dihydroergotamine (DHE 45, Migranal)	Contraindicated in peripheral vascular disease, coronary heart disease, hypertension, and hepatic or renal disease. Intravenous route preferred when rapid relief is desired. Migranal is a nasal spray.
Antiemetics Metoclopramide Prochlorperazine	Adverse effects: extrapyramidal side effects, fatigue, restlessness, sedation, dizziness.
NSAIDs Ibuprofen (Advil, Motrin) ASA (aspirin) Naproxen sodium (Aleve, Naprosyn)	For mild to moderate pain. Increased risk of gastrointestinal (GI) bleed with alcohol. Adverse reactions: GI upset, GI bleed
Combination analgesics Butalbital 50 mg/acetaminophen 325 mg/ caffeine 40 mg (Fioricet) Butalbital 50 mg/ASA 325 mg/caffeine 40 mg (Fiorinal)	For tension or muscle contraction headache. Potentiation with alcohol. Adverse effects: drowsiness, dizziness, GI disturbances. Use of butalbital-containing medications is not recommended as first-line treatment for migraine headaches; avoid if possible.
Opiates Morphine Oxycodone	Adverse effects: sedation, respiratory failure, constipation, addiction. Use of opiates is not recommended as first-line treatment for migraine headaches; avoid if possible.

Drugs Commonly Prescribed 6.1: Migraine Headache: Adults—cont'd

DRUG	ADVERSE REACTIONS AND PRESCRIBING CONSIDERATIONS
Prophylactic Medications	
Beta blockers	Preferred if patient is hypertensive or has angina
Propranolol (Inderal) Timolol (Blocadren)	Contraindicated in asthma, sinus bradycardia, second or third atrioventricular block Potentiated by alcohol
Metoprolol (Lopressor, Toprol)	May cause weight loss, asthenia, mental fuzziness
Atenolol (Tenormin) Nadolol (Corgard) ***Antidepressants*** Venlafaxine (Effexor XR) Nortriptyline Amitriptyline	
Calcium channel blockers Verapamil (Calan)	May take several months to be effective Contraindicated in pregnancy Adverse effects: extrapyramidal effects, bradycardia, fatigue, weight gain, constipation, nausea, edema, muscle pain
Anticonvulsant agents Topiramate (Topamax) Gabapentin (Neurontin)	Adverse effects: dizziness, somnolence, tremor, weight gain, teratogenic effects, paresthesias, kidney stones Adverse effects: Somnolence, dizziness, asthenia. Preferred for patients with seizure disorders or diabetic peripheral neuropathy.

Complementary Therapies 6.1: Headaches

Acupuncture/acupressure
  Aroma and herbal therapy

- Apply lavender oil to the temples (women).
- Apply peppermint oil to the temples (men).
- Use eucalyptus for sinus headaches.
- Drink rosemary tea or mix the essential oil in hot water and inhale.
- Take evening primrose oil 500 mg.
- Apply cold black tea bags to the eyes for 15 minutes.
- Take *Ginkgo biloba* 120–240 mg of dried extract in two to three doses daily.
- Take valerian *(Valeriana officinalis)* 2–3 g one to three times per day.

  Biofeedback
  Diet therapy

- At the first sign of a migraine, drink one to two cups of strong coffee to prevent vessel dilation (effective for some individuals) or a glass of carrot or celery juice.
- To reduce throbbing and contractions, eat foods high in magnesium such as dark, leafy greens, fresh seafood, sea vegetables, nuts, whole grains, and molasses.
- Eat vitamin C–rich foods such as broccoli, hot and bell peppers, sprouts, cherries, citrus.
- Drink green tea.
- Avoid foods known to trigger headache: additive and chemical-based foods (monosodium glutamate, sulfites [red wine], condiments, nitrates [aged and smoked meats]; pickled fish and shellfish; caffeine-containing foods, including chocolate; cultured foods [e.g., yogurt]; refined sweeteners); red meats;

dairy products (cheese); soft drinks (the phosphorus binds up magnesium); alcohol; salty, sugary, and wheat-based foods.
  Exercise
  Massage

- Massage the temples for 5 minutes.
- Do 10 neck rolls.
- Pull ear lobes for 5 seconds.
- Rub back of ear and all around ear shell.
- Apply an ice pack to the back of the neck to reduce vasodilation or put feet in a cold water bath.
  Poultices
- Rub capsaicin (Zostrix) cream on the forehead.
- Apply onion or horseradish poultices to the nape of the neck or soles of the feet.
  Reflexology
- Apply pressure to the inside base of the foot and big toe three times for 10 seconds each.
  Relaxation therapy
- Perform deep breathing.
  Vitamin therapy
- Take magnesium citrate 800 mg daily.
- Take niacin 100–500 mg daily.
  Other
- Avoid smoking and secondhand smoke.
- Taking a coffee enema may relieve the migraine.

with a nonrebreathing facial mask at 7 to 15 L/min. Most patients will obtain relief within 15 minutes.

FOLLOW-UP AND REFERRAL

A neurologic referral should be considered for any patient with episodes of transient neurologic deficits, increasing frequency and severity of unilateral headaches, or atypical auras, as well as changes in personality, excessive sleepiness, and new onset of progressive deficits suggesting a mass lesion, hemorrhage, or structural disorder. GCA must be carefully considered in a middle-aged or older patient who presents with a new and unexplained headache. Surgical referral may be necessary for a temporal artery biopsy and definitive diagnosis or possible use of chronic steroid therapy.

Patient Education: Migraine Headache

The management of migraine is a team effort in which the patient plays an equal role. Patients must be convinced of the practitioner's interest in their complaints and commitment to their treatment. Realistic outcomes should be discussed because treatment is often ineffective or can be used for only a short period of time. Patients should be educated about the nature of migraine and given additional literature. Patients should keep a diary of any events that may be associated with an attack. This helps to identify and avoid triggers associated with a single episode and distinguish them from triggers that lead to an increase in the frequency and severity of attacks. Although clinicians may not help patients deal with endogenous triggers (e.g., endocrine factors, genetic tendencies, and psychological depression), they may help the patient identify other triggers. Exogenous triggers include foods, for example, red wine and other alcoholic beverages, aged cheese, monosodium glutamate, aspartame (dietary sweetener), and chocolate; the frequency and pattern of light; and oral contraceptives. Environmental triggers include stress and stressful family events, air travel, weather changes, odors (bad and good), and meteorological depression. Having an awareness of the triggers may help the patient avoid them, which should diminish the frequency and intensity of the attacks. The clinician should explain the importance of warming up before exercise and avoiding tight-fitting goggles, sunglasses, helmets, or other headgear and suggest that regular exercise may prevent or decrease the headaches. If exercise is found to trigger an attack, discuss the importance of adequate nutrition and fluids before and after such activities.

Women who have migraines with aura have a higher risk of stroke with the use of estrogen-containing contraceptives compared with those without migraine. Alternative forms of birth control should be used. When discussing migraine therapy with women of childbearing age, the clinician should ask what method of birth control the individual is using.

Stress-management strategies and relaxation techniques are commonly taught to patients to manage frequently unavoidable family- or work-related stress and emotional problems. When pharmacologic treatment is necessary, the family should fully understand the treatment. Impaired judgment may occur with severe attacks, and the patient may not remember what drugs or dosages were used. The patient should understand each medication type, its proper use, and adverse effects of the medications, including interactions with other medications and any contraindications, such as pregnancy. The patient should be asked to record in a headache diary the medications used (including any OTC or other medications), dosages, response to medication, and evaluation of treatment, including adverse effects. Clinicians should advise patients not to take headache medications other than those prescribed. Excessive use of other analgesics may reduce their effectiveness. Using triptans and analgesics frequently can lead to rebound headaches or chronic daily headaches. Adverse effects are common, and the patient must keep the practitioner informed in case changes in medicine are needed. Patients should discuss with the practitioner if they desire to become or are pregnant.

PARESTHESIA AND PARESIS

Paresthesia is an abnormal sensation described as numbness or tingling, cramping, or pain without a known stimulus, felt along peripheral nerve pathways. *Paresis* is weakness. It may be local to a single extremity or the face, or it may involve more than one extremity. Paresis may develop suddenly or gradually and may be permanent or transient. Feelings associated with paresthesia are annoying "pins and needles" sensations that often cause the patient to touch or rub the affected area. Paresthesia is a common complaint, especially in patients with certain systemic diseases or those taking certain medications.

DIFFERENTIAL DIAGNOSIS

Paresthesia is usually due to damage or irritation to the parietal lobe, thalamus, spinothalamic tract, or the spinal or peripheral nerves that are the usual pathways for transmission and interpretation of sensory stimuli. It is important to explore the symptom of paresthesia by asking the patient to describe when it first began; the character, duration, and distribution of the paresthesia; and any other associated signs and symptoms such as sensory or motor loss. A medical history may reveal neurologic, cardiac, vascular, endocrine, renal, or inflammatory diseases the patient may have had or still has. Recent trauma, surgery, or invasive procedures may reveal possible causes of peripheral nerve injury. The physical examination should focus on the neurologic system, assessing level of consciousness; cranial nerve function; reflexes; motor strength; and touch, pain, and temperature sensations. Skin color and the quality of all pulses should also be noted. If the patient has diabetes, symptoms of diabetic neuropathy such as a bilateral loss of pain sensation and diminished touch, temperature sensation, and proprioception may be present. They may present in a stocking-glove distribution.

The most common diagnoses associated with paresthesia symptoms are arterial occlusion, arteriosclerosis obliterans, nerve entrapment syndrome, neuropathy, TIAs, and herpes zoster (Fig. 6.5).

Arterial occlusion is a surgical emergency. An acute occlusion may be either an arterial embolism or a thrombosis. Immediate embolectomy is the treatment of choice in early emboli in the extremities and is preferably performed within 4 to 6 hours of the embolic event.

Arteriosclerosis obliterans is a disorder that involves the pathologic process of atherosclerosis, which causes progressive narrowing of the arteries with subsequent obstruction of blood flow, resulting in diminished or decreased flow of blood to the legs and feet.

Nerve entrapment syndrome results from compression of a nerve pathway along the root of the nerve, which results in paresthesia or weakness. Trauma causing compartment syndrome or bruising, rheumatoid arthritis, edema, infection, prolonged standing or sitting, and tight clothing can all cause entrapment of the nerve. The compression diminishes blood supply and can result in cellular changes to the nerve pathway.

Neuropathy is usually the result of underlying diseases such as diabetes, renal failure, multiple sclerosis, cancer, collagen disease, vasculitis, thyroid disease, ingestion of toxins, or nutritional deficiency. Afferent nerve fibers conduct impulses from the skin to the brain. Alterations along these nerve pathways because of disease pathology can cause paresthesia. The majority of the diseases listed involve peripheral nerves.

Herpes zoster is caused by the varicella-zoster virus, which causes an acute vesicular eruption in adults, especially in immunocompromised patients. An early symptom of herpes zoster is paresthesia, which occurs as a result of infection, inflammation, and compression along the dermatomal distribution of a spinal nerve.

A TIA is a sudden loss of neurologic function caused by impaired blood flow to the brain. The loss of function can last from a few minutes to 24 hours; after a TIA, normal function returns. If some residual weakness remains, the patient has had a stroke.

TREMORS

Tremors are rhythmic involuntary muscle movements that result from alternate contraction and relaxation of opposing muscle groups. They are typically evident in patients with cerebellar or extrapyramidal disorders. They are also seen as side effects with certain drug regimens. Tremors are sometimes classified into seven groups: physiological, essential, toxic, cerebellar, parkinsonian, resting, and intentional. A *resting tremor* occurs in a relaxed and supported extremity and ends with purposeful movement, whereas an *intentional tremor* occurs when the patient attempts voluntary movement. Essential tremors are typically underreported because many persons do not seek treatment for mild tremors. It is estimated that at least 10 million persons in the United States have essential tremor. As the most common movement disorder, it is apparent in 1 in 20 Americans older than age 40 and 1 in 5 older than age 65. These patients, when they do present, should be referred to a neurologist.

DIFFERENTIAL DIAGNOSIS

A complete history and physical examination are necessary to obtain important subjective data that will provide information on the tremor's characteristics, including duration, onset of action, progression, alleviating factors, and associated symptoms (such as memory loss, agitation, and nausea). It is important to note when the tremor is present (e.g., with rest or activity), what part of the body is affected, whether it is bilateral, and the type of movement produced by the tremor (e.g., flexion or extension, pronation, supination, or pill-rolling). The patient's muscle tone should also be assessed to determine whether it is normal or increased (cogwheel rigidity). The patient's speech, gait, and posture all must be assessed. A thorough drug history is essential, including a list of any OTC drugs the patient is taking. The clinician should note whether the tremors affect the patient's activities of daily living and if there is any history of family members having tremors. A review of systems may disclose a history of endocrine, metabolic, or neurologic disorders. A complete musculoskeletal and neurologic examination must be done to assess range of motion, mental status, strength and sensitivity, cranial nerve function, deep tendon reflexes, and gait. Figure 6.6 presents common differential diagnoses of tremor.

Diagnostic Reasoning Algorithm: Paresthesia and Paresis

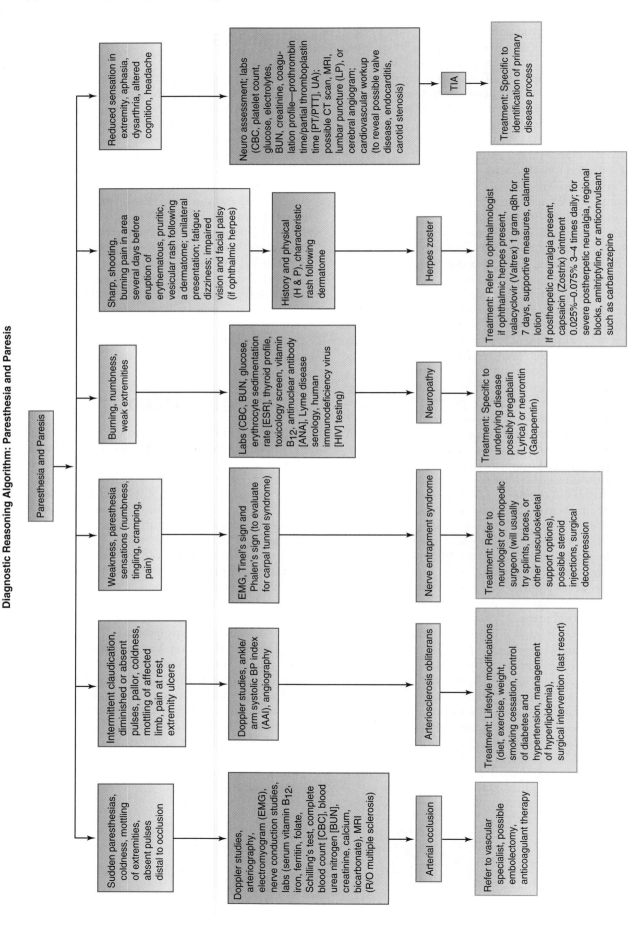

Figure 6.5 Diagnostic reasoning algorithm: paresthesia and paresis.

Diagnostic Reasoning Algorithm: Tremors

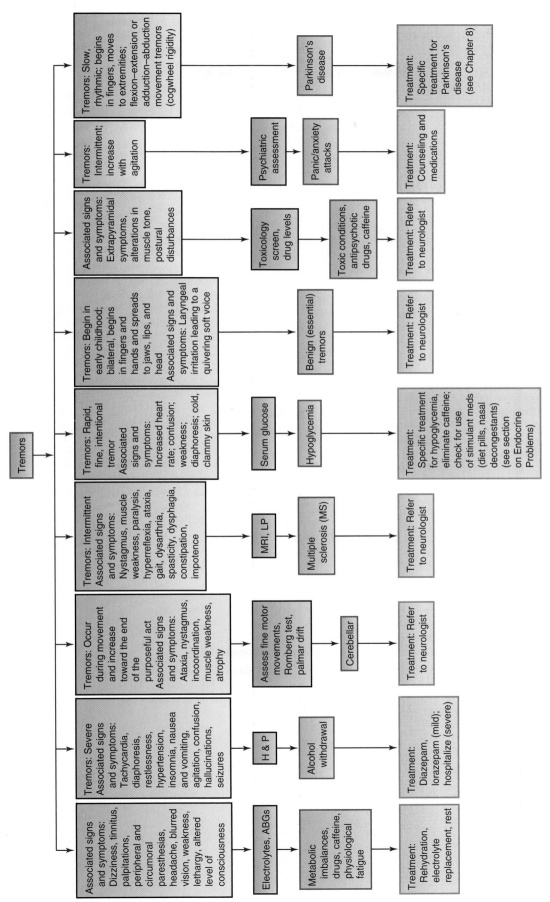

Figure 6.6 Diagnostic reasoning algorithm: tremor.

REFERENCES

Delirium and Dementia

Alzheimer's Association. Delirium or dementia—do you know the difference? http://www.alz.org/norcal/in_my_community_17590.asp. Accessed May 5, 2014.

American Psychiatric Association. *Diagnostic and statistical manual of mental disorders*. Washington, DC: American Psychiatric Association; 2013.

Blazer DG, van Nieuwenhuizen, AO. Evidence for the diagnostic criteria of delirium. *Curr Opin Psychiatry*. 2012;25(3):239–243.

Borson S, Scanlan JM, Chen P, Ganguli M. The Mini-Cog as a screen for dementia: validation in a population-based sample. *J Am Geriatr Soc*. 2003;51(10):1451–1454.

Clevenger, CK. Memory maker: Clinical management of early and midstage dementia. *Adv NPs PAs*. 2012;3(9):14–17.

Corbett A, Burns A, Ballard C. Don't use antipsychotics routinely to treat agitation and aggression in people with dementia. *BMJ*. 2014;349:g6420.

Filippi M, et al.; European Federation of the Neurologic Societies. EFNS task force: The use of neuroimaging in the diagnosis of dementia. *Eur J Neurol*. 2012;19(12):1487–1501.

Halloran L. Cognitive impairment: Pearls for practice. *J Nurse Pract*. 2013;9(4):254–255.

Hendry K, Quinn TJ, Evans J, et al. Evaluation of delirium screening tools in geriatric medical inpatients: a diagnostic test accuracy study. *Age Ageing*. 2016;45(6):832–837.

Medscape. Delirium and dementia at the end of life. http://www.medscape.org/viewarticle/499458. Accessed May 5, 2014.

Montreal Cognitive Assessment. https://www.parkinsons.va.gov/consortium/moca.asp.

Office of Disease Prevention and Health Promotion. Dementias, including Alzheimer's disease. *Healthy People 2020*. https://www.healthypeople.gov/2020/topics-objectives/topic/dementias-including-alzheimers-disease. Accessed February 19, 2017.

Segal-Gida F. Cognitive screening tools. *Clin Rev*. 2013;23(1):12–18.

St. Louis University Mental Status (SLUMS) Exam (SLUMS). http://www.globalrph.com/slumsCalc.htm.

Tariot PN, et al. Memantine treatment in patients with moderate to severe Alzheimer disease already receiving donepezil: A randomized controlled trial. *JAMA*. 2004;291(3):317–324.

Tombaugh TN, McIntyre NJ. The mini-mental state examination: a comprehensive review. *J Am Geriatr Soc*. 1992;40(9):922–935.

Tucci DL. Dizziness and vertigo. Merck manual—professional version. http://www.merckmanuals.com/professional/ear,-nose,-and-throat-disorders/approach-to-the-patient-with-ear-problems/dizziness-and-vertigo#v943820. Published 2016. Accessed February 25, 2017.

University College London (UCL) Institute of Neurology. Queen Square Brain Bank. www.ucl.ac.uk/ion/departments/molecular/themes/neurodegeneration/brainbank. Updated March 22, 2013.

Wei LA, Fearing MA, Sternberg EJ, Inouye SK. The confusion assessment method (CAM): A systematic review of current usage. *J Am Geriatr Soc*. 2008;56(5):823–830.

Headaches

Anderson P. New headache classification system published. The International Headache Congress (IHC). July 3, 2013. http://www.medscape.com/viewarticle/807334#vp_2. Accessed May 11, 2017.

Beithon J, et al. *Diagnosis and treatment of headache*. Bloomington, MN: Institute for Clinical Systems Improvement; 2013.

Curtis KM, Tepper, NK, Jatlaoui, TC, et al. U.S. medical eligibility criteria for contraceptive use, 2016. *MMWR Recomm Rep*. 2016;65(3):1–103.

Hain, TC. Migraine headache in women. http://www.dizziness-and-balance.com/disorders/central/migraine/migraine%20in%20women.html. Published 2016. Accessed July 25, 2017.

Hammond A, Holcomb M. Exploring treatment options for migraine headache. *Clin Advisor*. 2015;18(8):35-43.

Martelletti P, Birbeck GL, Katsarava Z, et al. The Global Burden of Disease survey 2010: Lifting the burden and thinking outside-the-box on headache disorders. *J Headache Pain*. 2013;14(1):13.

McCarthy M. Practical evaluation and treatment of headaches. Lecture presented at Pri-Med. Ft. Lauderdale, FL. February 5, 2017.

Migraine.com. Migraines statistics. https://migraine.com/migraine-statistics/. Published 2010. Accessed May 11, 2017.

Olesen J. International Headache Society classification of headache disorders. 3rd ed. Updated 2016. https://www.ichd-3.org/. Accessed June 29, 2017.

Silberstein SD, Holland S, Freitag F, Dodick DW, Argoff C, Ashman E. Evidence-based guideline update: Pharmacologic treatment for episodic migraine prevention in adults: Report of the Quality Standards Subcommittee of the American Academy of Neurology and the American Headache Society. *Neurology*. 2012;78(17):1337–1345.

RESOURCES

Dementia

Alzheimer's Association
http://www.alz.org

Headache

National Headache Foundation
1-888-NHF-5552
http://www.headaches.org

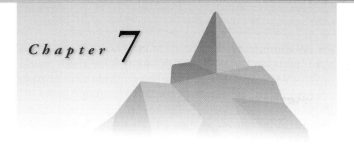

Chapter 7

Seizure Disorders

Jill E. Winland-Brown, EdD, APRN, FNP-BC

Sarah Horn, MD

The term "seizure" refers to a sudden change in behavior caused by abnormal, synonymous electrical activity within the brain. Seizures can be provoked by an underlying medical condition or unprovoked. A provoked seizure may never recur nor require treatment beyond treating the underlying medical condition. Causes of provoked seizures include febrile-related seizure in infancy, trauma, hypoglycemia, hyponatremia, hypocalcemia, drug abuse, and alcohol withdrawal. Provoked seizures are most often generalized tonic-clonic seizures. *Epilepsy*, by definition, is a condition in which an individual is predisposed to seizures and has had two or more unprovoked seizures during their lifetime. Seizure disorders referred to in this chapter include the diagnosis of epilepsy. *Status epilepticus* is defined as a seizure lasting longer than 30 minutes or multiple seizures without return to baseline in a 30-minute period. This is a medical emergency; discussion of management of status epilepticus is beyond the scope of this chapter.

A *seizure* occurs when an abnormal electrical discharge in the brain causes a sudden, involuntary, typically time-limited alteration in behavior. The manifestations of a seizure can be quite varied and relate to the area of the brain affected by the seizure. Seizures can cause the changes in the following functions:

- Motor activity—jerking or stiffening of a limb
- Autonomic function—tachycardia or sweating
- Vision—seeing colored shapes
- Olfaction—smelling strange odors
- Language—aphasia
- Psychological feeling—déjà vu
- Sensation—paresthesias in one area of the body
- Consciousness

Seizures can be focal (affecting just one part of the brain) or generalized (affecting the entire brain). Individuals with epilepsy, however, tend to be have stereotypical seizures; they look the same every time. Figure 7.1 presents the different types of seizures.

Focal onset seizures are those in which the first clinical and electroencephalographic (EEG) changes of the seizure are limited to one part of the cerebral hemisphere. Focal onset seizures are typically caused by an underlying focal lesion or abnormality in the brain that acts as an epileptogenic seizure focus. A seizure focus can lie in any area of the cerebral cortex and thus, different patients' seizures can vary quite dramatically from one another, depending on the area of brain affected. A focal onset seizure is further classified on the basis of whether consciousness is impaired during the attack. There may or may not be motor involvement, such as repetitive and rhythmic jerking or one limb. Focal seizures with impaired awareness, previously called complex partial seizures, are the most common type of seizure in adults with epilepsy. Typically,

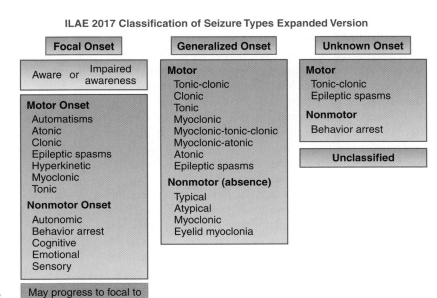

Figure 7.1 International League Against Epilepsy (ILAE) classification of seizure types. Source: *Fisher RS, Cross JH, D'Souza C, et al. Instruction manual for the ILAE 2017 operational classification of seizure types. Epilepsia. 2017;58(4):531–542.*

patients appear awake, although they are not aware of their surroundings and do not respond appropriately to others. These seizures may be associated with repetitive behaviors called automatisms, such as chewing, lip smacking, repeating words, or gestures. Focal seizures with impaired awareness may begin with a focal seizure with preserved awareness, also called a *seizure aura* or a *simple partial seizure*. Focal onset seizures may progress to a generalized seizure, called a *focal to bilateral tonic-clonic* seizure.

Generalized onset seizures are those that begin with generalized abnormal electrical activity. Examples include generalized tonic-clonic, absence, myoclonic, tonic, and atonic seizures. Generalized onset seizures are often associated with childhood onset generalized epilepsy syndromes. Since both hemispheres are involved, consciousness is typically briefly impaired (except in myoclonus). Motor manifestations are bilateral. The EEG shows bilateral and widespread seizure activity in both hemispheres.

An *absence seizure* is a nonmotor seizure that causes a sudden interruption of ongoing activities, typically with a blank stare. If the patient is speaking, speech will be slowed or interrupted; if the patient is walking, he or she will stand transfixed; if eating, the food will be stopped on the way to the mouth. The attack typically lasts a few seconds.

Tonic-clonic seizures, which used to be referred to as *grand mal seizures*, are the most frequently encountered generalized seizures. There is a sudden, tonic stiffening of muscles, often associated with stridor or an ictal cry, and the patient falls to the ground in the tonic state. The patient lies rigid; during this state, tonic contraction inhibits respiration and cyanosis may occur. The tongue may be bitten, and urine may be voided involuntarily. The tonic stage then leads to clonic convulsive movements lasting a variable period of time. At the end of this stage, deep respiration will occur and all muscles will relax. In the postictal period (the stage following a tonic-clonic seizure), the patient will have a depressed level of conscious. The individual frequently goes into a deep sleep and may have a significant headache when awakened. Tonic-clonic seizures may be generalized onset, meaning that the seizure begins as a tonic-clonic seizure, or of focal onset that then progresses to a bilateral tonic-clonic seizure.

Myoclonic jerks are sudden, brief, shock-like contractions, which may be generalized or confined to the face and trunk or to one or more extremities. They may occur predominantly during sleep and are associated with certain generalized epilepsy syndromes.

Atonic seizures cause a sudden loss of muscle control. *Tonic* seizures cause sudden muscle stiffening. Both are also associated with generalized epilepsy syndromes and cause "drop attacks" (sudden falls without warning). These types of seizures typically begin in childhood and can lead to injuries.

Psychogenic nonepileptic seizures (PNES) are paroxysmal seizure-like events that arise from psychological disturbances rather than abnormal electrical brain activity. Up to 80% of PNES are associated with early sexual abuse, especially in females. The previously used term "pseudoseizures" has fallen out of favor in the neurology community. Because these may mimic true seizures, confirming the diagnosis is key. PNES often can be distinguished from epileptic seizures by history and examination during an event, but EEG monitoring usually is required for accurate diagnosis. History may reveal that the events are triggered by stressful events. Features of the seizure-like events may be atypical for epileptic seizures and may include preserved consciousness despite having bilateral motor involvement; lack of response to antiepileptic medications; variation of events over time; nonrhythmic movements; and lack of typical associated features such as incontinence, tongue biting, and postictal period. During a nonepileptic seizure, the EEG will be normal. PNES are often comorbid with epilepsy and can be considered to be a type of conversion disorder. It can cause significant morbidity including repeated hospitalizations and intensive care unit admissions. Typically, psychotherapy and use of psychiatric medications are used to treat this condition.

EPIDEMIOLOGY AND CAUSES

Seizures are common and affect 8% to 10% of people during their lifetime. Each year, approximately 300,000 individuals in the United States seek medical attention because of a first-time seizure, representing an incidence of 120 per 100,000. The majority of patients are younger than age 5 and present with a febrile seizure.

Epilepsy is among the most common neurologic conditions, affecting more than 2.5 million people in the United States, with a cumulative lifetime incidence of approximately 3%. Each year, 50 per 100,000 individuals in the United States are diagnosed with epilepsy, which is approximately 125,000 new cases each year. Although epilepsy may start at any age, the incidence is bimodal with the highest frequency in young children and persons older than age 65.

In most newly diagnosed cases, no specific cause is identified. Many factors have been implicated in the etiology of seizure disorders, such as severe head trauma, central nervous system (CNS) infections, mesial temporal sclerosis, and stroke. Children with brain injury present from birth, such as those with cerebral palsy, have an increased risk of seizures. Children who are intellectually challenged and who may or may not have genetic disorders may have an increased risk for a seizure disorder. When both conditions coexist, 50% or more of patients affected can be expected to develop a seizure disorder by age 20. Although most children with a history of febrile seizures do not develop epilepsy, there is a slight increased risk for developing a seizure disorder during their lives.

Seizure disorders frequently occur in families. The parents, siblings, and offspring of a patient with a seizure disorder are more likely (3%–5%) than the general population to have a seizure as a result of both genetic and environmental causes.

PATHOPHYSIOLOGY

A seizure is an uncontrollable paroxysm caused by abnormal, synchronous, repetitive firing of neurons in the brain. The motor cortex, the hippocampal formation, and the amygdaloid complex are regions that are especially susceptible to seizures.

Many disorders can initiate seizures, including drug overdose (e.g., from antihistamines, cholinesterase inhibitors, methylxanthines, muscarinic agonists, and tricyclic antidepressants), drug withdrawal (e.g., from alcohol, benzodiazepines, barbiturates), head trauma, strokes, degenerative brain diseases, mesial temporal sclerosis, infections, tumors, and developmental brain defects (e.g., cortical dysgenesis and vascular malformations). The common epileptogenic feature of all these disorders is that they can cause populations of brain neurons to become hyperexcitable.

One category of disorders that cause hyperexcitable neurons includes systemic problems—fever, infection, sleep deprivation, and metabolic imbalances (hypocalcemia, hypoglycemia, hyponatremia, and hypoxia). These problems cause ionic changes throughout the body. For example, hyponatremia causes a relative increase in extracellular potassium concentrations systemically. In the CNS, increased extracellular K^+ at the neuron cell membrane lowers the threshold for triggering axon potentials, and for this reason, acute hyponatremia (typically at levels less than 120 mEq/L) leads to seizures.

The excitability of neuron cell membranes is regulated by intramembrane molecular complexes that either actively move molecules from one side to the other (i.e., ion pumps) or control gated ion channels. Genetic defects in the structure of ion pumps or ion channels can cause seizures. Some of the uncommon heritable epilepsies (e.g., *generalized epilepsy with febrile seizures* and *benign familial neonatal convulsions*) are known to be caused by genetic defects in ion channels. It is believed that other heritable seizure disorders are caused by as-yet-unidentified genetic defects in ion pumps or ion channels.

The antiepileptic drugs phenytoin (Dilantin), carbamazepine (Tegretol), and lamotrigine (Lamictal) reduce the hyperexcitability of neuron cell membranes by slowing the activation of sodium channels; ethosuximide (Zarontin) decreases the activity of certain calcium channels.

Much of the excitatory activity throughout the brain occurs via glutamatergic synapses, and increasing the amount or the effect of glutamate in the brain predisposes a person to seizures. Normally, the amount of extracellular glutamate in the brain is minimized by astrocytes, which selectively take up glutamate. Experimental studies have shown that seizures will occur if astrocytes cannot efficiently clear extracellular glutamate from the vicinity of synapses.

Glutamate depolarizes neurons by activating specific receptors that open channels for small cations, such as Na^+ and K^+. These are called *ionotropic receptors*, and the CNS contains at least three different ionotropic glutamate receptors. High brain concentrations of agonists, such as the street drugs cocaine and angel dust (phencyclidine) may induce seizures. These agonists (chemicals) bind to a receptor and activate it to produce a biological response (the seizure).

Much of the inhibitory transmission throughout the brain is via gamma-aminobutyric acid (GABA)ergic synapses. In general, neurons use the neurotransmitter GABA to prevent the spread of abnormal bursts of neuronal discharges. Reducing the availability of GABA predisposes a person to seizures. Drugs that interfere with the synthesis of GABA, such as 3-mercaptopropionic acid, cause seizures. Vitamin B_6 (pyridoxine) is required for the biosynthesis of GABA, and genetic forms of vitamin B_6 deficiency can cause epilepsy. Drugs that interfere with GABA receptors or with GABA binding to receptors can also cause seizures; such drugs include bicuculline, penicillin, and picrotoxin.

GABA agonists have the opposite effect: they counteract a person's tendency to have seizures. Benzodiazepines (e.g., diazepam [Valium], lorazepam [Ativan]) are GABA agonists and are used to treat seizure disorders. Gabapentin (Neurontin) and pregabalin (Lyrica) are drugs that increase GABA. Barbiturates, which potentiate the actions of both GABA and benzodiazepines, are antiepileptic drugs. Likewise, the antiepileptic drugs tiagabine and vigabatrin both work by enhancing GABA-mediated inhibitory the circuitry. Besides the GABAergic pathways, noradrenergic circuits (originating mainly in the reticular formation of the brainstem) also appear to play an antiseizure role, because damage to noradrenergic pathways can predispose a person to seizures.

During a seizure, brain metabolism accelerates in the affected areas. Oxygen consumption, glucose use, and lactate levels increase; free fatty acids are released into the blood; extracellular concentrations of neurotransmitters rise; and cerebral blood flow increases. Between seizures, metabolism in the affected areas drops below normal. Prolonged seizures increase the local transcription of certain genes and the synthesis of certain proteins (although the synthesis of most proteins declines). The abnormal metabolic activities associated with repeated seizures produce long-term changes in brain circuitry that make further seizures more likely, a phenomenon referred to as *kindling*. One reason for controlling epilepsy is to prevent these lasting increases in neural sensitivity.

CLINICAL PRESENTATION

Subjective

The patient may or may not be aware of a seizure. He or she may wake up slightly confused, on the floor, or in a different position. The patient may have been incontinent. If an aura was present at the start of a seizure, the patient may know that a seizure took place.

Objective

In evaluating a presumed seizure, it is important to determine whether the event in question was a seizure or another type of condition that mimics seizure (such as syncope, PNES, or a panic attack). Not all events associated with abnormal body movements are seizures. Some events may be mistaken for seizures on initial presentation, but accurate diagnosis is essential for successful treatment. Careful and detailed history-taking remains the cornerstone of accurate diagnosis of a seizure. Epilepsy is primarily a historical diagnosis; the initial assessment and approach to management is based on the patient's clinical history, especially on an accurate description of the event in question. It is important to ask the patient for a description of the event in chronological order, for example: What circumstances surrounded the seizure? Did any factors bring it on? What did you feel before, during, and after the seizure? These chronological questions may reveal the presence of an aura at the start. The patient also should be asked about the last attack witnessed, the first seizure, presence of risk factors, and provoking factors. The setting in which the attacks occurred may be significant for differential diagnosis. A careful review of the events occurring days before the seizure is important. Points of particular interest include relation of events to the sleep–wake cycle, concurrent infections, or other factors that lower the seizure threshold. It is important to determine if the seizure was provoked by an underlying medical condition, such as alcohol withdrawal. Questions need to be asked to determine whether the patient experienced an aura or other focal feature at onset, which indicates the seizure is probably focal onset. Obtaining a history of the patient's social, behavioral, and cognitive functioning, as well as a previous health history including prior CNS insults (such as trauma, infections, stroke), history of febrile seizures, and family history of seizure disorders or neurologic disorders, is crucial because this may reveal risk factors for the development of epilepsy. History of postictal behaviors should also be elicited; for example, how long did it take to return to normal function?

The physical examination should take into account the interval since the patient's most recent seizure. If the examination is performed within minutes or hours of an attack, the practitioner should look for postictal signs, including confusion, depressed level of consciousness, or Todd's paralysis, which is a transient hemiparesis following some seizures. When the examination is performed after some time has elapsed since the last seizure, the practitioner's main objective is to determine whether there are signs of baseline neurologic dysfunction indicating evidence of a focal brain lesion, favoring a diagnosis of symptomatic epilepsy due to an underlying brain lesion. A full neurologic examination should be performed to evaluate for focal neurologic signs. The examination may also reveal papilledema indicating elevated intracranial pressure or evidence of drug toxicity. A general medical examination should also be performed to detect the presence of a heart arrhythmia or murmur or other abnormalities, which may suggest an alternate diagnosis such as syncope.

DIAGNOSTIC REASONING

Diagnostic Tests

Initial tests should be done to assess for provoking factors and seizure mimics. Tests may include electrocardiogram, complete blood count (CBC) with differential; blood glucose level; serum electrolytes; liver function tests; serum calcium, urinalysis; a drug screen or blood alcohol level, if appropriate; and blood levels to assess target levels if the patient is on antiseizure medications. Serum prolactin, white blood cell count, creatine kinase, and lactate levels assessed soon after a seizure may be elevated, although these findings are nonspecific and are not recommended for the routine evaluation of seizure.

All patients who present with a first-time seizure should have brain imaging, either with a computed tomography (CT) scan or magnetic resonance imaging (MRI) to evaluate for a structural lesion, such as a hemorrhage or tumor, as the cause of the seizure. A brain MRI provides a more detailed view of the brain than CT scan and may reveal more subtle seizure foci, such as mesial temporal sclerosis, that can be missed on CT scan. EEG is helpful in the evaluation of patients with seizures. Between seizures, an EEG can support a diagnosis of epilepsy if epileptiform discharges are present. An EEG also can help differentiate between focal onset and generalized onset epilepsy. A lumbar puncture should be done if a CNS infection is suspected.

Differential Diagnosis

Two of the most common seizure mimics include syncope and PNES. Benign sleep myoclonus, breath-holding spells in children, movement disorders, migraine aura, parasomnias, hemifacial spasm, and tic disorders can also be mistaken for seizures. Additional differential diagnoses are included in Differential Diagnosis 7.1.

MANAGEMENT

The main principle of seizure management is to prevent the recurrence of seizures with anticonvulsant medications while avoiding adverse effects from the drugs. The clinician should refer the patient to a neurologist, who should make the decision to start treatment after a complete review of the risk of further seizures is discussed with the patient. Before initiating treatment, the type of seizure the patient experiences should be identified and classified accordingly. In adults presenting with a first-time unprovoked seizure, the risk of recurrent seizure is greatest in the first 2 years after the seizure (21%–45%). Typically, after a single, isolated seizure, a work-up is

Differential Diagnosis 7.1: Seizures

Type of Disorder	Specific Conditions Associated With Seizure
Cerebrovascular disorders	Transient ischemic attack (carotid artery, vertebrobasilar), cerebrovascular accident (paramedian thalamic nuclei, fusiform gyrus, right parietal lobe), Moyamoya disease
Diencephalic and brainstem disorders	Decorticate and decerebrate posturing, diencephalic attacks, nonepileptic paroxysmal laughter, peduncular hallucinosis, Kleine-Levin syndrome
Headaches	Classic migraine (with aura), basilar artery migraine, cluster headache, chronic paroxysmal hemicrania, icepick headache, trigeminal neuralgia
Infant and pediatric disorders	Jitteriness, shuddering, esophageal reflux (Sandifer's syndrome), breath-holding attacks, alternating hemiplegia
Miscellaneous	Idiopathic drop attacks of older adults, transient global amnesia, flumazenil-responsive recurring stupor, paroxysmal attacks in multiple sclerosis
Movement disorders	Habit spasm, tic, paroxysmal kinesogenic choreoathetosis, paroxysmal dystonia, paroxysmal ataxia, tremor, chorea, segmental dystonia
Nonepileptic myoclonus	Hypnic jerks, myoclonus (spinal, reticular, palatal, essential), myoclonus and asterixis in toxic-metabolic states
Psychiatric disorders	Psychogenic nonepileptic seizures, depersonalization, psychogenic amnesia, psychogenic fugue, panic attacks, hyperventilation anxiety attacks, intermittent explosive disorder (episodic dyscontrol), schizophrenia
Sleep disorders	Pavor nocturnus, jactatio capitis nocturna, confusional arousals, somnambulism, periodic leg movements of sleep or nocturnal myoclonus, sleep apnea syndrome, narcolepsy, other hypersomnias, rapid eye movement behavior disorder
Startle disorders	Startle reaction, startle disease (hyperekplexia), jumping Frenchman, Malay latah, etc.
Syncope disorders	Vasovagal syncope, convulsive syncope, cardiac syncope (Stokes-Adams attack, tachyarrhythmias, prolonged QT syndrome aortic stenosis, hypertrophic cardiomyopathy), orthostatic syncope (idiopathic orthostatic hypotension, Shy-Drager syndrome, autonomic neuropathy), deliberate syncope ("fainting lark"), syncope in specific situations (micturition syncope, tussive syncope, carotid sinus hypersensitivity, glossopharyngeal neuralgia)
Toxic-metabolic or infectious disorders	Alcoholic blackouts, hallucinogens (LSD, mescaline), strychnine and camphor poisoning, tetanus, rabies, hypoglycemia, porphyria, pheochromocytoma, carcinoid syndrome, mastocytosis

done to identify the cause of the seizure, but antiepileptic therapy is usually not required unless the patient experiences recurrent seizure activity or an underlying disorder with a high predisposition to future seizures is revealed. Some structural lesions are clearly associated with recurrent seizures. These include brain tumor and arteriovenous malformation (AVM). When these conditions are diagnosed after a single seizure, patients usually begin pharmacologic treatment; however, a more common situation is one in which the initial evaluation fails to reveal a specific causative factor for the seizure. Then the neurologist must carefully evaluate the risk of subsequent seizures. The choice of antiepileptic therapy must often be individualized for each patient. Choice of therapy is contingent on comorbid conditions, medication interactions, adverse side effects, patient age, and type of seizure.

If the decision to treat is made, accurate identification of the seizure type is helpful in choosing the drug for the best outcome. Drugs Commonly Prescribed 7.1 presents suggested medications based on the different types of seizures. Although it is not a complete list, it includes the more commonly prescribed antiepileptic medications. These can be used as monotherapy or in combination. If a patient has uncontrolled epilepsy requiring multiple antiepileptic drugs, consultation with a neurologist should be considered. Some neurologists choose to begin long-term therapy with anticonvulsant medications after a single seizure in the following situations: if an MRI or EEG shows evidence of a structural lesion such as a brain tumor, AVM, or infection; if there is a history of a seizure disorder in a sibling; or if there is a history of a brain injury or stroke. It is worth noting that in 2008, the Food and Drug Administration issued a warning about a possible increased risk of suicidality linked to antiepileptic drugs. Thus, patients who are taking an antiepileptic drug should be monitored for notable changes in behavior that could indicate new or worsening depression or suicidal thoughts.

Once the appropriate drug has been chosen based on the seizure type, baseline CBC, electrolytes, and liver function tests may be done. Depending on the agent chosen, monitoring of serum drug levels and trending of the laboratory test results also may be done.

Drugs Commonly Prescribed 7.1: Seizure Disorders (Monotherapy Only)

DRUG	INDICATION	ADVERSE REACTIONS AND PRESCRIBING CONSIDERATIONS
Benzodiazepines: Clonazepam (Klonopin), clobazam (Onfi), lorazepam (Ativan), diazepam (Valium)	Focal and generalized onset seizures *Lorazepam and diazepam generally used in the acute setting to abort seizures *Clonazepam and clobazam can be used for chronic epilepsy treatment (although typically not used in monotherapy)	Formulations: PO and IV (lorazepam and diazepam) May cause sedation, fatigue, ataxia, nystagmus, depression, dependence, withdrawal seizures with abrupt discontinuation; potentiates CNS depression with alcohol
Carbamazepine (Tegretol)	Focal onset seizures May worsen generalized onset seizures	Recommended therapeutic range is 4–12 mg/L Formulation: PO Adverse reactions: hyponatremia, nausea, headache, dizziness, sedation, cognitive impairment, leukopenia, weight gain, decreased bone density, rare aplastic anemia, teratogenicity, rash, hepatotoxicity. With elevated levels: blurry vision, double vision, nystagmus, gait unsteadiness, incoordination, tremor Inducer of liver enzymes
Ethosuximide (Zarontin)	Absence seizures	Formulation: PO Adverse reactions: nausea, anorexia, vomiting, diarrhea, dizziness, insomnia, fatigue, behavioral changes, rash, Stevens-Johnson syndrome, headaches, psychosis, depression, hallucinations, thrombocytopenia, rare aplastic anemia
Gabapentin (Neurontin)	Focal onset seizures *May worsen absence and myoclonic seizures	Formulation: PO Adverse events: weight gait, peripheral edema, behavioral changes, dizziness, ataxia
Lacosamide (Vimpat)	Focal onset seizures	Formulations: PO and IV Adverse reactions: PR interval prolongation (obtain baseline and steady-state ECG), dizziness, nausea, vomiting, headache, diplopia, fatigue
Lamotrigine (Lamictal)	Focal and generalized onset seizures	Formulation: PO Adverse reactions: Stevens-Johnson syndrome, rash (requires slow titration to avoid), hepatic and renal failure, disseminated intravascular coagulation, tics, insomnia, dizziness, blurry vision, unsteadiness, diplopia, headache, tremor Note: interaction with valproic acid necessitates lower doses when used in combination
Levetiracetam (Keppra)	Focal and generalized onset seizures	Formulations: PO and IV Adverse reactions: irritability and behavior change, depression, dizziness, somnolence
Oxcarbazepine (Trileptal)	Focal onset seizures *May worsen generalized onset seizures	Formulation: PO Adverse reactions: hyponatremia, rash, drowsiness, headache; high doses can cause dizziness, blurry vision, diplopia, nausea, vomiting, and ataxia
Phenobarbital	Focal or generalized onset seizures *May worsen absence seizures	Formulations: PO and IV Recommended therapeutic range is 15–40 mg/L Adverse reactions: respiratory depression, irritability, folate deficiency, sedation, nystagmus, cognitive function, long-term connective tissue effects, teratogenicity Formulations: IV and PO Inducer of liver enzymes

Drugs Commonly Prescribed 7.1: Seizure Disorders (Monotherapy Only)—cont'd

DRUG	INDICATION	ADVERSE REACTIONS AND PRESCRIBING CONSIDERATIONS
Phenytoin/fosphenytoin (Dilantin)	Focal onset seizures *May worsen absence and myoclonic seizures	Recommended therapeutic range is 10–20 mg/mL Formulations: PO and IV Adverse reactions: ataxia, cognitive effects, incoordination, dysarthria, nystagmus, diplopia, rash, rare Stevens-Johnson syndrome; long-term use can cause gingival hyperplasia, acne, hirsutism, cerebellar atrophy, decreased bone density, anemia, and peripheral neuropathy; hypotension, local reactions, and arrhythmias using IV formulation Inducer of liver enzymes
Topiramate (Topamax, Trokendi XR)	Focal and generalized onset seizures	Formulation: PO Adverse reactions: weight loss, cognitive slowing and language dysfunction, paresthesias, kidney stones, glaucoma, hypohidrosis, metabolic acidosis, fatigue, ataxia, depression, birth defects
Valproic acid (Depakene, Depakote)	Focal and generalized onset seizures	Recommended therapeutic range is 50–100 mcg/mL Formulations: PO and IV May cause depression, hair loss, weight gain, peripheral edema, highest risk of birth defects among anticonvulsants, pancreatitis, thrombocytopenia, coagulopathy, upset stomach, tremor, elevated ammonia, rare severe hepatotoxicity Inhibitor of liver enzymes; interacts with lamotrigine
Zonisamide (Zonegran)	Focal and generalized onset seizures	Recommended therapeutic range is 10–40 mg/L Formulation: PO Adverse reactions: kidney stones, hypohidrosis, irritability, weight loss, photosensitivity, rash, dizziness, nausea, cognitive slowing, rare Stevens-Johnson syndrome, metabolic acidosis; avoid if history of sulfonamide allergy

Abbreviations: CNS, central nervous system; ECG, electrocardiogram; IV, intravenous; PO, by mouth.

Surgery may be performed to treat partial epilepsy. The portion of the brain that triggers the seizure is removed. This is the only potential cure for epilepsy.

FOLLOW-UP AND REFERRAL

If the seizures are controlled, the clinician can monitor the patient routinely for side effects and seizure control. Drug levels are routinely available for some antiepileptics and can be helpful to assess compliance and whether symptoms of toxicity arise. If the seizures are not controlled with adequate doses and levels of the medication, the clinician should refer the patient to a neurologist for a second opinion and possible combination therapy. Patients may be taken off medications after a few years in some types of epilepsy, while other types may require lifelong therapy. If attempting to discontinue antiepileptics, medications should be weaned gradually.

Patient Education: Seizure Disorders

Education about seizure disorders can provide the patient with understanding and a sense of control over the illness. It

is necessary to recognize that to the affected individual, this condition is more than seizures. The patient and his or her family may be overwhelmed by thoughts of disability and impaired quality of life. Such factors as age at onset, duration of seizure activity, frequency, seizure type, associated neurologic abnormalities, and associated environmental factors contribute to the degree of disability in each patient. Education is ongoing and should be constantly reinforced. Patients and their families should be referred to seizure literature available through the Epilepsy Foundation of America as soon as they are diagnosed, because the well-informed patient is the best advocate for his or her own care. Using the Circle of Caring model and coming to know the patient and what matters most to him or her will assist in helping the patient reach his or her highest potential.

Other treatments for refractory epilepsy include the ketogenic diet and vagal nerve stimulator implantation. A diet high in fat and low in carbohydrates has helped reduce the burden of seizures in the pediatric population. Several studies have shown this diet reduces or prevents seizures in some children who could not be controlled by medications alone. A vagal nerve stimulator is an implanted device used in the treatment of patients with refractory epilepsy. These treatments should typically be done in consultation with a neurologist.

Box 7.1 Emergent Care for Seizures

Partial Seizures

The patient may resemble an intoxicated or drugged person. He or she may stare without focusing or speaking, appear to be fidgeting, make chewing movements, or smack the lips.

During the seizure:

- Do not attempt to restrain the patient.
- Gently move the patient away from dangerous objects.

After the seizure:

- Stay with the patient until the patient is fully alert.
- Reassure others that the behavior was medically caused.

Generalized Seizures

The patient may have a warning sign, cry out or scream, then fall down, and rhythmically jerk arms and legs in a strong movement that cannot be stopped.

Before or during the seizure:

- Remove the patient's glasses (if wearing) and help the patient lie down on their side, but do not restrain.
- Clear the area of dangerous objects.
- Loosen tight clothing around the patient's neck.
- Do not put any object into the patient's mouth.

After the seizure:

- Stay with the patient until he or she is fully awake.
- If the patient has a known seizure disorder, it may not be necessary to call for medical help depending on the preference of the patient and family unless an injury has occurred, the seizure lasts longer than 3 minutes, a second seizure occurs, or the patient requests help.

A patient with a seizure disorder lives with the fear that a seizure may strike at any moment. Persons with a seizure disorder fear dying during a seizure. They also fear personal injury. This fear is justified; therefore, health-care providers need to counsel patients regarding safety issues. Persons with a seizure disorder should take showers instead of baths to reduce their risk of drowning. If they take a bath, they should only do it with the door unlocked and when someone else is home. Automatic safety devices that adjust water temperature and shut off water when the shower drain is blocked can be installed. They should swim only with a partner who is aware of their diagnosis and knows what to do if a seizure occurs (Box 7.1). When cooking, patients should be instructed to use the microwave or back burners on the stove and keep pot handles turned inward. They should be encouraged not to smoke, but if they must, they should never smoke when alone. Their home should be evaluated to identify any safety hazards and to develop a risk-reduction plan. Families, friends, and coworkers need to be taught what to do in case of a seizure. They should avoid climbing ladders or doing other activities that could be dangerous if a seizure occurs.

Patients with a seizure disorder and their caregivers should be apprised of the risks of harm. Compared with the general population, children and adolescents with seizure disorders have a 1,000-fold greater risk of drowning during bathing and a 70-fold greater risk of drowning while swimming. Burns tend to occur in the home and are most commonly associated with cooking, showering, and use of space heaters. Driving needs to be discussed at length. The loss of driving privilege is serious because it restricts a patient's mobility and, therefore, his or her independence. Each state has different laws governing the granting of driver's licenses for individuals with a seizure disorder that will dictate a period of time patients must refrain from driving after having a seizure. At the federal level, the U.S. Department of Transportation has regulations that bar anyone with a history of seizures from being licensed to drive in interstate trucking. The purpose of the driving restrictions is obvious: to protect the public. Although only six states require health-care providers to report patients who have been diagnosed with seizure disorder, all practitioners have the responsibility to advise their patients of the medical risks, legal requirements, and recommendations regarding driving. Educational and support materials are available through the Epilepsy Foundation of America.

REFERENCES

Abou-Khalil BW. Antiepileptic drugs. *Continuum (Minneap Minn)*. 2016;22(1 Epilepsy):132–156.

Annegers JF, Hauser WA, Lee JR, Rocca WA. Incidence of acute symptomatic seizures in Rochester, Minnesota, 1935–1984. *Epilepsia*. 1995;36(4):327.

Fisher RS, Cross JH, D'Souza C, et al. Instruction manual for the ILAE 2017 operational classification of seizure types. *Epilepsia*. 2017;58(4):531–542.

Goldenberg MM. Overview of drugs used for epilepsy and seizures etiology, diagnosis, and treatment. *P T*. 2010;35(7):392–415.

U.S. Food and Drug Administration. Information for healthcare professionals: suicidal behavior and ideation and antiepileptic drugs. https://www.fda.gov/drugs/drugsafety/postmarketdrugsafetyinformationforpatientsandproviders/ucm100190.htm.

RESOURCES

Epilepsy Foundation
1-800-EFA-1000
   www.epilepsyfoundation.org

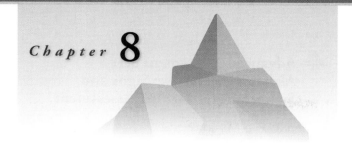

Chapter **8**

Degenerative Disorders

Sarah Horn, MD

Jill E. Winland-Brown, EdD, APRN, FNP-BC

ALZHEIMER'S DISEASE

Alzheimer's disease (AD) is a progressive, neurodegenerative condition and the most common form of dementia (60% to 80%) in the older population. One in three elderly individuals dies with AD or another form of dementia. AD accounts for about $100 billion per year in medical and custodial expenses, with approximately $27,000 per year for each patient for medical and nursing care. In 2016, more than 15 million caregivers provided an estimated 18.2 billion hours of unpaid care, valued at more than $230 billion (Alzheimer's Association, 2017).

AD is characterized by an insidious onset; slow, progressive cognitive decline; and an array of emotional and behavioral problems that result from cognitive decline. The cognitive decline in AD manifests as an impaired ability to learn new information or recall previously learned information and one or more additional cognitive disturbances in language (aphasia), function (apraxia), perception (agnosia), or executive function. Recent advances in understanding AD have modified both diagnostic and treatment choices. Most cases are sporadic, although there are rare familial forms of the disease.

AD was named after Dr. Alois Alzheimer, who in 1906 noticed changes in the brain tissue of a woman who had died of an unusual mental illness. She had symptoms of memory loss, language problems, and inappropriate behavior. On autopsy, he found abnormal clumps and tangled bundles of fibers in her brain. These findings are called amyloid plaques and neurofibrillary tangles.

EPIDEMIOLOGY AND CAUSES

The incidence of the sporadic form of AD in the general population increases rapidly with age. As many as 5.5 million Americans are currently living with AD. It affects an estimated 1 in 10 people older than age 65 years. AD is projected to affect nearly 16 million people in 2050, of whom 60% will be older than 85 years.

Additional risk factors that have been identified include lower educational and occupational levels, family history, head injury, Down syndrome, and vascular disease. Because onset is insidious, it is difficult to accurately predict duration or survival time with the disease. For 60- to 70-year-old individuals with AD, the average life expectancy is 7 to 10 years after diagnosis. AD is the sixth leading cause of death overall and the fifth leading cause of death for individuals older than 65 years. More than 60% of patients with AD are expected to die before age 80 years compared with 30% of people without AD. However, it is not just a disease of old age. Early-onset AD affects approximately 200,000 individuals under age 65.

The rare familial form of AD typically has an earlier onset. Inheritance is autosomal dominant; if a parent has the familial form of AD, offspring have a 50% chance of developing the disease.

PATHOPHYSIOLOGY

AD is a progressive and irreversible neurodegenerative syndrome. The disease depletes the cerebral cortex of neurons, causing generalized cortical atrophy. Neurons that use the neurotransmitter acetylcholine are especially susceptible to the disease; for example, the nucleus basalis, a set of large cholinergic neurons in the telencephalon beneath the basal ganglia, is selectively depopulated of neurons. Cortical areas that are especially affected include the hippocampus, the amygdala, the temporal cortex, the olfactory system, and intercortical connections.

Pathologic changes seen in brains of patients with AD include neuritic plaques and neurofibrillary tangles. Neuritic plaques are macroscopic spherical lesions found throughout the cortex (although they are relatively sparse in the primary motor and sensory areas), hippocampus, and amygdala. Each plaque has a core of beta-amyloid, an insoluble peptide. The core is surrounded by swollen and degenerating neurites, which are encased in a layer of microglia and astrocytes. Excess beta-amyloid is also found diffusely throughout the cerebral cortex, cerebellar cortex, and basal ganglia, especially in and around blood vessels.

Neurofibrillary tangles are microscopic collections of intertwined cytoskeletal fibers that form inside neurons. The tangles are best seen in silver-stained tissue, and their density correlates with the degree of the patient's dementia. One major protein in these tangles is an aberrant form of *tau* protein (which, in its normal form, stabilizes microtubules), and patients with AD have elevated concentrations of *tau* proteins in their cerebrospinal fluid. The formation of neurofibrillary tangles immobilizes or otherwise deactivates the neuron's normally dynamic cytoskeleton and leads to the cell's death. The tangles are insoluble and remain after the neurons have degenerated.

The central biochemical problem in AD appears to be a defect in the metabolism of *beta-amyloid precursor protein,* leading to accumulation of beta-amyloid. Normally,

105

many types of cells, including neurons, make beta-amyloid precursor protein, the function of which is not yet fully understood. When this protein is broken down, the by-products include beta-amyloid peptides. In AD, beta-amyloid peptides accumulate in the brain. One current theory proposes that beta-amyloid deposition is the primary problem in AD and that intracellular neuro-fibrillary tangles are the consequence of the toxic effects of beta-amyloid on neurons.

CLINICAL PRESENTATION

Subjective

The patient usually presents initially with complaints of memory problems. Often it is a family member who mentions this because patients with AD do not typically have insight into their memory difficulties. Recognition of cognitive difficulty on the part of the patient or family is often related to a change in pattern: getting lost in familiar places, inability to accomplish a demanding task at work, or increasingly slow response to any cognitive challenge. Difficulties with balancing the checkbook, preparing dinner, traveling alone, or maintaining employment are frequent problems reported by family members when the disease has progressed to the point where it is noticeable to others. In the later stages, the person needs help dressing, bathing, and staying continent. Eventually, the person loses the capacity to converse, walk, sit, or hold up the head. Eighty percent of patients in nursing homes with AD have behavioral problems. These may include hostility, aggression, suspiciousness and paranoia, delusions, agitation, sundowning, incontinence, and inappropriate or impulsive sexual behavior.

Objective

Concern about cognitive decline expressed by the patient or family or changes in behavior or cognition are noted that should trigger an initial assessment for dementia. Cognitive assessment is central to diagnosis and management of dementias and should be performed in all patients. Routine social conversation and questions that can be answered automatically will not elicit symptoms of early AD. Instead, the clinician should probe the patient's memory further with such questions as "Do you remember what you did last Sunday?" or "What did you have for breakfast this morning?" The importance of maintaining the patient's dignity by examining the patient alone before interviewing others cannot be overemphasized. The patient should be informed if others are to be interviewed. It is also important to be alert to the possibility that family members at times may minimize or exaggerate their report of symptoms, depending on their motives. Family members can report on the patient's ability to perform independent activities of daily living (ADLs) using the Functional Activities Questionnaire (FAQ) (see Advanced Assessment 8.1 for further assessment).

 Advanced Assessment 8.1:
Alzheimer's Disease: Signs and Symptoms for Further Assessment

LEARNING AND MEMORY

The patient becomes repetitive; has trouble remembering recent conversations, events, appointments; or frequently misplaces objects. These problems disrupt daily life.

HANDLING COMPLEX TASKS

The patient has trouble following a complex set of tasks that require many steps, such as organizing bills or following a recipe.

REASONING ABILITY

The patient is unable to respond with a reasonable plan to challenges at work or home, such as knowing what to do if the kitchen sink is plugged; shows poor judgment.

SPATIAL RELATIONSHIPS

The patient has trouble remembering directions or driving to what once was a familiar place, organizing objects around the house, unfamiliarity with familiar objects and places.

SPEECH

The patient has increasing difficulty with finding the words to express him or herself and following along with conversations.

CHANGES IN BEHAVIOR

The patient appears less social and responsive; is more irritable, depressed, anxious, and suspicious than usual.

The clinician should take a focused history documenting signs and symptoms related to the dementia, chronology of the problem (including onset, duration, and stepwise vs. continuous progression), and family history. Other causes of cognitive impairment, such as medication side effects, thyroid disease, low levels of B_{12}, depression, anxiety, and sleep issues, should be evaluated for and addressed. The physical examination should include a neurologic evaluation and evaluation of any factors contributing to delirium and evidence of neglect or abuse (see Chapter 6). Formal neuropsychologic testing can pinpoint the types and severity of impairments in language, reasoning, visuospatial, and memory deficits.

An easily administered bedside test for cognition is the Montreal Cognitive Assessment (MoCA; U.S. Department of Veterans Affairs, 2004). Asking the patient to name the months of the year backward or spell the word "world" backward are two easy tests to evaluate attention. Functional assessment tests are also very basic screening tools. These may include the timed "get up and go," a gait assessment, or the FAQ (see Advanced Assessment 8.2), which may be performed by the clinician. The FAQ

Advanced Assessment 8.2: Functional Activities Questionnaire

The Functional Activities Questionnaire (FAQ) is an informant-based measure of functional abilities. The caregiver or informant provides a score of dependent (3); requires assistance (2); has difficulty but does by self (1); or normal (0) on 10 functional items. Other responses include the following: never did the activity but couldn't do it now (0) and never did the activity but would have difficulty now (1).

The 10 activities are as follows:

1. Maintains financial records.
2. Collects information for IRS purposes.
3. Shops alone for necessities.
4. Does an intellectual activity.
5. Heats water and turns off the stove.
6. Cooks a healthy meal.
7. Has knowledge of what is going on in the world.
8. Carries on a conversation about something in the media.
9. Remembers medications and significant dates.
10. Arranges own travel for activities.

The sum of scores for the 10 items ranges from 0 to 30. The higher the score, the poorer the function.

For a complete discussion and instructions for administering this test, see Pfeiffer Pfeffer, RI; Kurosaki, TT; Harrah, CH; Chance, J M Filos, S., et al. Measurement of functional activities of older adults in the community. *J Gerontol.* 1982;37(3):323–329.

is also a useful measure that is reported to discriminate well at higher functional levels. One of the easiest tests to administer and informative of various areas of cognition is the clock-drawing test. The patient is asked to draw a clock face with all the numbers in place within a specific timeframe. The drawing can be placed in the patient's record, and the test can be repeated periodically. Asking the patient to name items, follow commands, repeat a phrase, and write a sentence tests language function. These tests are appropriate for initial assessment. The results also provide a baseline from which any further decline can be quantitatively compared. The clinician should refer the patient to a memory disorder center or a specialist in dementing diseases if the initial assessment is suggestive of AD, particularly when atypical presentation, severe impairment, or complex comorbidities are present. Other assessment tests are listed in Chapter 6.

DIAGNOSTIC REASONING

Diagnostic Tests

Laboratory tests (complete blood count, electrolytes, blood glucose, serum calcium, thyroid-stimulating hormone level, and vitamin B_{12}) may be used to rule out other conditions that impair brain function. Structural

imaging should be used in the diagnostic evaluation of every patient suspected of dementia. Noncontrast computed tomography can be used to identify surgically treatable lesions and vascular disease. For increased sensitivity, magnetic resonance imaging (MRI) should be used. Single-photon emission computed tomography (SPECT) imaging measures blood flow and activity patterns and can be used to differentiate AD from other possible causes. Positron emission tomography (PET) imaging may be used to detect amyloid deposits. Studies show that this test is 86% accurate in predicting which individuals will develop AD within 2 years and 92% accurate in ruling out the likelihood of developing AD. AD-related brain changes may occur 20 years before symptoms begin.

An individual with early brain changes has preclinical AD or mild cognitive impairment (MCI) due to AD. Two categories of serum biomarkers are being studied to determine relevance as diagnostic criteria. The first are biomarkers showing the level of beta-amyloid accumulation in the brain; the second are biomarkers indicating the level of injury or degeneration of neurons in the brain. These biomarker tests could be used in the future to determine whether individuals with MCI have brain changes that put them at high risk for developing AD. These biomarkers could also be important in evaluating the effectiveness of treatment. Genetic testing is available in patients with a family history, although less than 1% of AD cases are caused by the three known genetic mutations.

Differential Diagnosis

To some extent, the diagnosis of AD is still a process of excluding other causes of cognitive impairment (Fig. 8.1). Medical conditions and drug-related adverse effects need to be ruled out in patients suspected of AD. Infection, structural central nervous system (CNS) lesion, traumatic conditions, metabolic derangements, and vitamin B_{12} deficiency need to be considered. In addition, depression, drug and alcohol abuse, drug-induced delirium, and psychosis need to be ruled out. Other common causes of dementia to consider include vascular dementia, frontotemporal dementia, and Lewy body dementia.

Patients may present with a combination of issues. Delirium or depression may be superimposed on AD; vascular dementia (or other dementia) can also coexist with AD, causing a mixed dementia.

Depression can mimic AD and is frequently mistaken for AD in older adults. Information from multiple sources—patient self-report, family members, healthcare provider observations, and patient history—should be considered when making a diagnosis.

The Alzheimer's Disease Management Council Clinical Consensus Panel and Scientific Roundtable proposed that the following signs are highly suggestive of the diagnosis of AD:

- Absence of a precipitating medical illness
- Absence of a drug-related phenomenon

Diagnostic Reasoning Algorithm: Alzheimer's Disease

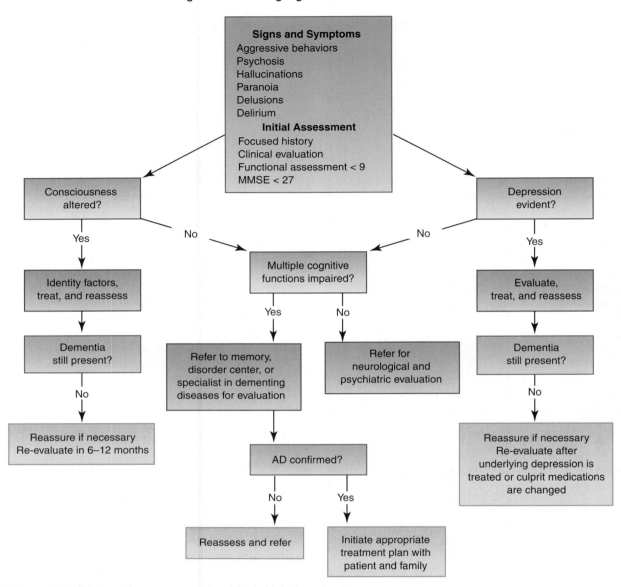

Figure 8.1 Diagnostic reasoning algorithm: Alzheimer's disease.

- Presence of objective, well-documented, progressive, and worsening deficits in new learning and memory
- Signs of functional impairment

MANAGEMENT

The principles of management of AD are directed toward slowing progression of the disease pharmacologically, protecting physical health, providing emotional support, and maintaining optimal function through prevention or reduction of excess disability. Maintaining as much normalcy as possible in relationships and everyday activities may be the most effective way to prevent the development of excess disability, defined as the difference between the observed function and the actual underlying impairment.

Family members have reported that sensitivity to their distress, acknowledgment of their contributions, and information about the disease and its management have not always been dealt with adequately in encounters with primary-care providers. Both patient and family need assistance in understanding and coping with a diagnosis of AD. Most patients are eager to try approved and research-stage drugs. Support group attendance can be helpful but should be relevant to the stage of the disease. Anxiety and depression should be recognized and treated vigorously. Legal and financial planning and discussion of future care options should take place early in the disease course.

Medications may improve cognitive function in mild to moderate AD. Treatment with cholinesterase inhibitors should be considered at the time of diagnosis, taking into account expected therapeutic benefits and potential safety issues (see Drugs Commonly Prescribed 8.1). The dosages for the following drugs are adjusted gradually as tolerated: donepezil (Aricept), galantamine (Reminyl), and rivastigmine (Exelon). An *N*-methyl-D-aspartate receptor antagonist, memantine (Namenda and Namzaric), has been effective in moderate to severe AD by improving cognitive function and has additive effects to cholinesterase inhibitors.

Donepezil does not prevent progression of AD, but it seems to slow the rate of decline. Patients who stop and restart donepezil will not reach the level of function that they had before stopping the drug. Therefore, if the drug is tolerated, it should be continued because there are no clear guidelines about when to stop it. Antidepressant drugs have shown to be effective in patients with depressive symptoms. Anxious and agitated behavior may respond to anxiolytic drugs; however, use of pharmacologic agents for noncognitive symptoms such as anxiety, depression, and insomnia should be reserved for instances where behavioral intervention is ineffective.

Because of their side effects, antipsychotics should be used with caution and reserved for patients who exhibit persistent disruptive or dangerous behavior. Precautions include avoidance of drugs that have even a moderate anticholinergic effect and drugs that sedate, affect balance, or are known to cause confusion in older individuals. Atypical antipsychotic medications—risperidone (Risperdal), olanzapine (Zyprexa), and quetiapine (Seroquel)—are usually well tolerated. Federal regulations require that if antipsychotic agents are used in nursing homes, an effort should be made to reduce the dosage at least every 6 months. Alpha-tocopherol (vitamin E) may help to slow progression of AD in some patients.

The failure to institute timely pharmacologic management in patients with AD may result in a more rapid need for institutionalization, an increase in aggression, further difficulty with ADLs, and further cognitive decline.

Given the advanced age, compromised brain function, and frequent presence of other chronic conditions in most patients with AD, close monitoring of response to any drug regimen is advisable. In addition, as the patient becomes less able to communicate physical or emotional distress, more careful observation of general health and well-being is needed.

Attention to good nutrition, exercise, and preventive care (immunizations, dental, vision, and hearing care) should not be reduced. Patients and their families also need continued support and assistance related to changes that occur as the disease progresses. Recognition of and respect for the patient's humanity can be difficult to maintain in the face of declining cognition, leading to the unfortunate temptation to care for family members while ignoring the patient.

FOLLOW-UP AND REFERRAL

Referral to a memory disorder center is usually warranted. These centers offer multidisciplinary services ranging from differential diagnosis and access to experimental medications to counseling and support groups. They are excellent sources of accurate information about AD. Most cities have local chapters of national organizations for patients with AD and caregivers that usually offer referrals and support groups as well. Respite care, both at home and overnight in participating health-care facilities, and adult day centers provide social outlets for people with AD and a break in the constant care demands for family members. Family members must be cared for as well; if the clinician is unable to support them, it is essential to find social service agencies that will be able to help.

Patient Education: Alzheimer's Disease

Both patient and family members need to understand the disease, its ramifications, its future course, and treatment options. Memory aids and environmental modifications can prolong independent function. Specialized communication techniques, memory training, exercise, training in independent and basic ADLs, and therapeutic recreational activities can all contribute to improved function and quality of life as the disease progresses. Patients need information on legal and financial issues related to the capacity to make decisions, including end-of-life decisions. Driving and living alone are safety issues that arise in the earlier stages; wandering and falls become issues in the later stages. Both patient and family must deal with changes

---

⊙ **Drugs Commonly Prescribed 8.1: Alzheimer's Disease**

DRUG	ADVERSE REACTIONS AND PRESCRIBING CONSIDERATIONS
Cholinesterase Inhibitors	
Donepezil (Aricept) Galantamine (Reminyl) Rivastigmine (Exelon) (oral as well as patch) Galantamine (Razadyne)	For mild to moderate AD Side effects include nausea, diarrhea, anorexia, weight loss. Use with caution in patients with mild to moderate hepatic impairment.
N-Methyl-D-Aspartate Receptor Antagonist	
Memantine (Namenda, Namzaric)	For moderate to severe AD. Can be used in conjunction with the above. Contraindicated in patients with renal and hepatic impairment. Use with caution in patients with cardiac conduction abnormalities and peptic ulcer.

Abbreviation: AD, Alzheimer's disease.

in ability, lifestyle, and relationships with others. Finally, family members need to learn how to help the patient while taking care of themselves as well. There are negative consequences of caregiving such as depression, anxiety, and failure to care for self.

Many patients with advanced disease are taking as many as 8 to 10 medications daily, and many of these medications have side effects that affect cognition and result in falls. Fall precautions need to be taken at home, as well as in long-term care facilities, and clinicians should educate families regarding these at every visit (see Evidence-Based Nursing Practice 8.1).

PARKINSON'S DISEASE

Parkinson's disease (PD) is a chronic, progressive, degenerative disorder of the basal ganglia in the CNS. The disease usually begins insidiously and eventually leads to disability. *Parkinsonian syndrome* is any disorder that manifests symptoms of parkinsonism, which include rest tremor, rigidity, bradykinesia, postural instability, flexed posture, and freezing. Idiopathic PD is the most common cause of parkinsonism, but numerous other causes include parkinsonism-plus syndromes, secondary parkinsonism, certain genetic disorders (such as Wilson's disease) and other causes of atypical parkinsonism. Patients with idiopathic PD make up the largest subgroup, which represents 78% of the affected population. Parkinsonism-plus syndromes are caused by degeneration of multiple systems and are characterized by neurologic signs and symptoms in addition to parkinsonism. Examples in this category include progressive supranuclear palsy, multiple systems atrophy,

---

Evidence-Based Nursing Practice 8.1

Yueh-Feng Y, Ellis J, Yang Z, et al. Satisfaction with a family-focused intervention for mild cognitive impairment dyads. *J Nurs Scholarsh.* 2016;48(4);334–344.

This study describes the satisfaction that persons with mild cognitive impairment and their caregivers had with the Daily Enhancement of Meaningful Activity (DEMA) intervention. A randomized study compared satisfaction with DEMA to an information support group (both patients and caregivers) as well as to a control group. Six biweekly sessions were given. Data analysis included descriptive statistics, independent-sample *t* tests, and content analysis. Results documented patients' satisfaction with their caregivers and intervention of DEMA. The study findings provide preliminary support of DEMA as a means to improve quality of life by helping to support patient and caregiver engagement in meaningful activities and problem-solving.

---

and corticobasal degeneration. Secondary parkinsonism is parkinsonism that is symptomatic of an underlying cause of the disorder, such as cerebrovascular disease, drugs, infections, trauma, or exposure to toxins. Common causes of secondary parkinsonism include exposure to dopamine-blocking medications, such as antipsychotics or certain antiemetics. There are numerous rare hereditary causes of parkinsonism. One of the more common causes is Wilson's disease, which causes an abnormal accumulation of copper. This disease should be ruled out in all young patients presenting with a movement disorder because it is easily treatable.

EPIDEMIOLOGY

PD is the second most common neurodegenerative disorder in the elderly after AD. It typically affects people in middle to later life, with a mean age of onset of 57 years. The incidence is slightly higher in men, with a 3:2 ratio of men to women. People in all ethnic groups, countries, and socioeconomic classes are affected. Age is the greatest risk factor for PD, and it is estimated that approximately 2% of the population will be affected by the age of 80 years (Fahn et al., 2011). The annual cost of PD in the United States is estimated to be approximately $11 billion. The Centers for Disease Control and Prevention's National Center for Health Statistics reports that complications from PD constituted the 14th leading cause of death in the United States in 2014. Persons with PD do not die from the disease itself but from secondary complications, such as pneumonia and injuries resulting from falls. Patients with PD have an increased risk of developing dementia in their lifetime (Fig. 8.2).

The morbidity and mortality rate for PD is higher than the general population. An estimated 9% of patients become disabled or die within 1 to 5 years, 21% in 6 to 10 years, and almost 38% in 11 to 15 years.

Michael J. Fox, the actor, was first diagnosed with young-onset PD at age 30 and has raised public awareness for the disease. His foundation for PD research has funded more than $700 million to find a cure for PD (see michaeljfox.org).

PATHOPHYSIOLOGY AND CAUSES

PD is a degenerative disease of the nervous system. Its neurologic effects include tremor at rest, muscular rigidity, slow movements, and difficulty maintaining a steady posture. Characteristically, the motor problems of PD improve when a patient is treated with levodopa. Pathologically, PD causes abnormal accumulation of Lewy bodies and degeneration of the pigmented dopaminergic cells of the substantia nigra (located in the brainstem). Lewy bodies are spherical, eosinophilic inclusions in the cytoplasm consisting primarily of alpha-synuclein.

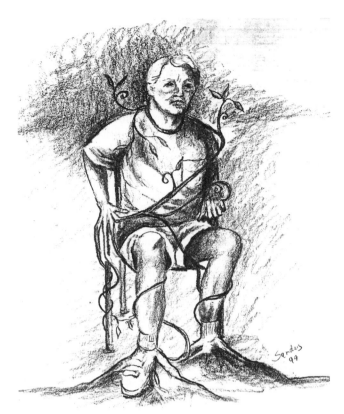

Figure 8.2 One man's depiction of having Parkinson's disease. (Illustration by Christine Sanders.)

The substantia nigra is part of the basal ganglia, a group of subcortical nuclei with strong connections to the cortex, thalamus, and brainstem. The main components of the basal ganglia include the caudate, putamen, globus pallidus, subthalamic nucleus, and substantia nigra. It is a critical part of the motor system, through its interactions with the motor pathways of thalamus and cortex.

The main input to the basal ganglia is from the cerebral cortex, and these inputs are mostly excitatory, using the neurotransmitter glutamate. The main output of the basal ganglia is to the thalamus; these outputs are mostly inhibitory and use the neurotransmitter GABA (gamma-aminobutyric acid). Within the basal ganglia lie intrinsic excitatory and inhibitory connections named the direct pathway and indirect pathway, respectively. Aberrations in these pathways lead to hyperkinetic and hypokinetic movement disorders. PD depletes the dopaminergic neurons of the substantia nigra. Dopamine has both excitatory effects in the direct pathway and inhibitory effects in the indirect pathway. Thus, loss of dopaminergic neurons in PD causes a blanket inhibition of the motor activity passing through the thalamus. Clinically, this leads to the rigidity and bradykinesia seen in PD.

In addition to cell loss in the substantia nigra, PD also causes Lewy body accumulation and destruction of cells in other areas of the nervous system, leading to other associated signs and symptoms seen in PD. Cortical Lewy

bodies can lead to dementia, either dementia with Lewy bodies or PD dementia. Differentiation between these conditions depends on the timing of dementia onset as it relates to the development of parkinsonism and can be somewhat arbitrary given they are variations of the same pathologic disorder.

The cause of sporadic idiopathic PD is unknown. The pathogenesis is thought to be multifactorial, resulting from a combination of genetic predisposition, exposure to possible environmental toxins, and endogenous factors. Research indicates that oxidative stress, mitochondrial dysfunction, and accumulation of toxic proteins play a role. A positive family history increases the lifetime risk of developing PD from 2% to 4%. Numerous genes have been found that cause a hereditary form of PD, although this type is rare.

CLINICAL PRESENTATION

Subjective

Presentation of the disease is variable. The patient may present with one or more of the six cardinal features of PD: tremor at rest, rigidity, bradykinesia or hypokinesia, flexed posture, loss of postural reflexes, and the freezing phenomenon. The major manifestations of tremor, rigidity, akinesia (or bradykinesia), and postural disturbances form the mnemonic "TRAP."

A tremor may be the reason the patient or family first seeks care and is recognized as the first symptom of PD in 70% of patients at initial diagnosis. The classic rest tremor of PD is a low-frequency tremor that appears distally in the extremities when the extremity is motionless and at rest. It can mimic the motion of rolling an object between the thumb and forefinger fingers and because of this is also called a "pill-rolling tremor." This resting tremor disappears with action but reemerges as the limbs maintain a posture. A resting tremor is most common in the hands but can also be present in the jaw and feet. The resting tremor of the hands tends to increase when the patient is walking and may be an early sign of PD before other signs are visible. Stress tends to worsen the tremor, and it is absent during sleep.

In addition to tremor, patients may present with a variety of nonspecific symptoms, including generalized stiffness, pain, or paresthesia of the limbs; constipation; sleeplessness; and reduced voice volume (Przuntek, 1992). A variety of nonmotor symptoms are common in PD including cognitive decline, anxiety and other mood symptoms, apathy, orthostatic hypotension, urinary frequency and incontinence, fatigue, drooling, concentration difficulty, constipation, loss of sense of smell, and REM sleep behavior disorder (an abnormal acting out of dreams during REM sleep; Barone et al., 2009). Constipation, REM sleep behavior disorder, and anosmia frequently predate symptoms of PD by several years (Postuma et al., 2012). Progressive bradykinesia may contribute to slowness and difficulty in the performance of ADLs. Swallowing problems may be prominent in advanced disease, causing aspiration and choking. These nonmotor symptoms can have a major impact on patients with PD.

Objective

The three cardinal manifestations of PD are bradykinesia, rigidity, and rest tremor. Parkinsonism is defined as bradykinesia (slowness of movement) in combination with rest tremor and/or rigidity (Postuma et al., 2015). A standardized approach to examination of parkinsonism is presented in the Unified Parkinson's Disease Rating Scale (UPDRS; 1987) and allows for objective quantification of parkinsonism.

Bradykinesia is defined as slowness of movement and decreased amplitude or speed of movements. This can be evaluated by assessing finger and toe tapping. Rigidity is a state of increased muscle tone felt when the clinician passively moves a patient's neck and limbs when they are completely relaxed. The muscles feel stiff, making the extremities difficult to move. This resistance is independent of velocity (as opposed to spasticity, which increases with increased velocity). Rigidity is equal in all directions. "Cogwheeling," a ratchet-like quality to the rigidity, is also commonly found on examination in patients with PD and is caused by an underlying tremor, even in the absence of a visible tremor. When another limb is engaged in voluntary movement, rigidity of the passive limb increases. Rest tremor is a low-frequency, 4- to 6-Hz tremor in a fully resting limb that is suppressed by active movement. Of note, although postural instability is a feature of parkinsonism, it is not part of the diagnostic criteria for PD because it is typically a later manifestation and its presence early in the disease process suggests a parkinsonism-plus disorder (Postuma et al., 2015). The clinician can assess postural reflexes with the pull test, in which the examiner stands behind the patient; gives a sudden, firm pull on the patient's shoulders; and checks for retropulsion.

Particularly late in the disease process, a patient with PD may have a flexed posture that involves the entire body. The head is bowed, the trunk is bent forward, and the back posture is kyphotic. Extreme truncal flexion is called camptocormia; this trunk flexion resolves when in the supine position. There may be a "striatal hand" deformity including ulnar deviation, fingers flexed at the metacarpophalangeal joints, and extension of interphalangeal joints. Walking is slow, with a shortened stride length and tendency to shuffle. Freezing, also called "motor block," is the transient inability to perform active movements. Most often, the legs are affected and become stuck to the floor when trying to walk, but it may also involve eyelid opening, speaking, and writing. Freezing is transient and occurs suddenly. It typically occurs when the patient begins to walk (start-hesitation), attempts to turn while walking, or approaches a destination (target-hesitation). The patient may be fearful about the inability to handle perceived barriers such as elevator doors and heavily trafficked streets.

Other common manifestations of PD are drooling as a result of decreased frequency of swallowing, dysphagia secondary to the neuromuscular incoordination of the hypopharyngeal musculature, excessive perspiration as a result of a disorder of the hypothalamic heat-regulating mechanism and impairment of perspiration controls, constipation secondary to hypomotility of the gastrointestinal tract, orthostatic hypotension as a result of deterioration of the peripheral autonomic nervous system, and urinary urgency secondary to autonomic dysfunction. The patient may also demonstrate a "masklike" face (hypomimia), soft speech (hypophonia), slurred speech (dysarthria), and small, slow handwriting (micrographia).

Many patients with PD exhibit behavioral changes. Personality changes become apparent as the patient becomes fearful, dependent, and anxious. Passivity, lack of motivation, and decreased attention span are common. There may also be confusion, agitation, hallucinations, and mania—all of which can be side effects of dopaminergic PD medications as well. More than 50% of patients with PD experience depression, and this may precede motor symptoms.

Patients with PD commonly experience cognitive decline. The MoCA (U.S. Department of Veterans Affairs, 2004; see also Chapter 6) is a 10-minute screening tool for mild cognitive dysfunction. It is effective in determining which patients need treatment for MCI.

The patient may be slow to answer questions and may be unable to change mental set rapidly. There may also be sensory and autonomic dysfunctions such as pain, burning, and tingling. The patient may report that these sensations diminish or disappear on moving. Autonomic dysfunctions such as cool skin, constipation, inadequate bladder emptying, difficulty obtaining an erection, and orthostatic hypotension may be present.

DIAGNOSTIC REASONING

Diagnostic Tests

Usually the history and physical examination lead the clinician to the diagnosis of PD. Diagnosis requires the presence of parkinsonism (bradykinesia plus rigidity and/or rest tremor) and absence of exclusion criteria, which include cerebellar abnormalities, vertical supranuclear gaze palsy, treatment with antidopaminergic medication and time course consistent with drug-induced parkinsonism, absence of response to high-dose levodopa, signs of cortical dysfunction on examination, and normal functional neuroimaging of the presynaptic dopaminergic system. Red flags that indicate an alternative diagnosis include rapid progression of gait impairment, absence of progression over years, severe early bulbar dysfunction, severe early autonomic failure, recurrent early falls, and symmetric signs (Postuma et al., 2015).

Genetic testing may be used in the diagnosis of PD along with other specific features such as family history and early age of onset. An MRI of the brain may be performed to exclude structural brain lesions but not to demonstrate pathological changes indicative of PD. A SPECT scan and a PET scan may show a pattern of reduced dopaminergic activity in the basal ganglia and may help in diagnostic accuracy. Levodopa may be given on a trial, as the patient's response to levodopa is helpful diagnostically. Patients with PD usually have improvement in rigidity, bradykinesia, and tremor with levodopa, whereas patients with other forms of parkinsonism are less likely to respond.

Differential Diagnosis

PD may be mistaken for *essential tremor,* although the latter is characterized by postural and action tremor, not resting tremor. Idiopathic PD needs to be differentiated from parkinsonism-plus syndromes. In progressive supranuclear palsy (Steele-Richardson-Olszewski syndrome), parkinsonism is accompanied by a supranuclear disorder of eye movements, pseudobulbar palsy, and axial dystonia. Multiple system atrophy (previously known as Shy-Drager syndrome, striatonigral degeneration, or olivopontocerebellar atrophy) causes a combination of parkinsonism, cerebellar signs, and autonomic symptoms. Reversible parkinsonism may be caused by dopamine-blocking or dopamine-depleting medications such as antipsychotics, metoclopramide (Reglan), and reserpine (Serpasil). Vascular disease, other causes of dementia, Wilson's disease, and Huntington's disease can have features of parkinsonism. It is important to recognize Wilson's disease because it is treatable. Onset of symptoms usually occurs in childhood or early adulthood. It also causes psychiatric and liver disease. Signs include gray-green Kayser-Fleischer rings in the cornea, chronic hepatitis, and increased concentrations of copper. Patients with Huntington's disease can also present with rigidity and bradykinesia, but the cardinal clinical manifestation is chorea (dance-like movements), which will be absent in untreated PD.

MANAGEMENT

The principle of management is to control the symptoms of PD because no drug or surgical approach has been found to definitively prevent the progression of the disease. Each patient has a unique set of signs, symptoms, and responses to medications, so treatment must be individualized. Patients also have social, occupational, and emotional needs to be considered. Treatment is lifelong; the goal is to keep patients functioning independently for as long as possible.

The decision of when to initiate symptomatic treatment for PD should be individualized. In early PD when symptoms are mild and not disrupting daily activity, treatment may be deferred. When PD symptoms begin to interfere with activities, treatment should be initiated. Numerous

medications are available. Levodopa is the most efficacious drug for PD. However, over time, patients can develop motor fluctuations with wearing off and dyskinesia, which can affect quality of life. Some patients feel the need to keep increasing their dosage to feel at their best. Often, other medications are used before and in combination with levodopa to delay and treat these complications. Neurologists may consider adding dopamine agonists, an monoamine oxidase (MAO)-B inhibitor, or catechol-*O*-methyltransferase (COMT) inhibitors.

Medications prescribed for the management of PD are presented in Drugs Commonly Prescribed 8.2. Levodopa, a dopaminergic agent, is considered the most effective antiparkinsonian. Some experts prefer using dopamine agonists first if the patient is younger with milder deficits, although these agents can have cognitive side effects and lead to compulsive behaviors.

Once levodopa therapy is started, the rule of thumb is to administer the lowest dosage that controls symptoms. An adequate trial with a reasonably high dose should be tried before deciding a patient does not respond to levodopa. With more advanced disease, patients may also experience the "on–off" phenomenon. After 2 to 5 years of treatment, more than 50% of patients experience fluctuations in their response to levodopa with dyskinesia (extra hyperkinetic choreiform movements) at peak doses and recurrence of parkinsonism as the medication wears off. Rasagiline is an MAO-B inhibitor that initially showed promising data as a neuroprotective agent (Olanow et al., 2009) in PD. However, additional studies have questioned its effectiveness, and its utility as a neuroprotective agent that slows disease progression is controversial (Ahlskog & Uitti, 2010). It has fewer side effects than levodopa, but the effects tend to be only moderate. Because it provides only inadequate symptomatic therapy as the disease progresses, rasagiline typically is not used as monotherapy.

Dopamine agonists presumably act directly on striatal dopamine receptors and do not require metabolic conversion to an active product to exert effects. They are slightly less effective than levodopa but are alternative first-line agents for PD. Anticholinergic agents are centrally acting drugs and are often used to treat PD. These drugs are typically prescribed for patients aged 70 years or younger in whom tremor is the dominant clinical feature and whose cognitive function is preserved. These agents are useful for treating resting tremors; however, adverse effects, including memory impairment, hallucinations, and confusion, are common with these drugs. Adverse CNS effects of drugs used to treat PD include dysphagia, sedation, and dyskinesia. These drugs should always be tapered gradually.

Peripheral COMT inhibitors such as tolcapone (Tasmar) and entacapone (Comtan) can be used as adjunctive therapies to levodopa. These drugs increase the bioavailability of levodopa, thereby extending the duration of levodopa's effect. COMT inhibitors have

Drugs Commonly Prescribed 8.2: Parkinson's Disease

DRUG	ADVERSE REACTIONS AND PRESCRIBING CONSIDERATIONS
Monoamine Oxidase (MAO)-B Inhibitors	
Selegiline (Eldepryl) Rasagiline (Azilect)	Adverse effects include nausea, headache, confusion, hallucinations, insomnia. When given with levodopa, can increase dopaminergic effects.
Dopaminergic Medications	
Carbidopa/levodopa (Sinemet, Sinemet CR, Rytary) Duopa (gel form for use with gastrostomy tube) Parcopa (oral disintegrating table)	Gradually titrate to relief of symptoms. Can use Parcopa if swallowing dysfunction is present. Duopa requires placement of gastrostomy tube. Adverse effects include nausea, headache, orthostatic hypotension, somnolence, hallucinations, psychosis.
Dopamine Agonists	
Pramipexole dihydrochloride (Mirapex ER) Ropinirole (Requip) Apomorphine (injectable) (Apokyn)	Apomorphine can be used as rescue therapy because of its quick onset of action. Adverse effects include nausea, sleepiness, orthostatic hypotension, confusion, hallucinations, peripheral edema, compulsive behavior.
Comt (Catechol-O-Methyl Transferase) Inhibitors	
Tolcapone (Tasmar) Entacapone (Comtan)	Only beneficial in combination with carbidopa/levodopa. Helpful in patients with motor fluctuations and with wearing off. Adverse effects include diarrhea, orange urine, elevation in liver enzymes (rare severe hepatotoxicity in tolcapone), and can worsen adverse effects of levodopa.
Anticholinergics	
Trihexyphenidyl (Artane) (Trihex) Benztropine mesylate (Cogentin)	Adverse effects include confusion, hallucinations, dry mouth, urinary retention.
Antiviral Medications	
Amantadine (Symmetrel)	Unknown mechanism of action in PD. Can treat dyskinesia. Adverse effects include ankle edema, confusion, hallucinations.

been shown to be effective in both nonfluctuating and fluctuating patients.

Patients with severe symptoms, such as tremor, that are refractory to medications may require referral to a movement disorder neurologist or neurosurgeon to discuss deep brain stimulation. This therapy can be helpful in patients with refractory tremor or significant motor fluctuations with levodopa. In deep brain stimulation, electrodes are placed in subthalamic nuclei or globus pallidus.

For PD dementia, cholinesterase inhibitors such as rivastigmine or donepezil can be helpful. Hallucinations can be exacerbated by medications used to treat PD, particularly dopamine agonists and anticholinergics. If an antipsychotic needs to be used to treat psychosis in PD patients, the drugs of choice include quetiapine, clozapine, or pimavanserin because they are less likely to worsen parkinsonism.

FOLLOW-UP AND REFERRAL

The frequency of follow-up and visits is based on the patient's response to treatment, adverse effects of medications, and disease progression. Follow-up should be early and repeated initially, especially during the introduction of a new medication or dose change. The decision for referral to a specialist should be made based on the practitioner's knowledge level and comfort treating PD and on the severity of symptoms. As the disease progresses, especially in the area of tremor, it may become necessary to refer the patient to a movement disorder neurologist or to a stereotactic neurosurgeon.

Rating scales are frequently used to evaluate and monitor a patient's response to medications. The UPDRS is a comprehensive evaluation tool that assesses mental, historical, and motor features and the complications of dopaminergic therapy. A subscale of the UPDRS is the Activities of Daily Living Scale, which assesses speech, salivation, swallowing, handwriting, cutting food, handling utensils, hygiene, turning in bed, falling, freezing, walking, tremor, and sensory symptoms.

Patient Education: Parkinson's Disease

Speech therapy may be beneficial to increase the voice volume; affect speech pattern modification; and assist with breathing, memory, and vocal range of motion exercises. Occasional swallowing assessments and therapies may be needed to assist with problems of dysphagia and drooling.

Patients should be educated on all issues of the disease, medications, adverse effects, complications, progression of the disease, diet, sleep, and exercise. Patients with PD should be encouraged to exercise regularly, and a referral to physical therapy may be indicated. Nutrition in patients with PD is an important component in care, particularly if they develop swallowing difficulties. The patient should also be assessed for physical and psychological problems, which may interfere with eating and nutrition. Functional capacity may be limited, hindering the patient's ability to prepare meals.

Patients must also be instructed to continue routine health maintenance and screenings. In addition, both patient and caregiver must be educated about the risk for falls in patients with decreased mobility, as well as other home safety issues. There is an increase in mortality from influenza and pneumonia among patients with PD, so guidance for immunizations must be given. Patient and caregivers may benefit from referral to a support group.

AMYOTROPHIC LATERAL SCLEROSIS (LOU GEHRIG'S DISEASE)

Amyotrophic lateral sclerosis (ALS) is a progressive neurologic disorder that involves destruction of motor neurons. Both upper motor neurons (located in the motor cortex) and lower motor neurons (located in the anterior horn of the spinal cord and the motor nuclei of cranial nerves in the brainstem) are affected, distinguishing ALS from other motor neuron diseases. The etiology is not known, although approximately 10% of cases are genetic. Researchers are studying possible causes, which may include abnormal RNA processing, mitochondrial dysfunction, viral infection, disorganized immune response, toxicity, and others (Peters et al., 2015). Slightly more men than women have ALS. Age, family history, and possibly tobacco use are the only known risk factors (Armon, 2009). It is universally fatal with a median survival of 3 to 5 years.

Symptoms typically start in one limb or region in the spinal cord ("limb onset"), although in 20% of patients the symptoms begin in the cranial nerve nuclei ("bulbar onset"). Bulbar onset portends a poorer prognosis because swallowing and breathing functions are affected sooner. Presentations may vary considerably between patients, as motor functions of any area of the body may be affected.

A patient may present with a foot drop or other localized motor symptom. Over time, weakness will spread to other areas of the body. Signs of both upper and lower motor neuron dysfunction affecting multiple regions of the body occur, which is the hallmark of ALS. Diagnostic criteria are defined by the El Escorial World Federation of Neurology (ALS Association, n.d.):

- Signs of degeneration of lower motor neurons (spinal cord and brainstem)
- Signs of degeneration of upper motor neurons (brain)
- Progressive spread of signs
- Other disease processes excluded

Bowel and bladder control are usually not affected. There may be comorbid development of frontotemporal dementia in approximately 15% of patients. The diagnosis is clinical, although it can be confirmed with electromyography and nerve conduction studies. There is no treatment to reverse ALS; however, treatment may slow the progression of symptoms. The only medication that has been shown to improve survival in ALS is riluzole (Miller et al., 2012). The mechanism of action is unknown, but it may be related to a reduction in excitotoxicity caused by a chemical messenger in the brain called glutamate. Other treatments are aimed at managing the symptoms of the disease.

REFERENCES

Alzheimer's Disease

Alzheimer's Association. 2017 Alzheimer's disease facts and figures. https://www.alz.org/documents_custom/2017-facts-and-figures.pdf. Published 2017.

Langman N. Caregivers of dementia patients: Mental health screening & support. *Clin Rev.* 2016;26(6):42–49.

Shanley A. Is it Alzheimer disease? Guidelines for evaluating patients with mild memory loss. *Consultant.* 2016;56(12):1074–1078.

Yueh-Feng Y, Ellis J, Yang Z, et al. Satisfaction with a family-focused intervention for mild cognitive impairment dyads. *J Nurs Scholarsh.* 2016;48(4);334–344.

Amyotrophic Lateral Sclerosis

ALS Association. (n.d.). El Escorial World Federation of Neurology Criteria for the Diagnosis of ALS. http://www.alsa.org/assets/pdfs/fyi/criteria_for_diagnosis.pdf. Accessed July 18, 2017.

Amyotrophic lateral sclerosis (ALS). S http://www.mayoclinic.org/diseases-conditions/amyotrophic-lateral-sclerosis/diagnosis-treatment/treatment/txc-20247219. Accessed April 27, 2017.

Armon C. Smoking may be considered an established risk factor for sporadic ALS. *Neurology.* 2009;73(20):1693–1698.

Miller RG, Mitchell JD, Moore DH. Riluzole for amyotrophic lateral sclerosis (ALS)/motor neuron disease (MND). *Cochrane Database Syst Rev.* 2012. 2012;(3):CD001447

Peters OM, Ghasemi M, Brown RH Jr. Emerging mechanisms of molecular pathology in ALS. *J Clin Invest.* 2015;125(5):1767–1779.

Sanofi-Aventis, U.S. LLC. Survival rates of patients with ALS treated with Rilutek (riluzole). [Drug insert study.] http://products.sanofi.us/rilutek/rilutek.pdf. Published 2012.

Parkinson Disease

Ahlskog JE, Uitti RJ. Rasagiline, Parkinson neuroprotection, and delayed-start trials: Still no satisfaction? *Neurology.* 2010;74(14):1143–1148.

Barone P, Antonini A, Colosimo C, et al. The PRIAMO study: A multicenter assessment of nonmotor symptoms and their impact on quality of life in Parkinson's disease. *Mov Disord.* 2009;24(11):1641–1649.

Dancis A, Cotter VT. Diagnosis and management of cognitive impairment in Parkinson's disease. *J Nurse Pract.* 2015;11(3):307–313.

Fahn S, Jankovic J, Hallett M. *Principles and practice of movement disorders.* 2nd ed. Philadelphia, PA: Elsevier Health Sciences; 2011.

Kaufman DM, Truong D. Parkinson's disease: Making an evidence-based diagnosis. *Clin Advisor.* 2017;20(2):27–34.

Kochanek KD, Murphy SL, Xu J, Tejada-Vera B. Deaths: Final data for 2014. *Natl Vital Stat Rep.* 2016;65(4):1–122.

Medifocus Guidebook on Parkinson's Disease. A comprehensive patient guide to symptoms, treatment, research, and support. http://www.medifocus.com/parkinsons/?assoc=Bing&keyword=parkinsons. Updated January 22, 2017. Accessed May 1, 2017.

Movement Disorder Society Task Force on Rating Scales for Parkinson's Disease. The Unified Parkinson's Disease Rating Scale (UPDRS): Status and recommendations. *Mov Disord.* 2003;18(7):738–750.

U.S. Department of Veterans Affairs. Parkinson's disease research, education and clinical centers. Montreal Cognitive Assessment (MoCA). https://www.parkinsons.va.gov/Consortium/MoCA.asp. Published 2004. Accessed May 11, 2017.

Olanow CW, Rascol O, Hauser R, et al. A double-blind, delayed-start trial of rasagiline in Parkinson's disease. *N Engl J Med.* 2009;361(13):1268–1278.

Postuma RB, et al. MDS clinical diagnostic criteria for Parkinson's disease. *Mov Disord.* 2015;30(12):1591–1601.

Postuma RB, Aarsland D, Barone P, Ziemssen T. Identifying prodromal Parkinson's disease: Pre-motor disorders in Parkinson's disease. *Mov Disord.* 2012;27(5):617–626.

Press, D. Parkinson's disease: Diagnosis and treatment. Lecture from Pri-Med conference. Ft. Lauderdale, FL. February 3, 2017.

Przuntek H. Early diagnosis in Parkinson's disease. *J Neural Transm Suppl.* 1992;38:105–114.

Unified Parkinson's Disease Rating Scale. In Fahn S, Elton R, Members of the UPDRS Development Committee. In: Fahn S, Marsden CD, Calne DB, Goldstein M, eds. *Recent developments in Parkinson's disease*; vol Florham Park, NJ: Macmillan Health Care Information; 1987, 153–163, 293–304. http://img.medscape.com/fullsize/701/816/58977_UPDRS.pdf. Accessed May 1, 2017.

RESOURCES

Alzheimer's Disease

Alzheimer's Association
1-800-272-3900
    www.alz.org
Alzheimer's Foundation of America
1-866-232-8484
    http://alzfdn.org

Amyotrophic Lateral Sclerosis

Amyotrophic Lateral Sclerosis (ALS) Association
Washington, DC
    www.alsa.org

Parkinson's Disease

Parkinson's Disease Foundation
1-800-457-6676
    www.pdf.org
National Parkinson Foundation, Inc.
1-800-327-4545
    www.parkinson.org
United Parkinson Foundation
833 West Washington Blvd.
Chicago, IL 60607
1-312-733-1893

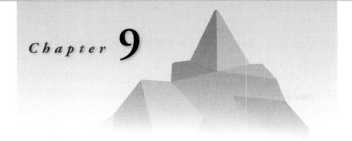

Chapter 9

Cerebrovascular Accident (Stroke)

Sarah Horn, MD

Jill E. Winland-Brown, EdD, APRN, FNP-BC

Stroke, also referred to as a *cerebrovascular accident (CVA),* causes acute onset of neurologic deficits caused by decreased blood flow or bleeding in a localized area of brain tissue. Although the incidence of stroke has decreased in the past 25 years because of risk-factor management and improved treatment, it has continued to be a significant public health problem in terms of both mortality and permanent disability. Stroke is a leading cause of disability in adults, incurring major economic burdens on the patient, family, and public as a result of direct medical costs and lost employment. The impact of cerebrovascular disease as a major health problem with demands on health care and other support systems will continue to grow as the number of stroke survivors living with disabilities increases and the population continues to live longer. The need for continued improvement in stroke prevention, the control of risk factors, and acute management of stroke is critical.

There are two kinds of strokes: *hemorrhagic* and *ischemic.* Approximately 80% of strokes are ischemic and 20% hemorrhagic. Ischemic stroke, also called an *ischemic cerebral infarct,* is caused by decreased blood flow to a localized part of the brain supplied. Etiologies include embolism, thrombosis, and hypoperfusion. A transient ischemic attack (TIA) is a temporary episode of focal cerebral ischemia that resolves spontaneously and does not leave permanent damage. People who have had a TIA are at higher risk for future stroke.

Hemorrhagic strokes can be further classified as intracerebral hemorrhage (hemorrhage into the brain parenchyma itself), subarachnoid hemorrhage (bleeding into the cerebrospinal fluid (CSF) in the subarachnoid space surrounding the brain), epidural, and subdural.

EPIDEMIOLOGY AND CAUSES

Stroke is the fifth leading cause of death in the United States after heart disease, cancer, chronic lower respiratory diseases, and accidents. The rate of stroke is highest in the southeastern United States. Although there are approximately 130,000 deaths from stroke annually in the United States (1 in every 20 deaths), an estimated 795,000 people have a stroke each year. About 610,000 are new strokes. Every 40 seconds, someone has a stroke. Someone dies from stroke every 4 minutes. More women than men (about 3:2) die from a stroke. In reviewing long-term survival, 25% of people who have an initial stroke die within 1 year and two-thirds die within 12 years.

Health costs associated with stroke are significant. The average health-care costs per person (inpatient and outpatient) for strokes have been estimated to be between $8,000 and $16,500. These numbers do not include the additional costs of morbidity-related expenses (lost time from work, additional nursing care, etc.). The direct and indirect costs to the nation are an estimated $33 billion.

Age, sex, race, ethnic origin, and heredity have been identified as nonmodifiable risk factors for stroke, helping to identify those at greatest risk. Compared with whites, young African Americans are at two to three times greater risk of stroke and are 2.5 times more likely to die of one. A higher incidence of stroke is also noted in Hispanics and Asians, particularly Chinese and Japanese, than in white Americans. For people older than age 55 years, the incidence of stroke more than doubles in each successive decade. Thirty-four percent of people who suffer a stroke are younger than age 65 years. An increased incidence of stroke in some families has been noted, probably because of a genetic tendency and familial exposure to similar environmental or lifestyle risks.

Important modifiable risk factors for stroke include hypertension, cardiac disease, diabetes, hypercholesterolemia, smoking, illicit drug use, and lifestyle factors. There is a fourfold increase of stroke when a patient is hypertensive with a blood pressure (BP) greater than 160/95 mm Hg. Studies show that with treatment for hypertension, there is a 38% reduction in strokes and a 40% reduction in mortality from strokes. Atrial fibrillation is associated with a threefold to fivefold increased risk for stroke. Other cardiac diseases related to increased risk for stroke include artificial cardiac valves, cardiac structural abnormalities such as patent foramen ovale (PFO), and heart failure with low ejection fraction. People with diabetes are more prone to develop atherosclerosis, thus increasing the risk of stroke.

PATHOPHYSIOLOGY

Pathologically, two categories of stroke are recognized: ischemic and hemorrhagic.

Cerebral Ischemia

Cerebral ischemia is caused by a reduction in blood flow to the brain, particularly the cerebrum. Neurons will stop functioning after less than 10 seconds of insufficient blood flow, but they can recover fully if circulation is restored promptly. After a few minutes without oxygen and glucose, however, neurons begin to die. The specific neurologic deficits caused by cerebral ischemia reflect the functions of the brain affected by the ischemia. Ischemia can be subdivided into three subtypes: thrombosis, embolism, and hypoperfusion.

Thrombosis

Thrombosis refers to local obstruction of an artery. Common causes include atherothromboses, dissection of an artery, or other disease of the arterial wall. Atherosclerosis produces atheromatous plaques—gummy bulges that protrude from the inner walls of arteries. Atheromatous plaques are masses of lipids, cell debris, collagen, fibrin, platelets, and blood cells, covered by smooth muscle cells, macrophages, and lymphocytes. Plaques that erode can also initiate local blood clotting. When the clot sticks to the plaque, it often grows, occludes the arterial lumen, and leads to ischemia in the areas of brain supplied by that occluded artery.

Embolism

Embolism refers to fragments of debris that travel downstream and occlude smaller arteries and arterioles, producing areas of ischemia. Occlusive emboli can be generated upstream some distance from the cerebral arteries. The two most common emboli are cardioembolic and artery to artery. Atrial fibrillation, prosthetic heart valves, valve vegetations, and myocardial infarcts can generate cardioembolic emboli. Artery-to-artery emboli are caused by clots and fragments of atherosclerotic plaque that form in the aorta, internal carotid arteries, or the vertebral arteries that dislodge and are carried into more distal brain arteries, which then become occluded. Paradoxical embolism occurs when a venous thromboembolism passes through a PFO to enter the arterial system. Embolism of clots and clumps of platelets formed during conventional angiography procedures and cardiac surgery can also become occlusive emboli. Hypercoagulability syndromes, elevated levels of blood platelets, calcified fragments of plaque and tissue, air, fat, cholesterol crystals, tumor fragments, bacterial vegetations, and foreign material (such as talc and cornstarch injected with illicit drugs) can all clog brain arteries either via embolism or thrombosis.

Decreased Brain Perfusion

Transient global low cerebral blood flow causes syncope (fainting). If brain perfusion remains low, such as during shock or cardiac arrest, neurons begin to die, starting in the watershed areas—that is, at the borders between regions supplied by the major cerebral arteries. Watershed areas are located at the border between the areas supplied by the anterior cerebral artery and medial cerebral artery (MCA) as well as between the MCA and posterior cerebral artery (PCA) territories. Watershed infarcts are often bilateral and affect the brain more diffusely. In addition, certain hippocampal neurons are especially sensitive to loss of cerebral perfusion, and this may explain the memory deficits that occur after the hypoperfusion caused by even a brief cardiac arrest.

Cerebral Hemorrhage

The neurologic symptoms of a cerebral hemorrhage result from the pressure of a hematoma. In some cases, this pressure causes infarcts in the compressed tissue. In others, there is less cell death so that when the hematoma is resorbed, the neurologic deficits resolve to some degree. As a rule, the larger the hematoma, the greater and more permanent the damage.

Epidural Hematomas

Epidural bleeding is caused by severe head injuries. Epidural hematomas are most common along the temporal cranial wall and result from tears in the middle meningeal artery. The leaking arterial blood rapidly creates a hematoma between the dura and bone. This increases the overall intracranial pressure, which in turn reduces the cerebral blood perfusion. As the hematoma enlarges, it presses on adjacent brain tissue, causing contralateral hemiparesis. Next, the increasing pressure affects the diencephalon, and the patient becomes lethargic and drowsy. When the midbrain becomes compressed against the dural rim of the tentorium, patients develop ipsilateral oculomotor nerve palsy and an enlarged pupil. Continued expansion of the hematoma compresses the contralateral cerebral peduncle, leading to hemiplegia. Eventually, the diencephalon and ipsilateral temporal lobe can be pushed down through the tentorial notch; such herniations compress the PCAs, press on the brainstem, and can be fatal.

Subdural Hematomas

Subdural bleeding is usually caused by blunt trauma that knocks the brain against the skull. Movement of the brain relative to the skull tears the thin superior cerebral veins (the bridging veins), which drain the external cerebral veins into the superior sagittal sinus. Minor repeated injuries can cause chronic venous leakage. Venous subdural hematomas expand more slowly than the higher-pressure arterial epidural hematomas. Small, self-limited subdural hematomas are often absorbed spontaneously, but subdural hematomas can also continue to enlarge slowly without severe or clear-cut neurologic symptoms, especially in the elderly. An untreated subdural hematoma can lead to permanent severe neurologic deficits or death.

Intracerebral Hemorrhage

Also known as *intraparenchymal hemorrhage* (IPH), intracerebral hemorrhage refers to bleeding within the brain parenchyma. One of the most common causes of IPH is hypertension. Sudden increases in cerebral BP or cerebral blood flow can rupture intraparenchymal arteries, especially when the arteries have been weakened by chronic hypertension, aneurysms, or vascular malformations. Hypertensive IPHs most often develop from ruptures of arteries to the basal ganglia and thalamus, although hematomas can also form elsewhere in the cerebral lobes, cerebellum, and pons. Other etiologies include trauma, amyloid angiopathy, underlying tumor, clotting disorders, low platelet counts, anticoagulant drugs, vasoconstrictors (including amphetamine or cocaine use), and eclampsia during pregnancy. Hemorrhages from amyloid angiopathy tend to be in lobar locations (i.e., located more peripherally toward the cortex of the brain) as opposed to hypertensive hemorrhages, which tend to be located within deep structures in the brain.

The neurologic symptoms of an IPH reflect the specific location of the hematoma—for example, a basal ganglia hematoma pressing on the internal capsule will cause contralateral motor weakness.

Subarachnoid Hemorrhage

Subarachnoid hemorrhages are caused by tears in the arteries running along the subarachnoid space at the surface of the brain. Ruptured arterial aneurysms are the most common source of subarachnoid bleeds. In the brain, these aneurysms usually occur at branch points of the large arteries, especially in the circle of Willis. Other causes include congenital vascular malformations, trauma, amyloid angiopathy, and bleeding diathesis.

CSF circulates through the subarachnoid space, and blood from a subarachnoid hemorrhage will spread quickly throughout the CSF surrounding the brain and spinal cord. In such cases, a lumbar puncture (LP) produces CSF that contains red blood cells. In this case, the CSF often assumes a yellowish tinge referred to as xanthochromia. Xanthochromia occurs as a result of the breakdown of hemoglobin in the CSF by enzymes producing yellow-pigmented bilirubin. Ruptures of arteries in the subarachnoid space cause a sudden increase in intracranial pressure and produce severe headache, vomiting, and drowsiness.

CLINICAL PRESENTATION

Subjective

A stroke should be suspected when a patient presents with sudden onset of focal neurologic signs and symptoms. Particularly with ischemic strokes, maximum neurologic deficits tend to occur at the onset and then improve over time as a patient recovers. Patients may complain of weakness or numbness on one side of the body depending on the location of the stroke. Impairment may be seen in cognitive abilities, level of consciousness, vision, sensation,

extraocular muscle functioning, coordination, and gait as well. They may or may not complain of a headache.

Unilateral weakness or numbness in a stroke is caused by damage to the opposite side of the brain that controls those functions. A variety of cognitive changes can be exhibited by patients, depending on the location of the brain affected by the stroke. A common cognitive change seen in a stroke affecting the right brain hemisphere, particularly in the territory of the right middle cerebral artery, is left-sided neglect. With this, patients lose awareness of the left side of their bodies. They may not realize they have weakness or numbness on the left side of their body. In severe cases, they may not be able to recognize their own left hand. Lesions in the left middle cerebral artery territory commonly cause aphasia (language difficulty) in addition to right-sided weakness. Other possible cognitive changes include impairment of memory, decreased ability to concentrate on and attend to tasks, alexia (reading problems), and agraphia (difficulties in writing). Strokes in the brainstem tend to cause cranial nerve (CN) abnormalities (such as double vision from extraocular movement abnormalities) in addition to weakness and/or numbness on one side of the body. Strokes in the PCA territory, which supplies the occipital lobes, can cause an isolated visual field deficit.

The primary-care practitioner (PCP) should ask about a history of cardiovascular risk factors, such as hypertension, hyperlipidemia, smoking history, diabetes, coronary artery disease (CAD), cardiac valvular disorders, atrial fibrillation, and recent myocardial infarction (MI). A list of current medications should be obtained, including prescribed, over-the-counter, and recreational (illicit) drugs. The PCP should be especially attentive to the use of anticoagulant, antiplatelet, and illegal drugs, which may provide clues to the cause of the stroke or affect treatment.

In brain hemorrhage, a severe headache of abrupt onset ("thunderclap headache"), possibly with a decreased level of consciousness, raises concern for subarachnoid hemorrhage. In subdural hematoma, headache is the single most common symptom and is more common in older adults. A subdural hematoma is often accompanied by focal neurologic symptoms. IPH presents with focal neurologic signs and symptoms similar to those seen in ischemic stroke.

Objective

Information obtained during the history and physical examination assists in identifying the area of the brain involved, the etiology of the stroke, and in determining whether the stroke is hemorrhagic or ischemic. Relevant aspects of the history include the nature of the onset, the timing, and duration of the neurologic deficit, and whether the deficit is static, improving, or worsening. It is important to inquire specifically about the patient's activity when the symptoms began; how the symptoms progressed; the severity of the symptoms; and whether they have worsened, improved, or remained the same. The hallmark of stroke is the sudden onset of symptoms, regardless of etiology. Headache is more common in hemorrhagic strokes, but is also seen in ischemic strokes. The only definite way to differentiate between ischemic and hemorrhagic strokes is with brain imaging, typically computed tomography (CT) of the head. It is important to determine whether the symptoms are transient, which could indicate a TIA. To differentiate TIA from a stroke, the patient should undergo brain magnetic resonance imaging (MRI), which will indicate whether permanent damage to the brain has occurred. The causes of TIAs are the same as the causes of stroke. Expedited work-up and treatment of TIAs is important because the risk of stroke is elevated after a TIA. Table 9.1 presents the different etiologies of TIA and ischemic stroke.

Neurologic examination aids in localization of the stroke. Signs and symptoms exhibited by the patient typically localize to a specific area of the brain (Table 9.2). Hemiparesis (i.e., weakness on one side of the body) indicates involvement of the motor pathway on the opposite side of the brain. Weakness may be evident in the lower face (a flattened nasolabial fold and asymmetrical smile), arm, and leg on one side of the body. This is often accompanied by sensory deficits as well. Aphasia typically localizes to the left middle cerebral artery territory. Left-sided neglect typically localizes to the right middle cerebral artery territory. Assessment of visual fields may identify deficits such as vertical defect (homonymous hemianopsia), blindness in one or both eyes, bitemporal hemianopsia, or homonymous quadrant defect. A visual field deficit helps localize the stroke along the visual pathways. Presence of CN abnormalities occur in brainstem strokes. A review of the CNs may indicate

TABLE 9.1	Pathologies of Ischemic Stroke and TIA		
Etiology of Stroke and TIA	*Signs and Symptoms*	*Physical Examination*	*Diagnostic Tests*
Carotid artery pathology	Paresthesia Weakness of hand, arm, face Aphasia Dysarthria Unilateral neglect Transient blindness or blurred vision in one eye Cognitive/behavioral changes (rare)	Neurologic examination Assess for carotid bruits Assess for retinal emboli (refer for complete ophthalmologic examination) Cardiac auscultation	Laboratory tests: CBC, platelets, electrolytes, lipid panel, diabetes screen, syphilis serology, toxicology screen, coagulation studies, hypercoagulability screen (antiphospholipid antibodies, PT/PTT, Russell's viper venom time for lupus anticoagulant, anticardiolipin antibodies, beta 2 glycoprotein, ESR, ANA) CT scan of the head MRI brain (more sensitive than CT) Vessel imaging: Doppler studies of carotid vessels, magnetic resonance angiography, or CT angiography Echocardiography and Holter monitoring to evaluate for cardiac sources of emboli
Small cerebral vessel pathology	Pure motor hemiparesis Pure sensory stroke Ataxic hemiparesis Dysarthria—clumsy hand syndrome Sensorimotor stroke	As above	As above
Vertebrobasilar system pathology	Ataxia Dizziness, vertigo Dysarthria Alteration in consciousness, Diplopia, hemianopia, or bilateral vision loss Unilateral or bilateral sensory or motor systems	As above	As above
Cardioembolic	May cause any of the above symptoms. May also cause multiple areas of infarct.	As above	As above

Abbreviations: ANA, antinuclear antibodies; CBC, complete blood count; CT, computed tomography; ESR, erythrocyte sedimentation rate; MRI, magnetic resonance imaging; PT/PTT, prothrombin time/partial thromboplastin time; TIA, transient ischemic attack.

TABLE 9.2 Signs and Symptoms of Occlusion of Specific Areas of the Brain

Common Stroke Syndrome	Area of Brain	Signs and Symptoms of Occlusion
Right ICA, MCA, ACA	Right anterior hemisphere	Left-sided weakness Left-sided numbness Left-sided neglect Left visual field deficit Difficulty with leftward gaze
Left ICA, MCA, ACA	Left anterior hemisphere	Right-sided weakness Right-sided numbness Right visual field deficit Aphasia Difficulty with rightward gaze Difficulty with reading, writing, and calculations
PCA	Occipital lobe, thalamus, medial temporal lobes	Contralateral homonymous hemianopia Let PCA lesion: alexia without agraphia, impaired color naming
Vertebrobasilar system	Cerebellum and brainstem	Contralateral hemiplegia Bilateral motor, sensory, and visual complaints Vertigo Diplopia Dysphagia Ataxia Dysconjugate gaze Crossed signs Horner's syndrome (ptosis of upper eyelid, slight elevation of lower lid, constriction of pupil, anhidrosis)
Pure motor stroke Ataxic hemiparesis	Small vessel occlusion ("lacunar infarct"): Internal capsule Base of the pons	Weakness in the face, arm, and leg on one side of the body May be accompanied by ataxia on the side of the weakness Absence of other abnormalities on neurologic examination
Pure sensory stroke	Thalamus	Numbness in the face, arm, and leg on one side of the body. Absence of other abnormalities on neurologic examination

Abbreviations: ACA, anterior cerebral artery; ICA, internal carotid artery; MCA, middle cerebral artery; PCA, posterior cerebral artery.

difficulties with eye movements (CNs III, IV, VI), facial sensation and chewing (CN V), facial weakness involving both the upper and lower face (CN VII), vertigo or impaired hearing (VIII), dysphagia and absent gag reflex (CNs IX and X), or impaired tongue movement (CN XII). Vertigo and unilateral ataxia typically indicate involvement of the cerebellum or brainstem. Alteration of consciousness indicates involvement of the reticular activating system and is typically caused by strokes in the upper brainstem or bilateral thalami. The degree of infarction following a stroke varies depending on the arteries involved, the duration of ischemia, and the adequacy of cerebral collateral circulation. The National Institutes of Health Stroke Scale (NIHSS; see Resources) is a standardized neurologic examination designed to quickly identify the examination abnormalities caused by a stroke.

The physical examination can help discern the etiology of the stroke. An irregular heartbeat points toward atrial fibrillation. Severe hypertension often accompanies a hypertensive intracerebral hemorrhage. Patients with carotid atherosclerotic disease may have a carotid bruit. Detecting the presence of a bruit is significant. Not only

does it indicate atherosclerosis and ischemic heart disease, but it may also increase the risk for a stroke. In caring for a patient with asymptomatic carotid bruit, the PCP should begin with a thorough history for the presence of coronary and peripheral vascular occlusive disease. It is important to identify and manage stroke risk factors.

DIAGNOSTIC REASONING

Diagnostic Tests

Patients who present within the first few hours of stroke symptom onset may be eligible for acute stroke treatment with intravenous tissue plasminogen activator and require emergent evaluation in an emergency department. Evaluation should include vital signs, NIHSS, blood glucose level, head CT, and assessment of contraindications. Ideally, a neurologic consultation should also be available within 30 minutes of the patient's arrival. In the clinician's physical and neurologic examination and management of the stroke, the time at onset of symptoms is particularly important to determine the proper use of thrombolytic therapy.

It is strongly recommended that emergency CT be the initial brain imaging study for the emergency evaluation of a suspected ischemic stroke. Practice guidelines of the American Heart Association Stroke Council recommend the use of noncontrast CT of the head in patients with suspected acute stroke to exclude a nonvascular lesion as the cause of the signs and symptoms and to assess for an intracranial hemorrhage. Signs of an ischemic stroke may not be initially apparent on a head CT. Detection of an acute ischemic stroke by CT depends on the location, extent, and duration of the infarct. Even large infarcts may not be apparent for several hours after onset. Some early infarct signs on head CT include hyperdensity in a segment of a blood vessel (representing clot at that location), loss of the "insular ribbon," loss of gray-white matter differentiation, hypoattenuation of the deep nuclei, and cortical edema. Eventually, an infarcted area appears hypodense on head CT. A CT during the first hours of symptoms can differentiate between a hemorrhagic and ischemic stroke and facilitate the decision to use early thrombolytic therapy. Acute blood appears hyperdense on head CT. Other imaging techniques can help with diagnosis but should not delay treatment.

MRI is generally recommended for patients with stroke because it is more sensitive than CT for identifying small ischemic lesions, particularly in the acute period. It also can also help identify the etiology of ischemic and hemorrhagic strokes. Abnormalities in MRI diffusion and perfusion sequences occur within minutes of ischemic stroke onset.

Pregnant women are at higher risk of stroke compared with the general population. There are no specific imaging recommendations for pregnant women other than those related to radiation precautions. There is a potential risk of radiation-induced defects during the first trimester, when the patient may be unaware of pregnancy.

After a stroke is diagnosed, it is important to discern the cause of the stroke because this will affect management. In ischemic stroke, large artery atherosclerosis, cardioembolic infarcts, and small-vessel occlusion are common etiologies. A basic stroke work-up for patients with ischemic stroke includes obtaining laboratory test results, electrocardiogram (ECG) and cardiac monitoring, brain MRI, vessel imaging, and echocardiogram. Patients with ischemic stroke should be screened for diabetes and hyperlipidemia. An ECG will detect the presence of risk factors, increasing the probability of stroke, including a recent MI, atrial fibrillation, or left ventricular hypertrophy. Cardiomegaly may be seen on a chest x-ray. All patients with ischemic stroke should undergo cardiac monitory for underlying paroxysmal atrial fibrillation, a common cause of embolism. Vessel imaging is important to identify sources of artery-to-artery embolism and demonstrate large vessel occlusions amenable to mechanical thrombectomy in the acute setting. Angiography is considered the test of choice. Magnetic resonance angiography, CT arteriogram, color duplex ultrasound, and transcranial Doppler are acceptable, noninvasive techniques to screen patients for vascular abnormalities in the setting of stroke. A cardiac echocardiogram should be obtained, preferably with a bubble study (which helps evaluate for a PFO), in patients with ischemic stroke to assess for cardioembolic source. A hypercoagulability screen may be warranted in cases of unexplained stroke. This can include laboratory testing and screening for underlying malignancy.

Patients with hemorrhagic stroke should also be evaluated to determine the etiology. BP must be closely monitored and severe hypertension treated. Angiography can assess for vascular abnormalities. Laboratory data may reveal a decreased platelet count or prolonged prothrombin time or partial thromboplastin time, which may indicate a bleeding disorder or use of anticoagulants, respectively. If the etiology is unclear, brain MRI can evaluate for evidence of underlying amyloid angiopathy, tumor, or hemorrhagic transformation of an ischemic infarct. The brain MRI may need to be repeated in several weeks after the blood resorbs if vascular malformation or tumor is suspected but not evident on initial imaging. An LP may be an additional test used to diagnose subarachnoid hemorrhage if the head CT is negative. Contraindications to this procedure include mass effect on head imaging, thrombocytopenia, and coagulation disorders.

Differential Diagnosis

Common conditions with similar signs and symptoms of stroke and TIA include focal seizure and complex migraine aura, both of which can cause focal neurologic signs and symptoms. However, in seizure and migraine, these symptoms are transient and the timing is different. In a stroke or TIA, the onset of symptoms is very sudden; in seizure, the symptoms can progress over seconds, and in migraine aura, the symptoms tend to progress over minutes.

Brain tumors can mimic stroke and cause focal neurologic signs. Headache is often present, and patients may also develop seizures. Vomiting and papilledema may be present. Brain abscess, encephalitis, and meningitis can also cause focal neurologic signs, although these are typically accompanied by headache and fever.

MANAGEMENT

The main principle in the management of stroke is prevention and early recognition and treatment. Patients with symptoms of a possible stroke require immediate referral to an emergency department for evaluation, CT scan of the brain, and possible use of thrombolytic therapy. Evans et al. (2017) cited multiple studies that have changed the landscape of acute stroke care by highlighting the efficacy of mechanical thrombectomy for treatment of acute stroke.

Initial management of a stroke is focused on addressing the patient's airway, breathing, and circulation to maintain adequate tissue oxygenation. Anaerobic metabolism with depletion of energy stores can increase the extent of brain injury and worsen the outcome. In the prehospital setting, special attention is given to monitoring the patient's oxygen status through pulse oximetry and the use of supplemental oxygen as needed. Maintaining an adequate airway is crucial, and intubation with mechanical ventilation is initiated when there is decreased level of consciousness or evidence of apparent hypoventilation. Hypotension is treated to maximize cerebral blood flow and minimize complications. Aggressive treatment of hypertension in the prehospital setting is not done in patients with known ischemic disease, because lowering the BP may precipitate hypoperfusion and injury. There is a permissive level of hypertension allowed in the days after the stroke as well. Prehospital evaluation and transport time can account for significant delays in initiation of thrombolytic therapy for patients with acute ischemic stroke who require it. Aggressive stroke protocols and educational programs keyed to emergency medical services can markedly reduce the time from stroke onset to initiation of treatment.

Once the clinical presentation, laboratory data, and results of the CT scan are completed and diagnosis of acute ischemic stroke is suspected, thrombolytic agents must be considered. The patient and/or family should understand that thrombolytic therapy carries at least a 6.4% risk of intracerebral hemorrhage. Intravenous thrombolytic therapy is effective in reducing the neurologic deficits in some patients without CT evidence of intracranial hemorrhage within 3 hours after symptom onset. Although the 3-hour "rule" has been accepted, several studies extend this timeframe for thrombolytic therapy. Contraindications to thrombolytic therapy include recent head trauma in the last 3 months, previous intracranial hemorrhage, recent intracranial or intraspinal surgery, active internal bleeding, known brain tumor or intracranial vascular malformation, seizure at stroke onset, evidence of intracranial bleed on CT scan, international normalized ratio greater than 1.7, and a platelet count of less than 100,000.

It is important for the clinician to treat and reduce sources of fever, which can accompany an infectious complication of a stroke, to prevent recurrent seizures with anticonvulsants, and to prophylactically administer heparin, low-molecular-weight heparin, or heparinoids (Lovenox) to prevent deep vein thrombosis. The use of corticosteroids is not indicated in the management of cerebral edema and increased intracranial pressure due to stroke.

Edema in large territory infarcts can lead to herniation and be life-threatening. This is often referred to as a "malignant" stroke. Large strokes in the cerebellum are particularly dangerous because swelling can compress the brainstem. Treatment options include hyperosmolar therapy and decompressive surgery.

Early ambulation and preventive measures against aspiration, malnutrition, pneumonia, deep vein thrombosis, pulmonary embolism, decubitus ulcers, contracture, and joint abnormalities are important goals in managing the patient with a stroke.

It is important to investigate the etiology of the stroke because this affects management. Typically, either an antiplatelet or anticoagulant will be used for secondary stroke prevention. In patients with a cardioembolic source of stroke, such as atrial fibrillation, anticoagulation is typically recommended. If a PFO is discovered on echocardiogram, it should prompt investigation for deep vein thrombosis. Sometimes PFOs are surgically closed. Patients with high-grade carotid artery stenosis ipsilateral to the side of a TIA or stroke may be referred for surgical management, in addition to aggressive medical management of vascular risk factors. Carotid endarterectomy is established as effective for symptomatic patients with 70% to 99% internal carotid artery stenosis. Carotid endarterectomy should not be considered for symptomatic patients with less than 50% stenosis.

A significant number of patients with carotid artery disease have concomitant CAD, and serum cholesterol in patients with CAD should be evaluated and treated. The hydroxymethylglutaryl–coenzyme A reductase inhibitors, or statins, reduce the risk of both nonfatal and fatal strokes, demonstrating a significant protective effect similar to that conferred by antiplatelet agents. Medical management is preferred to carotid endarterectomy for symptomatic patients with less than 50% stenosis.

One of the most significant changes in the approach to the medical management of patients with CAD with respect to stroke risk reduction has been the use of antiplatelet drugs, principally daily aspirin therapy (acetylsalicylic acid or ASA) and clopidogrel (Plavix). Clinicians disagree as to whether high or low doses of aspirin are more efficacious; recommended dosages range from 81 to 325 mg per day. The recommended dosage of clopidogrel for stroke prevention is 75 mg daily.

In brain hemorrhage, severe hypertension must be treated. If the patient is taking anticoagulants, reversal agents must be given, if available. Evidence-Based Nursing Practice 9.1 describes a large prospective multicenter chart review that shows poor prognosis in warfarin-associated intracranial hemorrhage despite the reversal of anticoagulation.

FOLLOW-UP AND REFERRAL

Follow-up and rehabilitation focus on the return of the patient's optimal level of functioning. Following treatment and stabilization, the patient should be assessed for the potential for rehabilitation and transferred to a rehabilitation unit. The rehabilitation process involves six major areas of focus:

1. Prevention, recognition, and management of comorbid illness and medical complications

Evidence–Based Nursing Practice 9.1

Dowlatshahi D, Butcher KS, Asdaghi, N. Poor prognosis in warfarin-associated intracranial hemorrhage despite anticoagulation reversal. *Stroke.* 2012;43:1812–1817.

This prospective multicenter chart review of 141 patients was aimed to determine outcomes in patients with anticoagulant-associated intracranial hemorrhage (aaICH) treated with prothrombin complex concentrates (PCCs). Patients with aaICH presented with larger hematoma volumes, higher risk of hematoma expansion, and worse outcomes than patients with a spontaneous intracranial hemorrhage. The researchers examined clinical, imaging, and laboratory data, including thrombotic events after therapy. Although PCC therapy rapidly corrected the international normalized ratio (INR) in the majority of patients, mortality and morbidity rates remained high. They determined that rapid INR correction alone may not be sufficient to alter prognosis after aaICH.

2. Training for maximum independence
3. Facilitating psychosocial coping and adaptation by the patient and family
4. Prevention of secondary disability by promoting community reintegration, including resumption of home, family, and vocational activities
5. Enhancing quality of life in view of residual disability
6. Prevention of recurrent stroke and other vascular conditions, such as MI, that occur with increased frequency in patients with stroke

Patient Education

Adjustments may need to be made in the home environment before discharge, such as building a ramp or removing a door to accommodate a wheelchair. Specific areas of teaching involve exercise and ambulation techniques, dietary requirements, recognition of symptoms of another stroke, and an understanding of the emotional lability and depression that commonly accompany strokes. Also important are knowledge of appropriate use of medications and the time, place, and frequency of occupational and physical therapy activities. To help prevent caregivers at home from becoming overburdened, clinicians should teach caregivers to plan for respite or time away from caregiving activities on a regular basis. Information regarding community, state, and national resources can be a welcome source of support to patients and their families. The National Stroke Association has resource information, including referral services and a quarterly newsletter. The American Heart Association provides a large variety of information regarding risk factors and referrals for assistive devices. The Easter Seal Society also may provide assistance with wheelchairs or other assistive devices. Some communities have organizations to help with meals or transportation, along with self-help groups.

Education regarding the modification and reduction of risk factors plays a significant role in the reduction in the incidence of stroke and TIA. Risk factor reduction measures include control of hypertension, the use of ASA for prophylaxis in patients with a moderate to high risk of stroke or TIA, and the use of anticoagulants in patients with atrial fibrillation. In a summary of 17 treatment trials of hypertension throughout the world with nearly 50,000 patients, there was a 38% decrease in all strokes and a 40% decrease in fatal strokes after treatment of hypertension (Kaplan, 2001). In the Framingham study, smoking cessation promptly reduced the risk of stroke, with the major risk reduced within 2 to 4 years. Heavy use of alcohol also should be avoided. Moderate and intense levels of physical activity have been associated with a decrease in chronic incidence of stroke. Physical activity is believed to exert a beneficial influence on the risk factors for atherosclerotic disease by decreasing blood pressure, weight, and pulse rate; raising high-density lipoprotein cholesterol and lowering low-density lipoprotein cholesterol; decreasing platelet aggregability; increasing insulin sensitivity and improving glucose tolerance; and promoting a lifestyle conducive to changing diet and cessation of cigarette smoking. A diet low in fat, sodium, and cholesterol and high in fiber, fruits, and vegetables should be encouraged. Patients should also be encouraged to exercise modestly, to avoid weight gain, and to use stress reduction techniques. If the patient has atrial fibrillation, anticoagulant therapy should be initiated to prevent pooling of the blood in the atria that could promote potential emboli.

Because treatment within 3 to 4.5 hours of onset of a stroke is critical, successful treatment depends on educating the patient and the family to recognize stroke symptoms and to contact and secure access to medical care by calling 911. Delay in treatment has been known to occur for patients who call their PCP instead of 911, live alone, have onset of stroke while asleep, have onset at home rather than work, and who experience milder stroke symptoms. Studies have documented that 38% of patients and their families did not know a single warning sign of a stroke and that 28% could identify only one sign of seizures. They may attribute tingling or numbness of the fingers or mild gait clumsiness to a problem with the arm or leg. Patients may also feel they have dust in their eyes, when in fact they are experiencing amaurosis fugax. Patients may think such symptoms are trivial and may not seek attention, or if they do, they may not mention these symptoms to their PCP. Older adults may simply forget that any symptoms occurred.

Education of the patient and family should include the importance of reporting any new neurologic symptoms. Thorough education of high-risk patients and their families about the warning signs of a stroke, along with frequent evaluation and a careful review of symptoms by the PCP, will assist in detecting a problem and initiating treatment as soon as possible.

See the Iceberg of Stroke for the intense interactions that need to occur for a patient recovering from a stroke to achieve his or her highest potential.

The Iceberg of Stroke

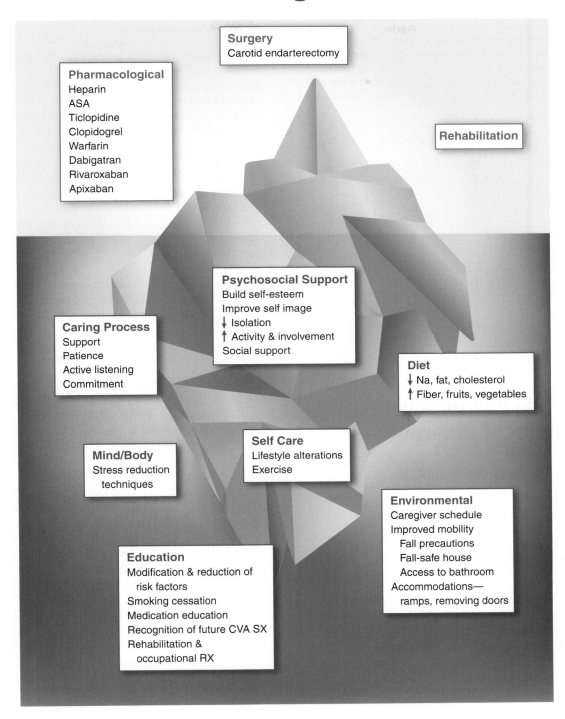

Surgery
Carotid endarterectomy

Pharmacological
Heparin
ASA
Ticlopidine
Clopidogrel
Warfarin
Dabigatran
Rivaroxaban
Apixaban

Rehabilitation

Psychosocial Support
Build self-esteem
Improve self image
↓ Isolation
↑ Activity & involvement
Social support

Caring Process
Support
Patience
Active listening
Commitment

Diet
↓ Na, fat, cholesterol
↑ Fiber, fruits, vegetables

Mind/Body
Stress reduction
    techniques

Self Care
Lifestyle alterations
Exercise

Environmental
Caregiver schedule
Improved mobility
    Fall precautions
    Fall-safe house
    Access to bathroom
Accommodations—
    ramps, removing doors

Education
Modification & reduction of
    risk factors
Smoking cessation
Medication education
Recognition of future CVA SX
Rehabilitation &
    occupational RX

REFERENCES

American College of Emergency Physicians; American Academy of Neurology. Clinical policy; use of intravenous tPA for the management of acute ischemic stroke in the emergency department. *Ann Emerg Med.* 2013;61(2):225–243.

Centers for Disease Control and Prevention. Stroke facts. https://www.cdc.gov/stroke/facts.htm. Updated December 30, 2016. Accessed May 8, 2017.

Centers for Disease Control and Prevention/National Center for Health Statistics. Leading causes of death. https://www.cdc.gov/nchs/fastats/leading-causes-of-death.htm. Published 2017. Accessed May 8, 2017.

Ennen KA. Taking a second look at stroke in women. *Am Nurse Today.* 2013;8(5):12–15.

Evans MRB, White P, Cowley P, Werring DJ. Revolution in acute ischaemic stroke care: a practical guide to mechanical thrombectomy. *Pract Neurol.* 2017;17(4):252–265.

Jauch EC. Acute management of stroke. Medscape. http://emedicine.medscape.com/article/1159752-overview#a2. Updated May 19, 2016. Accessed May 8, 2017.

Kaplan RC. Treatment of hypertension to prevent stroke: translating evidence into clinical practice. *J Clin Hypertens (Greenwhich).* 2001;3(3):153–156.

National Heart, Lung, and Blood Institute. Stroke. https://www.nhlbi.nih.gov/health/health-topics/topics/stroke/diagnosis. Published 2017. Accessed May 8, 2017.

Wolf PA, D'Agostino RB, Kannel WB, Bonita R, Belanger AJ. Cigarette smoking as a risk factor for stroke. The Framingham Study. *JAMA.* 1988;259:1025–1029.

RESOURCES

American Stroke Association
1-800-242-8721
   www.strokeassociation.org
National Institutes of Health Stroke Scale.
   https://en.wikipedia.org/wiki/National_Institutes_of_Health_Stroke_Scale.
National Stroke Association
1-800-STROKES
   www.stroke.org

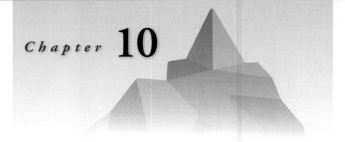

Chapter **10**

Infectious and Inflammatory Neurological Disorders

Jill E. Winland-Brown, EdD, APRN, FNP-BC

Sarah Horn, MD

MENINGITIS

Meningitis is an inflammation of the meninges (which includes the pia, arachnoid, and dura) surrounding the structures of the central nervous system (CNS). It can be acute, subacute, or chronic, depending on the etiology. Causes include infection, neoplastic, autoimmune, and drug induced. The common factor shared by all types of meningitis is an increase in the number of white blood cells (WBCs) in the cerebrospinal fluid (CSF), typically with symptoms and signs of meningeal irritation.

Although most cases of infectious meningitis are caused by viral infections, bacterial and fungal infections also occur. Acute bacterial meningitis is a life-threatening infection. The most common organisms are *Streptococcus pneumonia*, *Neisseria meningitidis*, and *Haemophilus influenza* type B. When routine bacterial cultures are negative, meningitis is called *aseptic meningitis*, which

has a very broad differential diagnosis. Viral infection is the most common cause of aseptic meningitis. Table 10.1 reviews the types of meningitis.

EPIDEMIOLOGY AND CAUSES

The incidence of meningitis is 15 per 100,000, with a prevalence of 5 cases per 100,000. Since the initiation of the widespread use of antibiotics in the 1950s, the mortality figures have remained steady at 10% to 15%. About one in five of those who do survive experience chronic long-term problems, such as brain damage, kidney disease, hearing loss, or limb amputations. Susceptibility differs with the causative organism, but generally young people, elderly people, and immunocompromised patients are at greatest risk. Bacterial meningitis affects more than 4,000 persons in the United States annually; 500 of those affected die from the disease. Fifteen percent of all cases involve adolescents and young adults. In adolescents, one in seven cases results in death. According to the National Meningitis Association, many adolescents do not receive the meningococcal serogroup B vaccine because it was only permissively recommended by the Centers for Disease Control and Prevention in 2015.

The majority of cases of infectious meningitis are attributed to bacteria and viruses, with a much smaller occurrence caused by fungi or parasites. Among the viral causative agents, enteroviruses are the most common. Meningitis has a seasonal occurrence, with a higher incidence in the spring and fall. Infants and young children are particularly susceptible because of a lack of immunity and the higher rate of fecal-to-oral transmission that takes place in this age-group. Arboviral infection is another common source during warm months when insect vectors are in abundance. The mumps virus can also be a causative factor in unimmunized populations. Various

TABLE 10.1	Types of Meningitis			
Major Type	**Description**	**Organism**	**Diagnostic Tests**	**Treatment**
Bacterial	Rapid onset: hours or days after exposure	**Age 3 months–18 years:** *H. influenzae* *N. meningitidis* *S. pneumoniae* **Age 18–50:** *S. pneumoniae* *N. meningitidis* **Age 50 or older:** *S. pneumoniae* *N. meningitidis* *Listeria monocytogenes* Gram-negative bacilli	CSF Gram stain analysis CSF culture (positive in 70%–85%) CSF PCR (putative transmembrane protein) for specific pathogenesis	**Age 3 months–18 years:** cefotaxime **or** ceftriaxone **Age 18 or older:** cefotaxime **or** ceftriaxone **plus** vancomycin ampicillin or amoxicillin if *Listeria* is suspected
Chronic/ subacute	Symptoms develop over weeks to months; less acutely ill	*M. tuberculosis* Fungi Spirochetes Virus Neoplastic Sarcoid systemic lupus erythematosus Behçet's disease Vasculitis Drug-induced (NSAIDs, IV Ig)	CSF analysis (cell count, differential, glucose, protein) Culture PCR for specific pathogens	**Tuberculosis:** isoniazid, rifampin, pyrazinamide, and a fluoroquinolone **Fungi:** amphotericin flucytosine **Spirochetes:** penicillin G for syphilis. Ceftriaxone for Lyme
Viral	More benign type; self-limited syndrome caused primarily by viruses	Herpes simplex virus Enterovirus Varicella zoster HIV EBV	CSF analysis (cell count, differential, glucose, protein) Culture PCR for specific pathogens	Supportive care in most cases Acyclovir can be used for HSV, VZV

Abbreviations: CSF, cerebrospinal fluid; EBV, Epstein-Barr virus; HSV, herpes simplex virus; IV IgG, intravenous gamma globulin; PCR, polymerase chain reaction; VZV, varicella-zoster virus.

herpes viruses cause meningitis and recurrent genital herpes can be associated with recurrent aseptic meningitis called Mollaret's meningitis.

Although anyone can get meningitis at any age, those most susceptible include the following groups:

- Infants younger than 1 year of age
- Adolescents and young adults (especially those living in crowded settings, such as dorms or barracks)
- Visitors outside the United States (such as the meningitis belt in Africa)
- Laboratory personnel who may have been exposed to meningococcal disease during an outbreak

PATHOPHYSIOLOGY

Meningitis is an inflammation of the brain's meningeal membranes, most often caused by infection. Acute bacterial meningitis is a purulent infection that develops within the subarachnoid space. Signs and symptoms include fever, headache, and stiff neck, usually accompanied by vomiting, lethargy, confusion, seizures, or coma.

Bacteria enter the host via the nasopharynx where they can enter the underlying blood vessels. *S. pneumoniae* and *N. meningitidis* are both encapsulated bacteria, and their capsules protect them from phagocytosis in the bloodstream.

From the circulation, bacteria enter the CSF through the choroid plexuses in the ventricles and through injured or leaky areas of the blood–brain barrier. Bacteria can multiply rapidly in the subarachnoid space because normal CSF has few WBCs, no immunoglobulin M antibodies, and low concentrations of the complement components C3 and C4. Local monocytes, macrophages, astrocytes, and microglia react to components in the bacterial cell walls by releasing inflammatory molecules, which increase the permeability of the blood–brain barrier and attract polymorphonuclear leukocytes from the systemic circulation. Large numbers of WBCs enter the CSF and form a purulent exudate in the subarachnoid space. Meningeal irritation from the exudate causes nuchal rigidity (the neck resists passive flexion), and lumbar puncture (LP) in bacterial meningitis produce CSF with a high WBC count. The pus can reduce the flow of CSF and lead to increased intracranial pressure. LPs of patients with bacterial meningitis yield high CSF pressures.

CLINICAL PRESENTATION

Subjective

Subjective symptoms of meningitis include headache, photophobia, and neck pain and stiffness (nuchal rigidity).

Objective

Objective signs include fever, tachycardia, and tachypnea. Signs of meningeal irritation include photophobia, pain with eye movement, Brudzinski's sign (hip and knee flexion when the neck is flexed) and Kernig's sign (inability to fully extend the legs). Occasionally, opisthotonus (severe back spasm, causing arching) is observed. Bacterial meningitis can cause hydrocephalus, altered level of consciousness, and seizures. Cranial nerve dysfunction can occur, resulting in possible diplopia, deafness, facial weakness, and pupillary abnormalities.

History taking may yield clues to possible causative agents or risk factors for meningitis. Major areas to emphasize in taking the history include pertinent exposures, recent infectious symptoms, evidence of immunocompromise, underlying systemic disorders, and travel history.

DIAGNOSTIC REASONING

Diagnostic Tests

Initially, routine blood studies may show marked elevation of WBCs (neutrophils) in bacterial meningitis or mild elevation in viral meningitis. Electrolytes should be monitored. Hyponatremia may occur from a common complication of meningitis, the syndrome of inappropriate antidiuretic hormone secretion (SIADH).

If the clinical signs and symptoms indicate the possibility of meningitis, an LP should be done to obtain CSF studies. Treatment of bacterial meningitis should not be delayed while awaiting LP. CSF in bacterial meningitis is typically cloudy with elevated WBCs, elevated pressure, greater than 80% polymorphonuclear neutrophils, low glucose, and elevated protein. Gram stain and culture of CSF may assist in detecting causative organisms. A computed tomography (CT) examination of the head should be performed before LP in cases of an abnormal neurologic examination (alteration of consciousness, focal findings, papilledema) to assess risk for herniation with LP.

Imaging studies such as a CT or magnetic resonance imaging (MRI) may reveal meningeal enhancement, basilar exudate, hydrocephalus, and associated focal lesions.

Any other contributing abnormalities such as skin, lung, or sinus lesions should be investigated.

Differential Diagnosis

Many infectious and noninfectious conditions may mimic meningitis. Headache and alteration of consciousness are both nonspecific with many differential diagnoses. Subarachnoid hemorrhage can cause meningeal irritation and headache. Meningitis should be differentiated from encephalitis, which affects the brain parenchyma. It is also important to establish the etiology of meningitis because this affects management.

MANAGEMENT

Meningitis can be life-threatening. If meningitis is suspected, the primary-care practitioner should refer the patient to the collaborating physician for immediate hospitalization and extensive diagnostic examination and treatment. The principal goals for managing meningitis include eliminating infection, symptomatic care, and prevention or treatment of complications.

The first goal and priority is to eliminate infection. This is achieved through the judicial use of specific antimicrobial therapy if the meningitis is bacterial in origin. If the diagnosis of bacterial meningitis is suspected, the administration of empiric antibiotics should not be delayed. Blood cultures and an LP should be performed immediately, and empiric antibiotic therapy should be initiated without delay. Antibiotic therapy should not be withheld if there is a delay in the performance of the LP. The choice of empiric therapy is based on the demographics of the patient (age, immunocompromised state, medical comorbidities). The patient's antibiotic regimen can be narrowed based on the results of cultures of the CSF. The usual course of intravenous (IV) antimicrobials is 10 to 14 days. Some treatment regimens are included in Table 10.1. Adjunctive corticosteroids have been used in adolescents and adults with bacterial meningitis and have been shown to reduce hearing loss and mortality.

Chronic meningitis treatment is based on the underlying etiology. Symptomatic treatment includes reduction of fever with acetaminophen, headache management with analgesics, and treatment of nausea and vomiting with an antiemetic such as Zofran. Oversedation should be avoided because it may mask increasing intracranial pressure. Other supportive treatment includes rest in a quiet, darkened room; adequate liquids; and a nutritious diet as tolerated.

Several vaccines are available for the more common forms of meningitis. In some cases, prophylaxis is advised for documented exposure.

Of major concern as a complication of meningitis is increasing intracranial pressure caused by cerebral edema or hydrocephalus. Early signs include drowsiness, headache, double vision (from cranial nerve six palsy), and confusion. Later signs include decreasing levels of consciousness; hemiparesis; pupillary changes; and Cushing's triad of hypertension, bradycardia, and respiratory changes. This serious complication requires emergent neurosurgical consult and intensive care unit admission, often with ventilatory support. Techniques to reduce intracranial pressure include hyperventilation, hyperosmolar therapy, and neurosurgical procedures such as drain placement.

FOLLOW-UP AND REFERRAL

All patients who are suspected of having any form of meningitis should be referred to the emergency department for urgent work-up and treatment. When the patient's condition is stable, the patient may be released to the care of the primary health-care practitioner to continue follow-up care, which consists of completion of the antibiotic regimen and monitoring of blood work. Any indication of a complicated course warrants close follow-up and neurologic referral. Cases of uncomplicated acute meningitis such as aseptic meningitis may require only supportive care or home IV antibiotic therapy after discharge. Patients with chronic meningitis or with neurologic deficits require rehabilitation and continuous follow-up. Choice of facility depends on the nature of the patient's needs and family resources.

Patient Education: Meningitis

Education regarding prevention of meningitis through available immunization or chemoprophylaxis, as well as observance for clues to impending complications, should be provided. The meningococcal vaccine is routinely recommended for all children and adolescents aged 11 to 18 years. If not administered in childhood, adults should also be vaccinated if they are college students leaving home to live in dorms, military personnel living in barracks, laboratory workers exposed to specimens containing meningococcus isolates, traveling to high-risk areas, or are immunocompromised.

Home management after hospital discharge includes assessing the need for assistance with routine activities while recovering. The patient should be encouraged to have frequent rest periods and to gradually increase activities while looking for signs (e.g., shortness of breath, increased pulse) that the activity is too strenuous. The diet should be well balanced and nutritious. Soft foods may be better tolerated. Plenty of fluids should be encouraged unless other conditions are present, such as congestive heart failure or kidney disease. Two tablets of acetaminophen (Tylenol) may be given every 4 to 6 hours for pain or headache. The patient may feel more comfortable initially in a darkened, quiet room, which will prevent discomfort related to photophobia. The importance of completing the full course of antibiotic or antiviral medications exactly as prescribed must be stressed to the patient and family. The

patient needs to avoid close contact with others to whom he or she may transmit the infection orally. The patient should be taught about potential complications and when it is necessary to call the health-care provider, for example, if he or she has any signs of an upper respiratory infection, any change in alertness or wakefulness, any recurrent fever, or any other sign of a worsening illness.

ENCEPHALITIS

In contrast to meningitis, which is inflammation of the meninges surrounding the brain, encephalitis is an inflammation of the parenchymal brain tissue. Symptoms and signs include fever and other systemic signs of infection, depressed level of consciousness, seizures, and focal neurologic signs. Often, there are associated signs of meningeal irritation as well such as headache and neck stiffness. Whereas bacterial meningitis can cause signs of brain parenchyma involvement (new-onset seizures, focal neurologic signs, and depressed level of consciousness), aseptic meningitis does not. Both conditions frequently occur together, which is referred to as meningoencephalitis. Viruses are a common cause, although nonviral agents, such as bacteria, parasites, chemicals, and autoimmune reactions are also possible etiologies.

EPIDEMIOLOGY AND CAUSES

There are more than 100 infectious, postinfectious, and immune-mediated conditions known to cause encephalitis (Parpia et al., 2016). It remains a public health concern with approximately 20,000 cases of encephalitis occurring annually in the United States (Vora, 2014). Viral pathogens are most common when a cause is identified, with herpes simplex virus (HSV) being by far the most common cause of sporadic encephalitis. With overall mortality due to encephalitis averaging between 5% and 20% and with residual neurologic deficits occurring in an additional 20% of cases, treatment and supportive care become important (Schmidt, 2011). Although most cases of encephalitis are viral, there are many nonviral agents responsible for encephalitis including syphilis, *Rickettsia rickettsii* (responsible for Rocky Mountain spotted fever), mycoplasma, *Cryptococcus neoformans*, Lyme disease (*Borrelia burgdorferi*), and *Mycobacterium tuberculosis*. Worldwide, the cause of encephalitis is unknown for 37% to 85% of encephalitis cases.

Encephalitis may occur at any age, but very young children and older adults are at the highest risk. The incidence of encephalitis has been reduced, especially in children, by the elimination of smallpox and vaccines against mumps, measles, and rubella. There is no significant ethnic predisposition, and encephalitis occurs equally among men and women. Arboviruses (carried by arthropods, such as mosquitos) can cause seasonal epidemic encephalitis. These agents include Zika, West Nile virus, and the Eastern and Western equine encephalitis viruses.

PATHOPHYSIOLOGY

Patients typically present with encephalopathy, infectious symptoms, and diffuse or focal neurologic symptoms. Encephalitis is usually accompanied by inflammation of the meninges; therefore, headache and nuchal rigidity are also frequent symptoms. Encephalitis can produce a range of focal neurologic problems, including seizures, muscle weakness or paralysis, and isolated cranial nerve palsies. Sometimes the inflammation disrupts the hypothalamic-pituitary axis, which can lead to diabetes insipidus, SIADH, or the inability to maintain a normal body temperature. When the infective agent is the HSV, the encephalitis has a predilection for the temporal lobes and therefore can cause memory problems, hallucinations, aphasia, and seizures.

Encephalitis is usually caused by a virus (in the United States, the most common cause is HSV), and the neurologic signs and symptoms of encephalitis are usually preceded by other signs of viral infection, such as fever, malaise, muscle aches, rashes, gastrointestinal disturbances, or respiratory symptoms. Encephalitis viruses enter the body through a number of routes: HSVs are transmitted through person-to-person contact, enteroviruses are swallowed and invade through the gut, arboviruses are introduced by bites of insects, rabies enters through bites of mammals, and varicella-zoster viruses are inhaled. In most cases, the viruses replicate, a viremia develops, and virus particles enter the CNS from the bloodstream. Some viruses (rabies, HSV, and varicella-zoster), however, are carried into the CNS in a retrograde fashion via axons.

The brain areas that sustain the most damage vary, and different causative agents have specific predilection for certain areas of the brain. Signs and symptoms also vary depending on the areas of brain affected. Seizures are common. When the brainstem becomes infected, coma or respiratory failure can result.

CLINICAL PRESENTATION

Subjective

Patients commonly present with confusion, alteration in level of consciousness, symptoms of meningeal irritation (headache, neck stiffness, photophobia), lethargy, behavioral or personality changes, amnesia, and/or lethargy.

Herpes simplex encephalitis caused by HSV may be heralded by bizarre behavior, aphasia, or hallucinations as the temporal and frontal lobes are selectively attacked by the virus. Other types of infectious agents (other herpes viruses, Lyme disease, varicella-zoster virus, *R. rickettsii*)

may produce a cutaneous rash in addition to neurologic signs such as headache, seizures, or nuchal rigidity. The rash is a typical feature of many viral diseases.

Objective

Physical examination may reveal a fever, nuchal rigidity, hemiparesis, cranial nerve palsy, ataxia, movement disorders, focal seizures, encephalopathy, systemic signs of infection, and rash.

DIAGNOSTIC REASONING

Diagnostic Tests

Epidemiological clues and assessment of risk factors to identify potential etiological agents should be sought in all patients with encephalitis. When encephalitis is suspected, the patient should be referred to the collaborating physician and to a neurologist. Cultures of body fluid specimens (e.g., from blood, stool, nasopharynx, or sputum), if clinical and epidemiological clues are suggestive, should be performed to identify various viral, bacterial, and fungal etiologies of encephalitis. CSF testing reveals increased WBCs and an increased protein level. A Gram stain of CSF is useful to assess for bacterial meningitis as the cause of the symptoms. Polymerase chain reaction (PCR) tests of numerous common viral pathogens are commercially available and may identify the viral type. Serum antibody testing performed early in the infectious course and compared with a specimen drawn 1 to 3 weeks after onset of illness can reveal a significant increase in the antibody titer. Brain imaging is helpful to assess parenchymal involvement and rule out other causes of focal neurologic signs (such as stroke and hemorrhage). Imaging can also provide clues to etiology. On examination, HSV encephalitis commonly causes hemorrhagic necrosis in the frontal and temporal lobes. However, normal brain imaging does not rule out encephalitis.

Because changes in the CSF may not be apparent at the beginning of the infection, a repeat LP may be indicated if the first is negative and suspicion remains high. Electroencephalogram is nonspecific in establishing an etiology but has a role in identifying seizures, including nonconvulsive seizure activity, in patients who are confused, obtunded, or comatose.

Differential Diagnoses

There is significant overlap between organisms that cause aseptic meningitis and encephalitis. Therefore, patients often present with meningoencephalitis, with features of both meningeal irritation and brain parenchymal involvement. To differentiate meningitis from encephalitis (or meningoencephalitis), one must assess for signs of brain involvement such as confusion, seizures, or focal signs on examination. Encephalitis can also be postinfectious or autoimmune in etiology. Postinfectious encephalitis is part of acute demyelinating encephalomyelitis, which causes areas of demyelination in the brain and spinal cord after an infection. Autoimmune encephalitis is often, but not always, part of a paraneoplastic process. Identification and treatment of the underlying tumor is important for diagnosis and treatment. Anti-*N*-methyl-D-aspartate receptor encephalitis is one of the most common of the autoimmune encephalopathies and is typically associated with ovarian teratomas. Psychiatric manifestations are common early in the course of the disease. Seizures are also common in this population (Lancaster, 2016).

MANAGEMENT

A suspicion of encephalitis requires referral and patient hospitalization for definitive neurologic diagnosis and treatment. Treatment includes antimicrobials, supportive care, and preventing complications.

If viral encephalitis is suspected, patients should be promptly started on treatment with IV acyclovir while awaiting further work-up because empirical treatment reduces both morbidity and mortality in HSV encephalitis.

Seizures should be treated with anticonvulsants like phenytoin (Dilantin), levetiracetam (Keppra), or other antiseizure meds. Safety must also be a consideration with these patients. Padding should be used to prevent seizure injury. Acetaminophen (Tylenol) is used to reduce hyperthermia and may be given as a rectal suppository if needed. Cerebral edema resulting in increased intracranial pressure is an ominous complication of encephalitis and can be treated with hyperosmolar therapy, hyperventilation, or neurosurgical intervention.

FOLLOW-UP AND REFERRAL

Patients suspected of having encephalitis are referred to the emergency department for urgent work-up and treatment and to a neurologist for definitive care and follow-up. When the patient is stabilized, the neurologist will release the patient's care to the primary-care provider. The relative degree of neurologic deficit determines the nature of follow-up care.

Patient Education: Encephalitis

Prevention of infection vectors through mosquito control and insect repellents should be one important focus of patient and community education. Early detection and proper removal of ticks is another important aspect. For convalescence, the importance of bedrest, fluids, and nutrition is emphasized, as well as clues to impending complications. The patient should be encouraged to take frequent rest periods and to increase activities gradually while looking for signs that the activity is too strenuous, for example, shortness of breath and increased pulse. The patient should be instructed to eat a balanced diet to ensure the inclusion of nutrients such as protein and vitamin C. Fluids should be encouraged unless contraindicated. Acetaminophen may be used for pain or a headache. The patient may feel more comfortable in a darkened, quiet room if photophobia is present. The importance of taking the antibiotics or antiviral medications exactly as prescribed should be stressed to the patient. Patients should be instructed to avoid close contact with others who may be harboring germs. If they notice any signs of an upper respiratory infection, they should seek help from their health-care provider immediately. Patients and families should be instructed to inspect the skin for ticks and to remove them intact. They should wear protective clothing to prevent tick bites. Last, patients should be instructed when to call the health-care provider—for example, if there are any changes in their level of consciousness, recurrent fever, or any other signs of a worsening illness.

HERPES ZOSTER

Herpes zoster, commonly known as shingles, is an infection by the varicella-zoster virus occurring along dermatomal pathways and resulting in a vesicular skin rash.

EPIDEMIOLOGY AND CAUSES

Varicella-zoster virus becomes latent in the neurons of sensory ganglia after a primary infection of chickenpox; it then reactivates later in life in a dermatomal area as herpes zoster (shingles). One in three individuals in the United States will develop shingles. An estimated 1 million cases occur each year. Children may get shingles; however, the risk of disease increases with age; approximately one half of all cases occur in men and women aged 60 and over. Four percent of patients with herpes zoster experience a second episode but rarely a third episode. Immunocompromised patients are at a significantly increased risk for developing shingles and also have a higher incidence of complications.

PATHOPHYSIOLOGY

Varicella-zoster virus, which causes chickenpox, is also responsible for a number of neurologic disorders, including encephalitis, meningitis, polyneuritis, multiple cranial neuropathies, and myelitis. Varicella-zoster virus initially infects people through the mucosa of the upper respiratory tract or the conjunctivae of the eyes. Within a week, the virus spreads throughout the body via the bloodstream, and approximately 1 week later, infections of the capillaries of the skin produce the vesicular lesions of chickenpox.

Once the lesions appear, virus particles are retrogradely transported inside sensory axons to dorsal root ganglia, where the viruses remain latent for the life of the patient. Varicella-zoster virus is most often found in the sensory ganglia of the ophthalmic division of the trigeminal nerve and in the dorsal root ganglia of the mid to lower spinal cord (ganglia T3 to L2). If viruses in a ganglion are reactivated, they replicate, destroy ganglion nerve cells, and migrate through the nerves to the innervated dermatomes, where they again produce vesicular skin lesions.

The destruction of sensory neurons in a ganglion produces pain in the innervated dermatome. This pain usually precedes the skin lesions by a few days, although sometimes pain is the only symptom. Typically, viruses are reactivated in only a single ganglion at a time; therefore, the symptoms are unilateral and affect a single dermatome. When the pain does not resolve within a few weeks, the syndrome is called postherpetic neuralgia (PHN). The pain of PHN can be either constant or intermittent and worsens at night and during temperature changes. Varicella-zoster virus that has been reactivated in the ophthalmic division of the trigeminal nerve can cause eye problems, including lesions of the cornea.

It is not known what triggers the reactivation of latent varicella-zoster viruses. The likelihood of developing this reactivation syndrome (called "herpes zoster" or "shingles") increases as a person ages and when a person's immune system becomes compromised. Herpes zoster is a frequent complication of HIV infection.

CLINICAL PRESENTATION

Subjective

Initially, the patient with herpes zoster may present with unexplained pain. The pain is described as constant or intermittent and may have a tingling or stabbing quality. The pain occurs along the involved dermatome, usually 48 to 72 hours before eruption of the classic vesicular skin rash. Pain acuity differs among individuals, but many patients say the pain becomes progressively worse at night or with changes in temperature. Herpes zoster ophthalmicus is a common complication of shingles in the V1 distribution of the trigeminal nerve. This condition can cause blindness and requires immediate referral to an ophthalmologist for evaluation and treatment. Ocular involvement is more common in patients who have concurrent lesions at the tip of the nose, referred to as Hutchinson sign. Lesions located inside of the mouth and in the external ear opening are often associated with unilateral facial weakness, vertigo, and hearing loss due to involvement of the VIIth and VIIIth cranial nerves; this is referred to as Ramsay-Hunt syndrome.

Another major characteristic of the disease is the occurrence of acute neuritis along the path of the rash dermatome. PHN occurs in approximately 25% to 50% of patients older than age 60. The constant or intermittent stabbing pain worsens at night or with temperature changes.

Objective

Herpes zoster is characterized by a unilateral vesicular rash along a dermatome, most commonly a thoracic or lumbar dermatome. The rash begins as erythema, then changes to papular lesions that rapidly form vesicles. The vesicles rupture, releasing infectious fluid, and then form scabs. Occasionally, the vesicles coalesce to form bullae. The skin lesions usually continue to develop for 3 to 5 days, and the entire disease course usually lasts 10 to 15 days. In some individuals, the skin lesions can persist for 30 days or longer. The pain caused by PHN may last much longer and at times may be permanent.

DIAGNOSTIC REASONING

Diagnostic Tests

Diagnosis is made after careful review of data obtained from the history and physical examination. The characteristic appearance and distribution of the lesions along with a history of preceding neuropathic pain help establish the diagnosis of herpes zoster. Usually the history and physical examination are all that is needed to make a definitive diagnosis.

If the diagnosis is questionable, a PCR assay, which detects the DNA sequence of the virus, may be done, along with an antibody titer (which requires more than one test for comparison). CSF analysis may be needed when CNS involvement is suspected.

Differential Diagnosis

Other conditions that cause similar rashes need to be ruled out. Impetigo may present as vesicles around an area of broken skin. The scrapings of these lesions can be sent for a Gram stain, which will reveal Gram-positive cocci if herpes zoster is present. Viral cultures may be done to rule out HSV or Coxsackie viral infections that can appear in a dermatomal region. Cellulitis, bites and stings, candidiasis, and drug eruptions should all be ruled out.

MANAGEMENT

The principal goals are to manage the healed vesicles, obtain pain relief, and prevent secondary infection and other complications. Initial management of herpes zoster involves the use of antiviral agents. They reduce the impact of herpes zoster by diminishing neuritis and speeding the healing of the skin lesions. Early intervention in the treatment of herpes zoster produces the best results. Famciclovir (Famvir), acyclovir (Zovirax), or valacyclovir (Valtrex) may be used. Systemic corticosteroids such as prednisone may assist in reducing acute pain when given in conjunction with the antiviral therapy. Lotions such as calamine and dressings soaked with Burow's solution may be used to soothe the lesions and prevent scratching or rubbing, thereby improving healing time, decreasing pain, and preventing secondary infection. Some patients find that corticosteroid cream helps as well. Some report that the pain of lesions in the thoracic area can be diminished by using a tight wrap of the chest to produce a splinting effect. The practitioner should use this method with care, especially in older adult patients or those with pulmonary disease, because the restriction (splinting) of normal breathing patterns could promote pulmonary stasis of secretions and increase the incidence of pulmonary infections. Patients with ophthalmic herpes affecting the first branch of the trigeminal nerve must be referred to an ophthalmologist because this condition may result in blindness.

PHN is a persistent pain resulting from shingles that lasts more than 3 months after the disease has run its course. PHN rarely occurs in individuals younger than age 40, is more severe in individuals older than age 50, and may occur in up to one-half of untreated people over age 60. Even with treatment, PHN may occur. Some clinicians think that administering systemic corticosteroids at the earliest onset of the rash reduces the risk of developing PHN. Analgesics (from nonnarcotic to narcotic agents in doses individualized for the patient) are supportive in reducing neuritis and PHN. If PHN is present, the use of tricyclic antidepressants such as amitriptyline taken each night may help if simple analgesics are ineffective. For additional pain relief, gabapentin (Neurontin) may help. Topical capsaicin cream is approved by the U.S. Food and Drug Administration (FDA) for relief of PHN. Topical lidocaine patches may be helpful. If pain is persistent, chronic PHN may respond to a regional block with or without corticosteroids. Ideally, the patient should be referred to a pain center because PHN can have devastating effects (see The Patient's Voice 10.1.)

FOLLOW-UP AND REFERRAL

It is essential that any patient with ophthalmic herpetic lesions be referred to an ophthalmologist. Additional follow-up includes a return visit if skin lesions become infected or if PHN is present. Referral to a neurologist may be required at any time if the patient does not respond to primary treatment plans. Patients should be referred to a pain center if PHN results in chronic persistent pain.

Patient Education: Herpes Zoster

Because herpes zoster is usually treated on an outpatient basis, patient and family education is important. The clinician should encourage patients to complete the course of the antiviral agent, even if they feel the disease has abated, or especially if they feel the treatment is not as effective as they had hoped it would be. Patients should be informed that elimination of the disease could take longer than anticipated, and careful medication administration and follow-up care could mean fewer complications in the long run. Patients should be instructed that the medication may be better tolerated if taken with food. If adverse effects from the treatment plan occur, patients need to keep the practitioner informed so adjustments can be made. Education on the potential for spread of the herpes zoster virus via fluid from ruptured vesicles is important. Patients should be instructed that before the rash crusts, it can release fluid that will cause an infection in others. Patients must be careful in handling dressings, linens, towels, and clothes that they have

---

 The Patient's Voice 10.1: Postherpetic Neuralgia

My mother died of postherpetic neuralgia (PHN).

My mother was 80 years old and had recently won the golf championship at her club. She had been a widow for 25 years and decided that she wanted to move in with me, her daughter, and her only granddaughter (age 3). We lived 4 hours away. At first she was very independent, driving around by herself and going shopping while I worked. That only lasted a few months. Then the decline began. First, she broke a wrist, which incapacitated her, and then she got pneumonia, which weakened her. Then she got "shingles" (herpes zoster), which did her in. She was diagnosed at the earliest onset of pain, yet treatment wasn't started until the vesicles erupted. She had ophthalmic herpes, so her vision was affected. She developed PHN very early, and due to the persistent pain, she became reclusive. She stopped going out, retreating to her room, and eventually wouldn't get out of

bed. Nothing helped the pain. I'm convinced it was because preventive treatment wasn't started early. As she became more depressed and stayed in bed, she got weaker and weaker and just gave up. She complained of shooting pain over half of her head that was worse at night, so she'd be awake all night, and sleep all day. Nobody could help—not her primary-care provider, neurologist, ophthalmologist, psychologist, or me. She died in her sleep, and I'm convinced it was the result of PHN.

I've learned three things from this experience. First, if older persons are optimally functioning, don't move them out of their familiar supportive environment. Second, treat all cases of herpes aggressively, as you don't know who is going to develop PHN. As my mom used to say, "An ounce of prevention is worth a pound of cure." This leads to the third, probably most important lesson: get every older adult vaccinated!

used. They should not be around children who have not been vaccinated for chickenpox or those who have not had chickenpox yet; contact with pregnant women should also be avoided. Patients need to know that scratching the rash can lead to an infection. The clinician should pursue ways to relieve the pruritus, as mentioned previously. Patients should be instructed about the nature of the rash so that when they see it in varying stages of progression, they will not think that it is not healing. Again, the importance of completing all prescribed medications needs to be stressed. Patients need to know the reason they are taking other medications, for example, antidepressants (which can treat PHN), so they will continue taking them. Research has shown that the shingles vaccine Zostavax has reduced the occurrence of shingles in people aged 60 and older and offers more than 50% protection. In addition, it reduces the incidence of PHN by almost 70%. The Advisory Committee on Immunization Practices (2017) recommends a single dose of Zostavax for adults aged 60 and older, even if they have already had shingles. The FDA has approved the vaccine for persons older than age 50 years. Immunocompromised individuals should not receive the vaccine. Shingrix (Zoster Vaccine Recombinant, Adjuvanted) has proven to be more effective (at 97%) than Zostavax. It is recommended for those over age 50 years for the prevention of herpes zoster. It is given intramuscularly once, followed by another injection in 2 to 6 months. It may also be given to patients who have already received Zostavax (Westmead Institute for Medical Research, 2018).

TRIGEMINAL NEURALGIA

Trigeminal neuralgia is a distressing, painful idiopathic disorder of the trigeminal nerve (cranial nerve V). It is also known as tic douloureux. This excruciating facial pain is paroxysmal and usually lasts less than 3 seconds. For many individuals, the severity of the pain is disabling, and patients will do almost anything to prevent triggering an episode.

The lancinating, sharply cutting pain occurs along one or more of the three branches of the trigeminal nerve. Characteristically, the painful episodes occur when specific trigger zones are stimulated by touch, chewing, talking, shaving, or environmental temperature changes. Patients often describe the pain as "electric" or "stabbing" and penetrating. The pain of trigeminal neuralgia is chronic. Although patients may experience periods of spontaneous pain remission that may last weeks or months, the pain returns.

EPIDEMIOLOGY AND CAUSES

Trigeminal neuralgia occurs more frequently in women than in men and more often in individuals older than age 50. The incidence is 12 per 100,000 of the general population per year. A higher incidence of risk occurs in individuals with hypertension and multiple sclerosis (MS).

These at-risk individuals are much younger than the characteristic age of patients with trigeminal neuralgia.

PATHOPHYSIOLOGY

Trigeminal neuralgia is sometimes caused by compression by the basilar artery and secondary demyelination of axons in the fifth cranial nerve, the trigeminal nerve. It is also associated with demyelination caused by MS. The trigeminal nerve has three main branches: V_1, the ophthalmic branch, which transmits sensation from the eye region and forehead; V_2, the maxillary branch, which transmits sensation from the midface and upper jaw; and V_3; the mandibular branch, which transmits sensation from the lower jaw. The neuron cell bodies for the sensory axons in these nerves are located in the trigeminal ganglion, which is inside the skull along the floor of the middle cranial fossa.

Trigeminal neuralgia most often affects the mandibular or maxillary branch of the trigeminal nerve. The problem tends to occur in middle-aged and elderly people. Patients with MS, another demyelinating syndrome, are affected by trigeminal neuralgia with a higher frequency than the rest of the population.

Although it is extremely painful, trigeminal neuralgia produces no obvious neurologic deficits. On the other hand, patients with trigeminal neuralgia have a general sensory hypersensitivity of the face, and 90% of sufferers have trigger points on their faces that will set off paroxysms of pain.

CLINICAL PRESENTATION

Subjective

The patient with trigeminal neuralgia presents with complaints of severe paroxysmal pain, most commonly on one side of the face. The pain lasts for a few seconds, with no ache or pain between occurrences, and follows the trigeminal nerve distribution. The patient's history includes the onset of a painful event after trigger points have been stimulated by chewing, talking, brushing teeth, touching the face, or, in some cases, after physical activity, lowering of the head, and wind touching the face. The patient's history may include periods of remission with or without medical treatment.

During periods of exacerbation, the patient may be totally disabled by the severity of the pain. Patients may report refraining from eating, sleep deprivation, depression, and even suicidal thoughts, which reflect their willingness to go to great extremes to escape the severe paroxysmal pain.

Objective

On physical examination, the cranial nerves, specifically the trigeminal nerve, have normal motor and sensory function; facial muscle strength and reflexes are normal.

Clinically, the cardinal signs of idiopathic trigeminal neuralgia are elicited when a facial trigger point is stimulated; the patient experiences a sharp, electric-type pain that follows the distribution of the trigeminal nerve and lasts for only a few seconds, and the patient's face grimaces. After the painful attack, there is no residual ache or pain. Facial pain that is continuous and varies in intensity must be further evaluated for atypical trigeminal neuralgia that is caused by trauma, tumor, or previous facial surgery, however. Because of the many pathological and etiological theories regarding trigeminal neuralgia, the clinician must be alert to the characteristic symptoms of typical (idiopathic) trigeminal neuralgia. These are short periods of paroxysmal pain associated with trigger zones, pain limited to the distribution of the trigeminal nerve branches, and a normal neurologic examination.

DIAGNOSTIC REASONING

Diagnostic Tests

Idiopathic trigeminal neuralgia can often be diagnosed based on clinical history that describes paroxysmal pain episodes triggered by specific activities in patients characteristically older than age 50.

Patients who have prolonged episodes of pain that increases in intensity and occurrence and are younger need to be evaluated for secondary causes including tumors, trauma, MS, and vascular compression. The tests most frequently used for the diagnosis of atypical trigeminal neuralgia are a CT scan and an MRI. MRI is the method of choice in differential diagnoses of trigeminal nerve pathology.

Differential Diagnosis

There are many causes for the general presentation of orofacial pain. These conditions can usually be categorized as inflammatory (e.g., dental pathology, sinusitis, parotitis, sialolithiasis, temporal arteritis, HSV), neurologic (e.g., trigeminal, glossopharyngeal, or paratrigeminal neuralgia; cluster or migraine headaches; meningiomas; posterior fossa tumors), or musculoskeletal (e.g., temporomandibular joint pain, myofascial pain dysfunction syndrome). It is important, therefore, to identify whether the clinical presentation is either typical trigeminal neuralgia or some other orofacial pain.

MANAGEMENT

The major principles in the management of trigeminal neuralgia are to (1) elicit a remission by drug therapy, (2) prevent adverse effects in patients resulting from prescribed medications, and (3) help the patient avoid triggering painful episodes. Trigeminal neuralgia is a chronic condition that results in the need for the patient's chronic pain to be managed. In addition to interventions related to establishing remission and avoidance of painful episodes, the patient's psychological needs—related to depression, isolation, and possible suicidal thoughts—are significant areas in the plan of care.

Initially, pharmacologic management is to initiate remission of the pain. Carbamazepine or gabapentin can be effective for neuropathic pain. If the patient experiences good pain relief from the medication, it should continue for several months. Tricyclic antidepressants such as amitriptyline can also be used to treat pain.

Follow-up for complications of drug therapy with anticonvulsants is essential in the pharmacologic management of typical trigeminal neuralgia. Carbamazepine has many adverse effects, including nausea, vomiting, dizziness, diplopia, skin rash, blood dyscrasias (aplastic anemia, agranulocytosis, thrombocytopenia, and leukopenia), fever, and chills.

Other therapies for trigeminal neuralgia include acupuncture, transcutaneous electrical nerve stimulation (TENS), and topical application of capsaicin (Zostrix).

Patients with trigeminal neuralgia who have few or no periods of remission should be referred for surgical evaluation. The unrelenting paroxysmal pain associated with trigeminal neuralgia is frequently associated with compression of the trigeminal nerve root. Microvascular decompression is performed to relieve the compression, although recurrence in 1 to 2 years is common after surgery, regardless of the surgical method chosen.

Some patients have benefitted from acupuncture and TENS.

FOLLOW-UP AND REFERRAL

Because of the intense and chronic pain associated with trigeminal neuralgia, the patient may experience depression, social isolation, and suicidal tendencies. The clinician must recognize these effects of the disease and reinforce coping mechanisms the patient may use during periods of exacerbation. Referral for counseling may be required if the patient is not able to cope with the chronicity and severity of the pain. The patient experiences pain when eating and washing the face and frequently avoids these and other activities. The patient begins to lose weight and becomes dehydrated, and hygiene becomes a problem.

Patient Education: Trigeminal Neuralgia

The goals of patient instruction are the avoidance of triggering painful events, pharmacologic management, and coping with chronic, severe pain. Nutritional counseling should encourage intake of soft or pureed, high-caloric foods, along with increased fluids. For hygiene, the use of soft washcloths and mouthwashes should be encouraged. Patients should be educated about adverse reactions (e.g., dizziness, sleepiness, ataxia, nausea, and vomiting) to their medications and about the necessity for follow-up blood studies to detect any blood dyscrasias. Intense counseling and supportive education are a continuous process in caring for the patient with trigeminal neuralgia. Recognition of the patient's educational needs based on his or her coping mechanisms, search for pain treatment, and the status of the neuralgia will direct the clinician in establishing an individualized plan.

BELL'S PALSY

Bell's palsy is an idiopathic cranial nerve seven palsy causing lower motor neuron facial paralysis, typically occurring on one side of the face. The peripheral facial palsy is self-limiting and complete recovery usually occurs in a few weeks or months in 80% to 86% of patients. Initially, the facial paralysis may be incomplete and then worsen within 48 hours after onset. The sudden experience of facial paralysis can be frightening to the patient, who usually seeks medical care immediately.

EPIDEMIOLOGY AND CAUSES

The cause of Bell's palsy most likely to be viral, typically from HSV infection. Approximately 40,000 individuals each year in the United States are affected by Bell's palsy. Men and women are affected equally, but it is less common in persons younger than age 15 years or older than age 45 years. A higher incidence is seen in individuals with diabetes, hypertension, trauma, toxin exposure, Lyme disease, HIV, pregnancy, and those with upper respiratory ailments.

Recovery from facial paralysis usually occurs over 3 to 6 months. Persons at risk for incomplete recovery are those older than age 55 or who have hypertension, experience pain other than ear pain, have complete facial paralysis, or have changes in lacrimation.

PATHOPHYSIOLOGY

Cranial nerve VII—the facial nerve—is mainly a motor nerve innervating the muscles of facial expression. It also has a small sensory component proving taste to the anterior two-thirds of the tongue and sensation to part of the external auditory canal. Its preganglionic, parasympathetic axons innervate the lacrimal and nasopalatine glands and all the salivary glands except the parotid.

The various classes of axons in the facial nerve peel off group by group as the nerve makes its way through the bony canals of the skull; therefore, pressure on or lesions of the nerve at different locations will produce different deficits. Inside the skull, the facial nerve runs with cranial nerve VIII, and lesions here may cause hearing loss and vestibular problems in addition to deficits in all the motor and sensory components of the facial nerve. Within the skull wall, the facial and vestibulocochlear nerves separate. After this, the first components to leave the facial nerve are the lacrimal and nasopalatine axons; therefore, damage to the facial nerve distal to this juncture will not affect a patient's ability to produce tears. The chorda tympani branch, which includes taste axons and the axons to the salivary glands, branches off next; therefore, damage to the facial nerve distal to this juncture will cause unilateral paralysis of all the muscles of facial expression but will not affect taste or the production of saliva. Most cases are thought to be caused by a reactivated herpes simplex infection of the geniculate ganglion, which leads to inflammation and swelling of the nerve inside its restrictive bony canal. Reactivated varicella-zoster virus can also cause Bell's palsy; this type also causes a rash in the external auditory canal or palate and can involve cranial nerve VIII, leading to hearing loss and vertigo.

CLINICAL PRESENTATION

Subjective

Patients with Bell's palsy present with an acute onset of partial or total paralysis on one side of the face that may worsen over a couple days. The patient has normal ocular movements. They may experience loss of taste (dysgeusia) on their ipsilateral tongue, postauricular pain, abnormal sensitivity to sound (hyperacusis), and a heavy feeling in the face.

Objective

On physical examination, the motor and sensory functions along the entire facial nerve should be assessed. Hallmarks of Bell's palsy are its acute onset and the fact that no other CNS symptoms exist. The physical assessment characteristically reveals side the absence of forehead wrinkles on the affected, wider palpebral fissure of the eye with weakness of eye closure, decreased corneal reflex, Bell's phenomenon (the eyeball turns upward when the patient tries to close the eyelid), flattening of the nasolabial fold, and loss of taste on the anterior two-thirds of the tongue. Lacrimation may or may not be affected. During the history, it is important to ask about pregnancy, diabetes, any recent infection, and rash.

A patient with Bell's palsy typically is unable to make these movements on the affected side on request: raise the eyebrow, wrinkle the forehead, close the eyelid, whistle, or smile. When talking, the patient's cheek puffs out and there is an inability to clearly pronounce words that require pursing of the lips. There appears to be a deviation of the tongue because of mouth paralysis on the affected side (although tongue deviation is not present when comparing tongue protrusion relative to the teeth).

The patient is unable to suck or hold fluids in the mouth but is able to swallow.

Close inspection of the patient's ears and palate is done to assess for herpes zoster lesions that would indicate Ramsay Hunt syndrome, which is herpes zoster affecting the facial and auditory nerves, causing facial palsy and cutaneous herpes zoster lesions of the external ear, palate, and/or tympanic membrane. Associated symptoms include tinnitus, vertigo, and deafness (Sweeney & Gilden, 2001).

DIAGNOSTIC REASONING

Diagnostic Tests

Diagnosis is based primarily on patient history and clinical examination. If the history and physical examination are inconclusive for Bell's palsy, the patient should be referred for further diagnostic work-up. A CT scan or MRI with contrast can rule out a tumor, stroke, MS, or other structural lesions.

Documentation of the extent of facial function at the time of initial diagnosis and at subsequent assessments is important to evaluate the course of the disease. The progression or lack of progression of the symptoms is important to differentiate Bell's palsy from other pathology.

Differential Diagnosis

Tumors, infections (HIV, infectious mononucleosis, Lyme disease), GBS, trauma, stroke, sarcoidosis, and other inflammatory conditions can cause unilateral facial weakness that may appear similar to Bell's palsy. The history and physical examination are important to exclude other causes of facial weakness.

Damage to the facial nerve inside the skull wall can be caused by skull fractures, hemangiomas, tumors, and inflammation. When the facial nerve is damaged and no structural problems are found, the condition is called Bell's palsy. Bell's palsy always produces unilateral facial paralysis, and depending on the location of the nerve lesion(s), it may also include deficits in functions of the other components of the facial nerve.

In addition, a Bell's palsy–like facial paralysis is the most common neurologic problem caused by Lyme disease, although this is often bilateral.

MANAGEMENT

The majority of patients with Bell's palsy will recover without treatment, although treatment with steroids starting within the first few days of symptom onset improves recovery and is recommended. Treatment with antiviral medications is controversial. Some practitioners prescribe antiviral medications in cases of particularly severe Bell's palsy and in cases of Ramsay Hunt syndrome.

Because Bell's palsy causes weakness of eye closure, it is important to protect the eye from injury, particularly during sleep. Loss of the ability to blink and close the eyelid subjects the cornea to drying and ulceration. The patient is instructed to keep the eye moist by topical application of artificial tears frequently during the day and use of an ocular lubricant ointment and eye patch at night. An ophthalmologist should be consulted if the patient experiences any signs of corneal irritation or injury.

Ear sensitivity can be treated with acetaminophen (Tylenol) and ibuprofen (Advil, Motrin). Rest and decreased auditory stimulation may lessen the effects of hyperacusis.

FOLLOW-UP AND REFERRAL

The patient should be examined at regular intervals to assess for resolution or deterioration of Bell's palsy symptoms and adverse effects of medication, if prescribed. Special attention should be given to effectiveness of eye care by the patient. If the patient's symptoms do not improve, worsen beyond the acute setting, or if other neurologic signs are evident, the patient should be referred to a neurologist.

Patient Education: Bell's Palsy

The clinician should provide essential teaching that supports the recovery process. Reassurance that Bell's palsy is usually a short-term and benign condition will allay some anxiety. Drinking from a plastic, spouted bottle may be easier than drinking from a cup or glass because liquid can be squeezed into the back of the mouth.

In addition to meticulous eye care, the patient should be taught to perform oral hygiene vigorously because food becomes trapped and there can be a reduced amount of saliva. Foods may also need to be spicier than normal to compensate for loss of taste. The clinician should encourage the patient to eat soft foods of high nutritional value because patients often avoid eating because of difficulty holding food in the mouth.

GUILLAIN-BARRÉ SYNDROME

EPIDEMIOLOGY AND CAUSES

Guillain-Barré syndrome (GBS) is an acute monophasic immune-mediated polyradiculoneuropathy. It is usually an ascending paralysis most often beginning in the legs and then progressing in an ascending fashion. Sensation can be involved, and patients usually report tingling in the extremities. Back pain and autonomic dysfunction are also common. It affects only about one to two persons per 100,000 individuals, peaking in young adults aged 14 to 20 years and older adults aged 70 to 74 years, with a higher incidence in winter. There are many variations of GBS (Wakerley et al., 2014). The Miller Fisher variant causes brainstem symptoms such as ataxia and eye-movement abnormalities, in addition to loss of reflexes. GBS is often postinfectious, and there is a strong association with the gastric *Campylobacter* infection. It is caused by the production of antibodies that attack nerves because of molecular mimicry. GBS can be mild or severe, causing respiratory failure. Most individuals reach the stage of greatest weakness within the first 2 to 3 weeks after the symptoms appear, and 90% will reach this point by the third week. Almost 30% of patients will experience residual weakness even after 3 to 5 years.

DIAGNOSISTIC REASONING

The diagnosis is made by history and physical examination. Spinal fluid analysis can be helpful to exclude alternate diagnoses and typically reveals elevated protein with little or no pleocytosis. Nerve conduction studies and electromyography can also help aid in the diagnosis. MRI with contrast of the spine may show enhancement of the nerve roots.

MANAGEMENT

The treatment involves IV gamma globulin or plasmapheresis. All patients suspected of having GBS, even if the case is mild, must be referred to the emergency department because respiratory failure can develop quickly and become life-threatening.

MYASTHENIA GRAVIS

EPIDEMIOLOGY AND CAUSES

Myasthenia gravis (MG) is a disorder of the neuromuscular junction. It is an autoimmune disease in which an antibody targets the receptor for acetylcholine at the neuromuscular junction. More women are affected than men, and it occurs in approximately 5 to 15 individuals per 100,000. Younger women, with peak onset at age 31 to 40, and older men older than age 60 are most commonly affected.

MG causes muscle fatigue and weakness associated with use. Eye movements and speech are commonly affected. Weakness is usually worse later in the day, and the symptoms will usually ameliorate with rest.

DIAGNOSTIC REASONING

The diagnosis is usually made be demonstrating fatigable weakness on examination (weakness that develops or worsens with muscle activation). Diagnosis can be supported with the Tensilon test, in which use of edrophonium chloride results in resolution of the weakness. However, given the risk for systemic side effects, this test is less commonly used in practice. Electromyography can confirm the diagnosis.

MANAGEMENT

Symptomatic treatment is with anticholinesterase agents, which afford temporary relief. The major side effect is gastrointestinal irritability. Immunosuppressant drugs, IV immunoglobulins, and plasmapheresis are also used to reduce antibody levels. Because MG is associated with thymoma, all patients should be screened for this condition; in some patients, thymectomy can be curative.

MULTIPLE SCLEROSIS

Multiple sclerosis (MS) is a chronic and potentially disabling demyelinating disease of the CNS that begins most commonly in young adulthood. Common symptoms include visual changes (unilateral vision loss, double vision), weakness and numbness, and loss of balance.

MS is the most common cause of disability in young adults. It causes demyelination of the nerves in the brain and spinal cord, which can be seen on MRI. MS is thought to be a disorder of the T and B lymphocytes in which the body's immune system attacks the myelin coating of the nerves in the CNS.

There are three classifications of MS that differ with pattern of progression:

- *Relapsing–remitting* MS is characterized by acute attacks, with recovery (either partial or full between episodes.
- *Primary progressive* MS has a steady disease progression from onset, with possibly some plateaus and remissions.
- *Secondary progressive* MS is a combination of the first two types, beginning as a relapsing–remitting disease but then transitioning to a progressive course.

MS phenotypes can be further described by disease activity. MS is active if there are clinical relapses or if contrast enhancement (which demonstrates active inflammation) is seen on MRI (Lublin et al., 2014).

The clinical course of MS varies between patients. Prognosis is a common concern. Although there are no definitive prognostic indicators, the following are general guidelines. Good prognostic indicators include minimal disability after 5 years of onset, complete and rapid remission of initial symptoms, onset at age 35 or younger, only one symptom during the first year, acute onset of the first symptoms, brief duration of most recent exacerbation, long first remission, optic neuritis, or sensory symptoms. Poor prognostic indicators include late onset, chronic progressive course, motor symptoms, polysymptomatic onset, and vertigo. After 15 years, 50% to 60% of patients with MS remain ambulatory, 10% to 20% need assistance devices to ambulate, and 15% to 30% are bedridden.

EPIDEMIOLOGY AND CAUSES

MS occurs worldwide, but there are differences in both incidence and prevalence on the basis of race, sex, genetics, geographic location, and age at the time of probable exposure to a virus or other infectious agent. MS is most commonly diagnosed between ages 20 and 50 years, with a median onset at age 30. The first symptoms of the disease usually occur between ages 20 and 40. If the disease is diagnosed after age 50, it tends to have a more progressive course. The disease affects two to three times more women than men. It is more common among Caucasians and people of northern or central European descent. Asians and persons of African descent are at lower risk. About 450,000 people have MS in the United States.

Although the exact cause of MS is unknown, it is likely to be multifactorial. Some epidemiological findings suggest a relationship between MS and an unknown environmental factor, possibly a viral exposure during childhood. This exposure may lead to the entry of immune cells into the CNS, where a population of T cells becomes sensitized to a CNS antigen. After years of latency, an environmental agent may lead to an upregulation of circulating mediators or T-cell activation that may trigger an episode of demyelination and clinical disease. Other possible causes include genetic susceptibility, autoimmune mechanisms, and viral infections. One leading hypothesis is that of a cell-mediated immunopathological response directed against myelin in genetically predisposed persons.

The possibility that susceptibility to MS is inherited is supported by its higher incidence in twins and in certain families. The major histocompatibility complex (MHC) on chromosome 6 has been identified as one genetic determinant for MS. Although genetic factors may contribute to an individual's susceptibility, they are neither sufficient nor necessary for development of MS. Clinical expression of the disease is likely to require additional exposure to one or more environmental factors, which are as yet undefined.

There is evidence of autoimmune mechanisms in the pathogenesis of MS. In a normal immune response, foreign antibodies are processed and presented to helper T cells by antigen-presenting cells and macrophages. These T-helper cells recognize foreign peptides bound to MHC molecules, become activated, and release various cytokines, tumor necrosis factor, and interleukins that augment the immune response to a particular antigen. These particular class II MHC molecules are usually found only on cells involved in an immune response. In MS, class II MHC induction has been shown to occur in CNS tissue. In peripheral blood of patients with MS, several nonspecific changes are seen that are similar to those in other autoimmune diseases. Suppressor T lymphocytes are decreased in both function and number. Excessive immunoglobulin is present, especially high levels of immunoglobulin G (IgG). Suppressor cell inducers are decreased in many patients with progressive disease.

PATHOPHYSIOLOGY

MS is a disease of the CNS stemming from progressive, patchy demyelination of axons. In MS, local immune reactions destroy CNS myelin and cause the death of oligodendrocytes, the cells that make myelin. Astrocytes react to these injuries by proliferating. At the same time, many of the axons remain intact.

MS is most commonly characterized by neurologic problems that periodically flare up and then abate. The symptoms reflect repeated episodes of demyelination in new parts of the white matter throughout the CNS. The specific neurologic deficits of an MS patient depend on the regions of the CNS that have been affected. For example, lesions in the optic nerve produce blindness, lesions in the corticospinal tracts produce weakness, lesions in the posterior column of the spinal cord produce unusual sensations or numbness, lesions in the medial longitudinal fasciculus produce double vision, and lesions in the vestibular pathways produce dizziness.

Areas of MS damage form sharply defined plaques, which are typically found around venules. MS plaques tend to be large (greater than 6 mm in diameter) and oval shaped; over time, the plaques become more widely distributed. Newly forming plaques, in which demyelination is not yet complete, are filled with lymphocytes, plasma cells, and macrophages. Older plaques have no myelin in their centers and contain only fibrous astrocytes and unmyelinated axons. Axon damage inevitably follows, but this appears to be a secondary phenomenon and occurs slowly. Between the plaques, myelin is also affected, although here the damage is not as dramatic.

MS plaques are the result of immune reactions, and the state of the disease is reflected in the immune indicators in the CSF. When the disease flares up, the CSF has an increased number of lymphocytes (although usually less than 50/mcL). The CSF will also contain elevated levels of immunoglobulins, the majority of which are IgG. Oligoclonal bands are found in the CSF, regardless of the current state of the disease symptoms.

CLINICAL PRESENTATION

Subjective

The most common presenting symptoms in MS include weakness of the legs, bladder and bowel dysfunction, ataxic gait, paresthesias in the extremities, and optic neuritis. Seventy-five percent to 95% of patients with MS experience MS-related fatigue. Exacerbations and remissions occur, and signs and symptoms may localize to more than one lesion. The clinical course is variable. The subjective complaint at any one presentation depends on the location of the active lesion. Optic neuritis causes unilateral blurred vision, dulling of colors, or sometimes even blindness in one eye. Transverse myelitis (spinal cord inflammation) causes bilateral weakness, numbness, spasticity, and bladder dysfunction. Brainstem lesions can cause double vision, tremor, ataxia, and dizziness. When a patient presents with symptoms that may be from MS, it is important to ask about previous transient neurologic symptoms. The diagnosis of MS requires demonstrating multiple lesions over time affecting different areas of the CNS.

Objective

Symptoms may begin to manifest over a period of hours to days. The clinician should assess the patient for common visual symptoms, including diplopia, blurred vision, diminution or loss of visual acuity unilaterally or bilaterally, and visual field defects. A patient with unilateral optic neuritis will have a relative afferent pupillary defect on examination. They may also have red desaturation, decreased visual acuity in one eye, and pain with eye movements. Demyelination in the brainstem of the fifth cranial nerve can cause trigeminal neuralgia. Limb weakness is a common sign of MS, presenting as monoparesis, hemiparesis, or tetraparesis, and is typically caused by spinal cord lesions (myelitis). Over time, myelitis leads to hyperreflexia and spasticity. In patients with severe spasticity, there may be extensor or flexor spasms either spontaneously or on attempted movement. Spasticity may cause pain, interfere with sleep, or prevent movement. Cerebellar or brainstem involvement causes dysarthria, scanning speech, tremor, gait ataxia, and incoordination of limbs and trunk.

Bladder symptoms are common, including incontinence and frequency or urgency. Patients may have a small-capacity, spastic bladder or a large, flaccid bladder with overflow incontinence. Bladder dysfunction from myelitis may become chronic, requiring self-catheterization. Loss of libido and erectile dysfunction are common in men with MS; in women with MS, sexual dysfunction most commonly involves lack of lubrication and failure to reach orgasm. Although bowel incontinence is less common, constipation may occur.

Sensory impairment and paresthesias are common. Patients may complain of tingling or numbness in the face, limbs, or trunk. A sensation of "electricity" down the back after passive or active neck flexion, called Lhermitte's sign, is indicative of a lesion in the posterior column in the cervical spinal cord. Pain is common in MS. Pain may be associated with trigeminal neuralgia, flexor–extensor spasms, tonic spasms of the limbs, and local pain syndromes such as constricting pain around a limb, burning pain, pseudoradicular pain, foreign body sensation, headache, neuralgic pain, and pain caused by pressure sores.

Patients may experience depression, euphoria, subtle aphasic manifestations, or cognitive changes. Patients may have difficulty with tasks that require processing new information rapidly, recalling newly acquired knowledge, and problem-solving. Attention deficits may be present early in MS, even before the onset of physical symptoms. In general, the longer the history of MS, the greater the attention impairment. Memory and abstract reasoning may be affected, as well as the capacity to direct attention.

DIAGNOSTIC REASONING

Diagnostic Tests

The diagnosis of MS requires the demonstration of multiple CNS lesions that develop over time and in different locations. Diagnosis is based on patient history, neurologic examination, and diagnostic tests. A history of several MS relapses is supportive. Abnormalities on examination localizing to multiple areas of the CNS are also supportive. The examiner should assess for increased muscle tone in legs, paraparesis, changes in visual acuity, red desaturation, relative afferent pupillary defect, clonus of ankles, positive Babinski's sign, and a decreased appreciation of vibration or position sense in arms and legs.

For a diagnosis of MS to be made, two or more areas of the CNS must be involved at two different periods of time. Locations of common CNS lesions and the functional areas that they affect include the following:

- Optic nerve—vision
- Corticobulbar system—speech, swallowing
- Corticospinal system—muscle strength
- Cerebellar system—gait, coordination
- Medial longitudinal fasciculus system—eye movement (causes internuclear ophthalmoplegia, with diplopia and nystagmus)
- Spinocerebellar system—balance
- Posterior columns—position

An LP with an evaluation of CSF for the presence of lymphocytes and oligoclonal IgG bands may provide supportive data for a diagnosis of MS and help exclude other disorders with similar signs and symptoms.

Cortical-evoked responses or evoked potentials are of value in demonstrating clinically unsuspected lesions. Visual responses are abnormal in 75% to 97% of patients with MS. Somatosensory responses are abnormal in 72% to 87%, and brainstem responses are abnormal in 50% to 70% of patients with MS.

MRI is a sensitive, objective measure of plaques and is used to measure the outcomes of treatment. Periodic recording of the volume and number of lesions detected in the brain by MRI can assist the clinician in monitoring the extent of the disease. Areas of contrast enhancement observed by MRI correlate with active inflammatory damage. In addition, the MRI should be obtained as soon as possible in all patients presenting with an isolated demyelinating syndrome involving the CNS to exclude other possible neurologic conditions.

The McDonald criteria are used for definitive diagnosis of MS (Polman et al., 2011). A clinically definitive diagnosis of MS requires either (1) evidence from history of two episodes at least 1 month apart, signs of one lesion on examination, and evidence from evoked responses or MRI of other lesions or (2) evidence from both history and neurologic examination of more than one lesion. A laboratory-supported definitive diagnosis of MS requires evidence from two lesions in either history or neurologic examination. If only one lesion is evident on examination or history, at least one more lesion must be evident in MRI or evoked response testing. The CSF IgG pattern and content should also be abnormal. A clinically probable diagnosis of MS requires that either history or examination, but not both, provides evidence of more than one lesion. If only one lesion is evident by history or neurologic examination, MRI or evoked responses may provide evidence of additional lesions. If the collaborating neurologist is uncertain of the MS diagnosis, reevaluation of the patient may be needed.

If only one clinical event can be demonstrated, the patient cannot be diagnosed with MS, but may have clinically isolated syndrome. Patients with clinically isolated syndrome are at risk for developing MS in the future if they develop another attack. Patients with evidence of demyelinating plaques consistent with MS on MRI but no clinical symptoms are described as having radiologically isolated syndrome.

Differential Diagnosis

Other CNS diseases may resemble MS clinically or radiologically, including tumors such as lymphoma or glioma; infections such as Lyme, HIV, and other causes of encephalitis and/or myelitis; collagen vascular disease such as systemic lupus erythematosus, Behçet's disease, and sarcoidosis; leukoencephalopathies; and other autoimmune demyelinating diseases of the CNS such as neuromyelitis optica and acute disseminated encephalomyelitis.

MANAGEMENT

The principles of management include three major goals: to delay the progression of the disease, manage chronic symptoms, and treat acute exacerbations. There is no known cure for MS. Disease-modifying therapies are available; treatment decisions should be individualized, balancing the risks of the medications and the potential benefits. Disease-modifying medications include oral, injectable, and infusion methods. See Drugs Commonly Prescribed 10.1 (Freedman, 2013). Follow-up should be based on progression of disease and the treatment of symptoms and exacerbations.

Glucocorticoids are the mainstay of treatment for acute exacerbations. Glucocorticoids have both immunomodulatory and anti-inflammatory effects, which restore the blood–brain barrier, decrease edema, and may improve axonal conduction. The decision to treat an acute exacerbation depends on the functional limitations of the patient,

the level of patient discomfort, and objective evidence of neurologic dysfunction on examination. If symptoms of an exacerbation are severe enough to require treatment, IV methylprednisolone (Depo-Medrol) with or without an oral prednisone taper is administered.

Patients with relapsing–remitting MS may benefit from early aggressive treatment with disease-modifying agents. Disease-modifying agents can reduce the frequency of MS exacerbations but do not necessarily decrease long-term disability. Side effects vary. Medications with higher efficacy in preventing MS relapses may increase the risk of opportunistic infections, which can be deadly. Progressive multifocal leukoencephalopathy is a CNS infection caused by the John Cunningham (JC) virus that can cause significant morbidity and mortality. JC antibody titers must be monitored when patients are taking certain disease-modifying medications. Patients with MS should be referred to a neurologist for treatment with disease-modifying medications.

Physicians who prescribe these medications must be thoroughly familiar with dosage, possible adverse effects, and management of those adverse effects. Patients must be educated about side effects, injection techniques, storage, and care of the medications. Once appropriate drug therapy has been stabilized, the clinician may monitor the patient as described under Follow-up and Referral.

Symptomatic management and therapy are important in MS. Spasticity is a major cause of disability in 55% of patients with MS. Antispasmodics may be effective. If other noninvasive therapeutic measures for spasticity have failed, the patient may be referred to a neurosurgeon for evaluation of an implantable drug infusion pump to administer baclofen (Lioresal) intrathecally. This is highly effective because the drug can cross the blood–brain barrier. Adverse effects are minimal, and a test dose is administered intrathecally before implantation as part of the screening process for candidates.

Selective chemodenervation may be beneficial for localized spasticity in a single muscle or limb. This may be accomplished through administration of botulin *(Clostridium botulinum)* toxin type A (Botox). Only a specialist familiar with the use, adverse effects, and injection sites for botulinum toxin should administer this medication.

The tremors associated with MS are usually cerebellar outflow tremors. Medications such as clonazepam (Klonopin) and primidone (Mysoline) may be effective.

Fatigue is a common problem in patients with MS. The existence of sleep apnea, pain, spasms, restless leg syndrome, and sleep quality and patterns should all be assessed. Other medical problems that may cause fatigue should be excluded. Patients should be instructed to take a daytime nap and remain in a cool environment and should be educated in energy conservation techniques. A referral for occupational therapy may be beneficial.

Neuropathic pain may be treated with antiepileptics such as gabapentin and/or antidepressants such as duloxetine and nortriptyline.

Drugs Commonly Prescribed 10.1: Multiple Sclerosis

DRUG	INDICATION	ADVERSE REACTIONS AND PRESCRIBING CONSIDERATIONS
Injectables		
Methylprednisolone (Depo-Medrol)	Acute exacerbation	• Side effects: glaucoma, cataracts, secondary infections, hypokalemia, hypocalcemia, hypernatremia, hypertension, psychotic disorders, myopathy, osteoporosis, peptic ulcer, dermal atrophy, increased intracranial pressure, glucose intolerance • Caution as some patients experience depression or suicidal thoughts
Glatiramer acetate (Copaxone)	Relapsing–remitting multiple sclerosis (MS)	• Side effects: reaction at injection site, flushing, sweating, shortness of breath, palpitations, chest tightness, anxiety
Daclizumab (Zinbryta)	Relapsing–remitting MS	• Humanized monoclonal antibody • Subcutaneous injection every 4 weeks. • Contraindicated in patients with liver impairment. • Side effects include headache, upper respiratory infection, malignancies
Ocrelizumab (Ocrevus)	Relapsing–remitting MS; primary progressive MS	• Monoclonal antibody • Contraindicated in patients with active hepatitis B virus infection • Infusions: two IV infusions 14 days apart, which are administered every 6 months • Side effects include infusion reactions and infection
Natalizumab (Tysabri)*	Relapsing–remitting MS	• Infusion every 28 days • Monitor for progressive multifocal leukoencephalopathy (PML) • May cause infusion-related symptoms, hypersensitivity reactions
Alemtuzumab (Lemtrada)*	Relapsing–remitting MS	• Monoclonal antibody • Initial infusion for 5 consecutive days; repeat 12 months for 3 days • Common side effects include infusion-related reactions • Secondary autoimmune diseases and development of cancer seen in trials • May cause immune thrombocytopenia and kidney damage
Oral Medications		
Teriflunomide (Aubagio)	Relapsing–remitting MS	• Avoid using in patients with any infection or PML • Use with caution in patients with liver disease, hypertension, immunosuppression, peripheral neuropathy, and respiratory problems
Symptomatic Medications		
Baclofen (Lioresal)	Symptomatic treatment for spasticity	• May cause drowsiness and confusion
Tizanidine (Zanaflex)	Spasticity	• May cause drowsiness • Do not use with clonidine (Catapres)
Diazepam (Valium)	Spasticity	• Contraindicated with acute narrow-angle glaucoma; potential for abuse

*Natalizumab (Tysabri) and alemtuzumab (Lemtrada) are available through restricted distribution through a Risk Evaluation Mitigation Strategy called the TOUCH Prescribing Program.

Providers should be aware of issues related to complementary therapies that may be raised by patients with MS. Complementary and alternative medicine (CAM) is used by up to 70% of persons affected with MS due to the progressive and debilitating nature of the disease. The following are frequently used complementary therapies for patients with MS: acupuncture, hypnotherapy and imagery, massage, biofeedback, tai chi, therapeutic touch, Reiki, bioelectromagnetic therapy, and chiropractic therapy. If referring a patient with MS to complementary therapy providers, it is important to suggest those who are experienced in treating people with MS. Relaxation, meditation, as well as yoga and spiritual practices may all be of benefit the persons living with MS. Other CAM therapies need to be further researched.

FOLLOW-UP AND REFERRAL

Follow-up and referral should occur soon after diagnosis and repeated initially at monthly intervals or more often as symptoms appear. During follow-up visits, the patient's level of functioning and effectiveness of medications should be assessed and dosage adjustments made if needed. The patient should be instructed to contact the clinician immediately if symptoms appear that may signal an exacerbation. Periodic MRIs are typically obtained to trend disease progression.

Patient Education: Multiple Sclerosis

Patients should be educated about all aspects of the disease, including medications and adverse effects, complications, progression, fatigue management, pain management, diet, and exercise. The weakness that results from MS may be amenable to strengthening exercises. Range-of-motion exercise is important to prevent contractures and joint restriction. Referral to a physical therapist experienced in the treatment of patients with MS may be beneficial. Regular exercise may change the course of the patient's response to illness by minimizing the deconditioning process and maintaining optimal levels of physical activity and functioning. The beneficial effects of prolonged activity are well documented; it can help prevent muscular atrophy and weakness, fatigue, loss of flexibility, cardiovascular deficits, depression, and sleep disturbances. It is important to balance activity and exercise to prevent fatigue. There is no conclusive scientific evidence that any diet or nutritional therapy affects the course of MS. Many of the diets available are not harmful but may be tiring because of the attention to detail required, while offering no benefit. A generally well-balanced diet is recommended. Patients who have been diagnosed with MS may experience a wide range of emotions, ranging from euphoria to depression, including helplessness, lack of hope, mental confusion, stress, and anxiety. These emotions can affect marital relationships and increase child-rearing stress. The chronic nature of MS and the inability to predict level of dysfunction contribute to difficulty in coping with chronic illness and symptoms disruptive to daily living. Patients may also experience job loss, embarrassment, exhaustion, and the feeling of loss of contribution to society. It is important to teach patients health-promotion behaviors to emphasize emotional and social well-being.

Patients and families should also be educated in coping with possible behavior changes and mood swings. Patients with MS have reported feelings of hopelessness, loss of control, conflict, fear, loss, and uncertainty. Education in the management of problems related to sexual dysfunction may also need to be addressed. Caregivers should be educated not to neglect their own health because coping with a chronic illness may change and stress the dynamics both within a family and within other individual relationships. The complexity of issues surrounding caring for a person with MS is highlighted in the Evidence-Based Nursing Practice 10.1.

 Evidence-Based Nursing Practice 10.1

Rollero C. The experience of men caring for a partner With multiple sclerosis. *J Nurs Scholarsh.* 2016;48(5);482–489.

ABSTRACT

Purpose: The aim of the study was to explore the experience of male caregivers with a partner with MS.

Design and Methods: A qualitative study was conducted with a grounded theory approach. Twenty-four partners of a man or woman diagnosed with MS were interviewed in depth. A thematic analysis of the narratives was done.

Findings: Five major themes emerged: caregiving as a full-time job, changes in the couple, the importance of social support and social life, gender specificities, and fear of the future.

Conclusions: Results highlight the complexity of issues surrounding this specific form of caregiving. Social expectations referring to the marital relationship and to gender norms play a central role.

Clinical Relevance: Findings may help in developing ad hoc interventions to support male spousal caregivers to care for their partners.

 For additional resources please visit
https://davisedge.fadavis.com/

REFERENCES

Bell's Palsy

Sullivan F, Daly F, Gagyor I. Antiviral agents added to corticosteroids for early treatment of adults with acute idiopathic facial nerve paralysis (Bell Palsy). *JAMA.* 2016;316(8):874–875.

Encephalitis

Lancaster E. The diagnosis and treatment of autoimmune encephalitis. *J Clin Neurol.* 2016;12(1):1–13.

Parpia A, Li Y, Chen C, Dhar B, Crowcroft NS. Encephalitis, Ontario, Canada, 2002–2013. *Emerg Infect Dis.* 2016;22(3):426.

Tunkel AR, Glaser CA, Bloch KC, et al. The management of encephalitis: clinical practice guidelines by the Infectious Diseases Society of America. *Clin Infect Dis.* 2008;47(3):303–327.

Vora NM, et al. Burden of encephalitis-associated hospitalizations in the United States, 1998–2010. *Neurology.* 2014;82(5):443–451.

Guillain Barré Syndrome

McGrogan A, Madle GC, Seaman HE, de Vries CS. The epidemiology of Guillain-Barré syndrome worldwide. A systematic literature review. *Neuroepidemiology.* 2009;32(2):150–163.

Wakerley BR, Uncini A, Yuki N. Guillain-Barre and Miller Fisher syndromes—new diagnostic classification. *Nat Rev Neurol.* 2014;10(9):537–544.

Herpes Zoster

Centers for Disease Control and Prevention. What everyone should know about shingles vaccine. Vaccines and preventable diseases. https://www.cdc.gov/vaccines/vpd/shingles/public/index.html. Published 2016. Accessed June 8, 2017.

Davis TL. Postherpetic neuralgia. *Adv NPs PAs.* 2012;3(9):29–31.

Janniger CK. Herpes zoster. Medscape. http://emedicine.medscape.com/article/1132465-overview. Updated February 26, 2013.

Johnson BH, Palmer L, Gatwood J, Lenhart G, Kawai K, Acosta CJ. Annual incidence rates of herpes zoster among an immunocompetent population in the United States. *BMC Infect Dis.* 2015;15:1–5.

Sweeney CJ, Gilden DH. Ramsay Hunt syndrome. *J Neurol Neurosurg Psychiatry.* 2001;71(2):149–154.

Meningitis

Castelblanco RL, Lee M, and Hasbun R. Epidemiology of bacterial meningitis. *Lancet Infect Dis.* 2014;14(9):813–819.

National Meningitis Association. Statistics and disease facts. http://www.nmaus.org/disease-prevention-information/statistics-and-disease-facts/. Accessed June 3, 2017.

U.S. Department of Health and Human Services. Meningococcal vaccine. https://www.vaccines.gov/diseases/meningitis/index.html. Published 2016. Accessed August 15, 2017.

Multiple Sclerosis

Dunmore FR. Fatigue in multiple sclerosis. *Adv NPs PAs.* 2013;4(4):23–25.

Freedman MS. Present and emerging therapies for multiple sclerosis. *Continuum (Minneap Minn).* 2013;19(4 Multiple Sclerosis):968–991.

Lublin FD, et al. Defining the clinical course of multiple sclerosis: the 2013 revisions. *Neurology.* 2014;83(3):278–286.

Polman CH, Reingold SC, Banwell B, et al. Diagnostic criteria for multiple sclerosis: 2010 revisions to the McDonald criteria. *Ann Neurol.* 2011;69(2):292–302.

Rollero C. The experience of men caring for a partner with multiple sclerosis. *J Nurs Scholarsh.* 2016;48(5):482–489.

Rutecki GW. What we know today: multiple sclerosis. *Consultant.* 2015;55(8):649.

Sammarco CL. Treatment strategies for multiple sclerosis. *Nurse Pract Perspect.* 2016;3(2):12–14, 28.

Myasthenia Gravis

Smith C, Stickler D. A collaborative approach to myasthenia gravis. *Clin Advisor.* 2012;15(12):20–27.

Trigeminal Neuralgia

National Institute of Neurological Disorders and Stroke. Trigeminal neuralgia fact sheet. https://www.ninds.nih.gov/Disorders/Patient-Caregiver-Education/Fact-Sheets/Trigeminal-Neuralgia-Fact-Sheet. Accessed June 9, 2017.

RESOURCES

Encephalitis

Nemours Foundation—Encephalitis (for children and teenagers) https://kidshealth.org/en/teens/encephalitis.html

Schmidt A, Buhler R, Muhlemann K, Hess CW, and Tauber MG. Long-term outcome of acute encephalitis of unknown aetiology in adults. *Microbiol Infect.* 2011;17:621–626.

Herpes Zoster

Centers for Disease Control and Prevention—Shingles (Herpes Zoster) https://www.cdc.gov/shingles/index.html

Westmead Institute for Medical Research (2018, March 7). Why the latest shingles vaccine is more than 90 percent effective. https://www.sciencedaily.com/releases/2018/03/180307095243.htm. Accessed September 2018.

Meningitis

Centers for Disease Control and Prevention—Meningitis https://www.cdc.gov/meningitis/clinical-resources.html

National Institute of Neurological Disorders and Stroke—Meningitis and Encephalitis https://www.ninds.nih.gov/Disorders/All-Disorders/Meningitis-and-Encephalitis-Information-Page

Multiple Sclerosis

National MS Society https://www.nationalmssociety.org/

Myasthenia Gravis

Myasthenia.org www.ninds.nih.gov

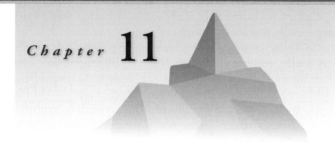

Chapter **11**

Common Skin Complaints

Susan Garnett, *MSN, APRN, FNP-BC*

Jill E. Winland-Brown, *EdD, APRN, FNP-BC*

Brian Oscar Porter, *MD, PhD, MPH, MBA*

ALOPECIA

Alopecia (baldness) is considered an autoimmune disease, which may be genetic in etiology with an environmental trigger. It can occur anywhere on the body where hair is present, although it is commonly associated with absence of hair on the scalp area. Scalp hair loss can occur in patches (*patchy alopecia or alopecia areata*) or over the entire scalp and face (*alopecia totalis*). Hair loss can also occur over the entire body (*alopecia universalis*) and can be either a temporary or permanent condition.

Hair loss is a gradual process; it is estimated that up to 50% of scalp hair can be lost before the loss becomes clinically apparent. Alopecia may be accompanied by psychological distress, even if the hair loss is temporary (*alopecia areata*). The most common cause of permanent hair loss is *androgenetic alopecia* (AGA) or male-pattern baldness (common baldness). AGA has a polygenic inheritance pattern; thus, it is inherited from both parents, not only through maternal genes, which is a common myth. Another common misconception is that AGA is more common in men; in reality, it occurs in both sexes and all ethnicities.

Factors that influence normal hair development and cycling include estrogens, growth hormone, glucocorticoids, thyroid hormone, retinoid, prolactin, and androgens; these factors can be adversely affected by certain medications. The most important hair growth factors are the androgens testosterone and its active metabolite,

dihydrotestosterone. During puberty, when androgen secretion starts, hair follicles become enlarged in certain areas of the body such as the beard area, chest, and extremities. Androgens have the opposite effect on the hair follicles of the scalp region; they cause a decrease in the size of the hair follicles (miniaturization) and can alter the hairline over the bitemporal region and the vertex area.

There are four cycles of scalp hair growth. The growth phase (*anagen*) of scalp hair is the longest cycle, lasting from 2 to 6 years. The majority of hair on the scalp (90% to 95%) is in the anagen phase. The latent or involution phase (*catagen*) is the shortest cycle, which lasts only 2 to 3 weeks. The resting phase (*telogen*) lasts from 2 to 3 months. Hair is shed during the fourth phase (*exogen*). An average person loses 50 to 150 hairs daily, and the cycle is repeated. Both topical and systemic medications for hair loss affect some or all of the phases of hair growth.

Thirty-five million men in the United States experience hair loss, and 21 million women do as well. For men, 40% have noticeable hair loss by age 35 years, 65% by age 60 years, 70% by age 80 years, and 80% by age 85 years. Women tend to develop AGA 10 years later than men. Thirteen percent of women develop AGA before menopause, and 75% develop it postmenopausally (International Society of Hair Restoration Surgery, 2016).

In reversible cases of nonscarring alopecia, regrowth of hair usually takes several months. Patients who are reassured of this important fact will have lessened anxiety about their condition. Two important factors that the clinician should address in the evaluation of alopecia are (1) whether it is scarring or nonscarring alopecia and (2) whether hair loss is in a small, well-circumscribed area (alopecia areata or trichotillomania) or generalized (AGA). On the basis of these two general categories, the differential diagnosis is made easier for the clinician. Scarring alopecia (*cicatricial alopecia*) causes permanent hair loss and is not reversible. Hair loss from nonscarring alopecia (*noncicatricial alopecia*) can be either temporary or permanent.

DIFFERENTIAL DIAGNOSIS

A thorough history is important in the evaluation of alopecia. Information regarding family members—both male and female—with hair loss should be elicited. Because some medications affect hair growth, the patient's medication history should be reviewed. Drugs that cause

Differential Diagnosis 11.1: Alopecia

Type of Alopecia	Differential Diagnosis
Scarring alopecia (cicatricial alopecia)	Trauma (chemical, physical, heat) Kerion formation in tinea capitis Chronic discoid lupus erythematosus Scleroderma Excessive radiation to scalp Lichen planopilaris Bacterial infection of scalp
Nonscarring alopecia (noncicatricial alopecia)	Alopecia areata Drug-induced hair loss Trichotillomania (hair pulling) Telogen effluvium (after pregnancy, major surgery, major emotional stress) Androgenetic baldness Tinea capitis (with no kerion formation) Hypothyroidism (Hashimoto's thyroiditis) Systemic lupus erythematosus Addison's disease

hair loss include hormones, anticonvulsants, anticoagulants, oral contraceptives, beta blockers, antimetabolites, antithyroid drugs, and excessive amounts of vitamin A or topical Retin-A (see Differential Diagnosis 11.1).

A potassium hydroxide and Wood's light examination is helpful in the diagnosis of tinea capitis in cases of patchy hair loss. Although most cases of tinea capitis do not fluoresce, a fungal culture can provide definitive proof of fungal infection and should be performed if suspicion is high.

Some dermatologists use the telogen count, in which 100 hairs (only 50 hairs are needed for accuracy) are removed from different areas of the scalp and the number of hairs in telogen is counted. Telogen hairs are recognized because of the large white club on the end of each hair. The appearance of the skin on the scalp will give the primary-care practitioner (PCP) clues about the type of alopecia that is involved. In nonscarring alopecia, the scalp will have normal texture and color. In contrast, the scalp of a patient with scarring alopecia has no visible hair follicles (or no follicular openings) and is atrophied and smooth. The affected area of the scalp (or the entire scalp) is sometimes hypopigmented or hyperpigmented. Obvious scarring is seen in some patients, and some have erythema and scaling (in these cases, it is important to rule out fungal infection). Look for fine pitting of the dorsal nail plate (with the appearance of "hammered brass") on the physical examination.

Nonscarring Alopecia

Nonscarring alopecia has both systemic and nonsystemic causes. Nonsystemic causes of alopecia include hair pulling (*trichotillomania*), excessive traction of the frontal

and temporal areas of the scalp (from tight cornrows or tight ponytails), trauma (both physical and chemical), radiation therapy to the head, local bacterial infection, and local fungal infection. Trichotillomania (compulsive hair pulling) is more commonly seen in children and teens. It is usually on the same side as the dominant hand and may include other more than just scalp hair (e.g., eyelashes, eyebrows hair, and beards, although those hairs are usually not long enough to pull).

Systemic causes of nonscarring alopecia include alopecia areata, telogen effluvium (TE), androgenetic baldness (common baldness), vitiligo, Hashimoto's thyroiditis, Addison's disease, systemic lupus erythematosus (SLE), hypothyroidism or hyperthyroidism, secondary syphilis, severe herpes zoster of the scalp, drug-induced alopecia (common in patients on cyclophosphamide therapy), iron-deficiency anemia, and pituitary insufficiency.

TE—excessive shedding of scalp hair that results from an increased number of hair follicles entering the resting stage (telogen)—can be caused by fever and certain drugs; therefore, a search for these possible causes should be included in the history taking. TE may also be caused by stress, pregnancy and/or childbirth, extreme weight loss, and general anesthesia. TE is almost nonexistent in men. In contrast, the classic signs of androgenetic baldness are thinning hairs of various diameters and lengths ("miniaturized" hairs) located in typical areas of the scalp, which differ in men and women. In men, hair loss usually starts on the hairline and around the temples (bitemporal area) and at the vertex or crown (top of the head). In women, hair loss is much more diffuse and occurs mostly on top of the head. Hair loss is sometimes harder to recognize in women because of hairstyles that are used to camouflage the problem.

Alopecia areata is a common condition in primary care practice. The typical patient will present with well-circumscribed patches of hair loss on the scalp or sometimes on the face, in areas such as the eyebrows or the beard area. Occasionally only one patch is seen, although multiple patches of hair loss may be apparent. *Alopecia areata* can occur once in a lifetime, or it can be a recurrent problem. Some cases become recalcitrant and are best treated by specialists. Because gray hair is spared, patients may complain of going gray overnight. When the scalp is examined closely with a magnifying lens, short, stubby hairs with tapered ends ("exclamation point hairs") are seen on the periphery of the bald patch (or patches). Alopecia areata is associated with autoimmune endocrinopathies such as Hashimoto's thyroiditis, Addison's disease, and pernicious anemia.

Hair regrowth occurs after several months, with new hairs that look thinner and finer than the original hair. There is no cure for alopecia areata, but in most patients hair usually regrows spontaneously after several months. The prognosis for alopecia areata is good if it occurs after puberty, as studies have found that up to 80% of these patients will regrow hair. Occasionally, a case of persistent alopecia areata that is unresponsive to treatment is seen; these cases are best referred to dermatologists for management.

Scarring Alopecia

Etiology of scarring (cicatricial) alopecia can include trauma (physical or chemical), severe bacterial or fungal infections of the scalp, scleroderma, discoid lupus erythematosus, lichen planopilaris, and excessive radiation. Early recognition and treatment of bacterial or fungal infections can help prevent or minimize the incidence of scarring. Severe local infection with either bacteria or fungi can permanently damage hair follicles and cause a patchy (and scarring) alopecia that is permanent.

When an autoimmune disease is suspected, laboratory tests include antinuclear antibodies to rule out lupus or autoimmune disorders, rheumatoid factor, and erythrocyte sedimentation rate (ESR), a nonspecific marker for inflammation. The rheumatology profile or "arthritis panel" may help in the diagnosis of autoimmune disorders that can cause alopecia, such as SLE and scleroderma. Scleroderma (progressive systemic sclerosis) is a systemic and multisystem inflammatory disorder associated with sclerotic changes in the body, including the skin. The skin becomes diffusely thickened with frequent telangiectasia (small dilated blood vessels) visible at the skin surface. A scalp biopsy is reserved for difficult and recalcitrant cases of alopecia.

In addition, serum testosterone, dehydroepiandrosterone, iron, total iron-binding capacity, and thyroid function tests, along with a complete blood count (CBC), will identify most other causes of hair thinning in premenopausal women.

A biopsy is useful in diagnosing scarring alopecia, but specimens must be obtained from the active border rather than from the scarred central zone.

MANAGEMENT

Medical treatment is available but is not a permanent solution for alopecia. Patients should be educated that total return to previous levels of hair growth is not possible, but cosmetically acceptable hair coverage is possible. Medical treatments must be used daily to maintain regrown hair. Stopping treatment will result in shedding of hair and a return to the previous levels of alopecia. Hair shedding is seen rapidly in a matter of days after stopping minoxidil (Rogaine), but is more gradual over several months with finasteride (Propecia).

Treatment options for alopecia are determined by the patient's age and severity of hair loss. For patients with hair loss of less than 50%, treatment options include intralesional corticosteroid injections, anthralin cream or ointment, topical minoxidil solution and foam, or topical corticosteroid creams. Topical treatment with a potent corticosteroid is preferred by PCPs because it is not invasive and is simple to use, although it is not as effective as intralesional injections (Bolduc, 2017). Small amounts of triamcinolone acetonide (Kenalog) 5 mg/mL may be injected intralesionally into the mid-dermal layer, spaced approximately 1 cm apart on bald patches and given every 4 to 6 weeks. Hair growth is usually seen in 4 weeks. One side effect of corticosteroid use that patients and PCPs should monitor for is atrophy of the skin. Unfortunately, these injections are only a temporary solution and do not alter the underlying pathophysiology of hair loss.

Treatments for more extensive (50% or greater) hair loss include oral corticosteroids, topical immunotherapy, and immunomodulators. Oral corticosteroid therapy is known to have significant side effects with long-term use. In topical immunotherapy, chemicals such as diphenylcyclopropenone, dinitrochlorobenzene, and squaric acid dibutylester cause contact dermatitis when applied to the scalp, which modulates the autoreactive immune reaction driving hair loss. Immunomodulators such as Janus kinase inhibitors are also being studied in clinical trials.

Nonmedical options include hair weaves, toupees, and wigs. Wigs are either worn on top of the head or are interwoven into existing hair as a "weave." As the existing hair (to which the weave is anchored) grows, the weave must be readjusted periodically, which may impart increased stress on hair follicles. Surgical approaches to the treatment of extensive alopecia include hair transplantation and surgical scalp restoration techniques.

Finasteride

Finasteride is U.S. Food and Drug Administration (FDA) approved for men only. Systemic treatment for alopecia with finasteride should not be used in women of reproductive age because this drug can cause abnormalities of the external genitalia of male fetuses. In women of non–childbearing age, finasteride does not appear to be effective in treating AGA. Therefore, finasteride once daily is approved for the treatment of androgenetic baldness in men only, while any use in women for female pattern baldness (with or without elevated androgen levels) is considered off-label and not FDA approved.

Finasteride blocks the effects of 5-alpha reductase, an enzyme that converts dihydrotestosterone to testosterone and reduces the total amount of testosterone in the body. Because it is metabolized in the liver, finasteride should be used with caution in patients with liver disease. In men aged 60 years or older, finasteride may be less effective than in younger men because of decreased 5-alpha-reductase activity that occurs with age. Adverse effects include decreased libido (1.8%), erectile dysfunction (1.3%), and ejaculatory dysfunction (1.2%). In most men, these sexual side effects gradually resolve with prolonged treatment (Merck & Co, Inc., 2011).

Minoxidil

Topical treatments for men and women containing minoxidil are available over the counter (OTC). Treatments for men include minoxidil 5% extra strength solution (Rogaine) and minoxidil 5% unscented foam, applied twice daily. Topical treatments available for women include minoxidil 5% foam applied once daily and 5% solution applied twice daily. At higher doses, oral minoxidil is a vasodilator and is used to treat hypertension. Topical minoxidil has not been found to cause lowering of systolic or diastolic blood pressure and pulse rate.

The best candidates for treatment with topical minoxidil are patients with recent onset of alopecia (less than 5 years), those younger than age 50 years, and patients with smaller areas of hair loss. Up to 40% of patients who use topical minoxidil for a period of 1 year or more will experience moderate to dense hair regrowth (Gupta & Foley, 2014). Minoxidil 2% solution has been consistently shown to reduce hair loss and induce new hair growth in females with female pattern hair loss. Because the 2% solution is used twice per day, the once daily 5% minoxidil foam approved by the FDA in 2014 for use in women is more effective because of improved compliance and patient-reported satisfaction, as well as milder side effects. Adverse effects include irritation, itching, dryness, scaling, and redness of the scalp; sometimes minoxidil can cause contact dermatitis. An adverse effect that is more common in women is hypertrichosis (excessive hair growth on the body).

PIGMENTATION CHANGES

The skin is the largest and most visible organ of the body. For most people, skin color is an important part of their identity as an individual. Because of the skin's visibility, conditions affecting the skin cause not only physical discomfort but also have emotional overtones. Pigmentation disorders seen in primary care include both hyperpigmentation and hypopigmentation. Either condition can be a sign of disease, or it can be considered a normal finding, depending on the clinical picture.

Melanin is a skin pigment produced by melanocytes that determines skin color. Although there is no difference in the number of melanocytes among different ethnic groups, the ability of the melanocytes of darker-skinned people to produce and retain melanin (from melanosomes) is much greater than in people with lighter skin. Research has found that melanosome size is directly related to skin color: the larger the size of the melanosomes, the darker the skin color. Asians and Caucasians (those considered to have "white" skin) have fewer and smaller melanosomes compared to individuals with darker skin, especially people of African descent considered to have "black" skin, whose melanosomes

are much larger and more numerous. Darker skin gives protection from ultraviolet (UV) radiation. Studies of people with darker skin have shown that dark skin has a sun protection factor between 5 and 13. Because of the protective aspect of darker skin, the incidence of nonmelanoma skin cancer in blacks or people of African origin is much less than in whites. Studies have shown that basal cell carcinomas are extremely rare in individuals with darker skin.

Skin bleaching (or lightening) creams and ointments may be used by some patients wanting to lighten their overall skin tone, particularly those from darker-skinned ethnic groups, such as Asians, African Americans, and Hispanics. These creams, typically not prescribed, are sold OTC and may be prone to misuse or overuse. In turn, their active ingredients are largely unregulated, and some preparations have been known to contain potential toxins, such as heavy metals. Patients should, therefore, be cautioned against the use of such nonprescription bleaching creams. The clinician should be sensitive to the fact that such discussions may also extend to the larger societal implications of skin color valuation as perceived on a personal level by the patient.

Normal Variations of Pigmentation

Pigmentation disorders presenting in the primary setting care may include misclassifications of normal variations in skin color related to ethnic differences (e.g., oral hyperpigmentation in people with darker skin). Normal variations in pigmentation are commonly seen in patients with darker skin. In patients with dark skin or those of African descent, oral hyperpigmentation is considered a normal variant, but underlying pathology should be ruled out. One exception is newborn infants, in whom oral pigmentation should not be present at this early stage. The most common site of normal oral hyperpigmentation is the gingivae (the gums), but other sites, such as the inside of the cheeks (buccal mucosa) and the tongue, can be involved as well. The hyperpigmented areas can range from bluish black to deep brown in color. Another pigmentation change that is considered a normal variant in blacks or people of African descent is hypopigmentation of the midsternal area. This type of hypopigmentation is usually seen in up to 70% of black children and in up to one-third of adults and is more common in males.

Voigt or Futcher lines are seen in up to one-fourth of blacks or people of African descent and less frequently in Asians. These distinct lines appear down the length of each arm symmetrically, dividing lighter-colored skin anteromedially from darker colored skin, with the lighter shade of skin touching the trunk. The nails of people with darker skin can also be pigmented, with involvement of the entire nail plate or in longitudinal bands or streaks of darker color. Normal nail pigmentation should be bilateral and symmetrical. Any asymmetry or new onset of pigmentation should arouse the clinician's suspicion for underlying disease, including acral melanoma. Pigmentation changes in people with darker skin do not necessarily point to pathology, but the clinician should not neglect the possibility of a disease process.

DIFFERENTIAL DIAGNOSIS

Pigmentation disorders can be clinical manifestations of diseases including endocrine, genetic, metabolic, or nutritional disorders or malignancy. Differential diagnoses to consider with oral hyperpigmentation include Peutz-Jeghers syndrome, pigmented tumors such as melanoma, Addison's disease, heavy metal exposure, and side effects of antimalarial medications. Peutz-Jeghers syndrome is an inherited disorder that presents with pigmented (dark brown–colored) macules on the lips and inside the mouth on the mucous membranes. It is associated with multiple hamartomatous polyps in the stomach, the small intestine, and large bowel, causing abdominal pain and other gastrointestinal symptoms. Patients who are suspected of having this disease need to be referred to a gastroenterologist for further evaluation.

Vitiligo

Vitiligo, or the total loss of skin color in patchy areas of the body (rarely over the entire body), is recognized clinically as white macules or patches that are usually located on sun-exposed areas, such as the face, lips, arm, hands, and feet. Mucous membranes and the retina may also be affected, and premature graying of the hair may occur. Uveitis may be an associated symptom. Vitiligo most often occurs in the mid-20s, although it may present at any age. It occurs equally in both sexes and in all races. It is relatively common and affects 0.5% to 1% of the population (Stoppler, 2016).

Vitiligo is thought to be an autoimmune disorder in which the body produces antibodies against its own melanocytes. There is also some evidence that vitiligo may be inherited. Another theory of causation is related to trigger events, such as emotional stress, a skin rash or sunburn, or other skin trauma, but this theory is not scientifically supported. In support of an autoimmune etiology, vitiligo occurs more often in individuals with autoimmune diseases such as hyperthyroidism, adrenal insufficiency, alopecia areata, and pernicious anemia. It is also associated with (autoimmune) diabetes mellitus type 1 but not with diabetes mellitus type 2. (Vitiligo, 2017).

The diagnosis of vitiligo is based on family history; a history of skin trauma, rash, or sunburn to the affected area; a family or personal history of other autoimmune disease; and physical examination. Biopsy may be done to confirm the absence of melanocytes in affected skin. Laboratory studies include a CBC and peripheral smear (to detect pernicious anemia), thyroid function studies, and an antinuclear antibody test. An eye examination to rule out uveitis may be considered.

Current treatments for vitiligo include topical corticosteroids, light therapy, psoralen (oral or topical) with UVA therapy (PUVA) and more recently with UVB light, depigmentation with topical creams, and surgical approaches, including skin grafting. Topical corticosteroids may cause skin thinning and striae; light therapy, including excimer laser treatments, may require repeated sessions and may not have permanent results. The side effects of oral psoralen include sunburn, nausea, vomiting, hyperpigmentation, pruritus, and abnormal hair growth; oral psoralen with UVA may also cause skin cancer. Depigmentation may be a viable choice for those with greater than 50% skin involvement. Side effects of depigmentation creams may include redness, swelling, pruritus, or xerosis (dry skin). Surgical therapies are reserved for those who have not had success with other therapies.

Chloasma and Melasma

A physiological hyperpigmentation condition called *chloasma* ("the mask of pregnancy") is caused by increased levels of estrogen-, progesterone-, and melanocyte-stimulating hormone during pregnancy. Chloasma may also occur in up to 25% of women taking oral contraceptives (Aguirre, 2017). Areas commonly affected include the face (especially the malar region and jawline), nipples, genitals, and the linea nigra extending midline down the abdomen from the umbilicus to the pubis. The hyperpigmentation is worsened by exposure to sunlight, and patients should be advised to avoid sun exposure, use sunblock such as clear zinc oxide or titanium dioxide, and wear wide-brimmed hats and high UV protection factor sun-protective clothing. Diagnosis of chloasma and the extent of epidermal/dermal involvement is determined by performing a Wood's lamp examination to visualize excess melanin in the epidermis.

Treatment of chloasma can include retinoic acid, hydroquinone cream, tretinoin and corticosteroids with hydroquinone ("triple" cream), azelaic acid or kojic acid creams, glycolic acid peels, microdermabrasion, galvanic or ultrasound facials, and various laser and intense pulsed light photorejuvenation treatments. Because hydroquinone is not recommended for women who are pregnant or planning to become pregnant, patients should be referred to an obstetrician for management. Chloasma can be difficult to treat in Asian and Hispanic clients. (Aguirre, 2017). A 24-hour skin patch test to rule out allergy to any bleaching agent should be done before use. The cream can be applied twice a day for 2 months. The patient should be advised to avoid the eye area and to use the cream cautiously in sensitive areas such as the nose and the lips.

Although dark patches on the face that develop during pregnancy are referred to as chloasma, *melasma* is a more general term referring to hyperpigmentation of certain areas of the skin regardless of pregnancy status, as a result of sun exposure and hormonal influences. It is usually more common in women than in men. First-line treatments are prescription skin bleaching creams (hydroquinone) and strict sun avoidance. Studies are being done to examine the benefit of laser therapy and salicylic acid peels every 2 to 8 weeks (American Academy of Dermatology, 2012; Arif, 2015).

Drug-Induced Hyperpigmentation

Drugs that are known to cause diffuse hyperpigmentation (melanosis) include zidovudine and cyclophosphamide. Skin discoloration has also been reported in patients who have been taking amiodarone, chlorpromazine, and certain antimalarial drugs. Photosensitivity reactions resulting in hyperpigmentation after sun exposure can also be caused by citrus oils that are present in fruits or certain perfumes.

Addison's Disease

Addison's disease is caused by inadequate secretion of corticosteroids as a result of partial or complete destruction of the adrenal glands; 70% of cases are due to an autoimmune mechanism. Addison's disease can cause a diffuse generalized hyperpigmentation, especially on skin creases, because of increased levels of adrenocorticotropic hormone (ACTH) from the pituitary. Classic areas where hyperpigmentation is seen are skinfolds; palmar creases; pressure points such as the elbows, knees, or knuckles; the inside of the mouth on the cheeks (buccal area); vaginal and perianal mucosa; and on scars. Symptoms of Addison's disease include generalized weakness, fatigue, poor appetite, weight loss, amenorrhea, and loss of axillary hair in women. Gastrointestinal symptoms may include nausea, vomiting, and diarrhea. Laboratory findings in Addison's disease include elevated serum potassium and calcium, low serum sodium, anemia, and an elevated ACTH level. Screening laboratory tests to detect autoimmune diseases include thyroid-stimulating hormone (TSH), antinuclear antibody, ESR, random blood glucose levels, vitamin B_{12} level, rheumatoid factor, and a CBC.

Skin Cancer

In patients with pigmented nevi (moles), the presence of certain unusual colors on the nevi, such as blue, gray, pink, white, and black (or a variegation of color), should raise suspicion in the clinician. Benign moles are usually small in size (less than 6 mm)—smaller than a pencil eraser—and have a well-defined border. Benign moles should be only a single shade of color—either brown, beige, or pink.

When evaluating nail pigmentation changes, symmetry and bilateral involvement of the nails and a history of stable pigmentation with no changes in color is reassuring. A variegated color or very dark color on one solitary nail should arouse suspicion for acral melanoma. Melanomas in people with darker skin are more likely to present on the extremities (acral areas) rather than on the trunk. The nailbeds, the palms, and the soles are sites where acral melanoma is more likely to be seen in darker-skinned people. The differential diagnoses of nail pigmentation change include acral melanoma, Peutz-Jeghers syndrome, a subungual nevus, gold therapy, Addison's disease, hemochromatosis, and a history of taking antimalarial medications. If acral melanoma is suspected, referral to a dermatologist for a nail biopsy and definitive diagnosis is imperative.

Malignant melanoma, the deadliest of all skin cancers, requires a high index of suspicion. Factors that can precipitate the appearance of acquired melanocytic nevus include immunosuppression, pregnancy, puberty, and sun exposure. Any asymmetry and changes in pigmentation, size, or surface of a mole require referral to a dermatologist. Moles that are larger than 5 mm are more likely to be atypical. Persons at higher risk for skin cancer include patients with numerous moles (50 or more), atypical and large (more than 5 mm) moles, and a family history of melanoma. The American Cancer Society mnemonic to help detect skin cancer is ABCDE: A—Asymmetry, B—Border (irregularity), C—Color (variegation), D—Diameter (greater than 6 mm), and E—Elevation or Evolving. Any patient with a suspicious mole should be referred to a dermatologist for definitive diagnosis and treatment.

PRURITUS

Pruritus—the sensation of itching accompanied by the urge to scratch—is perceived as unpleasant; therefore, people often seek help in the primary care setting for this problematic symptom. Pruritus is a frequent symptom of dermatological disease; it can be acute or chronic and is sometimes so severe as to interfere with sleep and daily life activities.

Pruritus is generally caused by either a local (e.g., insect bite, contact dermatitis) or systemic (e.g., chronic renal failure, hyperbilirubinemia with skin deposition of bile salts) etiology. Pruritus is the most common skin complaint in people aged 65 years and older (Cohen et al., 2012). Rashes or other skin lesions generally accompany the sensation of itching on the skin, although in some cases of systemic etiology, no external findings on the skin are ever identified. Therefore, the finding of skin lesions or rashes is most useful in classification of the differential diagnosis of pruritus (see Differential Diagnosis 11.2).

◈ Differential Diagnosis 11.2: Pruritus

Condition	Differential Diagnosis
Pruritus—rash present	Atopic dermatitis (eczema) Bullous pemphigoid Burrowing insects/larvae (scabies) Contact dermatitis Dermatitis herpetiformis Dermatographism (Darier's disease) Drug eruptions Ecthyma Erythroderma Folliculitis Impetigo Insect bites/pediculosis Lichen planus Malignancy (cutaneous T-cell lymphoma) Miliaria (heat rash) Neurotic excoriation Pityriasis rosea Pregnancy-induced Prurigo nodularis Psoriasis Seborrheic dermatitis Tinea (capitis, corporis, pedis, cruris) Transient acantholytic dermatosis (Grover's disease) Urticaria (hives)
Pruritus—no rash present	Chronic renal disease, especially with hemodialysis Cholestatic liver disease Delusions of parasitosis Hyperparathyroidism Hodgkin's lymphoma Polycythemia vera

DIFFERENTIAL DIAGNOSIS

A thorough and careful history is an important step in the evaluation of pruritus. If skin findings suggest an external causation (such as the linear striations characteristic of contact dermatitis), the history should be directed toward eliciting an external etiology. If the patient complains of generalized itching with no skin lesions, an internal or systemic etiology is more likely. The presence of a generalized rash should also arouse the clinician's suspicion of a drug reaction. Some systemic causes of pruritus include conditions such as allergies, drug reactions, malignancy (lymphomas and leukemias), chronic renal disease (especially with hemodialysis), and pruritus from obstructive biliary disease due to elevated blood levels of unconjugated bilirubin (see Focus on History: Pruritus).

Focus on History: Pruritus

History of contact with insects:

- Have you had any exposure to mosquitoes, fleas, sand flies, ticks, or spiders? (Brown recluse and black widow bites have necrotic centers.)

History of contact with the outdoors:

- Have you been to the beach, at a picnic, gone camping or swimming, or attended a sporting event (especially outdoors)?

History of contact with plants:

- Have you been in contact with plants or done any gardening?

History of contact with jewelry/metals:

- Any new watches, belts/belt buckles, earrings, necklaces? Any contact with metals?

History of occupation:

- What is your occupation? (Gardeners and employees of prisons, day-care centers, and schools have the potential for scabies, pediculosis, or impetigo exposure.)

History of hobbies and sport participation:

- Any exposure to hobby paints and glues?
- Do you participate in any sports? (Weight lifters and athletes are prone to fungal skin infections.)

History of chemical exposure:

- Any use or exposure to pesticides, herbicides, fertilizers, household cleaners?

History of medications:

- Any use of topical medications such as Neosporin ointment, Benadryl topical lotion, anti-itch lotion or spray? If so, did it reduce the itching? (This would be consistent with contact dermatitis.)
- Any prescription medicines, over-the-counter, herbals, or vitamins?

Family history:

- Any family members or intimate friends with the same symptoms? (This raises suspicion for scabies, pediculosis, or tinea infections.)

Social history:

- Any history or current alcohol or drug abuse, emotional distress, or psychiatric illness?

Pruritus is a symptom and should elicit an investigation of its potential cause. External causes of pruritus include insect bites, insect infestations (scabies, pediculosis), pinworms (more common in children with perianal pruritus), larva migrans, contact dermatitis, fiberglass dermatitis, sea bather's eruption, and bacterial folliculitis. It is not uncommon for patients to deny the knowledge of insect bites (especially if the event occurred during sleep) because some insects do not have painful bites. The patient should be asked about any history of medication use, including prescription drugs, hormones, vitamin supplements, and the use of nutritional or protein supplements. The history should include a review of all detergents, soaps, creams, moisturizers, cosmetics, and perfumes. A history of alternative medicines should also be included, including herbs, homeopathic remedies, and oils for aromatherapy. The use of recreational substances, including chewing tobacco, marijuana, and illicit drugs, should be considered as a potential cause of pruritus. Psychiatric illness as a cause of pruritus is a diagnosis of exclusion. With a psychogenic etiology, skin markings are seen more often on the extremities, and the urge to scratch even in the absence of itch is sometimes reported. The clinician should search for symptoms of depression or mood disorder. There is frequently a history of increased stress because of personal, financial, or familial problems.

The most predominant and disturbing symptom of scabies is pruritus, especially nighttime pruritus. The clinician needs to have a high index of suspicion for scabies because it frequently does not manifest in its classic presentation. If the clinician is looking for the mites' burrows, which the patient can obliterate by scratching, the diagnosis can easily be missed. Frequently, the rash has secondary changes, including excoriation, scaling, lichenification, and occasionally nodules (nodular scabies) due to the intense inflammatory response from the mites. Even if skin lesions do not resemble those typically associated with scabies, the clinician should consider the diagnosis if the location of the rash is on the axilla, under the breast, on the waistline, on the penis, or between the fingers. The clinician should not assume a lack of scabies infestation just because the classic rash on the interdigital webs is not seen. Scabies is more common in group homes and nursing homes. The management and treatment of scabies are discussed in depth in Chapter 12.

If a pruritic rash does not respond to symptomatic treatment, a work-up for systemic diseases is in order. Laboratory tests that should be ordered if systemic disease is suspected include a CBC with differential, ESR, fasting blood sugar, liver and renal function tests, a thyroid profile including TSH level, and a viral hepatitis profile. If the pruritic area is in the anus, an examination for external hemorrhoids should be done. In children or in adults with small children, a stool sample to check for ova and parasites, or a Scotch tape test, is recommended when pinworm infestation is suspected.

Dry skin, or *xerosis,* is a common finding in the elderly. It is also seen in young adults who are overly meticulous with personal hygiene. Use of strong deodorant soaps or daily hot baths can precipitate dry skin and worsen pruritus.

Systemic causes of pruritus to consider include atopic dermatitis (eczema), psoriasis, drug reactions, urticaria (from exposure to any substance, including airborne allergens), urticarial eruptions of pregnancy, lichen planus, lichen simplex chronicus, prurigo nodularis, and malignancies such as Hodgkin's lymphoma (with pruritus seen in approximately 35% of cases), cutaneous T-cell lymphoma (mycosis fungoides), and leukemia. A history of similar pruritic lesions in the past (especially if at the same location) should suggest an atopic history or urticaria. Atopic skin diseases that present predominantly with pruritus include atopic dermatitis (eczema) and psoriasis. The presence of hives or a history of hives to a known trigger is sufficient to diagnose urticaria. It is often seen with dermatographism, which can be elicited by rubbing a blunt object or finger on the skin firmly. An immediate response is seen, with formation of whealing that resolves within a few hours.

Lichen planus can mimic psoriasis; its cause is unknown. The lesions appear with shiny flat tops that are a red to violaceous color (red-violet tinged). Other presentations include small, flat-topped papules and a netlike lesion on the buccal mucosa (reticular lichen planus), penis, and external female genitalia. Malignant oral lesions occasionally occur, but oral carcinoma is rare. Lichen planus may have several presentations and locations. Lesions may be generalized, or they may be located on the arms, trunk, mouth, and genitalia. This disease may last for months to years; it does not have a cure and is best managed by a dermatologist.

MANAGEMENT

The treatment of pruritus depends on the correct diagnosis. The goal of treatment of pruritus is to relieve the itch, break the itch–scratch cycle, and maintain the barrier protection of the skin. Patients should be educated to avoid scratching, to use cool compresses and apply pressure to itchy areas, and to keep fingernails trimmed.

Symptomatic treatment for dry skin consists of avoidance of strong soaps; taking shorter, tepid showers (10 to 20 minutes) instead of hot baths; and the use of effective emollients. Mild bland soaps such as Dove, Basis, Purpose, Cetaphil, and Neutrogena are recommended. The patient should be educated to gently towel dry the skin after showering because rubbing the skin stimulates pruritus. To seal moisture in the skin, applying a bland emollient such as Eucerin, Lubriderm, or Alpha-Keri immediately after dabbing the skin with a towel to partially pat dry is helpful. Waiting too long (more than 5 minutes) after finishing a bath or shower allows moisture to evaporate. The strongest emollients are ointments that are petrolatum based, followed by creams (oil in water), and then lotions (powder in water). Gels are alcohol based; they should not be used for pruritus associated with dry skin because of their drying effect. Severe cases of dry skin may be treated using the "soak and smear" technique by wetting the skin for 20 minutes and then applying ointment directly to wet skin.

Pruritus of the scalp caused by seborrheic dermatitis (with dandruff and fine scales at the hairline, by the nares, and at the ears) should be treated with ketoconazole 2% shampoo (Nizoral shampoo). The rash of seborrheic dermatitis on the hairline, nares, and ears is best treated with hydrocortisone 1% (OTC) used two to three times a day. Fluorinated topical steroids should not be used on the face because of the risk of skin atrophy. If the etiology is an irritating external agent (such as fiberglass insulation), elimination of the agents may provide clinical relief of pruritus. Treatment of scabies infection is discussed in Chapter 12.

Symptomatic treatment of pruritus includes systemic and topical treatments, or combinations of both. Systemic medications include classic oral H_1 antihistamines such as hydroxyzine (Vistaril), one of the most effective treatments for pruritus, given three to four times per day. Cyproheptadine is used two to three times per day. OTC antihistamines include loratadine, desloratadine, cetirizine, and fexofenadine, which can all be taken once daily. In addition, older-generation agents such diphenhydramine, brompheniramine maleate, and chlorpheniramine maleate can be taken every 4 to 6 hours as needed. Newer-generation agents, cetirizine, fexofenadine, and desloratadine, cause less (or no) sedation when taken at their approved doses.

Any patient who is on antihistamines should be warned of possible drowsiness and should be cautioned against driving or operating dangerous machinery until the effects of the antihistamine are known. Alcohol and other central depressants worsen this effect. First-generation antihistamines with anticholinergic properties, such as diphenhydramine, cyproheptadine, brompheniramine maleate, and chlorpheniramine maleate, should be avoided in the elderly.

Other systemic treatments for persistent pruritus may include antidepressants such as doxepin and mirtazapine, as well as anticonvulsant/nerve pain therapy such as gabapentin (Neurontin). The antinausea/antiemetic aprepitant (Emend) has also been shown to be effective in treating the itch of atopic dermatitis.

Topical treatments for pruritus include topical anesthetics such as lidocaine 2.5% and prilocaine 2.5% cream (EMLA) and pramoxine (ProctoFoam, Sarna Sensitive, Gold Bond Anti-Itch, Pramox). Topical antihistamines and capsaicin may provide relief from itching; topical immunomodulators (pimecrolimus [Elidel], tacrolimus [Prograf]) may be used for atopic dermatitis. For anogenital pruritus, treatment includes the use of hydrocortisone and pramoxine cream 1% or 2.5% (Pramosone) on the anogenital area. Pramoxine preparations are effective and have a low incidence of sensitivity reactions compared with topical antihistamines and benzocaine. They are effective not only for anogenital pruritus but also for short-term relief of urticaria, insect bites, pruritus vulvae, and nummular eczema. Use of fluorinated and potent topical steroids on the anogenital area is not recommended because it can lead to atrophy and striae. Lichen planus is treated with antihistamines, topical and systemic steroids and retinoids, cyclosporine, psoralens with PUVA, and tacrolimus or pimecrolimus topical preparations. The treatment of lichen planus is best managed by dermatologists.

If Hodgkin's lymphoma is suspected, the clinician should perform a thorough physical examination and should especially look for painless and enlarged lymph nodes and constitutional symptoms such as generalized pruritus, weight loss, night sweats, and fever. Cutaneous T-cell lymphoma (mycosis fungoides) is a malignancy of the helper T cells of the immune system. Onset of lesions may take many years; sometimes, intractable pruritus may be the only presenting symptom. The lesions are sometimes misdiagnosed as psoriasis or as nummular dermatitis (eczema) because of their similar appearance. The lesions go through several stages and can present as red and scaly plaques that mimic the appearance of psoriasis. Nodules and tumors can be present, sometimes with ulceration. Diagnostic laboratory testing for suspected malignancy can include a CBC with differential, a peripheral smear, liver and renal function tests, ESR, a chest x-ray film, and computed tomography (CT) scan. Patients with suspected malignancy should be referred to cancer specialists.

RASH

The word *rash* refers to any pink or red-colored skin eruption, although rash colors may differ depending on underlying skin color. Words that are synonymous with rash include *exanthem* and *eruption*. Rashes are clinical manifestations of inflammation and have multiple etiologies.

Skin cells (keratinocytes) originate in the basal layer of the epidermis. These cells take approximately 28 days to mature and migrate to the surface (*stratum corneum*). The epidermis has no blood supply of its own and is dependent on the dermis for its circulation. It is stratified into two main layers—the inner viable layer (*stratum germinativum*) and the outer layer of dead, anucleated cells (*stratum corneum* or the horny layer). The stratum corneum consists of up to 25 layers of flat and tightly packed anucleated cells filled with keratin, a tough and durable protein that limits the passage of molecules into and out of the skin. This tough outer layer is relatively impermeable to many external substances and prevents the evaporation of bodily fluids. It is also a protective barrier against numerous microorganisms.

When the stratum corneum is damaged by inflammation (rash), it becomes more permeable to external substances, including microorganisms and chemicals. Not only do these substances and microorganisms have a greater chance of gaining entrance into the body, but therapeutic topical creams and ointments applied to inflamed skin also are more likely to be absorbed and thus have an increased chance of toxicity.

The dermis, which gives the skin its elasticity and strength, is made up primarily of a complex network of collagen and elastic fibers interspersed with blood vessels, cutaneous nerves, apocrine glands, eccrine glands, lymphatics, and pilosebaceous units of the skin. The *dermoepidermal junction* (the topmost section of the dermis) is the interface between the epidermis and the dermis. A defect in the dermoepidermal junction results in separation of these layers and the formation of bullae. Inherited autoimmune diseases of the skin resulting from abnormalities of the dermis include bullous pemphigoid and epidermolysis bullosa.

Gram-positive bacterial infections such as *Staphylococcus aureus* (the causative agent of toxic shock syndrome [TSS]) present with systemic symptoms such as fever, malaise, and an erythematous rash. Drug reactions can also present with a rash (e.g., erythema multiforme, urticaria). Autoimmune disorders that can cause a rash include SLE (butterfly rash), erythema nodosum, and Kawasaki disease (seen in children).

Viruses are responsible for many cases of rash and are usually self-limited in patients with intact immune systems. Viral infections that manifest with rash and systemic symptoms such as fever and malaise include measles, rubella (German measles), hand-foot-mouth disease, erythema infectiosum, herpes simplex infection, herpes zoster, varicella-zoster (chickenpox), and roseola infantum (also known as exanthema subitum) in children.

Rashes are more difficult to see in patients with darker skin because the red to dark pink color that is associated with rash becomes less visible. Instead of the pink to red color, a rash in a person of African descent with darker skin might appear as a dark brown color. Thus, rashes on patients with darker skin can sometimes go unnoticed unless the patient complains of the problem to the clinician. The clinician must learn to use other dermatological clues besides skin color to differentiate rashes in this population. These include the history of the rash and associated symptoms; the type of lesions present (macule, papule, pustule); the texture of the lesions (flat, raised, rough); and the pattern of distribution (central vs. on the extremities) (see Focus on History: Rash).

DIFFERENTIAL DIAGNOSIS

Because the differential diagnoses of rash are so numerous, this section focuses on rashes that are associated with serious health consequences. Primary-care clinicians should become familiar with these rashes because of the potential for serious sequelae, including death, if the diagnosis is missed.

Focus on History: Rash

Onset of skin lesions:

- When did the skin lesion(s) first appear?
- How did the skin lesion appear at onset?
- Where did the skin lesion first appear?

Spread of skin lesions:

- Have the skin lesions spread? Where?

Change in skin lesions:

- Has the appearance of the skin lesions changed over time?
- Have the skin lesions gotten better or worse?

Symptoms associated with the skin lesion:

- Are there any associated symptoms, such as itching, burning, or pain?
- Are there any systemic symptoms such as fever, anorexia, malaise, pharyngitis, or myalgia?

History of treatment:

- What type of self-treatment have you attempted?
- Have you seen another health-care provider for the skin lesions? What type of treatment was given? Was it effective?

History of food:

- Do you have any food allergies or sensitivities, such as dairy, seafood, peanuts, other nuts, strawberries, tomatoes, alcoholic drinks (such as red or white wine, beer, or mixed drinks)?

History of medications:

- Are you taking any prescription medications (e.g., antibiotics such as penicillin or sulfa drugs or pain medications such as codeine) and/or OTC medications such as aspirin, NSAIDs, cold medicines, or vitamins?
- Do any of these medications contain artificial colors or preservatives?

Alternative medicine:

- Are you taking any herbal medicines or teas, homeopathic remedies, aromatherapy, juices, or other alternative medicines?

Atopic history:

- Do you have a history of the same rash before? What was the diagnosis? How was it treated?
- Do you have a family history of skin conditions or rash?
- Have you or a family member ever been diagnosed with eczema, psoriasis, skin allergies, asthma, or allergies?

Infectious disease exposure (any exposure up to 2 weeks before onset of rash):

- Are you exposed to other people with the same symptoms?
- Are you exposed to small children, day care, or schools?
- Have you had sexual activity with a new partner (known for less than 3 months)?

Systemic symptoms (infectious, autoimmune, malignancies, metabolic):

- Do you have any systemic symptoms, such as sore throat and rhinitis (viral etiology), fever, fatigue, myalgia, joint pain, nausea, night sweats, weight loss (malignancy), or weight gain (diabetes mellitus)?

Cancers such as mammary Paget's disease present with a rash that looks like eczematous dermatitis of the nipple and areola. Although it is an uncommon intraepithelial adenocarcinoma, the clinician should be careful not to overlook this diagnosis. The onset is gradual, ranging from several months to years. Early in its course, the disease is asymptomatic except for a rash. During the later stages, it is accompanied by symptoms such as pruritus, discharge, bleeding, and ulceration. The sizes of lesions can range from less than 1 cm in diameter to several centimeters. Sometimes an underlying breast mass is palpable during the later stages of the disease—a worse prognosis is associated with this ominous finding. Patients with suspected mammary Paget's disease should be referred to a breast specialist.

The usual location of the classic rash of mammary Paget's disease is on one nipple (or areola); rarely, it is seen on both breasts. The skin lesion appears as an oval-shaped, erythematous scaling plaque with sharp margins. Because of the similarity in appearance, this lesion can be misdiagnosed as eczema, psoriasis, contact dermatitis, or impetigo. Usually, the lesions of eczematous dermatitis involve both breasts and last from 2 to 3 weeks; the lesions respond to treatment with topical steroids. Contact dermatitis usually involves only one breast (sometimes both); again, the rash usually resolves in 2 weeks and responds to topical steroids. If a rash on the nipple or areolar region lasts longer than 2 weeks and does not resolve with topical steroids, a high index of suspicion is imperative and the patient should be referred to a breast specialist for further evaluation.

TSS is an acute illness caused by toxin-producing *S. aureus.* In the United States, TSS occurs in both male and female patients, with an overall incidence of 0.52 per 100,000; however, among menstruating women between 15 and 25 years of age who use tampons, its incidence is 1 to 3 per 100,000. Fifty percent of TSS cases are nonmenstrual in etiology; males compose 25% of these cases. Risk factors for menstrual TSS include tampon use in general, using tampons regularly during the menstrual cycle, and leaving tampons inserted for extended periods of time. Cases of menstrual TSS have progressively declined over the past 20 years after superabsorbent tampons were taken off the market (Venkataraman, 2016). In these cases, symptoms begin in nearly all patients within days of the onset of the menstrual period in women who have used tampons. Nonmenstrual TSS can occur after childbirth or abortion or as a result of surgical wounds, nasal packs, burns, catheters, and use of birth control methods such as the sponge, diaphragm, and cervical cap. The amount of time a diaphragm or cervical cap remains in the vagina—particularly if greater than 30 hours—seems to be a factor in the development of TSS, as well as if pieces of a sponge are retained in the genital tract. Women younger than age 19 account for one-third of TSS cases, and these women are prone to recurrence. The mortality rate for nonmenstrual cases is 18%, and 5% for menstrual-related TSS. Severe group A beta-hemolytic *Streptococcus* (GABHS) infection can mimic TSS, except that GABHS is also associated with necrotizing fasciitis and has a higher mortality rate (30%).

TSS presents with a sudden onset of high fever (higher than 102°F [38.8°C]) and vomiting. It is associated with a tingling sensation of the hands and feet, myalgia, weakness, headache, and diarrhea. In severe cases, it is associated with confusion, hypotension, and shock. It is accompanied by a bright red, fine maculopapular (scarlatiniform) rash and is sometimes accompanied by petechiae and bullae. The skin on the palms of the hands and the soles of the feet is very erythematous, and in 1 to 2 weeks the palms and soles start to desquamate. Abnormal laboratory results include leukocytosis, thrombocytopenia, abnormal liver function tests, elevated levels of creatinine, and abnormally low levels of platelets (thrombocytopenia).

Complications of TSS include multisystem failure, including adult respiratory distress syndrome, acute renal failure, metabolic acidosis, disseminated intravascular coagulation, septic shock, and death. A high index of suspicion and early recognition of serious causes of rash are important to avoid potential sequelae. Patients with suspected TSS should be referred immediately to a physician or to an emergency department. Menstruating women who are using a tampon should be advised to remove the tampon immediately. Treatment consists of hospitalization in the intensive care unit for aggressive systemic antibiotic treatment and supportive therapy.

URTICARIA

Urticaria (hives or wheals) is a common problem seen in primary care. It affects 15% to 20% of the population at least once (Joshi & Ferri, 2018). *Urticaria* is defined as a sudden generalized eruption of pale, evanescent wheals or papules associated with severe itching. *Angioedema* is urticaria that involves not only edema of the dermis, as in uncomplicated urticaria, but the subcutaneous tissues as well. Angioedema and urticaria can be part of a life-threatening immunoglobulin E (IgE)–dependent anaphylactic reaction, which involves bronchospasm, laryngeal edema, and shock. If anaphylaxis is not treated and reversed immediately with subcutaneous epinephrine, it can be fatal. Angioedema associated with chronic urticaria is rarely life-threatening. In these cases, the patient will report a history of angioedema but without significant compromise of the throat or airway.

Urticarial wheals (hives) and angioedema are produced by the degranulation of mast cells when an offending allergen to which the patient has been sensitized is encountered. Degranulated mast cells release inflammatory factors, including histamines, that increase vascular permeability and cause pruritus. On microscopic examination, the edema on the dermis is manifested by the wide separation of dermal fibers in cells from urticarial lesions, along with dilation of the venules and lymphatics. Urticaria is also associated with non–IgE-dependent reactions involving the complement cascade of the immune system. Chronic urticaria may be a symptom of an autoimmune condition.

DIFFERENTIAL DIAGNOSIS

The typical patient with urticaria will present with a complaint of numerous, intensely pruritic hives or wheals that appear regularly at certain times of the day, then spontaneously resolve within a few hours (and typically within no more than 24 hours), only to reappear again the next day. The wheals typically enlarge and coalesce, forming round or irregular shapes. Most cases of acute urticaria resolve spontaneously in 1 to 2 weeks. As a result, some authorities recommend waiting at least 2 weeks before initiating an extensive (and expensive) laboratory workup. Laboratory results are usually normal when testing is done.

Urticaria that lasts longer than 6 weeks is classified as *chronic idiopathic urticaria*. Studies of patients with chronic urticaria have found clinically relevant changes in quality of life, including sleep deprivation, social isolation, and mood changes that are on the same level as in patients with ischemic heart disease.

Urticaria is classified into several categories. *Cholinergic urticaria* accounts for one-third (34%) of all cases of physical urticaria. Factors that trigger cholinergic urticaria include exercise, anxiety, elevated body temperature (e.g., fever, exercise, sweating), and hot baths or showers. The lesions usually resolve within 30 minutes after the offending activity is stopped. The hives are small (2 to 4 mm), highly pruritic, surrounded by erythema, and appear on the upper trunk and arms. *Physical urticaria* accounts for 17% to 20% of all cases of urticaria (English et al., 2017). It occurs immediately or shortly after exposure to physical stimuli such as pressure, cold, heat, exercise, sunlight (solar urticaria), water (aquagenic urticaria), vibrations, or in response to increased body temperature. Urticarial episodes resulting from exposure to these stimuli are usually of short duration; most last only 2 hours. Dermatographism occurs in 2% to 5% of the normal population and can occur with other forms of urticaria. A dermatographic reaction can be elicited by applying friction to the skin with a dull object and watching for wheal formation. The wheal (hive) typically lasts for a few hours, then resolves.

Some pregnant women develop an extremely pruritic eruption known as pruritic urticarial papules and plaques of pregnancy (PUPPP) or polymorphic eruption of pregnancy. It occurs in 1 in 160 pregnancies (Pierson, 2017). These lesions appear as erythematous urticarial papules and plaques (striae distensae) that usually start on the striae of the abdomen and spread to the thighs, buttocks, and, occasionally, arms. The lesions can start at any time during the third trimester, but they are frequently seen during the last 2 to 3 weeks of pregnancy. The cause is unknown. PUPPP is not associated with increased maternal or fetal morbidity and usually resolves after delivery of the fetus. Risk factors for the development of PUPPP include pregnancies with male fetuses (70% of pregnancies developing PUPPP), first pregnancies, multiple pregnancies, and women with hypertension (Pierson, 2017). Treatment during the last trimester of pregnancy involves the use of a moderate-potency topical corticosteroid, such as triamcinolone acetonide cream 0.1% (Aristocort, Kenalog), applied two to three times daily on the skin lesions. With topical treatment, improvement of the lesions should be seen in a few days. Topical corticosteroids should not be applied to rashes that are suspected to be of viral etiology (such as herpes simplex or varicella zoster) because corticosteroids can worsen them. Severe cases are best referred to an obstetrician for possible treatment with systemic corticosteroids. Antihistamines have been shown to provide little relief in PUPPP, and there are no antihistamines that are considered completely safe in pregnancy. However, first-generation antihistamines such as diphenhydramine, hydroxyzine, chlorpheniramine, and dexchlorpheniramine are considered by many sources to be the safest antihistamines to recommend in pregnancy due to their long history of availability and use during pregnancy.

MANAGEMENT

The treatment for urticaria is to find the cause of the skin rash and to stop exposure to the sensitizing allergen. Certain drugs, such as aspirin, angiotensin-converting enzyme inhibitors, and NSAIDs, should be avoided in patients with urticaria. Tight clothing should be avoided because wheals tend to occur in areas with increased pressure or friction. Showering or bathing with hot water should be avoided because this worsens itching. Cool environmental temperatures in the home are helpful and aid in inducing sleep.

Allergens that can cause both acute and chronic urticaria include drugs, foods, food preservatives, insect bites, and bacterial, fungal, viral, or parasitic infections. If the patient is taking vitamins, herbs, and supplements that are not critical, they should all be stopped; even "natural" vitamins and herbs should not be exempt. The patient can start a trial of eliminating certain highly allergenic foods such as eggs, strawberries, tomatoes, chocolate, citrus fruits, peanuts and other nuts, all vinegars and wines (due to allergenic sulfites), alcoholic beverages, and shellfish, although this is cumbersome and bothersome for most patients. In addition, broad food elimination in children by concerned parents or overzealous health-care providers increases the risk of malnutrition and social isolation. Chronic urticaria can also be caused by food dyes or additives, including sulfites (found in dried fruit, wines, and vinegar). Food allergens can be occasionally confirmed by an antigen-specific radioallergosorbent test or by skin-prick tests performed by allergists. Viral infections that have been implicated in causing urticaria include herpes, hepatitis, acute mononucleosis, and rubella. Bacterial infections such as sinusitis and fungal infections have also been implicated.

In chronic urticaria, the clinical evaluation should look for underlying disease, although the etiology in most cases of chronic urticaria is never found. A careful history (including international travel) and a thorough physical examination should assess for signs of chronic disease such as chronic sinusitis, tooth abscess, low-grade fungal infection (candidiasis), intestinal parasites, or chronic hepatitis. Some screening tests that may be helpful (depending on the patient history) include a stool sample for ova and parasites, sinus x-rays or CT scan, ESR or C-reactive protein, CBC, liver function tests, a hepatitis profile, urinalysis, and a urine sample for culture and sensitivity. In most cases of chronic urticaria (which is more common in women aged 30 to 60 years), the cause is never determined. Up to one-half of the cases of chronic urticaria and angioedema resolve spontaneously after a period of 5 years.

First-line therapy for urticaria includes second-generation (nonsedating) H_1 antihistamines. Fexofenadine, loratadine, and cetirizine are available OTC, whereas desloratadine and levocetirizine are available by prescription. First-generation antihistamines, such as hydroxyzine, diphenhydramine, and cyproheptadine, are faster acting but have greater effects of sedation. The timing of administration of the antihistamine is important and should be tailored individually so that the bloodstream levels of the drug will peak during the time of day when urticarial lesions are most likely to occur, which will differ among individuals. All antihistamines, even the so-called nonsedating antihistamines, have the potential for sedation, particularly at high doses. Susceptible patients, especially elderly patients and children, are at higher risk for sedation and somnolence. Patients should be educated regarding drowsiness as a potential adverse effect of antihistamine use and should be warned against driving or operating heavy machinery until the effects of the medication on the patient are known. The combination of antihistamines with other central nervous system depressants, such as alcohol, tranquilizers, and certain antidepressants will increase the risk of sedation.

Different classes of H_1 antihistamines should be tried until adequate relief is achieved, as some patients will respond better to one type of antihistamine than another. A combination of H_1 and H_2 antihistamines (e.g., cimetidine, famotidine, ranitidine) may be used by some clinicians, but the evidence does not support using these combinations versus H_1 antihistamines alone. Some antihistamines (such as diphenhydramine) tend to cause more sedation than others; diphenhydramine is the main ingredient in OTC sleep aids. For patients who can tolerate its sedating effects (or avoid the problem by taking it at bedtime), diphenhydramine can be taken at 25 to 50 mg every 4 to 6 hours (maximum 300 mg daily). Due to its anticholinergic effects, diphenhydramine should be avoided in the elderly. The classic prescription antihistamine used for pruritus and urticaria is hydroxyzine. Hydroxyzine can be given as a bedtime dose of 50 mg to reduce the risk of daytime sedation. Cetirizine is 13% less sedating than hydroxyzine and has a rapid onset of action. The dose of cetirizine is 10 mg once daily given at bedtime. Cetirizine has been found to be especially useful for delayed pressure urticaria. Cetirizine does not cause cardiac toxicity when it is combined with other drugs, such as erythromycin, imidazole antifungals, or other hepatically metabolized drugs. Fexofenadine, a nonsedating antihistamine, is given as 60 mg every 12 hours or 180 mg daily. For treatment of cold urticaria, cyproheptadine (Periactin) can be prescribed in a dosage of 4 mg three times daily. The use of cyproheptadine is contraindicated in angle-closure glaucoma, prostatic hypertrophy, with concurrent use of monoamine oxidase inhibitors, and in elderly or debilitated patients. Because of its atropine-like actions, caution should be taken in patients with asthma, increased intraocular pressure, heart disease, hypertension, or hyperthyroidism.

Patients with specific types of urticaria should be referred to a specialist (allergist or dermatologist), including urticaria associated with angioedema of the tongue or throat, peanut allergy, latex allergy, and urticaria that persists beyond 6 weeks (chronic urticaria). The anti-IgE monoclonal antibody therapy omalizumab (Xolair) has been used for severe persistent asthma and is now being used for the treatment of chronic idiopathic urticaria in symptomatic patients who do not respond to H_1 antihistamine treatment. It is given by subcutaneous injection every 2 to 4 weeks. Doxepin, an antidepressant antihistamine, has been shown to be effective in resistant cases of urticarial. Short-term oral corticosteroids have also been effective in the treatment of acute urticaria.

Teledermatology is the practice of dermatology from a distance by remote health-care providers. Skin lesions are photographed, and the images are sent to a consultant dermatologist or other specialist to determine whether treatment is indicated. A biopsy may be performed and sent for further diagnostic studies if indicated.

REFERENCES

Alopecia

Bolduc C. Alopecia areata treatment & management. http://emedicine. medscape.com/article/1069931-treatment?pa=QgXLCrVEeLkb wLJsFdw3RdCdksWkI%2F6P2fOEOmFK5NA2yAq9sCCttZn hioHw1cFqaBSWBtBwCPfIOCh2JAZ0ZqMMvXjUcyZ8uhF NFUtVAb4%3D#d12. Published 2017. Accessed June 22, 2017.

Gupta AK, Foley KA. 5% minoxidil: Treatment for female pattern hair loss. *Skin Ther Lett.* 2014;19(6):5–7.

International Society of Hair Restoration Surgery. About your hair loss and what causes it. http://www.ishrs.org/content/about-your-hair-loss-and-what-causes-it. Published 2016. Accessed July 7, 2017.

Merck & Co, Inc. Proscar (finasteride) tablets prescribing information. Whitehouse Station, NJ; 2011.

Pigmentation Changes

Aguirre C. An introduction to hyperpigmentation. Dermascope. http://www.dermascope.com/disorders/an-introduction-to-hyperpigmentation-may-2017#.WUw6eyMrL9A. Published May 2017. Accessed June 22, 2017.

American Academy of Dermatology. Lasers lighting the way for enhanced treatment of melisma and tattoo removal. https://www.aad. org/media/news-releases/lasers-lighting-the-way-for-enhanced-treatment-of-melasma-and-tattoo-removal. Published 2012. Accessed June 22, 2017.

Arif T. Salicylic acid as a peeling agent: A comprehensive review. *Clin Cosmet Investig Dermatol.* 2015;8:455–461.

Stoppler MC. Vitiligo facts. http://www.medicinenet.com/vitiligo/article.htm. Published 2016. Accessed June 22, 2017.

Pruritus

Butler DF. Pruritus and systemic disease. http://emedicine.medscape. com/article/1098029-overview. Published March 8, 2016. Accessed March 21, 2017.

Cohen KR, Frank J, Salbu RL, Israel I. Pruritus in the elderly: Clinical approaches to the improvement of quality of life. *P T.* 2012;37(4):227–232, 236–239.

English J, Reddy K, Gonzalez-Estrada G, Bajaj K. Physical urticaria. *BMJ Case Rep.* http://casereports.bmj.com/content/2017/bcr-2017-220286.full. 2017;2017.

Yosopovitch G, Hundley JL. Practical guidelines for the relief of itch. *Dermatol Nurs.* 2004;16(4):325–328.

Rash

Medicine.net. Group A streptococcal (GAS) disease (strep throat, necrotizing fasciitis, impetigo). http://www.medicinenet.com/script/main/art.asp?articlekey=60947. Published 2017. Accessed June 22, 2017.

Venkataraman R. Toxic shock syndrome. https://emedicine.medscape. com/article/169177-overview. Published August 11, 2016. Accessed March 27, 2017.

Urticaria

Joshi S, Ferri FF. *Ferri's clinical advisor.* Philadelphia, PA: Elsevier; 2018:1326–1327, e2.

Kaplan A. A 34 year old man with a 1 year history of itchy hives. *Clin Advisor.* 2016;19(8):49–53.

Kar S, Krishnan A, Preetha K, Mohankak A. A review of antihistamines used during pregnancy. *J Pharmacol Pharmacother.* 2012;3(2):105–108.

Pierson JC. Polymorphic eruption of pregnancy. http://emedicine. medscape.com/article/1123725-overview#a5. Published 2017. Accessed June 22, 2017.

Wong HK. Urticaria. http://emedicine.medscape.com/article/762917-overview#a1. Published June 2, 2016. Accessed March 29, 2017.

RESOURCES

General

American Academy of Dermatology
    www.aad.org
American Society of Dermatology
    www.asd.org

Alopecia

American Cancer Society
    www.cancer.org
National Alopecia Areata Foundation
    www.naaf.org
National Institute of Allergy and Infectious Disease
    www.niaid.nih.gov
National Institute of Arthritis, Musculoskeletal and Skin Diseases
    www.niams.nih.gov
National Institutes of Health
    www.nih.gov
The National Eczema Society
    www.eczema.org

Skin Cancer

The Skin Cancer Foundation
    www.skincancer.org

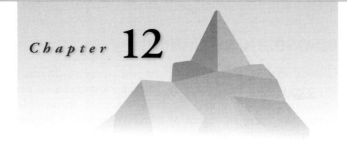

Chapter **12**

Parasitic Skin Infestations

Jill E. Winland-Brown, EdD, APRN, FNP-BC

Brian Oscar Porter, MD, PhD, MPH, MBA

SCABIES

Scabies is a highly contagious mite infestation that occurs mainly in children, young adults, health-care workers, and institutionalized persons of all ages. It is characterized by generalized intractable pruritus, often with minimal cutaneous manifestations. The diagnosis of scabies infection is easily missed and should be considered in patients of any age with persistent and severe pruritus. Scabies can develop into a chronic condition.

EPIDEMIOLOGY AND CAUSES

Human scabies is caused by the itch mite *Sarcoptes scabiei* var. *hominis,* which infects human skin. The adult female measures 0.3 to 0.5 mm long and has a rounded body with four pairs of short legs. Scabies infestations occur worldwide, are endemic in most parts of the world, and affect people of all races and social classes. Epidemics are historically associated with war, conditions of poverty, overcrowding, poor hygiene, malnutrition, and sexual promiscuity. The World Health Organization estimates that there are about 300 million cases of scabies in the world each year. Some studies suggest 6% to 27% of the general population has scabies, but other surveys find a lower prevalence. Close personal contact is the major mode of transmission for scabies, although casual contact such as nursing care may be sufficient for transmission to occur. Institutional epidemics have been reported in which caregivers were infested. Live mites have been discovered in dust samples from the homes of infested persons, suggesting fomite (shared objects, such as furniture or linens) transmission as a possibility.

PATHOPHYSIOLOGY

The scabies itch mite is an aerobic organism and thus requires exposure to surface air to survive. The male mite dies shortly after mating, but the female mite may live 4 to 6 weeks. As an obligate parasite, the scabies mite burrows into the skin shortly after contact. It both resides and reproduces in human skin. The female mite can lay two to three eggs per day (up to 10 to 25 total) in burrows created at the base of the stratum corneum of the epidermis, traveling up to 2 mm per day. Burrows average 5 mm in length, allowing for continued exposure to surface air, but soon after egg laying is completed, the female mite dies. Eggs hatch, and larvae emerge in 72 to 84 hours, molting at least three times before reaching adulthood. Mating of these new mites, thus, occurs after approximately 17 days.

Interestingly, sensitivity to *S. scabiei* must take place for pruritus to occur. Initial sensitivity takes several weeks to develop after primary infection and is caused by a foreign body inflammatory reaction to either the mite itself or its feces. In persons who are experiencing reinfestation, pruritus may occur within 24 hours because the immune system has been previously sensitized. Individuals who are immunocompromised or have a neurologic disorder, such as Down syndrome, stroke, dementia, neuropathy, or spinal cord injury, may be predisposed to a variant of scabies known as crusted scabies (*scabies crustosa;* previously known as "Norwegian scabies"). Scabies crustosa is characterized by scaly lesions at the sites of invasion that soon become warty and encrusted, creating a protective barrier for these mites. The number of mites infesting a patient with scabies crustosa can exceed more than a million, whereas infestation with classic scabies is usually limited to 10 mites or fewer. One-half of patients with crusted scabies do not experience pruritus, reflecting the absence of key inflammatory mediators seen in classic scabies. A nodular form of scabies also exists in which firm, erythematous, dome-shaped lesions roughly 0.5 cm in size develop over the groin, buttock, and axillary areas. Nodular scabies represents the body's reaction to the infestation and is not itself a different type of scabies infestation. Histamine-mediated urticarial lesions may accompany this rash, which is intensely pruritic. In all forms of scabies, if rashes go untreated, bacterial superinfection by *Staphylococcus* species may result, worsening acute inflammation.

CLINICAL PRESENTATION

Subjective

The typical patient usually presents with a complaint of intense itching that is usually described as being more severe at night. Mothers may report changes in feeding patterns of children and that they are more tired and irritable than usual. Itching may be widespread but is commonly located in the interdigital web spaces, wrists, anterior axillary folds, periumbilical skin, pelvic girdle, penis, and ankles. The palms, soles, face, neck, and scalp are more frequently involved in small children. The pruritus is usually described as not responding to treatment.

Many patients will complain of a rash, whereas others experience itching for months with no apparent rash. Patients are often aware of similar symptoms in family members and/or in sexual contacts. Patients presenting with the described symptoms should be screened for possible scabies infestation.

Focus on History: Scabies

If scabies is suspected:

- Do you live or work in a nursing home or group home, in a school, or in a prison?
- Do you have any family members or sexual partners that have similar symptoms?
- Are young children displaying increased signs of fatigue or irritability?
- Have the eating patterns of children changed?

If patient complains of pruritus:

- Where is the itching worse?
- What part of your body is itching?
- Is the itching worse at night?
- Does itching interfere with your ability to sleep?
- How long have you been itching?
- Is the itching relieved by anything? If so, what?
- Are any family members who live with you also complaining of itching?

Objective

The earliest physical signs of scabies are small, 1 to 2 mm, red papules located in areas of the body that are most attractive to mites. Because of the intense itching, excoriations from repeated scratching, with crusting and scaling, may also be present. It may be difficult to visualize scabies mites on the skin, and the patient may complain only of incessant itchiness. Skin lesions occur at the sites of mite infestation or result from a hypersensitivity reaction to the scabies mite. Secondary skin lesions including lichenification and excoriations are the result of chronic rubbing or scratching of lesions. Secondary bacterial infections present with increased symptoms, pruritus, and crusting of lesions (secondary impetigo).

The classic scabies skin lesion is the intraepidermal burrow. Each female mite produces one burrow. In light-skinned people, burrows have a whitish color with black specks caused by fecal particles. The female mite resides at the blind end of the tunnel and can burrow 2 to 3 mm per day. Burrows are usually distributed in areas where there are few or no hair follicles and where the stratum corneum is thin and soft.

Burrows are sometimes seen on the top of early scabetic nodules that occur in 7% to 10% of patients with scabies. Nodules vary in color from pink to brown and are 5 to 20 cm in diameter. They may become more visible after treatment.

DIAGNOSTIC REASONING

Clinical diagnosis of scabies is almost never made until hypersensitivity has occurred. The diagnosis is based on epidemiological history, the occurrence of intractable itching, and an assessment of the distribution of lesions and pruritus.

Diagnostic Tests

The clinician should search for the presence of mites. The highest yield of mites is in burrows located on the finger webs, penis, or wrists. The Burrow Ink Test is performed by rubbing a felt-tip pen over the suspected burrow (blue and green markers work best because they do not interfere with microscopic results). Excess ink is removed with an alcohol wipe, while the remaining ink concentrates in the tunnel, indicating the location of the burrow.

Once a burrow has been located, the clinician should place a drop of mineral oil over it, then scrape off the burrow using a number 15 scalpel blade. The scrapings should be placed on a slide with a drop of oil, then sealed with a cover slip. The identification of the *S. scabiei* mite, its eggs, or fecal pellets is diagnostic of scabies. There are no serologic tests currently available for scabies.

Failure to identify mites, their eggs, or burrows does not rule out scabies infestation. If scabies infestation is suspected because of clinical symptoms, empirical treatment should be tried. Resolution of symptoms within a few days is indicative of previous scabies infection.

Differential Diagnosis

The diagnosis of scabies can be easily missed. Although there are common skin findings (e.g., burrows), the clinical picture of scabies can be extremely variable, depending on the duration of the infection and the severity of the sensitivity reaction. Variants of scabies in immunocompromised persons and persons with neurologic disorders further cloud the diagnosis. An accurate diagnosis is essential for effective treatment. It should be noted that it is possible for patients to have preexisting skin problems in addition to scabies. A thorough history can help minimize diagnostic pitfalls (see Differential Diagnosis 12.1).

MANAGEMENT

With proper adherence to treatment regimens, cure rates for scabies approach 100%. However, application of medicated creams or lotions is insufficient for an affected person if the entire household is not treated and if all environmental reservoirs of the scabies mite (such as bedding, clothing, or towels) are not sufficiently cleaned with hot water and detergents. Therefore, effective care

Differential Diagnosis 12.1: Scabies

Scabies	Atopic dermatitis (eczema)
	Bullous pemphigoid
	Chronic renal disease, especially with hemodialysis
	Cholestatic liver disease
	Delusions of parasitosis
	Contact dermatitis
	Dermatitis herpetiformis
	Dermatographism (Darier's disease)
	Drug eruptions
	Ecthyma
	Erythroderma
	Folliculitis
	Hyperparathyroidism
	Hodgkin's lymphoma
	Impetigo
	Insect bites/pediculosis
	Lichen planus
	Malignancy (cutaneous T-cell lymphoma)
	Miliaria (heat rash)
	Neurotic excoriation
	Pityriasis rosea
	Polycythemia vera
	Pregnancy-induced
	Prurigo nodularis
	Psoriasis
	Pyoderma
	Seborrheic dermatitis
	Tinea (capitis, corporis, pedis, cruris)
	Transient acantholytic dermatosis (Grover's disease)
	Urticaria (hives)
Nodular scabies	Darier's disease
	Insect bites
	Prurigo nodularis
	Secondary syphilis
	Urticaria pigmentosa (in young child)
Crusted scabies	Eczematous dermatitis
	Erythroderma
	Psoriasis
	Seborrheic dermatitis

of patients with scabies involves treating the patient, his or her close personal contacts, and the surrounding environment. Treating the source of the infestation and any secondary complications, such as bacterial infection (e.g., secondary impetigo) or dermatitis, should also be included in the management plan.

Initial management of the patient diagnosed with scabies is directed at killing all live mites (see Drugs Commonly Prescribed 12.1). Lotions containing scabicides (such as permethrin, lindane, crotamiton, or sulfur) are commonly used. Permethrin is the first-line treatment. Antihistamines and topical steroids are helpful for pruritus. Of the products containing scabicides, lindane is the most toxic. It is rapidly absorbed through the skin and has been associated with central nervous system (CNS) symptoms such as irritability, seizures, and, in cases of ingestion or overdose, death. Older patients, young children, and pregnant and lactating women have the greatest risk of toxicity. Therefore, the choice of scabicide should be based on the age of the patient, pregnancy status, resistance patterns, degree of toxicity, and severity of infestation. High mite populations, the presence of crusts, and decreased immune status of the host make treating crusted scabies more difficult. It may be necessary to remove crusts that protect mites from scabicides before treating.

The majority of patients require only medical treatment with a topical scabicide. However, some patients experience hypersensitivity to the mite and mite products and may require systemic corticosteroids for the relief of severe pruritus. Ivermectin 200 mcg/kg is used as a single dose and followed by another dose 1 to 2 weeks later. This should be used in conjunction with a topical cream or lotion. Some patients may delay treatment until a secondary bacterial infection has occurred, necessitating the additional use of an antistaphylococcal antibiotic. Cephalexin or dicloxacillin for 7 to 10 days may be prescribed.

In addition, patients with extensive dermatitis lesions may obtain relief with topical corticosteroids, such as triamcinolone 0.1% cream twice daily for 7 days. Fluorinated steroids must not be used on the face or on skinfolds (e.g., intertriginous areas) because of the increased risk of skin atrophy. Management must include a strict isolation protocol for scabies crustosa.

FOLLOW-UP AND REFERRAL

Uncomplicated scabies infestations should be followed up 1 week after the initial treatment. If generalized itching persists, hypersensitivity to the remaining dead mites and mite products should be considered. It may be necessary to repeat the scabicide treatment, however. Patients who experience persistent scabetic nodules or scabies crustosa may require advanced management and should be referred to a dermatologist.

Patient Education: Scabies

Patient education is an integral part of successfully treating scabies. Patients should be instructed to trim their fingernails to reduce the possibility of harboring mites and reinfesting themselves or passing the infestation to others. Safety information regarding the use of scabicides should be stressed, such as not exceeding recommended exposure times, reporting characteristic toxicity symptoms, and the secure storage of treatment

Drugs Commonly Prescribed 12.1: Scabies

DRUG	INDICATION	ADVERSE REACTIONS AND PRESCRIBING CONSIDERATIONS
Topical		
Permethrin cream 5% (Elimite)	Presence of live mites (scabicide)	Mite resistance has been reported. Safe for use in children 2 months and older. May also need to treat head and neck. Apply to all areas of body from the neck down. Leave on for 8–12 hours. Repeat application in 1 week. May repeat a third time 1 week later.
Lindane 19% (gamma-benzene hexachloride)	Presence of live mites (scabicide)	Potential CNS toxicity. Rapidly absorbed through skin. Do not use on infants or young children, pregnant or lactating women, or if history of seizures. Mite resistance has been reported. May also need to treat head and neck. *Adults:* apply thinly to all areas of the body from the neck down. Wash off thoroughly after 8 hours. Do not retreat.
Crotamiton cream 10% (Eurax)	Presence of live mites (scabicide)	Reported failure rates of up to 50%; may need to be repeated. Shake well before using. Apply to all areas of the body from the chin down for two consecutive nights. Change clothing and bed linen the morning after each application; wash these articles in hot water with a strong cleanser to avoid reinfection.
Sulfur ointment 8%–10%	Presence of live mites (scabicide)	Extensive use suggests it is safe to use on pregnant and lactating women and infants. Malodorous and stains clothing. Adults: apply to all parts of the body from the neck down for three consecutive days. Children: may need to treat head and neck also.
Systemic		
Ivermectin (Stromectol)	Presence of live mites (scabicide)	Reported to be effective for common scabies refractory to topical treatment and crusted scabies in conjunction with topical cream/lotion. Given twice over a 7- to 10-day period. Can pass into breast milk.
Others		
Antihistamines	Eczematous dermatitis	Helps patient to sleep at night. Hydroxyzine, diphenhydramine: 25–50 mg at bedtime.
Topical corticosteroid ointments	Extensive dermatitis	For mild to moderate pruritus. Apply to areas of extensive dermatitis.
Systemic corticosteroids	Severe hypersensitivity reaction	For severe pruritus. Prednisone: tapered course for 1–2 weeks.
Systemic and topical antibiotics	Secondary bacterial infection	*Staphylococcus* and *Streptococcus* species are common pathogens. Risk of acute poststreptococcal glomerulonephritis in severe cases Systemic: 7- to 10-day course.

products to prevent accidental ingestion by children. Patients should be informed that itching may continue for up to a week after successful treatment due to local irritation.

Patients should also receive instruction about treating their home environment to avoid reinfestation; they should be reminded that the scabies mite lives on humans, so environmental spraying of pesticides is ineffective and not recommended. Bedclothes and clothing should be washed in hot, soapy water. Except in cases of crusted scabies, extensive decontamination of the environment is not necessary. Children in day care or school can return after treatment.

PEDICULOSIS

Pediculosis (infestation by lice) in humans has been documented for thousands of years. It is difficult to document the number of lice cases occurring annually in the United States because reporting is not required in most states. It is estimated that 6 to 12 million American children are infested with head lice each year.

EPIDEMIOLOGY AND CAUSES

Pediculosis infestations occur worldwide and are endemic in most parts of the world. Only three species of lice are known to infest humans: *Pthirus pubis* (the crab louse), *Pediculus humanus capitis* (the head louse), and *Pediculus humanus corporis* (the body or clothing louse). Lice infestations occur in people of all ages. Head lice are commonly seen in school-age children, whereas pubic lice are most often seen in sexually active young adults. Children aged 3 to 12 years are most commonly affected by head lice, with more frequent occurrences in girls. Lice are blood-obligate parasites that obtain all their nutritional requirements from the host. Both *Pediculus capitis* and *P. pubis* lice reside and reproduce on the human host. The *P. humanus corporis* louse feeds on the human host but resides and lays its eggs in clothing fibers. Body lice are increasingly rare in the United States but can be seen in communities of persons who are homeless or among persons who live in crowded conditions without the ability to wash and change clothing. Body lice are the only lice associated with disease transmission. Infected feces of the body louse can transmit typhus, trench fever, and relapsing fever. However, lice-borne outbreaks of these diseases have not been seen for many decades in the United States.

Although epidemics of pediculosis in the United States are relatively rare, outbreaks of head lice are common in elementary school settings. Outbreaks usually occur at the start of the school year and after winter and spring breaks. One explanation for the timing of these outbreaks is that they occur after children have spent extended time in the community. Close personal contact is the major mode of transmission for all types of pediculosis.

The cost of treatments, lost wages, and school expenses related to lice outbreaks total an estimated $1 billion annually, making pediculosis a major public health concern and an economic burden on families.

PATHOPHYSIOLOGY

Pediculosis infestation may be asymptomatic or cause few symptoms in the first 2 weeks following exposure. Sensitivity to lice must take place before pruritus occurs. Therefore, in individuals who have never before been exposed to a lice infestation, it can take several weeks before clinical symptoms (e.g., pruritus) develop during the initial infestation. A foreign body inflammatory reaction is caused by lice saliva injected into the skin during the insect's bite. In individuals with a reinfestation, pruritus occurs rapidly, within 24 to 48 hours, due to key inflammatory mediators including histamine.

Head lice infestation averages about 10 lice per patient. However, in severe cases, they can number in the hundreds. Head lice are transmitted through close contact rather than by fomites; they survive for approximately 2 days away from a human host, at which time they die from dehydration. Both males and females are equipped with specialized mouth parts adapted for sucking blood, as well as legs capable of adhering to human hairs. Each female head louse may lay from 7 to 10 eggs per day for a month. Pubic lice ("crab lice") lay relatively fewer eggs (up to three per day) that incubate for 1 week before hatching. Severe lice infestations may be complicated by bacterial superinfection from *Staphylococcus* species that normally colonize the skin.

CLINICAL PRESENTATION

Subjective

Patients may present with complaints of intense itching in areas of the body preferred by the particular type of infesting louse. The itching is usually described as being more severe at night. Mothers may report changes in feeding patterns and that their children are tired and irritable. School-age children may become inattentive and restless in class, with frequent scratching of the scalp. Some cases of pediculosis are asymptomatic or present with few symptoms.

Objective

The earliest physical signs of lice infestation are small (2 to 3 mm), red erythematous macules or papules that may be pruritic. Skin lesions may appear within minutes or several days after initial infestation. Some patients develop an allergic, hivelike reaction, with typical wheal-and-flare formation after lice infestation.

Pruritus is the hallmark of all types of pediculosis. Because of the intense itching, excoriations on the scalp, body, or pubic area (depending on the type of lice) with crusting and scaling may also be present. Fresh nits (lice eggs) on hair shafts are thought to be deposited closer to the scalp. As the hair grows (0.5 mm daily on the scalp), the nit moves further away from the scalp. Therefore, if nits are found at varying distances on the hair shafts, the infestation has been present for several weeks to months. Individual lice are difficult to see on the scalp and hair strands. They appear as six-legged, wingless insects from 1 to 4 mm in length that move extremely fast. When engorged with blood, the insect's abdomen appears dark red.

Nits (eggs) are much easier to see than live lice: the teardrop-shaped eggs are attached securely to the hair shaft by the female louse. Newly laid eggs may be tan to coffee colored and are difficult to see. Hatched lice eggs are whitish in color and appear shiny. The cap (operculum) of the egg faces away from the scalp. Distribution of lice, itching, and lesions provides clues to the type of louse present on the host. Head lice (*P. humanus capitis*) prefer the scalp, and crab lice (*P. pubis*) infest the pubic and perianal region. However, head lice can be found in facial hair such as eyebrows, beards, and mustaches. Crab lice and their nits can also be found in such areas as the eyelids, mustache area, axillae, or on the scalp. Combing the hair to visualize the lice or nits is almost four times more effective than simple visual inspection. Visual inspection may actually miss up to half of the infestations. Using a magnifying glass may be helpful.

DIAGNOSTIC REASONING

Clinical diagnosis of pediculosis, body lice, or pubic lice is based on both the history of pruritus (because of a hypersensitivity reaction to the lice) and the finding of white nits or lice on the hair shaft. Sometimes, a lice infestation may be picked up during a routine physical examination or a precamp screening inspection.

Diagnostic Tests

The clinician should search for lice and nits on the area of the body where the patient is complaining of pruritus. Lice and their nits can be seen with the naked eye or with a handheld magnifying lens. Gloves should be worn during this procedure. Microscopic examination is generally not required. A Wood's light examination can be done for mass screening (or individual screening), but it requires a darkened room and protective eyewear for both the clinician and the child. When the light is directed at the scalp, live nits appear with a pearllike fluorescence, whereas empty nits do not fluoresce. The Wood's light examination is impractical in school settings and not recommended for use with young children

who might be afraid of the dark. If secondary bacterial infection (impetigo) is suspected, bacterial cultures should be done with a standard Culturette swab.

Failure to identify the presence of lice or nits does not rule out lice infestation. When suspicion is strong, based on history and clinical presentation, the patient should be treated empirically; the relief of signs and symptoms is indicative of lice infestation. Treatment for head lice should be limited to persons who are experiencing an active infestation, which is defined as the presence of live lice. Because pubic lice are considered a sexually transmitted disease (STD), patients with this type of infestation should be screened for other STDs, including syphilis, gonorrhea, chlamydia, and HIV infection.

Differential Diagnosis

The diagnosis of pediculosis may be easily confirmed. However, "pseudonits" (hair casts, dandruff, or sebaceous plugs) can be mistaken for nits, resulting in inappropriate treatment. A hallmark of nits is that they are firmly cemented in place and, therefore, do not slide easily on the hair shaft, compared with dandruff scales. Sebaceous plugs result from plugged oil glands on the scalp and (unlike nits) do not originate on the hair shaft. Secondary bacterial infection can also complicate the diagnosis. Secondarily infected skin lesions resemble impetigo lesions, with crusting and erythema (see Differential Diagnosis 12.2).

MANAGEMENT

Effective care of patients with pediculosis involves treating not only the patient but also his or her close personal contacts who have been diagnosed with an active infestation. Treatment involves both medication and environmental control measures. It is important to screen all close contacts for head lice, keeping in mind that the contacts may be asymptomatic and have a small number of live lice. Treating the source of the infestation (if identified) and any secondary complications, such as secondary bacterial infection (impetigo) or dermatitis, should also be included in the management plan. Patients need to be reevaluated after 1 week. If live lice are present or if fresh eggs (nits) are seen close to the scalp, retreatment is necessary.

Initial management of patients who are diagnosed with pediculosis is directed at killing and/or removing lice and their nits. Shampoos, cream rinses, and lotions containing benzyl alcohol, ivermectin, permethrin, spinosad, pyrethrin, and malathion are commonly used to kill lice. Lindane is a second-line treatment due to possible CNS toxicity (see Drugs Commonly Prescribed 12.2). Treatment history should be explored with the patient or caregiver. It is common for persons with head lice to delay seeking professional help until three to five

---

⁙ Differential Diagnosis 12.2: Pediculosis

Rash present	Atopic dermatitis (eczema)
	Bullous pemphigoid
	Burrowing insects/larvae (scabies)
	Contact dermatitis
	Dandruff
	Dermatitis herpetiformis
	Dermatographism (Darier's disease)
	Drug eruptions
	Ecthyma
	Erythroderma
	Folliculitis
	Impetigo
	Insect bites
	Lichen planus
	Malignancy (cutaneous T-cell lymphoma)
	Miliaria (heat rash)
	Neurotic excoriation
	Pityriasis rosea
	Pregnancy induced
	Prurigo nodularis
	Pyoderma (impetigo)
	Psoriasis
	Scabies
	Seborrheic dermatitis
	Tinea (capitis, corporis, pedis, cruris)
	Transient acantholytic dermatosis (Grover's disease)
	Urticaria (hives)
No rash present	Chronic renal disease, especially with hemodialysis
	Cholestatic liver disease
	Delusions of parasitosis
	Hyperparathyroidism
	Hodgkin's lymphoma
	Polycythemia vera

self-treatment failures have occurred. Products resulting in treatment failure should not be tried again.

Of these products, lindane is the most toxic. Lindane is rapidly absorbed through the skin and has been associated with CNS symptoms such as irritability, seizures, and, in cases of ingestion or overdose, death. Lindane should not be used on older patients, any patient with a history of seizure, infants and children younger than 2 years old, or pregnant or lactating women due to an increased risk of toxicity. The pediculicide of choice should be based on the age of the patient, resistance patterns, degree of toxicity, treatment history, and, in reproductive-aged females, pregnancy status.

Manual delousing and nit removal using a fine-toothed comb are gaining popularity in light of increasing reports of resistance to available pediculicides. Electronic combs are available that electrocute the lice. They are safe for children and should be used on clean, dry hair. The coated lice comb tips protect the scalp. Many of these products are battery operated.

In children with respiratory allergies, asthma, or compromised immune status, manual delousing methods should be considered as an initial form of treatment. Petroleum jelly, mayonnaise, tea tree oil, or olive oil may be used as topical agents to suffocate the lice, as the product is massaged into the scalp and left on overnight with a shower cap in place.

Numerous nonpesticidal treatment options have recently become available. There is limited empiric evidence, however, to support their efficacy and safety. Clinicians should caution patients against the use of home remedies that include kerosene and agricultural-grade or veterinary pesticides—such remedies are unsafe and potentially fatal. The majority of patients with pediculosis require only pediculicide treatment or manual delousing. Some patients may delay treatment until secondary bacterial infection has occurred, necessitating the use of topical or systemic antibiotics. Complicating staphylococcal bacterial superinfection may be treated by cephalexin or dicloxacillin for 7 to 10 days.

Children who present with pediculosis pubis (infestation by *P. pubis*) in their eyelashes or hair should alert the clinician to the possibility of sexual abuse, although intimate (genital to face) contact is not the only mode of transmission. Eyelash infestation can be treated by applying petroleum jelly to the eyelid margins twice daily for 10 days. *Pediculosis ciliaris* (eyelash infestation) may also be treated with physostigmine ophthalmic ointment 0.25% to 1% twice daily for 8 to 10 days, but this treatment may cause eye spasms in younger adults. Lice and nits should also be manually removed from the eyelashes by gently sliding them off the hairs.

FOLLOW-UP AND REFERRAL

Uncomplicated pediculosis infestations do not require follow-up. In some areas, however, the American head louse has demonstrated resistance to pyrethrin and permethrin, as well as to lindane, resulting in increased treatment failures. Follow-up in 1 week is recommended if symptoms persist; the patient or the parent of an affected child can call the clinic to report any further symptoms. The National Pediculosis Association recommends manual delousing methods at the first sign of medical treatment failure. Because of toxicity concerns and known resistance patterns, lindane should be used only as a last resort, and prescriptions should not be written with refills. Referrals for pediculosis infestations are usually not required.

⊘ Drugs Commonly Prescribed 12.2: Pediculosis

DRUG	INDICATION	ADVERSE REACTIONS AND PRESCRIBING CONSIDERATIONS
Topical		
Permethrin 1% lotion or 5% cream OTC (Nix)	Presence of lice/nits; may use on children older than 2 months	May need to reapply in 7–14 days. Use nit-remover products before application of permethrin. Apply to towel-dried, affected area; leave on 10 minutes, then wash off.
Pyrethrin 0.3% with piperonyl butoxide shampoo or gel OTC (RID, R&C shampoo)	Presence of lice/nits	May need to reapply in 7–14 days. Use shampoo for head or pubic lice, gel for body lice. Contraindicated in persons sensitive to ragweed. Apply to dry hair until wet; leave on 10 minutes, then wash off.
Lindane 1% shampoo	Presence of lice/nits; second-line therapy only	Possible central nervous system toxicity. Not recommended for children younger than 12 years or pregnant or lactating women. Apply to dry hair; leave on 4 minutes, then wash off thoroughly.
Malathion 0.5% lotion or gel (Ovide)	Presence of live head lice (not approved for other lice species) Lotion for use on children older than 6 years; gel safe to use on children older than 2 years	No reported resistance. Product contains 78% isopropyl alcohol and is flammable. Apply to dry hair; use sufficient amount to thoroughly wet hair and scalp (cover all lice on the hair and scalp). Rinse off after 10 minutes, and allow to air dry. Shampoo hair after 8–12 hours. Repeat in 1 week.
Benzyl alcohol 5% (Ulesfia) lotion	Use in patients older than 6 months Pregnancy category B	Leave on hair and scalp for 10 minutes. May repeat in 7 days if live lice are still present.
Ivermectin 0.5% lotion	May use on children 6 years of age and older	Apply to dry hair for 10 minutes. May repeat after 7 days.
Spinosad (Natroba) 0.9% Topical suspension	May use on patients 4 years of age and older	Apply to dry hair for 10 minutes; rinse, then shampoo. May repeat after 7 days.
Systemic		
Ivermectin (Stromectol)	Resistant pediculosis Not FDA approved but some recommend "at your own risk"	For cases resistant to permethrin and malathion, 200–400 mcg/kg by mouth as a single dose, followed by another dose in 1–2 weeks.
Trimethoprim-sulfamethoxazole (Bactrim)	Not FDA approved but some recommend "at your own risk'	10 mg/kg/day in two divided doses. Potential to cause Stevens-Johnson syndrome reaction.

Abbreviation: FDA, U.S. Food and Drug Administration.

Patient Education: Pediculosis

Patient education is an integral part of successfully treating pediculosis. Patients and parents should be instructed not to share hats, combs, scarves, headsets, towels, and bedding. Following removal of hair and debris, combs and brushes should be washed in hot, soapy water, rinsed in hot water, and allowed to air dry.

Safety information regarding the proper use of pediculicides should be stressed, including information about not exceeding recommended exposure times, possible toxicity symptoms that should be reported, and the safe storage of treatment products to prevent accidental ingestion by young children. When using head lice products, patients should be instructed to cover the eyes and rinse products over a sink (not in the shower or bathtub) to reduce unnecessary pesticide exposure. Patients should be informed that itching may continue after successful treatment for up to 1 week because of the slow resolution of the inflammatory reaction caused by the lice infestation.

Patients should also receive instruction on cleaning the environment. With the exception of the body louse, lice live only on humans; therefore, treatment of pets is not necessary. Excessive decontamination of the environment is also not necessary. Environmental spraying of pesticides is ineffective, may be dangerous, and is therefore not recommended. Bedclothes and clothing should be washed in hot soapy water and dried in a hot dryer. Normal vacuuming of carpets, rugs, upholstery, mattresses, cars, and car seats should be sufficient.

Parents should devote their energy to removing lice and nits. Children in day care or school can return after treatment. Some schools have a "no-nit" policy that requires parents to remove all lice and nits before a child may reenter the classroom, but these policies are changing, as they have not been demonstrated to reduce the spread of lice at school. Parents should be instructed to screen children once a week for head lice as part of their regular hygiene routine. Early detection of lice infestation results in fewer transmissions and more successful treatment regimens.

REFERENCES

General

Kimberlin DW, Brady MT, Jackson MA, Long S. *Red Book, 30th edition. 2015 Report of the Committee on Infectious Diseases.* Elk Grove Village, IL: American Academy of Pediatrics; 2015.

Pediculosis

Brody JE. Parents, relax. Don't keep them from school. It's just lice. *The New York Times.* September 20, 2010. http://www.nytimes.com/2010/09/21/health/21brody.html. Accessed June 27, 2017.

Centers for Disease Control and Prevention. Pediculosis. DPDx—laboratory identification of parasitic diseases of public health concern. https://www.cdc.gov/dpdx/pediculosis/index.html. Published 2016. Accessed July 6, 2017.

Scabies

Centers for Disease Control and Prevention. Parasites—scabies. https://www.cdc.gov/parasites/scabies/index.html. Published 2010. Accessed January 30, 2017.

Simon MW. Update on the diagnosis and treatment of head lice. *Clin Advisor.* 2016;19(9):43-51.

Stoppler MC. Scabies. MedicineNet.com. http://www.medicinenet.com/scabies/article.htm. Published 2017. Accessed July 6, 2017.

World Health Organization. Lymphatic filariasis: scabies. http://www.who.int/lymphatic_filariasis/epidemiology/scabies/en/. Accessed June 27, 2017.

RESOURCES

American Academy of Dermatology
    www.aad.org
American Society of Dermatology
    www.asd.org
Centers for Disease Control and Prevention
    www.cdc.gov
National Institute of Allergy and Infectious Disease
    www.niaid.nih.gov
National Institutes of Health
    www.nih.gov
National Pediculosis Association
    www.headlice.org

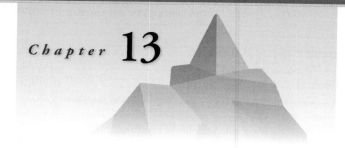

Chapter 13

Fungal Skin Infections

Susan Garnett, MSN, APRN, FNP-BC

Jill E. Winland-Brown, EdD, APRN, FNP-BC

Brian Oscar Porter, MD, PhD, MPH, MBA

CANDIDIASIS

Candidiasis (also known as moniliasis and candidosis) is defined as an infection with the organism *Candida*. *Candida* is an opportunistic pathogen that causes not only superficial mucocutaneous infections but also serious disease that can be fatal, especially in immunocompromised patients. *Candida* belongs to the yeast family of fungi. There are more than 20 species of *Candida* that can cause infection in humans, the most common of which is *Candida albicans*. *Candida* is part of the normal flora of both the oropharynx and gastrointestinal (GI) tract. In addition, up to 20% of women who are asymptomatic test positive for vaginal *Candida*.

Favorable environmental factors and a weakened immune system are the two most important factors contributing to candidal infections. Certain areas of the body are also more prone to infection, such as those that tend to trap heat and moisture.

Risk factors for serious disease include conditions that alter cellular immunity, such as AIDS, diabetes mellitus, corticosteroid treatment, bone marrow transplant, chemotherapy, and invasive parenteral catheterization (parenteral feeding catheters are considered high risk), and invasive monitoring devices in intensive care units. Broad-spectrum antibiotic therapy, including antibiotics following major surgery in normal hosts, can increase the risk of candida infection. Only superficial cutaneous infections are discussed in this chapter.

Cutaneous infections caused by *Candida* include the following:

- Infections of infancy: thrush, diaper dermatitis
- Oral infections: oral candidiasis (thrush), angular cheilitis
- Genital infections: vulvovaginitis, balanitis
- Intertriginous (skinfold) infections: cutaneous candidiasis of the inframammary area, groin, axillae, web spaces of the fingers or toes, perianal area
- Other infections: folliculitis, candidal paronychia, subungual candidiasis (beneath the nail)

EPIDEMIOLOGY AND CAUSES

Although *C. albicans* is the most common (60% to 90%) of all yeast isolates found in the oropharynx and on the genitalia, other types of *Candida* coexist in the body, including *C. tropicalis*, *C. glabrata*, *C. krusei*, *C. rugosa*, and other yeast strains. Unfortunately, some candidal species (*C. krusei*, *C. glabrata*) are less responsive to the common antifungal agent imidazole and have developed resistance. *Candida* infection can occur at any age and in either gender. A higher incidence of thrush is seen among patients with AIDS and in infants. A higher prevalence of vulvovaginal candidiasis occurs in women of reproductive age and African American ethnicity. Areas in the body where there is skin-to-skin contact are more prone to candidal infection. These include areas under the breast (inframammary candidiasis), between the fingers (interdigital candidiasis), between the toes, the groin, the axillae, and the genital area. Infections in these areas are collectively called *intertrigo* or intertriginous infections.

Cellular immunodeficiency states increase the risk of mucocutaneous disease. Conditions such as AIDS, diabetes mellitus, corticosteroid therapy, and immunosuppressive therapy increase an individual's susceptibility to infection with *C. albicans*. Infants, who have immature immune systems, can easily become infected with *Candida* through the birth canal or through oral contact with an infected caregiver. In infants (as opposed to adults), oral candidiasis (thrush) and diaper candidiasis are considered benign findings. In adults, however, mucocutaneous candidiasis is the most common AIDS-defining condition seen. In women with AIDS, one of the earliest and most frequent opportunistic infection is vaginal candidiasis. Frequent episodes of vaginal candidiasis that are not accompanied by an underlying condition (e.g., diabetes mellitus, antibiotic use, pregnancy, or oral contraceptive use) should prompt the clinician to consider HIV infection in the differential diagnosis, although most cases of candidal vaginal infections occur in normal hosts.

Vaginal infection with *C. albicans* is common; it occurs in up to 75% of women at some point in their lifetime (pregnant women and patients with diabetes are at increased risk). If left untreated, candidal vaginitis will either resolve spontaneously or will become a chronic low-grade infection. Men with diabetes, especially if uncircumcised, are at higher risk for candidal infections of the glans penis (balanitis). The uncircumcised foreskin holds heat and moisture and increases the risk of candidal overgrowth. Males may become infected with *Candida* organisms from female or male sexual partners through either vaginal, anal, or oral intercourse. In candidal paronychia, the patient will report a history of hangnail or minor trauma in the cuticle area prior to the infection. Dishwashing or frequent water exposure may be the culprit.

PATHOPHYSIOLOGY

Candida organisms cause a strong inflammatory response on the skin, which accounts for the intense erythema and pruritus commonly seen with this infection. Microscopic examination of *Candida* lesions reveals a pseudomembrane composed of masses of yeast organisms that invade the superficial layer of the epithelium. Satellite lesions are small colonies of *Candida* that have spread beyond the main lesion, which eventually enlarge and become confluent, resulting in large erythematous patches. Normal commensal flora and intact cellular immunity mediated primarily by cytotoxic T cells are the body's primary defenses against fungal overgrowth and invasive candidal infection. The use of systemic antibiotics has the potential for clearing normal microbial skin flora, and both oral and inhaled corticosteroids, HIV infection and AIDS, malignancy, chemotherapy and other immunosuppressant drugs, diabetes mellitus, and senescence all contribute to decreased helper and cytotoxic T-cell function, increasing the likelihood of candidal skin infection.

CLINICAL PRESENTATION

Subjective

Oral Candidiasis (Thrush)

The patient will complain of a severe sore throat. Pain or difficulty is noted during swallowing (dysphagia), especially with acidic foods such as citrus. (See Chapter 21 for more information.)

Vaginal Candidiasis

The patient, usually ranging in age from adolescence to middle age, typically complains of burning, itching, and irritation, either on the vulva or both the vulva and vagina (vulvovaginitis). Burning may be noted during intercourse (dyspareunia) or urination (dysuria). The vaginal discharge is reported as white in color, with a "cottage-cheese" or thick texture (see Chapter 51 for more information).

Balanitis

The typical patient is a sexually active adult man who complains of a reddish rash and itching on the glans penis. It is sometimes accompanied by penile burning after intercourse, although no burning is usually felt with urination. Some patients will report having a female sexual partner who is being treated for a yeast infection or who has irritative vaginal symptoms or a male sexual partner with anogenital or perianal candidiasis. (See Chapter 51 for more information.)

Intertriginous Candidiasis

The typical patient is an obese adult who complains of a red, itchy rash that is occasionally "weepy" (draining tissue fluid) and moist. It is sometimes accompanied by burning. The location of the rash may be in the inframammary area, the groin, the perianal area, or the interdigital spaces of both the hands and feet.

Candidal Paronychia

The typical patient is an adult who complains of an extremely painful fingertip that is red, hot, and swollen. A history of frequent water immersion of the hands is common.

Subungual Candida

No pain or itching is associated with this infection. The typical patient is an adult who reports one or several discolored, yellow fingernails for several weeks to months. A history of excessive contact with water from dishwashing, bartending, or other occupations is frequently present.

Objective

A cardinal sign of cutaneous candidal infections is a bright red rash with macules or satellite lesions seen on the borders. A cardinal symptom is pruritus and sometimes burning.

Oral Candidiasis (Thrush)

The anterior and posterior pharynx (including the tongue) is frequently involved. White creamy patches are seen and can be easily scraped off with a tongue blade, leaving behind erythematous patches. The affected areas are tender to palpation and may bleed with minor trauma. In adults, the buccal mucosa, tongue, and lips may also be involved and may extend to the angles of the mouth (perlèche).

Vaginal Candidiasis

The vulva and, in some patients, the surrounding area appear erythematous and irritated. During speculum examination, the vaginal tissue appears erythematous, with white, curdlike patches pasted on the vaginal walls. The posterior fornix of the vagina may be full of thick white discharge.

Balanitis

The glans penis has small erythematous and eroded patches that are tender to touch. A different presentation demonstrates small white round lesions with a red base on the glans.

Intertriginous Candidiasis

Any area of skin on the body where there is maceration (i.e., skin rubbing against skin) or increased heat and moisture can become easily colonized by *Candida*. These areas include the inframammary area, axilla, groin, perianal area, and interdigital areas between the fingers and toes. In some extremely obese patients, macerated skin may occur in other areas as well. The lesions appear as bright red patches with satellite lesions. The skin will appear eroded and moist and is tender to touch.

Candidal Paronychia

The area around the nail (the paronychium) is bright red, swollen, and extremely tender. A purulent pocket of discharge is sometimes present; when fluctuant, this abscess will rupture and drain pus.

Subungual Candida

The nail is discolored and yellow in color. The nail may be deformed and partially or totally separated from the nailbed. No pain is associated with this condition, in contrast to candidal paronychia.

DIAGNOSTIC REASONING

Diagnostic Tests

Skin infections caused by *Candida* are generally diagnosed by their classic appearance. *Candida* yeasts are normally present in the mouth, vagina, sputum, or stool. Candidal cultures can be obtained from the skin or mucous membranes with a Culturette. Because *Candida* is part of the normal flora, a positive culture from the mouth or vagina is of limited value unless confirming signs and symptoms accompany it. For vaginal candidal infections, a saline wet mount, pH paper, and potassium hydroxide (KOH) test are helpful in the diagnosis (see Advanced Assessment 13.1). The whiff test will be negative, and the vaginal pH is normal (acidic) at 4.5 or less.

Advanced Assessment 13.1: KOH Examination

When assessing for candidiasis, a saline wet mount of vaginal discharge or a potassium hydroxide (KOH) examination of vaginal discharge or superficial scrapings from a suspected focus of infection may be performed. The KOH slide examination is necessary to visualize *Candida* and tinea fungus; however, a KOH examination is not necessary to see yeast forms in vaginal infections. The saline wet mount works well and is faster to prepare than a KOH examination.

The KOH examination is used to determine the presence of mycelial fragments or budding yeast cells in a skin lesion. The test involves adding KOH solution to a small amount of vaginal discharge on a glass slide, covering the slide, and applying gentle heat. The slide is then examined microscopically for fungal elements.

PERFORMING A SALINE WET MOUNT MICROSCOPIC EXAMINATION

1. Take a small amount of vaginal discharge from the posterior fornix of the vagina with either a long, cotton-tipped applicator or from the end of a speculum.

2. Place a small amount of the vaginal discharge in the middle of a clean, dry glass slide.
3. Add one to two drops of normal saline solution to the vaginal discharge and stir/mix to produce a thin, milky mixture.
4. Add a cover slip.
5. View the specimen first under low power and then at 40x magnification. Look for pseudohyphae, spores, and leukocytes.

PERFORMING A POTASSIUM HYDROXIDE (KOH) MICROSCOPIC EXAMINATION

1. Scrape an area of the suspected area (e.g., skin rash) with the edge of a clean glass slide or a no. 15 sterile scalpel blade moistened with tap water to contain scales. Transfer the scraped tissue onto a slide and add a small droplet of plain water. A slide may also be prepared with a small amount of vaginal discharge.
2. Add one or two drops of KOH 10% solution onto the specimen slide, place a cover slip, and warm the slide carefully for 15 to 30 seconds using a match, small candle, or Bunsen burner (do not place the slide directly in the flame).
3. Examine the specimen under low power with minimal illumination.
4. Look for pseudohyphae and/or spores. Identify hyphae—thin tubular structures, often branching strands of uniform diameter.
5. Switch to high dry (40x to 43x) magnification to confirm findings.

NOTE: Although a positive examination establishes the diagnosis, a negative test does not rule out the disease.

MICROSCOPY TIPS: SALINE WET MOUNT AND KOH EXAMINATIONS

- Do not confuse a piece of hair or thread on the slide with pseudohyphae. Hair or threads will appear as black opaque lines, whereas hyphae are translucent and colorless.
- Pseudohyphae or hyphae (the stems) have thin translucent walls that have septa dividing each segment (like a bamboo stem).
- Spores are small and oval to round in shape, seen either alone or in clusters.
- Leukocytes are round to oval and are the size of nuclei in epithelial cells.
- A large number of leukocytes are seen in candidal and trichomonal infections because of the inflammatory response.
- Few leukocytes are seen in bacterial vaginosis (which does not cause significant inflammation) unless there is concurrent infection with *Candida* or *Trichomonas*.
- Epithelial cells are the largest cells found on the slide. Superficial epithelial cells are the most numerous (about 90%) and appear as squares with rounded corners and edges.
- The presence of immature epithelial cells (from the basal and parabasal layer) indicates severe inflammation. The immature cells are smaller and have larger nuclei than superficial (mature) epithelial cells.
- Bacteria are too small to be visualized clearly with a regular light microscope. They will appear as extremely small dark "specks" on the slide, under both low- and high-power magnification.

Of note, although systemic *Candida* infection is not covered in this chapter, there is a rapid diagnostic test for *Candida* infections of the bloodstream that may reduce patient mortality from 40% to 11% by diagnosing candidemia 25 times faster than a blood culture and quickly identifying the *Candida* species that is causing the infection. The test, T2 Candida, uses a polymerase chain reaction (PCR) assay to amplify *Candida* DNA in the blood.

Differential Diagnosis

The location of the skin lesions determines the differential diagnoses to be considered. Contact dermatitis lesions can appear similar to candidal lesions. Fungal infections caused by dermatophytes may affect a variety of sites include the nails (tinea unguium causing onychomycosis), groin (tinea cruris), scalp (tinea capitis), foot (tinea pedis), and body (tinea corporis or "ringworm") (see Differential Diagnosis 13.1).

MANAGEMENT

Most cases of mucocutaneous and vaginal candidal infections (and tinea infections) respond well to topical treatment with antifungal creams that are available over the counter (OTC) or by prescription. The formulation of the topical antifungal used will depend on the site of the infection and whether the rash is moist or dry. Powders work well with moist, macerated lesions. Creams work well on drier lesions. Solutions and sprays are alcohol based and cause burning on inflamed or macerated skin; therefore, they should be avoided on these areas. Preparations in ointment form are more adherent than liquid, lotion, or cream formulations and tend to work best for intertriginous areas. Oral formulations include suspensions and troches.

Pharmacologic Therapy

Topical antifungals such as nystatin (Nyamyc, Pedi-Dri, Nystop; effective for *Candida* only), clotrimazole (Lotrimin), miconazole (Monistat-Derm), naftifine (Naftin), terbinafine (Lamisil), and ciclopirox (Loprox) are effective. Most topical antifungal creams are applied twice per day for at least 2 weeks (and up to 4 weeks). The patient should be instructed to apply creams sparingly because too much cream will cause skin maceration, especially in intertriginous areas. The cream is massaged gently into the rash and the surrounding area. The patient is advised that mild improvement in the rash may be seen in a week, but it frequently takes 2 to 4 weeks until the rash is cleared. Adverse reactions are usually mild and may include erythema, local irritation, itching, burning, and dryness. In some patients, sensitization occurs, and a contact dermatitis results. (If this occurs, the medication should be discontinued.)

For topical treatment of severe cases of candidal vulvovaginitis, cream formulations often yield better results than vaginal suppositories. Women should be cautioned that topical treatments may weaken latex condoms and diaphragms. Vaginal suppositories can become dislodged from the vagina when the patient is voiding or during defecation. For mild to moderate cases, suppositories work well and are available as 3-day treatment regimens. In recurrent candidal vaginitis, both partners may need treatment. Partners should abstain from sexual intercourse until both have finished treatment. Pregnant women with vulvovaginal candidiasis should be treated with topical azole therapy for 7 days.

Some experts discourage the use of systemic therapies for cutaneous candidiasis because of the potential for adverse effects and an increase in resistance. Studies have found that the increased use of imidazoles for systemic therapy has been associated with an increase in the strains of *Candida* species resistant to the systemic antifungal fluconazole (Diflucan). Less common candidal species such as *C. glabrata* and *C. tropicalis* are also more likely to be resistant to treatment with topical imidazoles. If the patient is immunocompromised, has severe vaginal or perianal candidiasis, or is unresponsive to topical medications, systemic antifungal therapy may be justified. Drug interactions may occur with many oral systemic antifungals that are available by prescription when given with warfarin (Coumadin), phenytoin (Dilantin), and rifampin. There is limited evidence that topical miconazole may potentiate warfarin. Serious adverse events that may occur with oral systemic antifungals include hepatotoxicity, angioedema,

---

⁂ Differential Diagnosis 13.1: Cutaneous Candidiasis

Type of Candidiasis	Differential Diagnosis
Thrush (oral candidiasis)	Milk curd (infants) Pharyngeal exudate (bacteria/viral)
Intertrigo (skinfolds)	Contact dermatitis Bacterial intertrigo (erythrasma)
Vaginal candidiasis	Trichomoniasis Bacterial vaginosis Contact dermatitis
Balanitis (glans of penis)	Flat genital warts Erythroplasia of Queyrat (Bowen's disease of the penis) Contact dermatitis Balanitis plasma cellularis (Zoon's balanitis)
Candidal paronychia (tissue surrounding the nail)	Bacterial paronychia (*Pseudomonas, Proteus*) Herpetic whitlow
Subungual *Candida* (under nail)	Tinea unguium (onychomycosis)

and anaphylaxis. For significant skin infections resistant to extended topical therapy, systemic antifungal treatment options include fluconazole for 10 to 14 days or itraconazole for 2 to 3 weeks. Skin infections resistant to this treatment should be reevaluated for a nonfungal or noncandidal etiology or infection by a fluconazole-resistant candidal strain in need of alternative oral or even IV antifungal treatment such as voriconazole, amphotericin B, or caspofungin. These treatments are not prescribed in the primary-care setting because they require highly specialized care and observation.

First-line treatment for mild oral candidiasis is clotrimazole troches 10 mg five times a day or miconazole 50 mg buccal tablet once a day for 7 to 14 days, applied to the upper gum over the incisor. Oral candidiasis (thrush) may also be treated with nystatin, which is available in suspension, pastilles, or troches. Nystatin is available in a 100,000 units/mL suspension, and 4 to 6 mL (or one teaspoon) is given (one-half dose on each side of the mouth) four to five times daily. The patient should be advised to retain the suspension inside the mouth as long as possible before swallowing. Nystatin is available in pastille form (200,000 units); the patient should be told to allow one or two pastilles to dissolve slowly inside the mouth five times a day for 14 consecutive days. Clotrimazole (Mycelex) troches are also indicated for prophylaxis of thrush at a dosage of one troche three times daily. Oral fluconazole 100 to 200 mg daily for 7 to 14 days is recommended for the treatment of moderate to severe oropharyngeal candidiasis. Itraconazole solution (10 mg/mL) is indicated for oral candidiasis that is unresponsive to fluconazole and is available in cherry and caramel flavors. The patient is instructed to swish 10 mL (100 mg) twice daily in the mouth for several seconds before swallowing; treatment should continue for 2 to 4 weeks. Itraconazole oral antifungal medications are contraindicated in women who are pregnant or could become pregnant. Relapse frequently occurs after treatment of thrush in immunocompromised patients.

In candidal paronychia, a warm compress on the affected fingertip will enhance drainage of purulent discharge and help relieve the pain. Incision and drainage of purulent material may speed resolution and provide relief. Candidal infections of the nailbed (subungual candida) are best treated with systemic antifungals.

FOLLOW-UP AND REFERRAL

The patient should be seen in 2 weeks to monitor response to treatment. If there is no response to treatment, the initial diagnosis should be reconsidered, or the patient should be referred to a dermatologist. If a partial response is seen, treatment can be continued for another 1 to 2 weeks and the patient is reevaluated. If there is poor response at that time, the patient needs a referral to a dermatologist.

Patient Education: Candidiasis

Patients must be taught to decrease favorable environmental conditions for *Candida* such as moisture, warmth, and poor air circulation of affected areas (e.g., tight clothing). To prevent diaper rash, infants should be kept as dry as possible, and the use of rubber or plastic pants and undergarments should be discouraged. Baby powder with cornstarch should not be used because it will worsen the infection (*Candida* can utilize the cornstarch as a nutrient).

For obese patients, one method of keeping deep folds of skin apart is by using clean, dry, white tissues between the folds of skin. Educate the patient on the importance of keeping the affected area dry to assist in healing and to prevent future candidal infections. Patients may be instructed to use a hair dryer to dry moist areas but stress that it must be kept on the "low" setting. Patients with candidal paronychia should be advised to minimize exposure of hands to water and the prolonged use of rubber gloves. If a fluctuant abscess is present, the patient should apply a warm compress to the involved finger two to three times per day to assist in drainage.

DERMATOPHYTOSES

Dermatophytoses, or *tinea*, are superficial skin infections caused predominantly by three fungal species: *Trichophyton*, *Epidermophyton*, and *Microsporum*. Transmission occurs primarily through direct contact with an infected person or animal (dogs, cats). Other modes of transmission include contact with asymptomatic carriers who can infect family members and close contacts, or contact with soil (which contains a large number of fungal spores). Although this route of transmission is controversial, fomites (shared objects, such as combs or hats) have been implicated in spreading tinea infections. It is not uncommon to find two (or more) tinea infections in one patient. Tinea manuum often occurs in the "one hand, two feet" distribution. Tinea pedis ("athlete's foot") can occur simultaneously with both tinea unguium (onychomycosis) and tinea corporis (ringworm), as well as with other combinations. Multiple tinea infections are caused by spreading infection from one area of the body to another through scratching.

Environmental and host factors play an important role in the development of tinea infections. Favorable environmental factors that increase the risk of tinea infection include heat, moisture, and poor air circulation. Host factors include age, broken skin, broken hair shafts, and excessive moisture on the skin or nails. Tinea infections are classified by their location on the body; different types include the following:

- Tinea capitis or ringworm of the scalp
- Tinea corporis or ringworm of the body, also known as tinea circinata

- Tinea cruris or ringworm of the groin, also known as "jock itch"
- Tinea pedis or "athlete's foot"
- Tinea manuum or tinea of the hands
- Tinea versicolor, also known as pityriasis versicolor
- Tinea unguium (onychomycosis; covered in a separate section)

Although tinea versicolor is caused by the yeast *Pityrosporum orbiculare (Malassezia furfur)* and is not considered a classic dermatophytosis, it is also discussed in this section.

EPIDEMIOLOGY AND CAUSES

The estimated lifetime incidence of tinea infections is between 10% and 20%. Tinea infections are more common in warmer climates. Individuals with diabetes are at higher risk for tinea and yeast infections. Tinea pedis, or "athlete's foot," is the most common fungal infection in the United States. Acute tinea pedis is caused by *Trichophyton mentagrophytes* var. *interdigitale,* and chronic tinea pedis, which is more common, is caused by *Trichophyton rubrum.* Tinea cruris (jock itch) is more common in men, and *T. rubrum* is the typical agent. Tinea capitis (ringworm of the scalp) is more common in children until puberty when, for unknown reasons, the incidence markedly decreases. Tinea unguium (onychomycosis) occurs more frequently in adults and elderly patients.

The most contagious of all dermatophytoses is tinea capitis (scalp ringworm). It has been known to cause epidemics in crowded conditions such as schools and group homes and as outbreaks among family members. Tinea capitis infections are more common in toddlers and school-age children from urban areas. Tinea capitis is easily transmitted because *Trichophyton tonsurans* tends to produce large numbers of infectious spores called arthroconidia. *T. tonsurans* causes up to 90% of all cases of tinea capitis in the United States and Western Europe. A minor cause of tinea capitis in the United States is *Microsporum canis,* a zoophilic fungus from dogs. Less common causes are *Microsporum audouinii* and *T. rubrum.*

Tinea barbae, an infection of the beard area, is more common in men who work with animals. Tinea manuum (tinea manus), or tinea of the hand(s), is relatively rare compared with other tinea infections. Tinea manuum infection frequently occurs with tinea pedis infection. The patient infects the hand by touching or scratching an infected foot. Unlike tinea pedis, in which both feet usually become infected, in tinea manuum infection, only one hand is usually involved. Tinea versicolor (pityriasis versicolor) infection is caused by the yeast *P. orbiculare* (which causes round lesions) or *Pityrosporum ovale* (which produces oval lesions); it is more common in the summertime. Tinea versicolor becomes more obvious during the summer, when tanning exposes hypopigmented macules that do not tan.

PATHOPHYSIOLOGY

Three types of parasitic fungi are implicated in causing dermatophytic or tinea infections. *Microsporum* and *Epidermophyton* species both cause infections of the skin and nails. *Trichophyton* species cause infections not only of skin and nails but also of the hair. These fungal infections are superficial because all three types metabolize keratin, the protein that comprises the topmost layer of body surface epithelium, which normally serves as a protective barrier against microbial infection. The clinical presentation of tinea infections depends on their anatomical location and the species of fungi. Asymptomatic carriers do not show symptoms of disease but infect susceptible hosts through direct contact or by possibly depositing spores onto fomites such as combs, brushes, or hats. Acute tinea pedis is usually caused by *T. mentagrophytes* var. *interdigitale* whereas chronic tinea pedis is caused by *T. rubrum* and is more common. For tinea cruris (jock itch), *T. rubrum* is the most common causal agent.

Microscopic examination of tinea lesions reveals either acute or chronic inflammation and a spongelike texture in the infected tissue, appropriately termed *spongiosis.* Fungal hyphae are seen on the superficial keratin layer of the epidermis. In tinea capitis, infection occurs either inside (endothrix) or outside (ectothrix) the hair shaft. In ectothrix infections, fungal hyphae and spores invade the hair shaft, leading to destruction of the hair cuticle. Ectothrix infections are caused by *Microsporum* species (*M. canis* and *M. audouinii*). In contrast, endothrix infections are caused by *Trichophyton* species (*T. tonsurans* in North America) and occur inside the hair shaft, leaving the hair cuticle intact. Spores (also called arthroconidia) are found inside the hair shaft, rather than on skin scrapings of surface scale. This type of infection is most common in African American children, and coiling of the hair shaft may play a role in susceptibility to infection.

Kerion formation sometimes results from an endothrix infection and is associated with severe inflammatory changes of the scalp, consisting of nodules and boggy, exudative tissue. Secondary staphylococcal infection may complicate kerion, causing purulent drainage, with infection possibly spreading to draining lymph nodes and causing painful lymphadenitis. When it heals, it typically results in scarring and alopecia. A variant of endothrix infection that is uncommon in North America but more common in South Africa and the Middle East is favus infection, a severe form of tinea capitis that results in extensive hair loss and scarring.

CLINICAL PRESENTATION

Subjective

Tinea Capitis

The typical patient with tinea capitis is a toddler or school-age child. The parent often reports a painless bald spot. If kerion formation accompanies the infection, the child will show signs of discomfort or will complain of pain. Systemic symptoms such as fever or malaise are not associated with kerion formation.

Tinea Corporis

The typical patient will report a history of an erythematous round and elevated pruritic lesion that grows in size and starts to clear in the center—the classic shape of "ringworm." Sometimes, there is a history of another family member with the same infection, and patients may report a history of prior infection. The clinician should inquire about possible exposure through close contact with domesticated animals, such as cats or dogs.

Tinea Cruris

The typical patient is an obese adult man who complains of a pruritic rash on the groin that spreads to the medial inner aspect of the upper thigh. Sometimes, the rash is not associated with pruritus.

Tinea Pedis

The typical patient is usually a male teenage athlete or an adult who comes to the clinic complaining of "athlete's foot" and strong foot odor. Most patients do not have pain with this infection unless it becomes secondarily infected with bacteria, causing cellulitis. The patient reports areas of macerated soft, whitened skin between the toes. Some patients will complain of concurrent infections on the hand (tinea manuum), on the body (tinea corporis), or under the toenails (tinea unguium).

Tinea Versicolor

Most cases of tinea versicolor are recognized in the summer because the hypopigmented spots become more visible at that time of year, as they do not tan. Tinea versicolor is asymptomatic and has a gradual onset. Rarely, a patient will complain of mild pruritus. The typical patient is a teen or young adult, although tinea can occur at any age. People of African descent with tinea will complain of either light-colored (hypopigmented) or dark-colored (hyperpigmented) spots. In adults, the usual sites are on the back, upper chest, arms, and sometimes the neck and face. In children, the rash is more likely to be on the face or forehead.

Objective

Tinea Capitis

Three clinical presentations are seen with tinea capitis infections. One presentation is "black dot" tinea capitis caused by *T. tonsurans*. The child with "black dot" tinea capitis presents with painless patchy alopecia (either in single or multiple patches). The skin on the scalp does not have erythema; the "black dot" appearance results from broken hair stubbles that remain on the scalp.

Another presentation is called "gray patch" tinea capitis. The child with this condition also presents with patchy alopecia, but the bald patches are covered with fine gray-white scales. The patch is made up of thick, keratinized skin that is grayish-white in color. Broken hair shafts of different lengths are present on the surface. Because the inflammatory response is so minimal in both "gray patch" and "black dot" tinea capitis, pain, erythema, nodules, and kerion are not present.

An extremely painful and inflammatory presentation of tinea capitis is known as a kerion. A kerion appears as a large, bright red, boggy "bump" on the scalp with alopecia. Purulent drainage can be expressed out of the kerion by gentle pressure, and pus can be seen oozing out of its tiny follicular openings. Kerion formation can result in scarring alopecia. The affected hair follicles atrophy and become permanently damaged; hair does not grow back, even when the scalp is healed. A permanent bald patch can result from this tinea infection if it is not treated aggressively or if the patient does not present early enough during the course of the disease.

Tinea Corporis

This infection presents as the classic "ringworm" infection—it is easy to recognize in the clinical setting. The patient will present with ringlike lesions with a bright red elevated border (collarette) that is covered with scales. Tinea corporis can occur in any age group from child to adult, and the size of the lesions can range from small to large. The patient or parent will report that the lesion is getting bigger. Some patients have only one lesion, whereas others have numerous lesions. The lesions are usually very pruritic, but sometimes they are asymptomatic.

Tinea Cruris

Tinea cruris ("jock itch") is more common in men in the summer or during warm weather. It is usually extremely pruritic, and most lesions will show some lichenification from chronic scratching. The typical lesion is round to a half-circle and will spread to the inner medial upper thigh but spare the scrotum. In contrast, candidal intertrigo can affect not only the groin and thigh but also the penis and scrotum. The color of the lesion, depending on whether it is chronic or acute, can vary from bright red to a dull discoloration. The lesions can become macerated from infection and scratching; they may become secondarily infected with bacteria or *C. albicans*.

Tinea Pedis

This infection can be seen in up to five clinical presentations. Tinea pedis is usually asymptomatic, although the patient will sometimes complain of pain from a secondary bacterial infection. The most common cause of tinea pedis is *T. mentagrophytes*. The infection usually starts in the third or fourth interdigital web space and sometimes spreads to all toe webs and the soles of the feet. Other fungi that cause tinea pedis (but are less common) include *T. rubrum*, *C. albicans*, and *Epidermophyton floccosum*.

The most common presentation of tinea pedis is macerated white skin between the web spaces of the toes; the infection is pruritic with occasional painful fissures and can be accompanied by an unpleasant foot odor. If it becomes infected with bacteria (usually *Staphylococcus aureus*), a tender cellulitis with redness and ulceration can develop in the web space. This condition is called ulcerative tinea pedis. Moccasin-type tinea pedis is seen more often with *T. rubrum* infection. Scaling and thickening of the skin is seen in a moccasin distribution on both feet.

Another presentation of tinea pedis is a dermatophytid or "id" eruption. Acute id eruptions are caused by a hypersensitivity reaction to the fungus. The id eruption presents as vesicles on the sides of the fingers and/or the palms of the hands. The vesicles do not contain fungus but rather are sterile. The patient may or may not be aware of a concurrent tinea pedis infection.

Another vesicular type of tinea pedis (*T. mentagrophytes*) is associated with burning pruritus and sometimes pain. It is more likely to flare up during warm weather, forming multiple vesicles and bullae. It can become secondarily infected with bacteria, resulting in cellulitis or even lymphangitis.

Tinea Versicolor

Tinea versicolor is usually asymptomatic; it is not associated with pruritus. The patient will present with oval to round, pink or hypopigmented or hyperpigmented macules, located mainly on the back, chest, arms, and sometimes the neck and face. Tinea versicolor in children is more likely to present on the face, especially on the forehead. Sometimes very fine scales are visible, especially if the patient has not showered or bathed for several days; otherwise, daily bathing usually eradicates the scales.

DIAGNOSTIC REASONING

Diagnostic Tests

Tinea infections are usually diagnosed by their clinical presentation. The classic "ringworm" lesions are easy to recognize. The diagnosis can be confirmed via microscopy in the clinic or a specimen (skin scraping) can be sent to the laboratory in a sterile plastic cup. Fungal culture is usually not necessary except in cases where the diagnosis is in doubt or in resistant cases, or before treatment of onychomycosis (tinea unguium) and tinea capitis is initiated. Because of the length of treatment and the potential for adverse reactions from systemic antifungals, positive proof by fungal culture is necessary. Fungal cultures can take up to 2 weeks for results to become available, although if done on Sabouraud's agar or with dermatophyte test medium, results may be obtained in 3 days. PCR assays may also be used to identify fungus in nails.

A fungal culture is recommended for onychomycosis (tinea unguium) and for tinea capitis. Because these two tinea infections require long-term therapy with systemic antifungals (with a high potential for serious side effects), physician consultation is recommended. Proof of the causative agent must be provided by a positive fungal culture. Fungal cultures are also useful if the clinician is unsure of the diagnosis or if the infection does not respond to treatment. Hair bulbs and broken hair, along with scales from the active lesion, should be cultured. Specimens from the affected site should include scales and hair roots. It is important to look for spores and hyphae on the hair shaft, inside the hair shaft (endothrix), and outside the hair shaft (ectothrix) using microscopy.

To obtain a fungal culture for suspected tinea capitis, the clinician should use a dry toothbrush to brush the areas of alopecia and then impregnate the culture media with the bristles. Another method is to use a wet cotton swab, wipe it over the areas of alopecia, and then implant it on the media. Growth is usually seen in 10 to 14 days of culture.

Microscopy is the most useful diagnostic tool for tinea in the primary-care setting. A small piece of skin from the active edge of the lesion or a nail fragment is placed on a glass slide. A drop of 10% KOH is placed on the sample, which is then heated gently with a lighter or match. The slide should not be placed too close to the flame or the KOH will get too hot and boil off. The heating accelerates the effect of the KOH on keratinized fungal cell walls. If the KOH contains dimethyl sulfoxide, the sample does not require heating. When the sample is ready, the hyphae will be easier to see because the cell walls have already been lysed by the KOH. If KOH is not used in this test, the examiner will not be able to see the hyphae because the keratinized cells are too thick. A Wood's light examination should be used on any area of alopecia and hypopigmentation. Some fungi fluoresce when examined under Wood's light, which emits ultraviolet light (black light). The examining room should be darkened for this examination. A characteristic color that is associated with two minor causes of tinea capitis is a blue-green or bright green color from *M. canis* or *M. audouinii*. *T. tonsurans*, the most common cause of tinea capitis, does not fluoresce under a Wood's light examination.

If the tinea infection is resistant to treatment, a fungal culture is mandatory. If a secondary bacterial infection is suspected, a sample of the exudates must be taken for culture and sensitivity using a sterile culture tube.

Differential Diagnosis

Almost all tinea infections tend to have a slow and gradual onset, producing low levels of inflammation. Low levels of inflammation do not typically produce bothersome symptoms such as pruritus and pain. In turn, some tinea infections have been present for months to years before the patient reports them to a health-care provider. Sometimes, tinea infections are an incidental finding during a routine physical examination.

Some tinea infections, such as tinea manuum and tinea unguium (onychomycosis), are usually asymptomatic and are tolerated by the patient for many years. Tinea infections such as tinea cruris and tinea corporis tend to be more symptomatic; the severe pruritus associated with this infection usually drives the patient to seek medical care. Because onychomycosis is so prevalent, it is discussed separately in a subsequent section (see Differential Diagnosis 13.2).

MANAGEMENT

Most cases of tinea infections (except tinea infections of the scalp and nails) respond well to a 2- to 4-week course of topical treatment with azole-class drugs, such as those listed in Drugs Commonly Prescribed 13.1. These agents should be continued for at least 1 week after the lesions have cleared. They should be applied a few centimeters beyond the edges of the skin lesions. Other drugs, including systemic formulations, are also included in the Drugs Commonly Prescribed box as well.

As noted previously, for all patients who are on systemic antifungals, physician consultation is recommended because systemically absorbed antifungal drugs can cause hepatotoxicity. A baseline liver function profile should be done initially and repeated again in 4 weeks

⁂ Differential Diagnosis 13.2: Tinea Infections

Location	Differential Diagnoses
Scalp (tinea capitis, tinea of the scalp)	Psoriasis, seborrheic dermatitis Alopecia areata
Body (tinea corporis, "ringworm")	Atopic or contact dermatitis Psoriasis
Hands (tinea manuum)	Atopic dermatitis Dyshidrotic eczema
Groin (tinea of the groin, "jock itch")	Erythrasma Contact dermatitis
Feet (tinea pedis, "athlete's foot")	Candidal or bacterial intertrigo Psoriasis Candidal intertrigo Contact dermatitis Dyshidrotic eczema Impetigo
Nails (tinea unguium, onychomycosis)	Candidal nail infection Psoriasis of the nail Pseudomonal nail infection
Tinea versicolor (pityriasis versicolor)	Vitiligo Pityriasis alba Pityriasis rosea

☯ Drugs Commonly Prescribed 13.1: Tinea Infections

DRUG	INDICATION	DOSAGE	COMMENTS
Topical Agents			
Miconazole 2% cream (Lotrimin AF, Micatin, Monistat Derm)	Tinea: pedis, cruris, and corporis Cutaneous candidiasis Vaginal candidiasis	Twice daily for 2 weeks Vaginal candidiasis: once at bedtime for 3–7 days	Tinea pedis needs longer treatment, for 4 weeks.
Clotrimazole 1% cream and solution (Lotrimin)	Tinea: pedis, cruris, and corporis Tinea versicolor	Twice daily for 2–8 weeks	Tinea pedis should be treated for 4 weeks.
Betamethasone 0.05% and clotrimazole 1% cream and lotion (Lotrisone)	Fungal skin infections	Apply sparingly twice daily for 1 week and reevaluate Maximum: 2 weeks	Contraindications: varicella, herpes, vaccinia, other viral infections. Do not use on face. Can cause atrophic skin changes with prolonged use. Do not use for diaper dermatitis.
Terbinafine 1% cream (Lamisil AT)	Tinea: cruris, corporis, pedis Moccasin-type tinea pedis (or plantar tinea pedis)	Tinea cruris/corporis: once daily for 1 week Tinea pedis between toes: twice daily for 1 week Plantar tinea pedis: twice daily for 2 weeks	Improvement may continue to be seen for up to 2–6 weeks after therapy.

Drugs Commonly Prescribed 13.1: Tinea Infections—cont'd

DRUG	INDICATION	DOSAGE	COMMENTS
Terbinafine 1% solution (Lamisil solution)	Tinea: versicolor (pityriasis), pedis, cruris, corporis	Versicolor/pedis: twice daily for 1 week Tinea cruris/corporis: once daily for 1 week	Alcohol-based solution. Use only for 1 week. Apply on dry skin. Do not use on face or mucous membranes; avoid broken or irritated skin.
Ciclopirox 0.77% cream, lotion (Loprox)	Cutaneous candidiasis and fungal skin infections (tinea pedis, corporis, cruris, versicolor)	Twice daily for 2–4 weeks	Do not use in children younger than 10 years. Avoid occlusion.
Ciclopirox 1% shampoo	Seborrheic scalp dermatitis	Shampoo and leave on for 3 minutes, then rinse; repeat twice weekly, at least 3 days apart	Not recommended for children younger than 16 years. Avoid eyes and mucous membranes.
Ciclopirox 8% topical solution (Penlac nail lacquer)	Onychomycosis of fingernails and toenails	Apply thin coat once daily at bedtime	Remove with alcohol once per week; repeat for up to 1 year. Do not use nail polish.
Efinaconazole 10% topical solution (Jublia)	Onychomycosis	Apply once daily	Use for 48 weeks.
Tavaborole 0.5% topical solution (Kerydin)	Onychomycosis	Apply once daily	Use for 48 weeks.
Ketoconazole 2% cream, shampoo (Nizoral)	Tinea: pedis, cruris, corporis, versicolor Cutaneous candidiasis Seborrheic dermatitis	One to two times daily for 2–4 weeks or until clinical clearing	Contains sulfites. Treat tinea pedis for 6 weeks. Seborrheic dermatitis: use shampoo or cream for 2 weeks or until clear. Tinea versicolor: use shampoo (1 application); apply to damp scalp, leave on for 5 minutes, then rinse.
Econazole 1% cream, foam (Spectazole) (Ecoza)	Tinea: pedis, cruris, corporis, versicolor Cutaneous candidiasis	Tinea: once daily Cutaneous candidiasis: twice daily	Treat tinea pedis for 4 weeks and other types for 2 weeks.
Sulconazole 1% cream, solution (Exelderm)	Tinea: cruris, corporis, versicolor, cream only: tinea pedis	Tinea pedis: twice daily for 4 weeks; others: once or twice daily for 3 weeks	Reevaluate if no improvement within 4–6 weeks.
Sertaconazole 2% topical cream, tablet (Ertaczo)	Tinea pedis Vaginal candidiasis	Apply twice daily for 4 weeks Single-dose tablet	Reevaluate if no improvement.
Oxiconazole cream, lotion (Oxistat)	Tinea pedis, corporis, cruris Tinea versicolor	Tinea pedis: apply one to two times daily for 4 weeks; others: one to two times daily for 2 weeks Apply once daily for 2 weeks	Reevaluate if no improvement.
Naftifine 1% cream, gel (Naftin)	Tinea: pedis, cruris, corporis	Cream: once per day Gel: twice daily for up to 4 weeks	Reevaluate if no improvement within 4 weeks. Wash hands after application. Not recommended for children.

Continued

Drugs Commonly Prescribed 13.1: Tinea Infections—cont'd

DRUG	INDICATION	DOSAGE	COMMENTS
Luliconazole 1% cream (Luzu)	Tinea pedis Tinea corporis and cruris	Once daily for 2 weeks Once daily for 1 week	Wash hands after application.
Nystatin cream (Mycostatin)	Cutaneous candidiasis (intertrigo)	Twice daily for 2–4 weeks	Apply liberally to affected area.
Nystatin powder (Bio-Statin)	Candidiasis, especially moist lesions (under breast, groin, shoes, feet, body folds)	Two to three times a day for 2–4 weeks	Good for weeping lesions under breast, in groin, and bodily folds. Irritation is rare.
Nystatin suspension (Mycostatin)	Thrush (oral candidiasis)	4–6 mL (one tsp.) four times daily for at least 2 weeks	Retain in mouth as long as possible before swallowing.
Systemic Agents			
Itraconazole (Sporanox PulsePak) (Sporanox)	Onychomycosis of toenail or fingernail, histoplasmosis, blasto-mycosis Tinea: capitis, corporis; recalcitrant tinea pedis infections	Toenail: 200 mg daily for 12 consecutive weeks Fingernail: total of two "pulses"; 200 mg twice daily for 1 week, then 3 weeks off; repeat pulse Repeat 200 mg two times daily again for 1 week Recalcitrant tinea pedis: 200 mg daily for 2 weeks or 400 mg daily for 1 week Tinea corporis/severe cruris: 200 mg once daily for 1–2 weeks	Take with food; suspension form is better absorbed. Hypoglycemia with oral hypogly-cemics. Numerous drug interactions; check before prescribing. Check liver function tests before, during, and after treatment. Black box warning: heart failure.
Terbinafine (Lamisil)	Onychomycosis of toenail or fingernail due to tinea unguium Tinea corporis and cruris	Toenail: 250 mg once daily for 12 weeks Fingernail: 250 mg once daily for 6 weeks 250 mg once daily or every 12 hours in divided doses for 2–4 weeks	Check liver function/renal function. Use with caution in patients with liver/renal disease. Clinical cure not apparent for months.
Fluconazole (Diflucan)	Oropharyngeal, esopha-geal, vaginal, systemic candidiasis; tinea versicolor	All doses once daily: Thrush: 200 mg on day 1, then 100 mg/day for at least 2 weeks Esophageal: 200 mg on day 1, then 100 mg/day for at least 3 weeks Vaginal: 150 mg single dose, or every 72 hours for 3 doses Recurrent vaginal: 150 mg by mouth daily for 10–14 days followed by 150 mg once weekly for 6 months Tinea versicolor: 150–300 mg single weekly dose for 2–4 weeks, or 300 mg weekly for 2 weeks	Check liver function tests. Contraindicated in patients with liver disease.
Posaconazole oral suspension (Noxafil)	Oropharyngeal candidia-sis, and oropharyngeal candidiasis refractory to itraconazole and/or fluconazole	Loading dose: 100 mg (2.5 ml) twice a day on first day Maintenance dose: 100 mg (2.5 mL) once a day for 13 days Refractory: 400 mg (10 mL) twice a day	

Drugs Commonly Prescribed 13.1: Tinea Infections—cont'd

DRUG	INDICATION	DOSAGE	COMMENTS
Griseofulvin (microsize and ultramicrosize) Grifulvin V	Tinea capitis, onychomycosis, severe recalcitrant tinea cruris, pedis, and corporis	Tinea corporis, cruris or capitis: Microsize—500 mg once daily for 2–4 weeks Ultramicrosize—375 mg daily Tinea pedis or unguium: Microsize—1000 daily in single or divided doses every 12 hours for 1–2 weeks Ultramicrosize—250 mg every 8 hours Onychomycosis, fingernail or toenail: Microsize—1,000 mg daily in two to four doses for 6 months Ultramicrosize—660–750 mg/day in two to four divided doses for 6 months	Ultramicrosize formulation better absorbed. High rate of resistant strains of tinea capitis. Use with caution in patients with liver and renal disease. Monitor renal, hepatic, and hematopoietic function. Decreases effectiveness of oral contraceptives, oral anticoagulants, and barbiturates. Avoid sunlight.

and periodically thereafter during the course of treatment. Griseofulvin can cause leukopenia and granulocytopenia. A baseline complete blood count (CBC) and another repeated in 4 weeks are recommended. Thereafter, a follow-up CBC can be done at 4- to 6-week intervals.

The patient should be told to report symptoms such as anorexia, nausea, vomiting, malaise, dark urine, jaundice, and rash to the clinician. If the clinician suspects hepatoxicity, the offending drug should be stopped and consultation with the supervising physician is recommended.

Tinea Capitis

In tinea capitis, a kerion that looks like a honeycomb may be observed. It is an inflammatory boggy mass containing broken hairs and oozing purulent material from follicular orifices. This rare, delayed hypersensitivity reaction to fungal antigens may result in permanent hair loss. Kerion rarely needs to be treated with concurrent antibiotics, as a noninfected kerion may appear exudative. It should be treated with antibiotics only if a secondary staphylococcal infection is apparent. Tinea infections of the hair and nails do not respond to topical treatment, unlike other tinea infections. Tinea capitis should be treated with oral systemic antifungals, along with a topical antifungal for localized scalp lesions. A Wood's light examination should be done in all cases of scalp alopecia. Although some infections will fluoresce (*M. canis, M. audouinii*), others do not (*T. tonsurans, T. violaceum*). A fungal culture is necessary not only to help in the diagnosis but also to classify the species of fungi. It is important to examine the patient's close contacts, including family members (especially other children) and schoolmates. Fungal cultures of close contacts are recommended, if possible. Asymptomatic cases of tinea capitis can be treated with selenium sulfide shampoo

(e.g., Selsun Blue). There is no need to wait for results of the fungal culture (which take 2 weeks) before initiating treatment, especially if there is kerion formation (see Drugs Commonly Prescribed 13.1).

The treatment of choice for tinea capitis is griseofulvin (Grifulvin V) 250 to 500 mg by mouth twice per day for severe cases in adults or once per day for children weighing more than 50 pounds. For children who weigh 30 to 50 pounds, 125 to 250 mg daily is recommended. Treatment duration is from 2 to 4 months or at least 2 weeks after negative cultures are obtained. Some authorities recommend against griseofulvin as a first-line drug because of its potential adverse effects. Other effective alternatives used to treat tinea capitis are oral terbinafine or itraconazole. Female patients must be cautioned that oral contraceptives may be less effective with griseofulvin and to use alternate birth control during treatment and for 1 month after treatment. Male patients on griseofulvin should be advised that this drug affects sperm (it is teratogenic) and to avoid fathering a child for at least 6 months after stopping the drug. Concurrent treatment with selenium sulfide shampoo three times per week is used as adjunctive therapy to systemic antifungals.

Tinea Corporis

Topical antifungal therapy generally works well for tinea corporis. The patient must be reminded to apply the topical agent for at least 1 week after the resolution of the lesions and to apply the cream a few centimeters beyond the edges of the affected area. Concomitant short-term treatment with a mild corticosteroid such as hydrocortisone 1% (available OTC) is effective in helping to relieve itch and inflammation. In severe cases, systemic antifungals such as itraconazole or terbinafine daily are effective.

Tinea Cruris

Topical antifungal therapy is effective for the treatment of jock itch. Concomitant short-term treatment with a mild corticosteroid such as hydrocortisone 1% (OTC) is effective in helping to relieve itch and inflammation. If weeping areas are present, compresses made from Burow's solution are helpful. Use of OTC antifungal powders helps prevent future recurrences. For severe cases, a short course of a systemic antifungal such as itraconazole (Sporanox) or terbinafine (Lamisil) is effective.

Tinea Pedis and Tinea Manuum

Tinea pedis and tinea manuum are both treated with topical antifungals. Treatment of tinea pedis should emphasize moisture control; drying foot powders (miconazole, tolnaftate) are very helpful. If weeping areas are present, compresses made from Burow's solution are beneficial. The feet should be exposed to air as much as possible; during warm weather, the use of airy sandals or going barefoot is helpful. If socks are worn, cotton or a synthetic "wicking" blend is the best material. Socks should be changed once a day; changing socks twice a day is indicated if the patient's feet become wet within the next 4 hours. An antiperspirant spray on the soles of the feet (to be applied on normal skin only) can help patients with excessively sweaty feet. Severe tinea pedis can be treated with oral agents such as itraconazole or terbinafine daily. After a short course of systemic therapy, the patient should be placed on maintenance topical therapy with an antifungal powder or a spray (miconazole, tolnaftate) to prevent recurrences.

Tinea Versicolor

Tinea versicolor is treated with topical selenium sulfide lotion (Selsun) applied daily for 7 days from neck to waist daily ("lathered" on with a small amount of water and left on for 10 minutes) before rinsing thoroughly. Treatment is repeated once a week for 1 month and then once a month for maintenance. Ketoconazole (Nizoral) shampoo can also be used weekly for maintenance. The clinician should advise patients that treatment will eradicate the infection but will not remove the hypopigmented spots from the skin, which take longer to resolve. Patients should also be warned of the high rate of recurrence, because *P. orbiculare* (*M. furfur*) is a normal inhabitant of the skin. Exposing the hypopigmented lesions to sunlight can speed up the process of resolution in some patients. For patients who want more aggressive treatment, fluconazole and itraconazole are the drugs of choice. Fluconazole 150 to 300 mg weekly for 2 to 4 weeks is considered the safest choice for systemic treatment. Fluconazole may also be given once monthly for 6 months. As an alternate treatment, itraconazole may be prescribed at 200 mg daily for 7 days. The patient should be advised that there is a risk of hepatotoxicity with systemic antifungals and that treatment does not prevent recurrence. Because tinea versicolor is a superficial benign disease, this fact should be given serious consideration. Some success has also been reported with the use of photodynamic therapy for tinea versicolor.

FOLLOW-UP AND REFERRAL

The patient should be seen for initial follow-up 2 weeks after the start of therapy. For resistant cases, the clinician should confirm the diagnosis with a fungal culture or the diagnosis should be reevaluated. Resistant cases should be referred to a dermatologist for reevaluation or for more aggressive treatment with systemic antifungals. If the patient was initially placed on topical therapy only, systemic therapy can be considered. Severe tinea corporis and tinea pedis respond well to oral terbinafine or itraconazole.

Some tinea infections have higher recurrence rates than others. Tinea versicolor (pityriasis versicolor)—although not a true tinea (because it is caused by a yeast)—has a high recurrence rate because *P. orbiculare* and *P. ovale* are normal colonizers of the skin. Tinea pedis also tends to reoccur, so meticulous attention should be given by the patient to eradicating favorable environmental conditions for fungal growth (see discussion of tinea pedis for preventive measures). Maintenance therapy for tinea pedis with topical OTC agents in powder or spray form (miconazole, tolnaftate) is effective in helping to prevent recurrences.

If the clinician suspects that a secondary bacterial skin infection (cellulitis) is complicating tinea infection, a culture should be done on the purulent discharge. Empiric therapy for mild cellulitis, which is usually caused by gram-positive bacteria such as *Staphylococcus* or group A beta-hemolytic *Streptococcus*, includes oral antibiotics such as cephalexin or dicloxacillin for 7 to 14 days. For patients with penicillin allergy, either erythromycin or clarithromycin is an appropriate alternative. Toe web infection (ulcerative type) can be due to gram-negative bacterial infection (e.g., *Pseudomonas aeruginosa*, *Escherichia coli*, *Proteus*) and must be treated with systemic fluoroquinolones (e.g., ciprofloxacin). Patients with moderate or severe cellulitis should be referred to a physician for more aggressive treatment, including IV antibiotics.

Patient Education: Antifungal Therapy

Patients who are taking systemic antifungal therapy must be informed of the risk of hepatotoxicity and educated on the signs and symptoms of acute hepatitis, such as anorexia, nausea, vomiting, malaise, dark urine, jaundice, and rash. For all patients on systemic antifungals, consultation with a physician is recommended. A baseline liver function profile and CBC should be obtained before treatment is initiated and repeated in 4 weeks and periodically thereafter.

Griseofulvin decreases the effectiveness of certain drugs, such as oral anticoagulants, and barbiturates. Any woman of reproductive age who is on oral contraceptives and is prescribed griseofulvin should be warned that the contraceptive will become less effective and therefore her risk of pregnancy will be increased. The patient should be advised to see her gynecologist about using another effective method of birth control. If a patient who is on a barbiturate or an oral anticoagulant feels strongly about starting antifungal treatment, the patient should consult the physician who prescribed the original medication before starting treatment with systemic antifungals. Terbinafine is potentiated by cimetidine and is antagonized by rifampin. Itraconazole (Sporanox) is contraindicated if the patient is taking any drug that is metabolized in the liver by the CYP3A system. Itraconazole increases the blood levels of triazolam (Halcion), diazepam (Valium), digoxin, dihydropyridine calcium channel blockers (Norvasc, Procardia), and several other drugs. Adverse reactions to these agents include gastrointestinal upset, abdominal pain, dizziness, headache, hepatotoxicity, rash, and taste disturbance (associated with terbinafine). Blood dyscrasias including granulocytopenia and leukopenia, a lupus-like syndrome, and proteinuria are also possible adverse effects of griseofulvin.

For patients interested in complementary therapies, they may try *Melaleuca alternifolia* (tea tree oil) and apply twice daily to the affected areas. Although sufficient research has not been done on this therapy, no adverse side effects are known.

The following measures should be recommended to help prevent spread or recurrence of tinea infections:

- Tinea capitis: Family members should be advised not to share combs, hats, or any headgear.
- Tinea corporis: The patient should be advised to control excessive sweat and body moisture by wearing looser clothing and to change clothing when it becomes wet or damp. After bathing, a hair dryer on the low setting may be used to dry intertriginous skinfolds.
- Tinea cruris: Cotton boxer shorts are better at preventing infections than tight briefs. The patient should avoid wearing tight jeans, pantyhose, or tight shorts made of close-fitting materials such as Spandex (e.g., biker shorts).
- Tinea corporis: Given its colloquial name, some patients (especially children) may incorrectly think that an actual worm is the cause of "ringworm" infections. Reassuring these patients that the infection is a fungus can significantly allay anxiety.
- Tinea pedis: The patient should be advised to avoid scratching the feet because the infection can spread to the hands (tinea manuum) and the body (tinea corporis). The patient should avoid tight shoes and moist socks, especially socks made out of synthetic material, unless they are designed to wick away moisture. Patients who are prone to "athlete's foot" should change socks two or three times a day and

expose their feet to air; they should use sandals if possible in warm weather. Absorbent nonsynthetic socks are preferred. Feet should be washed daily and dried thoroughly (a hair dryer on a low setting is helpful). Use of antiperspirant spray on the soles of the feet may decrease sweating. Patients should also be advised to clean their shower stalls with bleach and to wash all white sheets with bleach. When showering away from home, shower shoes should be worn.
- Tinea versicolor: Advise the patient that exposure to sunlight will help in repigmentation of hypopigmented areas.

ONYCHOMYCOSIS

Onychomycosis (Tinea unguium) is a benign superficial infection of the toenails and fingernails, which negatively affects their appearance and may lead to dystrophic changes. Most patients tolerate mild to moderate forms of tinea nail infections for many years. Patients who seek treatment are usually younger adults who are disturbed by the cosmetic effects of the infection. The most common etiology for onychomycosis is infection with dermatophytic fungi, but molds, yeast, and nondermatophytic fungi may be causative agents as well. Factors that increase the risk of onychomycosis include wearing occlusive shoes, diabetes mellitus, participation in sports, increasing age, and poor circulation of the lower extremities.

EPIDEMIOLOGY AND CAUSES

Onychomycosis is more common in adults and elderly patients than in children. The combination of poor circulation in the lower extremities as a result of peripheral vascular disease and the immunocompromising effects of advanced age makes this a common problem in older adults. Toenails are more likely to become infected than fingernails. Onychomycosis is a common infection worldwide; the incidence of disease is variable and is dependent on many factors. In the United States, 20% of all adults have onychomycosis. Onychomycosis is sometimes caused by the yeast *C. albicans*. Dermatophytic species of fungi commonly implicated in this tinea infection are *Trichophyton* species: *T. rubrum*, *T. mentagrophytes*, *T. schoenleinii*, and several others. A zoophilic fungus that is normally found in animal species and can cause onychomycosis is *T. verrucosum*.

Like many infections, onychomycosis frequently has a multifactorial etiology, including both fungal exposure and decreased immunity. The development of onychomycosis cannot be attributed solely to the presence of the offending organism because most causative yeasts and fungi are ubiquitous in the environment. Molds, for example, are plentiful in soil, and the soil mold *Scopulariopsis brevicaulis* is the most common nondermatophytic cause of onychomycosis. Other molds implicated in onychomycosis include *Aspergillus* and *Alternaria* species. In addition, *C. albicans* can be part of the normal flora of the mouth, GI tract, or vagina.

PATHOPHYSIOLOGY

Onychomycosis is classified as either a primary or secondary infection. *Primary onychomycosis* involves invasion of the healthy nail plate. In *secondary onychomycosis*, diseased nails (e.g., from psoriasis or trauma) are predisposed to developing infection. Factors that increase the risk of onychomycosis include a decrease in circulation, resulting from either a chronic process such as peripheral vascular disease, or an acute traumatic process, such as fracture of the lower extremity. Abnormal enervation due to spinal trauma has also been implicated. Tinea unguium can result from an extension of an infection with tinea pedis, tinea manuum, or tinea corporis.

Nail invasion can proceed in several ways. In proximal subungual onychomycosis, the pathogen enters the nailbed through the posterior nail and cuticle area, then migrates to the proximal nailbed. This form of onychomycosis is most commonly seen in immunocompromised individuals who exhibit suboptimal T-cell function. In distal and lateral subungual onychomycosis, infection starts at the distal or lateral margins of the nail. The infection then moves toward the center of the nail until the entire nail is affected. Distal subungual onychomycosis is almost always caused by *T. rubrum.* Superficial white onychomycosis involves infection of the nail surface only and is caused mainly by *T. mentagrophytes.* Total dystrophic onychomycosis is associated mostly with chronic candidiasis, which is seen in severely immunodeficient states such as AIDS.

CLINICAL PRESENTATION

Subjective

The typical patient who seeks treatment for onychomycosis is either a young or middle-aged adult who is bothered greatly by the negative cosmetic effects of the infection. The duration of the infection can range from a few weeks to many years. Onychomycosis is an asymptomatic infection, and there should be no pain involved. Some patients report having tried several OTC remedies with no result. The patient may complain of thickened dystrophic nails or nails with cloudy, white-colored patches. Some report nail discoloration, ranging from yellow to green or brown to black. In more severe forms, some patients complain of nails that are partially detached from the nailbed (onycholysis).

Objective

Onychomycosis has several presentations, and in some patients, multiple types can occur simultaneously. Superficial infections are more responsive to treatment with prescription topical antifungals (naftifine gel) than subungual types, in which infection occurs beneath the nail. Superficial white onychomycosis involves only the nail surface but may occur with either distal or lateral subungual onychomycosis. Subungual onychomycosis may involve distal, lateral, and proximal sites of infection. The first or fifth toenail is more likely to become infected than the other toes. The infected nail typically appears dry and has an opaque white patch with sharp borders that start on the distal, lateral, or proximal subungual portion, or is limited to the nail surface (superficial white onychomycosis). As the infection persists, the nail becomes brittle and thickened. The area underneath the nail accumulates chalky material made up of hyperkeratotic debris that can be scraped off easily for fungal cultures. In some patients, the white opaque areas become discolored—either yellow or brown. A green-black color suggests complication with a bacterial *Pseudomonas* infection.

DIAGNOSTIC REASONING

Diagnostic Tests

All cases of presumed onychomycosis must be confirmed by laboratory findings. A positive result on fungal culture, which includes proper identification of the fungus species involved, is necessary to start treatment with systemic antifungals. Findings of the KOH examination typical of fungal infection are hyphae and spores with a classic "spaghetti and meatballs" appearance. Under the microscope, hyphae appear as long translucent tubes with septae (separate sections), while spores are small round to ovoid shapes.

Fungal Culture

Fungal cultures done on Sabouraud's agar or with Dermatophyte test medium produce results in up to 3 days. The area where the samples are to be taken should be cleansed with 70% alcohol and allowed to dry before specimen collection. Skin should be taken from the active border of the lesion. Nail samples should be taken from the subsurface of the infected nail. To obtain samples from underneath the nail, a scalpel can be used to scrape the underside of the infected nail. In proximal subungual onychomycosis, the affected part of the nail is at the proximal fold and cannot be sampled without nail removal. Nail removal is done with a bilateral digital nerve block and is contraindicated if the patient has a bleeding disorder. The patient should be referred to a podiatrist for nail removal and treatment.

KOH Examination

A laboratory examination using KOH is necessary for diagnosis, because only 50% of dystrophic nails are due to dermatophytosis. A drop of 10% KOH is placed on the sample of nail clippings and is heated gently with a lighter or match. The heating accelerates the effect of the KOH on the keratinized cell walls, but the slide should not be placed too close to the flame, or the KOH will get too hot and boil off. When the sample is ready, the hyphae will be easier to see because the cell walls will have been lysed by the KOH.

Differential Diagnosis

The differential diagnosis of onychomycosis includes psoriasis of the nail, reactive arthritis (postinfectious), trauma to the nail, and congenital nail abnormalities. Onychomycosis accounts for only 50% to 60% of abnormally appearing or dystrophic nails. Lichen planus, eczematous conditions, and senile nailbed ischemia all may result in similarly appearing nails; however, fungal infection does not underlie such conditions, and antifungal medications would be inappropriate in such cases.

MANAGEMENT

In the past, onychomycosis of the toenail required long-term treatment with systemic antifungals and had a high recurrence rate. With the advent of newer antifungals (e.g., itraconazole, terbinafine), the cure rates for onychomycosis have greatly improved. Fluconazole (Diflucan) has consistently been shown to be less effective than either itraconazole or terbinafine, however, and is not typically recommended. Alternative therapies include laser treatment, photodynamic therapy, and chemical or surgical nail removal.

Fingernail infection is easier to cure and has a lower rate of recurrence than toenail infection. The decision to treat onychomycosis aggressively must be considered carefully because it is predominantly a benign cosmetic infection. The patient's desires for treatment and his or her health history are probably the strongest determinants in deciding whether to treat with systemic antifungals. Other important factors include the presence of any preexisting medical problems and the past medical history. Patients who have liver disease should avoid systemic antifungal drugs because of the high risk of hepatoxicity and liver failure. A history of infection with viral hepatitis can result in chronic infection with hepatitis B or C, and a history of excessive alcohol use can result in cirrhosis of the liver or elevations in liver function tests—all of which are considered high-risk conditions for starting systemic antifungal therapy.

Medication interactions are also problematic. Drugs metabolized by the cytochrome p450 3A enzyme system interact with systemic antifungals. Itraconazole potentiates the effects of many common prescription drugs, including diazepam (Valium), digoxin (Lanoxin), triazolam (Halcion), anticoagulants (Coumadin), HIV protease inhibitors (e.g., indinavir, ritonavir), methylprednisone, and verapamil. Patients who are taking vinca alkaloids (used in cancer chemotherapy) should not take itraconazole.

In addition, itraconazole requires a low gastric pH (acidic) to be absorbed. Therefore, H_2 blockers and antacids must be avoided within 2 hours of taking the drug.

Topical Therapy

Topical treatment of onychomycosis is generally not very effective (cure rates of 10% or less), but it is worth an attempt because it is not typically associated with any serious side effects. Good candidates for topical treatment are motivated patients with only mild involvement (i.e., one half or less of distal nail plate infected) or with surface involvement only (superficial white onychomycosis). Also, patients unable to take systemic antifungals may benefit from topical formulations. A topical solution such as ciclopirox nail lacquer 8% (Penlac) applied twice daily for 6 to 18 months or either efinaconazole 10% topical or tavaborole 0.5% solution applied once daily for 48 weeks may be effective when it is applied consistently to toenails. Efinaconazole and tavaborole should be applied once daily over the entire nail surface and under the nail. Ciclopirox 8% (Penlac) is indicated for mild to moderate onychomycosis of the fingernails and toenails (without lunula involvement). Initial improvement may take up to 6 months, and treatment can continue up to 48 weeks. Penlac should be applied evenly on the affected nail and surrounding 5 mm of skin once daily, preferably at bedtime. It should be applied over previous coats, then removed with alcohol once a week. Nail polish should not be used during treatment.

Systemic Therapy

For patients who desire treatment for onychomycosis, most authorities recommend systemic therapy. If concurrent tinea pedis, tinea manuum, or tinea corporis is present, it should be treated with topical antifungals, so that the source of infection is eradicated. Fingernails are easier to treat than toenails and have a higher cure rate from 50% to 70%. See Drugs Commonly Prescribed 13.1 for recommended systemic medications.

Itraconazole and terbinafine are better choices for toenail infections, which are more difficult to treat. Patients who are on H_2 blockers can also take these drugs. There is no role for griseofulvin in the treatment of toenail onychomycosis because up to 80% to 90% of patients will relapse with this drug.

FOLLOW-UP AND REFERRAL

After initiation of therapy, liver function tests should be rechecked every 4 weeks. The first follow-up visit is scheduled during the fourth week to monitor for symptoms of hepatoxicity, adverse reactions, and compliance with treatment and to obtain a liver function panel. Thereafter, the patient should be seen for follow-up every 4 to 6 weeks with liver function tests done. Resistant cases of onychomycosis should be referred to a dermatologist. Nail growth should be monitored until the nails become clinically normal.

Patient Education: Onychomycosis

The patient should avoid tight, ill-fitting shoes because they traumatize nails, especially the first toenail. Cotton socks that become moist should be changed. Patients should be encouraged to air dry their feet and wear open-toed slippers or sandals. Some patients have also had some success with *Melaleuca alternifolia* (tea tree oil) when applied to the affected nail twice daily.

Patients on itraconazole and terbinafine should be advised that although mycological cure has been achieved, normal nails might not be clinically apparent until regrowth in 3 to 12 months.

REFERENCES

Candidiasis

Centers for Disease Control and Prevention. 2015 sexually transmitted disease treatment guidelines: Vulvovaginal candidiasis. https://www.cdc.gov/std/tg2015/candidiasis.htm. Accessed April 17, 2017.

Pappas PG, Kauffman CA, Andes DR, et al. Clinical practice guideline for the management of candidiasis: 2016 update by the Infectious Diseases Society of America. *Clin Infect Dis.* 2016;62(4):e1–e50.

Scheinfeld NS, Lambiase MC. Cutaneous candidiasis. http://emedicine.Medscape.com/article 1090632. Published February 5, 2016. Accessed April 20, 2017.

Sobel JD. Candida vulvovaginitis: Clinical manifestations and diagnosis. https://www.uptodate.com/contents/candida-vulvovaginitis-clinical-manifestations-and-diagnosis. Published October 12, 2016. Accessed April 20, 2017.

Onychomycosis

Tosti A. Onychomycosis. Emedicine.medscape.com/article/1105828. Published June 30, 2016. Accessed April 24, 2017.

Tinea

Crouse LN. Tinea versicolor. emedicine.medscape.com/article/1091575. Published March 9, 2017. Accessed April 23, 2017.

Handler MZ. Tinea capitis. emedicine.medscape.com/article 1091351. Published May 13, 2016. Accessed April 24, 2017.

Lesher JL. Tinea corporis. emedicine.medscape.com/article/1091473. Published August 8, 2016. Accessed April 24, 2017.

Robbins CM. Tinea pedis. emedicine.medscape.com/article/1091684. Published August 5, 2016. Accessed April 24, 2017.

Wiederkehr M. Tinea cruris. emedicine.medscape.com/article/1091806. Published August 5, 2016. Accessed April 23, 2017.

RESOURCES

American Academy of Dermatology
    www.aad.org
Centers for Disease Control and Prevention
    www.cdc.gov
National Institute of Allergy and Infectious Disease
    www.niaid.nih.gov
National Institutes of Health
    www.nih.gov
Information on dermatologic drugs:
Drugs, herbs, and supplements
    https://medlineplus.gov/druginformation.html

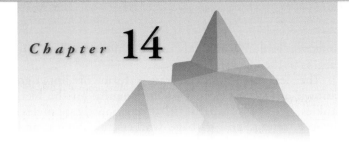

Chapter **14**

Bacterial Skin Infections

Susan Garnett, MSN, APRN, FNP-BC

Jill E. Winland-Brown, EdD, APRN, FNP-BC

Brian Oscar Porter, MD, PhD, MPH, MBA

IMPETIGO

Impetigo is a highly contagious, superficial vesiculopustular infection of the skin that is commonly seen in infants and children. Impetigo spreads readily through direct contact among family members, children in classrooms or play groups, and during contact sports or via fomites (shared objects such as clothing or furniture). Impetigo infection in adults is not as contagious as impetigo infection in infants and younger children. Impetigo infection typically demonstrates a mixed flora of gram-positive bacteria that includes *Staphylococcus aureus* and group A or group B beta-hemolytic *Streptococcus*. Two forms of impetigo are commonly seen in clinics: bullous and nonbullous (vesiculopustular). Bullous impetigo occurs primarily in newborns and infants. Nonbullous impetigo is the more common form, constituting approximately 70% of impetigo cases; it is caused solely by *S. aureus*.

EPIDEMIOLOGY AND CAUSES

Impetigo primarily affects infants in hospital nurseries and young children aged 2 to 5 years, especially those with poor hygiene and who are in day-care groups; however, patients of all ages are susceptible. Impetigo makes up nearly 10% of skin complaints in pediatric practices. It is the most prevalent bacterial skin infection and the third most common skin condition that occurs children. Impetigo is more common in hot, humid weather, when biting insects and mosquitoes are most pervasive. The trauma caused by these insect bites favors bacterial growth on moist skin. There is an increased incidence of impetigo in lower socioeconomic groups due to several factors, including overcrowding, inadequate personal hygiene, and a higher incidence of anemia and malnutrition. In addition, any preexisting skin disease that goes untreated (e.g., atopic dermatitis) may also predispose individuals to secondary infection. Staphylococcal impetigo may be associated with immunodeficiency disease.

PATHOPHYSIOLOGY

The infectious process in impetigo is limited to the stratum corneum. The presence of numerous neutrophils within the blister (subcorneal blister) and the presence of gram-positive cocci are characteristic of impetigo infections. Etiologic agents may be found alone or in combination.

In cases of impetigo caused by a combination of gram-positive bacteria, symbiosis promotes the growth of both bacteria and produces more rapid spread. *Staphylococcus* bacteria are usually noted during the early stages of the lesions, whereas *Streptococcus* bacteria tend to predominate in the later stages. In recent years, epidemiologists have noted an etiologic shift in which *S. aureus,* either alone or in combination with group A *Streptococcus,* has replaced the latter as the most common causative organism. Thus, chronic skin colonization with either *S. aureus* or group A *Streptococcus* predisposes an individual to impetigo. Infected lesions typically result from sites of previous injury, such as insect bites. Blister formation is caused by the action of epidermolytic (exfoliative) exotoxins produced by the bacteria; blisters are the result of local separation (acantholysis) of keratinocytes in the underlying epidermal layer that form the floor of the blister. Group A *Streptococcus* is the primary etiologic agent for a rare, severe, ulcerative form of impetigo known as ecthyma. Ulcer formation is also aided by coagulase-positive *Staphylococcus*.

Bullous impetigo is caused by *S. aureus* infection in newborns and young children. In this condition, exfoliative toxin A causes loss of cellular adhesion in the superficial epidermis normally mediated by the protein desmoglein. This results in large blistering lesions known as bullae, which eventually drain, leaving thin, nonpurulent crusts over the affected skin area.

Methicillin-resistant *S. aureus* (MRSA) has increasingly been identified as a causative agent in primarily nonbullous impetigo. In recent years, impetigo has more frequently been caused by strains of community-acquired MRSA and gentamicin-resistant *S. aureus*.

CLINICAL PRESENTATION

Subjective

The most common symptom of both types of impetigo is pruritus from the lesions. The parent of a young or school-age child may report a red, crusty rash that is spreading or getting larger in size. The rash is usually located on the face or on the extremities. Parents or the child may report that a close friend or classmate of the patient has the same rash.

The provider should ask about the location, onset, and duration of the lesions and any associated symptoms. The clinician should also inquire if any other family member has been affected and if treatment has been effective.

185

Fever is unusual in impetigo, but if present, it should prompt investigation for a deeper infection.

Objective

The plaques of impetigo begin as vesicles. The roofs of these vesicles break down, leaving shallow erosions with yellowish crusts. The lesions may be discrete or confluent in their distribution and are usually seen on the face. Early impetigo may resemble many vesicular skin conditions, such as herpes simplex.

The bullous form of impetigo may present with bullae that begin as small (1 to 2 mm) superficial vesicles with fragile roofs that rupture easily. The parent or patient may deny seeing bullae because the vesicles rupture so quickly that they are not recalled by the patient or the parent. The serous fluid inside the ruptured vesicles develops into a thin, transparent, and varnish-like crust. Hence, the vesicles become pustular in a matter of hours. The bullous type of impetigo is usually caused by *Staphylococcus* bacteria; it commonly occurs on the face, elbows, and knees.

In the nonbullous or vesiculopustular form, the lesions are characterized by thick, adherent, dirty yellow–colored crusts that have erythematous margins. This type of impetigo occurs more often in older children. Both bullous and nonbullous types produce symptoms such as burning and pruritus. In addition, regional lymphadenopathy is seen. When the face is involved, the cervical lymph nodes (and sometimes the preauricular and submandibular nodes) are enlarged; when the lesions are present on the upper extremities, the axillary nodes become enlarged.

A variant of bullous impetigo that is caused exclusively by *S. aureus* is known as "staphylococcal scalded skin syndrome." Exotoxins produced by the bacteria lead to bullous, sheetlike necrosis of the epidermis and cause the epithelium layer of the skin to peel off in large pieces. The "scalded skin" thus mimics a thermal burn. This serious infection is more commonly seen in children and usually begins in the intertriginous areas.

The less common, ulcerative form of impetigo known as *ecthyma* occurs predominantly on the feet, ankles, legs, and thighs. It affects mostly homeless people, sewage and garbage workers, alcoholics, and neglected elderly individuals. It is a deeper form of impetigo and often results from a neglected or poorly treated superficial abrasion or from infected insect bites. Itching is common, and autoinoculation from scratching may cause satellite lesions that are annular in form. Ecthyma presents as pruritic and tender red vesicles or pustules that are surrounded by erythema and eventually ulcerate. Because this process is superficial, healing often occurs spontaneously in the center of the lesion and results in scarring. The inflammatory process involves both dermal and epidermal layers. See Table 14.1 for the clinical presentation of the different types of impetigo.

During physical assessment, a thorough examination of the skin should search for erosions that are covered with moist, honey-colored crusts. The physical assessment should include an examination of the head, ears, pharynx, and neck, and the regional lymph nodes should be noted for lymphadenopathy. Firm and dry or dark crusts with surrounding erythema are characteristic of *ecthyma*.

DIAGNOSTIC REASONING

Diagnostic Tests

Diagnosis may be based solely on medical history and clinical presentation. Initial testing for impetigo may also include a bacterial culture and sensitivity analysis from the moist crusts of the lesions. The results of the culture and sensitivity help to assess for antibiotic resistance of the responsible pathogen. Resistance patterns can vary from

TABLE 14.1 Types of Impetigo		
Types of Impetigo	*Causative Agent*	*Clinical Presentation*
Bullous impetigo	*Staphylococcus aureus*	Lesion starts as 1–2 mm superficial vesicle with fragile roof, easily ruptured; ruptured vesicle forms thin, transparent, varnish-like or classic "honey-colored" crust. Becomes pustular in a matter of hours; pruritic; burning sensation.
Staphylococcal scalded skin syndrome	*S. aureus*	Variant of bullous impetigo: epidermal necrosis caused by bacterial exotoxins, resulting in the epithelial layer peeling off in large, sheetlike pieces; mimics scalded-skin thermal burn.
Nonbullous impetigo	*Streptococcus, S. aureus*	Lesions are thick, adherent; recurrent with dirty yellow–colored crusts and erythematous margins; pruritic; burning sensation.
Ecthyma	*S. aureus, Streptococcus;* other infective organisms may be observed	Pruritic, tender, red vesicles or pustules surrounded by erythema; rash eventually ulcerates. Deeper impetigo resulting from inadequately treated or neglected skin infections; also seen in infected insect bites or abrasions.

community to community. In addition, a Gram stain can be obtained; if the lesions are caused by impetigo, the stain will reveal gram-positive cocci. If herpes simplex is suspected, a viral culture can be obtained. If the patient is febrile or has systemic symptoms, a complete blood count (CBC) with differential should be obtained.

DIFFERENTIAL DIAGNOSIS

The typical dirty-looking, honey-colored crust is almost pathognomonic of bullous impetigo, so much so that cultures are not necessary before treatment is started. Bullous impetigo should be differentiated from other vesicular and pustular skin conditions. Many skin diseases with weepy lesions may resemble impetigo, such as varicella-zoster virus, herpes simplex virus, eczematous dermatitis (atopic dermatitis), bullous pemphigus/pemphigoid, and contact dermatitis. The history, distribution, and morphological features of the primary skin lesions provide the best information to help in the differential diagnosis of other skin conditions.

Varicella-zoster infection (herpes zoster or chickenpox) produces a rash with widely distributed papules and vesicular lesions. The onset of the rash typically starts on the head and neck area. The lesions of herpes zoster follow a dermatomal pattern that consists of a group of uniform 2- to 3-mm vesicles on an erythematous base.

A localized group of vesicles located on a single anatomical site, with clear to cloudy fluid on an erythematous and edematous base, helps to characterize herpes simplex lesions. These lesions are usually preceded by a prodrome of burning and tingling before the lesions erupt.

Bullous pemphigus and bullous pemphigoid are autoimmune diseases affecting the skin and causing bulla that can become eroded and infected. They should be included in the differential diagnosis for any vesicular or bullous skin disease.

Acute nummular eczema manifests as pruritic, coin-shaped plaques or patches on an erythematous base; the lesions may become exudative and crusted. Candidiasis lesions are bright red; this rash forms satellite lesions along with macerated moist patches. Candidiasis is often accompanied by pruritus and burning in the macerated areas.

MANAGEMENT

There are two principles of therapy in the management of impetigo: (1) nonpharmacologic measures are used to enhance resolution and to reduce bacterial colonization on the skin surface, and (2) antibiotics are prescribed to help eradicate the responsible pathogen and to prevent recolonization and complications. Even without treatment, impetigo usually heals within 2 to 3 weeks. With appropriate treatment, lesions usually resolve after 7 to 10 days. The key to treating and preventing impetigo

is practicing good personal hygiene and maintaining a clean environment.

Nonpharmacologic Management

Nonpharmacologic management of impetigo involves the use of solutions or substances to debride the impetiginized lesions and to expose the skin surfaces where the bacteria are present. Exudative impetigo lesions may benefit from drying compresses to remove thick crusts and desiccate (dry out) the lesions. Normal saline, plain tap water, or Burow's solution may be applied for 10 to 20 minutes, three to four times daily. Although the dehydrating effect of the compresses may help to improve the appearance of the skin lesions, disinfectant solutions are not particularly effective in treating the underlying condition.

Pharmacologic Management

Pharmacologic treatment of impetigo includes the use of both topical and oral antibiotics. Mild cases of bullous and nonbullous impetigo can be treated effectively with a topical antibiotic, combined with cleansing and debridement. One topical agent is mupirocin 2% cream or ointment (Bactroban) applied twice daily for 5 days. This is equivalent in efficacy to oral cephalexin. However, *S. aureus* and MRSA have developed resistance to mupirocin. Washing with chlorhexidine (Hibiclens) is a valuable adjunct because of its bactericidal properties. The patient should be instructed to wash the affected skin area with the bactericidal soap two to three times a day before the mupirocin cream is applied.

Another topical ointment belonging to the pleuromutilin antibiotic class is retapamulin (Altabax). It is effective against mupirocin-resistant strains. Retapamulin is applied twice daily for 5 days. However, it is not intended for mucosal use and is not Food and Drug Administration approved for the treatment of MRSA or the prevention of nasal carriage. New topical treatments that are in development for the treatment of impetigo include minocycline foam and ozenoxacin cream.

Systemic antibiotics are indicated for impetigo when there are systemic symptoms such as fever or toxicity, if a large area of the skin is involved, or within the context of athletic teams or child-care or family clusters. Antibiotic therapy should cover *S. aureus* and group A beta-hemolytic *Streptococcus*. The prevalence of MRSA and macrolide-resistant *Streptococcus* is a recent challenge. MRSA has been cited as the causative agent for nearly 80% of all community-acquired staphylococcal skin and soft-tissue infections. Penicillin therapy is recommended for streptococcal impetigo. Antibiotics effective against *S. aureus* such as dicloxacillin or cephalexin are given for 7 days. If MRSA is suspected, the choice of antibiotic should be doxycycline, clindamycin, or trimethoprim-sulfamethoxazole (TMP-SMX). Newer antibiotics prescribed for MRSA include dalbavancin (Dalvance) and tedizolid phosphate (Sivextra); however, they are not indicated for use in children.

Empirical treatment depends on the prevalence and sensitivities of MRSA in the patient's geographical area. Patients with penicillin hypersensitivity should take doxycycline or clindamycin. Because oral antibiotics have far more gastrointestinal and systemic side effects than topical therapy, topical treatment is often preferred for mild to moderate infections.

In addition to topical and systemic antibiotic therapy, antihistamines may be prescribed if pruritus is problematic to prevent skin trauma from excoriation and decrease the potential for spreading the infection. Second-generation antihistamines are preferable, given once daily at bedtime, in order to minimize associated sedation.

FOLLOW-UP AND REFERRAL

Follow-up for the patient with an uncomplicated case of impetigo should occur in 10 to 14 days after initiation of therapy. Patients who have a fever should be followed closely; consultation with or referral to a physician is recommended. Development of acute glomerulonephritis (acute nephritic syndrome), typically as a result of streptococcal infection, requires referral to a nephrologist; symptoms include the abrupt onset of proteinuria, hypertension, edema, azotemia, and red blood cells in the urine.

The majority of cases of both types of impetigo (bullous and nonbullous) resolve uneventfully after 10 days of treatment. Patients with recurrent impetigo should be tested for nasal carriage of *S. aureus* with a culture of the anterior nares. If the culture is positive, treatment of the nares with topical mupirocin (Bactroban) is effective. Repeat culture should be done to confirm the patient's status. Chronic nasal carriers may be treated with mupirocin three times a day for 5 days of each month. In the event of treatment failure, consultation with an infectious diseases specialist should be considered. Bullous impetigo typically resolves even without antibiotic treatment. Nonbullous impetigo generally has a good prognosis, although poststreptococcal glomerulonephritis is a possible complication of this infection.

Patient Education: Impetigo

The clinician plays a pivotal role in the treatment and prevention of this highly contagious skin infection through patient education and counseling. Good hand washing and personal hygiene are strongly recommended to reduce the likelihood of bacterial spread. The fingernails should be kept short so that there is less likelihood of spread to other areas of the body through self-inoculation.

Children and family members should be educated about the contagious nature of impetigo. They should be told to refrain from participation in any contact sport or activity that might spread the infection. Children should not attend day care or school for 24 hours after antibiotic therapy is started. Family members should not share clothing or personal hygiene items such as towels, robes, razors, and shavers. Bed linens should be washed with soap and hot water.

The patient should be instructed to gently clean the crusts from the lesions with antibacterial soap before applying mupirocin 2% cream or retapamulin. Nighttime application is also advised. If occlusive dressings are used, they should be discarded carefully to prevent the spread of infection. If the patient is taking oral antibiotics, the side effects and potential adverse reactions of the drug should be explained, as well as the importance of completing the course of antibiotic therapy to prevent the possible complication of poststreptococcal glomerulonephritis. Patients should be informed that good personal hygiene and cleanliness, along with prompt attention to skin trauma, may help prevent future breakouts of impetigo. Patients should not visit hospitals or nursing homes until the infection is resolved. If MRSA is involved, patients should stay at home and not handle food until they have been on antibiotics for 24 hours.

FOLLICULITIS

Folliculitis is a superficial to deep skin infection of the hair follicles. Lesions can range from minute white-topped pustules in newborns to large, yellow-white tender pustules in adults. Bacteria infect the hair follicle at a superficial level, leading to erythematous papules and pustules. Although the main pathogens are gram-positive bacteria, occasional cases are caused by a fungus or by gram-negative bacilli. Folliculitis represents the start of a continuum of skin infections. Deeper infections (as complications of folliculitis) can include the furuncle (boil) or carbuncle (multiple boils), which are covered in depth elsewhere in this chapter.

EPIDEMIOLOGY AND CAUSES

Folliculitis is often caused by bacteria; in particular, it is frequently caused by coagulase-negative *Staphylococcus*. Predisposing factors include diabetes, obesity, a chronic carrier state of *Staphylococci* (present in the nares, axillae, or perineum), poor hygiene, hyperimmunoglobulin E (Job's syndrome, a primary immunodeficiency disorder), exposure to chemicals and solvents (cutting oils), and chronic skin friction. However, folliculitis may have other etiologies as well. Gram-positive resident flora of the nasal mucosa and adjacent facial skin become suppressed by long-term oral antibiotic therapy and are replaced by gram-negative rods, namely *Klebsiella* and *Escherichia coli*. Thus, gram-negative folliculitis may develop in patients who are on long-term tetracycline therapy for acne or rosacea, as well as in older men with seborrhea. Patients whose sebaceous follicles of the perioral and perinasal areas have become colonized by gram-negative bacteria can become infected due to trauma (e.g., from shaving), resulting in a suppurative process within the hair follicle. This type of folliculitis is usually seen on the upper lip in men. In addition, antibiotic use also increases the risk of *Candida* folliculitis, due to clearance of the normal bacterial skin flora. Exposure to wet environments, such as whirlpools or inadequately chlorinated pools, which contributes to *Pseudomonas aeruginosa* infection, also predisposes to folliculitis. In addition, chronic steroid use that compromises T-cell immunity contributes to folliculitis by *Candida albicans*.

Folliculitis most commonly occurs among middle-aged individuals (aged 40 to 60 years) and children, especially if they are immunocompromised or spend an extended amount of time in a prone position due to impaired mobility. Studies have found that folliculitis may be spread by fomite transmission. Intensive care units (ICUs) are the frequent origin of nosocomial outbreaks in the hospital setting. The higher incidence of folliculitis in the ICU is the result of trauma from invasive procedures performed on immunocompromised or severely ill patients. Impairment of host resistance increases a patient's risk of contracting folliculitis in the presence of virulent pathogens such as gram-negative coliform bacilli. Stethoscopes have been known to harbor many organisms (Shiferaw et al., 2013).

Folliculitis may occur anywhere on the skin as a result of trauma or damage to the hair follicle from chronic irritation due to friction from clothing or blockage of the hair follicle. Occlusion of the skin with tight-fitting nylon clothing promotes infection, and symptoms may occur abruptly within 1 to 3 days of wearing such garments. Occlusive therapy (plastic wrap) used for other diseases such as severe psoriasis or eczema allows for significant bacterial multiplication in a moist environment, which can also lead to folliculitis. Spread of bacterial infection to the surrounding skin may develop from exudative or transudative discharge from wounds, abscesses, or any type of draining lesion.

Eosinophilic folliculitis (EF) is a form of noninfectious sterile folliculitis. On histological examination, the hair follicle in EF is invaded by eosinophils and lymphocytes. Three types of EF have been identified. Eosinophilic pustular folliculitis, or Ofuji disease, generally occurs in Japanese men in their 30s. Another form of pustular EF is associated with immunosuppression and presents in patients with HIV/AIDS with low CD4 T-cell counts. A third type presents in infants, most commonly males. Rather than antibiotics, EF is treated with anti-inflammatory agents. First-line therapy for EF is systemic indomethacin, in addition to topical corticosteroids.

Acne is another noninfectious form of folliculitis. Currently, acne is theorized to be a primary inflammatory condition. Acne is discussed in depth in Chapter 17.

PATHOPHYSIOLOGY

Infection of the hair follicle with *Staphylococcus* or *Streptococcus* is marked by suppuration and liquefaction necrosis of the follicular base, thus termed a *pyodermal* infection. It is usually localized and results in abscess formation. Liquefaction necrosis develops when lytic enzymes released by polymorphonuclear leukocytes (PMNs) digest bacteria and cellular material. Thus, a competent immune system is required for such a response, as large numbers of PMNs are found in the central area of the abscess, along with necrotic debris. Because this inflammatory response is localized, however, folliculitis rarely causes systemic manifestations in the immunocompetent individual. Interestingly, HIV-positive patients do not display this neutrophilic response because they typically experience an eosinophilic perifollicular pustular folliculitis, as described previously.

CLINICAL PRESENTATION

Subjective

Generally, the patient will present with a "bumpy rash," which can appear on any area of the body. The rash can be located on the hair follicles of the face, forehead, back of the earlobes, neck, shoulders, buttocks, torso, or extremities. Usually, the rash is not accompanied by itching. Often there is no history of previous skin eruptions or of pertinent medical history such as diabetes. The patient is usually concerned about the cosmetic effect of the lesions. The patient may report a history of hot tub use or of borrowing a shaver or razor from a friend. The clinician should inquire about the onset, duration, and location(s) of the rash, its appearance, and whether purulent drainage was present. The patient should also be asked about any associated systemic symptoms of fever and chills.

Objective

The primary lesions in folliculitis are small pustules surrounded by 1 to 2 mm of erythema located over the pilosebaceous orifice or the ostium of the hair follicle. There is no involvement of the surrounding skin. The eyelids, face, scalp, and extremities are the most typical sites. A hair in the center of the pustule sometimes perforates the lesion. This presentation is a hallmark for diagnosis. The pustules resolve into red macules, which fade to leave postinflammatory hyperpigmented scars in susceptible persons. Folliculitis is usually asymptomatic, but it can be very pruritic and is sometimes accompanied by burning. During the physical examination, checking vital signs, including temperature, is important to help rule out systemic involvement. The practitioner should inspect the lesion for signs of inflammation and suppuration (erythema, swelling, pustules) and palpate the surface of the pustule for fluctuance. It is also important to palpate the adjacent lymph nodes for evidence of spreading lymphadenitis

Folliculitis is divided into two main types—*superficial folliculitis* and *deep folliculitis.* Follicular impetigo (Bockhart's impetigo) is a superficial form of folliculitis that presents as small, dome-shaped pustules that occur over the opening of the hair follicle. It is more common on the scalps of children. When follicular impetigo becomes chronic, it may lead to follicular destruction and consequent permanent patchy alopecia.

The distinctive forms of deep folliculitis include barber's itch, pseudofolliculitis barbae, and *Pseudomonas* folliculitis. In addition, newer diagnoses have been established based on the histological characteristics of the skin eruption, such as EF (e.g., HIV-EF) and nosocomial folliculitis.

Barber's itch (sycosis barbae) is a chronic and recurrent staphylococcal infection of the hair follicles on the bearded area of the face in men (usually the upper lip). It is aggravated by shaving and is most commonly seen in black men. It is usually propagated by the autoinoculation of bacteria caused by shaving. Tinea barbae is similar to barber's itch, but the tinea infection is caused by a fungus. Pseudofolliculitis barbae, another differential diagnosis for sycosis barbae, is caused by hair in the beard area and posterior scalp and neck that curls toward the skin, causing an inflammatory reaction that can mimic folliculitis. It is more common in men of African ancestry due to the curliness of the hair. This can become a chronic problem, and the hair follicles involved can become infected with any variety of bacteria.

Pseudomonas folliculitis presents as follicular erythematous papules, pustules, or vesicles over the back, buttocks, and upper arms. Associated features include pruritus, malaise, low-grade fever, sore throat and eyes, and axillary lymphadenopathy. This type of folliculitis usually resolves spontaneously within 10 days.

Folliculitis decalvans is a rare disease that tends to occur in individuals who have coarse, bristly hair. The predisposing factors of this disease are still unknown. The infection begins as a localized area of follicular pustules or papules. Exudation or suppuration soon follows; as the crust accumulates, the hair are shed. New follicles become involved at the periphery, while at the center the process eventually subsides, with scarring and permanent hair loss.

Hot tub folliculitis is caused by *Pseudomonas aeruginosa,* which withstands temperatures of up to 107°F (41.6°C) and chlorine levels of up to 3 mg/L. The lesions of this variant of folliculitis are found on the trunk and lower extremities of patients who have a recent history of hot tub use. Superhydration of the stratum corneum softens this protective layer and allows the bacteria to cause infection.

There are documented cases of superficial actinic folliculitis characterized by recurrent skin eruptions occurring within 6 to 24 hours after sun exposure.

Histologically, there is perivascular lymphocytic infiltration and intrafollicular accumulation of neutrophils in the upper infundibulum of the follicle; these findings indicate the presence of an inflammatory response and suppurative process.

DIAGNOSTIC REASONING

Diagnostic Tests

A Gram stain and culture of purulent discharge is obtained by rupturing a pustule and taking samples of the exudate. The culture is useful to distinguish staphylococcal infections from other bacterial or fungal infections, as well as from epidermal and pilar cysts that are sterile lesions. The Gram stain is usually positive for clusters of gram-positive cocci (*S. aureus*) along with large numbers of PMNs. With deeper forms of folliculitis, the presence of systemic symptoms or positive blood cultures require referral to a physician for hospitalization and IV antibiotics.

If fungal infection is suspected, a fungal culture or potassium hydroxide (KOH) microscopic examination is helpful; if results are positive, treatment should change to an antifungal agent.

Differential Diagnosis

Superficial folliculitis is differentiated from tinea barbae by performing a KOH examination (see Advanced Assessment 13.1) of the affected hair or by a fungal culture. Acne vulgaris and bullous impetigo may occasionally mimic folliculitis, but the patient's age (i.e., nonadolescent) and the absence of comedones (blackheads or whiteheads) suggest a diagnosis of folliculitis. The lesions of bullous impetigo are usually larger and rupture easily, and the exudate is serous, not purulent. Approximately 50% of HIV-infected persons with scabies have coexistent *S. aureus* folliculitis.

Occasionally, follicular lesions extend more deeply, forming abscesses. Rarely, follicles covering an area several centimeters across become infected, forming large violaceous plaques. The plaque may be studded with pustules and have deep sinus tracts connecting infected follicles. Rarely, an abscess of the muscles (pyomyositis) may occur due to extension of the infectious process.

MANAGEMENT

Patients rarely consult a health-care provider for minor cases, except for infections that become recurrent and persistent. The goal of treatment of superficial and deep folliculitis is to make the skin inhospitable to pathogens. This includes both nonpharmacologic and pharmacologic approaches (see Drugs Commonly Prescribed 14.1).

Gentle cleansing by washing the skin twice a day with antibacterial soap (e.g., Lever 2000, Safeguard, Dial) is

Drugs Commonly Prescribed 14.1: Folliculitis

DRUG	TYPE	ADVERSE REACTIONS AND PRESCRIBING CONSIDERATIONS
Topical Antibiotics		
Mupirocin (Bactroban)	2% ointment or cream Three times a day for 5–14 days	Consider for secondarily infected skin lesions.
Retapamulin (Altabax)	Twice daily for 5 days	Do not use alone, due to antibiotic resistance. Lotion less irritating. May cause diarrhea. Avoid in patients with colitis.
Clindamycin	1% solution, lotion, gel, pledget— twice daily until lesions clear	
Erythromycin	2% solution, lotion or gel, twice daily until lesions clear	
Other		
Ketoconazole (Nizoral)	Topical—cream, shampoo, foam, gel Tablets	Prescribed for fungal forms of folliculitis. Topical formulations are safer than systemic formulations. Multiple U.S. Food and Drug Administration precautions. Use only when other antifungal treatment is ineffective. Monitor hepatic function before and during therapy. Check for numerous drug interaction warnings.

as important as prescription antibacterial medicines. Large pustular lesions with necrotic areas should first be cleansed with a weak soap solution, followed by soaking of (or the use of compresses on) the affected skin with saline or aluminum subacetate twice daily. When the skin is softened, the clinician can gently open the large pustules and trim away necrotic tissue.

Clearance of nasal colonization of *S. aureus* by mupirocin treatment twice daily for 5 days has been shown to reduce significantly the incidence of recurrent folliculitis. Systemic anti-staphylococcal antibiotics may be ordered if the infection is resistant to local treatment or if the scalp is involved. Usually, however, systemic antibiotics are not helpful or advantageous over topical treatments.

FOLLOW-UP AND REFERRAL

A patient who does not respond to therapy should be evaluated for possible diabetes mellitus or for chronic carriage (in the nares, axillae, or perineum) of *S. aureus*. Cultures of the anterior nares, axillae, and perineum are recommended. Topical mupirocin 2% (Bactroban) should be applied twice daily for 5 to 7 days to the sites that yielded a positive culture. Because most strains of MRSA are resistant to topical mupirocin, in cases of MRSA colonization, retapamulin (Altabax) should be applied twice daily for 2 weeks.

More severe forms of folliculitis and rare skin eruptions such as HIV-EF should be referred to a physician. Systemic IV antibiotics may be necessary. Referral for patients with recurrent or persistent infections that do not respond to a standard treatment regimen is recommended.

Patient Education: Folliculitis

The clinician should emphasize to the patient that good hygiene is essential in treating this condition. Effective hand-washing technique is the best approach in preventing the spread of folliculitis. Patients who are prone to folliculitis should be advised to use an antibacterial soap and to wash the affected areas twice a day with antibacterial soap before applying topical agents. Patients should also be informed that any source of friction can predispose to a recurrence of folliculitis.

In hospitals (especially the ICU), emphasis on proper hand washing and proper cleaning of patient care equipment such as stethoscopes can help prevent the spread of infection.

Men who are prone to recurrent sycosis barbae should be advised to avoid shaving during treatment to allow complete healing. A preventive approach is the best treatment for this condition. When shaving is resumed, an electric shaver may cause fewer breaks in the skin than a razor. Patients should be cautioned to avoid borrowing or using old razor blades when shaving infected areas.

FURUNCLES AND CARBUNCLES

A *furuncle (boil)* is a deep bacterial infection of a hair follicle with abscess formation. Furuncles are caused almost exclusively by gram-positive *S. aureus*. Furuncles are extremely tender to the touch and appear as bright red color. The most common locations for furuncles are the scalp, neck, axilla, buttocks, groin, and thighs. Furuncles frequently become fluctuant. With the application of warm compresses, most furuncles drain pus and resolve spontaneously.

A *carbuncle* is a large, multiloculated abscess comprising multiple furuncles in a contiguous area. Carbuncles, which are less common than furuncles, appear as large, red, painful lumps on the skin, with multiple follicular openings. Some carbuncles can be quite large—up to 10 cm in size. Eventually, a carbuncle spontaneously drains pus.

EPIDEMIOLOGY AND CAUSES

Furuncles and carbuncles are usually caused by *S. aureus* and rarely by other pathogens. In some patients, especially those who are immunocompromised, infection can be due to MRSA. Conditions predisposing patients to formation of furuncles and carbuncles include diabetes mellitus, poor hygiene, incarceration, obesity, and immune system defects. Chronic staphylococcal carriage in the anterior nares, axilla, and perineum also increase the risk of infection and should be explored in cases of recurrent infections. Favorable environmental conditions that predispose the individual to furuncle and carbuncle formation include areas of moisture, friction, or occluded skin. Any area of skin that is subject to friction, such as the axilla, buttocks, groin, or thighs, is at increased risk of infection.

PATHOPHYSIOLOGY

Both furuncles and carbuncles evolve from superficially infected hair follicles (folliculitis), mediated primarily by *S. aureus*. Thus, all factors that contribute to folliculitis also predispose to furunculosis and carbuncle formation. As this superficial infection extends along the hair shaft, a small, painful inflammatory nodule is formed at the follicular base that is termed a *furuncle*. Eventually, a series of abscesses form along the hair shaft involving dermal and subcutaneous layers, ultimately coalescing into a fluctuant, subcutaneous mass that develops a soft, pointed necrotic center. When the furuncle ruptures, it results in the extrusion of pus and a necrotic plug at the entrance to the follicle. A small opening or cavitation remains that eventually heals with scarring. Thus, the affected hair follicle is destroyed and does not regenerate, resulting in destruction of the hair itself.

Carbuncles ("boils") undergo a similar process, except on a larger scale. Carbuncles are comprised of several furuncles that form into a large, multiloculated abscess with multiple follicular openings that eventually drain pus. Carbuncles are significantly larger than furuncles, typically involving deeper skin layers. Both carbuncles and furuncles are considered boils. They are more likely to occur on thicker skin, in areas such as the nape of the neck and upper back. A systemic response including fever resulting from the production of pyogenic cytokines is more common with carbuncle formation than furunculosis.

Certain risk factors are associated with furunculosis and carbuncle formation. Obesity results in thick skinfolds that are closely approximated. This creates a moist environment in which bacteria are prone to reproduce. Impaired immune function from chronic steroid use, underlying systemic disease such as HIV or diabetes mellitus, or impaired neutrophil function also predispose to this condition. The presence of a bacterial virulence factor known as the Panton-Valentine leukocidin in certain strains of *S. aureus* has been associated with particularly aggressive skin infections.

CLINICAL PRESENTATION

Subjective

The typical patient will complain of a hot, tender, bright red bump or "boil" of several days' duration that becomes progressively larger. Some furuncles will "come to a head" or become fluctuant and will drain spontaneously on their own. Some patients will report a history of manipulation of the furuncle or carbuncle, either by squeezing it or by puncturing it with a needle. Some patients will report a past history of boils and other skin infections.

Objective

Both furuncles and carbuncles are extremely tender to the touch and are a bright red color. A furuncle initially appears as a small (0.5 to 1.0 cm), red, indurated nodule. As the nodule grows in size, it starts to develop a yellow-colored central plug. It begins to appear conical, with a central "nipple" that is covered by thinning skin. The pus, which is yellow to green in color, gives the "nipple" its characteristic color. Most furuncles eventually spontaneously rupture and drain pus, which hastens their resolution. As the necrotic material and pus are discharged, a small cavitation is left that heals with minimal scarring. Carbuncles initially appear as multiple furuncles that develop into a large, erythematous lump that eventually starts to drain pus from multiple follicular openings. Patients with darker skin can have permanent hyperpigmentation changes as a result of severe inflammation.

DIAGNOSTIC REASONING

Diagnostic Tests

Although most cases of furuncles and carbuncles are caused by *S. aureus,* a Gram stain and culture of the fluctuant lesion is still recommended, because MRSA strains may be identified. A CBC with differential is not necessary unless the patient has a severe case with an underlying immunocompromising disease, such as diabetes, or shows systemic symptoms such as fever.

No subsequent testing is necessary unless a patient is a staphylococcal carrier. The nares and anogenital region should be recultured after treatment with topical mupirocin (Bactroban) is finished. In resistant cases where no response is seen after 1 week of therapy, a repeat culture should be done.

Differential Diagnosis

Some skin conditions to consider in the differential diagnosis of furuncles include an epidermal inclusion cyst that is acutely inflamed. Epidermal inclusion cysts are usually located in areas of the body where there is thicker skin and a large number of sebaceous glands, such as on the back and upper shoulders. The patient with an epidermal inclusion cyst will report a history of the cyst on the same site for months to years. In contrast, furuncles are an acute process, taking only several days to form. Another characteristic of an epidermal inclusion cyst is a cheesy white discharge with a strong odor when it is expressed. A furuncle or carbuncle will have a purulent yellow to green-colored discharge when it ruptures.

Another differential diagnosis for a furuncle is a deep fungal infection of the soft tissue called *sporotrichosis.* It is more common in gardeners and other agricultural workers and is usually seen on the hands or arms. It is caused by injury from a thorn or wood splinter that has been contaminated with the common soil fungus *Sporothrix schenckii.* Because it is usually asymptomatic, patients tend to ignore it.

If the furuncle or carbuncle is located on the axilla, a differential diagnosis to consider is hidradenitis suppurativa. The lesions of hidradenitis suppurativa are also extremely tender and inflamed. Patients with this condition report a chronic history of recurrent infection in the axilla, groin, or anal region. It is a chronic disease of the apocrine glands of the axilla and groin and is associated with severe hypertrophic scarring and sinus tracts, which are not seen in furuncles or carbuncles. The classic finding in hidradenitis suppurativa that differentiates it from a furuncle or carbuncle are numerous hypertrophic scars and sinus tracts that are found on the affected skin.

MANAGEMENT

Carbuncles usually must drain before healing will take place, and this typically occurs spontaneously within 2 weeks. Application of warm compresses will promote the localization and spontaneous rupture and drainage of a furuncle. If a furuncle has not come to a head by the time the patient is seen, the patient should be instructed to apply warm compresses two to three times per day until it becomes fluctuant. However, randomized controlled trials have failed to consistently show the benefit of such treatment. Treatment with topical antibiotics with sufficient gram-positive coverage (e.g., mupirocin [Bactroban], retapamulin [Altabax], or neomycin–polymyxin B [Neosporin]), applied twice per day until resolution.

Treatment with systemic antibiotics is not necessary in a healthy patient if no surrounding cellulitis is present. Antibiotic therapy should be considered for immunocompromised patients, the very young or elderly, those with systemic symptoms such as fever, as well as patients with more than one lesion and when incision and drainage does not lead to improvement. For furuncles or carbuncles in an immunocompromised patient (or one who is at risk for bacteremia because of a preexisting condition), systemic antibiotics are always mandatory, and physician referral is recommended. In addition, incision and drainage will hasten the resolution of infection. Preexisting immunocompromising conditions such as diabetes or chronic steroid use predispose a patient to more complications. These patients should be monitored closely or referred to a physician. An occasional patient with furuncles or carbuncles will have bacteremia as a complication, with possible hematogenous spread to the heart valves (endocarditis), kidneys (perinephric abscess), joints, spine, and long bones (osteomyelitis).

A furuncle (especially if it is located on the upper lip or the central area of the face) or a carbuncle located on the neck, face, or scalp should be treated with physician consultation or referred to a physician for management. A furuncle located on the central face can spread via venous drainage to the cavernous sinus and result in cavernous sinus thrombosis or meningitis.

Fluctuant furuncles are ideally treated with incision and drainage. A sterile 18-gauge needle can be used to puncture the thin skin on top of a small furuncle to allow for adequate drainage of pus. For larger furuncles that are fluctuant, incision and drainage is indicated. The cavity formed by the furuncle if often packed with iodoform or petroleum jelly (Vaseline)-impregnated gauze; however, packing results in more discomfort and has not been shown to enhance healing. Rather, covering with a sterile dry dressing is recommended. After a furuncle has been incised, the patient should be instructed to use warm compresses twice daily to encourage the drainage of pus. Carbuncles frequently need incision and drainage as well to aid in recovery.

Systemic antibiotics and physician referral are always indicated for the treatment of carbuncles. Empiric treatment for moderate infections or for methicillin-sensitive *S. aureus* (MSSA) include dicloxacillin, cephalexin, TMP-SMX, or doxycycline. Severe MSSA infections may be treated with nafcillin, cefazolin, or clindamycin.

Moderate infections of community-acquired MRSA are susceptible to TMP-SMX. However, severe infections with MRSA or Panton-Valentine leukocidin–expressing strains of *Staphylococcus* may require inpatient IV antibiotic therapy (e.g., vancomycin, linezolid, daptomycin, telavancin, or ceftaroline) to ensure adequate treatment. Vancomycin or clindamycin is substituted for daptomycin and telavancin for treatment in children. Linezolid is typically used only under close physician supervision, given its potential for inducing thrombocytopenia, anemia, and neutropenia. Thus, antibiotic susceptibility testing is critical in these cases to most appropriately direct therapy. Newer antibiotics approved for both MSSA and MSRA treatment include tedizolid and dalbavancin.

If a patient has a history of frequent infections, a search for staphylococcal carriage is recommended. Cultures should be taken from the patient's nares, the perineum, and the anogenital region. If a patient is found to be a *S. aureus* carrier, a daily shower with chlorhexidine wash is recommended. Mupirocin ointment (Bactroban) or retapamulin (Altabax) should be applied twice a day to the anatomical sites from which *S. aureus* was cultured (nares, body folds, perineum, anogenital region) for 5 days. A repeat culture should be done to document clearance of the bacteria. This program will eliminate the staphylococcal carrier state and reduce the incidence of recurrence. There is some evidence that vitamin C supplementation (1 g/day for 4–6 weeks) may also help prevent recurrent skin infection in persons with impaired neutrophil function.

FOLLOW-UP AND REFERRAL

The patient should be seen for initial follow-up within a few days to 1 week to monitor response to therapy, compliance with treatment, and any adverse reactions. A subsequent visit can be scheduled in 7 to 10 days to monitor for continuing progress and resolution of the lesions. For carbuncles or multiple furuncles on immunocompromised patients (or patients at risk for bacteremia because of pre-existing disease), a physician referral is recommended.

In addition, if a patient has systemic signs such as fever or appears toxic, physician consultation or referral is recommended. These patients frequently need multiple laboratory tests, including blood cultures, which can be done in a hospital setting, in addition to treatment with parenteral antibiotics.

Patient Education: Furuncles and Carbuncles

The patient should be warned not to pop, squeeze, or to manipulate furuncles in any way, especially those that are located on the mid to upper lip or near the border of the nasolabial folds, given the risk of cavernous sinus thrombosis, which may be fatal.

CELLULITIS

Cellulitis is a bacterial infection of the skin involving both the dermis and subcutaneous tissue, which in certain cases may result in death. Most cases of cellulitis are caused by group A beta-hemolytic *Streptococcus* or by *S. aureus* (gram-positive bacteria). Less common bacteria that can cause cellulitis include *Haemophilus influenzae* (more common in children), *Eikenella corrodens* (human bites), *Pasteurella multocida* (cat bites), *Capnocytophaga canimorsus* (dog bites), and *Vibrio* species (seawater-exposed injuries).

The typical lesion of cellulitis is a wide, diffuse area of erythematous skin that is warm and tender to palpation. Infection is occasionally accompanied by severe edema. Systemic symptoms such as fever, chills, and malaise may accompany some cases as well. A cellulitic infection can occasionally result in the loss of a limb.

Cellulitis may become a life-threatening event that is heralded by systemic inflammatory response syndrome: fever, tachypnea, tachycardia, white blood count greater than 12,000 cells/μcL, and hypotension. Toxic shock syndrome (TSS) and multiple organ failure resulting from both streptococcal and staphylococcal infections have been reported. The clinician must learn to differentiate between a severe case of cellulitis that is potentially life-threatening and an uncomplicated case that can be treated on an outpatient basis. Special types of cellulitis that have potentially serious consequences discussed in this chapter include erysipelas, necrotizing fasciitis, and periorbital cellulitis (Box 14.1). Severe cases of cellulitis, such as necrotizing fasciitis, must be treated with surgical debridement in addition to parenteral antibiotics to stop the spread of rapid tissue destruction; such patients require hospitalization. Periorbital cellulitis, an emergent condition, should also be treated aggressively with parenteral antibiotics and hospitalization to prevent permanent vision loss and extension of infection into deep cranial structures.

EPIDEMIOLOGY AND CAUSES

There is usually an obvious portal of entry into the skin or mucous membranes, such as an insect bite or a wound, although in some cases there is no obvious point of entry (this is more common with recurrent cellulitis). Cellulitis may occur at any age, but some organisms are more common in certain age-groups. *Haemophilus influenzae* type B infections are more common in children. In adults and elderly patients, *S. aureus* and *Streptococcus pyogenes* are more common. In patients with diabetes mellitus or who are otherwise immunocompromised, unusual bacterial pathogens may include *Escherichia coli* and other enteric species (e.g., *Enterobacter*), as well as *Proteus mirabilis*, *Pseudomonas aeruginosa*, *Acinetobacter*, *Mycobacterium fortuitum*, and *Cryptococcus neoformans*.

Any break on the skin or mucous membranes is a potential portal of entry for bacterial pathogens. Skin breaks can

Box 14.1	**Types of Cellulitis**
Erysipelas	Erysipelas is a streptococcal infection of the superficial layers of skin that does not involve the subcutaneous layers, unlike more typical cellulitis. An older name for erysipelas is "St. Anthony's fire." Despite the superficial nature of this infection, erysipelas should not be taken lightly, because it can be fatal if it is not treated promptly—especially in the very young and the elderly. Before the advent of antibiotics, this infection was associated with a high mortality rate. Most cases of erysipelas are caused by group A beta-hemolytic *Streptococcus pyogenes* and sometimes develops after an episode of streptococcal pharyngitis (strep throat). The most common sites of involvement are the face (especially the cheeks) and lower legs. Patients usually have systemic symptoms such as high fever, chills, and malaise. Erysipelas on the face first appears as a bright red lesion by the nares that can spread rapidly within a few hours to days. An enlarging shiny, bright red, indurated plaque develops that is warm to the touch and has sharp, distinct borders, as opposed to cellulitis, which has more diffuse, flat borders. The affected skin appears shiny and taut because of the edema from the infection. Skin streaking and regional enlarged nodes indicate lymphatic involvement.
Necrotizing fasciitis	The hallmark of this infection is its rapid progression with tissue destruction and the severity of the symptoms. The progress of the infection is measured in terms of hours instead of days, as the border can be seen literally spreading in just a few hours. This infection is caused by "flesh-eating bacteria," and loss of life or limb is a potential complication. Most cases of necrotizing fasciitis are caused by group A *Streptococcus pyogenes*, although several kinds of bacteria have been implicated in these rapidly progressive infections, including *Staphylococcus aureus*, *Clostridium perfringens*, *Bacteroides fragilis*, and *Aeromonas hydrophila*. During the early phase of the infection, the lesion appears as bright red in color with edema that progresses to purpuric changes (indicated by a purple color change), including gangrene (indicated by a black color change). The symptom that differentiates necrotizing fasciitis from cellulitis is severe pain at the affected site, which may be out of proportion to the appearance of the skin lesion. This pain is due to involvement of the fascia around the muscle and sometimes of the muscle itself (myositis). Pressure on the skin may reveal crepitus due to gas production by the anaerobic bacteria *Clostridium perfringens*. Gangrene can present in just a few hours, with hypotension and mental status changes regarded as particularly ominous signs. Other indications of severe infection include violaceous bullae, hemorrhage, sloughing of the skin, and localized sensory loss.
Periorbital cellulitis	Periorbital cellulitis is a potentially life-threatening form of cellulitis that should be treated as an emergent condition. The typical patient is a young child with erythema and edema over the affected periorbital area. The edema can be so severe that the entire affected side of the face is puffy. Symptoms include pain with certain eye movements due to inflamed extraocular muscles. Other symptoms include high fever, tachycardia, lethargy or mental status changes, and other systemic symptoms. On physical examination, the involved eye will lose the ability to move into certain quadrants (i.e., lateral or downward gaze) and the examination of cranial nerves III, IV, and VI that control extraocular movements will be abnormal.

be caused by surgical incisions, skin tears and wounds, trauma, insect bites or stings, and animal or human bites. Preexisting skin conditions such as stasis ulcers, dermatitides (eczema, psoriasis, contact dermatitis), viral skin infections (herpes simplex, herpes zoster, or varicella zoster), superficial bacterial infections (acne, folliculitis), and bullous diseases (bullous pemphigoid, pemphigus vulgaris, burns) all have the potential for secondary bacterial infection. The likelihood and severity of cellulitis is affected by three important factors: (1) virulence of the pathogen, (2) host immune status, and (3) depth of infection.

Risk factors that predispose an individual to cellulitis include the following conditions that affect cellular immunity and lymphatic drainage:

- Diabetes mellitus
- Lymphatic blockage
- History of recurrent cellulitis
- Postmastectomy
- Postsaphenous vein grafting
- HIV infection and AIDS
- Chronic steroid use
- Cancer chemotherapy
- Drug or alcohol abuse
- Peripheral vascular disease

PATHOPHYSIOLOGY

The skin and subcutaneous tissue respond to bacterial invasion with an acute inflammatory process. An increase in vascular permeability of the microcirculation of the skin allows protein-rich fluids to leak into the interstitial tissue. This results in tissue edema, which may become chronic in recurrent cellulitis. Agents that are released into the tissue and increase vascular permeability include histamine, cytokines, platelet-activating factor, bradykinin, complement proteins, and arachidonic acid metabolites, including leukotrienes and prostaglandins. Vasodilation also occurs, giving cellulitis its characteristic bright red color and indistinct borders. In addition, during the cellular phase of inflammation, leukocytes accumulate at the site of injury and engulf particulate material such as bacteria, cellular debris, and antigen–antibody complexes. Engulfed bacteria and other cellular debris are digested inside phagolysosomes by potent hydrolytic enzymes. Interestingly, the bacterial burden in cellulitis may be low, except in cases where abscesses or skin ulcers are present.

The most predominant leukocyte during the cellular inflammatory phase is the PMN (or neutrophil) and, to a lesser extent, basophils, mast cells, and platelets. PMNs express at least three types of granules containing proteolytic enzymes. Necrosis of normal tissue may occur during the inflammatory process due to these proteolytic enzymes and reactive oxygen metabolites. Some aggressive cases of cellulitis may progress to TSS in which certain strains of *Staphylococcus* and *Streptococcus* produce toxins that stimulate a massive release of inflammatory cytokines. This in turn can result in shock, multiorgan failure, and ultimately death if untreated. In addition, bacterial exotoxins have been shown to potentiate hypersensitivity responses to fungal antigens such as *Trichophyton,* the primary agent involved in tinea pedis or "athlete's foot" infection. Such responses have been shown to contribute to the pathogenesis of cellulitis in certain individuals.

CLINICAL PRESENTATION

Subjective

The typical adult patient with cellulitis will complain of a tender, warm, and erythematous area of skin that is usually located on the face, neck, or extremities. The patient will usually report a precipitating condition such as an insect bite or small cut that "got infected." The patient might already have a preexisting skin condition such as acne, tinea pedis, or chronic eczema with breaks in the skin that serve as the portal of entry for bacteria, although this may not be apparent to the patient. In cases of recurrent cellulitis of the lower leg, the patient will frequently deny any trauma or injury but will report a history of repeated infections on the same leg. The size of involvement can vary from a few centimeters to a larger area, including the entire limb. The patient will report a history of the lesion or plaque getting progressively larger over several days, but in the case of necrotizing fasciitis, the border will literally spread in just a matter of hours. Some cellulitis patients will complain of tender and enlarged lymph nodes near the affected area. Patients with more severe cases of cellulitis or with specific types such as necrotizing fasciitis, erysipelas, and periorbital cellulitis are more likely to complain of systemic symptoms such as fever and chills, lethargy, and malaise.

Objective

In adults, the lower leg is usually the most common site of infection. In cases of lower extremity cellulitis, the clinician should search for signs of tinea pedis and areas of macerated or peeling skin in the interdigital areas of the toes. A chronic tinea pedis ("athlete's foot") infection can become a point of entry for bacteria. In children, and occasionally in adults, the cheeks and the periorbital area are common sites of involvement. In lighter-skinned patients, the area of infected skin will have a bright red color that is warm and tender to touch. In darker-skinned patients, the color will be a darker red. Sometimes extensive edema will be present, especially if the arm or leg is involved.

The red borders seen in cellulitis are flat and diffuse, compared with the distinct raised border seen with an erysipelas infection. Serious signs of systemic toxicity to look for include high fever, hypotension, tachycardia, marked leukocytosis, and associated lymphangitis. If these signs are present, the patient must be treated aggressively with hospitalization and parenteral antibiotics. Referral to a physician is recommended for severe or certain highly morbid cases of cellulitis, as described earlier.

DIAGNOSTIC REASONING

Diagnostic Tests

Most cases of mild to moderate cellulitis are diagnosed by clinical presentation and history. In most cases of acute cellulitis, there is usually no discharge or obvious wound present; therefore, obtaining cultures is difficult. If an open wound or purulent discharge is present, a culture and Gram stain should be obtained. For patients who appear ill or have systemic symptoms such as fever, a CBC and consultation with a physician is necessary. If periorbital cellulitis is suspected due to swelling and redness of the eyelids, limited spontaneous extraocular movements (EOMs), or fever, formal testing for the full range of EOMs should be done, along with other tests of cranial nerve function. Leukocytosis is seen in periorbital cellulitis, as well as in necrotizing fasciitis and erysipelas.

Differential Diagnosis

The site of the infection helps guide the clinician in searching for a differential diagnosis. If a lower limb is affected, deep vein thrombosis (DVT) should be considered. It may be difficult to make the distinction between DVT and cellulitis. DVT presents as a swollen and warm limb with erythema that is tender to the touch and can be similar in presentation to acute cellulitis. A history of recent surgery, bedrest, or prolonged immobility points more toward DVT; however, DVT can also occur after cellulitis, although rarely. There are usually no systemic symptoms such as fever associated with DVT. If fever is present, it points more toward a diagnosis of cellulitis. If crepitus is noted on palpation or if violaceous bullae and intense pain are present, the clinician should rule out necrotizing fasciitis. Serious systemic symptoms that point to severe infection include hypotension, lethargy (or any change in mental status), nausea and vomiting, severe pain (which points to possible fascial involvement), and a toxic appearance. If these signs are present, immediate consultation with a physician or referral to the emergency department is necessary.

MANAGEMENT

Treatment of cellulitis should take into consideration several factors: severity of the infection, site of the infection, presence of underlying disease, and virulence of the pathogen. Patients with diabetes are known to have a higher incidence of complications from skin infections because of chronic hyperglycemia that adversely affects the immune system and the microcirculation. Patients who are under long-term treatment with corticosteroids or chemotherapy are also at increased risk because of immune system depression. Previous surgical procedures, such as a mastectomy or saphenous vein graft, predispose the affected limb to cellulitis because of defective lymphatic drainage. Some sites of the body, such as the hands, feet, and the face, must be treated more aggressively to prevent any potential loss of future function. Particular care must be taken with soft-tissue infections of the hand because a compartment-like syndrome can ensue, in addition to destruction of complex structures.

Human bite wounds are known to have a higher rate of infection because of the large amounts of anaerobic bacteria present in the mouth. Because of increased vascularity, the face and neck areas are less likely to become infected than the hands and feet. Closed-fist injuries of the hand are more likely to become infected, probably because exposed tendons and tissue that become contaminated with oral flora (during a punch to the mouth) retract back into the skin under anaerobic conditions and allow bacteria to proliferate. Cat bites (30% to 50%) are more likely to become infected (with *Pasteurella multocida*) than human bites. To a lesser extent, some dog bites (only 5%) become infected with *P. multocida* or *Capnocytophaga canimorsus*. In addition, any injury that occurs in salty or brackish water has the potential for infection with *Vibrio* species of bacteria. Periorbital cellulitis is potentially life-threatening and should be regarded as an emergent condition. It is seen more commonly in children than in adults.

Although *Streptococcus* and *Staphylococcus* cause most cases of skin infections, it is still important to establish the specific etiology of any infection. If purulent discharge or an open wound is present, a culture and Gram stain should be obtained. Because it is difficult to culture most cases of cellulitis, diagnosis is based mostly on clinical presentation. Empirical treatment for cellulitis must provide good coverage for both *Staphylococcus* and *Streptococcus*. Good choices for uncomplicated cases of cellulitis that are not associated with human or animal bites include penicillin VK, dicloxacillin, clindamycin, or cephalexin for 5 days or longer if insufficient improvement is seen over the first several days of therapy.

Patients with penicillin allergy are prescribed clindamycin, azithromycin, or clarithromycin. Infected human and animal (cat or dog) bites are best treated with amoxicillin–clavulanic acid (Augmentin) for at least 2 weeks. Physician consultation or referral is recommended in complicated cases of cellulitis. Prophylaxis (not treatment) for fresh, uncomplicated human and animal bites (less than 6 hours old) to prevent infection is amoxicillin–clavulanic acid for 3 to 5 days.

Management of cellulitis infection of the lower extremities requires bedrest (with bathroom privileges) and elevation of the infected leg. Patients who are at increased risk of thrombus formation should be referred to a physician for possible anticoagulation therapy.

Erysipelas is treated in the hospital with parenteral antibiotics. Necrotizing fasciitis is a medical emergency and must be treated aggressively in the hospital with parenteral antibiotics, surgical debridement, and fluid replacement.

Patients with underlying diseases such as AIDS, diabetes, alcoholism/injection drug use, neuropathy, arterial insufficiency, lymphatic drainage abnormalities, intermittent claudication, a history of recent trauma of the same affected body part, or those who are receiving chemotherapy or chronic corticosteroids are more prone to complications of cellulitis and infection with unusual bacterial pathogens (e.g., gram-negative bacteria, anaerobes) and must be treated more aggressively. These cases frequently require referral and consideration for hospitalization. Unusual pathogens that may cause cellulitis include *E. coli, Klebsiella, Enterobacter,* and *Pseudomonas,* which are more common in patients with impaired immune systems. Cellulitis of vital structures such as the hand, foot, or face also requires close follow-up.

Patients suspected of having a complicated case of cellulitis, including, for example, bacteremia (with fever and chills), periorbital cellulitis, necrotizing fasciitis, or erysipelas, require immediate consultation with a physician or referral to an emergency department. The clinician should not rely solely on laboratory results (such as leukocytosis) to diagnose a serious cellulitis infection because clinical presentation and symptoms are more helpful in guiding the management of cellulitis than any laboratory test result.

For oral therapy, cefuroxime (Ceftin) can be used when *Haemophilus influenzae* is suspected. Azithromycin or clarithromycin is preferred as a macrolide over erythromycin for penicillin-allergic patients with suspected *H. influenzae*. If gram-negative microorganisms are suspected, fluoroquinolones such as levofloxacin are typically chosen for complicated skin infections in adult patients. Clindamycin may be added to extend the spectrum of gram-positive coverage. Importantly, however, *Clostridium difficile* colitis is associated with clindamycin usage. *Vibrio* infections from seawater-associated injuries are best treated with doxycycline plus ceftazidime, whereas cellulitis related to freshwater injuries must cover *Aeromonas* infection and include a fluoroquinolone such as ciprofloxacin combined with doxycycline. Diabetics are typically treated with Augmentin, although this may produce significant gastrointestinal effects such as loose stools. Table 14.2 lists medications used for pharmacologic management of skin and soft-tissue infections in primary care.

Other broad-based regimens for hospitalized patients with moderate infections include IV penicillin, clindamycin, cefazolin, or ceftriaxone. For severe infections, vancomycin with either piperacillin-tazobactam or a carbapenem such as imipenem or meropenem is recommended. If tinea pedis infection is concurrent with cellulitis, treatment for this must be initiated using terbinafine or itraconazole (covered in Chapter 13). For information on community-acquired MRSA infection, refer to the previous discussion about furuncles and carbuncles regarding selected oral agents, such as TMP-SMX (Bactrim). For more serious MRSA infections, IV vancomycin may be used.

FOLLOW-UP AND REFERRAL

Most cases of uncomplicated cellulitis resolve with adequate antibiotic treatment. Improvement is usually obvious within 48 hours, although some cases might take 72 hours before improvement is seen. If the patient is responding to treatment, follow-up can be done on an outpatient basis. Recurrent infections of cellulitis on a lower extremity can result in chronic nonpitting edema, and the patient should be advised of this potential complication. Diabetic patients should be advised to adhere to dietary and lifestyle changes (in addition to diabetic medications) to control their blood glucose levels. Consistent diabetic control is associated with fewer and less serious complications of infection, including potential vascular, kidney, or eye damage.

Initial follow-up for cellulitis should be done within 48 hours or sooner for sicker patients. Improvement in signs and symptoms should be seen, including a decrease in swelling, erythema, and pain of the affected area. The borders of erythema should be receding and

TABLE 14.2 Pharmacologic Management of Skin and Soft-Tissue Infections in Primary Care

Purulent (Furuncle/Carbuncle/Abscess)	Nonpurulent (Cellulitis/Erysipelas /Necrotizing Infection)
Mild* Incision and drainage	*Mild** Oral treatment: Penicillin VK *or* Cephalosporin *or* Dicloxacillin *or* Clindamycin

Moderate**
 Incision and drainage
 Culture and sensitivities
 Empirical treatment:
   Trimethoprim-sulfamethoxazole *or* doxycycline
 Defined treatment:
   MRSA: trimethoprim-sulfamethoxazole
   MSSA: dicloxacillin *or* cephalexin
	Moderate**
	 Emergency department referral for IV antibiotic treatment

Severe*** Requires immediate physician consultation/emergency department referral for hospitalization and IV antibiotic treatment	*Severe**** Emergency department/surgical referral for evaluation/debridement

Abbreviations: MRSA, methicillin-resistant *Staphylococcus aureus*; MSSA, methicillin-sensitive *Staphylococcus aureus*.
Purulent: *Mild infection—no systemic signs of infection; **Moderate infection—systemic signs of infection (temperature >38°C, tachycardia, tachypnea, white blood cell count >12,000 cells/mcL), immunocompromised; ***Severe infection—systemic signs of infection; no improvement with incision and drainage and oral antibiotic treatment.
Nonpurulent: *Mild infection—cellulitis, erysipelas with no purulence; **Moderate infection: systemic signs of infection; ***Severe infection: systemic signs of infection; no improvement with oral antibiotic treatment; immunocompromised; signs of deep infection (e.g., bullae, sloughing of skin), ↑ blood pressure, organ failure.
Source: Stevens DL, Bisno AL, Chambers HF, et al. Practice guidelines for the diagnosis and management of skin and soft tissue infections: 2014 update by the Infectious Diseases Society of America. *Clin Infect Dis.* 2014;59(2):e10–e52.

getting smaller at follow-up. The clinician can use a marking pen (with the patient's permission) to mark some of the borders during the initial visit; this will make any changes in size easier to notice at subsequent follow-up visits. If the patient's response is satisfactory, the next follow-up visit is usually done in 1 week (or sooner, if closer follow-up is necessary). Thereafter, the patient can be seen on a weekly basis until the cellulitis is largely resolved.

If the patient does not respond to treatment with oral antibiotics after 48 to 72 hours or starts to appear toxic, a CBC and consultation with a physician (or referral to the emergency department) is necessary.

Patient Education: Cellulitis

The clinician should instruct the patient to call his or her health-care provider if the infection worsens or if fever persists despite antibiotic treatment for at least 48 hours. The patient should also call the clinic in 3 days to report the progress of uncomplicated cellulitis. The patient should be advised to elevate the affected limb as much as possible to decrease swelling. If the patient has chronic tinea pedis ("athlete's foot"), an OTC antifungal powder or spray should be used daily to prevent a recurrence of secondary infection with bacteria.

REFERENCES

General

Burns DA, Breathnach SM, Cox N, Griffiths CEM. *Rook's textbook of dermatology.* 8th ed.; 4 vols. New York, NY: John Wiley & Sons; 2013.

Shiferaw T, Beyene G, Kassa T, Sewunet T. Bacterial contamination, bacterial profile and antimicrobial susceptibility pattern of isolates from stethoscopes at Jimma University Specialized Hospital. *Ann Clin Microbiol Antimicrob.* 2013;12:39.

Cellulitis

Herchline TE. Cellulitis. Medscape drugs and diseases. http://emedicine.medscape.com/article214222. Updated August 15, 2016. Accessed June 7, 2017.

Erysipelas

Davis, L. Erysipelas. Medscape drugs and diseases. http://emedicine.medscape.com/article/1052445. Updated June 29, 2016. Accessed June 7, 2017.

Folliculitis

Satter EK. Folliculitis treatment and management. Medscape drugs and diseases. http://emedicine.medscape.com/article/1070456. Updated March 23, 2017. Accessed June 2, 2017.

Impetigo

Hartman-Adams H, Banvard C, Juckett, G. Impetigo: Diagnosis and treatment. *Am Fam Physician.* 2014;90(4):229–235.

Lewis LS. Impetigo treatment and management. Medscape drugs and diseases. http://emedicine.medscape.com/article/965254-treatment#aw2aab6b6b3. Updated May 04, 2016. Accessed April 27, 2017.

Necrotizing Fasciitis

Edlich RF. Necrotizing fasciitis. Medscape drugs and diseases. http://emedicine.medscape.com/article/2051157. Updated April 14, 2017. Accessed June 9, 2017.

Periorbital Cellulitis

Zonnook, B. Periorbital infections. Medscape drugs and diseases. http://emedicine.medscape.com/article798397. Updated November 22, 2016. Accessed June 9, 2017.

Skin and Soft-Tissue Infections

Stevens DL, Bisno AL, Chambers HF, et al. Practice guidelines for the diagnosis and management of skin and soft tissue infections: 2014 update by the Infectious Diseases Society of America. *Clin Infect Dis.* 2014;59(2):e10-e52.

RESOURCES

American Academy of Dermatology
　　www.aad.org
Centers for Disease Control and Prevention
　　www.cdc.gov
National Institute of Allergy and Infectious Disease
　　www.niaid.nih.gov
National Institutes of Health
　　www.nih.gov

Others

American Society of Dermatology
　　www.asd.org
Information on dermatological drugs
　　www.nsc.gov.sg/brochures.html

Chapter 15

Viral Skin Infections

Susan Garnett, MSN, APRN, FNP-BC

Jill E. Winland-Brown, EdD, APRN, FNP-BC

Brian Oscar Porter, MD, PhD, MPH, MBA

WARTS

Warts (verruca vulgaris, plantar warts, flat warts) are contagious skin lesions formed by infected keratinocytes, caused by human papillomavirus (HPV). Warts are identified based on their morphology (flat, mosaic, digitate, or filiform) or anatomical location (e.g., the plantar, anogenital, or palmar areas).

EPIDEMIOLOGY AND CAUSES

Warts are a common skin disease throughout the world. Infection is more prevalent in children, with the highest incidence between the ages of 12 and 16 years. Individuals who walk barefoot, handle raw meat as an occupation, and/or bite their nails are at increased risk of acquiring warts. In addition, children and teens who use public showers and pools have a greater risk of developing warts, as do those with family members and schoolmates who have warts. Immunosuppression is an additional risk factor, as is having a preexisting atopic condition such as eczema (atopic dermatitis). Warts occur equally in men and women and in all ethnicities; however, common warts occur with twice the frequency among Caucasians compared with all ethnicities.

HPV is a small, double-stranded DNA virus that infects epithelial cells and causes hyperproliferation of these cells. HPV is species specific and infects only humans, with a particular tropism for epithelial cells (such as keratinocytes) and the mucous membranes. There are more than 150 genetically distinct HPVs (including HPV subunits) that are distinguished as separate serotypes. Common warts (verruca vulgaris) are primarily caused by HPV serotypes 1 to 5, 7, 27, or 29, whereas HPV serotypes 3, 10, 28, and 29 cause flat warts. HPV serotypes 1 to 4, 27, 29, and 57 typically causes plantar warts, whereas HPV serotypes 6 and 11 cause anogenital warts. Certain HPV serotypes are also associated with anogenital malignancies, including cervical intraepithelial neoplasia and invasive cervical cancers. Oncogenicity of HPV appears to be determined by the viral gene products E6 and E7 proteins, which are necessary for host cell immortalization. HPV serotypes 6 and 11 are considered either inactive or weakly capable of transformation, whereas E6 and E7 proteins in HPV serotypes 16 and 18 are capable of producing progressive squamous epithelial neoplasia in experimental studies with mice.

In general, HPV and resultant warts can be transmitted by touch, by trauma to skin tissue such as from nail biting or shaving, and by fomites. HPV enters through breaks in the skin or mucosa. Viral particles contained within skin cells serve as the vehicle for person-to-person transmission. Plantar warts occur at points of maximum pressure (e.g., at the heads of metatarsal bones and heels) as a thick, painful callus forms in response to the pressure. Anogenital warts are usually transmitted by genital-to-genital contact; penetrative intercourse is not necessary for transmission.

PATHOPHYSIOLOGY

Warts consist of infected keratinocytes, which form a mass in the epidermis that does not extend into the dermis or subcutaneous layers. It is a common misconception that warts have roots, as the underside of a wart is usually smooth and round. Several types of warts form tightly fused cylindrical projections resulting in a uniform mosaic pattern that is unique to warts. This pattern is a useful diagnostic sign. The black dots seen on the surface of common warts are thrombosed capillaries that become trapped in the cylindrical, fingerlike projections.

CLINICAL PRESENTATION

Subjective

Patients typically complain of a wart or small "bump" (or group of bumps) that has been present for several weeks to many months and sometimes for years. Some patients report the same wart being treated before and then recurring in the same area. Many adult patients with common warts attempt self-treatment with over-the-counter (OTC) wart remedies with limited to no success. Warts are usually asymptomatic but may be cosmetically undesirable. Plantar warts may cause discomfort with weight-bearing.

Objective

Warts are small or large, fleshy or firm growths or lumps, which can be raised, fairly flat, single, or multiple, isolated, or clustered together to form a cauliflower-like shape. There are no skin lines crossing the surface, and examination with a hand lens reveals centrally located capillaries (black dots) that bleed with paring.

Varieties of warts include common warts (verruca vulgaris), filiform warts, flat warts (verruca planae), periungual warts, plantar warts, and deep palmoplantar warts. Common warts initially begin as smooth, flesh-colored papules. As they grow, they become dome-shaped, gray-brown hyperkeratotic masses with black dots on the surface. Although common warts can be found on any part of the body, the hands and knees are the most frequent sites of involvement. Filiform and digitae warts are fingerlike, flesh-colored projections that protrude from a narrow or broad base, usually on the face. Flat warts (verruca planae) are small (0.1–0.3 cm), slightly elevated, flat-topped papules. They are usually numerous and involve the forehead, mouth, chin, eyes, back of hands, shins, and shaved areas. Scratching may produce a line of flat warts on shaved surfaces. Flat warts range in color from pink or light brown to light yellow.

Deep palmoplantar warts occur on the plantar surfaces of the hands and around or under the fingernails. They extend deeper than other warts and are, therefore, more painful. Mosaic warts are a group of plantar warts that form a plaque. Plantar warts occur at the heads of metatarsal bones and the heels (i.e., points of maximal pressure), appearing as thick, painful calluses. This may lead to repositioning of the foot while walking, causing a distortion in posture as well as producing pain in other parts of the foot, leg, or back.

Cutaneous HPV infections (serotypes 1, 2, 4, and 7) are more likely to be seen in children and young adults, with an incubation period of 2 to 6 months. As an individual reaches adulthood, the prevalence of cutaneous warts decreases, probably because of improved host immunity. Because these infections are usually benign, they are rarely brought to the attention of health-care providers. HPV serotypes 5 and 8 are closely linked with a rare form of hereditary skin cancer called epidermodysplasia verruciformis.

DIAGNOSTIC REASONING

Diagnostic Tests

If the clinician is unable to distinguish the lesion as a wart, a small specimen can be sent to the laboratory for identification.

Differential Diagnosis

Corns may be mistaken for warts and can be differentiated from warts by paring them with a number 15 scalpel blade. Skin lines are absent on warts, and the black dots that are interspersed in the center of the wart will bleed with additional paring. Its mosaic pattern can be easily identified under a handheld lens. Whereas corns have a painful, hard, translucent core, warts do not. In addition, the pain in corns is relieved when the hard central kernel is freed from the corn.

It is important to differentiate between the surface of the foot that is healing from a recent trauma and warts (black warts) that are undergoing spontaneous resolution. The black dots (thrombosed capillaries) seen on the plantar surface of a foot that has sustained a shearing injury may be confused with the black color of warts that are healing. It is hypothesized that the black color of warts that are spontaneously healing may be part of the process of regression and may represent a specific cell-mediated immune response to HPV-infected keratinocytes.

MANAGEMENT

There is no known cure for HPV infection. Studies suggest that one-half of warts resolve without treatment within 1 year, and two-thirds resolve within 2 years. Therefore, first-line therapy for new warts is watchful waiting with no treatment. Initial management for established warts should be geared toward relieving pain and pressure and minimizing skin trauma and scarring caused by available therapies. Although filiform and digitate warts are relatively easy to treat, flat warts present a unique therapeutic challenge. Their duration is prolonged, and they may be resistant to treatment. Because flat warts may be located in areas that are cosmetically important, treatment modalities that produce scarring should be avoided. It is important to note that several treatments for warts are contraindicated in pregnant women; however, salicylic acid applied to a small area of the skin for a short duration and liquid nitrogen cryotherapy are considered safe during pregnancy.

The treatment plan must be individualized because available therapies may produce unwanted effects such as pain, hyperpigmentation, scarring, damage to normal tissue, sun sensitivity, chemical sensitization, toxicity, and potential harm to pregnant women. In addition, it is important to identify previous treatment failures and successes, as well as the patient's risk factors (such as immunosuppression or lapses in therapy compliance) that may account for the failure of first-line therapy. Treatment intervals usually range from 1 to 2 weeks, but other patients may require prolonged therapy to eradicate more resistant lesions.

Treating cutaneous warts with a duct tape regimen was previously considered effective; however, recent studies have demonstrated little or no effectiveness with duct tape therapy alone. Duct tape occlusion is still used in combination with salicylic acid and 5-fluorouracil (Efudex 5%) in some treatment regimens. First-line treatments for warts include 17% salicylic acid, as well as cryotherapy with liquid nitrogen.

Pharmacologic Treatments

Keratolytic therapy in the form of salicylic acid plasters (Mediplast) or solution (DuoPlant, Occlusal) is a safe, nonscarring, moderately effective, and low-cost OTC treatment of common warts, which patients can apply at home. First, the wart is pared with a number 15 scalpel blade, pumice stone, or emery board, and then the area is soaked in warm water to soften the surface and to facilitate penetration of the solution. In the case of salicylic acid solution, one drop or more is applied with an applicator to cover the surface of the wart. The surface is allowed to dry and covered with a piece of adhesive tape, duct tape, or bandage. This will enhance the penetration of the solution.

Tape occlusion may precipitate inflammation and soreness and may necessitate periodic interruption of treatment. The patient may prefer to apply the solution at bedtime. Within a few days, a soft white keratin layer will form; this layer should be pared or abraded until pink skin is exposed. This procedure may be better accomplished by an occasional office visit. When applying keratolytic plasters (40% salicylic acid), the patient may use the same procedure. The plaster is more useful when treating mosaic warts (i.e., a large cluster of warts). Once the plaster is cut to the size of the wart, the backing is removed, and the adhesive surface is attached to the wart and secured with adhesive tape. The plaster should be removed in 24 to 48 hours, and the surface should be pared or abraded as outlined earlier; a new plaster should then be applied to the area. Although this treatment may take several weeks to fully treat the wart, it is less irritating than salicylic acid solution.

Chemicals such as bichloracetic acid (BCA) or trichloroacetic acid (TCA) are caustic agents that destroy warts by chemical coagulation of the proteins. These chemicals are frequently used for recurrent warts or sometimes as initial therapy. The clinician should pare the excess calloused skin and apply petrolatum to the surrounding area before applying the acid with a cotton-tipped applicator. BCA or TCA should be applied sparingly because both are caustic agents that can damage adjacent normal tissue. These acids are self-neutralizing, but any excess amount can be wiped away with gauze. Repeat applications may be necessary every 7 to 10 days. A change of therapy should be considered if the patient has not improved substantially after three provider visits or if the warts have not cleared after six treatments.

Verruca plana (flat warts) are especially difficult to treat. Treatment includes applying tretinoin cream 0.025%, 0.05%, or 1% (Retin-A) at bedtime over the entire area, applied twice daily for 4 to 6 weeks. The frequency of application should be adjusted to elicit a fine scaling and mild erythema. If other treatment options fail, 5-fluorouracil (Efudex 5%) can be applied with tape occlusion one or two times a day for 3 to 5 weeks. Hyperpigmentation and recurrent warts at the site of inflammation are limitations of this therapy.

Podophyllin resin 10% to 25% in a compound tincture of benzoin can be used for external warts. Because of the potential complications associated with systemic absorption and toxicity, it is recommended that the treatment area be limited to 10 cm per session, using 0.5 mL or less of solution. To minimize irritation, the area should be allowed to dry and then washed off 1 to 4 hours after application. Podophyllin is not used for cervical warts or dysplasia and is primarily reserved for exophytic lesions. It is contraindicated for use by pregnant or lactating women.

Surgical Treatments

Although cryosurgery with liquid nitrogen is effective for common and genital warts, it may produce severe pain around the palms, feet, and nail areas. Thermal injury to nerve tissue, epithelial cells, and melanocytes can occur and cause changes in pigmentation. Therefore, light applications of liquid nitrogen are preferable. More aggressive applications have been shown to be more effective; however, they may also cause more pain and blistering. Liquid nitrogen can be stored in 1- to 2-gallon tanks for approximately 10 days. Applications can be repeated every 1 to 2 weeks. OTC home-based cryotherapy kits are now available without a prescription for use on small, isolated warts in easily accessible areas, such as the hands and fingers. Directions for these kits must be followed closely to avoid damage to surrounding normal skin and tissue. These kits should not be used for warts located in highly sensitive areas, such as the face or genitalia; consultation with a health-care provider is warranted in such cases.

Surgical techniques such as blunt dissection or electrosurgery usually render patients wart free with a single visit; however, scarring may result and recurrence has been reported. Additional clinical training, equipment, and longer patient visits are necessary for these procedures. Blunt dissection is relatively painless if performed on areas other than the plantar or palmar surface. After preparation with local anesthesia, a plane of dissection is established by inserting the tip of a pair of blunt-tipped scissors between the wart and normal skin. The wart is cut circumferentially and the lesion is separated from the normal tissue with short, firm strokes. After the lesion is removed, the blunt dissector is moved firmly back and forth over the area of excision, to ensure that no tissue fragments remain. Liquid nitrogen should be applied to the base using a cotton-tipped applicator. Liquid nitrogen will destroy any remaining virus. Table 15.1 summarizes various treatment strategies for warts.

FOLLOW-UP AND REFERRAL

For the majority of common wart cases, a satisfactory response occurs after several treatments. For warts that are unresponsive or are recalcitrant to treatment, more aggressive treatment options are available, which are best administered by a dermatologist.

TABLE 15.1 Treatment of Warts

Type of Wart	*Description*	*Treatment Considerations*
Common warts (verruca vulgaris)	Small, hardened growths of keratinized tissue. Warts usually grow around nails, on fingers, and the backs of hands, but can appear anywhere on the body.	• Salicylic acid solution/plasters • Cryotherapy with liquid nitrogen • Surgical excision
Flat warts (verruca plana)	Pink, light brown, or yellow; slightly elevated papules: 0.1–0.3 cm. Numerous sites: mouth, forehead, backs of hands, shaved areas (e.g., legs or beard area); may recur despite treatment. Frequently undergo spontaneous remission.	• May resolve without treatment • Avoid potentially scarring therapies • Tretinoin cream 0.025%, 0.05%, or 0.1%. Apply to involved areas daily; adjust treatment to produce fine scaling and mild erythema; may require weeks to months • Cryotherapy with liquid nitrogen • 5-fluorouracil (Efudex 5%) once or twice daily for 3–5 weeks. Produces dramatic results, but may produce persistent hyperpigmentation (use ointment to minimize this adverse effect)
Filiform/digitate warts	Fingerlike, flesh-colored projections emanating from a narrow or broad base. Common sites include the mouth, eyes, and ala nasi.	• Easiest to treat, but recur • Shaving spreads the lesions • Retract skin and use curette drawn across base to remove wart • May use light electrocautery • Cryotherapy with liquid nitrogen
Plantar warts	Lesions appear at maximum point of pressure (e.g., heads of metatarsal bones or heels) or anywhere on plantar surface; a thick, painful callus forms around lesion. Pain is elicited on indirect pressure.	• More refractory to treatment • Remove surrounding callus with pumice stone or paring, after soaking feet in warm water to soften skin • Daily application of salicylic acid liquid, film, or plaster after soaking
Black warts	Warts become black when spontaneously healing; black heel caused by sheared capillaries usually associated with trauma.	• Confirm spontaneous healing • Differential diagnosis for black heel: normal skin lines present; when area is pared with no. 15 blade, skin underneath is soft and bleeds
Oral warts	Can be located on hard/soft palate or oral mucosa. Usually transmitted through oral–genital contact.	• Cryotherapy with liquid nitrogen • Surgical excision

Intralesional administration of interferon (natural or recombinant) is more effective than systemic treatment. The Centers for Disease Control and Prevention (CDC) does not recommend this treatment as first-line therapy because of the need for frequent office visits and the high frequency of systemic side effects. In addition, the cure rate is similar to that of other available therapies.

When other treatments fail, intralesional bleomycin sulfate may be considered. Bleomycin is mixed with 5 mL of sterile water and 10 mL of lidocaine to form a solution, and then this solution is reconstituted with normal saline. Using a 30-gauge needle, the solution is injected into the lesion to achieve blanching. The size of the wart will determine the amount of solution injected. Larger warts may require repeat injections. Leakage of the solution is unavoidable during the procedure. The cure rate is 48% (for plantar warts) to 71% (for periungual warts). A multiple-puncture method can result in a 92% cure rate. Responsive warts produce hemorrhagic eschars that heal without scarring.

Intralesional injection of a skin antigen such as candida or mumps has been shown to be effective in the treatment of recalcitrant warts. Pretesting is recommended to demonstrate an immune response prior to attempting treatment.

Another treatment modality that has been reported to be effective for refractory warts is photodynamic therapy with aminolevulinic acid, a photosensitizer. This treatment is costly and administered only by dermatologists. The need for referral to a dermatologist is determined by several factors, including a lack of response to standard treatments, possible cosmetic consequences (especially with warts on the face and eyelids), and the clinician's knowledge, experience, and comfort in identifying and treating specific types of warts. If the clinician is unsure of the diagnosis or if the wart is resistant to multiple treatments, the patient should be referred to a dermatologist.

There have been isolated anecdotal reports of seemingly coincidental remission of cutaneous warts following administration of HPV vaccine (Gardasil). Prospective randomized and controlled clinical trials are needed to establish whether the HPV vaccine may provide preventive or therapeutic solutions for cutaneous warts.

Patient Education: Warts

The clinician should educate the patient on the prevention of self-inoculation and the routes of transmission for common warts. These measures include limiting shaving of the affected area until warts are eradicated, strategies to control nail biting, and avoidance of scratching and rubbing warts. Wearing protective foot coverings in wet public areas such as showers, locker rooms, and pools and keeping warts dry are additional approaches to prevent infection (Box 15.1).

HERPES SIMPLEX INFECTIONS

Herpes simplex viruses (HSVs) are part of the Herpesviridae family and the Alphaherpesvirinae subfamily. HSV infections are caused by two types of viruses, HSV-1 and HSV-2, and can result in a wide range of clinical manifestations across age groups, depending on location (Table 15.2). HSV-1 is associated primarily with oral infections, whereas HSV-2 is associated mainly with genital infections. HSV-1 genital infections are becoming more common, however, as are HSV-2 oral infections, probably due to oral–genital sexual contact. Herpes viral infections are lifelong; although there are effective antiviral medications for outbreaks, to date there is no known cure. Clinical studies on the development of herpes virus vaccines and topical microbicides are ongoing.

Box 15.1   Basic Patient Information About Warts

About the Disease

- Warts are small growths or tumors produced by infection of normal skin tissue by human papillomavirus (HPV). The most common areas where warts are found include the plantar and palmar surfaces, nailbeds, hands, face, mouth, penis, vulva, cervix, and anus.
- One in four people are infected with HPV. Despite treatment, most warts will recur. Broken or abraded skin may facilitate transport of the virus. Lesions can be spread by skin-to-skin contact, including touch, vigorous rubbing, shaving, nail biting, and sexual intercourse.
- Contrary to popular belief, warts do not have roots. The underside of a wart is smooth and round. The black dots found in the center of a wart represent broken small blood vessels (capillaries).
- Strategies to prevent spreading warts:
  Avoid touching warts.
  Avoid nail biting.
  Wear waterproof foot coverings in public showers, locker rooms, and around pools.
  Keep warts dry, as wetness facilitates spreading.
- Immunosuppression caused by diseases such as HIV or cancer, organ transplantation with antirejection therapy, and certain medications may reduce the efficacy of treatment. Cigarette smoking weakens the immune system and enhances the expression of HPV; therefore, smoking should be discontinued.

About Treatments

- For self-management of warts at home, refer to the American Academy of Dermatology for video instructions: https://www.aad.org/public/diseases/contagious-skin-diseases/warts.

- Treatment often involves more than one session at 1- to 2-week intervals, and therapy may be prolonged.
- To minimize inflammation, do not apply medicated solutions, ointments, gels, creams, or plasters beyond the recommended duration.
- Cryotherapy may be available in a doctor's office or as an OTC wart freezing and removal kit for home use. Directions must be followed closely with home-based kits to avoid excessive damage to normal surrounding tissue.
- To improve efficacy, plasters should be cut to the size of the wart and kept in place with an adhesive for 24 to 48 hours. Pare or use a pumice stone to abrade the area and then reapply the plaster. The process may take several weeks to produce results.
- Podophyllin is applied only to external warts, and the area of application should be limited to 10 cm per session. To minimize irritation, the area should be allowed to dry and washed off after 1 to 4 hours of therapy.
- Caustic acids, such as bichloracetic acid or trichloracetic acid, are very effective but may damage normal tissue if not allowed to dry properly. Repeat applications may be necessary every 7 to 10 days.
- With any topical treatment, wash the treated area after the recommended waiting period, and always check for signs and symptoms of infection, such as pus, severe pain, heat, redness, and swelling.
- For mild to moderate pain, take OTC analgesics.
- Pursue stress reduction activities, such as exercise, imagery, biofeedback, meditation, and yoga, and maintain a healthy diet. Decreasing stress will boost the immune system and improve healing, as well as reduce the desire to smoke, overeat, and nail bite.

TABLE 15.2 Herpes Simplex Infections

Infection	Location	Commonly Affected Age Group
Oral–labial herpes simplex	Lips, oral cavity	Children age 2–5 years, adults
Herpetic keratoconjunctivitis	Eyelids, periorbital area, cornea	Newborns, adults
Herpetic tracheobronchitis	Pharynx, trachea, bronchi	Older adults
Herpes simplex encephalitis	Temporal lobe of the brain	Any age, primarily immunocompromised adults
Herpes gladiatorum	Shoulder, neck, knuckles, areas of contact	Age 14 years and older (commonly seen in wrestlers)
Herpetic whitlow	Fingertip	Age 1 year and older
Lumbosacral herpes	Trunk or back	Adult
Herpes simplex of the buttocks	Buttocks	Adult women
Genital herpes	Labia minora, labia majora, vagina, cervix, urethra, penis, rectal area	Young and older adults, 1% of pregnant women
Eczema herpeticum	Face or any area of active or recently healed atopic dermatitis	Infants, children, and adults, commonly with a history of atopic dermatitis
Erythema multiforme	Extremities, palms, soles of feet	Age 20–30 years; more commonly seen in men than women

EPIDEMIOLOGY AND CAUSES

Both types of HSV produce identical patterns of infection. The World Health Organization (WHO) estimates that 3.7 billion people worldwide are infected with HSV-1 and 417 million people worldwide have HSV-2. The WHO further estimates that 67% of people younger than age 50 years are infected with HSV-1. According to the CDC, about 50 million people in the United States are thought to be infected with HSV-2, and there are 776,000 new cases of HSV-2 each year. The prevalence of HSV-2 in women is nearly double that of men, with a 48% prevalence in black women in particular. People with HSV-2 are also three times more likely to acquire HIV. HSV is not a nationally reportable infection; thus, most people do not know they have HSV infection.

PATHOPHYSIOLOGY

HSV infection has two phases: primary infection and secondary or recurrent infection. During the primary infection, the virus enters keratinocytes in the epidermis, eventually migrating to nerve endings. The virus then ascends via peripheral nerves to the dorsal root ganglion, where it enters a latent stage without active viral replication, which can last for days to years. The trigeminal ganglia are the targets of oral herpes strains, whereas the sacral ganglia are the targets of genital herpes strains. Infection of the ganglia may occur within 24 hours of initial viral exposure and is essentially lifelong.

The majority of primary infections with HSV-1 and HSV-2 are subclinical and asymptomatic, and most HSV transmission occurs during periods of asymptomatic viral shedding. The severity of the viral infection increases with age, and herpes infection may markedly compromise nutritional intake in the elderly. HSV is spread by direct contact with active lesions, saliva, semen, or cervical secretions. Viral replication in the gingival epithelia facilitates oral shedding of the virus.

Symptoms may occur from 2 to 21 days after exposure. Tenderness, pain, mild paresthesias, or burning can occur before the onset of lesions at the site of inoculation. Headache, fever, muscle aches, localized pain, and tender lymphadenopathy may occur as part of the prodrome, although some patients have no prodromal symptoms. Herpes infections may occur anywhere on the skin. After several days, grouped vesicles on an erythematous base appear, followed by ulcers or erosions that crust over with a characteristic honey color. Eventually there is a loss of crusts and reepithelialization occurs. In the moist genital region, crusts may not form; however, exudate may accumulate. Lesions typically heal in 7 to 10 days without scarring but may last up to 6 weeks or longer if they become secondarily infected with bacteria. Vesicles in primary HSV infection are more numerous and scattered than they appear in recurrent infection.

Tissue destruction in HSV infection is mediated directly by viral replication within keratinocytes and other epithelial cells. A mononuclear and lymphocytic cellular infiltrate occurs at sites of infection, consisting primarily of CD4+ T cells early on, but eventually involving equal numbers of CD8+ T cells, as well as macrophages and cytotoxic natural killer cells that attempt to clear infected host cells. The cytokines interferon-γ and interleukin-6 are primary mediators of cytotoxic killing mechanisms. Interestingly, in animal models, nonclassical T cells endogenous to the skin and mucosal surfaces that express γ-δ rather than α-β antigen receptors have been shown to protect against severe mucocutaneous and encephalitic HSV infection.

Recurrent disease typically occurs at or near the site of primary infection. Physical and emotional stress, fever, exposure to ultraviolet light, chapping or abrasion of the skin, immune suppression, menses, or fatigue may cause reactivation of the virus, which descends spontaneously along sensory nerve axons to the skin surface. The anatomical site of infection and virus type affect the frequency of recurrence. Genital herpes recurs six times more frequently than oral–labial herpes. Genital HSV-2 infections recur more frequently than genital HSV-1 infections. However, oral–labial HSV-1 infections recur more often than oral-labial HSV-2 infections.

CLINICAL PRESENTATION

Subjective

HSV infections are usually oral or genital; however, any area of the body can be infected. The most common manifestation of HSV infection is oral–labial herpes (cold sores). Primary infection with HSV may present as herpetic gingivostomatitis in children and young adults, although most commonly children aged 2 to 5 years are affected. The patient may present with fever, sore throat, hypersalivation, and painful vesicles and ulcers on the tongue, palate, gingivae, buccal mucosa, and lips. In genital herpes, early symptoms may include pain in the legs, buttocks, or genital area, genital burning or itching, vaginal discharge, and lower abdominal pressure. Within a few days, lesions appear at the site of infection. With the first episode of genital herpes, fever, headache, muscle aches, painful or difficult urination, and inguinal lymphadenopathy may occur.

In elderly patients, primary infection or reactivation of oral–facial HSV-1 can be extensive. Painful oral lesions make eating difficult and can compromise nutritional status. Superinfection with bacteria or *Candida* may further complicate HSV infection in the elderly. Of major concern in older adults is autoinoculation of the eye, resulting in keratoconjunctivitis, which is the most frequent cause of corneal blindness. Signs and symptoms include unilateral excessive lacrimation, edema, chemosis, photophobia, and purulent exudate. Decreased visual acuity is a poor prognostic sign.

Herpetic whitlow is an HSV infection of the fingertip. This disorder was common among health-care practitioners before the use of gloves in universal precautions. Now, herpetic whitlow is commonly found in children with a recent history of gingivostomatitis and in women with genital herpes. Transmission apparently results from autoinoculation. Vesicles with a red halo may erupt on the finger, and lymphangitis may accompany generalized symptoms of chills, fever, and feeling ill.

A patient with a history of atopic dermatitis who presents with vesicles on the face or areas that have recently healed is likely to have eczema herpeticum. A patient who recently had an HSV infection but now presents with iris-shaped lesions on the palms and soles of the feet most likely has erythema multiforme. HSV lesions on the back are often misdiagnosed as varicella-zoster virus (VZV), and the correct diagnosis is often not made until there is a recurrence. The primary difference on clinical evaluation is that HSV vesicles are uniform in size, whereas varicella-zoster lesions vary in size.

Both HSV-1 and HSV-2 infection can cause encephalitis, in which patients present with an altered level of consciousness, personality changes, fever, and seizures. Patients may also experience olfactory and gustatory (taste) hallucinations and aphasia. Herpetic encephalitis is a medical emergency that requires immediate hospitalization and treatment with IV acyclovir (Zovirax). Herpes infections in immunocompromised patients are more severe, as frequent HSV recurrences often result in chronic and nearly continuous ulcerations. Focus on History lists key questions for eliciting information on HSV infection.

Objective

Lesions must be examined for their characteristic location, appearance, and distribution. Depending on the site of lesions, the anterior and posterior cervical chains, submental or inguinal lymph nodes should be evaluated for lymphadenopathy. Grouped vesicles on an erythematous base occurring in the mouth or on the face or genitals are most likely the result of HSV infection. Vesicles on the eyelid, chemosis, or the presence of corneal dendrites requires prompt referral to an ophthalmologist.

DIAGNOSTIC REASONING

Diagnostic Tests

Viral culture and DNA studies such as polymerase chain reaction (PCR) testing are the standard methods of diagnosis. HSV can be cultured from vesicle fluid or from scrapings at the base of an erosion. Sampling must be done early (during the first 72 hours) in the course of an outbreak. The initial viral culture may be negative, but clinical evaluation and subsequent recurrence with early culture can verify HSV infection. Viral culture differentiates between HSV-1 and HSV-2 with high sensitivity. The Tzanck smear is rapid, easily performed, and can be used to identify multinucleated giant cells in vesicular fluid, before the results of viral cultures becoming available. The Tzanck smear does not, however, differentiate among HSV-1, HSV-2, or VZV and is not considered reliable for this purpose. HSV antibodies can be detected in blood using type-specific serologic tests based on the HSV glycoproteins G1 and G2, and PCR is useful in the diagnosis of central nervous system and systemic infections. However, viral culture remains the gold standard for the diagnosis of HSV infection when there is a lesion to sample.

Because persons with HSV-2 are three times more susceptible to infection with HIV, additional testing for HIV and other sexually transmitted infections is advisable in all HSV-infected patients. The U.S. Preventive Services Task Force does not recommend routine screening for HSV infection.

Focus on History: Herpes Simplex Virus Infections

General Questions

- When did the sores first appear?
- Have you ever had sores on the same area before?
- Before the appearance of the sores, did you experience burning, tingling, pain, or numbness?
- Do you have muscle aches, fever, and/or weakness?
- Are you able to swallow?
- Have you ever had this happen to you before? If so, when and how was it treated?
- Have you been around any person who may have had these same symptoms?
- Do you have a history of any skin problem?

Specific Questions for Genital Herpes

- How old were you at first sexual intercourse?
- How many total sex partners have you had?
- How long have you been with your present sexual partner (if applicable)?
- Have you ever had a sexually transmitted infection or a STD?
- Do you use latex condoms? If so, do you use them correctly and consistently?
- Do you engage in oral sex? Vaginal sex? Anal sex? Are you a man who has sex with other men?
- If you are a woman, have you ever had an abnormal Pap smear?

Differential Diagnosis

History and clinical presentation are the best guide to diagnosis, as several other conditions, both infectious and noninfectious, can mimic HSV infection. Aphthous stomatitis differs from HSV infection in that ulcerations of nonkeratinized mucosa occur. Therefore, lesions rarely appear on the gingivae or hard palate, as do herpetic ulcers. Also, no fever or lymphadenopathy occurs. In addition, an aphthous stomatitis ulcer is usually solitary and larger than a herpetic ulcer. Herpangina can also mimic HSV infection. Herpangina is seen predominantly in children and infrequently in adults; treatment is symptomatic. Hand-foot-and-mouth disease (caused by coxsackievirus) presents with red macules that progress to vesicles on an erythematous base. However, in this infection, the extremities, in particular the hands and feet, as well as the mouth develop lesions. The characteristic target lesions of erythema multiforme can result from a hypersensitivity reaction to HSV or *Mycoplasma* infection or from a drug reaction. Treatment is based on the underlying cause, which may be directed to the infection or by removing exposure to the offending agent. Pemphigus is an autoimmune disorder that usually occurs in middle-aged patients (aged 40 to 60 years) in which erosions of the oral mucosa may mimic HSV infection. However, these are followed by distinctive bullae (large blisters) all over the body, due to the formation of autoantibodies against desmoglein, a protein that mediates attachments between adjacent epidermal cells.

MANAGEMENT

No cure for herpes exists; however, recurrences tend to be milder and of shorter duration than the primary infection. Therapy is primarily symptomatic and supportive, although oral antiviral medications are also used, especially in immunocompromised patients. Nutritional intake is important, especially in elderly patients, who may also benefit from using anesthetic mouth rinses for symptomatic relief. The goals for management include the reduction or elimination of pain, decreased viral shedding, and healing of tissue. In cases of frequent recurrence of herpetic lesions, suppressive therapy may be needed.

Initial therapy is palliative and promotes healing. The primary-care practitioner can initiate management with pharmacotherapy and self-help techniques, based on the location and extent of HSV infection. Acetaminophen can be used to control fever and pain. Lesions on the lip (if small) may require nothing more than applications of ice and lip ointments such as Blistex. OTC docosanol 10% cream (Abreva) applied five times daily may improve lesions. If lesions are more extensive, penciclovir 1% cream (Denavir) applied to the affected area every 2 hours while awake for 4 days promotes healing, shortens the course of the illness by several days, and substantially decreases viral shedding. Extensive oral lesions may require the use of oral anesthetics such as viscous xylocaine 2% (Lidocaine) or dyclonine hydrochloride 0.5% to 1% to control pain. In addition, acyclovir suspension 200 mg/5 mL can be used to treat oral lesions directly by rinsing the mouth with one teaspoon and swallowing five times a day for 7 days.

Initial treatment of genital herpes requires the use of oral antiviral drugs. Valacyclovir and famciclovir have greater bioavailability and require less frequent daily dosing than acyclovir, which makes them preferable. Comfort measures such as warm compresses or an oatmeal sitz bath several times a day can relieve pain and promote healing. A patient with genital or urethral herpes may find it easier to urinate into warm bath water. All patients with HSV infection benefit from increased fluid intake and rest.

The need for subsequent management is based on the recurrence of symptoms. A patient with a negative initial viral culture should be told to return to their primary-care practitioner for another viral culture within the first 72 hours if symptoms recur. After the initial occurrence, a patient with genital herpes can be given a prescription for an antiviral drug and instructed to take the medication should he or she experience the beginning of symptoms in the future, such as tingling or burning at the site of previous lesions. A patient with genital herpes who experiences six or more recurrent episodes per year should be offered suppressive therapy (see Drugs Commonly Prescribed 15.1). Suppressive therapy will reduce recurrences by 70% to 80%, with approximately a 50% reduced risk of transmission. Long-term suppressive therapy is safe, and after a period of 5 to 7 years, many patients discontinue such therapy with no relapses. In addition to suppressive therapy, correct and consistent condom use and abstaining from sexual activity during outbreaks are important to reduce the incidence of HSV transmission.

Pregnant women with preexisting HSV infection or infection acquired during pregnancy may be prescribed suppressive therapy to prevent transmission to the neonate during delivery, avoiding the need for a caesarean delivery. No evidence of fetal harm has been demonstrated with the use of antivirals during pregnancy, whereas neonatal herpes may result in severe neurologic disability or death.

Herpetic keratoconjunctivitis (herpes simplex keratitis) is an intraocular HSV infection that requires immediate referral to an ophthalmologist to prevent blindness. Treatment may include topical optic antiviral preparations and gentle epithelial debridement of the eye to remove infectious organisms and viral antigens that induce an ocular inflammatory response, as well as oral antiviral drugs, such as acyclovir.

FOLLOW-UP AND REFERRAL

Follow-up should be early and repeated, depending on the extent of disease. Lesions confined to the lip area may not need to be seen in follow-up unless they do not resolve. However, extensive oral or genital lesions should be seen on a weekly basis until resolution. As previously mentioned, herpetic lesions of the eye must be referred to an ophthalmologist immediately. Patients with herpes zoster ophthalmicus should be instructed to return to the practitioner if they experience a recurrence until they feel comfortable in handling subsequent episodes on their own. A patient with genital herpes may benefit from referral to a local herpes health advocacy organization for counseling and emotional support.

Patient Education: Herpes Simplex Infections

Patient education is an integral component of the management of HSV infection. Most patients achieve relief of symptoms within 4 to 7 days of beginning therapy. Self-care techniques and instructions on the proper use of pharmacotherapy are vital. Box 15.2 provides basic information and guidelines about herpes infection.

Drugs Commonly Prescribed 15.1: Herpes Simplex Infections

DRUG	INDICATION	ADVERSE REACTIONS AND PRESCRIBING CONSIDERATIONS
Topical		
Docosanol 10% cream (Abreva)	Recurrent oral–facial herpes simplex Over the counter	Begin at earliest sign or symptom five times/day
Penciclovir 1% (Denavir)	Recurrent herpes labialis on the lips and face	Every 2 hours while awake for 4 days
Systemic Therapy		
Famciclovir (Famvir)	Acute herpes zoster, treatment or suppression of recurrent genital herpes, and treatment of recurrent herpes labialis in immunocompetent patients	No evidence of fetal harm if used during pregnancy Check prescribing reference or CDC guidelines for dosage regimens for initial outbreaks, recurrent episodes, and suppressive therapy
Valacyclovir (Valtrex)	Treatment of herpes zoster, herpes labialis, and varicella (chickenpox) Treatment or suppression of genital herpes in immunocompetent patients	As above
Acyclovir (Zovirax)	Genital herpes, herpes zoster, varicella, herpes labialis, herpetic whitlow	As above

Box 15.2 Basic Patient Information About Herpes Simplex Infection

- Fever, stress, sunlight, and menses can trigger recurrence of lesions.
- Burning and tingling at the site may signal recurrence of the infection. If antiviral therapy was prescribed, begin it at the first sign of infection. If symptoms persist beyond 10 days, see your primary-care practitioner.

Treatment

General:

- Apply penciclovir (Denavir) 1% cream to affected area while awake, every 2 hours for 4 days or until symptoms resolve.
- Frequent hand washing, rest, and increased fluid intake are needed during a herpetic outbreak.

Lip lesions:

- Apply gel ice pack to lip lesions for 10–15 minutes as needed to relieve pain and decrease swelling.
- Lip balm (e.g., Blistex) may be used on the lips to prevent drying of sores and to reduce pain.
- Apply lip balm sunscreen (e.g., Chapstick) with an SPF of 15 to lips before sun exposure.

Oral lesions:

- Apply a dental protective paste (e.g., Orabase) four times a day to prevent irritation of lesions by the teeth.
- An equal mixture of diphenhydramine (Benadryl) syrup (12.5 mg/5 mL) and unflavored Maalox can be used as an oral rinse every 2 hours, then expectorated. Viscous xylocaine 2% (Lidocaine) 5 mL can be added to the mixture or used alone as an oral rinse before meals to decrease pain and facilitate eating.
- For those with orolabial lesions, there should be no sharing of towels, silverware, or glasses; avoid oral contact until lesions are healed.

Genital, anal, and/or buttocks lesions:

- To soothe lesions, apply warm compresses or take a warm oatmeal sitz bath for 20–30 minutes as needed.
- A blow dryer placed on the cool setting can be used to thoroughly dry genital lesions.
- Avoid sexual activity until lesions are healed. A latex condom must be used correctly and consistently during sexual intercourse to decrease viral spread, and not just during herpetic outbreaks.

REFERENCES

Herpes Simplex Infections

Ayoade FO. Herpes simplex. Medscape drugs and diseases. http://emedicine.medscape.com/article/218580. Updated March 09, 2017. Accessed June 28, 2017.

Centers for Disease Control and Prevention. 2015 sexually transmitted diseases treatment guidelines. Genital HSV infections. https://www.cdc.gov/std/tg2015/herpes.htm. Accessed July 14, 2017.

U.S. Preventive Services Task Force; Bibbins-Domingo K, Grossman DC, Curry SJ, et al. Serologic screening for genital herpes infection: US Preventive Services Task Force Recommendation Statement. *JAMA*. 2016;316(23):2525–2530.

World Health Organization. WHO guidelines for the treatment of genital herpes simplex virus. http://www.who.int/reproductivehealth/publications/rtis/genital-HSV-treatment-guidelines/en. Accessed July 17, 2017.

Human Papillomavirus

Gearhart, PA. Human papilloma virus. Medscape drugs and diseases. http://emedicine.medscape.com/article/219110. Updated January 5, 2017. Accessed June 28, 2017.

Warts

Aldahan AS, Mlacker S, Shah VV, et al. Efficacy of intralesional immunotherapy for the treatment of warts: a review of the literature. *Dermatol Ther*. 2016;29(3):197–207.

American Academy of Dermatology. Warts. https://www.aad.org/public/diseases/contagious-skin-diseases/warts. Accessed July 10, 2017.

Kreuter A, Waterboer T, Wieland U. Regression of cutaneous warts in a patient with WILD syndrome following recombinant quadrivalent human papillomavirus vaccination. *Arch Dermatol*. 2010;146:1196–1197.

Mulhem E, Pinelis S. Treatment of non-genital cutaneous warts. *Am Fam Physician*. 2011;84(3):288–293.

Shenefelt PD. Nongenital warts. Medscape drugs and diseases. http://emedicine.medscape.com/article/1133317. Updated April 10, 2017. Accessed June 28, 2017.

Sterling JC, Gibbs S, Haque Hussain SS, Mohd Mustapa MF, Handfield-Jones SE. British Association of Dermatologists' guidelines for the management of cutaneous warts 2014. *Br J Dermatol*. 2014;171(4):696–712.

Venugopal SS, Murrell DF. Recalcitrant cutaneous warts treated with recombinant quadrivalent human papillomavirus (types 6, 11, 16, and 18) in a developmentally delayed, 31 year old white man. *Arch Dermatol*. 2010;146:475–477.

RESOURCES

American Academy of Dermatology
  www.aad.org
Centers for Disease Control and Prevention
  www.cdc.gov
Online Resource for Herpes and HPV
  www.herpes.org
National Institute of Allergy and Infectious Disease
  www.niaid.nih.gov
National Institutes of Health
  www.nih.gov

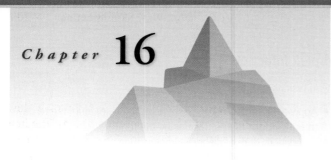

Chapter **16**

Dermatitis

Donna Maheady, APRN, CPNP, EdD

Jill E. Winland-Brown, EdD, APRN, FNP-BC

Brian Oscar Porter, MD, PhD, MPH, MBA

ATOPIC DERMATITIS

Atopic dermatitis (eczema) is not considered a distinct disease entity but is a descriptive term for a group of skin disorders characterized by pruritus and inflammation whose distinct cause is unknown. *Eczema* is a more general term that is often used collectively to describe skin of an erythematous and inflamed appearance, reflective of a superficial pathological process. Currently, the terms *eczema* and *dermatitis* are often used synonymously in the clinical arena in a nonspecific sense. The use of the term *eczematous rash,* although also indistinct, may be helpful both diagnostically and therapeutically because eczematous dermatitis may be classified into two major etiological categories—atopic dermatitis and contact dermatitis. Early in its presentation, atopic dermatitis is erythematous in appearance, with papulovesicular lesions that may ooze and crust. At its later stages, the rash becomes a red-purple color, dries, and develops scaling and lichenification, which is exacerbated by scratching resulting from its highly pruritic nature.

EPIDEMIOLOGY AND CAUSES

Atopic dermatitis is an inherited skin reaction that usually begins in infancy. Interestingly, children born to older women are more likely to develop eczema than children born to younger women. For unknown reasons, the prevalence of atopic disease has risen steadily over the past 30 years. Statistics vary, but overall the prevalence is estimated at 1 in 18 or 5.5%, which amounts to 15 million people in the United States. About 10% of the U.S. population will have atopic dermatitis at some point in their lifetime. It occurs across all ethnic groups and equally in both sexes.

Atopic dermatitis presents more severely in childhood. Onset during the first year of life occurs in up to 50% of patients, and in 85%, onset occurs before the age of

5 years. Up to 5% of all children are affected by atopic dermatitis, although most cases (40%) resolve by adulthood. The remainder of patients with atopic dermatitis are affected with a chronic disease course that is characterized by acute exacerbations (often during times of stress) and intermittent remissions.

The cause of atopic dermatitis is unknown, although family history is positive for atopy in two-thirds of all cases. A genetic predisposition toward allergic reactivity may be the most important etiological factor in all atopic conditions. A personal or family history of all or part of the "atopic triad"—asthma, allergic rhinitis, and eczema—is often present. It has been proposed that individuals with any of these three conditions have a preferential production of allergen-specific immunoglobulin E (IgE) and that the presence of such antibodies should be a mandatory criterion for the diagnosis of atopic dermatitis. Such a diagnostic test, however, only establishes the diagnosis of *atopic syndrome* and not atopic dermatitis. Any patient with a history of hives (urticaria), hay fever, or rashes should be considered to have an atopic history.

All atopic individuals seem to have itchier skin, yet what seems to be unique about the atopic patient's skin is its hypersensitivity. Many factors that do not make nonatopic individuals itch will make the atopic person feel itchy. Atopic patients are known to itch seconds after experiencing a stressful event. This type of reaction is thought to be caused by neuropeptide-induced vasodilation, which produces an increase in skin temperature and erythema. Symptoms are triggered or exacerbated through the interaction between genetic predisposition and environmental factors. Environmental factors that trigger atopic dermatitis include dust mites, animal dander, pollen, microbes, pollutants, climate, and emotional stress.

Excessively hot or cold climates or excessively dry or moist environments are particularly suitable for setting the stage for the atopic process. Anything that dries the skin can aggravate symptoms. Common triggers include excessive bathing, hand washing, lip licking, sweating, or swimming. Contact with irritants such as solvents, detergents, deodorants, tobacco, cosmetics, soap, and both wool and synthetic fabrics can precipitate an exacerbation of atopic dermatitis. Improperly fitting clothes can create friction and irritate the skin, thereby precipitating a flare-up. Other skin conditions or infections can also lead to an exacerbation of atopic dermatitis. Heat and sweat may also be aggravating factors for atopic dermatitis, including practices that generate an increase in body temperature, such as hot showers or baths, overdressing, use of heating pads, and electric blankets. Patients with atopy often are intolerant of heat, have difficulty with thermal sweating, and are more likely to develop heat exhaustion. It is thought that perspiration retention might be a complicating factor in atopic patients. Excessive humidity may also be a factor because it interferes with normal evaporation of sweat from the body.

PATHOPHYSIOLOGY

The inflammatory process in eczema causes erythema of the skin as a result of dilated blood vessels that are surrounded by inflammatory cells that migrate into the epidermis, resulting in edema both inside and in between the epidermal cells (spongiosis). The epidermal cells malfunction as a consequence, resulting in thickening of the epidermis (acanthosis), excess production of keratin, and scaling. The outer epidermal layer of the skin, the stratum corneum, normally forms an impermeable barrier that protects the living cells beneath from environmental irritants and toxins. In atopic dermatitis, this outer barrier is impaired. There is an increase in the water loss and a decrease in water binding, which has been attributed to decreased functionality of filaggrin proteins in the skin, which leads to a brittle outer barrier. This condition is made worse by environmental factors such as physical trauma from scratching, cycles of wetting and drying, and the chemical erosion that is caused by detergents and solvents.

In addition, superinfection of eczematous skin by bacterial (e.g., *Staphylococcus aureus*) or fungal (e.g., *Malassezia furfur*) species and irritation from dust mites and their excrement is an important factor that worsens atopic dermatitis by potentiating the immune response. Superinfection is also much more likely in atopic dermatitis than in other forms of dermatitis, such as psoriasis. Thus, infection may be thought of as both a trigger and a complication of atopic dermatitis.

Immunological abnormalities are key to the pathophysiology of the atopic response. These abnormalities can include elevated serum IgE levels (seen in 85% of affected individuals), hypereosinophilia, reduced cell-mediated immunity and antibody-dependent cellular cytotoxicity, slowed chemotaxis of neutrophils and monocytes, a relative increase in the number of CD4-positive (CD4+) Th2 helper T cells that secrete interleukin (IL)-4, and a decrease in CD4+ T helper cells that secrete interleukin-2 (IL-2). Interestingly, however, in later stages of the immune reaction, Th1 helper T-cell activity, which enhances cell-mediated immunity, appears to play an increasing role. In addition, the impairment of essential fatty acid metabolism has been identified as a causative factor of atopy.

Recently, Th17 cells and their associated cytokines (e.g., IL-17A) have also been implicated in this disease process, including in the protection against infection/colonization with superficial skin fungi (e.g., *Candida*) and bacteria (e.g., *Staphylococcus*) containing superantigens that are thought to trigger dysregulated immune responses, thereby resulting in eczematous lesions. However, reports in the literature are conflicting and have implicated Th17 cells in both proinflammatory and antiinflammatory roles.

CLINICAL PRESENTATION

Subjective

Atopic dermatitis is characterized by an extremely low threshold for pruritus and has been referred to as "the itch that rashes." Almost always, the itch occurs before the rash appears, and scratching the rash worsens it clinically. In fact, the cardinal sign of atopic dermatitis is severe pruritus, which is often extremely distressing in both the acute and chronic stages. In turn, the diagnosis of atopic dermatitis cannot be made without a history of pruritus, and if pruritus is absent, alternate diagnoses should be sought.

The patient may report a personal or family history of other atopic conditions (e.g., asthma, allergic rhinitis). In addition, the patient usually reports a history of episodic exacerbation of similar symptoms or a childhood rash or eczema. Often, the rash is reported as better in the warmer months and worse in the fall and winter. The clinician should inquire about any exposure to known or unknown common antigens and irritants, regardless of the history. Individuals with atopic dermatitis may also develop contact dermatitis; in fact, they are more susceptible to irritant reactions because of the impaired barrier function of their epidermal skin layer.

Objective

Atopic dermatitis usually begins as infantile eczema, with lesions affecting the cheeks, face, and upper extremities. Erythema is often seen before pruritus, and the acute lesions are excoriated, maculopapular, and inflamed. In infancy and early childhood, oozing and crusting usually characterize the erythema. As the child becomes older, the disease can go into remission or change to a flexural distribution (i.e., occurring in the antecubital fossae and neck area). Flexural eczema usually lasts until about age 4 to 10 years but may continue into adulthood.

In adults, eczema presents with symmetrical lesions that are crusting and excoriated. In its early stages, lesions may be erythematous, papulovesicular, edematous, and weeping. Later the rash becomes crusted, scaly, thickened, and lichenified. The classic locations for lesions are noted to correspond to areas that are most accessible to rubbing and scratching. In addition, the typical flexural sites are more susceptible because they are areas that are more likely to be hot and moist (see Advanced Assessment 16.1). Intergluteal involvement is uncommon and should raise suspicion of another diagnosis.

DIAGNOSTIC REASONING

Diagnostic Tests

Laboratory tests are usually not useful in the diagnosis of atopic dermatitis, but they can be helpful in ruling out other disorders or to confirm that a patient is prone

Advanced Assessment 16.1: Atopic Dermatitis

DISTRIBUTION

Infants: trunk, face, extensor surfaces, scalp
Children: antecubital fossae, popliteal fossae
Adults: face, neck, upper chest, genital area, hands

STAGES

Acute

Erosions with serous exudate
Intense pruritus
Papules and vesicles on an erythematous base
Pain, heat, tenderness

Subacute

Scaly, excoriated
Pruritus (may be intense)
Papules or plaques over an erythematous base
Secondary infection possible

Chronic

Lichenification, pigmentary changes (increased or decreased)
Pruritus
Excoriated papules and nodules
Dryness, fissuring

OTHER CLINICAL MANIFESTATIONS

Keratosis pilaris ("chicken skin"): asymptomatic follicular papules, particularly on the posterolateral aspects of the upper arms and lateral thighs
Lichenification of the skin, with a predilection for flexural creases
Ichthyosis vulgaris: hyperlinearity of the palms and soles and fishlike scales, especially on the lower legs
Dennie-Morgan lines (infraorbital folds) caused by edema
Excessive fissuring of the earlobes, palms, soles, and fingers
Pityriasis alba: hypopigmented asymptomatic areas on the face and shoulders
Allergic "shiners": facial pallor and infraorbital darkening
Anterior capsular cataracts
Keratoconus: a cone-shaped cornea may develop in the second or third decade of life (in severe cases)
Facial erythema, dry skin, history of wool intolerance, nonspecific hand dermatitis, and a tendency for skin infection (commonly impetiginization of excoriated skin)

to atopy (allergic reactions), as the etiology of the rash. Alterations in cell-mediated immune responses contribute to an increased susceptibility of atopic patients to cutaneous viral infections, such as herpes simplex virus, vaccinia, and molluscum contagiosum. Thus, if a viral etiology of the rash is suspected, a viral culture should be done on the exudate and moist parts of the rash. If atopy (allergy) is suspected, skin prick testing or serum radioallergosorbent test (RAST) may be done to identify antigen-specific mast cell activation or to quantify levels of allergen-specific IgE, respectively.

The RAST test is usually available to primary-care practitioners, whereas skin prick (scratch) testing is typically done only by board-certified allergists. However, interpretation of RAST results requires specialized knowledge of the specificity and sensitivity of the assay because false-positive results are not uncommon. Thus, RAST should not be ordered arbitrarily or as a general atopic screening tool; instead, serum IgE testing should be directed by a detailed patient history. Commonly available RAST panels often include not only antigen-specific IgE levels but also antigen-specific IgG and IgM levels, which are not helpful in the diagnosis of atopic disease (hypersensitivity) and are therefore prone to misinterpretation.

A RAST panel may include testing for antigen-specific IgE to dust mites, mold, ragweed, animal dander, tree pollen, and many other allergens. RAST panels also exists for food allergens, which are often highly relevant in pediatric patients; however, true IgE-mediated food allergies are far less common in adults. Thus, RAST testing is useful for patients suspected of having an atopic history if directed by the patients' presenting signs, symptoms, and environmental exposures. An atopic or allergic tendency manifests as chronic or recurrent symptoms (in addition to dermatitis), which might include a history of allergic rhinitis (e.g., nasal congestion, chronic postnasal drip, sneezing, itchy nose) and asthma during childhood. Some patients will deny any allergic tendency but will report a history of frequent "sinus problems." RAST is usually positive in patients with a history of symptoms of atopic dermatitis, but it often does not correlate well with clinical symptoms. Results appear to vary with the type of allergen being tested. Another potentially helpful marker for atopy is the serum IgE level. Serum IgE levels are usually elevated during acute periods of dermatitis but may decrease during periods of remission. Higher levels of total serum IgE, however, also increase the tendency toward false-positive allergen-specific RAST test results.

Allergen skin prick testing is considered useful because it is a direct functional test of a patient's allergic response, as it is based on antigen-specific IgE in the skin binding to mast cells and triggering an immediate hypersensitivity response. Patients should be advised to stop all antihistamines for at least 2 weeks before undergoing allergen skin testing, because these medications will interfere with skin prick test outcomes and may lead to false-negative results. In addition, delayed-type hypersensitivity responses to epicutaneously applied antigens (as used in scratch and skin-prick tests) may be blunted in atopic skin during periods of disease activity, so scratch tests should be avoided during flare periods to avoid uninterpretable results.

If the diagnosis proves elusive or if serious pathology (e.g., mycosis fungoides) is suspected, a skin biopsy can provide important information. The skin biopsy of atopic skin will reveal a thickened and hyperkeratoid epidermis, along with perivascular inflammation of the dermis. Patients with pustular superinfection should have their lesions cultured for antibiotic sensitivities if they do not heal in response to empiric therapy.

Differential Diagnosis

Both common and rare skin disorders can mimic atopic dermatitis. Common disorders include contact dermatitis, tinea infections (dermatophytosis), seborrheic dermatitis, and the early stages of mycosis fungoides (cutaneous T-cell lymphoma [CTCL]). In contact dermatitis, the characteristic linear or asymmetrical distribution of skin lesions helps to distinguish this condition from atopic dermatitis. The location and characteristic ringlike erythematous lesions with central clearing distinguish tinea corpora infections (ringworm) from atopic dermatitis. Mycosis fungoides skin lesions do not respond to topical corticosteroids; therefore, suspicious lesions in adults that do not respond to topical corticosteroids after a minimum of 2 weeks of treatment should be considered for skin biopsy.

If none of the common skin disorders apply, rare systemic diseases and skin disorders that can produce rashes that mimic atopic dermatitis include gluten-sensitive enteropathy, acrodermatitis enteropathica, phenylketonuria, hyper-IgE syndrome, Wiskott-Aldrich syndrome, X-linked agammaglobulinemia, selective IgA-deficiency, and Letterer-Siwe disease (see Differential Diagnosis 16.1).

Differential Diagnosis 16.1: Atopic Dermatitis

Scabies
Seborrheic dermatitis
Allergic contact dermatitis
Tinea infections
Psoriasis
Ichthyosis
Dermatitis herpetiformis
Mycosis fungoides (cutaneous T-cell lymphoma)
Netherton's syndrome
Wiskott-Aldrich syndrome
Acrodermatitis enteropathica
Neurodermatitis
HIV infection (especially in children)
Phenylketonuria (if symptoms appear during the first year of life)
Hyper-immunoglobulin E syndrome
Dermatomyositis

MANAGEMENT

The primary aim in the management of atopic dermatitis is to control signs and symptoms because no cure exists at present. The management of dermatitis embodies the fundamental principles of dermatology: precipitating factors should be eliminated, wet lesions should be dried, dried lesions should be hydrated, and inflammation should be treated with corticosteroids. Crucial to management is a careful and systematic assessment of trigger factors. The goals of management are to decrease pruritus, prevent secondary infection, and educate patients so that they can control the disease themselves. For example, atopic patients should be warned of their increased susceptibility to viral infections and encouraged to avoid exposure to infected individuals.

The critical importance of skin hydration cannot be overstated, as the chronic use and overuse of corticosteroids while neglecting sufficient skin hydration carries significant iatrogenic risks, including both local adverse effects (e.g., skin atrophy, local irritation, telangiectasias) and the potential adverse effects of systemic absorption (e.g., cataract formation, growth impairment, bone demineralization, adrenal suppression). The benefits of moisture barrier-restoring therapies are highlighted in Evidence-Based Nursing Practice 16.1.

 Evidence-Based Nursing Practice 16.1

Valdman-Grinshpoun, Y.; Ben-Amitai, D; & Zvulunov, A. Barrier-restoring therapies in atopic dermatitis: current approaches and future perspectives. *Dermatol Res Pract.* 2012;2012: 923134.

Atopic dermatitis is a multifactorial, chronic relapsing, inflammatory disease characterized by xerosis, eczematous lesions, and pruritus. The latter usually leads to an "itch–scratch" cycle that may compromise the epidermal barrier. Skin barrier abnormalities in atopic dermatitis may result from mutations in the gene encoding for the protein filaggrin, which plays an important role in the formation of cornified cytosol. Barrier abnormalities render the skin more permeable to irritants, allergens, and microorganisms. Treatment of atopic dermatitis must be directed to control itching, suppress inflammation, and restore the skin barrier. Emollients, both creams and ointments, improve the barrier function of the stratum corneum by providing it with water and lipids. Studies on atopic dermatitis and barrier repair treatment show that adequate lipid replacement therapy reduces inflammation and restores epidermal function. Efforts directed at developing immunomodulators that interfere with cytokine-induced skin barrier dysfunction provide a promising strategy for the treatment of atopic dermatitis. Moreover, an impressive proliferation of more than 80 clinical studies focusing on topical treatments in atopic dermatitis has led to growing expectations for better therapies.

Nonpharmacologic Management

To avoid excessive irritation and skin dryness, the patient should use mild emollients (e.g., Cetaphil) as a substitute for soap. Controversy surrounds best bathing practices. Despite the chronic dryness of eczematous skin, showering has paradoxically been implicated in worsening the lesions of atopic dermatitis, possibly due to the physical trauma of strong water streams on the skin. Thus, soak baths are preferred, provided they are followed by the liberal application of moisturizers after partially patting dry the skin. This approach is referred to as "soak and smear." Soaps containing perfumes, coloring agents, or strong scents can be particularly irritating. If patients insist on the use of soap for cleanliness, glycerin soaps have been well tolerated and should be limited to the axilla, groin, and feet.

Excessive bathing can be detrimental in the eczematous patients because bathing effectively removes the skin's protective oils. Older patients should take short, lukewarm showers with a mild water stream and avoid long, hot baths, which are extremely desiccating. The use of bubble baths and fragrance-containing oils should be discouraged. Bath oils are of minimal benefit because whatever oil remains on the skin after bathing is generally wiped off with toweling. Minimizing contact with cosmetics, deodorants, detergents, and solvents should be stressed. Moisturizers are useful in helping to prevent water loss and are most effective when applied immediately after patting the skin partially dry after a short shower or soak bath. Atopic dermatitis patients should be cautioned against using lotions and gels that contain alcohol, preservatives, and fragrances. Patients with atopic dermatitis should not use agents that contain lactic acid or other alpha-hydroxy/glycolic acids that can aggravate the condition.

Ointments (which contain petroleum jelly) form an occlusive layer and are more effective in preventing water loss than lotions, solutions, or creams. For less severe conditions or in hot, humid areas, creams that do not contain fragrance and have few preservatives are acceptable (e.g., Cetaphil cream, Eucerin, Dermabase, Unibase). Humidifiers are most helpful in maintaining skin hydration in cold and dry climates, but they can inadvertently contribute to an environment that is conducive to increased dust mite and mold growth. Acaricide is an insecticide that is effective against dust mites; it may be used on all fomites (pillows, beds, sofas, etc.). After application, thorough vacuuming, preferably with a high-efficiency particulate air–filtered apparatus, must be done to remove the insecticide. Antifungal cleaners for wet and damp areas are recommended for patients who are sensitive to mold. However, acaricide and other pesticides/chemical treatments have not been shown to be consistently helpful and are not first-line preventive treatments.

Pharmacologic Management

If the skin lesions are wet, inflamed, or have an exudate, wet soaks or compresses with cool tap water, Burow's (aluminum acetate) solution (1:40 dilution), saline (1 teaspoon per pint of water), or silver nitrate solution (1%–10%) can be used to dry the lesions and provide comfort. Burow's solution can be applied as a compress for 20 to 30 minutes four to six times throughout the day. Over-the-counter (OTC) topical corticosteroids should be immediately applied to inflamed areas after the soak. Prescription corticosteroid cream may be needed for more severe cases.

Given that dry skin lesions are most common with atopic dermatitis, petrolatum or other emollients (e.g., Aquaphor healing ointment, Eucerin cream, Keralac lotion) should be applied not only to dry eczematous lesions but also to all noninflamed areas of the skin to maintain hydration. Colloidal oatmeal baths (Aveeno) are soothing and may also be helpful with more generalized lesions.

Although antihistamines are often used to relieve pruritus, they are usually ineffective in atopic dermatitis because histamine is not the only factor responsible for the mediation of pruritus in atopic dermatitis. The sedative effect of antihistamines may be more beneficial than their antipruritic properties if used at night. Individuals with atopic dermatitis have a tendency to scratch in their sleep, so sedation at bedtime may decrease the amount of scratching during sleep. First-generation H_1 blockers, such as ethanolamines (diphenhydramine) and phenothiazines (promethazine), are very sedating. Of note, sedating antihistamines are generally not recommended in children because they have been shown to lead to daytime drowsiness and impair school performance, as well as have a paradoxical effect of inducing hyperactivity in some children. Thus, sedating patients at night for severe atopic dermatitis, urticaria, or other forms of pruritus only applies to adults.

Some tricyclic antidepressants, such as doxepin (Sinequan), have potent antihistaminic activity as well and are useful in urticarial, atopic dermatitis, and other forms of pruritus. An added benefit to using an antidepressant agent is the relief of depression that may accompany severe atopic dermatitis.

Montelukast sodium (Singulair) 5 to 10 mg daily may contribute to the relief of atopic dermatitis in a patient with other forms of concurrent atopy. Montelukast is a leukotriene-receptor antagonist and inhibits eosinophil infiltration in the skin, a major histological characteristic of atopic dermatitis. Of note, however, montelukast is not approved by the Food and Drug Administration (FDA) for the treatment of atopic dermatitis.

Corticosteroids are effective anti-inflammatory agents and are usually considered first-line pharmacotherapy for atopic dermatitis, although their use must always be preceded by optimal moisturization, since restoring skin hydration is the most important step in breaking the itch–scratch cycle of atopic dermatitis. In addition, the use of emollients (e.g., petroleum jelly, Eucerin, Lubriderm) will enhance the absorption and effectiveness of topical corticosteroids. Applying topical corticosteroids after hydrating the skin (after a brief shower or bath) may increase their absorption up to 10-fold. A weak coal tar preparation applied over a corticosteroid ointment can also reduce itching at night.

Acute exacerbations of atopic dermatitis can be treated with a potent to mid-strength topical corticosteroid for a few days to quickly control acutely inflamed skin lesions, but the patient should switch to a weaker-strength agent once the lesion is under control. Medium- to high-potency topical corticosteroids should not be used on the face or neck area because of potential adverse effects such as local irritation, atrophy of the skin, and formation of telangiectasias. Skin atrophy is more likely to occur when potent topical corticosteroids are applied repeatedly to thin and highly absorptive inflamed skin. In some instances, hypopigmentation has been associated with the use of topical corticosteroids, especially in darker-skinned individuals, such as African Americans. Most cases of pigmentation changes are related to the underlying dermatitis, however, rather than the use of topical corticosteroids. Topical corticosteroids may also complicate treatment by masking underlying bacterial or fungal infections or impairing healing processes. Topical corticosteroids should never be used on ulcerated skin.

Systemic corticosteroids are rarely necessary for the treatment of chronic atopic dermatitis, but they may be useful for an incapacitating acute exacerbation or when large numbers of weeping lesions are present. In these rare instances, the patient may benefit from a short course of oral prednisone (40 to 60 mg/day for adults and 1 mg/kg/day for children). Short-term therapy with prednisone does not require tapering if it is limited to 5 to 7 days and the patient does not have a history of recent oral prednisone use. As the lesions dry, topical corticosteroids may be started. Of note, given the significant adverse effects associated with systemic corticosteroid use, such regimens should be considered a last resort and not used regularly. In some instances, the decision to use systemic corticosteroids to treat atopic dermatitis may signify the need for inpatient care to gain control of a debilitating exacerbation, particularly in pediatric patients.

When the acute inflammation subsides after 2 to 3 weeks, the patient should decrease the frequency of the topical corticosteroids and focus primarily on emollients such as petroleum jelly or Eucerin cream. The chronic use of topical corticosteroids (mid to low strength) should be limited to twice-weekly applications to any given area and should not be continued indefinitely.

Topical tacrolimus (Protopic) and the related agent pimecrolimus (Elidel), applied twice per day, have been shown to be effective and safe for use as second-line agents in atopic dermatitis. These are immunomodulating calcineurin inhibitors. Most patients experience a dramatic reduction of pruritus within 3 days of initiating treatment and have significant improvement in quality of life. When used as long-term maintenance therapy, topical preparations reduce the number of flares of atopic dermatitis and the requirement for corticosteroid treatment. Of note, given limitations in long-term safety data for these agents, including rare reports of malignancy, the FDA has issued a black box warning for tacrolimus and pimecrolimus, warning clinicians against continuous long-term use of these agents in any age-group and highlighting the lack of approval of these agents in children younger than 2 years.

Aggressive treatment of refractory atopic dermatitis may also include cyclosporine A, an immunomodulatory drug, which may be as effective as corticosteroids, with fewer adverse effects. It may be used in patients who have failed to respond to at least one systemic therapy or in patients for whom other systemic therapies are contraindicated or are intolerable. Its use can be highly beneficial in severe cases, but renal function must be closely monitored, and treatment courses must be restricted to 8 to 12 weeks. Azathioprine (Imuran) may also be used for maintenance therapy, but hematological and hepatic functions must be monitored, given its potential toxicity. As with systemic corticosteroids, the use of a systemic immunosuppressant, such as cyclosporine A or azathioprine (Imuran), for atopic dermatitis would strongly suggest the need for inpatient care to adequately control such an exacerbation.

Omalizumab (Xolair), an anti-IgE antibody, that has been developed as an immunotherapeutic biological agent, has shown benefit in reducing atopy in highly allergic individuals, although it is not FDA approved to treat atopic dermatitis. In severe cases of atopic dermatitis, phototherapy with ultraviolet B radiation or PUVA (psoralens with ultraviolet A radiation) photochemotherapy may be used as an adjunct therapy. Lesions of patients with pustular superinfection should be cultured for antibiotic sensitivities if they do not heal in response to empiric therapy, as bacterial or fungal superinfections must be treated appropriately.

Complementary Therapies

There is limited evidence that mind–body relaxation techniques (e.g., yoga, meditation) may help improve symptoms of atopic dermatitis, particularly in the pediatric population. However, clinical studies of these therapies have not been methodologically rigorous.

Studies indicate that certain plants and herbs may be of value in the treatment of dermatological conditions. These include chamomile, arnica, calendula, hamamelis (witch hazel), aloe vera, cardiospermum, *Mahonia aquifolium,* oak bark, bittersweet stalk, and capsicum. Use of these herbs should be reserved for experienced practitioners in alternative health medicine because of the potential for allergic reactions. Complementary Therapies 16.1 lists herbs that are used in the treatment of eczema.

Complementary Therapies 16.1: Herbal Treatments for Eczema

HERB	COMMENTS
Chamomile (*Matricaria recutita*)	Topical application Anti-inflammatory properties Contraindicated in patients with ragweed allergy
Evening primrose (*Oenothera biennis*)	Should not be taken with phenothiazines
Marigold (*Calendula officinalis*)	Topical application—ointment or cream Anti-inflammatory properties
Goldenseal (*Hydrastis canadensis*)	Topical application Powdered root mixed with water to make a paste and applied to rash
Licorice (*Glycyrrhiza glabra*)	Topical application Anti-inflammatory properties
Turmeric (*Curcuma longa*)	Topical application Anti-inflammatory properties

FOLLOW-UP AND REFERRAL

If basic management of atopic dermatitis fails, specialty referral to an allergist or dermatologist should be prompt. More aggressive treatment by a specialist is necessary for patients who have severe and extensive lesions or who do not respond to usual treatment with topical or systemic corticosteroids. Atopic skin is very susceptible to bacterial and viral infections. These patients may develop a widespread herpetic skin infections known as eczema herpeticum, which may be life-threatening in children. Thus, patients with atopic dermatitis should avoid contact with people with active herpetic lesions. During an exacerbation, patients may contract secondary bacterial infections, and empiric therapy with erythromycin or penicillinase-resistant penicillins is sometimes necessary.

Patient Education: Atopic Dermatitis

Patients with atopic dermatitis should be educated to be vigilant in watching for the signs of secondary bacterial infection and report them immediately so that an oral antibiotic can be prescribed. Education about the importance of environmental measures in the prevention of disease exacerbation should be emphasized. House dust mites, animal dander, and pollen may all be identified as potential triggers based on antigen-specific IgE antibodies in the bloodstream, and avoidance of these triggers should be addressed when educating patients. Patients can also be counseled to reduce sweating, which may exacerbate wet lesions, such as by limiting the amount of bedclothes at night, avoiding hot occlusive garments, and keeping living areas cool. Patients should be encouraged to recognize their stress "triggers" and to find measures to reduce their stress level, such as exercise.

Because *S. aureus* colonizes the skin of more than 90% of patients with atopic dermatitis (compared with only 5% of persons without the disease), fingernails should be kept short, smooth, and clean. This may prevent trauma from scratching that exacerbates skin inflammation and allows microbes to be introduced into the skin. Bleach baths may also be used as a means of reducing bacterial colonization of the skin. Patients can be instructed to add a half cup of unscented laundry bleach to a full bathtub of lukewarm water and soak for 20 minutes, followed by the standard application of a copious amount of moisturizer after partially patting dry the skin. These bleach baths may be done one to two times per week.

Patients should be informed that a change in seasons will cause exacerbations of their disease, especially during the fall. Patients can be reminded to use extra effort in taking care of their skin at this time by upgrading to stronger moisturizers (e.g., from lotions to petroleum jelly). Refills of medications should be ordered before the recurrence of symptoms to allow for prompt treatment of acutely inflamed lesions. The provider can assist the patient in developing a simple regimen of topical corticosteroid therapy for acute exacerbations. Patients with frequent exacerbations of skin lesions on their hands should avoid occupations that require repeated hand washing, immersion in water, or other wet conditions.

Food allergies are a common aggravating factor in up to 20% of patients with atopic dermatitis and are more common in children. Food sensitivities may be assessed through the judicious use of skin prick testing or RAST panels, provided interpretation of the results is done by an adequately trained clinician with the specialized knowledge to execute and interpret these tests. A dietitian should then be consulted when patients are eliminating foods from their diet because unsupervised food restriction may lead to malnutrition.

CONTACT DERMATITIS

Contact dermatitis is a common condition categorized as either *irritant dermatitis* or *allergic dermatitis*. Although both these conditions can have similar presentations, the etiology of each disease is what differentiates the two dermatitides. *Allergic contact dermatitis* is immunologically mediated, whereas *irritant contact dermatitis* is the result of repeated "insults" to atopic skin from caustic, irritant, or detergent-type substances.

EPIDEMIOLOGY AND CAUSES

Almost any substance may induce a cutaneous reaction depending on its concentration, the duration of contact, and the condition of the exposed skin. The etiology of allergic contact dermatitis may be from antimicrobials such as neomycin, antihistamines, anesthetics such as benzocaine, hair dyes, preservatives, latex, nickel, or adhesive tape. The etiology of irritant contact dermatitis may be from soaps, detergents, or organic solvents. Irritant contact dermatitis accounts for about 80% of all cases of contact dermatitis.

Delayed-type hypersensitivity reactions are immunological responses to contact allergens that occur in sensitized individuals. One of the most frequent causes of allergic contact dermatitis is from plants in the *Rhus* genus, which includes poison ivy, poison oak, and poison sumac. Other common topical sensitizers include ragweed pollen, dust mites, ethylenediamine (a stabilizer in many topical creams), potassium dichromate, paraphenylenediamine (dyes), nickel (10% of females are allergic to nickel often found in inexpensive jewelry, belt buckles, or metal fasteners on clothing), rubber compounds, and benzocaine (an OTC topical anesthetic for itching or pain). It is estimated that there are more than 6 million chemicals in the environment and that approximately 3,000 of them are potential sensitizers.

Contact dermatitis accounts for 4% to 7% of all dermatology consults. Hand dermatitis affects 2% of the population at any given time, and 20% of female patients will be affected at least once in their lifetime. Contact dermatitis is more common in adults than in children, and effects are more extreme in elderly patients. Women are twice as likely as men to develop dermatitis and are at highest risk after childbirth. White Americans are affected more frequently, and fair-skinned redheads are the most vulnerable population.

PATHOPHYSIOLOGY

Contact dermatitis is considered either allergic or irritant induced. A delayed-type hypersensitivity response (type IV immune reaction) elicits a non–IgE-mediated allergic response to specific antigens when applied to the skin, producing a local reaction characterized histologically by epidermal changes, including intracellular edema, spongiosis, and vesiculation. On initial contact with the offending agent, the antigen is taken up and processed by epidermal antigen-presenting cells known as Langerhans cells. These cells present antigens to naïve, antigen-specific CD4+ and CD8+ T lymphocytes, located in regional lymph nodes that drain the affected areas of skin. Over approximately 10 to 14 days, sensitized T cells migrate from the lymph nodes to sites of antigenic exposure, where subsequent re-exposure to the same antigen results in an allergic reaction mediated by cytokine release. This response with notable skin surface changes typically occurs within 12 to 48 hours of re-exposure to the antigen.

Irritant contact dermatitis is the result of a direct cytotoxic effect of an irritant on the cells of the epidermis, with a subsequent inflammatory response in the dermis. The main pathological feature of contact dermatitis is intracellular edema of the epidermis, which may result in intraepidermal vesicles and bullae formation in the acute phase. In chronic cases, papules, scaling, and lichenification occur. Irritants penetrate and disrupt the stratum corneum and injure the underlying epidermis and dermis as various immune cells congregate around dilated capillaries, contributing to the inflammatory process.

Rubber-glove dermatitis demonstrates the spectrum of pathophysiological mechanisms involved in contact dermatitis. Chemical irritants used in the glove manufacturing process (e.g., thiram, mercapto derivatives) may cause an allergic dermatitis via a delayed-type T-cell–mediated hypersensitivity reaction. In addition, rubber glove components may result in a direct irritant effect on the moist skin of glove wearers. Finally, the natural rubber protein *latex*, once widely used in medical products, may elicit a profound IgE-mediated immediate hypersensitivity response, leading to systemic anaphylaxis and even death.

Interestingly, people with venous stasis (i.e., impaired venous return with pooling of blood in distended veins, particularly in the lower extremities) are more susceptible to irritant contact dermatitis, particularly from wood alcohols such as lanolin, fragrances, topical antibiotics such as neomycin, and methylparaben preservatives. Correctly diagnosing this condition is often difficult in these patients because contact dermatitis may be confused with stasis dermatitis.

CLINICAL PRESENTATION

Subjective

The cardinal symptom of contact dermatitis is a pruritic erythematous rash. Often, the patient is not aware of a previous history, but there may have been periodic episodes of pruritic rash that resolved spontaneously. The patient may or may not be able to describe the conditions or substances contributing to the dermatitis, but exposure history to known or unknown common antigens and irritants should be sought by the clinician. In allergic contact dermatitis (in contrast to atopic dermatitis), the inflammatory reaction on the skin occurs much faster, typically within 6 to 12 hours of re-exposure. In contrast to allergic contact dermatitis, irritant reactions do not always occur immediately after contact with the offending substance. The response time between the initial contact with the irritant and the symptoms is variable, and the severity of the reaction depends on the concentration, amount, and length of exposure to the irritating substance. The stages of contact dermatitis are listed in Box 16.1.

Objective

Contact dermatitis presents with inflammation of the epidermis and is manifested by erythema (as in all types of dermatitis), but it does not present with the smooth, intact epidermal surface that characterizes hives (urticaria). The epidermal inflammation seen in acute contact dermatitis results in rough, reddened patches, but without the skin thickening and discrete demarcation of psoriasis. The acute presentation of contact dermatitis is characterized by weeping lesions with numerous tiny vesicles on an erythematous base that is pruritic or has a burning or stinging sensation. The surrounding area in severe cases is also erythematous, with edema and increased heat in the area, making it difficult to rule out secondary bacterial infection in some cases.

Lesions in nonallergic and delayed-type hypersensitivity contact dermatitis present in similar fashion, but the typical distribution and the lack of an atopic history are the most helpful factors in the diagnosis. Often the location of the rash gives the clinician the best clue as to

the possible etiological agent (see Advanced Assessment 16.2). Usually the area of skin that has been the most heavily contaminated will break out first, followed by areas of lesser exposure.

For example, a patient with a rash on the scalp and the back of the neck might report a history of using a new shampoo, hair dye, or other scalp or hair treatment. A clothing- or detergent-related cause should be suspected if the lesions are generalized and primarily affect the borders of the axillae, waist, and upper thighs. Lesions in an area where jewelry has been worn recently (e.g., neck, wrist, earlobes) or where metal fasteners contact the skin (e.g., the infraumbilical area for belt buckles or snaps on denim pants) may indicate hypersensitivity to nickel. Reactions to toxic plants (e.g., *Rhus* or *Toxicodendron* species) are common on the extremities and follow a history of exposure. The characteristic rash is vesicular and linear (often asymmetrical) and is frequently found on the hands and ankles. *Rhus* dermatitis lesions may also be found on the facial area if the patient has inadvertently scratched the face with contaminated fingers.

DIAGNOSTIC REASONING

Diagnostic Tests

The diagnosis of contact dermatitis is based on the history of exposure to an irritant or allergen and the subsequent appearance of a rash on the exposed skin, either rapidly or one or more days after exposure (delayed hypersensitivity). If scabies is suspected, skin scrapings can be examined under a microscope to rule out that infestation. If

---

Box 16.1   Stages of Contact Dermatitis

Acute

Erythema and edema
Clear, fluid-filled vesicles or bullae
Exudate, clear fluid
Distinct margins

Subacute

Lessening edema
Formation of papules
Less distinct margins

Chronic

Minimal edema
Scaling skin
Lichenification
Minimal erythema

Advanced Assessment 16.2: Contact Dermatitis

STAGES

Acute

Erythema and edema
Clear, fluid-filled vesicles or bullae
Exudate, clear fluid
Distinct margins

Subacute

Lessening edema
Formation of papules
Less distinct margins

Chronic

Minimal edema
Scaling skin
Lichenification
Minimal erythema

tinea (corporis, cruris, pedis, capitis, manuum) infection is suspected, skin scrapings should be treated with potassium hydroxide (KOH) and gently heated on a glass slide; subsequent microscopic examination for tinea infection should search for septate hyphae and spores. If bacterial infection (impetigo) is suspected, cultures should be taken from the moist areas of the rash or from the discharge. Viral cultures can be done to rule out suspected viral etiology (herpes simplex, herpes zoster).

Laboratory tests that are done by specialists (e.g., allergists, dermatologists) include the scratch (skin prick), patch, and intradermal tests. These tests should not be done during an acute episode of contact dermatitis, however, because of an increased rate of false-positive reactions. The patch test is useful in identifying specific irritants in patients with histories that are suggestive of acute contact dermatitis. Allergens that are commonly responsible for such reactions are fixed in dehydrated gel layers or mixed in a small amount of petroleum jelly) and taped against the skin of the patient's back for 48 hours and then removed. A negative control patch with only the vehicle without antigen should also be applied to rule out nonspecific reactions. A final reading done at 72 to 96 hours after initial application will usually reveal any evidence of contact dermatitis. In some patients, a complete blood count (CBC) with differential will show eosinophilia, but this blood test is neither sensitive nor necessary for the diagnosis. Skin biopsy is rarely necessary for diagnosis, particularly with a convincing contact exposure history.

Differential Diagnosis

The differential diagnosis of contact dermatitis is similar to that of atopic dermatitis and includes both common and rare disorders. Common disorders that have a similar presentation to contact dermatitis include seborrheic dermatitis, impetigo, and herpes zoster. Seborrheic dermatitis rashes, although erythematous, have a greasy and scaly appearance and appear only in certain areas of the body, such as the hairline, ears, scalp, and face. Impetigo, which is caused by gram-positive *Staphylococcus* or *Streptococcus* bacteria, is more common in children. A honey-colored crust is seen on top of erythematous lesions; impetigo also does not have a linear appearance like the rash of contact dermatitis. Herpes zoster is more common in older patients, and the lesions appear as multiple small vesicles on an erythematous base. Although herpes zoster has a linear distribution, it is more likely to occur on the trunk area (contact dermatitis occurs more often on the hands or face) and will follow the path of a dermatome.

MANAGEMENT

The clinical challenge in the treatment of contact dermatitis is to provide symptomatic relief to the patient while attempting to identify the underlying allergic precipitant. Identifying the antigen or irritant in contact dermatitis is critical, both to eliminate or minimize the current contact and to avoid future exposure. The responsible irritant should be identified and eliminated to prevent the cycle of itching, scratching, and skin disruption, which can lead to chronic changes in the skin. A careful history of exposures is key, in addition to a thorough skin examination. The effects of *Rhus* dermatitis (from poison ivy, poison oak, or poison sumac) may be lessened if the exposed skin is thoroughly rinsed in soap and water or with isopropyl alcohol as soon as possible after exposure. Exposed clothing should be discarded.

For localized contact dermatitis with weeping lesions, treatment with moist compresses and simple drying agents or antipruritic lotions (e.g., Burow's aluminum acetate solution, calamine lotion) applied several times a day is usually effective. For more extensive and severe cases, potent topical corticosteroids in cream form (avoid the use of ointments on wet lesions because they can cause skin maceration) can be applied twice daily for the first few days to help decrease pruritus and inflammation. If treatment is necessary beyond 2 weeks, a less potent (mild or moderate) topical corticosteroid may be used twice daily until the rash resolves. High-potency corticosteroids should not be used on the face or in bodily folds (intertriginous areas) because of their ability to thin the skin and cause hypopigmentation.

Oral systemic corticosteroids may be indicated in acute and particularly severe cases of contact dermatitis, offering relief within 12 to 24 hours. For example, relatively high doses of oral prednisone can be given for 10 to 14 days (or up to 21 days in the most severe cases). However, abrupt cessation of high-dose systemic corticosteroids given for more than 1 week should be avoided, with tapering used for regimens lasting longer than this to decrease the risk of adrenal suppression. Potential adverse effects of oral corticosteroid therapy are more likely with long-term use and may include any of the following: suppression of the hypothalamic-pituitary-adrenal (HPA) axis, hypokalemia, hypocalcemia, masking or worsening of infection, increased likelihood of secondary infection, carbohydrate intolerance and worsening of diabetes, glaucoma, cataracts, osteoporosis, dermal atrophy, skin hypopigmentation, and psychiatric disorders including depression, euphoria, or acute psychosis. It should also be noted that even systemic corticosteroids will likely prove ineffective if exposure to the offending allergen or irritant is not limited.

FOLLOW-UP AND REFERRAL

Follow-up and referral are determined by the patient's condition and response to therapy. Although most cases of contact dermatitis are effectively managed by the primary-care practitioner, with at least one follow-up visit after a week to assess therapeutic response (thereby confirming the diagnosis), severe cases should be referred to a dermatologist or an allergist.

Patient Education: Contact Dermatitis

The provider should teach the patient and family about the disease course, how to recognize triggers (i.e., exposure to allergen or irritant 24–72 hours before the onset of rash) and prevent future contact, the appropriate use of medications, and signs of an exacerbation that should prompt the patient to seek care. The mainstay of prevention is helping patients identify the agents causing the dermatitis and teaching them to avoid exposure, to use protective clothing and gloves, and to prevent the spread of contact allergens by avoiding scratching, trimming the fingernails, and thorough hand washing.

SEBORRHEIC DERMATITIS

Seborrheic dermatitis is one of the most common skin conditions seen in primary care among adults and the elderly. It is a chronic condition that is characterized by remissions and exacerbations and may be a sign of more serious underlying pathology, such as immune suppression. The rash of seborrheic dermatitis is seen on skin that is rich in sebaceous glands, such as the scalp, forehead, eyebrows, and the area surrounding the nose and ears.

EPIDEMIOLOGY AND CAUSES

Seborrheic dermatitis affects approximately 2% to 5% of the adult population. It runs in families and has a known genetic component. It may be an inflammatory reaction to *Malassezia furfur* yeasts. The occurrence of seborrheic dermatitis is most common during early infancy on the scalp ("cradle cap"), after the second decade of life, and in the elderly or immunocompromised patients. A strong association with HIV infection and AIDS is well established, and severe or resistant cases of seborrheic dermatitis should prompt investigation for the risk factors of HIV infection. Emotional stress has also been associated with acute flares.

PATHOPHYSIOLOGY

This type of dermatitis was originally defined by excess oil secretion from the sebaceous glands and is thus found on areas of the body where such glands are most concentrated. In decreasing order, these include the scalp, face, chest, upper back, pubic area, and axillae. Interestingly, however, overproduction of sebum is not seen in all cases of seborrheic dermatitis, nor is the composition of sebum, the main factor in this condition. The condition is not thought to be an allergic reaction nor the result of poor hygiene. Skin biopsies typically reveal parakeratotic scale heaped around hair follicles and an inflammatory

lymphocytic infiltrate. Thus, mild epidermal hyperproliferation has been cited as a contributing factor.

M. furfur commonly colonizes affected individuals. However, it is not known whether seborrheic dermatitis occurs in response to infection by saprophytic skin fungi or if the disease process creates conditions that may predispose affected skin to superficial fungal infection. Of note, the recurrence of symptoms has been linked to an increase in the number of *M. furfur* organisms found on the skin surface, and fungal-specific stains of affected skin reveal large numbers of fungal spores within the stratum corneum, the uppermost skin layer.

CLINICAL PRESENTATION

Subjective

The typical patient is an adult man who complains of a pink, scaling rash located on the face and scalp. Seborrheic dermatitis can also be an incidental finding, as some patients, especially elderly patients, are not bothered by the cosmetic effect of the rashes. The lesions are usually asymptomatic in most patients, but pruritus may be present and is aggravated by perspiration, especially in scalp lesions.

Objective

Seborrheic dermatitis presents as scaly patches that may be slightly papular; each patch is surrounded by erythema. The affected skin is pink, edematous, and covered with yellow to brown scales and crusts. The lesion borders are poorly defined, and the scales may appear greasy. The most frequently involved area is the scalp, and the condition is differentiated from common dandruff (pityriasis sicca) by the appearance of erythema, which may be minimal or moderate. Commonly affected areas include the forehead at the hairline, eyebrows, nasal folds, and the retroauricular and presternal areas. In more severe cases, intertriginous areas, the external ear canal, or the umbilicus may be involved. These rashes may be more difficult to recognize in fastidious patients because daily bathing removes some of the scale.

DIAGNOSTIC REASONING

Diagnostic Tests

The diagnosis of seborrheic dermatitis is based on clinical findings and the medical history. Dermatologists and allergists can test for *M. furfur* using antigen-specific skin prick or serum RAST testing. Fifteen percent to 65% of patients with seborrheic dermatitis have positive responses to skin prick tests with *Malassezia* extracts. *Malassezia* antibodies have also been found in young adults with head and neck dermatitis.

Fungal-specific periodic acid Schiff and Gomori methenamine silver stains identify hyphae and spores in skin scrapings or biopsy samples; however, these specialized stains typically require specialist referral and are not commonly used in the primary-care setting. Rather, the diagnosis of seborrheic dermatitis is most frequently based on the characteristic appearance and distribution of the rash, as well as its response to empiric therapy.

Differential Diagnosis

Skin conditions that mimic seborrheic dermatitis include impetigo, atopic dermatitis, psoriasis, scabies, tinea capitis, and Langerhans cell histiocytosis. A history of the same rash recurring at characteristic locations on the body (e.g., the scalp and hairline, sides of the nose and upper lip, eyebrows and eyelashes, cheeks, or ears) will give the clinician the best clues to identify seborrheic dermatitis accurately.

Impetigo, a bacterial infection of the skin caused by *Staphylococcus* or *Streptococcus* bacteria, has an acute onset and tends to occur on the extremities such as the sides of fingers (a location not seen in seborrheic dermatitis) or on the face under the nose (due to repeated wiping of nasal secretions with the hands). The most useful distinguishing feature between atopic dermatitis and seborrheic dermatitis is the increased number of lesions on the forearms in the former, compared with the increased number of lesions in the axillae in the latter. The erythema of seborrheic dermatitis typically has a pinkish hue, rather than the bright-red appearance of psoriasis.

Seborrheic dermatitis is also associated with several chronic conditions including Parkinson's disease, HIV infection and AIDS, phenylketonuria, cardiac failure, zinc deficiency, and epilepsy. This association is not specific, however, as other dermatological disorders, such as acne vulgaris, rosacea, and psoriasis, may also be associated with these diseases. Importantly, florid manifestations of seborrheic dermatitis may be an early cutaneous indicator of HIV infection, and these patients may demonstrate extensive symptoms that are often resistant to therapy.

MANAGEMENT

The high incidence and chronic benign nature of seborrheic dermatitis present a therapeutic challenge. Mild to moderate cases do not seem to bother some patients, especially elderly patients who frequently refuse treatment or are noncompliant. In contrast, younger patients who are bothered by the cosmetic effects of the rashes on the face frequently request treatment. The therapeutic approach is aimed at managing symptoms and reducing the yeast count on the skin.

The regular use of an OTC antidandruff shampoo is sufficient to control most scalp lesions. The preparation must remain on the scalp for at least 5 to 7 minutes to be effective. Commonly used ingredients in these products include selenium sulfide, zinc pyrithione, coal tar, salicylic acid, sulfur, or ketoconazole. Zinc pyrithione and selenium sulfide are classified as keratolytic agents. They appear to be both fungicidal and cytostatic. The combination of sulfur and salicylic acid has keratolytic, antifungal, and antiseptic actions. Coal tar shampoo should be used with caution in persons with light-colored or dyed hair because changes in hair color may occur while the product is being used.

Resistant seborrheic dermatitis may require a prescription shampoo. A 2.5% selenium sulfide shampoo and a ketoconazole (Nizoral) shampoo are available. Ketoconazole shampoo and similar products are recommended to be used every other day for resistant cases. When there is facial or chest involvement, ketoconazole 2% cream may be applied to the affected areas twice daily. Topical ketoconazole (Nizoral 1%) is available OTC. Keratolytic or oil-based lotions are recommended to soften heavy crusts.

A topical corticosteroid may be necessary when significant erythema is present. Hydrocortisone cream 0.5% to 1.0% (OTC) for the face or betamethasone valerate 0.1% for the scalp should be applied after cleansing. Facial application and long-term use of topical corticosteroids should be avoided because of the risk of telangiectasia and dermal atrophy. These risks are not present with the topical use of ketoconazole (Nizoral 1%). Exudative lesions may require compresses of Burow's solution applied for 30 minutes three times daily.

Calcineurin inhibitors that decrease the activity of the immune system may be effective for recalcitrant cases, although these drugs are not FDA approved for seborrheic dermatitis. Such agents include tacrolimus (Protopic) and pimecrolimus (Elidel), which are available in topical formulations. As indicated for second-line therapy in atopic dermatitis, the FDA cautions against the chronic use of these medications in any age group, given concerns over their long-term safety, including rare reports of malignancies.

Once symptoms resolve, maintenance therapy may be required with a once to twice a week application of a topical product for prophylaxis, such as ketoconazole (Nizoral) shampoo or an OTC anti-dandruff shampoo. For a superinfection of gram-positive skin bacteria, an appropriate antibiotic course is indicated, as guided by the patient's allergy history (e.g., cephalexin given for 7 to 10 days in patients without penicillin allergy). Similarly, given the strong association with HIV infection and AIDS, treating a patient's underlying HIV infection with effective antiretroviral therapy is often the key to resolution of the patient's skin findings.

FOLLOW-UP AND REFERRAL

Although uncomplicated forms of seborrheic dermatitis are readily managed by the primary-care practitioner, repeated secondary infections or resistance to standard management requires a prompt referral to a dermatologist. In addition, underlying exacerbating factors, such as immune suppression or neurodegenerative disorders that have an impact on self-care, also require appropriate referrals.

Patient Education: Seborrheic Dermatitis

Patients should be reassured that seborrheic dermatitis in and of itself is neither contagious nor progressive. They must understand the chronic nature of the condition and the need for continued management, as well as the potential for this condition to be associated with more serious underlying disorders, such as immunosuppression, poor self-care, or superinfection. The role of emotional stress in acute flare-ups should also be noted and addressed with self-relaxation techniques. If topical corticosteroids are used, the patient needs to be instructed in their proper application and the potential adverse effects of indiscriminate use. A list of effective OTC preparations should be provided, so each patient can select one that meets his or her personal preferences. Daily shampooing of oily hair is recommended for the first week, and then decreasing to two or three times a week as maintenance therapy.

PSORIASIS

Psoriasis is a chronic relapsing disorder of keratin synthesis that is characterized by well-circumscribed, raised, erythematous papules and plaques, covered with silvery-white scales, usually involving extensor areas in adults such as the elbows and knees, the scalp, and, in some forms, the flexural surfaces of the body. The phrase "heartbreak of psoriasis" was coined because of the physically and emotionally disabling effects of the disease.

The more commonly seen variants of psoriasis are plaque, guttate, inverse, pustular, and erythrodermic psoriasis. Plaque psoriasis is the most common form in young adults, which presents as erythematous lesions with well-demarcated margins, topped with a thick, silvery scale. Plaque psoriasis accounts for approximately 80% of all cases of psoriasis. Guttate psoriasis is more common in children, presenting as an acute eruption of multiple, smaller plaques (less than 1 cm). Inverse psoriasis is characterized by localization of psoriatic plaques to flexural (intertriginous) surfaces. Pustular psoriasis is the most serious form of the disease and is characterized by widespread scaling with a sheet of superficial pustules. Erythrodermic psoriasis may be considered a separate entity or as the most severe form of pustular psoriasis, which may be life-threatening and is associated with chronic immunosuppression (e.g., HIV infection). Bright-red erythema affecting a large portion of the skin surface is the most prominent feature of erythrodermic psoriasis, which may present with variable keratotic scale and the presence of pustules.

EPIDEMIOLOGY AND CAUSES

Psoriasis is universal in occurrence, but the prevalence varies according to geography, race, and ethnicity. Approximately 7.5 million people in the United States have psoriasis, as well as 2% to 4% of the population worldwide. Geographic variations in prevalence (e.g., almost no cases in South Americans living in the Andes to nearly 3% of the population in Denmark) reflect the influence of both genetic and environmental factors. Psoriasis is less frequent among Asians and among North and South American native peoples, compared with people of European ancestry. It is also less frequent among West Africans, which may help explain the low prevalence of psoriasis among African Americans. Prevalence is highest among Scandinavians, with rates slightly higher in northern rather than southern Sweden, further supporting the role of climate and sunlight exposure in the expression of the disease.

Adult men and women are affected with equal frequency. The two peak ages of onset are during the late teens to early 20s and in the late 50s to early 60s. Women and adolescent girls tend to have an earlier onset than males, and earlier onset is associated with a more severe disease. There is little to no epidemiological evidence that psoriasis is mediated by infectious agents.

Psoriasis has a strong genetic influence, with one-third of patients with psoriasis reporting having a relative with the disease. In family studies, when one parent is affected, 8% of offspring develop psoriasis and tend to have an earlier onset. When both parents have psoriasis, the percentage increases to approximately 40%. The mode of genetic transmission is not yet defined, however.

Environmental factors are known to precipitate the disease among genetically predisposed patients and include trauma to normal skin that results in psoriasis in areas of repeated friction (Köbner phenomenon), infections (upper respiratory infections, *Streptococcus pyogenes,* HIV), stress, fatigue, a warm and humid climate, sunlight, and certain drugs (e.g., systemic corticosteroids, lithium, beta-adrenergic blockers, NSAIDs, and antimalarials). Risk factors for psoriasis are listed below.

Risk Factors: Psoriasis

Trauma to normal skin (in patients with preexisting psoriasis) that develops into new psoriatic lesions (Köbner phenomenon)
- Physical, chemical, electrical, surgical, infective, or inflammatory insults

Infections
- HIV, *Streptococcus*

Endocrine and metabolic factors
- Postpartum period
- Hypocalcemia (e.g., after dialysis and parathyroidectomy)

Weather-related factors
- Extreme cold weather
- Prolonged exposure to sunlight* or hot, humid weather (more exacerbations occur in summer)

Medications
- Systemic corticosteroids
- Lithium
- Beta-adrenergic blockers
- Antimalarial drugs
- NSAIDs

Psychogenic factors
- Stress
- Mood disorders, e.g., depression

Other factors
- Fatigue
- Alcoholism
- Smoking

*Controlled exposure to sun/ultraviolet light can be therapeutic—see discussion in text.

Despite intensive investigation, the cause of psoriasis remains unknown, but it is thought to be a multifactorial disease, with genetic, environmental, biochemical, and immunological origins. Formerly theorized as an idiopathic skin disease, psoriasis is now known to be a genetically controlled, immune-mediated chronic disease.

Because the cutaneous lesions of psoriasis were thought to result from unregulated hyperproliferative activity in the epidermis, past treatment for psoriasis has been primarily directed toward normalizing the hyperkeratinocytic activity. Currently, the speculation is that genetically predisposed persons may experience clonal T-cell activation in response to antigenic stimulation. Proponents of this theory advance this view based on evidence that affected persons have an increase of various human leukocyte antigens (HLAs), particularly certain class I HLAs such as HLA-B27, which is also seen in patients with psoriatic arthritis, a form of inflammatory arthritis with redness and painful swelling of peripheral joints that may co-occur with psoriasis. Although not all patients with psoriatic arthritis will have active skin manifestations, a personal or family history of psoriasis is required for diagnosis. In addition, psoriatic plaques have high numbers of activated T lymphocytes that are capable of both cellular proliferation and inflammation.

Current research is focused on the role of T cells and the ability of cytokines to influence the dermal immune response to an as yet unidentified antigen. This focus is based on the finding that the immunomodulatory agent cyclosporine is capable of improving psoriatic symptoms, which led to a rethinking of disease pathogenesis. The genetic component of the disease has been the subject of extensive research, as a primary goal of current psoriasis research is to elucidate the interplay of genetic and environmental influences on the errant cellular effects seen in the disease. A genetic region linking susceptibility to psoriasis in some individuals has been isolated on chromosome 6, and the first non–chromosome 6 gene marker was identified on chromosome 17q. Subsequent research identified possible DNA loci on chromosomes 4, 8, and 16.

PATHOPHYSIOLOGY

Microscopic examination of psoriatic plaques typically reveals a thickened stratum corneum with hyperplasia of the epidermis and little inflammation. The basic histopathology of psoriasis is the uncontrolled hyperkeratinization of the stratum corneum layer of the skin. Hyperproliferation of keratins 6 and 16 (common to reactive and healing skin) predominates, whereas expression of keratins 1 and 10 (typically found in normal skin) is reduced. The psoriatic pathophysiologic process occurs in varying degrees and results in a wide range of clinical symptoms. If increased mitosis or hyperkeratinization predominates, the result is a thick, silvery scale because of the separation of corneocytes with the presence of air in between. Despite this epidermal hyperplasia and parakeratosis, however, the granular layer of the epidermis is significantly thinned or absent. In contrast, if vasodilation predominates, the result is a presentation of diffusely reddened, hot, and slightly scaling skin. Of note, these two processes may coexist.

There are three stages to the psoriatic process: (1) an increased mitotic rate that results in rapid cellular turnover and shortened transit time from the basal layer to the stratum corneum or epidermis (3 to 4 days vs the normal 28 days); (2) dilation of upper dermal capillaries with intermittent extravasation of T cells and polymorphonuclear neutrophils into both the dermis and epidermis, leading to (3) the faulty keratinization and accumulation of the stratum corneum, which clinically presents as raised papules and plaques covered with white, silvery scales.

Multiple growth factors (e.g., epidermal growth factor, transforming growth factor–alpha) and cytokines (e.g., interferon-γ, IL-2, IL-6, IL-8, and IL-17A) are overexpressed in psoriatic skin. Moreover, in plaque-type psoriasis, the T cells localized to the epidermis appear to express specific clonalities with regard to their antigenic receptors, implicating unrestrained T-cell replication in the pathogenesis of the disease. Interestingly, however, psoriasis is also associated with many causes of chronic immunosuppression and may be the presenting finding in newly diagnosed HIV infection—particularly the severe erythrodermic form.

Most recently, the importance of a novel subset of CD4 T helper T cells, known as Th17 cells, has been highlighted in the autoimmune pathogenesis of psoriasis, as they have also been isolated from psoriatic skin plaques. Activated Th17 cells produce multiple cytokines, including IL-17, IL-21, and IL-22, and proliferate in response to IL-23. Several studies have demonstrated the importance of Th17 cells in fighting infection by extracellular bacteria and fungi. Thus, one theory is that dysregulated Th17 function leads to an exuberant immune response to skin flora and ultimately the characteristic hyperkeratinization of psoriasis.

Drug-induced exacerbations of psoriasis can be unpredictable and severe. They are often delayed and may occur months after the start of drug use. Associations with specific drugs have offered some insights into the pathogenic mechanisms of psoriasis. Lithium is believed to act by enhancing the release of inflammatory mediators from neutrophils. Beta blockers lead to psoriasis by decreasing cyclic adenosine monophosphate-dependent protein kinase—an inhibitor of cellular proliferation. NSAIDs cause a buildup of the proinflammatory mediator arachidonic acid by inhibiting the enzyme cyclooxygenase. Antimalarials, the antifungal terbinafine (Lamisil), and angiotensin-converting enzyme inhibitors are also associated with exacerbations of psoriasis, although these mechanisms are unclear.

CLINICAL PRESENTATION

Subjective

Patients with psoriasis usually present to the practitioner with concern over "itchy, red, inflamed and dry, scaly plaques that have gotten worse." Statements about the onset and course of the disease are highly variable among patients. Symptoms usually begin gradually and are confined to only a few areas (e.g., one or both elbows, the knees, buttocks, or scalp), but psoriasis can also be explosive in onset.

One cause of rapid-onset, explosive psoriasis is a preceding streptococcal throat infection, which can lead 2 to 3 weeks later to multiple, small, guttate lesions developing in a generalized distribution over the body. Once the disease appears, it follows an irregular, chronic, and unpredictable course, as it may remain localized to a few areas or cause intermittent or continuous generalized lesions.

Itching is usually not a problem in most cases of psoriasis, but it may be severe in some patients. These patients often notice bloodstains on bed sheets from traumatic, inadvertent scratching of the plaques during sleep. Lesions often occur at sites of trauma (Köbner phenomenon). A family history of psoriasis is elicited in one-third of patients, and 50% of these patients have an affected parent.

Three tools commonly used to assess the severity of psoriasis are as follows:

1. The Psoriasis Area and Severity Index combines the assessment of plaque severity (erythema, induration/thickness, and scaling) and the extent of skin surface area affected; it is the most widely used assessment tool for psoriasis in clinical research and practice settings.
2. The Dermatology Life Quality Index has the patient self-rate the impact of the condition on important aspects of his or her life.
3. Affected body surface area is an assessment of the overall skin area involved by percentage.

A Web site for accessing and automatically calculating disease severity scores using these tools is listed in the Resources section at the end of the chapter.

Psoriasis patients are known to be at greater risk for depressive symptoms, which may progress to suicidal ideation or behavior. The impact of psoriasis on one's quality of life and emotional state cannot be overgeneralized because this is largely dependent on the individual patient's coping skills. Thus, all psoriasis patients should undergo a screening mental health assessment for depression and suicidal ideation, regardless of the severity of disease.

Objective

Physical examination reveals erythematous plaques surrounded by a thick, silvery scale (which is not easily removed), resembling mica. When these micaceous scales are traumatically removed, multiple small sites of bleeding appear (Auspitz's sign). In intertriginous areas, maceration and moisture prevent dry scales from accumulating, but the lesions remain red and sharply defined.

Lesions usually are distributed symmetrically over areas of bony prominences such as the elbows and knees. Scaly plaques also occur frequently on the trunk, scalp, intergluteal cleft, and umbilicus. The latter three areas are frequently overlooked by the patient and clinician but are important in making the diagnosis, especially in patients with associated psoriatic arthritis and limited skin lesions. In fact, the nature of such inflammatory arthritis may only become apparent after typical psoriatic skin lesions are recognized.

A thorough examination of the entire skin surface is therefore crucial to the diagnosis and treatment of a patient with suspected psoriasis. Another helpful diagnostic feature is the Köbner phenomenon, in which physical trauma (e.g., at flexural surfaces) induces the formation of new skin lesions. Such isomorphic lesions can also be induced on the palms of patients whose hands are exposed to friction.

Nail involvement may include stippling or pitting of the nail plate or a yellow to red-brown coloring ("oil-staining") of the nails (nail psoriasis). An accumulation of yellow debris under the nails, simulating a tinea infection (tinea unguium), is seen in some patients. Swelling, redness, and scaling of the paronychial margins occur often and are associated with arthritis of the distal interphalangeal joints. The clinical course of this disease is characterized by chronicity and seasonal fluctuations, with improvement in the summer (due to sun exposure) and worsening in the winter as dry skin leads to epidermal injury.

Up to 10% to 20% of patients with psoriasis may also have an inflammatory arthritis known as psoriatic arthritis, although the most common form of arthritis seen in psoriasis patients, as in the general population, is osteoarthritis. The inflammatory joint manifestations of psoriatic arthritis may occur when psoriatic skin lesions are present, or they may precede initial skin manifestations, with psoriatic arthritis being suspected in a patient with inflammatory joint disease due to a family history of psoriasis. Associated inflammatory arthritis seen in psoriasis patients typically involves the distal interphalangeal joints of the hands and feet but may also involve the vertebrae of the spine, as seen with another form of seronegative (i.e., rheumatoid factor–negative) arthritis known as ankylosing spondylitis.

The clinical characteristics of common variants of psoriasis (plaque, pustular, guttate, inverse, and erythrodermic) are discussed in greater detail in Differential Diagnosis 16.2.

Differential Diagnosis 16.2: Psoriasis

Type of Psoriasis	Clinical Presentation	Differential Diagnosis	Distinguishing Differential From Psoriasis
Plaque psoriasis	• Plaques with white silvery scales • Seen on knees, elbows, neck, scalp, between buttocks, or on back	Seborrheic dermatitis	Sharply marginated yellowish-red to brown patches with sharp borders and greasy scales. Seen on the scalp (especially the hairline), central face, eyebrows, eyelids, nasolabial folds, and external ear. Can be pruritic.
	• Usually bilateral involvement • Intertriginous areas may be involved, but scales are absent	Nummular eczema	Pruritic, coin-shaped plaques or papulovesicles on an erythematous base with uniform scaling; may become exudative and crusted. Typically seen on legs, upper extremities, and trunk.
	• Positive Auspitz sign and Köbner phenomenon	Lichen planus	Pruritic, flat, irregular purple papules with fine white lines and scales. Commonly seen on flexor surfaces, nails, and scalp.
	• Gradual onset, chronic course	Pityriasis rubra pilaris	Generalized erythematous, red-orange lesions with diffuse thickening, interspersed with areas of normal skin. The palms and soles are usually affected.
		Atopic dermatitis	Severe pruritus, palmar markings, increased creasing of infraorbital folds. The sides of the neck, hands, and flexural surfaces are most commonly affected after age 12 years.
		Mycosis fungoides (cutaneous T-cell lymphoma)	Sharply demarcated, scaly, raised plaques to violaceous nodules that may ulcerate.

Continued

✤ Differential Diagnosis 16.2: Psoriasis—cont'd

Type of Psoriasis	Clinical Presentation	Differential Diagnosis	Distinguishing Differential From Psoriasis
Pustular psoriasis	• Lesions may be localized, appearing on the hands and feet (Barber's disease), or involve the entire skin surface (Von Zumbusch's disease). • Onset is sudden. • Pustules appear on the edges of existing psoriatic plaques and on the palms. • Pruritus and intense burning sensation are present. • Patient may have a fever and systemic symptoms; systemic complications include pneumonia, congestive heart failure, and hepatitis.	Pustular dermatitis	Persistent or recurrent dry red and scaly rash; first appearance in infancy, with history of dry skin since birth.
Guttate psoriasis	• Characterized by small, red papules (<1 cm in diameter)	Secondary syphilis	Base of lesion (ulcer) is clean and smooth; edges are raised and well circumscribed. Usually occurs in genital region or on lips.
	• Discrete lesions, seen in a raindrop- or shower-like distribution, usually on the trunk and extremities • Triggered by streptococcal infection • May see Köbner phenomenon	Pityriasis rosea	Well-demarcated, salmon-colored herald patch, forming a collarette of fine scaling, followed by other lesions on trunk and proximal extremities. Christmas-tree distribution on exposed areas.
Inverse psoriasis	• Involves the flexural areas (e.g., armpits, groin)	Candidiasis	Erythematous, macerated patches with sharp, scaling border. Satellite lesions (papules and pustules that are tender and pruritic) are common.
Erythrodermic psoriasis	• Severe form of pustular psoriasis • Generalized distribution • Erythema with variable scale and fluid and electrolyte loss • May experience chills	Drug eruption	Massive superficial dermal edema that lifts off the epidermis, developing necrosis that appears as violaceous plaques or bullae, later healing with postinflammatory hyperpigmentation (e.g., Stevens-Johnson syndrome, toxic epidermal necrolysis).
		Pityriasis rubra pilaris	Fine to thick scales on the palms or soles; orange-red lesions with diffuse thickening.
		Eczematous dermatitis	See preceding descriptions for nummular eczema and atopic dermatitis.
		Mycosis fungoides	See description above for cutaneous T-cell lymphoma.

DIAGNOSTIC REASONING

Diagnostic Tests

Initial laboratory studies include routine testing with a CBC with differential to assess for infection and a serum chemistry profile with a serum uric acid level. Laboratory tests are generally within normal limits in psoriasis, except for the serum uric acid level, which may be elevated (hyperuricemia). In more severe variants of psoriasis, other specific tests may be ordered. Throat culture is appropriate if *Streptococcus pyogenes* infection is suspected as the precipitating factor (as in guttate psoriasis). Immunoglobulins are generally normal, but selective IgA and IgG deficiencies are observed in some patients. In pustular psoriasis, leukocytosis and hypocalcemia are seen. An elevated erythrocyte sedimentation rate and decreased albumin levels, along with anemia, can be observed in chronic disease.

X-ray studies of the hands are sometimes helpful to search for associated psoriatic arthritis in patients who complain of joint pains in their hands. X-ray of patients with psoriatic arthritis will show extensive erosion and luxation of distal interphalangeal or metatarsophalangeal joints bilaterally, with characteristic "pencil-in-cup" erosive abnormalities of the interphalangeal joints. In these abnormalities, the distal head of a bone becomes pointed like a sharp pencil, while the adjacent articular surface becomes rounded, like a cup.

Biopsy is seldom necessary because the clinical features of psoriasis are so distinctive. Only in unusual circumstances (severe or unusual forms of the disease) are histological studies necessary to diagnose psoriasis. Biopsies should be planned to yield maximal information. When performing a biopsy, nonexcoriated intact lesions should be sampled. If there are lesions at different stages of eruption, more than one sample is necessary. Biopsies can include partial dermal thickness procedures, such as shave or curettage biopsy, or full-thickness sampling with punch or excisional biopsy.

A skin biopsy is done with the use of a local anesthetic to obtain sufficient tissue for an accurate diagnosis. Skin biopsy is a "clean" procedure and should be done simply and quickly. A standard 4-mm punch biopsy is often used and recommended because minimal scarring is the desired end result. It may be useful to take two or more samples at the first examination of complex cases. However, a biopsy should not be performed on infected skin, on any patient with a bleeding disorder, or on any individual who is allergic to local anesthetics. The key to an informative biopsy is careful selection of the sample based on experience. Clinicians who are not experienced in this procedure should refer the patient to a dermatologist (see Therapeutic Procedure 16.1).

Of note, the sudden onset of psoriasis, in particular erythrodermic forms, may be associated with HIV; thus, the presence of underlying HIV infection should be ruled out in such patients, if unknown.

Therapeutic Procedure 16.1: The Skin "Punch" Biopsy

- Prep the area around the lesion that has been carefully selected.
- Inject 1% lidocaine slowly and superficially at several sites around the lesion, for rapid effect and minimal injury. Epinephrine may be used to control bleeding except at certain distal sites, given the risk of tip necrosis (nose, ears, fingertips, toes, penis).
- Punch into the skin with the punch biopsy tool around the lesion at a 90-degree angle to the plane of the skin, with a quick back-and-forth twisting motion, reaching in fast.
- Carefully lift out the plug and snip it at the base with sharp tissue scissors.
- Place the tissue plug in a formalin solution.
- Apply pressure with sterile gauze for hemostasis.
- Lose with two sutures (4.0 or 5.0 size). (Suture removal will be determined according to the location—sutures on the face should be removed sooner than those on the extremities.)

NOTE: Nerve damage can occur in areas where nerves are located superficially, such as the lateral aspects of fingers and the ulnar groove of the elbows. Any lesions in these areas (including the face for cosmetic reasons) should be referred to a dermatologist for biopsy, if needed.

Differential Diagnosis

It is not uncommon to see a patient with more than one variant of psoriasis at the same time, and the pattern may change over time. Often, psoriasis is mistaken for other dermatological conditions. Thus, other skin diseases should be ruled out by evaluating for characteristic clinical presentations (see Differential Diagnosis 16.2), especially in atypical cases that are complicated by systemic manifestations. The differential diagnosis for psoriasis includes the following: atopic dermatitis, nummular eczema, CTCL, tinea corporis, lichen planus, seborrheic dermatitis, drug eruptions, and secondary syphilis.

Eczematous rashes may be mistaken for psoriasis, but several distinguishing characteristics may be noted. Hyperkeratotic eczema of the palms is a common cause of misdiagnosis, as psoriasis may also present in a palmoplantar distribution, but eczematous rashes tend to be more pruritic than psoriasis. Atopic dermatitis frequently has its first presentation in infancy or childhood, and the patient may report a persistent or recurrent dry, red, scaly, pruritic rash and a history of dry skin since birth. Atopic dermatitis at times develops a psoriasiform appearance, especially on the legs. Nummular eczema has a characteristic morphology that helps to distinguish it from other eczematous eruptions. Initially, nummular eczema presents with tiny papules and vesicles and then assumes its characteristic clinical appearance of coin-shaped plaques. It is typically seen on the legs, but it can also appear on the upper extremities and trunk; the lesions are pruritic, erythematous, and surrounded with uniform scaling.

CTCL can be difficult to diagnose in its early stages. Early on, the rash may appear as a single or multiple erythematous, scaly macules. In its subsequent stage, which may occur anywhere from 6 months to 6 years later, the development of sharply demarcated, scaly, elevated, red to violaceous plaques, known as mycosis fungoides, occurs. These plaques may coalesce to form larger plaques with annular, circinate, or serpiginous borders, or they may completely regress. The disease may further progress to brown or purplish red dermal nodules (tumors). The nodules often occur on the face, the body folds, and the inframammary area in women. The tumors can progress further to exfoliative erythroderma. Through much of this process, CTCL may resemble atopic dermatitis with diffuse erythema and scaling; a definitive diagnosis can be made by skin biopsy.

Tinea corporis (ringworm) presents as erythematous patches and plaques with central clearing and peripheral scales, crusts, vesicles, and pustules; this fungal infection may spontaneously resolve or worsen with topical corticosteroid treatment. In seborrheic dermatitis, the lesions are lighter in color, less well defined, and covered with a dull yellow scale. Lesions commonly occur in a similar psoriatic distribution, including face, scalp, and central chest. Lichen planus presents a diagnostic challenge if it presents as hypertrophic lesions on the legs, as penile lesions, or on the hands, which result from excessive scratching. In pityriasis rosea, a single herald patch occurs first; subsequent smaller eruptions follow skin lines in a Christmas-tree pattern. Pityriasis rubra pilaris presents as generalized erythematous lesions with areas of normal skin; the palms and soles are usually affected.

Drug eruptions resulting from beta blockers, methyldopa, and gold preparations can produce psoriatic-type lesions. Intertriginous psoriasis may appear similar to candidiasis but in most cases would be distinguishable through Wood's lamp examination and KOH wet mount testing. Mycosis fungoides lesions progress to violaceous, indurated plaques and nodules, which typically begin on the thighs, buttocks, and trunk.

MANAGEMENT

The goal of therapy for psoriasis is to control the disease so that the patient no longer feels physically or psychologically hindered by the skin lesions. For sparse or mild lesions that do not bother the patient, no treatment may be needed. When treatment is indicated, however, the disease is controlled by decreasing epidermal proliferation and underlying dermal inflammation through the use of topical corticosteroids and other immunomodulatory agents, along with phototherapy in some patients. Systemic agents are reserved for moderate to severe or recalcitrant cases.

The chronic course of psoriasis and the lack of cure can be both discouraging and challenging for the patient and the clinician. Patients should be reassured that the therapeutic options today are much broader than in the past, and several new therapeutic approaches and medications, including highly effective biological therapies, are now available, as well as improvements in phototherapy and photochemotherapy.

Some patients find the presence of even a few small plaques highly objectionable because the location of the plaques in highly visible areas of the body is disfiguring or may hinder physical activity. Other patients are willing to accept the condition as bothersome but not overly impairing, particularly when they realize there is no cure. A long-term individualized plan of disease management is therefore helpful for patients with psoriasis to help deal with exacerbations, which cause frustration or discouragement.

Psoriasis is not simply localized skin disease. Its pathophysiology is characterized by systemic inflammation, in which other bodily systems, such as the cardiovascular network, may be affected by inflammation and subsequent high-risk events. In turn, the National Psoriasis Foundation (NPF) has established recommendations for comorbidity screening of adults with psoriasis. These include guidance on cardiovascular disease and metabolic syndrome, obesity, depression, infections, malignancy, and other immune-mediated inflammatory diseases such as Crohn's disease and inflammatory psoriatic arthritis. Similarly, the Pediatric Dermatology Research Alliance and the NPF have also collaborated to develop evidence-based guidelines for comorbidity screening for patients with pediatric psoriasis. Appropriate therapy must be directed toward comorbidities identified by such screening.

Topical Therapy

Topical agents are first-line pharmacotherapeutics for psoriasis that are usually effective. If less than 20% of the body (e.g., no more than the elbows, knees, ears, and scalp) is involved, topical agents are usually sufficient. However, if more than 20% of the body is affected and manifestations are moderate to severe, systemic therapy may be warranted, and referral to a dermatologist is recommended. For stubborn, persistent, and widespread lesions, ultraviolet (UV) light treatment should be strongly considered. Systemic therapy in psoriasis is usually used as a last resort because the significant effectiveness of biological agents must be weighed against their high cost and side-effect profile.

Widely used topical agents are available both as OTC and prescription formulations. OTC emollient creams or ointments applied to the skin at least twice daily are helpful in preventing cracking and fissuring of lesions, especially those on the palms and soles. Keratolytic agents, such as 1% to 5% salicylic acid preparations, may be combined with emollients to enhance the absorption of other drugs, such as topical corticosteroids, through thick psoriatic lesions. Keratolytic agents may be applied twice daily.

Topical corticosteroids are widely used because they are relatively easy to apply. Those with intermediate and strong potency should be applied no more than once or twice daily. Topical corticosteroids are an appropriate treatment in cases involving 10% or less of the body surface (e.g., the face, neck, flexural surfaces, and genitalia). Psoriatic plaques usually blanch and thin in response to the treatment. More potent corticosteroids may be applied to achieve complete clearing of psoriasis and are helpful in treating exposed areas of the body. However, caution is needed in corticosteroid usage, because they can cause skin atrophy and suppression of the HPA axis, resulting in a Cushingoid syndrome.

An effective treatment approach for exacerbations of psoriasis is to initially use "superpotent" topical corticosteroid preparations (e.g., Diprolene, Psorcon, Temovate, Ultravate) for 2 weeks and then decrease to a lesser potency agent for maintenance therapy. Superpotent corticosteroids should not be used for more than 2 weeks. Once symptoms are under control, other topical agents or a weaker corticosteroid may be substituted after gradually tapering the dose (see Box 16.2).

The penetration and absorption of topical corticosteroids will increase with occlusive dressing, but some superpotent corticosteroids should not be applied with occlusion because of increased risk of HPA suppression from systemic absorption. Ointment preparations are preferred over creams or lotions if the psoriatic scale is thick. When heavy scaling is present, gentle brushing of the psoriatic scales after warm soaks or during warm baths before applying the topical agents will increase absorption. Hard scrubbing should be avoided, however, because skin trauma can exacerbate the psoriasis.

Topical corticosteroid therapy has several drawbacks. Remission periods are often relatively short. Prolonged use produces striae and thinning of skin (atrophy), and the rebound effect can worsen the existing symptoms, possibly converting "stable" disease to an "unstable" state, if the dose of corticosteroid is suddenly discontinued. Prolonged use of corticosteroids has been associated with suppression of the HPA axis and a Cushingoid syndrome, as noted previously, due to suppression of endogenous glucocorticoid production.

Topical tar and anthralin are agents that can be used once daily in combination with topical corticosteroids. Scalp involvement may benefit from use of a tar shampoo (e.g., Zetar, Sebutone, Pentrax) before the application of a topical corticosteroid. The tar shampoo is gently massaged on the scalp and left on for a few hours

---

Box 16.2 Potency of Topical Corticosteroids for Atopic Dermatitis

Extremely High Potency

Betamethasone dipropionate, augmented 0.05%
Clobetasol propionate 0.05%
Fluocinonide 0.1%
Flurandrenolide 4 mcg/cm^2 (tape)
Halobetasol propionate 0.05%

High Potency

Amcinonide 0.1%
Betamethasone dipropionate 0.05%
Desoximetasone 0.05%, 0.25%
Diflorasone diacetate 0.05%
Fluocinonide 0.05%
Halcinonide 0.1%
Triamcinolone acetonide 0.5%

Intermediate Potency

Betamethasone valerate 0.05%, 0.12%
Clocortolone pivalate 0.1%
Desonide 0.05%
Desoximetasone 0.05%
Fluocinolone acetonide 0.025%
Flurandrenolide 0.025%, 0.05%
Fluticasone propionate 0.005%, 0.05%
Hydrocortisone probutate 0.1%
Hydrocortisone butyrate 0.1%
Hydrocortisone valerate 0.2%
Mometasone furoate 0.1%
Prednicarbate 0.1%
Triamcinolone acetonide 0.05%, 0.1%, 0.2%

Low Potency

Alclometasone dipropionate 0.05%
Fluocinolone acetonide 0.01%
Hydrocortisone base or acetate 1%, 1.85%, 2%, 2.5%
Triamcinolone acetonide 0.025%

---

and then rinsed off. Softened scales are gently removed. The scalp should be gently dried before application of the corticosteroid lotion. Wearing a shower cap after corticosteroid application enhances absorption and improves results. Excessive combing after washing the hair should be avoided to prevent trauma.

Anthralin (0.1% or 3.0% ointment) belongs to the class of trihydroxyanthracene compounds; it is used topically for psoriasis. Anthralin is an antimitotic agent capable of inhibiting DNA synthesis. Anthralin is applied once or twice daily and should be washed off after 10 to 30 minutes. It produces quick remission of plaques after several weeks of use but has a tendency to irritate and stain adjacent skin and clothing, making it less preferable than other treatment options. Paradoxically, if topical corticosteroids are added to an anthralin regimen, there may be an increased risk of early relapse.

Another topical treatment includes calcipotriene (Dovonex), a vitamin D ointment derivative. Calcipotriene produces keratinocyte differentiation and controls proliferation. It is superior to a superpotent corticosteroid and is the best treatment for mild to moderate disease. It is a major alternative to topical corticosteroid therapy for plaque-type psoriasis. Studies have found it to be effective in nearly three-quarters of patients with plaque psoriasis, with relatively minor side effects. Pulse therapy utilizes calcipotriene for 5 days and then a moderate- to high-potency topical corticosteroid for 2 days.

A topical agent with similar action to calcipotriene is tazarotene (Tazorac). It interferes with excessive differentiation and proliferation of epidermal cells and also limits the migration of inflammatory mediators to the areas of hyperkeratinization. It achieves a 60% to 70% response rate and long remissions of up to 12 weeks. It is available as an ointment, cream, or lotion preparation. Like other receptor-selective retinoids, tazarotene is considered teratogenic and should not be used by pregnant women.

The topical calcineurin inhibitors tacrolimus (Protopic) and pimecrolimus (Elidel), applied twice per day, may be effective. These treatments have been particularly helpful for psoriasis in the facial and intertriginous areas where topical corticosteroid treatments (other than low-potency agents) should be avoided, given the risk of dermal atrophy. Exposure to natural sunlight improves psoriasis and permits a more enduring remission than does the use of topical corticosteroids. In some patients, topical corticosteroids may even be suspended during the summer. Although sun exposure to the point of mild erythema is helpful, sunburn exacerbates psoriasis and should be avoided.

In 1925, W. H. Goeckerman, a physician at the Mayo Clinic, achieved encouraging results with experimental use of midrange ultraviolet B (UVB) light and coal tar ointment for patients whose psoriasis did not respond to topical therapy. With some modifications of the sunbeam spectrum and combined with topicals, the traditional Goeckerman program is still being used. Crude coal tar of 1% to 2% in gel or ointment form is applied at night to the psoriatic plaques and is followed by UVB treatments. UVB treatment is continued for 4 to 6 weeks and causes remission (for up to 4 months) in 60% to 90% of patients without evidence of increased risk of skin cancer. Guttate psoriasis, in particular, responds well to UVB therapy.

A more aggressive treatment approach is photochemotherapy or PUVA. It has been reported to achieve an 80% to 90% rate of remission on otherwise recalcitrant severe forms of psoriasis, such as the pustular form. The treatment inhibits mitosis by stopping DNA replication and is administered two to three times per week. PUVA involves ingestion of an oral psoralen compound (methoxsalen)

before light exposure. Psoralen may be taken orally or it can be added to a bath, but "bath PUVA therapy" is not widely used in the United States. Psoralen is inactive in the body, but on the skin it is activated by UVA (long-wavelength UVA light). The eyes must be protected during exposure to UVA light because of the potential for cataract formation. Because of the significant occurrence of nausea, body malaise, phototoxic erythema, premature aging of the skin, and pruritus following administration of psoralens, the attrition rate of this treatment is high.

Although it can clear chronic plaque psoriasis in 6 to 8 weeks, overexposure to UVA light can cause acute sunburn in the short term; in the long term, it can cause nonmelanoma skin cancer. Since the mid-1980s, the use of phototherapy has been shown to be associated with squamous cell carcinoma, and in 1991, some cases of melanoma began to surface among patients who had received more than 250 courses of treatment. Therefore, careful follow-up of patients who have had PUVA therapy is crucial. Patients considered at increased risk for skin cancer (those with fair skin who are easily sunburned or individuals who have had previous x-ray therapy to the skin) should not receive PUVA, although PUVA in combination with topical agents is extremely effective.

Systemic Therapy

Systemic therapy is reserved for patients with severe incapacitating disease—pustular, guttate, and/or arthritic psoriasis. It is administered only by expert specialists such as rheumatologists or dermatologists who regularly use systemic antimitotic agents, including methotrexate, etretinate, and cyclosporine.

Methotrexate (Rheumatrex) is a folic acid antagonist and a cytotoxic agent that inhibits cellular proliferation. It is used as chemotherapy for cancer, but it is also useful in patients with moderate to severe psoriatic arthritis. Oral regimens include every other day and once-weekly dosing. If nausea is significant, intramuscular administration can be used. A therapeutic response is usually seen within 2 to 3 weeks, at which time the dosage or dosing interval should be reduced. With prolonged use, cumulative doses of methotrexate could result in hepatotoxicity, nephrotoxicity, and bone marrow depression. Coadministration of folic acid 1 mg by mouth daily effectively protects against many of the minor side effects associated with this treatment, such as stomatitis. Methotrexate is contraindicated in patients with cirrhosis of the liver, immunodeficiency syndromes, or a history of alcoholism.

Monitoring of blood counts, including platelets, should be done weekly in patients taking methotrexate, followed by monthly testing. Renal and liver function tests (baseline and follow-up studies) should be done. Intermittent liver biopsies may be needed with chronic dosing because hepatic fibrosis may occur with prolonged use. Methotrexate is teratogenic and should not be given to those who are pregnant or who want to become pregnant.

Apremilast (Otezla) has been approved to treat moderate to severe plaque psoriasis. This oral drug inhibits the enzyme phosphodiesterase-4, which plays a role in the inflammation of psoriasis. Taken once daily, there is no requirement for ongoing laboratory monitoring or initial laboratory testing with apremilast. Of note, this drug contains a labeled warning for an association with an increase in depression and suicidal ideation.

Cyclosporine (Gengraf, Neoral) is an immunosuppressant that was originally used for the prevention of organ rejection in organ transplant recipients. Its efficacy in severe erythrodermic and psoriatic arthritis was discovered serendipitously while the drug was being tested for rheumatoid arthritis. Significant improvement and even total clearing of psoriasis becomes evident within days of administration in some patients, whereas withdrawal of cyclosporine is associated with relapse within weeks. Hypertension and nephrotoxicity can develop during cyclosporine treatment, although in the vast majority of patients, renal function subsequently normalizes. Treatment with cyclosporine for more than 1 year is not recommended because it may cause prolonged immunosuppression and myalgias. Serum creatinine levels should be monitored throughout the duration of treatment because cyclosporine can cause interstitial fibrosis and tubular atrophy. Other systemic immunosuppressants such as hydroxyurea (Hydrea), azathioprine (Imuran), and tacrolimus have also been used, although these systemic agents all carry significant safety risks and their use is reserved only for cases of sufficient severity.

An oral systemic agent, Acitretin (Soriatane), is a retinoid that can be beneficial for patients with resistant and severe pustular and erythrodermic variants of psoriasis. About 50% of patients who are refractory to PUVA alone improve when a retinoid is added. Female patients who are treated with acitretin (Soriatane) should be advised not to become pregnant for 3 years after ceasing treatment, because retinoids are teratogenic. Patients treated with this drug must also not donate blood for at least 3 years after taking it. Careful monitoring of blood counts, plasma triglycerides, and liver function tests is required.

The most significant development in the psoriasis treatment armamentarium in recent years has been the array of immunomodulatory injectable biological agents used for moderate to severe plaque psoriasis, psoriatic arthritis, and refractory disease. These initially included alefacept (Amevive), a recombinant CD2 antagonist fusion protein that inhibits T-cell activation, and efalizumab (Raptiva), a humanized monoclonal antibody against CD11a. However, efalizumab was withdrawn from the market by the FDA in 2009 due to its association with fatal cases of progressive multifocal leukoencephalopathy, and alefacept was voluntarily withdrawn from the market by its manufacturer in 2011.

Currently, the most widely used class of biologic agents for psoriasis are the tumor necrosis factor–α (TNF-α) antagonists, which include the TNF receptor fusion protein etanercept (Enbrel), the human monoclonal antibodies adalimumab (Humira) and golimumab (Simponi), the human-murine chimeric monoclonal antibody infliximab (Remicade), and the monoclonal TNF-α-specific Fab fragment formulation certolizumab (Cimzia). These biological agents have been revolutionary in the treatment of moderate to severe and refractory psoriasis. However, they require laboratory monitoring and carry the risk of significant side effects, including a black box warning for serious infections and certain malignancies such as lymphoma. In addition, given their significant cost, these and other biologic agents are typically considered second-line therapeutics when UV light therapy or other systemic agents fail.

More recently, alternative classes of biologic agents have been developed to treat moderate to severe psoriasis, such as the anti–IL-12/IL-23 human monoclonal antibody ustekinumab (Stelara), which is specific for the shared cytokine subunit p40 and has proven highly effective. In addition, given the key role of Th17 cells in psoriasis, biologic agents blocking the IL-17 pathway have been developed that are not approved to treat moderate to severe psoriasis in adults. These include the IL-17A-specific human monoclonal antibody secukinumab (Cosentyx), the IL-17A-specific humanized monoclonal antibody ixekizumab (Taltz), and the human monoclonal antibody brodalumab (Siliq), which blocks the IL-17 receptor A and, therefore, multiple isoforms of IL-17 (IL-17A, IL-17F, IL-17C, IL-17A/F, IL-25). Because of their effects on the immune system, patients using these treatments may be at increased risk for infections. Suicidal ideation and behavior were also noted to have occurred in clinical trials of brodalumab; therefore, labeling for Siliq includes a black box warning and is available only through a restricted program under an FDA-mandated Risk Evaluation and Mitigation Strategy.

Complementary Therapies

Utilization of complementary therapies for psoriasis is growing. Therapies include dietary modifications, herbs and supplements, mind–body therapies (e.g., aromatherapy, yoga, meditation), physical therapy, exercise, acupuncture and tai chi. Much of the evidence supporting the use of complementary therapies for psoriasis and psoriatic arthritis is anecdotal, however, and certain practices such as dietary restrictions may actually be harmful, if key nutrients are removed from the diet.

FOLLOW-UP AND REFERRAL

Newly diagnosed patients and patients who have moderate to extensive skin involvement or severe disease (e.g., pustular psoriasis) should be referred to a dermatologist or psoriasis specialty treatment center. Patients with recalcitrant or frequent flare-ups should be referred to a dermatologist for UV light therapy and/or systemic treatment. An ophthalmology consultation is necessary before UV therapy to rule out the presence of cataracts. Patients with inflammatory arthritis should be referred to a rheumatologist for specialty care.

Patients with severe psoriasis are usually followed every 2 months by a specialist or more often as required by their particular treatment regimen. Patients who exhibit symptoms of depression or poor coping skills will benefit from referral to a psychiatrist, psychologist, or other mental health professional for psychological evaluation and therapy. Patient support groups that offer social support within the context of a shared patient experience may also be of great psychological help, regardless of the type of treatment initiated. In addition, as psoriasis and psoriatic arthritis patients have higher overweight and obesity rates than the general population, applicable patients may benefit from dietary counseling and/or referral to a nutritionist.

Patient Education: Psoriasis

Psoriasis presents many challenges to both the patient and the health-care provider. For patients with disfiguring and difficult-to-control psoriasis, education and support are central to the treatment process. The patient should be informed of available community resources and support groups. Explanation of the disease process and treatment, including potential adverse effects of medications, is helpful. A newly diagnosed patient and his or her family should be reassured that the disease is not contagious or infectious. Patients need to understand that psoriasis may be an added risk for health problems in the future, such as cardiovascular and psychological comorbidities. Overweight and obese patients should also undergo dietary counseling.

Although the genetic aspects of psoriasis are complex and incompletely characterized, it may be explained to family members of a patient that if neither of the patient's parents has psoriasis, the chances are less than 10% that another child will develop the disease. If one parent is affected, the chance of a child developing psoriasis increases to 15%. If both parents are affected, the chance increases to approximately 60% that one or more children will have the disease.

The clinician should educate the patient that there are several ways of remaining in remission, once treatments have taken effect. Patients with psoriasis should avoid skin trauma and should keep the skin relatively dry to decrease pruritus, scratching,

and scaling. They should avoid photosensitizing medications such as tetracyclines, sulfa drugs, or phenothiazines. If drugs of these types are necessary, patients should be advised to inform the prescribing physician of their psoriasis and to ask for a possible alternative. Although photosensitizing drugs should be avoided, controlled sun exposure during the summer is beneficial, although patients should be advised to use a high-SPF sunscreen to prevent sunburns. Patients should also be informed to seek treatment immediately for streptococcal infections (e.g., skin infections, sore throats), and that other aggravating factors for psoriasis include increased stress and alcohol.

The clinician should explain to the patient that dietary manipulations do not appear to play a role in treating psoriasis. However, healthy eating habits support a strong immune system, and nutritionists recommend a low-fat, high-fiber diet for patients. Naturopaths recommend many herbal medicines to improve psoriasis and to control or provide relief from the disturbing effects of these flare-ups (e.g., capsaicin, tea tree oil, turmeric). Although many persons subscribe to these therapies, there is a lack of data from randomized clinical trials to confirm their effectiveness.

REFERENCES

General

Pickett H, O'Callaghan M. Shave and punch biopsy for skin lesions. *Am Fam Physician.* 2011;84(9):995–1002.

Atopic Dermatitis

Eichenfield LF, Tom WL, Chamlin SL, Feldman SR, Hanfin JM, Simpson EL, et al. Guidelines for the management of atopic dermatitis. *J Am Acad Dermatol.* 2014;70(2):338–351.

Cardona ID, Stillman L, Jain N. Does bathing frequency matter in pediatric atopic dermatitis? *Ann Allergy Asthma Immunol.* 2016; 117(1):9.

Valdman-Grinshpoun Y, Ben-Amitai D, Zvulunov A. Barrier-restoring therapies in atopic dermatitis: Current approaches and future perspectives. *Dermatol Res Pract.* 2012;2012:923134.

Contact Dermatitis

Fonacier L, Bernstein DI, Pacheco K. Contact dermatitis: a practice parameter—update 2015. *J Allergy Clin Immunol Pract.* 2015; 3(suppl 3):S1–39.

Johnston GA, Exton LS, Mohd Mustapa MF. British Association of Dermatologists' guidelines for the management of contact dermatitis. *Br J Dermatol.* 2017;176(2):317–329.

Psoriasis

Alexa K, Gladman D, Gelfand. National Psoriasis Foundation clinical consensus on psoriasis co-morbidities and recommendations for screening. *J Am Acad Dermatol.* 2008;58(6):1031–1042.

Armstrong A, et al. From the Medical Board of the National Psoriasis Foundation: Treatment targets for plaque psoriasis. *J Am Acad Dermatol.* 2017;76(2):290–298.

Armstrong A, Aldredge L, Yamauchi P. Managing patients with psoriasis in the busy clinic. *J Cutan Med Surg.* 2016;20(3):196–206.

Cottrill RR. Psoriasis: A review of diagnosis and management. *Adv NPs PAs.* 2013;4(5):20–26.

Hjalte F, Steen Carlsson K, Schmitt-Egenolf M. Sustained PASI, DLQI and EQ-5D response of biological treatment in psoriasis: 10 years of real-world data in the Swedish National Psoriasis Register. *Br J Dermatol.* 2018;178(1):245–252.

Menter A, Korman NJ, Elmets CA. Guidelines of care for the management of psoriasis and psoriatic arthritis. Section 5. Guidelines of care for the treatment of psoriasis with phototherapy and photochemotherapy. *J Am Acad Dermatol.* 2010;62(1):114–135.

National Clinical Guideline Centre. Psoriasis: Assessment and management of psoriasis. London, UK: National Institute for Health and Clinical Excellence (clinical guideline no. 153). Published October 2012.

Osier E, Tollefson MM, Wang AS, Eichenfield, LF. Pediatric psoriasis comorbidity screening guidelines. *JAMA Dermatol.* 2017; 153(7):698–704.

Vaughn A, Branum A, Sivamani RK. Effects of turmeric (*Curcuma longa*) on skin health: A systematic review of the clinical evidence. *Phytother Res.* 2016;30:1243–1264.

Yamauchi P, Bissonnette R, Texeira HD, Valdecantos, WC. Systematic review of efficacy of anti–tumor necrosis factor (TNF) therapy in patients with psoriasis previously treated with a different anti-TNF agent. *J Am Acad Dermatol.* 2016;75(3):612–618.

Young M, Aldredge L, Parker P. Psoriasis for the primary care practitioner. *J Am Assoc Nurse Pract.* 2017;29(3):157–178.

Seborrheic Dermatitis

Borda LJ, Wikramanayake TC. Seborrheic dermatitis and dandruff: A comprehensive review. *J Clin Investig Dermatol.* 2015;3(2):10.

Gupta AK, Versteeg SG. Topical treatment of facial seborrheic dermatitis: A systematic review. *Am J Clin Dermatol.* 2017; 18(2):193–213.

RESOURCES

American Academy of Dermatology
www.aad.org
American Society of Dermatology
www.asd.org
Information on dermatological drugs
www.nsc.gov.sg/brochures.html
https://www.psoriasis.org/treating-psoriasis/complementary-and-alternative/herbal-remedies
National Psoriasis Foundation (USA)
www.psoriasis.org
Psoriasis Association (UK)
https://www.psoriasis-association.org.uk
The National Eczema Society
www.eczema.org

Psoriasis Assessment Tools

Case presentations to educate practitioners—International Dermoscopy Society (IDS)
www.dermoscopy-ids.org
Dermatology Life Quality Index (DLQI)
www.dermatology.org.uk/quality/dlqi/quality-dlqi-questionnaire.html
Free dermoscopy training is also available at:
www.dermlite.com/cms/en/learn/for-professionals/video-course.html
http://dermoscopic.blogspot.com
http://dermnetnz.org/procedures/dermoscopy.html
Psoriasis Area Severity Index (PASI) Calculator
http://pasi.corti.li

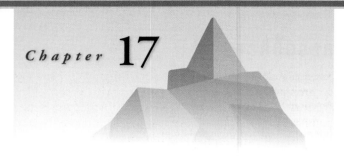

Chapter **17**

Skin Lesions

Jill E. Winland-Brown, EdD, APRN, FNP-BC

Brian Oscar Porter, MD, PhD, MPH, MBA

BENIGN LESIONS

ACNE VULGARIS

Acne vulgaris (commonly called "acne") is the most common skin condition in the United States and one of the most common skin conditions that a clinician will see in the primary-care setting. Sixty million Americans have active acne, and Americans spend an average of more than $3 billion annually on acne treatment.

EPIDEMIOLOGY AND CAUSES

Acne is derived from the Greek word *acme* meaning "prime of life" because it is a disease primarily of adolescence, although it may continue into adulthood. Acne vulgaris has the highest incidence among individuals aged 12 to 25 years, with incidence peaking at 15 years of age. Twenty percent of all adults have active acne, and 85% will experience acne at some point in their lives. Even after resolving in adolescence, acne can recur during adulthood, which is called *adult-onset acne*. Adult-onset acne is more commonly seen in women who are in their mid-20s to 40s in age, although an increasing number of women have acne in their third to fifth decades of life and beyond. Overall, however, the incidence of acne markedly decreases with age.

Although 80% of cases occur in women, acne is often more severe in males. Fifty percent of adult women have premenstrual flares of acne, and many women have their first flare, or worsening of existing acne, during pregnancy. Racial and ethnic differences in presentation have also been noted. The average age of onset of acne is 16 years for Hispanics, 19 years for Asians, and 20 years for African Americans, and Hispanic teenagers have the highest incidence of acne and resultant scarring.

The etiology of acne is interdependent with several factors, including the following:

- An increase in production of sex hormones (androgens) in puberty and adolescence
- An increase in sebum production resulting from activation of the sebaceous glands (during puberty and adolescence) and genetic factors
- A disorder of epithelial cell "stickiness" (keratinization) and sheddingedu (desquamation), leading to keratin plug formation
- Proliferation of *Propionibacterium acnes* bacteria inside the hair follicles
- The host inflammatory response

PATHOPHYSIOLOGY

Acne is an inflammatory disorder of the sebaceous gland and accompanying hair follicle (known collectively as a pilosebaceous unit). Approximately 5,000 pilosebaceous units are present in the human body. Most of them are located on the face, back, chest, and upper arms, the most common sites for acne. Acne lesions include comedones, papules, nodules, and cysts. Painful nodules and cysts are found in severe forms of acne.

Comedones are the primary lesions of acne and are caused by a defect in desquamation at the opening of the pilosebaceous follicle. Instead of regular cellular shedding, desquamation is reduced, and shed epithelial cells become "sticky," forming plugs that block follicular openings in a process known as retention hyperkeratosis. It takes about 2 months for the accumulated shed epithelial cells, sebum, and keratin to produce a comedone. Comedones are noninflammatory lesions and are classified into two types: *closed* comedones ("whiteheads") and *open* comedones ("blackheads"). The black color of open comedones is caused by the oxidation of tyrosine, a substance normally present in the plug material, to melanin. Tyrosine is an amino acid precursor of melanin.

Enlargement of the sebaceous glands and increased sebum production triggered by adrenarche during adolescence provides a rich growth medium for the overgrowth of *P. acnes* bacteria within the pilosebaceous follicles. *P. acnes* is an anaerobic diphtheroid that is part of the normal skin flora in humans and is responsible in large part for the inflammatory response observed in acne vulgaris. *P. acnes* bacteria utilize triglycerides as their primary source of nutrients by breaking down the sebum inside the affected hair follicle into its basic units—fatty acids and glycerol. Free fatty acids act as irritants and produce a sterile inflammatory response inside the sebaceous follicles. *P. acnes* also causes a direct inflammatory response by releasing proteolytic enzymes such as hyaluronidase, as well as chemotactic factors that attract neutrophils to the site of infection.

These neutrophils extrude lysozyme, which further degrades surface epithelia, leading to rupture of the previously closed comedone. When a comedone ruptures, its contents, which include sebum, bacteria, keratin, and free fatty acids, enter the dermis and elicit a severe inflammatory response. This results in the formation of deep abscesses, which present on the skin surface as nodules and cysts. Although androgen excess may lead to acne formation, most individuals with acne do not overproduce androgens. However, their pilosebaceous glands are likely hypersensitive to these hormones and more prone to retention hyperkeratosis. Some studies have shown that the production of sebum is increased in patients with acne compared with control subjects of similar age, thus suggesting a possible genetic predisposition for acne vulgaris.

CLINICAL PRESENTATION

Subjective

The typical patient is an adolescent boy or girl who has already tried self-treatment for several months with over-the-counter (OTC) products without much success. The patient might present to the primary-care practitioner not only with numerous acne lesions but also with dry, irritated skin—a common side effect of many topical acne medications. Female patients are more likely to verbalize emotional distress over their appearance. Male patients are more likely to wait until their acne is severe before they will seek treatment from a clinician. Some patients with severe acne complain of pain and tenderness from multiple deep pustules, nodules, and cysts. Mild to moderate acne normally does not cause pain.

Objective

Mild Acne

In mild acne, lesions are primarily noninflammatory comedones with occasional small papules. Commonly, there is a mixture of both types of comedones. The location of the comedones and papules may vary, from predominantly facial involvement to other locations, such as the chest, back, and the upper outer arms. Closed comedones are small papules 1 to 3 mm in size that are the same color as the surrounding skin, sometimes with a visible white plug. Occasionally, a closed comedone can get irritated from trauma (e.g., scratching, scrubbing) and become inflamed. Open comedones have a black-colored central plug. The hard plug on some comedones can be removed easily by putting firm pressure on the sides of the lesion. See the figure of the Iceberg of Acne to appreciate all the issues involved.

Moderate Acne

In moderate acne, lesions are mainly inflammatory lesions such as papules and pustules. The papules range in size from a few millimeters to one-half centimeter. The color of the acne papules in light-skinned patients ranges from light pink to bright red. Papules in darker-skinned patients can be red to shades of brown. Pustules are easier to recognize; they appear like pointed papules, with yellow to green-colored tops. When pustules become fluctuant, they rupture spontaneously, providing relief from pain. Resolution of a pustule is usually rapid after rupture. Scarring is more likely with larger and deeper pustules. Postinflammatory hyperpigmentation can be problematic, especially in patients with darker skin; patients with olive-toned complexions and darker skin tones are more likely to have this problem. Patients who are prone to hyperpigmentation should be advised to avoid sun exposure to the face and to use oil-free sunblock on the face.

Severe (Nodulocystic) Acne

In severe acne, or nodulocystic acne, lesions are mainly nodules and cysts. This form of acne always results in scar formation. The severity of acne scars is variable, from numerous atrophic pits ("pockmarks") to large, depressed scars. In patients with darker skin, keloids and hypertrophic scars can result. Severe acne is more common in males. Occasionally, fistula formation is seen in some patients. Nodules are inflammatory lesions that appear bright to dark red (or brown), depending on the patient's shade of skin. Nodules are smaller and feel harder than acne cysts. In addition, some darker-skinned patients develop permanent hyperpigmentation changes secondary to severe inflammation, with brown to black-colored macules on the skin.

Acne conglobata is severe cystic acne in which nodules, cysts, and abscesses develop; lesions are predominantly located on the trunk area instead of the face. Females with acne conglobata should be evaluated for polycystic ovary syndrome (PCOS). *Acne fulminans* is rare and is seen in young adolescent males. This condition is characterized by acute onset of multiple painful, ulcerated acne lesions, along with systemic symptoms such as fever, chills, malaise, and generalized joint and muscle aches.

DIAGNOSTIC REASONING

Diagnostic Tests

Acne is diagnosed by its classic location and characteristic lesions. A complete history is crucial to the diagnosis and supplants the importance of most diagnostic tests, which are only needed when an underlying predisposing condition is suspected or for cases refractory to standard treatments. For acne fulminans, a complete blood count (CBC), blood chemistry panel, urinalysis, and erythrocyte sedimentation rate (ESR) can be helpful. Abnormal laboratory results seen in cases of acne fulminans include leukocytosis, an elevated ESR, anemia, and hematuria.

If an endocrine disorder such as PCOS is suspected (e.g., in a hirsute overweight woman with moderate to severe acne and amenorrhea or irregular menses), an evaluation for excessive androgen production should be done. A complete physical examination, along with laboratory tests that include serum total and free testosterone and dehydroepiandrosterone sulfate, is recommended. A pelvic ultrasound should be ordered to assess for enlarged and polycystic ovaries.

The Iceberg of Acne

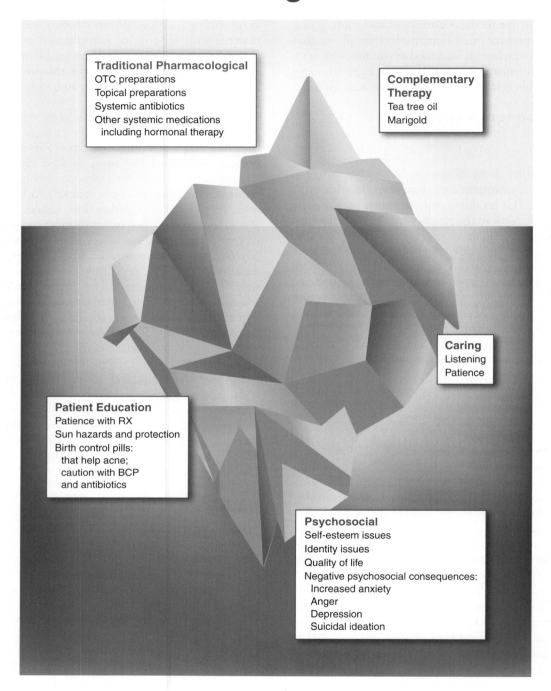

Traditional Pharmacological
OTC preparations
Topical preparations
Systemic antibiotics
Other systemic medications
  including hormonal therapy

Complementary Therapy
Tea tree oil
Marigold

Caring
Listening
Patience

Patient Education
Patience with RX
Sun hazards and protection
Birth control pills:
  that help acne;
  caution with BCP
  and antibiotics

Psychosocial
Self-esteem issues
Identity issues
Quality of life
Negative psychosocial consequences:
  Increased anxiety
  Anger
  Depression
  Suicidal ideation

Differential Diagnosis

Rosacea, previously termed "acne rosacea," should be ruled out. Rosacea is more common in adults and older patients and is located more centrally on the face, cheeks, chin, and nose. Comedones are never found in rosacea. There is a tendency for easy flushing in response to alcohol or heat. Telangiectasias (dilations of small groups of superficial blood vessels) may be present at the skin surface. Rosacea can be accompanied by eye complaints such as excessive

dryness and irritation, and it is more common in patients of Irish, Scottish, or English descent. Chronic rosacea can result in rhinophyma (hyperplasia of nasal tissue) and is seen more often in older men, requiring medical (see the following section on management) or more commonly surgical treatment (e.g., scalpel shaving, laser resurfacing, cryosurgery, dermabrasion) to remove excess tissue.

Other differential diagnoses include "hot tub folliculitis" (folliculitis lesions caused by *Staphylococci*), which appears within 1 to 4 days after hot tub use, due to insufficient temperature and inadequate chlorination of the water. Patients will complain of small red pustules that are occasionally pruritic. Folliculitis is located on the areas of the body that were immersed in the water, such as the lower torso, buttocks, and legs. Perioral dermatitis is another similar presentation that appears as small, erythematous papules occurring around the mouth area and nasolabial folds, which is the main diagnostic clue. It is more common in adult women (usually 20 to 30 years old); treatment is similar to that for rosacea except that topical corticosteroids are not indicated.

MANAGEMENT

In the United States, of the 60 million individuals who have acne, 20 million will have lesions severe enough to cause scarring. However, only 10% of individuals with acne seek advice or treatment from a health professional. Although acne is not a life-threatening illness, it has the potential for causing physical scars as well as emotional trauma. The primary-care practitioner should not ignore the impact of acne on self-esteem and identity, which are closely tied to physical appearance during the adolescent period. Research suggests that more than 90% of persons with acne have felt depressed and 14% have considered suicide.

Most cases of acne can be treated safely in the primary-care setting. For pediatric patients, treatment options should be offered to both the affected teen and his or her parents during routine wellness visits, as well as during episodic visits. Many adolescents are reticent to discuss this health-care issue, and the primary-care practitioner should be proactive about treatment to prevent disfiguring scarring and to address any associated mental health issues.

The primary goal of acne treatment is to prevent and/or minimize scarring and permanent pigmentation changes. Patient education is important in acne management and should not be neglected. Mild acne is treated with topical medications only, whereas systemic antibiotics may be used in moderate cases that are unresponsive to topical agents and in severe cases (see Drugs Commonly Prescribed 17.1). Of note, numerous misconceptions regarding acne treatment abound in the community. Many patients and their parents think that antibiotic treatment can result in a "quick cure." However, the response rate from acne treatment tends to be slow compared with most infections treated with antibiotics and can take up to 4 to 6 weeks before visible results are detected.

Drugs Commonly Prescribed 17.1: Acne and Rosacea

DRUG	INDICATION	ADVERSE REACTIONS AND PRESCRIBING CONSIDERATIONS
Topical Anti-Inflammatory and Antibiotic Formulations		
Azelaic acid (Azelex) cream 20%	Acne vulgaris and inflammatory rosacea	Both bacteriostatic and bactericidal. Avoid mouth, eyes, and mucous membranes. Watch for hypopigmentation on darker-skinned patients. Wash hands after use.
Sulfacetamide (Rosula) gel, wash, and cream	Acne vulgaris, rosacea, and seborrheic dermatitis	Avoid mucous membranes.
Benzoyl peroxide (Benzac) gel, wash, lotion, and foam	First-line therapy for acne	2.5% as effective as 10% and less irritating. Use water-based rather than alcohol-based.
Metronidazole (MetroGel) 1% gel	Rosacea	Will not cure rosacea but reduces inflammatory lesions.
Clindamycin 1% solution, lotion, gel, and pledget	Acne vulgaris and rosacea	Do not use alone, due to antibiotic resistance. Lotion less irritating. May cause diarrhea; avoid in patients with colitis.
Combination Topical Anti-inflammatory + Antibacterial Therapy		
Clindamycin + benzoyl peroxide (BenzaClin)	Acne vulgaris	Safety and efficacy in patients younger than 12 years has not been established. Risk of severe pseudomembranous colitis; discontinue use if significant diarrhea occurs. May bleach fabrics. Avoid eyes and mucous membranes. Caution in pregnant or breastfeeding women.

Continued

Drugs Commonly Prescribed 17.1: Acne and Rosacea—cont'd

DRUG	INDICATION	ADVERSE REACTIONS AND PRESCRIBING CONSIDERATIONS
Erythromycin + benzoyl peroxide (Benzamycin)	Acne vulgaris	Safety and efficacy in patients younger than 12 years has not been established. Risk of severe pseudomembranous colitis; discontinue use if significant diarrhea occurs. May bleach fabrics. Avoid eyes and mucous membranes. Transient skin discoloration. Caution in pregnant or breastfeeding women.
Topical Retinoids Not recommended for use in pregnancy unless otherwise stated.		
Tretinoin (Renova) 0.05% cream	Acne vulgaris and rosacea	Not recommended for children younger than 10 years. Do not use on sunburned skin.
Tretinoin (Retin-A) cream, gel, and liquid	Acne vulgaris	Allow effects of other topical agents to subside before using.
Tazarotene (Tazorac) 0.1%	First-line therapy for all acne variants	Women of childbearing potential should have a negative pregnancy test 2 weeks before starting and must use effective birth control. Do not breastfeed while using.
Adapalene (Differin)	First-line therapy for all acne variants	Less sun sensitivity than tretinoin.
Isotretinoin (Amnesteem)	Severe recalcitrant nodular acne or rosacea, unresponsive to conventional therapy (including antibiotics)	Teratogenic—must register patients in iPLEDGE program to avoid pregnancy. Avoid sun. Monitor lipids, glucose, complete blood count, liver enzymes. Take with meals.
Combination Topical Retinoid + Antibacterial Therapy		
Adapalene plus benzoyl peroxide (Epiduo gel)	Acne vulgaris	Ideal for teenage boys because they may be more likely to use just one topical product. Apply a thin film once daily after washing.
Systemic Therapies—Antibiotics		
Minocycline (Minocin)	Severe acne and rosacea	Take on an empty stomach with fluids.
Doxycycline (Vibramycin)	Severe acne and rosacea	Monitor blood, renal, and hepatic function with long-term use.
Doxycycline (Oracea) 40 mg	Inflammatory acne	Sub-antibacterial dose acts as an anti-inflammatory agent.
Hormonal Therapy		
Norgestimate and ethinyl estradiol (Ortho Tri-Cyclen and others)	Oral contraceptive pills (OCPs) for moderate acne vulgaris in female patients older than 15 years	See Chapter 46 for precautions accompanying OCP use.
Norethindrone acetate and ethinyl estradiol (Estrostep FE) (Loestrin) (Loestrin FE)	Moderate acne vulgaris in female patients older than 15 years	See above.
Drospirenone and ethinyl estradiol (Gianvi, Loryna, Nikki, Ocella, Syeda, Vestura, Yasmin, Yaz, Zarah)	Moderate acne vulgaris in female patients older than 15 years	See above.

A combination of several types of acne lesions in a single patient is not uncommon, but the most predominant lesions present will help in the determination of treatment choices. Other factors that help guide the choice of treatment include a higher risk of pigmentation changes (more common in patients with darker skin), a patient's refusal of systemic antibiotic treatment, and the severity of the acne. Parental permission is necessary to treat patients younger than 18 years.

Topical Treatment of Comedonal Acne

Comedones respond well to topical retinoids, which are derivatives of vitamin A and are available in multiple vehicles in a wide variety of concentrations. Synthetic retinoids such as tretinoin (Retin-A) and adapalene gel (Differin) decrease comedone formation by increasing cell turnover and decreasing epithelial cell cohesiveness. Mild adverse effects of tretinoin include dryness, erythema, scaling, and burning. Adapalene gel seems better tolerated on sensitive skin than tretinoin, but patients with extremely sensitive skin can still develop skin irritation. Adapalene 0.1% is a Food and Drug Administration (FDA) approved prescription strength retinoid that is OTC.

Tretinoin has been shown to cause thinning of the top layer of epidermis during the first 4 weeks of treatment and can result in dryness and irritation. During this period, patients may notice more skin sensitivity to the elements (cold air, wind, sun) and an increase in skin photosensitivity. Sunscreen or sunblock should be used during the entire treatment period, especially at this time. The thickness of the epidermis returns to normal after 4 to 6 weeks. It is important to warn patients and parents that tretinoin and, to a lesser extent, adapalene gel will cause a worsening of acne lesions during the first 4 to 6 weeks of treatment, as preexisting comedones will continue to surface during this time. Improvement should become visible by 6 to 8 weeks; however, a trial period of 2 months is generally recommended for topical retinoids, unless the patient develops contact dermatitis or other problems with the medicine.

To avoid excessive skin irritation, the patient should wait for at least 10 to 15 minutes after washing and should allow the skin time to dry before applying topical acne agents. Patients with a history of eczema or with sunburned skin should not use this medicine. The patient should avoid the eyes, mouth, angles of the nose, and mucous membranes when applying this medicine. Adverse reactions include excessive skin irritation, an apparent exacerbation of symptoms, transient pigmentation changes, stinging on application to the skin, and dry skin. The effects of other topical acne agents, such as benzoyl peroxide, sulfur, resorcinol, and salicylic acid, should be allowed to subside before the application of topical retinoids (see Box 17.1). Given their teratogenic effects, retinoids should not be used by pregnant or nursing women or children. The popular media have suggested

> **Box 17.1   Initiating Tretinoin Therapy**
>
> Start with tretinoin 0.025% (Retin-A) cream (the least irritating formulation). Apply three to four times per week at bedtime on clean dry skin for the first 2 weeks until the patient can tolerate a daily dose. Wait 20 to 30 minutes after cleansing the face and ensure the face is completely dry before applying the cream. Give this dose a trial of 6 to 8 weeks.
>
> - Gradually increase to a 0.05% cream or 0.025% gel if patient can tolerate the initial regimen above and needs a stronger dose (i.e., if no reduction in acne lesions seen after 8 weeks).
> - If there is still improvement of acne lesions, escalate to the 0.1% cream.
>
>   NOTE: The most potent and irritating dose of tretinoin is the 0.05% liquid formulation. Tretinoin 0.05% (Renova) has been shown to decrease the effects of solar damage and is approved by the U.S. Food and Drug Administration for the treatment of fine wrinkles, mottled hyperpigmentation, and tactile roughness of the skin. Remind the patient that acne breakouts may occur with up to 4 to 6 weeks of treatment, after which the skin will begin to clear.

that tretinoin has been associated with psychotic or suicidal behavior in teens, but this has not been substantiated by rigorous epidemiological data.

Topical Treatment of Inflammatory Acne

Patients with predominantly inflammatory lesions may respond well to topical antibiotics such as erythromycin or clindamycin, benzoyl peroxide, or a combination of benzoyl peroxide and erythromycin. Other good candidates for nonretinoid topical acne therapy include patients who cannot tolerate tretinoin or adapalene gel or patients who have concurrent eczema. All topical antibiotics are applied once or twice daily and must be refrigerated when stored. The most common side effects include mild erythema or burning. Because topical antibiotic solutions use an alcohol base, they can cause excessive skin dryness. To avoid this problem, the clinician should tell the patient to start use gradually on a once-daily basis for 2 weeks.

Monotherapy with topical antibiotics may lead to bacterial resistance with a resultant slower therapeutic effect. Switching the patient to a combination of antibiotics and benzoyl peroxide has shown increased efficacy and a reduction of antibiotic resistance in *P. acnes*. The combination products, available in gel form, include 1% clindamycin–5% benzoyl peroxide (BenzaClin) and 3% erythromycin–5% benzoyl peroxide (Benzamycin). Azelaic acid (Azelex), a dicarboxylic acid with bacteriostatic and keratolytic properties, is approved for acne as a 20% cream formulation. It is particularly effective in treating patients with postinflammatory hyperpigmentation or concomitant melasma.

Systemic Antibiotic and Hormonal Treatment of Moderate to Severe Acne

Topical acne medicines are a safer alternative than oral antibiotics, as they have less potential for adverse effects. Topical therapy has its limitations, however. Oral antibiotic treatment should generally be continued for 4 to 6 months, and maximal clinical results may not be evident before 3 to 4 months.

Good candidates for oral antibiotic treatment include patients who

- have not responded to topical medications after a trial of at least 2 to 3 months.
- are unable to tolerate topical acne treatment.
- have large numbers of inflammatory lesions after several months on topical treatment.
- have severe nodulocystic acne.
- have large numbers of inflammatory lesions located on the back or upper outer arms (hard-to-reach areas).
- want quick relief from inflammatory acne.
- are at increased risk of pigmentation changes or scarring.

Oral antibiotics are the standard of care in the management of moderate to severe acne and treatment-resistant forms of inflammatory acne. *P. acnes* is a biofilm-forming organism, and topical treatment is recommended along with oral antibiotics. Oral antibiotics used in the treatment of inflammatory acne include doxycycline and minocycline, which are more effective than tetracycline. There is evidence that minocycline is superior to doxycycline in exerting not only an antibacterial effect against *P. acnes* but a direct anti-inflammatory effect as well. Trimethoprim-sulfamethoxazole and trimethoprim alone are also effective in instances where other antibiotics cannot be used.

The starting dose of minocycline (for tetracycline-resistant acne) is 50 mg at bedtime for 1 week; the dose is then gradually increased to 100 mg at bedtime. Once improvement is seen at 4 to 6 weeks, the dose can be decreased gradually every 6 to 8 weeks. The maintenance dose of minocycline is 50 mg once daily. The safety of minocycline has not been established for longer than 12 weeks. Adverse effects of minocycline include vertigo, dizziness, and ataxia (due to its effects on the vestibular apparatus of the inner ear). This effect can be avoided or decreased by starting the patient on a lower dose. Rare cases of blue-gray discoloration of the skin are sometimes seen in minocycline use. Other adverse effects associated with tetracycline antibiotics include serum sickness, hepatitis, and a lupus-like syndrome.

Doxycycline and minocycline are lipophilic and can be taken with food without affecting most of the drug's activity. Doxycycline should be taken with a full glass of water (if the pill becomes lodged in the esophagus, it can cause ulceration). Adverse reactions to doxycycline include photosensitivity, gastrointestinal upset, enterocolitis, rash, blood dyscrasias, and hepatotoxicity. If the patient's occupation or hobbies include plenty of sun exposure, another drug besides doxycycline should be considered. The patient must use strong sunscreen or sunblock while on this drug, in addition to avoiding excessive sun exposure.

Adverse reactions to tetracyclines in general include nausea, dizziness, rash, blood dyscrasias, pseudotumor cerebri, photosensitivity, and hepatotoxicity. Antacids, dairy products, and iron or magnesium-containing vitamins will inactivate tetracyclines due to binding of the drug with those substances. Tetracyclines should not be used in pregnant women or patients younger than 9 years of age because of the risk of tooth discoloration and inhibited skeletal growth. In addition, tetracyclines reduce the effectiveness of oral contraceptives. Thus, patients on oral contraceptives should use a reliable second method of birth control, such as condoms.

Erythromycin is a macrolide antibiotic that prevents the production of bacterial proteins. Although erythromycin is effective, its use should be limited to patients who cannot use tetracyclines (e.g., pregnant women or children younger than 9 years of age, due to the potential for damage to the skeleton or teeth). Adverse reactions to erythromycin include nausea, gastrointestinal upset, abdominal pain, anorexia, candidal vaginitis, hepatic dysfunction, rash, superinfection (overgrowth of nonsusceptible bacteria or fungi), and pseudomembranous colitis (rare). The development of bacterial resistance by *P. acnes* is also more common with erythromycin treatment. Thus, erythromycin is usually considered a second-line agent, with doxycycline being an effective treatment for patients who develop erythromycin-resistant *P. acnes* infection.

In addition to antibiotic treatment, certain combination progestin plus estrogen hormonal therapies used for birth control are also approved for moderate acne in women aged 15 years or older and have acne that is unresponsive to topical medications. The patient should have no known contraindications to hormonal therapy, such as a history of thrombophlebitis or thromboembolic disorders, cerebrovascular or cardiovascular disease, breast or other estrogen-dependent neoplasms, hepatic tumors, or undiagnosed genital bleeding. Norgestimate/ethinyl estradiol (Ortho Tri-Cyclen) is available with different doses of the progestin component (norgestimate), and Estrostep Fe is available with different doses of the estrogen component (ethinyl estradiol). Drospirenone/ethinyl estradiol (Beyaz) combines the estrogen component with an artificial form of progestin. Although thromboembolism is an established risk for all forms of hormonal birth control, birth control pills containing the synthetic progestin drospirenone may have an increased risk for thrombus formation compared with combination pills containing other types of progestins.

Severe Acne

Individuals with severe acne should be referred to a dermatologist for aggressive treatment with isotretinoin, a vitamin A derivative indicated for severe recalcitrant nodular acne that has not responded to conventional therapy (including oral antibiotics). Tretinoin and isotretinoin are confused by some patients as the same medication. Tretinoin is the active ingredient in Retin-A and is a topical medication. Isotretinoin is an oral acne medication that is the only treatment that works on all causes and types of acne. The most familiar brand name of this drug was Accutane, which has not been marketed in the United States since 2009 due to lawsuits related to inflammatory bowel disease claims. However, isotretinoin is now available generically under many brand names worldwide, include Sotret, Amnesteem, Claravis, and Roaccutane.

Isotretinoin induces sebaceous gland atrophy, normalizes follicular keratinocytes, reduces *Propionibacterium acnes* colonization, and has direct anti-inflammatory effects. It is a highly potent teratogen and carries significant medicolegal implications for the clinician when prescribed to female patients of reproductive age. The manufacturers of isotretinoin require all prescribers to join the iPLEDGE program to minimize fetal exposure to the drug. The primary-care practitioner should refer any woman of reproductive age who is a candidate for isotretinoin therapy to a dermatologist for management, as physician consultation is highly recommended. The risk and the benefits of therapy should be discussed with the female patient, including the possibility of pregnancy and contingency plans if she becomes pregnant (including a discussion regarding pregnancy termination, if this is an option). Two negative pregnancy tests must be obtained within 1 week of prescribing the isotretinoin, and two reliable forms of contraception must be used (unless abstinence is the chosen method). Monthly pregnancy tests must be ordered thereafter. The patient must have maintained effective contraception for at least 1 month before, during, and after therapy.

The dose usually starts at 0.5 mg/kg daily in two divided doses and may be increased gradually, depending on effect, to 1 mg/kg daily in two divided doses. Isotretinoin should generally be taken with food, although some formulations do not carry this recommendation. Only a 1-month supply of the drug should be prescribed at each visit, and it can be discontinued early if the patient's acne nodule count decreases by 70% or more. Isotretinoin will induce long-term remissions of acne in up to 40% of patients. After a period of 2 months or more off therapy, if persistent or recurrent severe nodular acne recurs, referral to a dermatologist is recommended.

The most frequent adverse effect of isotretinoin is cheilitis, which occurs in up to 90% of patients. Other common adverse effects include dry skin, dry nose, dry mouth, pruritus, epistaxis, and an increase in skin fragility. Patients who complain of headache should be evaluated for pseudotumor cerebri or benign intracranial hypertension. If the patient complains of moderate to severe myalgia, the medication should be discontinued immediately and a creatine phosphokinase should be done. Corneal opacities and decreased night vision have also been reported in patients taking isotretinoin. The link between isotretinoin and depression, psychosis, and suicide remains controversial, and some clinicians prefer not to prescribe this medication in patients with this type of psychiatric history.

The incidence of hypertriglyceridemia is high (25%), and some patients develop elevated liver transaminases. Elevated blood sugar levels have also been seen in patients, as well as new-onset diabetes, although a causal association is unclear. Baseline laboratory testing, such as a fasting lipid panel and liver function tests, should therefore be done before starting treatment and weekly or biweekly thereafter until the patient's response to therapy is determined, after which laboratory monitoring can be done monthly.

Patients with acne fulminans present a particularly challenging situation because of the severity of the condition and the high potential for scarring. Patients should be referred as soon as possible to a dermatologist and treated with prednisone for its anti-inflammatory effects in combination with isotretinoin, which is the treatment regimen of choice for this condition, although other anti-inflammatory and immunosuppressant compounds (e.g., dapsone, cyclosporine A) have also been used.

Other Medical Therapies

Nonpharmacologic therapies may be used in place of or in conjunction with medications to assist in the overall treatment of patients with acne. The surgical procedure of comedone extraction is common for the treatment of comedonal acne and may be used along with topical retinoids. Beta-hydroxy acid peels may also be effective against comedonal acne. To reduce acne scarring, Fraxel laser resurfacing, dermabrasion, and subcision (subcuticular cutting of fibrous scare tissue under the skin surface using a tri-beveled hypodermic needle inserted via a small puncture in the skin) or punch grafting (replacement of small plugs of scar tissue with punch grafts of healthy skin removed from an inconspicuous area, such as behind the ear) may be effective. In addition, dermal augmentation (soft-tissue fillers) with autologous or nonautologous tissue may improve the appearance of atrophic scars. Photodynamic therapy with the use of a blue light or intense pulsed light and aminolaevulinic acid may be given every other week. Results are usually apparent after the second treatment.

FOLLOW-UP AND REFERRAL

Patients should be reevaluated in 4 to 6 weeks to monitor for response and any potential adverse effects of acne medication. Noncompliance issues should be addressed. In particular, female patients on oral antibiotics or isotretinoin should be monitored for their continued use of reliable methods of birth control. By the third month of treatment, clinical improvement of acne lesions should be visible. If no improvement is seen or if the acne worsens, topical treatment with two agents or systemic therapy should be considered. However, the risk of skin irritation is increased when two topical agents are combined, and therapy should be started slowly to minimize these effects. Systemic oral antibiotic treatment should generally be continued for a period of 4 to 6 months.

There is no need to wait until acne becomes severe before considering referral to a dermatologist. Moderate to severe acne that is unresponsive to conventional treatment should be referred to a dermatologist for more aggressive treatment to minimize scarring. Without treatment, acne lesions can persist for months to years.

Patient Education: Acne

Appropriate education regarding the causes and treatment of acne can help prevent disappointment in angry and discouraged patients who might become noncompliant due to a loss of trust in both the treatment and the health-care provider. In particular, patient education is needed to correct many common misconceptions about acne. For example, no connection has been found between the ingestion of specific foods and the risk of acne, despite the folklore surrounding certain foods, such as chocolate and fried foods.

Patient education is a vital component of acne treatment because of the long duration of treatment required and the potential for adverse effects, including serious ones (see Box 17.2 for key information). Patients and parents of patients younger than 18 years should be warned of the potential adverse effects of acne medications (as discussed under Management). For example, topical retinoids frequently cause skin dryness and irritation if not started gradually or if used incorrectly. Most patients are not willing to try them again after they experience skin irritation and the temporary flare-up of acne typically seen within 4 to 6 weeks of starting therapy.

Patients should also be encouraged to read consumer information labels on skin products and to only use noncomedogenic (non–acne-causing) products, such as makeup, moisturizers, and sunscreens. Patients on oral contraceptives for acne therapy should be aware of potential drug interactions, which include a decrease in their efficacy when used in conjunction with certain antimicrobials, such as tetracyclines. In general, oral contraceptives should not be used in breastfeeding patients, given their potential to impact milk production and a theoretical risk to the infant from the transfer of hormones in breastmilk.

Complementary therapies suggested for acne include marigold (*Calendula officinalis*) as a topical application (e.g., soap), which has anti-inflammatory properties, and tea tree oil (*Melaleuca alternifolia*) as a topical application twice daily.

Box 17.2   Key Information for Patients With Acne

- Wash the face gently at least twice a day with an antibacterial soap (Dial, Lever 2000) or with a very mild soap (Dove).
- Wait at least 30 minutes after washing the face before applying topical acne medications in order to minimize the chance of skin irritation.
- Topical acne medications should not be used on sunburned or irritated skin, abrasions, cuts, or on eczematous skin. If these conditions are present, the medication can be temporarily stopped for a few days.
- Avoid contact with the eyes, lips, angles of the nose, and the mucous membranes when applying topical acne medicines.
- Sunscreen should be used with all acne medications, especially in sunny climates and during the summer.
- Avoid oily makeup or oily hair conditioners or scalp products.
- Avoid excessive handling of the face and cradling phones on the chin.
- Avoid excessive scrubbing of the face.

ROSACEA

Rosacea is a chronic and progressive skin disorder in middle-aged and older adults that resembles acne. Rosacea and acne may respond to the same treatments and can coexist in the same patient.

EPIDEMIOLOGY AND CAUSES

It is estimated that rosacea affects more than 16 million Americans. Despite its high prevalence, fewer than 10% are diagnosed because patients confuse the symptoms with acne, sunburn, flushing, or a temporary rash. Rosacea is most common in persons aged 30 to 60 years who are of Irish, English, Scottish, Welsh, or eastern European ancestry. Patients sometimes have one or more close relatives with the condition. Women are three times more likely to develop rosacea than men, particularly cutaneous vascular manifestations that lead to erythema of the central face.

Rosacea is idiopathic with no recognizable causes, other than certain exacerbating triggers. Rosacea is a lifelong condition that is usually worsened by sun exposure. Other environmental triggers include hot or cold weather, wind, overheating during exercise, excessive alcohol ingestion, hot beverages, spicy or aged food products such as cheese, emotional stress, irritating cosmetics, hot baths, saunas, hot tubs, smoking, caffeine, and excessive washing of the face. Several researchers have suggested that *Helicobacter pylori*, a bacteria found in the stomach, may possibly be a cause, as well as the *Demodex* species of mite, which has been found in the hair follicles of patients with rosacea. However, these hypotheses are controversial.

PATHOPHYSIOLOGY

Rosacea is characterized by flare-ups that include three cutaneous components, which may occur individually or concurrently. The first component is vascular in nature, with persistent erythema that primarily involves the central face. This may be followed after a period of time by the development of telangiectasias or clusters of small, superficial blood vessels. In addition, flushing episodes may occur spontaneously as part of these vascular manifestations. The second component is cutaneous and involves the development of recurrent acneiform, erythematous papules and pustules around the central face. The third component consists of connective tissue hyperplasia around the central face with discrete sebaceous gland hyperplasia, consisting of persistent yellow papules particularly around the nose. In some patients, the nose may become swollen and bumpy from excess tissue in a condition called rhinophyma. This condition is what gave the late comedian W.C. Fields his trademark bulbous nose. Blepharoconjunctivitis may also result if there is ocular involvement, which has been considered a distinct fourth component by some.

At present, the underlying pathogenesis of the vascular dilation characteristic of rosacea is not fully understood. Inflammation, rather than infection, appears to be the primary mechanism, as shown through several lines of indirect evidence. For example, studies have failed to show consistent differences in *H. pylori* seropositivity between patients with rosacea and unaffected control subjects. Moreover, the ability of amoxicillin-metronidazole-bismuth treatments to clear *Helicobacter* infection and improve rosacea symptoms has been attributed to the anti-inflammatory effects of metronidazole, rather than the anti-infective effects of this regimen. This was similarly shown with tetracycline treatment of rosacea associated with *Demodex* mite infestations. Mite counts were not decreased with this treatment, although symptomatic improvement was evident. Moreover, the anti-inflammatory effects of tetracycline antibiotics have been well documented in the treatment of acne vulgaris.

CLINICAL PRESENTATION

Subjective

Patients with rosacea usually do not seek out care because they mistakenly think they have acne, a sunburn, or a temporary rash. They usually present because they become intolerant of the persistent burning, itching, or stinging sensations on the face, in particular. Patients with ocular rosacea complain of watery, irritated, or bloodshot eyes.

Objective

Initially the patient's forehead, cheek, nose, or chin may have a rosy hue without comedones. This is the central third of the face and is referred to as the "flush/blush" area. There may be inflammatory papules, pustules, and telangiectasias. Scarring is usually unapparent unless the patient also has concomitant acne. Although the lesions tend to be symmetrical bilaterally, they may appear on only one side. Seborrhea may also be seen. If there has been ocular involvement resulting in blepharoconjunctivitis, there will be redness of the eyelids and conjunctiva.

With prerosacea, the clinician will note a rosy-cheeked, ruddy complexion on a patient who never develops the full clinical spectrum of the disease. There is no effective treatment for prerosacea, nor is any needed. Patients should just be observed for signs of developing rosacea and encouraged to use sunscreen.

There are four subtypes of rosacea classified by the pattern and grouping of symptoms:

- Subtype 1: erythematotelangiectatic rosacea—flushing and persistent redness, which may include visible blood vessels
- Subtype 2: papulopustular rosacea—persistent redness with transient bumps and pimples
- Subtype 3: phymatous rosacea—skin thickening usually with hyperplasia of the nose, resulting in a large, bumpy, and bulbous appearance
- Subtype 4: ocular rosacea—ocular manifestations with dry eye, tearing and burning, erythematous eyelids, recurrent styes, and possible vision loss from corneal damage

DIAGNOSTIC REASONING

Diagnostic Tests

There is no diagnostic test for rosacea; physical assessment is the key to diagnosis. Although there is no cure for rosacea, if treatment is started early, some of the cutaneous manifestations may be prevented.

Differential Diagnosis

Differential diagnoses include adult acne, perioral dermatitis, seborrheic dermatitis, the "butterfly" rash of systemic lupus erythematosus, and corticosteroid-dependent facial dermatoses. Acne may be a concomitant condition along with rosacea, but acne is characterized by the presence of comedones, a lack of facial flushing or telangiectasias, and a broader distribution around the face than the limited central distribution of rosacea. Perioral dermatitis is typically seen in young women, although it may occur in women aged 15 to 40 years. Multiple acneiform papules are seen around the mouth with a clear area spared directly around the lips; the small erythematous papules or pustules of perioral dermatitis lack telangiectasias.

Seborrheic dermatitis usually has a scaly appearance not seen in rosacea; the erythema is without acneiform lesions and may be distributed throughout the nasolabial area, eyebrows, and scalp. The "butterfly" or malar rash of systemic lupus erythematosus lacks papules and pustules, and laboratory evaluation typically verifies the presence of antinuclear antibodies. Importantly, long-term topical corticosteroid use on the face can also result in burning erythema, sometimes associated with erythematous papules and/or scaling. When topical corticosteroids are abruptly discontinued, a rebound flare-up of this condition typically occurs.

MANAGEMENT

The key to management is early diagnosis and avoidance of triggers because rosacea is a chronic condition with no known cure. Topical treatments should be the mainstay of therapy, with oral antibiotics used only for breakthrough flare-ups. Potent topical corticosteroids should be avoided because they may worsen the condition.

Topical Therapy

Metronidazole cream is the mainstay of therapy but it may take up to 6 to 8 weeks for a therapeutic response to be seen. If metronidazole (0.75% or 1%) is not effective, other topical antibiotics may be tried. Topical ointments such as tretinoin and azelaic acid are also recommended (see Drugs Commonly Prescribed 17.1). The same therapy is used for perioral dermatitis and topical corticosteroid–induced rosacea.

Systemic Therapy

Antibiotics should be reserved for flare-ups or when initiating therapy with topical medications, after which antibiotics should be discontinued. Clinicians should taper the dose as soon as possible; typically patients can readily learn how to taper the dosage at home. Treatment with tetracycline, minocycline, or doxycycline typically delivers a rapid therapeutic response. Antibiotic therapy is usually effective in reducing acneiform lesions, and this helps confirm the diagnosis of rosacea. These antibiotics typically work more as anti-inflammatory agents rather than as anti-infectives. The flushing and flat telangiectasias of rosacea tend to persist and do not respond well to antibiotic therapy. In refractory cases, isotretinoin may succeed when other measures have failed.

Other Therapies

Electrocautery with a small needle may be used to destroy small telangiectasias. Larger telangiectatic vessels may require laser treatment (intense pulsed light therapy). For men with rhinophyma, surgical reduction may be used to reduce the bulbous appearance of the nose.

FOLLOW-UP AND REFERRAL

If rosacea results in telangiectasias, patients can be referred to a dermatologist for electrodesiccation or laser treatment for cosmetic purposes. A dermatologist may also treat patients with diffuse facial erythema due to rosacea with pulsed light therapy.

Patient Education: Rosacea

Patients should be taught about the events or circumstances that can trigger a rosacea flare-up and learn how to avoid them. Sunscreen with a sun protection factor of at least 15 should be used on all exposed skin surfaces when outdoors. Patients should stay cool on hot days and protect their face from cold air and wind by using a scarf. Caution should be used when exercising, and patients should be encouraged to exercise for shorter, more frequent intervals, using a cool towel around the neck and taking frequent water breaks. Gentle cleansing with fragrance-free facial cleansers should be encouraged. Proper use of topical creams and lotions should be stressed, along with the use of minimal antibiotics.

SEBORRHEIC KERATOSIS

Seborrheic keratosis is one of the most common noncancerous skin growths seen in older adults. It is characterized by benign, warty-appearing growths that are usually found on the trunk, but they may also be seen on the hands and face. They develop in both sun-exposed and sun-protected areas.

EPIDEMIOLOGY AND CAUSES

Seborrheic keratosis is extremely common. It has been found in 88% of persons older than 65 years. Of this group, approximately 50% develop 10 or more lesions. In fact, for some individuals, lesions may number into the hundreds. A predisposition for seborrheic keratosis appears to be inherited in an autosomal dominant pattern.

PATHOPHYSIOLOGY

Seborrheic keratosis lesions are superficial epithelial growths that originate from the horny layer of the epidermis and are the result of a benign proliferation of immature keratinocytes. Inspection of the lesions may reveal dark keratin plugs or firm, horny cysts on their surface. These are epidermal tumors, but they are not considered malignant or premalignant because they do not undergo transformation into cancerous lesions.

However, a condition known as Leser-Trélat sign is characterized by the sudden development of multiple seborrheic keratotic lesions, along with skin tags, and acanthosis nigricans (a darkening and mild thickening of the skin in characteristic intertriginous areas). Although the skin lesions in this condition are not considered malignant, Leser-Trélat sign is associated with various types of cancer, including lung and gastrointestinal cancers, and is thus considered a neoplastic syndrome. In addition, seborrheic keratosis has also been observed in association with certain skin malignancies such as BCCs, occurring at various skin sites.

CLINICAL PRESENTATION

Subjective

Although seborrheic keratosis occurs in both men and women, the typical patient is an older white woman who complains of the cosmetic effects of the lesion. The patient typically complains of the unsightliness of the lesion, itching, and constant irritation from friction or clothing. The lesions are sometimes called the "barnacles of aging."

Objective

Lesions found on sun-exposed areas rarely increase in size, whereas seborrheic keratotic lesions in protected areas tend to be darker, have a more crumbly appearance, and may enlarge in size. Seborrheic keratosis is more prevalent in persons with lighter-colored skin. The lesions are typically raised, well-defined, scaly, hyperpigmented, and brownish-gray, with a warty or "stuck-on" appearance. Lesions look as if they could literally be "picked off" the skin surface and are most often found on the trunk, face, and arms.

Seborrheic keratotic lesions tend to grow slowly and are round to oval in shape. The lesions occasionally appear as smooth papules. The color of the lesions can range from flesh tone to dark brown in lighter-skinned patients. In darker-skinned individuals, the lesions also appear as smooth, round to oval black papules on the upper part of the face (dermatosis papulosa nigra).

DIAGNOSTIC REASONING

Diagnostic Tests

No laboratory testing is necessary to diagnose seborrheic keratosis. However, if the patient presents with an atypical lesion and the diagnosis is uncertain (especially if melanoma cannot be ruled out), the patient should be referred to a dermatologist for further evaluation, and a skin biopsy should be done for a more definitive diagnosis.

Differential Diagnosis

The diagnosis of seborrheic keratosis is based on the appearance of the lesion and on patient demographics (especially age). Skin lesions that can mimic seborrheic keratosis include any pigmented papule or nodule. The differential diagnoses for seborrheic keratosis include benign pigmented nevi, pigmented basal cell carcinoma (BCC), and malignant melanoma. See Table 17.1 for information about other skin lesions, including nevi, skin tags (acrochordons), and lipomas.

Pigmented nevi appear as smooth, round macules or papules that do not have a warty appearance. Nevi (moles) are also seen in younger patients as well as in adults, unlike seborrheic keratosis, which appears most commonly in patients aged 30 years and older. Pigmented BCCs usually have a waxy surface with dilated blood vessels. They may be ulcerated during later stages, a feature not seen in seborrheic keratosis. Malignant melanomas can appear in younger patients; melanomas may be nodular but usually do not have a warty, stuck-on appearance. A malignant melanoma's borders can be irregular, and it can have a variegation (inconsistency) of color. Most patients with melanoma will also report a history of a changing mole.

MANAGEMENT

Most seborrheic keratoses do not require treatment, but removal is warranted for lesions that are symptomatic, unsightly to the patient, or become easily irritated (i.e., from shaving or from clothing rubbing against them). Seborrheic keratoses may be removed using liquid nitrogen therapy or mechanical methods. Results obtained with cryosurgery (liquid nitrogen) are slightly superior to those obtained using electrodesiccation with curettage; however, the choice is generally the practitioner's preference. Liquid nitrogen may produce transient hyperpigmentation or hypopigmentation. Mechanical methods of removal include curettage and snip or shave excision (see Therapeutic Procedure 17.1).

FOLLOW-UP AND REFERRAL

A follow-up visit is generally not necessary unless the liquid nitrogen does not completely remove the lesion. A biopsy should be performed on any seborrheic keratosis that fails to respond to liquid nitrogen to confirm the diagnosis. Infection following the application of liquid nitrogen is rare. However, should the removal of a lesion by cryotherapy from the dorsa of the hands result in blistering, the patient should return to have the blister drained. This is accomplished by puncturing one edge of the blister with a sterile needle or with a number 11 scalpel; the top of the blister should not be removed.

A biopsy or referral to a dermatologist should be done if the diagnosis is unclear and the clinician wants to rule out a pigmented BCC or malignant melanoma. A high index of suspicion is necessary in the diagnosis of melanoma because of its aggressive and malignant

TABLE 17.1	Other Skin Lesions		
Lesion	*Description*	*Clinical Presentation*	*Management*
Lipoma	A lipoma is a benign, subcutaneous tumor that consists of adipose tissue. Lipomas are most commonly found in older adults; usually asymptomatic. Cause is unknown.	• Rubbery smooth and round mass of adipose tissue that is compressible and has a soft to very firm texture • May have symptoms of irritation, such as redness and tenderness • Commonly occurs on back of the neck, trunk, and forearms	• Observe for changes, rapid growth • Excision or liposuction • Referral to dermatologist if indicated
Nevi	Nevi (moles) are circumscribed areas of pigmentation. Types include congenital, acquired, or atypical or dysplastic (>5 mm in diameter, with color variation and irregular borders).	• Flat or raised circumscribed area of pigmentation • Assess for suspected melanoma (check ABCDEs: asymmetry, irregular borders, variations in color, diameter >6 mm, elevation above the surface of the skin)	• Excision • Referral to dermatologist if melanoma is suspected
Skin tags	Skin tags (acrochordons) are benign overgrowths of skin, commonly seen after middle age. Cause is unknown.	• Overgrowths of normal skin that have formed soft, polyp-like lesions that have a stalk • Usually found on the neck, axilla, groin, upper trunk, and eyelid	• Usually none unless patient is bothered by the cosmetic effect or irritation • If treatment is required, may include snip excision, electrocautery, or cryosurgery • Referral to dermatologist if skin tag is located on the eyelids or face, if the patient has a history of keloid formation, diabetes, or infection, is on high-dose corticosteroid therapy, or if there is the possibility of a malignant lesion

 ## Therapeutic Procedure 17.1: Removal of Seborrheic Keratoses

NOTE: Treatment is for patient comfort or for cosmetic reasons only.

LIQUID NITROGEN

• Spray the area with liquid nitrogen or apply the liquid nitrogen with rayon–wool tipped applicators. Special care must be taken not to contaminate the reservoir of liquid nitrogen. If using applicators, dip the applicator into the reservoir only once, apply, and discard the applicator.

• It is generally preferable to lightly freeze (underfreeze) the lesion than to freeze it too deeply and risk scarring. A second application may be applied at a follow-up visit if necessary.

NOTE: Hyperpigmentation and hypopigmentation are possible sequelae of liquid nitrogen treatment (cryotherapy); reactive hyperpigmentation is more common in Asians. Care must be taken when treating areas where nerves are relatively superficial and can be damaged, such as the lateral aspects of the fingers and the ulnar groove of the elbows.

CURETTAGE

• Anesthetize the area with 1% lidocaine and cleanse the area.
• Stretch the skin surrounding the lesion with the fingers of one hand.
• Using a 5- or 6-mm curette, scrape off the base of the keratosis with short, clean strokes.

NOTE: If the lesion is in a critical area such as the face, lateral aspects of the fingers, ulnar groove in elbow (superficial nerve present), or if the diagnosis is uncertain, referral to a dermatologist is recommended. If the lesion is in the hairline or groin, styptics or aluminum chloride may be used to control bleeding.

SNIP OR SHAVE EXCISION

• Anesthetize the area with 1% lidocaine and cleanse the area.
• Using iris scissors, snip off the lesion, or using a number 11 or number 15 scalpel, shave off the lesion.

NOTE: Control bleeding using pressure, gel foam, styptics, or aluminum chloride, if needed.

nature. Any pigmented lesion for which the primary-care practitioner suspects melanoma should be evaluated by a dermatologist.

Patient Education: Seborrheic Keratoses

The clinician should inform the patient that seborrheic keratoses are a harmless and common occurrence as people age. Some people develop many lesions, whereas others will have only a few. These lesions are not caused by chronic exposure to sunlight and may develop on any exposed or protected area of the body. Color changes in these lesions are harmless, but if the clinician is unsure about the exact nature of the lesion, referral to a dermatologist is recommended.

When evaluating any patient with a skin issue, the clinician should take the opportunity to teach about the ABCDEs of malignant melanoma. The mnemonic for characteristic features of melanoma is as follows:

A = asymmetry
B = border irregularity
C = color change
D = diameter larger than a pencil eraser (greater than 6 mm)
E = an evolving lesion (changing over time); may also be used for elevated, as in a raised lesion

PREMALIGNANT LESIONS

ACTINIC KERATOSIS

Actinic keratosis (AK), also called solar keratosis and senile keratosis, is the most common precancerous skin lesion found in lighter-skinned (white) patients. They are found on sun-exposed areas of skin that have been damaged by cumulative sun exposure. Estimates of progression to squamous cell carcinoma (SCC) vary widely from 0.1% to 20%. The progression to SCC (the second most common skin cancer) usually occurs within an average of 2 years. However, up to 25% of actinic keratoses spontaneously regress without treatment. Therefore, aggressive treatment of these premalignant lesions remains controversial.

EPIDEMIOLOGY AND CAUSES

Up to 58 million Americans have these premalignant lesions. Actinic keratoses are more common in men, probably as a result of occupational exposure (i.e., working outdoors). The most susceptible individuals are lighter skinned, with a history of frequent sun exposure and evidence of other signs of sun damage, such as freckles, senile lentigines (liver spots), wrinkles, and uneven

pigmentation. Actinic keratoses are found predominantly in older adults (older than age 50 years); however, occasionally they are seen in young adults with fair skin. These patients usually are of Celtic (Irish, Scottish, English) descent and are light-haired (blond or red haired) and blue-eyed. Susceptible individuals are sun sensitive and tend to freckle and sunburn easily.

AK is caused by the accumulation of damage to epithelial skin cells caused by chronic sun exposure. Renal transplant patients, as well as others who are immunocompromised, also have an increased tendency to develop AK. Individuals who work with compounds that contain polycyclic aromatic hydrocarbons (PAHs), such as coal or tar (e.g., roofers, road construction workers), are at a higher risk as well.

PATHOPHYSIOLOGY

Cumulative exposure to ultraviolet (UV) radiation in sunlight causes damage to the DNA of epithelial cells. With further UV light exposure, continued cumulative DNA damage may lead to malignant transformation of epidermal cellular clones. AKs that progress to SCC tend not to be aggressive unless they occur on the lip.

CLINICAL PRESENTATION

Subjective

The typical patient complains of an irritated rough or scaly rash. Some patients also complain of pruritus, tenderness, or a burning, stinging sensation in one or several lesions. Their lips may constantly feel dry. In contrast, some patients are asymptomatic and mention cosmetic concerns or worry about a potential malignancy.

Objective

AKs are small (0.2 to 5.0 mm) papules that can be flesh colored or slightly hyperpigmented. The primary lesions of AK consist of macules or plaques that are poorly circumscribed. Secondary lesions appear erythematous, scaly, and slightly raised. Areas of skin that have AK feel rough and uneven to the touch due to hyperkeratosis and have been likened to feeling like sandpaper. The hyperkeratosis of these lesions is characteristically hard or spiny.

Actinic keratoses are found in areas of skin that have been chronically exposed to the sun, such as the face (cheeks and forehead), ears, back of the neck, neckline, forearms, dorsal surfaces of the arms and hands, and (in women) the dorsal surfaces of the legs. In older men, lesions are predominant on the ears and balding scalp.

DIAGNOSTIC REASONING

Diagnostic Tests

The diagnosis can usually be made by history and physical examination. Palpating the lesion is key to the diagnosis by feeling for the typical scaly, rough, uneven sandpaper-like texture, as lesions may be more readily recognized by palpation rather than visual inspection. Fluorescence with the use of a photosensitizing drug (e.g., methyl ester of 5-aminolevulinic acid) can be used as a diagnostic tool for AK, because areas of involvement emit a pink fluorescence with a Wood's lamp or photodynamic therapy lamp.

Differential Diagnosis

Skin lesions that can mimic AK include SCC, seborrheic keratosis, and verruca plana (flat warts). SCC is characterized by an indurated plaque or nodule that is eroded or ulcerated and has a thickened scale. The lesion is found on sun-exposed skin, as is AK; however, what differentiates SCC from AK is the induration and ulceration of the former. Seborrheic keratosis lesions are highly pigmented (brown to black) and have a warty, stuck-on appearance. They can appear on both sun-exposed and protected skin. Verruca plana are caused by the human papillomavirus (HPV) and appear as multiple flesh-colored to light brown warts that are from 1 to 5 mm in size. Their color and smaller size distinguish them from AK.

MANAGEMENT

There is no solid evidence that removal of all of an individual's AK lesions prevents skin cancer. Indeed, some estimates are that only 1 in 1,000 actinic keratoses will progress to SCC. However, it is standard dermatological practice to remove most AK lesions. Because the lesions reside in the epithelium, therapies that separate the epidermis from the dermis are most effective and do not leave scars. Two methods are currently available to the primary-care practitioner: topical therapy and surgical destruction of the lesion. Treatment may also include a combination of both methods.

Topical Therapy

Topical application of fluorouracil cream (Fluoroplex, Carac) may eradicate AK, given its selective effects on sun-damaged cells. The cream is used for an average of 3 weeks. The eyelids, nasal folds, and lips should be avoided. Complete healing takes from 1 to 2 months after completion of therapy through the replication of epidermal cells. Patients treated with fluorouracil frequently become noncompliant with the treatment because the inflammatory effect (destruction of the lesion) leaves raw, tender, reddened skin in its place. If the lesion or lesions do not respond to one treatment course, these lesions must be evaluated for potential carcinoma via skin biopsy. Some evidence shows that tretinoin (Retin-A), when used in combination with fluorouracil, may increase effectiveness and shorten length of therapy. The safety and efficacy of fluorouracil during pregnancy have not been established.

Imiquimod cream (Aldara) is an immune response modifier. It may be used on face and scalp lesions and is applied two times weekly for 16 weeks. Side effects may include erythema, pruritus, rash, and xerosis (dry skin). Another topical cytotoxic agent, ingenol (Picato), may also be used, which works by killing rapidly growing cells, such as the abnormal cells associated with AK. For the face and scalp, ingenol 0.015% gel is usually applied once a day for 3 days in a row. On the torso or extremities, 0.05% gel is applied once a day for 2 consecutive days.

Another treatment for AK is photodynamic therapy, which uses a light-sensitizing compound that uniquely accumulates in AK cells, where it may then be activated by the appropriate wavelength of light. Delta-aminolevulinic acid (Levulan Kerastick) is a component of the heme biosynthetic pathway that accumulates in dysplastic cells. Once inside the cells, it is enzymatically converted to a potent photosensitizer. With exposure to either blue or red light of an appropriate wavelength, oxygen free radicals are generated and cell death results. These specialized treatments typically give improved cosmesis over the more commonly used method of cryosurgery and may be preferred for facial lesions. In addition, they only require a 2-day course of therapy.

Cryosurgery

Cryosurgery (freezing) with liquid nitrogen is used most frequently for patients with solitary or few lesions as a rapid and effective treatment for eradicating AK (see Therapeutic Procedure 17.2). As with all surgical interventions, informed consent must be obtained from the patient before cryosurgery is performed. With cryosurgery, the clinician must rely entirely on a clinical diagnosis because the tissue is destroyed by freezing. Therefore, there is no specimen available for confirmatory pathological analysis. The liquid nitrogen probe should be applied firmly to the lesion for 10 to 15 seconds and repeated twice in one visit. The lesion will crust over and generally disappear in 10 to 14 days. A possible drawback to this procedure is the potential for hypopigmentation because a white spot may appear at the treated site.

Therapeutic Procedure 17.2: Cryosurgery for Actinic Keratoses

- Liquid nitrogen applied with a cotton-tipped applicator is preferred because it causes minimal damage to the dermis.
- Using liquid nitrogen, freeze each lesion for 10 to 15 seconds. It may be necessary to repeat the freezing cycle a second time. The more pressure is applied to the cotton swab, the deeper the point of freeze contact or "freeze ball" will be.
- The "freeze balls" should be approximately 1.5 times as wide as they are deep.
- If in doubt, it is better to underfreeze and to retreat lesions than to overfreeze them and leave a scar or hypopigmentation (if damage to the dermis is avoided, scarring should not occur).
- Any lesion that does not respond to liquid nitrogen must be biopsied.

   NOTE: If diagnosis of any skin lesion is in doubt, refer to a dermatologist for possible skin biopsy. The treated area will become red and swollen a few hours after treatment. A serous or blood-filled blister forms and will subsequently crust and disappear in 10 to 14 days. The patient should be advised not to cover the blister with any bandages and not to touch or manipulate the blister because it will protect the treated area until it is healed.

Other Surgical Techniques

Lesions that are isolated and thick may be amenable to surgical curettage, shave excision, or conventional excision, particularly when located on the dorsal surfaces of the upper extremities. However, there are few data that speak to the efficacy of this approach, and these techniques are typically not considered first-line interventions. Importantly, however, surgical resection is the only method of AK removal that produces an intact biopsy sample available for histological examination and diagnostic confirmation. In addition, this method may be more appropriate for immunocompromised patients or for lesions suggestive of invasive cancer. Such surgical procedures require referral to a dermatologist.

FOLLOW-UP AND REFERRAL

Patients on fluorouracil should be followed up in 2 to 3 weeks or upon completion of treatment. Adverse effects of the medication, compliance issues, and effectiveness of treatment should be noted at this time. Any skin lesions that remain after treatment with fluorouracil cream for 2 to 3 weeks must be biopsied for pathological examination. Patients treated with cryosurgery are reevaluated in 2 weeks. Patients who have had excision biopsy by a dermatologist are usually seen again in 2 weeks.

Any AK lesion that does not respond to treatment should be referred to a dermatologist for further evaluation, including the need for a skin biopsy, even for superficial lesions. A dermatologist may remove multiple superficial lesions with a topical acid formulation followed by pulsed light laser therapy or photodynamic therapy. This is effective on the face and does not result in the hypopigmentation that may result from cryotherapy. An added benefit is one of esthetic skin rejuvenation.

Patient Education: Actinic Keratosis

Regardless of the method of treatment, the patient should be educated regarding the need for using sunscreen and wearing protective clothing in the sun, such as a hat, pants, and a shirt with long sleeves. An important aspect of actinic keratosis management is prevention—avoidance of excessive sun exposure is key to avoiding development of these premalignant lesions and their cancerous sequelae. In addition, the patient should also be taught the signs and symptoms of melanoma screening by using the ABCDE mnemonic (A, asymmetry; B, border irregularity; C, color change; D, diameter larger than a pencil eraser (greater than 6 mm); E, elevation from a flat lesion to a raised or evolving lesion).

Patients treated with fluorouracil should be warned that exposure to sunlight during treatment can exacerbate the inflammatory effect of the medicine. The clinician should instruct the patient that if erosions develop while using fluorouracil cream, petroleum jelly can be applied to provide comfort, but the treatment must be continued for 10 to 14 days. Patients should be warned to avoid prolonged sunlight exposure during and after treatment. A high-SPF sun block should be worn after treatment to prevent future damage to the skin.

Patients treated with cryosurgery should be informed that bandages are not necessary after treatment and actually impede healing. If blister formation results, the patient should be instructed to return to the office to assess whether the blister should be drained, but not to manipulate or remove the blister. The patient should be advised to avoid irritation of the treated lesion with clothing or jewelry, although showering and the use of makeup are permissible. The patient should be taught to monitor for the signs and symptoms of infection (e.g., redness, purulent discharge, heat). Infection is a rare occurrence after cryosurgery.

MALIGNANT LESIONS

MALIGNANT MELANOMA

Malignant melanoma is the most deadly of all skin cancers. *Melanoma* is a malignancy that arises from epidermal melanocytes, most commonly found in the skin. Melanocytes produce *melanin*, a brown-black pigment that is responsible for skin, hair, and eye color. Almost all melanomas arise from the skin (more than 90%), but a few melanomas originate from the eye (uveal melanoma), and a small number (less than 4%) do not have an identifiable primary site.

Although the majority of skin cancers in the United States are BCC (the most numerous type) and SCC, melanoma is responsible for 75% of all skin cancer deaths. Melanoma, if discovered early, is highly curable, but if the melanoma extends beyond 4 mm in depth, the prognosis is extremely poor. A 75% mortality rate is associated with this depth of invasion. Therefore, the role of the primary-care practitioner in screening for this skin cancer cannot be overemphasized. Screening programs that result in early diagnosis are important weapons in the armamentarium against this disease. The American Cancer Society's ABCDE mnemonic, explained in the section on skin pre-malignancies, is an easy tool for the clinician to use and to teach patients to recognize potential melanomas and dysplastic nevi, the precursor lesion of melanoma, at an early stage.

EPIDEMIOLOGY AND CAUSES

The incidence of melanoma in the United States has been increasing in both men and women over the past decade, with rates of melanoma increasing annually for both lighter-skinned men and women of European descent, although rates have remained steady for African Americans, Hispanics, Asians, and Native Americans, in whom melanoma is much less frequent. In 2016, of all the skin cancers, an estimated 76,380 were invasive melanomas, with about 46,870 in men and 29,510 in women. In 2017, an estimated 87,110 new cases of invasive melanoma will be diagnosed and an estimated 9,730 individuals will die from melanoma. Of the seven most common cancers in the United States, melanoma is the only type of cancer in which incidence is consistently increasing, and although it is not the most common type of skin cancer, melanoma causes the most deaths.

It is estimated that 1 in 10 individuals with a melanoma has a family history of the disease. In adults aged 25 to 29 years, melanoma is the most common form of cancer and the second most common among 15 to 19 year olds. One contributing factor is the use of tanning beds among young people. One indoor tanning session has been estimated to increase a person's risk of developing melanoma by 20%, and each additional session during the same year increases that rate by another 2%.

Several factors have been identified that increase an individual's risk of melanoma (see Risk Factors: Malignant Melanoma). Exposure and sensitivity to sunlight remain two of the most widely recognized risk factors. A disproportionate number of melanoma deaths occur among lighter-skinned individuals who sunburn easily.

Whites (Caucasians) who are at highest risk come from Celtic (Irish, Scottish, English) backgrounds and have light hair (especially red hair), light eyes, and freckles. The ability of the skin to freckle in response to sun exposure is thought to be a marker of susceptibility to melanoma, although stronger risk factors for melanoma exist.

Risk Factors: Malignant Melanoma

Age: risk increases with age
Skin, Eye, Hair Color: light, blue or green eyes, red or blond hair
Personal History
   History of skin cancer (any type)
   History of dysplastic nevi
   History of congenital nevi greater than 20 mm
   History of blistering sunburn before age 20 years
   History of immunosuppression
Family History
   History of melanoma
Environmental History
   Excessive outdoor exposure to ultraviolet radiation
   Exposure to indoor tanning

Research into the genetic components of melanoma and dysplastic nevi (precursor lesions) has found a relationship between dysplastic nevi, family history, and the development of melanoma. The finding of a dysplastic nevus (atypical mole) or any other type of skin cancer (such as BCC or SCC) is thought to increase the risk of melanoma. The number of nevi (moles) normally peaks during young adulthood (ages 20 to 25 years), then gradually decreases after age 50 years. Large numbers of nevi on an individual who is older than 50 years is considered to be a strong marker for increased risk of melanoma. It is estimated that 7% of the white population has at least one atypical nevus, and many individuals have numerous nevi that should be monitored closely.

All melanomas should be tested for mutations in *BRAF,* a gene involved in cell growth signaling, because such mutations appear in about half of all metastatic melanomas. Although *BRAF* is the official symbol designation, the gene is also known as *B-Raf* or *v-Raf murine sarcoma viral oncogene homolog B1.* As with other proto-oncogenes, a mutation in this gene has the potential to cause normal cells to become cancerous. The benefit of identifying this mutation may be beneficial in the treatment of melanoma, because at least two small molecule inhibitor drugs, vemurafenib (Zelboraf) and dabrafenib (Tafinlar), are used to treat *BRAF* mutation–positive melanomas. These drugs are discussed in more detail in the section on melanoma management.

The combination of having a first-degree relative with melanoma and the presence of one or more dysplastic nevi increases the risk of developing melanoma by up to 50% compared with the general population. Individuals with these traits tend to develop multiple primary lesions at a younger age compared with other individuals with melanomas. In addition, large-sized nevi (greater than 20 mm) are believed to be associated with increased melanoma risk. Currently, lifetime risk within the entire population is estimated at 1 in 75, with fully one-third of all cases occurring in persons aged younger than 45 years. However, this risk ranges widely depending on ethnic background and skin color, with a lifetime risk as high as 1 in 40 for lighter-skinned (white) individuals and as low as 1 in 1,000 for darker-skinned individuals, such as African Americans.

Pediatric overexposure to UV rays, especially a history of one or more blistering sunburns before the age of 20 years, has been linked to a dramatic increase in lifetime risk of developing melanoma. However, the incidence of malignant melanoma in children is low. It is thought that the effect of accumulated sunburns in addition to genetic predisposition is not seen until years later. Intermittent intense sun exposures (e.g., those that may occur in occupational groups such as farmers) that result in blistering sunburns appear to be more significant in terms of increased melanoma risk than chronic sun exposure.

PATHOPHYSIOLOGY

Malignant melanoma can be divided into several subtypes:

- *Superficial spreading* (70% to 85%): characterized by extensive lateral or radial growth before vertical invasion
- *Nodular* (15% to 30%): characterized by vertical growth only
- *Lentigo maligna* (5%): an in situ form that may persist for years before vertical extension
- *Acral lentiginous* (2% to 8%): a particularly aggressive form most common in darker-skinned patients, especially when appearing on the hands or feet

A combination of UV exposure and genetic susceptibility is believed to be the most common mechanism for developing melanoma. Studies have linked UV radiation, particularly UVB rays, to genetic mutations in DNA in susceptible individuals, resulting in the development of abnormal pigmented lesions (dysplastic nevi). Genetic predisposition to melanoma appears to be the result of the presence of a mutated or absent tumor suppressor gene. Abnormalities have been mapped to chromosomes 1 and 9. In particular, mutations in chromosomal region 9p21, which encodes the tumor suppressor gene *CDKN2A* that produces the protein p16, have been observed in a large proportion of both familial and spontaneous melanomas, as well as the previously discussed mutations in the *BRAF* gene, which are seen in over half of all melanomas.

Germline mutations in the gene *CDK4* have also been observed. Individuals in these susceptible groups tend to develop melanoma at multiple primary sites at an earlier age. Another strong genetic association is observed in the autosomal recessive condition xeroderma pigmentosum. Persons affected with this inherited disorder lack a critical DNA repair mechanism that corrects UV light–associated cross-linked DNA nucleotides. This results in multiple DNA breaks in response to cumulative UV light exposure and a resultant high level of sun-associated skin cancers.

Atypical nevi are precursors to malignant melanoma. They differ histologically from benign nevi in that they are disorganized and carry higher potential for transformation into malignant tissue. Initially, the tumor remains confined to the epidermis. If left untreated, it spreads into the subcutaneous fat. Microscopic lesions of superficial spreading-type melanoma have large, atypical pigmented cells of variable colors in the epidermis and the papillary dermis and lymphocytes. Nodular melanoma lesions have multiple tumor cells that form a nodule in the dermis, with invasion to the deeper dermal layers. Metastases to distant sites result when tumors invade through dermal lymphatics or blood vessels. Thus, metastasis occurs in the regional lymph nodes and occasionally at distant sites such as the bone, viscera, and especially the lungs, liver, and brain, which are the most commonly affected organs.

In the absence of metastasis, the four primary prognostic factors of melanoma are patient age, gender, tumor thickness, and tumor location. Worse prognoses are seen in older men with thicker tumors located in an axial distribution, as opposed to on the extremities. In addition, the relative importance of certain prognostic factors also depends on tumor stage. In earlier disease limited to the skin, tumor thickness and the presence of ulceration are key. However, in more advanced disease, along with the presence of ulceration, the degree of lymph nodal involvement is the most important factor.

CLINICAL PRESENTATION

Subjective

There are usually no symptoms associated with melanoma; however, some patients present with a pruritic, ulcerated, or bleeding mole. The typical patient is an adult who is concerned about a large mole that has changed in appearance. A change in characteristics of a mole is a frequent observation made by melanoma patients, while other patients seek care in response to a concerned family member, such as a spouse, who has advised them to have a mole checked. The patient typically will report having had the same mole for many years prior to its change in appearance. A family history of melanoma or skin cancer may be reported by some patients.

Objective

Most melanomas appear on sun-exposed areas of skin. The back and the neck are the most common sites in men, and the legs are more common in women. In African Americans and Asians, the feet, fingers, nailbeds, eyes (uveal tract), and mucous membranes are more common sites.

Melanoma often presents as an asymmetrical lesion with an irregular border, notching, and a diameter greater than 6 mm. The tumor often exhibits variegation in color, with admixtures of blue, red, tan, brown, black, and white. Rarely, tumors may be amelanotic. Early nodular tumors, for example, are typically flat and may lack most of the typical characteristics of melanoma. As the tumor advances, however, an increase in thickness causes elevation into a firm nodule (nodular melanoma).

Atypical nevi bear many of the same characteristics of a true melanoma, including irregular ill-defined borders, color variegation, and a large size (more than 6 mm). However, the emphasis on larger lesion size as an increased risk factor for melanoma is not always accurate because early melanomas can be smaller than 6 mm in diameter. Distinguishing between malignant melanoma and benign nevi can be difficult and often requires a skin biopsy.

Nailbed or subungual melanoma may be observed in older patients and is most commonly found on the thumb or great toe. This variant of acral lentiginous melanoma may present similarly to an ungual fungal infection, because discoloration of the nailbed known as longitudinal melanonychia may distort the nail itself. Posterior nailbed involvement called Hutchinson's sign is an ominous physical finding associated with advanced disease.

DIAGNOSTIC REASONING

Diagnostic Tests

Following a thorough physical examination including full-body skin inspection, suspicious lesions should be biopsied under local anesthesia by a dermatologist. Excisional biopsy is the preferred method if melanoma is suspected because a measurement of thickness can be made along with staging, as a predictor of prognosis and a guide for treatment. Thickness or depth of the melanoma is one of the critical factors in determining both prognosis and choice of therapy. Traditionally, the Breslow depth classification system has been used as a prognostic factor, complemented by the Clark staging system of tumor invasiveness, as described in Table 17.2. In addition, the American Joint Committee on Cancer classification system has been developed to take into account tumor thickness, mitotic rate, ulceration, and invasiveness (localized tumor versus nodal or distant metastases) as key prognostic factors.

TABLE 17.2   Skin Cancer Classification Systems

Malignant Melanoma

The American Joint Committee on Cancer (AJCC) has an ongoing collaborative staging system in process.

The TNM (tumor, node, metastasis) system adopted by the AJCC uses both Clark and Breslow's methods to clinically stage malignant melanomas. The extent of the tumor is determined only after excision.

The presence or absence of lymph node involvement is the most important predictor of survival.

Clark's Levels

This method describes the lesion based on the invading depth into the dermis and subcutaneous fat and is related to the prognosis and metastatic potential of the lesion. Clark's levels are not used as often today because of the subjectivity of describing the lesions.

Level I (in situ)	Confined to epidermis
Level II	Extends through the basement membrane and into the papillary dermis (upper portion)
Level III	Extends into the papillary dermis
Level IV	Extends into the reticular dermis
Level V	Invades the deep subcutaneous tissue

Breslow's Method

This method describes tumor thickness by measuring the distance from the dermis to the deepest level of involvement. The thicker the lesion, the higher the incidence for metastasis. Measured in millimeters (mm).

Breslow thickness	Estimated 5-year survival rate
Less than 1 mm	92%–97%
1.01–2 mm	81%–92%
2.01–4 mm	70%–81%
More than 4 mm	53%–70%

A patient diagnosed with melanoma should be referred to a dermatologist or an oncologist for excision of the melanoma and its margins. However, if biopsy pathology reveals only atypical nevi, removal of the lesion by excisional biopsy is sufficient treatment. A patient who has dysplastic nevi should receive regular skin surveillance. Skin examinations are usually done at 6-month intervals by a dermatologist.

Subsequent testing may include a lymph node biopsy via computed tomography (CT)–guided needle aspiration. Lymphatic drainage mapping and sentinel node biopsy have been shown to identify occult metastases by employing a technique that identifies the lymph node specifically draining the area of skin that contains the melanoma. This node, called the *sentinel node,* is excised and examined for melanoma cells. If any cancer cells are present, the remaining nodes in the area are dissected. If biopsy of the sentinel node is negative, metastasis is unlikely and recurrence rates are low. If metastatic disease is suspected, however, a thorough physical examination, laboratory tests, x-ray studies, and CT scans are done to evaluate for distant metastases.

Differential Diagnosis

Differentiating between melanoma and benign or pre-malignant lesions can prove challenging, even for dermatologists. Although the majority of atypical nevi and melanomas fit the ABCDEs of melanoma, an occasional lesion will escape early detection. The differential diagnosis for melanoma includes pigmented skin lesions such as benign nevi, solar lentigines, and seborrheic keratoses. Seborrheic keratoses are benign lesions that are common in elderly and older adult patients. The lesions are light to dark brown and appear as soft, wart-like growths, located mainly on the trunk. In contrast, melanoma is usually located on sun-exposed areas such as the neck, the back, or the legs. Solar lentigines (liver spots) are pigmented (light to dark brown) macules that appear on sun-exposed areas such as the dorsum of the hands and arms. Benign nevi (moles) are round to oval, with regular borders; most are less than 5 mm in diameter. The color is evenly distributed in a benign nevus, which is asymptomatic.

MANAGEMENT

A high index of suspicion is necessary because it is often difficult to distinguish atypical nevi from melanoma or normal nevi. If a clinician suspects possible melanoma or dysplastic nevi, referral to a dermatologist is necessary. In the United States, when a melanoma is detected early, there is an estimated 5-year survival rate of 98%. However, this survival rate falls to 62% when the melanoma extends into the lymph nodes and 18% when it metastasizes to distant organs.

There are four treatments available for melanoma, which may be used in combination: Mohs surgery (or other type of excision), chemotherapy, radiation therapy, and biological therapy. If the melanoma lesion is discovered early enough, the chance of a complete cure with excision is good. Management will depend on the staging of the lesion (see Table 17.2). In situ melanomas require excisional margins of at least 0.5 cm. Melanomas measuring less than 2 mm in thickness require at least a 1-cm circumferential surgical margin, whereas thicker tumors need at least 2-cm margins. Lymph node dissection is required when there is evidence of draining lymph node involvement on clinical examination, but its ability to improve outcomes is unclear when performed empirically.

Nonmetastatic melanomas that have not spread beyond their site of origin are often curable. Melanomas with a Breslow thickness of 2 mm or more are curable in a significant proportion of patients, but the risk of lymph node and/or systemic metastasis grows with increasing thickness of the primary lesion. Some melanomas that have spread to regional lymph nodes may be curable with wide local excision of the primary tumor and removal of the affected regional lymph nodes.

In addition to excision of the lesion with its margins, patients with metastatic disease are treated with several other modalities. One of the main treatments is chemotherapy with dacarbazine (DTIC), cisplatin, and vincristine or a combination of these agents. Temozolomide, an oral agent resembling DTIC, is FDA approved for brain cancer and is being used off-label for melanomas that have spread to the central nervous system. Only 15% to 30% of patients respond to chemotherapy with a reduction in tumor size. Unfortunately, the response to chemotherapy is typically short term, and fewer than 5% of patients will experience a remission of their disease. If the melanoma is located on a limb, high-dose chemotherapy via isolated limb perfusion is available. In this technique, the circulation of the affected limb is isolated by tourniquet at the root of the limb. High-dose chemotherapy is infused and is limited to the affected limb only, minimizing the adverse systemic effects from the chemotherapy.

External beam radiation to treat melanoma is usually reserved for palliative treatment. For metastatic lesions of the lung, brain, or viscera that cause pressure on tissue, radiation therapy is used to reduce the tumor's size and provide relief from pain.

Administration of biological therapy such as high-dose interferon and interleukin-2 in high-risk patients (to prevent recurrence) has shown some promise. In addition, therapies directed at specific gene mutations have been developed. Although melanomas that have spread to distant sites are rarely curable, the small molecule serine/threonine protein kinase inhibitors vemurafenib (Zelboraf) and dabrafenib (Tafinlar), as well as the fully human monoclonal antibody therapy ipilimumab (Yervoy), which is an antagonist of the cytotoxic T-cell inhibitory factor CTLA-4, have demonstrated improvements in progression-free survival of metastatic melanoma patients in large studies. Combination therapy with both biological therapy and chemotherapy continues to be studied. In addition, vaccines that stimulate immune function against melanoma tumors are being developed.

FOLLOW-UP AND REFERRAL

Patients at increased risk for developing melanoma should be referred to a dermatologist for increased surveillance, including regular physical examinations and full skin and mucosal surface inspection. Ophthalmological examination may also be indicated in the metastatic patient without a readily identifiable primary tumor (e.g., a patient with melanomatous liver metastases but no primary skin tumor), given the propensity for melanoma to develop in the pigmented uveal cells of the eye. The patient who wishes to participate in clinical trials for melanoma can obtain information on current studies from an oncologist. For the patient with an inoperable melanoma or extensive distant metastases, hospice and palliative care should be offered to the patient and his or her family.

Patient Education: Melanoma

Prevention of all skin cancers should start early during infancy, especially in individuals with a Celtic background or with a positive family history for skin cancer. Prevention remains the most important intervention, and early diagnosis significantly improves treatment outcomes. Early detection of melanomas is made easier to remember with the ABCDE mnemonic, as discussed earlier.

A person's risk of melanoma doubles if he or she has had more than five sunburns. Thus, teaching patients about the proper use of sunscreen cannot be overemphasized. Studies have shown that with daily, rather than discretionary, use of sunscreen, the risk of developing squamous cell carcinoma was reduced by approximately 40%, the risk of developing any melanoma by 50%, and the risk of invasive melanoma by 73%. Thus, patients should avoid staying under the sun during the hottest part of the day, high-SPF sunscreens should be applied on a daily basis, and hats or headgear should be worn to protect the scalp and back of the neck. Wearing loose-fitting long-sleeved shirts and pants provides some protection from the sun and is equivalent to wearing sunscreen if the skin is entirely covered.

The hazards of tanning beds need to be discussed with all patients. Because more than 419,000 cases of skin cancer in the United States each year are linked to tanning beds, in 2014, the FDA reclassified tanning beds from Class I (no risk) to Class II (moderate risk). In the United States, at least 45 states restrict minors of some age from using indoor tanning beds, and some countries (e.g., Brazil, Australia) have banned indoor tanning beds altogether, as a result of the World Health Organization declaring tanning beds a Level I carcinogen. Some research indicates that more people have developed skin cancer due to tanning beds than have developed lung cancer due to smoking (Wehner et al., 2014).

Survivors of melanoma need to be informed of their increased risk of a second primary tumor or of recurrence of the previous lesion. Any change in an existing lesion or any new pigmented skin lesion should be reported to the patient's primary-care practitioner and dermatologist. Likewise, patients should be urged to report any swelling in the lymph nodes of the neck, axilla, or groin area.

NONMELANOMATOUS SKIN CANCERS

The two most common forms of nonmelanomatous skin cancer in humans are basal cell carcinoma and squamous cell carcinoma. *Basal cell carcinoma (BCC)* is a malignant tumor of the skin that originates in the basal cells of the epidermis. It is a slow-growing and locally invasive tumor that rarely metastasizes. It represents the beginning of a continuum of skin cancers in both severity and mortality. *Squamous cell carcinoma (SCC)*, a malignant tumor originating from keratinocytes, can invade the dermis and occasionally metastasize to distant sites. Avoidance of excessive sun exposure is an important factor in preventing these skin cancers. In addition, screening programs are important in the early recognition and diagnosis of these cancers, because they are highly curable when discovered in their early stages.

EPIDEMIOLOGY AND CAUSES

The incidence of BCC and SCC is expected to rise in the United States over the next decade because of the increase in the older adult population and a longer overall life expectancy. More than one of three new cancers is a skin cancer, with BCC being the more common of the two nonmelanomatous skin cancers and the most common type of skin cancer overall. Each year, more than 4 million cases of BCC are diagnosed in the United States.

Rarely, BCC results from basal cell nevus syndrome, an inherited autosomal dominant disorder. Patients with this disorder tend to have multiple sites of BCC at a younger age. It is associated with bone cysts, palmar skin pits, and frontal bossing (a protuberance of the bones of the skull—particularly those under the skin of the forehead).

SCC is the second most common skin cancer, accounting for an estimated 20% of all skin cancers. Every year in the United States, there are more than 1 million persons diagnosed with SCC. Over the past 30 years, the incidence of SCC has increased up to 200%, and as many as 8,800 individuals die from SCC annually. This increase is due in part to the use of tanning beds. One variant of the disease that affects mostly older white men is Bowen's disease, an intraepidermal SCC that can be induced by exposure to inorganic trivalent arsenic or inhaled mustard gas, in addition to chronic sun exposure.

The most important risk factor for both BCC and SCC is chronic accumulated sun exposure. Therefore, these skin cancers are typically seen in older adults and elderly patients. In particular, midrange UV light in the UVB part of the spectrum is believed to be more cancer-inducing than UVA rays. Individuals most at risk are those of Celtic background (Irish, Scottish, English) who are light-haired (e.g., red-haired or blond), blue-eyed, freckled, and who sunburn easily. In addition, men are twice as likely to develop BCC and three times as likely to develop squamous skin cancers compared with women.

Other conditions that increase the risk of SCC include immunosuppression, a history of exposure to ionizing radiation, exposure to arsenic and PAHs (paint thinners, organic solvents), treatment with psoralens and UV light (therapy used for psoriasis), and infection with oncogenic HPV. SCC is also seen with increased frequency in areas of skin damage due to chronic inflammation, burns, old scars, or chronic ulcers (see Risk Factors: Nonmelanomatous Skin Cancer).

Risk Factors: Nonmelanomatous Skin Cancer

Age: risk increases with age

Sex: Male

Skin, Eye, Hair Color
Lighter—tendency to tan poorly and burn quickly
Blue eyes, red or blond hair

Personal History
History of skin cancer
History of basal cell nevus syndrome
History of precancerous lesions, including actinic keratosis
History of burn scars or areas of skin damaged by chronic inflammation or ulcers
History of immunosuppression

Environmental History
Excessive exposure to UV radiation (sunlight)
Exposure to arsenic, polycyclic aromatic hydrocarbons, or radiation

---

PATHOPHYSIOLOGY

The majority of BCCs and SCCs are the result of DNA damage in skin cells that have been exposed to many years of UV radiation from sunlight. The damage is cumulative and is mediated primarily by defects in DNA repair mechanisms in response to mutational cross-linking by UV light. Such cumulative damage is particularly important in the development of BCC, particularly within skin containing a high concentration of sebaceous glands.

Several forms of BCC are seen clinically, including nodular, sclerosing, and superficial forms. The noduloulcerative type is the most common, with well-differentiated tumor cells that may extend from the dermal–epidermal interface into the dermis and subcutaneous fat. Superficial BCC appears similar to dermatitis, with erythema and scaling bordered by a fine rim. The origins of these tumors appear to be multifocal, with multiple small nodules arising from different epidermal foci. The sclerosing, or morpheaform, type of BCC is highly aggressive with a high rate of recurrence, presenting as a white plaque with palpable fibrosis and poorly circumscribed margins. Histologically, these tumors consist of spindle cells invading the dermal skin layer.

If not treated, BCC continues to grow and invade surrounding cartilage, bone, and soft tissues. BCC rarely metastasizes to distant sites, however.

In contrast, SCC is considered more dangerous than BCC because of its faster rate of growth and tendency to metastasize. The precursor lesion of most SCC is AK, a relatively common finding in older lighter-skinned patients. As discussed in the section on skin premalignancies, AK results from accumulated chronic sun exposure and is found only on sun-exposed skin. Actinic keratoses are premalignant lesions involving the uppermost layer of the epidermis that have been shown in some studies to have a low potential for development into malignancy (as low as 0.1%), although other studies have suggested rates as high as 20%, especially when one considers the risk becomes additive for individuals with more than one AK on the body, which is not unusual.

In situ SCC (Bowen's disease) involves the full thickness of the epidermis and is the earliest form of SCC. Interestingly, in contrast to BCC, more recent excessive UV light exposure, rather than cumulative lifetime exposure, correlates best with the development of squamous cell skin cancer, particularly in areas with few sebaceous glands. Invasive SCC is characterized by penetration through the epidermis and into the dermis, with a rate of metastasis of approximately 5%, primarily to the regional lymph nodes. Lesions that metastasize at a higher rate include those located on the lips, the ear, or at sites of trauma such as old scars and chronic wounds (ulcers), as well as larger lesions (more than 2 cm in diameter or more than 4 mm in depth). Patients on immunosuppressive therapy also have a higher rate of metastasis.

As observed in melanoma, any underlying condition affecting DNA repair increases the risk of developing BCC and SCC. For example, in the rare autosomal recessive condition xeroderma pigmentosum, individuals lose the ability to repair UV light–induced DNA cross-linking damage, resulting in multiple DNA breaks and malignant transformation of skin cells. UV light exposure has also been correlated with mutations of specific oncogenes and tumor suppressor genes, including *p53* (seen in more than half of all BCC and up to 90% of SCC) and the human patched gene. Such mutations result in dysregulated programmed cell death (apoptosis) and uncontrolled proliferation of epidermal cellular clones.

Several other mechanisms also contribute to the development of keratinocyte and basal cell skin cancers. Epidermal antigen-presenting Langerhans cells suffer direct damage from UV radiation, compromising the ability of the immune system to recognize and clear tumor antigen-expressing cancer cells. Systemic glucocorticoids also contribute to immunosuppression and have been shown in some studies to more than double the risk of developing nonmelanomatous skin cancer. In fact, intact immunosurveillance is key to the prevention of cutaneous carcinomas, as BCC is 10 times more likely to develop in chronically immunosuppressed organ transplant recipients, while SCC is up to 250 times more likely to occur. Although these tumors tend to develop at least 2 years after the transplant, they are more aggressive, more likely to occur at multiple sites, and begin to develop at a younger age than in non-transplanted, immunocompetent individuals.

Several types of proinflammatory cytokines have been identified in skin affected by cutaneous carcinomas, including tumor necrosis factor–alpha and IL-10. Prostaglandin synthesis also appears critical to this process, and selective cyclooxygenase-2 inhibitors have been shown to confer a protective effect against BCC and SCC in mouse models. Infection with HPV is associated with the development of anogenital SCC—particularly serotypes 16 and 18. In immunosuppressed individuals, the development of cutaneous warts and nonmelanomatous skin cancers appears to be correlated. In addition, kerato-acanthoma (a fast-growing hyperkeratotic nodular lesion indistinguishable from well-differentiated SCC) has also been associated with HPV infection. However, the specific role of HPV in additional forms of keratinocyte skin cancers remains controversial, and further research to explore this relationship is ongoing.

CLINICAL PRESENTATION

Subjective

A typical patient with nonmelanomatous skin carcinoma is an adult or elderly patient who presents with complaints of a spot or a bump that is getting larger or a sore that is not healing. Often the lesion appears as a thick, rough patch that may bleed if scratched or scraped. Some patients think they are warts with a raised border and crusted surface. The skin lesion may be pruritic or asymptomatic.

Objective

BCC typically appears in areas of skin that are chronically exposed to the sun, such as the face, ears, cheeks, nose, and the neck. Nodulo-ulcerative BCC is characterized by elevated papules that have a pearly appearance, with some crusting. When the crusts are removed, a small amount of bleeding ensues. On close examination, telangiectatic blood vessels are seen on the border of the lesion. A central ulceration is seen during the later stages of BCC lesions. BCC lesions may be the same color as the patient's skin or have areas of variegated color such as blue, black, or brown.

SCC is typically found on sun-exposed areas, such as the lips, the tips of ears, the nose, the upper cheeks, the scalp (in bald men), the dorsa of the hands and forearms, and the shins in women. Smokers are prone to cancerous lesions on the lips and tongue. The most common presentation of SCC is a firm papule with a scaly (keratotic) rough surface with irregular borders. These lesions may even present as cutaneous horns, with columnar hyperkeratosis atop

an erythematous base. Later, the surfaces of SCC lesions tend to bleed easily (become friable) with minor trauma and appear eroded with ulcerations. The typical lesion of Bowen's disease appears as a solitary, slowly enlarging erythematous, red-brown hyperkeratotic plaque that has a slight scaling and minimal crusting. Similar lesions in the anogenital region known as Bowenoid papulosis have been associated with oncogenic HPV strains.

DIAGNOSTIC REASONING

Diagnostic Tests

Suspicious lesions (if not located on the face) can be biopsied by an experienced primary-care practitioner or referred to a dermatologist. Because BCC rarely metastasizes, staging of the lesions is not necessary. SSC, however, has a higher rate of metastasis and may require staging based on the pathologist's report. Other important factors that determine staging include tumor characteristics, spread to regional lymph nodes, and metastasis to other organs.

Differential Diagnosis

The differential diagnoses of nonmelanomatous skin cancer include seborrheic keratosis, atopic dermatitis (eczema), solar lentigo, and AK. The presence of AK lesions on patients is considered a marker for excessive sun exposure. Recognition of AK, a precancerous skin lesion, is important because treatment during this stage is very simple. Typical AK lesions appear on sun-exposed surfaces and are pink to red or sometimes brown. In contrast to BCC, in which only one or a few lesions are present at a time in most patients, AK lesions are typically present in greater numbers. Lesions vary in size from 2 mm to 1 cm in diameter. These numerous lesions are also located on chronically sun-exposed areas such as the face and the head, the back of the neck, the dorsum of the hands and arms, and the upper shoulders.

In contrast to BCC and SCC, seborrheic keratosis lesions predominantly appear on non-sun-exposed areas of the body, such as the trunk in older adult patients, and do not appear erythematous or scaly. A patient with atopic dermatitis will report an atopic history and the recurrence of lesions in the same location that resolve with 1 to 2 weeks of treatment with topical corticosteroids. Solar lentigo lesions are found in older adults on sun-exposed areas of skin; these "liver spots" appear as multiple smooth, flat brown macules (like enlarged freckles) that are from 1 to 3 cm in size.

MANAGEMENT

Management of nonmelanomatous skin cancers is dependent on several factors: size and depth of the invasion, location, cosmetic concerns, and metastasis to other sites. Almost all cases of BCC and most cases of SCC require only simple excision under local anesthesia. Some primary-care practitioners and dermatologists elect excisional biopsy at the time of initial diagnosis; this procedure is both diagnostic and curative. Alternative methods for removal of small BCC and SCC lesions include electrodesiccation and curettage, cryosurgery (liquid nitrogen), and laser surgery. SCC has an overall rate of remission of up to 90% after therapy.

Mohs microsurgery has the highest cure rate for both BCC and SCC. This precise technique involves the surgical removal and simultaneous microscopic examination of small layers of skin, with removal of only the smallest amount of tissue necessary to eradicate the tumor (until disease-free margins are confirmed). This technique involves less scarring and is particularly suited for treatment of tumors in places of cosmetic importance, such as the face. Skin grafting may be necessary in addition to tumor removal.

In addition to surgical excision, lymph node dissection and systemic chemotherapy are used to treat large and invasive SCC lesions that have metastasized. External beam radiation is used as the primary treatment on tumors that are large or located in areas of skin that make surgery difficult, or in elderly or debilitated patients who are poor surgical candidates. External beam therapy is also used as adjuvant therapy in lesions with a high risk of recurrence or in cancers that have metastasized.

Topical therapies are also used for superficial forms of basal BCC, including imiquimod cream (used five times weekly), topical 5-fluorouracil (5-FU), and photodynamic treatment (used for both nodular and superficial forms) utilizing a photosensitizer with blue wavelength phototherapy to create reactive oxygen species. Similar approaches are being used for SCC. For example, imiquimod is used for in situ Bowen's disease. Premalignant AK is also typically treated with topical chemotherapy (e.g., 5-FU cream) or cryotherapy with liquid nitrogen. Other treatment options include dermabrasion, shave excision, electrodesiccation and curettage, and laser therapy.

Recurrence rates for both BCC and SCC after treatment vary with tumor characteristics and the treatment modality selected. Most recurrences occur within 3 years of treatment. Mohs microsurgery is an option for recurrent lesions, as it has a particularly high cure rate for lesions that have recurred after other types of treatment. Metastasis following SCC usually occurs where there is a chronic inflammatory skin condition, such as on the ears, nose, lip, or in mucosal areas such as the mouth, nose, or genitals.

FOLLOW-UP AND REFERRAL

Referral to a dermatologist or oncologist is necessary for all suspicious skin lesions, including nonmelanomatous skin cancers. The majority of patients require only simple excision of the skin lesion, with follow-up by the dermatologist or the clinician who performed the procedure to monitor skin healing. Subsequent follow-up includes complete physical examinations with full skin examinations every 6 to 12 months or more often if there are any signs of new or changing skin lesions or recurrence of a lesion at the primary site. The patient who has been diagnosed with any type of skin cancer is at increased risk of developing more skin lesions in the future, including recurrences of the original primary lesion.

Patient Education: Basal Cell and Squamous Cell Carcinomas

Although the U.S. Preventive Services Task Force states there is insufficient evidence to recommend screening for skin cancer by clinicians, the American Cancer Society recommends skin examinations both by clinicians and patients (self-examination). Patients of all ages should be taught the importance of monthly skin self-examinations and to report any changes in preexisting skin lesions (see Table 17.3). Moreover, the importance of careful examination of the skin on an annual basis by a trained health professional cannot be overemphasized for certain patients. These include patients with a family history of melanoma, multiple nevi, a history of sunburns, frequent sun exposure, and persons who work in certain high-risk occupations or avocations, such as farmers, gardeners, and sailors. Unfortunately, research has shown that a large proportion of primary-care practitioners do not routinely document findings related to the skin on physical examination.

Survivors of nonmelanomatous skin cancer should be informed of their increased risk of developing a second lesion or of recurrence of the original lesion. Thus, these patients in particular should be instructed to report any changes in existing moles or the development of new or rapidly growing lesions.

Approximately 80% of lifetime exposure to UV radiation occurs before the age of 20 years in the majority of patients. Therefore, *Healthy People 2020* has several objectives to increase the proportion of adolescents and adults who follow protective measures that may reduce the risk of skin cancer. Strategies to avoid sun exposure should be discussed with all patients at every physical examination, particularly with the parents of infants, young children, and adolescents. Patients and their families should be advised of the following preventive strategies:

- Avoid sun exposure from 11 a.m. to 4 p.m., the period of the most intense UV radiation.
- Wear protective clothing (tight-weave fabric, long-sleeve shirt, and a wide-brimmed hat). Men frequently get lesions on the top of the ear.
- Wear large-framed, wraparound sunglasses with 99% to 100% UV absorption.
- Apply a sunscreen with an SPF of at least 15 as directed, even on hazy days; reapply sunscreen as needed.
- Avoid the use of tanning beds and sun lamps.
- Learn the ABCDEs of malignant melanoma.

TABLE 17.3   Patient Education: Skin Self-Examination

Once a month, perform a skin self-examination. Record your initial examination, then note any changes with each subsequent examination. Use the following table as a guide.

Head	Looking in a mirror, carefully inspect your head. Using a comb or hair dryer, carefully part your hair and inspect your scalp.
Face and neck	Looking in a mirror, carefully inspect your entire face and neck, including the nose, lips, and ears.
Arms and hands	Holding up each arm, carefully inspect each arm and hand, including the underarms and back of your upper arms (a mirror may be needed). Holding up each hand, carefully inspect the front and back of each hand and wrist, including the areas between each finger and the fingernails.
Chest, torso, and front of the legs	Standing and looking in a full-length mirror, carefully inspect your chest (including breasts), torso, and front of the legs.
Back, buttocks, and back of the legs	Standing and looking in a full-length mirror, turn so that you can carefully inspect your full back, buttocks, and back of the legs (a hand mirror may also be needed).
Ankles and feet	Sitting and propping each foot on a chair or stool at a comfortable height, carefully inspect the tops and bottoms of both ankles and feet, including the areas between the toes and the toenails.
Genitalia	Sitting and using a hand mirror, carefully inspect the genitalia.

 For additional resources please visit
https://davisedge.fadavis.com/

REFERENCES

Acne Vulgaris

American Academy of Dermatology. Acne. https://www.aad.org/public/diseases/acne-and-rosacea/acne#treatment. Published 2017. Accessed July 1, 2017.

Palmer A. What is the difference between tretinoin and isotretinoin? https://www.verywell.com/difference-between-tretinoin-and-isotretinoin-15647. Published 2016. Accessed July 1, 2017.

PubMed Health. Which birth control pills can help reduce acne? https://www.ncbi.nlm.nih.gov/pubmedhealth/PMH0072393/. Published 2013. Accessed July 2, 2017.

Society for Investigative Dermatology and the American Academy of Dermatology Association, Statistic Brain Research Institute. Acne statistics—papule, pustule, nodule. http://www.statisticbrain.com/acne-statistics-papule-pustule-nodule/. Published 2016. Accessed July 1, 2017.

Actinic Keratosis

Drugs.com. Fluorouracil cream. https://www.drugs.com/cdi/fluorouracil-cream.html. Published 2017. Accessed July 4, 2017.

DUSA Pharmaceuticals. Statistics on actinic keratoses. http://www.dusapharma.com/actinic-keratoses2.html?gclid=CMnL5MmW8NQCFeYy0wod530FfA. Published 2017. Accessed July 4, 2017.

Malignant Melanoma

The Skin Cancer Foundation. Skin cancer facts & statistics. http://www.skincancer.org/skin-cancer-information/skin-cancer-facts. Published 2017. Accessed July 4, 2017.

U.S. Preventive Services Task Force. Screening for skin cancer: U.S. Preventive Services Task Force recommendation statement. http://www.guideline.gov/summary/summary.aspx?doc_id=13695&nbr=007029&string=. Published 2009.

Nonmelanomatous Skin Cancers

American Family Physician. (2016). Screening for skin cancer: Recommendation statement. *Am Fam Physician.* 2016;94(6):479–481.

DiChiara T. Clark level and Breslow thickness: What do these measures mean? https://www.verywell.com/melanoma-staging-what-it-means-and-reveals-3010755. Published 2017. Accessed July 8, 2017.

Healthy People.gov. Skin CA objectives. https://www.healthypeople.gov/2020/data-search/Search-the-Data#srch=skin. Accessed June 30, 2017.

Skin Cancer Foundation. Basal cell carcinoma (BCC). http://www.skincancer.org/skin-cancer-information/basal-cell-carcinoma. Published 2017. Accessed July 8, 2017.

Rosacea

Kumar PR. Rosacea. http://www.rkskinclinichyderabad.com/rosacea-en-in.htm. Published 2017. Accessed July 2, 2017.

National Rosacea Society. Tools for the professional. https://www.rosacea.org/physicians/index.php. Published 2017. Accessed July 2, 2017.

Seborrheic Keratosis

American Academy of Dermatology. Seborrheic keratosis. https://www.aad.org/public/diseases/bumps-and-growths/seborrheic-keratoses. Published 2017. Accessed July 2, 2017.

Skin Cancer Foundation. Squamous cell carcinoma (SCC). http://www.skincancer.org/skin-cancer-information/squamous-cell-carcinoma. Published 2017. Accessed July 8, 2017.

Wehner M, Chren M-M, Nameth D, et al. International prevalence of indoor tanning: A systematic review and meta-analysis. *JAMA Dermatol.* 2014;150(4):390–400.

RESOURCES

American Academy of Dermatology
    www.aad.org
American Cancer Society
    www.cancer.org
National Cancer Institute
    www.nci.nih.gov
National Institutes of Health
    www.nih.gov
Skin Cancer Foundation Skin Cancer Staging
    http://www.skincancer.org/skin-cancer-information/melanoma/the-stages-of-melanoma/guide-to-staging-melanoma

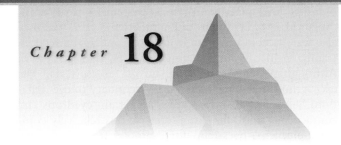

Chapter **18**

Common Eye Complaints

Ruth McCaffrey, DNP, APRN, FNP-BC, GNP, FAAN, FAANP

Lynne M. Dunphy, PhD, APRN, FNP-BC, FAAN, FAANP

Brian Oscar Porter, MD, PhD, MPH, MBA

DRY EYE

Dry eye syndrome (DES), also known as keratoconjunctivitis sicca or keratitis sicca, is a multifactorial disease of the tears and the ocular surface that results in discomfort, visual disturbance, and tear film instability with potential damage to the ocular surface. Essentially, dry eye occurs when the quantity and/or quality of tears fails to keep the surface of the eye adequately lubricated. It is a relatively common syndrome that affects approximately 5 million people in the United States, especially those older than 40 years. Prevalence estimates range between approximately 10% and 30% of the population. An estimated 3.23 million women and 1.68 million men aged 50 years and older are affected. Because the population is aging, DES is expected to increase in prevalence and thus impose a growing burden on ophthalmologic practices.

In a healthy eye, lubricating tears called basal tears continuously bathe the cornea, the clear, dome-shaped outer surface of the eye. With every blink of the eye, basal tears flow across the cornea, nourishing its cells and providing a layer of liquid protection from the environment. When the glands nearby each eye fail to produce enough basal tears, or when the composition of the tears changes, the health of the eye and vision are compromised. Vision may be affected because tears on the surface of the eye play an important role in focusing light. Tears are a complex mixture of fatty oils, water, mucus, and more

than 1,500 proteins keep the surface of the eye smooth and protected from the environment, irritants, and infectious pathogens. Tears form in three layers:

1. An outer, oily (lipid) layer, produced by the Meibomian glands, keeps tears from evaporating too quickly and helps tears remain on the eye.
2. A middle (aqueous) layer contains the watery portion of tears as well as water-soluble proteins. This layer is produced by the main lacrimal gland and accessory lacrimal glands. It nourishes the cornea and the conjunctiva, the mucous membrane that covers the entire front of the eye and the inside of the eyelids.
3. An inner (mucin) layer, produced by goblet cells, binds water from the aqueous layer to ensure that the eye remains wet. Eighty-six percent of patients with DES also have signs of meibomian gland dysfunction.

Dry eye can greatly affect an individual's quality of life. It most commonly affects both eyes and may be described as a feeling of "sand in the eyes," especially when blinking. The eyes may feel hot, irritated, gritty and may redden. The patient may present with complaints of blurred vision and lack of tears, or, in some cases, with excessive tearing as the eyes attempt to compensate. Patients may also complain of burning, itching, foreign body sensation, sensitivity to light, and loss of the glossy appearance of the cornea. Some patients with dry eye may also complain of feeling as if their eyelids are "heavy." Dry eye may be an indication of underlying systemic disease, such as autoimmune disorder, and the health-care practitioner should always be alert to these possibilities.

Symptoms typically worsen with smoky or dry environments, hot-air heating systems, and windy conditions, as all may contribute to tear evaporation. Risk factors include advancing age because of declines in tear production that can occur with aging, and the female sex. Prolonged computer usage may cause a decrease in blinking; seasonal allergies can contribute to symptoms worsening; autoimmune disorders such as Sjögren's syndrome, lupus, scleroderma, and rheumatoid arthritis and other disorders such as diabetes, thyroid disorders, and vitamin A deficiency are associated with dry eye, and autoimmune diseases are also more common in woman. Medications including antihistamines, decongestants, antidepressants, birth control pills, hormone replacement therapy to relieve symptoms of menopause, and medications for anxiety, Parkinson's disease, and high blood pressure have all been associated with dry eye. Rosacea (an inflammatory skin disease) and blepharitis (an inflammatory eyelid disease) can disrupt the function of the Meibomian glands, which in turn effect tear composition and production.

DIFFERENTIAL DIAGNOSIS

The differential diagnosis of dry eye includes the following conditions:

- Conjunctivitis
- Blepharitis
- Contact lens complications
- Exophthalmos
- Ectropion
- Bell's palsy
- Medication-related side effects
- Sjögren's syndrome
- Age-related changes
- Hormonal changes
- Vitamin A deficiency

DES is essentially a clinical diagnosis that is made by combining information obtained from the history and physical examination and performing one or more diagnostic tests to lend additional objectivity to the diagnosis. No single test is sufficiently specific to permit an absolute diagnosis of DES. Symptom questionnaires can be used to help establish a diagnosis of DES and to assess the effects of treatments or to grade disease severity. At least 14 questionnaires are available; among the most commonly used and validated include the following:

- Ocular Surface Disease Index
- System for Patient Evaluation of Eye Dryness
- Visual analog scale
- McMonnies Dry Eye Index
- Symptom Assessment in Dry Eye

Studies that may be used in the work-up include impression cytology to monitor the progression of ocular surface changes, measurement of tear breakup time, the Schirmer test, and quantification of tear components through analysis of tear proteins or tear-film osmolarity. Serology for circulating autoantibodies may be indicated.

EXCESSIVE TEARING (EPIPHORA)

Excessive tearing is defined as the overflow of tears from one or both eyes and can occur continuously or intermittently. Excessive tearing may be a result of (1) a paradoxical response to dry eye, (2) exposure to an irritant, (3) or from an obstruction of the nasolacrimal duct. It is an especially common complaint in elderly patients and in individuals

with allergies. A healthy eye is a wet eye; however, a continuously wet eye with uncontrolled tearing signals a malfunction due to a variety of possible causes.

The complaint of excessive tearing may be related to dry eye, such as in cases of lacrimal apparatus malfunction or dysfunction in neurologic control of the tearing process. Excessive tearing may also occur secondary to a blockage in the lacrimal drainage system from the accumulation of discharge from conjunctivitis. The eyes may also water secondary to an irritant (e.g., allergy, infection, trauma, pain, or structural abnormalities, as in ectropion). Although patients may complain of "excess tears," the excess fluid is actually a discharge secondary to eye irritation. Sensitivity to preservatives in certain eyedrops and contact lens solutions can also cause this relatively common problem. Eyestrain, for example, from prolonged computer use, may lead to a decrease in blinking, which may then lead to compensatory and excessive tearing.

Excessive tearing may also occur secondary to a blockage in the lacrimal drainage system from the accumulation of discharge from conjunctivitis. Frequently, excess tearing will lead to increased irritation and even more tearing, so it is necessary to break this cycle to treat this symptom effectively.

Tearing in one eye is not uncommon and is commonly related to foreign body, corneal irritation and/or inflammation, superficial infections, and irritation from contact lens.

DIFFERENTIAL DIAGNOSIS

The differential diagnosis of epiphora includes the following conditions:

- Allergens
- DES
- Viral or bacterial conjunctivitis
- Blocked lacrimal duct
- Ectropion
- Trauma (e.g., foreign body or corneal abrasion)
- Environmental pollutants
- Glaucoma
- Uveitis
- Orbital inflammatory disease
- Orbital cellulitis

EYE PAIN

One of the most important aspects in the management of eye pain and eye problems in general for the primary-care practitioner to know is when to refer the patient to an ophthalmologist. The risks related to liability and complications, such as permanent damage to a patient's vision, are high. Table 18.1 presents conditions associated with eye pathology that require immediate referral to an ophthalmologist.

TABLE 18.1 Conditions Requiring Immediate Referral to an Ophthalmologist

Patient complains of severe and sudden vision loss or sudden severe nontraumatic eye pain.

Physical examination reveals:

- Corneal ulceration
- Suspected herpes zoster ophthalmicus
- Hazy or opaque cornea
- Irregular pupil shape
- Elevation of fundus on funduscopic examination
- Papilledema
- Limbal flush
- Muscle paresis

Management issues:

- Conditions requiring corticosteroid therapy
- Patient not improving with conservative therapy

The most common cause of eye pain is trauma. However, because of the subjective nature of the pain experience, the presentation of eye pain may reflect a variety of underlying conditions. Thus, it is important to differentiate whether the pain is coming from the eye itself or from one of the surrounding structures.

DIFFERENTIAL DIAGNOSIS

The differential diagnosis of eye pain includes the following conditions:

- Referred pain may occur from trauma, headache, sinusitis, temporomandibular disorder, herpes zoster ophthalmicus, postherpetic neuralgia, tumors, stroke, or trigeminal neuralgia
- Eyelid disorders (e.g., hordeolum, trauma, blepharitis)
- Conjunctivitis, corneal abrasions, ulcerations, foreign body irritation, ultraviolet light overexposure, overuse of contact lenses, or prolonged computer use
- Orbital cellulitis (pain with swelling)
- Scleritis or episcleritis (pain with eye movement)
- Uveitis or glaucoma (deep pain)

RED EYE

Red eye, a common ophthalmic problem encountered in both acute and primary-care settings, is a nonuniform redness of the conjunctiva from hyperemia, which can be diffuse, localized, or peripheral or may encircle a clear cornea. The most common cause is the benign condition known as viral conjunctivitis ("pink eye"). Other causes of red eye include bacterial infection, allergies, chemical irritants, or minor eye irritation from inadequate sleep, overuse of contact lenses, environmental irritants, or excessive

rubbing of the eyes. Some conditions are benign, whereas others may threaten the vision and require the immediate attention of an ophthalmologist.

DIFFERENTIAL DIAGNOSIS

The differential diagnosis of red eye includes the following conditions:

- Conjunctivitis
- Hordeolum (stye)
- Glaucoma (acute angle closure)
- Iritis
- Corneal abrasions
- Dry eye (keratitis sicca)
- Subconjunctival hemorrhage
- Orbital cellulitis, scleritis, or episcleritis

Table 18.2 compares selected characteristics that may be helpful in assessing the differential diagnosis of red eye.

VISUAL DISTURBANCES AND IMPAIRED VISION

Patients often present to the primary-care setting with symptoms related to changes in vision. The list of differential diagnoses of impaired vision is lengthy; however, a number of conditions occur commonly and should be well known to the primary-care provider.

Common visual disturbances include "floaters" and flashing lights. These subjective complaints usually have different causes. The visualization of floaters is usually due to contraction of the vitreous humor. These degenerative vitreous changes are a common sequela of the aging process, called syneresis. Floaters may also result from tear-film debris or other material in the vitreous. Floaters are usually unilateral and are often seen when looking at a bright background. Floaters that appear gradually and become less noticeable over time are usually benign and require no treatment. However, floaters that appear suddenly, especially if bilateral, may warrant further evaluation.

Photopsia (i.e., flashing lights) is the subjective sensation of sparks or flashes of light induced by mechanical or electrical retinal stimulation. Any patient who complains of seeing flashing lights should be evaluated immediately for retinal tear or detachment. Monocular photopsia may occur secondary to cataracts, migraine headaches, epilepsy, vertebral basilar insufficiency, retinitis, retinal hole, detachment of the retina, or retinal microembolization. In addition, a condition seen especially among women aged 55 to 65 years is vitreal detachment, which causes a fluid-filled, optically empty space to form between the vitreous and the retina.

TABLE 18.2   Selected Causes of Red Eye

Assessment	Bacterial Conjunctivitis	Allergic Conjunctivitis	Viral Conjunctivitis	Iritis	Acute Glaucoma
Discharge	Purulent, thick; crusted lids in morning	Stringy mucoid	Watery	Rare	None
Visual acuity	Normal	Normal	Normal	May be decreased if iritis is severe	Decreased
Pain	Sandy, gritty feeling	Itching and burning	Itching	Moderate pain	Severe pain
Conjunctival abnormalities	Moderately heavy, diffuse	Mild, diffuse	Moderate, diffuse	Moderate, around cornea	Anterior chamber may appear narrow with penlight examination
Pupillary abnormalities	None	None	None	Poor light reflex	Mid-dilated; nonreactive or sluggish
Photophobia	No	No	No	Yes	Mild
Bilateral involvement	Sometimes	Usually	Often	No	Sometimes
Intraocular pressure	Normal	Normal	Normal	Normal	Increased
Preauricular lymph nodes	Not palpable	Not palpable	Palpable	Not palpable	Not palpable
Other symptoms	Occurs in fall and winter	Rhinorrhea, sneezing, watery eyes; occurs in the fall and spring	Highly contagious; associated with upper respiratory infection	Associated with connective tissue disease	Nausea, vomiting, and headache

DIFFERENTIAL DIAGNOSIS

The differential diagnosis of impaired vision includes the following conditions:

- Refractive errors
- Cataracts
- Glaucoma
- Diabetic retinopathy
- Macular degeneration
- Retinal detachment
- Vitreous hemorrhage
- Central retinal artery or vein occlusion

The various etiologies of impaired vision are compared in Table 18.3.

TABLE 18.3   Selected Causes of Impaired Vision

Diagnosis	Typical Patient Age	Subjective Assessment	Objective Assessment	Urgent Treatment and Immediate Referral Required?
Myopia	Teenager	Painless progressive loss of vision (PPLV)	No change in fundal examination	No
Presbyopia	Older than 40 years	PPLV; may have blurred vision	No change in fundal examination	No
Cataracts	Older adults	PPLV	Vision decreased; opaque or cloudy lens may be apparent; decreased view of the fundus	No
Macular degeneration	Older adults	PPLV; decreased central vision	Decreased central vision; blood or lipid exudates on fundal examination	Usually not
Diabetic retinopathy	Related to length of time patient has had diabetes and any comorbid conditions	PPLV	Vision will usually not improve with pinhole test; vision varies with stages of retinopathy; dot-blot hemorrhages, micro-aneurysms, lipid exudates, or infarcts in nerve fiber layer may be apparent	Usually not

TABLE 18.3   Selected Causes of Impaired Vision—cont'd

Diagnosis	Typical Patient Age	Subjective Assessment	Objective Assessment	Urgent Treatment and Immediate Referral Required?
Chronic glaucoma	Usually older than 40 years, but may occur in younger patients	PPLV; halos seen around lights	Decreased peripheral field of vision, decreased central vision is a later sign; increased intraocular pressure and increased cup-to-disc ratio with normal chamber angle	Usually not
Acute glaucoma	Usually age 50–85 years	Sudden onset of severe eye pain, vomiting, and headache	Conjunctiva may be infected; steamy cornea; pupil may be fixed and partially dilated with narrow chamber angle	Yes

REFERENCES

General

American Academy of Ophthalmology. Preferred practice patterns guidelines. https://www.aao.org/about-preferred-practice-patterns. Accessed September 2018.

Dry Eye

Al Houssien AO, Al Houssien RO, Al-Hawass A. Magnitude of diabetes and hypertension among patients with dry eye syndrome at a tertiary hospital of Riyadh, Saudi Arabia—a case series. *Saudi J Ophthalmol*. 2017;31(2):91–94.

Javadi M-A, Feizi S. Dry eye syndrome. *J Ophthalmic Vis Res*. 2011;6(3):192–198.

Kim WS, Wee SW, Lee SH, Kim JC. Angiogenin for the diagnosis and grading of dry eye syndrome. *Korean J Ophthalmol*. 2016; 30(3):163–171.

National Eye Institute. Facts about dry eye. https://www.nei.nih.gov/health/dryeye/dryeye. Published 2017. Accessed August 31, 2017.

Schultz C. Safety and efficacy of cyclosporine in the treatment of chronic dry eye. *Ophthalmol Eye Dis*. 2014;6:37–42.

Epiphora

Welch K. Epiphora (excessive tearing). American Rhinologic Society. http://care.american-rhinologic.org/epiphora. Published 2015.

Eye Pain

Collier SA, Gronostaj MP, MacGurn AK, et al. Estimated burden of keratitis--United States, 2010. MMWR Morb Mortal Wkly Rep 2014;63:1027.

Galor A, Levitt RC, Felix ER, et al. Neuropathic ocular pain: An important yet underevaluated feature of dry eye. *Eye (Lond)*. 2015;29(3):301–312.

Lim CH, Turner A, Lim BX. Patching for corneal abrasions. *Cochrane Database Syst Rev*. 2016;7:CD004764.

Roque MR. Scleritis. http://emedicine.medscape.com/article/1228324-overview. Published 2017.

Verma A. Corneal abrasion. http://emedicine.medscape.com/article/1195402. Published 2016.

Wakai A, Lawrenson JG, Lawrenson AL, et al. Topical non-steroidal anti-inflammatory drugs for analgesia in traumatic corneal abrasions. Cochrane Database Syst Rev 2017;5:CD009781.

Waldman N, Winrow B, Densie I, et al. An Observational Study to Determine Whether Routinely Sending Patients Home With a 24-Hour Supply of Topical Tetracaine From the Emergency Department for Simple Corneal Abrasion Pain Is Potentially Safe. Ann Emerg Med 2018; 71:767.

Red Eye

Azari AA, Barney NP. Conjunctivitis: A systematic review of diagnosis and treatment. *JAMA*. 2013;310(16):1721–1729.

Cronau H, Kankanala RR, Mauger T. Diagnosis and management of red eye in primary care. *Am Fam Physician*. 2010;81(2):137–144.

Herretes S, Wang X, Reyes JM. Topical corticosteroids as adjunctive therapy for bacterial keratitis. Cochrane Database Syst Rev 2014; :CD005430.

Sheikh A, Hurwitz B, van Schayck CP, et al. Antibiotics versus placebo for acute bacterial conjunctivitis. *Cochrane Database Syst Rev*. 2012;9:CD001211.

RESOURCES

Aging Eye (National Eye Institute)

https://nei.nih.gov/sites/default/files/health-pdfs/AgingAndEyeHealth_Tagged.pdf

https://nei.nih.gov/sites/default/files/nehep-pdfs/NEHEP_VisionAging_Infographic.pdf

Vision and Aging: See Well for a Lifetime Toolkit (National Eye Institute)

https://nei.nih.gov/nehep/programs/visionandaging/toolkit

Blepharitis

https://nei.nih.gov/health/blepharitis/blepharitis

Dry Eye

https://nei.nih.gov/health/dryeye

Eyelid Disorders

https://www.nei.nih.gov/faqs/eyelid-disorders-chalazion-stye

Red Eye

https://nei.nih.gov/health/pinkeye/pink_facts

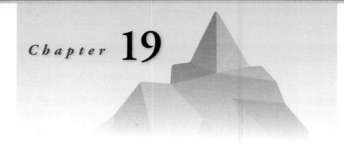

Chapter 19

Lid and Conjunctival Pathology

Humberto Reinoso, PhD, FNP-BC, ENP-BC

Lynne M. Dunphy, PhD, APRN, FNP-BC, FAAN, FAANP

Brian Oscar Porter, MD, PhD, MPH, MBA

BLEPHARITIS

Blepharitis is an inflammation of the eyelids and their margins. There are two forms of blepharitis: (1) a nonulcerative form associated with seborrhea of the face and greasy scaling at the eyelid margins and (2) an ulcerative form that may involve the eyelash follicles and the Meibomian glands of the eyelid. Secondary infections may develop with either form, and recurrences are common and frequently persistent. Both types may coexist.

EPIDEMIOLOGY AND CAUSES

Blepharitis is a common ocular disease, affecting males and females equally. Nonulcerative blepharitis is occasionally seen in those with trisomy 21 and tends to affect people with psoriasis, seborrhea, eczema, allergies, and lice infestations. Poor hygiene is implicated, as well as poor nutritional status, immune suppression, rosacea, and yeast infections. Exposure to chemical or environmental irritants, as well as the use of eye makeup and contact lenses, may contribute to the development of this disorder.

PATHOPHYSIOLOGY

Although difficult to discern without a full ophthalmological examination, the localization of blepharitis assists in identifying which structures are affected. Anterior blepharitis typically affects the eyelash hair follicles along the eyelid's anterior lamella, whereas posterior blepharitis involves inspissation and inflammation of the Meibomian gland orifices (meibomianitis) along the tarsal plate. Seborrheic gland dysfunction, along with accelerated shedding of skin cells, appears to be the primary insult resulting in nonulcerative inflammation, in which an oily crust envelops individual eyelash cilia (seborrheic blepharitis).

The inflammatory, noninfectious skin disorder known as rosacea, which commonly affects the central face, is another common etiology of blepharitis in young adults. Blepharitis may also be a manifestation of an allergic process, such as a contact dermatitis caused by a foreign irritant. In contrast, underlying infection by skin flora, most notably *Staphylococcus aureus,* produces an ulcerative form that may become chronic, extending to the conjunctivae and cornea, known as blepharoconjunctivitis, a condition with a strong potential to affect eyesight.

CLINICAL PRESENTATION

Subjective

Both forms of blepharitis may present with complaints of itching, burning, and foreign body sensation in the eye. Sensitivity to bright light and tearing may also be present. Presentation may be unilateral or bilateral.

Objective

Lid margins are edematous and erythematous. Closer visual inspection with a magnifying glass or Wood's lamp may reveal scaling, erythema, or ulcerations. Nonulcerative blepharitis may present with scales along the lid margins that are easily removed. With ulcerative blepharitis, there may be pustules at the base of the hair follicles that may crust and bleed. The lashes become thin and break easily. The eyelids and the lid margins should be palpated for masses and preauricular lymphadenopathy.

DIAGNOSTIC REASONING

Diagnostic Tests

With any eye problem, it is vital to evaluate visual acuity in both the affected eye and the unaffected eye. Additionally, visual acuity of both eyes with and without corrective lenses should be documented. Any alteration in visual acuity may indicate a potentially serious underlying problem that warrants further investigation. If discharge is present, culture and sensitivity testing should be considered. Immediate referral for patients with blepharitis should occur in the following situations: visual loss, moderate to severe eye pain, and corneal involvement. Chronic redness of the eye, recurrent blepharitis, and/or a failure to respond to treatment also warrants an ophthalmology referral. Persistent inflammation and thickening of the eyelid margin may indicate squamous cell, basal cell, or sebaceous cell carcinoma. Sebaceous cell carcinoma has a 23% mortality rate; up to one-half of potentially fatal sebaceous cell carcinomas resemble chronic, benign inflammatory disease, particularly chalazion and blepharoconjunctivitis. Patients with chronic inflammation or thickening of the eyelid should be referred to a specialist for possible biopsy.

Differential Diagnosis

Persistent inflammation and thickening of the eyelid margin may indicate squamous cell, basal cell, or sebaceous cell carcinoma masquerading as blepharitis. Carcinoma may also mimic a stye or chalazion. Other differentials diagnoses include hordeolum, conjunctivitis, retained foreign body, herpes zoster, orbital cellulitis, and dacryocystitis (infection or inflammation of the nasolacrimal sac).

MANAGEMENT

Box 19.1 describes the management of various forms of blepharitis. Any swelling or inflammation of the eyelid that does not resolve promptly (within 1 month) with treatment should be evaluated further.

FOLLOW-UP AND REFERRAL

The clinician should reevaluate the patient in 2 weeks; if symptoms are improving, the patient should then be reevaluated in 2 months. In contrast, if there is no resolution in 1 month, the patient should be referred to an ophthalmologist. Vision changes and pain in the eye also warrant referral. Blepharitis may be difficult to treat, and recurrences are common. Hordeolum, loss of eyelashes, misdirection of the eyelashes (trichiasis), scarring, and corneal infection may occur.

Patient Education: Blepharitis

Patients should be encouraged to wash their hands often and dry them with clean towels to prevent reinfection or the transfer of bacteria or viruses to other persons. In addition, patients should be advised to avoid environmental irritants, to use hypoallergenic soap and makeup, and to exercise care in the use of contact lenses. The clinician should educate the

Box 19.1	Treatment for Blepharitis	
Type	**Treatment Goal**	**Treatment Description**
Nonulcerative blepharitis	This type of blepharitis may be persistent, and treatment is aimed at improving hygiene.	Eyelid cleaning with a diluted 1:1 mixture of no-tears shampoo (baby shampoo) and water, using a soft washcloth or cotton balls. Warm, moist compresses provide comfort, open meibomian glands, and facilitate drainage. The patient should apply compresses for 10–15 minutes, then rest for at least 1 hour. Patients should be advised that eyelid hygiene may be required for life, and symptoms may recur if treatment is discontinued. Advise the patient to discontinue the use of eye makeup and contact lenses until the condition is completely resolved. Once resolved, only new hypoallergenic makeup products and new contact lenses should be used to avoid reinfection.
Staphylococcal blepharitis/ ulcerated lesions	Infectious blepharitis should be treated with topical antibiotic ointments that adhere to the eyelid margins more effectively than eye drops.	Bacitracin or erythromycin 0.5% ointment can be prescribed and applied on the eyelids one or more times daily or at bedtime after gentle cleansing and using warm compresses. Treatment may continue for 7–10 days. The frequency and duration of treatment should be guided by the severity of the blepharitis.
		For resistant staphylococcal infections, a quinolone antibacterial ointment is appropriate or a sulfacetamide/corticosteroid combination that, like erythromycin, has been shown to be effective against *Staphylococcus*. The corticosteroid component is useful in decreasing both inflammation and eye symptoms. Use of the two agents combined has been shown to increase patient compliance. Blephamide is available in an ophthalmic suspension and in an ointment, both containing the same concentrations of active ingredients (10% sulfacetamide/0.2% prednisolone).
Severe blepharitis	Associated with rosacea; treatment is aimed at curing the infectious process with systemic antibiotic therapy.	Oral doxycycline 100 mg by mouth twice daily or tetracycline 250 mg by mouth four times daily is appropriate. These are prescribed for several weeks and then tapered. Continue hygienic measures as described above.

patient about the chronic and recurrent nature of this disorder and the need for strict adherence to the treatment plan until the blepharitis is completely resolved. Long-term eyelid hygiene—gently cleansing with diluted baby shampoo daily—is required to control this disorder. Eye makeup should not be used until resolution of the disorder, and then the patient should switch to hypoallergenic makeup. A blepharitis fact sheet is available at the American Ophthalmological Society (see Resources).

HORDEOLUM AND CHALAZION

A *hordeolum,* also known as a *stye,* is an acute, erythematous, tender lump within the eyelid. This condition is caused by inflammation or infection of the eyelid margin affecting the hair follicles of the eyelashes (external hordeolum) or the Meibomian glands (internal hordeolum), which may evolve into a *chalazion.* A chalazion is a granulomatous infection of a Meibomian gland that presents as a a painless swelling on the eyelid. Initially, a chalazion may be tender and erythematous before evolving into a nontender lump. Blepharitis is frequently associated with a chalazion. The primary difference between a chalazion and hordeolum is that chalazia are a result of inflammation and hordeola or styes are infectious.

EPIDEMIOLOGY AND CAUSES

Both disorders are common and affect men and women equally. The cause is often a blockage in a duct of the Meibomian gland leading to the eyelid surface; secondary infection may be present, again, commonly with *Staphylococcus.* This ductal obstruction results in inflammation that may manifest as infection of the sebaceous glands of the eyelash (external hordeolum), infection of posterior margin of the eyelid (internal hordeolum), or progression to a hard, granulomatous mass (chalazion). Previously unresolved blepharitis, poor hygiene, immunosuppression, and underlying chronic diseases all contribute to the development of these eyelid disorders. Skin conditions, such as rosacea or seborrheic dermatitis, may also predispose the patient to development of a hordeolum.

PATHOPHYSIOLOGY

Hordeolum and chalazion are various manifestations of an inflammatory response in the eyelids, exhibiting both microscopic (accumulation of fluid and cells at the inflammatory site) and macroscopic (redness, swelling, heat, pain, and loss of function) hallmark signs of inflammation. An internal hordeolum is a suppurative infection of the oil-secreting Meibomian glands within the tarsal plate of the eyelid that may evolve into a chalazion. An external hordeolum occurs with infection of the more superficial anteriorly located glands of Zeis or Moll

found at the eyelid margin. With a stye (hordeolum), the eyelid may show a classic inflammatory reaction; however, a chalazion results from an obstruction of the Meibomian gland with a granulomatous response and is typically painless. The blockage of the gland's duct at the eyelid margin results in the release of the gland's contents into the surrounding soft tissue, and a lipogranulomatous reaction ensues, producing a pea-sized nodule within the eyelid. Occasionally, a chalazion may also become secondarily infected with *S. aureus.*

CLINICAL PRESENTATION

Subjective

A hordeolum presents as a localized tender inflammation of the eyelid (external) or redness at the margin of the eyelid with swelling (internal). Patients may experience itching or scaling of the eyelid, chronic redness, and eye irritation, leading to localized tenderness and pain. A chalazion commonly presents as a slow-developing, painless, hard mass, with inflammation and possible involvement of the surrounding tissue.

Objective

As with all eye complaints, the clinician should evaluate visual acuity. With a chalazion, inversion of the eyelid will reveal a red, elevated mass that may become quite large and press against the eye, causing nystagmus and distortion of vision. With a hordeolum, there is erythema and localized tenderness with palpation; there may also be drainage from the lesion on the margin of the lid. The clinician should also palpate for preauricular adenopathy.

DIAGNOSTIC REASONING

Diagnostic Tests

Hordeolum and chalazion are usually diagnosed by their appearance. If drainage is present, it should be cultured. If the conditions persist, referral for biopsy may be indicated.

Differential Diagnosis

As noted previously, patients with inflammation or swelling that does not resolve with conservative therapy should be referred to an ophthalmologist. Basal cell or sebaceous cell carcinoma may mimic other disorders of the eyelid, so differentiating these disorders is key. Sebaceous cell carcinoma, according to some reports, has a 23% mortality rate, and up to one-half of these potentially fatal carcinomas may initially resemble benign inflammatory disorders.

MANAGEMENT

Box 19.2 describes the various treatment options for hordeolum and chalazion.

Box 19.2	Treatment for Hordeolum/Chalazion
Initial treatment of hordeolum	At the first sign of inflammation and pain, warm compresses should be applied increase blood supply and potentiate spontaneous drainage. Gently scrub the eyelids with a 1:1 dilution of baby shampoo and warm water two to four times a day, or directly apply diluted baby shampoo with a cotton-tipped applicator and then rinse with warm water. Follow with gentle massage of the eyelid. The hordeolum (stye) should not be squeezed. Blepharitis, if present, should be treated. Eye makeup should be discontinued until the infection resolves. Contact lenses should not be used during treatment. Once the condition is resolved, a new pair of contact lenses and new hypoallergenic eye makeup may be resumed.
Infection or inflammation	Erythromycin ophthalmic ointment or sulfacetamide (Sulamyd) ophthalmic ointment can be applied four times a day or ciprofloxacin ointment (Ciloxan, Cipro) can be applied three times a day. Use a thin application to the eyelid margin with a cotton-tipped applicator.
Resistant or recurrent hordeolum *Basal cell carcinoma or sebaceous cell carcinoma of the eyelid can be misdiagnosed clinically and should be included in the differential diagnosis for recurrent hordeolum or chalazion.*	A course of oral antibiotics that is effective against *Staphylococcus* and *Streptococcus*, such as cephalexin (Keflex, Keftabs), can be prescribed.
Chalazion (unresolved) *A chalazion that persists for more than 4 weeks needs referral to an ophthalmologist for incision and drainage, biopsy, or local injection directly with glucocorticoids.*	Warm compresses and gentle massage of the swelling in the eyelid with a 1:1 dilution of baby shampoo and warm water may help to open the blocked Meibomian duct.

FOLLOW-UP AND REFERRAL

Patients with vision changes or pain should be referred to an ophthalmologist. Recurrence of hordeolum or chalazion is likely without proper eyelid hygiene. If there is no improvement with conservative therapy, the clinician should refer the patient to an ophthalmologist for further evaluation.

Patient Education: Hordeolum and chalazion

The patient should understand the recurrent nature of the disorder and the need for vigilance. Treatment should be initiated at the first sign of recurrence. Infections with *S. aureus* are contagious; therefore, patients and family members should not share towels, washcloths, or eyewear such as sunglasses. The patient should use a clean cloth each time a compress is applied to the eye and should wash his or her hands frequently.

DRY EYE

Lacrimal disorders may be acquired or congenital. Acquired disorders may be systemic, such as Sjögren's syndrome; may reflect a more local infectious process, as in some forms of conjunctivitis; or may be related to trauma or facial nerve (cranial nerve VII) palsy. It has been shown that patients with chronic dry eye demonstrate increased activation of T cells. These T cells produce cytokines that may result in a neural signal to the lacrimal gland that disrupts the production of natural tears. This process leads to a decrease in the patient's own tears, which in turn may cause tissue damage in the lacrimal glands and on the ocular surface, recruitment of additional T cells, and increased cytokine production.

Certain medications, such as anticholinergic agents, beta-adrenergic blockers, and antihistamines with anticholinergic side effects, decrease tear production because the lacrimal gland is stimulated by the parasympathetic nervous system. Mucin deficiency may also be caused by certain medications, vitamin A deficiency, chronic conjunctivitis, or as a result of the aging process. Tear production decreases with aging, especially in women during menopause. In addition, patients who use a computer or microscope may have a diminished blink rate, which can cause evaporative loss of natural tears

EPIDEMIOLOGY AND CAUSES

Dry eye is a common disorder affecting approximately 10% to 30% of the population, especially those older than 40 years. In the United States, an estimated 3.23 million women and 1.68 million men aged 50 years and older are affected. The frequency of this condition globally closely parallels that of the United States. However, the frequency and clinical diagnosis of dry eye are greater in the Hispanic and Asian populations.

Keratoconjunctivitis sicca (KCS) associated with Sjögren's syndrome is a type of dry eye that affects 1% to 2% of the population; 90% of those affected are women. Approximately 1% of the U.S. population is affected with Sjögren's syndrome, and it occurs in 15% of patients with rheumatoid arthritis.

PATHOPHYSIOLOGY

A genetic predisposition to Sjögren's syndrome–associated KCS is evidenced by a high prevalence of human leukocyte antigen (HLA)-B8 in these patients. A high level of HLA-B8 is associated with a chronic inflammatory state, in which autoantibodies (e.g., antinuclear antibodies, rheumatoid factor) are produced. In addition, this condition is associated with inflammatory cytokine release and focal lymphocytic infiltration (CD4 T cells and B cells) of the lacrimal and salivary glands, with eventual degeneration and apoptosis of the lacrimal glands and conjunctiva. The result is dysfunction of the lacrimal gland, decreased tear production, loss of response to neural stimulation, and less reflex tearing. Cytokine release inhibits neural function and may also convert androgens into estrogens, resulting in Meibomian gland dysfunction. Both androgen and estrogen receptors are located in the lacrimal and Meibomian glands. At menopause, there is a decrease in circulating sex hormones, possibly affecting the secretory function of the lacrimal gland. Deficiency of mucin-synthesizing genes may be a factor in dry eye syndrome as well. Vitamin A deficiency, Stevens-Johnson syndrome, and ocular cicatricial pemphigoid may contribute to the loss of goblet cells and promote dry eye syndrome.

CLINICAL PRESENTATION

Dry eye commonly affects both eyes and is often described as "a feeling of sand in the eyes," especially when blinking. The eyes feel hot, irritated, and gritty and may become reddened. The patient may present with complaints of blurred vision, lack of tears, burning, itching, foreign body sensation, sensitivity to light, and loss of glossy appearance of the cornea. The triad presentation of burning, itching, and a foreign body sensation in the eye is characteristic of KCS. This symptom is frequently associated with the diagnosis of Sjögren's syndrome, a systemic disorder affecting the function of all secretory glands that is associated with rheumatoid arthritis.

Untreated or severe KCS may result in inflammation, erosion, and eventually keratinization of the cornea and/or conjunctiva, which may ultimately may lead to blindness. A correlation does not always exist, however, between the failure of tear production, leading to dry eye, and inflammatory or degenerative changes to the surface of the eye. Accessory glands in the palpebral conjunctiva may secrete sufficient tears to prevent corneal damage.

Subjective

A careful history (see Focus on History: Eye Complaints) includes inquiries about current medication usage, especially the overuse of artificial tears, in which the ocular surface develops toxicity to active ingredients or preservatives in lubricant formulations. Symptoms of vision-threatening conditions, such as cataracts, macular degeneration, and glaucoma, must be considered. Past medical history or family history about coexisting connective tissue disorders, rheumatoid arthritis, Parkinson's disease, rosacea, and thyroid abnormalities are pertinent positives that will help the clinician to formulate a diagnosis. Dry mouth (xerostomia), muscle or joint pains, and heat or cold intolerance are significant findings because they are often associated with comorbid inflammatory disorders.

Focus on History: Eye Complaints

The following questions should be asked when evaluating a patient presenting with eye complaints:

- When did the symptoms start? Was onset sudden or gradual?
- Do you have changes in vision? If yes, were the changes sudden or gradual?
- Do you have any pain?
- Are you experiencing photophobia or seeing floaters?
- Did you sustain an injury to your eyes? If so, please describe.
- Do you have any discharge? If yes, please describe its characteristics.
- Do you wear contact lenses? If yes, describe the type, wearing schedule, and care.
- What current medications are you taking?
- Do you have a history of eye problems?
- Have you had any new or past exposures to cosmetics, contact with person with an eye infection, smoking, or pollution? Have you traveled recently? What is your occupation? What type of environment do you live and work in?
- Do you have any systemic complaints (fever, genital discharge, rash, joint pains, etc.)?
- Do you have a family history of eye problems?

Objective

The physical examination of the eyes must always include visual acuity, which may be normal. The examination may reveal a mechanical, infectious, and/or traumatic cause for the complaint of dry eyes. If one of these conditions is revealed, once it is treated, the dry eye complaint should resolve. The conjunctiva may be infected and dull, and the eyelids and surrounding tissues may be erythematous due to frequent rubbing. The lacrimal apparatus will be nontender, and in the case of KCS or Sjögren's syndrome, the mucous membranes of the mouth will also be dry. Examination of the eyes by a trained professional with fluorescein staining and a slit lamp may reveal punctuate lesions of the conjunctiva or a secondary abrasion.

DIAGNOSTIC REASONING

The complaint of dry eye is frequently a subjective finding with few or no cues in the physical examination; therefore, a clinical diagnosis will require referral to a specialist for examination and testing. Occasionally, the patient will complain of excessive tearing (epiphora) or inappropriate tearing, which may be reflexive due to poor neural control of the lacrimal apparatus from dry eyes.

Diagnostic Tests

In addition to a slit-lamp examination, a Schirmer test to quantify lacrimal secretions may be done. Laboratory tests to rule out an autoimmune disease that include an erythrocyte sedimentation rate, antinuclear antibodies, and rheumatoid factor may be indicated. If discharge is associated with the complaint, a culture with sensitivity testing may be helpful.

Differential Diagnosis

Differential diagnosis includes conjunctivitis, blepharitis, contact lens complications, exophthalmos, ectropion, Bell's palsy, medicamentosa, Sjögren's syndrome, age-related and hormonal changes, corneal abrasion, and systemic vitamin A deficiency.

MANAGEMENT

Elimination of systemic medications that may have contributed to the condition should be considered. Reports in the literature have associated the relief of dry eye symptoms with the initiation of hormone therapy in postmenopausal women. Most cases of dry eye are best managed symptomatically. However, when the complaint of dry eye is persistent and unrelieved by self-care measures, referral is necessary. Also, it is not unusual for patients to need adjustment of their contact lens prescription or a review of their self-care regimen.

The principles of treatment for dry eye are based on the severity of the condition (International Dry Eye Workshop, 2007). The first level of treatment provides education and includes environmental and dietary modifications, such as elimination of offending systemic medications, the introduction of artificial tear substitutes, lubricants, gels, and ointments, and possibly eyelid therapy. Wearing wraparound sunglasses to keep wind from drying the eye surface, using a humidifier in the home, and avoiding rubbing the eyes may all help reduce the symptoms of dry eye. Specific topical treatments include the application of ocular lubricants such as an ophthalmic ointment of petrolatum, lanolin, and mineral oil (Duratears Naturale) as needed, which is especially helpful for use with soft contact lenses, or one or two drops of 1% polyvinyl alcohol preservative-free ophthalmic solution (HypoTears) as needed. Sodium chloride 2% or 5% hypertonic ophthalmic solution (MURO 128) may be used (one to two drops) every 3 to 4 hours, reducing frequency as inflammation subsides.

A second level of care is instituted if the first level is not effective. This includes the use of specific pharmacologic measures, including not only ocular lubricants and nonpreserved artificial tear substitutes, but also anti-inflammatory and immunomodulatory agents such as topical corticosteroids, topical or systemic omega-3 fatty acids, or topical cyclosporine A. Topical cyclosporine ophthalmic emulsion (Restasis) is used to treat chronic dry eye. It contains a very small concentration of cyclosporine, which is believed to inhibit the activation of T cells. T cells disrupt normal tear production in the lacrimal glands, and improving lacrimal gland function through T-cell inhibition is believed to result in increased tear production and relief of inflammation and further damage. Temporary punctal plugs may be warranted after inflammation has resolved. Punctal plugs are painlessly inserted and act as a dam that prevents tears from draining into the puncta and nasolacrimal duct. Several studies have demonstrated subjective and objective improvement with punctual plugs in the treatment of dry eye syndrome.

The third level of treatment is instituted when the previous levels have failed to adequately control symptoms. The therapies at this level consist of use of autologous serum, special contact lenses, and permanent punctual occlusion, as well as systemic anti-inflammatory agents and possibly surgical intervention to correct abnormalities of the lid. Other surgical procedures may include grafting of mucous membranes or possible transplantation of a salivary gland duct. See "Dry Eye" in Chapter 18 for new directions in research and treatment for this disorder.

FOLLOW-UP AND REFERRAL

Supportive measures such as listening to the patient's fears associated with vision changes or the possible systemic causes of dry eye are both therapeutic and compassionate. A patient with chronic complaints of dry eye or conjunctivitis may need to be referred to an ophthalmologist. Arranging for prompt referral for accurate diagnosis and specialized treatments promotes a patient's confidence in the primary-care practitioner.

Patient Education: Dry Eye

In general, the prognosis for visual acuity in patients with dry eye syndrome is good. However, complications of decreased visual acuity and blindness can occur, and patients need to seek medical advice should visual changes occur or if the current regimen has lost effectiveness or symptoms worsen. Box 19.3 summarizes several environmental modifications that patients can make to minimize the symptoms and recurrence of dry eye.

Box 19.3   Ocular Self-Care for Dry Eye

Keep home humidity between 30% and 50%.

Cleanse humidifier frequently with dilute 1:10 bleach/water solution. Rinse well with fresh water.

Wear wraparound sunglasses, especially on windy days.

Wear goggles when swimming.

Use a preservative-free artificial tears preparation or bathe eyes in an herbal therapy solution made with Eyebright (*Euphrasia officinalis*) when irritated.

Avoid blowing hot air from hair dryer in the eyes.

Take frequent rest periods away from computers, handheld electronic devices (e.g., smart phones), or microscopes.

Stop smoking to eliminate direct exposure to ocular irritants in tobacco smoke.

Omega-3 fatty acid deficiency, especially reduced levels of docosahexaenoic acid (DHA) and eicosatetraenoic acid (EPA), have been linked to dry eye syndrome. Dietary intake of these compounds is generally lower than the recommended daily intake; therefore, it is important to encourage patients to increase their dietary intake of DHA- and EPA-rich foods (e.g., salmon, tuna, mackerel, anchovy, halibut, and scallops). Regular use of lubricating drops or ointments and consistent use of prescribed ocular medications should be stressed.

EXCESSIVE TEARING (EPIPHORA)

Excessive tearing is often a case of paradoxical tearing as a response to dry eye. It is an especially common complaint in elderly patients and individuals with allergies. A healthy eye is a wet eye; however, a continuously wet eye with uncontrolled tearing signals a malfunction due to a variety of possible causes. Frequently, excess tearing will lead to increased irritation and even more tearing, so it is necessary to break this cycle to treat the symptom effectively.

EPIDEMIOLOGY AND CAUSES

Epiphora is a common problem and will become more widespread as the population ages. Because epiphora is frequently associated with "dry eye" as a paradoxical and compensatory response, the epidemiologic statistics are similar, with elderly and allergic patients being particularly predisposed.

Anatomical abnormalities, such as ectropion, entropion, lower lid laxity, and lacrimal pump weakness due to Bell's palsy, may lead to structural and functional problems in the distribution and drainage of tears. Lacrimal obstruction that limits normal drainage into the lacrimal ducts is a significant contributor to the problem. Obstruction can be associated with thickened discharge secondary to infection, tumor, trauma, or autoimmune diagnoses. The eye may water excessively secondary to irritation from contact lenses, medications, or environment irritants as a protective mechanism. Excessive tearing may also be related to allergy, infection, trauma, or pain. The patient may complain of "excess tears" when in reality the tears are a discharge secondary to some form of red eye. Sensitivity to preservatives in certain eyedrops and contact lens solutions can also cause this relatively common problem.

PATHOPHYSIOLOGY

Tears are made up of several layered components, with each layer playing a role in the maintenance of stable tear film. The outer layer is composed of lipids, which form the superficial layer of the tear film. The intermediate layer is an aqueous layer derived from the main lacrimal gland. The inner layer is a mucin layer derived from goblet cells. During blinking, a suction effect draws the tear film into the lacrimal apparatus. In the case of facial nerve palsy, the loss of the blink reflex allows tearing to occur without any physiologic tear pumping and drainage. This is also an issue with prolonged computer use accompanied by a decreased blink reflex; the eyes become dry and may reflexively tear excessively. A malfunction of the lacrimal apparatus or neural control of the lacrimal apparatus may also cause eyes to water inappropriately.

CLINICAL PRESENTATION

Subjective

A complete history, which should include any trauma and infections that could threaten vision, should be elicited. If the patient complains that clear tears run down the cheek, it may signal that there is an obstruction of the lacrimal system. If the complaint is of "watery eyes," with tears collecting or welling up in the lower eyelid pouch, the problem may be associated with poor tear quality or poor tear distribution. Blurred vision, diplopia, photophobia, or eye pain may indicate a serious condition. Allergic causes for excessive tearing are common, and frequently the source of the allergen is identified during the history. Past medical history of seasonal allergies, asthma, or other atopic diseases, as well as a family history of atopic conditions, helps in making an accurate diagnosis. The review of systems should address systemic symptoms such as fever, headache, upper respiratory complaints, sore or scratchy throat, cough or wheeze, dizziness, malaise, and skin changes.

Objective

The physical examination includes as assessment of visual acuity and careful examination of the structures in the eye and the surrounding tissues, evaluating for edema, redness, discharge, rashes, and any structural abnormalities. Careful examination for foreign bodies or corneal irritants is essential. Many primary-care clinics have access to a Wood's lamp and fluorescein staining, while specialists will use the slit lens of an ophthalmoscope to demonstrate damage in the anterior structures of the eye. In addition, signs of allergies such as pale, boggy mucous membranes in the nose, dry skin, or eczematous changes may be present.

DIAGNOSTIC REASONING

Diagnostic Tests

Diagnostic testing is rarely done in the primary-care setting, with the exception of a Wood's lamp examination. Ophthalmologists use a variety of other tests to determine tear quality, quantity, and flow. The dye disappearance test is one such test. A drop of fluorescein dye is placed in both eyes in the inferior fornix, and the tear meniscus height is measured after 5 to 10 minutes. This is an easy test for assessing the presence of an excretory problem with excessive tearing. Other dye tests evaluate whether fluid drains properly into the inferior meatus and lacrimal sac. Lacrimal irrigation and probing can demonstrate a punctal or canalicular problem. Occasionally, computed tomography scanning of the lacrimal drainage system can be done.

Differential Diagnosis

Presentation of acute unilateral epiphora with red eye and pain suggests foreign body or corneal abrasion. Irritating bilateral epiphora may be due to allergies, dry eye syndrome, environmental pollutants, glaucoma, or viral conjunctivitis. Blocked lacrimal duct and bacterial conjunctivitis are usually unilateral. Ectropion may be unilateral or bilateral, whereas the development of lid laxity associated with aging is usually bilateral.

MANAGEMENT

Treatment of excessive tearing secondary to trauma or infection includes the use of topical antibiotics. Corticosteroid eye drops and anesthetic drops should not be used because they may block healing and increase the risk of infection. If a foreign body is visualized on physical examination, it should be removed by saline irrigation using a Morgan Lens or by direct removal with a moist cotton swab. Eye rest is important, but patching may be too uncomfortable and is not recommended.

Treatment of allergic causes of excessive tearing (i.e., allergic conjunctivitis) consists of cold compresses for comfort and relief of itch, topical antihistamines, topical NSAIDs, mast cell stabilizers, and systemic antihistamines. Occasionally, consultation with an allergy specialist is necessary for allergy testing to identify trigger agents to avoid.

See Drugs Commonly Prescribed 19.1 for approved medications to treat allergic and infectious forms of conjunctivitis that typically lead to excessive tearing and watery eyes. In patients who wear contact lenses and develop excessive tearing due to a corneal abrasion with signs of bacterial conjunctivitis, an anti-*Pseudomonas* antibiotic (e.g., ciprofloxacin [Ciloxan], gentamycin, ofloxacin [Ocuflox]) should be used and the contact lens use discontinued. Clinical trial data are lacking, but it is recommended that contact lenses be avoided until the abrasion is healed and the antibiotic course is completed.

FOLLOW-UP AND REFERRAL

Any foreign body that cannot be promptly removed in the primary-care setting should be referred to an ophthalmologist or an emergency department within 24 hours, given the risk of corneal abrasion and infection. Corneal abrasions that cause acute excessive tearing should also be reevaluated in 24 hours. If corneal erosion is suspected or there has been no relief in the excess tear production and the pain level is unchanged or worsened, the patient needs to be referred immediately for evaluation by an ophthalmologist. It is important to communicate this information to the patient because timely referral to a specialist is essential to avoid vision loss.

The patient with chronic epiphora should have an ophthalmologic consultation to evaluate and consider treatment with possible surgical correction. Individuals with conjunctivitis should be reevaluated after a course of antibiotic therapy or after 2 weeks of instituting pharmacologic measures for allergic problems. As noted, referral to an allergist may be appropriate.

Patient Education: Epiphora

Patients need to be attentive to changes in eye pain, tearing, or discharge and should understand general expectations as to how quickly symptoms should resolve. In addition, they should be alert as to when to seek medical intervention. Vision loss is a very concerning issue, and problems of red eye with visual changes must be addressed promptly. Hygienic measures, such as washing hands, using separate washcloths, and disposing appropriately of dressings, should be stressed. Washing hands before applying eye drops or topical ointments is essential to prevent infection or cross-contamination of a bacterial infection. Patients need to know that there are surgical options to manage changes in eyelid structure that occur with aging and lead to epiphora. If the excessive tearing is paradoxically associated with "dry eye," consistent use of topical cyclosporine emulsion will eventually bring both symptoms under control, although it may take several weeks for the full effect to be realized.

Drugs Commonly Prescribed 19.1: Conjunctivitis

TYPE OF CONJUNCTIVITIS	DRUG CATEGORY	DRUGS
Allergic Conjunctivitis		
	Mast Cell Stabilizers Block a calcium channel essential for mast cell degranulation, stabilizing the cell and thereby preventing the release of histamine and related mediators.	Iodoxamide 0.1% (Alomide) Nedocromil 2% (Alocril) Pemirolast 0.1% (Alamast)
	Antihistamines Combat the histamine released during an allergic reaction by blocking the action of the histamine on the tissue.	Emedastine 0.05% (Emadine) Levocabastine 0.05% (Livostin)
	Combination Mast-Cell Stabilizers and Antihistamines	Olopatadine 0.1% (Patanol) Azelastine 0.05% (Optivar) Ketotifen fumarate 0.025% (Zaditor) Epinastine 0.05% (Elestat)
	Nonsteroidal Anti-Inflammatory Agents The mechanism of their action is thought to be due to the ability to inhibit prostaglandin biosynthesis, thereby having an analgesic and anti-inflammatory action.	Ketorolac 0.5% (Acular)
Bacterial Conjunctivitis		
Usual organisms: *Streptococcus pneumoniae, Haemophilus influenzae,* Group A *Streptococcus, Staphylococcus aureus,* pseudomonads	**Antibiotics** First-line therapy: Treat empirically with broad-spectrum topical agents. High levels of the agent are delivered directly to the site of infection. The level of concentration exceeds what is normally achieved in body tissues by oral or parenteral routes. Most agents available as ointments or solutions.	Sodium sulfacetamide (Bleph 10, Cetamide, AK-sulf) Erythromycin ointment (E-Mycin) Azithromycin ophthalmic (AzaSite) Bacitracin (AK-Tracin, Baciguent) Ciprofloxacin (Ciloxan) Trimethoprim and polymixin B (Polytrim) Tobramycin (Tobrex) Neomycin (Mycifradin) Ofloxacin (Ocuflox) Levofloxacin (Quixin) Besifloxacin (Besivance) Gentamicin (Genoptic, Ocumycin)
Chlamydial Conjunctivitis		
	Antibiotics *Systemic antibiotics in addition to topical agents are necessary.* Sexual partners should be evaluated for infection and treated simultaneously.	Azithromycin 1 g as a single dose or doxycycline 100 mg twice daily for 7 days
Viral Conjunctivitis		
	Antibiotics Usually not recommended unless there is a secondary bacterial infection. **Lubrication for comfort**	Ocular lubricants: artificial tears (Refresh, Celluvisc, Murine) one to two drops four to eight times a day
	Antiviral Agents Herpes simplex conjunctivitis requires systemic or topical antiviral agents. *Any patient with HSV or herpes zoster ophthalmicus (varicella zoster virus) eye disease needs to be seen by an ophthalmologist.*	Pyrimidine (thymidine) ophthalmic sol. *(may have toxic reaction)* Oral antivirals: acyclovir (Zovirax) PO. *Start therapy within 72 hours to prevent postherpetic neuralgia*

RED EYE/CONJUNCTIVITIS

Conjunctivitis is an inflammation of the conjunctiva (mucous membrane) covering the front of the eye. The conjunctiva protects the eye against foreign materials and microorganisms. "Pink eye" refers to non-*Neisseria* bacterial conjunctivitis. Although most conjunctivitis is self-limiting, a few types may lead to permanent vision impairment if not promptly diagnosed and treated. It is essential for the clinician to be able to distinguish different types of conjunctivitis (see Chapter 18).

EPIDEMIOLOGY AND CAUSES

Conjunctivitis is the most common of all eye disorders, affecting all ages. Males and females are equally affected; there are no specific ethnic predispositions. Risk factors are numerous, including trauma from wind, heat, smoke, cold, chemicals, or foreign bodies. Common causes of conjunctivitis include infectious agents (which may be bacterial, viral, or fungal), as well as toxicity (from an inciting agent) and allergy. Sexual transmission and ophthalmia neonatorum (vertical transmission from mother to child of eye infection during passage through the birth canal) are associated with *Chlamydia, Neisseria gonorrhoeae,* and herpes simplex virus (HSV) type 1.

Trachoma, the leading cause of blindness in developing nations, is caused by *Chlamydia trachomatis*; it is spread by direct contact with eye, nose, and throat secretions from affected individuals or via contact with fomites (infectious inanimate objects), such as towels or washcloths, that have had contact with such secretions. Flies can also be a route of mechanical transmission. Untreated, repeated trachoma infections result in entropion—a painful cause of permanent blindness in which the eyelids turn inward, causing the eyelashes to repeatedly scratch the cornea. Children are the most susceptible to infection because they are more likely to come into contact with contaminated inanimate objects and less likely to practice hand washing. However, the blinding effect and more severe symptoms are often not realized until adulthood.

Most forms of conjunctivitis, depending on the causative organism, may be transmitted by contaminated towels, washcloths, or the patient's own hands (autoinoculation). Noninfectious conjunctivitis may be drug-induced as a result of chronic irritation from the use of eye medications over a long period of time. Chronic inflammatory conjunctivitis may similarly develop secondary to irritation from contact lens use, seen most commonly with soft lenses but also occasionally with hard lenses. A family history of atopy is a risk factor for allergic conjunctivitis.

PATHOPHYSIOLOGY

A hallmark of conjunctival inflammation is hyperemia of the ocular and palpebral surfaces with engorged, superficial capillaries. This vascular injection gives the eye the typical angry, red appearance of conjunctivitis. Contact with viruses, bacteria, or allergens is the most common cause of inflammation of the conjunctiva. There is also an idiopathic form of conjunctivitis associated with certain systemic diseases, such as thyroid disorders and reactive arthritis (formerly known as Reiter's syndrome).

The most common causes of bacterial conjunctivitis include *S. aureus, Streptococcus pneumoniae,* and *Haemophilus influenzae. N. gonorrhoeae, Moraxella catarrhalis,* and *Chlamydia* which are responsible for a particularly virulent hyperacute bacterial conjunctivitis. Viral agents frequently implicated in viral conjunctivitis include adenovirus serotypes 3, 4, and 7 (which cause pharyngitis with conjunctivitis); adenovirus serotypes 8 and 19 (which cause epidemic keratoconjunctivitis); adenovirus 11; coxsackievirus A24; enterovirus 70 (which causes acute hemorrhagic conjunctivitis); primary or recurrent HSV (usually type 1); and herpes zoster (which spreads down the optic nerve) as well as the poxvirus *Molluscum contagiosum. Chlamydia trachomatis* infection (trachoma) causes adult inclusion conjunctivitis, as well as ophthalmia neonatorum. *Chlamydia oculogenitalis* (which causes inclusion conjunctivitis) and *Chlamydia lymphogranuloma* (which causes lymphogranuloma venereum) are also sexually transmitted causative agents. *Chlamydia trachomatis* (which causes both STIs and non-sexually transmitted infections, including adult inclusion conjunctivitis, ophthalmia neonatorum, Chlamydia oculogenitalis, and trachoma) and *Chlamydia lymphogranuloma* (which causes lymphogranuloma venereum) are also sexually transmitted causative agents.

Allergic (atopic) conjunctivitis may be linked to a systemic humoral or local histaminic response to an inciting environmental allergen. Forms of allergic conjunctivitis include (1) seasonal (hay fever conjunctivitis), which is usually caused by grass pollens in May and June and by ragweed pollen in August and September; (2) vernal keratoconjunctivitis, which usually occurs in childhood through young adulthood in individuals with a personal or family history of atopy, is recurrent in warm weather, and is associated with epithelial hyperplasia in the eye and large "cobblestone" papillae lining the posterior pharynx in chronic cases; or (3) atopic keratoconjunctivitis that usually occurs in the late teen years. Certain autoimmune phenomena such as Sjögren's syndrome or Wegener's granulomatosis may also involve conjunctivitis.

CLINICAL PRESENTATION

Subjective

Symptoms vary with the cause, but cardinal symptoms of conjunctivitis are itching, watering, and redness of the eye. There may be a foreign body sensation and/or a sense of fullness around the eyes. Bacterial infections, such as with *Staphylococcus aureus,* may produce significant thick, yellow, sticky exudates at the eyelids. This profuse exudate is especially apparent in the morning, and patients may complain that their eyelids "are stuck together" when they wake, which is known as matting. Bacterial infections usually begin unilaterally, whereas viral infections often appear in both eyes at once.

Adenoviral conjunctivitis causes a foreign body sensation, minimal pruritus and exudate, but profuse tearing. This type of conjunctivitis is often bilateral; preauricular adenopathy is common, along with systemic symptoms typical of a viral infection, such as fever and myalgia. Other family members may be affected, as it is highly contagious. Associated symptoms of upper respiratory tract infection or gastroenteritis may point to a viral cause. Visual loss, photophobia, and severe eye pain may suggest corneal involvement. The clinician should ask the patient about any history of allergens and potential contacts, including mention of symptoms of sexually transmitted diseases. Chlamydial infections tend to present bilaterally, with minimal pruritus and moderate to profuse tearing and exudate. Allergic conjunctivitis also presents bilaterally, with severe pruritus, moderate tearing, and no exudate.

Objective

The first step in the examination is testing of visual acuity in both eyes, as well as in each eye individually. Upon inspection of the eyes, there will be hyperemia and tearing. The clinician needs to determine the extent of inflammation, and it is important to note if the inflammation involves the pupil, whether it is local or diffuse, and whether it is symmetrical or asymmetrical in one or both eyes. If exudate is present and is thick and copious, the cause is probably bacterial or chlamydial.

There may be eyelid swelling, and the clinician should examine the eyelids, lashes, and surrounding skin for abnormalities. Areas of lymphoid tissue hyperplasia that appear as dome-shaped elevations with blood vessels on their surface are called follicles; these are present in many types of conjunctivitis. If follicles are prominent in the upper tarsus, this is usually indicative of a viral etiology, such as adenovirus or *Chlamydia*. Minute elevations with vascular cores that may coalesce to form large papillae occasionally form secondary to an inflammatory process. These may be present on the superior tarsal plate in cases of vernal keratoconjunctivitis, adenovirus, or HSV infection. Preauricular nodes often represent a viral etiology, such as HSV or adenovirus, and may also be present in caused by *Chlamydia* and *N. gonorrhoeae* infections. These nodes are less prominent but more tender to palpation in patients with conjunctivitis of bacterial etiology. Subconjunctival hemorrhage may be seen in bacterial conjunctivitis or enterovirus 70 conjunctivitis.

Pupillary response should be assessed for equality and reactivity to light and accommodation, as failure of the pupil to react appropriately is indicative of a more serious problem, and patients with this sign require quickly referred to an ophthalmologist for evaluation.

Corneal involvement, which often manifests with eye pain, decreased visual acuity, and photophobia, may be present and appear as punctate epithelial lesions. The potential for corneal involvement is increased in cases of vernal keratoconjunctivitis, adenovirus, and *N. gonorrhoeae* infection. The presence of a membranous film that covers and adheres to the entire surface of the conjunctival epithelium is usually associated with epidemic keratoconjunctivitis or infection with HSV, *S. pneumoniae,* and *N. gonorrhoeae.* If the membrane is removed, a bleeding surface is left behind.

DIAGNOSTIC REASONING

Diagnostic Tests

The clinician should always check visual acuity first. A dilated pupil examination should be performed by a trained professional in patients with hyperemia accompanied by proptosis, optic nerve dysfunction, decreased visual acuity, diplopia, or anterior chamber inflammation. Fluorescein staining may be indicated to rule out corneal involvement or keratitis, and Blue penlight illumination can be used to check for corneal scratches, corneal dendrites (which occur in HSV infection), or corneal ulceration. The clinician should use anesthetic drops before staining the eye. If *N. gonorrhoeae* is suspected, the conjunctivitis has failed to respond to treatment, or in cases of ophthalmia neonatorum, membranous conjunctivitis or prolonged, severe conjunctivitis, Gram stain and culture should be done of conjunctival secretions or exudate. In cases of suspected *Chlamydia* or herpes, the clinician should perform specific cultures and/or a fluorescent antibody test.

In persistent cases of conjunctivitis, referral to an ophthalmologist is essential so that scrapings, cultures, and smears can be taken for further diagnostic work-up. Conjunctival biopsy is occasionally useful in refractory or atypical conjunctivitis and is always done in cases of suspected neoplasm. When a hypopyon (a layer of white blood cells) or hyphema (a layer of red blood cells) in the anterior chamber is detected on examination, an immediate referral to an ophthalmologist is required because this may reflect infectious keratitis, endophthalmitis, or penetrating eye trauma.

Differential Diagnosis

The task at hand for the primary-care practitioner is to determine which type of conjunctivitis is involved, as an essential first step prior to initiating treatment. See Differential Diagnosis 18.1 for a comparison of selected differential diagnoses for red eye.

In *allergic conjunctivitis,* there is bilateral itching, with a watery discharge. The patient or his or her family may have a history of atopy. The conjunctiva and lids are swollen and reddened. This is a seasonal occurrence, most commonly seen in the fall and spring, which may be accompanied by sneezing, rhinorrhea, and a scratchy throat.

In *bacterial conjunctivitis,* signs and symptoms include itching and tearing, either bilaterally or unilaterally, with a moderate amount of mucopurulent (yellow-green) discharge. There is a moderate amount of conjunctival hyperemia, with a shiny red appearance to the lower lids. There is typical no focal pain nor visual disturbances. The cornea is clear, and there is usually minimal no preauricular adenopathy, although if present, lymph nodes may be painful to palpation. Bacterial conjunctivitis most commonly occurs in the winter and fall.

Viral conjunctivitis should also be ruled out. The patient with this type of conjunctivitis typically complains of itching, burning, and increased tearing. The conjunctiva is brilliant red, diffuse, and peripheral. There is a watery mucoid discharge, with a moderate amount of mucoid debris. The patient may also have conjunctival edema, follicles on the palpebral conjunctiva, and eyelid edema. Preauricular adenopathy may also be present. There are usually signs of an upper respiratory tract infection or a history of recent contact with another person with red eye.

In *iritis,* the patient presents with marked conjunctival injection, mainly around the cornea; it is unilateral and without discharge. The patient may have moderate to severe pain and photophobia. Vision is blurred, pupils are constricted, and the pupillary response to light is poor. Iritis requires prompt referral to an ophthalmologist.

In *keratoconjunctivitis,* the lack of an adequate tear film to cover and protect the cornea and conjunctiva results in a nonspecific irritation, with burning, redness, dryness, the sensation of foreign body, and generalized eye pain.

Blepharitis, as discussed earlier in this chapter, is an inflammation involving the structures of the eyelid margin, with redness, scaling, and crusting. It commonly affects older adults and is usually secondary to either chronic staphylococcal infection or seborrheic dermatitis. Treatment includes warm eyelid compresses and eyelid scrubs with dilute baby shampoo two to four times per day. Chronic cases may require antibiotic ointment.

Pterygium, a conjunctival degeneration that results in an opacity that partially covers the cornea, is most commonly seen at the 3- and 9-o'clock positions. There is conjunctival hyperemia and tear filming; the opacity is usually slow growing and may eventually obstruct the vision. Pterygium is most commonly seen in persons with excessive exposure to ultraviolet light, windy conditions, or dusty surroundings. Treatment includes artificial tears to alleviate irritation, protective eyewear that should be worn when outside, and surgical removal of the opacity if visual disturbance occurs.

Subconjunctival hemorrhage, the sudden onset of painless red eye without any other associated symptoms, is usually caused by trauma, excessive straining, coughing, or hypertension. No treatment is needed if the cause can be found. The patient should be reassured that the condition resolves in 2 to 4 weeks.

The signs and symptoms of *herpes zoster ophthalmicus* include eye pain (which may be severe), tearing, photophobia, mucoid discharge, and moderate conjunctival hyperemia. The cornea may be clear or cloudy. Vesicles may or may not be present. Symptoms are usually the result of reactivation of latent zoster infection because of stress or infection. Patients with herpes zoster ophthalmicus should be immediately referred to an ophthalmologist.

Signs and symptoms of *corneal abrasion* include pain, foreign body sensation, photophobia, conjunctival hyperemia, and acute profuse tearing. The patient will usually have a history of scratching the eye, contact lens irritation, or actual trauma. The clinician should stain the eye with fluorescein and use a cobalt blue filter light or slit lamp to inspect the eye for foreign objects or scratches. Treatment includes antibiotic eye drops or ointment for 5 days. Patching is not usually necessary. The patient should avoid wearing contact lenses until the abrasion heals.

With acute closed-angle *glaucoma,* the patient will have a sudden onset of severe pain and blurred vision, with nausea and vomiting. The patient will report seeing rainbow halos around lights. There will be corneal cloudiness, with diffuse conjunctival hyperemia. The pupil of the affected eye will be moderately dilated and completely unresponsive to light. Any patient with glaucoma should be referred to an ophthalmologist immediately. The patient who presents with acute glaucoma is usually older, more visual loss is present, pain is more severe, and there may also be headache and nausea.

Uveitis (iritis, iridocyclitis, choroiditis) usually presents with severe eye pain, photophobia, blurred vision, injection in the limbus area, and deposits in the cornea. All of these conditions are ocular emergencies, and patients should be referred to an ophthalmologist immediately to avoid permanent vision loss.

MANAGEMENT

Treatment depends on etiology and impact on visual acuity. Any purulent material or debris should be removed from the conjunctival area. Lubrication of the eye with artificial tears is recommended, or frequent cleansing by lavage. Although corticosteroids sometimes help with conjunctival irritation, clinicians should not routinely order topical corticosteroids, as there is a risk their immunosuppressive effects could worsen infection.

With blepharitis or conditions that are accompanied by conjunctival discharge, the patient should be instructed to clean the lid margins with a dilute no-tears shampoo and discontinue wearing contact lenses (if any). Compresses are often effective for local relief; they should be warm in cases of infective conjunctivitis and cold in cases of allergic or irritative conjunctivitis. Patching of the eye is not typically warranted.

Pharmacologic therapy for conjunctivitis depends on the identified etiology and/or suspected causative agent (see Drugs Commonly Prescribed 19.1).

FOLLOW-UP AND REFERRAL

Given the potential for unresolved conjunctivitis to threaten vision, patients with red eye that does not resolve as expected with standard therapy should be referred to an ophthalmologist in a timely fashion for further diagnostic studies and therapeutic management, especially if there is an ulcer, keratitis, or suspected herpes infection or if the conjunctivitis worsens within 24 hours.

Patient Education: Conjunctivitis

The clinician should explain that secretions may remain infectious for at least 48 hours after the start of treatment. Conjunctivitis is highly contagious; therefore, the patient should take care when coming into contact with other members of the household, especially infants, children, older adults, and pets. The spread of conjunctivitis may be prevented by effective hand washing, avoiding touching the eyes, and not sharing towels and washcloths. The clinician should instruct the patient to avoid autoinoculation by not touching the medication applicator to the eye and using separate eyecups for each lavage. The patient should be taught to instil topical medication in the outer aspect of the lower eyelid. It may be best to use ophthalmic solution during the daytime and then apply a thin film of ointment before sleep. Contact lenses should not be used until the infection is resolved.

REFERENCES

General

Robinson A. Managing common eye problems in general practice. http://www.prescriber.co.uk/article/managing-common-eye-problems-general-practice. Published 2017.

Blepharitis

Lowery S. Adult blepharitis. http://emedicine.medscape.com/article/1211763-overview. Published 2016.

Dry Eye

American Academy of Ophthalmology Cornea/External Disease Panel, Preferred Practice Patterns Committee. Dry eye syndrome. www.guidelines.gov/summary/summary.aspx?doc_id=13503. Published 2008.

Bhargava R, Kumar P, Kumar M, Mehra N, Mishra A. A randomized controlled trial of omega-3 fatty acids in dry eye syndrome. *Int J Ophthalmol.* 2013;6(6):811–816.

Chiva A. Dry eye and clinical disease of tear film—diagnosis and management. *Eur Opthalmol Rev.* 2014;8(1):8–12.

Foster S. Dry eye syndrome (keratoconjunctivitis sicca). http://emedicine.medscape.com/article/1210417-overview. Published 2017.

Gupta A, Sadeghi PB, Akpek EK. Occult thyroid eye disease in patients presenting with dry eye symptoms. *Am J Opthalmol.* 2009;147(5):919–923.

International Dry Eye Workshop. The definition and classification of dry eye disease: Report of the Definition and Classification Subcommittee of the International Dry Eye Workshop (2007). *Ocul Surf.* 2007;5:75–93.

Management and therapy of dry eye disease: Report of the Management and Therapy Subcommittee of the International Dry Eye Workshop. *Ocul Surf.* 2007;5(2):163–178.

Nilufer I et al. Is there a relationship between pathologic myopia and dry eye syndrome? *Cornea.* 2014;33(2):169–171.

Pflugfelder SC. The VIEW II: Halting progression of dry eye disease. 2009. http://cme.medscape.com/viewarticle/704768.

Rocha EM, Mantelli F, Nominato LF, Bonini S. Hormones and dry eye syndrome: an update on what we do and don't know. *Curr Opin Opthalmol.* 2013;24(4):348–355.

Shultz C. Safety and efficacy of cyclosporine in the treatment of chronic dry eye. *Ophthalmol Eye Dis.* 2014;6:37–42.

Epiphora

Nordqvist C. Causes and treatments for watering eyes. http://www.medicalnewstoday.com/articles/169397.php. Published 2017.

Verma A, Singh D. Corneal abrasion treatment & management. http://emedicine.medscape.com/article/1195402-treatment. Published 2016.

Hordeolum and Chalazion

Ansari AS, de Lusignan S, Arrowsmith B, Hinton W, McGovern A. Is diabetes really a risk factor for acute eye infection? Clinical care and other categories posters: lesser known complications. *Diabet Med.* 2017;34.

Cheng K, Law A, Guo M, et al. Acupuncture for acute hordeolum. *Cochrane Database Syst Rev.* 2017;2:CD011075.

Kabat AG, Sowka JW. Stye vs. stye. Rev Optometry. https://www.reviewofoptometry.com/article/stye-vs-stye. Published 2016. Accessed August 31, 2017.

Lindsley K, Nichols JJ, Dickersin K. Interventions for acute internal hordeolum. *Cochrane Database Syst Rev.* 2017;9:CD007742.

Red Eye/Conjunctivitis

Graham R. Red eye. http://emedicine.medscape.com/article/1192122-overview. Published 2017.

La Rosa M, Lionetti E, Reibaldi M, et al. Allergic conjunctivitis: A comprehensive review of the literature. *Ital J Pediatr.* 2013;39:18.

Narayana S, McGee S. Bedside diagnosis of the "red eye": A systematic review. *Am J Med.* 2015;128(11):1220–1224.

Scott IU, Luu K. Viral conjunctivitis (pink eye). http://emedicine.medscape.com/article/1191370-overview. Published 2017.

Yeung K. Bacterial conjunctivitis (pink eye). http://emedicine.medscape.com/article/1191730. Published 2017.

RESOURCES

Digital Atlas of Ophthalmology (New York Eye and Ear Infirmary of Mount Sinai)
http://www.nyee.edu/health-professionals/digital-atlas-of-ophthalmology

Blepharitis
https://www.aao.org/eye-health/diseases/what-is-blepharitis

Chalazia
https://www.aao.org/eye-health/diseases/what-are-chalazia-styes

Dry Eye
https://www.aao.org/eye-health/diseases/what-is-dry-eye

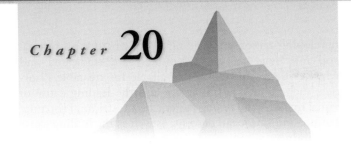

Chapter **20**

Visual Disturbances and Impaired Vision

Brian Oscar Porter, MD, PhD, MPH, MBA

Lynne M. Dunphy, PhD, APRN, FNP-BC, FAAN, FAANP

Cathleen Provins, RN, MSN, PhD, CCRN-K, NE-BC, ACNP-BC

REFRACTIVE ERRORS

Normal vision is dependent on a clear image being projected through the cornea, aqueous humor, lens, and vitreous humor, and then onto the retina. All of these structures must be healthy to provide a clear retinal image, and the optic nerve must be able to transmit an accurate image to the visual cortex in the occipital lobe of the brain. Refractive errors result in blurred vision due to aberrations in how external light is reflected into the eye.

EPIDEMIOLOGY AND CAUSES

Refractive errors that are uncorrected or incompletely corrected are a common cause of visual impairment. Refractory errors include myopia, hyperopia, astigmatism, and presbyopia. Although more prevalent in older persons, refractive errors are common in all age groups.

PATHOPHYSIOLOGY

To transmit an external image into the eye, parallel rays of light enter the cornea, which are bent by the cornea and lens to converge on the retina. The macula of the retina is responsible for central visual acuity and is thus the most important portion of the retina for distinguishing visual details, such as when reading. The patient perceives a blurred image when light rays do not converge on a common point on the retina. Light ray convergence in front of the retina causes myopia, or near-sightedness. If light rays converge posterior to the retina, the patient is hyperopic, or farsighted. If light rays focus on two separate lines rather than a single point, the patient has astigmatism.

CLINICAL PRESENTATION

Subjective

Patients may present with a chief complaint of a change in vision; they may report that their current eyeglasses are not effective in correcting their vision. They may also present with a complaint of recent headaches suggestive of eye strain. Refractive errors have a gradual onset and are not usually accompanied by pain or redness. Refractive errors may be found on screening during a routine examination. Patients may be unaware of a change in vision because they have become accustomed to it; this is especially true when the error is in only one eye.

Objective

Visual acuity on examination with a Snellen eye chart will be less than 20/20 and worsened from previous examinations. A simple "pinhole test" can be administered in the primary-care setting to determine whether the diminished visual acuity is the result of a refractive error or the presence of organic disease. A pinhole test is performed by creating pinholes 0.5 to 2 mm in diameter in a stiff paper card. The patient is asked to look through one of the pinholes one eye at a time. If the visual acuity improves without the use of corrective lenses, the diminished acuity is a refractive error improvement. Improvement occurs because light rays are being focused through the pinhole, and the pinhole card blocks peripheral light waves. If there is no improvement, the diminished acuity is organic.

DIAGNOSTIC REASONING

The role of the primary-care provider is to evaluate the patient for the need for emergent or routine referral to an ophthalmologist or optometrist. Refractory errors are not life-threatening but do require timely referral to prevent secondary injury from accidents or falls related to poor visual acuity.

Diagnostic Tests

The hallmark of diagnostic assessment of refractory errors is examination of visual acuity, which is typically done in the primary-care setting using a properly distanced Snellen eye examination wall chart or hand-held printed card. Although these office-based tests can quantify refractive errors on a gross level and generally characterize the visual defect as far-sightedness or near-sightedness, more detailed examinations will be required by an appropriate referral to an optometrist for corrective lenses or an ophthalmologist for more serious eye pathology.

Differential Diagnosis

A thorough history and physical examination will reveal if the vision change is acute or progressive, as well as associated signs or symptoms. Vision-threatening conditions requiring emergent referral to an ophthalmologist should be ruled out.

MANAGEMENT

Corrective lenses are used to compensate for refractive errors. Accurate prescriptions for such lenses may be obtained from an optometrist or ophthalmologist. Some patients may be candidates for and benefit from vision correction procedures, such as LASIK eye surgery.

FOLLOW-UP AND REFERRAL

Accurate diagnosis and characterization of refractive errors requires referral to an optometrist or ophthalmologist, who have the appropriate equipment to measure refractive errors. These referrals are needed to obtain prescriptions for effective corrective lenses, as well as to screen for other common eye problems, which may contribute to decreased visual acuity. The timing of follow-up is determined by the presence of more significant eye pathology; simple refractive errors that are adequately addressed with corrective lenses may not require more than annual follow-up to assess for a progressive component.

Patient Education: Refractive Errors

Patients should be encouraged to use corrective lenses for all activities that require optimal visual acuity, such as reading, driving, or operating machinery. Proper care of eyeglasses and contact lenses should be discussed with all patients.

CATARACTS

A *cataract* is any opacity of the lens of the eye. They may or may not be associated with visual impairment or functional consequences and may form in one or both eyes. The decreased visual acuity associated with cataracts is caused by degradation of the optical quality of the crystalline lens, thereby affecting vision.

EPIDEMIOLOGY AND CAUSES

Epidemiologic models estimate that there are approximately 30 million blind people in the world, 50% of whom are blind due to cataracts. The pattern and rate of blinding disorders is different in developed and developing nations depending upon whether nutritional and infectious causes of blindness are eradicated and whether there are resources available for treatable disorders such as cataract. They are also the leading cause of visual impairment among Americans of African, Hispanic/Latino, and European descent, as well as the leading cause of blindness among Americans of African descent over age 40 years. The number of Americans with cataracts is expected to double by 2050. The incidence of cataracts increases with age. Risk factors for cataract formation include diabetes mellitus, long-term corticosteroid use, prior intraocular surgery, cigarette smoking, excessive exposure to sunlight (UVB rays), trauma, and a low level of formal education. Avoidance of these risk factors is key to cataract prevention, including smoking cessation and the wearing of protective eye gear, especially when engaged in high-risk activities for cataract formation or ocular injury, such as the use of tanning beds or welding.

PATHOPHYSIOLOGY

The lens is a transparent, biconvex structure located behind the cornea and supported by zonules. Contained within the lens capsule is a central nucleus surrounded by a cortex. The lens is avascular, deriving its metabolic needs from the aqueous and vitreous humors. Early in life, the lens is pliable and can change its shape as connecting zonules anchored to ciliary bodies place varying degrees of stress on the lens through involuntary contraction and relaxation. These changes in lens shape result in accommodation, allowing objects to come into focus at varying distances.

The transparency of the human lens results from the highly ordered nature of its composite stratified epithelia, which contain a high density of cytoplasmic proteins called crystallins.

Aging alters the biochemical and osmotic balance required for lens clarity, as do comorbid disease processes, such as diabetes mellitus. Unlike the other endothelia in the body, the lens cannot shed nonviable cells. Thus, as the lens ages, it loses both its pliability and its clarity. These changes are thought to occur because of damage from oxidation, a biochemical process set in motion when a highly reactive form of oxygen (an oxygen radical) forms within the cells of the lens itself. Over time, the crystalline lens becomes fibrotic, hardened, and dehydrated, causing progressive opacification that eventually results in a cataract. Healing fibrosis from ocular trauma is a primary etiology of acquired cataracts, whereas secondary cataracts may result from other forms of ocular inflammation that extend to the lens, including uveitis, topical anticholinesterase preparations, and radiation therapy used to treat ocular tumors.

There are three subtypes of cataracts, categorized by anatomical location. The size, density, and location of the cataract determine its effect on vision and the most appropriate method of surgical intervention/lens replacement. Many patients have a combination of these subtypes:

1. Nuclear cataracts are characterized by significant near-sightedness and a slow, indolent course.
2. Cortical cataracts do not significantly impair vision.
3. Posterior cataracts create a subcapsular haze and a severe glare in bright light. They are strongly associated with systemic corticosteroid use and progress much faster than the nuclear form (over months rather than years).

Regardless of anatomical type, immature cataracts are those that do not obscure the red retinal light reflex on fundoscopy. In contrast, mature cataracts obscure the red reflex with significant visual impairment, and hypermature cataracts are characterized by liquefaction of the cortical lens with mobility of the nucleus.

CLINICAL PRESENTATION

Subjective

The patient with cataracts may present with visual changes and/or functional impairment; however, asymptomatic cataracts (without a perception of vision loss) may be found on routine examination. Cataracts produce a gradual, painless, and progressive loss of vision, although many patients are unaware of any vision problems due to the gradual nature on onset. For example, with monocular (asymmetrical) cataracts, reduced vision may only be apparent when the unaffected eye is covered. Age-related cataracts tend to be bilateral in nature and may manifest as blurred or distorted vision, with complaints of a glare when driving at night or in bright light. Because of the increase of yellow-brown pigment in the lens, color perception is also affected.

The increased density of the lens nucleus results in near-sightedness that may require frequent changes in a patient's eyeglass prescription. Myopia (near-sightedness) may result from nuclear cataracts. The term "second sight" refers to older adults who abandon their reading glasses related to this phenomenon; however, as the cataract worsens, so does their near vision. Mononuclear diplopia (double vision in one eye) is a cardinal refractive error associated with cataracts.

The Lens Opacities Classification System III is a widely used subjective grading to assess the cataract severity. Decision making for cataract surgery also includes assessment of the visual functional status, especially limitations in the ability to do daily activities. These aspects can be measured with clinical history or with formal instruments or questionnaires, such as the Catquest-9SF questionnaire, or the Visual Functioning Index-14, which was designed to assess patient-reported visual functioning.

Objective

In some patients, lens opacity will be apparent on inspection, but this is not always the case. Decreased visual acuity is the most common objective finding associated with cataracts.

A detailed ophthalmic examination by an ophthalmologist or optometrist would include visual acuity testing, refraction, intraocular pressure, slit-lamp examination, and fundus assessment to rule out other ocular comorbidities. Mature or "ripe" cataracts eventually produce a gray or white pupillary reflex known as leukocoria, although a dense posterior subcapsular cataract may produce reduction in vision without altering the pupillary reflex. The best direct visualization of cataracts may be obtained by slit-lamp evaluation after pupillary dilation. Other tests that might be used include B-scan ultrasonography if direct visualization of the retina is not possible because of dense cataract, and contrast sensitivity and glare tests in selective patients.

DIAGNOSTIC REASONING

Diagnostic Tests

A detailed history and physical examination are vital to proper diagnosis, including visual acuity with current corrective lenses, measurement of best-corrected (distance) visual acuity, external eye examination, ocular alignment and motility, glare test, pupillary function, intraocular pressure measurement, slit-lamp examination, and dilated examination of the lens, macula, peripheral retina, optic nerve, and vitreous humor.

A detailed ophthalmic examination might include visual acuity testing, refraction, intraocular pressure, slit-lamp examination, and fundus assessment to rule out other ocular comorbidities that could affect the postoperative prognosis. Other tests that might be used include B-scan ultrasonography if direct visualization of the retina is not possible because of dense cataract, and contrast sensitivity and glare tests in selective patients. The Lens Opacities Classification System III is a widely used subjective grading to assess the cataract severity. Decision making for cataract surgery also includes assessment of the visual functional status, especially limitations in the ability to do daily activities. These aspects can be measured with clinical history or with formal instruments or questionnaires, such as the Catquest-9SF questionnaire, or the Visual Functioning Index-14, which was designed to assess patient-reported visual functioning.

There is no single eye test or examination that can describe fully the effects of a cataract on a patient's visual status or functional ability, nor is there a single test that establishes the need for cataract surgery. The decision to have surgery is based on the patient's quality of life and perception of visual deficits as well as the size and maturity of the cataracts.

Differential Diagnosis

The following causes of visual impairment should be ruled out in patients suspected of having cataracts: refractive errors, glaucoma, retinopathy, and age-related macular degeneration (AMD). Any sudden change in vision or sudden vision loss should be treated as an emergency and referred to an ophthalmologist immediately.

Cataracts are gradual in onset and develop over time. Macular degeneration also presents with a slow, progressive loss of vision, but this impairment is focused centrally, by virtue of its effects on the macula. In addition, macular degeneration may also manifest with symptoms of acute vision loss and distortion (metamorphopsia), resulting from leakage of exudative fluid or bleeding from abnormally proliferative subretinal vessels. Open-angle glaucoma produces a slow and painless visual field loss that usually begins peripherally and often (although not always) presents with increased intraocular pressure and/or an increased cup-to-disc ratio (>0.6), termed cupping of the optic nerve. Diabetic retinopathy may also result in vision loss; funduscopic examination will usually reveal dot-and-blot hemorrhages, microaneurysms, exudates, dilated and torturous ocular blood vessels, and neovascularization of the disc and retina.

MANAGEMENT

There is currently no nonsurgical treatment for cataracts. Surgery should be discussed when changes in eyeglasses no longer correct vision sufficiently and quality of life is jeopardized. Cataract surgery is a relatively safe outpatient procedure that has been shown to be highly cost-effective, given the reduction in comorbidities and injuries associated with progressive visual impairment. Patients who are scheduled for cataract surgery may be referred to their primary-care practitioner for a preoperative health assessment. However, healthy adult patients scheduled for cataract surgery under local anesthesia do not typically require preoperative medical testing.

For patients with risk factors or comorbid medical conditions, a physical examination, electrocardiogram, electrolytes, and urinalysis may be ordered. Causes for concern include the presence of diabetes mellitus, hypertension, ischemic heart disease, certain pulmonary disorders, and the use of anticoagulants. Any patient with uncontrolled diabetes is at risk of postoperative vision loss related to diabetic macular edema, which causes the retinal vessels to leak, leading to swelling of the visual center (macula). Anticoagulant therapy should be discontinued before surgery. This includes over-the-counter supplements such as high doses of fish oil or omega-3 fatty acids that have been associated with prolonged bleeding. Systemic hypertension may also place the patient at risk for intraocular hemorrhage during or after surgery.

The standard of care in cataract surgery in the United States is a small-incision phacoemulsification with foldable intraocular lens implantation. The procedure is safe and affords improved vision with decreased dependence on corrective eyewear for distance, intermediate, and near vision. Two surgical techniques are currently used—phacoemulsification and extracapsular cataract extraction. In both types of surgery, an incision is made into the eye, and the central anterior lens capsule is removed. In phacoemulsification, the surgeon makes a 2- to 4-mm incision and inserts an ultrasonic vibrating needle that breaks the cataract into small pieces, which are then aspirated through the needle's central bore. The smaller incision and smaller sutures used in phacoemulsification make it the preferred method for cataract removal. In extracapsular surgery, the surgeon makes a 10- to 14-mm incision, and the entire lens nucleus is loosened from the cortex and removed through the incision. In both cases, the surgery continues with removal of the residual lens cortex and insertion of a replacement intraocular lens. The incision may be self-sealing or closed with sutures.

There is little evidence from randomized controlled studies that evaluates the optimal regimen of antibiotics and/or corticosteroids postoperatively. There is more evidence demonstrating that intracameral antibiotics reduce the risk of postoperative bacterial endophthalmitis. Postoperative straining of the eyes (from reading small print, prolonged computer, or smart phone use, etc.) should be avoided until the patient receives clearance from an ophthalmologist. Bilateral cataract surgery is common and often indicated because of better visual acuity outcomes, although optimal timing of the second surgery remains controversial.

FOLLOW-UP AND REFERRAL

Patients need early referral and monitoring by an ophthalmologist, although education about the advances in surgical techniques and reassurance may be important aspects of care before referral. A patient who has undergone cataract removal surgery should be reevaluated by the ophthalmologist within 48 hours of the procedure. Approximately 4 weeks after surgery, the patient should be evaluated for the need for corrective lenses.

Patient Education: Cataracts

Modification of dietary intake and nutritional supplements have demonstrated minimal to no effect in the prevention or treatment of cataracts; however, there is some conflicting evidence of their utility. A Cochrane review found no evidence supporting high doses of vitamin E, vitamin C, or beta-carotene in preventing the formation or progression of cataracts. In fact, some studies have found high doses of vitamin C to increase age-related cataract development, and there is also conflicting evidence regarding vitamin E. Daily lutein has shown no significant impact, and there is little research to support high-dose antioxidants. There is moderate evidence, however, that multivitamins and mineral supplements may decrease the risk of nuclear cataracts.

GLAUCOMA

Glaucoma is defined as a group of diseases characterized by progressive damage to the optic nerve, resulting in optic nerve atrophy and blindness, most typically associated with elevated intraocular pressure. Glaucoma is classified as open-angle glaucoma and angle-closure glaucoma (classically referred to as closed-angle or narrow-angle glaucoma). These classifications are based on the anatomy of the anterior chamber. Both types of glaucoma may be present in the same eye (referred to as combined-mechanism glaucoma). Glaucoma is further differentiated as primary or secondary (associated with an ocular condition or a systemic process). There is also a congenital form of glaucoma seen in infants.

Open-angle glaucoma is the most common type and is characterized as a chronic form of the disorder that, before loss of peripheral visual fields, is asymptomatic. It has an excellent prognosis if treated early and appropriately. Angle-closure glaucoma, on the other hand, may have subacute and chronic components, but it is most often associated with acute episodes of significant eye pain, redness, and acute visual loss, which, if untreated, may rapidly lead to permanent blindness.

EPIDEMIOLOGY AND CAUSES

Glaucoma affects approximately 4% of all individuals older than age 40. There is an increasing prevalence of glaucoma in adults older than 65 years in the United States and an increased prevalence of open-angle glaucoma in African Americans older than age 75. Primary open-angle glaucoma (chronic glaucoma) is the most prevalent form of glaucoma and accounts for 90% to 95% of all cases. Angle-closure glaucoma (acute glaucoma) is not as common; it affects approximately 100 per 100,000 of the population (approximately 0.1%). Glaucoma is the second leading cause of blindness among white Americans and the most common cause of blindness in African Americans. Angle-closure glaucoma tends to occur in people aged 55 to 70 years. Angle-closure glaucoma is more prevalent in people of Asian descent, as well as in those with Eskimo ancestry, especially among the Inuit. Chronic open-angle glaucoma occurs equally in males and females. Angle-closure glaucoma occurs more frequently in females.

Increased intraocular pressure, positive family history, older age, and African American descent place an individual at increased risk for glaucoma. Older African Americans have a higher prevalence of glaucoma and a more rapid progression of the disease. Specifically, myopia (near-sightedness) and diabetes may both contribute to the development of chronic open-angle glaucoma, whereas hyperopia (far-sightedness) eyes and a small cornea contribute to angle-closure glaucoma.

Glaucoma may also develop secondarily as a result of several ocular and systemic diseases or medication use.

The use of steroid therapy (topical, inhaled, or systemic) may lead to increased intraocular pressure. Antidepressant drugs or other anticholinergic drugs and emotional stress may contribute to an acute episode, as may childbirth, sneezing, laser therapy or surgery, and IV overhydration. Increased pressure in the anterior chamber that is uncorrected will, over time, impair peripheral visual fields, destroy central vision, and ultimately destroy the optic nerve. Increased intraocular pressure, optic nerve atrophy, and visual field loss make up the classic triad of glaucoma.

PATHOPHYSIOLOGY

The ciliary body of the eye produces aqueous humor, which circulates from the posterior chamber to the anterior chamber and then exits through the trabecular meshwork. In primary open-angle glaucoma (in which no secondary cause is identified), elevated intraocular pressure is almost always caused by obstruction of the outflow channels, especially the trabecular meshwork; however, overproduction of aqueous humor may also occur. The manner in which the trabecular meshwork is obstructed is a matter of debate, but it probably involves changes in the biochemical makeup of the cells lining this meshwork. These changes appear to occur with aging. In addition, secondary glaucoma may result from increased intraocular pressure caused by ocular trauma or inflammation such as uveitis, chronic steroid use, vasoproliferative retinopathy, and recurrent retinal hemorrhages.

The specific mechanism by which increased intraocular pressure leads to optic nerve atrophy is also debated. One theory is that increased intraocular pressure causes direct mechanical damage and loss of retinal ganglionic cell axons known as "cupping." Others theorize that increased intraocular pressure impairs the small-vessel circulation that provides nutrients to the optic nerve and extracellular matrix. Glutamate toxicity and processes involving apoptosis leading to axonal loss are also currently being investigated.

It is critical to recognize, however, that optic atrophy may occur in the absence of increased intraocular pressure. Traditionally, elevated intraocular pressure has been defined as greater than 21 mm Hg. Ocular hypertension has also been identified in the absence of optic nerve atrophy. Thus, other pathophysiological processes leading to progressive, irreversible vision loss also function in primary open-angle glaucoma; increased intraocular pressure by itself must be considered only a risk factor, rather than the definitive glaucomatous etiology. Work is also underway to identify the gene products and functions associated with inherited forms of open-angle glaucoma, which typically occur before the age of 40 years, known collectively as juvenile glaucoma.

Angle-closure glaucoma, which may be either acute or chronic, is less common than open-angle glaucoma. It is caused by anatomical narrowing of the anterior chamber angle, a factor that is fundamentally determined by genetics and becomes more likely with advanced age. This narrowing is primarily related to the size of the eyeball and lens. Specifically, angle-closure glaucoma results from the forward displacement of the iris toward the cornea, with narrowing of the iridocorneal angle resulting in an obstruction of outflow from the anterior chamber. Acute angle-closure glaucoma occurs when there is an acute closure of the iridocorneal angle with a sudden, severe rise in intraocular pressure, often well above 40 mm Hg, which is highly symptomatic. Permanent vision loss may result if this condition is not treated within 24 hours of onset.

CLINICAL PRESENTATION

Subjective

Generally, patients are asymptomatic until optic nerve damage is quite advanced. Chronic open-angle glaucoma has a gradual onset, with slow, painless bilateral peripheral vision loss and poor night vision. Frequent changes in refractory prescription may be a common presenting symptom. In later stages, symptoms may include seeing halos around lights and further visual loss. Acute angle-closure glaucoma has a rapid onset, with unilateral pain and pressure, blurred vision, seeing halos around lights, and photophobia, followed by loss of peripheral vision, subsequently followed by central vision loss. A headache may be present and possibly nausea and vomiting as well. Chronic angle-closure glaucoma is as insidious in onset as open-angle glaucoma. Its fundamental mechanism relates to the anatomical narrowness of the anterior chamber angle. Often patients have a history of vague discomfort about the eyes and intermittent blurring of vision.

Objective

The physical examination in most patients with chronic glaucoma will most likely be unremarkable. In later stages, the eyeball may be hardened. Visual acuity may or may not be affected. Visual field abnormalities to confrontation will be present usually only in the later stages of severe cases. A Marcus Gunn pupil (afferent pupillary defect) may be present.

In acute angle-closure glaucoma, intraocular pressure rises rapidly to very high levels. The eye becomes red and painful, the cornea may have a "steamy" appearance, and vision is severely blurred. There may be a pupil that is mid-dilated and immobile. Findings on funduscopic examination may show a pale optic disc with excavated cupping and a shallow anterior chamber; there may be an increased cup/disc ratio related to atrophy and asymmetry on comparison with the other eye. Visual acuity is severely affected because visual field defects are common. In many cases, the clinician can detect a shallow anterior chamber and narrow angle with the flashlight test: in this test, a penlight is held at the temporal limbus of the eye and the degree of illumination is noted. A narrow angle is suggested if the nasal half of the iris is in the shadow. Dilation of the pupil with mydriatic agents tends to narrow the angle further, which can lead to an acute attack, as can dim light or darkness, and physical or emotional stress. The primary-care provider should closely monitor patients with a family history of angle-closure glaucoma or hyperopia accompanied by a history of eye ache, headache, and blurred vision.

DIAGNOSTIC REASONING

At the present time, guidelines for glaucoma screening by the primary-care practitioner have not been firmly established. The U.S. Preventive Services Task Force concludes that the evidence of effectiveness of screening for glaucoma on clinical outcomes is lacking and that the balance of benefits and harms therefore cannot be determined. Improvement in the diagnostic skills for the early detection of glaucoma in the primary-care setting, coupled with clear guidelines for referral to an ophthalmologist, will have significant economic and health implications. Diagnosis of primary open-angle glaucoma is based on a combination of tests showing characteristic degenerative changes in the optic disc and defects in visual fields (often loss in peripheral vision). Although increased intraocular pressure was previously considered an important part of the definition of this condition, it is now known that many persons with primary open-angle glaucoma do not have increased intraocular pressure and not all persons with increased intraocular pressure have or will develop glaucoma. Therefore, screening with tonometry alone may be inadequate to detect all cases of primary open-angle glaucoma.

Measurement of visual fields can be difficult. The reliability of a single measurement may be low; several consistent measurements are needed to establish the presence of defects. Specialists use dilated ophthalmoscopy or slit-lamp examination to evaluate changes in the optic disc; however, even experts have varying ability to detect glaucomatous progression of the optic disc. In addition, no single standard exists to define and measure progression of visual field defects. Most tests that are available in a primary-care setting do not have acceptable accuracy to detect glaucoma. Multiple testing methods requiring specialized equipment and training are available, including pneumotonometry, which uses a puff of air against the eyeball, or the more accurate method of applanation tonometry, in which the cornea is directly observed while pressure is placed against it.

Diagnostic Tests

The diagnosis of glaucoma is not made on the basis of a single test but on the finding of characteristic degenerative changes in the optic disc and defects in visual fields. Tonometry to measure intraocular pressure is essential, although not diagnostic. In chronic, closed-angle glaucoma, there may or may not be elevation of intraocular pressure. Normal intraocular pressure is 12 to 22 mm Hg. In chronic, open-angle glaucoma, there may be normal or elevated intraocular pressure, whereas in an acute exacerbation of angle-closure glaucoma, intraocular pressure may be as high as 40 to 80 mm Hg. However, increased intraocular pressure alone is not required for the diagnosis of glaucoma because many patients with open-angle glaucoma consistently have intraocular pressure within the normal range.

Physical diagnosis relies on gonioscopic evaluation of the angle by an ophthalmologist. Gonioscopy determines the angle of the eye's anterior chamber and thus enables the examiner to differentiate between open-angle and angle-closure glaucoma; the angle is normal in open-angle glaucoma, although this often narrows with aging. Visual inspection of the angle is done using a special lens (goniolens) at the slit-lamp biomicroscope. The two primary types of disease, open-angle glaucoma and angle-closure glaucoma, are classified according to the anatomy of the anterior chamber angle. Both types of the disease may be present in the same eye.

The appearance (e.g., color and contour) of the optic nerve and findings on visual field examination are the most important clues to diagnosis. Pathognomonic changes indicate glaucoma. Funduscopic examination of the optic nerve reveals changes in the cup and neuroretinal rim relatively early in the disease, indicating the possibility of open-angle glaucoma. Particularly significant are the size of the cup relative to the optic nerve, any thinning or nicking of the disc rim, and the presence of disc hemorrhages. Visual field examination, which requires specialized equipment, detects defects in the field of vision that are characteristic for glaucomatous damage to the optic nerve relatively early in the disease.

Testing of visual fields using confrontational finger motions to assess the location of the patient's fields compared with the examiner's is unreliable for diagnosing glaucoma. Specialized tests can be performed by an ophthalmologist or optometrist for visual field assessment, including automated perimetry, Goldmann perimetry, or tangent screen testing. Pachymetry, which is a method of measuring corneal thickness, may also be done by an ophthalmologist. Thinner corneas are at higher risk for the development of primary open-angle glaucoma.

Differential Diagnosis

Patients with conjunctivitis and uveitis usually have visual changes that should alert the clinician to these diagnoses. Vascular disease may also produce funduscopic changes; however, these changes will be more hemorrhagic in nature. Medications such as steroids, amphetamines, and chlorpromazine can all increase intraocular pressure. Many ocular

and systemic conditions are associated with the development of glaucoma; in addition, the use of topical, systemic, and inhaled corticosteroids may increase intraocular pressure, depending on dose and duration of treatment.

MANAGEMENT

Once nerve damage has occurred, it is irreversible; thus, the goal of treatment is to prevent progression of damage and to protect the optic nerve from pressure. Glaucoma is a disease of pressure; adequate lowering of intraocular pressure by one means or another almost always stops optic nerve damage.

Traditionally, open-angle glaucoma is managed pharmacologically for as long as possible, with laser or surgical treatment reserved for glaucoma that cannot be controlled by medication alone. The choice of medication regimen is usually made by an ophthalmologist. The goal of pharmacologic therapy is to decrease and control intraocular pressure (see Drugs Commonly Prescribed 20.1)

First-line therapy is usually a beta blocker, but sometimes prostaglandin analogs may be used as first-line therapy or added soon after beta blockers are started. Treatment compliance with multiple doses of eye drops daily is often poor in open-angle glaucoma; however, newer topical agents require less frequent dosing (once daily for prostaglandins). If medications do not control pressure, surgical options include laser or external trabeculectomy. Laser therapy is often effective only in the first several years after surgery and then the pressure begins to build again. The timing of surgery has not been shown to influence visual outcomes, and surgery imparts greater risk for future cataracts; therefore, medications should be tried first. Target intraocular pressure that therapy attempts to achieve must be decided on an individual basis. If one medication is not sufficient to lower the intraocular pressure, a second medication from a different class may be added. It should be noted that occasionally localized or systemic reactions to the medication may occur and the patients should be instructed as to what to look for. Other systemic medications that the patient may be taking must be taken into consideration.

Medications are administered during the acute attack to lower intraocular pressure so that surgical intervention can occur. Acetazolamide (Diamox) and intravenous mannitol with a topical miotic, such as pilocarpine, may be administered, followed by laser iridotomy or peripheral iridectomy. Bedrest should be maintained until the attack is broken.

FOLLOW-UP AND REFERRAL

Patients with glaucoma should be referred to and followed by an ophthalmologist. Nonetheless, as the primary-care provider, the clinician needs to understand what medications the patient is receiving as well as how often

Drugs Commonly Prescribed 20.1: Glaucoma

DRUG	MECHANISM OF ACTION	ADVERSE EFFECTS
Cholinergic Agents		
Pilocarpine (Isopto, Pilocar, Pilostat)	Constrict pupils to open the angle and allow aqueous humor to escape.	Contraindicated in conditions in which pupillary constriction should be avoided.
Beta Blockers		
Timolol (Timoptic), betaxolol (Betoptic), levobunolol (Betagan), carteolol (Cartrol), metipranolol (Betanol)	Reduce the production of aqueous humor.	Additive effect in patients who are also taking an oral beta blocker. Contraindicated in asthma, sinus bradycardia, second- or third-degree atrio-ventricular block, overt congestive heart failure.
Prostaglandin analogs bimatoprost (Lumigan), latanoprost (Xalatan), travoprost (Travatan)	Decrease intraocular pressure by increased ureoscleral outflow (drainage).	Can cause conjunctival hyperemia, iris pigment color changes, uveitis, and macular edema.
Carbonic Anhydrase Inhibitors		
Brinzolamide (Azopt), dorzolamide (Trusopt), echothiophate (Phospholine), physiostigmine (Eserone sulfate ophthalmic)	Reduce aqueous humor production.	Caution in patients with nephrolithiasis, diabetes, hepatic disease, and a history of sulfonamide sensitivity.
Alpha-Adrenergic Agonists		
Epinephrine and dipivefrin (Propine), apraclonidine (Iopidine), brimonidine (Alphagan)	Inhibit aqueous humor production.	Avoid in patients with grade 2 or 3 heart block, congestive heart failure, chronic obstructive pulmonary disease, asthma, or pulmonary edema.
Systemic Medications		
Acetazolamide (Diamox), dichlorphenamide (Sulfonamide), metazolamide (Sulfonamide)	Reduce production of aqueous humor.	

the patient should be monitored by an ophthalmologist (every 3 to 4 months for life). The clinician needs to be alert to possible signs and symptoms of exacerbation. There is always potential for loss of vision and possible blindness if acute glaucoma attacks are not treated promptly and consistently.

Patient Education: Glaucoma

Careful and lifelong follow-up is essential for patients with glaucoma, especially periodic checks of intraocular pressure and eye examinations. The need to take medications as ordered, to be aware of adverse effects of medications prescribed, and to recognize changes (such as sudden changes in vision) that warrant a call to the health-care provider are essential for all patients with glaucoma. The clinician may need to teach the patient how best to instill the eye drops. If vision is severely compromised, a caregiver will need to be taught as well. Any sign of eye infection, especially fever, should be reported. In addition, the knowledge that certain medications, such as systemic steroids, may interfere with glaucoma control is essential. Support and counseling may also be necessary. In the case of open-angle glaucoma, patients need to know that they will most likely need bilateral treatment because the second eye is at risk for the same disease process.

DIABETIC RETINOPATHY

Diabetic retinopathy is a noninflammatory disorder of the retina that develops in patients with diabetes mellitus. It is typically divided into three stages: (1) background diabetic retinopathy, (2) preproliferative diabetic retinopathy, and (3) proliferative diabetic retinopathy. The initial evaluation for a patient with diabetes mellitus should include a referral to an ophthalmologist for a comprehensive eye evaluation, with particular attention to the aspects relevant to diabetic retinopathy.

EPIDEMIOLOGY AND CAUSES

Approximately 6.6% of the population aged 20 to 74 have diabetes mellitus; approximately 25% of individuals with diabetes have some form of diabetic retinopathy. Most patients with diabetes will eventually develop some form of retinopathy. Diabetic retinopathy accounts for approximately 10% of new cases of blindness each year and is the leading cause of new cases of legal blindness among Americans aged 20 to 64.

The peak incidence of type 1 diabetes mellitus is between ages 12 and 15; the peak incidence of type 2 diabetes mellitus is between ages 50 and 70. Almost all patients with diabetes will develop background diabetic retinopathy after they have had diabetes for at least 20 years. Two-thirds of patients with type 1 diabetes who have had the disease for at least 35 years will develop proliferative diabetic neuropathy, and one-third will develop macular edema. The proportions are reversed for patients with type 2 diabetes.

Diabetes mellitus type 1 occurs about equally in males and females, whereas type 2 is more common in women. Predilection for type 1 diabetes is higher among Anglo Americans (African Americans have the lowest incidence); however, certain groups, such as the Pima Indians, have a 35% incidence rate of diabetes mellitus type 2.

The longer the patient has had diabetes mellitus, the greater the likelihood that he or she will develop retinopathy. In addition, poor glycemic control translates into end-organ damage, including retinopathies, in patients with either type 1 or type 2 diabetes. Pregnancy, renal disease, systemic hypertension, smoking, and elevated serum lipid levels (associated with an increased risk of retinal lipid deposits) are all risk factors for the development of retinopathy.

PATHOPHYSIOLOGY

The key insult driving diabetic retinopathy is uncontrolled hyperglycemia. The precise mechanism by which this causes retinal damage is unclear, but there are several prevailing hypotheses that likely contribute to varying degrees. Hyperglycemia is known to contribute to the dysregulation of retinal blood flow. In the setting of systemic hypertension, increased shear stress on retinal blood vessels drives the release of vasoproliferative factors (e.g., vascular endothelial growth [VEGF] factor, insulin-like growth factor-1, basic fibroblast growth factor, hepatocyte growth factor) that stimulate neovascularization of the retina, optic nerve, and iris. The buildup of sorbitol (a by-product of glucose metabolism by the enzyme aldose reductase) in retinal cells is believed to increase intracellular osmolality, causing fluid shifts (cellular edema) and subsequent retinal damage. In hyperglycemic states, free amino acids, serum, and tissue proteins may all become irreversibly glycosylated. These end products are thought to cross-link with collagen fibers within the extracellular space, initiating microvascular complications. Retinal microthromboses composed of platelets and fibrin have also been proposed to stimulate neovascularization, as the body attempts to compensate for decreased retinal blood flow. Moreover, several other risk factors have been identified, including certain genetic predispositions and enzymatic allelic variants, serum hypertriglyceridemia, anemia, and hormonal fluctuations associated with pregnancy.

In the case of background diabetic retinopathy, retinal pericytes and the microvascular endothelium are damaged early in the disease process, leading to vascular permeability and basement membrane thickening (similar to the histopathological changes seen in diabetic nephropathy). This predisposes retinal capillaries to microaneurysms and the retinal surface to thickening with deposits of proteinaceous and lipid material (hard exudates). If the macula is affected (i.e., macular edema occurs), vision may gradually blur and progress to profound visual loss if left untreated. In the preproliferative phase, multiple cycles of cellular death and renewal lead to venous beading, tortuous venous dilation, and intraluminal cellular proliferation, along with platelet, erythrocyte, and fibrinogen aggregation, which ultimately results in vascular occlusion. Upstream of such lesions, flame shaped and blot hemorrhages occur; downstream, microvascular infarcts present as "cotton wool spots" or soft exudates on fundoscopy. Finally, the proliferative phase is characterized by neovascularization on the retinal surface, optic nerve, and iris. These fragile vessels may be venous or arterial in origin and may extend into the vitreous chamber, attaching to the posterior pole of the vitreous in a fine fibrous mesh. This network places stress on the retinal surface as the fibers contract. As a result, hemorrhage into the vitreous body and even retinal detachment may occur, requiring both vitrectomy and laser photocoagulation.

CLINICAL PRESENTATION

Subjective

The patient will complain of visual changes as the disease progresses but is usually asymptomatic in the early stages.

Objective

Changes will be noted on funduscopic examination. In background diabetic retinopathy, microaneurysms, intraretinal hemorrhage, macular edema, and lipid deposits may be apparent. As the disease progresses, nerve fiber layer infarctions ("cotton wool" spots), venous beading and dilation, edema, and, in some cases, extensive retinal hemorrhage will be noted. In the proliferative form of diabetic retinopathy, new blood vessel proliferation (neovascularization) may be seen on the retinal surface, optic nerve, and iris.

DIAGNOSTIC REASONING

Diagnostic Tests

A thorough eye examination should be done, including an assessment of visual acuity and documentation of the status of the iris, lens, vitreous, and fundus. Fluorescein angiography will demonstrate retinal nonperfusion, retinal leakage, and proliferative diabetic retinopathy.

Differential Diagnosis

A history of diabetes, especially if present for more than 10 years, correlated with observable changes on funduscopic examination, establishes the diagnosis. Other causes of retinopathy include hypertensive retinopathy, radiation retinopathy, and retinal venous obstruction.

MANAGEMENT

The first goal for patients at risk for microvascular complications, including diabetic retinopathy, is prevention. Risk is significantly increased for patients with blood sugar levels above 200 mg/dL. The most significant preventive measure is to keep blood sugar under control. The American Diabetes Association sets an acceptable level of glycated hemoglobin or HgbA1C at less than 7%. In patients who have their blood sugar under adequate control, the incidence of diabetic retinopathy is far lower and the onset in those who do develop this disease is later. All patients who carry the diagnosis of diabetes mellitus must be referred to ophthalmology on diagnosis.

Similarly, patients with diabetes and hypertension should strive to maintain as normal a blood pressure as possible to prevent the development of end-organ damage. Because many patients have both disorders, vigilance is especially important in this subset of patients.

The only pharmacologic agent that has been found to slow the progression of diabetic retinopathy is lisinopril, an angiotensin-converting enzyme inhibitor.

Laser surgery is recommended for patients with proliferative diabetic retinopathy and for patients with clinically significant macular edema.

Diabetic retinopathy patients should be followed by an ophthalmologist, who can decide when to treat the disorder with laser treatment (focal and panretinal photocoagulation); in certain cases, cryoretinopexy can be used to decrease the neovascular stimulus and to treat proliferative diabetic retinopathy. Vitrectomy may be considered for patients with severe proliferative diabetic retinopathy, traction retinal detachment involving the macula, and nonclearing vitreous hemorrhage (this surgical option should be considered after 1 month for a vitreous hemorrhage that has decreased the vision to the 5/200 level or worse).

FOLLOW-UP AND REFERRAL

All patients with diabetes mellitus should be monitored annually by an ophthalmologist. The patient with background retinopathy should be followed at least every 6 months, and patients with proliferative retinopathy should be seen at least every 3 to 4 months. Patients with active proliferative retinopathy should be seen approximately every 8 weeks.

Glaucoma, cataracts, retinal detachment, vitreous hemorrhage, and disc edema (papillopathy) are all common in patients with diabetic retinopathy, even in its early stages. Cataracts, especially, are common in patients with diabetes. If the patient has retinopathy, he or she should try to postpone the cataract surgery as long as possible because cataract surgery can sometimes worsen diabetic retinopathy.

Patient Education: Diabetic Retinopathy

Patients with diabetes, as well as those with hypertension, need to be educated regarding the need to keep their disease under maximal control to decrease the incidence of complications. Creating an alliance with the patient and family is essential in encouraging lifestyle changes. Working with the patient over time and being there for the patient are essential. Patients should be educated about the importance of ophthalmological evaluation and follow-up. Patience, advocacy, and commitment are all important qualities in working with these patients. Optimism and emphasis on the possibility for change, even if just to prevent further disease progression, are essential characteristics.

MACULAR DEGENERATION

Macular degeneration, or low vision, as it is sometimes referred to, is a disease of aging and is the leading cause of blindness in patients older than 60 years. Risk factors associated with macular degeneration are shown in the accompanying text.

Risk Factors: Macular Degeneration

- Caucasian race
- Female gender
- Age older than 60
- Cigarette smoking
- Family history
- Macular degeneration gene (complement factor H)

Other risk factors that are unproved, but documented in some studies, include the following:

- High serum cholesterol/obesity
- Low serum carotenoid levels
- Exposure to ultraviolet light
- Hypertension
- Light-colored eyes
- Far-sightedness
- Past cataract surgery

Macular degeneration is a condition characterized by slow, progressive atrophy and degeneration of the retina. This condition is called "dry" macular degeneration. Occasionally, new blood vessels develop under the retina in the macula, causing a sudden distortion or loss of central vision. This condition is known as "wet" AMD; it presents as a sudden decrease in vision that requires immediate referral to an ophthalmologist. There is often a progression from "dry" to "wet" macular degeneration.

EPIDEMIOLOGY AND CAUSES

The macula is the most sensitive and central portion of the retina, a nerve-rich area essential for sight. For largely unknown reasons, after age 60, the macula begins to break down. As it degenerates, central vision and fine detail perception deteriorate. Patients typically cannot read well (if at all), see facial details, or perform ordinary daily visual activities.

A recent study reported that 30% of individuals aged 75 and older have some form of AMD, and 7% of those aged 75 and older have an advanced form. Recent studies estimate that 8 million Americans are at risk for developing advanced AMD in the next 5 years, and 1.75 million are currently affected with the advanced form of the disease. AMD is the leading cause of blindness in older North Americans.

PATHOPHYSIOLOGY

Research in mice has provided a few genetic-based clues to the pathogenesis of AMD and has suggested that inflammatory dysfunction may have a role in pathogenesis. Growth factor, choriocapillary endothelial damage, and inflammatory cytokines are likely involved. Most recently, genetic research has shown that mutations in the gene for complement factor H on chromosome 1 are strongly associated with AMD, supporting a possible inflammatory etiology.

CLINICAL PRESENTATION

Subjective

The clinician's main task is to determine whether the problem is acute and requires referral for immediate treatment, or a more routine one. Determining whether the onset of the visual impairment is acute or gradual will assist the clinician in making this determination. Likewise, the severity of the visual loss is also important. Severe and sudden visual loss requires immediate referral to an ophthalmologist. Vitreous hemorrhage, retinal detachment, uveitis, retrobulbar optic neuritis, and vascular occlusion generally present in this manner. A gradual progressive change suggests a changing refractive error, cataract, glaucoma, diabetic retinopathy, and macular degeneration.

Objective

First, visual acuity must be evaluated, with the patient wearing any assistive lenses. If vision is less than 20/20, it should be checked by the pinhole test. Vision that corrects with the pinhole test implies an uncorrected refractive error. The clinician should then evaluate the external structure of the eye. The lids, conjunctivae, pupils, and extraocular movements should be checked. Acute angle-closure glaucoma presents with an unreactive pupil, for example. A Marcus Gunn pupil implies damage to the optic nerve. In addition, conjunctival injection is present with trauma, corneal problems, iritis, acute angle closure, glaucoma, and hyphema.

The fundoscopic examination is normal in patients with refractive errors. If dense, cataracts may make it hard to visualize the retina, but otherwise the examination is normal. Patients with glaucoma have increased cupping of the optic disc (a normal cup-to-disc ratio is 0.5 or less). Increased cupping is cause for referral to an ophthalmologist. Retinal hemorrhages, hard exudates, "cotton wool" spots, or neovascularization indicates diabetic retinopathy. If the fundus is difficult or impossible to view, suspect vitreous hemorrhage, especially in diabetic patients with sudden visual loss. Yellow round spots (drusen) may be indicative of early macular degeneration. Clumps of pigment irregularly interspersed with depigmented areas of atrophy in the macula are more typical of a later phase of the disorder.

DIAGNOSTIC REASONING

Diagnostic Tests

Analysis of central vision may be done with an Amsler grid to locate macular blind spots and areas of distortion and wavy lines. Measurement of contrast sensitivity with specially designed tests for low vision may reveal the degree of loss of retinal sensitivity (contrast) and indicate the potential success or failure of optical magnifying devices.

Differential Diagnosis

As previously discussed, visual impairment may be associated with a variety of conditions. The task of the clinician is to know when to refer for ophthalmology evaluation and treatment and which conditions can be treated in primary care. The characteristics of the associated symptoms and physical findings in the problem of visual loss require focused history and excellent physical examination skills. A recent study of primary-care providers found that approximately 25.0% of eyes deemed to be normal based on dilated eye examination by primary eye-care physicians had macular characteristics that indicated AMD revealed by fundus photography and trained raters. A total of 30.0% of eyes with undiagnosed AMD had AMD with large drusen that would have been treatable with nutritional supplements had it been diagnosed. Improved AMD detection strategies may be needed in primary eye care as more effective treatment strategies for early AMD become available in the coming years (Neely et al., 2017).

MANAGEMENT

There are no proven strategies for preventing AMD, nor are there any treatments for the initial stage of early disease. Some evidence has shown that in the intermediate stage of the disease, oral intake of high-dose antioxidant vitamins and zinc supplements modestly decreased the risk of developing severe vision loss. Recent evaluation of the evidence supports using genetic testing to guide selection of ocular vitamin use. This approach will avoid using supplements that could speed the progression of AMD in vulnerable patients, avoid using supplements that will have little to no effect in others, and result in appropriately using supplements in those that are likely to derive meaningful benefits.

Thermal laser photocoagulation may be used to treat certain forms of wet AMD. However, its use is of limited value for lesions in the central macula area. Wet AMD is also treated with injections directly into the eye (intravitreal) by a retinal specialist or ophthalmologist (see Drugs Commonly Prescribed 20.2). There is a recent literature review published in the United Kingdom of positive reports of nurse-led ranibizumab intravitreal injections in wet AMD. The medication used belongs to the class of drugs called anti-VEGF therapies. These drugs reduce the growth of abnormal blood vessels and may slow leakage from blood vessels. Large-scale clinical trials have demonstrated that these drugs preserved and even improved visual acuity. There are four drugs in this class: the monoclonal antibodies ranibizumab (Lucentis) and bevacizumab (Avastin), the nucleic acid VEGF inhibitor pegaptanib (Macugen), and the receptor fusion protein aflibercept (Eylea). These drugs are expensive and may not readily be covered by medical insurance. As the number of cases increase with the growing aging population, strategies that incorporate cost-effective methods that may include treatments provided by specialized nurse practitioners may become a trend.

Several clinical trials are also investigating potential alternative treatments for AMD, such as submacular surgery, photodynamic therapy, and irradiation. Antioxidants and other plant chemicals (phytochemicals) have been shown to protect against the development of macular degeneration.

FOLLOW-UP AND REFERRAL

The patient should be referred to a rehabilitation source where the outcome of the disease can be evaluated, daily living needs can be assessed, and visual aids offered. Sources may include ophthalmologists who provide low-vision services in their practices; optometrists who are trained to offer low-vision remediation; agencies for the visually impaired (either private or state supported); institutions that offer services for veterans; and organizations such as the American Academy of Ophthalmology, the American Optometric Association, the National Eye Institute, and Lighthouse International. A team approach is useful in rehabilitation, and the primary-care provider is part of the team. Because the loss of vision can be especially debilitating, quality of life needs to be assessed during routine primary-care visits.

Vision loss increases the risk of falls and may limit the patient's ability to live on his or her own. Depression rates are high in cases of vision loss, and screening in primary care for signs of depression is important. A psychosocial assessment with a multidisciplinary team should be arranged to explore resources and monitor quality of life.

Drugs Commonly Prescribed 20.2: Wet Acute Macular Degeneration

DRUG	INDICATION	DOSAGE	ADVERSE EFFECTS
Vascular Endothelial Growth Factor (VEGF)-Receptor Fusion Protein			
Aflibercept (Eyla)	Wet AMD (FDA approved)	2-mg intravitreal injection once a month for 3 months, then every 2 months	*Severe:* Allergic reaction including hives, difficulty breathing, and facial swelling; retinal detachment; endophthalmitis
Anti-VEGF Monoclonal Antibody			
Bevacizumab (Avastin)	Wet AMD (unapproved)	1.25-mg intravitreal injection once a month (off-label use)	*Moderate:* Eye pain; eye redness; sudden vision changes, including flashes of light; photophobia; severe headache with confusion
Nucleic Acid VEGF Inhibitor			
Pegaptanib (Macugen)	Wet AMD (FDA approved)	0.3-mg intravitreal injection every 6 weeks	*Mild:* Watery eyes; blurred vision; pain at injection site; edema of eyelid
Anti-VEGF Monoclonal Antibody			
Ranibizumab (Lucentis)	Wet AMD (FDA approved)	0.5-mg intravitreal injection every month	

Abbreviations: AMD, age-related macular degeneration; FDA, Food and Drug Administration.

Nursing Situation: Living With Severe Visual Impairment

Mr. Nesbitt is a 78-year-old widower who has been in your practice for 15 years. You have managed his hypertension and mild congestive heart failure for the past 5 years, and he has been following all your advice, including walking 1 mile every day, weather permitting. He was recently diagnosed with AMD, and his visual loss has been progressive. He has always been very active in community events since the death of his wife and spends several hours each day at the local senior center where he entertains the other seniors by playing the piano during lunchtime. He usually drives himself the 2 miles across town to the center and has been doing all of his own grocery shopping, cooking, and tending to his house and yard. He has a large garden and shares his produce with his neighbors. He tearfully admits that his children have been after him to stop driving and to give up his home and move to an assisted living facility. He says he has not had any accidents and that he stays close to the center line when he drives and knows the route by heart. "I could get there blindfolded," he jokingly remarks. As to moving he says, "Why would I do that? I know where everything is, and I haven't had any problems. My kids can help me. If they put me in a home, I might as well be dead." Mr. Nesbitt has two sons aged 50 and 49. Both of these men have jobs that take them out of town a good portion of the week. Both work in the family business started by their father. One son is divorced with two teenage boys, and the other is married with four children and one grandchild.

This past week both sons called asking you to bring Mr. Nesbitt to his senses and to take away his car keys, relating that he has had two near misses in the past 2 weeks. They say that he refuses to listen to reason and that his reason for the near misses is that he "got distracted by a pedestrian jaywalking and by a school bus."

Some of the issues in this case were addressed in a small study by Moore and Miller (2003) that focused on older men's experiences of living with severe visual impairment. In this study, a phenomenological approach was used to investigate the experience of severe visual impairment in eight older men with macular degeneration. Six central themes that emerged were as follows: (1) abilities and inabilities, (2) cherishing of independence, (3) creating strategies, (4) acknowledging the progression of visual impairment, (5) confronting uncertainties and fears, and (6) persisting with hope and optimism.

One interesting finding in this study was that the theme of uncertainty encompassed skepticism about their diagnosis and treatment. Acceptance of the fact that there is no successful treatment for AMD is hard for most individuals, and persisting with hope and optimism needs to be supported in the face of severe progressive visual loss and mistrust of how their case is managed. A recent study (Emsfors et al., 2017) conducted patient interviews that revealed important information about nursing actions that created a sense of good nursing care in patients with wet AMD. Nurses acknowledged people as individuals and created trust by building partnerships and sharing decision making. To address each patient's concerns, nurses need to prioritize patients' narrative and participation by documenting agreements in their medical record.

Gopinath et al. (2015) investigated caregivers of those with advanced AMD. A high prevalence of caregiver distress related to caring for persons with advanced AMD was observed. Level of dependence on the caregiver and presence of comorbid chronic illnesses were independent predictors of the caregiver experiencing psychological distress. More than one in two caregivers reported a negative state of mind.

Patient Education: Age-Related Macular Degeneration

Recognition of the signs of advanced AMD is crucial for the success of treatment in preventing visual loss. Self-monitoring of central vision in both eyes using an Amsler grid may be useful in detecting subtle visual changes or distortion, as well as monitoring changes in vision once they have been detected. A hallmark of AMD is visual difficulties in low light.

Smoking cessation and improvement of cardiovascular risk factors are important variables in the progression of AMD. Patients should be instructed as to rehabilitation resources in the community and encouraged to take advantage of programs specifically targeted for AMD.

Optical aids include spectacles with and without prisms, hand magnifiers, stand-mounted magnifiers, and telescopes. As with any type of rehabilitation, time and patience are needed to determine the appropriate remedial lens for the patient. Working with the patient until he or she understands how to use the device is an important part of patient education. In addition, patients may be taught skills such as folding money in such a way that the denomination is more apparent, as well as techniques for grooming and for identifying medications. The goal is to use "practical approaches tailored to individual's specific needs" (see The Patient's Voice 20.1).

The Patient's Voice 20.1: Macular Degeneration

My mother, who is 78, called me in a panic because she could not see out of one eye. The ophthalmologist agreed to see her right away. When we met with the doctor after her examination, he told us that she had been diagnosed with macular degeneration 4 years ago. She had never told a soul! "I couldn't stand the thought of being a burden." That's what she told me. If only I'd known, maybe we could have done more to slow down the disease. Now, if anything happens to her other eye, I don't know what we'll do. This will change everything about how my mother lives and will affect everyone in the family.

REFERENCES

General

Bostock-Cox B. Red flag eye conditions: A guide for the practice nurse. *Practice Nurse.* 2017;47(2):28–32.

Final Recommendation Statement: Impaired visual acuity in older adults: screening. Rockville, MD: Agency for Healthcare Research and Quality; March 1, 2016. https://www.uspreventiveservices taskforce.org/Page/Document/RecommendationStatement Final/impaired-visual-acuity-in-older-adults-screening. Accessed September 29, 2018.

Cataracts

Age-Related Eye Disease Study 2 (AREDS2) Research Group; Chew EY, SanGiovanni JP, Ferris FL, et al. Lutein/zeaxanthin for the treatment of age-related cataract: AREDS2 randomized trial report no. 4. *JAMA Ophthalmol.* 2013;131(7):843–850.

Christen WG, Glynn RJ, Ajani UA, et al. Smoking cessation and risk of age-related cataract in men. *JAMA.* 2000;284(6):713–716.

Christen WG, Glynn RJ, Gaziano JM, et al. Age-related cataract in men in the selenium and vitamin E cancer prevention trial eye endpoints study: A randomized clinical trial. *JAMA Ophthalmol.* 2015;133(1):17–24.

Chylack LT Jr, Wolfe JK, Singer DM, et al. The Lens Opacities Classification System III. *Arch Ophthalmol.* 1993;111(6):831–836.

Day AC, Donachie PH, Sparrow JM, Johnston RL; Royal College of Ophthalmologists' National Ophthalmology Database. The Royal College of Ophthalmologists' National Ophthalmology Database study of cataract surgery: Report 1, visual outcomes and complications. *Eye.* 2015;29:552–560.

Glaser TS, Doss LE, Shih G, et al. The association of dietary lutein plus zeaxanthin and B vitamins with cataracts in the age-related eye disease study: AREDS report no. 37. *Ophthalmology.* 2015; 122:1471.

Gupta VB, Rajagopala M, Ravishankar B. Etiopathogenesis of cataract: An appraisal. *Indian J Ophthalmol.* 2014;62(2):103–110.

Juthani VV, Clearfield E, Chuck RS. Non-steroidal anti-inflammatory drugs versus corticosteroids for controlling inflammation after uncomplicated cataract surgery. *Cochrane Database Syst Rev* 2017;7:CD010516.

Keay L, Lindsley K, Tielsch J, et al. Routine preoperative medical testing for cataract surgery. *Cochrane Database Syst Rev* 2012;2:CD007293.

Kessel L, Andresen J, Erngaard D, et al. Indication for cataract surgery. Do we have evidence of who will benefit from surgery? A systematic review and meta-analysis. *Acta Ophthalmol.* 2016;94:10–20.

Lai FH, Lok JY, Chow PP, Young AL. Clinical outcomes of cataract surgery in very elderly adults. *J Am Geriatr Soc.* 2014;62(1):165–170.

Lewallen S, Mousa A, Bassett K, Courtright P. Cataract surgical coverage remains lower in women. *Br J Ophthalmol.* 2009;93:295–298.

Lindblad BE, Håkansson N, Wolk A. Smoking cessation and the risk of cataract: A prospective cohort study of cataract extraction among men. *JAMA Ophthalmol.* 2014;132:253.

Liu Y-C, Wilkins M, Kim T, Malyugin B, Mehta JS. Cataracts. *Lancet.* 2017;390:600–612.

Lundström M, Barry P, Henry Y, Rosen P, Stenevi U. Evidence-based guidelines for cataract surgery: Guidelines based on data in the European Registry of Quality Outcomes for Cataract and Refractive Surgery database. *J Cataract Refract Surg.* 2012;38:1086–1093.

Mathew MC, Ervin AM, Tao J, Davis RM. Antioxidant vitamin supplementation for preventing and slowing the progression of age-related cataract. *Cochrane Database Syst Rev.* 2012;13:CD004567.

McAlinden C, Gothwal VK, Khadka J, et al. A head-to-head comparison of 16 cataract surgery outcome questionnaires. *Ophthalmology.* 2011;118:2374–2381.

O'Day DM. (1995). Socioeconomics viewpoint: the need for an update of the clinical practice guideline on cataract. *Arch Ophthalmol.* 1995;113(6):718–720.

Olson RJ, Braga-Mele R, Huang Chen S, et al. Cataract in the adult eye preferred practice pattern®. *Ophthalmology.* 2017;124(2):P1–P119.

Schein OD, Cassard SD, Tielsch JM, Gower EW. Cataract surgery among Medicare beneficiaries. *Ophthalmic Epidemiol.* 2012;19:257–264.

Schein OD, Katz J, Bass EB, et al. The value of routine preoperative medical testing before cataract surgery. Study of medical testing for cataract surgery. *N Engl J Med.* 2000;342:168–175.

The Royal College of Ophthalmologists. Commissioning guide: cataract surgery, 2015. https:www.rcophth.ac.uk/wp-content/uploads/2015/03/Commissioning-Guide-Cataract-Surgery-Final-February-2015.pdf. Published 2015.

Virendrakumar B, Jolley E, Gordon I, Bascaran C, Schmidt E. Availability of evidence on cataract in low/middle-income settings: A review of reviews using evidence gap maps approach. *Br J Ophthalmol.* 2016;100(11):1455–1460.

Young B, Wu C, Wu A, Margo C, Greenberg P. Are clinical practice guidelines for cataract and glaucoma trustworthy? *Am J Med Qual.* 2015;30(2):188–190.

Zhao LQ, Li LM, Zhu H. The effect of multivitamin/mineral supplements on age-related cataracts: A systematic review and meta-analysis. *Nutrients.* 2014;6(3):931–949.

Diabetic Retinopathy

American Academy of Ophthalmology Retina/Vitreous Panel. Preferred Practice Pattern® Guidelines. Diabetic retinopathy. San Francisco, CA: American Academy of Ophthalmology. https://www.aao.org/preferred-practice-pattern/diabetic-retinopathy-ppp-updated-2017. Published 2017.

American Diabetes Association. Standards of medical care in diabetes—2017. *Diabetes Care.* 2017;40(suppl 1):S1–135.

Cheung N, Mitchell P, Wong TY. Diabetic retinopathy. *Lancet.* 2010;376(9735):124–136.

Mohamed Q, Gillies MC, Wong TY. Management of diabetic retinopathy: A systematic review. *JAMA.* 2007 22;298(8):902–916.

Perente I, Alkin Z, Ozkaya A, et al. Focal laser photocoagulation in non-center involved diabetic macular edema. *Med Hypothesis Discov Innov Ophthalmol.* 2014;3(1):9–16.

Solomon SD, Chew E, Duh EJ, et al. Diabetic retinopathy: A position statement by the American Diabetes Association. *Diabetes Care.* 2017;40(9):412–418.

Glaucoma

Boland MV, Ervin AM, Friedman D, et al. Treatment for glaucoma: comparative effectiveness (comparative effectiveness review no. 60; AHRQ publication no. 12-EHC038-EF). Rockville, MD: Agency for Healthcare Research and Quality; April 2012.

Boland MV, Ervin AM, Friedman DS, et al. Comparative effectiveness of treatments for open-angle glaucoma: A systematic review for the U.S. Preventive Services Task Force. *Ann Intern Med.* 2013;158(4):271–279.

Canadian Ophthalmological Society Glaucoma Clinical Practice Guideline Expert Committee; Canadian Ophthalmological Society. Canadian Ophthalmological Society evidence-based clinical practice guidelines for the management of glaucoma in the adult eye. *Can J Ophthalmol.* 2009;44(suppl):S7–93.

Ervin AM, Boland MV, Myrowitz EH, et al. Screening for glaucoma: Comparative effectiveness (comparative effectiveness review no. 59; AHRQ Publication No. 12-EHC037-EF). Rockville, MD: Agency for Healthcare Research and Quality; April 2012.

Feder RS, Olsen TW, Prum BE Jr, et al. Comprehensive adult medical eye evaluation. Preferred Practice Pattern(®) Guidelines. *Ophthalmology.* 2016;123(1):P209–236.

Friedman DS, Jampel HD, Muñoz B, West SK. The prevalence of open-angle glaucoma among blacks and whites 73 years and older: The Salisbury Eye Evaluation Glaucoma Study. *Arch Ophthalmol.* 2006;124(11):1625–1630.

Lee PP, Feldman ZW, Ostermann J, Brown DS, Sloan FA. Longitudinal prevalence of major eye diseases. *Arch Ophthalmol.* 2003;121(9):1303–1310.

Prum BE Jr, Herndon LW Jr, Moroi SE, et al. Primary angle closure Preferred Practice Pattern(®) Guidelines. *Ophthalmology.* 2016;123(1):P1–P40.

Prum BE Jr, Lim MC, Mansberger SL, et al. Primary open-angle glaucoma suspect Preferred Practice Pattern® Guidelines. *Ophthalmology.* 2016;123(1):P112–151.

U.S. Preventive Services Task Force. Final update summary: Glaucoma: Screening. https://www.uspreventiveservicestaskforce.org/Page/Document/UpdateSummaryFinal/glaucoma-screening. Published September 2016.

Macular Degeneration

American Academy of Ophthalmology. Retina/vitreous panel. Age-related macular degeneration. Preferred Practice Pattern® Guidelines. San Francisco, CA: American Academy of Ophthalmology; 2015. https://www.aao.org/preferred-practice-pattern/age-related-macular-degeneration-ppp-2015.

Chakravarthy U, Evans J, Rosenfeld PJ. Age related macular degeneration. *BMJ.* 2010;340:c981.

Christen WG, Glynn RJ, Manson JE, et al. Effects of multivitamin supplement on cataract and age-related macular degeneration in a randomized trial of male physicians. *Ophthalmology.* 2014;121(2):525–534.

Donoso L, Vrabec T, Kuivaniemi H. The role of complement Factor H in age-related macular degeneration: A review. *Surv Ophthalmol.* 2010;55(3):227–246.

Emsfors Å, Christensson L, Elgán C. Nursing actions that create a sense of good nursing care in patients with wet age-related macular degeneration. *J Clin Nurs.* 2017;26(17/18):2680–2688.

Ferris FL III, Wilkinson CP, Bird A, et al. Clinical classification of age-related macular degeneration. *Ophthalmology.* 2013;120:844–851.

Finger RP, Wiedemann P, Blumhagen F, Pohl K, Holz FG. Treatment patterns visual acuity and quality of life outcomes of the WAVE study. *ACTA Ophthalmol.* 2013;91(6):540–546.

Gopinath B, Kifley A, Cummins R, Heraghty J, Mitchell P. Predictors of psychological distress in caregivers of older persons with wet age-related macular degeneration. *Aging Ment Health.* 2015;19(3):239-246.

Gregg E. Nurse-led ranibizumab intravitreal injections in wet age-related macular degeneration: A literature review. *Nurs Stand.* 2017;31(33):44–52.

Kaldenberg J, Smallfield S. *Occupational therapy practice guidelines for older adults with low vision.* Bethesda, MD: American Occupational Therapy Association; 2013.

Kauppinen A, Paterno J, Blasiak J, Salminen A, Kaarniranta K. Inflammation and its role in age-related macular degeneration. *Cell Mol Life Sci.* 2016;73:1765–1786.

Klein R, Klein BE, Knudtson MD, et al. Prevalence of age-related macular degeneration in 4 racial/ethnic groups in the multi-ethnic study of atherosclerosis. *Ophthalmology.* 2006;113:373–380.

Lim LS, Mitchell P, Seddon JM, Holz FG, Wong TY. Age-related macular degeneration. *Lancet.* 2012;379(9827):1728–1738

Moore LW, Miller M. Older men's experiences of living with severe visual impairment. *J Adv Nurs.* 2003;43(1):10–18.

Moore LW, Miller M. Driving strategies used by older adults with macular degeneration: Assessing the risks. *Appl Nurs Res.* 2005;18:110–116.

Neely DC, Bray KJ, Huisingh CE, et al. Prevalence of undiagnosed age-related macular degeneration in primary eye care. *JAMA Ophthalmol.* 2017;135(6):570–575.

Rojas-Fernandez CH, Tyber K. Benefits, potential harms, and optimal use of nutritional supplementation for preventing progression of age-related macular degeneration. *Ann Pharmacother.* 2017;51(3):264–270.

Sharts-Hopko N. Low vision and blindness among midlife and older adults: A review of the nursing literature. *Holis Nurs Pract.* 2009;23(2):94–100.

Stein JD, Newman-Casey PA, Mrinalini T, et al. Cost-effectiveness of bevacizumab and ranibizumab for newly diagnosed neovascular macular degeneration. *Ophthalmology.* 2014;121:936-45.

Tufail A, Patel PJ, Egan C, et al. Bevacizumab for neovascular age related macular degeneration (ABC trial): Multicentre randomized double masked study. *BMJ.* 2010;340:c2459.

Refractory Errors

Chew EY. Nutrition effects on ocular diseases in the aging eye. *Invest Ophthalmol Vis Sci.* 2013;54(14):42–47.

Chou R, Dana T, Bougatsos C, Grusing S, Blazina I. Screening for impaired visual acuity in older adults: Updated evidence report and systematic review for the US Preventive Services Task Force. *JAMA.* 2016;315(9):915–933.

Davila E, Caban-Martinez A, Muennig P, et al. Sensory impairment among older U.S. workers. *Am J Public Health.* 2009;99(8):1378–1385.

Okwen M, Lewallen S, Courtright P. Primary eye care skills scores for health workers in routine and enhanced supervision settings. *Public Health.* 2014;128(1):96–100.

World Health Organization. Vision 2020 the right to sight: Global initiative for the elimination of avoidable blindness. http://www.who.int/blindness/Vision2020_report.pdf. Published 2007. Accessed June 5, 2016.

RESOURCES

American Diabetes Association—Retinopathy
http://www.diabetesforecast.org/diabetes-101/retinopathy-eye-disease
American Macular Degeneration Foundation
http://www.glaucoma.org/
Cleveland Clinic
https://my.clevelandclinic.org/health/articles/age-related-macular-degeneration

Glaucoma Research Foundation
   http://www.glaucoma.org/

National Eye Institute

Age-Related Macular Degeneration
   https://nei.nih.gov/health/maculardegen/armd_facts
Cataract
   https://nei.nih.gov/health/cataract

Diabetic Eye Disease
   https://nei.nih.gov/sites/default/files/health-pdfs/Refractiveerrors.pdf
Glaucoma
   https://nei.nih.gov/health/glaucoma/
Refractive Errors
   https://nei.nih.gov/sites/default/files/health-pdfs/Refractiveerrors.pdf

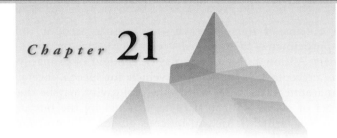

Chapter **21**

Common Ear, Nose, and Throat Complaints

Ruth McCaffrey, DNP, APRN, FNP-BC, GNP, FAAN, FAANP

Lynne M. Dunphy, PhD, APRN, FNP-BC, FAAN, FAANP

Brian Oscar Porter, MD, PhD, MPH, MBA

EAR PAIN (OTALGIA)

Ear pain, also known as *otalgia*, is a common clinical complaint. Ear pain can be caused by an infection. However, in the absence of physical signs in the structures of the ear, other causes of ear pain need to be ruled out, such as dental abscesses, sinus infections, temporomandibular joint disease, or mastoiditis. Otalgia can be bilateral or localized to one ear. Ear pain may become more prevalent in the summer months due to otitis externa (swimmer's ear) or sinus infections, which can be more common during peak allergen season. Ear pain associated with acute and chronic otitis media is frequently associated with eustachian tube dysfunction, especially in the pediatric population.

DIFFERENTIAL DIAGNOSIS

Otalgia is defined as ear pain. Two separate and distinct types of otalgia exist. Pain that originates within the ear is primary otalgia; pain that originates outside the ear is referred otalgia.

Primary otalgia is typically caused by are external otitis, otitis media, mastoiditis, and auricular infections. When an ear is draining and accompanied by tympanic membrane perforation, simply looking in the ear and noting the pathology can make the diagnosis. When the tympanic membrane appears normal, however, the diagnosis becomes more difficult. Otalgia may also be referred by other locations (referred otalgia). Although many entities can cause referred otalgia, their relationship to ear pain must be identified. A categorical discussion of the work-up, treatment, prognosis, demographics, and other issues is beyond the scope of this text because the various pathologies responsible for creating referred otalgia are so diverse.

The differential diagnosis of ear pain includes the following disorders:

- Otitis externa
- Acute otitis media
- Otitis media with effusion
- Eustachian tube dysfunction
- Barotrauma (pressure changes in the immediate atmosphere, such as when flying)
- Cerumen impaction
- Dental disease
- Temporomandibular joint dysfunction
- Perforated tympanic membrane
- Sinus disease
- Cervical lymphadenopathy

IMPAIRED HEARING

Hearing loss is the decreased ability or complete inability to hear, which may be temporary or permanent. It may involve the middle ear, which indicates a mechanical or conductive problem (usually implying a reversible issue), or the inner ear, which indicates a nerve or sensorineural issue. In fact, hearing loss may have both conductive and sensorineural components.

One of the first assessments to identify the cause of hearing loss should be to check for cerumen (ear wax) impaction, which can decrease hearing. Once the impaction is removed, hearing may return to normal. Many types of hearing loss can be improved with hearing aids; however, only 10% to 15% of patients who could benefit from a hearing aid actually use one. The most common reasons for not wearing a hearing aid include background noise, poor fit and discomfort, care and maintenance requirements, expense (including initial cost and maintenance and battery costs), increased risk of ear infections and cerumen impaction, and tinnitus.

Hearing loss is a universal phenomenon of aging, with an increased incidence in individuals with a family history of hearing loss. In particular, sensorineural hearing loss increases with age, with degenerative decline starting at age 20 years, without regard to ethnicity or gender. The prevalence of hearing loss increases after age 40 years, affecting approximately 25% of all adults aged 65 to 74 years and 50% of all adults older than age 85 years.

DIFFERENTIAL DIAGNOSIS

The differential diagnosis of hearing loss includes the following disorders:

- Presbycusis
- Noise exposure
- Ototoxic drugs
- Eustachian tube dysfunction
- Cerumen impaction
- Chronic middle ear infection, effusion
- Otosclerosis
- Tympanosclerosis
- Cholesteatoma
- Trauma
- Congenital disorders

TINNITUS

Tinnitus is a subjective ringing or buzzing sound in the ear. It may be intermittent, continuous, or pulsatile (i.e., synchronous with the heartbeat). It has been variously described as the sound of escaping air or running water; the sound heard inside a large seashell; or a buzzing, ringing, or humming noise. Tinnitus also has been described as a roaring or musical sound. It may be unilateral or bilateral. Tinnitus can be a minor irritation for some or a debilitation for others. It can be caused by different diseases or drug toxicities, and the underlying cause should be addressed to reduce the tinnitus.

Recent estimates suggest that as many as 40 million Americans are affected by tinnitus. Approximately 90% of patients with hearing loss experience some tinnitus, and approximately 1% of the population has chronic tinnitus.

DIFFERENTIAL DIAGNOSIS

The differential diagnosis of subjective tinnitus includes the following disorders:
- Otologic: hearing loss, Ménière's disease, acoustic neuroma
- Ototoxic medications or substances
- Neurologic: multiple sclerosis, head injury

- Metabolic: thyroid disorder, hyperlipidemia, vitamin B_{12} deficiency
- Psychogenic: depression, anxiety, fibromyalgia

MOUTH SORES

Problems of the oral cavity and throat account for approximately 20% of visits to primary-care practitioners. Although the mouth may be thought of primarily as a receptacle for food and a vehicle for speech, several anatomical structures within the oral cavity may be the foci of disease. The oral cavity is lined by the buccal mucosa, which is rich in mucous glands. The mucous glands of the lips open into the oral cavity. The mouth cavity communicates with the pharynx posteriorly. The floor of the mouth contains the tongue and the openings of the submandibular and sublingual salivary glands.

Specific lesions of the oral and buccal mucosa may be immunogenic, inflammatory (most commonly aphthous ulcers), traumatic, or caused by a localized malignancy. Painful inflammatory lesions may occur in isolation, or they may be associated with a generalized disorder of other mucous membranes or the skin. The patient's medical history is important because it indicates whether the lesions are acute or chronic, single or multiple, and primary or recurrent.

DIFFERENTIAL DIAGNOSIS

The differential diagnosis of mouth sores includes the following:

- Food or drug allergies
- Chemical irritation
- Dry mouth
- Mechanical or thermal injury, such as braces or dentures
- Infections (bacterial, viral, fungal)
- Host immunosuppression
- Nutritional deficiency

HOARSENESS

Hoarseness is a common complaint; the term describes a voice with a harsh quality and low pitch. Hoarseness suggests an abnormality in voice production at the level of the larynx. It is a common symptom that may occur in both men and women at any age. Changes in the voice are part of the natural process of aging. In elderly men, the voice becomes weaker and higher in pitch as a result of muscle atrophy and increased stiffness of tissues. In women, the same changes occur, but the pitch of the voice becomes lower because during menopause, mucoid edema accumulates in the submucosa of the vocal folds. More severe edema and polyps may occur in women who smoke. The prevalence of hoarseness is 41% in adults aged 50 to 79 years, with no significant difference in gender. However, hoarseness is a cardinal sign of laryngeal cancer, which is most commonly seen in men aged 50 to 70 years.

DIFFERENTIAL DIAGNOSIS

Differential Diagnosis 21.1 categorizes the differential diagnoses of hoarseness.

SORE THROAT

Sore throat (pharyngitis) is defined as discomfort or pain in the throat that is most intense when swallowing. It can be associated with a sore mouth, especially if caused by a viral infection such as herpes simplex virus (HSV) that erupts as lesions that can cause soreness in both anatomical locations. Sore throat can be part of a generalized upper respiratory infection or a specific infection localized in the pharynx. The most common causes of sore throat are streptococcal or viral infections, such as from rhinovirus. Each year in the United States, pharyngitis is responsible for 40 million visits to healthcare providers, as adults typically experience at least two sore throats per year. Viral pharyngitis is one of the most common causes of absence from work or school.

DIFFERENTIAL DIAGNOSIS

The differential diagnosis for sore throat includes the following conditions:

- Streptococcal pharyngitis
- Tonsillitis
- HSV infection
- *Gonococcus*
- Candidiasis
- Aphthous ulceration
- Influenza virus
- Rhinovirus, adenovirus, Epstein-Barr virus, coxsackievirus
- Mycoplasma infection

Differential Diagnosis 21.1: Hoarseness

Infectious and Inflammatory

- Viral laryngitis
- Bacterial tracheitis or laryngitis
- Papillomatosis
- Chronic allergies
- Postnasal drip

Neurologic

- Dystonia
- Neuromuscular disease (e.g., vocal cord paralysis)
- Laryngeal nerve involvement by thyroid, pulmonary, or esophageal causes

Traumatic

- Smoke inhalation
- Chronic cough
- Esophageal reflux
- Overuse of the larynx (from yelling, singing, or prolonged speaking)
- Throat muscle atrophy (i.e., from aging)
- Gastroesophageal reflux disease

Neoplastic

- Vocal cord nodules or polyps
- Vocal cord cancer
- Supraglottic cancer with muscle invasion

REFERENCES

Ear Pain

Djalilian HR. Symptoms: Ear infections and joint pain. *Hearing J.* 2015;68(4):16–20.

Hui CP; Canadian Paediatric Society, Infectious Diseases and Immunization Committee. Acute otitis externa. *Paediatr Child Health.* 2013;18(2):96–98.

Wade T, Sames E, Beach MJ, Collier SA, Dalfour AP. The incidence and health burden of earaches attributable to recreational swimming in natural waters: A prospective cohort study. *Environ Health.* 2013;12:67.

Worrall G. Acute earache. *Can Fam Physician.* 2011;57(9):1019–1021.

Hoarseness

U.S. Preventive Services Task Force. *Screening for oral cancer: Recommendation statement.* Rockville, MD: Agency for Healthcare Research and Quality. http://www.ahrq.gov/clinic/3rduspsf/oralcanrs.htm. Published November 2013.

Impaired Hearing

Dalton DS, Cruickshanks KJ, Klein BE, et al. The impact of hearing loss on quality of life in older adults. *Gerontologist.* 2003;43(5):661–668.

Oh IH, Lee JH, Park DC, et al. Hearing loss as a function of aging and diabetes mellitus: A cross sectional study. *PLoS One.* 2014;9(12):e116161.

Owen D. High-tech hope for the hard of hearing. *New Yorker Magazine.* April 3, 2017. http://www.newyorker.com/magazine/2017/04/03/high-tech-hope-for-the-hard-of-hearing.

Williams TR, Alam S, Gaffney M; Centers for Disease Control and Prevention. Progress in identifying infants with hearing loss—United States, 2006–2012. *MMWR Morb Mortal Wkly Rep.* 2015;64(13):351–356.

Mouth Sores

Altenburg A, El-Haj N, Micheli C, Puttkammer M, Abdel-Naser MB, Zouboulis CC. The treatment of chronic recurrent oral aphthous ulcers. *Dtsch Arztebl Int.* 2011;111(40):665–673.

Scully C. *Aphthous ulcers treatment & management.* http://emedicine.medscape.com/article/867080-treatment. Published 2017.

Tarakji B, Gazal G, Al-Maweri SA, Azzeghaiby SN, Alaizari N. Guideline for the diagnosis and treatment of recurrent aphthous stomatitis for dental practitioners. *J Int Oral Health.* 2015;7(5):74–80.

Tinnitus

Joo Y-H, Han K-D, Park KH. Association of hearing loss and tinnitus with health-related quality of life: The Korea National Health and Nutrition Examination Survey. *PLoS One.* 2015;10(6):e0131247.

Lindblad A-C, Rosenhall U, Olofsson Å, Hagerman B. Tinnitus and other auditory problems – occupational noise exposure below risk limits may cause inner ear dysfunction. *PLoS One.* 2014;9(5):e97377.

Møller AR. Sensorineural tinnitus: Its pathology and probable therapies. *Int J Otolaryngol.* 2016;2016:2830157.

Weaver J. First evidence-based tinnitus guideline shines light on treatment. *Hearing J.* 2014;67(12):19, 22–24.

Sore Throat

Brook I. Treatment challenges of group A beta-hemolytic streptococcal pharyngo-tonsillitis. *Int Arch Otorhinolaryngol.* 2017;21(3):286–296.

Choi HG, Park B, Sim S, Ahn SH. Tonsillectomy does not reduce upper respiratory infections: A national cohort study. *PLoS One.* 2016;11(12):e0169264.

Stelter K. Tonsillitis and sore throat in children. *GMS Curr Top Otorhinolaryngol Head Neck Surg.* 2014;13:Doc07. http://www.egms.de/static/en/journals/cto/2014-13/cto000110.shtml.

RESOURCES

American Academy of Otolaryngology
www.entnet.org

American Tinnitus Association
https://www.ata.org/

Better Hearing Institute
www.betterhearing.org

National Institute on Deafness and Other Communication Disorders
https://www.nidcd.nih.gov/

NursesLabs: Impaired Verbal Communication
https://nurseslabs.com/impaired-verbal-communication

Oral Cancer Foundation
www.oralcancerfoundation.org

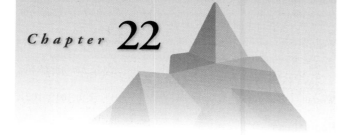

Chapter **22**

Hearing and Balance Disorders

Ruth McCaffrey, DNP, APRN, FNP-BC, GNP, FAAN, FAANP

Lynne M. Dunphy, PhD, APRN, FNP-BC, FAAN, FAANP

Brian Oscar Porter, MD, PhD, MPH, MBA

HEARING LOSS

Hearing loss may be acute or insidious. While rapid hearing loss typically triggers a patient to seek medical care, many forms of hearing impairment are slowly progressive and may not be perceptible by the patient until he or she can no longer compensate effectively for this sensory loss (i.e., an inability to understand others' speech).

EPIDEMIOLOGY AND CAUSES

Approximately 17% (36 million) of American adults aged 45 to 64 years have hearing impairment. Aging is a factor in hearing loss, with degeneration of delicate inner ear structures over time. In turn, among older Americans, hearing impairment is present in 30% of adults aged 65 to 74 years and 47% of adults aged 75 years and older. Men are more likely than women to experience hearing loss, and for some adults, heredity plays a role in hearing loss through the genetic susceptibility to ear damage.

Chronic middle ear infections (otitis media) are a contributing factor to the development of hearing loss, especially if they are recurrent, due to the scarring that can affect middle ear structures from repeated bouts of inflammation and healing. A ruptured tympanic membrane occurring as a complication of advanced otitis media or from direct physical trauma can lead to hearing loss, which may improve with uncomplicated healing. Acoustic trauma or exposure to loud noises, either occupationally or recreationally, is also a risk factor for hearing loss, as are ototoxic drugs (e.g., aminoglycoside antibiotics, aspirin, quinine). Allergies, cerumen impaction, and other causes of eustachian tube obstruction may also contribute to hearing loss. Risk factors for cerumen impaction specifically include ear canal hairs, hearing aids, bony growths secondary to osteophytes or osteomas, and previous episodes of impacted cerumen.

PATHOPHYSIOLOGY

Sensorineural hearing loss is defined as a lesion in the organ of Corti or in the central neural pathways of the ear, including the cranial nerve (CN) VIII and auditory cortex. Age-related hearing loss, termed *presbycusis,* is a form of sensorineural hearing loss. After age 50, otic hair cells in the organ of Corti tend to degenerate, and the *stria vascularis,* a capillary-fed layer of stratified epithelium that secretes endolymph and promotes the sensitization of hair cells in the cochlea, may atrophy. These changes first affect perception of high-frequency sounds, which then progresses to affect the detection of lower-frequency tones. Sensorineural hearing loss may also be a result of Ménière's disease or be noise-induced from repeated acoustic trauma.

Conductive hearing loss results when the passage of sound waves through the tympanic membrane and inner ear is impaired. Sound waves travels from the external environment through the ear canal to the tympanic membrane, where the vibrations are transmitted across the middle ear by three delicate bones known as the ossicles (malleus, incus, stapes). Conductive hearing loss may occur at any age due to factors that reduce the flow of sound waves through the ear canal, across the tympanic membrane, and to the middle ear ossicles. However, conductive hearing loss is often reversible (see Differential Diagnosis 22.1).

▓ Differential Diagnosis 22.1: Causes of Sensorineural Hearing Loss and Conductive Hearing Loss

Causes of Sensorineural Hearing Loss	Causes of Conductive Hearing Loss
Presbycusis	Cerumen impaction
Ménière's disease	Perforation of the tympanic membrane
Tumors (e.g., acoustic neuroma)	Chronic ear infections
Medications (e.g., aminoglycosides, aspirin, quinine)	Congenital abnormalities
Trauma	Otosclerosis or tympanosclerosis
Diseases (e.g., syphilis, viral infections such as mumps)	Temporal bone fractures or other injures

CLINICAL PRESENTATION

The most important task for the clinician, and frequently a difficult one, is to determine whether hearing loss is sensorineural (which is usually irreversible) or conductive (which is often reversible). Another important determination is whether the hearing loss is unilateral or bilateral. Presbycusis produces a typical high-frequency hearing loss that is bilaterally symmetrical. Ménière's disease causes fluctuating hearing loss, usually unilateral, associated with tinnitus and vertigo. Acoustic neuroma (schwannoma), a rare tumor of CN VIII, causes unilateral constant or progressive hearing loss, possibly associated with headache. With a tumor of the acoustic nerve, there will most likely be neurologic changes, such as facial weakness and tingling and loss of taste and dysphagia, in addition to hearing loss.

Subjective

Hearing loss is not a distinct clinical entity; it is a symptom or sign of multiple medical conditions. Patient complaint terminology is more diversified than for many other medical conditions. A patient may report having "difficulty hearing," which may be associated with pain, pressure, discomfort, vertigo, or loss of balance. The patient may also complain of tinnitus, dizziness, blockage, popping, pressure, crackling, distant sounds, or stiffness. The clinician should question the patient about how long he or she has noticed a hearing loss and whether it is partial or complete. Does the patient think both ears are affected? Is there a family history of hearing loss? The clinician should inquire whether the patient has ever had any injury or surgery to the ears and if he or she has had any serious illnesses or infection, such as tuberculosis or sepsis, which might have required treatment with ototoxic antibiotics.

The review of systems should focus on the neurologic system, including CN function (e.g., facial weakness or tingling, loss of taste, or dysphagia). The social and occupational history should include specific questions regarding noise or toxin exposure and any blast-related injuries, including a history of hunting and/or target shooting. A complete history of prescription and over-the-counter medication use should be obtained.

Objective

The physical examination should include otoscopic examination to inspect the external auditory canal and middle ear. The clinician should note any redness, foreign objects, discharge, scaling, lesions, and cerumen (ear wax). There may be a significant accumulation of cerumen in the ear canal, especially in elderly patients. The tympanic membrane should have no perforations and should be a translucent pearly gray. Changes in the tympanic membrane may be consistent with conductive hearing loss.

The clinician should perform Weber, Rinne, and Schwabach tests to determine whether hearing loss is primarily conductive or sensorineural. Unexpected findings from the three tuning fork tests must be integrated to differentiate clinically the nature of the hearing loss. Conductive hearing loss occurs when sound transmission is impaired through the external or middle ear. Sensorineural hearing loss occurs because of a defect in the inner ear that leads to the distortion of sound and misinterpretation of speech.

For office testing, the Weber test is done first. A vibrating 512-Hz (or higher-frequency) tuning fork is placed midline on the patient's skull. Normally, the sound should be heard equally in both ears. In sensorineural loss, the sound in the unaffected (or less affected ear) is louder. In conductive loss, the sound is louder in the affected ear.

The Rinne test can also be done in the office. A vibrating tuning fork is placed on the mastoid process. When the sound fades away, the fork is promptly placed (without restriking it) over the external auditory meatus. Normally, via air conduction, the sound can be heard for twice as long as via bone conduction. In sensorineural loss, the ratio remains the same, whereas in conductive loss, the ratio is closer to 1:1, or even reversed.

In the Schwabach test, a vibrating tuning fork is placed over the mastoid process of the patient and then the examiner (assuming the examiner has normal hearing) and the results are compared. In sensorineural loss, the patient's bone conduction is present for a shorter time than the examiner's bone conduction; in conductive loss, the patient's bone conduction persists for a longer time than the examiner's bone conduction.

DIAGNOSTIC REASONING

Diagnostic Tests

Often, the patient needs to be referred for audiometry. Audiometry includes pure tone and speech testing, as well as impedance (middle ear pressure) testing. Both types of hearing loss may fluctuate, making audiometric results variable from test to test. Marked conductive loss on one ear may be difficult to exclude (mask) when testing the opposite ear. Computed tomography (CT) and magnetic resonance imaging (MRI) scans are used to detect tumors, such as acoustic neuromas and tympanic paragangliomas (formerly called glomus tumors), as well as damage from traumatic injuries.

Various mechanical obstructions, such as wax, tumor, or fluid associated with infection/inflammation, that lead to conductive hearing loss may be visualized. CT scan and/or MRI may be needed to demonstrate tumors and cholesteatoma (a destructive growth of keratinizing squamous epithelium) in the middle ear. Cholesteatoma may also sometimes be identified by a perforation located near the margin of the eardrum.

Differential Diagnosis

To treat hearing loss, the etiology must be accurately identified. The differential diagnosis for hearing loss includes conditions that cause either sensorineural or conductive hearing impairment. Aging is associated with sensorineural loss of hearing (presbycusis). However, other possible conditions need to be ruled out. Sensorineural hearing loss may also have an etiology of ototoxicity, exposure to loud noises, an autoimmune disorder, an acoustic neuroma, or possibly Ménière's disease. Conductive hearing loss may be explained simply by cerumen accumulation or impaction (ceruminosis) or a foreign body in the external canal, otitis externa, chronic otitis media, middle ear effusion, otosclerosis, a vascular anomaly, or cholesteatoma.

MANAGEMENT

Many types of conductive hearing loss are reversible, while sensorineural causes tend to be irreversible. In cases of conductive hearing loss caused by cerumen buildup, cerumen disimpaction may be necessary. The recommended procedure is to place a 1:1 mixture of 3% hydrogen peroxide and warm mineral oil in the external ear canal and for 1 hour, followed by lavage with warm saline. The saline should be directed toward the canal wall and not toward the eardrum. An alternative method is to put three drops of warm olive oil in each ear to soften the wax, and then flush with warm 3% hydrogen peroxide. Cerumenolytic agents such as 6.5% carbamide peroxide (Debrox) are effective; docusate sodium liquid may also be used. These agents should not be used in the presence of a perforated tympanic membrane or infection, however. After instilling the cerumenolytic, the clinician should press gently but firmly behind the ear and then in front of the ear. The ear lobe is pulled up and down to work the wax out, after which the ear canal may be dried with a hair dryer set to low heat. Advise the patient who has cerumen buildup but may not be complaining of hearing loss to use Debrox for 1 week before returning for ear canal irrigation as described.

If not performed properly, cerumen removal may cause damage to the external auditory meatus, perforation of the tympanic membrane, or otitis media. If trauma to the canal occurs, a combination corticosteroid/antibiotic otic solution (Cortisporin otic; four drops three to four times daily for 5 to 7 days) should be prescribed. In recurrent or resistant cases, a cerumenolytic may be installed two times daily for 5 days per month, but disimpaction of the ear should not be done if tympanic membrane perforation is present.

If hearing loss is caused by an infection, treat as appropriate (see the sections on otitis media and otitis externa in Chapter 23). The cause of the hearing loss in cases of sensorineural impairment must also be identified correctly to treat it properly. Noise damage is a common cause of hearing loss in the United States. Although this type of hearing loss is not reversible, it is preventable. Hearing loss related to the use of ototoxic medications (especially certain antibiotics, such as aminoglycosides) must be recognized; this etiology should be suspected if hearing loss, dizziness, and tinnitus occur during the course of treatment with certain medications. In this case, the patient should stop the medications. Salicylate toxicity, for example, is reversible. In cases resulting from metabolic causes, such as hypothyroidism, the underlying disorder should be treated. For cases of sudden sensorineural hearing loss with no apparent cause, high doses of corticosteroids (80 mg/day of prednisone or equivalent) are sometimes used.

FOLLOW-UP AND REFERRAL

Any patient who presents with sudden sensorineural hearing loss should be referred to a otorhinolaryngologist for further diagnosis and treatment. Patients should be referred to an ear, nose, and throat specialist if perforation of the tympanic membrane is present, as well as in cases of damage to the ossicles, tympanosclerosis, otosclerosis, tumor, and temporal bone injury. Referral to an audiologist for further evaluation may be appropriate. Patients who are suspected of having Ménière's disease should be referred to an ear, nose, and throat specialist and an audiologist for appropriate diagnostic testing and treatment. In the case of perilymphatic fistula, diagnosis should be based on evidence or history of injury to the ear (including barotrauma during diving), and referral to a specialist is indicated. Acoustic neuromas should be referred for surgical evaluation and potential resection.

Patient Education: Hearing Loss

Although no specific treatment will reverse the process, in cases of presbycusis it is important to educate and support the patient so that no further damage will occur; for example, exposure to excessive noise and ototoxic drugs should be avoided. Severe nerve deafness, particularly when associated with tinnitus, may produce severe depression and isolation and may even be a risk factor for suicide. Clinicians should inquire as to daily activities and social interaction, refer the patient to learn lip-reading if appropriate, and instruct family members to speak clearly while facing the patient. The purchase of hearing aids should be encouraged, and telephone companies may be requested to provide special audio equipment for the hearing impaired.

Permanent hearing loss is common with a sensorineural etiology and may even occur with conductive hearing loss. Patients need to be counseled about follow-up with audiometry and the use hearing aids. Middle ear problems may progress to chronic ear problems, such as perforations or cholesteatomas, which will adversely affect hearing.

As a prevention strategy in cases of hearing loss due to occupational or recreational acoustic trauma (excessive noise exposure), the patient must be counselled to always use protective ear devices. It is also important to teach the patient to equalize ear pressure when diving and to chew gum when landing in airplanes. As needed (but not excessive) decongestant use may be indicated during flights and, if an upper respiratory infection is present, the patient should avoid flying and/or diving until the infection is resolved.

TINNITUS

Tinnitus is a subjective perception of noise (ringing or buzzing) when no environmental noise is present. It may be intermittent, continuous, or pulsatile (synchronous with heartbeat). Risk factors include hearing loss, labyrinthitis, Ménière's disease, otitis media, otitis externa, otosclerosis, ear-canal blockage (from ear wax or a foreign body), a history of high or low blood pressure, head trauma, anemia, hypothyroidism, hyperthyroidism, or allergies. Chronic exposure to noise, especially high-pitched sounds, may damage the cilia and auditory hair cells, causing tinnitus. Certain medications may contribute to tinnitus, some with reversible effects (salicylates, quinine, alcohol, and indomethacin [Indocin]) and others with irreversible effects (kanamycin, streptomycin, gentamicin, and vancomycin).

EPIDEMIOLOGY AND CAUSES

Recent estimates suggest that as many as 40 million Americans are affected by tinnitus. Approximately 90% of patients with hearing loss experience some tinnitus, and approximately 1% of the population has chronic tinnitus. Tinnitus is strongly associated with aging. Experts estimate that 15% of Americans have experienced tinnitus that lasts longer than 5 minutes and that 155 million have sought medical care for tinnitus. About 6% of that number report being incapacitated by tinnitus. The peak range of patients with tinnitus is 40 to 70 years of age. Patients in their seventh decade of life have a 25% to 30% risk of developing tinnitus. Men have a higher risk of developing tinnitus, and whites experience tinnitus in greater numbers than blacks.

PATHOPHYSIOLOGY

Tinnitus is classified in several ways. Tinnitus may be divided into vibratory and nonvibratory classifications. Vibratory tinnitus is caused by transmission to the cochlea of vibrations from adjacent tissues or organs. Nonvibratory tinnitus is produced by biochemical changes in the neural mechanisms of hearing. Subjective tinnitus, which is more common, is heard only by the patient. Objective tinnitus can be heard by an examiner through a stethoscope placed over the head and neck structures near the ear.

The causative mechanism of tinnitus is poorly understood. Theories include injured cochlear hair cells discharging repetitively and stimulating auditory nerve fibers in a continuous cycle, spontaneous activity in individual auditory nerve fibers, hyperactivity in the auditory nuclei in the brainstem, or a reduction in the usual suppressive activity of the central auditory cortex on peripheral auditory nerve activity.

CLINICAL PRESENTATION

Subjective

Patients have variously described tinnitus as the sound of escaping air, running water, the sound heard inside a large seashell, or as a buzzing, ringing, or humming noise. Tinnitus also has been described as a roaring or musical sound. It may be unilateral or bilateral. Most patients are not bothered by tinnitus when they are surrounded by the typical ambient sounds of daily life. However, when they are in an unusually quiet location, the perception of tinnitus may be profound. In more extreme cases, tinnitus may interfere with their lives, affecting concentration and sleep and causing severe depression in the worst cases. Tinnitus that manifests as a continuous and unbearably loud sound has led some patients to self-harm.

Other presentations commonly seen include a stiff neck and pain aggravated by activity that produces the tinnitus and accompanied by vertigo, nystagmus, hearing loss, and pain that radiates down the arms. Weakness, confusion, and feelings of unsteadiness (orthostatic hypotension) may also occur, especially when the patient stands up quickly. These symptoms may be indicative of atherosclerosis as a causative factor.

Complaints of ear fullness, itching, and hearing loss, along with tinnitus, may be caused by a foreign body obstruction, such as cerumen (ear wax) impaction; thus, obstruction should always be ruled out. Bilateral, high-pitched tinnitus may occur with severe hypertension (diastolic blood pressure exceeding 120 mm Hg). The patient may have associated symptoms of headache, numbness, nausea, and vomiting. If the patient describes the sudden onset of vertigo, unilateral or bilateral hearing loss, dizziness, nausea or vomiting, and nystagmus, labyrinthitis should be considered.

Objective

In addition to standard vital sign assessments, blood pressure should be evaluated via orthostatic measurements. Physical examination should include gross hearing tests, as well as the Weber and Rinne tuning fork tests to detect conductive or sensorineural hearing loss, and a thorough otologic examination should be done. If tinnitus is unilateral or asymmetric, auscultation of the upper part of the neck proximate to the affected ear may detect a bruit, and

palpation may reveal a weak pulse. In turn, cardiovascular studies may need to be considered, including Doppler ultrasound examination of the carotid arteries to assess for stenosis and an electrocardiogram to detect changes associated with atherosclerotic disease. A neurologic examination should be done to rule out other deficits of the nervous system (including the CNs) that suggest a neurologic etiology.

DIAGNOSTIC REASONING

Diagnostic Tests

Laboratory studies are necessary to confirm possible underlying causes of tinnitus. A complete blood count should be done to rule out anemia or infection. Metabolic studies need to be done to rule out thyroid disease, hyperlipidemia, vitamin B_{12} deficiency, zinc deficiency, or electrolyte abnormalities. If drainage from the ear canal is evident, a culture should be obtained. MRI may reveal ear-related pathology in detail, and this is currently the diagnostic procedure of choice. If the patient cannot tolerate MRI due to the enclosed space, CT scan with dye enhancement is an alternative. Special tests to determine the presence of middle ear fluid may be considered, such as tympanometry, acoustic reflex measurement, or acoustic reflectometry. Because of the association of depressive disorders in severe tinnitus, screening for psychologic disorders should also be done.

Differential Diagnosis

Accompanying symptoms in the patient with tinnitus may alert the primary-care practitioner to the underlying cause. For example, tinnitus may be associated with presbycusis, or it may present as a somatic symptom of acute anxiety. In addition, hearing loss and tinnitus accompanied by vertigo, facial paralysis, headaches, nausea, vomiting, and papilledema may occur due to an acoustic neuroma. A characteristic early symptom of an acoustic nerve (CN VIII) tumor is unilateral tinnitus.

Tinnitus may also arise from systemic cardiovascular disorders. Bilateral, high-pitched tinnitus may occur with severe hypertension (diastolic blood pressure exceeding 120 mm Hg), with the patient experiencing associated symptoms of headache, numbness, nausea, and vomiting. Occasionally, anemia may produce mild, irreversible tinnitus. In this case, the patient may complain of dim vision, syncope, and the associated signs of anemia, such as fatigue, weakness, exertional dyspnea, and tachycardia that accompany the tinnitus.

In Ménière's disease, low-pitched tinnitus, along with vertigo and fluctuating hearing loss, may occur. Tinnitus accompanied by bleeding from the ear canal can be caused by trauma. Purulent drainage and pain with tinnitus may be caused by infection, in which other presenting symptoms may include fever, chills, and dizziness.

MANAGEMENT

Elimination of possible offending medications (such as aspirin-containing products and other NSAIDs) is a priority. Tinnitus usually cannot be treated successfully. However, management of symptoms and treatment of the underlying causative disorder (if one can be identified) may help. Overall, learning to cope with the tinnitus is the best approach. Avoidance of risk factors, such as excessive noise, is advised whenever possible. Some experts suggest supplementation with vitamin A, vitamin C, cyanocobalamin, and nicotinic acid or with magnesium or copper, but data from randomized controlled trials supporting this practice are lacking.

Protective earplugs may need to be worn. Alternatively, tinnitus-masking devices can match the frequency range and intensity of the tinnitus, producing a level of noise that will help block out the tinnitus without interfering with hearing. The device fits in the ear like a hearing aid and presents a more pleasant sound to the patient. Regular relief may be obtained by masking the tinnitus with background noise from an external "white noise" machine. Hearing aids are also helpful in tinnitus suppression, as they help to amplify environmental sounds, thereby obscuring tinnitus. For patients who find the noise of tinnitus intolerable, biofeedback may be needed to help with psychological problems that can develop from the near-constant feeling of distress.

Although there is no medication to help tinnitus, oral antidepressants have proved to be effective in reducing symptoms. Nortriptyline (Elavil), at an initial dose of 50 mg orally at bedtime, may be considered. Meclizine HCl (Antivert, Bonine) is the most commonly used vestibular suppressant. Diazepam (Valium), usually in low doses such as 2 mg, may be a valuable adjunctive therapy for patients with tinnitus caused by an acute attack of vertigo, as well as for patients with anxiety. If chronic vertigo and dizziness accompany the tinnitus, vestibular rehabilitation (an exercise program to improve balance and reduce dizziness; see Resources) should be considered.

Patients with tinnitus related to otitis media or other infections should be treated with antibiotics for an adequate duration, with careful monitoring of serum peak and trough levels. This will help minimize the loss of vestibular function and deafness from antibiotic therapy with aminoglycosides. If medical management does not resolve ear infections, surgical intervention, with myringotomy and possible ear tube placement, should be considered, in which case, referral to an otorhinolaryngologist should be initiated.

FOLLOW-UP AND REFERRAL

Referral to an audiologist should be initiated for a patient with tinnitus and hearing loss. If vertigo, nausea, and vomiting accompany the tinnitus, the patient should be referred to an otorhinolaryngologist. Other specialty referrals will be driven by the underlying etiology, if identified. Given the chronic nature of most tinnitus cases, regular follow-up may occur over an extended period, as patients adjust to the therapeutic recommendations and physical interventions (e.g., hearing aids, tinnitus-masking devices) designed to minimize the distress caused by tinnitus.

Patient Education: Tinnitus

General measures the patient may take to minimize symptoms include playing background music during the daytime and before sleep to mask the noise of tinnitus, as well as stopping smoking and decreasing the intake of caffeine, chocolate, alcohol, and salt, which are suggested by some experts to exacerbate the condition, potentially due to their effects on inner ear fluid volume and composition. Fatigue may also increase tinnitus; therefore, patients need to be instructed in proper sleep hygiene and encouraged to rest during the course of the day. Chewing gum or swallowing should be encouraged during descent on airplanes to promote eustachian tube opening and equalization of middle ear pressure through deglutition (swallowing).

MÉNIÈRE'S DISEASE

Ménière's disease (Ménière's syndrome, endolymphatic hydrops) is a peripheral sensory disorder of both the labyrinth (semicircular canal system) and cochlea of the inner ear. Endolymphatic volume and, in turn, inner ear pressure are increased due to unknown etiology, resulting in both vestibular (proprioceptive, balance-related) and auditory dysfunction, characterized by recurrent attacks of tinnitus (ringing or buzzing in the ears), vertigo (a sense of whirling or spinning in space), and progressive hearing loss. Although Ménière's disease is not life-threatening, if untreated, acute attacks typically recur over the course of many years.

EPIDEMIOLOGY AND CAUSES

Well-documented incidence figures for Ménière's disease are not available, but it is estimated that 46 new cases per 100,000 occur annually in the United States. Prevalence is estimated at 1,150 per 100,000. Age at onset is between 30 and 60 years, with most cases developing during the fifth decade of life. The disease is rare both in young children and in adults older than 70 years of age. Some studies indicate that white Americans of European descent are at an increased risk of developing the disease. Both sexes are affected nearly equally, but some studies have reported slightly higher rates in women.

There are multiple risk factors for Meniere's disease, which include stress; allergies; high salt, caffeine, and alcohol intake; hormonal changes; changes in barometric pressure; and exposure to high noise levels for periods of many years. There is a reported 20% familial history with this disease. An associated condition is a history of migraines, which is also a differential diagnosis.

PATHOPHYSIOLOGY

The precise cause of Ménière's disease is not fully established, but marked edema of the membranous labyrinth is typically observed at autopsy, and endolymphatic hydrops has been established as the defining pathological finding in the disease. Theories have implicated the inflammatory response of the inner ear to a variety of insults, including blunt trauma, viral infection, allergies, reduced or negative middle ear pressure, and various vascular, endocrine, and lipid disorders. Migraine headache and autoimmune conditions, including systemic lupus erythematosus, rheumatoid arthritis, and certain thyroid disorders, also predispose to Ménière's disease. A genetic predisposition has also been identified in 8% of people affected.

Dilation of the endolymphatic system may lead to rupture of the membranous labyrinth. This engorgement has been associated with excessive endolymph production, decreased resorption of fluid in the endolymphatic sac, and hypoplasia of the vestibular aqueduct. Resultant mixing of the endolymph and perilymph is thought to cause degeneration of both vestibular and cochlear neuroepithelial sensory hair cells, which are particularly sensitive to ionic changes from the potassium-rich endolymph. This may result in vertigo, tinnitus, and hearing loss characteristic of Ménière's disease. Compression of the vestibular portion of CN VIII by an enlarged blood vessel is yet another etiological theory.

CLINICAL PRESENTATION

Subjective

Acute episodes of Ménière's disease last anywhere from 20 minutes to 3 hours and are characterized by sudden attacks of nausea, emesis, pallor, diaphoresis, dizziness (spatial disorientation), vertigo, roaring tinnitus, and increased pressure, fullness, and hearing loss in the affected ear. Patients typically refer to any vestibular symptomatology as "dizziness." Rapid movement aggravates all proprioceptive symptomatology, and patients often report a history of falls or accidents during acute episodes.

The frequency and severity of attacks may decrease over time, and hearing may improve immediately after an acute attack. However, some episodes may last for more than 24 hours. Overall, low-frequency hearing loss is typically progressive, with bilateral involvement in 10% to 50% of cases. Patients may also experience motion-related imbalance without vertigo between acute attacks. Complete hearing loss in advanced cases of Ménière's disease is associated with a cessation of vertiginous episodes.

Objective

Upon inspection, otoscopic examination typically demonstrates no apparent abnormalities, unless underlying otitis media is present. Dilation of the inner ear endolymphatic system is apparent only at autopsy. Spontaneous nystagmus is often observed after preventing eye fixation by having the patient wear 40-diopter glasses (Frenzel lenses) during the period of observation.

DIAGNOSTIC REASONING

Diagnostic Tests

Diagnosis of Ménière's disease is based on a careful history, neurologic assessment, and response to empiric therapy, because no specific diagnostic testing exists. Diagnostic criteria requires two distinct episodes of rotational vertigo lasting at least 20 minutes each, along with sensorineural hearing loss and either tinnitus or a perception of aural fullness. Thus, both the Weber and Rinne tests typically elicit findings characteristic of a sensorineural hearing defect. Sound lateralization to the nonaffected ear occurs when a 512-Hz tuning fork is placed midline on the top of the head (Weber test), and air conduction is superior in duration and volume to bone conduction (positive Rinne test).

Audiometry demonstrates low-frequency sensorineural hearing loss, as well as impaired speech discrimination. Both cold and warm caloric responses are typically reduced in the affected ear, as demonstrated by electronystagmography or direct patient observation (while wearing 40-diopter Frenzel lenses); the direction of the fast phase of nystagmus is variable. These findings are not diagnostic for Ménière's disease, however. Vestibular function tests are used to evaluate CN VIII function; however, these findings are questionable in patients taking sedative drugs of any kind.

Differential Diagnosis

Ménière's disease is a diagnosis of exclusion; thus, if a distinct cause is identified, the condition should no longer be termed Ménière's disease. In turn, numerous disorders that mimic its clinical presentation must first be ruled out. For example, otitis media is evaluated using otoscopic examination and culture of otic fluid. If middle ear infection is present, the tympanic membrane is typically erythematous and either edematous or retracted, with altered bony landmarks and a diminished cone of light reflex. Bubbles or an air-fluid level may be seen directly behind the membrane, and mobility is reduced or absent on insufflation with a pneumatic otoscope.

Otitis media and Ménière's disease are not mutually exclusive conditions, however, as negative middle ear pressure associated with serous otitis media may be a contributing factor to Ménière's disease. Otitis media may also precipitate a viral infection of CN VIII known as vestibular neuritis (benign recurrent vertigo), which presents as recurrent vertiginous episodes lasting for several hours, which may be accompanied by severe vomiting and nausea. Vestibular neuritis may also be idiopathic, but in these patients (unlike in those with Ménière's disease), auditory impairment is rarely noted.

Secondary or tertiary syphilis can also affect CN VIII and is ruled out using a variety of immunological tests specific for its causative agent *Treponema pallidum,* such as the microhemagglutination, fluorescent treponemal antibody, and Treponema immobilization assays. Acute viral or bacterial infection of the labyrinth may also present with similar symptoms; however, pathogenic microorganisms are not associated with Ménière's disease because it is not of infectious etiology. Discrete lesions of the central nervous system (CNS), such as tumors or infarcts of the brain and cerebellum, as well as degenerative nervous disorders such as Parkinson's disease, multiple sclerosis, and Alzheimer's disease, may be ruled out via CT and MRI. Hypothyroidism may also mimic Ménière's disease and is ruled out through measurement of both free and protein-bound thyroid hormone levels (thyroxine and triiodothyronine), as well as pituitary thyroid-stimulating hormone.

Benign positional vertigo (benign paroxysmal vertigo) is a more common diagnosis of vestibular dysfunction than Ménière's disease in elderly patients who complain of dizziness. It is characterized by paroxysmal vertigo accompanied by nystagmus when lying down, turning over in bed, or tilting the head backward. The Nylen-Bárány maneuver is used to make this diagnosis: the patient is reclined rapidly from a sitting to supine position with the head tilted to one side, and the neck is hyperextended 30 degrees below the horizontal for at least 10 seconds, off the end of the examination table. The maneuver is then repeated with the head tilted to the opposite side. In this benign condition, nystagmus lasting between 15 and 45 seconds is observed after each maneuver, following a brief 1 to 5-second latent period. In contrast to Ménière's disease, benign positional vertigo does not present with hearing loss or tinnitus.

Presbycusis, the most common cause of sensorineural hearing loss in the elderly, is distinguished by high-frequency rather than low-frequency hearing loss, as revealed by audiometric testing. Serum glucose levels should be evaluated to rule out hypoglycemic disorders, and hemoglobin and hematocrit are measured to assess anemic conditions, if suspected. Lipid disorders affecting cerebral blood flow and, in turn, vestibulocochlear function may be ruled out via serum lipid studies. Other cerebral and cardiovascular disorders, such as transient ischemic attacks, vertebrobasilar ischemia, or subclavian steal syndrome, may lead to CNS ischemia and vertigo, thus mimicking Ménière's disease. However, syncope (fainting) and generalized weakness are also usually observed. Angiography is used to rule out such disorders, if suspected.

Another common cause of vestibular and auditory dysfunction is iatrogenic, drug-induced ototoxicity from many commonly used drugs, including aspirin; potent diuretics; quinine; tetracyclines (particularly minocycline); many cancer chemotherapies (e.g., *cis*-platinum); and aminoglycoside antibiotics, including gentamicin, neomycin, kanamycin, and streptomycin. If use of these medications is not prolonged, ototoxicity may be reversible once drug intake has stopped. Sedative side effects of many medications, as well as undesirable multidrug interactions, are a common cause of dizziness that often accompanies tinnitus, especially in elderly patients, who are at an increased risk of polypharmacy-related sequelae.

In the adult patient, acoustic neuroma causing compression of the auditory portion of CN VIII is one of the most important diagnoses of auditory dysfunction to rule out because these tumors may be life-threatening if untreated. MRI and auditory brainstem response audiometry are used to detect such neoplasms.

Finally, psychiatric diagnoses should be a major consideration if examination and laboratory findings rule out systemic disease and specific organ involvement as the cause of vestibulocochlear dysfunction. Psychiatric illness is the second most common etiology of dizziness in elderly patients after peripheral nervous system disorders. Common conditions include depression, anxiety, panic attacks, somatization disorders, alcoholism, and other forms of substance abuse. A proper psychiatric evaluation, which may include drug screens of the urine and blood, is necessary to rule out such illnesses.

MANAGEMENT

The first step in management of an acute attach of Ménière's disease is to rule out all other causes of the symptoms. Sometimes, dizziness and loss of balance, which are first assessed as a Ménière's outbreak, are simply due to a cerumen impaction. There is no proven cure for Meniere disease and current therapy is mainly palliative, with a focus on reducing symptoms. Actual acute attacks of Ménière's are best treated by rest with the eyes closed and protection from falling. Attacks rarely last longer than 4 hours. Conservative treatment is reported to be effective for managing vertigo in the majority of patients, such as dietary modifications, specifically restriction of sodium, caffeine, and alcohol, but avoid severe sodium restriction for patients treated with diuretics. Compliance with reduced sodium diet may reduce vertigo spells, and compliance to caffeine-free diet may improve function. Also, vestibular rehabilitation may reduce symptoms specifically for unilateral peripheral vestibular dysfunction; there are a variety of self-management booklets and/or symptom control booklet that may improve symptoms in some cases. Medications can help control symptoms during acute attacks and help to prevent attacks.

Vestibular sedatives, for example, buccal or intramuscular prochlorperazine, can be used to treat severe nausea and vomiting. A trial of an antihistamine, specifically betahistine (suggested dosing regimen 16 mg orally three times/day), can be considered to reduce frequency and severity of vertigo attacks. Diuretics are widely used in the treatment of Meniere's disease but may have adverse effects, especially in older patients, and strong evidence for efficacy is lacking. Intratympanic dexamethasone may be considered for patients with vertigo refractory to lifestyle changes, especially if an underlying autoimmune disorder is present.

As a last resort, if Ménière's disease progresses bilaterally, streptomycin or gentamicin ablation therapy may be appropriate to reduce unbearable vestibular symptoms. An aminoglycoside antibiotic is administered over a course of several days to weeks to intentionally damage the neuroepithelium of the vestibular centers in the inner ear, thus reducing related symptomatology. However, hearing must be carefully monitored both during and after this treatment to avoid damage to auditory structures.

Disabling symptoms of Ménière's disease may require surgical intervention, typically used in 5% to 10% of all cases. For patients with normal hearing ability, decompression of the endolymphatic sac may be accomplished by surgically draining excess endolymph into the mastoid or subarachnoid spaces. Alternatively, the vestibular nerve may be transected intracranially. For patients whose hearing ability has degenerated and is deemed unsalvageable, the cochlea itself may be decompressed (via cochleocentesis) or directly perfused with streptomycin. A more radical surgery is labyrinthectomy of the affected ear, a procedure that entirely ablates vestibular function.

FOLLOW-UP AND REFERRAL

If symptoms do not worsen, patients may return for follow-up in 3 to 6 weeks. However, patients should return for reevaluation immediately if disabling symptoms such as tinnitus, vertigo, nausea, or emesis persist. Hearing loss, in particular, must be carefully monitored for progression because this is a telltale sign of an underlying, potentially life-threatening acoustic neuroma. Patients often report that previously consulted clinicians failed to take this condition seriously when they first presented with symptoms. Thus, close follow-up care of the patient with Ménière's disease provides emotionally beneficial validation as well.

Progressive bilateral hearing loss may result from Ménière's disease, leading to chronic tinnitus, deafness, and disabling vertigo. Accidental injuries, including falls, related to vestibular dysfunction may occur in the work or home setting, and patients often report an increasing inability to function productively at their present jobs in the face of progressive disease. Failing to diagnose

an underlying acoustic neuroma is a potentially life-threatening complication.

Referral to a specialist is necessary if symptoms worsen with treatment. Advanced diagnostic procedures such as electronystagmography or specialized vestibulocochlear function tests require referral to a neurologist. A physician consultation is also needed in cases involving persistent emesis, seizures, syncope, or fever. New, unexplained symptoms (which are often due to multidrug interactions or adverse effects of medications) also require referral to a specialist for diagnosis and treatment. Streptomycin ablation therapy and surgical interventions should be directed by a qualified specialist only, because the risk of serious sequelae is significant, including permanent hearing loss.

Patient Education: Ménière's disease

Patients must be encouraged to stop smoking because this aggravates all otic disorders. Stress levels should be monitored and controlled. Salt intake should be reduced to a maximum of 1 g/day to lessen the severity of future attacks. Reductions in caffeine and alcohol are also recommended. Additionally, vestibular rehabilitation through development of self-management techniques and a symptom log have been shown to be effective in some cases. All ototoxic medications should be avoided, and polypharmacy (multiple prescription drug use) should be evaluated with the aid of a specialist.

Patients should be instructed to return for further evaluation if symptoms worsen or acute episodes increase in frequency. Patients need to understand that treating Ménière's disease pharmacologically is difficult, and acute attacks are best managed with quiet bedrest and careful protection from falls. To avoid accidental injuries and minimize symptoms, patients should not drive, climb ladders, work near or operate dangerous machinery, walk without assistance, read, or look at glaring lights during these episodes. Food intake should also be reduced during acute attacks to lessen nausea and vomiting.

REFERENCES

General

Williams ME. Examining the ears, nose, and oral cavity in the older adult patient. http://cme.medscape.com/viewarticle/556144. Published 2007.

Hearing Impairment

Bainbridge KE, Wallhagen MI. Hearing loss in an aging American population, extent, impact and management. *Annu Rev Public Health*. 2014;35:139–152.

Balachandran R, Reda FA, Noble JH, et al. Minimally invasive image-guided cochlear implantation for pediatric patients: Clinical feasibility study. *Otolaryngol Head Neck Surg*. 2014;150(4):631–637.

Fitzpatrick E, McCrae R, Schramm D, et al. A retrospective study of cochlear implant outcomes in children with residual hearing. *BMC Ear Nose Throat Disord*. 2006;6:7.

Hillier S, McDonnell M. Is vestibular rehabilitation effective in improving dizziness and function after unilateral peripheral vestibular hypofunction? An abridged version of a Cochrane Review. *Eur J Phys Rehabil Med.* 2016;52(4):541–556.

Hillier SL, McDonnell M. Vestibular rehabilitation for unilateral peripheral vestibular dysfunction. *Cochrane Database Syst Rev.* 2011;(2):CD005397.

Ibekwe TS, Nwaorgu OG, Ijaduola TG, et al. Correlating the site of tympanic membrane perforation with hearing loss. *BMC Ear Nose Throat Disord.* 2009;9:1. http://www.ahrq.gov/professionals/clinicians-providers/guidelines-recommendations/index.html.

National Guideline Clearinghouse. *Guideline summary: ACR Appropriateness Criteria® hearing loss and/or vertigo.* Rockville, MD: Agency for Healthcare Research and Quality; 2013. https://www.guideline.gov. Accessed August 19, 2017.

National Guideline Clearinghouse. *Guideline summary: American College of Medical Genetics and Genomics guideline for the clinical evaluation and etiologic diagnosis of hearing loss.* Rockville, MD: Agency for Healthcare Research and Quality; 2014. https://www.guideline.gov. Accessed August 19, 2017.

National Guideline Clearinghouse. *Guideline summary: Clinical practice guideline: sudden hearing loss.* Rockville, MD: Agency for Healthcare Research and Quality; 2012. https://www.guideline.gov. Accessed August 19, 2017.

National Guideline Clearinghouse. *Guideline summary: Screening for hearing loss in older adults: U.S. Preventive Services Task Force recommendation statement.* Rockville, MD: Agency for Healthcare Research and Quality; 2012. https://www.guideline.gov. Accessed August 19, 2017.

Nguyen S, Cloutier F, Philippon D, Côté M, Bussières R, Backous DD. Outcomes review of modern hearing preservation technique in cochlear implant. *Auris Nasus Larynx.* 2016;43(5):485–488.

Stachler RJ. Clinical practice guidelines: Sudden hearing loss. *Otolaryngol Head Neck Surg.* 2012;146:1–35.

Valentino RL. Chronic dysfunction of the eustachian tube. *Clin Advisor.* 2009;21–25.

Ménière's Disease

Bartels L, Danner C, Allen K. Office-based Ménière's disease management. *Operative Tech Otolaryngol Head Neck Surg.* 2016;27(4):225–234.

Cruz MD. Ménière's disease: a stepwise approach. *Med Today.* 2014;15(3):18-26.

Lopez-Escamez JA, Carey J, Chung WH, et al.; Classification Committee of the Barany Society; Japan Society for Equilibrium Research; European Academy of Otology and Neurotology (EAONO); Equilibrium Committee of the American Academy of Otolaryngology-Head and Neck Surgery (AAO-HNS); Korean Balance Society. Diagnostic criteria for Ménière's disease. *J Vestib Res.* 2015;25(1):1–7.

Morrison AW, Bailey ME, Morrison GA. Familial Ménière's disease: clinical and genetic aspects. *J Laryngol Otol.* 2009;123(1):29–37.

Muller I, Kirby S, Yardley L. Understanding patient experiences of self-managing chronic dizziness: A qualitative study of booklet-based vestibular rehabilitation, with or without remote support. *BMJ Open.* 2015;5(5):e007680.

National Guideline Clearinghouse. *Guideline summary: Vestibular rehabilitation for peripheral vestibular hypofunction: An evidence-based clinical practice guideline.* Rockville, MD: Agency for Healthcare Research and Quality; 2016. https://www.guideline.gov. Accessed August 19, 2017.

Radtke A, von Brevern M, Feldmann M, et al. Ménière's disease. http://medscape.com/viewarticle/509085.

Radtke A, et al. Screening for Ménière's disease in the general population—the needle in the haystack. *Acta Otolaryngol.* 2008;128(3):272–276.

Ray J, Carr SD, Popli G, Gibson, WP. An epidemiological study to investigate the relationship between Meniere's disease and migraine. *Clin Otolaryngol.* 2016;41(6):707–710.

Rossi-Izquierdo M, Santos-Pérez S, Soto-Varela A. What is the most effective vestibular rehabilitation technique in patients with unilateral peripheral vestibular disorders? *Eur Arch Otorhinolaryngol.* 2011; 268(11):1569–1574.

Seemungal B, Kaski D, Escamez J. Early diagnosis and management of acute vertigo from vestibular migraine and Ménière's disease. *Neurol Clin.* 2015;33(3):619–626.

Tassinari M, Mandrioli D, Gaggioli N, Roberti di Sarsina P. Ménière's disease treatment: A patient-centered systematic review. *Audiol Neurootol.* 2015;20:153–165.

Tsukamoto HF, Costa Vde S, Silva RA Jr, et al. Effectiveness of a vestibular rehabilitation protocol to improve the health-related quality of life and postural balance in patients with vertigo. *Int Arch Otorhinolaryngol.* 2015;19(3):238–247.

Weinreich HM, Agrawal Y. The link between allergy and Ménière's disease. *Curr Opin Otolaryngol Head Neck Surg.* 2014;22(3):227–230.

Yardley L, Donovan-Hall M, Smith HE, et al. Effectiveness of primary care-based vestibular rehabilitation for chronic dizziness. *Ann Intern Med.* 2004;141(8):598–605.

Tinnitus

Fuller TE, Haider HF, Kikidis D, Lapira A. Different teams, same conclusions? A systematic review of existing clinical guidelines for the assessment and treatment of tinnitus in adults. *Front Psychol.* 2017;8:206–212.

Langguth B, Kreuzer PM, Kleinjung T, Ridder D. Tinnitus: Causes and clinical management. *Lancet Neurol.* 2013;12(9):920–230.

National Guideline Clearinghouse. *Guideline summary: Clinical practice guideline: Tinnitus.* Rockville, MD: Agency for Healthcare Research and Quality; 2014. https://www.guideline.gov. Accessed August 19, 2017.

Walker DD, Cifu AS, Gluth MB. Tinnitus. *JAMA.* 2016;315(20):2221–2222.

RESOURCES

American Academy of Otolaryngology-Head and Neck Surgery
http://www.entnet.org/
American Tinnitus Association
https://www.ata.org/understanding-facts
Hearing Loss Association of America
http://www.hearingloss.org/
National Institute on Deafness and Other Communication Disorders
https://www.nidcd.nih.gov/

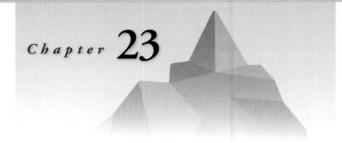

Chapter 23

Inflammatory and Infectious Disorders of the Ear

Brian Oscar Porter, MD, PhD, MPH, MBA

Lynne M. Dunphy, PhD, APRN, FNP-BC, FAAN, FAANP

Humberto Reinoso, PhD, FNP-BC, ENP-BC

OTITIS EXTERNA (SWIMMER'S EAR)

Otitis externa (also called *swimmer's ear* because of its common presentation) is an inflammation of the membranous lining of the auditory canal and/or contiguous structures of the outer ear. The term refers to a wide spectrum of both acute and chronic inflammatory processes that may be diffuse, localized, or invasive in nature. This disorder is largely benign and self-limiting, albeit painful. Invasive otitis externa (malignant otitis externa, necrotizing otitis externa) is a potentially life-threatening disease, however, if left untreated.

EPIDEMIOLOGY AND CAUSES

Ear pain, in general, is a common clinical complaint, accounting for 2% to 3% of all family practice office visits. Specifically, otitis externa is 10 to 20 times more likely to occur during the warmer summer months than in cooler seasons. No ethnic predispositions to otitis externa have been documented. Men and women are affected equally.

Immunocompromised persons on corticosteroid therapy or individuals with chronic conditions such as diabetes mellitus are at a greater risk for developing infectious otitis externa and, in particular, invasive disease. Deep tissue invasion may be related to decreased polymorphonuclear neutrophil function and/or microvascular disease associated with diabetes. Corticosteroid use specifically increases the likelihood of otomycosis, which is significantly more prevalent in the tropics and southeastern United States; however, in general, environmental changes are the most common risk factors for otitis externa.

When the pH of the auditory canal shifts from acidic to alkaline or an increase in temperature and/or humidity

occurs, the auditory canal becomes conducive to pathogenic colonization. In fact, excess moisture from any cause may predispose the external ear to infection. *Pseudomonas* infections, in particular, commonly result from the mild ear canal trauma associated with excessive swimming in hot, humid weather, especially in polluted water, hence the common name "swimmer's ear." Highly chlorinated pool water can also contribute to this disorder because it can dry out the ear canal, creating a potential portal of entry for bacteria and fungi.

Inadequate cerumen (earwax) production removes another critical nonspecific barrier to infection. In addition, patients with seborrhea have an increased risk of otitis externa resulting from seborrheic dermatitis caused by their excess sebum production. Manual picking of the ear; foreign bodies in the auditory canal; and the prolonged use of ear plugs, hearing aids, or cotton swabs may all contribute to local irritation of the external ear, as well as predispose to infection. Other risk factors include previous ear infections, as well as skin allergies, particularly those sensitivity to hair sprays and dyes that may enter the ear canal and cause contact dermatitis. In fact, dermatitic processes often precede microbial infection of the auditory canal because they create a potential portal of entry through the skin for pathogens.

PATHOPHYSIOLOGY

Inflammation of the external ear is most commonly caused by microbial infection. Pathogenic colonization of the external ear is prevented by a number of immune and anatomical mechanisms. The keratinizing squamous epithelia of the ear canal continually sloughs, and the hair follicles that line the outer third of the canal rhythmically sweep laterally, acting as a natural cleansing mechanism and mechanical barrier to the accumulation of matter in the auditory canal. The production of viscous, hydrophobic cerumen in the auditory canal maintains an acidic pH and repels moisture, both of which antagonize bacterial growth. In addition, the presence of competing, nonpathogenic endogenous microbial flora inhibits the overgrowth of more virulent bacteria along the auditory canal. If any of these protective mechanisms is compromised, pathogenic colonization by bacteria or fungi normally found in the auditory canal may occur, resulting in acute otitis externa.

Bacterial agents of infectious otitis externa include *Pseudomonas aeruginosa*, which is the most common cause of diffuse infection and accounts for nearly all cases of invasive otitis externa, and *Staphylococcus aureus*, which typically causes a localized lesion stemming from an infected hair follicle, although it may cause the diffuse form as well. In addition, group A *Streptococcus pyogenes* is associated with localized disease, presenting as a folliculitis or, more frequently, as outer ear erysipelas. Polymicrobial infection has also been noted in up to one-third of cases of diffuse disease, and the anaerobic bacteria *Bacteroides* and *Peptostreptococcus* have been cited in up to one-fourth of cases. Commonly identified fungal agents include *Aspergillus niger* (which typically causes focal lesions but may occasionally lead to invasive disease with bony involvement in immunocompromised patients), *Malassezia pachydermatis*, and *Candida albicans*. Hyperkeratotic processes such as eczema, psoriasis, and contact or seborrheic dermatitis can also lead to outer ear inflammation. Chronic otitis externa may result from inadequately treated OM with continuous serous or exudative drainage from the middle ear into the auditory canal.

Additional risk factors, if not direct causes of otitis externa, include local skin maceration and traumatic injury. The anatomy of the outer ear, which includes the tragus and conchal cartilage, serves as a physical barrier to foreign body entry into the outer ear canal. However, excessive cleaning of the ear with cotton swabs or other devices may leave small pieces of foreign matter in the canal, where they eventually disintegrate due to the canal's acidic pH, serving as a nidus of infection. This irritation in turn leads to pruritus, and excessive scratching of the ear canal only aggravates this cycle of epithelial damage and infection by creating physical access through this protective barrier. Excessive moisture in the external canal, particularly associated with swimming or humid environments, acts in a similar manner, leading to maceration and breakdown of the skin with subsequent bacterial infection.

Necrotizing otitis externa (formerly known as malignant otitis externa) is the most severe infectious form of external otitis in which bacterial infection extends from the skin of the auditory canal into the soft tissues, cartilage, and bone in the temporal region or base of the skull (i.e., skull osteomyelitis). Multiple cranial nerves may become involved, increasing morbidity, and death may result from septic thromboemboli to vessels of the brain if inadequately treated. *P. aeruginosa* remains the most common infectious agent in such severe disease, although invasive fungal disease in immunocompromised individuals may also extend to multiple tissues.

CLINICAL PRESENTATION

Subjective

The most common presenting complaint of patients with otitis externa is an acute, often severe otalgia of sudden or gradual onset, which may present bilaterally. Pain may worsen at night and disturb sleep, and it is exacerbated by pulling the pinna or earlobe or by applying pressure to the tragus. In severe cases, chewing may also elicit otic pain. Severe pain is common in invasive disease. In its early stages, the affected ear may feel full or obstructed, and a temporary conductive hearing loss related to luminal occlusion on the affected side is common if edema is severe. The affected ear may also be pruritic. A purulent discharge may be evident in bacterial disease, and systemic

symptomatology such as fever or chills, although rare, may accompany cases of infectious etiology. Chronic otitis externa usually presents with dryness and pruritus of the ear canal. The ear canal may be slightly red and edematous, and there is usually an absence of cerumen.

Objective

A classic sign of acute otitis externa is tenderness on traction of the pinna and/or pain on applying pressure over the tragus. The clinician should instill several drops of benzocaine/antipyrine (Auralgan) otic solution before attempting examination in patients in acute distress. This solution should not be used in cases of suspected ruptured tympanic membrane, however.

On otoscopic examination, the auditory canal typically appears edematous and erythematous, preventing full visualization of the external canal and tympanic membrane; there also may be accumulation of purulent drainage in cases of bacterial infection. Diffuse cases present with nearly complete involvement of the auditory canal, whereas localized processes are recognized as focal lesions (pustules or furuncles) anywhere along the auditory canal or external ear structures. Sebaceous secretions in the ear canal are usually evident in patients with seborrhea, but cerumen production among patients is variable, depending on etiology.

Fluid may be apparent in infectious cases. *Pseudomonas* infection produces a copious green exudate, whereas *Staphylococcus* infection presents as a yellow crusting in the midst of a purulent exudate. Fungal infections present as a fluffy white or black malodorous carpet of growth, and allergic reactions are characterized by scaly, cracked, and/or weepy tissue. Granulation tissue spreading out from the primary site of infection and eroding into the temporal bone, outer auricle, or through a perforated tympanic membrane is indicative of frank invasive disease.

Except in invasive disease or cases related to chronic otitis media (OM), head and neck lymphadenopathy typically is not detected. Invasive disease may also be accompanied by tenderness of the temporomandibular joint (TMJ).

DIAGNOSTIC REASONING

Diagnostic Tests

Laboratory tests are rarely needed if symptomatology clearly fits the classic clinical picture of otitis externa. However, any fluid from the ear may be cultured and, if microorganisms are detected, tested for antibiotic sensitivity. This may be particularly important in determining alternative treatment approaches for patients who do not respond promptly to empirical antibiotic therapy or those with chronic otitis externa, particularly with purulent exudates indicative of bacterial infection. Cultures and antibiotic sensitivity testing are also important for immunocompromised patients because their disease may be caused by rare pathogens or even by endogenous, typically nonpathogenic microbial flora. Fungi and mycobacteria should be ruled out.

The erythrocyte sedimentation rate may be elevated, although this finding has not been thoroughly studied. Soft tissue or bony involvement in malignant disease may be assessed by computed tomography (CT) and magnetic resonance imaging (MRI) scans. The temporal bone is the first bone to be affected. It is important to remember that at least one-third of bone mineral must be lost before radiological changes become apparent. Plain films and gallium or technetium-99 bone scans may also detect bony involvement, but these imaging techniques are less desirable because they lack specificity and, in the case of x-ray films, sensitivity.

Differential Diagnosis

In the absence of visible changes in the auditory canal and tympanic membrane, otalgia from referred pain associated with other disorders must be ruled out. These disorders include TMJ dysfunction, dental disease, neurologic disorders such as trigeminal and glossopharyngeal neuralgia, parotitis secondary to mumps (paramyxovirus infection) secondary to mumps, or, rarely, tumors of the middle ear and auditory meatus. Chondrodermatitis chronicus helicis may cause an otalgia similar to otitis externa in elderly patients, manifesting as an extremely tender nodule of the inner ear helix. TMJ dysfunction and dental disease may be specifically ruled out via dental x-ray films to demonstrate alterations in joint morphology or dentition. Mumps may be diagnosed serologically by measuring antibody titers. In general, a thorough head and neck examination, complete with cranial nerve testing, typically will typically differentiate among the aforementioned causes of ear pain.

OM may be distinguished from otitis externa by changes in the tympanic membrane that are characteristic of middle ear infection, including erythema, edema, and a significant lack of mobility on insufflation with a pneumatic otoscope. Moreover, movement of the tragus fails to elicit pain in middle ear infection. OM should be suspected if continuous discharge from the middle ear is evident for more than 10 days, and x-ray films may aid in ruling out this diagnosis. Otitis externa and OM may occur concurrently. A systemic dermatological condition, such as seborrheic dermatitis, psoriasis, or erythroderma, may manifest as otitis externa.

Otoscopic examination may rule out alternative pathologies including other dermatological disorders such as impetigo, herpes zoster infection, and even insect bites. Serious cranial infections requiring aggressive therapy must also be considered. Mastoiditis is characterized by fever, spontaneous rupture of the tympanic membrane, tenderness, edema, and erythema posterior to the auricle, as well as by palpable preauricular and anterior cervical lymph nodes. The mastoid process is exquisitely painful in mastoiditis, but not in unlike otitis externa. Meningitis typically presents with fever, diffuse headache, altered mentation, vomiting, and cervical stiffness. A recent history of upper respiratory tract infection (URI) may be a clue to these and other infectious processes, including sinusitis and OM.

Blood in the auditory canal may indicate temporal bone fracture or the presence of an invasive tumor. Carcinoma should be ruled out if invasive disease is suspected through the biopsy of apparent granulation tissue, which in otitis externa will demonstrate necrotizing vasculitis with no evidence of malignant cells. Other noninfectious diagnoses that may be ruled out through biopsy include primary skin and cartilage disorders such as sarcoidosis, discoid lupus, and trauma-related perichondritis of the pinna. Perichondritis may also be of infectious origin caused by *P. aeruginosa*, as confirmed by culture. Excessive cerumen buildup may also lead to a feeling of fullness or stuffiness in the ear, as well as pain and hearing loss. Otoscopic examination performed before and after irrigation of the auditory canal will rule out cerumen impaction. Gouty tophi may also affect the external ear, but they are usually painless. Rarer infectious conditions that should be ruled out by special stains, cultures, and antigen/antibody tests in refractory cases include tuberculous otitis and leprosy (both diagnosed by acid-fast stain for *Mycobacteria*) and syphilitic otitis (diagnosed by rapid plasma reagin [RPR] and Venereal Disease Research Laboratory [VDRL] tests and dark-field microscopy to identify the causative agent, *Treponema pallidum*).

MANAGEMENT

Because the predominant symptom of otitis externa is pain, alteration in comfort is a primary focus of care. Medical management of the disease should focus on alleviating pain promptly, which includes the following measures:

- Local application of heat to the outer ear can offer some relief of pain.
- Some patients get relief with application of an ice pack to the outer ear.
- Nonprescription pain relievers such as aspirin or acetaminophen (325 to 650 mg by mouth [PO] every 4 hours as needed; maximum daily dose 4,000 mg/day) or an NSAIDs such as ibuprofen (400 to 600 mg PO every 4 to 6 hours as needed to a maximum dose of 1.2 g/day) are first-line agents.
- In cases of extreme pain, acetaminophen/codeine (Tylenol #3) 325 mg/5 mg one to two tablets PO every 6 hours or acetaminophen/hydrocodone (Vicodin) 325 mg/5 mg PO every 8 hours may be prescribed for the first 24 to 48 hours, but these medications carry an abuse potential.

Patients should be instructed to keep the ear dry and to avoid swimming or submersion of the ear under water for 4 to 6 weeks.

Treatment of otitis externa to facilitate healing involves three basic steps:

1. Gentle cleaning of the ear canal to remove all cerumen, exudate, and epidermal debris using a cotton pledget or irrigation with warm tap water; irrigation

should be done cautiously until tympanic membrane perforation has been ruled out. The ear must then be kept dry, with no swimming or submersion of the ear under water for 4 to 6 weeks.

2. Evaluation of otic discharge and edema of the auditory canal and tympanic membrane.

3. Selection of an appropriate local medication once the etiology has been identified. For example, corticosteroids such as 0.1% triamcinolone solution or cream may be applied three or four times daily to relieve eczematous or psoriatic lesions.

Diffuse bacterial otitis externa may be treated empirically with topical antibiotics and anti-inflammatory otic drops that may also serve to restore the protective acidic pH level of the ear canal. Several preparations are available for use (see Drugs Commonly Prescribed 23.1). Occasionally, the pustules or furuncles associated with localized otitis externa may require surgical drainage before initiating pharmacotherapy, and more serious infections refractory to topical treatment may require systemic antibiotic therapy.

Common topical otic preparations approved by the U.S. Food and Drug Administration include acetic acid/aluminum acetate, acetic acid/hydrocortisone, ciprofloxacin/hydrocortisone, ciprofloxacin/dexamethasone, neomycin/polymyxin B/hydrocortisone, and ofloxacin. Liquid ophthalmic preparations of gentamicin and tobramycin may be used otically to cover both *P. aeruginosa* and *S. aureus*. If the ear is edematous, a small cotton plug soaked in an otic preparation should be inserted. An absorptive 1-inch cotton wick or sponge may be inserted into a highly edematous ear canal by gentle twisting if luminal occlusion prevents the passage of otic preparations. Antibiotic drops may then be placed on the wick for the first 2 to 3 days of treatment, until swelling subsides. After this, drops should be placed directly into the ear canal.

Cases that are refractory to initial therapy or involve auricular cellulitis require systemic antibiotic treatment covering both *Staphylococcus* and *Pseudomonas*. Systemic antibiotics are also indicated in the case of specific host factors such as diabetes or in an immunosuppressed patient. Diffuse and localized otitis externa may need to be treated with multiple various systemic antibiotic choices:

- First-generation cephalosporins or penicillins with relatively narrow coverage, such as cephalexin (Keflex) 250 to 500 mg PO four times daily and dicloxacillin 250 to 500 mg PO four times daily.
- Second-generation cephalosporins with broader-spectrum coverage, such as cefuroxime (Ceftin) 250 to 500 mg PO two times daily or cefdinir (Omnicef)

🌀 Drugs Commonly Prescribed 23.1: Bacterial Otitis Externa

DRUG	INDICATION	PRESCRIBING CONSIDERATIONS AND ADVERSE REACTIONS
Drugs Safe to Use With Perforated Tympanic Membrane (TM)		
Ciprofloxacin 0.3% and dexamethasone 0.1% (Ciprodex Otic)	Antibiotic and steroid corticosteroid	Not recommended for age: 6 months
Ofloxacin 0.3% (Floxin otic)	Antibiotic	Age 6 months–13 years: five drops in affected ear daily for 7 days Adults: 10 drops in affected ear for 7 days
Drugs Not Safe to Use With Perforated TM		
Chloroxylenol 1 mg Pramoxine HCL 10 mg Hydrocortisone 10 mg/mL (Cortone B aqueous)	Antibacterial/antifungal + topical anesthetic + steroid corticosteroid	Children: three drops in affected ear three times daily for 7 days Adults: four to five drops in affected ear three times daily for 7 days
Chloroxylenol 1-mg pramoxine HCl 10-mg hydrocortisone 10 mg/mL (Cortane B aqueous)	Antibacterial/antifungal + topical anesthetic + steroid corticosteroid	Children: three drops in affected ear three times daily for 7 days Adults: four to five drops in affected ear three times daily for 7 days
Colistin 3 mg Neomycin 3.3 mg, hydrocortisone Acetate 10 mg Thonzonium bromide 0.5 mg (Cortisporin-TC Otic)	Antibiotic + steroid corticosteroid + surfactant	Five drops in affected ear three to four times daily for 10 days only

300 mg PO two times daily, or beta-lactamase–resistant penicillins such as amoxicillin/clavulanate (Augmentin XR) 1,000 mg PO two times daily based on the amoxicillin component, which have broader-spectrum coverage.

- Ceftazidime (Ceftaz, Fortaz) 2 g IV every 8 to 12 hours or a combination of tobramycin (1–1.5 mg/kg IV every 8 hours, with dosage adjusted by monitoring serum levels and renal function) and ticarcillin (3 g IV every 4 hours). These regimens, however, carry a significant risk of nephrotoxicity, ototoxicity, and bleeding diatheses

An alternative to IV therapy is the oral quinolone ciprofloxacin (Cipro) administered at a higher dose of 750 mg two times daily, which is generally well tolerated and has a high cure rate in complicated disease. Fluoroquinolones should be reserved for those who have no alternative treatment options, as the serious adverse effects associated with fluoroquinolones may outweigh the benefits for patients with otitis externa. Patients who are immunocompromised from systemic corticosteroid therapy or who have chronically immunosuppressive disorders such as diabetes, as well as patients with invasive bony involvement, may require surgical debridement of the affected area to drain abscesses and remove sequestered collagen. This therapy is usually followed by 4 to 6 weeks of IV antipseudomonal therapy. Steroidal therapies such as 0.1% triamcinolone solution or cream may be applied three or four times daily to relieve eczematous or psoriatic lesions. When otitis externa has been determined to be secondary to OM, therapy should be directed toward the underlying middle ear infection. Pharmacotherapy for chronic otitis externa is directed by extensive antibiotic sensitivity testing after the infectious organisms have been cultured and identified in the laboratory. In the overwhelming majority of patients who present with chronic otitis externa, the condition is caused by persistent fungal infection, in which the ears are often dry and scaling.

The treatment of fungal infections differs mainly in the choice of antimicrobials. Before antimicrobial administration, the auditory canal must be carefully cleaned. A single dusting of sulfanilamide powder is then applied, followed by an otic suspension such as hydrocortisone/acetic acid otic (VoSol) solution, or acetic acid/aluminum acetate (Otic Domeboro). Four drops are placed in each affected ear four times daily for 7 to 10 days.

Topical fungicide preparations containing nystatin or clotrimazole are increasingly accepted, although these agents are not available solely as otic preparations. If this treatment is planned, a referral to an ear, nose, and throat (ENT) specialist should be considered. In chronic cases of otitis externa from fungal infection, systemic antifungals such as fluconazole, ketoconazole, or griseofulvin may be considered. Clotrimazole solution is available over the counter and should be used as four drops in each ear daily. Ketoconazole cream may be placed into the external canal by a trained specialist using an operating microscope and a syringe with a blunt needle. About 1 inch of cream is needed to fill the canal, and it should be removed a week later. In chronic cases of otitis externa from fungal infection, systemic antifungals such as fluconazole, ketoconazole, or griseofulvin may be considered. Pharmacotherapy for chronic otitis externa is directed by extensive antibiotic sensitivity testing after the infectious organisms have been cultured and identified in the laboratory.

FOLLOW-UP AND REFERRAL

Acute otitis externa is commonly cured after 7 to 10 days of treatment. A follow-up appointment to assess the effects of treatment may be scheduled after 1 week of therapy for uncomplicated cases. If an ear wick has been placed, the patient should return in 2 days for removal and canal cleaning. The patient should be instructed to call if symptoms do not begin to subside in 48 hours.

Immunocompromised patients with invasive disease and any patients receiving IV antibiotic therapy require daily follow-up during hospitalization, and periodic appointments are recommended for up to 1 year after the discontinuation of treatment. Otherwise healthy patients with invasive disease who do not respond to treatment promptly should also be monitored closely, and these patients should undergo further evaluation and diagnostic procedures as necessary. Results of CT and MRI scans remain abnormal for many months after clinical resolution of invasive disease; thus, serial nuclear medicine scans (gallium scans) may be preferable in evaluating treatment efficacy during follow-up because recurrence of infection may be as high as 10% within 6 months after of treatment.

A common complication in the management of otitis externa is dermatitis medicamentosa. Neomycin, an antibiotic commonly found in otic preparations, is known to cause skin reactions and ototoxicity; however, these complications may be minimized by limiting the duration of pharmacotherapy. The use of neomycin-containing agents in cases in which the tympanic membrane is ruptured is controversial because neomycin may be toxic to middle ear structures if applied directly. Otitis externa may also lead to severe furunculosis (boil formation) or cellulitis (deep-tissue infection) within the ear canal. Invasive otitis externa is a potentially life-threatening complication of poorly treated diffuse and localized disease that must be detected early. Fever, excruciating pain, and the presence of friable granulation tissue are ominous signs of this sequela. Other serious cranial infections may result from inadequately treated otitis externa, including meningitis, mastoiditis, parotitis, and osteomyelitis of either the temporal bone or the base of the skull. Cranial nerve (CN) palsies affect 20% to 30% of patients with invasive disease, most commonly involving CN VII and, if disease progresses unchecked, CNs IX, X, XI, and XII.

Invasive otitis externa, cellulitis, bony involvement, and all complicating cranial infections must be referred to a specialist for immediate treatment. Patients who are immunocompromised from steroid therapy, diabetes, or other chronic illnesses should be referred to an otorhinolaryngologist to fully evaluate the extent of disease.

Patient Education: Otitis Externa

Patients should avoid getting water in the ears for at least 4 to 6 weeks after symptoms subside because moisture from any source can trigger a recurrent episode of infection. Shower caps or earplugs should be worn when bathing, and swimming should be prohibited entirely for at least 1 month after an acute episode (cotton balls impregnated with petroleum jelly may be used as temporary ear plugs). For persons who are particularly susceptible to repeated infections, a 2% acetic acid solution may be used prophylactically to acidify the ear canal (two to three drops in each ear, two times daily and after any contact with water in which the ears become wet).

Patients should be instructed in the proper method of cleaning the ears (with a soft cotton pledget) and warned never to use swabs, sticks, or chemical agents to clean the auditory canal. Patients should understand that a small amount of earwax is necessary to prevent infection in the auditory canal and that excessive cleaning can be harmful. Clinicians should instruct patients and/or family members in how to instill topical otic drops.

The importance of keeping the ear canals dry for at least 4 to 6 weeks, both during and after an acute episode, should also be stressed. The clinician should also discuss the importance of avoiding strong jets of water from showerheads or dental water-jet systems. Alternative or complementary therapies such as candling have not been shown to be efficacious and may in fact cause harm.

OTITIS MEDIA

Otitis media (OM) is an inflammation of the structures of the middle ear. Less common in adults, 75% of children experience at least one episode of OM by the age of 3 years, and almost half of these children will have three or more episodes of OM during this age. Acute OM (AOM), also referred to as suppurative OM or purulent OM, denotes the presence of pus in the middle ear in association with local or systemic infection, including otalgia, otorrhea, and fever. OM with effusion (OME) involves the transudation of plasma fluid from middle ear blood vessels, leading to chronic effusion in the absence of the signs and symptoms of acute infection. Recurrent OM is characterized by the clearance of middle ear effusions between acute episodes of otic inflammation.

Chronic OM is present when inflammation persists for more than 3 months, typically related to tympanic membrane perforation with either intermittent or persistent otic discharge.

Measures to prevent AOM in infants and young children should be discussed with parents at well-child visits. Preventive measures include avoidance of tobacco exposure, exclusive breastfeeding for the first 6 months of life or longer, annual influenza vaccine for all children 6 months of age and older (and all adults), pneumococcal 13-valent protein-conjugate vaccine (Prevnar-13) for all children 6 weeks of age and older (and all adults), and pneumococcal 23-valent polysaccharide vaccine (Pneumovax-23) for high-risk children 2 years of age and older (and high-risk adults of all ages and all adults 50 years of age and older), according to the updated immunization schedules. However, although OM is primarily a disease of infants and young children, it can also affect adults, and the same recommendations of tobacco avoidance and appropriate vaccinations apply.

EPIDEMIOLOGY AND CAUSES

Ear pain, in general, is a common clinical complaint, accounting for 2% to 3% of all family practice office visits. Specifically, the incidence rate of OM increases during the winter months, when the climate is colder and more time is spent indoors. Although AOM is most common in very young children, older adults also have an increased risk of developing the condition because of decreases in immune functioning. Native Americans, particularly Navajos and Native Alaskans, have higher prevalence rates of OM than the general population (Hoffman et al., 2013; Kaur et al., 2017; Pumarola et al., 2017). A smaller increase in rate is also seen in white Americans of European descent. Men and women are affected equally, although OM still tends to be rare in adults.

Factors contributing to eustachian tube dysfunction leading to OME include allergies, sinusitis, rhinitis, and pharyngitis, all of which cause swelling of the membranous lining of the eustachian tube. However, the most significant precipitating event is a recent or concurrent URI, attributed most often to influenza type A (family Orthomyxoviridae), respiratory syncytial virus (*Pneumovirus*, in family Paramyxoviridae), or adenovirus. URI is thought to contribute to host immunosuppression and the loss of ciliated epithelium in the eustachian tube. In turn, bacterial adherence to the membranous lining is increased.

Differences in the anatomy of the eustachian tube among infants and young children may predispose them to OM. Anatomical abnormalities that can lead to direct blockage of the eustachian tube include hypertrophy or chronic inflammation of the adenoids (pharyngeal tonsils), cleft palate, deviated nasal septum, and nasopharyngeal tumors. Perforation of the eardrum from direct blunt trauma, swimming or diving accidents, or sudden outward pressure or suction (such as from a kiss over the ear) may create a portal of entry for bacteria directly into the middle ear. Certain genetic conditions such as Down syndrome (trisomy 21) also predispose individuals to middle ear infections. Both active and passive smoking have been associated with an increased risk of all forms of OM, and crowded or unsanitary living conditions, exposure to wood-burning stoves, along with a family history of OM (particularly in the same household), are also contributing factors.

PATHOPHYSIOLOGY

AOM results when bacterial infection by nasopharyngeal microorganisms follows eustachian tube dysfunction, in which the narrowest portion of the tube (the isthmus) becomes obstructed. Inflammation results primarily in response to bacterial products, including endotoxins and cell-wall components, creating in effect a middle ear abscess. Pressure from this buildup of pus may impinge on the fine blood vessels supplying the tympanic membrane, weakening its structure, reducing tensile strength, and eventually causing perforation or rupture of the eardrum to facilitate draining of inner ear fluid. Fortunately, in the absence of underlying immunocompromise, the tympanic membrane typically begins to heal spontaneously within hours and may be fully healed by 1 or 2 weeks, with complete restoration of baseline hearing capacity.

OME is caused by a transudation of plasma fluid through engorged blood vessels resulting from the loss of eustachian tube patency, caused either by swelling of the membranous lining or direct anatomical blockage of the eustachian tube. Swelling of the mucosa is particularly common in the presence of an antecedent viral URI or acute allergy attack. Effective drainage of middle ear fluid is thus prevented, and negative pressure develops in the middle ear cavity, further drawing in fluid.

Streptococcus pneumoniae (implicated in 40% to 50% of AOM cases) is the most frequent pathogen isolated from middle ear effusions in adults. The currently available polyvalent streptococcal vaccines cover only 60% to 70% of these isolates. However, several studies have suggested the incidence of AOM infections due to *Streptococcus* strains covered by the originally developed 7-valent protein-conjugate vaccine (Prevnar-7) and the second-generation 13-valent vaccine (Prevnar-13) has decreased since their introduction as recommended immunizations in pediatric populations, although the methodology of some of these studies have been criticized (Wasserman & Gerber, 2017). A recent 2017 study (Kaur et al., 2017) concluded that the epidemiology (distribution of causative organisms) but not the risk factors for AOM has undergone substantial changes since the introduction of pneumococcal conjugate vaccines.

Other common organisms include nontypeable *Haemophilus influenzae* (10% to 30% of cases), which are not covered by the *Haemophilus influenzae* type b (Hib) vaccine, and *Moraxella (Branhamella) catarrhalis,* the vast majority of which express the beta-lactamase gene and are resistant to first-line penicillin and cephalosporin antibiotics. These organisms are thought to reach the middle ear from the upper respiratory tract via aspiration or reflux. *S. aureus* and *Streptococcus pyogenes* are far less common causative agents, particularly since the introduction of sulfonamide antibiotics such as trimethoprim-sulfamethoxazole (Bactrim).

Up to one-half of AOM cases are attributed to viral infections originating in the nasopharynx and extending to the middle ear via the eustachian tube, including rhinovirus, adenovirus, coronavirus, influenza, and respiratory syncytial virus. In fact, nearly 40% of documented influenza cases in children younger than 3 years are complicated by AOM, adding to the impetus for widespread flu vaccination. *Mycoplasma* and *Chlamydia pneumoniae* are rarer causes of OM. *Chlamydia trachomatis* is typically seen only in infants younger than 6 months. In developing countries, unusual agents such as *Mycobacteria tuberculosis, Corynebacterium diphtheriae,* parasites (e.g., *Ascaris*), or fungi (e.g., *Blastomycoses, Candida, Aspergillus*) may be identified.

OME may be viral in origin but is usually attributed to beta-lactamase–producing bacterial strains that are resistant to first-line antibiotic therapies. Importantly, middle ear effusions often last for weeks to months after an AOM clears; thus, OME may simply reflect part of the natural history of a resolved episode of AOM. Recurrent OM typically results from bacterial infection due to anatomical abnormalities that repeatedly compromise eustachian tube patency. Chronic OM may also be caused by any of the bacteria associated with AOM, as well as *Escherichia coli* and *Proteus,* but *P. aeruginosa* and *S. aureus* are the most commonly isolated pathogens in chronic suppurative OM.

CLINICAL PRESENTATION

Subjective

The patient with OME will typically complain of stuffiness, fullness, and a loss of auditory acuity in the affected ear only. Pain is rare, but patients may describe popping, crackling, or gurgling sounds when chewing, yawning, or blowing the nose. Very rarely, patients may experience vertigo (a sense of whirling or spinning in space) or ataxia, if inner ear complications such as labyrinthitis are present. Although patients are typically afebrile, a recent history of viral URI or either allergic or vasomotor rhinitis is common.

In contrast, AOM usually presents with marked "deep" ear pain and fever, as well as unilateral hearing loss, otic discharge, and a recent history of URI. Some patients may also experience dizziness (space disorientation), vertigo, tinnitus (ringing in the ears), vomiting, or nausea. Pain typically subsides if the tympanic membrane ruptures because this relieves middle ear pressure. In these cases, patients also usually complain of otic discharge. Recurrent OM is characterized by the clearance of middle ear effusions between acute episodes of inflammation.

Chronic OM typically presents with a history of repeated bouts of AOM, followed by a period of continuous or intermittent otorrhea lasting for more than 3 months. Pain is seldom a complaint, and hearing loss (related to tympanic membrane perforation) is the primary concern. Risk factors for AOM include enrollment of a child in day care, presence of tobacco smoke in the home, and residing in communities where antibiotic-resistant forms of *S. pneumoniae* are endemic.

Objective

Examination of the external ear in patients with OME is typically unremarkable; however, the mucous membranes of the nasal and oral cavities may be infected or edematous, confirming a recent history of URI. The eardrum may be dull but usually is not bulging, and eardrum mobility typically decreases on pneumatic otoscopy. When examining a patient with AOM, the use of Auralgan otic solution (a combination analgesic and anesthetic agent, contraindicated in cases of perforated eardrum) may be needed to facilitate the examination if the patient is experiencing pain. The tympanic membrane may be amber or yellow-orange, or the membrane may be infected and pinkish gray to fiery red in color. The tympanic membrane is typically full or bulging in acute cases, with absent or obscured bony landmarks and cone light reflex.

Although the auditory canal usually shows no abnormalities, a discharge from the middle ear may be present if the tympanic membrane has perforated as a result of the collection of middle ear fluid and subsequent inflammatory response. Otorrhea may be purulent or mucoid, depending on the stage of inflammation; polymorphonuclear neutrophils are prominent in the early stages of bacterial infection. Otoscopic examination in chronic OM usually reveals a perforated, draining tympanic membrane and possibly invasive granulation tissue. Chronic, foul-smelling otorrhea is typical of anaerobic bacterial infection, and a chronic, grayish-yellow suppuration may indicate the development of a cholesteatoma from the degenerative products of invasive epithelialization (involuted squamous epithelia and keratin debris) at the site of infection. In rare cases, bullae formed between layers of the tympanic membrane (bullous myringitis) caused by certain viruses or *M. pneumoniae* are seen; multiple perforations of the tympanic membrane are characteristic of tuberculous otitis.

On palpation, in cases of acute infection, lymphadenopathy of the preauricular and posterior cervical nodes is common. If OM is complicated by an acute mastoiditis, tenderness over the mastoid will be elicited because the bony architecture of the middle ear is continuous with the mastoid process.

DIAGNOSTIC REASONING

Diagnostic Tests

Laboratory tests are rarely needed if symptomatology clearly fits the classic clinical picture of OM. However, if confirmation is desired, pneumatic otoscopy will demonstrate decreased or absent tympanic membrane mobility in serous, acute, or chronic OME. Tympanometry may be useful if fluid buildup behind the middle ear is suspected in the absence of other clinical signs; a flat tympanogram is consistent with restrictive disease of the middle ear cavity. A complete blood count is usually not indicated; however, patients with AOM may demonstrate a leukocytosis, particularly if they are febrile.

Cultures of tympanocentesis fluid are not indicated in serous OM and are of little practical value in acute disease, unless the patient is immunocompromised or infectious complications such as mastoiditis are evident. In subacute, recurrent, or chronic cases of OM, however, cultures and antibiotic sensitivity testing are helpful in guiding alternative treatment approaches. If cultures are obtained, fungi and mycobacteria should be specifically ruled out.

Conventional sinus x-ray films and CT scans (which can reveal mucosal thickening in the middle ear space) may be helpful in evaluating patients with effusion and particularly patients with recurrent infection. Pure-tone audiometry may be helpful both before and after treatment; Weber and Rinne tuning-fork tests typically will reveal conductive, as opposed to sensorineural, hearing loss. Sound lateralization to the affected ear occurs when a 512-Hz tuning fork is placed midline on the top of the head (Weber test), and bone conduction is superior in duration and volume to air conduction (negative Rinne test).

Differential Diagnosis

OM must be distinguished from otitis externa, which is inflammation of the auditory canal and/or external ear, including the pinna and tragus. These structures are usually not affected in OM, and otitis externa typically does not involve the tympanic membrane. Otitis externa resulting from furunculosis, local skin maceration, trauma from a foreign body, or direct blunt force must be ruled out. Exacerbated pain on manipulation of the tragus, pinna, or earlobe is a telltale sign of external ear inflammation. Rarer infectious conditions that may cause OM that must be ruled out by special stains, cultures, and antigen/antibody tests, include tuberculous otitis and leprosy (requiring an acid-fast stain for *Mycobacteria*) and syphilitic otitis (requiring RPR and VDRL tests and then dark-field microscopy to identify the causative agent *Treponema pallidum*).

TMJ syndrome pain is similar to the pain of AOM. Patients may complain of ear pain when in fact the pain is being referred from the TMJ. Mastoiditis presenting without middle ear infection should also be considered when no physical signs of middle ear involvement are evident. Referred otalgia from TMJ dysfunction or dental abscesses may be ruled out by dental x-rays. Parotitis secondary to mumps (paramyxovirus infection) may be ruled out via serology studies (antibody titers), if suspected.

Other noninfectious causes of OM include nasopharyngeal neoplasm that must be ruled out through biopsy in cases of unilateral recurrent, chronic, or refractory OM. Excessive earwax buildup (cerumen impaction) with or without infection may also lead to a feeling of fullness or stuffiness in the ear, as well as pain and hearing loss; otoscopic examination is performed before and after irrigation of the auditory canal to rule out this disorder. Barotrauma may also mimic OM, with transient middle ear effusion resulting from air travel or drastic increases in altitude, such as when driving up mountains.

MANAGEMENT

Uncomplicated cases of OM are likely to be self-limited and may not require any specific intervention other than pain and symptomatic relief (see Drugs Commonly Prescribed 23.2). However, pharmacologic treatment of complicated or recurrent OM is indicated to prevent permanent anatomical changes of the middle ear and subsequent hearing loss. Changes in characteristics of auditory stimuli related to middle ear pathology lead to sensory or perceptual alterations. In the unfortunate instance when middle ear infection leads to permanent comorbidity, loss of auditory perception may affect a patient's lifestyle, communication patterns, socialization, and self-concept. Other identifiable clinical problems include alteration in comfort and an increased potential for injury related to hearing loss. Thus, interventions should focus on

Drugs Commonly Prescribed 23.2: Acute Otitis Media (AOM) in Adults

INDICATION	DRUG	DOSE	PRESCRIBING CONSIDERATIONS
Otherwise healthy pediatric patients with mild symptoms	Acetaminophen (Tylenol)	10–15 mg/kg/dose PO by mouth every 4 hours as needed (maximum 75 mg/kg/day [infants/children])	For ages 6–24 months, observation with the use of systemic analgesics *without* the use of antibacterial agents is an option for selected children with uncomplicated AOM based on diagnostic certainty, age, illness. Evaluation at 48–72 hours and discontinue medication if symptoms do not persist. If signs and symptoms of AOM persist despite systemic analgesic, use for 48–72 hours, reassess and consider treatment with antibiotic.
	ibuprofen (Motrin, Advil)	5–10 mg/kg/dose PO every 6–8 hour as needed (maximum 40 mg/kg/day [6 months–11 years old])	
No day-care attendance and no antibiotics within the past 90 days	Amoxicillin	Standard dose: 40–45 mg/kg/day PO in two divided doses for 10 days	No risk factors should be present that increase the risk of penicillin-resistant *Streptococcus pneumoniae*.
Day-care attendance or antibiotics within the past 90 days	Amoxicillin	High dose: 80–90 mg/kg/day (maximum 1,000 mg/dose) PO in two divided doses for 10 days	Amoxicillin retains the most activity of all oral β-lactam agents against *S. pneumoniae*, including penicillin-intermediate resistant strains.
β-Lactam allergy	Of note, penicillin allergy without clinical confirmation is over-reported, and the incidence of cephalosporin cross-reactivity with penicillin allergy is <2%; thus, consider allergy testing when infection resolves to confirm penicillin allergy.		
Penicillin allergy (mild, nonanaphylactic)	Cefuroxime axetil	30 mg/kg/day (maximum 1000 mg/day) PO in two divided doses for 10 days	Due to bad taste of cefuroxime suspension, recommend tablets if possible, which can be crushed and put into a palatable fluid.
	Cefprozil	30 mg/kg/day (maximum 1,000 mg/day) PO in two divided doses for 10 days	Compared with cefuroxime, liquid cefprozil has a better taste but inferior coverage of *Haemophilus* and penicillin-intermediate resistant *S. pneumonia*.
Penicillin allergy (severe, anaphylactic) or cephalosporin allergy	Clarithromycin (Biaxin)	15 mg/kg/day in two divided doses for 10 days	Macrolides are inferior options, due to high resistance rates and clinical failure rates.

Drugs Commonly Prescribed 23.2: Acute Otitis Media (AOM) in Adults—cont'd

INDICATION	DRUG	DOSE	PRESCRIBING CONSIDERATIONS
	Trimethoprim/ sulfamethoxazole (TMP/SMX; Bactrim)	TMP 6–12 mg/kg/day (maximum 320 mg/day TMP) PO in two divided doses for 10 days	TMP/SMX is an inferior option, due to high resistance rates and clinical failure rates. Consider referral to otorhinolaryngologist for tympanocentesis.
	Azithromycin (Zithromax)	10 mg/kg/day PO on the first day and 5 mg/kg/day PO for 4 days	Macrolides are inferior options, due to high resistance rates and clinical failure rates.
Failure of Initial AOM Treatment in Pediatric Patients			
Failure of standard-dose amoxicillin	Amoxicillin-clavulanate (7:1 formulation) (Augmentin)	Amoxicillin 45 mg/kg/day PO in two divided doses for 10 days	The combination is recommended to provide a high dose of amoxicillin (for penicillin-intermediate resistant *S. pneumoniae*) and a regular dose of clavulanate (for coverage of β-lactamase–producing *H. influenzae* and *Moraxella catarrhalis*) without excessive (>10 mg/kg/day) clavulanate exposure that could lead to increased incidence of diarrhea.
Failure of high-dose amoxicillin	Amoxicillin-clavulanate (4:1 formulation) (Augmentin)	40 mg/kg/day PO in three divided doses for 10 days (based on amoxicillin component)	Excessive (>10 mg/kg/day) clavulanate exposure could lead to increased incidence of diarrhea.
	Cefuroxime axetil	30 mg/kg/day PO in two divided doses for 10 days	Due to bad taste of cefuroxime suspension, recommend tablets if possible, which can be crushed and put into a palatable fluid.
	Cefprozil	30 mg/kg/day PO in two divided doses for 10 days	
β-Lactam (penicillin) allergy	Clarithromycin (Biaxin)	15 mg/kg/day PO in two divided doses for 10 days	Therapeutic options for these patients are very limited; consider referral to otorhinolaryngologist for tympanostomy.
	Trimethoprim/sulfamethoxazole (TMP/SMX; Bactrim)	TMP 6–12 mg/kg/day PO in two divided doses for 10 days	TMP/SMX is less efficacious than amoxicillin-clavulanate.
	Azithromycin (Zithromax)	10 mg/kg PO first day then 5 mg/kg/day × 4 days	Macrolides are less efficacious than amoxicillin-clavulanate; there is significant macrolide resistance in *S. pneumoniae*.
Treatment of AOM in Adults			
AOM	Amoxicillin	500 mg every 8 hours OR 875 mg two times daily for 10 days	
β-Lactamase–resistant	Amoxicillin-clavulanate (Augmentin) Cefixime (Suprax)	875 mg two times daily for 10 days 400 mg daily for 7 days	
Penicillin-allergic patients	Macrolides Azithromycin (Zithromax) Clarithromycin (Biaxin)	500 mg on day 1, then 250 mg daily for 4 days 500 mg every 12 hours for 7 days	

Continued

Drugs Commonly Prescribed 23.2: Acute Otitis Media (AOM) in Adults—cont'd

INDICATION	DRUG	DOSE	PRESCRIBING CONSIDERATIONS
Drugs to Avoid in AOM, Unless Otherwise Indicated			
Cephalexin	No activity against penicillin-intermediate resistant *S. pneumoniae* No activity against *H. influenzae/M. catarrhalis*		
Cefaclor	No activity against penicillin-intermediate resistant *S. pneumoniae* Marginal activity against *H. influenzae/M. catarrhalis*		
Cefixime (Suprax)	No activity against penicillin-intermediate resistant *S. pneumoniae* Excellent activity against *H. influenza*		
Ceftriaxone (Rocephin)	Routine use not recommended due to potential for increased resistance to third-generation cephalosporins. May be an option in severe cases that have failed therapy, in immunosuppressed patients, or in neonates. **Note: 3 days of IM/IV therapy recommended** (single dose not as effective in eradicating penicillin-resistant *S. pneumoniae*)		
Clindamycin	No activity against *Haemophilus/Moraxella* spp. (may be an option for *S. pneumoniae* in severe penicillin-allergic patients)		
Erythromycin	Poor activity against *H. influenzae* Significant macrolide resistance in *S. pneumonia*		

Abbreviations: IM, intramuscultar; PO, by mouth.

moving the patient toward acceptance, identifying effective communication patterns, and recognizing support mechanisms and resources for coping with hearing loss. Fortunately, the vast majority of OM cases never reach this advanced stage.

In cases of OME, watchful waiting is indicated, with monthly examinations to monitor for resolution. If the effusion is unresponsive to medical treatment and persists for longer than 12 weeks, a 10-day course of an antibiotic should be considered, in addition to a referral to an otorhinolaryngologist. Antibiotic choice needs to be individualized; however, for the patient who is not penicillin allergic and has not recently been exposed to antibiotics, amoxicillin (80 to 90 mg/kg/day; maximum 1,000 mg/dose) is a reasonable choice. For patients who have had antibiotics in the past month, a beta-lactamase resistant agent (e.g., amoxicillin/clavulanate) or a second- or third-generation cephalosporin is an appropriate choice. Studies have indicated that prolonged (more than 10 days) treatment of OME has not shown an advantage over a 10-day course of therapy.

Some studies suggest the addition of prednisone; however, the most recent recommendations from the American Academy of Otolaryngology suggest that antibiotics, oral corticosteroids, and intranasal corticosteroid preparations are not recommended for the treatment of OME in a child of any age (Roditi et al., 2017). Studies have not borne out the effectiveness of decongestants or antihistamines, although these may be of some benefit in patients with comorbid allergic rhinitis.

Although there is an increasing trend to observe uncomplicated AOM in children for the first 48 to 72 hours, rather than prescribe early antibacterial treatment in the hopes of self-limited resolution, antimicrobial therapy in adults is largely the norm. Selection of an agent to treat AOM requires consideration of several factors, including the patient's age, OM history, drug hypersensitivity, prior antimicrobial response, and associated illnesses. For children aged 6 to 24 months, observation and systemic analgesics without the use of antibacterial agents is an option for selected children with uncomplicated AOM based on diagnostic certainty, age, severity of illness, and assurance of follow-up. In children older than 24 months, many cases of AOM may resolve and do not require antibiotics, as long as the symptoms are manageable with systemic analgesics, the child has access to reevaluation at 48 hours, and symptoms do not persist. If signs and symptoms of AOM persist for 48 to 72 hours in spite of using systemic analgesics, the child should be reassessed, and antibiotic treatment should be considered. Given that the majority of AOM cases occur in pediatric patients, pharmacotherapeutic approaches for AOM in both children and adults are summarized in Drugs Commonly Prescribed 23.2. It should be noted that according to the Centers for Disease Control and Prevention, approximately one-third of children with AOM do not receive the recommended first-line antibiotic (Table 23.1).

TABLE 23.1 Percent of Patients Receiving the Recommended First-Line Antibiotic by Condition, the United States, 2010–2011

	Adults (≥20 years)	Children (0–19 years)
Sinus infection	37%	52%
Pharyngitis (sore throat)	37%	60%
Middle ear infection	N/A	67%

Abbreviation: N/A, not available.

*Based on the prevalence of allergy to first-line antibiotics and estimated treatment failures after first-line antibiotics, at least 80% of patients presenting with these conditions should receive first-line antibiotics. Analysis is based on NAMCS and NHAMCS data.

Source: Centers for Disease Control and Prevention. *Antibiotic use in the United States, 2017: Progress and opportunities.* Atlanta, GA: Centers for Disease Control and Prevention, U.S. Department of Health and Human Services; 2017.

FOLLOW-UP AND REFERRAL

Patients with AOM should be seen for follow-up in 48 to 72 hours if symptoms have not resolved. Otherwise, a follow-up appointment may be scheduled several days after the completion of pharmacotherapy. Most patients experience spontaneous closure of a ruptured tympanic membrane and recovery of normal hearing within 4 weeks of treatment. Otoscopic examination should be done 4 weeks after diagnosis. If symptoms persist, consider changing the antibiotic regimen to cover beta-lactamase–producing organisms. Patients with OME should be reevaluated at 4 to 6 weeks after treatment because the full clinical course of the disease may last up to several weeks. Monthly otoscopic or tympanometric examinations should be done as long as OME persists. Chronic OM requires monthly follow-up to assess the efficacy of treatment and monitor for recurrence of infection.

Nursing Situation: Otitis Media in Children

J.S. is a 2-year-old child who presents to the pediatrician's office with a temperature of 101.8°F. Her mother reports that for the past 2 days, she has been tugging on her right ear and producing a moderate amount of yellow nasal drainage and has been very irritable. On physical examination, you discover that the tympanic membrane is erythematous, is bulging, and has decreased mobility. The mother states that the child's appetite is normal and denies any vomiting or diarrhea. The child's history is negative for previous ear infections, congenital syndromes, and prematurity. Immunizations are up to date, and no one else in the family has experienced these symptoms. The mother states that the child started attending day care 2 weeks ago.

Your diagnosis is acute otitis media. Recommendations from the American Academy of Family Physicians in 2013 and published as part of the *Choosing Wisely* initiative of the American Board of Internal Medicine Foundation in partnership with *Consumer Reports* that seeks to advance a national dialogue on avoiding wasteful or unnecessary medical tests, treatments, and procedures is as follows:

Don't prescribe antibiotics for otitis media in children aged 2 to 12 years with nonsevere symptoms where the observation option is reasonable. The "observation option" refers to deferring antibacterial treatment of selected children for 48 to 72 hours and limiting management to symptomatic relief. The decision to observe or treat is based on the child's age, diagnostic certainty, and illness severity. To observe a child without initial antibacterial therapy, it is important that the parent or caregiver has a ready means of communicating with the clinician. There also must be a system in place that permits reevaluation of the child.

(http://www.choosingwisely.org/clinician-lists/american-academy-family-physicians-antibiotics-for-otitis-media-in-children/).

If medical management does not clear the infection, inner ear effusion persists, or OM episodes recur, referral to an ENT specialist for potential surgical evaluation is indicated. Common surgical procedures include myringotomy (incision of the eardrum to allow draining and relieve fluid buildup in the middle ear) or tympanostomy (insertion of tubes across the eardrum into the inner ear to drain pus or serous fluid). Tonsillectomy and/or adenoidectomy may also be used as secondary prevention measures. All infectious sequelae of contiguous cranial structures, as well as invasive complications requiring excision such as a cholesteatoma, require referral to a specialist.

OME can lead to irreversible conductive hearing loss if middle ear structures are permanently damaged from effusion-related pressure changes. If AOM is poorly treated or is present in an immunocompromised patient, it may lead to OME, chronic OM, otitis interna (labyrinthitis), vertigo, ataxia, or several acute, subacute, and chronic infections of adjacent cranial structures (e.g., including mastoiditis, petrositis, meningitis, and epidural, subdural, or brain abscesses). Other complications include perforation of the tympanic membrane, cholesteatoma, facial nerve palsies, lateral sinus thrombophlebitis, and otitic hydrocephalus.

Although the clinical course of OME may last for several weeks, patients should be referred to a specialist for impedance audiometry testing and further evaluation to rule out nasopharyngeal tumors and other anatomical eustachian tube obstructions, if hearing loss persists beyond 6 weeks, extends bilaterally, or reaches more than 20 decibels. Patients with AOM may require referral to a specialist if vertigo or ataxia develops, if a ruptured tympanic membrane fails to close, if symptoms worsen after 3 to 4 days of treatment, or if significant hearing loss is present.

Patient Education: Otitis Media

Swimming should be avoided until OM clears because immersion in water may lead to otitis externa, complicating the middle ear infection. The ear canal should be kept as dry as possible. Tympanic membrane perforation can be avoided by not using cotton swabs or sharp objects of any kind to clean the ears. Traumatic injuries to the middle ear should be avoided as well to prevent perforation. In all cases, especially those in which the tympanic membrane is perforated, blowing of the nose should be avoided. If the nose must be blown, it should be done as gently as possible. Nasal saline may be used to liquefy nasal secretions and facilitate drainage.

All patients and their families should be encouraged to stop smoking because smoking aggravates all forms of otic inflammation. Folk remedies such as "sweet oil" should also be avoided. Patients should be instructed to return to the clinic for further evaluation after 48 hours if symptoms of AOM have not ameliorated. Explain that OM per se is not contagious but that predisposing URIs may be passed from person to person. Bedrest or reduced activity may be suggested in severe cases until fever and pain subside, and the importance of completing the full regimen of all antibiotic therapies should be emphasized. Instruct patients to keep the ear canal dry during the course of infection, and demonstrate the proper method of cleaning the ear canal without chemical agents, sharp objects, cotton swabs, or a finger.

REFERENCES

Otitis Externa

Centers for Disease Control and Prevention. Estimated burden of acute otitis externa—United States, 2003–2007. *MMWR Morb Mortal Wkly Rep.* 2011;60(19):605–609.

Chawdhary G, Pankhania M, Douglas S, Bottrill I. Current management of necrotising otitis externa in the UK: Survey of 221 UK otolaryngologists. *Acta Otolaryngol.* 2017;137(8):818–822.

Gruber M, Sela E, Doweck T, et al. Management of malignant (necrotising) otitis externa. *J Laryngol Otol.* 2011;125(12):1212–1217.

Gruber M, Sela E, Doweck I, et al. The role of surgery in necrotizing otitis externa. *Ear Nose Throat J.* 2017;96(1):E16–E21.

Hasibi M, Ashtiani MK, Zarandi MM, et al. A treatment protocol for management of bacterial and fungal malignant external otitis: A large cohort in Tehran, Iran. *Ann Otol Rhinol Laryngol.* 2017;126(7):561–567.

Llor C, McNulty CA, Butler CC. Ordering and interpreting ear swabs in otitis externa. *BMJ.* 2014; 349:g5259.

Munguia R, Daniel SJ. Ototopical antifungals and otomycosis: A review. *Int J Pediatr Otorhinolaryngol.* 2008;72:453–459.

Rosenfeld RM, Schwartz SR, Cannon CR, et al. Clinical practice guideline: Acute otitis externa executive summary. *Otolaryngol Head Neck Surg.* 2014;150(2):161–168.

Schaefer P, Baugh RF. Acute otitis externa: An update. *Am Fam Physician.* 2012;86(11):1055–1061.

Vennewald I, Klemm E. Otomycosis: Diagnosis and treatment. *Clin Dermatol.* 2010;28:202–211.

Otitis Media

Austrian R, Howie VM, Ploussard JH. The bacteriology of pneumococcal otitis media. *Johns Hopkins Med J.* 1977;141:104–111.

Benninger MS. Acute bacterial rhinosinusitis and otitis media: Changes in pathogenicity following widespread use of pneumococcal conjugate vaccine. *Otolaryngol Head Neck Surg.* 2008;138: 274–278.

Block SL, Hedrick J, Harrison CJ, et al. Community-wide vaccination with the heptavalent pneumococcal conjugate significantly alters the microbiology of acute otitis media. *Pediatr Infect Dis J.* 2004;23:829–833.

Brownlee RC Jr, DeLoache WR, Cowan CC Jr, Jackson HP. Otitis media in children. Incidence, treatment, and prognosis in pediatric practice. *J Pediatr.* 1969;75:636–642.

Casey JR, Pichichero ME. Changes in frequency and pathogens causing acute otitis media in 1995–2003. *Pediatr Infect Dis J.* 2004; 23:824–828.

Celin SE, Bluestone CD, Stephenson J, et al. Bacteriology of acute otitis media in adults. *JAMA.* 1991;266:2249–2252.

Centers for Disease Control and Prevention. *Antibiotic use in the United States, 2017: Progress and opportunities.* Atlanta, GA: Centers for Disease Control and Prevention, US Department of Health and Human Services; 2017.

Eskola J, Kilpi T, Palmu A, et al. Efficacy of a pneumococcal conjugate vaccine against acute otitis media. *N Engl J Med.* 2001; 344:403.

Harmes KM, Blackwood RA, Burrows HL, et al. Otitis media: Diagnosis and treatment. *Am Fam Physician.* 2013;88(7):435–440.

Hersh AL, Fleming-Dutra KE, Shapiro DJ, et al. Frequency of first-line antibiotic selection among US ambulatory care visits for otitis media, sinusitis, and pharyngitis. *JAMA Intern Med.* 2016;176(12):1870–1872.

Hoffman HJ, Daly KA, Bainbridge KE, et al. Panel 1: Epidemiology, natural history, and risk factors. *Otolaryngol Head Neck Surg.* 2013;148(suppl 4): E1–E25.

Hwang SY, Kok S, Walton J. Balloon dilation for eustachian tube dysfunction: Systematic review. *J Laryngol Otol.* 2016;130(suppl 4): S2–6.

Karma PH, Penttilä MA, Sipilä MM, Kataja MJ. Otoscopic diagnosis of middle ear effusion in acute and non-acute otitis media. I. The value of different otoscopic findings. *Int J Pediatr Otorhinolaryngol.* 1989;17:37–49.

Kaur, R, Morris, M, Pichichero, ME. Epidemiology of acute otitis media in the postpneumococcal conjugate vaccine era. *Pediatrics.* 2017;140(3):e20170181.

Lee KY. Pediatric respiratory infections by *Mycoplasma pneumoniae.* *Expert Rev Anti Infect Ther.* 2008;6(4):509–521.

Leskinen K, Jero J. Acute complications of otitis media in adults. *Clin Otolaryngol.* 2005;30:511–516.

Lieberthal AS, Carroll AE, Chonmaitree T, et al. The diagnosis and management of acute otitis media. *Pediatrics.* 2013;131(3):e964–e999.

Mittal R, Lisi CV, Gerring R, et al. Current concepts in the pathogenesis and treatment of chronic suppurative otitis media. *J Med Microbiol.* 2015;64(10):1103–1116.

Morris P. Chronic suppurative otitis media. *BMJ Clin Evid.* 2012;2012:0507.

National Guideline Clearinghouse. *Guideline summary: Clinical practice guideline: otitis media with effusion (update).* Rockville, MD: Agency for Healthcare Research and Quality; February 1, 2016. https://www.guideline.gov. Accessed September 14, 2017.

Prymula R, Peeters P, Chrobok V, et al. Pneumococcal capsular poly-saccharides conjugated to protein D for prevention of acute otitis media caused by both *Streptococcus pneumoniae* and nontypable *Haemophilus influenzae:* A randomised double-blind efficacy study. *Lancet.* 2006;357:740–748.

Pumarola F, Marès J, Losada I, et al. Microbiology of bacteria causing recurrent acute otitis media (AOM) and AOM treatment failure in young children in Spain: Shifting pathogens in the post-pneumococcal conjugate vaccination era. *Int J Pediatr Otorhinolaryngol.* 2013;77(8):1231–1236.

Qureishi A, Lee Y, Belfield K, Birchall JP, Daniel M. Update on otitis media—prevention and treatment. *Infect Drug Resist.* 2014;7:15–24.

Roditi RE, Rosenfeld RM, Shin JJ. Otitis media with effusion: Our national practice. *Otolaryngology.* 2017;157(2):171–172.

Rosenfeld RM, Schwartz SR, Pynnonen MA, et al. Clinical practice guideline: Tympanostomy tubes in children. *Otolaryngol Head Neck Surg.* 2013;149(suppl 1):S1–35.

Rosenfeld RM, Shin JJ, Schwartz SR. Clinical practice guideline: Otitis media with effusion executive summary (update). *Otolaryngol Head Neck Surg.* 2016;154(2):201–214.

Rovers MM, Glasziou P, Appelman CL, et al. Antibiotics for acute otitis media: A meta-analysis with individual patient data. *Lancet.* 2006;368:1429–1435.

Samuels MA, Gonzalez RG, Kim AY, Stemmer-Rachamimov A. Case records of the Massachusetts General Hospital. Case 34-2007. A 77-year-old man with ear pain, difficulty speaking, and altered mental status. *N Engl J Med.* 2007;357:1957.

Schilder AG, Chonmaitree T, Cripps AW, et al. Otitis media. *Nat Rev Dis Primers.* 2016;8;2:16063.

Schwartz LE, Brown RB. Purulent otitis media in adults. *Arch Intern Med.* 1992;152:2301.

Smith-Vaughan H, Byun R, Nadkarni M, et al. Measuring nasal bacterial load and its association with otitis media. *BMC Ear Nose Throat Disord.* 2006;6:10.

Sun D, McCarthy TJ, Liberman DB. Cost-effectiveness of watchful waiting in acute otitis media. *Pediatrics.* 2017;139(4):e20163086.

Vernacchio L, Vezina RM, Mitchell AA, et al. Management of acute otitis media by primary care physicians: Trends since the release of the 2004 American Academy of Pediatrics/American Academy of Family Physicians Clinical Practice Guideline. *Pediatrics.* 2007;120(2):281–287.

Walton L. Otitis externa. *BMJ.* 2012;344:1756–1833. doi: 10.113/bmje3623

Waseem H, Aslam H. Otitis media treatment and management. Medscape. **http://emedicine.medscape.com/article/994656-treatment.** Accessed May 4, 2017.

Wasserman, RC, Gerber JS. Acute otitis media in the 21st century: What now? *Pediatrics.* 2017;140(3):e20171966.

Yano H, Okitsu N, Hori T, et al. Detection of respiratory viruses in nasopharyngeal secretions and middle ear fluid from children with acute otitis media. *Acta Otolaryngol.* 2009;129(1):19–24.

RESOURCES

Choosing Wisely: Otitis Media
    http://www.choosingwisely.org/clinician-lists/#keyword=otitis_media

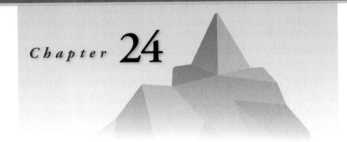

Chapter 24

Inflammatory and Infectious Disorders of the Nose, Sinuses, Mouth, and Throat

Humberto Reinoso, **PhD, FNP-BC, ENP-BC**

Lynne M. Dunphy, **PhD, APRN, FNP-BC, FAAN, FAANP**

Brian Oscar Porter, **MD, PhD, MPH, MBA**

RHINITIS

Rhinitis (coryza) is an inflammation of the nasal mucosa characterized by nasal congestion, rhinorrhea, sneezing, pruritus, and/or postnasal drainage. Its etiology is varied, but it is generally categorized as either allergic or nonallergic rhinitis. Allergic rhinitis may be either seasonal or perennial. Nonallergic rhinitis may be (1) infectious, (2) irritant related (often in the workplace), (3) vasomotor, (4) hormone related, (5) associated with medication use or overuse (rhinitis medicamentosa), or (6) atrophic (seen primarily in geriatric patients). It may be acute or chronic, but the most common forms are viral rhinitis and perennial or seasonal ("hay fever") allergic rhinitis.

Although rhinitis is often a benign and self-limited disorder, poorly controlled allergic rhinitis may contribute to sleep loss, absenteeism from work or school, secondary daytime fatigue, learning impairment, decreased overall cognitive functioning, decreased long-term productivity, and decreased quality of life. In addition, poorly controlled rhinitis may lead to the development of other related disease processes, such as sinusitis, nasal polyps, otitis media (OM), hearing impairment, aggravation of underlying asthma, sleep apnea, and may include secondary bacterial infections. "Rhinosinusitis" (also known as sinusitis) is a term that encompasses disorders affecting both the nasal passages and paranasal sinuses and has overlapping but distinct symptoms from pure rhinitis. Symptoms of sinus involvement may include nasal congestion, posterior nasal drainage (which is often purulent), facial pressure and/or pain, headache, and in some cases, reduced sense of smell. Rhinosinusitis is included under "Sinusitis" later in this chapter.

EPIDEMIOLOGY AND CAUSES

Although the actual prevalence of acute rhinitis is undocumented, it is extremely common, occurring at least as frequently as the common cold. Moreover, an estimated 40 to 50 million U.S. adults suffer from some form of chronic rhinitis; some sources quote cumulative frequencies of 42% of the population of the United States by age 40 years. Specifically, the incidence of seasonal allergic rhinitis parallels pollen production, increasing in the fall and spring and peaking in the winter, although many individuals have pollen allergies that predominate in the summer months, such as to grasses. Other forms of rhinitis may last year-round if they are caused by perennial allergens such as dust or house mites. Allergic rhinitis occurs in all age groups, most commonly in adults aged 30 to 40 years, but it is rare in adults older than 50 years. The onset of symptoms typically occurs between ages 10 and 20 years.

Nonallergic infectious rhinitis may be acute or chronic. Acute rhinitis is usually viral and self-limited, whereas chronic rhinitis may be associated with bacterial sinusitis and may have associated allergic or mucociliary disturbances as predisposing factors. Rhinitis medicamentosa affects primarily young to middle-aged adults (correlating with medication use), and atrophic rhinitis affects primarily older adults, although the onset of symptoms may begin as early as puberty.

Most forms of rhinitis appear to have no ethnic predispositions; however. Hispanic, Asian, and African American individuals seem to be particularly susceptible to atrophic rhinitis. In contrast, the incidence of this form of rhinitis is low in natives of equatorial Africa. Viral and atrophic rhinitis affect women more often than men, whereas most other forms affect both sexes equally.

Viral upper respiratory tract infections (URIs) occur more frequently in families with young children, whereas exposure to offending allergens is the primary risk factor for allergic rhinitis. The most common irritants implicated in the seasonal form are pollen and mold spores. Dust mites, insect debris (cockroaches, locusts, fish food), tobacco smoke, animal dander, dried saliva, and urine are the most common offending agents for the perennial form of allergic rhinitis.

Immunosuppression secondary to illness or medication use and a family history of allergic disease (e.g., atopic dermatitis, asthma) are also risk factors for allergic rhinitis. Vasomotor rhinitis is aggravated by low humidity, sudden temperature or pressure changes, cold air, strong odors, emotional stress, cigarette smoke, and other nasal irritants. Use of nasal decongestants more frequently than every 3 hours or for periods longer than 3 weeks is the primary risk factor for rhinitis medicamentosa.

In some patients, certain drugs may precipitate rhinitis. Antihypertensive agents are the most frequently cited culprits. Angiotensin-converting enzyme inhibitors, beta-adrenergic antagonists, certain NSAIDs, guanethidine (Ismelin), clonidine (Catapres), hydralazine (Apresoline), prazosin (Minipress), chlordiazepoxide (Librium), amitriptyline (Elavil), or even aspirin can be contributing factors. Oral contraceptive use and hormone therapy for menopause have also been implicated as risk factors for rhinitis, along with a family history of rhinitis and septal/anatomical obstruction. In addition, ingestion of certain foods (e.g., spicy foods) may precipitate rhinitis in susceptible individuals. Illicit drug use such as cocaine snorting may also precipitate rhinitis.

PATHOPHYSIOLOGY

Viral rhinitis stems from an acute catarrhal response caused by viral replication in the nasopharynx, resulting in varying degrees of nasotracheal inflammation. Strongly associated with viral URI ("common cold"), the primary etiological agents of viral rhinitis include rhinovirus, influenza virus, parainfluenza virus, respiratory syncytial virus, coronavirus, adenovirus, echovirus, and coxsackievirus. When viral sinusitis is also present, the condition is collectively referred to as rhinosinusitis. The vast majority of rhinosinusitis is due to viral infection, but bacterial superinfection may complicate a small percentage of these cases. Anatomical defects or obstructions anywhere along the nasopharyngeal tract may predispose to infection by impairing physiological nasal drainage.

In contrast, allergic rhinitis results from immunoglobulin E (IgE)–mediated type I hypersensitivity to airborne irritants affecting the eyes, nose, sinuses, throat, and bronchi. IgE antibodies, elicited by repeated allergen exposure, bind to eosinophils and basophils in the bloodstream and their mucosal counterparts known as mast cells. These leukocytes subsequently degranulate, releasing chemoinflammatory substances, including histamine, leukotrienes, prostaglandins, slow-reacting substance of anaphylaxis, and erythrocyte chemotactic factor, which results in increased vasodilation, capillary permeability, mucus production, smooth muscle contraction, and eosinophilia. In a small percentage of cases, food allergies (referred to in some sources as "gustatory") may be the cause. In addition, chemical or particulate airborne irritants may cause direct mucosal inflammation in the absence of IgE production or immune hypersensitivity.

Vasomotor rhinitis is a chronic, noninfectious process of unknown etiology without accompanying eosinophilia, characterized by periods of abnormal autonomic responsiveness and vascular engorgement unrelated to specific allergens. Fluctuations and reductions in estrogen levels associated with menses, hormonal birth control preparations, pregnancy, and menopause may all predispose to nonallergic rhinitis. Rhinitis medicamentosa is a rebound condition secondary to medication overuse. In some patients, it is caused by certain antihypertensive medications via undefined mechanisms, but most often mucosal inflammation results from the use of topical nasal decongestants such as phenylephrine (Neo-Synephrine) or oxymetazoline (Afrin) for greater than 3 to 4 days, which leads to secondary vasodilation, repeated small-vessel coagulation, and eventual fibrosis. Bacterial infection is thought to play a role in the development of atrophic rhinitis, in which the nasal epithelia and bones progressively atrophy, resulting in distinct morphological changes.

CLINICAL PRESENTATION

Subjective

Viral rhinitis is typically accompanied by malaise, headache, sore throat, and occasionally fever. Patients with allergic rhinitis usually complain of itching in the nasal passages, conjunctivae, and roof of the mouth, as well as epiphora (excess tearing with stringy, watery ocular discharge). Sneezing, coughing, and a sore or burning throat commonly present in both viral and allergic rhinitis.

In contrast, patients with vasomotor rhinitis (noninfectious rhinitis without eosinophilia) rarely display any of the aforementioned symptoms. However, watery rhinorrhea, nasal congestion, "nasal" speech, and forced mouth breathing are common complaints of patients with viral, allergic, vasomotor, or medication-related rhinitis. The onset of congestion is rapid in vasomotor rhinitis; patients typically complain of a pronounced, watery postnasal drip, as well as persistent nasal obstruction that may switch sides with each attack. Rhinitis medicamentosa patients may present with increased heart rate and elevated blood pressure because of the effects of sympathomimetic decongestants. Patients with atrophic rhinitis may complain of nasal congestion, a thick postnasal drip, frequent clearing of the throat, anosmia (impaired olfaction), a constant foul odor in the nose, and severe epistaxis (nosebleeds).

Objective

On inspection, the nasal mucosa typically appears erythematous in viral rhinitis, and throat inspection may reveal pharyngitis or laryngitis, characterized by erythematous and edematous pharyngeal mucosa or vocal cords.

The nasal mucosa appears particularly friable, and if present, nasal polyps are typically soft, edematous, and nontender. If the viral rhinitis is complicated by a secondary bacterial infection, the nasal discharge may be greenish yellow, which is indicative of purulence.

In allergic rhinitis, the mucosa are pale and boggy (edematous) and may take on a bluish hue. Yellowish, gray, or erythematous mucosa may also be seen. Gray-blue to yellow-tan nasal polyps may present with chronic perennial rhinitis. The conjunctivae are usually inflamed (allergic conjunctivitis), with the palpebral conjunctiva being particularly edematous (chemosis) and "cobblestoned" in appearance, owing to chronically injected blood vessels. Dark circles under the eyes ("allergic shiners") may be apparent, along with excess wrinkles under the lower eyelid (Dennie lines). In both viral and allergic rhinitis, the external nose may appear erythematous, and the nasal turbinates and palatine or pharyngeal tonsils (adenoids) may also be enlarged. The external nose may be tender from repeated sneezing in patients with viral and allergic rhinitis. On auscultation, wheezing breath sounds may reflect concurrent asthma associated with allergic rhinitis.

The nasal mucosa in patients with vasomotor rhinitis will range from bright red to bluish in hue, and again, the nasal turbinates may be swollen. The mucosa in patients with rhinitis medicamentosa is also injected and edematous, with some patients presenting with dry and rubbery mucosa. In contrast, the mucosa in patients with atrophic rhinitis usually appear crusted with dried mucus or blood from repeated bouts of epistaxis, although the nasal passages typically remain patent.

DIAGNOSTIC REASONING

Diagnostic Tests

Laboratory tests are not typically indicated for uncomplicated cases of viral rhinitis, allergic rhinitis, or rhinitis medicamentosa. However, if an exudate is present as a colored or translucent nasal discharge, a Giemsa- or Wright's-stained smear should be prepared, along with a complete blood count (CBC) to characterize the disease process. Leukocytosis or the presence of polymorphonuclear neutrophils in the discharge reflects an infectious disorder other than a typical viral URI. Eosinophilia in the discharge is indicative of allergic rhinitis. Peripheral eosinophil count and serum IgE levels have low predictive values; however, intradermal skin testing of minute amounts of allergens (skin prick testing) may be helpful if the diagnosis of allergic rhinitis is in doubt.

Vasomotor rhinitis tends to be a diagnosis of exclusion because nasal smears and skin tests are typically negative, and no family history of allergic disorders is expected. Hormonally related rhinitis and rhinitis medicamentosa are diagnosed primarily through patient history once other common forms of rhinitis have been excluded.

Atrophic rhinitis may be confirmed by nasal mucosal biopsy. Histopathology will demonstrate transformation of ciliated pseudostratified columnar epithelia into the stratified squamous form. In addition, the lamina propria will be decreased in thickness and vascularity. Bacterial culture of nasal secretions may be helpful if bacterial infection is expected, although the nares are expected to have colonization of mixed normal flora.

Differential Diagnosis

Acute or chronic sinusitis resulting from bacterial infection of the facial sinuses may also inflame the nasal mucosa and is referred to as "rhinosinusitis" in many sources. Sinus x-ray films demonstrating mucosal thickening, air–fluid levels, or opacification are effective at ruling out this disorder, as are cultures or smears of sinus aspirates to identify the infectious organisms present. Physical examination may rule out nasal foreign bodies, nasal polyps, or a deviated septum as causes of mucosal inflammation or congestion. Cocaine snorting, inhalant abuse (sniffing, huffing), and other forms of substance abuse should also be ruled out through a detailed patient history and, if indicated, urine or serum drug screens.

Chronic inflammatory conditions such as sarcoidosis may be ruled out via biopsy, which would reveal granulomatous (histiocyte/macrophage) inflammation of the nasal mucosa. Hormonal changes associated with pregnancy and hyperthyroidism or hypothyroidism may also lead to nasal vasodilation and inflammation. Such conditions are ruled out through a careful physical examination, detailed patient history, and serum hormone screens.

MANAGEMENT

With all types of rhinitis, much of the treatment regimen will focus on the relief of symptoms and self-care measures, although environmental triggers must also be addressed. Viral rhinitis is mostly treated symptomatically because viral URIs are predominantly self-limited.

The following list outlines adult dosages of common medications used for symptoms relief:

- Fever and headache may be treated with acetaminophen 325 to 650 mg by mouth (PO) every 4 hours as needed (daily maximum dose 4,000 mg/day). Aspirin is not recommended because it may increase viral shedding. Rhinorrhea may be treated with oral decongestants such as pseudoephedrine (Sudafed) 30 to 60 mg PO every 3 to 4 hours as needed or topical preparations such as phenylephrine (Neo-Synephrine) 0.25% to 0.5% nasal spray one to two sprays in each nostril every 3 to 4 hours as needed for no more than 3 to 4 days.
- Intranasal ipratropium (Atrovent) 0.03% two sprays in each nostril two to four times daily as needed may also relieve excessive runny nose.
- Persistent cough may be treated with dextromethorphan 15 to 30 mg PO every 3 to 4 hours as needed,

but prescription codeine 10 to 15 mg PO every 3 to 4 hours as needed usually proves to be the only consistently effective cough suppressant.

For allergic rhinitis, avoidance or reduced exposure to offending allergens is the primary method of treatment because acute attacks are typically self-limited if not continually aggravated by allergen. Newergeneration oral antihistamines designed to be less sedating are now the first-line short-term treatment of choice for allergic rhinitis. These work best for early symptoms of allergy such as sneezing, watery eyes, and ocular pruritus. However, intranasal corticosteroids have traditionally been considered the most effective means of controlling the longer-term symptoms of allergic rhinitis, including nasal congestion and discharge, and meta-analyses have suggested that intranasal corticosteroids are the best overall first-line treatment for allergic rhinitis. It should be stressed, however, that intranasal corticosteroid therapy may require 2 or more weeks of continuous daily use before symptomatic relief is apparent. Systemic corticosteroids have significant side effects and tend to be discouraged for such a common condition. Leukotriene receptor antagonists are also approved for allergic rhinitis, and randomized controlled studies have shown montelukast (Singulair) to be as effective as loratadine (Claritin) in the symptomatic relief of allergic rhinitis.

Vasomotor rhinitis is also treated symptomatically, albeit at times unsatisfactorily, with environmental humidification using a vaporizer or humidified central heating system. Rhinorrhea may be treated with systemic oral decongestants such as pseudoephedrine (Sudafed) 30 to 60 mg three or four times daily as needed. Congestion may also improve with topical saline nasal sprays. Thorough cleaning of the nose and restoration of nasal patency may be achieved using a powered device such as a Grossan nasal irrigator or a manual nasal irrigation system, such as a Neti pot. Intranasal ipratropium (Atrovent) 0.03% two sprays in each nostril two to four times daily as needed or azelastine (Astelin) two sprays in each nostril twice daily may also relieve symptoms.

Rhinitis medicamentosa or "rebound rhinitis" is characterized by nasal congestion without rhinorrhea following the short-term use of topical vasoconstrictive medications. This condition can be remedied by immediately stopping all topical decongestant use. The condition typically resolves after 2 to 3 weeks. Treatment of rhinitis medicamentosa, if needed, may include:

- Oral antihistamine-decongestant preparations or short courses of topical nasal corticosteroids may provide symptomatic relief.
- A short course of systemic corticosteroids such as prednisone 30 mg PO daily for 5 days may be needed if other treatments prove ineffective.

Atrophic rhinitis may be treated with bacitracin ointment applied intranasally two or three times daily until the nasal crusting and foul odor are eliminated. Expectorants such as guaifenesin 400 mg PO every 4 hours as needed, physiological saline solutions as a nasal spray, regular use of a Neti pot or other means of nasal douching, or electric nasal irrigators (e.g., Grossan) may provide symptomatic relief. Menopausal women may be helped by systemic estrogens (see Drugs Commonly Prescribed 24.1 for more information).

Desensitizing immunotherapy ("allergy shots" or "allergy vaccines") may be an option for allergic rhinitis

Drugs Commonly Prescribed 24.1: Rhinitis

DRUG	INDICATION	DOSAGE	PRESCRIBING CONSIDERATIONS
Antihistamines—First Generation			
Diphenhydramine (Benadryl)	Allergic rhinitis	Adults: 25–50 mg PO every 4–6 hours; maximum 300 mg/day	Must use 3–5 hours before anticipated allergen exposure or on a regular basis. **Adverse effects:** Use with caution in older adults. May cause central nervous system (CNS) sedation, gastrointestinal (GI) upset, anticholinergic effects (dry mouth, blurred vision, confusion in elderly), additive CNS-depressant effects with alcohol, sedatives, or hypnotics. *Use with caution in older adults.*
Chlorpheniramine maleate (Chlor-Trimeton)	Allergic rhinitis	Adults: 2–4 mg by mouth (PO) every 4–6 hours	Must use 3–5 hours before anticipated allergen exposure or on a regular basis. **Adverse effects:** CNS sedation, GI upset, anticholinergic effects (dry mouth, blurred vision, confusion in elderly), additive CNS-depressant effects with alcohol, sedatives, or hypnotics. *Use with caution in older adults.*
Azelastine HCl (Astelin)	Seasonal allergic rhinitis	Adults: 137 mcg/spray: two sprays per nostril twice daily	Intranasal spray **Adverse effects:** Bitter taste, somnolence, CNS sedation, GI upset, anticholinergic effects (dry mouth, blurred vision, confusion in elderly), additive CNS-depressant effects with alcohol, sedatives, or hypnotics. *Use with caution in older adults. Only use in pregnancy if potential benefits justify potential risks to fetus.*
Antihistamines—Second Generation			
Desloratadine (Clarinex, Clarinex RediTabs)	Seasonal allergic rhinitis	Adults: 5 mg PO daily dissolved on the tongue	**Adverse effects:** Pharyngitis, dry mouth, somnolence, headache, fatigue. *Only use in pregnancy if potential benefits justify potential risks to fetus. Not recommended for nursing mothers.*
Loratadine (Claritin)	Seasonal allergic rhinitis	Adults: 10 mg PO daily	**Adverse effects:** Headache, mild drowsiness. Less effective than first-generation antihistamines; use in patients who cannot tolerate sedation.
Cetirizine (Zyrtec)	Seasonal allergic rhinitis	Children: <2 years: not recommended 2–6 years: 2.5 mg PO daily; maximum 5 mg/day >6 years: 5–10 mg PO daily Adults: 10 mg PO daily	Somewhat more sedating than other second-generation antihistamines, but less than first-generation. Less effective than first-generation antihistamines; use in patients who cannot tolerate sedation. **Adverse effects:** Drowsiness, somnolence, dry mouth, pharyngitis. *Not recommended for pregnant women or nursing mothers.*

Continued

Drugs Commonly Prescribed 24.1: Rhinitis—cont'd

DRUG	INDICATION	DOSAGE	PRESCRIBING CONSIDERATIONS
Fexofenadine (Allegra)	Seasonal allergic rhinitis	Adults: 60 mg PO twice daily or 180 mg PO daily	Less effective than first-generation antihistamines; use in patients who cannot tolerate sedation. **Adverse effects:** Headache, back pain, viral infection, dizziness. *Only use in pregnancy if potential benefits justify potential risks to fetus.*
Olopatadine (Patanase)	Seasonal allergic rhinitis	Adults: 665 mcg/spray: Two sprays per nostril twice daily	Avoid eyes. Monitor for nasal mucosal changes. **Adverse effects:** Bitter taste, headache, epistaxis, throat pain, nasal ulceration, somnolence. *Only use in pregnancy if potential benefits justify potential risks to fetus.*
Decongestants (Monotherapy)			
Pseudoephedrine HCI (Sudafed)	Nasal congestion	30–60 mg PO every 4–6 hours; maximum four doses/day	Should not be used for longer than 3–4 days. **Adverse effects:** Can cause CNS excitation, hypertension, and palpitations. *Use with caution in elderly patients and those taking beta blockers. Contraindicated in patients with diabetes, benign prostatic hyperplasia (BPH), hypertension, cardiac disease, and those taking monoamine oxidase (MAO) inhibitors.*
NSAID and Decongestant (Combination Therapy)			
Ibuprofen 200 mg and pseudoephedrine HCI 30 mg (Advil Cold and Sinus)	Rhinorrhea, sinusitis, flu	One to two tablets every 4–6 hours; maximum 6 tablets/day	Should not be used for longer than 3–4 days. Take with food. *Use with caution in patients with hypertension, diabetes, glaucoma, BPH, and those taking beta blockers.*
Antihistamine and Decongestant (Combination Therapy)			
Diphenhydramine HCI 25 mg and pseudo-ephedrine HCI 60 mg Tavist NightTime Allergy, Benylin Multi-Symptom, Benadryl Allergy Decongestant, Actifed Allergy Day/Night	Rhinorrhea, nasal congestion	One tablet every 4–6 hours	Should not be used for longer than 3–4 days. Potentiates the effects of alcohol, sedatives. *Do not use with MAO inhibitors or in patients with broncho-spasm, hypertension, diabetes, BPH.*
Loratadine 10 mg and pseudoephedrine 50 mg (Claritin-D 24 Hour)	Rhinitis, sinusitis with congestion, allergic rhinitis	One tablet daily	Should not be used for longer than 3–4 days. Do not crush or chew. *Use with caution in elderly patients and those taking beta blockers. Contraindicated in patients with glaucoma, BPH, hypertension, coronary artery disease.*

Drugs Commonly Prescribed 24.1: Rhinitis—cont'd

DRUG	INDICATION	DOSAGE	PRESCRIBING CONSIDERATIONS
Fexofenadine HCl 60 mg and pseudo-ephedrine 120 mg (Allegra-D 12HR) Fexofenadine HCl 180 mg and pseudo-ephedrine 240 mg (Allegra-D 24HR)	Seasonal allergic rhinitis with nasal congestion	One tablet twice daily Extended release: One tablet once daily	Should not be used for longer than 3–4 days. Avoid giving with food.

Intranasal Corticosteroids

DRUG	INDICATION	DOSAGE	PRESCRIBING CONSIDERATIONS
Beclomethasone dipropionate (Beconase AQ)	Decrease nasal inflammatory reaction	42 mcg/spray: one to two sprays per nostril twice daily	Available in aerosol and metered pump. May eliminate need for antihistamines or decongestants. Must be used regularly; onset of action may require 1–2 weeks several days of regular use; use decongestant before application if necessary. **Adverse effects:** Local irritation, increased rhinorrhea, localized fungal infection.
Budesonide (Rhinocort Aqua)	Decrease nasal inflammatory reaction	32 mcg/spray: two sprays per nostril daily; maximum four sprays per nostril daily	Aerosol. May eliminate need for antihistamines or decongestants. Must be used regularly; onset of action may require several days of regular use; use decongestant before application if necessary. **Adverse effects:** Local irritation, increased rhinorrhea, localized fungal infection. Caution with CYP3A4 inhibitors (e.g., ketoconazole). *Only use in pregnancy if potential benefits justify potential risks to fetus.*
Ciclesonide (Omnaris)	Decrease nasal inflammatory reaction	50 mcg/spray: two sprays per nostril daily	Aerosol. May eliminate need for antihistamines or decongestants. Must be used regularly; onset of action may require 1–2 days of regular use; use decongestant before application if necessary. **Adverse effects:** Local irritation, increased rhinorrhea, headache, pharyngitis, localized fungal infection. Worsening of tuberculosis or other existing infections. *Only use in pregnancy if potential benefits justify potential risks to fetus.*
Fluticasone propionate (Flonase)	Decrease nasal inflammatory reaction	50 mcg/spray: two sprays per nostril daily or one spray per nostril twice daily; maximum two sprays per nostril daily	Available in metered pump. Maintain regular regimen. Monitor for visual changes. Onset of action may require several days of regular use. **Adverse effects:** Local irritation, increased rhinorrhea, localized fungal infection. Caution with CYP3A4 inhibitors (e.g., ketoconazole). *Only use in pregnancy if potential benefits justify potential risks to fetus.*
Triamcinolone acetonide (Nasacort)	Decrease nasal inflammatory reaction	55 mcg/spray: two sprays per nostril daily	Available in aerosol or metered pump. Maintain regular regimen. Monitor for visual changes. Onset of action may require several days of regular use. **Adverse effects:** Headache, viral infections. It is unknown whether drug accumulates in breast milk; however, other corticosteroids are excreted in breast milk. *Nursing mothers should use with caution. Only use in pregnancy if potential benefits justify potential risks to fetus.*

Continued

Drugs Commonly Prescribed 24.1: Rhinitis—cont'd

DRUG	INDICATION	DOSAGE	PRESCRIBING CONSIDERATIONS
Mometasone furoate (Nasonex)	Decrease nasal inflammatory reaction	50 mcg/spray: two sprays per nostril daily	Begin 2–4 weeks before start of pollen season. Maintain regular regimen. Monitor for visual changes. Onset of action may require several days of regular use. **Adverse effects:** Local irritation, increased rhinorrhea, localized fungal infection. Caution with CYP3A4 inhibitors (e.g., ketoconazole). *Only use in pregnancy if potential benefits justify potential risks to fetus.*
Anticholinergic Drugs			
Ipratropium bromide nasal spray 0.03% or 0.06% (Atrovent)	Prevention of rhinorrhea	21 mcg/spray: two sprays per nostril two to three times daily 42 mcg/spray: two sprays per nostril two to three times daily	Does not relieve itching or nasal blockage. **Adverse effects:** Epistaxis, pharyngitis, nasal dryness. *Avoid in patients with BPH and glaucoma. Only use in pregnancy if benefits outweigh the risks.*
Mast Cell Stabilizer			
Cromolyn sodium 5.2 mg (Nasalcrom)	Prevention and relief of nasal allergy symptoms	5.2 mcg/spray: one spray per nostril three or four times daily; maximum six sprays/ nostril/day	Regular use required. Do not use to treat sinus infection or asthma.
Leukotriene Receptor Antagonist			
Montelukast (Singulair)	Seasonal rhinitis	6–23 months: one packet of 4 mg oral granules 2–5 years: one 4 mg chewable tablet or one packet of 4 mg oral granules 6–14 years: one 5 mg chewable tablet ≥15 years: one 10 mg tablet	Monitor with potent CYP450 inducers and with drugs metabolized by CYP2C8. **Adverse effects:** Upper respiratory infection

that is refractory to pharmacologic treatment. Patients receive subcutaneous injections of purified allergen weekly at a dosage that increases with each treatment. The interval between injections is lengthened once a maintenance dose is reached. This treatment regimen may last up to 3 to 5 years, but it should not be continued past 12 months if symptoms are not improving; cure rates may be as low as 20%, although many patients experience long-lasting relief for many years, even after immunotherapy is stopped. In addition, to reduce the risk of anaphylactic reactions, antigen injections must never be given intravenously.

Occasionally, surgery is recommended if the etiology of refractory or recurrent rhinitis is anatomical, including nasal polypectomy for obstructing lesions or septoplasty if septal deviation is significant enough to interfere with the benefits of medication.

FOLLOW-UP AND REFERRAL

A return visit should be scheduled in 2 to 3 weeks to review patient education, adherence to the treatment plan, and effectiveness of prescribed treatments. After this, quarterly or biannual visits are recommended, depending on the patient's comfort level and general state of health.

Complications of infectious rhinitis include serous OM (extension of nasal infection into the ear), acute or chronic sinusitis (rhinosinusitis), and repeated or disseminated respiratory infections. Allergic rhinitis may lead to restless sleeping and chronic fatigue, and asthma may complicate allergic attacks. Rhinitis medicamentosa may be complicated by physical addiction to topical nasal decongestants, because relief periods shorten and the severity of rebound congestion increases with each use. Thus, stopping the use of nasal decongestants becomes especially difficult for the addicted patient.

Physician referral may be necessary for allergen skin testing, allergen immunotherapy, or nasal irrigation. The diagnosis and treatment of certain sequelae such as chronic sinusitis or high fever may also require physician referral. Surgical referral is necessary if anatomical obstructions of the nasal cavity (e.g., nasal polyps or a deviated septum) are causative or complicating factors.

Patient Education: Rhinitis

Viral rhinitis is best avoided by limiting exposure to persons with an acute URI, and all patients should be instructed to arrange for further evaluation if clear rhinorrhea becomes purulent. Similarly, allergic flare-ups are best prevented by avoiding exposure to environmental irritants. Many preventive steps may be taken. Windows and doors should be kept closed to reduce pollen entry into the household, and high-efficiency particulate air (HEPA) filters are helpful in removing allergens from ambient air. Pet traffic from outdoors should be minimized because this may transport pollen indoors, and patients should avoid being outside on excessively sunny or windy days. Patients who are allergic to animal dander should bathe their pets often and restrict them from the bedroom or from the house altogether.

Patients with allergic rhinitis should be taught not only to avoid allergens but also to observe the onset, duration, and progression of symptoms so that they can correlate their flare-ups to environmental exposures and, thus, better guide self-treatment. Emphasize all preventive and prophylactic measures, particularly the importance of keeping bedrooms allergen free. Allergic attacks to mold spores can be prevented by avoiding piles of leaves during the fall months, by wiping down household surfaces where mold grows with bleach solutions, using HEPA filters, and reducing ambient humidity to 30% to 40%. Allergic attacks caused by perennial antigens such as dust or dust mites can be minimized by thoroughly cleaning or removing all carpets, drapes, curtains, and fabric-covered or stuffed furniture from the house, as well as by damp mopping, floor waxing, and dusting of all surfaces with a damp cloth. Stuffed animals, feather pillows, mattresses, and box springs should be either covered with plastic or removed and replaced with synthetic materials, such as polyester. Chenille bedspreads, quilts, or comforters should be avoided, and bedding should be washed weekly. The use of air-conditioning with frequent filter changes, rather than open windows, to cool automobiles or homes is recommended.

Vasomotor rhinitis is also best avoided by limiting exposure to environmental triggers, and rhinitis medicamentosa can be prevented by diligently monitoring and limiting topical nasal decongestant use. Patients with all forms of rhinitis should understand the reasoning behind limiting nasal decongestant use, as well as the appropriate use of prophylactic cromolyn sodium sprays.

Prophylactic use of 4% cromolyn sodium nasal spray (one spray in each nostril three to six times/day at regular intervals) before known antigen exposure may prevent allergic flare-ups but is ineffective once an attack is underway. Ophthalmic cromolyn sodium preparations are also available for the symptom of itchy eyes (one to two drops can be instilled in each eye four to six times/day). Patients taking combination therapies, such as combined decongestants and antihistamines, must be educated on the individual ingredients in these combinations and warned of the possibility of inadvertent double-dosing with other over-the-counter remedies with different brand names that contain the same active ingredients. It is also critical to explain that peak symptomatic relief from topical nasal corticosteroid preparations may not be evident until several days to a week into therapy.

RHINOSINUSITIS

Sinusitis is an inflammation of the mucous membranes of one or more of the paranasal sinuses: frontal, sphenoid, posterior ethmoid, anterior ethmoid, and maxillary, with the latter two sinuses most often affected. The term "rhinosinusitis" is often used because inflammation of the sinuses rarely occurs without concurrent inflammation of the nasal mucosa. This inflammation may be classified as (1) acute, which is characterized by an abrupt onset of infection and post-therapeutic resolution of symptoms, lasting no more than 4 weeks; (2) subacute, in which a purulent nasal discharge persists despite therapy and lasts from 4 to 12 weeks; or (3) chronic, which occurs with episodes of prolonged inflammation with repeated or inadequately treated acute infection, with symptoms lasting greater than 12 consecutive weeks. These classifications are based on both symptom duration as well as etiology and clinical manifestations.

EPIDEMIOLOGY AND CAUSES

Researchers have estimated that 0.5% of all URIs are complicated by bacterial infection of one or more of the paranasal sinuses. Acute bacterial rhinosinusitis (ABRS) accounts for 16 million clinical visits annually, whereas chronic sinusitis is classified by the U.S. Public Health Service as the most common chronic disease in the United States and is estimated to account for more than $2 billion a year in health-care costs. Rhinosinusitis affects adults of all ages, males and females equally, with no specific ethnic predisposition.

Mucosal inflammation and congestion caused by a viral URI that lasts more than 7 to 10 days is a key risk factor for acute viral rhinosinusitis (AVRS; especially for maxillary sinus involvement), particularly during the autumn, winter, and spring seasons. Individuals with URIs who travel in an airplane may increase their risk of developing sinusitis. Smoking, exposure to air pollution, persistent coughing, sneezing against a closed mouth, exposure to cold and damp outdoor weather or dry indoor heat, sudden changes in temperature, injury to the nose or sinuses from foreign bodies (e.g., nasogastric tubes or nasotracheal intubation) or trauma, nasal polyps, and chronic use of over-the-counter (OTC) or prescription decongestants may all impair mucociliary function, which can lead to mucosal inflammation, blockage of the sinus ostia, hypo-oxygenation of the sinuses, and transudation of fluid due to negative sinus pressure. Dental abscesses with oroantral fistulae extending into the paranasal sinuses can introduce pathogenic microorganisms; this etiology is associated with 10% to 15% of acute rhinosinusitis cases. In addition, particularly during the summer months, airborne allergens, as well as swimming, diving, and jumping into contaminated water without holding the nose, are common mechanisms for developing rhinosinusitis. Allergic rhinitis is seen in 25% of sinusitis cases.

Recurrent or persistent bacterial infection resulting from blockage of nasociliary sinus drainage via the sinus ostia has been particularly associated with subacute and chronic sinusitis/rhinosinusitis. Mechanical blockage may result from anatomical abnormalities such as a deviated septum, adenoidal hypertrophy, nasal polyps, reduced ostial diameter, and sinus or nasal neoplasms. Half of all asthmatic patients suffer from some form of sinusitis as a result of their inflammation-prone, hypersensitive airways. Furthermore, mucosal immunoglobulin A deficiency, immobile cilia syndrome (Kartagener's syndrome), and cystic fibrosis also contribute to decreased mucociliary clearance and persistent sinus infection resulting from stasis. Chronic inflammatory diseases such as sarcoidosis and Wegener's granulomatosis also predispose patients to mucosal inflammation. In particular, patients who are diabetic, have HIV infection, are malnourished, or are otherwise chronically immunocompromised may develop severe, invasive sinus disease.

PATHOPHYSIOLOGY

Infection by nonendogenous pathogens and bacterial invasion of the sinuses by normal nasal or pharyngeal microbial flora are the primary causes of acute rhinosinusitis. The vast majority (>95%) of acute rhinosinusitis cases are caused by the same viruses associated with uncomplicated URIs. However, many of these patients do not seek primary-care interventions. AVRS is most commonly caused by the following five viruses, which collectively account for 80% of all URIs: rhinovirus (30%), coronavirus, adenovirus, echovirus, and coxsackievirus, as well as respiratory syncytial virus, parainfluenza virus, and influenza virus.

Viral rhinosinusitis is the main predisposing factor for acute bacterial sinusitis, which complicates about 2% of all cases. During these episodes, mucosal secretions from sinus goblet cells increase in volume and viscosity. The nasal mucosa also swells in response to viral replication, creating an anatomical barrier to the steady outflow of

nasal secretions. Nasal polyps, foreign bodies, allergen-induced mucosal swelling, and altered sensorium affecting nasal clearance and coordinated swallowing reflexes are other potential mechanisms of impaired nasal outflow.

In addition, the act of sneezing creates tremendous pressure in the nasopharynx of up to 60 to 80 mm Hg, which is capable of forcing fluid not only out the nares but from the nasal cavity into the sinuses as well, transporting viruses and bacteria into these environments that are ideal for microbial replication. Here the normally ciliated pseudostratified columnar epithelium lining the sinuses is eroded as infecting organisms proliferate, resulting in a loss of mucociliary clearance through the sinus ostia (bony openings) and the ostiomeatal complex located in the anterior ethmoid region, which serves as a common drainage pathway for the frontal, maxillary, and ethmoid sinuses. Blockage of the ostiomeatal complex and/or impairment of ciliary function is thought to underlie all forms of sinusitis.

The only consistently reliable method of identifying causative organisms in acute rhinosinusitis is direct sinus aspiration, which typically is performed only in controlled research trials or by specialists because of its invasive nature. The most common bacterial pathogens isolated in acute sinusitis are *Streptococcus pneumoniae*, seen in nearly 40% of all cases, particularly during the summer and fall; *Haemophilus influenzae*, implicated in nearly 30% of all cases, especially in winter and spring; and, to a lesser extent, *Moraxella (Branhamella) catarrhalis*, which is more common pathogen in children. Thus, the infectious agents of sinusitis closely pattern those of acute OM. *Streptococcus pyogenes* (especially group A beta-hemolytic *Streptococcus*) and *Staphylococcus aureus* have each been identified in 5% of sinusitis cases studied, with *S. aureus* most frequently isolated in intracranial complications.

The specific role of bacteria, fungi, and viruses in chronic sinusitis is hotly debated. *S. aureus*, gram-negative rods, and, in up to half of cases, anaerobic bacteria (including *Peptostreptococcus* and *Bacteroides*) are most often implicated. Polymicrobial infection is also more common in chronic than acute sinusitis. *S. aureus* and *Pseudomonas aeruginosa* are the most common causes of cystic fibrosis–related and nosocomial sinus infection associated with nasal or endotracheal intubation and nasogastric feeding tubes.

In the immunocompromised host, gram-negative aerobic bacteria must be considered, as well as the fungi *Aspergillus fumigatus* and *Mucor* species, both of which may cause severe, rapidly invasive sinusitis in diabetic or otherwise chronically immunocompromised patients. More common than invasive fungal sinusitis, however, is allergic fungal sinusitis occurring in atopic individuals in which the nasal and sinus mucosa undergo an IgE-mediated type I hypersensitivity response to airborne fungal spores or fungal proliferation facilitated by obstructed sinus outflow. Dematiaceous (brown-pigmented) molds account for more than 75% of these cases, and *Aspergillus* is implicated in 10% to 20% of cases. The sinuses become filled with allergic mucin consisting of necrotic cellular debris, eosinophils, and fungal hyphae. If neither a hypersensitivity response nor an invasive sinusitis ensues, fungal colonization may result in unilateral chronic sinusitis characterized by formation of a dense fungal ball with sclerosis of the surrounding bone.

CLINICAL PRESENTATION

Subjective

During the early stages of rhinosinusitis, patients typically report a gradual onset of symptoms, including recurrent or chronic dull, constant pain over the affected sinuses (because of expanding purulent inflammation); as sinusitis progresses, pain increases and becomes characteristically throbbing. Typically, pain over the cheeks and upper teeth is correlated with maxillary sinus involvement; pain over the eyebrows indicates frontal sinus involvement; and pain over or behind the eyes indicates ethmoid sinusitis. Pain is exacerbated by coughing and sudden head movements. Specifically, frontal sinus pain may worsen with recumbency, whereas maxillary sinus pain may worsen when the patient is erect. Ethmoidal sinusitis is associated with retro-orbital pain. Notably, however, subacute and chronic sinusitis are often painless, as are some cases of acute sinusitis. These cases typically develop after at least 2 weeks of viral URI symptoms (e.g., cough from postnasal drip, purulent nasal discharge, headache).

All types of sinusitis may present with nasal congestion (stuffiness), mucopurulent rhinorrhea (runny nose), a feeling of pressure inside the head, cough (in some cases), sore throat (in some cases), eye pain from ethmoid involvement, malaise, and fatigue. In particular, acute sinusitis is strongly predicted by maxillary toothache, a poor response to nasal decongestants, and a colored nasal discharge. Such patients usually report yellow-green or even blood-stained rhinorrhea, voice nasality, anosmia because of edematous nasal turbinates, early morning periorbital edema, fever and chills (in 25% to 50% of cases), and a headache that is worse in the morning or when bending forward. These patients also sometimes report a nonproductive cough and disturbed sleep.

Subacute or chronic sinusitis patients typically report a persistent cough or coldlike symptoms that may last from several weeks to several months, as well as a headache or feeling of pressure specifically across the cranial midline. Fever is less common, and most patients have a past history of responding poorly to sinusitis pharmacotherapy. Other symptoms include a thick postnasal discharge (postnasal drip), "popping" ears, excessive tearing, toothache-like cheek pain, difficulty chewing, and halitosis. Immunocompromised patients may present with more subtle signs and symptoms because leukopenia may limit the inflammatory response to infection.

Objective

On inspection, purulent nasal secretions (recognized by polymorphonuclear neutrophils in a Giemsa-stained nasal smear) and total opacification of affected sinuses on transillumination (e.g., through the supraorbital or maxillary bony ridges) are strongly predictive of acute sinusitis. Although only one in four patients with decreased transillumination typically has a sinus infection, complete light transmission rules out an active sinus infection. A nasal speculum should be used to examine the anterior nasal passages. A red, swollen nasal mucosa indicates infection; a pale mucosa that appears swollen, with watery secretions, points to allergic sinusitis or rhinitis. Purulent secretions seen coming from inside the middle meatus are characteristic of sinusitis. Black or necrotic material may be seen in mucormycosis-related rhinorrhea in immunocompromised patients. Ethmoid sinus involvement may result in chemosis (eyelid mucous membrane edema), proptosis, conjunctival injection, extraocular muscle palsy, or orbital fixation.

On palpation, the affected sinuses may be exquisitely tender to palpation. Sphenoid sinusitis presents as tenderness over the vertex or mastoids, ethmoid sinusitis as retro-orbital or nasal bridge tenderness, maxillary sinusitis as cheek or dental tenderness, and frontal sinusitis as tenderness of the forehead. In the event of maxillary sinusitis related to a dental abscess, percussion over the affected sinus will produce marked tenderness in the teeth and gums.

DIAGNOSTIC REASONING

Diagnostic Tests

It is important for the clinician to focus on clinical signs and symptoms for initial diagnosis and avoid unnecessary diagnostic tests. Although laboratory tests and x-ray films are not needed for typical presentations of sinusitis, anteroposterior, lateral, and particularly occipitomental sinus x-ray examinations can be done if symptoms show no improvement after 4 to 5 days of pharmacotherapy. Air–fluid levels, mucosal thickening beyond 4 mm, or complete opacification of the sinuses on any of these views is strongly suggestive of sinusitis. However, mucosal thickening and impaired sinus transillumination on physical examination have both been observed in healthy, asymptomatic individuals who do not meet the criteria for acute sinusitis. In turn, the positive and negative predictive values of these diagnostic tests have consistently been questioned in the scientific literature.

A CBC to detect leukocyte elevation may be indicated if an infectious etiology is suspected in acute sinusitis; however, leukocytosis is rarely observed in chronic sinusitis. Stains or cultures of nasal and throat secretions do not correlate with the causative agents of sinusitis because the nasopharyngeal mucosa is widely colonized by a diverse array of endogenous, nonpathogenic microbial flora. However, the presence of at least 10,000 organisms per milliliter on Gram stain of sinus aspirates may confirm the presence of local sinus infection. Allergic skin testing may be necessary if the patient history suggests allergic disease (e.g., allergen exposure, seasonal attacks). These patients often demonstrate peripheral eosinophilia and elevated total or allergen-specific IgE levels. Culture and microscopic examination of sinus aspirates, sinus mucosal biopsy, or flexible fiber-optic rhinoscopy by a well-trained specialist is typically needed only for sub-acute, chronic, or suspected fungal sinusitis cases that are refractory to several courses of empiric pharmacotherapy or when intracranial extension is suspected. Chronic sinusitis, in particular, is characterized by a morphological change of the ciliated sinus epithelia to a hypertrophied, stratified squamous form that is evident on biopsy.

Although sinus computed tomography scans may demonstrate mucosal thickening and ostiomeatal occlusion in a large number of people with uncomplicated viral URI, this type of imaging may be helpful in cases of chronic sinusitis, infection that has spread into orbital or intracranial regions (e.g., orbital cellulitis or brain abscess), or in patients who are immunocompromised to fully evaluate the disease process. Sinus magnetic resonance imaging (MRI) is superior for soft tissue discrimination but is poor at visualizing bony structures. Thus, MRI tends to be reserved for suspected sinus neoplasia or extension of sinus disease into intracranial soft tissues.

Differential Diagnosis

Myofascial pain that is unrelated to infectious causes may mimic the pain from acute sinusitis, but pain from other myofascial disorders is typically more diffuse and does not progressively worsen. Uncomplicated dental abscesses may produce similar pain, but the pain will not extend into the maxillary sinus on physical examination. Patients with migraine, cluster headache, or trigeminal neuralgia also present with facial and cranial pain, but the sinuses will be nontender to palpation, and the accompanying signs and symptoms of inflammation will not be observed in these patients. Allergic rhinitis, vasomotor rhinitis, rhinitis medicamentosa, mechanical nasal airway obstruction, acute viral URI (persistent viral rhinitis), and chronic inflammatory conditions such as sarcoidosis or Wegener's granulomatosis may all present with nasal congestion or pain. If these cases are uncomplicated by sinusitis, no signs of sinus inflammation will be detected on examination.

If a patient has had an URI for at least 7 days, the presence of two or more of the following signs and symptoms will confirm the diagnosis of sinusitis: colored nasal drainage, a poor response to decongestants, facial or sinus pain (particularly if aggravated by postural change or Valsalva maneuver), and headache. In addition, a documented history of prior episodes of sinusitis, a fever higher than 102°F (38.9°C), and tooth pain accompanying these findings all support a diagnosis of sinusitis. Viruses may produce all of the clinical manifestations described; however, patients who meet the 7-day criteria described in the preceding text are more likely to have ABRS than a viral URI.

MANAGEMENT

Because the vast majority of acute rhinosinusitis cases are caused by viruses rather than bacteria, antibiotics are largely unhelpful. Their indiscriminate use for symptom complexes failing to meet the aforementioned diagnostic criteria for bacterial sinusitis offers no medical benefit, wastes financial resources, and is potentially harmful in that it encourages widespread antibiotic resistance in common nasopharyngeal flora. With this in mind, antimicrobial therapy usually cures ABRS, although recurrence is not uncommon.

Adjunctive measures may also be used to enhance mucociliary clearance, countering the main risk factor for the development of sinusitis. Saline nasal spray may be helpful in improving sinus drainage, but dedicated sinus irrigation two or more times a day with an adequate volume of saline to fully flush the sinuses has been shown to significantly relieve symptoms even without antimicrobial therapy. Patients are instructed to infuse their sinuses using a warm isotonic or hypertonic saline-filled bulb syringe expressed into each nostril, followed by immediate drainage of the liquid over a sink to remove both infectious organisms and excess mucus. A number of commercial saline sinus irrigation systems with balanced salt solutions are currently available. However, homemade preparations may be made by mixing one teaspoon of salt with 8 ounces of warm water; noniodized salt should be used, because iodine is a known mucosal irritant. A cool-mist, ultrasonic humidifier (cleaned daily with a 1:10 solution of bleach and water) may also assist in thinning sinus secretions and facilitating drainage. Smoke and other environmental pollutants should be avoided. Fluid intake should be increased, and heated mist from a facial sauna, steam bath, shower, or hot, moist towels wrapped around the face may help relieve sinus and nasal pain by liquefying secretions.

Oral analgesics may also be used for pain (e.g., ibuprofen [Motrin, Advil] 400 to 600 mg every 6 to 8 hours as needed, acetaminophen [Tylenol] 650 mg every 4 to 6 hours as needed, or a stronger combination of acetaminophen 300 mg/codeine 30 mg [Tylenol #3] one to two tablets every 4 to 6 hours as needed). In general, nonprescription medicated nose drops and sprays should be avoided, and prescription decongestant nasal sprays should be taken no longer than 3 to 4 days at a time because long-term use can lead to rebound nasal congestion (rhinitis medicamentosa) and addiction. Phenylephrine (Neo-Synephrine; one to two upright sprays in each nostril three to four times daily as needed) or the stronger oxymetazoline (Afrin; one to two upright sprays in each nostril two to three times daily as needed) may be helpful in adults. Pseudoephedrine (Sudafed) 30 to 60 mg every 4 to 6 hours as needed is an oral alternative but tends to be less effective than topical preparations.

Expectorants such as guaifenesin 200 to 400 mg every 4 hours as needed or iodinated glycerol 30 to 60 mg PO four times daily as needed are used to liquefy sinus secretions and facilitate drainage. Prescription use of anti-inflammatory topical corticosteroids in nasal spray preparations such as fluticasone 0.05% (Flonase), mometasone (Nasonex), or triamcinolone (Nasacort), all at two sprays in each nostril daily, used for 2 to 3 weeks is becoming more common; however, randomized controlled trials have been inconsistent with regard to their effectiveness in rhinosinusitis. In fact, corticosteroid therapy has actually been shown to increase viral load in AVRS. Oral antihistamines should be avoided unless an allergic component is evident because they tend to dry the mucosa, thicken purulent sinus fluids, and slow mucosal drainage, although some studies have suggested their efficacy in symptomatic relief of uncomplicated viral URIs.

ABRS occurs in only 0.5 to 2.0 percent of episodes of acute rhinosinusitis. ABRS occurs when bacteria secondarily infect an inflamed sinus cavity. Patients with ABRS tend to have symptoms that last longer (>10 days) or are more severe. In randomized trials, 60 percent of adults with symptoms persisting 7 to 10 days had a bacterial etiology identified when sinus aspirate was performed. Purulent discharge early in the disease course suggests bacterial infection. Purulent nasal discharge, nasal obstruction, and facial pain/pressure/fullness have relatively high sensitivity and specificity for ABRS, particularly when they occur concurrently and when symptoms persist for more than 10 days.

Although localized sinus infection may be self-limited, antibiotic and symptomatic therapy may be considered appropriate for suspected ABRS to prevent disease progression and complications. Empiric antibiotic therapy for 5 to 10 days covering the most common etiological agents should be instituted before the identification of causative organisms because symptoms may progress while awaiting laboratory confirmation. In adults, common choices include narrow-spectrum antibiotics such as amoxicillin (Amoxil) 500 mg to as high as 1 g PO three times daily, trimethoprim/sulfamethoxazole (Bactrim) 160 mg/800 mg, one Double Strength tablet PO twice daily, or doxycycline 100 mg PO twice daily.

In light of increasing resistance of *S. pneumoniae*, *H. influenzae* (up to 50% of strains), *M. catarrhalis*, and virtually all *S. aureus*, one of the following beta-lactamase–resistant alternatives may be considered:

- Amoxicillin/clavulanate (Augmentin XR) 1,000 mg/ 125 mg PO twice daily
- Clarithromycin (Biaxin XL) 1,000 mg PO daily
- Cefaclor (Ceclor; second-generation cephalosporin) 500 mg PO every 6 hours
- Cefpodoxime (Vantin; third-generation cephalosporin) 200 mg PO twice daily
- Cefdinir (Omnicef; third-generation cephalosporin) 600 mg PO daily
- Levofloxacin (Levaquin) 750 mg PO daily (should not be a first-line choice)

- Moxifloxacin (Avelox) 400 mg PO daily (should not be a first-line choice)

Current treatment guidelines for ABRS in adults consider first-line therapy to be amoxicillin either with or without clavulanate, depending on whether risk factors for antibiotic resistance are present (e.g., high endemic rates of penicillin-resistant *S. pneumoniae*, antibiotic use within the past 30 days, severe infection with systemic symptoms such as fever ≥102°F (39°C), age >65 years, recent hospitalization, or immunocompromised status).

Oral fluoroquinolone or trimethoprim/sulfamethoxazole is usually considered first-line treatment for penicillin-allergic or cephalosporin-allergic patients. Fluoroquinolones should be reserved for those who have no alternative treatment options as the serious adverse effects associated with fluoroquinolones generally outweigh the benefits for patients with ABRS. Immunocompromised patients typically require broad-spectrum coverage for gram-positive and gram-negative organisms and possibly empiric antifungal therapy. Tetracyclines do not cover *S. pneumoniae*, however, and erythromycin, penicillin, and first-generation cephalosporins do not cover *H. influenzae*. Acute infections that fail to clear after one course of antibiotic therapy are often treated with a second course from a separate antibiotic class for 14 days.

A minority of patients require parenteral therapy for CRS. Parenteral antimicrobials are indicated in patients who are seriously ill, undergoing surgery, or in whom compliance is questionable. Sinus cultures should be obtained from patients requiring parenteral therapy. Parenteral antibiotics effective against both anaerobes and aerobes include ampicillin-sulbactam, ticarcillin-clavulanate, piperacillin-tazobactam, clindamycin, moxifloxacin, the carbapenems (imipenem, meropenem, ertapenem), and the second-generation cephalosporins (cefoxitin and cefotetan). If *P. aeruginosa* is suspected, the preferred antibiotics include a fluoroquinolone (e.g., moxifloxacin or levofloxacin); a third- or fourth-generation cephalosporin with antipseudomonal activity (ceftazidime or cefepime); an aminoglycoside; or the carbapenems imipenem or meropenem (but not ertapenem, which lacks activity against *Pseudomonas*). There is currently a black box warning for fluoroquinolones as of 2016. In certain situations, however, fluoroquinolones may still be the best course of treatment. Risks and benefits of this treatment should be carefully evaluated, and infectious disease consultation may need to be initiated as well as pharmacist input.

Metronidazole may also be given parenterally to cover anaerobes in combination with an agent with aerobic activity. The absorption of oral metronidazole and the fluoroquinolones (e.g., moxifloxacin) are excellent, so these should only be given parenterally if the patient is unable to take oral medications. Parenteral antimicrobials effective against methicillin-resistant *Staphylococcus aureus* (MRSA) include vancomycin, linezolid, and daptomycin. The use of these and other agents for the treatment of invasive MRSA infections are discussed separately. (See "Methicillin-resistant *Staphylococcus aureus* in adults: Treatment of bacteremia.")

Antibiotics against anaerobic organisms such as *Peptostreptococcus* and *Bacteroides* are typically required for subacute and chronic sinusitis, with regimens lasting up to 3 to 4 weeks or even as long as 6 weeks for refractory chronic cases. Antibiotic regimens include amoxicillin/clavulanate (Augmentin XR) 1,000 mg/125 mg PO every 12 hours or cefuroxime (Ceftin; second generation cephalosporin) 250 to 500 mg PO twice daily. For penicillin-allergic patients, antibiotics include clarithromycin (Biaxin XL) 500 mg PO daily or clindamycin (Cleocin) 300 mg PO every 6 hours. For documented gram-negative infection, one of the fluoroquinolones (e.g., levofloxacin or moxifloxacin) should be prescribed at the doses mentioned previously. As always, a careful risk/benefit analysis of use of these drugs should be carefully considered; in certain cases, they are still the best—and possibly only—available choice. Patients requiring three or more antibiotic courses will likely benefit from referral to an otorhinolaryngologist for further diagnostic work-up. Similarly, serious invasive fungal sinusitis often requires surgical debridement and inpatient intravenous antifungal therapy with amphotericin B (1 mg/kg IV daily) or, if not tolerated due to rigors, chills, or hypotension, a liposomal amphotericin preparation (Abelcet 5 to 7.5 mg/kg IV daily). In contrast, allergic fungal sinusitis calls for sinus drainage and systemic corticosteroids for 2 to 4 weeks followed by topical corticosteroid therapy because the benefits of antifungal therapy have not been clearly demonstrated. Fungal balls associated with sinus colonization must be removed surgically because neither corticosteroids nor antifungals have been shown to be effective in relieving obstruction.

Maxillary sinus puncture and aspiration may be needed to relieve pain in any form of sinusitis that fails to subside following pharmacotherapy, and patients with subacute or chronic sinusitis may require surgery to remove damaged mucosal tissue or to correct anatomical obstructions of the sinus ostia such as recurrent nasal polyps. In addition, complementary therapies may be considered in the treatment of patients with chronic sinusitis. Several studies indicate that vigorous exercise, for example, has been shown to improve nasal function (through vasoconstriction and decreased nasal resistance) in healthy patients, as well as those with allergic rhinitis. The same benefits may also result in patients with chronic sinusitis. Some patients with particularly severe chronic disease have reported trying acupuncture, herbal therapies, biofeedback, and self-help groups.

Prompt treatment of all respiratory infections can prevent acute sinusitis complications, and surgery to correct anatomical blockages of the sinus ostia (e.g., deviated septum or nasal polyps) may prevent chronic sinusitis. When sinus inflammation is connected with an allergy, desensitization by a trained allergist should be considered. Recurrent attacks of sinusitis can sometimes be prevented by the routine use of a humidifier and/or air-conditioner. Nose drops or sprays should be discarded after use during an acute episode, however, and should never be shared to avoid person-to-person transmission of infectious organisms.

FOLLOW-UP AND REFERRAL

Patients should be reevaluated for symptomatic improvement in 48 to 72 hours, and a return visit should be scheduled for 10 to 14 days from the initial assessment. If symptoms fail to improve with pharmacotherapy, the patient should be evaluated for antibiotic resistance, allergic contributions, or immunological abnormalities. Sinus x-ray films may remain abnormal for up to 2 months after the resolution of acute sinusitis; thus, follow-up films to document improvement are not usually indicated until at least 6 weeks after initial therapy. Immunocompromised patients with sinusitis should be monitored daily in an inpatient setting.

Although complications are relatively uncommon, visual impairments, ophthalmoplegia, orbital or facial cellulitis, severe fever, aphasia, abducens palsy (cranial nerve VI deficit), seizures, altered mental status, osteomyelitis of the frontal or maxillary bones, and focal swelling over the frontal bone are all reflective of localized extensions of bacterial infection. Rare but potentially life-threatening complications that require a high index of suspicion include meningitis, subdural empyema, epidural abscess, cavernous sinus thrombosis, and other central nervous system complications.

Patients should be referred to a specialist if their sinusitis is allergic or immunological, refractory to antibiotic therapy, recurrent, associated with unusual opportunistic infections, or when the infection is adversely affecting their quality of life. In addition, when sinusitis is associated with chronic OM, bronchial asthma, nasal polyps, recurrent pneumonia, immunodeficiency, allergic fungal disease, granulomas, or multiple antibiotic resistances, the patient should be referred to an allergist or an otolaryngologist.

Patient Education: Rhinosinusitis

Patients should be instructed to be wary of worsening symptoms after the institution of pharmacotherapy. Patients should also be informed of potential complications and should be instructed to contact the practitioner at once if telltale signs such as periorbital swelling develop. The clinician should stress the importance of avoiding contact with all contributing factors (e.g., cigarette smoke or airborne allergens), as well as the exacerbating side effects of nonprescription antihistamine use. Patients should make sure that OTC decongestant preparations do not contain antihistamines, and they should drink plenty of fluids to thin nasal secretions.

STOMATITIS AND GLOSSITIS

Stomatitis is a generalized inflammation of the oral mucous membranes characterized by erythema and/or vesicular or ulcerative lesions. *Glossitis* is an acute or chronic inflammation of the tongue that shares many of the same etiologies as stomatitis. Either of the two may present alone, although glossitis often accompanies stomatitis, and clinicians often group the two conditions together under the latter designation. In general, both disorders are classified according to their etiology, which is extremely variable.

EPIDEMIOLOGY AND CAUSES

A variety of types of stomatitis are seen in adults, including oral candidiasis, aphthous stomatitis (aphthous ulcers or "canker sores"; those that recur are called recurrent aphthous stomatitis [RAS]), secondary herpetic stomatitis/herpes labialis, Vincent's stomatitis (acute necrotizing ulcerative gingivitis or "trench mouth"), allergic stomatitis, nicotinic (cigarette-related) stomatitis, denture-related stomatitis, angular stomatitis, pseudomembranous stomatitis, and parasitic glossitis (anthracosis linguae or "black hairy tongue"). Glossitis is also a common symptom of systemic skin diseases such as erythema multiforme (Stevens-Johnson syndrome) and pemphigus vulgaris. Herpetic stomatitis and RAS occur commonly, as do nicotinic and denture-related stomatitis. Other causes are less commonly seen.

Herpes simplex virus (HSV) infection is widespread in the United States. According to recent estimates, up to 20% of the adult population may be secreting herpes simplex type 1 or 2 virus at any given time. The prevalence of HSV-specific antibodies indicative of past or dormant HSV infection is up to 30% in higher socioeconomic strata and may approach 100% in lower socioeconomic groups. In general, prevalence of infection is estimated to be between 20,000 and 70,000 cases per 100,000 people. Oral candidiasis most commonly occurs in immunocompromised adults, such as patients with HIV infection or in cancer patients after chemotherapy and/or radiation therapy. Nicotinic stomatitis and denture-related stomatitis are common. Most other forms are rare among adults. Mouth sores may affect adults of all ages. Specifically, Vincent's stomatitis is seen among adolescents and adults aged 20 to 40 years, whereas denture-related stomatitis affects primarily elderly patients.

Chronic mouth breathing dries the tongue and oral mucosa, and hot foods or beverages may lead to thermal injury in the mouth. Chemical irritation may result from spicy, acidic, or salty foods such as potato chips and pickles, as well as from peroxide-containing mouthwashes, toothpaste, and other dental care products. Viral, bacterial, and fungal infections, prolonged radiation or chemotherapy treatments, long-term corticosteroid or antibiotic use, chronic metabolic diseases such as diabetes, emotional or physical stress, anxiety, depression, premenstrual tension, advanced age, low socioeconomic status, and malnourishment may all contribute to host immunosuppression and lead to the development of stomatitis/glossitis. Systemic autoimmune or inflammatory diseases also predispose patients to these conditions,

while pregnancy has been associated with erythema multiforme.

Tobacco smoking and chewing ("dipping snuff") clearly can lead to nicotinic stomatitis, whereas ill-fitting dentures, recent dental work, repeated biting during convulsive seizures, and poor oral/dental hygiene contribute to mechanical injury–related inflammation of the oral cavity and tongue. Occupational or domestic exposure to chemical irritants or allergens are risk factors, as are resective gastrointestinal surgery involving the ileum and malabsorptive disorders of the ileal mucosa such as sprue (villous atrophy), both of which impair vitamin B_{12} absorption and thereby contribute to angular and other vitamin deficiency–related forms of stomatitis. Anemia of any type is a risk factor. Repeated emesis secondary to bulimia may inflame the oral mucosa and erode the posterior (lingual) surfaces of the teeth because of repeated exposure to stomach acid in the vomitus. In addition, anorexia, bulimia, and off-and-on ("yo-yo") dieting may lead to malnourishment, vitamin deficiencies, or immunosuppression.

Prior HSV infection is the primary risk factor for all secondary manifestations of herpes simplex infection. In addition, any factors that lead to immunosuppression may be considered contributing factors. Specifically, fever, physical and/or emotional stress, excess sun exposure, menstruation, common colds, gastrointestinal upset, dental work that excessively stretches the mouth, and underlying systemic illnesses may be considered precipitating factors. Intercourse with multiple sexual partners and unprotected sex (failure to use barrier protection, e.g., condoms, during intercourse or oral sex or latex dental dams during oral sex) increase the likelihood of HSV transmission from infected sexual partners.

PATHOPHYSIOLOGY

In general, excessive dryness of the oral cavity; food and drug allergies; chemical irritation; mechanical or thermal injury; bacterial, fungal, and viral pathogens (e.g., coxsackievirus causing hand-foot-and-mouth disease, varicella-zoster virus causing oral and lingual vesicular lesions, primary HIV infection); host immunosuppression; and nutritional deficiencies of iron, folate, riboflavin (B_2), niacin, pyridoxine (B_6), and cyanocobalamin (B_{12}) are all risk factors that can cause stomatitis and glossitis.

Aphthous ulcers are one of the most common types of oral lesions, yet their pathogenesis is poorly defined. Stress, hormonal fluctuations, inflammatory bowel disease, and antimetabolite chemotherapies all predispose a patient to aphthae. Specifically, the spirochete *Borrelia vincentii* and certain fusiform *Bacillus* bacterial species are strongly associated with Vincent's stomatitis, although some cases are of indeterminate etiology. If complicated by HIV infection and left untreated, this condition may progress to necrotizing stomatitis. Nicotinic stomatitis results directly from the chemical irritants in tobacco. Denture-related stomatitis results from the mechanical injury caused by ill-fitting dentures. Angular stomatitis is symptomatic of the vitamin deficiencies discussed in the preceding text, and pseudomembranous stomatitis has been associated with numerous chemical irritants and bacterial pathogens.

Parasitic glossitis is caused by several mycoses of the tongue, including *Cryptococcus linguae-pilosasae* and *Nocardia lingualis* coinfection. The use of systemic antibiotics is well known to clear normal microbial flora from the oral cavity and, in fact, the entire gastrointestinal tract, thus facilitating fungal overgrowth caused by the lack of endogenous microbial competition. In addition, both oral and inhaled corticosteroids are known to compromise cellular immunity within the oral cavity—the main defense mechanism against fungal overgrowth and infection. HIV infection and AIDS, malignancy, chemotherapy, diabetes mellitus, and age-related decreases in natural immunity may contribute to immune suppression as well, increasing the likelihood of fungal overgrowth and viral reactivation of HSV.

Erythema multiforme is a widespread immune-mediated inflammatory reaction of the skin and in the advanced stages can involve the mucous membranes, including the oral cavity. This condition may be caused by different types of infectious agents (e.g., HSV, *Mycoplasma*, *S. pyogenes*), drug allergies (e.g., anticonvulsants, sulfonamides, allopurinol), as well as collagen vascular disorders. However, oral involvement in erythema multiforme, as well as its extreme forms (Stevens-Johnson syndrome, toxic epidermal necrolysis) will never be isolated to stomatitis because these are systemic, life-threatening conditions.

In contrast, the etiology of pemphigus vulgaris is unknown, but flaccid bullae typically begin in the oropharynx as superficial epidermal layers separate from their base. A similar appearing blistering disorder, bullous pemphigoid, only rarely presents with isolated oral lesions; but as this disease progresses, roughly one-third of individuals may demonstrate oral involvement. A number of inherited disorders of the epidermis and dermis known collectively as epidermolysis bullosa may also involve the oral mucosa in their moderate and severe forms. Finally, a wide array of autoimmune disorders such as systemic lupus erythematosus may also present with mucosal ulcerative lesions.

CLINICAL MANIFESTATIONS

Subjective

In general, patients with stomatitis may complain of excessive dryness of the mouth; halitosis; difficulty speaking or swallowing; minor to severe oral pain; or bleeding, swollen, or erythematous gums; they may also describe constitutional symptoms (including fever, malaise, headache, and weight loss) that may be secondary to infection or malnourishment. Patients with Vincent's stomatitis may complain of excess salivation. In cases of allergic

stomatitis, patients may also report itching and burning in the mouth. In contrast, parasitic glossitis is usually painless, whereas anemia and niacin deficiency lead to lingual pain.

Patients with secondary herpetic stomatitis usually report a 24- to 48-hour prodrome consisting of a burning sensation in the mouth, followed by the appearance of 1- to 2-mm vesicular lesions, which start as fluid-filled bullae and then evolve into ulcerated lesions that eventually crust over the course of several days. These frequently appear around the lips. Although most patients report only one to two recurrences per year, 5% to 25% of patients suffer more than one attack per month.

Objective

The mouth and the tongue (if also inflamed) often appear bright red and swollen, either at the tip and edges (from vitamin deficiencies or mechanical injury) or over the entire glossal surface. Depending on the cause of inflammation, the tongue may be ulcerated (from niacin deficiency, streptococcal infection, erythema multiforme, or pemphigus) or smooth and pale (from iron, folate, or B_{12} deficiencies). Vincent's stomatitis causes necrotic ulceration of the interdental gingival papillae and oral mucous membranes, characterized by a purulent, gray exudate. Allergic stomatitis causes intense, shiny erythema and slight swelling of the mucosa and tongue. Nicotinic stomatitis presents with centrally erythematous white nodular elevations, and pseudomembranous stomatitis produces a membranelike exudate coating the oral mucosa. Parasitic glossitis presents with hypertrophied (1-cm) filiform papillae that color the dorsum of the tongue dark brown or black. The lesions of pseudomembranous stomatitis cannot be scraped off with a tongue blade, whereas the lesions of parasitic glossitis are easily broken.

Syphilis and mouth breathing result in white patches on the tongue. Inflammation and external fissuring of the corners of the mouth are characteristic of angular stomatitis. Erythema multiforme presents with polymorphous disseminated macular, papular, nodular, vesicular, bullous, and target (bull's eye–shaped) lesions of the skin and mucous membranes. Pemphigus is characterized by disseminated thin-walled bullae throughout the skin and mucosa, which, when ruptured, leave raw patches.

Inspection of the oral mucosa of patients with HSV infection reveals individual or groups of 1- to 2-mm vesicular lesions that evolve into ulcers, apparent after the prodromal period (24 to 48 hours, characterized by pain, tingling, burning, and itching preceding vesicle formation), particularly on the gingivae, hard palate, buccal mucosa, and tongue. If observed at a later stage of healing (4 to 10 days after vesicle formation), oral lesions may appear ulcerated but crusted over. Herpes labialis presents as similar clusters of open vesicular lesions in the labial area, particularly at the mucocutaneous border, with erythematous bases and possibly crusting, if the lesions are in an advanced stage of healing. Palpation of the oral mucosa may demonstrate edema or tenderness, aiding in the identification and characterization of oral lesions. Anterior cervical or jaw lymphadenopathy may be felt with herpes infection, as well as in cases related to autoimmune or systemic inflammatory disease.

Although not directly related to HSV infection, back percussion over the posterior lung fields may reveal the dull tones of pulmonary consolidation characteristic of lung infections (e.g., tuberculosis) common to HIV infection, AIDS, or other immunocompromising disorders that often underlie the reactivation of HSV infection. Likewise, chest auscultation may reveal signs such as crackles, crepitus, or wheezing, which may indicate the presence of systemic inflammatory disease or pulmonary infections secondary to an underlying immune disorder.

Oral candidiasis may exhibit diverse clinical patterns, and some patients exhibit more than one form. Factors that affect clinical presentation are the immune status of the host, such as the presence of HIV or a history of organ transplant, as well as the oral mucosal environment, for example, the impaired salivary function seen in Sjögren's syndrome, postradiation xerostomia, or age-related atrophy, and whether the person is dentate or edentulous (more common) and a nonsmoker or smoker (more common). Pseudomembranous candidiasis, also known as "thrush," is recognized by the development of creamy white plaques that resemble cottage cheese or curdled milk. When these plaques are scraped off, an erythematous mucosal base is exposed.

Erythematous candidiasis, in which the oral mucosa appears fiery red and the mouth feels like it has been "scalded with a hot beverage," often follows broad-spectrum antibiotic therapy and is also associated with immunosuppression and xerostomia. Breath mints, cinnamon gum, mouthwash, or toothpaste can cause allergic reactions that mimic this form of candidiasis; thus, the patient's history is important in differentiating the clinical picture because treatment will vary accordingly.

Chronic hyperplastic candidiasis, or candidal leukoplakia, is the least common form of oral candidiasis. Patients have a white patch (leukoplakia) that cannot be scraped off. Some researchers believe that this is a candidiasis superimposed on a preexisting leukoplakia lesion. Hairy leukoplakia is associated with Epstein-Barr virus (EBV). These white mucosal lesions do not rub off and may appear as faint vertical streaks or thick, furrowed areas of leukoplakia. Hairy leukoplakia has been reported in organ and bone marrow transplant recipients and, on rare occasions, in immunocompetent patients. However, its presence strongly suggests HIV infection in an individual with no other signs of immune suppression. HIV patients with hairy leukoplakia frequently develop

AIDS within 2 years of the onset of lesions. *Candida* may be present in these cases without the tissue's normal inflammatory reaction to the fungus.

Other conditions leading to an inflamed appearance of the oral mucosa include systemic or local vasculitis and oral neoplasia; the latter (oral or glottic cancer) often presents as a single, painless lesion. Measles (roseola paramyxovirus infection) also leads to erythematous patches with bluish white centers on the lingual and buccal mucosa, known as Koplik's spots. However, this systemic infection is accompanied by a skin rash, cough, and coryza 24 to 48 hours after the appearance of these distinctive oral lesions.

DIAGNOSTIC REASONING

Diagnostic Tests

Stomatitis or glossitis may result from a myriad of causes, and detecting the primary underlying problem is key to effective management. A CBC may reflect bacterial infection if polymorphonuclear neutrophils are elevated or viral infection if lymphocytes and mononuclear leukocytes predominate. Biochemical tests, special cellular stains, and cultures are used to identify most causative microorganisms, along with certain serological tests such as rapid plasma regain for the syphilitic agent *Treponema pallidum*. Serum levels of iron, folate, riboflavin, niacin, or cyanocobalamin may reveal nutritional deficiencies that can cause stomatitis and glossitis. Autoimmune disorders are diagnosed through a wide array of serologies (e.g., antinuclear antibody test for systemic lupus erythematosus).

Herpetic stomatitis caused by HSV may be ruled out via serum levels of anti-HSV antibodies, viral culture, or a Tzanck smear of lesion scrapings, which will present as multinucleated giant cells with intranuclear inclusions. Concurrent genital lesions are common in herpetic infection, as is also the case with Behçet's disease, a neutrophilic inflammatory disorder treated with topical and systemic corticosteroids, which does not appear infectious. Non–*Candida*-related pseudomembranous stomatitis may be distinguished from oral candidiasis by negative findings for the fungus on Gram stain or more appropriately 10% potassium hydroxide wet mount of lesion scrapings. Oral candidiasis, as well as lichen planus, may resemble nicotinic stomatitis. Lichen planus may be ruled out by biopsy, which demonstrates hyperkeratosis, irregular acanthosis, and lymphocytic dermal band–like infiltrates. Biopsy is also indicated in the case of suspected neoplasia and should be considered for any lingual or mucosal lesions that are chronic or recurrent.

Viral culture and serological tests may rule out measles and other viral infections, including infectious mononucleosis (EBV infection), warts (papillomaviruses), prodromal primary HIV infection, and severe cases of chickenpox (varicella-zoster infection), which may also present with vesicular lesions of the oral cavity, pharynx, and larynx.

Differential Diagnosis

Because the etiology of these lesions is so variable, the primary goal of the differential diagnosis for mouth sores is to determine their precise cause to direct management most effectively. Although the serum testing may be used to detect specific pathogens or nutritional deficiencies, the signs and symptoms elicited from patient history and physical examination provide the most useful information in determining the cause of mouth sores. For example, self-induced vomiting associated with bulimic disorders should be ruled out through a careful patient history. Similarly, physical examination can rule out aphthous stomatitis, which unlike the other forms listed, produces characteristic shallow, grayish, nonvesicular ulcers surrounded by a ring of hyperemia and covered with a fibrinous yellow membrane.

Ludwig's angina should also be considered in the differential for patients who present with rapidly progressing gangrenous cellulitis of the soft tissues of the neck and floor of the mouth. Pregnancy epulis (pregnancy gingivitis) results from hormonal changes and may be confused with other forms of stomatitis. However, the characteristic gingival hyperplasia of this disorder is usually limited to the interdental papillae, and pyogenic granulomas may form. "Geographic tongue" (benign migratory glossitis), which may be confused with pathological forms of glossitis, presents as continuously changing areas of loss and regrowth of filiform papillae with thickened white borders surrounded by red patches, creating a maplike appearance of the tongue. Geographic tongue is considered to be a harmless, normal physical variant requiring no treatment.

MANAGEMENT

Most cases of stomatitis are effectively treated with outpatient care unless severe or resulting from an underlying disease requiring inpatient care (e.g., advanced syphilis). For example, if severe dehydration secondary to oral pain and dysphagia is present, parenteral fluids may be required.

The following steps can be taken to relieve the pain of stomatitis and glossitis and speed recovery:

- All behaviors or conditions contributing to lesion formation should be stopped or corrected (e.g., smoking, eating hot or spicy foods, wearing ill-fitting dentures).
- Underlying causative infections should be treated appropriately, but pharmacologic and other treatments specific to oral inflammation are primarily directed to symptomatic relief.

- Baking soda or salt water rinses three or more times a day (one-half teaspoon salt or sodium bicarbonate dissolved in 8 ounces of water) may be sufficient to relieve mild discomfort. Alternatively, oral rinses of half strength 3% hydrogen peroxide solution (1:1 with water) may be used.
- Liquid antacids such as attapulgite (Kaopectate), aluminum hydroxide (Amphojel), or magnesium hydroxide (Maalox) may effectively relieve pain when swished and swallowed four times daily.
- Equal amounts of antihistaminic elixirs such as diphenhydramine (Benadryl) may be mixed with liquid antacids (1:1) and used as an oral rinse to reduce inflammation.
- Nonprescription analgesics such as acetaminophen (Tylenol) 650 mg every 4 to 6 hours may be used to relieve mouth pain.
- A viscous solution of 2% lidocaine may be applied to oral lesions every 3 hours as a topical anesthetic or used as a gargle or swish and spit (15 mL) before meals and every 3 hours as needed.
- Severe attacks in adults may require topical gel–based 0.1% triamcinolone (Kenalog) or fluocinonide applied at bedtime and, if needed, three times daily after meals.
- Anti-inflammatory oral corticosteroid "bursts" may be appropriate in severe cases of stomatitis and glossitis, but all oral medications should be monitored for toxicity because significantly more absorption than expected may result from open oral ulcers. In addition, corticosteroids would not be indicated in immunosuppressed patients or those with viral infections, although antiviral medications such as amantadine (Symmetrel) may be appropriate.
- For cases of HSV, ice cubes applied locally for an hour to newly formed lesions may prove helpful; likewise, drinking cool liquids and sucking on frozen juice bars may reduce discomfort.
- Pharmacologic preparations for HSV may be helpful, such as valacyclovir (Valtrex) 1 g twice daily for 2 days or famciclovir (Famvir) 500 mg twice daily for 5 days.
- High fluid intake and antiseptic mouthwashes (without alcohol, which may be irritating and painful) may help prevent secondary bacterial infection.

In cases of oral candidiasis, antifungal agents should be used in conjunction with attentive oral hygiene:

- Nystatin (Mycostatin, Nilstat), a polyene antibiotic, is formulated for use as a pastille (lozenge) or suspension 400,000 to 600,000 units (of 100,000 units/mL suspension) PO (swish and swallow) four times daily. Because it is not absorbed across the gastrointestinal tract, nystatin must remain in contact with the organism and be reapplied several times a day to be effective.
- Clotrimazole (Lotrimin, Mycelex), an imidazole agent, is not well absorbed and must be administered at least four times daily as a 10 mg troche.

- Ketoconazole (Nizoral) 200 to 400 mg PO daily for 7 to 14 days, another imidazole, is absorbed across the gastrointestinal tract and provides systemic therapy by the oral route. It should not be used routinely for routine oral candidiasis, however, because of possible drug interactions and potential liver toxicity. Alternatively, the triazole agent fluconazole (Diflucan), given as 200 mg on the first day and then 100 mg daily for 7 to 14 days, is well absorbed systemically and only rarely causes liver toxicity, although other drug interactions, as well as drug resistance, have been documented.
- Hydrocortisone-iodoquinol (Vytone) cream can be used to ease the discomfort of angular cheilitis. It combines the anti-inflammatory and antipruritic effects of hydrocortisone with the antifungal and antibacterial properties of iodoquinol.
- In terms of oral hygiene, toothbrushes should be changed frequently, and a patient who wears dentures or partial dental appliances must also treat the appliances to combat the infection.

Treatment of erythema multiforme requires eliminating exposure to the offending agent in the case of drug hypersensitivity or specific treatment of the underlying infectious agent (e.g., acyclovir for HSV infection). Specialist care by a dermatologist and close inpatient observation are required for severe cases that risk progression to Stevens-Johnson syndrome or toxic epidermal necrolysis. Vincent's stomatitis requires oral penicillin V potassium (Pen-Vee K) 250 to 500 mg every 4 to 6 hours as well as significant fluid intake of at least four to six glasses of nonacidic fruit juice or water per day.

Severe gangrenous stomatitis requires IV antibiotic treatment and debridement of wounds. Autoimmune disorders such as systemic lupus erythematosus, bullous pemphigoid, and pemphigus vulgaris are primarily treated with systemic corticosteroids. The mucosal lesions of lupus may be treated with topical or intralesional corticosteroids if located on the lips, whereas lesions of the oral cavity respond to antimalarial medications, provided no drug hypersensitivity manifests. However, for recalcitrant cases, increasingly potent immunosuppressive medications may be necessary. Treatment of any of these disorders typically requires specialist care and rapid referral.

Dehydration and malnutrition can result from altered eating habits due to oral pain. Secondary bacterial infections may complicate any type of ulcerative oral lesion. Recent scarification of lesions may progress to facial space infection, tonsillar or cervical lymph gland infection, or involvement of the vocal cords, bronchial tubes, rectum, vagina, and even sepsis. Thus, oral surgery may be needed to trim away rough, highly inflamed, infected gum tissue. Glossitis may become chronic if inadequately treated, and severe gangrenous or necrotizing stomatitis seen in severe HIV-infected cases may lead to death if untreated.

FOLLOW-UP AND REFERRAL

Difficult to treat and refractory cases of stomatitis and glossitis due to underlying systemic disorders, such as autoimmune conditions, require specialist referral to guide further management.

Patient Education: Stomatitis and Glossitis

The importance of proper oral hygiene and healthful nutritional habits should be stressed to all patients. Patients should be instructed to brush their teeth with a soft-bristled toothbrush at least twice daily and to floss regularly (once a day, if possible). Patients should also wear protective headgear whenever bicycling, skating, or playing contact sports to prevent cases of trauma-related tongue injury. Increased fluid intake during treatment should be encouraged, as should maintaining the recommended medication regimen while avoiding hot, spicy, salty, or acidic foods, and carbonated or alcoholic beverages. Patients may be instructed to drink through a straw if lesions are particularly painful. A liquid diet may be recommended during the first 2 to 3 days of treatment if pain is severe. Milk, gelatin, yogurt, ice cream, and custard are usually well tolerated. Severe cases of Vincent's stomatitis may even call for at-home rest during the first few days of treatment.

Early treatment of viral, bacterial, and fungal infections may prevent stomatic and glossal involvement. The contagious nature of pathogen-related forms of stomatitis or glossitis should be emphasized. The most effective means of avoiding secondary manifestations of reactivated HSV infection, for example, is to refrain from behaviors that put the individual at risk of HSV infection or reinfection—most notably, unprotected sex with multiple partners and physical contact with persons who have active herpetic lesions. Kissing and oral sex should be avoided if an individual is actively infected, and frequent hand washing during active flare-ups of herpetic lesions will aid in preventing autoinfection and viral transmission. It is also helpful to inform patients of the high prevalence rate of HSV infection to reduce the stigma commonly associated with herpes. Early treatment of primary or secondary HSV infection may also help to prevent stomatic or labial involvement. Wearing zinc oxide–containing sunscreens on the lips and face helps to prevent herpes labialis flare-ups when exposed to excessive sunlight.

In the long term, the most effective means of avoiding stomatitis is to refrain from risk behaviors such as smoking, eating hot or spicy foods, drinking alcohol, and practicing poor dental hygiene. Avoiding exposure to affected persons, especially in the case of HSV, as well as avoiding exposure to allergens, chemical irritants, or foods that seem to trigger attacks, is also recommended. Care should be taken to fit all dentures and dental prostheses properly to prevent mechanical injury; for cases related to bruxism (tooth grinding), a nightguard prosthesis with removable splints to reduce biting pressure on tooth surfaces may reduce damage to dentition, in turn, preventing related inflammation.

PHARYNGITIS AND TONSILLITIS

Pharyngitis and *tonsillitis* denote generalized inflammatory processes of both infectious and noninfectious etiology, involving the pharynx and pharyngeal tonsils, respectively. Most virally related cases are self-limited, with spontaneous recovery, although other infectious cases may require antibiotic or antifungal therapy. Pharyngitis and tonsillitis may occur independently of one another; however, they often co-occur, sharing a common etiology, clinical course, and treatment regimen. Many cases of pharyngitis and virtually all cases of tonsillitis are contagious.

EPIDEMIOLOGY AND CAUSES

About 8% of all patient visits in the ambulatory care setting each year are for complaints of sore throat. Viral pharyngitis related to respiratory tract pathogens occurs most often in the colder fall and winter months. Influenza infection typically occurs in epidemics between December and April. The incidence of pharyngitis from group A beta-hemolytic streptococcal infection typically increases from 10% of cases reported in the fall to 40% in the winter and spring. Herpangina is known to peak in the summer and fall. Allergic pharyngitis may also peak seasonally during the summer months.

Although infectious (bacterial and viral) pharyngitis and tonsillitis tend to occur most frequently in young children aged 5 to 10 years, both conditions may occur at any age. Streptococcal infection most frequently affects patients younger than 25 years; however, it may occur sporadically in older adults. Infectious mononucleosis (primarily caused by EBV) is also common in adolescents and young adults and is rarely seen in the elderly. Pharyngitis associated with the postnasal drip of sinusitis most often affects adults. No ethnic predispositions have been reported for either pharyngitis or tonsillitis, and men and women are affected equally by both conditions.

URI is a common predisposing factor for the development of viral pharyngitis. The postnasal drip associated with URI or sinusitis may also contribute to irritant-related pharyngitis. The risk of all forms of infectious pharyngitis (viral, bacterial, and fungal) is increased in immunocompromised persons who are afflicted by chronic illnesses, including diabetes mellitus and white blood cell dyscrasias such as agranulocytosis or acute leukemia. Work-related stress and excessive alcohol consumption have also been implicated as a cause of decreased resistance to throat infection. In general, close living quarters, such as military barracks, schools, and day-care centers increase the risk of person-to-person transmission of the infectious agents that cause both pharyngitis and tonsillitis.

EBV transmission typically requires intimate person-to-person contact between susceptible persons and symptomatic viral shedders (hence its nickname of "kissing disease"). Young adults and adolescents from higher socioeconomic backgrounds in developed countries who have not been exposed to EBV in their childhood are most susceptible. Persons with pharyngitis related to *Neisseria gonorrhea*, *T. pallidum* (syphilis), *Chlamydia*, or herpes usually have a history of performing oral intercourse with an infected sexual partner. Sexual abuse may be a factor in these cases as well. Bisexual and homosexual men and patients with anogenital gonorrhea are the groups most frequently affected by gonorrheal pharyngitis.

Adult cases of *Corynebacterium diphtheriae* occur almost exclusively in nonimmunized individuals. Recent contact with a wild animal (especially through a bite) is the major risk factor for the development of *Francisella tularensis* infection. Excessive antibiotic use has been associated with candidal infection and an overgrowth of *Candida* in the oropharynx (thrush); tobacco and particularly marijuana smoking have also been implicated.

PATHOPHYSIOLOGY

In up to 40% of pharyngitis cases, no causative agent is identified. Definitive diagnosis of an infectious agent is difficult, because the nasopharynx is a nonsterile environment normally colonized by an array of nonpathogenic flora. However, the current literature suggests that in adults, upper respiratory tract viruses are the most common cause of infectious pharyngitis, accounting for 30% to 50% of all cases: rhinovirus, coronavirus, adenovirus, influenza viruses A and B, parainfluenza virus, coxsackievirus (herpangina and hand-foot-and-mouth disease), enterovirus, and respiratory syncytial virus. Rhinoviruses and influenza viruses inflame the oral and nasopharyngeal mucosa via direct invasion and colonization, but the specific pathogenic mechanisms of other viruses are not well understood. Members of the herpes family of viruses are also common causative agents, including EBV and in immunocompromised hosts, cytomegalovirus (CMV), HSV, and reactivated herpes zoster. EBV, which infects pharyngeal B-lymphocytes and disseminates throughout the entire lymphoreticular system, is the primary causative agent of infectious mononucleosis and accounts for 1% to 2% of all pharyngitis cases. However, CMV causes up to 20% of all infectious mononucleosis cases. Primary infection with HIV may also cause pharyngitis owing to rapid retroviral replication; thus, HIV risk factors should always be assessed.

Bacterial agents typically cause an exudative pharyngitis, which represents roughly 20% of all cases of sore throat. Group A beta-hemolytic *S. pyogenes*, which accounts for 10% to 20% of adult pharyngitis cases, invades and multiplies within the pharyngeal mucosa, causing an intense inflammatory response known as "strep throat." *Streptococcus* bacteria are characterized into groups based on cell-wall antigenicity. Clinically relevant groups include A, B, C, D, and G. Group A is the most important cause of pharyngitis because it may lead to the most serious complications, including heart valve damage that may occur many years after systemic infection, known as acute rheumatic fever.

More than 80 serotypes of *Streptococcus* have been identified. The most clinically significant strain is based on the M protein, which is the major virulence factor of group A beta-hemolytic *S. pyogenes*. M protein is antiphagocytic, because it blocks activation of the alternative complement pathway. An immune response to bacterial M protein stimulates long-lasting type-specific anti-M antibodies that adhere to individual bacteria and facilitate their phagocytosis (i.e., opsonization), protecting patients against subsequent exposure to bacteria of the same M-protein serotype. The amount of time needed for patients to mount a protective immune response is unclear. In the past, it had been suggested that treatment of group A *Streptococcus* be delayed so that a protective immune response could be mounted, but this practice has since been refuted, and rapid treatment is now the standard of care.

S. pyogenes strains are becoming increasingly virulent, and the incidence of subsequent acute renal insufficiency due to postinfectious glomerulonephritis has increased over the past 15 years. Reports of bacteremia, deep tissue cellulitis, and systemic toxic shock–like syndrome mediated by *Streptococcal* exotoxins are also well characterized, with pharyngitis often recognized as the presenting complaint.

Other bacterial agents of pharyngitis include *N. gonorrhoeae* (especially in young, sexually active adults), *H. influenzae*, *S. pneumoniae*, *T. pallidum*, *S. aureus*, and *C. diphtheriae* and *Corynebacterium hemolyticum* (both often associated with epiglottitis and a potentially obstructive fibrinous gray membrane adherent to the posterior pharynx). The relative importance of atypical organisms known to cause bronchitis, including *Chlamydia pneumoniae*, *Chlamydia trachomatis*, and *Mycoplasma pneumonia*, as causative agents of pharyngitis is controversial. Studies have demonstrated markedly varied prevalence rates (0% to 20%) with these agents, and nasopharyngeal colonization by these organisms may be asymptomatic.

Noninfectious etiologies of pharyngitis may include trauma, allergies, collagen vascular diseases such as Kawasaki's syndrome, autoimmune blistering diseases such as pemphigus, chemical or drug-induced damage, and severe dehydration. Tobacco and particularly marijuana smoking are major contributing factors to noninfectious pharyngitis related to chemical irritation, and exposure to allergens such as dust and pollen increases the risk of allergic pharyngitis, typically associated with a history or family history of atopy. Severe drug reactions mediated by both type I immediate hypersensitivity and type III antibody–antigen immune complex reactions may extend in their most serious form to the oropharynx,

as well as other mucosal sites. Both low humidity and mouth breathing may contribute to dehydration-induced mucosal inflammation.

In contrast, tonsillitis (which may involve the posterior pharyngeal tonsils as well as the more anterior adenoid glands) is foremost a disorder of infectious etiology. It is characterized by inflammation, swelling, and purulent exudation of these lymphoid tissue collections that directly drain the colonized or infected nasopharynx. The spectrum of causative agents in this disorder is similar to that described for pharyngitis, including bacteria and upper respiratory tract viruses. Acutely, it is most often caused by group A *Streptococcus* infection, and a chronic form may also result from repeated *Streptococcus* infections. Streptococcal tonsillar infection always has the potential for progressing to peritonsillar or tonsillar abscess, which requires aggressive management (incision and drainage, followed by antibiotic therapy).

CLINICAL PRESENTATION

Subjective

Most patients with pharyngitis and/or tonsillitis report mild to severe throat pain or the sensation of a "tickle" or pruritus in the throat. Infectious mononucleosis, adenovirus, and especially group A *Streptococcus* pharyngitis tend to cause the most painful sore throats, with fever. Many patients also describe their throats as feeling swollen, with a "lump" in the back of the throat that persists despite repeated swallowing. A history of dysphagia (difficulty swallowing) is also common with throat inflammation, particularly from *H. influenzae* infection, and hoarseness is often associated with *C. pneumoniae* infection.

Group A *Streptococcus* infection usually produces a fever higher than 101°F (38.3°C); the patient may be tachycardic, and there is usually a pharyngeal exudate. Chills and fever are common with bacterial infection, although cough and rhinorrhea are rarely present. In contrast, laryngitis and cough are commonly associated with viral infection, while fever occurs only occasionally, as systemic symptoms are uncommon in viral pharyngitis. However, as with viral infections, streptococcal symptomatology is rapid in onset. Allergic pharyngitis, in contrast, does not present with fever but is recognized most readily by a persistent postnasal drip, paroxysmal sneezing, itchy, watery eyes, rhinorrhea, and a mild sore throat that typically worsen with recumbency. Malaise, generalized aches and pains, and headache may be reported in both conditions.

Infectious mononucleosis is infamous for its gradual onset of low-grade fever, marked fatigue, and severe sore throat. Anorexia and nausea may also be present. Influenza infection is characterized by an abrupt onset of fever ranging from 100°F to 104°F (37.8°C to 40°C), myalgias, and headache, which last for about 3 days, followed by 3 to 4 days of cough, rhinorrhea, and pharyngitis, and finally a 1- to 2-week convalescent period with persistent cough and malaise. Geriatric patients with influenza may also present with gastrointestinal symptoms such as nausea, vomiting, and diarrhea. Reactivated herpes zoster infection is characterized by painful prodromes before active flare-ups. In contrast, HSV infection does not usually cause a sore throat. Moreover, primary or secondary syphilitic lesions tend to be painless. Gonococcal pharyngitis may be asymptomatic. Severe cases of tonsillitis may also present with ear pain and sometimes with cough or vomiting.

Objective

On inspection, the inflamed throat typically appears erythematous, although color may vary. Conjunctivitis is often associated with adenovirus and other respiratory viruses, whereas mucosal exudates and enlarged tonsils occur only occasionally. EBV-related infectious mononucleosis, however, may present with an exudative tonsillitis (in about 50% of cases), in addition to palatal petechiae and an exanthem. The 1- to 2-mm vesicular lesions of herpes simplex infection may extend from the pharynx to the lips, gingivae, buccal mucosa, and tongue. Reactivated herpes zoster infection typically presents with 2- to 4-mm vesicular lesions unilaterally on the tongue, lip, and buccal mucosa. Herpangina presents as 1- to 2-mm oral vesicles or ulcers on the pharynx, tonsils, soft palate, pillars, uvula, and posterior buccal mucosa. Hand-foot-and-mouth disease presents with oral lesions co-occurring with an exanthem on the hands and feet. Maculopapular rashes on the extremities of young adult patients may be indicative of many types of infection, including *C. hemolyticum*, HIV, enteroviruses, or *T. pallidum* (syphilis).

Exudates and enlarged tonsils are common findings in bacterial infections. Streptococcal infection produces a characteristic white to yellow exudate and may be accompanied by a sandpaper-like, scarlatiniform rash. *Mycoplasma*-related cases may be clinically indistinguishable from streptococcal infections. *C. diphtheriae* presents with a characteristic grayish pseudomembrane overlying the pharyngeal mucosa, tonsils, epiglottis, uvula, or even the nasal cavity. The nonvesicular lesions of primary syphilis are 5 to 15 mm in size and appear indurated or "healed up," extending to the lips, tonsils, or tongue. Secondary syphilitic nonvesicular lesions (2 to 10 mm) arise symmetrically on all parts of the oropharynx and mouth. Candidal infections produce thin, white, nonvesicular, diffuse or patchy (3 to 11 mm) exudative ulcers on all parts of the oropharyngeal mucosa. In most inflammatory conditions of the throat, the pharyngeal mucosa and tonsils are edematous, particularly with group A beta-hemolytic streptococcal infection. This is true of allergic pharyngitis as well, although erythema of the pharynx is minimal. Tonsillitis presents with readily noticeable swollen lymph glands located bilaterally between the fauces of the posterior pharynx.

Bacterial pharyngitis commonly presents with significant tender lymphadenopathy of the draining anterior cervical lymph nodes. This finding also occasionally occurs in viral infections such as infectious mononucleosis or primary HIV infection. However, 90% of infectious mononucleosis cases present with posterior cervical lymphadenopathy. Hepatosplenomegaly is also a common finding. Tonsillitis usually presents with swollen lymph glands on either side of the jaw.

DIAGNOSTIC REASONING

Diagnostic Tests

Most cases of pharyngitis and tonsillitis are self-limited; therefore, laboratory work-up and identification of causative organisms through culture are unnecessary if the patient's clinical picture is consistent with influenza, the common cold, or irritant-induced throat inflammation. However, bacterial and viral cultures of throat swabs may be appropriate for more complicated cases or those requiring pharmacotherapy, such as with herpes virus or streptococcal infection. Herpangina and hand-foot-and-mouth disease are diagnosed via Coxsackie-positive viral cultures and positive serologies.

For exudative cases of pharyngitis, the rapid (10-minute) streptococcal antigen (Rapid Strep) test is used to detect group A streptococcal antigens and diagnose infection. Increased antistreptolysin O (ASO) titers are also observed, but treatment may blunt this antibody response. Rapid strep tests are highly specific (90%) and sensitive (80% to 90%) when used judiciously. A rapid strep test to guide antibiotic therapy is considered appropriate for any patient with two or three of the following criteria: fever greater than 100.5°F (38.1°C), tonsillar exudate, tender anterior cervical lymphadenopathy, and the absence of cough. Patients meeting three or four of these criteria may be empirically diagnosed with group A *Streptococcus* and treated immediately. Throat swab cultures of the posterior pharynx and tonsils—the current gold standard test for the diagnosis of streptococcal infection—are sent (rather than using the rapid strep test) for patients meeting fewer criteria and considered to have a low pretest likelihood of infection less than 20%. Patients with an intermediate pretest likelihood of *Streptococcus* infection (20% to 50%) who present with sore throat and only two of the associated criteria are given the rapid strep test first and, if positive, may avoid a throat culture. However, if the result is negative, it must be followed up by a throat culture, which typically displays greater sensitivity than the rapid strep test.

During the summer and fall, the false-positive rates of rapid strep tests may approach 50%. In turn, the recommended diagnostic approach is less aggressive at this time than during the winter or spring. During the summer and fall, no testing is recommended for patients with a sore throat who meet only one of the associated criteria unless the patient is at high risk for *Streptococcus* infection (e.g., has an immunocompromising illness such as diabetes mellitus or HIV, has a history of rheumatic fever, or is presenting during a community outbreak of *Streptococcus* infection). If possible, household members should also be screened because treated patients may be reinfected via contact with asymptomatic carriers in the home.

Immunofluorescence staining or viral throat swab cultures are used to detect herpes virus infection. A special Tzanck smear of any ulcerative exudative lesion is used to diagnose HSV and herpes zoster; multinucleated giant cells with ballooning degeneration represent a positive finding. Infection by the many types of herpes viruses (including HSV, EBV, and CMV) may also be diagnosed by serological tests detecting virus-specific antibodies. Convalescent titers may be necessary for proper interpretation. Nonspecific heterophile antibody tests, such as the Monospot test, are used to diagnose infectious mononucleosis related to EBV, although this test decreases in sensitivity when used at the extremes of age.

Pharyngeal, endocervical, and urethral cultures on Thayer-Martin agar can specifically detect gonorrheal growth, if suspected in high-risk patients. Syphilis is diagnosed via serology and, if disease is in its secondary stage, by dark-field microscopy of lesion scrapings that demonstrates *T. pallidum* spirochetes. *C. pneumoniae* and *C. trachomatis* are typically evaluated via serology, although cultures and titers are not recommended initially, because the relative contribution of these pathogens to throat inflammation remains highly controversial. Suspected *Candida* infections are diagnosed via a potassium hydroxide wet mount or Gram stain of pharyngeal exudates, which will demonstrate spores and budding hyphal yeast forms, as well as by yeast cultures for speciation if needed.

A CBC may be done in any case of infectious pharyngitis. An increase in granulocytes indicates bacterial infection, and a documented lymphocytosis (50% lymphocytes, of which at least 10% show atypical morphology) strongly supports a viral etiology. The presence of eosinophils in a Gram stain of nasal secretions or a nasal mucosal scraping is strongly indicative of allergic pharyngitis. Radiological evaluation of the posterior pharyngeal wall may be appropriate to detect retropharyngeal processes if abscess formation is suspected.

Differential Diagnosis

Although the entire oropharynx may be involved during many infectious processes, certain microorganisms have a greater propensity for affecting the oral cavity, resulting in stomatitis, before pharyngeal involvement. Patients may be sicker and more febrile with bacterial infection, but this is not always the case. When challenged with an infectious agent, numerous factors are brought into play, including the host defense mechanisms, microbial virulence, quantity of infectious inoculum, and the host's susceptibility.

Epiglottitis due to *C. diphtheriae* is an important consideration in nonimmunized (or inadequately immunized) individuals; it should be ruled out carefully by history and general presentation, including an inability to swallow, with resultant drooling and an inability to speak. Importantly, examination of the oropharynx may trigger sudden glottic spasm and risk occlusion of the airway. Thus, examination of the throat should only ever take place in a facility that could support severe respiratory compromise that may result from dislodging the pseudomembrane from the posterior pharynx.

Infection with group A *Streptococcus* causes intense mucosal inflammation because of bacterial extracellular factors such as pyrogenic exotoxin and streptolysin O. A major virulence factor is the streptococcal cell wall M protein (with 80 serotypes), which has antiphagocytic properties; particular serotypes appear to correlate with the occurrence of rheumatic fever and glomerulonephritis, which can lead to acute renal failure. Streptococcal tonsillar infection, also referred to as tonsillopharyngitis due to *S. pyogenes*, also known as group A *Streptococcus* always has the potential for progressing to peritonsillar or tonsillar abscess; therefore, these two conditions should be included in the differential list.

Pharyngitis from postnasal drip secondary to rhinitis or sinusitis may be ruled out via nasal cavity examination and sinus x-rays. Pharyngeal or tonsillar malignancy requiring surgical removal of the affected tissues must be ruled out via biopsy if malignancy is suspected.

MANAGEMENT

Supportive and Pharmacologic Management

Most cases of pharyngitis and tonsillitis in otherwise healthy patients are manageable with home care and/or antibiotics. For allergy-related forms of throat inflammation, contact with environmental irritants including tobacco smoke should be minimized, and patients may be treated symptomatically with a combination of antihistamines and decongestants, as described for allergic rhinitis. For infectious forms, patients should limit their physical activity until symptoms of pharyngitis and tonsillitis have subsided. Daily fluid intake should be increased to 8 to 12 glasses (2 to 3 quarts) of fluids such as water or nonacidic juices. Bedrest is recommended if fever is present, and regular physical activity should be resumed only after 2 to 3 days of normal temperature readings.

Throat pain may be significantly relieved by the following measures:

- Voice rest
- Ambient humidification with a regularly cleaned, cool-mist, ultrasonic humidifier to increase ambient air moisture, which may relieve feelings of dryness or tightness in the throat

- Saline nasal sprays
- Various types of gargles taken as needed, including hot or cold double-strength tea or a warm saltwater solution (one teaspoon of noniodized salt in 8 ounces of water)
- Nonprescription throat lozenges or sprays (e.g., Cepastat, Chloraseptic) containing topical anesthetics such as phenol may also alleviate minor pain
- Nonprescription analgesics such as acetaminophen or aspirin (325 to 650 mg every 4 to 6 hours as needed) to relieve intermediate pain
- Viscous lidocaine (Xylocaine) throat preparations or possibly codeine preparations (30 to 60 mg PO every 4 to 6 hours as needed) for more moderate to severe pain
- Warm, moist compresses applied four times daily for at least 30 to 60 minutes at a time to relieve enlarged, tender cervical lymph glands.

Uncomplicated viral pharyngitis typically requires only symptomatic care, and antibiotics are never indicated, other than selected antiviral therapies. Influenza symptoms may be improved within the first 2 days of symptom onset by prescribing amantadine (Symmetrel; 100 mg PO twice daily) for documented cases of influenza A, but this drug may also cause insomnia, dizziness, drowsiness, or difficulty concentrating. Thus, the dosage for elderly patients is reduced to once a day. Oseltamivir (Tamiflu; 75 mg PO twice daily for 5 days) may be similarly given within the first 48 hours of symptom onset to reduce duration of illness and symptom severity, as well as prophylactically at once-daily dosing in high-risk individuals during peak flu season.

Many cases of bacterial pharyngitis are self-limited as well, such as those caused by atypical organisms. However, cases due to infection with group A *Streptococcus* or *N. gonorrhoeae* merit rapid antibiotic treatment to prevent significant sequelae in both the short and long terms. In addition, cases caused by *C. diphtheriae, H. influenzae,* or influenza virus may require hospitalization because of the risk of life-threatening complications. Fungal infections also typically require antimycotic therapy.

Antibiotic therapy for group A streptococcal pharyngitis has been shown to shorten the clinical course of disease and reduce lymphadenopathy, fever, and pain (after 1 to 3 days of therapy), prevent suppurative complications and autoimmune sequelae such as rheumatic fever, and decrease person-to-person spread of infection. Empiric antibiotic therapy may be instituted before receiving culture results in certain clinical situations to prevent cross-reactive autoimmune phenomena including rheumatic fever and other cardiac sequelae, as well as immune complex-mediated acute renal insufficiency due to poststreptococcal glomerulonephritis. However, studies have demonstrated that delaying treatment for 48 hours in anticipation of throat culture results does not significantly affect the reduction in autoimmune sequelae provided by antibiotic therapy.

In cases of fever below 100.5°F (38.1°C) without an associated tonsillar exudate or anterior cervical lymphadenopathy, neither throat swab culture nor antistreptococcal therapy is recommended because a false-positive culture may lead to unnecessary antibiotic therapy. If fever greater than 100.5°F (38.1°C) accompanies a tonsillar exudate and tender anterior cervical lymphadenitis, antistreptococcal therapy should be instituted immediately because a false-negative culture could delay critical treatment. This is especially important for patients younger than 25 years. If a similar fever occurs with only one of the other two physical signs, antibiotic therapy should be instituted only for culture-positive patients. High-risk factors that favor immediate empiric treatment include a history of acute rheumatic heart fever or related cardiac damage, a scarlatiniform rash, a diabetic or other immunocompromised state, documented exposure to group A *Streptococcus* within the past week, or the presence of a known epidemic within the community.

Adults are typically given a 10-day course of penicillin V potassium (Pen-Vee K; 500 mg PO twice daily or 250 mg PO four times daily) or benzathine penicillin (Bicillin; 1.2 million units IM once) as an alternative to prolonged oral medication. If the patient is allergic to penicillin, azithromycin (500 mg PO daily) is recommended for 5 days. If the patient fails to respond to antibiotic therapy, tests for infectious mononucleosis and streptococcal antibiotic sensitivity should be performed. A 10-day course of amoxicillin/clavulanate (Augmentin; 40 mg/kg PO daily based on the amoxicillin component, in divided doses twice daily), erythromycin ethyl succinate (50 mg/kg PO daily in divided doses three times daily), or erythromycin stearate (1 g PO daily) has been shown to be effective for penicillin-resistant β-lactamase–producing organisms, whereas tetracycline and trimethoprim-sulfamethoxazole preparations (Septra, Bactrim) should be avoided.

N. gonorrhoeae infection calls for ceftriaxone (Rocephin; 125 mg IM once), along with empiric treatment for *C. trachomatis* (azithromycin [Zithromax] 1 g PO once or doxycycline 100 mg PO twice daily for 7 days), given its propensity for coinfection. *M. pneumoniae* and *C. pneumoniae* are both treated with erythromycin 250 to 500 mg PO four times daily for 10 days, depending on the specific preparation. Extensive throat infection with *Candida albicans* (thrush, pharyngitis, esophagitis) requires antifungal treatment such as fluconazole 200 mg PO once, followed by 100 mg PO daily for 2 weeks total.

Surgical Management

Surgical removal of the pharyngeal tonsils (tonsillectomy) and/or adenoids (adenoidectomy) is absolutely indicated if tonsillar inflammation leads to airway obstruction associated with any of the following: cor pulmonale (right-sided cardiac hypertrophy), dysphagia, or weight loss. Tonsillectomy may also be indicated if active flares recur more than three times a year, if the patient experiences mild dysphagia, if the tonsils remain chronically hypertrophied after a bout of infectious mononucleosis, or if the patient has a history of rheumatic fever with heart damage due to recurrent tonsillitis. However, in these situations, the indication for surgical intervention is relative and must be evaluated further. It should also be noted that lymph glands normally swell during episodes of active inflammation as part of the body's normal immune response. In turn, tonsillectomy is not indicated for colds, asthma, allergic rhinitis, focal infections, fever of unknown origin, cervical lymphadenopathy, or enlarged tonsils without obstructive symptomatology.

FOLLOW-UP AND REFERRAL

Most cases of pharyngitis and tonsillitis are self-limited, and symptoms tend to improve in 2 to 3 days. If symptoms fail to improve within this time frame, patients should return for a follow-up appointment, in which throat cultures for *Streptococcus* may be repeated on completion of therapy to confirm resolution of any infectious processes. This is not recommended, however, for asymptomatic patients who have completed a 10-day therapeutic regimen for streptococcal infection or for patients whose symptoms improve within 5 days of antibiotic therapy because clinical resolution is typically the best measure of therapeutic success.

Group A *Streptococcus* pharyngeal or tonsillar infection may lead to scarlet fever or autoimmune rheumatic fever, if not treated with antibiotics or if antibiotic therapy is discontinued before a full 10-day course is completed. These patients should be referred to a specialist. In areas where group A streptococcal infection is endemic, the probability of developing rheumatic fever is 0.3%. With epidemic pharyngitis, the risk increases to 3%.

Rheumatic heart disease may develop after rheumatic fever in an adult patient with recurrent streptococcal infection or a history of poorly treated streptococcal pharyngitis as a child or young adult. This may lead to severe sequelae such as calcification of the mitral valve and/or other heart valves, as well as to the destruction of cardiac myocytes, which is attributed to cross-reacting antistreptococcal antibodies. Even when acute rheumatic fever is treated appropriately with prophylactic antibiotic therapy, 4% of patients may develop debilitating cardiac sequelae, and 1% may develop severe class IV rheumatic heart disease. Chest pain is a key indicator of cardiac complications. Hematuria resulting from poststreptococcal glomerulonephritis may occur 1 to 3 weeks after acute pharyngeal or tonsillar infection, as antibiotic therapy may not protect against this immune complex–mediated complication.

Cases caused by *C. diphtheriae*, if left untreated, may lead to epiglottitis, which can obstruct breathing and may prove fatal if the pseudomembrane dislodges and chokes the patient as it is inadvertently swallowed. Spread of infectious organisms from the pharynx to the lungs may lead to pneumonia and severe respiratory complications. Infections of the posterior oropharynx may also ascend to the nasopharynx, leading to sinusitis and rhinitis (inflammation of the mucous membranes of the sinus and nasal cavities). The middle ear is another possible target of disseminated pharyngeal infection because the nasopharyngeal (eustachian) tube acts as a conduit for the spread of microorganisms. OM may occur in more than 20% of adenovirus infections. A less common complication of bacterial pharyngitis is septic jugular vein thrombophlebitis, which may occur several days after the initial sore throat. Patients with this complication are typically teenagers or young adults who experience an increase in neck pain and tenderness, as well as swelling of the jaw angle.

Liver function tests (e.g., serum aspartate aminotransferase [AST], serum alanine aminotransferase [ALT], serum bilirubin, platelet count, and the Coombs autoantibody test) should be performed for all cases of suspected infectious mononucleosis to diagnose serious sequelae, including severe hepatitis (ALT or AST levels of more than 1,000 units/L; bilirubin levels >10 mg/dL), hemolytic anemia, granulocytopenia, and thrombocytopenia. Airway obstruction may also occur in patients with infectious mononucleosis as a result of pharyngeal swelling. Such complications may require treatment with a corticosteroid such as prednisone (60 to 80 mg PO daily in divided doses, tapered over 1 to 2 weeks). Splenic rupture related to trauma is also a serious risk for all patients with infectious mononucleosis who have marked hepatosplenomegaly (liver and spleen enlargement).

Tonsillitis that goes untreated or fails to resolve with treatment may lead to grossly swollen, suppurative cervical adenitis, OM, or a peritonsillar abscess of the surrounding throat area, characterized by increasing unilateral ear and throat pain ipsilateral to the affected tonsil, dysphagia, drooling, trismus, erythema, and edema of the soft palate with fluctuance on palpation. Suppurative sequelae such as these may require surgical drainage and/or tonsillectomy. Repeated attacks of acute tonsillitis may lead to a chronic condition with a recurrent sore throat and greatly enlarged tonsils, which may complicate breathing and become potentially life-threatening; these cases also require surgical intervention.

All patients developing suppurative or retropharyngeal sequelae should be referred to an otorhinolaryngologist. The physical examination and treatment of *C. diphtheriae* infection are also highly risky and must be supervised by a qualified specialist. Surgical interventions such as tonsillectomy or abscess drainage require surgical referral.

Patient Education: Pharyngitis and Tonsillitis

Both pharyngitis and tonsillitis may be prevented by avoiding contact with persons with actively inflamed throats, particularly with URIs. Throat swabs from household members of patients should also be cultured to identify and treat carriers simultaneously to prevent the development of clinical disease and prevent reinfection. Toothbrushes should be replaced as soon as a sore throat develops because they may harbor causative microorganisms, and all eating and drinking utensils should be cleaned thoroughly and should not be shared. Food and washcloths also must not be shared during a period of active infection.

It is critical to keep all immunizations up to date, particularly the diphtheria-pertussis-tetanus (DTaP, Tdap) vaccine that confers immunity against *C. diphtheriae*. If a sexual partner is suspected of being infected with a sexually transmitted agent, intimate sexual contact should cease until a proper diagnosis is made and any applicable treatment has been completed. In general, oral intercourse between persons of either gender should be performed only using a form of latex barrier protection, such as a condom during fellatio or a dental dam during cunnilingus, to avoid orogenital transmission of infectious organisms. Environmental irritants such as tobacco and marijuana smoke, pollution, dust and other allergens, as well as low-humidity environments should be avoided to prevent noninfectious forms of pharyngitis.

Warm compresses applied to relieve enlarged, tender cervical lymph nodes can be effective; however, patients must be cautioned not to burn the skin inadvertently. Although the use of aspirin during viral infections in adults has not been linked to the development of Reye's syndrome (as is the case in children), NSAIDs should be used cautiously if patients suffer from ulcers or other gastrointestinal disorders. Heavy lifting and contact sports must be prohibited for all patients with infectious mononucleosis because these activities carry a high risk of splenic trauma and rupture. Patients must be instructed to finish their entire course of antibiotics, antivirals, or antifungals to avoid complications from latent infection such as glomerulonephritis or myocarditis. In cases involving dysphagia, patients may be instructed on how to maintain a healthy liquid or soft food diet (e.g., milkshakes, soups, and high-protein diet or instant breakfast drinks) for several days until the pain subsides. Patients who demand prescriptions for antibiotics in the absence of a throat culture confirming disease of bacterial origin should understand the rationale for using antibacterial drugs versus other types of medication.

REFERENCES

Pharyngitis and Tonsillitis

Acerra JR. Pharyngitis workup. http://emedicine.medscape.com/article/764304-workup. Published 2017.

Aung K, Ojha A, Lo C. Viral pharyngitis. http://emedicine.medscape.com/article/225362-overview. Published 2017.

Centers for Disease Control and Prevention. Pharyngitis (strep throat). https://www.cdc.gov/groupastrep/diseases-hcp/strep-throat.html. Published 2016.

Centor RM, Samlowski R. Avoiding sore throat morbidity and mortality: When is it not "just a sore throat?" *Am Fam Physician.* 2011;83:26, 28.

Centor RM. Expand the pharyngitis paradigm for adolescents and young adults. *Ann Intern Med.* 2009;151:812–815

Cunha, BA. Epstein-Barr virus (EBV) infectious mononucleosis (mono). http://emedicine.medscape.com/article/222040-differential. Published 2017.

Linder JA. Sore throat: Avoid overcomplicating the uncomplicated. *Ann Intern Med.* 2015;162:311–312.

National Guideline Clearinghouse. *Guideline summary: Clinical practice guideline for the diagnosis and management of group A streptococcal pharyngitis: 2012 update by the Infectious Diseases Society of America.* Rockville, MD: Agency for Healthcare Research and Quality. http://www.ahrq.gov/professionals/clinicians-providers/guidelines-recommendations/index.html. Published September 9, 2012. Accessed August 19, 2017.

National Guideline Clearinghouse. Guideline summary: Pharyngitis. Rockville, MD: Agency for Healthcare Research and Quality. https://www.guideline.gov. Published May 1, 2013. Accessed August 19, 2017.

Quail G. The painful mouth. *Aust Fam Physician.* 2008;37(11):935–938.

Rosenfeld RM, Piccirillo JF, Chandrasekhar SS, et al. Clinical practice guideline (update): Adult sinusitis. *Otolaryngol Head Neck Surg.* 2015;152(suppl 2):S1–S39.

Russell PT, Bekey JR. Oral antibiotics and the management of chronic sinusitis: What do we know. *Curr Opin Otolarynogol Head Neck Surg.* 2014;22(1)22–26.

Simon HK. Pediatric pharyngitis. http://emedicine.medscape.com/article/967384. Published 2016.

Winters M. Evidence-based diagnosis and management of ENT emergencies. Retrieved from https://www.medscape.com/viewarticle/551650_1. Published 2007.

Rhinitis

Adriaensen GF, Fokkens WJ. Chronic rhinosinusitis: An update on current pharmacotherapy. *Expert Opin Pharmacother.* 2013;14(17):2351–2360.

Chow AW, Benninger MS, Brook I, et al. IDSA clinical practice guideline for acute bacterial rhinosinusitis in children and adults. *Clin Infect Dis.* 2012;2012:e1–e41.

Harris AM, Hicks LA, Qaseem A; High Value Care Task Force of the American College of Physicians and for the Centers for Disease Control and Prevention. Appropriate antibiotic use for acute respiratory tract infection in adults: Advice for high-value care from the American College of Physicians and the Centers for Disease Control and Prevention. *Ann Intern Med.* 2016;164:425.

King D, Mitchell B, Williams CP, Spurling GK. Saline nasal irrigation for acute upper respiratory tract infections. *Cochrane Database Syst Rev.* 2015;(4):CD006821.

National Guideline Clearinghouse. *Guideline summary: Allergic rhinitis.* Rockville, MD: Agency for Healthcare Research and Quality. https://www.guideline.gov. Published October 1, 2013. Accessed August 20, 2017.

National Guideline Clearinghouse. *Clinical practice guideline: Allergic rhinitis.* Rockville, MD: Agency for Healthcare Research and Quality. https://www.guideline.gov. Published February 1, 2015. Accessed August 20, 2017.

National Guideline Clearinghouse. *Guideline summary: Diagnosis and treatment of respiratory illness in children and adults.* Rockville, MD: Agency for Healthcare Research and Quality. https://www.guideline.gov. Published January 1, 2013. Accessed August 20, 2017.

National Guideline Clearinghouse. *Guideline summary: IDSA clinical practice guideline for acute bacterial rhinosinusitis in children and adults.* Rockville, MD: Agency for Healthcare Research and Quality. https://www.guideline.gov. Published April 1, 2012. Accessed August 20, 2017.

Sheikh J. Allergic rhinitis. http://emedicine.medscape.com/article/134825. Published 2017.

Sinusitis and Rhinosinusitis

Chow AW, Benninger MS, Brook I, et al. IDSA clinical practice guideline for acute bacterial rhinosinusitis in children and adults. *Clin Infect Dis.* 2012;2012:54:e72.

Fokkens W, Lund V, Mullol J; European Position Paper on Rhinosinusitis and Nasal Polyps Group. EP3OS 2007: European position paper on rhinosinusitis and nasal polyps 2007. A summary for otorhinolaryngologists. *Rhinology.* 2007;45:97.

Gwaltney JM Jr, Scheld WM, Sande MA, Sydnor A. The microbial etiology and antimicrobial therapy of adults with acute community-acquired sinusitis: A fifteen-year experience at the University of Virginia and review of other selected studies. *J Allergy Clin Immunol.* 1992;90:457.

Hadley JA, Mösges R, Desrosiers M, et al. Moxifloxacin five-day therapy versus placebo in acute bacterial rhinosinusitis. *Laryngoscope.* 2010;120:1057.

National Guideline Clearinghouse. *Guideline summary: Clinical practice guideline (update): Adult sinusitis.* Rockville, MD: Agency for Healthcare Research and Quality. https://www.guideline.gov. Published April 1, 2015. Accessed August 20, 2017.

National Guideline Clearinghouse. *Guideline summary: IDSA clinical practice guideline for acute bacterial rhinosinusitis in children and adults.* Rockville, MD: Agency for Healthcare Research and Quality. https://www.guideline.gov. Published April 1, 2012. Accessed August 20, 2017.

Rosenfeld, RM. Clinical practice. Acute sinusitis in adults. *N Engl J Med.* 2016; 375:962.

Rosenfeld RM, Piccirillo JF, Chandrasekhar SS, et al. Clinical practice guideline (update): Adult sinusitis. *Otolaryngol Head Neck Surg.* 2015;152(suppl 2):S1–S39.

Russell PT, Bekey JR. Oral antibiotics and the management of chronic sinusitis: What do we know. *Curr Opin Otolaryngol Head Neck Surg.* 2013;22:22–26.

U.S. Food and Drug Administration. *FDA drug safety communication: FDA updates warnings for oral and injectable fluoroquinolone antibiotics due to disabling side effects.* https://www.fda.gov/Drugs/DrugSafety/ucm511530.htm. Published 2016. Accessed September 16, 2017.

Venekamp RP, Thompson MJ, Hayward G, et al. Systemic corticosteroids for acute sinusitis. *Cochrane Database Syst Rev.* 2014;(3): CD008115.

Venekamp RP, Thompson MJ, Rovers MM. Systemic corticosteroid therapy for acute sinusitis. *JAMA.* 2015;313:1258.

Stomatitis and Glossitis

Akintoye SO, Greenberg MS. Recurrent aphthous stomatitis. *Dent Clin North Am.* 2014;58:281.

Bieber T, Chosidow O, Bodsworth N, et al. Efficacy and safety of aciclovir mucoadhesive buccal tablet in immunocompetent patients with labial herpes (LIP Trial): A double-blind, placebo-controlled, self-initiated trial. *J Drugs Dermatol.* 2014;13:791.

Chattopadhyay A, Shetty KV. Recurrent aphthous stomatitis. *Otolaryngol Clin North Am.* 2011;44(1):79–88.

Gasteyger C, Suter M, Gaillard RC, Giusti V. Nutritional deficiencies after Roux-en-Y gastric bypass for morbid obesity often cannot be prevented by standard multivitamin supplementation. *Am J Clin Nutr.* 2008;87(5):1128–1133.

Issrani R, Prabhu N, Keluskar V. Oral proliferative verrucous leukoplakia: A case report with an update. *Contemp Clin Dent.* 2013;4:258.

Messadi DV, Younai F. Aphthous ulcers. *Dermatol Ther.* 2010;23(3):281–290.

Mirowski GW. Aphthous stomatitis. http://emedicine.medscape.com/article/1075570-overview. Published 2017.

National Guideline Clearinghouse. *Guideline summary: MASCC/ISOO clinical practice guidelines for the management of mucositis secondary to cancer therapy.* Rockville, MD: Agency for Healthcare Research and Quality. https://www.guideline.gov. Published May 15, 2014.

Pentenero M, Meleti M, Vescovi P, Gandolfo S. Oral proliferative verrucous leucoplakia: Are there particular features for such an ambiguous entity? A systematic review. *Br J Dermatol.* 2014;170:1039.

Rigante D, Vitale A, Natale MF, et al. A comprehensive comparison between pediatric and adult patients with periodic fever, aphthous stomatitis, pharyngitis, and cervical adenopathy (PFAPA) syndrome. *Clin Rheumatol.* 2017;36:463.

RESOURCES

American Academy of Allergy Asthma and Immunology
https://www.aaaai.org/conditions-and-treatments/library/at-a-glance/rhinitis

American Academy of Family Physicians Patient Education Web site

Sore Throat

http://www.aafp.org/afp/2001/0415/p1565.html

Streptococcal Pharyngitis

http://www.aafp.org/afp/2016/0701/p24.html

Peritonsillar Abscess

http://www.aafp.org/afp/2017/0415/p501.html

Nongenital Herpes Simplex Virus

http://www.aafp.org/afp/2010/1101/p1075.html

American Academy of Otolaryngology—Head and Neck Surgery

http://www.entnet.org/content/sore-throats
http://www.entnet.org/content/post-nasal-drip

American Cancer Society

https://www.cancer.org/treatment/treatments-and-side-effects/physical-side-effects/mouth-problems/mouth-sores.html

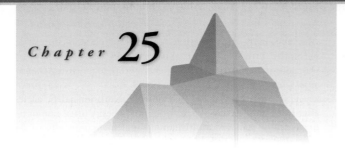

Epistaxis

Ruth McCaffrey, DNP, APRN, FNP-BC, GNP, FAAN, FAANP

Lynne M. Dunphy, PhD, APRN, FNP-BC, FAAN, FAANP

Brian Oscar Porter, MD, PhD, MPH, MBA

Commonly called a "nosebleed," *epistaxis* is a hemorrhage of the nasal mucosa resulting from the traumatic or spontaneous rupture of superficial veins and/or arteries, located most often on the anterosuperior portion of the nasal septum known as Little's area (Kiesselbach's triangle or Kiesselbach's plexus). Epistaxis is a physical sign rather than a disease. Therefore, after the initial management of bleeding, a thorough evaluation is essential to determine its underlying cause.

EPIDEMIOLOGY AND CAUSES

Epistaxis is an extremely common condition. In fact, 60% of the general population experiences at least one significant nosebleed over their lifetime. Epistaxis most commonly occurs in children younger than age 10 years and in adults older than 50 years. Men and women are affected equally by nosebleeds, although hemophilia, an inherited blood disorder that predisposes to nosebleeds, is expressed predominantly in males.

Excessive dryness of the nasal mucosa in poorly humidified environments or at high altitudes weakens nasal vessels, predisposing them to rupture. Septal deviation may thus contribute to epistaxis through the disproportionate exposure of one side of the nose to dry environmental air. Foreign bodies, especially common in children, lodged in the nasal airways are another common source of vessel injury. Prolonged use of nasal decongestant sprays is also a risk factor because it may lead to reflex inflammation of the nasal mucosa, known as rhinitis medicamentosa. An exceedingly rare cause of nasal bleeding is the presence of nasal ectopic endometrium (nasal endometriosis).

Malignant growths in the nasal cavity or paranasal sinuses may erode into blood vessels and present with epistaxis as their sole manifestation. Coagulopathies with resultant bleeding may be associated with chronic disorders such as cirrhosis, renal disease, cancer (especially Hodgkin's disease), and hemophilia. Familial blood dyscrasias such as hemophilia A (factor VIII deficiency), hemophilia B (factor IX deficiency or Christmas disease), and von Willebrand disease (the most common genetic bleeding disorder), as well as hereditary hemorrhagic telangiectasia (Osler-Weber-Rendu disease), are examples of inherited conditions that may be complicated by significant epistaxis. Medications such as warfarin (Coumadin) and heparin may also predispose to nosebleeds by inhibiting natural clotting pathways. Another risk factor is snorting powdered drugs such as cocaine or heroin, which can lead to septal perforation. Many nutritional deficiencies and febrile infectious disorders may also predispose to nosebleeds, including scurvy (caused by vitamin C deficiency) and rheumatic, scarlet, or typhoid fever.

PATHOPHYSIOLOGY

The majority of nosebleeds result from local irritation related to trauma or inflammation, occurring most often in the absence of any anatomical abnormality. Trauma to both nasal polyps and the well-vascularized watershed area of the nasal mucosa known as Kiesselbach's plexus is perhaps the most common direct cause of nosebleed, particularly from picking of the nose (epistaxis digitorum) or forcible injury related to blunt trauma. Kiesselbach's plexus marks the anastomosis of three major blood vessels of the nasal cavity: the septal branch of the anterior ethmoid artery, the septal portion of the superior labial branch of the facial artery, and the lateral nasal branch of the sphenopalatine artery. Similarly, posterior epistaxis most commonly originates from rupture of the posterior wall and choanal branches of the sphenopalatine artery.

CLINICAL PRESENTATION

Subjective

The patient with recurrent minor anterior epistaxis typically presents with a history of several episodes over several weeks. If blood loss has been extensive, patients may report weakness or other symptoms of anemia. Bleeding from the posterior portion of the nasal cavity may be asymptomatic or may present with hemoptysis (coughed-up blood), nausea, gastrointestinal upset, hematemesis (blood-streaked vomitus), or blackened stools (melena) from the swallowed blood.

Objective

Prominent blood vessels are typically seen traversing the anterior septum, and a small amount of clotted blood may be visible. If the patient is actively bleeding from the front of the nose, blood is typically bright red, and localizing the bleeding source may be difficult. The second most common site of hemorrhage after Little's area is the anterior end of the inferior nasal turbinate. Epistaxis originating deeper in the nose may produce either bright red or dark blood. Usually only one bleeding site exists, but if multiple sites or a diffuse ooze are evident, an underlying systemic bleeding disorder is likely.

If the source of hemorrhage is in the posterosuperior nasal cavity, the bleeding is termed *posterior epistaxis*. In these cases, blood loss into the pharynx will occur, and both clotted blood and brown to red throat discoloration may be evident. The most common sites of posterior bleeding are just under the posterior half of the inferior nasal turbinate or the roof of the nasal cavity. Patients with significant blood loss may demonstrate pallor, particularly in the face. Palpation of the paranasal sinuses may reveal tenderness if underlying sinusitis or malignancy is present. Likewise, percussion of the paranasal sinuses may demonstrate tenderness in sinusitis-related or malignancy-related cases.

DIAGNOSTIC REASONING

Diagnostic tests are rarely called for when nasal bleeding can be managed, and most episodes of epistaxis are not recurrent. A variety of diagnostic tests are helpful in determining the underlying cause of nasal hemorrhage. Laboratory tests exist for deficiencies of most clotting factors, but factor VIII and factor IX deficiencies are clearly the most commonly observed and tested for. Coagulation studies such as a prolonged prothrombin time (PT) or partial thromboplastin time (PTT) is characteristic of clotting factor disorders. Hemophilia A (factor VIII deficiency) and hemophilia B (factor IX deficiency) produce a prolonged PTT, whereas disorders of the extrinsic clotting pathway (factor VII deficiency) result in a prolonged PT. A complete blood count, including hemoglobin, hematocrit, and mean corpuscular volume, may offer insight into the chronicity of the condition. Radiological (x-ray) examination of the nasal cavity and paranasal sinuses may identify masses, including neoplasms or foreign bodies, as well as sinusitis if mucosal thickening or air–water levels are apparent. Computed tomography scan of the sinuses may also be done with greater sensitivity for detecting structural and soft-tissue abnormalities.

Differential Diagnosis

Differentiation among posterior epistaxis, hemoptysis, and hematemesis is critical. In the absence of respiratory or gastrointestinal findings, a diagnosis of posterior epistaxis can be assumed if visual evidence exists for a posterior source of bleeding,

MANAGEMENT

Initial interventions should be geared toward stopping the bleeding and alleviating anxiety. For recurrent nose bleeds, evaluation for an underlying cause should be conducted.

Initial treatment of uncomplicated anterior epistaxis consists of applying firm, continuous pressure for 10 to 15 minutes to both sides of the nose, immediately superior to the nasal alar cartilages. Ice packs may help. Patients should breathe through the mouth during this treatment period and must not release pressure to "sneak a peek" at the bleeding nares. To reduce vascular pressure, the patient should be seated upright with the head bent forward. Patients with no underlying medical problems may be treated at home, with directions to sit upright, minimize physical activity, and rest with the head elevated 45 to 90 degrees at night. Elderly or debilitated patients with epistaxis may require inpatient care, however, because of the increased risk of immunosuppression and anemia.

If bleeding is difficult to stop, pharmacologic agents may be of some help. A small piece of cotton or nasal pledget soaked in a topical vasoconstricting agent (such as 0.25% phenylephrine, 1:1000 epinephrine, 0.1% xylometazoline, or 4% cocaine solution) should be applied to the nasal vestibule and pressed against the bleeding site for 5 to 10 minutes. Epinephrine should be avoided in hypertensive patients or those with coronary artery disease, and cocaine should be avoided in children. Oxymetazoline (Afrin) nasal spray combined with direct pressure is often effective at stopping the bleeding.

If this treatment fails, chemical cauterization of the bleeding site may be necessary. The mucosa should first be anesthetized with a cotton ball soaked in 4% cocaine, 4% lidocaine, or 2% lidocaine viscous preparation, held over the bleeding site for several minutes. Alternatively, 2% lidocaine jelly may be used. A bead of chromic acid, 25% to 50% trichloroacetic acid solution, or a silver nitrate stick is then applied directly onto the bleeding vessels with firm pressure for 30 seconds, which will allow for limited, shallow cautery of the bleeding site. Thermal or bipolar electrocautery may be required in cases of deeper lesions involving larger vessels; however, indiscriminate cauterization of a large area should be avoided.

If bleeding does not stop, anterior nasal packing should be placed to fill the entire nasal fossa. Layers of .5- × 72-inch gauze impregnated with petroleum jelly should be inserted in folding layers with a nasal speculum and bayonet forceps, extending as far back as possible to the posterior nasal choanae, while retaining the gauze ends at the nares. Each layer should be pressed firmly against the preceding one without disturbing the walls of the nasal cavity, with the folded ends alternating front and back in an accordion pattern. Typically, the entire 72-inch strip will be accommodated, if properly placed. A 2- × 2-inch gauze pad is then taped over the nostrils to prevent the anterior packing from dislodging and to catch dripping blood. Commercially available nasal tampons may be inserted into the nares in desiccated form and rehydrated by bathing them in 10 to 20 mL of saline or an antibiotic-containing solution (e.g., bacitracin). The patient must be monitored during the packing procedure, as some patients may experience a vasovagal response to the procedure with syncope or a decrease in blood pressure.

Posterior sources of bleeding require more complex treatment, and consultation with an otorhinolaryngologist may be required. Treatments include posterior nasal packing, sphenopalatine ganglion nerve block, and even surgical ligation of the compromised vessels. Nasal balloon-packing systems are an alternative to nasal packing, but they must not be overinflated and should be removed in a timely fashion. Any form of nasal packing tends to be particularly painful for the patient once the local anesthetic has worn off, and analgesics should be considered. OTC analgesics such as acetaminophen are preferred. In contrast, NSAIDs, including aspirin, should be avoided because of their capacity to impair platelet function, which may lead to further bleeding. In patients requiring nasal packing, the use of antibiotics is controversial but reasonable in patients at greater risk for infection.

All underlying medical conditions that might contribute to epistaxis should also be appropriately treated. Concurrent use of blood thinning agents should be reevaluated in the presence of acute bleeding, and the decision to continue antithrombotic medications such as clopidogrel (Plavix), warfarin (Coumadin), or any other blood thinning agent should be discussed with a healthcare provider familiar with the prescribing indication.

FOLLOW-UP AND REFERRAL

Follow-up is not indicated for minor cases of nosebleed from local trauma or inflammation. However, if nasal packing is required, follow-up the next day is prudent to prevent infection. Excessive trauma during nasal packing or cauterization can result in septal hematoma, abscess, or perforation. External nasal deformities may also result from pressure necrosis from the anterior portion of nasal packing. Balloon-packing systems may result in mucosal pressure necrosis if the balloons are overinflated. Likewise, if the anterior portion of a two-balloon system breaks, the posterior balloon may migrate posteriorly down the airway and cause obstruction.

Individuals with recurrent anterior epistaxis that causes severe blood loss or that is refractory to vasoconstrictive or cauterization therapy should be referred to a specialist or emergency department, as appropriate. Hypovolemic or anemic patients require physician referral to evaluate the need for transfusion. Electrocautery for recurrent epistaxis caused by deep lesions should be performed only by a qualified specialist. The management of posterior epistaxis requires a specialist because treatment modalities may include ganglionic nerve blocks, posterior nasal packing, and vessel ligation. Coagulopathy-related and malignancy-related epistaxis require specialized treatment related to the underlying disorder.

Patient Education: Epistaxis

Patients who have been treated for epistaxis should not blow their nose and should avoid sneezing, rubbing the nose, or picking the nose after an acute episode to avoid dislodging the protective blood clot. Increased environmental humidity in the home also helps to prevent acute attacks, especially during the winter months. Petroleum jelly applied liberally to the nares promotes mucosal hydration, which helps prevent drying and cracking of the nasal mucosa. If nasal probing is persistent, the patient's fingernails should be cut to avoid mucosal trauma. Proper nasal pinching techniques should be demonstrated to enable patients to administer self-care at home for minor episodes of epistaxis. However, the importance of maintaining nasal mucosal hydration should be stressed, as well as the need to avoid nasal probing and vigorous blowing of the nose.

The ability of certain medications to contribute to bleeding disorders (e.g., antiplatelet effects of aspirin and other NSAIDs, anticoagulant therapies such as warfarin) should also be discussed. Patients should be told not to swallow blood because this may upset the stomach, resulting in nausea, vomiting, or "gagging" (inhalation of blood into the trachea and bronchi). Patients should be instructed not to spit blood from mouth but to allow the blood to drain by gravity into a container. This prevents disruption of any clot that may be forming. Patients should not talk during episodes of active bleeding for the same reason, and alcohol and hot liquids should be avoided after an acute attack.

REFERENCES

Abrich V, Brozek A, Boyle TR, et al. Risk factors for recurrent spontaneous epistaxis. *Mayo Clin Proc* 2014;89:1636.

Cohen O. Early and late recurrent epistaxis admissions: Patterns of incidence and risk factors. *Otolaryngol Head Neck Surg.* 2017;157(3)424–431.

Goddard JC, Reiter ER. Inpatient management of epistaxis: Outcomes and cost. *Otolaryngol Head Neck Surg.* 2005;132(5):707–712.

Min HJ, Kang H, Choi GJ, Kim KS. Association between hypertension and Epistaxis: Systematic Review and Meta-analysis. *Otolaryngol Head Neck Surg.* 2017;157:921.

Villwock JA, Jones K. Recent trends in epistaxis management in the United States: 2008–2010. *JAMA Otolaryngol Head Neck Surg.* 2013;139(12):1279–1284.

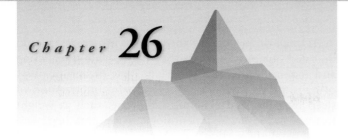

Chapter 26

Temporomandibular Disorders

Ruth McCaffrey, DNP, APRN, FNP-BC, GNP, FAAN, FAANP

Lynne M. Dunphy, PhD, APRN, FNP-BC, FAAN, FAANP

Brian Oscar Porter, MD, PhD, MPH, MBA

Temporomandibular joint (TMJ) *disease* is a collective term that refers to disorders affecting the masticatory musculature, the TMJ and associated structures, or both. The term *craniomandibular disorders* and *temporomandibular disorders* (TMDs) are synonymous with the more familiar term *temporomandibular joint (TMJ) disease*. Most current research favors the phrase *temporomandibular disorder* (TMD). Although TMD has been traditionally viewed as one syndrome, it is actually a cluster of related disorders in the masticatory system that has many features in common. The most common presenting symptom is pain in the muscles of mastication, the preauricular area, and/or the TMJ. Chewing, bruxism (clenching, grinding, or gnashing of the teeth during nonfunctional movements of the mandible), or other jaw functions tend to aggravate the pain.

EPIDEMIOLOGY AND CAUSES

It is estimated that 10% to 15% of adults are affected by TMD, 50% of whom seek medical treatment. TMD can be mild and self-limiting, or it may progress to chronic pain and discomfort, which will require consultation with multiple professionals over many years.

The incidence of TMD peaks from 20 to 40 years of age. Risk factors for TMD include being female and non-Hispanic Caucasian, although socioeconomic status does not seem to be related. There is an association between TMD and mood disorders and other psychiatric illness, as well as mechanical etiologies, such as bruxism. Patients with rheumatoid arthritis have a prevalence of TMD between 53% and 94%.

PATHOPHYSIOLOGY

The TMJ is one of the most complex joints in the body. It is a synovial, encapsulated joint that is stress bearing. The TMJ differs from other joints in the body in that its articular surfaces are covered with fibrocartilaginous tissue, rather than with chondrocartilage as found in other joints. The articular disc separates the upper and lower joint spaces. Pain from the TMJ arises from injury to the retrodiscal tissue or the capsular ligament. Locking of the joint may occur secondary to jaw malocclusion and, most commonly, anterior disc dislocation. However, several variations of articular disc displacement have been noted with this condition, as joint laxity from underlying connective tissue disorders and even asymmetrical body alignment from poor posture have been cited as risk factors. Dental manipulation of the jaw and degeneration of the TMJ from rheumatoid arthritis or osteoarthritis often underlie extracapsular joint dysfunction, because misalignment of the TMJ places pressure on nearby ear structures, resulting in otalgia (ear pain), tinnitus, vertigo, hearing loss, and tongue pain.

TMJ pain may also be intracapsular in origin and involve the masticatory musculature, known as TMJ myofascial pain syndrome or simply TMJ syndrome. Like all skeletal muscles, the TMJ muscles are susceptible to muscle splinting, spasm, or inflammation. Pain that originates in the orofacial area may be referred to other locations, such as the neck, shoulders, and head. TMJ syndrome often coexists with fibromyalgia; however, pain from the masticatory musculature is usually related to mandibular dysfunction.

CLINICAL PRESENTATION

Subjective

Patients may present with several complaints that lead to the suspicion of TMD or with only one symptom. The most common presenting symptoms are facial pain, ear discomfort or dysfunction, headache, and TMJ discomfort or dysfunction. The facial pain of TMD is usually unilateral with or without radiation to the ear, temporal region, angle of the jaw, or posterior neck. The facial pain is usually dull and may be constant or intermittent. Ear pain, fullness, and tinnitus are also common complaints of TMD that lead to referral. The typical headache of TMD is unilateral and described as a deep pain that is worse in the morning; however, variants of the headache are not uncommon. TMJ dysfunction manifests as clicking, popping, jaw deviation, or jaw locking, and again, with symptoms worse in the morning.

Objective

Because many of the presenting symptoms of TMD may be secondary to underlying medical conditions, a complete examination should be done to exclude dental, neurologic, immunological, musculoskeletal, and psychological causes. Special attention should be directed to observation of the patient's balance, gait problems, or unusual findings that would indicate an underlying systemic disease. The muscles of mastication and the TMJ should be palpated using a bimanual technique. Muscles to be palpated include the masseter, temporalis, medial pterygoid, digastric, and mylohyoid. Tenderness, enlargement, swelling, and unusual texture should be noted. Tenderness over the temporal artery region suggestive of giant cell (temporal) arteritis would be concerning, as would lesions suggestive of a herpetic etiology. Cervical muscle groups should also be palpated to differentiate craniocervical disorders. The oral examination may reveal ground-down teeth, which would indicate bruxism.

The TMJ should be examined with the mouth in the closed position, which will allow palpation of the lateral aspect. On opening of the jaw, assessment of mandibular range of motion and TMJ sounds can assist with diagnosis. A mandibular opening of less than 35 mm is considered restrictive, and the mandible may deviate to one side or the other when opened (asymmetrical opening). Pain may also be elicited with mandibular movement and should be noted. TMJ sounds may be described as clicking, popping, or crepitus.

DIAGNOSTIC REASONING

Diagnostic Tests

Initial testing for diagnosis of TMD should include ruling out other underlying medical conditions. Laboratory testing should include a complete blood count with differential, platelet count, serum chemistry panel, erythrocyte sedimentation rate, rheumatoid factor, and thyroid-stimulating hormone. Radiographic imaging (x-ray films) may be helpful in confirming a clinical diagnosis of TMD. The clinician must remember that even if anatomical changes are found, imaging results rarely have any bearing on clinical outcome. Panoramic imaging is best used to rule out any dental issues (e.g., abscesses) that may be causing the pain.

Subsequent testing should most appropriately be ordered by a dentist, otorhinolaryngologist, or oral surgeon on referral of the patient. This could include panoramic films, computed tomography (CT) scan, or magnetic resonance imaging (MRI). CT scan provides the clearest picture of osseous structures, and, with contrast, can help visualize the soft tissue of the head and neck; however, it is not useful in the diagnosis of disc displacement of the TMJ. MRI visualizes the soft tissues of the joint without radiation exposure or the need for contrast dye. MRI can be used to determine disc position and morphology. Therapeutic injections with local anesthetics or corticosteroids, synovial fluid analysis, or biopsy of suspicious areas by the specialist may be useful for differentiating TMD from similar diagnoses.

Differential Diagnosis

Because of the contributing factors and characteristic symptoms, it may be difficult to arrive at a diagnosis of TMD. Disorders of the intracranial structures should be ruled out early because they may be life-threatening and require immediate attention. New or abrupt onset of pain, progressively more severe pain, interruption of sleep by pain, and systemic symptoms such as weight loss, ataxia, fever, and neurologic symptoms (e.g., seizures, paralysis, vertigo) are characteristic of intracranial disorders. Differential Diagnosis 26.1 presents common differential diagnoses for TMD.

MANAGEMENT

The goals for management of TMD are similar to those of any musculoskeletal condition—reduction or elimination of pain and restoration of acceptable (mandibular) joint function. Complete resolution of TMD may not be a realistic expectation because this largely depends on the underlying cause. Initial management combines nonpharmacologic and pharmacologic modalities that are individualized to the patient. Nonpharmacologic options include self-care, biobehavioral pain management (including biofeedback, relaxation and imagery techniques, cognitive therapy), occlusal splints (bite guards), and physical therapy, as described subsequently.

Some of the most significant contributions toward management of TMD can be made by adjustment in dietary consistency, disease education, alteration of oral parafunctional habits, and the application of ice (for acute symptomatology) or moist heat (for chronic symptomatology). Wearing an intraoral appliance with an occlusal splint component may be recommended, generally by a dentist. Physical therapy may be employed, primarily as an adjunct to other therapeutic modalities, in an attempt to relieve pain of

 Differential Diagnosis 26.1: Temporomandibular Disorder (TMD)

- Sinusitis
- Dental abnormalities
- Otitis media and otitis externa
- Musculoskeletal pain
- Arthritis (rheumatoid arthritis, osteoarthritis, gout, septic arthritis, psoriatic arthritis, Lyme disease)
- Parotid gland pathology
- Mastoiditis
- Giant cell arteritis
- Trigeminal neuralgia
- Postherpetic neuralgia
- Headaches (cluster, migraine, tension, vascular)
- Psychogenic pain
- Mood disorders (e.g., depression, anxiety)
- Head and neck cancer pain

musculoskeletal origin and restore normal masticatory function. Physical therapy for TMD may include electromodalities and therapeutic exercises as prescribed by a physical therapist. Biobehavioral therapy is indicated for patients with behavioral and emotional problems and/or noxious habits that accompany TMD. Stress relief and pain control methods such as counseling, hypnosis, biofeedback, and guided imagery are safe and noninvasive.

Pharmacotherapy can be beneficial in controlling the pain and inflammation associated with TMD. Careful monitoring of the patient's tolerance to prescribed medications, as well as the effectiveness of these drugs, is key. A course of 10 to 14 days of NSAIDs is the initial treatment of choice. If there is pain on palpation of the muscles of mastication, short-term use of a short-acting muscle relaxant combined with an NSAID may benefit some patients. Tricyclic antidepressants are an option for long-term use, especially if TMD is associated with anxiety or depression. For patients with rheumatoid arthritis, treatment and control of the underlying disease is recommended, but neither corticosteroids nor hyaluronic acid is recommended for long-term use in these patients. In addition, the use of opioids or benzodiazepines is discouraged in TMD because of their abuse potential. Drugs Commonly Prescribed 26.1 presents the drugs commonly used to treat TMD disease.

For refractory cases, referral to a dentist or oral maxillofacial specialist for injection of trigger points with anesthetic agents may be beneficial. In rare cases, surgery such as arthroscopic arthrocentesis, open arthrotomy, or even reconstructive jaw surgery may be required.

For the majority of cases of TMD, subsequent management will necessarily be initiated and followed by a dentist, otorhinolaryngologist, or oral surgeon to whom the patient has been referred. (See The Iceberg of TMD.)

Drugs Commonly Prescribed 26.1: Temporomandibular Disorder (TMD)

DRUG	INDICATION	DOSAGE	COMMENTS
Nonopioid Analgesics			
Acetaminophen (Tylenol)	TMD (acute and chronic)	1,000 mg three times daily	Long-term use can cause liver disease.
Ibuprofen (Motrin, Advil)	TMD (acute and chronic): anti-inflammatory effect is desired.	400–800 mg three to four times daily with food	Contraindicated with aspirin allergy. Increased risk of gastrointestinal bleed with long-term use.
Naproxen (Aleve, Naprosyn)	TMD (acute and chronic): anti-inflammatory effect is desired.	220 mg every 12 hours with food	Contraindicated with aspirin allergy. Increased risk of gastrointestinal bleed with long-term use.
Muscle Relaxant			
Cyclobenzaprine HCl (Flexeril)	TMD (acute): to relieve muscle spasm	5–10 mg three times daily	Adverse effects include drowsiness, blurred vision, dry mouth, and dizziness. Cannot drive while taking. Pregnancy Category B.
Tricyclic Antidepressants			
Amitriptyline (Elavil)	TMD (chronic): especially helpful when underlying anxiety and/or depression are contributing factors.	25 mg three to four times daily or 75 mg at bedtime; begin with low nightly dose and increase	May result in decreased orofacial pain, improvement in sleep disorders, and promotion of muscle relaxation and decreased bruxism. Adverse effects include anticholinergic effects, drowsiness, dry mouth, and arrhythmias. Contraindicated within 14 days of use of monoamine oxidase inhibitors and acute postmyocardial infarction; monitor serum levels with concomitant use of drugs metabolized by CYP450.

The Iceberg of TMD

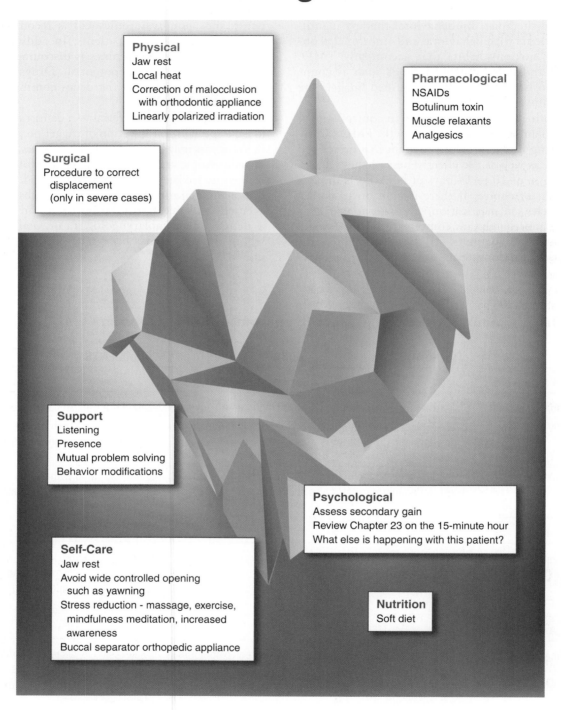

Physical
Jaw rest
Local heat
Correction of malocclusion
  with orthodontic appliance
Linearly polarized irradiation

Pharmacological
NSAIDs
Botulinum toxin
Muscle relaxants
Analgesics

Surgical
Procedure to correct
  displacement
  (only in severe cases)

Support
Listening
Presence
Mutual problem solving
Behavior modifications

Psychological
Assess secondary gain
Review Chapter 23 on the 15-minute hour
What else is happening with this patient?

Self-Care
Jaw rest
Avoid wide controlled opening
  such as yawning
Stress reduction - massage, exercise,
  mindfulness meditation, increased
  awareness
Buccal separator orthopedic appliance

Nutrition
Soft diet

FOLLOW-UP AND REFERRAL

The decision to refer a patient with TMD to a specialist should be based on the individual practitioner's knowledge level and comfort in treating TMD. If there is any uncertainty about the diagnosis, referral should be made to a dentist, otorhinolaryngologist, or oromaxillofacial surgeon who is knowledgeable in the treatment of TMD.

Once other systemic conditions have been ruled out, the primary-care practitioner may choose to begin initial management of TMD symptoms. Follow-up should be early and repeated (e.g., in 1–2 weeks initially and monthly thereafter), especially if pharmacotherapy is ordered. If initial therapy is unsuccessful or if advanced management is indicated, appropriate referrals should be undertaken.

Patient Education: Temporomandibular Disorder (TMD)

Home care and patient education are integral components in the management of TMD. The majority of patients achieve relief of symptoms with conservative therapy, including self-care techniques. Patient education for the management of TMD includes the following recommendations:

- Limit jaw function by eating softer foods, taking smaller bites, and not opening the mouth wide when eating. Avoid foods such as apples, corn on the cob, hard breads, raw vegetables, and steak or tough meats.
- To help reduce stress, strive for a nutritionally balanced diet and an active exercise program.
- Ice packs can be used for acute pain and muscle spasm; for chronic pain, moist heat should be used following the same guidelines.
- Disengage your teeth—the rule is "lips together, teeth apart."
- Do not chew gum or ice.
- Sleep on your back with a pillow under your knees and not on your stomach. Do not use firm, full pillows under your head; orthopedic pillows can be helpful in reducing head and neck pain.
- When talking on the telephone, do not support the receiver with your shoulder.
- Prevent wide-opening when yawning.
- Do not sit with your chin resting on your hand.

Practice good posture; if you must sit for long periods of time, stand and move around frequently to stretch your muscles.

REFERENCES

De Rossi SS, Greenberg MS, Liu F, Steinkeler A. Temporomandibular disorders: evaluation and management. *Med Clin North Am* 2014;98:1353–84.

Ferrando M, Andreu Y, Galdón MJ, et al. Psychological variables and temporomandibular disorders: distress, coping, and personality. *Oral Surg Oral Med Oral Pathol Oral Radiol Endod* 2004;98:153–60.

Gauer RL, Semidey MJ. Diagnosis and treatment of temporomandibular disorders. *Am Fam Physician.* 2015;24(6):378–386.

Mehta NR, Scrivani SJ, Correa L, Matheson JK. Sleep-Related Bruxism. In: Therapy in Sleep Medicine, Barkoukis TJ, Matheson JK, Ferber R, Doghramji K (Eds), Elsevier, Philadelphia 2012. p.324–27.

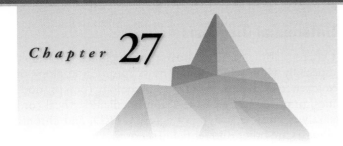

Chapter 27

Dysphonia

Ruth McCaffrey, DNP, APRN, FNP-BC, GNP, FAAN, FAANP

Brian Oscar Porter, MD, PhD, MPH, MBA

Lynne M. Dunphy, PhD, APRN, FNP-BC, FAAN, FAANP

Dysphonia, or *hoarseness,* is a common complaint; the term describes a voice with harsh quality and low pitch. The term can also indicate weakness, raspiness, or simply a change from usual voice quality. Hoarseness is the symptom, whereas *dysphonia* is the diagnostic term. Dysphonia suggests an abnormality in voice production at the level of the larynx. There are numerous causes of dysphonia; some are functional, and others are organic.

EPIDEMIOLOGY AND CAUSES

Dysphonia affects approximately 20 million people in the United States at any given time, and about one in three people will become hoarse at some point in their lifetimes. Dysphonia is frequently the result of a viral infection of the larynx (laryngitis). Usually, acute laryngitis affects individuals aged 18 to 40 years; however, children aged 3 years and older have been clinically observed with laryngitis. In women, the prevalence of hoarseness not associated with infection is 50% higher than it is in men.

Changes in the voice are part of the natural process of aging. In elderly men, the voice becomes weaker and higher in pitch as a result of muscle atrophy and increased stiffness of tissues. In women, the same changes occur, but the pitch of the voice becomes lower because during menopause mucoid edema occurs in the submucosa of the vocal folds. More severe edema and polyps may occur in women who smoke. Dysphonia is a cardinal sign of laryngeal cancer, which is most commonly seen in men 50 to 70 years of age.

PATHOPHYSIOLOGY

Vocal cord inflammation and edema as a result of an infectious process (usually viral) result in vocal fold movement that is asymmetrical with reduced mucosal waves and incomplete vibratory closure. In the process of phagocytosis, the vocal folds become more edematous and vibration is adversely affected. The phonation threshold pressure may increase to a degree that generating adequate phonation pressure in a normal fashion becomes difficult, thus eliciting hoarseness. Gastroesophageal reflux disease (GERD) may also contribute to inflammation and edema of the vocal cords.

CLINICAL PRESENTATION

Subjective

Onset of the problem is an important key to the diagnosis. A 1-day complaint is unlikely to be caused by cancer, whereas hoarseness persisting for more than several weeks is unlikely to be the result of an acute infection. Dysphonia that persists for greater than 2 weeks, without associated upper respiratory infection, requires a work-up.

Associated signs and symptoms should be ascertained. Shortness of breath, stridor, cough, hemoptysis, throat pain, difficulty swallowing, unilateral otalgia, and weight loss in a patient with voice symptoms raise concern for cancer. Chronic pain often suggests more serious underlying disease than acute onset of pain. Dysphagia or odynophagia accompanying hoarseness indicates the presence of disease affecting the pharynx or esophagus. Cough suggests irritation of the endolarynx or pulmonary disease. Fever and oral, nasal, or otologic discharge suggest an infectious process.

Voice use and lifestyle should be reviewed to assess for pertinent positives and negatives associated with the differential diagnosis. Overuse of the voice can cause hoarseness, as would be seen in singers. An individual who smoked two packs of cigarettes per day for 45 years may have irritation or malignancy. A scratchy throat the morning after eating spicy foods suggests a diagnosis of GERD. Previous head or neck surgery, tracheal intubation, or radiotherapy to the neck may be factors affecting the laryngeal nerve. The use of asthma inhalers and chronic exposure to pollutants may contribute to hoarseness as well.

Objective

A complete examination of the head and neck is necessary. Nasal drainage and excess mucus may indicate sinusitis. Tonsillar erythema or exudate indicates viral or bacterial infection. Ear canal erythema or exudate suggests infection. A normal ear examination, despite the complaint of otalgia, may be seen in patients with cancer of the pharynx or larynx. The clinician should inspect and palpate the oral cavity including the buccal mucosa, floor of the mouth, and tongue. The neck and lymph nodes should be palpated for masses. Infections often feel warm, tender, tense, or fluctuant. Malignancies typically are hard masses that may be fixed to underlying tissue.

Neck anatomy, including tracheal alignment, should be inspected and palpated. However, with dysphonia, it is important to note that a head, eyes, ears, nose, and throat examination may be normal.

DIAGNOSTIC REASONING

Diagnostic Tests

Infections cause elevated white blood cell counts. Culture and sensitivity of oral or otologic discharge can reveal the organism responsible for the infection and guide antibiotic therapy. Routine use of computed tomography or magnetic resonance imaging scans to evaluate hoarseness is not recommended.

If hoarseness persists for more than 2 weeks and is clearly not caused by infection, referral to an otolaryngologist for laryngoscopy is required. An adequate laryngeal examination should visualize the base of the tongue, epiglottis, pyriform sinuses, false vocal cords, subglottic larynx, and true vocal cords. Use of stroboscopy improves detection of small lesions by "freezing" the vocal cords (making them appear immobile) during vibration. Adequate examination of structures may require general anesthesia, which is necessary for palpation and biopsy of any abnormalities. Thyroid tumors are the most common cause of bilateral vocal cord paralysis; esophageal and pulmonary tumors are common causes of left-sided vocal cord paralysis.

Differential Diagnosis

Differential diagnosis of hoarseness includes infections, especially viral, which is the most common etiology of hoarseness. Overuse, vocal cord pathology (polyps, nodules, tumors), adverse effects from medicines, vocal cord paralysis, muscle atrophy of aging, GERD, and chronic allergies are other differential diagnoses.

MANAGEMENT

Management of the underlying cause is the key. Guidelines for the management of hoarseness recommended by the American Academy of Otolaryngology–Head and Neck Surgery Foundation, include the following:

- Review current medications that may be causing the symptom.
- Avoid vocal excess and irritants, such as inhaled smoke.
- Completely rest the voice. Avoid whispering because this strains the larynx.
- Avoid antihistamines because they serve to dry the mucous membranes.
- There is no benefit in using antibiotics to treat acute laryngitis.
- Imaging studies should not be performed before visualizing the larynx with laryngoscopy.

- Use of humidified air especially at night and during dry seasons may be helpful.
- Encourage increased oral fluids.
- Treatment with antireflux medication should not be undertaken in the absence of signs or symptoms of significant GERD and prior evaluation by laryngoscopy.
- Voice therapy, typically one or two sessions per week for 4 to 8 weeks, is a well-established intervention for patients of all ages who have hoarseness.
- Use of an amplifying device during heavy voice use can reduce hoarseness.
- Oral steroids are not routinely recommended. Oxymetazoline (Afrin) nasal spray should be avoided.

There is limited evidence that nimodipine, a calcium channel blocker, may speed recovery rates in acute hoarseness. There is also evidence that botulinum may be of benefit in spasmodic dysphonia (strained voice).

FOLLOW-UP AND REFERRAL

As noted, if dysphonia persists for more than 2 weeks, further evaluation by an otolaryngologist is warranted. For persistent or recurrent episodes of hoarseness, vocal hygiene and voice therapy should be considered, especially in professionals who must rely on their voice.

Patient Education: Dysphonia

Because hoarseness is generally self-limited, instructions to stop smoking and rest the voice are essential to facilitate improvement. Humidification and adequate fluid intake will help healing of inflamed tissues. Avoid cough and cold preparations that have antihistamines in the formulation because they will have a drying effect. Prevention strategies, for those at high risk of recurrence, should be emphasized.

For additional resources please visit
https://davisedge.fadavis.com/

REFERENCES

Pedersen M, McGlashan J. Surgical versus non-surgical interventions for vocal cord nodules. *Cochrane Database Syst Rev* 2012;CD001934. doi:10.1002/14651858.CD001934.pub2.

Remacle M, Lawson G. Diagnosis and management of laryngopharyngeal reflux disease. *Curr Opin Otolaryngol Head Neck Surg* 2006;14:143–149.

Ruotsalainen JH, Sellman J, Lehto L, et al. Interventions for treating functional dysphonia in adults. *Cochrane Database Syst Rev* 2007;CD006373.

Schwartz SR, Cohen SM, Dailey SH, et al. Clinical practice guideline: hoarseness (dysphonia). *Otolaryngol Head Neck Surg* 2009;141:S1–S31.

Wood JM, Athanasiadis T, Allen J. Laryngitis. *BMJ* 2014;349:g5827.

Zhukhovitskaya A, Battaglia D, Khosla SM, et al. Gender and age in benign vocal fold lesions. *Laryngoscope* 2015;125:191–196.

RESOURCE

American Academy of Otolaryngology-Head and Neck Surgery
http://www.entnet.org/

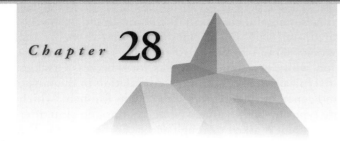

Chapter **28**

Common Respiratory Complaints

Jill E. Winland-Brown, EdD, APRN, FNP-BC

Brian Oscar Porter, MD, PhD, MPH, MBA

COUGH

Each year, more Americans seek medical treatment for cough than for any other complaint. In the United States, treatment costs are estimated to be more than $1 billion annually. Cough is the body's natural protective mechanism for clearing the airways of secretions and irritants and may affect psychological health. It often is caused by the following mechanisms associated with several conditions and diseases:

- Alteration of pulmonary secretions (chronic obstructive pulmonary disease [COPD], bronchiectasis, cystic fibrosis, bronchitis, pulmonary edema, postnasal drip)
- Increased sensitivity of the cough receptors and airways (asthma) or bronchial hyperreactivity from a postinfection (after a respiratory viral illness)
- Direct (aspiration) or indirect stimulation of cough receptors (gastroesophageal reflux disease [GERD])
- Infections (e.g., pneumonia, tuberculosis [TB], pharyngitis, sarcoidosis)
- Progressive disease, including lung cancer, tumors (bronchogenic or mediastinal), or interstitial lung disease (ILD)
- Other conditions such as cardiac tamponade, pulmonary embolism, heart failure, *Pneumocystis jirovecii*
- Occupational, environmental (air pollution, industrial dust, secondhand smoke), and psychogenic factors

Cough may also be an adverse side effect of certain hypertension medications that affect the bradykinin system, such as angiotensin-converting enzyme (ACE) inhibitors or angiotensin receptor blockers. A cough occurs in about 10% of these patients

In extreme cases of debilitation or in certain neuromuscular conditions, the cough mechanism may be impaired, which may predispose to respiratory infection. There are times when the cough mechanism should be supported to clear the airways of unwanted irritants and times when it should be suppressed. These issues are discussed in relation to the underlying condition that initiates the cough mechanism.

DIFFERENTIAL DIAGNOSIS

Patients who present with cough require a comprehensive medical history and assessment to determine appropriate treatment and management. One patient may present with the complaint of a dry, hacking cough of sudden onset *(acute cough)*, whereas another may present with a cough of longer duration. A *chronic cough* is defined as one that lasts longer than 8 weeks. Many patients try over-the-counter (OTC) measures for a chronic, nagging cough and delay seeking treatment or seek treatment only when the cough becomes productive or when there is blood in the sputum.

A diagnosis can be made about 80% of the time by taking a thorough history and exploring the following details regarding the onset and nature of the cough with the patient:

- When did the cough first start? What factors may have prompted the cough (e.g., recent respiratory infection, exposure to noxious agents, initiation of a new medication)? Is there a seasonal pattern? Is it related to work or hobbies?
- When does the cough occur—upon arising, at bedtime, during exercise, or throughout the night?
- What factors seem to stimulate the cough or make it worse? Is the cough aggravated by exposure to certain chemicals, body position, exercise, or cold air? Does the person have any reactive airway disease?
- Has the patient identified any factors that seem to provide relief from the cough, such as sitting upright or avoiding exposure to certain agents? What measures have been tried to alleviate the cough?

- What is the quality of the cough—is it dry and hacking, wet, raspy, deep, or throaty?
- Is the cough productive or unproductive? If the patient produces sputum with the cough, ask the patient to describe the amount of sputum produced per day (e.g., 1 tsp, 1 tbsp, etc.), the color (e.g., yellow, gray, green, brown, clear, white, blood-tinged), and consistency (e.g., thick, ropy, frothy, or tenacious). When is the productive cough most productive (e.g., morning, evening)?
- Does the patient cough more when lying supine? Is the cough constant throughout the day and night?

In addition, it is essential to find out whether the patient has signs and symptoms associated with cough, such as pedal edema, dizziness, chest pain or tightness (which may indicate reactive airway disease), fatigue, dyspnea, hoarseness, fever, tachypnea, chills, heartburn, wheezing, or hemoptysis. In describing dyspnea, ask the patient to rate the degree of dyspnea on a continuum scale of 0 to 10, similar to the pain scale, that compares today's dyspnea to previous dyspnea. Research indicates that a vertical analog scale is the most accurate way for a patient to rate dyspnea, and it also allows the patient to keep a diary or record of this until their next visit.

The patient should be asked to describe in detail the onset of the associated signs and symptoms. Standard data regarding the patient's medical history should be recorded, including hospitalizations, surgeries, and major illnesses, particularly recent illnesses and respiratory allergies. The patient's lifestyle should be explored, such as occupation and work history; hobbies; exposures to noxious agents; and use of alcohol, tobacco, and other substances. Patients should also be asked about the use of marijuana, especially since it is now legal in many states for medical and recreational use, as well as the use of electronic cigarettes that contain nicotine or other extracts. The most common cause of chronic cough is cigarette smoking, which triggers the cough reflex by direct bronchial irritation.

The patient should be asked about the use of prescription and OTC drugs. Certain antihypertensive drugs, such as ACE inhibitors and beta blockers, can cause hyperreactive airways, producing wheezing and a cough. Other drugs, such as nitrofurantoin (Macrobid, Macrodantin), or aminoglycosides (Gentamicin) may cause interstitial fibrosis and associated cough. All patients taking nitrofurantoin (Macrobid) should be monitored for changes in lung function. Some individuals who are at risk of certain autoimmune disorders seem to be more susceptible to lung disease after taking these antibiotics.

For the physical examination, focus on the following:

- Check the ears for cerumen or hairs impinging on the tympanic membrane, which may cause cough (Arnold reflex).
- Examine the nose for discharge, edema, polyps, and sinus tenderness. In the throat, look for cobblestoning of the oropharynx, which suggests postnasal drip.
- Palpate the neck, including both anterior and posterior cervical node chains, for enlarged lymph nodes or masses.

A complete assessment of the thorax and chest should be performed to rule out cardiac or pulmonary problems. If the patient has not coughed during the visit, ask the patient to reproduce the cough and listen to its sound and character. The lungs should be auscultated, especially for crackles (rales) and rhonchi. The patient should be asked to produce a forced expiration while the clinician checks for wheezes. Crackles are typically related to fluid accumulation in the lungs, and generally do not clear with cough. Rhonchi, which are typically due to mucus accumulation, do clear after the patient is asked to cough and clear the airways. The presence of heart murmurs, gallops, and carotid bruits should also be assessed.

In most cases with a cough, the underlying cause can be determined from a history and physical examination, but it may be necessary to consider the judicious use of one or more of the following diagnostic tests in conjunction with the differential diagnosis process. For example, if TB is suspected, a Mantoux purified protein derivative (PPD) tuberculin skin test (TST) should be administered and results read 48 to 72 hours later by qualified personnel at a second visit (information on interpreting PPD results is given in Chapter 30). A blood test that may be used to detect TB is an interferon-gamma release assay, such as the QuantiFERON-TB Gold Test, which only requires a single patient visit for one blood draw. A positive result on either screening test should be followed by a chest x-ray (CXR) film. For patients who are immunocompromised, the TST may need to be repeated because of T-cell anergy against TB antigens. The use of positive and negative control antigens alongside the TST has fallen out of favor, due to their poor predictive value in interpreting TST results.

Spirometry is helpful to determine the presence of obstructive or restrictive lung disease. A CXR film should be taken if there are signs and symptoms of pneumonia, TB, possible tumor, aspiration, foreign body, or ILD or even if the patient is not recovering as expected. This follow-up CXR may detect a hidden tumor that would otherwise have been missed. Sinus films may be useful to rule out sinusitis when the patient presents with a history of chronic postnasal drip or chronic sinus infections.

Computed tomography (CT) scanning of the chest can detect small peripheral lung nodules, evaluate coin lesions (solid, cystic, or calcified), and distinguish the chest wall from areas of pleural or parenchymal disease. Chest vessels can be separated from lymph nodes and other solid, nonvascular structures. The CT scan has replaced bronchography in diagnosing bronchiectasis. CT scan may help to better delineate endobronchial, parenchymal, or mediastinal masses. High-resolution chest CT scan, ventilation–perfusion scan, or pulmonary angiography is indicated when pulmonary thromboembolism is suspected. Sinus CT scans are also considered more sensitive than sinus plain films in detecting sinusitis, although findings of sinus inflammation on imaging may not correlate with clinical symptoms.

A complete blood count (CBC) with differential is helpful in diagnosing a bacterial infection. Fungal serology should be done to identify coccidiomycosis, histoplasmosis, or aspergillosis, if the history of exposure is positive or if the patient has AIDS or is immunosuppressed.

MANAGEMENT

Because a cough is a symptom, treatment should be directed toward resolving the underlying cause(s) and removing any identified triggers. In patients with chronic cough who are weak and debilitated, the goal is to reduce complications from uncontrolled, forceful coughing, such as fractured ribs, pneumothorax, aspiration, exhaustion, sleep deprivation, and post-tussive syncope.

With severe, acute coughing that disrupts sleep and causes pain or extreme fatigue and weakness, it may be necessary to treat with antitussives. However, because patients should be encouraged to expectorate during the day, these drugs have a limited role and should only be used on a short-term basis and only at night. Nonnarcotic agents such as dextromethorphan or pseudoephedrine/brompheniramine/dextromethorphan combination therapy may be used every 3 to 4 hours as needed. In addition, benzonatate (Tessalon) may be effective. When sleep or eating is interrupted by persistent cough, the preferred choice is codeine, 8 to 30 mg every 3 to 4 hours, but only on a short-term basis. (Patients with terminal lung cancer and patients with cystic fibrosis at the end of life should receive codeine in sufficient doses to keep them comfortable.)

Decongestants and antihistamines, alone or in combination, are indicated in cases of allergic rhinitis and postnasal drip. Antihistamines are useful for those who have allergic upper airway disease but should usually avoided in asthmatic individuals because they may thicken secretions and inhibit expectoration. Intranasal corticosteroid sprays or aerosols, such as beclomethasone (Beconase), fluticasone (Flonase), and mometasone (Nasonex), may also be useful when used on a consistent basis.

Expectorants are intended to decrease sputum viscosity and are used when the patient has a productive cough and needs help in clearing the airways. Suppression of a productive cough, however, may lead to complications such as obstructive pneumonia because the patient may not be able to clear the airways and lungs of sputum. Although expectorants may work in some cases, increasing the patient's water intake to 3 to 4 L/day is the most cost-effective means of helping to liquefy secretions, as long as the patient can manage the fluid volume and does not have heart failure or other disorder in which increased fluid intake could compromise health. Guaifenesin (Mucinex), which is available OTC, helps to break up mucus. Patients must be reminded to drink plenty of fluids when taking guaifenesin. Some clinicians prefer to give an expectorant during the day and a cough suppressant at night, so that the patient may sleep.

Two herbal remedies are currently used but have not been thoroughly researched in randomized controlled trials. Horehound has been suggested as a cough suppressant, and licorice has been said to calm coughs and have expectorant qualities. Licorice should be used with caution, because it may increase blood pressure.

Patients who smoke should be encouraged to stop smoking. Cigarette smoke destroys the mucociliary structures of the airway lining and reduces the body's natural ability to clear mucus and respiratory pathogens. A chronic cough may not disappear in ex-smokers for a year or more after smoking cessation. Smoking cessation techniques are discussed in Chapter 33.

Patients with GERD, whose cough reflex can be triggered by the reflux of acidic stomach contents usually respond to a course of antireflux therapy, which may include antacids, H2-receptor blockers, or proton pump inhibitors. The benefits may not be noticed for several weeks, however.

Educating the patient and family about potential environmental and occupational factors that precipitate cough is essential, including exploring ways to avoid exposure to irritants. If a family member smokes, the dangers of secondhand smoke should be explained to the patient and family. Adequate hydration (increasing fluids) and adequate ambient humidification may also help reduce coughing. Breathing in the steam from a hot shower may also be effective. Simple measures such as changing air filters may also be helpful in removing environmental irritants.

DYSPNEA

Dyspnea is one of the most common complaints for which patients seek help from health-care providers. Dyspnea, or shortness of breath, is estimated to be the third most frequent reason for seeking medical attention. Although dyspnea occurs primarily in patients with respiratory and cardiac disorders, it may also occur in other conditions such as lung neoplasms with metastasis, neuromuscular myopathies, neuropathies, spinal cord lesions, diaphragmatic disorders, and panic disorders. In patients receiving hospice care, it is the second most common symptom secondary to pain.

As with pain, *dyspnea* is a perceived sensation that may vary among patients, which is why the use of a scale from 0 to 10 is recommended. Patients with dyspnea usually describe a sense of difficult breathing or an inability to get sufficient air into or out of the lungs. Dyspnea may also be described as a feeling of breathlessness, suffocation or smothering, air hunger, or labored breathing. In many cases of dyspnea, the respiratory rate is rapid, and cough may be present, depending on the underlying disease or cause of the dyspnea. Dyspnea may be caused by several different health problems. Some individuals may experience exercise-induced dyspnea or exercise-induced bronchospasm. In older patients, dyspnea is the major atypical presentation for ischemic heart disease and myocardial infarction and is considered a frequent anginal equivalent. Dyspnea in aging patients may be difficult to evaluate when there are associated comorbidities.

DIFFERENTIAL DIAGNOSIS

In the majority of cases, dyspnea is a result of cardiac or pulmonary decompensation. There are several symptoms associated with dyspnea, such as tachypnea (rapid breathing), orthopnea (dyspnea relieved in a seated or upright position), and paroxysmal nocturnal dyspnea (sudden episodes of acute dyspnea at night). The causes of dyspnea are often complex. The common causes and precipitants of dyspnea follow:

- **Pulmonary:** COPD, asthma, pulmonary parenchymal disease, ILD, pulmonary hypertension, severe kyphoscoliosis, exogenous mechanical factors (ascites, morbid obesity, extensive pleural effusion)
- **Cardiac:** Congestive heart failure, pulmonary venous congestion (mitral stenosis, mitral regurgitation)
- **Hematological:** Severe chronic anemia
- **Psychogenic:** Anxiety and panic disorders

Dyspnea may be acute or chronic, and patients with COPD may have both acute and chronic dyspnea. It is important to do a complete work-up to determine the underlying cause of the dyspnea so that appropriate treatment can be initiated. Dyspnea caused by acute anxiety may mimic cardiopulmonary decompensation, and patients with pulmonary hypertension may have episodes that resemble anxiety-related dyspnea. Onset of dyspnea at rest, accompanied by a sense of chest tightness, a feeling of suffocation, and an inability to "get air in," is a common presentation of anxiety-related dyspnea. In the absence of heart and lung disease, a history of multiple somatic complaints, emotional difficulties, no activity limitations (exercise intolerance), and dyspnea unrelated to physical activity provides evidence for psychogenic dyspnea.

About 75% of cases of dyspnea are caused by respiratory conditions that may be acute or chronic. The majority of other causes of dyspnea are cardiac in origin. It is important to explore with the patient the details of the onset and character of the dyspnea. The clinician should note whether the patient has dyspnea at rest or on exertion. Standard questions include the following:

1. How many flights of stairs did the patient climb before dyspnea occurred (e.g., one-flight dyspnea)?
2. How many blocks did the patient walk before dyspnea occurred (e.g., one-block dyspnea)?
3. How many feet did the patient walk before dyspnea occurred (e.g., 100-feet dyspnea)?

The rate and clarity of the patient's speech during exercise can provide good clinical information.

Exploring when the dyspnea first occurred and what the patient was doing at the time is essential. Specific questions should be directed toward precipitating factors and factors that alleviate the dyspnea. Questions should explore potential environmental exposure (e.g., recent travel) or exposure to triggering agents (e.g., occupational exposure or hobbies) that aggravate the dyspnea. Paying attention to other signs and symptoms that may be associated with the dyspnea, such as cough, peripheral edema, dizziness, wheeze, fever, chest pain, heartburn, leg pain, and paresthesias, is also critical.

A complete physical examination should be done, with particular attention directed to the pulmonary and cardiovascular systems. The examiner should check for tachycardia, tachypnea, fever, and hypertension, and assess mixed venous oxygen saturation (SvO_2). The quality of breath sounds (increased, decreased, or absent) should be noted, along with the presence of crackles, rhonchi, wheezes, egophony, and fremitus. Bronchial lung sounds heard at other than the normal locations (tubular sounds) are common with acute bronchitis. Assessment should include checking for third and fourth heart sounds, murmurs, friction rubs, jugular venous distention, pedal edema, and calf tenderness. A visual analog scale (0 = *no dyspnea;* 10 = *worst dyspnea ever had*) or the Borg scale for perceived exertion with a score of 6 to 20 (6 = *no exertion;* 20 = *very, very hard exertion*) is useful in assessing the degree of dyspnea, as previously mentioned. The scales can be used again on the patient's next visit to compare the effects of treatment. The scales can also be used for patient self-management.

Diagnostic tests are guided by data from the history and physical examination and the suspected causes of the dyspnea. CXR films are useful in ruling out tumors, TB, pneumonia, and other major pulmonary disorders. A CBC with differential should be done to rule out anemia and infection. A blood chemistry profile should be ordered if metabolic acidosis is suspected and to differentiate anion-gap acidosis from non–anion-gap acidosis. Oximetry to measure the saturation level of oxygen may be useful in assessing whether the patient is hypoxic. If the O_2 saturation level is less than 90%, arterial blood gas (ABG) analysis should be done. Perceived levels of dyspnea have not been found to correlate well with physiological measures.

If carbon monoxide (CO) exposure is suspected, a carboxyhemoglobin (COHb) level should be obtained. COHb levels of 4% to 15% may be found in heavy smokers. Levels above 20% may cause dyspnea and headache; levels greater than 40% may cause seizures and death.

Peak expiratory flow rate is a simple, inexpensive test that can be done with a handheld flow meter in the office or at the bedside. This test determines the degree of expiratory airflow obstruction in patients with asthma and COPD. Full spirometry is useful in determining whether the patient has obstructive, restrictive, or mixed (obstructive and restrictive) lung disease. Diffusion capacity should be checked if ILD is suspected. If the patient uses a peak flow meter at home and notes an acute decrease in peak flow, he or she should be instructed to contact their health-care provider for further evaluation and possible treatment.

MANAGEMENT

Initial treatment is directed at helping the patient find relief from the shortness of breath by removing the underlying cause and contributing factors. Subsequent management is directed at prevention and assisting the patient with the management of chronic dyspnea in conditions such as COPD or ILD. In cases of dyspnea caused by hypoxemia, supplemental oxygen may be indicated. In cases of pulmonary shunting, the cause of the shunting must be corrected. For subsequent management, see the Chapter 31.

For the treatment of dyspnea related to cardiac disorders such as CHF, refer to Chapter 35. Appropriate diuretics to relieve fluid overload may improve breathing, and supplemental oxygen may be necessary in some cases.

For anxiety-related dyspnea, psychiatric referral may be needed if other measures, such as rebreathing exercises, have failed. Dyspnea caused by rapid overbreathing during anxiety attacks often can be corrected by teaching the patient breathing techniques. Until the patient learns a rebreathing technique, it may be helpful to prescribe short-term use of anxiolytics, such as buspirone HCl 20 to 30 mg/day.

HEMOPTYSIS

Hemoptysis is defined as the expectoration of blood. The patient often reports coughing up blood or sputum that is streaked or tinged with blood. In addition, hemoptysis may be manifested as fresh (bright red) or old (dark red or black) blood or, in the case of bleeding from an infected lung cavity, it may present as slow oozing or frank bleeding. In cases of profuse hemoptysis, blood clots may be expectorated. The patient should note whether the blood is from the nasal cavity, which may be from severe irritation or dehydration of the nasal mucosa.

DIFFERENTIAL DIAGNOSIS

About 80% of hemoptysis cases are related to inflammatory causes, such as bronchitis, bronchiectasis, pneumonia, and TB. Less common causes may include neoplasms that damage a pulmonary vessel or rupture a pulmonary artery. Use of pulmonary artery balloon catheters has increased the incidence of pulmonary artery rupture. Hemoptysis may also occur in patients with cystic fibrosis who have significant damage to the lung parenchyma. Cardiovascular causes of hemoptysis include left ventricular failure, mitral stenosis, pulmonary embolism or infarct, primary pulmonary hypertension, and aortic aneurysm. Clotting defects may also cause hemoptysis. Bleeding may occur anywhere along the respiratory tract, including the nose, sinuses, and mouth.

About 95% of pulmonary blood circulation is supplied by the pulmonary artery and its branches, which is a low-pressure system. Bronchial circulation, a high-pressure system, originates from the aorta and usually provides about 5% of the blood to the lungs, mostly to the airways and supporting structures. When bleeding occurs, it usually arises from the bronchial circulation, unless trauma or erosion has affected a major pulmonary vessel. Pulmonary venous bleeding is modest and occurs in pulmonary venous hypertension, especially in conjunction with left heart failure.

The patient usually presents with a complaint of "coughing up" blood. To most people, the presence of blood in the sputum or coughing up blood is a frightening experience, and most will seek immediate medical attention. Patients should be asked about hemoptysis, including its onset, amount of blood, aggravating and alleviating factors, and the presence of other associated symptoms such as dyspnea, cough, dizziness, fatigue, and chest pain. Bronchopulmonary bleeding may present as hematemesis (vomiting of blood). The patient may swallow blood during the night and may vomit blood upon arising.

The history and physical examination for hemoptysis are similar to those conducted for cough and dyspnea. In addition, if the examiner suspects that the hemoptysis is due to a pulmonary neoplasm, the examination should focus on the pulmonary system and lymph node enlargement.

Further diagnostic tests may be indicated, depending on the results of the history and physical examination. Common causes of hemoptysis will direct the laboratory tests. If hemoptysis occurs in patients aged 45 years or younger, it is likely caused by mitral stenosis, TB, bronchiectasis, or lung abscess. For patients older than age 45 years, common causes of hemoptysis include bronchogenic carcinoma, bronchitis, TB, and pulmonary embolus with infarction. In massive hemoptysis (loss of more than 600 mL of blood in 24 hours, which may occur in lung cancer, TB, bronchiectasis, and lung abscess), the condition is life-threatening and constitutes a medical emergency. There may be time to do only chest radiographs and a CBC before emergency surgery or bronchoscopy.

For nonemergency cases, in which the sputum is tinged or streaked with blood, there is time to do essential tests to identify the cause of hemoptysis. In addition to CXR films and a CBC, sputum should be cultured for acid-fast bacilli if TB is suspected. For suspected pneumonia or lung abscess, sputum culture and sensitivities should be done. Patients who present with hematemesis may also have hemoptysis caused by aspiration; a CXR film is indicated for these patients.

Patients with a history of thromboembolism may be taking anticoagulants. In these patients, clotting times should be assessed to rule this out as a cause of the hemoptysis.

Because of the exertion (forceful expiratory maneuvers) required by the patient during spirometry, measurement of lung volumes during periods of active hemoptysis is not recommended.

MANAGEMENT

Massive hemoptysis requires immediate treatment, surgery, or bronchoscopy. Prevention of aspiration and keeping the airway open are of utmost importance. Endotracheal intubation may be necessary. Supplemental oxygen and replacement of blood loss may be necessary, depending on the patient's blood pressure, pulse, ABG results, and hemoglobin level.

Treatment of chronic hemoptysis is directed toward the underlying cause. When the cause is inflammation, as in chronic bronchitis, TB, and bronchiectasis, the patient must be educated to stop smoking, comply with use of prescribed medications (e.g., antibiotics, bronchodilators), perform deep breathing and coughing exercises every 2 to 4 hours regularly, and avoid exposure to secondhand smoke and other noxious agents that might precipitate cough.

Education of the patient and family regarding the causes of the hemoptysis is essential. The patient should know what factors may precipitate the hemoptysis and how it can be prevented. The patient also should be taught to note any change in the color, amount, or consistency of the blood expectorated. Any sudden increase in the volume of blood expectorated or change in character of the hemoptysis should be reported to the health-care provider immediately for prompt medical attention.

REFERENCES

Dicpinigaitis PV. Angiotensin-converting enzyme inhibitor-induced cough: ACCP evidence-based clinical practice guidelines. *Chest.* 2006;129(suppl 1):169S–173S.

Goodenough E, Robinson TM, Zook MB, et al. Cryptic MHC class I–binding peptides are revealed by aminoglycoside-induced stop codon read-through into the 3' UTR. *Proc Natl Acad Sci U S A.* 2014; 111(15):5670–5675.

Longo DL, Fauci A, Kasper D, et al., eds. *Harrison's principles of internal medicine.* 19th ed. New York: McGraw-Hill; 2016.

National Heart, Lung, and Blood Institute. Cough. http://www.nhlbi. nih.gov/health/health-topics/topics/cough/. Published 2016. Accessed June 13, 2017.

Papadakis MA, McPhee SJ. *Current medical diagnosis and treatment.* New York: Appleton-Lange/McGraw-Hill; 2017.

Twilla J, Winton J. Nitrofurantoin pulmonary toxicity: A rare but serious complication. Patient Care. http://www.patientcareonline. com/respiratory-diseases/nitrofurantoin-pulmonary-toxicity-rare-serious-complication. Published 2010. Accessed June 13, 2017.

RESOURCES

American Lung Association: Living With Cough
    http://www.lung.org/lung-health-and-diseases/lung-disease-lookup/cough/living-with-cough.html
Medscape: Asthma
    http://www.medscape.com/resource/asthma
Medscape: Chronic Obstructive Pulmonary Disease
    http://www.medscape.com/resource/copd
National Institute of Allergy and Infectious Disease
    http://www.niaid.nih.gov
National Heart, Lung, and Blood Institute: Cough
    https://www.nhlbi.nih.gov/health/health-topics/topics/cough

Patient Education

Medline: Cough
    https://medlineplus.gov/cough.html

Chapter 29

Sleep Apnea

John Suen, MD

Jill E. Winland-Brown, EdD, APRN, FNP-BC

Sleep apnea is defined as a temporary pause in breathing during sleep that lasts at least 10 seconds. For a confirmed diagnosis, this should occur a minimum of five times an hour. The three patterns of apnea are central, obstructive, and mixed. *Central apnea* occurs when both airflow and respiratory efforts are absent. Central apneas are a result of an absence of neural output from the brainstem's respiratory control center, which leads to a lack of inspiratory effort. The respiratory center in the brain fails to respond to elevated carbon dioxide concentrations. In contrast, during *obstructive sleep apnea* (OSA), respiratory efforts persist although airflow is absent at the nose and mouth. Airflow obstruction occurs when the tongue and the soft palate fall backward and partially or completely obstruct the pharynx. Finally, many adult patients exhibit *mixed apnea*, in which both central and obstructive patterns occur.

Each type of apnea results in progressive asphyxiation until an arousal from sleep occurs, with a subsequent restoration of upper airway patency and airflow. A patient then usually returns to sleep quickly, resulting in another occlusion of the upper airway. Apnea and arousal cycles occur repeatedly, as many as 200 to 400 times during 6 to 8 hours of sleep in severe cases. Sleep hypopnea is a period of hypoventilation, or decreased airflow, defined as a 50% reduction in thoracoabdominal movements, with a 4% decrease in oxygen saturation lasting at least 10 seconds during sleep. OSA/hypopnea is present when the respiratory drive is intact, but the upper airway intermittently becomes obstructed during sleep.

The *apnea-hypopnea index* (AHI) may be used to define and quantify the severity of OSA. The AHI is obtained by dividing the total number of events (the number of apnea episodes plus the number of hypopnea episodes) throughout the entire night by the total sleep time in hours. The *respiratory disturbance index* (RDI), another commonly cited parameter, is defined as the AHI plus the average number of snoring-related arousals per hour. A diagnosis of OSA is confirmed with AHI and RDI scores as follows:

- AHI or RDI greater than or equal to 5 and less than 14 if comorbid factors such as excessive daytime sleepiness, hypertension, stroke, or heart failure are present, or
- AHI or RDI greater than or equal to 15 in the absence of comorbid factors.

In general, as the AHI increases, so does the severity of symptoms, although the condition may not become clinically significant until the score 20.

Patients with OSA may experience a number of potentially adverse physiological and neurobehavioral problems. Consequences of OSA result from daily exposure to abnormalities in breathing during sleep and may cause long-term neurobehavioral and cardiovascular morbidity. Sleep-disordered breathing is an independent risk factor for the development of hypertension and, subsequently, left ventricular dysfunction. The patient with combined coronary artery disease (CAD) and OSA may have an increased cardiac risk because of worsening of the relationship between myocardial oxygen demand and supply as a result of apnea-associated hypoxemia and activation of the autonomic nervous system (Box 29.1).

Cardiac dysrhythmias, usually occurring during apneic episodes, have been reported to be a significant complication of OSA. Atrial fibrillation, a common arrhythmia, is causally associated with OSA; treating OSA will improve the effectiveness of treatment of atrial fibrillation. People with sleep apnea have a higher risk of dying from sudden cardiac arrest. In addition, sleep quality may be influenced by apnea-associated activation of the central nervous system (CNS) (arousals) and ischemia-associated arousals. Timely diagnosis and treatment of CAD, as well as sleep apnea, is necessary for these patients.

OSA is also more prevalent in patients with chronic congestive heart failure. In these patients, treating OSA often will improve the heart failure.

OSA can cause mild pulmonary hypertension, even in the absence of pulmonary disease. Sustained pulmonary hypertension, often associated with clinical evidence of right ventricular failure, has been observed in approximately 20% of OSA patients. It is hypothesized that

---

Box 29.1 Possible Consequences of Sleep Apnea

Pulmonary hypertension
Systemic hypertension
Cardiac dysrhythmias
Right or left ventricular failure
Right ventricular hypertrophy
Myocardial infarction (increased risk of)
Stroke (increased risk of)
Nocturnal angina
Chronic obstructive pulmonary disorder (exacerbation of)
Insulin resistance
Endothelial cell dysfunction

repetitive hypoxemia during sleep may lead to vascular remodeling in susceptible patients and thus cause pulmonary hypertension during the day. In addition, because the patient with OSA is often obese or has pathologic lung function resulting in abnormalities of daytime arterial blood gas (ABG) values, pulmonary vasoconstriction is another mechanism inducing pulmonary hypertension.

EPIDEMIOLOGY AND CAUSES

Sleep apnea is an extremely common clinical disorder; as such, it has major public health implications. Unrecognized and untreated OSA is estimated to be 30% in the adult male population and to be 15% in the adult female population, most of whom are in the most productive period of their lives, and this contributes to significant and disabling psychomotor deficits. An estimated 40 million Americans are chronically ill with various sleep disorders, and 38,000 cardiovascular deaths annually are directly attributable to OSA; yet the majority of Americans with sleep disorders remain undiagnosed and untreated. This, in turn, costs billions of dollars in accidents in the home, at the workplace, and in traffic.

Approximately 15% of women and 30% of men have significant OSA. OSA is most prevalent in men older than age 50 and in postmenopausal women; in this latter group, OSA may be related to hormonal changes. OSA occurs in younger people as well. In general, men usually have a significantly higher pharyngeal and supraglottic resistance than women, which makes them more susceptible to pharyngeal collapse and OSA and may contribute to the male predominance of the syndrome. Pharyngeal resistance increases with age in normal men, possibly related to greater body weight. Although it is widely believed that the risk of developing OSA increases with age in men, this assumption is far from conclusive and requires further study. Clinicians should be aware that OSA also occurs in women and that women who present with typical signs and symptoms should be referred to sleep disorder centers.

Compared with OSA, central sleep apnea syndrome is uncommon. In most sleep laboratories, patients with central sleep apnea syndrome constitute fewer than 10% of patients tested. The division between central and obstructive sleep apnea is not as clear-cut as it might appear, because many patients with central sleep apnea present with clinical features more suggestive of OSA. It is possible that in some patients upper airway occlusion triggers a central, rather than an obstructive, apnea. Support for this notion comes from the finding that some patients with central sleep apnea can be successfully treated with nasal continuous positive airway pressure (CPAP).

The cause of OSA is poorly defined but appears to be multifactorial; upper airway tract malformation, oropharyngeal muscle dysfunction, and abnormal respiratory drive may play a role. A few recognized anatomical abnormalities are associated with narrowing of the upper airway and predispose patients to OSA. Conditions associated with facial dysmorphism or mandibular abnormalities that are associated with OSA include adenotonsillar hypertrophy, choanal atresia, micrognathia (small mandible), retrognathia, macroglossia, nasal septal deviation, and craniofacial dysostosis. Micrognathia is particularly associated with OSA because a small or retropositioned mandible places the base of the tongue closer to the posterior pharyngeal wall and interferes with the efficiency of the genioglossus muscle in keeping the tongue out of the narrowed pharynx.

There is increasing evidence that sleep apnea has a familial distribution. Relatives of a person with sleep apnea have approximately twice the normal risk of having sleep apnea. Most adult patients with OSA, however, have no specific skeletal or soft-tissue lesion obstructing the upper airway, but they often have a small, congested oropharyngeal airway. Symptoms of sleep apnea are present two to six times more frequently in family members of affected patients than in a control population.

Obesity and alcohol consumption are well recognized as aggravating factors. One possible explanation for the relationship between obesity and OSA is that the upper airway is narrowed in the obese patient as a result of increased fat deposition in the pharyngeal walls. Fat in the neck plays the largest role. Neck (or collar) size is the best indicator of the presence of sleep apnea. Approximately 30% of snoring males with a collar size larger than 17 inches will have OSA. Neck size in women is less well investigated, but when it is greater than 16 inches, it increases the risk for sleep apnea. Another possible explanation for the relationship between neck size and apnea is that the obese patient often has a smaller lung volume, particularly functional residual capacity, than the nonobese patient; this, in turn, can indirectly influence upper airway size and contribute to upper airway narrowing. About 15% of patients with sleep apnea, however, are not obese. Any factor that interferes with the arousal mechanism, such as alcohol consumption, could lead to more profound and prolonged apneas. Alcohol, which reduces upper-airway muscle tone, and sedatives or hypnotics, which reduce the arousal mechanism, exacerbate OSA.

PATHOPHYSIOLOGY

Sleep is divided into two states: rapid eye movement (REM) sleep and nonrapid eye movement (NREM) sleep. NREM sleep is further divided into three stages, based on changes in the electroencephalogram (EEG) pattern:

- Normal sleep begins with stage I, which is characterized by slow eye movements, usually preceding sleep onset.

- Stage II involves further slowing of the EEG, with the presence of sleep spindles and slow eye movements.
- Stage III is manifested by low-frequency, high-amplitude delta waves with occasional sleep spindles but no slow eye movements.
- REM sleep is characterized by desynchronized, low-voltage, fast activity that occurs about every 90 minutes beginning after 1 to 2 hours of NREM sleep. The normal adult alternates between NREM sleep and REM sleep approximately every 90 minutes throughout the night.

Typically, during the lighter stages of NREM sleep, the breathing pattern is irregular because of the decrease in respiratory drive associated with the stimulatory effect of wakefulness and decreased metabolic rate associated with sleep. In the deeper stages of NREM sleep, breathing is typically very regular; however, overall ventilation is reduced compared with that during wakefulness. During REM sleep, the respiratory drive is irregular because of the transient decrease in ventilatory response to chemical and mechanical stimuli. The influence of sleep on the upper airway is similar to its effects on other skeletal muscles, resulting in a general loss of muscle tone and a reduction in tidal volume and minute volume. The sleep structure of the patient with OSA is characterized by the loss of physiological REM/NREM alternation, as well as by a deficit of REM and slow-wave sleep. This can be caused by sleep fragmentation as a result of the high number of arousals related to respiratory events.

Central Sleep Apnea

Etiologic factors of central sleep apnea are linked mainly to disturbances in the respiratory control system in the brainstem. In most cases, however, the cause of these disturbances remains unclear. Central apneas are more common in individuals who live at high altitudes, where hypoxemia induces hyperventilation with associated alkalosis. Cheyne-Stokes respiration with central apneas may also occur in the patient with congestive heart failure. Neurologic diseases affecting the brainstem may cause breathing pattern disorders in sleep. Well-known neurologic diseases, such as arteriosclerosis in the older adult, stroke, tumors, hemorrhage, head trauma, encephalitis, poliomyelitis, and other infectious diseases, may cause central apnea during sleep with no evidence of breathing pattern abnormalities during wakefulness. If the neural pathways from medullary respiratory groups to motor neurons of the ventilatory muscles are interrupted, the metabolic control of breathing may be disturbed. This may occur after cervical cordotomy.

Obstructive Sleep Apnea

The underlying pathophysiology of sleep apnea is complex and not fully understood. However, it is generally accepted that patency of the upper airway is dependent on the action of oropharyngeal dilator and abductor muscles, which are normally activated in a rhythmic fashion during inspiration. The available evidence indicates that in OSA, the site of upper airway obstruction is the pharynx and that obstruction of the pharynx during sleep is a result of an imbalance between the forces that serve to dilate the pharynx and those that promote pharyngeal closure. The upper airway is subject to collapse when the force produced by these muscles for a given cross-sectional area of the upper airway is exceeded by the negative airway pressure generated by inspiratory activity of the diaphragm and intercostal muscles. Upper airway obstruction can occur if suction pressure is too high during inspiration or if the counteracting forces of the dilating muscles are too weak.

The subsequent obstructive apnea results in progressive and sometimes profound hypoxia and hypercapnia. These apnea-associated changes in PO_2 and PCO_2 stimulate ventilation, resulting in increasing inspiratory efforts. Eventually the progressive hypoxemia and hypercapnia and/or the associated increase in inspiratory effort result in arousal of the patient. During this usually transient arousal, augmentation of upper airway dilator muscle activity occurs to an extent proportionately greater than the simultaneous augmentation of diaphragm activity. This leads to de-occlusion of the pharynx and restoration of airflow. During the subsequent brief period of ventilation, PO_2 rises and PCO_2 falls. The rapid resumption of sleep, however, results in reocclusion of the upper airway. This cycle of events may recur hundreds of times each night, triggering repeated arousals that may contribute to many of the clinical features of OSA (Fig. 29.1).

CLINICAL PRESENTATION

Subjective

The diagnosis of OSA is not difficult to make; the symptoms are typical, and the major risk factors are relatively obvious. Patients with sleep apnea have both nighttime and daytime symptoms (Box 29.2). Hypersomnolence is the single most important presenting symptom of sleep apnea and frequently identifies which patient will require and accept specific therapy.

Hypersomnolence is not tiredness, fatigue, or lassitude; it is clear-cut, uncontrollable sleepiness. It develops over a long period and is first experienced by a patient as sleep onset when attention is not demanded (e.g., when watching television, sitting in a college lecture, or waiting at a traffic light). Eventually, situations requiring more attention are affected, such as long-distance driving or quiet conversation. Daytime symptoms include a morning headache (from hypercapnia) and neuropsychological disturbances, including falling asleep while performing purposeful activities. These episodes can occur during

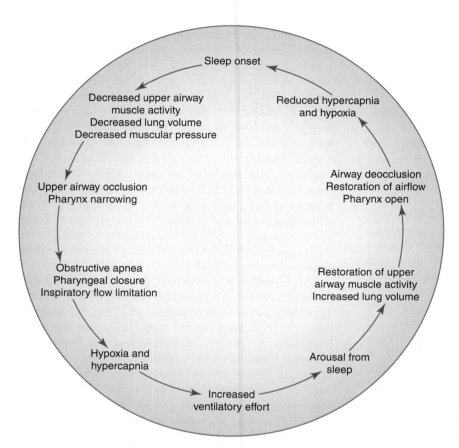

Sleep onset

Decreased upper airway
muscle activity
Decreased lung volume
Decreased muscular pressure

Reduced hypercapnia
and hypoxia

Upper airway occlusion
Pharynx narrowing

Airway deocclusion
Restoration of airflow
Pharynx open

Obstructive apnea
Pharyngeal closure
Inspiratory flow limitation

Restoration of upper
airway muscle activity
Increased lung volume

Hypoxia and
hypercapnia

Arousal from
sleep

Increased
ventilatory effort

Figure 29.1 Pathogenesis of obstructive sleep apnea.

Box 29.2   Conditions Presenting With Excessive Daytime Sleepiness

- Sleep apnea syndrome
- Narcolepsy
- Idiopathic hypersomnia
- Periodic limb movements in sleep
- Psychiatric disorders
- Drug and alcohol dependency
- Insufficient sleep syndrome
- Circadian disorders (jet lag, shift work)
- besity hypoventilation syndrome (Pickwickian syndrome)
- Hypothyroidism
- Seizure disorder
- Depression

work or social functions and can lead to embarrassment, domestic discord, decreased work productivity, loss of employment, and an increased incidence of accidents. The patient may complain of nocturnal restlessness, frequent urination or enuresis, and choking.

Often patients with hypersomnolence are conditioned to their excessive daytime sleepiness and are not aware of their symptoms. Additional history obtained from family members regarding excessive daytime sleepiness may be helpful.

Patients also may report impaired intellectual performance, such as decreased concentration, ambition, and memory loss. They may report limiting social contact because of their fear of sleepiness and falling asleep. Personality changes, such as irritability and moodiness, are seen in about 50% of patients, and more severe psychiatric disturbances such as major depression and psychosis have been reported. Sexual dysfunction is common (e.g., diminished libido, although men with apnea can obtain an erection). Persons with sleep apnea may note nocturnal palpitations or skipped heartbeats.

OSA is characterized by loud snoring that is repeatedly interrupted by episodes of complete upper airway obstruction and resolves with temporary arousal. The snoring of OSA is both loud (it can be heard in an adjacent room) and habitual (it occurs nightly). Hypoxemia and hypercarbia of varying degrees frequently accompany apnea or hypopnea. It is not uncommon for some patients to regularly desaturate to oxygen saturation levels below 70% and, occasionally, below 60%. Apneas and hypopneas often result in arousal from sleep, which then terminates the breathing disturbance and results in a surge in blood pressure. Once aroused, the CNS can respond appropriately to the partial or complete closure of the pharynx with a brief contraction of the pharyngeal dilating muscles. This restores upper airway patency and permits resumption of airflow, with subsequent reversal of the hypoxemia and hypercarbia. Arousals often last for only 1 to 3 seconds and are not recognized by the patient. Occasionally, during the arousal that terminates the apneic event, the bed partner may witness arm flailing or other gross movements.

On awakening in the morning, the patient is often completely unaware that he or she aroused several hundred times during the night. It is believed that recurrent arousals and the consequent sleep disruption are the causes of many of the daytime symptoms and effects of sleep apnea. Automobile accidents have been reported to occur 2.0 to 2.6 times more frequently among patients with OSA than among other individuals, a consequence that contributes to many unnecessary and costly days in the hospital.

Clinically, patients with central sleep apnea usually show less daytime sleepiness than do patients with other types of apnea. Sleep disruption, frequent awakening, shortness of breath after awakening, and signs of right-sided heart failure, such as peripheral edema, are frequently observed. The patient with central sleep apnea tends to have a normal body weight. Psychiatric symptoms such as depression may occur as well. As in OSA, oxygen desaturation and consequent hemodynamic disorders may be observed.

Objective

The predominant physical examination findings of OSA reflect the risk factors: obesity (particularly of the upper body), increased neck size, crowded oropharynx (tonsillar hypertrophy and enlargement of soft palate [uvula] and tongue). In addition, the patient may be hypertensive and have additional features of retrognathia and micrognathia.

DIAGNOSTIC REASONING

Diagnostic Tests

OSA should be suspected whenever hypersomnia and snoring coexist or even with new onset or poorly controlled hypertension. The recording of specific historical details from the patient and his or her spouse is crucial to the diagnosis, particularly because the patient sometimes does not realize the severity of the sleepiness. This is perhaps because he or she finds it socially unacceptable or the onset has been gradual. Initial testing may include determining how easy it is for a patient to fall asleep or, alternatively, how difficult it is for the person to remain awake. This type of testing may include both subjective and objective assessments. Two common subjective assessments of sleepiness are the Stanford Sleepiness Score (SSS) and the Epworth Sleepiness Scale (ESS). The SSS is used to record the degree of sleepiness experienced by a patient at a given time and does not necessarily relate to his or her overall

propensity to fall asleep. It is an introspective measure of sleepiness where the patient rates his or her alertness on a 7-point scale at different times during the day. If the score falls below a 3 when he or she should be feeling alert, a serious sleep deficit exists. The ESS measures sleepiness as a reflection of a patient's tendency to fall asleep during eight specific nonstimulating situations. Each situation is scored from 0 to 3. A total score of 10 is considered abnormal.

The definitive test for sleep apnea is an overnight polysomnogram. This all-night recording of the patient's sleep, performed in a sleep center, is the gold standard for identifying the presence, type, and severity of sleep apnea. Limitations of the test include its availability and its cost. Because the test must be performed in a specialized sleep centers, it may not be available to every patient. It is also expensive. The polysomnograph is a multichannel recorder that records the patient's eye movements, airflow, respiratory movements, leg movements, EEG readings, pulse oximetry, electrocardiograph (ECG) readings, and snoring. From such records, apneas, hypopneas, and snoring-related arousals are scored. The RDI is calculated from the number of apneas and hypopneas per hour added to the number of snoring-related arousals per hour. Recently, multichannel devices that record a limited number of parameters (e.g., respiratory movements, airflow, snoring, pulse oximetry, and ECG) have been introduced for home studies, which may be comparable to a full polysomnogram. However, the home sleep tests do not record actual sleep, only respiratory events; furthermore, the home sleep tests are often unattended and may be associated with loss of signal quality. Therefore, if a high clinical suspicion exists for sleep apnea, an attended sleep test (polysomnogram) should be considered even after a negative home sleep test.

The development of large numbers of limited diagnostic systems in recent years represents recognition of the logistical problems involved in gaining access to large sleep centers. Unfortunately, there is no uniformity among these devices, and the only consistent variable common to all such systems is the oxygen saturation level. Most offer some measure of respiration, based either on nasal flow or chest bands. In the patient with OSA, the polysomnogram demonstrates frequent episodes of apnea with corresponding periods of oxygen desaturation as demonstrated by pulse oximetry. The effort to breathe remains intact during the periods of OSA, as evidenced by the movement of the lower chest and abdomen.

If the polysomnogram is negative for OSA in the patient with significant daytime sleepiness, a multiple sleep latency test (MSLT) should be performed in a sleep center to evaluate for other disorders of hypersomnia, including narcolepsy and idiopathic hypersomnia. The MSLT is performed the day after the polysomnogram. The patient should not to take any medications such as sedatives and certain antidepressants for 2 weeks before the test. On the day of the test, the patient is instructed to take five 20-minute naps 2 hours apart. Healthy subjects have a sleep latency of greater than 7 minutes in the MSLT. A test is considered consistent with excessive daytime sleepiness if sleep onset occurs within 7 minutes. The presence of two sleep-onset REM episodes in the appropriate clinical setting is diagnostic of narcolepsy.

The syndrome of periodic limb movements (PLMs; also known as nocturnal myoclonus or periodic leg movements) consists of stereotypic periodic leg (or arm) movements during sleep that may or may not be associated with arousals. If enough arousals occur, sleep may be so fragmented that daytime sleepiness results. Because patients with narcolepsy frequently have PLMs, any patient with excessive daytime sleepiness and PLMs on a polysomnogram should be questioned carefully concerning narcoleptic manifestations.

An otolaryngological examination should be performed. In addition, screening with a home nocturnal pulse oximetry has a high negative predictive value if no desaturations are seen. Erythrocytosis is common. A hemoglobin level and thyroid function tests should also be performed.

Differential Diagnosis

Many disorders present with excessive daytime sleepiness (see Box 29.2). Drug addiction and depression can masquerade as sleep apnea, especially in the older adult patient. Certain diagnostic tests, such as ABGs, thyroid function testing, PFTs, ECG, and chest x-ray examination, may be indicated to determine the potential cause, presence, or severity of signs of hypoxic exposure occurring as the result of repetitive apneas during sleep. A recording of the patient's usual amount and pattern of sleep may be instructive.

MANAGEMENT

Obstructive Sleep Apnea

Currently, the treatments for OSA include the following:

- General measures: avoidance of alcohol, sedatives, narcotic pain medications, hypnotics; weight loss; and positional therapy to avoid the supine position
- Specific measures: position therapy, positive airway pressure (PAP), and oral appliances
- Surgical management: upper airway surgery may be considered as a treatment option in certain patient groups such as in children with OSA (adenotonsillectomy is often preferred over CPAP) and in adults intolerant to CPAP; however, surgical options for treating OSA in adults often have only about a 50% success rate and may need to be staged in multiple surgeries (from uvulopalatopharyngoplasty [UPPP] to mandibular advancement)

PAP can be delivered in three modes:

1. CPAP, which delivers PAP at a fixed rate during the respiratory cycle
2. Bilevel PAP (BPAP), which delivers PAP that is greater during the inspiratory cycle (explained in more detail later in the chapter)
3. Autotitrating PAP (APAP), which delivers PAP at fluctuating rates depending on the patient's breathing patterns

Although CPAP is the preferred method for treatment of OSA, BPAP or APAP may be considered in persons who for whatever reason cannot tolerate the CPAP machine. Note that supplemental oxygen is not routinely indicated for sleep apnea but is occasionally prescribed to treat hypoxia in patients who cannot tolerate CPAP or who remain hypoxic even with CPAP therapy. Nasal dilators have no role in the treatment of sleep apnea.

OSA and its treatment are highly dependent on patient behavior. Clinicians have both an opportunity and a responsibility to advise patients of the profound influence that their behavior can have on disease severity and outcome. For patients who cannot tolerate medical treatment or who do not desire long-term medical therapy, surgical treatment of sleep apnea should be considered.

Elimination of Risk Factors

A reasonable first step in the management of the patient with sleep-disordered breathing is to identify and subsequently eliminate the risk factors. The adverse effects of alcohol on upper airway stability during sleep and the arousal response to chemical stimuli mandate that the patient with OSA be instructed to abstain from alcohol. Although not invariably associated with OSA, obesity is usually present in this patient population. Weight reduction may result in significant improvement in OSA and sleep quality and obviate the need for further therapeutic interventions. Efforts in this regard represent a major, lifelong therapeutic challenge, best approached by using the multidisciplinary resources of the physician, nutritionist, psychologist, and a peer support system. It is difficult to accomplish and maintain weight loss, but it is very beneficial to patients with sleep apnea when they do so. Benefits of weight loss in obese patients with sleep apnea include reduced RDI, reduced blood pressure, and optimal CPAP pressure; improved pulmonary function, daytime ABGs, polycythemia, sleep structure, and oxygen saturation; elimination of snoring; and prevention of relapse after surgical treatment.

The relationship between sleep in the supine position and augmentation of snoring and sleep apnea in some patients is apparent. It has been hypothesized that the effects of gravity in promoting posterior movement of the tongue with apposition against the posterior pharyngeal wall are magnified in the supine position. Although manipulation of the sleeping position is not an effective therapy for the majority of patients with sleep-disordered breathing, it may be all that is needed in selected patients. It has been suggested that there may be a decreased incidence of sleep-disordered breathing events during sleep in the lateral decubitus position. Position therapy can be accomplished by sewing pockets for one or two tennis balls in the back of patients' sleeping attire to prevent them from assuming the supine position. Commercially available devices to facilitate sleeping in the nonsupine position exist. Devices to train people to sleep in the lateral position have been described.

Devices That Maintain Upper Airway Patency

CPAP administered through a nasal mask has become the most common treatment for OSA. Nasal CPAP also effectively reduces or eliminates mixed apneas, including both the central and obstructive components. A continuous flow of air is delivered from a blower unit to a tightly fitting nasal mask held in place by head straps. Nasal CPAP acts as a pneumatic splint preventing collapse of the upper airway in all phases of respiration. The device is used for the entire sleep period every night. The optimal CPAP pressure is determined by technologists during polysomnography. Typically, 5 to 20 cm H_2O is the pressure needed to abolish apneas, snoring, and oxyhemoglobin desaturations in all positions and during REM sleep. Although CPAP use is associated with few serious complications, it does elicit patient complaints. Minor adverse effects of CPAP include feelings of suffocation, nasal drying or rhinitis, ear pain, difficulty in exhaling, mask and mouth leaks, chest and back pain, and conjunctivitis. Most of these can be alleviated.

Newer automatic CPAP devices continuously adjust the positive pressure to the required levels. In the automatic CPAP mode, the positive pressure is maintained as long as ventilation remains stable; however, any respiratory disorder results in a progressive increase in pressure. If a breathing disturbance has not occurred for more than 4 minutes, the positive pressure decreases again.

For many patients who use it regularly, CPAP dramatically eliminates apneas and hypopneas, improves sleep architecture, and reduces daytime sleepiness, even for those with mild sleep apnea. The effectiveness of CPAP is limited, however, by incomplete patient compliance. About 25% of patients prescribed CPAP will not be compliant. Factors that help to improve CPAP compliance include patient education and regular follow-up with the health-care provider. CPAP is the only therapy for OSA that improves life expectancy and outcomes of hypertension and heart failure.

Oral Appliances

Oral appliances are an effective noninvasive alternative to CPAP in patients with mild to moderate sleep apnea. Although oral appliances are effective in some patients with OSA, they are not universally effective. There are major design differences in the numerous oral appliances that are now available, and this may have an impact on

their success and compliance rates. A novel anterior mandibular positioner has been developed with an adjustable hinge that allows progressive advancement of the mandible. This appliance may be an effective first-line treatment for the patient with mild to moderate OSA and may be associated with greater patient satisfaction than CPAP. For these devices to treat sleep apnea effectively, the mandible should be advanced to 50% to 75% of the maximal forward protrusion of the jaw. In most patients, dental appliances lessen but do not abolish OSA and snoring. In many patients treated with an oral appliance, the RDI remains high, with more than 20 events per hour after treatment. The side effects of oral appliances include excessive salivation, dental misalignment, and pain in, or damage to, the temporomandibular joint. To assess the efficacy of the oral appliance, a follow-up sleep test is useful to determine whether further forward advancement of the mandible would be helpful.

Surgical Management

Surgery for OSA is designed either to bypass the obstructing region of the upper airway or to modify the upper airway in a way that makes loss of patency less likely. Because upper airway obstruction is associated with a wide variety of structural aberrations, including nasal deformity, nasal polyps, hypertrophic tonsils and/or adenoids, craniofacial disproportion, and neoplasms, as well as with no detectable anatomical abnormalities, many different surgical procedures have been used in OSA patients.

Extensive excision of soft tissue in the oropharynx, termed *uvulopalatopharyngoplasty* (UPPP), was developed to improve pharyngeal function during sleep. The procedure involves a bilateral tonsillectomy and a submucosal resection of redundant tissue. A variable portion of the posterior margin of the soft palate and the uvula is also removed, and the palatopharyngeus muscle may also be resected. In the absence of weight gain or other confounding factors, a success rate of 50% has been sustained for at least 1 year postoperatively. However, even OSA patients in whom UPPP fails to resolve OSA often have substantial reduction in snoring after surgery, despite persistent apnea. A repeat polysomnogram is necessary to assess the therapeutic outcome of surgery. The success rate in patients undergoing UPPP appears to be partly related to the location of the obstructing tissue. Patients with retropalatal obstruction removal experience better results than those with retroglossal obstruction removal. The preoperative presence of tonsils has been associated with improved success of UPPP.

The patient undergoing surgical reconstruction of the airway for OSA, such as UPPP, often has coexisting medical problems, especially cardiovascular disease, which can complicate treatment. The uncertainty regarding the proper predictive parameters for surgical success greatly limits optimal patient selection. Further, a significant number of patients have difficulty at induction and intubation for general anesthesia. Men with increased neck circumference and associated skeletal deformities should be evaluated carefully and considered for fiber-optic intubation.

Laser-assisted uvulopalatoplasty is a procedure to treat snoring in the outpatient setting. The procedure entails reshaping the palate and tonsillar pillars in one to seven serial sessions under local anesthesia. Each session lasts approximately 15 minutes and is generally well tolerated; the incidence of complications is low. The procedure is successful in reducing snoring in 90% of patients. However, the success rate in patients with OSA is not yet clear.

A variety of maxillofacial and nasal surgical procedures may be performed to normalize the bony relationships of the maxilla and mandible to minimize the likelihood of airway collapse during sleep. Many of these procedures are preceded by UPPP, and if the results are unsatisfactory, a second stage involving mandibular advancement is undertaken. These procedures require a great deal of surgical and orthodontic expertise, along with careful consultation with anesthesia services and pulmonary medicine.

Nasal surgery has been performed on patients with OSA in an effort to reduce the predisposition to collapse during sleep. A nasal septoplasty is performed if gross nasal septal deformity is present. The definitive therapy is a tracheostomy. Because of the drastic nature of this procedure, it is limited to patients with life-threatening arrhythmias or severe disability who have not responded to conservative therapy.

A novel upper airway muscle stimulator has recently been approved in the United States for moderate to severe OSA intolerant to CPAP. A surgically implanted stimulator sends electrical signals to activate the genioglossus muscle (tongue) that are synchronized to respiratory activity as sensed by electrical signals from diaphragmatic muscle activation.

Central Sleep Apnea

Medical treatment may be ineffective in the patient with central sleep apnea. Some patients with central sleep apnea do respond to CPAP therapy. Implantation of a diaphragm-pacing device is an option, the efficacy of which has not been proven by long-term clinical trials. Diaphragm pacing may precipitate upper airway occlusion during sleep due to dyssynchrony between activation of the diaphragm and the upper airway and laryngeal dilators. Thus, tracheostomy is often performed concomitantly with diaphragm pacing. These difficulties, in conjunction with the resource-intensive nature of the procedure and subsequent care, have made this technique one that is infrequently employed in the clinical setting of central sleep apnea.

The use of a timed BPAP device may normalize blood gases during sleep. The BPAP prevents development of severe pulmonary artery hypertension during sleep. BPAP delivers a higher airway pressure during inspiration (when the airway is most likely to be occluded) and a lower airway pressure during expiration (patient exhales against less resistance). Cardiac dysrhythmias may decrease significantly. Improvement of the respiratory situation and of the hemodynamics using a timed BPAP device may reduce the mortality rate in these patients. Bilevel systems are more expensive than conventional CPAP systems, however, and the algorithms to adjust the inspiratory and expiratory pressures are essentially empiric. Consequently, bilevel systems are typically reserved for patients who cannot tolerate CPAP, especially for those who experience difficulties with exhalation or chest pain as a result of the hyperinflation produced by the applied positive pressure.

FOLLOW-UP AND REFERRAL

In recent years, chronic obstructive pulmonary disorder (COPD) and sleep apnea syndrome have been found to coexist in many patients, placing them at increased risk of respiratory insufficiency. The detection of small airway disease may be difficult in OSA patients because this syndrome is associated with various pulmonary function abnormalities resulting from obesity and upper airway obstruction. Both of these factors can be responsible for airway obstruction. Patients with both disorders frequently have marked hypoxemia, hypercapnia, and pulmonary hypertension, so they should be referred for investigation of both COPD and sleep apnea. The patient with this "overlap syndrome" is at a higher risk of developing respiratory insufficiency and pulmonary hypertension than the patient with "pure" OSA. Finally, hypoxemic stress is placed on the coronary circulation during sleep that may contribute to nocturnal mortality in the patient with COPD.

Patient Education: CPAP Use

Because CPAP is a safe and effective treatment of OSA, it is important to improve patient compliance with regular CPAP use. Only 75% of patients continue to use CPAP after 1 year, citing the noise, interference with positioning, and complaints of bed partners. Systematically collected data on family members' learning needs and descriptions of the psychosocial impact of CPAP technology treatments on family function and quality of life are essential to developing a comprehensive protocol for teaching and counseling for CPAP therapy. The effect of group patient education sessions on compliance with CPAP therapy has proved to be a simple and effective means of improving treatment of OSA. Nasal discomfort and lack of perceived benefit are possible characteristics of patients with poor compliance; these patients might benefit from education sessions and emotional support. The personal contact and teaching, along with interaction with other OSA patients, may provide an atmosphere of encouragement and support.

Counseling may be needed concerning the potential loss of employment because of poor performance or poor decision making related to profound fatigue from sleep deprivation. Problems of depression, extreme sleepiness, and the effects of hypoxia on cognition pose special difficulties for teaching these patients;

their family members must be educated. Family problem-solving skills for managing equipment, overcoming psychosocial barriers to regular nightly use, and eliminating the physiological side effects of CPAP such as oral dryness are important skills and knowledge for this patient population. Home follow-up programs could help patients to eliminate reported physiological adverse effects of CPAP treatments, monitor cardiac stability, and provide ongoing education and family function assessment as evidenced in other follow-up programs. A follow-up program would be cost-effective when quality of life is considered or compared with hospital admissions for traffic accidents or the severe cardiovascular sequelae associated with OSA.

Teaching must include nutrition counseling. Weight loss may be curative, but because 10% to 20% of body weight loss is required, many patients give up. Strict avoidance of alcohol and hypnotic medications must also be stressed. One of the developmental objectives from *Healthy People 2020* is to reduce the proportion of vehicular crashes caused by persons with excessive sleepiness. Educating patients to take corrective action is an important role of the health-care provider.

REFERENCES

American Academy of Sleep Medicine. *International Classification of Sleep Disorders.* 3rd ed. Darien, IL: American Academy of Sleep Medicine; 2014.

Epstein LJ, Kristo D, Strollo PJ Jr, et al. Clinical guideline for the evaluation, management and long-term care of obstructive sleep apnea in adults. *J Clin Sleep Med.* 2009;5(3):263–276.

Kryger MH, Roth T, Dement WC. *Principles and practice of sleep medicine.* 6th ed. Philadelphia, PA: Elsevier; 2016.

RESOURCES

American Sleep Apnea Association
   http://www.sleepapnea.org
American Sleep Association
   http://www.americansleepassociation.org
National Sleep Foundation
   http://sleepfoundation.org

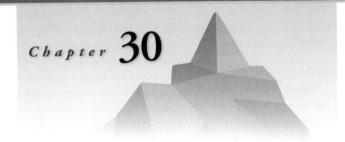

Chapter **30**

Infectious Respiratory Disorders

Jill E. Winland-Brown, EdD, APRN, FNP-BC

Brian Oscar Porter, MD, PhD, MPH, MBA

UPPER RESPIRATORY INFECTIONS

Upper respiratory infections (URIs) include some of the most common infectious diseases and account for millions of visits to health-care providers annually. Most URIs are caused by viruses. Bacteria cause about 25% of the cases. For the average adult, URIs are a source of discomfort, disability, and loss of productivity. For young children, the immunocompromised, and older adults,

these infections may be a cause of morbidity and serious illnesses. In children and older adults, as well as adults with underlying respiratory diseases, viral URIs are frequently complicated by bacterial superinfection.

EPIDEMIOLOGY AND CAUSES

Influenza ("the flu"), the common cold (viral rhinitis or acute coryza), and acute laryngitis are some of the more frequently occurring URIs that the practitioner will need to manage. Children younger than age 5 years are the most commonly affected. On average, children have approximately three to eight URIs per year, adolescents and adults two to four per year, and persons older than age 65 years have fewer than one URI per year. Most URIs are viral in origin with the most common agents being rhinoviruses, coronaviruses, adenoviruses, and Coxsackie viruses. For URIs caused by bacteria, the agents are similar to those causing otitis media. In decreasing order, they include *Streptococcus pneumoniae, Haemophilus influenzae, Moraxella catarrhalis,* and *Staphylococcus aureus.* Infections such as acute epiglottitis and respiratory syncytial virus (RSV) infection occur predominantly in infants and younger children but may occur as a life-threatening infection in adults. RSV infection can cause severe pneumonia and lower respiratory tract disease in older institutionalized adults and adults with suppressed immune status. Acute epiglottitis, a bacterial infection, can result in complete or partial airway obstruction (Box 30.1).

Influenza epidemics occur each year in the United States, with typically 5,000 to 250,000 cases annually. In some years with more severe outbreaks, as many as 40,000 deaths have occurred. Most of these deaths occur in older persons, particularly those with underlying pulmonary or cardiac disease. Infants and very young children also appear to be at greater risk for influenza-associated morbidity and mortality. Although influenza and colds may occur at any time, most cases occur during the winter and spring months. Acute laryngitis is generally associated with a viral URI and often persists for a week or more after other symptoms have cleared. The incubation period for most viral URIs is 1 to 4 days.

Box 30.1   Acute Epiglottitis

Acute epiglottitis is a life-threatening, rapidly progressive cellulitis of the epiglottis that may cause complete airway obstruction. Epiglottitis begins as a cellulitis between the tongue base and the epiglottis; the epiglottis is then pushed posteriorly. The epiglottis becomes swollen and threatens airway patency. Epiglottitis is more common and more severe in young children, but it may occur in older children and adults.

Clinical Manifestations

Epiglottitis in adults should be suspected when odynophagia (pain on swallowing) seems severe compared with pharyngeal findings. Other findings include dyspnea, drooling, and stridor.

Diagnostic Reasoning

Direct viewing of the epiglottis with a tongue blade and lighting should never be attempted because immediate laryngospasm and airway obstruction may result. It is recommended that children and adults be transported to the operating room (OR) while sitting up for visualization of the epiglottis with a fiberoptic laryngoscope, with preparations made for immediate airway control. The epiglottis will appear swollen and erythematous ("cherry red"), and an uncuffed endotracheal tube should be inserted.

Management

Acute epiglottitis requires emergency care for adequate airway control. No painful or stressful procedures should be performed on these patients unless preparations are in place for a planned intubation, such as in the OR.

The patient with epiglottitis will require hospitalization for IV antibiotics such as cefuroxime (Ceftin), ceftriaxone (Rocephin), or ampicillin/sulbactam (Unasyn). Dexamethasone (Decadron) should also be administered IV and tapered as signs and symptoms resolve. Continuous pulse oximetry and careful monitoring of the patient's airway are critical. Patients who develop hypoxemia and respiratory distress will require intubation.

Community-acquired respiratory tract infections caused by *Streptococcus* account for more than 20 million primary-care practitioner visits annually and are a major reason for work and school absenteeism.

PATHOPHYSIOLOGY

The common cold (coryza) is caused by viruses spread through direct inhalation of airborne droplet sprays aerosolized by the infected person while speaking, coughing, or sneezing, as well as hand-to-face transmission after handling fomites serving as reservoirs of infection. Hand-to-hand transmission, however, is probably the most common mode of transmission in adults, underscoring the importance of frequent hand washing in the prevention of new cases. Numerous serotypes of rhinoviruses, adenoviruses, coronaviruses, Coxsackie viruses, and parainfluenza viruses are associated with the common cold. The ability of these viruses to mutate readily ensures their ability to consistently evade host immune mechanisms. The number of rhinovirus serotypes, for instance, currently stands at more than 100. Following infection, individuals develop immunity to a specific viral strain but are susceptible to repeated infection by the same parent virus that has undergone only minor changes in surface proteins or polysaccharides.

Symptoms of congestion, rhinorrhea, and sneezing result directly from inflammation and edema of upper airway mucosal surfaces. The cough reflex may be triggered by this same mucosal inflammation in the posterior pharynx. After acute infection, postviral cough may persist for as long as 6 to 8 weeks due to postnasal drip—the persistent drainage of thin mucus into the posterior pharynx resulting in direct pharyngeal irritation.

Classic flu is caused by the orthomyxovirus influenza type A and, to a lesser extent, influenza type B. Both are enveloped RNA-based viruses. In addition to the viral rhinitis symptoms of the common cold, influenza infection causes generalized muscle aches and pains, fatigue, significant fever, and rigors (chills). Influenza infection may lead to viral pneumonia (lower airway infection), which may be further complicated by bacterial superinfection, particularly with *S. aureus*. These additional manifestations and high potential for complicated disease underscore the importance of widespread yearly vaccination against influenza.

The influenza virus frequently undergoes mutation of its major surface proteins, hemagglutinin and neuraminidase, which renders protein-specific host antibody defenses ineffective. Each year, a vaccine is developed using influenza proteins from the most likely serotype combination predicted to cause widespread infection for that year. The vaccine determination is made using complex disease modeling algorithms based on extensive Centers for Disease Control and Prevention (CDC) and World Health Organization (WHO) epidemiologic data. However, despite these data, the compilation of each yearly vaccine is a "best guess" that may or may not provide adequate protection against that year's primary strain. In addition, other strains of the virus not covered by the vaccine may also cause numerous infections in any given year.

Given concerns in recent years for the potential spread of other forms of influenza, including H5N1 influenza (avian or bird flu) and H1N1 influenza (swine flu), significant efforts are also being directed toward developing safe and effective vaccines against these forms of the disease. Throughout history, the most widespread and devastating flu-related pandemics have been traced back primarily to these novel forms of the virus (in particular, avian flu). On an annual basis, however, classic influenza results in far greater morbidity and mortality each year than these other forms. For the past 40 years, widespread pandemics of avian flu and H1N1 influenza have largely been avoided through multinational public health measures. Clinical trials are underway with an oral influenza vaccine tablet, although the long-term effects of this drug are not known.

Most cases of laryngitis (inflammation of the vocal cords with extreme hoarseness and temporary voice loss) and croup (any combination of laryngotracheobronchitis with edema leading to airway obstruction with characteristic stridor) are caused by parainfluenza virus, RSV, influenza virus, coxsackievirus, rhinovirus, and adenovirus. Laryngitis may also be caused by group A beta-hemolytic *Streptococcus pyogenes*, *H. influenzae*, and *M. catarrhalis*. These same viral and bacterial agents, along with *Neisseria gonorrhoeae* and Epstein-Barr virus (causing infectious mononucleosis), are also common causes of pharyngitis (see full discussion in Chapter 23).

RSV and influenza A (and less so influenza B) are the most common causes of bronchiolitis in children and adolescents, but adults tend to experience infection in the larger airways (i.e., acute bronchitis). Since the advent of widespread vaccination against *H. influenzae* type B (Hib vaccine) and *Corynebacterium diphtheriae* (DTaP vaccine), epiglottitis occurs only rarely in the United States (see Box 30.1). Bacterial tracheitis is a serious purulent infection of the subglottic trachea caused primarily by *S. aureus*, with a toxic clinical presentation requiring hospitalization and IV antibiotic therapy.

CLINICAL PRESENTATION

The onset of influenza is usually abrupt, with fever, chills, malaise, myalgia, headache, nasal stuffiness, sore throat, and sometimes nausea. A nonproductive cough is usually present and occurs early in the course of illness. The fever may be as high as 103°F (39.4°C) in adults and typically lasts 3 to 5 days. Subjective findings with the common cold include headache, myalgia, nasal congestion,

watery rhinorrhea, sneezing, foul breath, and a "scratchy throat." Laryngitis results in inflammation of the laryngeal mucosa and vocal cords. Symptoms include hoarseness, aphonia, and, occasionally, pain when swallowing. Physical findings in cases of URIs are usually minimal, with normal chest auscultation. Cervical lymphadenopathy may be present.

DIAGNOSTIC REASONING

Diagnostic Tests

Diagnosis of influenza tends to be more accurate during epidemics. A successful presumptive diagnosis requires appropriate symptoms at the right time of the year and knowledge of patterns of influenzal illnesses around the world. If necessary, the diagnosis can be confirmed via virology studies (e.g., nasal and pharyngeal cultures, cells from nasopharyngeal washings stained with monoclonal antibody fluorescence stains, and complement fixation studies on paired serum samples). Diagnosis of colds and laryngitis is typically based on the subjective presentation of the patient except when the etiologic agent in laryngitis is thought to be bacterial. In these situations, the practitioner should perform a throat culture to rule out group A beta-hemolytic streptococcal infection. Rapid strep tests have greater than 70% sensitivity and greater than 90% specificity. Leukocytosis found on a complete blood count (CBC) with differential may help diagnose a bacterial infection.

Differential Diagnosis

Conditions that need to be ruled out include allergic rhinitis, group A streptococcal pharyngitis, bacterial sinusitis, atypical *Mycoplasma* pneumonia, infectious mononucleosis, and possibly mumps, rubeola, and cytomegalovirus [CMV]. Close attention to epidemiologic patterns (e.g., current outbreak in the community) is important. The CDC or local health department can be helpful in determining the type of disease outbreak.

MANAGEMENT

Management of influenza and the common cold is generally symptomatic and is directed toward the relief of symptoms and prevention of secondary infections. Antibiotics are not indicated for influenza or common colds unless a secondary bacterial infection occurs. Mucopurulent rhinitis frequently accompanies the common cold and is not an indication for antimicrobial treatment. Although antibiotics are often viewed by the layperson as a necessary treatment for a cold or the flu, these drugs have no effect on viruses and if taken injudiciously may produce resistant organisms. In the past, clinicians ordered antibiotics in about half of all URI cases, which is thought to have contributed to the current antimicrobial-resistant crisis. Health-care providers continue to prescribe antibiotics in 50% or more of the time to adults and children with viral infections. Although most cases of acute rhinosinusitis (including bacterial sinusitis) resolve without antibiotics, if symptoms persist longer than 10 days, antibiotic therapy should be considered for 5 to 7 days.

Generally, most patients with influenza should rest at home until symptoms decrease in severity. The older patient or the patient with an underlying chronic illness may require hospitalization for influenza. In addition to rest and fluids, antipyretics and analgesics are recommended. Cough suppressants with codeine may be necessary for adequate cough control.

If the practitioner is reasonably confident that the virus in question is type A influenza, the patient may benefit from an antiviral drug. Widespread amantadine (Symmetrel) and rimantadine (Flumadine) resistance among influenza A virus strains has made this class of medications less useful clinically. Therefore, amantadine and rimantadine are not recommended for antiviral treatment or chemoprophylaxis of currently circulating influenza A virus strains. The majority of currently circulating influenza viruses are susceptible to the neuraminidase inhibitor antiviral medications oseltamivir (Tamiflu) and zanamivir (Relenza). Antiviral treatment is recommended as early as possible (within 48 hours of symptom presentation) for patients with confirmed or suspected influenza who have severe, complicated, or progressive illness; who require hospitalization; or who pose a risk for influenza-related complications, including pregnant women. Oseltamivir, either as a pill and in liquid form, is approved for the treatment of influenza in persons aged 2 weeks and older and for chemoprophylaxis to prevent influenza in patients 1 year of age and older. Zanamivir, given as a powder that is inhaled, is approved to treat flu in people aged 7 years and older and to prevent influenza in patients aged 5 years and older. Zanamivir is not recommended for persons with respiratory problems, such as asthma or chronic obstructive pulmonary disease (COPD). Both medications are usually prescribed for 5 days for individuals in a primary-care setting, although people hospitalized with the flu may need the medication for longer than 5 days. These medications should not be used in place of getting an annual flu vaccination, however, which is currently recommended for all individuals aged 6 months and older without contraindications (e.g., severe allergic reaction to any component of the vaccine).

Rest, fluids, and antipyretics are also useful in controlling the discomfort associated with a cold. Decongestants such as pseudoephedrine (e.g., Sudafed) are widely used and may help control rhinorrhea and nasal congestion. These medications should be used only for 3 days due to rebound effects and should not be used in the presence of hypertension. Nasal sprays such as phenylephrine (Neo-Synephrine) and oxymetazoline (Afrin) or ocular vasoconstrictor formulations of oxymetazoline (OcuClear, Visine LR) are rapidly effective. Patients should be cautioned to use them only for a few days, however, because chronic use leads to rebound congestion. Intranasal ipratropium (Atrovent) has also been approved for significant rhinorrhea associated with URIs. Nasal saline rinses and/or intranasal corticosteroids may also be considered. Vitamin C and zinc lozenges with echinacea are currently popular alternative treatments that are sold as over-the-counter therapies. Despite numerous randomized trials, the evidence of effectiveness of zinc lozenges in reducing the duration of colds is lacking. The efficacy of vitamin C supplements to decrease the incidence of colds or to shorten their duration has also not been demonstrated. An exception may be for the patient who has a possible vitamin C deficiency. Several small studies have shown that black elderberry syrup shortens the duration of flu-like illnesses by up to 4 days.

Treatment of laryngitis includes complete voice rest, steam inhalations, codeine or nonnarcotic cough suppressants for cough and pain, and a liquid or soft diet. If throat cultures are positive for group A beta-hemolytic *Streptococcus*, penicillin should be prescribed if the patient is not penicillin allergic. Erythromycin should be used for infections associated with *M. catarrhalis* or *H. influenzae*. For particularly toxic bacterial infections such as bacterial tracheitis, blood cultures may be appropriate to rule out bacteremia.

For the management of croup, racemic epinephrine and dexamethasone are indicated, and intubation may be needed in severe cases. Bacterial tracheitis requires IV antibiotic therapy with nafcillin or an appropriate cephalosporin, or, if methicillin-resistant *S. aureus* (MRSA) is suspected, vancomycin or linezolid. Because of impaired oral intake, all such infections other than the common cold may lead to dehydration requiring oral or IV rehydration therapy. In addition, hypoxemia based on pulse oximetry or blood gas analysis should be addressed with supplemental oxygen therapy. Bronchodilator therapy is often used as well, but randomized clinical trials do not consistently demonstrate its efficacy.

FOLLOW-UP AND REFERRAL

The duration of an uncomplicated case of influenza is 1 to 7 days; the prognosis is excellent. However, complications can occur, including acute sinusitis, otitis media, purulent bronchitis, and pneumonia. Influenza causes necrosis of some respiratory epithelium, predisposing the infected person to secondary bacterial infections. The interaction between bacteria and influenza is bidirectional, with bacterial enzymes activating influenza viruses. If a fever persists for more than 4 days, the white blood cell count rises to 12,000 cells/mcL or higher, or the cough becomes productive, bacterial infection should be ruled out or verified and treated.

The most common complication of influenza is pneumonia; most fatalities result from bacterial pneumonia. The patient with influenza with superimposed bacterial pneumonia may experience gradual improvement of symptoms for 2 to 3 days and then develop cough and purulent sputum. Pneumococcal pneumonia is the most common bacterial pneumonia associated with influenza, but staphylococcal pneumonia is the most serious. Primary viral influenza pneumonia is the least common but has a high mortality rate among pregnant women and patients with rheumatic heart disease. The patient develops symptoms of influenza that become increasingly severe. Respiratory distress is often sufficient to require mechanical ventilation.

Most cases of the common cold and laryngitis are self-limiting. Complications of a cold may include pharyngitis, sinusitis, otitis media, tonsillitis, and chest infections. Unless symptoms of these complications are present, antibiotic therapy is not indicated. The patient with laryngitis needs to maintain voice rest until hoarseness and aphonia have resided. Any vigorous use of the voice such as shouting or singing may foster the formation of vocal cord nodules.

Patient Education: Upper Respiratory Infections

There currently is no immunization for the prevention of colds. Research has demonstrated that the best method of preventing transmission of infected droplets is through frequent hand washing, particularly in day-care facilities and congregate adult living facilities. During the cold and influenza seasons, the person with a chronic illness or compromised immune status should be advised to avoid crowded settings and other persons who have obvious symptoms.

The Advisory Committee on Immunization Practices (ACIP) currently recommends an annual vaccination for all persons older than age 6 months. Trivalent influenza vaccine provides partial immunity (in approximately 86% of patients vaccinated) for a few months to 1 year. The vaccine's antigenic configuration changes yearly. It is based on the prevalent strains of the previous year, the viruses that are currently being seen in other parts of the world during the current year, and the estimated antibody response in persons previously infected with or vaccinated against these viruses. Vaccination in October or November of each year is recommended for all persons older than 6 months and particularly for those aged 65 years and older; nursing home residents; adults and children with underlying medical conditions, including cardiac, pulmonary, malignant, and some metabolic diseases; health-care workers; and pregnant women. High-risk children have a particularly low influenza vaccination rate annually, which is of significant

concern. Vaccination is also encouraged for the members of large groups who may be the principal vectors of influenza transmission in their communities such as schoolchildren, children in day care, college students, military personnel, and employees of large companies. Low-income minority populations typically have lower vaccination rates than other populations. Medicare covers the cost of influenza and pneumococcal vaccination. Recent research has shown that obtaining yearly influenza vaccination can be influenced by the health-care provider's recommendations and phone calls offering encouragement and reminders. *Healthy People 2020* set a goal of vaccinating 80% of noninstitutionalized adults aged 18 to 64 years annually; currently more than 40% receive the annual flu vaccine. More than 60% of individuals over age 65 received the vaccine in 2015. *Healthy People 2020* has also set a goal of vaccinating 90% of high-risk adults aged 18 to 64 years; currently 39% of this population receives the annual flu vaccine. For adults aged 65 years and older, the 2020 goal of annual vaccination is 90% (currently 67%). For health-care workers from 2012 to 2013, the vaccination rate was only 72%, although for health-care workers in occupational settings that require vaccinations, the rate was 96.5%. The practitioner may keep informed of current epidemiologic trends in influenza epidemics and changes in vaccine recommendations by accessing the CDC's flu Web site at https://www.cdc.gov/flu/index.htm.

PNEUMONIA

Pneumonia is typically an acute inflammation of the lung parenchyma, usually infectious in origin. The lung tissue typically becomes consolidated as alveoli fill with exudate. Gas exchange may be impaired as blood is shunted around nonfunctional alveoli. The timely diagnosis and appropriate management of pneumonia in patients is critical because of the morbidity associated with bacterial etiologies, as well as the increased mortality among older patients and those with underlying pulmonary disease. Community-acquired pneumonia (CAP) occurs outside the hospital or is diagnosed within 2 days after hospitalization in a patient who has not resided in a long-term care facility for 2 weeks or more before the onset of the symptoms.

EPIDEMIOLOGY AND CAUSES

It is estimated that in the United States almost 5 million people develop pneumonia annually. Of these, approximately 1.3 million persons with pneumonia are admitted to hospitals, and more than 90,000 die each year. Approximately 70% to 80% of patients who develop CAP are aged 60 years or older or have a coexisting medical condition. CAP remains one of the 10 leading causes of mortality among elderly people in the United States today and is frequently the terminal event in older adults and those debilitated by chronic diseases, particularly chronic respiratory disease. This population is increasing, thus making adequate treatment of pneumonia a health-care priority. Nosocomial (hospital-acquired) pneumonias account for approximately 15% of all hospital-associated infections; pneumonia is second only to urinary tract infections in terms of frequency among hospitalized patients. In addition, pneumonia is still the leading infectious cause of death in children younger than 5 years worldwide. The most common pathogens associated with CAP and nosocomial pneumonia are shown in Box 30.2.

Pneumocystis jiroveci (formerly *carinii*) pneumonia (PCP) remains one of the leading causes of death in patients with AIDS. However, widespread use of highly active antiretroviral therapy and antibiotic prophylaxis based on CD4 T-cell counts has led to a dramatic decline in PCP incidence over the last 10 years. For pneumonia in general, however, other vulnerable populations include infants younger than 6 months old, children younger than age 5 years, smokers, alcoholics, residents of nursing homes, young adults living in close quarters (e.g., college students and military recruits), and individuals with impaired swallowing capacity or cough reflex who is at risk for aspiration. Geographic location, the winter season, occupation, travel history, and pet or animal exposure are other factors associated with the development of pneumonia.

PATHOPHYSIOLOGY

Pneumonia is an infection of the alveoli, distal airways, and interstitium of the lungs and is therefore a predominantly a parenchymal disease. Pathogens, such as bacteria, viruses, fungi, or parasites, reach the lower respiratory tract in sufficient number or with sufficient virulence to overwhelm the innate defenses of the respiratory tract. An inflammatory response is initiated that increases capillary permeability and attracts neutrophils, lymphocytes, platelets, and fibrinogen to the site of infection. Tissue fluid extravasates into the interstitial space from the pulmonary capillary bed, forming an exudate with a higher protein content than typical transudative fluid. As this exudate develops, an increasing amount of cellular debris accumulates, impeding optimal oxygen diffusion from the alveoli to capillaries with resultant hypoxemia. Vital capacity, lung compliance, residual capacity, and total lung capacity are diminished, and ventilation–perfusion mismatch occurs.

The spongy consistency of the lung tissue becomes fluid filled and infiltrated by several lineages of white blood cells depending on the infective agent involved, including neutrophils, lymphocytes, and macrophages, as well as red blood cells and fibrin. Because of these changes, the area of pneumonia is often referred to as a consolidative focus, which is typically dull to percussion on physical examination. Pneumonia may be classified as lobar pneumonia, interstitial pneumonia, miliary pneumonia, or bronchopneumonia. Figure 30.1 shows some of the parenchymal changes in pneumonia. Lobar pneumonia involves an entire lobe of the lung, whereas interstitial pneumonia is a patchy or diffuse inflammatory process throughout regions of the interstitium. Miliary pneumonia consists of numerous discrete lesions resulting from hematogenous spread of infection, and bronchopneumonia is a patchy consolidation involving one or several lobes of the lung. Moreover, inflammation can also extend into the pleural space, causing a parapneumonic effusion or inflammation of the pleural membranes, known as pleuritis or pleurisy.

Possible routes of infection include aspiration, aerosolization, hematogenous spread from a distant infected site, and direct spread from a contiguous infected site. Aspiration pneumonia occurs most often in postoperative, stroke, comatose, or otherwise mentally altered patients with an impaired swallowing reflex. Although *S. pneumoniae* remains the most common causative agent in aspiration pneumonia, anaerobic bacteria and gram-negative bacilli (i.e., gastrointestinal flora) must also be considered. Hematogenous spread to the lungs can take place in endocarditis, from IV central catheter line infection, or from infection at other sites such as the urinary tract. Aerosolization, the most common means of infection, is the route by which most bacteria, *Mycobacterium tuberculosis,* fungi, and viruses reach the lungs.

Box 30.2 **Common Causes of Pneumonia**	
Community-Acquired Pneumonia (CAP)	**Nosocomial Pneumonia**
Streptococcus pneumoniae (70% of all cases of bacterial pneumonia) Pneumococcal pneumonia (25%–35% of all CAP) *Staphylococcus aureus* *Klebsiella pneumoniae* *Moraxella catarrhalis* (less common) Atypical pneumonias: *Mycoplasma pneumoniae* (second most common cause of CAP) *Legionella pneumophila* *Chlamydia pneumoniae* Fungi Oral anaerobes Viruses	Most are caused by gramnegative bacteria. Enteric aerobic gramnegative bacilli *Klebsiella pneumoniae* *Pseudomonas aeruginosa* *Staphylococcus aureus* (gram-positive) Oral anaerobes *Legionella pneumophila* (which grow in cooling systems, condensers, and shower heads)

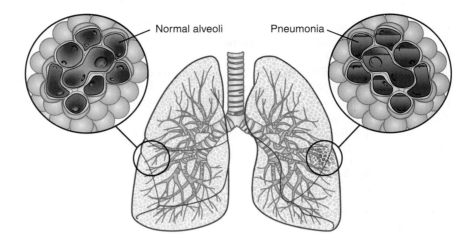

Figure 30.1 Parenchymal changes in pneumonia.

In adults, the most common organisms involved in CAP include viruses, *S. pneumoniae*, *M. catarrhalis*, *H. influenzae*, *Legionella pneumophila*, and methicillin-sensitive *S. aureus*. Nosocomial (hospital-acquired) pneumonia may be caused by *Pseudomonas aeruginosa* and MRSA. Of note, increasing numbers of community-acquired MRSA infections are being reported, particularly among elderly nursing home residents, resulting in severe cases of necrotizing pneumonia.

Streptococcus Pneumoniae

The most common cause of CAP is the gram-positive bacteria *S. pneumoniae,* also referred to as pneumococcal pneumonia. *S. pneumoniae* is one of the leading causes of illness and death worldwide for young children, older adults, and persons with chronic, debilitating pathology. The pathogenesis of pneumococcal pneumonia has been extensively studied and serves as a prototype for the management of other bacterial pneumonia.

Pneumococcal pneumonia occurs as a result of infected mucus or inhalation of organisms that have colonized the nasopharynx. *S. pneumoniae* can be recovered from the nasopharynx of approximately 40% of healthy adults. In the normal host, the bacteria are inactivated by opsonization with immunoglobulins and complement. Persons with defects in host defense mechanisms (e.g., inadequate immunoglobulin production or deficiency, impaired phagocytic function, autoimmune disease, immunosuppression, or impaired mucociliary clearance) have far greater susceptibility.

The lower lobes are most commonly infected because of the effects of gravity. Upon inhalation, the pneumococcus establishes itself in the alveoli, spreading rapidly through the pores of Kohn. Pneumococcal pneumonia typically includes four responsive stages of infection: engorgement, red hepatization, gray hepatization, and resolution. During engorgement, alveolar capillaries become congested, bacteria and exudate pour into alveoli from alveolar capillaries, and the bacteria multiply without inhibition. There is continued engorgement of the capillaries, with diapedesis of erythrocytes giving the lungs the gross appearance of liver (red hepatization). As the leukocyte count increases in the exudate, it compresses the capillaries and causes the lung tissue to assume a gray color (gray hepatization). At this point, phagocytosis ensues by polymorphonuclear leukocytes. The presence of opsonizing antibody enhances the ingestion of the bacteria. The stage of resolution is reached when the pneumococci have been destroyed and macrophages are seen within the alveolar spaces, where they lyse and absorb exudate. There may often be pleural involvement from contiguity to parenchymal lesions or by way of spread via the lymphatics. As in the alveoli, there is an outpouring of fluid, followed by polymorphonuclear leukocytes and fibrin. The structure of the pleural space has fewer surfaces suitable for phagocytosis than do the alveoli. Control of the infection in the pleural area is more dependent on heat-stable (specific antibody) than heat-labile (complement opsonins) antibodies.

Haemophilus Influenzae

H. influenzae, a gram-negative bacterium, is the cause of the second most common form CAP. It may occur in healthy individuals, as well as in patients with chronic debilitating diseases or chronic alcohol abuse. Development of *H. influenzae* pneumonia follows colonization of the upper respiratory tract. During viral infection epidemics, there is often an increase in the incidence of *H. influenzae* pneumonia.

Legionella Pneumophila

L. pneumophila, a gram-negative bacterium, was identified in 1976 as a causative agent of pneumonia (Legionnaires' disease) during an American Legion convention in Philadelphia. These bacteria thrive in aquatic environments. Sources of human infection has been associated with contaminated air-conditioning systems and showerheads. Within the hospital setting, contaminated respiratory tubing and equipment may serve as a source of *L. pneumophila*. The bacilli enter the lungs by aspiration, direct inhalation, and hematogenous dissemination. In the normal host, it is thought that the bacilli are cleared by the mucociliary process. This would explain the high incidence of the disease in patients with impaired mucociliary clearance (e.g., smokers, alcoholics, and older adults). Legionnaires' disease may occur in explosive outbreaks if large numbers of susceptible people are exposed to an infectious aerosol. Because of the low communicability of the disease, secondary cases typically do not occur.

Staphylococcus Aureus

S. aureus rarely causes pneumonia in healthy, young adults. Local pulmonary or systemic immune defenses must be compromised before the organism can produce pneumonia. *S. aureus* accounts for 2% to 9% of CAP in older adults or in patients with concomitant medical conditions, such as diabetes, chronic renal failure, bronchiectasis, or lung cancer, or with risk factors such as residence in a chronic-care facility or injection drug abuse. Infections may also occur in previously healthy adults following viral influenza with residual impaired bronchopulmonary anti-infective mechanisms.

Viral Pneumonia

Viral infections account for 5% to 15% of cases of adult CAP. Most viral infections are restricted to the upper respiratory system and tend to cause self-limited symptoms. Some patients, particularly those with influenza infections, may develop pneumonia. Influenza may result in a primary viral pneumonia or, more commonly, a secondary bacterial pneumonia; secondary pneumonia is most frequently caused by *S. pneumoniae* and *S. aureus*. Viral infections are transmitted by hand-to-hand contact or by aerosols (i.e., sneezing, coughing). The frequency of influenza as a precipitating factor of both CAP and nosocomial pneumonia increases in the winter months.

Mycoplasma Pneumonia

Mycoplasma pneumonia is also known as primary atypical pneumonia or "walking pneumonia" because of the predominance of constitutional symptoms. *Mycoplasma pneumoniae* is a class of bacterial L-forms, which are the smallest known free-living organisms. Children older than age 5 years and young adults are at greatest risk of developing *Mycoplasma* pneumonia. Outbreaks can occur in populations living in close proximity, such as colleges, military bases, and prisons. Because of the long incubation phase of 2 to 3 weeks and the relatively low communicability, *Mycoplasma* pneumonia tends to move through the community slowly.

Chlamydia Pneumoniae

Chlamydia pneumoniae was recognized as a pulmonary pathogen in 1983. *C. pneumoniae* is a gram-negative bacterium. Little is known about the mode of transmission and pathogenesis. The clinical features are similar to those caused by *M. pneumoniae*. Adult-onset asthma subsequent to infection with *C. pneumoniae* has been documented. Recurrent infection is common.

Anaerobic Pneumonia

Anaerobic pneumonia may occur in both the community and the hospital setting. *Prevotella melaninogenica*, anaerobic streptococci, and *Fusobacterium nucleatum* are commonly isolated anaerobic bacteria. Aspiration of oropharyngeal secretions normally occurs during sleep in healthy individuals but rarely causes disease. Individuals who are predisposed to aspiration of larger amounts of oropharyngeal secretions are at risk of anaerobic pneumonia. Alcoholism is the most frequent predisposing factor; others include dysphagia, cerebrovascular accidents, seizures, and general anesthesia. Periodontal disease, which increases the number of anaerobic bacteria, is also associated with anaerobic infection. Pneumonia typically develops in dependent lung zones. Although body position at the time of aspiration determines which lung zones are dependent, anaerobic pneumonia most often develops in the posterior segments of the upper lobes and the superior and basilar segments of the lower lobes. The onset of symptoms is usually insidious. Empyema, lung abscess, or necrotizing pneumonia may be present by the time the patient seeks medical attention.

Nosocomial Bacterial Pneumonia

Nosocomial bacterial pneumonia is most frequently caused by gram-negative organisms such as *Pseudomonas aeruginosa*, *Klebsiella pneumoniae*, *Escherichia coli*, *Serratia*, *Proteus*, and *Enterobacter*. However, *S. aureus* (especially MRSA), *S. pneumoniae*, and *H. influenzae* are frequently being reported among elderly nursing home residents. As in CAP, bacteria invade the lower respiratory tract by aspiration of oropharyngeal organisms, inhalation of aerosols containing bacteria, or hematogenous spread from a distant body site. Patients at high risk of nosocomial bacterial pneumonia include postoperative patients, particularly those undergoing thoracoabdominal procedures; patients with endotracheal incubation and/or mechanically assisted ventilation depressed level of consciousness an episode of large-volume aspiration or underlying chronic lung disease; and patient 70 years of age and older. Nosocomial pneumonia has a mortality rate of approximately 30%. Hospital-acquired pneumonia in patients on mechanical ventilation has a mortality rate of approximately 48%. Patients who develop acute respiratory distress syndrome have a mortality rate greater than 68%.

Pneumocystis Pneumonia

Pneumocystis pneumonia (PCP) is an AIDS-defining opportunistic infection that was once seen in as many as 65% of HIV-infected individuals and remains a major identifiable cause of death in AIDS patients. The causative agent, *P. jiroveci,* was originally classified as a protozoan named *P. carinii,* but it has since been reclassified as a fungus and renamed. Disease in adults represents reactivation of latent infection because almost all people are infected with *P. jiroveci* during the first decade of life. Most cases of PCP occur when the CD4-positive T-lymphocyte count has fallen below 200 to 250 cells/mcL. Pathologically, alveolar membranes become thickened, and mononuclear cell interstitial inflammation occurs as the disease progresses. PCP is discussed in more detail in Chapter 63.

Cytomegalic Inclusion Virus

Cytomegalic inclusion virus (CMV) is a causative agent of pneumonia in immunocompromised patients. CMV is a type of herpes virus that results in latent infections and reactivation with shedding of the infectious viruses. Pathologically, CMV produces an interstitial pneumonia that ranges from a mild disease to a fulminant course resulting in pulmonary insufficiency and death. CMV is discussed further in Chapter 63.

CLINICAL PRESENTATION

Although pneumonias may be classified as two syndromes, typical and atypical, according to the clinical presentation, they are very similar. However, the characteristics of the clinical manifestations do have some diagnostic value.

Subjective

The "typical" pneumonia syndrome is that which is seen in pneumococcal pneumonia, as well as in pneumonia caused by *H. influenzae* and *S. aureus* (Box 30.3). The syndrome is characterized by a sudden onset of fever, cough, chest pain, and fatigue. Generally, patients with a productive cough are more likely to have a bacterial infection. Patients with pneumococcal pneumonia produce sputum that has a characteristic rusty coloration; purulent sputum may also be evident. Fever may run as high as 106°F (41.1°C), with peaks observed in the afternoon or evening. The chest pain tends to be pleuritic in nature and increases in intensity during coughing or upon inspiration. Patients often feel cold; about half experience teeth-chattering, shaking, and chills. Myalgia is a common complaint and may extend to tenderness in the calves and thighs. Severe myalgia, particularly when accompanied by vomiting, strongly suggests the possibility of bacteremia. Respiratory and nonrespiratory symptoms are less commonly reported by older patients with pneumonia. Older patients may not show the typical febrile response (chills and sweats) or report pain (myalgia, headache, and chest pain). Although the older adult

Box 30.3	Typical Pneumonia Syndrome Associated With Pneumococcal Pneumonia
Subjective Findings	**Objective Findings**
Sudden onset of fever (may be blunted in older adults) Productive cough Rust-colored or purulent sputum Pleuritic-type pain Splinting Chills Myalgia	Crackles Dullness on percussion Bronchophony, egophony, whispered pectoriloquy Pleural friction rub (severe consolidation) Decreased or absent breath sounds Dense, homogenous shadows in one or more lobes on x-ray

may present with attenuated symptoms, this should not be misconstrued as an indication that such patients are less ill.

"Atypical" pneumonia is most commonly caused by *M. pneumoniae* but can also be caused by *L. pneumophila, C. pneumoniae, P. jiroveci,* and viruses. The atypical pneumonia syndrome is characterized by a more gradual onset of dry "hacking" cough, fever, and prominence of constitutional symptoms (e.g., pounding headaches, coryza, sore throat, shaking chills, and myalgia).

Pneumonias caused by anaerobic infections usually present with subacute or chronic constitutional and pulmonary symptoms. A chronic cough that produces purulent sputum is reported by the majority of patients. From 30% to 60% of patients report putrid sputum. This finding is considered to be virtually diagnostic of an anaerobic infection and is associated with the development of tissue necrosis and cavitary lesions. Patients also present with chest pain that is dull or pleuritic in nature, hemoptysis, anemia, leukocytosis, and weight loss.

Patients with PCP present with fever, sweats, weight loss, nonproductive cough, decreasing exercise tolerance, and dyspnea on exertion. The median duration of symptoms is 1 month. Tachypnea is common and is worsened by activity.

Objective

Physical examination of a person with typical pneumonia syndrome usually reveals an acutely ill patient who complains of chest pain and often splints on one side of the thorax. In some patients, crackles and dullness to percussion may be the only abnormality, particularly early in the disease. This finding may correspond with outpouring of fluid into the alveoli. A second group of patients shows the classic signs of consolidation: egophony, bronchophony, whispered pectoriloquy, bronchial breath sounds, and dullness on percussion. In patients with severe consolidation, crackles may be absent or minimal, and a leathery pleural friction rub may be heard over the area of chest tenderness. Finally, a third group of patients has one or more areas of dullness, inspiratory crackles, and diminished breath sounds, which are signs of mucous plugs in the smaller bronchioles.

Objective findings in atypical pneumonia tend to be less pronounced. Fine to medium crackles may be heard early or at the very end of the inspiratory cycle. Dullness on percussion and crackles or wheezing are more likely to be observed later in the disease course. Frank consolidation, pleural friction rubs, and pleural effusions are less common than in a typical pneumonia.

Although there is no "typical" syndrome of nosocomial pneumonia, one or more of the following clinical findings are present in most patients: fever, leukocytosis, purulent sputum, and a new pulmonary infiltrate on chest x-ray film. These findings must occur more than 48 hours after admission to the hospital to be considered suggestive of nosocomial pneumonia.

Auscultation of the lungs is generally negative in patients with PCP, although fine crackles may occasionally be heard. Mucocutaneous lesions such as oral thrush, hairy leukoplakia, and Kaposi's sarcoma are common and suggest the presence of underlying HIV-related immunodeficiency in previously undiagnosed individuals. Physiologically, patients manifest arterial hypoxemia.

DIAGNOSTIC REASONING

Diagnostic Tests

Initial Testing

Although a specific etiological diagnosis is optimal in the management of CAP, limitations in diagnostic testing make this difficult. The responsible microbe is not identified in approximately 50% of patients, even when extensive diagnostic tests are performed. The three most helpful tests used in the initial establishment of a diagnosis of pneumonia include chest radiograph, leukocyte count, and Gram stain of sputum specimens.

The chest x-ray study is important for three reasons. First, it may help distinguish whether the pneumonia is bacterial or viral in nature. Lobar infiltrates strongly suggest a bacterial infection. A bacterial pneumonia will show dense homogeneous shadows involving one or more lobes. Diffuse interstitial infiltrates are suggestive of a viral, *Mycoplasma*, or *Chlamydia* infection. Lateral and anterior-posterior views are necessary to evaluate lesions lying directly behind the heart.

A second reason for a chest x-ray study is to rule out a pleural effusion, a complication occurring in approximately one-third of pneumococcal pneumonia patients. It is important to note that chest x-ray films may be normal in patients who are unable to mount an inflammatory response or early in an infiltrative process. Follow-up chest

x-ray films are needed to see whether the infiltrate clears completely. Younger patients and those with only single-lobe involvement tend to have earlier resolutions.

Third, cavities may be seen on chest x-ray films in patients with pneumonia caused by anaerobes, *S. aureus*, *S. pneumoniae* serotype III, *M. tuberculosis*, aerobic gram-negative bacilli, and fungi. Cavities occur when necrotic material is discharged into airways, resulting in a necrotizing pneumonia (multiple small cavities, each less than 2 cm) or lung abscess (one or more cavities greater than 2 cm). Anaerobic abscesses are located in dependent segments, are most frequently seen in the right lung, and have air–fluid levels. Typical and atypical tuberculosis (TB) produce unilateral, well-drained, upper-lobe fibrocavitary disease. Cavities are rarely produced by *H. influenzae*, *M. pneumoniae*, viruses, and other serotypes of *S. pneumoniae*.

Although pulmonary infiltrates on x-ray films are considered suggestive of nosocomial pneumonia, findings tend to be very nonspecific. Conditions such as an atelectasis, pleural effusion, pulmonary thromboembolism, and pulmonary edema may mimic nosocomial pneumonia on x-ray evaluation.

It may not always be practical or feasible to obtain a chest x-ray study, so good clinical judgment is essential. Factors that have been found to be predictive of pneumonia infiltrates on chest films include fever above 100°F (37.8°C), tachycardia, locally decreased breath sounds, and sputum production. Chest x-ray films may be normal when the patient is unable to mount an inflammatory response (e.g., in agranulocytosis), is in the early stages of an infiltrative process, or in PCP associated with AIDS.

To help identify patients who need hospitalization, a CBC with differential should be done. The count may aid in differentiating between bacterial and viral pneumonia. Although there is no clear distinction, total white blood cell counts of more than 15,000 cells/μL suggest a bacterial infection. A differential cell count is not a reliable indicator of causation. Leukopenia may be seen in severe infections, as well as in alcoholics, older adults, and malnourished individuals. Blood cultures are indicated only for patients who require hospitalization or for cases of suspected nosocomial pneumonia.

A Gram stain of sputum is a widely available diagnostic tool for practitioners at the onset of therapy. Caution needs to be exercised in the evaluation of a sputum specimen because expectorated material is frequently contaminated by bacteria that normally colonize the upper and lower respiratory tracts. Large numbers of epithelial cells (more than 25 cells per low-power field) reflect contamination of the specimen with oral contents and mandate that another specimen be collected. If the sputum has been properly collected, polymorphonuclear leukocytes can be readily seen with a Gram stain. The characteristic lancet-shaped, gram-positive diplococci associated with pneumococcal pneumonia are generally seen in abundance. In contrast, Gram stains are seldom useful in patients with atypical pneumonia because sputum is scant and most organisms that cause this syndrome cannot be detected by a Gram stain. For example, acid-fast staining of sputum should be done when mycobacterial infection is suspected (see Advanced Assessment 30.1).

A sputum culture is less valuable than a Gram stain for providing a causal diagnosis in bacterial pneumonia. Approximately 50% of patients with pneumococcal pneumonia have negative sputum cultures, even when large numbers of organisms are present on Gram stain. Sputum cultures are also negative in 35% to 50% of cases of proven *H. influenzae* pneumonia. Isolation of the causative agent in atypical pneumonia is rare.

Sputum cultures may be valuable in the diagnosis of subacute and cavitary pneumonia. Mycobacteria grow well on culture media, and it has been estimated that sputum cultures can detect as few as 10 acid-fast bacilli (AFB) per milliliter of concentrated sputum. For a more in-depth discussion of the use of sputum cultures for the isolation of mycobacteria, refer to the section on tuberculosis.

The usefulness of fungal cultures varies with the organism and the stage of the disease. Chronic forms of coccidioidomycosis and blastomycosis may yield positive cultures in 70% to 100% of cases if multiple specimens are collected. Accurate positive cultures are not found in patients with histoplasmosis until the disease is in the chronic, cavitary stage. Fewer than 50% of patients with cryptococcosis have positive sputum cultures.

Expectorated sputum is usually collected in patients with a productive, vigorous cough, but may be scant in those with atypical pneumonia syndrome, in older adults, and in patients with altered mental status. If the patient is not producing sputum and can cooperate, respiratory secretions can be induced with ultrasonic nebulization of 3% saline solution. The use of more invasive procedures to induce sputum in the patient who is unable to produce a sputum specimen carries risks that must be weighed against the potential benefits. In patients who do not require hospitalization or in hospitalized patients who are not severely ill, the need to establish an accurate microbial diagnosis may not be crucial, and empiric therapy can be started on the basis of clinical and epidemiologic evidence alone. Patients who are hospitalized with CAP and are seriously ill or those who acquire a nosocomial pneumonia clearly need to have a specific causal diagnosis established. In these patients, it may be necessary to obtain specimens from the lower respiratory tract by fiberoptic bronchoscopy, transtracheal puncture, or percutaneous transthoracic lung puncture. Of these invasive procedures, fiber-optic bronchoscopy is currently the preferred technique for obtaining lower respiratory tract secretions. Specimens obtained by bronchoscopy should be tested with Gram and acid-fast stains, *Legionella* direct fluorescent antibody, and Gomori's methenamine silver stains and should be cultured for aerobic and anaerobic bacteria, *Legionella*, mycobacteria, and fungi.

Diagnostic testing for CAP caused by *S. pneumoniae* may include a pneumococcal urinary antigen test that can detect a protein common to all pneumococcal serotypes. Within 15 minutes, this test can demonstrate the presence of pneumococcus in unconcentrated urine. This can facilitate more immediate decisions about antibiotic therapy. However, the sensitivity of this test varies, and it should be used in addition to sputum and/or blood culture. Urinary antigen testing is also available for the gram-negative bacteria *L. pneumophila* (but only for serogroup 1, which may not capture all forms of the disease), as well as the fungus *Histoplasma*.

Subsequent Testing

If the pneumonia is severe enough to require hospitalization, at least two blood samples should be obtained for culture, as well as a CBC and serological analysis of sodium, urea, nitrogen, creatinine, and glucose. Liver and enzyme tests should be included if hepatic disease or malnutrition is suspected. Serological studies are sometimes helpful in defining the etiology of certain types of pneumonia. An immunoglobulin M or immunoglobulin G titer obtained by indirect immunofluorescence may be diagnostic of *M. pneumoniae* or *C. pneumoniae*. A *Legionella* titer or a urinary antigen test may help confirm Legionnaires' disease.

Pulse oximetry is indicated if the patient presents with respiratory distress, dyspnea at rest, or tachypnea or if the chest x-ray film shows multilobar pulmonary infiltrates. A blood gas analysis should be performed if the patient has known carbon dioxide (CO_2) retention,

---

⚛ Advanced Assessment 30.1: Sputum Staining

Sputum Stain	Organism
Gram stain	*S. pneumoniae* (gram-positive, lancet-shaped diplococci) *H. influenzae* (gram-positive coccobacilli) *S. aureus* (gram-positive tetrads and grapelike clusters)
Acid-fast stain	Mycobacterial infection
Direct fluorescent antibody stain	Viral respiratory culture
Fluorescent antibody: sensitivity diminished with concurrent use of inhaled pentamidine	*Legionella* infection
Wright-Giemsa stain: frequent false-positive and false-negative results	PCP
Gomori's methenamine silver	Fungal growth (living and dead organisms)
Periodic acid-Schiff stain	Fungal growth (living organisms only)

exacerbations of asthma, or COPD. Typically, an Sao_2 of less than 90% or a Pao_2 of less than 60 mm Hg indicates a need for supplemental oxygen. These threshold values must be modified if the patient is chronically hypoxemic.

Differential Diagnosis

Acute bacterial pneumonia should be differentiated from acute bacterial bronchitis. Both respiratory infections will cause fever and a productive cough. On auscultation, however, a patient with bronchitis will have clear lung sounds except for a few scattered rhonchi and possibly tubular sounds. In comparison, the patient with bacterial pneumonia will likely have crackles, dullness to percussion, and abnormal breath sounds. Cavitary forms of pneumonia need to be differentiated from pulmonary TB and systemic mycoses, particularly coccidioidomycosis and histoplasmosis. Likewise, the patient who presents with symptoms of PCP and a history of fever, weight loss, and pulmonary symptoms should be concurrently evaluated for TB, lymphomas, and brucellosis, in addition to HIV infection. Signs and symptoms secondary to central or endobronchial growth of a primary lung cancer will mimic those of a bacterial pneumonia (e.g., productive cough, fever, cough, dyspnea, hemoptysis). The practitioner needs to be aware of any occupational or environmental hazards to which the patient is exposed. For example, workers who develop berylliosis through exposure to beryllium (found in ceramics, high-technology electronics, and alloy manufacturing) may present with an acute pneumonia or, more commonly, with a chronic interstitial pneumonia. Exposure to moldy hay can result in symptoms of pneumonia (e.g., coughing, fever, chills, malaise, and dyspnea) within 4 to 8 hours after exposure. This disease (known as "farmer's lung") may become chronic.

Severe acute respiratory syndrome (SARS) should also be ruled out. Patients should be questioned about travel to an area with known transmission of SARS, as well as close contact with a person who has SARS. The causative agent is a coronavirus. Symptoms include a fever greater than 100.5°F (38°C), cough, or respiratory distress. The diagnosis is made via enzyme-linked immunosorbent assay or reverse transcriptase–polymerase chain reaction assays. Treatment is supportive care. The identification is critical from a public health standpoint rather than from the need of initiating SARS-specific care, which remains supportive.

MANAGEMENT

The initial task in the management of patients with CAP is to determine whether the person can be treated on an outpatient basis or whether hospitalization is required. The use of hospital services is costly and may further impair the patient's health because of the risk of nosocomial infections. The majority of patients with CAP with no comorbidity can be treated successfully as outpatients. Most patients, even those treated initially in a hospital, prefer outpatient treatment.

The decision to hospitalize a patient with CAP may be the single most important decision during the entire course of the illness. Scoring systems are helpful in determining the site-of-care decision. The CURB-65 criteria to determine the severity of CAP is an objective, easy tool to remember. The calculator takes into account **C**onfusion; BUN (blood **u**rea nitrogen); **R**espiratory rate; Systolic **B**P (blood pressure); and Age. The calculator for this may be found at www.mdcalc.com/curb-65-score-pneumonia-severity. The severity of illness will help determine in what setting treatment should take place. In addition, known risk factors for CAP-associated mortality and complications are summarized in the accompanying text.

Risk Factors for CAP-Associated Mortality and Complications

Age: Older than 65 years
Presence of coexisting illness:

- Chronic pulmonary disease
- Diabetes mellitus
- Chronic renal failure
- Congestive heart failure
- Chronic liver disease of any etiology
- Previous hospitalization within 1 year of the onset of pneumonia
- Suspicion of aspiration
- Altered mental status
- Postsplenectomy state
- Chronic alcohol abuse or malnutrition

Abnormal physical findings:

- Respiratory rate above 30 breaths/min
- Diastolic BP 60 mm Hg or below and/or systolic BP 90 mm Hg or below
- Temperature above 101°F
- Evidence of extrapulmonary sites of disease (e.g., septic arthritis, meningitis)
- Decreased level of consciousness or confusion

Abnormal laboratory findings:

- White blood cell count $<4 \times 10^9$/L or $>30 \times 10^9$/L
- Pao_2 <60 mm Hg or $Paco_2$ >50 mm Hg on room air
- Hemoglobin <9 g/dL
- X-ray showing more than one lobe involvement, pleural effusion, or evidence of rapid spreading
- Severe electrolyte or renal abnormality not known to be chronic (e.g., BUN >50 mg/dL, creatinine >1.2 mg/dL, sodium <130 mEq/L)

Antimicrobial therapy represents the mainstay of treatment for patients with suspected or confirmed pneumonia. Additional management is supportive and includes the use of analgesics for relief of chest pain and myalgia, antipyretics to control fever, increased fluid intake (typically at least 3 L over 24 hours), restricted activity or bedrest, a position of comfort (usually upright) to facilitate breathing, and humidified air to relieve irritated nares and pharynx. Expectorants may be indicated to decrease sputum viscosity and clear airways if a productive cough is present. Although many promote the use of expectorants, the most cost-effective way to liquify secretions for ease of coughing and elimination of secretions is hydration with water. Patients experiencing a dry, nonproductive cough may benefit from a cough suppressant with codeine if expectoration is not deemed necessary.

Patients requiring hospitalization need to have ongoing assessment for any indications of impaired respiratory status. Patients who manifest arterial hypoxemia will require supplemental oxygen therapy to attempt to maintain Po_2 above 80 mm Hg. In the past, chest physiotherapy had been widely used to mobilize secretions. However, percussion and postural drainage probably offer no added benefit to the patient who has an uncomplicated pneumonia without underlying pulmonary disease.

Treatment Guidelines for Community-Acquired Pneumonia

The Infectious Diseases Society of America has recommended specific therapy for CAP. Before initiating treatment, the clinician must determine whether the patient has had recent antibiotic therapy and any coexisting diseases that may be present, such as COPD or congestive heart failure. The Treatment Standards/Guidelines box summarizes the empiric treatment of the patient with CAP. In addition, treatment guidelines from 2016 are cited.

In the past, macrolides were used for monotherapy, but these medications are now avoided because approximately 25% of *S. pneumoniae* strains are naturally resistant to all macrolides. Highly penicillin-resistant *S. pneumoniae* strains are a rare cause of CAP because most *S. pneumoniae* strains remain susceptible to ceftriaxone. Preferred monotherapy for CAP includes doxycycline or a respiratory quinolone. These are the most cost-effective way to optimally treat CAP. They are well tolerated in oral and IV forms and are ideal for IV-to-oral switch monotherapy in terms of patient compliance, safety, and cost. Use of proton-pump inhibitors (PPIs) for gastric protection should be avoided when using respiratory quinolones for CAP drug therapy because they may alter drug levels. The PPI should be stopped, or a histamine-$_2$ receptor (H_2) blocker should

be used for the duration of therapy. However, there is conflicting evidence regarding the relative safety of PPIs and H_2 blockers.

Treatment regimens for community-acquired MRSA pneumonia should typically start with vancomycin until results of sensitivity testing are available, which may indicate susceptibility to Bactrim (sulfamethoxazole-trimethoprim). Most recently, guidelines have established linezolid (Zyvox) as an effective alternative therapy for susceptible vancomycin-resistant infections, including CAP.

 Treatment Standards/Guidelines: Empiric Antimicrobial Choices for Community-Acquired Pneumonia (CAP)

PATIENT PROFILE	ANTIMICROBIAL AGENT
Uncomplicated CAP	
Without recent antibiotic therapy (ATBX)*	Azithromycin (Zithromax) or clarithromycin (Biaxin) or doxycycline (Vibramycin)
With recent ATBX†	Respiratory fluoroquinolone moxifloxacin (Avelox) or levofloxacin (Levaquin) OR Azithromycin or clarithromycin PLUS High-dose amoxicillin (Amoxil) OR Azithromycin or clarithromycin PLUS High-dose amoxicillin–clavulanate (Augmentin)
Patient with CAP plus comorbidities: alcoholism; diabetes mellitus; lung/liver/renal diseases	Respiratory fluoroquinolone OR Beta-lactam IV/intramuscular ceftriaxone (Rocephin) or Cefuroxime (Ceftin) PLUS Macrolide
Patient with community-acquired methicillin-resistant *S. aureus* pneumonia	Vancomycin (Vancocin) OR Linezolid (Zyvox)

Source: Kalil, AC, Metersky, ML, Klompas, M, et al. Management of adults with hospital-acquired and ventilator-associated pneumonia: 2016 Clinical Practice Guidelines by the Infectious Diseases Society of America and the American Thoracic Society. *Clin Infect Dis.* 2016;63(5):e61–e111.

*ATBX antibiotic therapy within the last 3 months.

†Use a different class of antibiotic not chosen previously.

Subsequent Management

The advent of antimicrobial therapy has greatly decreased complications that were commonly seen before the use of antibiotics. Pneumonia that is associated with bacteremia, leukopenia, or multiple lobe involvement increases the likelihood of complications and death. The mortality rate for patients older than age 65 years with bacteremia and involvement of more than three lobes is approximately 60%. Complications are more frequently found in patients with underlying chronic diseases.

The radiographic resolution of CAP is complete in half of patients after 2 weeks and in two-thirds of patients after 4 weeks. Follow-up x-ray studies should be done within 3 to 6 months for all patients who smoke or who are older than age 40 years. If an abnormality has not cleared on follow-up films, the patient should be evaluated for a possible cancer.

Pleural effusion represents the most common complication seen in patients with pneumonia. Fluid can be detected radiographically in the pleural space of more than 40% of patients hospitalized with pneumonia. In most cases, the amount is so small that needle aspiration is unsuccessful. If fluid is removed, it is typically not purulent, nor can microbes be seen on Gram stain.

Fluid that is purulent and has a gram-positive stain or has a pH less than 7.1 is indicative of an empyema. *S. pneumoniae, S. pyogenes,* and anaerobic pneumonias are associated with most cases of empyema. It is critical that the infected material be removed from the pleural space by means of a thoracentesis, needle aspiration, or thoracotomy. If this treatment is delayed, the patient is likely to require a prolonged hospital stay. Lung abscesses develop infrequently in *S. pneumoniae* but often occur as complications of pneumonias caused by gram-negative bacteria (e.g., *Klebsiella*), anaerobic bacteria, and *S. aureus.* Drainage of the abscess is essential to prevent further necrosis of the lung tissue. Prolonged antimicrobial therapy is critical for the successful treatment of this complication.

Delayed resolution results from persistent infection and is seen on x-ray studies as residual consolidation. Delayed resolution occurs most often in the patient who is older, malnourished, alcoholic, or who has COPD. Progression of infiltrates despite antimicrobial therapy is a poor prognostic sign.

Metastatic infections that do occur tend to develop in the meninges, pericardium, heart valves, and skeletal system. Although these complications occur less frequently with antimicrobial therapy, persons with compromised health status remain at risk for the development of these infections. Possible metastatic infections include arthritis, pericarditis, endocarditis, and meningitis. Patients who develop arthritis will experience swollen, red, and painful joints. Purulent exudate may be aspirated from the joints. Meningitis caused by *S. pneumoniae* produces purulent cerebrospinal fluid. Patients with pneumococcal pneumonia who become disoriented, confused, or somnolent should have a lumbar puncture.

FOLLOW-UP AND REFERRAL

Patients considered well enough for outpatient treatment do not need to be closely monitored unless symptoms worsen despite antibiotic therapy. The patient should be contacted within 24 to 48 hours of starting therapy and should be scheduled for an office visit at 1 week and 4 to 6 weeks after the initial evaluation.

As mentioned, x-ray resolution of CAP is complete in 50% of patients after 2 weeks and in two-thirds of patients after 4 weeks. Examination at the second follow-up visit should include a chest x-ray film if clinical symptoms have not resolved. X-ray evaluations should be done for all patients who smoke. If an abnormality has not cleared on follow-up films, the patient should be evaluated for possible cancer.

Smoking cessation is essential if respiratory health is to be maintained. Patients may be most receptive to antismoking counseling while they are still ill or recovering from pneumonia. The follow-up examination provides an opportune time for patient education. Pneumococcal and influenza vaccines should also be given at this time if indicated.

Patient Education: Pneumonia

Annual influenza vaccine is strongly recommended for all individuals older than 6 months. The ACIP of the CDC recommends the pneumonococcal conjugate vaccine (13-valent Prevnar 13) for children younger than 2 years, adults older than 65 years, and persons aged 2 through 64 years with comorbidities. This vaccine should be followed by the 23-valent Pneumovax-23 one year later in all adults older than age of 65 years and those older than age of 2 years who are at high risk for pneumococcal disease due to comorbidities. The interval between vaccines depends on the order in which the vaccines are given (see the ACIP Interval Guidelines cited in the reference section).

The increasing prevalence of multiantibiotic-resistant pneumococci makes immunization of high-risk individuals of utmost importance. Vaccine use tends to increase when efforts are made to raise awareness and promote the benefits of vaccination. The practitioner may obtain current and relevant data on pneumococcal vaccines, incidence rates of CAP and hospital-acquired pneumonia, drug therapy, and other pertinent information by contacting the CDC, the National Institute on Aging, and the National Foundation for Infectious Diseases.

TUBERCULOSIS

Tuberculosis (TB) is one of the oldest human diseases. It is an infectious disease, most frequently caused by *M. tuberculosis* in humans. In early writings, TB was called "consumption" because of its tendency to produce great wasting in its victims. During the 18th and

19th centuries, it was known as the "white plague." TB is the leading cause of death worldwide from any single infectious agent. The pandemic of HIV infection and the emergence of drug-resistant TB strains have worsened the global problem of TB. One-third of the world's population is infected with TB, although not everyone infected with the mycobacteria become ill. Two conditions exist: latent TB infection (LTBI) and (active) TB. Active TB may be a primary infection or secondary reactivation. Individuals with LTBI who become immunocompromised may progress to active TB.

EPIDEMIOLOGY AND CAUSES

TB had once been considered to be under such good control that eradication of the disease in developing countries was considered an obtainable goal. Worldwide, the majority of infected persons are living in developing countries; about 75% of these infected people are younger than age 50 years. Each year, 1.8 million people worldwide die from the disease. TB is the most common HIV-associated opportunistic infection in many developing countries. Currently, the highest estimated case rates occur in India.

According to the CDC, in the United States the number of reported TB cases in 2016 (9,287) was the lowest recorded since national reporting began in 1953. Of these U.S. cases, just over 30% were U.S.-born individuals while almost 70% were foreign-born persons. The WHO recognizes 30 high TB burden countries; in 2015, the top four countries were Angola, Bangladesh, Brazil, and Cambodia. TB disproportionately affects patients belonging to racial and ethnic minorities, and the prevalence is three times higher in urban than rural populations. California, Florida, New York, and Texas each had more than 500 cases of TB in 2016, which account for more than 50% of the cases nationwide. These states, in addition to having large foreign-born populations, also have a relatively larger number of AIDS cases. African Americans continue to have a disproportionate share of the TB cases.

Overall, approximately 10% of persons infected with *M. tuberculosis* will develop clinical TB sometime during their lifetimes. About 5% of infected persons will manifest the disease within 1 year of infection. The remaining persons who develop the disease will have a delayed onset of TB, typically at a period of declined protective immunity, which can occur as a result of silicosis, diabetes mellitus, cancer, HIV infection, advanced aging, or with the use of immunosuppressive drugs. Susceptibility to TB is also greater during the first 2 years of life, at puberty, and during adolescence.

Outbreaks of drug-resistant TB (resistant to at least one anti-TB drug) and multidrug-resistant TB (resistant to isoniazid [INH] and rifampin [RIF]) have occurred in hospitals, prisons, shelters for the homeless, nursing homes, and AIDS patient residential facilities.

The genus *Mycobacterium* includes the causative agents of TB and leprosy. Mycobacteria are aerobic, asporogenous, nonmotile, acid-fast rods. Of the 58 species of the genus *Mycobacterium*, the members of the TB complex (*M. tuberculosis, Mycobacterium bovis, Mycobacterium africanum,* and *Mycobacteria microti*) are closely related, based on DNA homology studies. The TB complex depends on host transmission for its survival. *M. tuberculosis* is the major cause of human disease. Disease due to *M. bovis* is rare in the United States. *M. africanum* is a common cause of TB in Africa, and *M. microti* is a pathogen for rodents.

PATHOPHYSIOLOGY

M. tuberculosis strains vary in virulence due to differences in the bacteria's genetic makeup. Similarly, persons display varying susceptibility to TB infection due to genetically conferred resistance, age, and comorbid conditions (e.g., chronic illness, immunosuppression). *M. tuberculosis* is most commonly transmitted from person to person by droplet nuclei that are aerosolized by coughing, sneezing, or speaking. Person-to-person transmission is influenced by the intimacy and duration of contact, the degree of infectivity of the patient, and the shared contact environment. Patients with acid-fast staining organisms in their sputum are most infectious to others.

When *M. tuberculosis* organisms are first inhaled, some are expelled by the ciliated epithelium, and only a small fraction reaches the alveoli, leading to primary infection. There, alveolar macrophages attempt to phagocytose and contain the bacteria; however, virulent strains can multiply rapidly and overcome these macrophages by countering their oxidative bactericidal mechanisms. Nonetheless, activated macrophages react by releasing inflammatory mediators, such as interleukin-12 and tumor necrosis factor–alpha, which contribute to fever, anorexia, and weight loss. Macrophages also stimulate the recruitment of T lymphocytes to the area of infection. Helper T (CD4+) and cytotoxic killer T (CD8+) lymphocytes are also integral in the effort to kill mycobacteria. Activated macrophages and T lymphocytes form granulomas, or larger tubercles, in an effort to confine bacterial growth by walling off and containing the mycobacteria.

Within these tubercles, multiplication of the organisms is inhibited by low oxygen content and low ph. T lymphocytes release inflammatory mediators that neutralize the mycobacteria contained in the tubercle's central necrotic area known as the caseum because of its cheeselike appearance on gross inspection. In a minority of cases, highly virulent strains of *M. tuberculosis* may cause rapid infection, invading lung parenchyma, bronchioles, and blood vessels. Hemoptysis, a frequent clinical sign of active infection, may reflect the erosion of a granuloma into a pulmonary blood vessel. Old granulomas eventually calcify, identifiable as one or more Ghon complexes on a chest x-ray. Known as LTBI, viable bacteria may remain dormant in these lesions for decades, only to be reactivated when the balance between host immunity and bacterial pathogenesis is tipped in favor of the mycobacteria. This results in secondary infection known as reactivation TB, seen typically in chronically ill or otherwise immunosuppressed individuals. Secondary reactivation TB is typically the most lethal form of the infection.

Mycobacteria can also spread via the lymphatic system or bloodstream, resulting in disseminated infection. Extrapulmonary sites of TB infection include the lymph nodes, pleura, bones, meninges, peritoneum, pericardium, and genitourinary tract. Solid organs may be seeded at multiple tiny foci, approximately 2 mm in diameter, taking on a millet-seed–like appearance on gross inspection termed "miliary tuberculosis." Such pathological findings have been noted as far back as the 1700s. Today, the term miliary TB has been extended to encompass all forms of progressive, disseminated TB infection but is still seen most often in children younger than 1 year.

M. tuberculosis organisms are aerobic and, therefore, particularly attracted to the apical segments of the upper lung lobes where high oxygen concentrations favor their proliferation. Although the upper lung zone is the most common site of accelerated growth of the organisms, there may be later progression to distant sites in the body. The kidneys, brain, and bones are the most common sites of distant progression.

Individuals may continue to discharge mycobacteria into the environment from pulmonary tubercles until multiple-drug therapy is instituted to drive bacteria into a dormant state or eradicate infection completely. Although mycobacteria are almost always found in the bone marrow, liver, and spleen when disease occurs, uncontrolled multiplication of the mycobacteria in these organs is rare. Immunosuppressed individuals, particularly those with T-lymphocyte deficiencies and compromised cell-mediated immunity (e.g., persons living with HIV), are highly susceptible to TB.

CLINICAL PRESENTATION

Subjective

TB may mimic or occur concurrently with pneumoconiosis, pneumonia, bronchiectasis, sarcoidosis, lung abscess, neoplasm, or respiratory fungal infections. Onset commonly is insidious, with symptoms of anorexia, fatigue, digestive disturbances, slow weight loss, irregular menses, and lack of stamina. Persons may complain of being unable to complete a normal day's work. This pattern of symptoms at onset may continue for several weeks or even months, with a low-grade elevation of temperature that appears characteristically in the afternoon.

Pulmonary TB is characterized principally by a productive cough, purulent sputum, and repeated occurrences of coryza-like symptoms with rhinorrhea and nasal congestion. The cough progresses slowly over weeks or months to become more frequent and associated with the production of mucoid or mucopurulent sputum. The cough is usually due to sloughing of small caseous lesions with the presence of exudate in the bronchi. Sputum is characteristically yellow but is not tenacious or foul smelling. Hemoptysis is a common symptom in patients with necrotizing or cavitary lesions. Blood usually appears as small streaks in the sputum. Dyspnea is uncommon in pulmonary TB and usually indicates extensive parenchymal involvement, massive pleural effusion, or other underlying cardiopulmonary disease.

A less frequent pattern of onset is that of an acute febrile illness with an abrupt occurrence of high fever, chills, tachycardia, and weakness, accompanied by a productive cough with myalgia, and sweating. Erythema nodosum may occur with the acute onset of symptoms. Some patients may pay little attention to milder symptoms that precede the acute episode; this is a common occurrence in less educated persons, alcoholics, or older adults.

Less frequent modes of onset include pleuritic pain and hoarseness. Pleuritic pain, usually unilateral, tends to be accentuated by coughing or deep inspiration. Hoarseness is usually a result of involvement of the larynx and may be accompanied by severe pain. Constitutional symptoms tend to be general in nature and consist of night sweats, fatigue on exertion, weight loss, and malaise.

In obtaining the health history, the clinician must keep in mind the chronicity of TB and the insidious nature of the onset of symptoms. Patients should be questioned about exposure to anyone with an active case of TB. Potential sources of exposure include family and coworkers. Other significant disclosures obtained from a health history include a past diagnosis of pneumonia with recurrence, pleurisy, uncontrolled diabetes, alcoholism, malnutrition, and occupational exposures to quartz dust or silica. Additional risk factors include drug abuse, country of origin, corticosteroid use, and gastrectomy.

Objective

A complete examination of any patient suspected of having TB should always be performed. Examination of the chest usually reveals the primary indications of pulmonary TB. Rhonchi, crackles, wheezing, and bronchial breath sounds may be heard on auscultation but may have no radiographic counterparts. Dullness on percussion is commonly associated with pneumonic lesions. Persons with long-standing disease may manifest asymmetrical lung expansion, displacement of the trachea, and muscular atrophy. Although there are no specific changes related to pulmonary function, in patients with extensive parenchymal involvement, the vital capacity and other lung volumes may become decreased.

Although pulmonary TB is the most common form, the clinician should be alert to any indications of extrapulmonary TB. The patient should be examined for evidence of present or past extrapulmonary TB in structures such as the genitourinary tract, lymph nodes, bones

TABLE 30.1   Clinical Indicators of Extrapulmonary Tuberculosis

Extrapulmonary Sites	Clinical Manifestations
Genitourinary tract	Recurrent urinary tract infections with no growth of common pathogens Pyuria without bacteriuria Unexplained hematuria Irregular menses, amenorrhea, pelvic inflammatory disease, infertility Epididymitis Induration of the prostate
Bone and joints (lower spine and weight-bearing joints are most common sites)	Arthritis, osteomyelitis Fever and localized pain
Meninges	Headaches, convulsions Abnormal behavior
Peritoneum	Ascites, fever
Pericardium	Pericarditis
Lymph nodes	Hilar or mediastinal lymphadenitis Cervical and supraclavicular lymphadenopathy

and joints, peritoneum, larynx, eyes, abdominal organs, and neurologic system (Table 30.1). Physical findings may include hepatomegaly, splenomegaly, and generalized lymphadenopathy. Abnormal behavior, headaches, and seizures may indicate TB meningitis. Meningitis occurs frequently in infants and small children as a complication of early infection, but it may be seen in any age-group. Bone and joint involvement, most often seen in older adults, is often accompanied by fever and may result in arthritis, osteomyelitis, and localized pain. The lower spine and weight-bearing joints are most often affected by skeletal TB. Genitourinary TB may present as recurrent urinary tract infection with no growth of common pathogens, pyuria without bacteriuria, pelvic inflammatory disease, amenorrhea, infertility, or perianal fistulas.

DIAGNOSTIC REASONING

Diagnostic Tests

Initial Testing

The Mantoux tuberculin skin test (TST) is the most accurate and widely used method for TB skin testing. It involves injecting a small amount of mycobacterial antigen (purified protein derivative [PPD]) intradermally. Persons with previous exposure to or infection with TB organisms develop a positive cell-mediated (type IV) delayed-type hypersensitivity skin reaction as a result of previously sensitized helper T lymphocytes (CD4+) that are attracted to the testing site. Reactions of this type typically require 48 to 72 hours to develop and are classified based on the degree of skin induration at the site of injection in relation to specific population norms. Less invasive quantitative interferon-gamma release assays (IGRAs) also may be used to screen for TB. In these tests, T cells are collected by whole blood draw and subjected to ex vivo immunostimulation assays with TB-specific antigens. Both TB screening tests only assess for past exposure to TB and do not distinguish between LTBI versus active TB infection.

The TST is easily performed in an office or clinic setting. It is useful as an epidemiologic tool to identify infected (including recently infected) people for preventive therapy and contact tracing. The TST is the preferred TB screening test for children younger than 5 years. Persons for whom tuberculin testing is routinely indicated are listed in the Screening Recommendations/Guidelines.

⁘ Screening Recommendations/Guidelines: Guidelines for Tuberculin Screening

- Persons with signs and/or symptoms of current TB
- Close contact with known TB cases
- Persons with HIV infection
- Persons who inject illicit drugs
- Person from medically underserved or high-risk minority populations
- Resident or employees in prisons or long-term care facilities
- Employees in health-care facilities
- Infants, children, and adolescents exposed to adults in high-risk categories (use of IGRAs in children younger than 5 years is not established)

- Foreign-born persons arriving within 5 years from countries that have high TB incidence or prevalence (use IGRAs for persons with recent BCG vaccination)
- Persons on long-term high-dose corticosteroid therapy (use TST rather than IGRA)
- Persons on immunosuppressive therapy (use TST rather than IGRA)
- Persons with medical conditions that increase the risk of TB: chronic renal failure, diabetes, hematological disorders, cancer of the head or neck, body weight less than 10% of ideal body weight, silicosis, gastrectomy, jejunal bypass

Abbreviations: BCG, Bacillus Calmette-Guérin; IGRA, interferon-gamma release assay; TB, tuberculosis; TST, tuberculin skin test.

Sources: Lewinsohn DM, Leonard MK, LoBue PA, et al. Official American Thoracic Society/Infectious Diseases Society of America/Centers for Disease Control and Prevention Clinical Practice Guidelines: diagnosis of tuberculosis in adults and children. *Clin Infect Dis.* 2017;64(2):e1–e33; Centers for Disease Control and Prevention. Interferon-gamma release assays (IGRAs)-blood tests for TB infection. https://www.cdc.gov/tb/publications/factsheets/testing/igra.htm. Accessed May 4, 2016.

The TST must be administered correctly to avoid false-negative or false-positive results. Factors that may contribute to an inaccurate result include improper handling of the tuberculin, improper administration technique, and inaccurate reading of test results (e.g., by an inexperienced reader). To minimize reduction in potency by adsorption, tuberculin should never be transferred from one container to another, and the skin testing material should be placed soon after the syringe has been filled. Tuberculin should be kept refrigerated and stored away from light as much as possible. The TST (0.1 mL) should be injected into the volar or dorsal surface of the forearm, away from veins and into intact skin that is free of lesions. The injection should be made just beneath the surface of the skin, with a one-quarter to one-half-inch 27-gauge needle and a tuberculin syringe. A discrete, pale elevation of the skin (a wheal) 6 to 10 mm in diameter should be produced when the injection has been done correctly. If the test is improperly administered, another test dose can be given immediately, but at a site several centimeters from the original injection.

The reaction to intradermally injected tuberculin protein is a classic example of a delayed-type cellular hypersensitivity reaction. These reactions begin 5 to 6 hours after injection and are maximal at 72 hours. In older adults or in persons who are being tested for the first time, the reaction may develop more slowly and may not peak until after 72 hours. Older adults should be checked initially at 72 hours, and then 1 and 2 days later. Tests should be read 72 hours after the injection, using good lighting with the forearm slightly flexed at the elbow. Interpretation of the test result is based on the presence or absence of induration, which is determined by inspection and palpation. Erythema is not a factor in interpretation of the TST reaction. The diameter of the induration is measured transversely to the long axis of the forearm and recorded in millimeters (Table 30.2).

Factors that may cause a decreased ability to respond to tuberculin are listed in Box 30.4. The TST tends to have a strong positive predictive value but poorer negative predictive value due to the potential for anergy in immunosuppressed patients, who may have reduced delayed-type hypersensitivity responses. In addition, patients with previous exposure to Bacillus Calmette-Guérin (BCG) vaccine (commonly used in developing countries in childhood) may have false-positive results on TB skin tests. These factors do not negate testing, however, because only a fraction of infected persons with these conditions may have falsely nonreactive results. For example, because immunity from BCG vaccine wanes over time, if it has been many years since the vaccination, a TST may be performed and accurately read. To minimize the confounding of TB screening test results, however, the IGRA test is preferred in persons with a history of BCG vaccination (see subsequent discussion of IGRA).

TABLE 30.2 Interpretation of Tuberculin Skin Testing

Diameter of Induration	Positive Result
>5 mm	• Persons with HIV infection or persons with risk factors for HIV infection and unknown HIV status • Persons who were recently exposed to clinically active TB, persons with organ transplants • Persons with chest films indicating healed TB
>10 mm	• Recent arrivals (<5 years) • Foreign-born persons from high-risk countries in Africa, Asia, Latin America • Medically underserved low-income populations and high-risk racial or ethnic minority populations • Injection drug abusers • Residents and employees of high-risk congregate settings: prisons and jails, nursing homes and other residential settings for elderly people and/or AIDS patients, homeless shelters • Mycobacteriology laboratory personnel • Persons with medical conditions known to increase the risk for TB: diabetes, renal failure, silicosis, immunosuppressive therapy, hematological disorders (e.g., leukemia, lymphoma), gastrectomy, 10% or more below ideal body weight
>15 mm	• All other persons

Box 30.4 Factors Contributing to a Decreased Response to Tuberculin Skin Testing

Infections:

• Viral: measles, mumps, chickenpox, HIV infection
• Bacterial: typhoid fever, brucellosis, typhus, leprosy, pertussis, recent or overwhelming *M. tuberculosis* infection
• Fungal: South American blastomycosis
• Live virus vaccinations: measles, mumps, oral polio

Nutritional factors: severe protein depletion
Diseases affecting lymphoid organs: Hodgkin's lymphoma, chronic lymphocytic leukemia
Drugs: corticosteroids and other immunosuppressive agents
Age: newborns, older adults
Stress: surgery, burns, mental illness, graft-versus-host reactions

If the lack of reaction to the TST is suspected to be a false-negative response, a repeat TST should be done. If generalized inability to respond is suspected, it may be necessary to test delayed hypersensitivity using several other antigens to which the person has had a likely exposure. Anergy should be suspected if the person fails to respond to any of the antigens. Of note, many infectious disease specialists feel anergy testing is no longer useful because patients may have selective anergy to TB but not to other antigens, so this practice is not helpful in ruling out TB.

Persons with sensitivity to tuberculin are known as reactors. The definition of a tuberculin reaction size that is indicative of an infection with *M. tuberculosis* is influenced by the dose, dilution, and nature of the tuberculin preparation being used; immunologic factors of the patient; and the relative prevalence of tuberculin sensitivity resulting from infection with *M. tuberculosis* versus other mycobacteria in the population being studied. Reactions caused by infections with mycobacteria other than *M. tuberculosis* (cross-reactions) are common in many parts of the world. Generally, a reaction to *M. tuberculosis* will be larger than would be seen in a cross-reaction. Guidelines for the classification of reactions to intradermal Mantoux tests have established three categories of positive reactions based on the patient's immune status, risk factors for TB exposure, and probability of cross-reaction: 5-, 10-, and 15-mm induration (see Box 30.3). A positive reaction indicates only the presence of TB infection. In the United States, a positive TST without clinical evidence of TB infection (i.e., negative chest x-ray findings and no symptoms) reflects latent infection that should be treated to minimize the possibility of reactivation (secondary) TB.

In addition to the TST, an IGRA may be used. The QuantiFERON-TB Gold Plus and the T-SPOT are whole-blood tests that can aid in the diagnosis of TB but do not differentiate LTBI from active TB. IGRAs are less invasive and require only a single patient visit to conduct the test. Results can be available within 24 hours. Limited data are available on the use of IGRAs in children younger than 5 years and immunocompromised persons.

An additional advantage of IGRA is that it does not cause a false-positive test result in individuals who have received the BCG vaccine against TB. Many people born outside the United States receive BCG during infancy. Originally developed from *Mycobacterium bovis*, BCG has an estimated overall protection rate of approximately 50%, although it appears to be more effective in locations close to the equator. Vaccination with BCG may cause a false-positive reaction on the TST due to priming from the BCG vaccine antigens. In contrast, the IGRA and T-SPOT do not react against BCG antigens and typically do not give a false-positive results due to prior BCG exposure.

Subsequent Testing

In patients in whom there is a clinical suspicion of TB, the first diagnostic step should be a combination of a standard anterior-posterior and lateral chest x-ray film and a sputum examination for mycobacteria. The initial radiographic manifestation of a primary infection in an adult or child is usually parenchymal infiltration accompanied by ipsilateral lymph node enlargement. The parenchymal lesions may be seen in any portion of the lung but are seen most commonly in the apical and posterior segments of the upper lobes or in the superior segments of the lower lobes. Lesions may be dense and homogeneous, with lobar, segmental, or subsegmental distribution. Patients with HIV disease tend to have atypical radiographic findings; these patients tend not to have cavitations, and infiltrates are less likely to occur in the upper lobes. Cavitations are also seen infrequently in older patients and in patients who are immunosuppressed. Hematogenous TB is characterized by diffuse, finely nodular, uniformly distributed lesions on the chest x-ray film (military TB).

Chest x-ray films that show no change in findings over a 3- to 4-month interval can generally be interpreted as showing a past TB infection or another disease. The use of a single chest x-ray film as a guide to the nature or the stability of the underlying disease is questionable. The words "old" and "fibrotic" are not accurate terms to use when interpreting a single chest x-ray film. Any persistent infiltrate in an older person should be considered suggestive of TB. This form of TB is often missed in older adults, especially among patients residing in nursing homes.

In pulmonary TB, examination of sputum provides the most convenient method of identifying the presence of mycobacteria, in terms of low cost, widespread availability, ease of performance, and reliability. The patient must be instructed to produce material brought up from the chest by coughing. A series of at least three single specimens on different days should be collected from patients who have a productive cough. When a patient is unable to produce an adequate amount of sputum, it is possible to obtain by gastric lavage the bronchopulmonary secretions that the patient has unknowingly swallowed during the night. Gastric aspiration is done following a period of fasting for 8 to 10 hours; it should be performed before the patient arises. About 50 mL of gastric contents is required for this test, which is best performed in the hospitalized patient.

It is possible to induce sputum production by inhalation of hypertonic saline. These specimens will be thinner and more watery than sputum produced spontaneously. Inducing sputum by this method may produce a violent and uncontrolled cough, so special conditions to filter ambient air and minimize transmission may be indicated. Occasionally, a pooled specimen collected over a period of 10 to 24 hours may be helpful if the previous methods are not effective or appropriate. This type of specimen is more subject to contamination and is best collected in an institutional setting.

Bronchial washings obtained with fiber-optic bronchoscopy may be indicated in patients who are unable to produce sputum or in those who are thought to have TB despite negative sputum culture reports. When extrapulmonary TB is suspected, it is necessary to collect less common clinical specimens from sources such as urine; peritoneal, pericardial, and pleural fluids; bones and joints; or lymph nodes.

The detection of AFB in stained sputum smears examined by direct microscopy provides the first evidence of the presence of mycobacteria in a clinical specimen. It is estimated that 50% to 80% of patients with pulmonary TB will have positive sputum smears. The sputum smear is the easiest and quickest procedure to provide the practitioner with a preliminary confirmation of the diagnosis. The smear also provides the practitioner with a quantitative estimate of the number of bacilli being excreted by the patient. These estimates are described as rare, few, or numerous. The lowest concentration of organisms that can be detected by microscopic examination is 10 per milliliter of sputum. For direct microscopy of sputum, the most widely used method is the Ziehl-Neelsen staining method.

All clinical specimens suspected of containing mycobacteria must be inoculated onto culture media. Culture yield appears to be associated with the clinical presentation of the patient. One study reported that patients with cavitary disease tend to have a higher rate of positive cultures than do patients with focal infiltrates. The cultures should be incubated at 37°C and examined at weekly intervals. The time from the laboratory's receipt of the specimen to the report of the culture is usually 3 to 6 weeks. In rare situations, such as repeated contaminated specimens or patients with positive Gram stains and negative cultures, guinea pig inoculation may be necessary.

Susceptibility of tubercle bacilli to various anti-TB drugs may be determined via either the direct or the indirect test. The direct drug-susceptibility test is performed by using clinical specimens of AFB, which are inoculated directly onto a drug-containing culture medium. Growth is then compared with growth on a non–drug-containing medium. An indirect test is performed by using a subculture from the primary isolate as the inoculum. Although the direct test is preferred, because it is more representative of the bacterial population of the patient, the indirect test may be useful when the initial smear result is negative but the culture result is positive, when growth on the control medium is inadequate for a reliable test, or when a reference culture is submitted by another laboratory. In the past, the previously untreated patient with newly diagnosed TB was started on anti-TB therapy without prior drug-susceptibility testing. Recommendations for drug-susceptibility testing have been modified because of the emergence of drug-resistant bacilli and are discussed in the section on clinical management.

Differential Diagnosis

Difficulties in a differential diagnosis arise when the tubercle bacilli cannot be isolated by smear or culture and in situations in which other diseases such as carcinoma or pulmonary mycosis are present. Small pulmonary lesions, particularly a solitary nodule or coin nodule, need to be differentiated from early carcinoma of the lung, pulmonary infarction, localized pulmonary fibrosis, and pneumonia of fungal, viral, mycoplasmal, or bacterial origin with delayed clearing or resolution. In extensive forms of pulmonary TB, bronchopneumonia and lobar pneumonia must be considered. The acute cavitary forms of TB must be differentiated from lung abscess. Other chronic pulmonary diseases that frequently are characterized by cavity formations include systemic mycotic infections, particularly coccidioidomycosis, and histoplasmosis.

Pulmonary TB of hematogenous origin must be differentiated from other types of infection that may manifest in similar fashion: silicosis, berylliosis, asbestosis, sarcoidosis, diffuse interstitial fibrosis, scleroderma, metastatic neoplasms, or alveolar cell carcinoma. From the perspective of clinical manifestations, the clinician must consider other conditions that may cause prolonged or obscure fevers, such as lymphoma, brucellosis, and HIV infection.

MANAGEMENT

The development of specific chemotherapeutic agents has revolutionized the prognosis of TB infection, making the disease truly curable and preventable. Drug treatment of TB should be viewed as both a personal health measure intended to cure the ill patient and as a public health measure intended to interrupt transmission of tubercle bacilli in the community.

Initial Management

In patients in whom the clinical and radiographic findings suggest a diagnosis of TB and the sputum examination reveals the presence of mycobacteria, a working diagnosis can be made and anti-TB chemotherapy can be started. For patients in whom TB is suspected but whose sputum smear results are negative, an alternative is to begin therapy and wait for culture results. Initiating chemotherapy in the absence of a definitive diagnosis is a valid approach, but caution is needed for patients with HIV infection and multidrug resistance. X-ray findings of TB in patients with AIDS are often atypical and may be indicative of a range of diagnostic possibilities; thus, a presumptive diagnosis of TB in these patients may be more speculative.

The main goal of therapy is to eliminate all tubercle bacilli from the patient while avoiding the development of clinically significant drug resistance. Although individuals with LTBI do not have symptoms and cannot spread the TB bacteria to others, there is the possibility that the infection can become active; therefore, treatment of LTBI is essential for controlling and eliminating TB in the United States. For these individuals, a combination therapy in which both rifapentine and INH are given once a week for 12 weeks is recommended. Monotherapy regimens include daily INH alone for 6 to 9 months or daily RIF alone for 4 months.

For patients with active TB, treatment consists of administering multiple drugs that the organism is susceptible to, adding new drugs to the regimen when it is suspected that treatment is not working, providing the maximum therapy in the shortest amount of time, and ensuring patient compliance. While curing the individual patient, the transmission of *M. tuberculosis* to other persons also needs to be minimized.

The current minimal acceptable duration of treatment for all children and adults with culture-positive TB is 6 months. The initial phase of a 6-month regimen should consist of a 2-month course of INH, RIF, pyrazinamide (PZA), and ethambutol (EMB) or streptomycin in children who are too young to be monitored for visual acuity, This regimen is given until the results of drug-susceptibility studies are available, unless there is little possibility of drug resistance (e.g., less than 4% primary resistance to INH in the community and the patient has had no previous treatment with anti-TB medication, is not from a country with a high prevalence of drug-resistant TB, or has no known exposure to a drug-resistant case). Although there are 10 drugs currently approved by the Food and Drug Administration to treat TB, the preceding four drugs are first-line anti-TB agents that are the core of most treatment regimens. The second phase of therapy should consist of INH and RIF for a total of 4 months (daily treatment or three times per week). Therapy should be prolonged if the response is slow or otherwise suboptimal.

An alternative regimen for persons who cannot take PZA (e.g., pregnant women) consists of a 9-month regimen of INH and RIF. EMB should also be included until the results of susceptibility studies are available unless there is little possibility of drug resistance. Drug resistance is most common in HIV patients and immigrants. If INH resistance is confirmed, RIF plus PZA plus EMB should be continued for a minimum of 6 months. For RIF resistance, INH plus EMB should be used for 18 months or INH, PZA, and streptomycin for 9 months. In HIV-infected patients, rifabutin should always be used because RIF interacts with protease inhibitors and non-nucleoside retroviral inhibitors.

Adverse reactions and prescribing considerations for the most typically used TB drugs are shown in Drugs Commonly Prescribed 30.1. See Box 30.5 for a discussion of drug-resistant TB, both MDR-TB and XDR-TB.

Directly observed therapy (DOT) should be considered for all patients with active TB because of the difficulty in predicting which patients will adhere to a prescribed regimen. When TB is initially diagnosed, the practitioner should explain to the patient about the disease, required treatment, and the necessity of completing the recommended therapy. If DOT is indicated, the patient and the practitioner should agree on a method that ensures the greatest degree of adherence and maintains confidentiality. DOT may require an outreach worker to go into the community and administer each dose of medication to the patient. Many patients can, however, receive the treatment at a center agreed on by the practitioner and the patient. Common community settings include TB clinics, community health centers, migrant health clinics, homeless shelters, jails and prisons, nursing homes, schools, drug treatment centers, hospitals, HIV/AIDS clinics, or occupational health clinics. In some situations, a responsible person other than a health-care worker may be able to administer the chemotherapy. Possible resources in the community include correctional facility personnel, social and welfare caseworkers, clergy, teachers, and reliable volunteers. Adequate medication adherence is critical to the complete clearance of all infectious organisms and to the prevention of drug-resistant strains of TB.

HIV infection and other factors that compromise a patient's immune system are important considerations when selecting the most effective treatment RIF. These factors are particularly important with drug-resistant TB because of the potential for rapid disease progression and death when patients receive inadequate treatment. DOT and experienced TB/HIV caregivers are considered to be critical to the effective treatment of both conditions. Given the propensity for RIF to upregulate and induce the hepatic cytochrome p450 metabolic pathway, the dosage of several antiretroviral medications must be increased when administered with RIF. However, substituting rifabutin (Mycobutin) for RIF (Rimactane, Rifadin) allows for the concurrent administration of anti-TB and antiretroviral drug regimens, with no dosage adjustments in the latter. Currently, most guidelines indicate that HIV-infected patients should be treated for a total of 9 months and for at least 6 months after sputum conversion. In general, intermittent anti-TB therapy is not recommended for TB/HIV–coinfected patients. See the recommendations for the treatment of TB and antiretroviral dosage adjustments in HIV-infected patients in Chapter 63.

Effective therapy for TB is essential for pregnant women. Untreated TB represents a greater hazard to a pregnant woman and her fetus than does treatment of the disease. Initial treatment should consist of INH and RIF. EMB (Myambutol) should also be included unless primary INH resistance is unlikely. Streptomycin should not be prescribed for pregnant women because it may cause congenital deafness in the fetus. PZA is recommended by international TB organizations for use in pregnant women; however, in the United States, PZA is not currently recommended because it has not been determined whether there is a risk of teratogenicity. Breastfeeding does not need to be discouraged because the small concentrations of anti-TB drugs in breast milk are not adequate to produce toxicity in the newborn. TB during pregnancy is not an indication for a therapeutic abortion.

Drugs Commonly Prescribed 30.1: Tuberculosis

	ADVERSE REACTIONS AND PRESCRIBING CONSIDERATIONS
First-Line TB Drugs	All must be taken on an empty stomach to facilitate absorption—if unable to comply, may take medicine with food that does not contain fat or oils (may ease nausea).
Isoniazid (INH or H)	May cause peripheral neuropathy (pyridoxine may be given prophylactically). May be associated with increased risk of seizures in patients with epilepsy. May be hepatotoxic (potentiated by rifampin).
Rifampin (RIF, RMP, or R)	May cause thrombocytopenia. Commonly causes rash without itching during the first few weeks; usually resolves on its own. May cause an elevation in bilirubin, which usually resolves in 10 days; potentiates rifapentine and INH hepatotoxicity.
Pyrazinamide (PZA or Z)	May cause rash. May be hepatotoxic. If the patient will not take due to tablet size, pyrazinamide syrup may be substituted.
Ethambutol (EMB or E)	Periodic vision screens required, given ocular toxicity (optic neuritis).
Streptomycin (SM, STM, or S)	Use with caution in patients with mild to severe kidney problems. Periodic hearing screens required, given aminoglycoside-related ototoxicity.
Second-Line TB Drugs	Choice of agent should be guided by resistance testing.
Aminoglycosides (e.g., amikacin, kanamycin)	Use with caution in patients with mild to severe kidney problems. Chronic use may cause ototoxicity (audiologic and vestibular dysfunction).
Polypeptides (e.g., capreomycin, viomycin, enviomycin)	Capreomycin may cause nephrotoxicity.
Fluoroquinolones (e.g., ciprofloxacin, levofloxacin, moxifloxacin)	Commonly causes nausea, vomiting, or other gastrointestinal symptoms. May also cause tendinitis/tendon rupture. Associated with QTc prolongation.
Thioamides (e.g., ethionamide, prothionamide)	Gastrointestinal side effects may occur. Central nervous system and psychiatric effects.
Cycloserine (only antibiotic in its class)	Gastrointestinal side effects may occur.
p-aminosalicylic acid	Potential cause of drug-induced hepatitis.

Box 30.5 Drug-Resistant Tuberculosis (TB): MDR-TB and XDR-TB

MDR-TB

Multidrug-resistant TB: Tuberculosis resistant at least to isoniazid and rifampin

XDR-TB

Extensively drug-resistant TB: Tuberculosis resistant to both isoniazid and rifampin, as well as fluoroquinolones and at least one of the injectable second-line anti-TB agents (kanamycin, capreomycin, or amikacin)
Principles of treatment: The principles of treatment for both MDR-TB and XDR-TB are the same, focused on antimicrobial sensitivity testing and the selection of active agents.

Given resistance to second-line agents, XDR-TB has a higher mortality rate due to a reduced number of effective treatment options.

Treatment lasts for a minimum of 18 months and may last for years.

Regimens that are adequate for treating adults with pulmonary TB should also be effective in treating extrapulmonary disease. Bacteriological evaluation of extrapulmonary TB may be limited by the relative inaccessibility of the disease site to anti-infective chemotherapy. Response to treatment often must be judged on the basis of clinical and radiographic findings. Surgery may be necessary to obtain specimens for diagnosis and to treat certain complications, such as constrictive pericarditis. Corticosteroid therapy has been shown to be of benefit in preventing cardiac constriction from TB pericarditis and in decreasing the neurologic sequelae of TB meningitis.

Subsequent Management

Today, the majority of patients with TB may undergo treatment and remain in their home setting. There may be specific patient situations that mandate the need for hospitalization of the patient with TB. These include very ill patients who have no responsible person at home to provide care, patients with advanced pulmonary disease with highly positive sputum smears or severe extrapulmonary disease, or the presence of associated medical problems that require hospitalization.

Adults should have measurements of serum bilirubin, hepatic enzymes, BUN, and creatinine, and a CBC including platelet count, before starting chemotherapy for TB. Visual acuity and red-green color perception tests are recommended before initiation of EMB, and a serum uric acid level should be measured before starting PZA. Patients should be advised to report symptoms suggestive of drug toxicity. For INH-containing regimens, symptoms of concern are anorexia, nausea, vomiting, fatigue or weakness, dark urine, icterus, rash, paresthesias of the hands and feet, fever, and abdominal tenderness. Routine monitoring of laboratory tests for evidence of hepatic failure is not recommended, but monthly questioning for symptoms of drug toxicity is indicated. Patients with known liver disease or heavy drinkers may need to have periodic LFTs, however, as they are more prone to hepatic injury. Appropriate laboratory tests are mandatory if symptoms of drug toxicity develop.

Periodic examination of the patient is necessary to observe for changes in symptoms, signs, body weight, and temperature. The single most important laboratory test is the bacteriologic examination of bronchopulmonary secretions. A progressive decrease in the number of AFB in weekly or biweekly specimens is a good indicator of effective chemotherapy. Periodic laboratory checks of blood, urine, visual acuity, eighth cranial nerve (vestibulocochlear) function, renal function, and hepatic function are desirable based on the severity of the illness and the drugs being administered. Patients should be questioned carefully for any symptoms of drug toxicity, as well as the level of adherence to their treatment regimen.

It is not necessary to restrict physical activity or require bedrest of most patients. Bedrest may help make patients who are experiencing fever, night sweats, anorexia, or bouts of coughing more comfortable. Patients who present with a history of fever should have a normal temperature within 2 to 3 weeks after the initiation of chemotherapy. It may be necessary to suppress the cough reflex in patients who are experiencing severe coughing. Codeine and hydrocodone are the most useful for temporary treatment. If the patient is producing thick and tenacious secretions, suppression of the cough reflex is not desirable. These patients should be instructed in adequate hydration and air humidification and prescribed an expectorant. Chest pain may manifest if the patient develops pleuritis. Occasionally, chest pain may be caused by a fractured rib resulting from severe coughing. Instillation of a local anesthetic proximate to the rib fracture is preferred over the older method of strapping the chest. Coughing that results in occasional episodes of streaked or bloody sputum requires no specific treatment

other than managing the cough. There may be significant hemoptysis with bronchogenic spread of TB; however, this tends to be self-limited. In advanced chronic cavitary TB, fatal pulmonary hemorrhage or shock can occur if large pulmonary arteries ulcerate or a Rasmussen's aneurysm forms, which is a pulmonary artery aneurysm adjacent to or within a tuberculous cavity.

FOLLOW-UP AND REFERRAL

The response to anti-TB chemotherapy in patients with positive bacteriology is best evaluated by repeated sputum examinations. Sputum cultures should be done at least once monthly until sputum conversion is documented. After 2 months of treatment with regimens containing both INH and RIF, the majority of patients should convert to negative cultures. Patients whose sputum culture results have not become negative after 3 months of treatment should be carefully reevaluated and referred to a pulmonologist. Drug-susceptibility tests should be repeated and treatment should be administered or continued under direct observation. If organisms are found to be resistant, the treatment regimen should be modified to include at least two drugs to which the organisms are susceptible and administered using DOT. For patients whose sputum no longer contains *M. tuberculosis,* at least one further sputum smear and culture should be performed at the completion of therapy. X-ray evaluations during treatment are less important than sputum examination. A chest x-ray film at the completion of treatment will provide a baseline comparison for any future films.

Shortness of breath in a patient without underlying pulmonary disease is suggestive of complications of pulmonary TB and requires further diagnostic inquiry. Sudden breathlessness may be a symptom of acute pleurisy with pleuritic pain, pleural effusion, spontaneous pneumothorax, a massive extension of the TB, or atelectasis. Patients who have coexisting emphysema or pulmonary disease may become dyspneic with only minimal involvement of the lungs.

Preventive Therapy

The ATS has identified risk groups for whom preventive therapy is indicated (Table 30.3). Patients infected with *M. tuberculosis* who do not have active disease still harbor organisms. In turn, prophylactic or preventive treatment of LTBI significantly reduces the probability of reactivation TB later in life. INH given for 6 to 9 months is effective in asymptomatic adults (300 mg/day) or children (10 to 14 mg/kg/day, up to 300 mg/day) with LTBI demonstrated by a positive TB screening test but a negative diagnostic evaluation for active disease. Concurrent pyridoxine administration (25 to 50 mg/day in adults and 1–2 mg/kg daily in children) may reduce the potential for neuropathic complications associated with INH, and adjustments with intermittent dosing (900 mg twice

TABLE 30.3 Groups for Whom Preventive Therapy for Latent Tuberculosis (TB) Infection Is Recommended	
Group	*Comments*
The following high-risk groups should be given treatment if their reaction to the Mantoux tuberculin skin test (PPD) is ≥5 mm:	
1. Persons with known HIV infection and those suspected of having HIV infection (persons with risk factors for HIV infection whose status is unknown)	HIV-infected persons who are at high risk for TB but have negative skin tests should be considered for preventive therapy.
2. Close contacts of persons with newly diagnosed infectious TB 3. Persons with fibrotic changes on chest x-ray examination consistent with old TB	Household members and other close contacts have a 2%–4% chance of developing TB within the first year of exposure to the index case. The risk for very young children and adolescents may be twice that of adults. People who do not develop TB disease within the first year will continue to be at risk for the disease throughout their life. Children should be treated, even if their initial skin tests are negative. Skin testing should be repeated after 3 months of rifapentine and isoniazid (INH) therapy. If the skin test becomes positive, INH preventive therapy should be continued for a total of 9 months.
4. Recent tuberculin skin test converters	A skin test conversion is defined as an increase in induration of 10 mm or more within 2 years for those younger than age 35 years and 15 mm or more for those age 35 years or older.
5. Persons with medical conditions that increase the risk of TB with a PPD result of 10 mm or greater	
• Diabetes mellitus	The risk for this group may be two to four times that of the general population. Particularly at risk are poorly controlled insulin-dependent diabetics.
• Prolonged therapy with adrenocorticosteroids	TB that develops during corticosteroid therapy tends to be disseminated or presents in an obscure fashion. Prednisone (or equivalent) given daily at 15 mg or higher for 2–3 weeks markedly reduces tuberculin reactivity.
• Immunosuppressive therapy	Persons receiving other forms of immunosuppressive therapy are at an increased risk for TB.
• Hematological and reticuloendothelial diseases	Diseases such as leukemia and Hodgkin's disease may be associated with suppressed cellular immunity and an increased risk of TB.
• Injection drug users known to be HIV-negative	Persons injecting illicit drugs may be at increased risk of TB even if not infected with HIV.
• End-stage renal disease (ESRD)	Persons with ESRD are predisposed to developing extrapulmonary TB with disseminated disease. Because these patients may be anergic, a documented history or positive skin test is an indication for preventive INH therapy unless they have been treated previously.
• Clinical conditions associated with substantial rapid weight loss or chronic malnutrition	These conditions include intestinal bypass surgery for obesity (which carries an increased risk for disseminated TB), postgastrectomy, chronic peptic ulcer disease, chronic malabsorption syndromes, chronic alcoholism, and carcinomas of the oropharynx and upper gastrointestinal tract that prevent adequate nutritional intake. The postgastrectomy state may increase the risk of developing TB even without weight loss.
Persons in the following groups who are younger than age 35 years and have a positive tuberculin skin test (≥10 mm):	
• Foreign-born persons from high-prevalence countries	These countries include those in Latin America, Asia, and Africa that have a high prevalence of TB. Especially at risk are recent arrivals (<5 years).

TABLE 30.3   Groups for Whom Preventive Therapy for Latent Tuberculosis (TB) Infection Is Recommended—cont'd

Group	Comments
• Medically underserved low-income groups, especially high-risk racial or ethnic minority populations	These groups include African Americans, Native Americans, Hispanics, Asians, and Pacific Islanders.
• Residents of facilities for long-term care • Residents and staff of high-risk congregate settings (nursing homes, jails, homeless shelters)	These residents include those in correctional facilities, nursing homes, and mental health facilities. Staff of such facilities should also be considered for preventive therapy.
• Migrant farmworkers • Children younger than 4 years • Mycobacteriology laboratory personnel	
• Persons with clinical conditions that place them at high risk	HIV infection, substance abuse, recent infection with *M. tuberculosis* (within the past 2 years), previous TB, silicosis, prolonged immunosuppressive therapy, low body weight (<90% of normal), ESRD, chronic malabsorption
Persons with no known risk factors for TB may be considered for therapy if their reaction to the tuberculin test is ≥15 mm. This group should be given lower priority than the groups listed above.	

Source: Adapted from Chapter 6 of the CDC Curriculum: *Preventive therapy: treatment of TB infection.* www.cdc.gov/tb/education/corecurr/pdf/chapter6.pdf. Accessed July 1, 2013.

weekly) or an overall shortened duration (6 months) may be used for adult patients with medication adherence issues. For patients intolerant of INH or in whom INH-resistant LTBI is suspected, RIF may be used as an alternative in adults (600 mg/day for 4 months) or children (10 to 20 mg/kg/day for 6 months).

All persons with known HIV infection or suspected of having HIV who have positive TST results should receive preventive therapy for TB. HIV-infected persons who are at high risk for TB but have negative skin tests should also be considered for preventive therapy. Preventive regimens are similar to those for non–HIV-infected individuals. However, a full course of daily INH (9 months) or RIF (6 months) is recommended, with the latter reserved for suspected cases of INH-resistant, RIF-sensitive LTBI.

Household members and other close contacts have a 2% to 4% risk of developing TB within the first year of exposure to the index case. The risk for very young children and adolescents may be twice the risk in adults. People who do not develop active TB disease within the first year will continue to be at risk for developing the disease throughout their lives. Children should be treated even if their initial TTS results are negative. TTS should be repeated after 3 months of INH. If a skin test result becomes positive, INH preventive therapy should be continued for a total of 9 months.

Persons with medical conditions such as diabetes mellitus, long-term use of adrenocorticosteroids, use of immunosuppressive therapy, injection drug use, hematological disease, end-stage renal disease, and conditions associated with rapid weight loss or chronic malnutrition are also at risk for TB. Other risk groups include foreign-born persons from high-prevalence countries (e.g., in Asia, Africa, or Latin America); medically underserved groups, especially high-risk racial or ethnic populations (e.g., African Americans, Native Americans, Hispanics), and residents of long-term care facilities (e.g., prisons, nursing homes, mental health facilities).

For updates about current TB treatment recommendations, visit the Division of TB Elimination Web site at www.cdc.gov/nchstp/tb.

Patient Education: Tuberculosis

The necessity of educating the patient and the family about the disease, treatment, and importance of completing the recommended treatment regimen is critical to the management of TB. The patient and family should understand the information and continue to be provided with reinforcement and encouragement throughout the course of therapy. Patients should be offered the option of participating in DOT. For patients who are administering their own medications, strategies that may be helpful for improving adherence include use of a weekly pill dispenser, marking off each day on a calendar as medicine is taken, taking pills at the same time every day (e.g., with breakfast or during a coffee break), and asking a friend or family member to remind the patient to take his or her pills.

Patients are typically considered to be infectious for about 2 to 3 weeks after initiation of drug therapy. If the patient is being cared for at home, he or she should not go to work or school. These patients should be instructed about how to control the spread of tubercle bacilli in microdroplets by using good hygienic measures, appropriate ventilation, and avoiding close contact with family and friends. Patients should sleep in a separate room until no longer considered infectious (hospitalized patients are kept isolated in negative air flow rooms even after treatment is started, until their sputum smears consistently test negative for mycobacteria). Patients should be taught to always cover their mouths when they cough, sneeze, or laugh. Used tissues should be placed in a plastic or paper bag and discarded. If the weather is warm enough, patients should be instructed to place a fan in an open window to blow out air that may be contaminated with TB. Opening other windows in their room will help pull in fresh air.

Patients should be asked to identify any people who may need to be tested for TB infection, including coworkers, family members, and friends. All close contacts will need to undergo TB screening and may require preventive INH therapy. Assurance should be provided to the patient and family by stressing that the majority of properly treated patients with TB are cured.

Sometimes problems associated with TB and its treatment in foreign-born patients stem from communication barriers, cultural and cognitive dissonance between practitioners and patients, and gaps in provider training. Thus, education needs to be targeted to patients, providers, and community workers.

There are excellent TB control strategies available to the public from the CDC. Patients may access these guidelines at www.cdc.gov and obtain guidelines written in an easily understood manner. However, the problems of multidrug-resistant TB and issues of compliance with therapy among all populations remain a significant challenge for health-care providers. Practicing within a *Circle of Caring* enables the clinician to approach these problems in a meaningful way.

REFERENCES

Pneumonia

Donovan F. Community-acquired pneumonia empiric therapy. https://emedicine.medscape.com/article/2011819-overview. Published 2015. Accessed May 22, 2017.

Kobayashi M, Bennett NM, Gierke R, et al. Intervals between PCV13 and PPSV23 vaccines: Recommendations of the Advisory Committee on Immunization Practices (ACIP). *MMWR Morb Mortal Wkly Rep.* 2015;64(34):944-947. https://www.cdc.gov/mmwr/preview/mmwrhtml/mm6434a4.htm. Accessed May 22, 2017.

Tuberculosis

Centers for Disease Control and Prevention. Tuberculosis. https://www.cdc.gov/tb/topic/basics/default.htm. Accessed May 28, 2017.

Schmit KM, Wansaula Z, Pratt R, Price SF, Langer AJ. Tuberculosis—United States, 2016. *MMWR Morb Mortal Wkly Rep.* 2017;66: 289–294.

Upper Respiratory Infections and Influenza

Deutscher C, Johnson L. Influenza during pregnancy: The role of the nurse practitioner. *J Nurse Pract.* 2015;11(9):849–855.

Hammond A, Holcomb M. Managing patient perceptions of the influenza vaccine. *Clin Advisor.* 2015;18(12);41–48.

Kinaan M, Almukhtar T, Chaudhry A, Ali SK. Seasonal influenza: An overview and a treatment plan. *Consultant.* 2015;55(10):792–793, 798–800.

Meneghetti A. Upper respiratory tract infection. http://emedicine.medscape.com/article/302460-overview. Published 2017. Accessed May 19, 2017.

Tesfayesus B, Hill C, Chaney S. Influenza: Complications, diagnosis, and treatment. *Clin Advisor.* 2015;18(2):26, 28, 30, 32, 34, 36–37.

Ward BW, Clarke TC, Nugent CN, Schiller JS. Early release of selected estimates based on data from the 2015 National Health Interview Survey. National Health Interview Survey Early Release Program. https://www.cdc.gov/nchs/data/nhis/earlyrelease/earlyrelease201605.pdf. Accessed July 28, 2017.

RESOURCES

Centers for Disease Control and Prevention. National Center for HIV/AIDS, Viral Hepatitis, STD, and TB Prevention
https://www.cdc.gov/nchhstp/Default.htm

Centers for Disease Control and Prevention H1N1 Flu Web site
www.cdc.gov/h1n1flu

Centers for Disease Control and Prevention SARS Web site
www.cdc.gov/ncidod/sars/infectioncontrol.htm

CURB-65 Calculation Score for Pneumonia Severity
https://www.mdcalc.com/curb-65-score-pneumonia-severity

Patient Education

Key Facts About Influenza
https://www.cdc.gov/flu/keyfacts.htm

Basic TB Facts
https://www.cdc.gov/tb/topic/basics/tbinfectiondisease.htm

Influenza
https://medlineplus.gov/flu.html

Tuberculosis
https://medlineplus.gov/tuberculosis.html

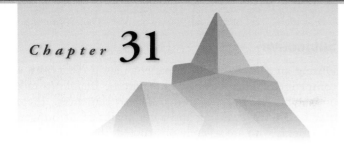

Chapter **31**

Inflammatory Respiratory Disorders

Jill E. Winland-Brown, EdD, APRN, FNP-BC

Barbara Beausejour, APRN, FNP-BC

Brian Oscar Porter, MD, PhD, MPH, MBA

ASTHMA

Asthma is a chronic, inflammatory, obstructive disease of the airways. It may occur at any age and may be characterized by wheezing due to airway spasms, tightness in the chest, breathlessness (dyspnea), and cough. The signs and symptoms may remit spontaneously or worsen in response to intrinsic (stress) or extrinsic (environmental) triggers. The severity of asthma is highly unpredictable, ranging from mild attacks to complete airway obstruction and death. Many pediatricians use the term *reactive airway disease* because the term "asthma" carries a negative connotation for some parents.

EPIDEMIOLOGY AND CAUSES

Asthma affects more than an estimated 100 million people worldwide, and the number is increasing rapidly. In the United States, more than 39.5 million Americans have been diagnosed with asthma at some point in their lives. It is estimated that 9.5% of children currently have asthma. African Americans have a prevalence rate 47% higher than Caucasians. Despite newer antiasthmatic drugs, asthma is responsible for more than 134 million days of restricted activity. The economic cost of asthma is staggering. More than $56 billion annually is lost due to direct medical costs from hospital stays and indirect costs due to lost school and work days.

There are more than 14 million ambulatory care visits related to asthma each year, along with more than 2 million emergency department visits. In the United States, 5,500 deaths each year are attributable to asthma. Despite current prevention efforts, the incidence of asthma continues to increase each year. The prevalence of asthma in adults is 35% higher in females. In children younger than 18 years, boys have a 16% higher incidence than girls. Children aged 5 to 17 years have the highest attack prevalence rates, whereas persons older than 65 years have the lowest.

Clinical practice guidelines were last updated in 2007 and reviewed in 2015 by the National Asthma Education and Prevention Program, which is part of the National Heart, Lung, and Blood Institute. This guidance document is known as the Expert Panel Report 3 (EPR-3). These evidence-based practice guidelines include ways to help patients control their asthma signs and symptoms and improve their quality of life.

Although the pathophysiology of asthma is multifactorial and involves many inflammatory pathways, from a practical perspective, three principal triggers for exacerbations of asthma have been identified:

1. Allergens and environmental factors: allergens may include inhaled substances, such as molds, pollens, dust, animal dander, cosmetics, and tobacco smoke; food additives with sulfite preservative agents; and medications, especially beta blockers and aspirin or aspirin-containing drugs.
2. Infections: upper respiratory tract infections are common precursors to an asthma attack, particularly viral infections.
3. Psychological factors: stressful events or crises at work or home may precipitate an asthma attack, although often stressors are overlooked or dismissed.

PATHOPHYSIOLOGY

Asthma is a chronic inflammatory disease characterized by reversible hyperreactivity of the bronchi and bronchioles to a variety of stimuli. Inflammation of the airways contributes to bronchial hyperreactivity, airflow limitation, and the resultant characteristic signs and symptoms of asthma: wheezing, breathlessness, chest tightness, and cough. The stage is then set for acute bronchoconstriction, airway edema, mucous-plug formation, airway narrowing, and bronchial obstruction.

Genetic predisposition, allergy, environmental factors, stress, and infectious agents are factors that play a role in the etiology of asthma. Immunologically mediated inflammation, the major pathological mechanism of this disease, involves mast cells, eosinophils, lymphocytes, neutrophils, and macrophages, which may directly infiltrate the airway at both smooth muscle and basement membrane layers. These cells release a variety of mediators that stimulate bronchoconstriction, vasodilation, edema formation, and increased mucus production, including histamine, interleukins (ILs), leukotrienes, tumor necrosis factor (TNF), bradykinin, thromboxanes, fibroblast growth factor, and prostaglandins.

The cascade of mediators in allergy-stimulated asthma is initiated when CD4+ T helper (Th) cells bearing a Th2 phenotype (which are predominantly involved in humoral immunity and are resistant to apoptotic killing) produce interleukin-3 (IL-3), IL-4, IL-5, and granulocyte-macrophage colony-stimulating factor in response to an allergen, which, in turn, upregulates the allergic response and airway hypersensitivity. Th1 T cells (predominantly involved in cell-mediated immunity) have been implicated to a lesser extent. Eosinophils are a rich source of leukotrienes that directly cause contraction of bronchial smooth muscle and increase vascular permeability. Activated B lymphocytes transform into plasma cells, synthesizing large amounts of immunoglobulin E (IgE) antibody that binds to and activates tissue mast cells and eosinophils. Mast cell-bound IgE molecules then become cross-linked by environmental allergens, which activate histamine release and further IL-4 and IL-5 production, thereby provoking bronchial smooth muscle contraction and vasodilation.

With each acute exacerbation of asthma, inflammatory mediators incite a structural remodeling of the airways. The alveoli remain largely unaffected, because asthma is not a parenchymal disease. Rather, airway remodeling involves thickening of the bronchial and bronchiolar mucosa, submucosa, and smooth muscle layers, which contributes to the persistence of disease. Increased collagen is deposited below the basement membrane, while the loose areolar connective tissue found between epithelial and smooth muscle layers undergoes hypertrophy. Therefore, prevention of acute episodes, which minimizes remodeling, is key to the proper treatment of asthma.

Asthma is an obstructive pulmonary disease with hypoxia as the universal finding during acute exacerbations. With acute bronchospasm, residual volume increases in the lungs and peak expiratory flow rate (PEFR) diminishes. Inflammation and constriction of the bronchioles increase airway resistance, decrease inspiratory capacity and expiratory volumes, and lead to ventilation–perfusion mismatching and altered arterial blood gas (ABG) concentrations. As a result of hyperventilation, respiratory alkalosis and hypocapnia are common findings with each episode. As an acute attack resolves, narrowing in the larger airways tends to reverse first, whereas the peripheral airways remain most constricted. If an attack progresses and fails to reverse, respiratory acidosis and an elevated arterial carbon dioxide concentration typically result, signaling impending respiratory failure. Severe irreversible bronchoconstriction and inflammation, termed "status asthmaticus," can be fatal.

CLINICAL PRESENTATION

The clinical presentation of asthma varies and depends on whether the patient is currently experiencing an acute attack or is seeking help to manage chronic asthma. It is important to note that not all people with asthma wheeze and that not everyone who wheezes has asthma.

Subjective

During an acute attack, the patient may present with a complaint of breathlessness and may be unable to talk or may be able only to blurt out short sentences. There may be profuse sweating and a complaint of air hunger. In patients who are severely obstructed, there may be no wheezing as only cough may be present.

The patient may present complaining of wheezing, persistent and recurrent cough, difficulty breathing, and/or tightness in the chest, particularly at night or in the early morning. Endurance problems during exercise may occur. Ninety percent of individuals with asthma report that exercise exacerbates their respiratory symptoms.

Any single symptom or combination of symptoms may occur, and symptoms are usually worse at night. The disease spectrum varies from a few mild episodes in a lifetime to daily debilitating symptoms. Food additives, particularly metabisulfite (used as a food preservative), certain dairy products, and, for some individuals, monosodium glutamate, may also cause symptoms. An extreme emotional state such as excessive laughing and/or crying may precipitate or exacerbate an attack.

Objective

Reversible airflow limitation and diurnal variation as measured by PEF constitute objective signs and symptoms of asthma. Variability between morning and evening PEF may reflect airway hyper-responsiveness and indicate instability and severity of asthma. Nasal discharge, mucosal swelling, frontal facial tenderness, nasal polyps, and allergic "shiners"—dark discoloration beneath both eyes—should be noted. The clinician should also check for manifestations of allergic skin conditions such as atopic dermatitis (eczema).

Audible inspiratory and expiratory wheezing may be present. The patient may be using accessory muscles of breathing (scalene and sternocleidomastoid) and sitting upright. Auscultation of the chest may reveal inspiratory and expiratory wheezes, if not already audible. Wheezing during forced exhalation is not considered a reliable indicator, as it may be absent between attacks and may be obscured during acute attacks due to diminished breath sounds.

DIAGNOSTIC REASONING

Expiratory airflow measurements are essential to the differential diagnosis of asthma. The essential elements to consider in making the diagnosis are listed in Box 31.1. In addition, asthma should always be considered as a possible etiology in a patient with a chronic cough.

Differentiating asthma from other respiratory diseases is usually not difficult, particularly with the aid of pulmonary function tests (PFTs), a complete history, and laboratory test

Box 31.1 Essential Elements to Consider When Diagnosing Asthma

History

- Cough (especially nocturnal)
- Recurrent wheeze (absence does not rule out asthma)
- Recurrent episodic dyspnea
- Recurrent chest tightness

Symptoms worsen in relation to specific factors

- Airborne chemicals or dust
- Animals with fur or feathers
- Changes in weather
- Exercise
- Gastroesophageal reflux disease
- Sensitivity to aspirin, other NSAIDs, and sulfites
- Dust mites in house (mattresses, furniture, carpets)
- Cockroaches
- Menses
- Mold/pollen
- Nighttime (patient awakens due to symptoms)
- Nonselective beta blockers
- Pollen
- Smoke (tobacco, wood, etc.)
- Strong emotional expression (laughing or crying)
- Viral infection, rhinitis, sinusitis

Reversible (at least partially) airflow limitations with diurnal variability

- Variation in peak expiratory flow rate of at least 20% between first morning measurement (before taking an inhaled, short-acting beta-agonist) and early afternoon measurement (after using inhaler)
- Exclusion of alternate diagnoses

results. Spirometry is recommended to confirm the diagnosis of asthma. A common feature of asthma is nocturnal awakening with one or more of the following symptoms: dyspnea, cough, and wheezing. Persistent wheezing localized to one area of the lung, with paroxysms of cough, is indicative of endobronchial disease such as foreign body aspiration, neoplasm, or bronchial stenosis. Acute left ventricular heart failure may initially present similarly to asthma (wheezing), but the findings of moist, basilar crackles, gallop rhythms, and other signs of heart failure exclude the diagnosis of asthma.

Allergic rhinitis and atopic dermatitis often accompany a diagnosis of asthma. Concurrent treatment for these conditions is critical. Effective treatment of allergic rhinitis (discussed in Chapter 24) is critical as another mode to prevent triggering acute asthma attacks.

Diagnostic Tests

To establish the diagnosis of asthma, episodic symptoms of airflow obstruction must be present, airflow obstruction must be at least partially reversible, and the provider must have ruled out any alternative diagnoses. Spirometry measurements are helpful in diagnosis and then evaluation and management of the disease. Forced vital capacity (FVC) and forced expiratory volume in 1 second (FEV_1) are helpful measurements. Prebronchodilator and postbronchodilator PFTs, including spirometry and diffusing capacity, to determine the response to bronchodilators are essential in the differential diagnosis and subsequent management of asthma. The diagnosis is made by demonstrating the reversibility of airway obstruction from the pre- and postbronchodilator PFTs. Reversibility is defined as a 10% or greater increase in the FEV_1 after two puffs of a short-acting beta-agonist (SABA) have been inhaled. When spirometry is nondiagnostic, bronchial provocation testing may be useful with histamine, methacholine, or exercise as a trigger of airway constriction. Contraindications to spirometry may include the following:

- Hypertension or hypotension
- Rapid atrial fibrillation
- Chest pain
- Recent heart attack (myocardial infarction)
- Recent eye, chest, heart, or abdominal surgery
- Presence of cerebral, thoracic, or abdominal aneurysm
- Active pulmonary infection, including tuberculosis
- Hemoptysis

Infections often precede an asthma attack. If infection is suspected (because of a productive cough with colored sputum), a sputum test for culture and sensitivity should be done. A complete blood count (CBC) should also be done. Levels of nasal eosinophils, serum eosinophils, and IgE are assessed to determine the allergic status of the patient. Intradermal skin testing may be indicated if the allergic status is significant. When persistent asthma is present, the EPR-3 recommends that skin testing or in vitro radioallergosorbent tests be done to determine sensitivity to allergens to optimize treatment and prevention.

A chest x-ray film may be negative or show only hyperinflation, although radiographs may also reveal thickening of bronchial walls and diminished peripheral lung vascular shadows. ABG analysis is included in the initial work-up to establish a baseline and to determine the degree of hypoxemia and the need for supplemental oxygen. The results of the ABG analysis and spirometry, along with the clinical history and findings on examination, are triangulated to classify the severity of the asthma, as shown in Table 31.1.

Differential Diagnosis

Airflow obstruction may result from foreign body aspiration or viral infections, as well as a variety of underlying pulmonary conditions, such as aspergillosis, tuberculosis, hypersensitivity pneumonitis, or habitual cough. Hyperventilation syndrome, panic disorder, vocal cord

5. RESPIRATORY PROBLEMS

TABLE 31.1 Classification of Asthma Severity	
Classification	**Clinical Features Before Treatment**
Intermittent	• Intermittent symptoms less than 2 days per week • Nighttime asthma symptoms less than twice per month • Asymptomatic and normal peak expiratory flow (PEF) between exacerbations • PEF or forced expiratory volume in 1 second (FEV$_1$) >80% predicted; PFT variability >20%
Mild persistent	• Symptoms more than 2 days per week but not daily; may be several times at night per month • PEF or FEV$_1$ >80% predicted; PFT variability 20%–30%
Moderate persistent	• Symptoms daily, but not continual; nighttime symptoms more than once a week, but not nightly • Exacerbations affect activity and sleep • PEF or FEV$_1$ 60%–80% predicted; PFT variability >30%
Severe persistent	• Continuous daily symptoms; frequent nighttime symptoms • Frequent exacerbations • Physical activities limited by asthma • PEF or FEV$_1$: <60% predicted; PFT variability >30%

Source: National Asthma Education and Prevention Program. Expert Panel 3 Summary Report 2007: Guidelines for the diagnosis and management of asthma (NIH publication no. 08-5846). Bethesda, MD: U.S. Department of Health and Human Services, Public Health Service, National Institutes of Health, National Heart, Lung, and Blood Institute. Reviewed 2015.

dysfunction (paradoxical closure of the vocal cords upon inhalation and/or exhalation), mitral valve prolapse, recurrent pulmonary emboli, congestive heart failure, and chronic obstructive pulmonary disease (COPD) may mimic asthma. In addition, for some sensitive patients, cough may be secondary to the use of certain drugs, such as angiotensin-converting enzyme inhibitors, beta blockers, aspirin, and NSAIDs. The key feature in the diagnosis of asthma is reversibility of the obstructive phenomenon.

MANAGEMENT

With initial diagnosis of asthma, the clinician may want to refer the patient to a pulmonologist. An aggressive approach to asthma management is recommended to improve short-term symptoms, prevent recurrence of symptoms, and/or manage a potentially chronic problem—all with the goal of improving the patient's quality of life by achieving and maintaining long-term control

of symptoms. The principles of management include the following:

- Identification of factors that exacerbate the condition
- Daily monitoring of PEF with a symptom record
- Written instructions on managing an acute asthma attack
- Intensive education and follow-up, emphasizing joint decision making

Initial and subsequent management of asthma is aimed at first removing all identified triggers or precipitants. Acute asthma attacks are treated with SABAs such as albuterol (salbutamol), administered via a metered dose inhaler (MDI) with a hydrofluoroalkane propellant or nebulized as an inhaled oral solution. MDIs containing chlorofluorocarbon propellants have been banned in the United States, due to their destructive effects on atmospheric ozone. Home-based rescue therapy for bronchospasm and shortness of breath typically calls for albuterol several times a day as needed, up to every 1 to 2 hours if necessary. If a patient must take rescue medication more frequently or for more than three consecutive doses, she or he should be instructed to seek further medical care. An individualized and detailed action plan may be developed between the care provider and patient to provide specific guidance for minimizing asthma exacerbations, preventing further progression, and educating about the dangers of medication overuse and when to seek medical care if rescue treatment thresholds are exceeded.

The prevention of asthma exacerbations through the use of daily controller medications for those with mild to severe persistent asthma remains the mainstay of effective asthma therapy, as a reduction in exacerbations and control of daily symptoms leads to improved quality of life. The stepwise therapy approach is a guide to assist the provider in working with the patient to make individually tailored treatment decisions that adequately address symptoms while avoiding medication overuse. As a rule, the highest appropriate therapeutic step should be used to gain early control. The therapy should be "stepped up" if control is not maintained. At each visit, the clinician should review the patient's medication delivery technique, treatment adherence, and control of asthma triggers. The stepwise approach, according to the severity of the asthma presentation, is shown in Figure 31.1.

In the management of chronic asthma, PFTs are done periodically to measure how well the patient is responding to treatment. The patient can be taught to use a handheld peak flow meter to measure the PEFR and gauge response to treatment. Several peak flow rate readings should be done when the patient is stable to establish a baseline (or "personal best"). This baseline can be used as a benchmark for guiding therapy. Once the patient's condition is stabilized, daily PEF monitoring can be done by the patient. If the PEF reading is less than 80% of the patient's personal best, adjustments in

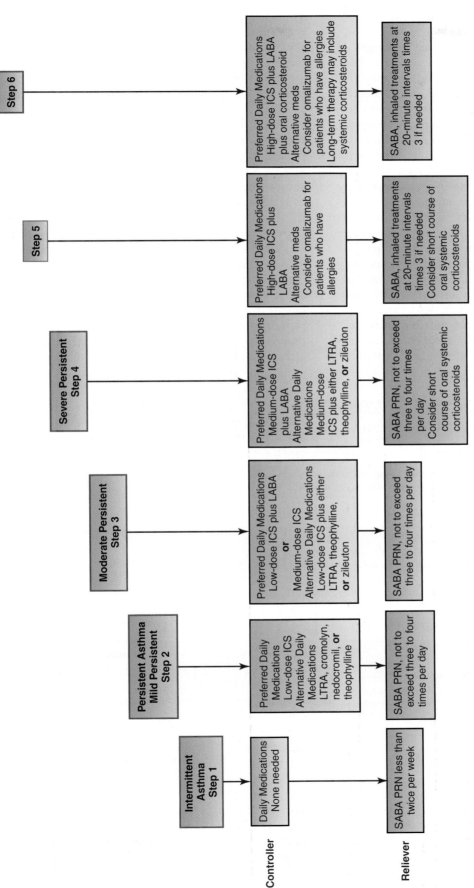

SABA = short-acting beta2-agonist

ICS = inhaled corticosteroid

LTRA = leukotriene receptor agonist

LABA = long-acting beta2-agonist

Step up to the next step if control is not achieved. First, however, review patient medication technique and prevention strategies (avoid all allergens or other trigger factors).

Step down to the next step when asthma is well controlled for 3 months.

Review RX every 3–6 months.

Adapted from the National Heart, Lung, and Blood Institute, Asthma Education and Prevention Program. Expert Panel Report 3 (EPR-3): Guidelines for the Diagnosis and Management of Asthma, 2007.

Figure 31.1 Treatment flowchart: asthma.

medications or lifestyle changes may be necessary to minimize asthma exacerbations (see Fig. 31.2).

Inhaled corticosteroids (ICS) are the treatment of choice as anti-inflammatory controller therapies, above other classes of inhaled medications and theophylline. Recent genetic and epidemiological studies suggest that certain individuals (especially those of African American ethnicity) have a negative reaction to long-acting beta-agonist (LABA) bronchodilators, such as salmeterol. These individuals seem to do worse on long-term beta-agonist therapy. Salmeterol (Serevent) is no longer used as a single agent because of safety concerns regarding increased morbidity and mortality if used without an accompanying corticosteroid. When used in combination with an ICS (Advair Discus, Symbicort, Dulera), however, such combinations are extremely effective at improving lung function in patients with moderate to severe asthma. See Drugs Commonly Prescribed 31.1 for a summary of medications for asthma.

Recently, monoclonal antibody biologic agents have been approved for more severe forms of persistent asthma, including the anti-IgE agent omalizumab (Xolair) for allergic asthma and the anti-IL-5 agent mepolizumab (Nucala), which are specifically approved for eosinophilic

asthma. The additional of such therapies to an asthma regimen requires referral to an asthma specialist and, in the case of omalizumab, requires close observation with dosing.

Bronchial thermoplasty is a therapeutic strategy used for adults aged 18 years and older with severe persistent asthma who remain symptomatic despite the use of high-dose ICS and a LABA. Bronchial thermoplasty reduces asthma attacks by delivering controlled therapeutic radiofrequency energy into the airway, heating the tissue and reducing the amount of smooth muscle present in the airway wall. As a result of less smooth muscle, less airway constriction occurs, thereby reducing asthma attacks.

Scant data exist on the prevalence of complementary therapy for asthma. Such therapies commonly used include breathing techniques, yoga, acupuncture, and herbal preparations. It is difficult to assess the safety and efficacy of these therapies, however, without well-designed clinical trials. Practitioners of herbal medicine recommend the fruit (soursop) and leaves of the graviola tree to relieve respiratory problems, such as cough and asthma, and for many other medical problems. Some

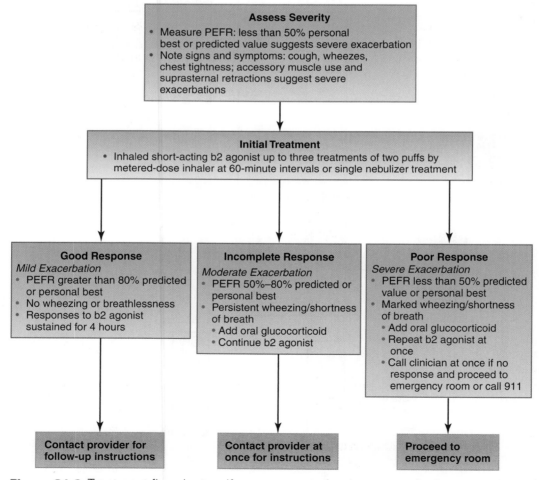

Figure 31.2 Treatment flowchart: self-management of asthma exacerbations.

Drugs Commonly Prescribed 31.1: Asthma

DRUG	INDICATION AND FORMULATION	ADVERSE REACTIONS AND PRESCRIBING CONSIDERATIONS
Short-Acting Beta-Agonists (SABAs)		
	First-line defense for acute attack; may be used prophylactically when necessary before exercise. Provide smooth muscle relaxation for bronchodilation. Increased need (usage) indicates need to change treatment regimen.	Adverse reactions: tachycardia, palpitations, tremor, hypokalemia. Use with caution in elderly patients.
Albuterol (Ventolin hydrofluoroalkane [HFA]; Proventil HFA; ProAir HFA; ProAir RespiClick inhalation powder)	Metered-dosage inhaler (MDI): 90 mcg/puff	Two puffs every 4–6 hours when necessary For exercise-induced asthma: two puffs 5 minutes before exercise
AccuNeb inhalation solution	Nebulizer: 2.5 mg (0.5 mL of 0.5% solution diluted to 3 mL with normal saline or 3 mL of 0.08% solution)	May be mixed with cromolyn or ipratropium solution when nebulized
Levalbuterol (Xopenex: L-isomer of albuterol)	0.63 mg in 3 mL or 1.25 mg in 3 mL	
Ventolin, Proventil	Syrup: 2 mg/5 mL	Adults: 2–4 mg orally three or four times a day
Anticholinergics		
	Not indicated for initial treatment of acute attacks where rescue therapy is required for rapid response; may be used as daily controller therapy or for rescue therapy in limited doses under medical supervision.	Adverse reactions: tachycardia, palpitations, cardiac arrest with overuse in asthma Do not give to patients with glaucoma or benign prostatic hypertrophy
Ipratropium bromide (Atrovent HFA)	MDI: 17 mcg/puff	Two puffs four times a day; maximum 12 puffs/day
(Atrovent solution)	Nebulizer: 0.02% (500 mcg in 2.5 mL of solution)	500 mcg two to four times a day
Leukotriene Receptor Antagonists (LTRAs)		
	Long-term controller medication; prophylaxis and treatment of chronic asthma; ineffective for acute attacks.	May allow gradual reduction of inhaled corticosteroids (not for abrupt substitution)
Montelukast (Singulair)	Prophylaxis and chronic treatment: 4- or 5-mg chewable tablets; 10-mg film-coated tablet; oral granules 4 mg/packet	Monitor with potent CYP450 inducers May take 10 mg/night
Inhaled Corticosteroids (ICS)		
	Long-term controller medication; prophylaxis and treatment of chronic asthma; ineffective for acute attacks.	Monitor for infections and susceptibility to oral candidiasis (rinse mouth after use) Avoid excessive use.
Mometasone furoate (Asmanex Twisthaler)	Dry powder for inhalation (DPI): 110–220 mcg/inhalation	Two inhalations twice daily
(Asmanex HFA)	MDI: 100–200 mcg	
Beclomethasone (QVAR)	40 or 80 mcg/inhalation	Twice daily
Budesonide (Pulmicort) (Pulmicort Flexhaler)	DPI: 90 or 180 mcg/inhalation (maximum 720 mg per day)	Twice daily

Continued

Drugs Commonly Prescribed 31.1: Asthma—cont'd

DRUG	INDICATION AND FORMULATION	ADVERSE REACTIONS AND PRESCRIBING CONSIDERATIONS
Fluticasone (Flovent)	MDI: 44, 110, 220 mcg/puff DPI: 50-, 100-, 250-mg dose	Twice daily (Not recommended for children younger than 4 years)
Combination Inhaled Corticosteroids and Long Acting (ICS + LABA)		
	Long-term controller medication for moderate to severe persistent asthma; prophylaxis and treatment of chronic asthma; ineffective for acute attacks.	Monitor for infections and susceptibility to oral candidiasis (rinse mouth after use) Avoid excessive use.
Fluticasone and salmeterol (Advair Diskus)	DPI: 100, 250, or 500 mcg fluticasone per dose plus 50 mcg salmeterol per dose	One puff twice daily One puff daily of 500 mcg/50 mcg formulation
Budesonide and formoterol (Symbicort)	MDI: 80 or 160 mcg budesonide per dose plus 4.5 mcg formoterol per inhalation	Two inhalations twice daily
Fluticasone furoate and vilanterol (BREO Ellipta)	DPI: 100 or 200 mcg fluticasone plus 25 mcg vilanterol per inhalation	One inhalation daily
Mometasone furoate and formoterol fumarate dihydrate (Dulera)	MDI: 100 or 200 mcg mometasone plus 5 mcg formoterol per inhalation	Two inhalations twice daily
Systemic Corticosteroids		
	For long-term treatment of severe persistent asthma that cannot be controlled with other medication classes, including ICS combined with LABAs. Short courses or "bursts" effective for establishing control when initiating therapy or during a period of gradual deterioration or as a supplement to rescue bronchodilator therapy during acute attacks to prevent late-phase bronchospasm. Ineffective as treatment for acute attacks.	Use with caution in patients with tuberculosis, hypothyroidism, cirrhosis, or ulcerative colitis May mask or increase risk of infection; may cause hypokalemia, hypernatremia, glucose intolerance, and bone demineralization Always titrate down to minimal effective dose
Methylprednisolone (Medrol)	2-, 4-, 8-, 16-, or 32-mg tablets	Give 7.5–60.0 mg once a day or every other day in a single dose or four divided doses for larger dosages, as needed for long-term control
Prednisolone (Orapred)	15-mg/5-mL solution	Short "burst" 40–60 mg/day as a single dose or in two divided doses over 3–10 days; tapering typically necessary if given for more than 10 days to prevent adrenal insufficiency
Prednisone	1-, 2.5-, 5-, 10-, 20-, or 50-mg tablets	
Methylxanthines		
	Long-term controller medication for moderate to severe persistent asthma (occasionally used for mild persistent asthma: Step 2); prophylaxis and treatment of chronic asthma; ineffective for acute attacks.	Multiple drug interactions with low therapeutic index; contraindicated in seizure disorders, arrhythmias, and active peptic ulcer disease
Theophylline (Theo-24)	100-, 200-, 300-, 400-extended-release capsules	One to two times daily Blood levels can be measured when dosed twice daily; to maintain steady state, keep serum levels between 5 and 15 mcg/mL (if on high dose, do not take within 1 hour of eating fatty foods) May have some anti-inflammatory properties

literature cites the use of eucalyptus (as a decongestant/cough suppressant), lycopene (for exercise-induced asthma), vitamin B_{12} and vitamin C, and goldenseal, but research needs to be done on their effectiveness, so caution should be exercised when discussing these with patients.

Nutritional therapies have been used in the treatment of asthma, although it is also known that certain foods may precipitate an asthma flare in the food allergic patient. To treat asthma, Moses Maimonides, the noted 13th-century physician, prescribed a spicy, herbal mixture of chicken broth that contained herbs such as fennel, parsley, oregano, mint, and onion. Onions and garlic have been known to have some protective effect against allergic reactions, and hydration from such a robust broth may also be a helpful component in asthma treatment. Strong coffee was a widely used treatment for asthma in 18th-century Europe and continues to be used as an effective bronchodilator today. Although drinking tea has never been particularly favored as an asthma treatment, tea leaves were the original source of theophylline, which means "tea leaf."

FOLLOW-UP AND REFERRAL

Therapy should be "stepped down" gradually if a review of the patient's status at 1- to 6-month intervals suggests that a reduction of treatment is warranted. Smoking cessation for patients with asthma is a must. (For more information on smoking cessation, see Chapter 33.) In addition, the patient should avoid exposure to secondhand smoke, and family members should be educated about the hazards of secondhand smoke. Regular visits to the primary-care provider can be combined with appropriate referrals to specialists (e.g., allergists, pulmonologists) as necessary.

The use of immunotherapy in asthma remains controversial, and its effectiveness has not been well established. For most patients, avoidance of the allergens and triggers that cause asthma attacks, along with the appropriate use of medications, is adequate therapy. If avoidance of certain allergens is impossible or controller medications fail, referral to an allergist for immunotherapy may be indicated. However, unless the patient's symptoms are exacerbated by exposure to specific allergens, which can be confirmed by skin-prick testing, it is unlikely that immunotherapy will be effective.

Patient Education: Asthma

A list of reasonable expectations for patients with asthma should be reviewed with the patient and family, including potential triggers that might be removed and problematic areas such as treatment noncompliance or improper use of inhalants (see Box 31.2).

Box 31.2 Reasonable Expectations for Patients With Asthma

When entering into a treatment plan, the patient with asthma expects the following:

- Be able to participate fully in any activity
- Be able to sleep through the night
- Be free of severe symptoms during the day and night
- Be satisfied with asthma care
- Have the best possible pulmonary function
- Need fewer or no emergency visits or hospitalizations due to asthma
- Not miss work or school because of asthma
- Use fewer medications with minimal adverse effects

The provider is responsible for the following:

- Asking patients about their concerns and issues at each visit
- Continually teaching and reinforcing key educational points
- Ensuring ongoing and open communication with the patient and family
- Reviewing short-term goals agreed on at the initial visit
- Reviewing the asthma action plan for worsening symptoms and exacerbations
- Reviewing the daily self-management plan and steps the patient needs to take
- Supplying patients with appropriate educational materials for self-management and prevention

---

The patient and family should be educated about the following aspects of self-care management:

- Basic asthma facts
- When and how to use a short-acting inhaler before exercising (some patients have only exercise-induced asthma)
- How to recognize early symptoms of an exacerbation and how to initiate a predetermined plan of action
- Role of medications (long-acting controller and short-term rescue therapy) and the critical role for anti-inflammatory controller medication regimens to reduce the rate of acute attacks
- Skills for proper inhaler use, including the use of spacers, and daily peak flow meter monitoring (for patients with moderate to severe persistent asthma); spacers are universally recommended for metered-dose inhalers to obtain maximum benefit (some medication delivery systems have "built-in" spacers)
- Use of a nebulizer if necessary; nebulizers may be needed if patients cannot take adequate breaths
- Environmental control for allergen reduction
- Avoidance measures for asthma triggers
- Importance of pneumococcal and annual influenza vaccination

Reinforcement of medication use and proper use of the handheld flow meter should be reviewed at each visit. It should be mentioned that rescue courses of systemic glucocorticoids may be needed at times to prevent late-phase reactions in acute attacks, although recurrent attacks indicate that a greater degree of controller medication is warranted. In addition, patient and family education is essential for control of asthma triggers and recognition of warning signals. An Asthma Attack Trigger Diary may be used to assist in identifying such triggers.

Patients may ask which ICS is the most effective. Research has shown that if equipotent doses are used, the efficacy of different agents is essentially the same; the key difference is in the delivery technique. With a dry powder inhaler device, age is a factor. Providers must spend time teaching the proper technique and observing a return demonstration. One of the adverse side effects of ICS is believed to be their effects on growth rate in children. Research has shown that this is a small but definable risk. Growth reduction is more pronounced in the first year of therapy. Daily use of ICS can cause a small reduction in height in children with persistent asthma up to age 18 years. Nonetheless, it must be cautioned that all individuals should be on the lowest dose of ICS possible. This small reduction in height must be weighed with the known benefit of ICS for asthma control (Zhang et al., 2014).

Another question commonly asked by asthmatic patients is which pets are hypoallergenic. There are many Web sites that promote costly specialty pets that are purported to be nonallergenic, but in reality, there are no hypoallergenic pets. Using commonsense measures such as keeping pets out of the bedroom and wiping down cats with a wet washcloth every night to help control dander may help; however, in some cases, removing pets from the home completely may be the only recourse, although asthmatic patients can still react to residual dander and hair in the environment.

The patient and family should be educated to the fullest extent possible to permit self-management and prevention of acute fatal attacks. Although asthma is a chronic disease, patients may die from a particularly severe acute asthmatic attack. The risk factors for fatal asthma are listed in Box 31.3.

Patients with any of these risk factors need additional teaching time so that they can learn self-management techniques to reduce their risk to the extent possible. It is extremely important that the patient be trained to use the handheld peak flow meter and learn to determine their predicted (personal best) PEF. During exacerbations, the patient should compare a current reading to the baseline PEF as a guide to determine how severe the attack is and to gauge medication use accordingly. The value of the green/yellow/red markers on the PEF meter as a guide for the patient and family as to when to seek emergency help should be emphasized.

A caring relationship among the provider, the patient, and family may prove pivotal to effective disease management and improved quality of life. Although self-care is an essential component of treatment, a family member should be educated about how to handle an acute attack, in case the patient becomes severely hypoxic and cognitively impaired.

Box 31.3 Risk Factors for Fatal Asthma

- Comorbidity (cardiovascular or pulmonary disease, such as chronic obstructive pulmonary disease)
- Current use of, or recent withdrawal from, systemic glucocorticoids
- Difficulty perceiving airflow obstruction or its severity
- History of sudden severe exacerbations
- Hospitalization or emergency care for asthma within the past month
- Illicit drug use
- Low socioeconomic status and urban residence
- Prior intubation for asthma
- Sensitivity to the fungus *Alternaria*
- Serious psychiatric disease or psychosocial problems
- Three or more emergency visits for asthma in the past year
- Two or more hospitalizations for asthma in the past year
- Use of three or more canisters of inhaled short-acting beta$_2$-agonists per month

---

CHRONIC BRONCHITIS AND EMPHYSEMA (CHRONIC OBSTRUCTIVE PULMONARY DISEASE [COPD])

There are two main forms of lung disease—obstructive and restrictive. Obstructive lung diseases are those in which the expiratory flow rate is impaired. Restrictive lung diseases are those in which the lung volumes are reduced due to musculoskeletal disorders, tumors, lung resection, or interstitial lung disease (ILD). Obstructive lung diseases are further classified as reversible (such as asthma) or irreversible (such as chronic bronchitis and emphysema). The American Thoracic Society (ATS) has defined *chronic bronchitis* as a clinical disorder characterized by excessive mucus secretion in the bronchial tree. It is manifested by chronic or recurrent cough (with or without sputum production), present on most days for a minimum of 3 months of the year, for at least 2 successive years. In addition, dyspnea with or without wheezing is present. Whereas more than 16 million Americans have been diagnosed with chronic obstructive pulmonary disease (COPD), an equal number are probably afflicted but not diagnosed.

EPIDEMIOLOGY AND CAUSES

Chronic bronchitis and emphysema are grouped together as COPD. The ATS defines COPD as a disease state characterized by the presence of airflow obstruction due to chronic bronchitis or emphysema. Asthma is not classified as COPD but is sometimes referred to as a reversible obstructive condition, whereas emphysema is irreversible. Chronic bronchitis is usually irreversible, but it may be partially reversible if there is a bronchospastic component and a significant response to bronchodilators. The prevalence and mortality rates for chronic bronchitis and emphysema increase with age. COPD is the third leading cause of death in the United States and the fourth leading cause of disability. There are more than 134,000 deaths annually due to COPD, and 52% of persons with COPD are women. The estimated direct medical costs of COPD annually are more than $29.5 billion. This fact highlights the economic importance of prevention and of interventions aimed at early diagnosis and delaying disease progression.

Morbidity and mortality are higher in persons with low incomes and less education. It is difficult to estimate the prevalence of chronic bronchitis because there is considerable overlap of various obstructive conditions, as many patients have some combination of aspects of all three conditions—asthma, chronic bronchitis, and/or emphysema. Several studies have established certain predisposing risk factors for morbidity and mortality from COPD. The established and probable risk factors for COPD are highlighted in the accompanying text.

Risk Factors for COPD

Established risks:

- Age
- Male gender
- Cigarette smoking
- Reduced lung function
- Occupational exposures
- Air pollution
- Alpha$_1$-antitrypsin deficiency phenotypes

Probable or possible risks:

- Infections of the respiratory tract
- Allergic conditions
- Bronchial reactivity
- Climate
- Poor socioeconomic resources
- Alcohol intake
- Poor diet and inadequate nutrition
- ABO (ABH) secretor cell phenotypes
- Impaired immune function
- Familial factors

Cigarette smoking is responsible for 80% to 90% of the cases of COPD, and it is also the risk factor most amenable to modification for preventing or delaying the development of COPD. Educational intervention at an early age can help reduce smoking and some other risk factors, such as occupational exposure, exposure to air pollution and allergens, and respiratory infections. If certain genetic risk factors are present, the patient should be educated about periodic baseline testing for pulmonary function and about routine checks to prevent respiratory infections and reduce risks to the extent possible. Smokers older than 40 years are at higher risk of developing CPOD. Stopping smoking at any age has some beneficial effect for lung function, although there may be permanent damage to lung tissue.

PATHOPHYSIOLOGY

COPD is a progressive disease characterized by airflow limitation that is not fully reversible. The disease process involves a combination of the pathological mechanisms of emphysema and chronic bronchitis. In addition, hyperreactivity of the airways is a common feature. Thus, COPD is a disease of both the lung parenchyma and the small airways (bronchioles).

Emphysema is characterized by destruction of alveolar walls due to an imbalance of proteinase–antiproteinase enzymatic activity. In healthy lung tissue, protective antiproteinases counteract protein-degrading enzymes secreted by white blood cells. A genetic condition called alpha-1 antitrypsin deficiency may play a role in causing COPD. People with this condition have low levels of alpha-1 antitrypsin, a protein made in the liver. Chronic inflammation, caused by long-term cigarette smoking or chronic exposure to lung irritants, for example, repeatedly recruits white blood cells to the alveoli. In contrast to the atopic processes of asthma, the lymphocytic infiltration of COPD consists predominantly of CD8+ T cells, rather than CD4+ Th cells. Neutrophil and monocyte-/macrophage-derived proteinases progressively degrade the alveolar walls, overcoming antiproteinase defenses. Overdistended, hyperinflated, and less elastic alveoli are the result of the recurring lung injury over time. Weak elastic recoil of alveoli leads to air trapping, increased residual lung volume, reduced expiratory flow, and retained carbon dioxide. Individuals experience hypercapnia but can maintain adequate oxygenation early in the disease process.

Desensitization of the central respiratory receptors to Pco_2 occurs with long-term hypercapnia. Under normal circumstances, Pco_2 accumulation in the blood stimulates individuals to breathe independently. However, persons who endure long-term states of hypercapnia lose this normal respiratory stimulus to breathe. Hypoxia becomes the stimulus for breathing instead of Pco_2. Hypoxia is sensed by peripheral chemoreceptors in the arteries, such as the carotid bodies. The individual with hypercapnia sustained over a prolonged period of time begins to rely on low oxygen levels to drive breathing. Consequently, supplemental oxygen must be used judiciously in these individuals because of their hypoxic drive to breathe. High levels of supplemental oxygen, as well as respiratory depressants of any kind (e.g., sedatives, narcotics), can suppress the hypercapnic individual's hypoxic drive to breathe independently.

Cigarette smoking is the major environmental risk factor for the development of COPD. Although smoking cessation slows progression of the disease, reversal of pathological changes does not occur. There is a proven causal relationship between cigarette smoking and COPD; however, there is marked variability in the pulmonary function of persons with similar smoking histories. This has led to investigation into genetic risk factors for COPD. As mentioned earlier, one such genetic risk factor is alpha-1 antitrypsin deficiency. Alpha-1 antitrypsin is a major antiproteinase enzyme that can counteract alveolar destruction. Individuals can inherit different genetic mutations that lead to variable degrees of deficiency of this enzyme. Individuals with complete absence of alpha-1 antitrypsin have an increased susceptibility to emphysema and develop the disease early in life.

Compared with emphysema, chronic bronchitis is the more common pathological mechanism involved in COPD. Airflow obstruction in chronic bronchitis is caused by bronchiolar edema, hyperplasia of mucus-producing goblet cells, and bronchiolar smooth muscle hypertrophy. Clinically, chronic bronchitis presents as a long-term cough or recurrent sputum production, primarily on morning awakening, extending over 3 months for a period of at least 2 years. Individuals with hypoxia and cyanosis have problems with ventilatory obstruction and suboptimal oxygenation of the blood. In chronic bronchitis, long-term hypoxia leads to pulmonary vasoconstriction, which can result in pulmonary hypertension. This increased pulmonary resistance against the right ventricle can lead to right ventricular failure or cor pulmonale. Chronic hypoxia also stimulates renal erythropoietin, which initiates and perpetuates red blood cell synthesis in the bone marrow, thereby increasing hemoglobin concentration and hematocrit, which makes the right ventricle hypertrophic from pumping more viscous blood into a constricted pulmonary artery.

Acute exacerbations of chronic bronchitis are highly characteristic of this disease. Increased purulent sputum production and worsened shortness of breath are the hallmark of such episodes, which may also be accompanied by fever and increased oxygen requirements for patients on supplemental oxygen. Although viral bronchitis requiring only supportive care is the most common etiology of such exacerbations, bacterial involvement must be considered with increased sputum production lasting more than a week or new chest x-ray findings. *Streptococcus pneumoniae* is the most common agent, followed by *Haemophilus influenzae* and *Moraxella catarrhalis,* similar to the causative agents of sinusitis and community-acquired pneumonia. Antibacterial therapy is often instituted empirically, however, without the need for cultures or Gram stain evidence.

The respiratory symptoms of COPD logically follow patterns of pulmonary neuromuscular anatomy because bronchiolar smooth muscle is innervated by beta-2 adrenergic and cholinergic nerve receptors. Bronchiolar constriction in COPD is largely cholinergically mediated. For this reason, blockade of cholinergic receptors by anticholinergic drugs enhances the ability of bronchioles to dilate in COPD. Increased mucus production is also counteracted by these agents. Similarly, beta-receptor activation mediates bronchodilation, as reflected in the therapeutic benefits of inhaled beta-agonist drugs. Inhaled and oral corticosteroids, on the other hand, function by decreasing overall airway inflammation mediated largely by T cells.

There is a normal age-related decline in pulmonary function in COPD; FEV_1 declines by 0.02 to 0.04 L per year. Cigarette smoking accelerates this decline by two- to threefold. Though smoking cessation slows the rate of decline, it will not reverse most pathological changes. Pulmonary function patterns and physical findings for various pulmonary conditions are shown in Table 31.2. PFT results reflect the underlying pathology of the condition.

It is common for patients to have mixed lung disease (both restrictive and obstructive). For example, patients with chronic bronchitis may also present with a restrictive ILD such as sarcoidosis. In cases like this, all lung volumes would be reduced, the diffusing capacity would be reduced, and the ABGs would be abnormal (showing hypoxemia and possibly carbon dioxide retention).

Age and FEV_1 are the strongest predictors of mortality in COPD (see Table 31.3). High mortality rates occur when COPD is complicated by respiratory infection (e.g., acute bronchitis exacerbations) or cor pulmonale from chronic pulmonary hypertension. These conditions increase the risk for ventilation–perfusion mismatch, hypoxemia, hypercapnia, respiratory acidosis, and respiratory failure.

CLINICAL PRESENTATION

Subjective

The typical smoker who develops COPD may be asymptomatic for 10 to 20 years except for frequent colds, persistent morning cough, and upper respiratory infections. Men, in particular, may wait until the dyspnea becomes severe before seeking medical help or may seek help only when they need antibiotics for a chronic productive cough. They may ignore symptoms of fatigue, shortness of breath, and cough because of embarrassment. Older persons may attribute the shortness of breath and fatigue to functional decline related to aging. The onset of COPD is typically in the fifth decade or later with a 20-pack-year smoking history (number of packs of cigarettes per day times number of years the person smoked).

With advanced disease in which chronic bronchitis predominates, pulmonary hypertension may result from chronic alveolar hypoxia, and cor pulmonale develops.

TABLE 31.2   Pulmonary Function and Physical Findings in Obstructive and Restrictive Lung Diseases

Parameters	Asthma	Chronic Bronchitis	Emphysema	Restrictive Disease
Forced vital capacity (FVC)	Normal	Normal to increased	Normal to increased	Decreased
Residual volume (RV)	Normal; increased during attacks	Increased	Increased	Decreased or normal
Total lung capacity (TLC)	Normal to increased	Normal	Normal to increased	Decreased
RV/TLC	Normal to increased	Increased	Increased	Normal
Expiratory flow rates	Normal to decreased	Normal to decreased	Normal to decreased	Normal to increased
FEV_1/FVC	Normal to decreased	Decreased	Decreased	Normal to increased
Bronchodilator response (% change)	>15%	0%–15%	None	None
Diffusing capacity	Normal to increased	Normal to decreased	Decreased	Normal or decreased (depends on type of disease)
PaO_2	Normal; decreased during attack	Decreased	Normal in mild to moderate disease; decreased in severe disease	Normal or decreased
$PaCO_2$	First decreased, then increased during acute attack	Increased	Normal until advanced disease, then increased	Normal or decreased; increased in very advanced disease
Breath sounds	Marked decrease during acute attacks If FEV_1 = 0.5 L or less: absent	If FEV_1 = 1 L: barely audible	Decreased	Normal or decreased in pneumonia, atelectasis
Crackles (rales)	Coarse crackles during infections	Coarse crackles during infections	Fine crackles may be present	Varies with type of restrictive disease
Wheezes (rhonchi)	High-pitched; continuous	Forced expiratory wheezes	No	No

TABLE 31.3   Severity of COPD Based on the Pulmonary Function Measures: FEV_1 Postbronchodilator

Stage of Severity	Pulmonary Function Measure (FEV_1) Postbronchodilator
Stage 1: mild COPD	FEV_1 ≥80% predicted
Stage 2: moderate COPD	FEV_1 >50% to <80% predicted
Stage 3: severe COPD	FEV_1 >30% to <50% predicted
Stage 4: very severe COPD	FEV_1 <30% predicted

Abbreviations: COPD, chronic obstructive pulmonary disease; FEV_1, forced expiratory volume in 1 second.
Source: Global Strategy for the Diagnosis, Management and Prevention of COPD. Global Initiative for Chronic Obstructive Lung Disease (GOLD). http://goldcopd.org. Published 2017.

Patients with these signs and symptoms are often called "blue bloaters" because of the edema and cyanosis that accompany their condition. A CBC with differential may reveal polycythemia secondary to the increased erythropoietin stimulation of increased red blood cells to compensate for chronic hypoxemia.

Patients who primarily have emphysema ("pink puffers") have severe dyspnea but usually present with relatively normal ABGs that are maintained because of high minute ventilation. As the disease progresses, dyspnea increases because diffusing capacity is severely reduced. These patients often appear very thin and may have the typical "barrel chest" resulting from hyperinflation of emphysematous lungs.

A patient with an acute exacerbation of chronic bronchitis may present with cough and increased sputum that is thick and colored (yellow, brown, gray, or green); fever may also be present. Sudden onset of cough with minimal sputum, chills, fever, and myalgia is more indicative of a viral infection. Older adults often have blunted responses to infection due to a decreased immune response.

Patients with COPD usually present with a complaint of chronic productive cough (chronic bronchitis) and increasing shortness of breath or dyspnea on exertion (emphysema). Associated symptoms may include fatigue, weakness, hemoptysis, loss of appetite, nausea, and dizziness. By the time there is dyspnea on exertion, the disease is usually well advanced. Patients may report having to sleep sitting up or with three or more pillows to relieve dyspnea. They may report awakening during the night with severe dyspnea (paroxysmal nocturnal dyspnea), which is relieved by sitting upright.

Objective

The physical findings will vary depending on the severity of the COPD. Physical findings are often not significant in mild to moderate COPD. In emphysema or mixed disease, the chest examination may indicate hyperinflation. Typically, a "barrel-chest" is noted. There may be flattening of the diaphragm, tachypnea, and the use of the accessory muscles of respiration (e.g., scalene, sternocleidomastoid). The patient often uses a "tripod" position to support function of the diaphragm and ease breathing. In hyperinflation, a predominant palpable or auscultatory cardiac contraction may be noted in the epigastrium rather than in the left intercostal space. On auscultation, breath sounds are distant and are not augmented much with deep breathing. End-expiratory wheezes may be heard on forced expiration. Patients with a bronchospastic component may have inspiratory and expiratory wheezes. Measurement of forced expiratory time is useful to determine if airway obstruction is present. When auscultating the lungs, have the patient take a full inspiration, then listen while the patient exhales through the mouth until airflow stops. The normal duration for full expiration is 3 seconds, but in COPD the time is prolonged because of airway obstruction.

Coarse lung crackles may be present during an acute COPD exacerbation. Neck vein distention, especially during expiration, may occur as a result of increased intrathoracic pressure. The patient's feet and ankles should be examined for edema that may occur as the disease progresses and cor pulmonale develops. The nailbeds should be examined for clubbing (i.e., hypertrophic osteoarthropathy), which often occurs in patients with pulmonary pathology. Other causes of clubbing are atrioventricular shunt, subacute bacterial endocarditis, inflammatory bowel disease, and biliary cirrhosis.

During the physical examination, the patient's ability to follow commands and respond to questions should be documented. Changes in mental status may be caused by hypoxemia or hypercapnia, rather than dementia. Fatigue is a common finding.

DIAGNOSTIC REASONING

The diagnostic approach to the patient is directed at assessment of the type of obstructive disease (primarily bronchitis, emphysema, or mixed) and whether it is reversible or irreversible. The possibility of underlying restrictive disease must be eliminated. Patients who have chronic bronchitis and have smoked for 20 years or longer should be evaluated for lung cancer.

Diagnostic Tests

Initial Testing

The initial diagnostic evaluation for COPD should include PFTs (spirometry, diffusing capacity, and ABGs). The standard PFTs should include prebronchodilator and postbronchodilator testing to determine if there is a significant response to bronchodilators. The diagnostic criterion for COPD is an FEV_1/FVC ratio of less than 70%. The FEV_1 (percent of predicted value) is the most useful parameter to assess severity of obstruction (see Table 31.3). The American College of Physicians' Guidelines recommend spirometry in the diagnosis of patients exhibiting symptoms but not in those who are asymptomatic.

Although bronchitis and emphysema usually occur together in most patients, it is important to distinguish the severity of the bronchitis and the emphysema and to identify how much of a bronchospastic component is present to direct treatment appropriately. In chronic bronchitis and emphysema, narrowing of the airways is present that usually results in an increase in airway resistance and a decrease in maximal expiratory flow rates. In emphysema, the loss of elastic recoil accounts for a decrease in the caliber of the airways (from loss of radial traction on the airways). The elastic recoil properties of the lung serve as a major determinant of the expiratory flow rates. Maximal expiratory flow rates represent a complex and dynamic interplay among airway caliber, elastic recoil pressures, and airway collapsibility. As a result of the altered pressure-airflow relations in COPD, the work of breathing is increased in bronchitis and emphysema. The maldistribution of inspired gas (through ventilation) and blood flow (through perfusion) is always present to a degree in COPD. When the mismatching is severe, it is reflected in the ABGs as hypoxemia or hypercarbia.

Chest radiography will appear normal in patients with early COPD. In patients with chronic bronchitis, chest x-ray films may reveal increased lung markings in the lower lobes and peribronchial thickening. In patients with emphysema, chest radiographs may show hyperinflation (i.e., a low flat diaphragm and enlarged retrosternal space), hypovascularity, areas of hyperlucency and bullae formation, and a small cardiac silhouette. Chest computed tomography (CT) scans are used to evaluate the extent and distribution of emphysematous cysts for possible surgery. In recurrent bronchitis, CT scans may be used to rule out bronchiectasis.

Laboratory tests should include a CBC and differential. The hemoglobin, hematocrit (Hct), and red blood cell count should be evaluated to rule out anemia or polycythemia. Serum alpha$_1$-antitrypsin levels should be checked in patients who develop COPD at an early age (younger than 45 years), those with clinical emphysema who have not smoked, and those with a family history of early-onset COPD. A blood chemistry profile is done to assess electrolyte balance (K, Na, Cl) and nutritional status (total protein, albumin), as well as rule out renal or liver problems.

For an exacerbation of chronic bronchitis, sputum should be tested via Gram stain. Sputum culture and sensitivity is done to confirm the findings of the Gram stain. The Gram stain is the best clinical method for diagnosing an acute exacerbation because the bacteria can be seen and quantified. Patients with COPD often are colonized by low numbers of bacteria, including *S. pneumoniae*, *H. influenzae*, and *M. catarrhalis*, which will grow in culture even though they are not present in sufficient numbers to be seen with Gram stain. If the Gram stain shows neutrophils but no bacteria in a patient with chronic bronchitis, the acute exacerbation is probably viral or chlamydial, even when the sputum culture yields *Haemophilus* or *Pneumococcus*. A negative Gram stain indicates that a positive culture result likely represents bacterial colonization rather than true infection.

An electrocardiogram (ECG) should be done if the patient has not had a baseline test, especially if there are signs of cardiac disease or in advanced COPD. Atrial arrhythmias are common in older adults and in pulmonary patients of any age. ECG changes in pulmonary disease include peaked P waves in leads II, III, and aV$_F$ and changes associated with right ventricular hypertrophy. Cardiac abnormalities may have implications for the drugs selected to treat the COPD.

Assessing degree of functional status and quality of life of patients with COPD should be done initially to determine the potential for rehabilitation and to direct appropriate therapy. The Rand SF-36 Health Survey is a valid and reliable tool used worldwide to assess physical and emotional health and is recommended for patients with chronic illnesses such as COPD.

Subsequent Testing

Annual spirometry, CBC with differential, chemistry profile, and chest radiographs should be done to measure the patient's decline in pulmonary function and to screen for other lung diseases that may be related to smoking. Gram stain, culture and sensitivity tests of sputum, and ABG analysis are done as needed during acute exacerbations. Pulse oximetry is a noninvasive test that can be done in the office to screen for hypoxemia. An oxygen saturation of 90% or less at rest

warrants monitoring ABGs. The ATS recommends ABG monitoring for hypoxemia and hypercapnia in patients with advanced COPD (i.e., those with an FEV$_1$ less than 50% of the predicted value).

Differential Diagnosis

Acute bronchitis, asthma, bronchiectasis, bronchogenic carcinoma, acute viral infection, heart failure, tuberculosis, normal aging of lungs, occupational asthma, sleep apnea, and chronic sinusitis are all conditions that need to be ruled out to make a diagnosis of COPD or emphysema. In young adults, cystic fibrosis needs to be ruled out. Patient history and PFT results (including decreased FEV$_1$ with a concomitant reduction in FEV$_1$/FVC ratio), as well as poor or absent reversibility, assist in making the diagnosis of COPD.

MANAGEMENT

Early diagnosis of COPD is essential. After the initial diagnosis is made, education of the patient and family is critical for therapy to be effective. The patient and family need to understand that although COPD is not a curable disease, with proper management and smoking cessation, symptoms can be controlled and quality of life improved. A nursing research study is provided that shares the importance of collaborative partnerships in caring for patients with COPD, due to the myriad problems experienced by these patients (see Evidence-Based Nursing Practice 31.1).

Smoking cessation improves declining lung function and is the single most important intervention to slow

---

 Evidence-Based Nursing Practice 31.1

Kirkpatrick P, Wilson E, Wimpenny P, et al. Research to support evidence-based practice in COPD community nursing. *Br J Community Nurs*. 2012;17(10):486, 488–492.

Implementing evidence-based practice (EBP) is a requirement of nurses in a bid to improve clinical practice. However, EBP may be difficult to achieve in the absence of rigorous evidence generation. This paper highlights an approach to generating evidence for enhancing community nursing services for patients with chronic obstructive pulmonary disease (COPD) through a collaborative partnership. A district nurse and two nursing lecturers formed a partnership to devise a systematic review protocol and perform a systematic review to enhance COPD practice. This paper illustrates the Joanna Briggs Institute systematic review process, the review outcomes, and the scope of practitioner learning. Collaborative partnerships among academics, researchers, and clinicians are a potentially useful model to facilitate enhanced outcomes in EBP and evidence application.

the rate of lung function decline, regardless of disease severity. After 5 years without cigarettes, lung function returns to almost that of a nonsmoker. Patients should be urged at each clinic visit to stop smoking; family members should also be encouraged to do the same if they smoke. For more information on smoking cessation, see Chapter 33.

Pharmacologic Therapy

Although only supplemental oxygen has been shown to improve the mortality associated with COPD (when oxygen levels are low at rest), pharmacotherapy has a significant role in reducing its associated morbidities and improving quality of life. The following general treatment guidelines are from the Global Initiative for Chronic Obstructive Lung Disease (GOLD).

 Treatment Standards/Guidelines: COPD

Source: From the Global Strategy for the Diagnosis, Management and Prevention of COPD. Global Initiative for Chronic Obstructive Lung Disease (GOLD). http://goldcopd.org. Published 2017.

The 2017 GOLD guidelines suggest the following medications for COPD:

- Long-acting bronchodilators (a long-acting beta agonist [LABA], a long-acting muscarinic antagonist [LAMA], or both)
- Inhaled corticosteroids (ICS), although not for monotherapy (with ICS plus a LABA for step-up therapy)
- An oral PDE$_4$ inhibitor as an add-on therapy for patients with COPD plus chronic bronchitis, if previously recommended medicines are ineffective or inadequate.

The 2017 GOLD Guidelines suggest using these medications according to the following grading scheme of clinical severity:

- COPD GOLD Grade A: any short- or long-acting bronchodilator
- COPD GOLD Grade B: a long-acting bronchodilator (LAMA or LABA) or both, if continued difficulty breathing with only one drug
- COPD GOLD Grade C: a long-acting muscarinic antagonist (LAMA), or if continued exacerbations occur, a switch to LAMA+LABA or LABA+ICS
- COPD GOLD Grade D: individualized management, possibly using a PDE4 inhibitor, roflumilast (Daliresp) and azithromycin (Zithromax); antibiotics are warranted in the presence of a prolonged illness, especially with purulent sputum.

Inhaled Beta$_2$-Agonists

Inhaled short-acting beta$_2$-agonists (SABAs) are the first line of therapy, as the major goals of therapy are to prevent bronchospasm with long-acting bronchodilators and to use a SABA "rescue" medication to alleviate acute episodes of bronchospasm. Each episode of acute bronchospasm causes permanent remodeling of the bronchioles; therefore, prevention of these episodes is critical. Inhaled SABAs (e.g., albuterol [Proventil, Ventolin] and pirbuterol [Maxair Autohaler]) are prescribed as "rescue" medications for intermittent symptoms of acute shortness of breath. Patients may experience adverse reactions from beta$_2$ agonists that include tremors, nervousness, and dysrhythmias. All patients who experience more than occasional dyspnea should be on long-acting bronchodilator therapy. LABA is not first-line therapy but is used for maintenance therapy to prevent acute bronchospastic episodes. Patients may either be on a LABA, a LAMA, or both.

Inhaled Muscarinic Antagonists

The short-acting muscarinic antagonist ipratropium may also be used as rescue therapy, although frequent use is not recommended, due to the potential for adverse effects and a plateau effect after several doses. Thus, short-acting muscarinic antagonists are typically used three times a day to confer antimuscarinic benefits throughout the day. Patients with more frequent episodes of dyspnea may benefit from a LAMA, such as tiotropium (Spiriva), which have the advantage of once-daily dosing. Tiotropium is the recommended therapy for GOLD Grade B disease, along with albuterol as a rescue medication. Typically, this combination produces a reduction in the use of rescue medication, as well as a reduction in COPD exacerbations.

Corticosteroids

The primary role of inhaled glucocorticoids in COPD is as an anti-inflammatory agent. The dosing of an ICS such as beclomethasone, budesonide (Pulmicort), or fluticasone (Flovent), among others, should be individualized. Proper inhaler technique with a spacing device and mouth rinsing after each use are advised to maximize medication delivery to the lungs and to avoid oral candidiasis. In rare cases, systemic corticosteroids may be used in the management of an acute COPD exacerbation for no more than 10 to 14 days. For acute COPD exacerbations, systemic corticosteroids are effective in reducing treatment failures. However, the potential risks associated with this treatment, including immunosuppression, hypertension, and hyperglycemia, necessitate that systemic corticosteroids be used with caution.

Some clinicians report that 15% to 20% of patients respond both subjectively (perceived dyspnea) and objectively (FEV$_1$ and improved exercise performance) to low-dose, long-term systemic corticosteroids, although this is not a widely accepted treatment. Rather, systemic corticosteroids should be used only when the other drugs have failed and when there is an acute exacerbation with a bronchospastic component to the COPD. Patients who are more likely to respond to corticosteroids are those who have blood and sputum eosinophilia, positive allergy skin test results, elevated levels of serum IgE, or a history of allergy and bronchodilator response. Before starting oral corticosteroids, baseline spirometry should be done; then the patient may take oral prednisone 40 mg daily for 1 to 2 weeks. An improvement in FEV_1 of at least 15% on repeat spirometry indicates a positive response. The dose should then be tapered to a low daily or alternate-day maintenance dose of 5 to 15 mg. The adverse effects of systemic steroids are well known (e.g., gastric ulcer, osteoporosis, masked infections, secondary infections), and the patient should be monitored carefully for adverse reactions.

Combination Therapy

A LABA may be combined with an ICS as effective combination therapy (Advair: salmeterol plus fluticasone; Symbicort: formoterol plus budesonide) in Grade B patients. Patients appear to do better when these two classes of agents are combined into a single delivery device, likely due to improved medication adherence. Typically, these combination agents are available with increasing doses of ICS, while the LABA dose is held constant, because higher LABA doses are associated with greater risks of adverse events, including death. Importantly, these combination agents are not to be used as rescue therapy.

The GOLD guidelines recommend that for Grade B or C disease (which represents the majority of people living with COPD), patients should utilize dual therapy including a LABA and LAMA. Tiotropium bromide plus olodaterol (Stiolto Respimat) or umeclidinium bromide plus vilanterol (Anoro Ellipta) are examples of LAMA/LABA combination therapies. Such combinations are also recommended for more severe Grade C and D disease, along with the addition of an ICS.

PDE₄ Inhibitors

Phosphodiesterase-4 inhibitors such as roflumilast (Daliresp) are indicated for patients with COPD and bronchitis who have exacerbations. They are not bronchodilators and are not indicated for the relief of acute bronchospasm but rather have anti-inflammatory effects on many inflammatory cell types. They should not be used in women who are anticipating pregnancy or in nursing mothers.

Xanthines

Aminophylline or theophylline may be used as a fourth-line drug if the combination of beta₂ agonists, muscarinic antagonists, and ICS prove ineffective. Xanthine preparations have a very narrow therapeutic index, and blood levels should be monitored closely for toxicity. The therapeutic levels are 5 to 15 mcg/mL. Their therapeutic benefit results from increased bronchodilation and decreased muscle fatigue, although these agents also have a stimulatory effect and can increase heart rate as well as blood pressure. Therapy should be initiated with low doses and then gradually increased, given the narrow therapeutic range. Xanthines interact with other drugs commonly taken by patients with COPD, including cimetidine (Tagamet), erythromycin, ciprofloxacin (Cipro), and beta blockers, among others. If the patient is taking a xanthine, it is safer not to use drugs of these classes to avoid drug toxicity.

Antibiotics

Antibiotics are often needed for acute exacerbations of chronic bronchitis when purulent sputum is present. There is little to no evidence for the use of chronic suppressive antibiotic therapy, and this practice has fallen out of favor. Most pulmonologists recommend the empiric use of antibiotics to treat acute episodes when the patient's cough increases and the character and the amount of sputum change (i.e., an increase in the amount, color, and/or consistency), even in the absence of fever, pulmonary infiltrates, or leukocytosis. For empiric therapy, the antibiotic should be effective against the three most common pathogens in chronic bronchitis (*S. pneumoniae*, *H. influenzae*, and *M. catarrhalis*), stable against the effects of beta-lactamase, and convenient to take with few adverse reactions. The choice of antibiotic should also depend on local bacterial resistance patterns and individual risk of *Pseudomonas aeruginosa* infection. Patients with COPD who have had a fairly stable course (i.e., few hospitalizations) and have not been exposed to many antibiotics typically respond well to therapy. Oral antibiotic options include doxycycline (100 mg every 12 hours), trimethoprim-sulfamethoxazole (160/800 mg every 12 hours), a cephalosporin such as cefpodoxime (200 mg every 12 hours), a macrolide such as azithromycin (500 mg the first day, followed by 250 mg daily for 5 days), and amoxicillin-clavulanate (875/125 mg every 12 hours). Some practitioners prescribe antibiotics for a period of 3 to 7 days. Some studies have shown that 5-day courses are as effective as 7-day courses with fewer side effects. Immunocompromised patients with a turbulent clinical course should be treated carefully with the most appropriate antibiotic (which may equate to newer and more expensive agents) to prevent respiratory failure and admission to an intensive care unit. Persistent gram-negative infection may require prolonged IV antibiotic administration.

Diuretics

Diuretics may be necessary when there is evidence of cor pulmonale (right heart failure). Often the triad of prerenal azotemia, hypernatremia, and low cardiac output develops in cor pulmonale, and loop diuretics may be used. Small doses of furosemide (Lasix) and potassium chloride supplements are used in conjunction with a sodium-restricted diet.

Mucolytics and Expectorants

Inhaled aerosols of water, saline, steam, or other agents do not improve mucociliary clearance or expectoration. Oral expectorants such as guaifenesin (Humibid, Mucinex, Robitussin) are usually ineffective. Chest physiotherapy and adequate hydration are the most cost-effective ways to clear the lungs.

Home Oxygen

Because hypoxia leads to pulmonary hypertension and increases the work of the right ventricle, low-flow oxygen may help prevent or deter development of cor pulmonale. In addition, of all the therapies mentioned, only supplemental oxygen has been shown to reduce the mortality rate associated with COPD. It is only recommended for severe resting hypoxia. Requirements for home oxygen include (1) a PaO_2 of 55 mm Hg or less or an oxygen saturation (SaO_2) below 88% and (2) a PaO_2 of 55 to 59 mm Hg if any of the following is present: erythrocytosis (Hct of 56% or more), cor pulmonale (P wave of more than 3 mm in leads II, III, and aV_F), edema, or congestive heart failure. The goal of therapy is a PaO_2 of 60 mm Hg or SaO_2 of 90%, which usually can be accomplished with 1 to 2 L of oxygen per minute for 15 hours per day. The patient should be reevaluated with ABGs or oximetry at 1, 3, and 6 months, and then annually. In advanced disease, supplemental oxygen has been shown to reduce the number of hospitalizations and increase the quality of life in individuals.

Surgery

Although surgery will not cure COPD, some patients have benefited from one of three surgical procedures with an improved quality of life. Because of the typically poor pulmonary state of the patient, any surgery is extremely risky and should be performed using epidural or spinal anesthesia rather than general anesthesia. A bullectomy involves resection of a bulla, which may be effective in reducing the patient's dyspnea. Lung volume reduction surgery involves resecting 20% to 30% of the lung to reduce hyperinflation. Exercise capacity may be improved, but it is highly unlikely that life expectancy would be improved because of the advanced nature of the disease at the point of requiring surgery. Lung transplant has been shown to improve quality of life, functional capacity, and exercise performance. The 1-year survival rate for lung transplantation is 80%, and the 5-year survival rate is more than 50%. The decision to undergo surgery should be made with a pulmonary specialist and may involve the entire family.

FOLLOW-UP AND REFERRAL

Patients who are unstable and those with severe disease should be seen by the primary-care provider on a monthly basis. If the patient is stable, an annual visit is the minimum requirement. If the patient is on theophylline, blood levels should be monitored every 6 to 12 months once the patient is on the desired dose. If the patient is on home O_2, ABGs should be checked whenever there is any change in clinical condition or, at a minimum, semiannually. It is also important to monitor oxygen saturation (pulse oximetry) more frequently with home O_2.

Follow-up for the patient with COPD includes the development of a close and supportive relationship with the health-care provider. Because smoking cessation is the single most effective way to slow the progression of COPD, the patient should be asked about this and supported in their efforts at every visit.

Patient Education: COPD

Use of inhaler devices and spacers requires patient education on proper technique. The clinician should observe the patient demonstrate proper inhaler technique for his or her specific medication, as there are differences in the technique used with each type of dispenser. Many patients have difficulty mastering the proper inhaler technique for optimal pulmonary delivery of medication. Spacers can be used with some inhalers to enable greater drug delivery. Nebulizers can also be used to facilitate the delivery of some inhaled medications in patients with poor inspiratory effort. Regardless of the method used, ongoing patient education is essential to reinforce adequate inhalation of the medication.

Patients with COPD should avoid extremes in environmental temperature and humidity when possible and limit their exposure to areas that have high levels of air pollution. Smoking should not be allowed in the home, car, or other confined places. Occupational exposure to fumes, vapors, dusts, and irritants may aggravate symptoms of dyspnea and bronchospasm. High altitudes and air travel can pose problems for hypoxemic patients. Arrangements can be made with commercial airline carriers in advance of travel for patients requiring oxygen therapy.

Respiratory therapy and oxygen equipment used in the home should be routinely cleaned to prevent bacterial colonization and subsequent infection. As most lung infections are viral, avoiding contact with crowds during flu season and limiting exposure to people with colds may help decrease the risk of lung infection. In the fall, patients with COPD should receive influenza immunizations with polyvalent vaccine from early October through mid-November. COPD patients with comorbid viral lung infection should be treated as soon as possible. Oseltamivir (Tamiflu) is an abortive antiviral that helps shorten the duration of infection and decrease the severity of influenza symptoms if used within the first 48 hours of symptom onset.

Polyvalent pneumococcal vaccine should also be given. The 13-valent protein conjugate pneumococcal vaccine should be administered first, before age 65 years in patients who are at risk for infection (e.g., those with other systemic disease). The 23-valent polysaccharide pneumococcal vaccine should be given at least 1 year after administration of the 13-valent vaccine. One or two doses of 23-valent vaccine may be needed in adults before age 65 years, depending on a patient's comorbidities.

The Iceberg of COPD

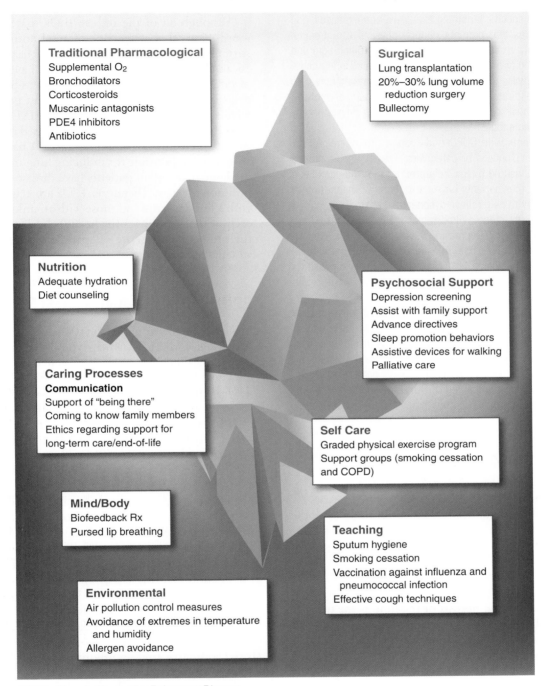

Traditional Pharmacological
Supplemental O_2
Bronchodilators
Corticosteroids
Muscarinic antagonists
PDE4 inhibitors
Antibiotics

Surgical
Lung transplantation
20%–30% lung volume
   reduction surgery
Bullectomy

Nutrition
Adequate hydration
Diet counseling

Psychosocial Support
Depression screening
Assist with family support
Advance directives
Sleep promotion behaviors
Assistive devices for walking
Palliative care

Caring Processes
Communication
Support of "being there"
Coming to know family members
Ethics regarding support for
long-term care/end-of-life

Self Care
Graded physical exercise program
Support groups (smoking cessation
and COPD)

Mind/Body
Biofeedback Rx
Pursed lip breathing

Teaching
Sputum hygiene
Smoking cessation
Vaccination against influenza and
   pneumococcal infection
Effective cough techniques

Environmental
Air pollution control measures
Avoidance of extremes in temperature
   and humidity
Allergen avoidance

COPD - Chronic Obstructive Pulmonary Disease
PDE - Phosphodiesterase

All adults older than 65 years are recommended to have received at least one dose of 13-valent vaccine and a repeat dose of 23-valent vaccine.

Pulmonary rehabilitation should be considered for all patients with functional impairment. This is defined as evidence-based, multidisciplinary, and comprehensive interventions and services that seek to improve quality of life for patients with chronic respiratory diseases and their families. Physical rehabilitation is recommended as a component because it not only deters functional decline but can also help the patient and family to maintain a positive outlook in the face of progressive disease. Often, the best exercise for patients with mild to moderate obstructive pulmonary disease is an individualized walking program. Physical therapy may also be beneficial, as the therapist may prescribe specific breathing exercises, arm exercises, and other modalities that promote general physical conditioning. Walking aids have been shown to support the diaphragm and ease the difficulty of breathing with ambulation. During acute respiratory attacks, use of slow, pursed-lip breathing may help to decrease respiratory rate, reduce bronchospasm, and relieve dyspnea. Effective cough techniques and chest physiotherapy are also recommended.

Many patients with COPD find support groups helpful for them and their spouses or caregivers. These support groups are usually sponsored by local chapters of the American Lung Association. Other patients have used forms of meditation or guided imagery to help relieve dyspnea and anxiety.

Patients with chronic illness such as COPD often are depressed. The Beck Depression Inventory can be used to screen for depression. Use of selective serotonin reuptake inhibitor antidepressants in patients with lung disease is considered safe and may improve sleep, quality of life, and functional status.

Health-care providers should have a frank discussion with patients and their families regarding end-of-life care, including the establishment of advanced directives, living wills, and health-care surrogates. Copies of all documents should be kept in the medical chart, as well as with patients' families and attorneys. See the Iceberg of COPD for additional patient education.

INTERSTITIAL LUNG DISEASE

Interstitial lung disease (ILD) encompasses nearly 200 clinical disorders that affect the epithelium, the endothelium, or both cell surfaces of alveolar wall and satellite structures, including terminal and respiratory bronchioles. ILD comprises a heterogeneous group of diseases that cause inflammation and fibrosis of the lower respiratory tract. The term "pulmonary fibrosis" is also applied to these diseases because fibrosis of the lung is the ultimate result of ILD. The term "interstitial" may be misleading in that most of these disorders have extensive alteration of alveolar and airway architecture as well. "Diffuse parenchymal lung disease" is perhaps a more appropriate descriptive term for this heterogeneous group of lung diseases because the term "interstitium" usually refers to the microscopic anatomical space bounded by the basement membranes of epithelial and endothelial cells. The entire lung parenchyma, however, is affected in ILD.

The ILDs have many common features, including similarity of patient symptoms, comparable appearance of chest x-ray films, consistent derangements in pulmonary physiology, and typical histological features. Four infections may be associated with the cause or onset of most of the various diseases: disseminated fungus (coccidioidomycosis, blastomycosis, histoplasmosis), disseminated mycobacteria, *Pneumocystis* pneumonia, and certain viruses.

Although all of the diffuse ILDs share the common morphological characteristic of an abnormal lung interstitium, a satisfactory classification has been elusive because about 150 individual diseases have a component of interstitial lung involvement, either as primary disease or as a significant part of a multiorgan process, such as a collagen-vascular disease. Generally, ILDs are classified according to the type of agent that caused the lung injury. About one-third of patients with ILD have an identifiable agent responsible for inducing lung injury; however, the large majority of patients have disease attributable to no known cause. Therefore, ILDs are classified as those with a known cause and those with an unknown etiology; each of these groups is further subclassified according to the presence or absence of granulomas in interstitial or vascular areas.

EPIDEMIOLOGY AND CAUSES

It is estimated that about 140,000 Americans have been diagnosed with ILD, which typically affects individuals between 50 and 75 years of age. There is a slightly younger age distribution associated with some ILDs (40 to 45 years for respiratory bronchiolitis–associated ILD and 45 to 55 years for nonspecific interstitial pneumonitis).

ILDs of known cause can be divided into several major subcategories. By far, the largest group comprises occupational and environmental inhalant diseases; these include diseases resulting from inhalation of inorganic dusts, organic dusts, gases, fumes, vapors, and aerosols. Other categories include ILDs caused by drugs, irradiation, poisons, neoplasia, and chronic cardiac failure. The major subgroups within the category of unknown causes are idiopathic pulmonary fibrosis (IPF) and connective tissue (collagen vascular) disorders with ILD, including rheumatoid arthritis (RA), systemic lupus erythematosus (SLE), progressive systemic sclerosis, polymyositis-dermatomyositis, and Sjögren's syndrome. Systemic vasculitides often have granulomas in tissue and include a variant of polyarteritis nodosa called allergic granulomatosis, lymphomatoid granulomatosis, and hypersensitivity vasculitis.

Seven major entities that are most frequently associated with diffuse ILD are (1) IPF, (2) bronchiolitis obliterans organizing pneumonia, (3) connective tissue (collagen vascular) diseases (SLE, RA, progressive systemic sclerosis [scleroderma], and polymyositis-dermatomyositis), (4) systemic granulomatous vasculitides (Wegener's granulomatosis, lymphomatoid granulomatosis, and allergic angiitis and granulomatosis), (5) drug-induced pulmonary disease, (6) sarcoidosis, and (7) hypersensitivity pneumonitis. These entities are briefly discussed further in Box 31.4.

Box 31.4 Interstitial Lung Diseases: Primary and Secondary Forms

Interstitial Pulmonary Fibrosis (IPF): A syndrome progressing from alveolitis to interstitial inflammation to fibrosis of the lungs.

Pulmonary Manifestations: Presents with dyspnea, cough, fatigue, adventitious crackles (sounding like Velcro), tachypnea, finger clubbing, abnormal pulmonary function tests (PFTs).

Management: No curative medical therapy; pirfenidone (Esbriet) and nintedanib (Ofev, tyrosine kinase inhibitor) both shown to improve lung function and approved to treat IPF; corticosteroids, immunosuppressants, antifibrotic agents (colchicine or D-penicillamine), recombinant tumor necrosis factor (TNF)-α antagonists, and other tyrosine kinase inhibitors are all being studied.

Bronchiolitis Obliterans Organizing Pneumonia (BOOP): A disease characterized by masses of granulation tissue in the lumens of small airways, with patchy organizing pneumonia distal to these obstructions.

Pulmonary Manifestations: Presents with cough, flu-like illness, inspiratory crackles, expiratory squeaks, restrictive ventilatory defect, and abnormal diffusing capacity; chest x-ray shows patchy alveolar infiltrates, often with a ground-glass appearance.

Management: Corticosteroid therapy.

Collagen Vascular Diseases

Systemic Lupus Erythematosus: Chronic, multisystem inflammatory disease of connective tissue that involves the skin, joints, serous membranes (pleura, pericardium), kidneys, hematological system, and central nervous system (CNS).

Pulmonary Manifestations: May present with pleuritis with or without effusion, diaphragmatic dysfunction with reduced lung volume, acute lupus pneumonitis, diffuse alveolar hemorrhage, diffuse interstitial disease, pulmonary hypertension, and pulmonary thromboembolism.

Management: The B-lymphocyte stimulator-specific inhibitor belimumab (Benlysta) is approved to treat lupus; NSAIDs, corticosteroids, disease-modifying antirheumatic drugs such as hydroxychloroquine and methotrexate, and other immunosuppressive agents such as cyclophosphamide (Cytoxan) are also used; plasmapheresis and stem cell therapy have also been tried but are not U.S. Food and Drug Administration approved.

Rheumatoid Arthritis: Chronic, systemic disease characterized by recurrent inflammation of the diarthrodial joints and related structures.

Pulmonary Manifestations: Presents with abnormal PFTs with reduced diffusing capacity and restrictive lung mechanics, pulmonary nodules, BOOP, pleuritis with or without effusion, interstitial lung disease (ILD).

Management: NSAIDS, COX-2 inhibitors, corticosteroids, methotrexate (Rheumatrex), biologic response modifiers:
- Non-TNF-α antagonists (e.g., abatacept [Orencia], rituximab [Rituxan])

- TNF-α antagonists (e.g., infliximab [Remicade], etanercept [Enbrel], adalimumab [Humira], golimumab [Simponi], certolizumab [Cimzia]
- Janus kinase inhibitors (e.g., tofacitinib [Xeljanz])

Progressive Systemic Sclerosis (Scleroderma): A disorder of connective tissue characterized by fibrotic, degenerative, and occasionally inflammatory changes in the skin, blood vessels, synovium, skeletal muscle, and internal organs.

Pulmonary Manifestations: Presents with dyspnea, bibasilar crackles, reduced lung compliance, pleural thickening, pulmonary fibrosis on x-ray, abnormal PFTs, pulmonary hypertension, recurrent aspiration pneumonia.

Management: Antifibrotic agents (e.g., D-penicillamine [Cuprimine]), immunosuppressants (e.g., azathioprine [Imuran], methotrexate [Rheumatrex]), and possibly stem cell therapy

Polymyositis-Dermatomyositis: A diffuse inflammatory myopathy of striated muscle, producing symmetrical weakness that is usually most severe in the proximal muscles.

Pulmonary Manifestations: The three types of lung disease classically described are interstitial pneumonitis, aspiration pneumonia due to esophageal dysmotility, and pneumonia secondary to hypoventilation as a result of respiratory muscle involvement.

Management: Corticosteroids, antineoplastic agents, and immunosuppressants (e.g., cyclophosphamide [Cytoxan]).

Systemic Granulomatous Vasculitis

Wegener's Granulomatosis: Characterized by a triad of (1) necrotizing granulomatous vasculitis of the upper and lower respiratory tracts, (2) glomerulonephritis, and (3) variable degrees of vasculitis of the small arteries and veins.

Pulmonary Manifestations: Upper respiratory tract lesions include sinusitis, otitis media, nasal septal ulceration; pulmonary manifestations vary from focal granulomatous vasculitis to diffuse alveolitis and capillaritis that may present as alveolar hemorrhage, with PFTs revealing a restrictive pattern.

Management: Immunosuppressants (e.g., cyclophosphamide [Cytoxan], azathioprine [Imuran], methotrexate [Rheumatrex]), corticosteroids, anti-TNF-α agents, or anti-B-cell therapies.

Lymphomatoid Granulomatosis: A systemic disease consisting of angiocentric lymphoid granulomatous vasculitis, primarily of the lungs, with frequent involvement of the kidneys and skin.

Pulmonary Manifestations: Presenting symptoms are usually cough and dyspnea; chest x-ray reveals multiple, bilateral, ill-defined, or nodular densities that may cavitate.

Management: Cyclophosphamide (Cytoxan) and corticosteroids; chemotherapy regimen if recurrence with malignant lymphoma; interferon treatment and stem cell therapy have also been used.

Continued

Box 31.4   Interstitial Lung Diseases: Primary and Secondary Forms—cont'd

Allergic Angiitis and Granulomatosis (Churg-Strauss Syndrome): A rare disorder characterized by necrotizing angiitis of the lungs, heart, skin, and CNS, with involved organs displaying infiltration with eosinophils.

Pulmonary Manifestations: Presents with an allergic history, often with asthma; chest x-ray abnormalities may range from patchy densities to large bilateral nodular infiltrates; lung cavitation is rare.

Management: Corticosteroids (e.g., prednisone), immunosuppressants (e.g., azathioprine [Imuran], cyclophosphamide [Cytoxan]), and plasma exchange have been used.

Drug-induced Pulmonary Disease: Iatrogenic and adverse complications of various drugs (cytotoxic agents, antibiotics, immunosuppressive drugs) can result in ILD.

Pulmonary Manifestations: Hypersensitivity pulmonary disease with dyspnea, nonproductive cough, lung crackles, tachypnea, diffuse linear streaks, and densities in lower lung zones on chest x-ray.

Management: Discontinuation of the drug or reduction in drug dosage, in conjunction with corticosteroid therapy.

Sarcoidosis: A multisystem syndrome of unknown etiology, involving complex cellular immune pathways, that most frequently affects the lung.

Pulmonary Manifestations: Lung most common organ affected; PFTs reveal a restrictive pattern and small lung volumes;

tissue biology demonstrates characteristic granulomas, with hilar lymphadenopathy typically seen on chest x-ray.

Management: Corticosteroids and other immunosuppressant drugs such as hydroxychloroquine (Plaquenil) and methotrexate (Rheumatrex).

Hypersensitivity Pneumonitis (Allergic Alveolitis): Caused by inhalation of a variety of organic dusts. These dusts can be derived from animal dander and proteins, from fungi that contaminate vegetables, wood bark, or water-reservoir vaporizers, or from dairy and grain products. Colorful, descriptive names for this disease underscore the frequent occupational nature of exposure.

Pulmonary Manifestations: In the acute form of disease, respiratory and systemic symptoms develop explosively within 4 to 6 hours after dust is inhaled, consisting of dyspnea, cough, chills, fever, and malaise; symptoms typically abate within 12 hours but with each re-exposure, the acute episode occurs again. The acutely ill patient is dyspneic with inspiratory crackles in the lower lung zones; chest x-ray shows fine, diffuse alveolar filling and variable interstitial streaks, and PFTs are abnormal.

Management: Avoidance of inhaled substance; corticosteroids (e.g., prednisone).

PATHOPHYSIOLOGY

ILD denotes a diverse group of conditions characterized by the common pathological finding of pulmonary fibrosis and a similar clinical presentation of restrictive lung findings (i.e., dyspnea on exertion and chronic nonproductive cough). The term "interstitial" used to describe this group of diseases is misleading because inflammation and fibrosis may affect bronchioles, alveoli, and capillary endothelia, as well as the interstitium of the lower respiratory tract. Thus, a more illustrative term for this disease is "pulmonary fibrosis." Sarcoidosis, hypersensitivity pneumonitis, pulmonary fibrosis in connective tissue disorders (e.g., SLE, RA, tuberous sclerosis, scleroderma), and occupational pulmonary diseases are all categorized as ILDs. Tissue injury and acute inflammation are believed to be the initial pathological processes. In some conditions, such as sarcoidosis, the inciting antigen is unknown, whereas occupational pulmonary diseases are caused by repeated inhalation of environmental irritants, inorganic and organic dusts, fumes, or gases. For most ILDs, including idiopathic conditions, cigarette smoking is a primary risk factor.

In the majority of ILDs, there is a perpetuation of the inflammatory process with repeated tissue injury and aberrant wound healing with subsequent remodeling of the lung architecture. Infiltration of the lung parenchyma by various combinations of immune cells mediates this process, including neutrophils, lymphocytes, plasma cells, eosinophils, basophils, mast cells, and alveolar macrophages. Cytokine production (e.g., granulocyte-colony stimulating factor, transforming growth factor–$\beta 1$, IL-1β, IL-8, TNF-α) drives these inflammatory and scarring (fibrotic) processes. Regions of chronic inflammation can develop granulomas consisting specifically of discrete masses of lymphocytes, macrophages, and fibroblasts. In turn, fibroblast proliferation and differentiation into myofibroblast forms (i.e., cells with both fibroblast and smooth muscle cell features) lead to fibrosis (collagen deposition) or scarring of the lungs and the development of cystic airspaces known as "honeycombing."

Such pathological pulmonary tissue becomes less compliant and increasingly rigid, with consequential impedance of ventilation and gas exchange, characteristic of a progressive, minimally reversible restrictive lung disease. Diffusion capacity of the lung (DLCO) also worsens with increasing fibrosis of the lung parenchyma. In turn, ventilation–perfusion mismatch, hypoxemia, and pulmonary vasoconstriction develop, and increased resistance on the right ventricle may lead to cor pulmonale (right ventriculomegaly). Hypercarbia typically manifests only in end-stage disease. Total lung capacity, functional residual capacity, residual volume, and FEV and FEV_1 are all commonly decreased on pulmonary function testing; however, because fibrotic lung tissue is stiffer with greater elastic recoil, rapid exhalation of a major portion of the overall expiratory volume may be seen, as reflected in a normal or increased FEV_1/FVC ratio on pulmonary function testing—a key feature distinguishing restrictive from obstructive pulmonary disease in which the FEV_1/FVC ratio is decreased.

Interestingly, recurrent dysregulated wound healing, rather than neutrophilic or immune cell–mediated inflammation, has been cited as the primary pathophysiological mechanism in ILD, potentially explaining the ineffectiveness of anti-inflammatory and immunosuppressive treatments in many forms of ILD. Lung tissue biopsy is not required for the diagnosis of ILD, which may be made from a combination of clinical and radiographic findings (including PFTs and certain serum markers of underlying connective tissue disease). However, the extent of lung fibrosis observed histopathologically is perhaps the most accurate prognostic indicator for this condition. In turn, much investigation has shifted toward antifibroblast therapies for ILD aimed at decreasing pulmonary collagen deposition.

CLINICAL PRESENTATION

The symptoms of ILD are similar regardless of the underlying cause. In addition, the symptoms of lung involvement are nonspecific and could suggest many other causes, including obstructive lung disease, heart disease, or pulmonary vascular disease. The first symptom of ILD is usually progressive dyspnea on exertion or a nonproductive cough. The patient initially notices dyspnea only during heavy exertion, but in very advanced stages of the disease, dyspnea occurs at rest.

The patient's breathlessness has no other obvious cause such as asthma, obstructive airway disease, bronchitis, or heart failure. Although emphasis is usually given to this most common presentation of patients with ILD, the provider must recognize the variability of clinical presentations. Dyspnea is a virtually constant finding in patients with IPF, but it is by no means consistent in other ILDs. Less common but important, and sometimes misleading, presentations include the following:

- Fatigue in the absence of dyspnea
- Dry cough without other respiratory symptoms
- Predominant systemic symptoms (e.g., fever, weight loss)
- Abnormal-appearing (90%) chest x-ray film in the absence of symptoms
- Incidental abnormalities of PFTs

Respiratory signs such as pleuritic chest pain, visceral chest pain, wheezing, or hemoptysis do not usually occur in most forms of ILD. One-half of patients have mucus hypersecretion and expectoration. This occurrence has been correlated with glandular hypertrophy in the airway mucosa and accumulated mucus in the airways. Patients with more advanced ILD may have clubbing and cyanosis. Clinical manifestations specific to the various types of ILD are discussed in Box 31.4.

DIAGNOSTIC REASONING

Assessment of History

The occupational and environmental history is the single most helpful tool to determine whether a respiratory problem may be related to an environmental exposure (see Focus on History: Taking an Occupational and Environmental History). A careful history must include a detailed chronological account of the patient's employment activities, social activities, travel, immune status, pets, hobbies, and typical environment. A thorough review of the patient's past medical history, along with current and previous medications, is also important. The goal of these questions is to determine whether the patient has been exposed to agents known to cause ILD. Many patients have an occupational history that includes exposure to one or a variety of toxic inhalation products; this may add uncertainty to the precise onset of symptoms and may suggest the contribution of several etiological factors. The temporal relationship to the exposure may be obvious in some cases, while in others, low-grade exposure may provoke chronic illness without acute flares after exposure. The latency may be extremely long (e.g., more than 20 years for asbestosis), so it is mandatory to take a detailed occupational history, including summer jobs and hobbies, in all patients with suspected ILD. Moreover, a history of smoking is associated with an increased risk for the development of IPF. Finally, the occurrence of familial cases of IPF suggests that genetic factors may modulate responses to causative agents.

Focus on History: Taking an Occupational and Environmental History

General health history

- Does the patient think symptom/problem is related to anything at work?
- When was the onset of symptoms, and how was this related to work?
- Has the patient missed any days of work and why?
- Prior pulmonary problems
- Medications
- Cigarette use

Current or most relevant employment

- Job or process: title and description
- Type of industry and specific work
- Name of employer
- Years employed

Exposure information

- General description of job process and overall hygiene
- Materials used by worker
- Ventilation/exhaust system
- Use of respiratory protection
- Are other workers affected?
- Industrial hygiene samples and Occupational Safety and Health Administration data

Environmental nonoccupational factors

- Cigarettes
- Diet
- Hobbies
- Pets

Specific workplace exposures

- Fumes/dust/fibers
- Gases
- Metals
- Solvent
- Other chemicals: plastics, pesticides, corrosive agents
- Infectious agents
- Organic dusts: cotton, wood
- Radiation
- Emotional factors, stress (helpful in ruling out other causes of difficulty breathing or chest pain, such as panic attacks)

Past employment

- List jobs in chronological order
- Job titles
- Military service

Dyspnea in the patient with ILD is the result of increased work of breathing caused primarily by the stiffness of the lungs and by excessive minute ventilation. Hypoxemia, often aggravated by exercise, may amplify the sensation of dyspnea by carotid body stimulation. Unfortunately, patients do not always know to which toxins they were exposed, and exposures to toxins may be easily overlooked so that considerable investigation may be required. For example, fungi in cooling systems or birds in the home may be a source of allergens that can elicit hypersensitivity pneumonitis. History of medication use is also critical to diagnosing ILD. Patients who have been using certain drugs (e.g., nitrofurantoin) for many years may not report them as medications on routine questioning. Mineral oil taken as a laxative or nose or ear drops also may not be reported as medications by patients.

Importance of Review of Systems

Diseases in other organs may present as ILD, so a detailed review of systems is important. With occupational lung diseases, the physical examination is generally unrevealing for a specific cause. It is most helpful in ruling out nonoccupational causes of respiratory symptoms or diseases related to cardiac or connective tissue disorders. Chronic heart disease may present as ILD with dyspnea, cough, crackles, and interstitial-type abnormalities on chest x-ray. Malignancies of virtually any organ system may spread to the lungs and present as ILD. The manifestations of collagen-vascular diseases (e.g., rashes, Raynaud's phenomenon, fevers, arthralgias, muscle weakness) may result in important clues on history taking. Dysphagia or regurgitation may relate to either recurrent aspiration or collagen-vascular disease, especially scleroderma. Connective tissue disease may be difficult to rule out because pulmonary manifestations occasionally precede the more typical systemic manifestations by months or years. Patients with AIDS complicated by pneumocystosis or lymphocytic interstitial pneumonia may first present with an insidious onset of dyspnea and fatigue, as in patients with other ILDs. Therefore, sexual orientation and other possible risk factors for AIDS should be identified.

Diagnostic Testing

Abnormalities on chest x-ray may be the first clue to the presence of ILD; however, the patient with ILD may be asymptomatic or symptomatic with either normal or abnormal chest x-ray results. The initial abnormality on the chest x-ray film is usually described as a ground glass or hazy appearance of the lungs. As disease progresses, diffuse abnormalities are found bilaterally. Pulmonary opacities (infiltrates) are usually described as small nodules (nodular), lines (reticular), or both (reticulonodular). Nodules are most commonly found in granulomatous diseases and hypersensitivity pneumonitis. The development of reticular densities is thought to be the result of edema, infiltration, or fibrosis of the septa in the periphery of the lung. A common characteristic of ILD is a progressive worsening of lung opacities, with the development of honeycomb lung. This honeycomb appearance is created by the cyst-like spaces that characterize the pathology of advanced ILD. Many ILDs have unique radiographic presentations. For example, Wegener's granulomatosis is associated with lower lobe cavities and nodules, whereas sarcoidosis is associated with swelling of the lymph nodes of the hilum of the lung (hilar lymphadenopathy). The hila are composed of the pulmonary arteries and their main branches, the upper lobe pulmonary veins, the major bronchi, and lymph nodes.

High-resolution computed tomography (HRCT) can evaluate ILD, as well as detect and localize pericardial and pleural fluid collections. HRCT examines only 1 mm of lung tissue at each level, thus revealing the lung parenchyma's delicate architecture. Several signs of ILD may be noted on HRCT. The most common are interface signs—the thickened and irregular appearance of the normally smooth interface of lung parenchyma with bronchi, blood vessels, and visceral pleura. Although HRCT is an exceptional tool for evaluation of parenchymal lung disease, it is important to note its limitations. It cannot be used to study the entire thorax, so conventional CT must be used to avoid missing abnormalities between images. Moreover, some HRCT findings may be difficult to interpret without a conventional CT image to use for reference.

Serological tests for antinuclear antibodies and rheumatoid factor are positive in 20% to 40% of patients, although rarely diagnostic. Antineutrophil cytoplasmic antibodies may be diagnostic in some settings.

A transbronchial biopsy is the leading invasive tool for evaluating and treating patients with a wide spectrum of pulmonary disorders. In addition, the technique of bronchoalveolar lavage through a fiber-optic bronchoscope into a segmental or smaller bronchus provides a means to sample both the cellular and soluble components of the lower respiratory tract. The area beyond the bronchoscope's reach is washed with saline, which is then aspirated back through the bronchoscope, containing a small number of cells. The cells that are recovered include many from the alveoli and are representative of the cells associated with the inflammatory process. This procedure has aided in the diagnosis of ILD and in the assessment of its pathogenesis and disease activity.

PFTs measure lung volumes and airflow with a spirometer. Whether the patient is symptomatic or not, PFTs should be performed to establish the presence of disease, determine its severity, and monitor response to treatment. The sensitivity and specificity of these tests to diagnose the various ILDs, however, is low. Routine spirometry values and lung volumes are often initially normal, as are resting blood gas measurements; only after exercise may some gas-exchange abnormalities become evident. The evaluation of the patient during exercise, although not constituting a direct measurement of respiration, gives more information than static measurements of lung volume or diffusing capacity regarding ventilation, blood flow, gas exchange, and control of breathing. PFTs usually show a purely restrictive defect in most patients with ILD. Obstructive lung disease develops gradually in some patients and more commonly in some diseases such as sarcoidosis and hypersensitivity pneumonitis.

The compliance of the lungs decreases as lung involvement progresses. This is caused, in part, by fibrosis of the pulmonary parenchyma and the formation of cystic airspaces. DLCO is a good reflection of alveolar capillary surface area. Destruction of lung parenchyma results in a reduction in DLCO as ILD progresses. An abnormal DLCO may be the earliest evidence of ILD found on standard PFTs.

The use of the thoracoscope in combination with standard surgical instruments is known as video-assisted thoracic surgery (VATS) or video-assisted thoracoscopy. VATS provides the same access to the hemithorax as both thoracoscopy and thoracotomy. VATS procedures are particularly useful for obtaining lung biopsies in patients with diffuse ILD. With VATS, the visualization

of the lung is better than it is with a limited thoracotomy because more areas of the lung can be sampled.

Transbronchial lung biopsy involves passing a forceps or needle through the bronchoscope. A specimen is obtained with forceps or aspirated through a needle. Pleural biopsy is useful in diagnosing granulomatous disease or malignancy of the pleura and should be performed only if these two diseases are suspected. If a specific diagnosis is not made by transbronchial biopsy, an open lung biopsy is indicated. Open lung biopsy is the most definitive way to diagnose and stage the disease so that appropriate prognostic and therapeutic decisions can be made. Depending on the age of the patient and the potential risks of the surgery in a compromised patient, empirical therapy may be initiated.

Differential Diagnosis

When confronted with a patient with unexplained dyspnea and fatigue, the differential diagnosis is immense. Pulmonary, cardiac, hematological, renal, neuromuscular, and even endocrine diseases may present with exercise intolerance or dyspnea. A complete work-up of these systems is required to determine the correct diagnosis. Some of the conditions that give rise to dyspnea, diffuse pulmonary infiltration, and a granulomatous reaction include extrinsic allergic alveolitis, asbestosis, silicosis, berylliosis, lymphoid granulomatosis, connective tissue diseases, certain drugs, miliary TB, lymphoma, leukemias, pneumocystis pneumonia, and coccidioidomycosis.

MANAGEMENT

Management of most ILDs is difficult, and different approaches are taken depending on the specific entity. Regardless of etiology, end-stage fibrosis is irreversible and untreatable. An extensive and aggressive diagnostic evaluation early on, even in the patient with relatively few symptoms, is recommended, as early clinical intervention in patients who are more likely to develop lung disease could be of considerable benefit for the patient. A good example is the identification and assessment of disease progression in diffuse lung disease found in systemic sclerosis.

The first course of action when faced with a patient with ILD is to determine whether exposure to environmental agents or drugs is the cause and to discontinue the exposure. Therapeutic dilemmas with certain classes of drugs, such as antiarrhythmic medications, arise because discontinuation of drugs such as amiodarone may result in life-threatening dysrhythmias. Second, the best chance for therapeutic success begins with the correct diagnosis. Finally, in cases in which specific medication is used, such as prednisone or cytotoxic agents, there is usually suppression rather than cure of the primary process. Many patients with ILD are older adults, so the decision to treat them with immunosuppressive drugs should not be taken lightly because the toxicity and adverse effects of these medications can be substantial. In addition, anti-inflammatory and immunosuppressive treatments may be ineffective because of recurrent dysregulated wound healing. Antifibroblast therapies for ILD are aimed at decreasing pulmonary collagen deposition. Stem cell therapy may also be considered in some cases.

Initial Management

Corticosteroids may be initiated as therapy for ILD. A trial of corticosteroids is reasonable, even for the patient who is in an advanced stage of the disease with relatively acellular and fibrotic changes in lung tissue. The best predictor of ultimate corticosteroid responsiveness and a better prognosis is early benefit following the initial 1 to 2 months of corticosteroid therapy. The dosage and duration of corticosteroid therapy depend on the specific disorder, but in general, relatively high doses are used for the first 6 weeks (1 to 2 mg/kg/day, or 60 to 100 mg/day) over the ensuing 3 months. A period of 3 to 6 months is often required to determine the corticosteroid responsiveness of fibrosing alveolitis, although patients with sarcoidosis and cryptogenic organizing pneumonia may respond much more quickly with lower dosages. Certain processes, such as IPF, commonly require therapy for 12 months or longer.

For IPF, nintedanib (Ofev) and pirfenidone (Esbriet, Pirfenex, Pirespa) may slow the progressive decline in lung function.

Subsequent Management

For the patient who is not well controlled with or responsive to corticosteroids, additional immunosuppressive therapy may be considered. Cyclophosphamide (Cytoxan), an alkylating drug, is a potent immunosuppressant and seems to be effective in patients with ILD who are not helped with corticosteroids. If improvement in the lung disease is documented after 3 months of this therapy, it should be continued for a 12-month interval. Azathioprine (Azasan, Imuran) has been used as an alternative to cyclophosphamide. Penicillamine (Cuprimine, Depen) has been used in some patients, with the rationale that it might prevent the cross-linking of abnormal collagen being synthesized in the interstitium and prevent or retard fibrosis. Exercise tolerance may be significantly improved with supplemental oxygen.

Because the pulmonary vascular bed is impaired by progressive fibrosis, pulmonary hypertension and cor pulmonale can develop; right-sided congestive heart failure can be difficult to control. Judicious use of diuretics is advised, for a significant decrease in intravascular volume may be deleterious for lung perfusion. Digitalis or antidysrhythmic drugs may be required, although adequate oxygenation is probably the best treatment for heart failure in this situation.

Some patients may also develop obstruction to air flow and be troubled with wheezing and coughing that may respond to bronchodilators. Because infection may occur during immunosuppressive therapy, it is important to maintain a high index of suspicion and to treat infection aggressively. Prophylactic use of pneumococcal and influenza vaccines is encouraged. Finally, lung transplantation may be an option for patients with refractory disease limited to the chest. See Box 31.4 for additional therapies for ILD.

FOLLOW-UP AND REFERRAL

Reassessment of disease activity is generally performed at 3, 6, 12, and 24 months or more often if needed. Responsiveness is defined as a decrease in symptoms: radiographic improvement; physiological improvement; or no further decline in clinical, radiographic, or physiologic parameters. The patient should be followed for signs of infection that are masked by immunosuppressive drugs, pneumothorax, or the development of lung cancer, which occurs in 5% to 10% of patients. The patient on corticosteroids must be monitored closely during times of illness or stress and during corticosteroid tapering or withdrawal. The patient should be encouraged to wear a medical identification bracelet. In view of exercise-related hypoxia, the patient should be assessed for the benefit of supplemental oxygen during exercise. Patients with a collagen vascular disorder must be regularly assessed for progression or exacerbations of their chronic illnesses. For example, patients with RA require rest, joint protection, daily heat and exercise, and psychological support. Community resources such as a home care nurse, homemaker services, and vocational rehabilitation may be considered. Self-help groups may be beneficial for the patient. These diseases require the collaborative and integrated approach as emphasized in the *Circle of Caring* model (see Chapter 1).

Specialized testing should be undertaken and the patient referred to a pulmonologist if no specific cause of dyspnea or cough can be found, if the symptoms exceed the physiological or radiographic abnormalities identified, if empiric management (with bronchodilators, diuretics, smoking cessation) results in an atypical or unsatisfactory clinical outcome, if the patient needs an impairment or disability evaluation for workers' compensation or other reason, if specialized cardiopulmonary testing (e.g., lung biopsy) is needed, or if a therapeutic immunosuppressive or cytotoxic drug trial is contemplated.

Patient Education: ILD

Patients with ILD must be educated about the nature of their illness, related diagnostic tests, and the treatment regimen for their particular type of lung disease (see Box 31.5). For example,

Box 31.5 Educational Content for the Patient With Interstitial Lung Disease

- Respiratory anatomy and physiology
- Pathophysiology of interstitial lung disease
- Respiratory diagnostic tests:
  Chest x-ray
  Pulmonary function tests
  Exercise tests
  Bronchoscopy
  High-resolution computed tomography
- Self-care measures:
  Pulmonary medications
  Diet
  Fluid intake
  Smoking cessation
  Environmental control
  Awareness of early signs of infection
- Chest therapy:
  Relaxation and guided imagery
  Breathing retraining
  Controlling dyspneic episodes
  Postural drainage
- Progressive exercise conditioning:
  Walking programs
  Treadmill or bicycle exercise training
  Arm or leg range-of-motion exercises
- Respiratory equipment:
  Oxygen therapy
  Handheld nebulizer

avoidance of exposure to antigens is paramount for those with hypersensitivity pneumonitis. All patients must be advised and assisted to stop cigarette smoking to prevent further lung damage. In many cases, the most comprehensive patient education occurs within the context of a pulmonary rehabilitation program.

The need to reduce repeated hospital and intensive care unit admissions necessitates an effective pulmonary rehabilitation program. The target population for these programs has traditionally been severely disabled patients with COPD or ILD, who require a broad range of comprehensive services to keep them clinically stable and out of the hospital for long periods of time. However, appropriate patients with all levels of respiratory impairment who could benefit from such programs, and not only the severely disabled, should be referred to pulmonary rehabilitation. These programs have criteria for referral that generally include the following patient characteristics: dyspnea on exertion, inability to carry out selected activities of daily living, repeated hospitalizations or need for home care services, time lost from work or school, and desire for educational update of self-care techniques. Moreover, the following laboratory features are inclusion criteria for pulmonary rehabilitation: reduced vital capacity in restrictive lung disease, reduced expiratory flow rate, hypercapnia, and hypoxemia at rest or during exercise.

REFERENCES

Asthma

Bernstein JA. Allergic rhinitis and asthma: How to help patients control environmental triggers. *Consultant.* 2012;52(7):508–514.

Bernstein, JA. Allergic rhinitis and asthma: Role of environmental determinants. *Consultant.* 2012;52(7):490–497.

Centers for Disease Control and Prevention. Asthma data, statistics, and surveillance. https://www.cdc.gov/asthma/asthmadata.htm. Accessed June 16, 2017.

Environmental Protection Agency. 2016 asthma facts. https://www.epa.gov/sites/production/files/2016-05/documents/asthma_fact_sheet_english_05_2016.pdf. Accessed June 16, 2017.

Langton, D; Sha, J; Ing, A; Fielding, D; & Wood, E. (2017). Bronchial thermoplasty in severe asthma in Australia. *Internal Medicine Journal* Oct. 27, 20017. https://www.researchgate.net/publication/312567659_Bronchial_thermoplasty_in_severe_asthma_in_Australia_Bronchial_thermoplasty_in_severe_asthma. Accessed 9/24/18.

National Asthma Education and Prevention Program. Expert Panel 3 Summary Report 2007: Guidelines for the diagnosis and management of asthma (NIH publication no. 08-5846). Bethesda, MD: U.S. Department of Health and Human Services, Public Health Service, National Institutes of Health, National Heart, Lung, and Blood Institute. Reviewed 2015.

Zhang L, Prietsch SO, Ducharme FM. Inhaled corticosteroids in children with persistent asthma: Effects on growth. *Evid Based Child Health.* 2014;9(4):829–930.

Chronic Bronchitis and Emphysema

American Lung Association. Trends in COPD (bronchitis and emphysema) morbidity and mortality. http://www.lung.org/assets/documents/research/copd-trend-report.pdf. Published 2013.

Breunig IM, Shaya FT, Scharf SM. Delivering cost-effective care for COPD in the USA. *Expert Rev Pharmacoecon Outcomes Res.* 2012;12(6):725–731.

Global Strategy for the Diagnosis, Management and Prevention of COPD. Global Initiative for Chronic Obstructive Lung Disease (GOLD). http://goldcopd.org. Published 2017.

Guarascio AJ, Ray SM, Finch CK, Self TH. The clinical and economic burden of chronic obstructive pulmonary disease in the USA. *Clinicoecon Outcomes Res.* 2013;5:235–245.

Kirkpatrick,P; Wilson,F & Wimpenny,P. Research to support evidence-based practice in COPD community nursing. *Br J Community Nurs.* 2012;17(10):486, 488–492.

Leader D. A comprehensive guide to chronic obstructive pulmonary disease (COPD). Lung transplant. http://www.healthline.com/health/lung-transplant#overview1. Accessed June 24, 2017.

Menn, P, Heinrich, J, Huber, RM.; KORA Study Group. Direct medical costs of COPD—An excess cost approach based on two population-based studies. *Respir Med.* 2012;106(4):540–548.

Rand Health. Rand 36-Item Health Survey. http://www.rand.org/health/surveys_tools/mos/36-item-short-form/survey-instrument.html. Accessed June 17, 2017.

Stanley T, Gordon JS, Pilon BA. Patient and provider attributes associated with chronic obstructive pulmonary disease exacerbations. *J Nurse Pract.* 2013;9(1):34–39.

U.S. Department of Health and Human Services. National Heart, Lung, and Blood Institute. COPD National Action Plan. https://www.nhlbi.nih.gov/health-pro/resources/lung/copd-national-action-plan. Published 2017. Accessed June 18, 2017.

Interstitial Lung Disease

American Lung Association. Learn about pulmonary fibrosis. http://www.lung.org/lung-health-and-diseases/lung-disease-lookup/pulmonary-fibrosis/learn-about-pulmonary.html. Accessed June 24, 2017.

Summerhill EM. Interstitial (nonidiopathic) pulmonary fibrosis treatment and management. Medscape. http://emedicine.medscape.com/article/301337-treatment?pa=vpG8EUX2yOl6dpVbvplV9oGC3Ew2Mt8mEAXF80ueBSthu%2BiRWl1NWE3RfotqhSGL6dJIMRX8tPuIe7Zc2ZeFleN5lPYw%2FtQ7Z8WOOzpssmw%3D. Published 2016. Accessed June 24, 2017.

RESOURCES

Asthma and COPD (selected Web sites)

Allergy, Asthma, and Immunology
http://allergy.mcg.edu/physicians/manual/manual.html
www.nhlbi.nih.gov/guidelines/asthma

American Academy of Allergy, Asthma, and Immunology
www.aaaai.org
American College of Allergy, Asthma, and Immunology
www.acaai.org
American Lung Association
www.lungusa.org
Asthma.com—a GlaxoSmithKline-sponsored Web site offering adult and pediatric asthma control test questionnaires
http://www.asthma.com/additional-resources/asthma-control-test.html
Asthma and Allergy Foundation of America
www.aafa.org
National Heart, Lung, and Blood Institute
www.nhlbi.nih.gov
National Institute of Allergy and Infectious Disease
www.niaid.nih.gov
National Library of Medicine
www.nlm.nih.gov

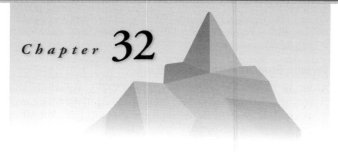

Chapter **32**

Lung Cancer

Jill E. Winland-Brown, EdD, APRN, FNP-BC
Brian Oscar Porter, MD, PhD, MPH, MBA

Lung cancer is the leading cause of death in the United States and accounts for 27% of all cancer deaths. Although the number of deaths from lung cancer has consistently declined each year since 2010, which may be due in part to massive education campaigns related to smoking cessation, approximately 156,000 people in the United States died from lung cancer in 2014. Approximately one-fourth of all patients diagnosed with lung cancer have no symptoms at diagnosis, and one-fourth of all lung cancer patients never smoked. Lung cancer in never-smokers accounted for approximately 56,000 deaths in 2016 and was the seventh leading cause of cancer deaths in the United States.

The diagnosis of lung cancer typically is made when a tumor is seen on a routine preoperative chest x-ray or a work physical chest x-ray. Approximately three-quarters of patients have a cough, which may be productive with bloody or rust-colored sputum.

Lung cancer arises from the epithelium of the respiratory tract. The four major histological types are (1) squamous-cell (epidermoid) carcinoma, (2) small-cell (oat-cell) carcinoma, (3) large-cell carcinoma (including giant-cell and clear-cell carcinoma), and (4) adenocarcinoma. Squamous-cell carcinoma is named for the resemblance of cells to the epidermis of the skin. These cells usually contain the skin protein keratin. Squamous-cell carcinomas arise most often from the bronchial lining and may grow to obstruct air passages. Adenocarcinoma, the most prevalent carcinoma of the lung in both sexes, resembles poorly formed glandular tissue. It may be difficult to determine whether an adenocarcinoma is a primary lung cancer or a metastatic tumor from elsewhere in the body. Fifty-five percent to 60% of adenocarcinomas are located in the periphery of the lung and are not obviously related to any bronchus. Many organs in the body can develop adenocarcinomas that may metastasize to the lungs. Large-cell carcinomas, also called undifferentiated carcinomas, are characterized by a collection of poorly formed large cells that have abundant cytoplasm. These tumors may exhibit a glandlike structure and produce mucin.

Small-cell lung carcinomas (SCLCs) (oat-cell, intermediate, and combined carcinomas) are characterized by very small cells with scant cytoplasm. SCLC is a very rapidly growing tumor that usually metastasizes to distant tissue while the tumor is quite small. The clinical effect of SCLC is much different from that of the other three forms of lung cancer, which is why lung cancers are usually classified in terms of SCLCs and non-SCLCs (NSCLCs) (Table 32.1).

Because the lung area is so large, tumors may go undetected for some time. Early symptoms such as coughing and fatigue are nonspecific, and patients often attribute these symptoms to causes other than lung cancer. For these reasons, early stage lung cancer (Stages I and II) is difficult to detect, and most patients are diagnosed at Stages III and IV.

EPIDEMIOLOGY AND CAUSES

Lung cancer is preventable, common, and lethal once it comes to clinical attention. It is also relatively resistant to current therapeutics. Lung cancer is the most frequent cause of cancer deaths in men and women in North America and accounts for 28% of all cancer deaths. In 2014, the American Cancer Society reported that more than 224,000 people were diagnosed with lung cancer, and there were more than 158,000 lung cancer deaths (American Lung Association, 2016). Eighty-six percent of lung cancer patients die within 5 years of diagnosis. In patients who have never smoked, the 5-year survival rate is 1%. This low survival rate may be explained by health-care professionals' lack of suspicion of lung cancer in nonsmokers, which prevents diagnosis early in the course of the disease.

The death rate for women due to lung cancer is now higher than from any other cancer because of increased cigarette smoking by women and because women may be more susceptible to the carcinogenic effects of tobacco smoke than men. In every ethnic group, men still have a higher lung cancer incidence and mortality rates than women, although women are rapidly closing the gap. African American men have the highest lung cancer incidence and mortality rates of any ethnic group. Lung cancer is the leading cause of cancer deaths in most racial and ethnic groups of women except for Native American, Filipino, and Hispanic women. New lung cancers and lung cancer deaths peak in individuals aged 55 to 65 years old.

Smoking still causes the majority of lung cancer cases. The risk of lung cancer increases with the duration of smoking, with earlier age at onset of smoking, and with smoking unfiltered or high-tar cigarettes. Of continued note are the effects of environmental tobacco smoke (ETS), also called secondhand smoke, side-stream smoke, involuntary smoke, or passive cigarette smoke. Exposure to ETS is thought to increase the risk of dying from lung cancer by 30%.

Lung cancer also occurs in association with occupational and environmental exposure to carcinogenic agents from sources other than smoking. Radon is the second leading cause of lung cancer deaths. Radon exposure causes almost 3,000 annual lung cancer deaths in nonsmokers. Other lung carcinogens include asbestos, radiation, certain heavy metals, and polycyclic aromatic hydrocarbons found in volcanoes, forest fires, burning coal, and exhaust fumes from cars. The combination of cigarette smoking and environmental exposure produces an additive effect, such that smokers exposed to asbestos increase their risk of lung cancer 92 times.

PATHOPHYSIOLOGY

The bronchial walls have three layers: an epithelial lining, a smooth muscle layer, and a connective tissue layer. The epithelial lining of the bronchi contains single-celled exocrine glands (i.e., mucus-secreting goblet cells) and ciliated cells. High columnar pseudostratified epithelium lines the larger airways, changing to columnar cuboidal epithelium in the bronchioles. It is hypothesized that at sites of segmental bronchial bifurcations, airflow and mucus production are altered and the bronchial epithelium becomes susceptible to injury. Carcinogenic agents, such as tobacco smoke, are likely deposited and absorbed in these areas. Particle size in ETS is smaller than in mainstream smoke, and inhaled particles may travel to peripheral lung regions more readily. This is thought to explain the excess of peripheral adenocarcinomas seen in passive smokers.

Cigarette smoke contains tumor initiators, promoters, and cocarcinogens. DNA-mutating agents in cigarettes produce alterations in both oncogenes (a class of genes that encodes proteins involved in normal cell-growth

TABLE 32.1 **Cellular Classification of Lung Cancer**	
Major Classification	*Subclassification*
Small-cell lung carcinomas	• Oat-cell carcinoma • Intermediate-cell carcinoma • Combined small-cell carcinoma (with squamous-cell carcinoma or adenocarcinoma)

• Non–small-cell lung carcinomas	• Squamous-cell (epidermoid) carcinoma
	  Well-differentiated
	  Moderately well-differentiated
	  Poorly differentiated
	• Adenocarcinoma
	  Well-differentiated
	  Moderately well-differentiated
	  Poorly differentiated
	  Bronchoalveolar
	• Large-cell carcinoma
	  Giant cell
	  Clear cell

processes) and tumor-suppressor genes. Multiple genetic events occur that result in cancer, first resulting in dysregulated growth and eventually in a malignant cell. These alterations include bronchial epithelial changes that progress from squamous-cell alterations, or metaplasia, to carcinoma in situ. Repeated carcinogenic insults to the bronchial epithelium may cause increased rates of cellular replication. Healthy ciliated cells are replaced with a proliferation of basal cells, resulting in hyperplasia, dysplasia, carcinoma in situ, and invasive carcinoma.

Small-Cell Lung Cancer

SCLC, which accounts for 15% of all lung cancers, invades the submucosa and is centrally located, developing around a main bronchus as a whitish-gray growth that compromises surrounding structures, eventually compressing the bronchi externally. SCLC results from smoking more so than NSCLC, grows more rapidly, and metastasizes earlier than NSCLC. SCLC is also more responsive to chemotherapy than NSCLC. The most striking difference between small-cell carcinoma and other forms of malignant lung neoplasms is the aggressiveness of this tumor, resulting in more rapid growth and early local and distant metastasis via the lymphatics and blood vessels.

There are three types of SCLC:

- Oat-cell carcinoma is composed of cells with round to oval nuclei. The tumors are soft in consistency and have shiny, gray-cut surfaces on examination.
- Intermediate cell-type SCLC is characterized by cells with larger, more vesicular, fusiform, or spindled nuclei.
- Combined cell-type SCLC is characterized by a combination of small-cell carcinoma cells and another cell type. The most important variant is the combination of small-cell and large-cell types, which is regarded as a small-cell carcinoma for treatment purposes. This variant lacks sensitivity to radiation and chemotherapy but retains the aggressiveness of "pure" small-cell carcinoma.

Non–Small-Cell Lung Cancers

NSCLCs comprise approximately 85% of all primary lung carcinomas in the United States. They comprise squamous-cell carcinomas, adenocarcinomas, and large-cell carcinomas.

Mutations in the tumor suppressor gene p53 are reported to be associated with human cancer more commonly than any other gene. A gene mutation is present in about 60% of all cases of NSCLC. The p53 gene encodes a protein with a central role in the regulation of transcriptional events in the cell nucleus, particularly in response to DNA-damaging agents, such as ionizing radiation

and a variety of other carcinogens. The central regulatory role of normal p53 protein has led to its description as the "guardian of the genome." Although many efforts to improve survival have focused on expanding NSCLC indications for both radiotherapy and surgery, little progress has been made.

Squamous-Cell Carcinoma

Squamous-cell carcinoma is the second most common lung cancer, accounting for 25% to 35% of cases. It is more common in men than in women and occurs almost entirely in cigarette smokers.

These tumors arise from the basal cells of the bronchial epithelium and usually present as masses in the segmental, lobar, or mainstem bronchi. The tumors tend to be bulky and invade cartilage and adjoining lymph nodes. On the basis of the degree of differentiation, these tumors are divided into three subtypes: well-differentiated, moderately well-differentiated, and poorly differentiated tumors. Well-differentiated tumors may show epithelial pearl formation, whereas poorly differentiated tumors are characterized by keratinization. Because squamous-cell carcinoma is a relatively slow-growing tumor, several years may elapse between the development of a carcinoma in situ and clinical detection. Metastases of squamous-cell carcinomas are initially to the hilar and mediastinal lymph nodes and then to the liver, adrenals, bones, and brain.

Adenocarcinoma

Adenocarcinoma, which represents 35% to 40% of all lung cancers, is the most prevalent carcinoma of the lung in both sexes and in nonsmokers. It forms acinar or glandular structures. Histologically, this tumor is divided broadly into well-differentiated, moderately well-differentiated, poorly differentiated, and bronchoalveolar subtypes. They arise from the bronchial epithelium and may form in lung scars or fibrous tissue. Adenocarcinoma usually presents as a NSCLC in the peripheral portion of the lungs, although rapidly progressive multifocal disease may be present at diagnosis. Although adenocarcinomas are usually slow-growing tumors, they may invade lymphatics and blood vessels early and thus produce early metastases; nearly half are considered to be unresectable at the time of diagnosis. Grossly, central cavitation is uncommon. Areas of metastasis commonly include the brain, liver, bone, and adrenal glands. Patients with adenocarcinomas may have an associated history of chronic interstitial lung disease such as scleroderma, rheumatoid arthritis, recurrent pulmonary infections, and other necrotizing pulmonary disease.

The bronchoalveolar subtype of adenocarcinoma represents approximately 2% to 4% of all lung cancers. Often, it is associated with prior lung disease leading to fibrosis, including repeated pneumonias, idiopathic pulmonary fibrosis, asbestosis, scleroderma, and Hodgkin's disease. There is little correlation between this type of cancer and smoking. Bronchoalveolar carcinoma commonly arises in the periphery of the lung and it grows in a scalelike fashion along the alveolar septa. Grossly, these tumors may be categorized as solitary, multinodular, or diffuse. The solitary, well-differentiated bronchoalveolar adenocarcinoma has a much better prognosis than the other forms; diffuse and multinodular forms usually are not amenable to therapy.

Large-Cell Carcinoma

Large-cell carcinoma, also called undifferentiated carcinoma, is the least common type of lung cancer, comprising approximately 10% of cases. It is classified into two types: clear-cell carcinoma and giant-cell carcinoma. Large-cell carcinomas include all tumors that show no evidence of differentiation to small-cell carcinoma, squamous-cell carcinoma, or adenocarcinoma. These tumors tend to form large, bulky, somewhat circumscribed and necrotic masses in the major or intermediate-sized bronchi or in the periphery, invade locally, and disseminate widely. The giant-cell variant of large-cell carcinoma is composed of huge, multinucleated, bizarre cells that are frequently associated with an extensive inflammatory cell infiltration. These tumors are usually large and peripheral and are very aggressive, highly malignant, and most often found at a late stage. These lesions are able to metastasize widely, with a predilection for the small intestine. Table 32.2 summarizes the disease characteristics of the various types of lung cancer.

CLINICAL PRESENTATION

Past history of a patient with suspected lung cancer should include an assessment of any history of chronic respiratory problems, as well as any prolonged exposure to environmental carcinogens. Habits must be explored

TABLE 32.2 Disease Characteristics of Lung Cancer

Lung Cancer Type	Tumor Type	Growth Rate	Metastasis	Manifestations	Treatment
Small-cell lung carcinoma	• 15%–20% • Neuroendocrine cells: oat-cell carcinoma Combined small-cell (with squamous-cell carcinoma or adenocarcinoma)	Very rapid	Very early, via lymphatics and blood vessels	Obstruction of main bronchus; associated with paraneoplastic syndrome	• Not resectable • Treated with chemotherapy and radiation
• Non–small-cell lung carcinomas	• Squamous-cell (epidermoid) carcinoma • 25%–35% • Keratin-producing cells: Well-differentiated Moderately well-differentiated Poorly differentiated	Slow	Hilar and mediastinal lymph nodes, liver, adrenals, bone, brain	Most often in cigarette smokers; bulky mass in mainstem bronchi	• Stages I and II: resectable • Stage III: chemotherapy and radiation • Stage IV: chemotherapy (refer to Table 32.5 for staging)
	• Adenocarcinoma • 35%–40% • Columnar cells: Well-differentiated Moderately well-differentiated Poorly differentiated Bronchoalveolar	Slow to moderate	Early and most frequently via lymphatics and blood vessels to brain, liver, bone, and adrenal glands	Form glandular structures in scar or fibrous tissue; single distal pulmonary nodule	• Stages I and II: resectable • Stage III: chemotherapy and radiotherapy • Stage IV: chemotherapy
	• Large-cell carcinoma • 5%–10% • Undifferentiated cells: Giant cell Clear cell	Rapid	Early and widespread to small intestine	Large, bulky necrotic masses in major or intermediate-sized bronchi or in periphery	• Stages I and II: resectable • Stage III: chemotherapy and radiotherapy • Stage IV: chemotherapy

to determine the patient's risk of developing lung cancer. Smoking history includes the age when smoking started, the average number of packs smoked per day, and the number of years smoked. The type of tobacco (cigar, cigarette, snuff, or chewing tobacco) used by the patient must also be determined. A positive family history of lung cancer may indicate that the patient is at a slightly higher risk of developing lung cancer. One study found a greater than two times higher likelihood of lung cancer in patients with a first-degree relative with lung cancer. A review of systems should reexamine all pertinent present and past symptoms that relate to the chief complaint and is needed to complete the health history.

Clinical manifestations of lung cancer depend on the location of the tumor and the extent of spread. Up to 25% of patients are asymptomatic at the time of diagnosis. However, if present, symptoms may be divided into four categories: intrathoracic or local–regional symptoms, nonspecific systemic symptoms, symptoms resulting from extrathoracic involvement, and paraneoplastic syndromes. Table 32.3 presents a summary of the clinical manifestations of lung cancer.

TABLE 32.3	Clinical Manifestations of Lung Cancer
Intrathoracic or local–regional manifestations	Cough Dyspnea Hemoptysis Wheezing Chest pain Stridor Hoarseness Vocal cord paralysis Hiccups Atelectasis Pneumonia Pancoast's syndrome Horner's syndrome Pleural effusion Pericardial effusion Superior vena cava syndrome
Nonspecific systemic manifestations	Weakness Fatigue Fever Anorexia Cachexia Anemia
Manifestations resulting from extrathoracic involvement	Bone pain Headache Dizziness Lymphadenopathy Central nervous system disturbances Gastrointestinal disturbances Jaundice Hepatomegaly Abdominal pain

Intrathoracic or Local–Regional Signs and Symptoms

The most common symptoms of local–regional disease are ambiguous and insidious; they include cough, sputum production, dyspnea, chest pain, hemoptysis, wheezing, postobstructive pneumonia, and pleural effusions. Cough resulting from bronchial irritation occurs in 60% of patients and often is attributed to a cold. The cough frequently goes away after a few days and returns intermittently. Cough may be produced by a small tumor acting as a foreign body or by ulceration of the bronchial mucosa. Severe paroxysms of coughing may lead to cough-induced rib fractures, rupture of an emphysematous bleb, or cough syncope. Cough and sputum production are not specific symptoms because the majority of lung cancer patients also have chronic bronchitis and emphysema due to cigarette smoking. However, a change in the character of the cough, a change in the quality and quantity of sputum, or unresponsiveness to previously effective therapy (e.g., bronchodilators, antibiotics, steroids) should raise the suspicion that a tumor is present.

Many patients with lung cancer experience dyspnea as a result of multiple disruptions in physiological function of the respiratory system. Dyspnea has been reported in 26% to 60% of patients presenting with NSCLC and is often an ominous development, signifying intrathoracic extension or dissemination. Some patients may have dyspnea resulting from underlying pulmonary disorders such as pulmonary fibrosis or chronic obstructive pulmonary disease (COPD). These patients may experience difficulties in airway clearance associated with excessive tracheobronchial secretions, thick tenacious secretions, muscle weakness, and chest pain. Central lung cancers cause dyspnea by means of obstruction, with or without postobstructive pneumonitis. Large pleural effusion or paralysis of the hemidiaphragm resulting from phrenic nerve involvement may also cause dyspnea. The assessment of dyspnea should include a description of the onset, duration, magnitude, and precipitating events. It is especially important to identify any interventions the patient has discovered that are helpful in relieving the dyspnea. Usually the chest radiograph in dyspneic patients demonstrates a sizable effusion, atelectasis of a lobe or entire lung, or clear evidence of intrapulmonary dissemination of the tumor.

Chest pain with deep inspiration or coughing may be reported, as well as fatigue and anorexia. Chest pain in lung cancer may indicate local invasion of the pleura, ribs, and nerves. Pain may be dull, constant, and debilitating or intermittent and sharp, varying with the respiratory cycle. It may localize to the chest wall, or it may radiate to the midback, scapula, shoulder, or arm on the side of the tumor. The pain is usually a dull intermittent ache lasting from minutes to hours on the same side as the tumor and is not related to cough or respiration. Intercostal retractions, supraclavicular retractions, and/or use of accessory muscles on inspiration indicate obstruction to air inflow, whereas bulging interspaces on expiration are associated with outflow obstruction; either may be indicative of a tumor. It is important to distinguish the chest pain that accompanies direct contiguous chest wall extension from painful rib metastases that are anatomically remote from the primary lesion.

Chest discomfort can be associated with atelectasis. Atelectasis develops in the patient with lung cancer secondary to mechanical obstruction of the airways, compression of lung tissue, and shallow breathing patterns. When the tumor obstructs the airway, it prevents or reduces alveolar ventilation to a region of the lung and produces atelectasis in that region. The size of the atelectatic area depends on the size of the obstructed airway and the degree of obstruction. Localized compression of lung tissue occurs with large tumors and with large pleural effusions secondary to metastases.

Hemoptysis is seen in up to 30% of patients and occurs when the tumor erodes the epithelial layer of the lung or invades a blood vessel. It occurs more often in squamous-cell carcinoma and large-cell carcinoma than in SCLC. Typically, hemoptysis consists only of blood-streaked sputum, which is sometimes erroneously attributed to chronic bronchitis. The quantity of blood is usually small, but it can become massive and life-threatening depending on the vessels affected. Hemoptysis usually prompts the patient to seek medical attention and is suggestive of an endobronchial tumor. Inspection seldom reveals any changes in the chest wall. Palpation may reveal lymph node enlargement.

Auscultation may reveal wheezing if an airway is partially obstructed. Wheezing is usually monophonic and localized and does not disappear after a cough. Wheezing may be heard on both inhalation and exhalation. Absent or decreased breath sounds can be heard when normal lung tissue is replaced by a tumor or when the patient has a pleural effusion. Percussion reveals diminished resonance over lung tissue affected by a large tumor, pleural effusion, or pneumonia (consolidation). Decreased tactile fremitus may be associated with pleural effusion and tumors of the pleural cavity, whereas increased tactile fremitus may indicate a lung mass.

The most frequent peripheral sign of lung cancer is clubbing of the fingers, which may be associated with generalized hypertrophic pulmonary osteoarthropathy (HPO), also known as Bamberger-Marie disease. HPO often resembles rheumatoid arthritis. The clinical syndrome consists of swelling of the soft tissues of the terminal phalanges, with curvature of the nails, pain and swelling of the joints, and periostitis of the long bones, with elevation of the periosteum and new bone formation. The incidence of HPO, which occurs almost exclusively in patients with NSCLC, has been reported from 2% to 12%. It occurs only rarely, if ever, in small-cell tumors. Its occurrence is distributed equally among the other three major cell types of NSCLC. Removal of the

pulmonary lesion may give dramatic remission of the arthralgia and peripheral edema.

Physical examination evidence for surgical nonresectability includes hoarseness, facial edema, arm pain, or changes in mental or emotional status. Hoarseness suggests vocal cord paralysis caused by recurrent laryngeal nerve compression by the tumor. Facial edema suggests compression of the superior vena cava by the tumor. Superior vena cava syndrome occurs when a lung tumor, usually SCLC, presses on the superior vena cava, partially or completely occluding it and impeding venous return from the head, neck, arms, and upper chest. Symptoms are related to venous obstruction, airway obstruction, and increased cerebral venous pressure. The most common symptoms include edema of the face, neck, arms, and upper torso. The conjunctiva may also be engorged. If the compression is untreated, neurologic symptoms related to increased intracranial pressure may ensue, including headache, dizziness, visual disturbances, and occasionally alterations in mental status. Associated upper airway obstruction or signs of cerebral edema are very poor prognostic signs.

Tumor compression of the cervical sympathetic nerve plexus causes Horner's syndrome, which consists of unilateral ptosis, miosis, and ipsilateral anhidrosis (lack of sweating due to extension of the tumor into the paravertebral sympathetic nerves). Horner's syndrome is often associated with radiographic evidence of destruction of the first and second ribs. Pancoast's syndrome, manifesting as arm and shoulder pain, suggests invasion of the brachial nerve plexus by a superior sulcus tumor. In addition, there may be muscular atrophy and decreased range of motion in the arm and shoulder; the patient may walk supporting the elbow of the affected arm.

Nonspecific Systemic Signs and Symptoms

Systemic symptoms of lung cancer include generalized weakness and fatigue, anorexia, cachexia, weight loss, and anemia. These nonspecific signs and symptoms are common in both SCLC and NSCLC. Weight loss, which is usually (but not always) accompanied by anorexia, occurs in more than one-half of patients, and generalized weakness occurs in one-third. Fever and anemia occur in about 20% of patients. Fever generally is not considered to be paraneoplastic in patients with lung cancer; if present, it usually is associated with a documented infection or liver metastases.

Signs and Symptoms Due to Extrathoracic Involvement

Extrathoracic metastatic spread most often occurs in the lymph nodes, brain, bones, liver, and suprarenal glands. Bone pain caused by metastasis occurs in approximately 25% to 40% of patients, although pathological fractures are rare. Neurologic symptoms resulting from intracranial metastases are present in 3% to 6% of patients. These include hemiplegia, epilepsy, personality changes, confusion, speech defects, gait disturbances, or only nonspecific headache. Symptoms that relate to liver involvement (right upper quadrant pain) are less common or nonspecific (e.g., nausea, weight loss, anemia). Rarely, jaundice, ascites, or an abdominal mass is the major complaint. Neck, muscle, or subcutaneous tissue masses are present infrequently. Involvement of adrenal glands often is asymptomatic, and most adrenal metastases are discovered incidentally, either during staging evaluation or at autopsy. If symptomatic, adrenal involvement presents with unilateral pain in the flank, abdomen, or costovertebral angle. Although adrenal metastases are fairly common, signs of adrenal insufficiency are rarely seen.

Paraneoplastic Syndromes

Associated with lung cancer are approximately 21 identified syndromes that meet the usual definition of the term "paraneoplastic" (Table 32.4). Approximately 2% of patients with lung cancer seek medical advice for systemic symptoms and signs of these paraneoplastic

syndromes. The major categories of paraneoplastic syndromes include endocrine, neurologic, cardiovascular, skeletal, and cutaneous manifestations.

Paraneoplastic syndromes are often the first indication of the presence of a tumor and may antedate identification of a clinically demonstrable tumor by a period ranging from months to years. SCLC is associated with paraneoplastic syndromes more frequently than the NSCLC. Most metabolic manifestations are the result of secretion of endocrine or endocrine-like substances by the tumor.

Hyperadrenocorticism, in association with ectopic secretion of adrenocorticotropic hormone, is a frequently observed hormonal syndrome in lung cancer, particularly in SCLC patients. It manifests as severe weakness, weight loss, edema, hypertension, hypokalemia, and hyperglycemia. The syndrome of inappropriate antidiuretic hormone secretion occurs in 5% to 10% of patients with SCLCs. It results from antidiuretic hormone secretion by the tumor and is associated with symptoms of water intoxication (e.g., anorexia, nausea, vomiting). Symptoms include hyponatremia and low serum osmolality, characterized by mental status changes, lethargy, seizures, and confusion. Hyponatremia resulting from the secretion of atrial natriuretic factor can also occur in some patients.

Hypercalcemia may be caused by bony metastases or excessive tumor secretion of parathyroid hormone–related protein, the so-called humoral hypercalcemia of malignancy. Although squamous-cell carcinoma is most commonly associated with hypercalcemia, other histological types can cause the syndrome as well. An accompanying hypophosphatemia is also frequently found. Clinically, the hypercalcemic patient may have somnolence, irritability, confusion, or coma, as well as anorexia, nausea, vomiting, constipation, and weight loss.

Eaton-Lambert myasthenic syndrome occurs in about 6% of patients with SCLC. This pseudomyasthenic syndrome is thought to be an autoimmune disorder in which the release of acetylcholine by the motor nerve terminals is impaired. Symptoms include proximal muscle weakness (especially in the pelvis, thighs, arms, and shoulders) and fatigue, peripheral paresthesia, dry mouth, dysphagia, diplopia, ptosis, difficulty chewing, and double vision.

DIAGNOSTIC REASONING

Early detection is the key to successful resection of NSCLC tumors, but mass screening programs have failed to affect mortality rates. The histological cell type and the stage of the disease are the major factors that influence choice of therapy for individuals. The currently accepted system for the staging of lung cancer is the tumor-node-metastasis (TNM) classification presented in Table 32.5. In this system, T denotes the extent of the primary tumor

TABLE 32.4 Paraneoplastic Syndromes Associated With Lung Cancer	
Type of Cancer	**Associated Paraneoplastic Syndrome**
Small-cell lung carcinoma	• Ectopic adrenocorticotropic hormone (Cushing's syndrome) • Inappropriate antidiuretic hormone secretion • Lambert-Eaton myasthenic syndrome • Atrial natriuretic factor • Hyperpigmentation
• Non–small-cell lung carcinomas	• Humoral hypercalcemia • Hypertrophic pulmonary osteoarthropathy • Nephrotic syndrome • Hypoglycemia • Gynecomastia • Nonbacterial thrombotic endocarditis
• All lung cancers	• Hypercoagulable state • Disseminated intravascular coagulation • Erythrocytosis • Granulocytosis • Neurologic and myopathic syndromes (dementia, limbic encephalitis, optic neuropathy, sensory neuropathy, sensorimotor peripheral neuropathy) • Dermatological syndromes (acanthosis nigricans, acquired ichthyosis, dermatomyositis)

TABLE 32.5 Lung Cancer Staging

Tumor-Node-Metastasis (TNM) Stage Grouping for Lung Cancer

Occult cancer	TX N0 M0
Stage 0	Tis N0 M0
Stage I	T1 N0 M0; T2 N0 M0
Stage II	T1 N1 M0; T2 N1 M0
Stage IIIA	T1 N2 M0; T2 N2 M0; T3 N0 M0; T3 N1 M0; T3 N2 M0
Stage IIIB	Any T N3 M0; T4 Any N M0
Stage IV	Any T Any N M1

TNM Definitions of Primary Tumor (T) Characteristics in Lung Cancer

Primary (T)	
TX	Primary tumor cannot be assessed or tumor proven by the presence of malignant cells in sputum or bronchial washings but not visualized by imaging or bronchoscopy
T0	No evidence of primary tumor
Tis	Carcinoma in situ
T1	A tumor that is 3.0 cm or less in greatest diameter, surrounded by lung or visceral pleura and without evidence of invasion more proximal than the lobar bronchus (e.g., not in the main bronchus) (*Note:* Uncommon superficial tumor of any size with invasive component limited to the bronchial wall, which may extend proximal to the main bronchus, is also classified as T1.)
T1a	Tumor of 2 cm or less in greatest dimension
T1b	Tumor more than 2 cm but less than 3 cm in greatest dimension
T2	A tumor with any of the following features of size or extent: more than 3.0 cm in greatest dimension; involving the main bronchus, 2.0 cm or more distal to the carina; invading the visceral pleura; associated with atelectasis or obstructive pneumonitis that extends to the hilar region but does not involve the entire lung
T2a	Tumor more than 3 cm but less than 5 cm in greatest dimension
T2b	Tumor more than 5 cm but less than 7 cm in greatest dimension
T3	Tumor of any size with direct extension to the chest wall (including superior sulcus tumors), diaphragm, mediastinal pleura, parietal pericardium; tumor in the main bronchus less than 2.0 cm distal to the carina but without involvement of the carina; associated atelectasis or obstructive pneumonitis of the entire lung
T4	Tumor of any size that invades any of the following: mediastinum, heart, great vessels, trachea, esophagus, vertebral body, carina; or tumor with a malignant pleural effusion
Regional Lymph Nodes (N)	
NX	Regional lymph nodes cannot be assessed
N0	No regional lymph node metastasis
N1	Metastasis in ipsilateral peribronchial and/or ipsilateral hilar lymph nodes, including direct extension
N2	Metastasis in ipsilateral mediastinal and/or subcarinal lymph node(s)
N3	Metastasis in contralateral mediastinal, contralateral hilar, ipsilateral or contralateral scalene, or supra-clavicular lymph node(s)
Distant Metastasis (M)	
M0	No (known) distant metastasis
M1	Distant metastases present; specify sites
M1a	Separate tumor nodule(s) in a contralateral lobe, tumor with pleural nodules or malignant pleural (or pericardial) effusion
M1b	Distant metastasis (in extrathoracic organs)

Note. Most pleural effusions associated with lung cancer are due to tumor; however, there are a few patients in whom multiple cytopathological examinations of pleural fluid are negative for tumor. In these cases, fluid is nonbloody and is not exudative. When these elements and clinical judgment dictate that the effusion is unrelated to the tumor, the effusion should be excluded as a staging element and the patient should be staged as T1, T2, or T3.

Used with the permission of the American College of Surgeons. The original source for this material is the AJCC Cancer Staging Manual, Eighth Edition (2017) published by Springer International Publishing AG.

(ranging from T0 to T4), N indicates the nodal involvement (ranging from N0 to N3), and M describes the extent of metastasis (M0 or M1). The stage of disease is based on a combination of clinical (physical examination, radiological, and laboratory studies) and pathological (biopsy of lymph nodes, bronchoscopy, mediastinoscopy, paramedian sternotomy, or other type of thoracotomy) factors.

The diagnostic approach for SCLC is the same as that for NSCLC, but the staging system is different. SCLC staging also focuses on disease extent but broadly classifies it as limited state (limited to one hemothorax with hilar and mediastinal nodes that can be included within a radiation therapy port) or extensive stage disease. The TNM staging system is not typically used for SCLC staging.

Diagnostic Tests

Initial Testing

A complete blood count (CBC) should be ordered because anemia may be associated with lung cancer, along with a basic metabolic panel and hepatic panel to check for abnormalities in Na, K, Ca, and liver enzymes, and a prothrombin time, partial thromboplastin time, and platelet count to assess for coagulopathies. An electrocardiogram should be done, as well as baseline pulmonary function tests.

Anterior-posterior and lateral chest x-ray films remain the simplest method for identifying patients with lung cancer. The heart and other thoracic structures obscure large portions of the lung tissue, so it is important to evaluate both a frontal and a side view. The chest x-ray film may demonstrate asymptomatic lung cancer and is almost always abnormal when the patient is symptomatic. A tumor nodule must be at least 2 to 3 mm before it is visible on the chest radiograph. Associated atelectasis, postobstructive pneumonitis, abscess, bronchiolitis, rib erosion, pleural effusion, or bulky mediastinal lymphadenopathy may be identified on radiographs, thus raising a suspicion of primary lung malignancy. The four most common types of lung cancer usually present with slightly different chest radiographic patterns, but there is so much overlap that only biopsy and histological examination provide reliable evidence of the cell type. Mediastinal changes on radiograph may suggest lymphadenopathy or pleural effusions, and an elevated diaphragm may be seen with phrenic nerve involvement.

A chest computed tomography (CT) scan with infusion of contrast material has become widely accepted as the primary cross-sectional imaging modality for evaluation of the thorax and is recommended to stage NSCLC. The CT scan should extend inferiorly to include the liver and the adrenal glands. Because of its earlier metastases and typical unresectability, staging for SCLC is less useful for treatment and prognosis. A contrast-enhanced chest CT scan will (1) characterize the size and location of the primary tumor and its relationship to other thoracic structures, (2) identify pathologically enlarged hilar and mediastinal lymph nodes, (3) identify satellite and other ipsilateral or contralateral pulmonary nodules, and (4) identify potential metastases to the liver and adrenal glands, both being common metastatic sites.

Cytological evaluation of sputum, bronchial washing, bronchial brushings, and fine-needle aspirations have a high diagnostic value, but the positive and negative predictive values of each, as well as their accuracy of diagnosis, depend on sampling error, tissue preservation, processing quality, and observer experience. Sputum cytology remains a simple test with a positive predictive value that can approach 100%, but it has a sensitivity rate of only 10% to 15%. If a diagnosis can be established through collective sputum cytology, invasive tests can often be averted. Automated sputum screening may play an increasingly important role in early diagnosis. The highest yield occurs in patients with large, centrally located tumors. It is much less helpful in diagnosing peripheral lesions because relatively few cells are released from the lesion, and those that are released rarely get to the central airways. Early morning sputum samples are collected for 3 to 5 days; deep coughing is recommended because coughing dislodges cancer cells into the sputum.

Flexible fiber-optic bronchoscopy is an essential and standard technique for the evaluation of patients with pulmonary neoplasms. It remains the most important procedure for determining the endobronchial extent of disease. The extent and operability of the tumor are assessed by observing the site of the tumor and extent of airway involvement. When lesions are visible endobronchially, bronchial washings have a diagnostic yield of approximately 90%; bronchial brushings and bronchial mucosal forceps biopsy samples provide a tissue diagnosis in nearly 98% of visualized tumors. Fluoroscopy is used to guide these sampling procedures. Transbronchial forceps biopsies, brushings, and washings can diagnose peripheral, parenchymal lesions up to 80% of the time. The visual assessment of the primary tumor can also provide a clinically useful estimate of the probability of tumor complications such as airway obstruction, postobstructive pneumonia, or hemoptysis.

Transthoracic percutaneous fine-needle aspiration (fine-needle aspiration biopsy) is used when lung lesions cannot be visualized by bronchoscopy but are accessible percutaneously. A needle guided by CT or fluoroscopy is inserted into the lesion for aspiration of cells. This procedure is most suitable for peripheral pulmonary nodules. Pneumothorax is the most common complication, with an increased risk in patients with COPD. A positive pleural fluid cytology proves the spread of malignancy to the pleural space. Thoracentesis and pleural biopsy combined provide up to a 90% diagnostic yield in patients with malignancy.

Mediastinoscopy is an invasive procedure used for the diagnosis and staging of lung cancer. A biopsy is recommended if mediastinal lymph nodes are found on chest

CT scan that are greater than 1.0 cm in size for the patient with clinically operable NSCLC. The patient with lymphadenopathy on chest CT scan will most likely have positive nodes on biopsy. Anterior cervical mediastinoscopy allows direct visualization and biopsy of mediastinal nodes with less risk than an exploratory thoracotomy.

Video-assisted thoracoscopic surgery is used for the staging and diagnosis of lung cancer when less invasive techniques fail to yield a diagnosis. Small thoracotomy incisions are made through which thoracoscopic instruments are inserted. Visualization of the chest and mediastinum and assessment of pleural effusions are superior to that achieved using older scopes, which may help improve diagnostic accuracy.

Thoracoscopy is useful for pleural evaluation but less useful for evaluating the inner segments of the lung. It is more than 90% sensitive for the diagnosis of pleural-based malignancies and peripheral lung nodules, with a specificity of 99%. With a thoracoscope, the mediastinum can be entered and nodes biopsied. Thoracoscopy affords the potential for more complete staging of patients with suspected mediastinal nodal spread, and it has become a valuable adjunct to cervical mediastinoscopy and anterior mediastinotomy. There is a concern, however, about seeding the thoracoscope entrance site with tumor cells.

Subsequent Testing

A head CT scan or brain magnetic resonance imaging, with and without infusion of contrast material, is recommended only in patients who have signs or symptoms of central nervous system disease. The finding of an isolated adrenal mass on ultrasonographic or CT examination requires biopsy to rule out metastatic disease, if the patient's tumor is considered to be potentially resectable. NSCLC metastasizes to the adrenal glands in 18% to 38% of cases. A bone scan should be performed only in patients who complain of bone pain or chest pain or who have elevated serum calcium serum alkaline phosphatase levels. It is estimated that between 9% and 15% of patients with newly diagnosed NSCLC have bony metastases at presentation, with the vertebral bodies most commonly affected. Finally, the finding of an isolated hepatic mass on ultrasonographic or CT examination requires a biopsy to rule out metastatic disease if the patient's tumor is otherwise considered to be potentially resectable.

Differential Diagnosis

The symptoms of lung cancer develop gradually in most cases and are often attributed by the patient to a smoker's cough or cold and by the patient's health-care provider to tracheobronchitis, pneumonia, influenza, pulmonary infarction, or lung abscess. Thus, it is common for a patient to delay seeking medical attention for several months from the first recognizable onset of symptoms. Several additional months of symptomatic treatment and antibiotic courses frequently pass before the health-care provider establishes the correct diagnosis. Much of the initial diagnostic task is to differentiate between a primary tumor and metastatic cancer, which is evaluated on biopsy. Other differential diagnoses include tuberculosis, lymphoma, *Mycobacterium avium* complex, sarcoidosis, or a foreign body aspiration that has been retained.

MANAGEMENT

The U.S. Preventive Services Task Force recommends annual screening for lung cancer with low-dose computed tomography in adults aged 55 to 80 years who have a 30 pack-year smoking history and currently smoke or have quit within the past 15 years. Screening should be discontinued once a person has not smoked for 15 years or develops a health problem that substantially limits life expectancy or the ability or willingness to have curative lung surgery.

Active patient participation in decision making respects the fundamental ethical and legal doctrine of autonomy and is especially important for the patient with unresectable NSCLC because the prognosis is often poor and symptom palliation is a central concern. Fewer than one-half of patients with lung cancer are candidates for resection, and only a small percentage of these are cured, so most patients with the disease require some form of palliation. Therapy should include efforts to slow the growth of the tumor and to treat complications as they arise, but above all, symptoms should be relieved.

Surgery

Surgical resection offers the best chance of cure for lung cancer. Stage I or II NSCLC is routinely resected via thoracotomy. Pneumonectomy (removal of a whole lung) and lobectomy (removal of a single lobe) are the most common of these surgical procedures. The nature of the tumor dictates the procedure, whereas pulmonary function determines if the patient can withstand the procedure. Pneumonectomy is required when a lung-conserving operation will not allow for complete resection, such as cases in which the tumor involves proximal structures or lymph nodes are affected. Lobectomy is the most common resection performed for lung cancer. This type of resection allows removal of the primary tumor, associated disease, and lymph node–bearing areas while leaving a significant amount of residual functional parenchyma. Survival is equivalent for patients undergoing lobectomy or pneumonectomy for all stages of disease when a complete resection is performed. For lesions close to the lobar orifice, an adequate margin of resection often cannot be achieved. In such circumstances, a portion of the main bronchus must be included with the resection. This type of resection is termed "sleeve resection," and it is performed as a parenchyma-sparing procedure, avoiding pneumonectomy.

Very limited resection in the treatment of lung cancer is reserved for patients with extremely poor lung function who can tolerate no more than minor resection because of their underlying medical condition or low pulmonary reserve. Limited resections include segmentectomy, wedge resection, or lumpectomy. Segmental resection is the removal of a lung segment, and wedge resection is the removal of a small, V-shaped wedge of lung tissue. Lesions that reside more deeply within the pulmonary tissue often are not amenable to wedge resection and may require precise, local excision with laser or electrocautery assistance (e.g., lumpectomy). These techniques are used to preserve as much lung tissue as possible, and they are performed for the removal of small tumors located close to the surface of the lung. The guiding principle of surgical therapy in lung cancer is to remove the tumor completely, leaving as much functional pulmonary tissue as possible. The aim of most operations is curative, and procedures that leave gross tumor are not warranted. Resection is abandoned if the tumor extends beyond the lung, when pleural seeding is evident, or when fixed mediastinal nodes are present.

Patients with Stage I disease have a 50% to 80% 5-year survival, and patients with Stage II disease have a 25% to 50% survival at 5 years. However, 75% of patients present with advanced disease and significant comorbidities. Treatment decisions should thus consider symptom control, quality of life, the patient's value or meaning of life, and the patient's perceptions and attitudes about a specific treatment.

Chemotherapy

Neoadjuvant chemotherapy involves giving antineoplastic drugs *before* surgery or radiation therapy. Adjuvant chemotherapy involves administering antineoplastic drugs *after* surgery or radiation therapy. Given that chemotherapy for advanced disease is marginally beneficial and noncurative, its use must be governed judiciously, with each treatment decision evaluated individually for each patient.

Current chemotherapeutic approaches consist initially of defining new combinations of established chemotherapeutic agents that may act synergistically. In addition, new drugs with novel mechanisms of action are also being investigated, both as single agents and, subsequently, as agents to be used in combination with established drugs. Drug developers have initiated many new studies, and it is predicted that eventually 30% of all chemotherapy drugs will be oral agents. Newer biologic immunotherapeutic agents are also being developed, such as the PD-1 (programmed cell death 1) inhibitor pembrolizumab (Keytruda), which was the first agent approved by the U.S. Food and Drug Administration for unresectable or metastatic solid tumors with certain genetic specifications, but without regard to tissue type or location. Standard chemotherapy consists of cisplatin or carboplatin along with pemetrexed, paclitaxel, or docetaxel. Bevacizumab (Avastin), an angiogenesis inhibitor, blocks the activity of vascular endothelial growth factor A is another option in some cases. Details on the use of these medications are beyond the scope of this text because referral to an oncologist is required to direct any chemotherapeutic regimens.

Non–Small-Cell Lung Cancer Chemotherapy

Chemotherapy modestly improves median survival with distant metastatic NSCLC compared with best supportive care, but it is not curative.

If a patient has Stage I disease, there is no agreement on the role of adjuvant chemotherapy. It is more widely used with patients with Stage II and IIIA disease. Patients with Stage I and N0 Stage II disease treated with multidrug platinum-based chemotherapy show improved survival of 3 months at 5 years. Because of the toxicity, risks versus benefits must be discussed with the patient and family. Newer drugs with less toxicity are currently being studied. With patients in advanced stages of disease, chemotherapy has shown to improve patients' quality of life by decreasing bothersome symptoms. For patients with Stage III lung cancer that cannot be removed surgically, chemotherapy is typically combined with definitive high-dose radiation treatments. In Stage IV lung cancer, chemotherapy is typically the main treatment, because radiation is used only for palliation of symptoms.

The newest developments in lung cancer treatment are targeted treatments. Whereas chemotherapy drugs cannot differentiate between normal cells and cancer cells, targeted therapies are designed specifically to attack cancer cells by attaching to or blocking targets that appear on cancer cell surfaces. Patients with advanced lung cancer with certain molecular biomarkers may receive treatment with a targeted drug alone or in combination with chemotherapy.

Small-Cell Lung Cancer Chemotherapy

Combination chemotherapy is capable of effecting high objective response rates in patients with SCLC. Furthermore, the simultaneous administration of multiple agents is superior to the sequential administration of the same drugs. Chemotherapy is most effective in SCLC with an 80% to 100% response in limited-stage disease (50–t0% complete response) and 60% to 80% response in extensive stage disease (15% to 40% complete response). Remissions last a median of 6 to 8 months. If the cancer recurs, the median survival time is 3 to 4 months.

Radiation

The basic indication for radiation therapy is inoperability; in addition, it is sometimes used as prophylactic cranial irradiation to help prevent metastasis to the brain. Radiation therapy can modify the natural course of the disease, relieve distressing symptoms, and produce an apparent cure in an occasional patient. Long-term results, however, have been generally disappointing. One-year and 5-year overall survival rates range from 25% to 55% and from 4% to 10%, respectively. Radiation is used as adjunctive therapy after surgery to improve tumor control, and it is used as palliative therapy to control symptoms in other cases.

Non–Small-Cell Lung Cancer Radiation

Radiation therapy is commonly offered to patients with inoperable NSCLC when the cancer has not spread beyond the thorax. In this case, the asymptomatic patient or the patient who is still functioning at a high level is most likely to benefit. In addition, radiation therapy is used to shrink the tumor and control symptoms in the patient with inoperable lung cancer and to prevent brain metastasis. Treating the tumor with radiation therapy may relieve hemoptysis, shoulder and arm pain, chest pain, and dyspnea. It can be used in superior vena cava obstruction to reduce the tumor size and alleviate obstruction. Although there are currently no data that demonstrate a survival advantage for postoperative adjuvant therapy in patients with completely resected Stage II disease, regardless of whether the patient receives radiation therapy alone or radiation therapy and chemotherapy, most of these patients are treated with postoperative radiation therapy to decrease local recurrence. Unfortunately, prevention of local recurrence has not been shown to translate into a survival benefit. The patient with a malignant pleural effusion or with distant metastatic disease is not appropriate for definitive thoracic radiotherapy.

Small-Cell Lung Cancer Radiation

SCLC is quite sensitive to both radiation and chemotherapy. In limited-stage SCLC, the addition of both radiation and chemotherapy can increase the 5-year survival rate from about 11% to 20%. Most oncologists consider thoracic radiation therapy in combination with chemotherapy for limited-stage disease to be the standard of care. The major contribution of thoracic irradiation is local tumor control, and local control of the intrathoracic tumor is a sine qua non for cure. Thoracic radiation therapy does reduce the risk of dying of SCLC but at the price of increased toxicity. Concurrent or alternating treatment schedules appear to improve response rates over sequential chemotherapy and radiation therapy, although toxicity is more intense with concurrent therapy. A summary of the treatment of NSCLC is shown in Figure 32.1.

FOLLOW-UP AND REFERRAL

When lung cancer is first detected, the patient should be referred to a specialist for staging and treatment decisions. The patient who has been successfully treated for lung cancer needs to be followed routinely. The goal of monitoring patients with unresectable lung cancer in complete remission is to detect symptomatic progression of their disease that may benefit from therapeutic intervention or symptom management. However, the great majority of patients with unresectable Stage III and Stage IV disease will not achieve a complete remission, or, if achieved, the duration of remission will be short.

A history and physical examination should be performed every 3 months during the first 2 years, every 6 months thereafter through year 5, and yearly thereafter. For the patient treated with curative intent, there is no clear role for routine x-ray evaluation in the asymptomatic patient and for those in whom no interventions are planned. A yearly chest x-ray film to evaluate for potentially curable second primary cancers may be reasonable. CT of the chest/abdomen, bronchoscopy, CBC, and routine chemistries, including liver function tests, should be performed only as indicated by the patient's symptoms because these tests do not appear to detect asymptomatic recurrent disease with a high frequency.

Patient Education: Lung Cancer

Assessment of learning needs and provision of information is likely to be of paramount importance for the patient at the time of initial biopsy, between diagnosis and definitive treatment, and at discharge. These are highly stressful times for patients, and they may be easily overwhelmed by the information regarding treatment options. It is important to assess what level of participation in the decision-making process is desired by the patient because that will help direct informational interventions and can reduce anxiety and psychological distress. This is particularly important for patients who have a choice between two treatment options or are deciding between participating in a clinical trial or receiving standard therapy.

Smoking cessation, never initiating smoking, and avoidance of occupational and environmental exposure to carcinogenic substances are recommended as effective interventions to reduce the risk of a second primary lung cancer in the curatively treated patient. For the patient with distant metastatic disease, the outlook is poor, and smoking cessation has little effect on overall prognosis but may improve respiratory symptoms. A tapering nicotine patch or other delivery system has been proven to increase the odds of smoking cessation when combined with behavioral interventions.

Additionally, patients with lung cancer who have never smoked may suffer from the stigma of lung cancer that is self-induced, whether accurate or not. These patients are likely to suffer from anxiety, depression, and social isolation, all of which call for increased support.

Recommendations for lifestyle modifications are the same for the patient with a history of lung cancer as for those who have no previous history of lung cancer. Epidemiological studies also suggest that people who consume relatively large amounts of fruits and vegetables have a lower risk of both cancer and cardiovascular disease. Antioxidant vitamins

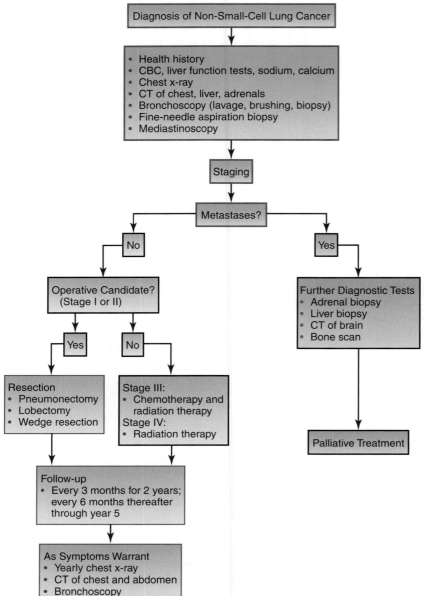

Figure 32.1 Treatment flowchart: non–small-cell lung cancer.

contained in fruits and vegetables prevent carcinogenesis by interfering with oxidative damage to DNA and lipoproteins; however, the use of antioxidants and/or chemopreventive agents for lung cancer (retinoic acid, beta-carotene, and selenium) is investigational.

When medical care for the patient with lung cancer shifts from curative to palliative, the patient and family must choose a care setting. Home or hospice care can provide familiar surroundings, feelings of normalcy, involvement of family, and a more comforting situation as they participate in readiness for the dying process. Although hospice has proved to be an extremely effective model for terminal care, referrals to hospice care are often not made until the final days of life.

The difficulty lies in predicting when death will occur because Medicare reimbursement requires that a hospice patient has a life expectancy of 6 months or less. Many states now have an "open access" model that allows for patients seeking curative care to still receive hospice services. Supportive resources for self-care should be provided as required by the individual situation. Patients will be able to manage less self-care as the disease progresses, and family members will require education with demonstration of care techniques and opportunities for questions and verbalization of feelings about caring for the one who is ill. Within the *Circle of Caring* model, collaborative planning is essential in helping the patient and family make informed choices and live in the moment.

REFERENCES

American Lung Association. Lung cancer fact sheet. http://www.lung.org/lung-health-and-diseases/lung-disease-lookup/lung-cancer/resource-library/lung-cancer-fact-sheet.html?referrer. Published 2016. Accessed July 8, 2017.

Office of Disease Prevention and Health Promotion. Cancer objective to reduce the lung cancer death rate. *Healthy People 2020.* https://www.healthypeople.gov/2020/data-search/Search-the-Data#objid=4061. Accessed May 28, 2017.

Sherry V. Lung cancer: Not just a smoker's disease. *Am Nurse Today.* 2017;12(2):16–20.

Thompson N, Christian A. Oral chemotherapy: Not just an ordinary pill. *Am Nurse Today.* 2016;11(9):16–20.

RESOURCE

American Cancer Society
www.cancer.org

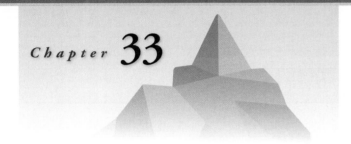

Chapter **33**

Smoking Addiction

Jill E. Winland-Brown, EdD, APRN, FNP-BC

Brian Oscar Porter, MD, PhD, MPH, MBA

A pack-a-day smoker takes more than 70,000 cigarette puffs per year. Each puff delivers various chemicals into the lungs and bloodstream, including nicotine, an addictive substance. The act of smoking reinforces cigarette addiction by establishing secondary reinforcers, such as the sight and smell of cigarettes, the lighting procedure, and association of cigarette smoking with a meal, a cup of coffee, or an alcoholic drink. Nicotine addiction fulfills all the criteria of a drug addiction: compulsive use, psychoactive effects, withdrawal symptoms, and drug-reinforcing behavior. Tolerance and physical dependence, manifested by an abstinence-mediated withdrawal syndrome, contribute to the strong control exerted by nicotine on smoking behavior. Although nicotine is the most likely reinforcing agent in tobacco, there are other possibilities, including tar and carbon monoxide (CO).

Tobacco use is the leading preventable cause of disease, disability, and death in the United States, particularly from cardiovascular disease, cancer, and lung disease. Table 33.1 lists the effects of cigarette smoke on the cardiovascular and respiratory systems. Cigarettes are responsible for one in every five deaths in the United States. In addition, 8.6 million people have a serious illness caused by smoking. For every person who dies from smoking, 20 more have at least one serious tobacco-related illness.

Besides the premature loss of life and the reduction in quality of life of smokers, billions of dollars in medical expenses per year can be directly attributed to cigarette smoking. These statistics are even more alarming when it is recognized that more than 50 years have passed since publication of the landmark U.S. Surgeon General's 1964 Report, "The Health Consequences of Smoking." Clinicians must do more to help patients refrain from or stop smoking. One of the objectives of *Healthy People 2020* is to decrease the percentage of adults of current smokers aged 18 years and older to 12%. The Centers for Disease Control and Prevention reports that in 2015, 36.5 million American adults (15.1%) were current cigarette smokers. It is hoped that this will eventually decrease to less than 12%, given the available modalities to assist patients with smoking cessation.

There are also significant hazards for nonsmokers who breathe the smoke of others' cigarettes (passive smoking or environmental tobacco smoke [ETS]). ETS is defined as a combination of the smoke emitted by a burning cigarette, cigar, or pipe and the smoke exhaled by smokers. Passive smoking is associated with a modestly increased risk of lung cancers and possibly other cancers and has been classified by the Environmental Protection Agency as a known human carcinogen. Exposure to ETS causes about 3,000 deaths from lung cancer per year in nonsmoking U.S. adults and damages the respiratory health of hundreds of thousands of children who live in homes with a parent who smokes cigarettes. It is estimated that between 150,000 and 300,000 cases of respiratory illness occurring in infants and children up to 18 months of age may be associated with exposure to ETS, which increases the risk of lower respiratory tract infections.

EPIDEMIOLOGY AND CAUSES

Substantial gains have been made in reducing smoking prevalence in the United States, although at present, almost one in five Americans still smoke. Notably, 90%

TABLE 33.1 Diseases Associated With Cigarette Smoking

Body System	*Disease or Condition*
Cardiovascular	• Atherosclerotic cardiovascular disease (CAD; carotid vascular disease; mesenteric, renal, iliac disease; abdominal aortic aneurysm) • Coronary artery spasm • Arrhythmias • Peripheral vascular diseases (thromboangiitis obliterans, deep vein thrombosis, pulmonary embolus)
Endocrine	• Altered hormonal secretion • Graves' disease • Antidiuresis • Goiter
Gastrointestinal	• Peptic ulcer disease (gastric, duodenal) • Gastroesophageal reflux disease • Chronic pancreatitis • Crohn's disease • Colonic adenomas
Genitourinary	• Glomerulonephritis • Benign prostatic hypertrophy
Rheumatologic/ musculoskeletal	• Rheumatoid arthritis • Osteoporosis
Infectious	• Tuberculosis • Pneumococcal infection • Meningococcal infection
Integumentary	• Skin wrinkling • Psoriasis
Malignancies	• Respiratory tract malignancies • Lung cancer (squamous cell, adenocarcinoma, large cell, small cell) • Laryngeal cancer • Oral cancer • Other cancers (esophageal, pancreatic, bladder, uterine, cervical, breast, renal, anal, penile, gastric, hepatic, leukemia)
Pediatric	• Effects on children of parental smoking (asthma, rhinitis, otitis, pneumonia, increased risk for child to begin smoking)
Psychiatric	• Depression • Schizophrenia
Reproductive	• Premature ovarian failure • Decreased sperm quality • Pregnancy-related diseases (prematurity, premature rupture of membranes, spontaneous abortion) • Fetal-/infant-related diseases (low birth weight, impaired lung growth, sudden infant death syndrome, febrile seizures, reduced intelligence, behavioral disorders, atopic diseases, asthma)
Respiratory	• Chronic obstructive pulmonary disorder • Asthma • Eosinophilic granuloma of the lung • Respiratory bronchiolitis • Goodpasture's syndrome • Sleep apnea • Pneumothorax
Sensory/head and neck	• Loss of olfaction • Loss of taste • Cataracts • Periodontal disease

of smokers start smoking before age 18 years. More than 430,000 deaths per year in the United States are attributed to tobacco use. At the current smoking rate, an estimated 5 million persons younger than 18 years will die prematurely from a disease related to smoking. At a cost of $50 billion per year in medical expenses, this problem is epidemic in proportion. The initiation of smoking by adolescents in middle school is now of great concern, and smoking has also become an important issue in women's health. Despite widespread public education about the health risks of smoking, women continue to start smoking, which persists at high rates.

Although the reduction in overall smoking prevalence represents a major victory for public health, there are several groups within the U.S. population that continue to smoke at disproportionately high rates. These groups have been less likely to experience the benefits of tobacco control efforts. For example, low socioeconomic status and low educational attainment are now the primary predictors of smoking status in the United States and Canada.

Unlike cigarette smoking, some forms of smokeless tobacco use (plug, leaf, and snuff) have actually increased. One of these forms is "dipping snuff," which involves placement of a coarse, moist tobacco powder between the cheek and gum that results in the direct absorption of nicotine and other carcinogens through the oral tissue. Oral cancer occurs more frequently among snuff dippers, as well as among pipe and cigar smokers, compared with nonusers of tobacco.

With the advent of electronic cigarettes (e-cigarettes) many concerns arise. The U.S. Food and Drug Administration is concerned about these products for the following reasons:

- They may increase nicotine addiction and may lead adolescents to smoke conventional cigarettes.
- E-cigarettes contain known toxins.
- Sufficient clinical studies have not been conducted regarding their safety.
- The use of tobacco products is a complex, learned behavior that is woven into the fiber of daily life and is linked to how the smoker deals with the world. Numerous daily activities, thoughts, and emotions serve as powerful cues to smoke. Such conditioned responses become paired with the positive neuroregulatory effects of nicotine to reinforce the addictive process. Personal characteristics, such as education level, belief in one's ability to change, and coping skills, are determinants of tobacco use. Similarly, environmental factors, such as the level of acceptance of smoking in the home, peer group, workplace, and community norms, influence smoking behavior.
- The tobacco industry's drive for profits is the root cause of why cigarette smoking continues to thrive in the United States, despite irrefutable evidence that it is a health hazard and a form of drug addiction. Millions

of dollars are spent every day on tobacco advertising. The estimated 3,450 children and youths who initiate smoking and become regular tobacco users each day ensure an enduring supply of adult smokers. Legislative initiatives to control cigarette smoking in the United States have gained significant ground in some states, such as California, but from a public health perspective are not as stringent as they should be nationally. Moreover, bans on smoking in the workplace and in restaurants have done little to discourage smokers from smoking in other private venues.

PATHOPHYSIOLOGY

When a cigarette is smoked, approximately 4,000 chemicals and gases are inhaled into the lungs. Many carcinogens have been isolated from cigarette smoke; 3,4-benzpyrene is the most dangerous. At least 43 other components have been identified as carcinogens, cocarcinogens, tumor promoters, tumor initiators, and mutagens. The primary active (and addictive) ingredient in tobacco is nicotine. In its purest state, nicotine is an extremely toxic, clear, oily liquid with a characteristic odor. At low doses, it acts as a stimulant; at high doses, it depresses the central nervous system (CNS).

Nicotine enters the body through a variety of routes. Inhalation of smoke from a cigar, cigarette, or pipe is perhaps the most common route. With cigarettes, some absorption of nicotine occurs through the membranes of the mouth, throat, and bronchi, as well as the alveoli of the lungs. With snuff and chewing tobacco, nicotine reaches the bloodstream by absorption through the mucosal linings of the mouth, nose, and throat.

Inhalation is the quickest and most effective delivery method of nicotine. It is estimated that 90% of the nicotine that reaches the alveoli of the lungs in each breath is absorbed into the bloodstream. Although an average cigarette contains 15 to 20 mg of nicotine, only 1 to 2 mg from each cigarette smoked is delivered to the lungs. About 25% of the nicotine is immediately carried to the brain, where it easily crosses the blood–brain barrier and affects normal brain biochemistry. In humans, 60 mg of nicotine can be a lethal dose.

Acute Effects of Nicotine Use

Outside the CNS, nicotine affects the transmission of nervous system signals by mimicking acetylcholine. It occupies receptor sites at the synapses and prevents the transmission of nerve impulses from neuron to neuron and from neuron to muscle cells. Smoking exerts its deleterious effects primarily on the cardiovascular and pulmonary systems (Box 33.1). Nicotine, a direct adrenergic agonist, causes the release of epinephrine, which increases heart rate, systemic vascular resistance, and blood pressure. Smoking directly increases coronary vascular resistance,

Box 33.1 Effects of Tobacco Smoke	
Cardiovascular Effects	**Respiratory Effects**
• Increased myocardial oxygen consumption • Increased heart rate • Increased systemic vascular resistance • Decreased myocardial inotropic activity • Decreased myocardial oxygen supply • Increased carboxyhemoglobin (reduced available hemoglobin) • Coronary artery vasospasm • Oxyhemoglobin dissociation curve shifted to the left	• Decreased mucociliary clearance • Bronchospasm • Cough • Sputum accumulation • Decreased circulating immunoglobulin levels • Decreased neutrophil chemotaxis • Decreased pulmonary macrophage count and adherence • Altered T-lymphocyte immunoregulatory activity • Decreased natural killer lymphocyte activity • Decreased function of alpha$_1$-antitrypsin

especially at sites of atherosclerotic plaques and stenosis. Inhaled cigarette smoke also exerts a negative inotropic effect on the myocardium, possibly due to the binding of CO to cytochrome oxidase and myoglobin, resulting in increased myocardial oxygen consumption and decreased oxygen delivery. These changes are accompanied by the constriction of the blood vessels beneath the skin, a reduction in the motility in the bowel, and a loss of appetite.

CO, a component of tobacco smoke, is present in cigarette smoke in concentrations similar to those in automobile exhaust. CO has a binding affinity for the hemoglobin molecule that is 250 times greater than that of oxygen, thereby reducing the smoker's oxygen-carrying capacity. In heavy smokers, as much as 15% of circulating hemoglobin may be bound to CO, reducing the oxygen-carrying capacity of the blood. In addition, CO shifts the oxyhemoglobin dissociation curve to the left, inhibiting the release of oxygen. The half-life of the carboxyhemoglobin (COHb) complex is 4 to 6 hours when the individual is breathing room air. The heart's need for oxygen is increased because of the sympathetic stimulatory effect of nicotine. Because the blood's oxygen-carrying capacity is reduced, the heart must pump more rapidly to adequately supply tissues with oxygen.

The effects of smoking on the respiratory system are diverse. The irritating effect of the smoke causes hyperplasia of cells, including goblet cells, which results in increased mucus production. Hyperplasia reduces airway diameter and increases the difficulty in clearing secretions. Smoking is known to disrupt mucociliary function and the ability to clear particles from the peripheral airways, even before any abnormality in pulmonary function can be detected, as smoking may cause actual loss of ciliated cells. Smoking also produces abnormal dilation of the distal air spaces with destruction of alveolar walls. Many cells develop large, atypical nuclei, which are considered a precursor to cancer. Smoking also alters pulmonary immune defense mechanisms by depressing neutrophil chemotaxis, decreasing immunoglobulin levels, reducing natural killer lymphocyte activity, decreasing macrophage adherence, and altering immunoregulatory T-lymphocyte activity.

In the CNS, nicotine activates receptors within the brain. Stimulation of the brain is evidenced by changes in EEG patterns, reflecting an increase in the frequency of electrical activity. This is part of a general arousal pattern signaled by the release of the neurotransmitters norepinephrine, dopamine, acetylcholine, and serotonin. Heavy tobacco use, resulting in high levels of nicotine in the bloodstream, eventually produces a blocking effect, as more and more receptor sites are filled. The result is generalized depression of the CNS. When the blood levels of nicotine reach a critical point, the brain's vomiting center may be activated.

Chronic Effects of Nicotine Use

Chronic effects of nicotine use include the development of tolerance and chemical dependence. The user will consume greater quantities of nicotine for longer periods than originally intended, further endangering his or her health. Dependence on nicotine is quickly established in the majority of users. Although psychological dependence may occur as well, the hallmarks of physical dependence—establishment of tolerance and presence of withdrawal symptoms—have all been demonstrated. Nicotine withdrawal symptoms include a dysphoric or depressed mood, insomnia, irritability, frustration, anger, anxiety, poor concentration, restlessness, decreased heart rate, and increased appetite.

To understand better the neuropsychopharmacologic basis of why people smoke, researchers have performed positron emission tomography scans on smokers and abstainers and found that smokers had a 40% decrease in levels of a brain enzyme known as monoamine oxidase B (MAO B) compared with nonsmokers. The mechanisms of MAO inhibition by cigarette smoke are not known. The enzyme breaks down dopamine, a neurotransmitter associated with feelings of pleasure. Because nicotine stimulates dopamine release and dopamine produces pleasurable effects, this mechanism may play a significant role in reinforcing and motivating smoking behavior. Therefore, smoking seems to create a self-perpetuating cycle: less MAO B leads to more dopamine, which leads to more pleasure, which leads to more smoking, which leads to less MAO B, and so on. The researchers proposed that reduction of MAO B activity may synergize with nicotine to produce the diverse behavioral and epidemiological effects of smoking.

CLINICAL PRESENTATION

Subjective

Demographic, anthropometric, physiological, and laboratory features that distinguish cigarette smokers from nonsmokers reflect both baseline differences between these groups and the effects of smoking. Smokers drink more alcohol, coffee, and tea than do nonsmokers. Their weight and blood pressures are slightly lower and their heart rates are slightly faster than those of nonsmokers. Women who smoke are at increased risk for early menopause, decreased bone density, and osteoporosis. Smoking has also been shown to decrease fertility in those attempting pregnancy and to impair uteroplacental function, which adversely affects the fetus during pregnancy. Sudden infant death syndrome is two to four times more common in infants whose mothers smoked during pregnancy. Smokers have impaired maximum exercise performance and impaired immune systems compared with nonsmokers. A markedly increased number of pulmonary alveolar macrophages is present in smokers, and the function and metabolism of these cells are abnormal. In smokers, the ratio of high-density lipoprotein cholesterol to low-density lipoprotein cholesterol is reduced.

A causal association has been well characterized between smoking and coronary heart disease, atherosclerotic peripheral vascular disease, cerebrovascular disease, lung and laryngeal cancer, oral cancer, esophageal cancer, COPD, intrauterine growth retardation, and low-birth-weight babies. In addition, smoking is considered by many to be the probable cause of or a contributing cause to many other conditions, including miscarriage, increased infant mortality, peptic ulcer disease, and cancers of the bladder, breast, pancreas, uterus, and kidney (see Box 33.1). Smokers are at increased risk for bone fractures, premature skin wrinkling, gingival recession, dental caries, periodontal disease, cataracts, and glaucoma. Depression is twice as common among those who smoke than in people who have never smoked and has been linked to increased smoking initiation and to failures in smoking cessation efforts. A strong association also exists between smoking and other substance abuse disorders, especially alcohol dependence. Clinical manifestations of these specific diseases, although beyond the scope of this chapter, are all directly or indirectly associated with cigarette smoking.

Objective

Smokers usually demonstrate many observable signs of tobacco addiction. The smell of tobacco smoke lingers on the individual's clothing and on his or her skin and hair. The breath and sputum often smell of stale tobacco, and the fingers and nails are often stained from tobacco use. Use of smokeless tobacco may manifest in periodontal disease, a condition that may lead to tooth loss; abrasive damage to the enamel of the teeth due to the effects of processed tobacco; and oral cancer. The patient may also have lumps in the jaw or neck area, color change in lumps inside the lips, or white, smooth or scaly patches in the mouth or throat or on the lips or tongue. Smokers may also present with a red spot or sore on the lips or gums or inside the mouth that does not heal or difficulty speaking or swallowing.

Signs of cardiopulmonary disease often accompany tobacco addiction. A productive cough, dyspnea, wheezing, and fatigue should alert the clinician to respiratory problems related to smoking. Frequent bouts of pneumonia, influenza, and bronchitis, as well as chronic diseases such as emphysema, interstitial lung disease, or chronic airway obstruction, often result from cigarette smoking. Cardiovascular signs of smoking including tachycardia, cardiac dysrhythmias, increased blood pressure, decreased peripheral blood flow, and angina must all be assessed to determine the risk for and extent of cardiovascular disease in smokers or those exposed to secondhand smoke.

Nicotine dependence is related to the amount and duration of smoking and can manifest as withdrawal symptoms. These signs and symptoms begin within a few hours of the last cigarette, peak 48 to 72 hours later, and return to baseline within 3 to 4 weeks of quitting. Criteria for nicotine dependence disorder are published in the *Diagnostic and Statistical Manual of Mental Disorders*. They include dysphoric or depressed mood, insomnia, irritability or anger, frustration, anxiety, concentration difficulties, decreased heart rate, and increased appetite or weight gain.

DIAGNOSTIC REASONING

Asking the patient about smoking status and recording this information in the medical record require only an additional 15 seconds and serve as a reminder to the practitioner to discuss the problem with each smoker. Despite this, only 20% of smokers receive medical advice on smoking cessation during visits to health-care providers. All patients, starting at adolescence, should be asked if they use tobacco and should have their tobacco use status documented on a regular basis as a new vital sign. This is the age group that all providers should try to reach with this information. Several questionnaires measuring self-reported tobacco dependence are available. The six-question Fagerström Test for Nicotine Dependence predicts the level of nicotine dependence and may help predict smoking cessation success, as well as inform nicotine replacement dosages as a function of the classification of dependence.

Diagnostic Tests

Laboratory assays of smoking-related biochemical compounds such as thiocyanate, cotinine, nicotine, and

COHb in urine, blood, breath, or saliva can be performed to verify smokers' reports of smoking status or abstinence

A urine sample can be assayed for the constituents of the cigarette smoke itself or for excretion products associated with the physiological effects of smoking. Nicotine excretion in smokers correlates well with the number of cigarettes smoked and inversely with the pH of the urine. Urine metabolites of epinephrine can also be measured; however, false-positive results related to severe anxiety are possible.

CO is found in the blood of smokers and combines with hemoglobin to form COHb. A value of 2% suggests that smoking has occurred. However, environmental and occupational sources of CO must be considered. Although the COHb level increases proportionally with the number of cigarettes smoked and varies with nicotine content, clinical judgment is necessary in interpreting the data.

The measurement of mean alveolar CO partial pressure makes it possible to determine the COHb levels in the blood with a high degree of correlation. Also, by subtracting expired CO from inspired CO, it is possible to determine whether a smoker is an inhaler. Smokers have higher levels of both expired CO and thiocyanate than nonsmokers. To measure CO, the patient is instructed to inhale deeply and to hold his or her breath for 10 to 15 seconds before expiring with full force through the inflow valve of the monitor (EC_{50} monitor). Levels of nine parts per million (ppm) or lower are considered to reflect nonsmoking status.

Cotinine is a major metabolite of nicotine and is a useful marker. A sample of at least 3 mL of unstimulated saliva is collected in a plastic cup. The presence of nicotine (as reflected in cotinine levels) in saliva can be determined by gas chromatography and an alkali flame ionization detector, but it is difficult to distinguish the pattern of smoking based on cotinine levels. Moreover, nonsmokers exposed to secondhand cigarette smoke may also have nicotine in their saliva.

Differential Diagnosis

The most accurate way to rule out differential diagnoses is to ensure that, for every patient at every clinic visit, tobacco-use status is queried and documented. The cause of a smoker's cough and dyspnea must be explored to rule out other explanatory causes, such as lung cancer, interstitial lung disease, allergies, and infections. Unfortunately, many patients with symptoms of cough, dyspnea, sputum production, and changes in pulmonary function testing are not only smokers but also suffer from some form of lung disease or disorder. Smokers tend to have unique laboratory findings, such as increases in HCT, total white blood cell count, and platelet count. They may also have decreases in leukocytes, vitamin C level, serum uric acid, and albumin.

MANAGEMENT

Changes in the system of health-care delivery in the United States indicate the need to incorporate smoking cessation as a regular part of clinical care, particularly in the current managed care environment. The Centers for Disease Control and Prevention's *Best Practices for Comprehensive Tobacco Control Programs* (2014) is an evidence-based guide that helps states plan and establish effective tobacco control programs to prevent and reduce tobacco use. Clinicians must also commit to making changes in clinical culture and practice patterns to ensure that every patient who smokes is offered smoking cessation treatment at every office visit. Brief but effective interventions are essential for all tobacco users at each clinical visit. Patients who are counseled to quit are 1.6 times as likely to attempt quitting as those who receive no counseling. Clinicians aiding patients in smoking cessation should remember the five A's: Ask, Advise, Assess, Assist, and Arrange. A treatment flowchart for smoking cessation is presented in Figure 33.1.

Initial Management

When a patient is identified as a smoker, the clinician should advise him or her of the need to quit. This advice should be give after the patient's chief complaint has been addressed. The patient's response will determine the proper strategy to pursue. The patient must be informed of how unhealthy and dangerous smoking is. Pregnant smokers should be strongly encouraged to quit throughout pregnancy. Because of the serious risk of smoking to the pregnant smoker and fetus, pregnant smokers should be offered intensive counseling treatment. Patients should choose a quit date, usually within the next 30 days, to allow patients to develop effective alternative behaviors to smoking. Periods of extreme stress or depression are not optimal times to attempt smoking cessation.

Smoking Cessation Programs

Most smokers move through five stages of behavioral change in their attempts at cessation (1) precontemplation, (2) contemplation, (3) preparation, (4) action, and (5) maintenance. The first step a provider should take in initiating a smoking cessation program with a patient is to find out which stage of cessation the patient is in. By understanding the smoker's stage of behavior and readiness to change, the clinician can better assist him or her to achieve successful cessation.

Smokers in the *precontemplation stage* have no desire to quit in the next 6 to 12 months. These individuals usually benefit from motivational interventions that increase awareness of the adverse effects of smoking. Smokers who seriously thinking about and express interest in quitting but are not yet ready to do so are in the *contemplation stage*. These smokers also benefit from motivational counseling emphasizing the negative effects of smoking.

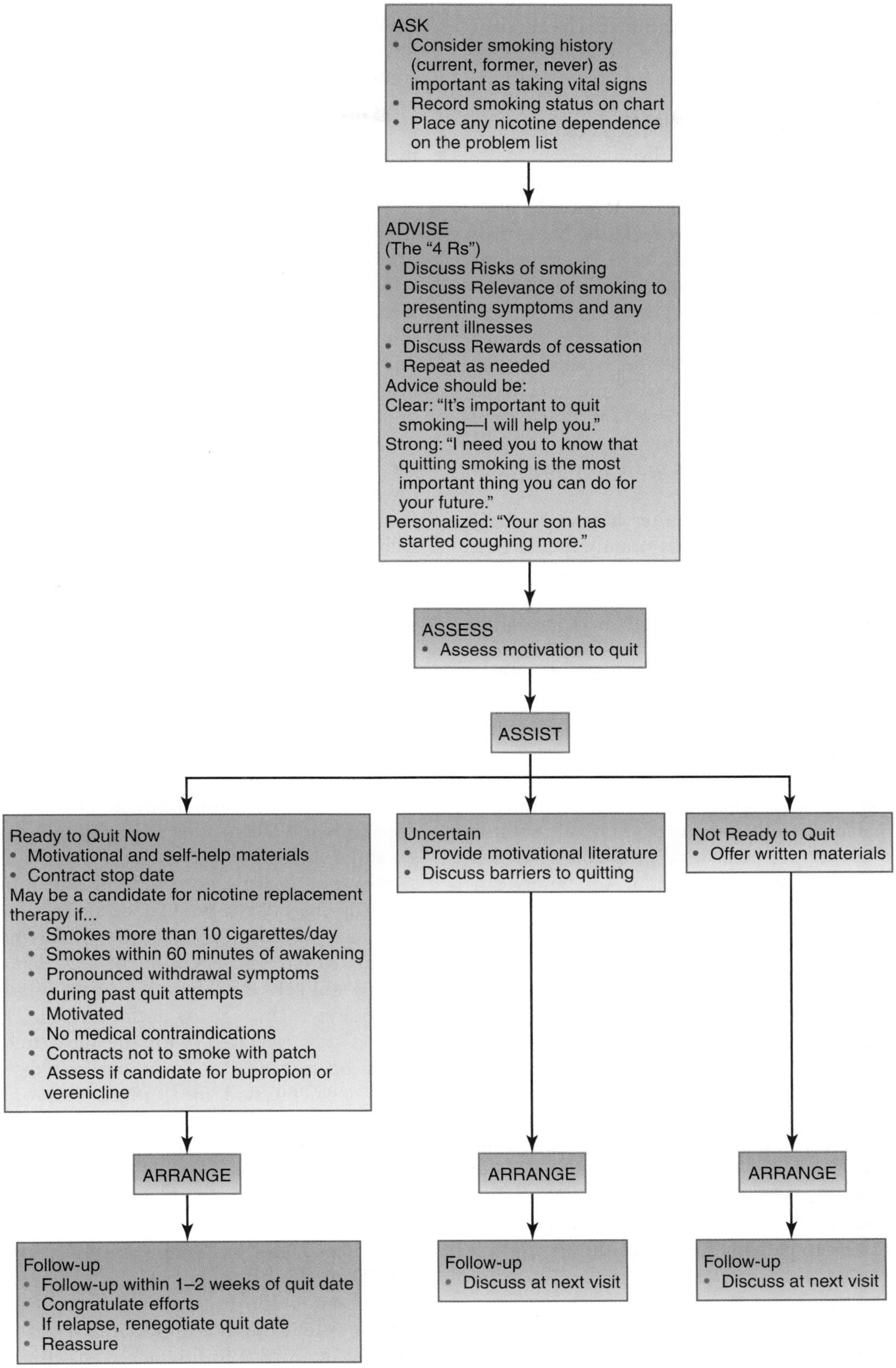

ASK
- Consider smoking history (current, former, never) as important as taking vital signs
- Record smoking status on chart
- Place any nicotine dependence on the problem list

ADVISE
(The "4 Rs")
- Discuss Risks of smoking
- Discuss Relevance of smoking to presenting symptoms and any current illnesses
- Discuss Rewards of cessation
- Repeat as needed

Advice should be:
Clear: "It's important to quit smoking—I will help you."
Strong: "I need you to know that quitting smoking is the most important thing you can do for your future."
Personalized: "Your son has started coughing more."

ASSESS
- Assess motivation to quit

ASSIST

Ready to Quit Now
- Motivational and self-help materials
- Contract stop date

May be a candidate for nicotine replacement therapy if...
- Smokes more than 10 cigarettes/day
- Smokes within 60 minutes of awakening
- Pronounced withdrawal symptoms during past quit attempts
- Motivated
- No medical contraindications
- Contracts not to smoke with patch
- Assess if candidate for bupropion or verenicline

Uncertain
- Provide motivational literature
- Discuss barriers to quitting

Not Ready to Quit
- Offer written materials

ARRANGE

ARRANGE

ARRANGE

Follow-up
- Follow-up within 1–2 weeks of quit date
- Congratulate efforts
- If relapse, renegotiate quit date
- Reassure

Follow-up
- Discuss at next visit

Follow-up
- Discuss at next visit

Adapted from Helping smokers quit. http://www.ahrq.gov/professionals/clinicians-providers/guidelines-recommendations/tobacco/5steps.html

Figure 33.1 Treatment flowchart: smoking cessation strategies.

Smokers who are serious about quitting and have taken the initial steps toward cessation are in the *preparation stage.* Individuals in this stage benefit from interventions that assist them in quitting. These interventions include providing information about nicotine replacement and developing behavior modification skills.

During the *action stage,* the smoker quits smoking. The action stage lasts from several weeks to 6 months after cessation, which is a common time of relapse. Because of the likelihood of relapse during this stage, interventions should address relapse prevention, including congratulating successes and rewarding positive behavioral changes with more frequent contacts by the clinician. When a smoker has abstained from cigarettes for 6 months, the *maintenance stage* begins. Most successful quitters relapse and recycle through these stages three or four times before attaining long-term abstinence; some may take several years to move through these stages until abstinence can be maintained.

Effective smoking cessation requires behavior modification. The behavior of smoking is usually linked to a variety of triggers (e.g., stress, foods or beverages, driving). When a patient recognizes the triggers, healthy alternative behaviors can be substituted. It is crucial to develop alternative coping strategies to overcome the urge to smoke. Such strategies include deep breathing and relaxation exercises, chewing gum, exercise, drinking water, sucking on a piece of sugarless candy, and eating carrots or celery sticks.

Patients quitting smoking need support from their clinicians, families, and other persons. The clinician can help the patient handle particularly difficult triggers and can treat underlying behavioral problems or mood disorders, such as anxiety or depression. The family can provide invaluable positive reinforcement to the patient during this time. If there are other smokers in the patient's household, the clinician should encourage them to quit smoking at the same time as the patient. It is difficult for a person to refrain from smoking in the long term when a spouse or other family member continues to smoke. Many patients benefit from support groups such as Nicotine Anonymous and Quintet. There are also online cessation programs, such as the American Lung Association's Freedom from Smoking program, the American Cancer Society's Freshstart program, Smokefree.gov, 1-800-QUIT-NOW, and quitnet.com. These online free customized smoking cessation programs should be mentioned at every visit to patients who smoke.

Hypnosis

The goal of hypnosis in smoking cessation is to enable the smoker to achieve an altered state of consciousness that enhances the ability to quit. However, the hypnotic state is generally not measurably different from that associated with deep muscle relaxation. The effects of hypnosis are often short lived. Controlled trials of hypnosis have generally not documented long-term efficacy for smoking cessation. Published quit rates range between 0% and 88%. Although it is of uncertain value, hypnosis remains a commercially popular stop-smoking method. The primary advantage of hypnosis is that it may be an attractive alternative for people who have failed to quit with other methods.

Aversion Conditioning

Aversion conditioning is based on the premise that smoking is a learned response that can be extinguished by creation of an association between smoking and a negative sensation. Among the aversion techniques used for smoking cessation are electric shock, nausea-inducing drugs, hot and smoky air treatments, and rapid smoking. High quit rates have been reported in some of the early smoking cessation trials using aversion conditioning. However, these high success rates may be attributed, in part, to factors related to patient selection because arguably only the most highly motivated persons are willing to undergo this type of therapy. In addition, aversion-conditioning techniques may represent a health hazard.

Subsequent Management

Pharmacologic Approaches

Although some smokers may need antidepressants or anxiolytics, it is difficult to predict who will benefit from these adjunctive therapies. Bupropion (Zyban) is an antidepressant and smoking deterrent. Bupropion is a weak inhibitor of the neuronal uptake of norepinephrine and dopamine but has no effect on serotonin. Its dopaminergic and noradrenergic activities are responsible for its efficacy in smoking cessation, with the dopaminergic activity affecting areas of the brain associated with the reinforcement activity affecting nicotine withdrawal. Bupropion appears to have no effect on patient depression scores, so it is unlikely that the mechanism for the efficacy of bupropion is through its antidepressant effects. Bupropion is well tolerated, with the most frequent adverse effects being headache, insomnia, and dry mouth. Like other antidepressant medications, bupropion is associated with a small risk of seizure and should not be given to patients with a seizure disorder. Moreover, patients with a history of severe head trauma, eating disorders, recent myocardial infarction, unstable heart disease, or active alcoholism should not take bupropion.

Bupropion for smoking cessation should be started 1 to 2 weeks before the patient's quit date. The initial dosage is 150 mg per day for 3 days followed by 150 mg twice a day. It is important for steady-state plasma levels of bupropion to be reached (usually within 8 days) before smoking cessation is begun. This dosing schedule has been found to lead to less weight gain during the medication phase. The duration of treatment is usually 7 to 12 weeks. For maintenance therapy, bupropion 150 mg twice a day for up to 6 months may be considered.

Behavioral modification therapy should be provided concurrently. For heavily addicted smokers, nicotine replacement therapy and bupropion can be coadministered.

Varenicline (Chantix) is a nicotinic acetylcholine receptor partial agonist used as a smoking cessation aid. It is recommended that therapy begin 1 week before a target quit date is set: 0.5 mg is given daily for the first 3 days, then 0.5 mg twice a day for 4 days, then 1 mg twice a day for 12 weeks. Adverse side effects include possible neuropsychiatric symptoms, particularly in those with a depressive or psychiatric history. Smoking cessation aids are listed in Drugs Commonly Prescribed 33.1.

Drugs Commonly Prescribed 33.1: Therapies for Smoking Cessation—Prescribing Considerations

DRUG	DOSAGE	ADVANTAGES	DISADVANTAGES
Transdermal Patch		Continuous Delivery	Expensive
NicoDerm CQ (worn 24 h/day)	21 mg/day for 4–6 weeks, then 14 mg/day for 2–4 weeks, then 7 mg/day for 2–4 weeks Consider starting with 14-mg patch if smoking less than 10 cigarettes/day	Less instruction required than nicotine gum	Risk of insomnia or nightmares; if this occurs, try wearing patch for 16 h/day while awake
Gum (nicotine polacrilex)		Useful on "as-needed" basis	Requires good dentition
Nicorette	2 mg/piece; maximum 30 pieces/day 4 mg/piece; maximum 24 pieces/day	Provides oral gratification Patient control Delayed weight gain	Risk of mouth irritation Dyspnea, nausea Risk of developing dependence Complicated usage guidelines
Nasal Spray		Useful on "as-needed" Basis	
Nicotrol (10-mL bottle)	0.5 mg/spray; two sprays; maximum 40 doses/day for 3 months	Rapid delivery	Risk of nasal and throat irritation Runny nose Watery eyes
Inhaler			
Nicotine inhaler	13 mcg/puff; 6–16 cartridges/day for up to 6 months	Mimics smoking behavior	Risk of cough, irritation of mouth and throat
Lozenge			
Commit	2 mg (if first cigarette smoked >30 min after waking) 4 mg (if first cigarette smoked within 30 min of waking) maximum 20 lozenges/day, dissolve over 20–30 min; minimize swallowing	First-line agent; effective in combination with patch	May cause hiccoughs, heartburn, nausea
Other			
Bupropion HCL (Zyban)	150 mg/day for 3 days, then 150 mg twice daily for 7–12 weeks (possibly up to 6 months)	Non-nicotine, less weight gain	Risk of seizures, headache, dry mouth, insomnia
Varenicline (Chantix)	0.5 mg/day for 3 days, then 0.5 mg twice daily for 4 days, then 1 mg twice daily for 12 weeks, take with a glass of water after eating	Non-nicotine, first-line agent	Nausea Risk of serious neuropsychiatric symptoms including depression, altered mood and behavior, suicidality

Nicotine Replacement Therapies

Nicotine patches, gum, and lozenges are available over the counter (OTC), and nicotine nasal spray and inhalers are available by prescription (see Drugs Commonly Prescribed 33.1). Increased access through OTC availability has substantially increased the number of people attempting to quit smoking in the United States. Evaluations of the efficacy of nicotine gum through 12-month follow-up suggest that the gum improves smoking cessation rates by approximately 40% to 60% compared with control interventions. Efficacy is increased when nicotine gum use is combined with an intensive psychosocial intervention. The efficacy of the nicotine patch overall appears to be somewhat stronger than that of nicotine gum. The patch has been found to double the 6- to 12-month abstinence rate over those of placebo interventions.

The cost of the patch continues to decrease each year, making it more available to smokers. Although the manufacturer of nicotine gum has developed a series of strategies for increasing access to nicotine replacement therapy among underserved populations, it is not clear if the penetration of such programs can match the need for an effective strategy among lower-income and other underserved groups. Many clinics now offer nicotine patches and gum free of charge through state-sponsored smoke-free initiatives.

The gum must be correctly chewed to a softened state (until a peppery taste or a tingling sensation is felt) and then placed in the buccal mucosa. Patients should not eat for 15 minutes before or during use of the nicotine gum. Initially, one piece is chewed every 1 to 2 hours over 6 weeks, with a maximum of 24 pieces in 24 hours. Time intervals for gum use are gradually increased to 2 to 4 hours for 3 weeks, then every 4 to 8 hours for 3 weeks. Fewer than 10% of patients will become dependent on the gum, although many will require long-term use (1 to 2 years) to maintain abstinence from smoking. Nicotine absorption is decreased by acidic foods and beverages, which should be avoided during use of nicotine gum. Irritation and trauma to the oral mucosa, teeth, and dental work can occur. Many patients experience jaw ache, gastrointestinal discomfort, hiccoughs, and increased heart rate.

Nicotine patches are applied every morning and worn continuously for 24 hours per day. Patches are usually indicated for 8 to 12 weeks to promote long-term abstinence. Patients should be instructed to change the application site daily to minimize skin irritation. The highest-dose patch should be considered if the patient smokes more than 10 cigarettes per day and has no active cardiovascular disease. Because there is a dose–response effect, researchers recommend that a higher nicotine dose is more effective for smoking cessation. Adverse effects include skin reactions, insomnia, vivid dreams, and myalgias. If vivid dreams or insomnia occur, the patient should be instructed to remove the patch before going to bed and then to apply a new patch on arising.

The nicotine nasal spray (Nicotrol nasal spray) delivers nicotine in a more rapid manner than the gum, patch, or inhaler (but less rapidly than cigarettes) and may therefore serve as a more effective substitute for smoking than other nicotine replacement systems. The device is similar to those used to administer nasal antihistamine sprays. The nasal spray delivers 0.5 mg of nicotine per spray. Smokers are instructed to use one to two doses per hour for up to 6 months at up to 40 doses per day. The nasal spray delivers nicotine rapidly, but less rapidly than cigarettes. Peak levels occur within 4 to 15 minutes and are about two-thirds of those associated with cigarettes. Patients may initially experience nasal and throat irritation, rhinitis, sneezing, coughing, and watering eyes. Tolerance to these effects develops in the first week. The spray may cause serious dysrhythmias, elevated blood pressure, and angina in postmyocardial infarction patients. Use of the spray is also not recommended in patients with other chronic diseases, including asthma, peptic ulcer disease, chronic nasal disorders, severe renal impairment, liver disease, diabetes, and hyperthyroidism.

Researchers have found that the use of a nicotine patch with a nicotine nasal spray is significantly more effective for long-term smoking cessation than with either alone. Studies suggest increased efficacy in the prevention of relapse with greater nicotine intake or by combining different types of nicotine replacement therapies. The combination of a nicotine patch and nicotine nasal spray may be successful not only because of the high level of substitution but also because of the opportunity to respond quickly to the smoker's cravings and physical needs. Researchers have suggested that using a patch for 5 months with a nicotine nasal spray for 1 year provides a more effective means of stopping smoking than using a patch alone.

The nicotine inhaler (Nicotrol inhaler) is a plastic rod with a nicotine plug that provides a nicotine vapor when puffed on. Each active cartridge contains approximately 10 mg of nicotine and 1 mg of menthol. The menthol is added to decrease the throat irritation caused by the nicotine. Although the device is designed as an inhaler, this label is a misnomer because the device does not deliver a significant amount of nicotine to the lungs; rather, the device delivers nicotine buccally. This occurs whether smokers use deep or shallow puffs. Each cartridge lasts about 20 minutes and provides the nicotine equivalent of about two cigarettes. Patients use 6 to 16 cartridges per day for 3 months, then taper for 6 to 12 weeks as needed. The most common adverse effects are cough and irritation in the mouth and throat.

The inhaler has the potential to assist in smoking cessation not only by providing nicotine replacement but also by mimicking the behavioral aspects of smoking. However, these devices may be problematic because they are closely related to cigarette smoking. In effect, the patient using these devices is brand switching (i.e., switching from his or her usual brand of cigarette to a smoke-free nicotine-delivery device), even though the effort required to obtain nicotine from the inhaler is greater than that required from a cigarette. Combining the nicotine inhaler with the nicotine patch may increase efficacy over using the patch alone because the inhaler serves to supplement the nicotine provided by the patch and mimic smoking behavior.

Two medications being used off-label for smoking cessation include nortriptyline (75 to 100 mg/day for 12 to 14 weeks) and clonidine (0.1 to 0.3 mg/day transdermal or 0.15 to 0.45 mg/day orally for up to 12 weeks). More research is needed, however, before they can be recommended as medications for smoking cessation

FOLLOW-UP AND REFERRAL

As with any serious medical problem, follow-up is essential after the initial intervention. A supportive phone call 1 week after the quit date can be made by a health-care worker with the reinforcement of the self-help materials that have been provided. Office follow-up by the clinician at 1 and 3 months after the quit date can assist the patient in coping with persistent exposure to triggers or smoking-associated situations; this support can help the patient who may have relapsed to get back on track. In the case of relapse, the client should be assisted to set another quit date, revisit the reasons for quitting, and begin the cessation process again. It is important to assure patients that stable abstinence is commonly achieved only after five or six cessation attempts.

Patient Education: Smoking Cessation

In the past, cigarette smoking was viewed as largely a social or psychological habit. As such, the ability to quit was considered a measure of personal motivation and willpower. Motivation to stop smoking, combined with sufficient psychological resources, was seen as a driving force behind successful smoking abstinence. Thus, if smokers could be educated about the health risks of cigarette smoking, they could theoretically become sufficiently motivated and psychologically empowered to quit.

Unfortunately, the anticipated benefits of achieving smoking cessation through health education were overoptimistic and simplistic. More than 80% of current smokers indicate they would like to quit but cannot. Educational programs to aid smoking cessation have produced disappointing results and high long-term failure rates. Only about 4% of smokers are able to quit each year. Nonetheless, it is helpful to give the patient age-specific smoking cessation literature. Training clinicians how to conduct tobacco cessation counseling is critical to reduce excess tobacco-related mortality (see Evidence-Based Nursing Practice 33.1).

In addition, health-care providers need to be aware of the nuances of smoking cessation. For example, individuals often experience constipation during smoking cessation, as the

 Evidence-Based Nursing Practice 33.1

VanDevanter N, Zhou S, Katigbak C, Naegle M, Sherman S, Weitzman M. Knowledge, beliefs, behaviors, and social norms related to use of alternative tobacco products among undergraduate and graduate nursing students in an urban U.S. university setting. *J Nurs Scholarsh*. 2016;48(2):147–153.

The purpose of this study was to assess nursing students' knowledge, beliefs, behaviors, and social norms regarding use of alternative tobacco products (ATPs). A survey was conducted among all students enrolled in a college of nursing, both undergraduates and graduates. It assessed knowledge and beliefs about ATPs (hookahs, cigars or cigarillos, bidis, kreteks, smokeless tobacco, electronic cigarettes) compared with cigarettes, health effects of ATPs, personal use of ATPs, and social norms. Nursing students demonstrated very low levels of knowledge about ATPs and their health consequences, despite high rates of ATP personal use. Nurses' lack of knowledge about the emerging use and health threats associated with ATPs may undermine their ability to provide appropriate tobacco cessation counseling. As nurses play critical roles in counseling their patients on tobacco cessation, further nursing research and education about the risks presented by ATPs are critical to reducing tobacco-related mortality.

gastrointestinal system adjusts to withdrawal from the stimulating effects of nicotine. The use of a bulk-forming agent such as Metamucil, increased dietary fiber, and increased fluids will alleviate the problem. A form of exercise, such as walking, is an effective and affordable stress reliever. A walking program also assists with reducing the expected mean weight gain of 5 to 7 pounds that occurs with smoking cessation. Nicotine is an appetite suppressant, and once its effects have cleared from the body, food will taste better.

It is important to understand the meaning of smoking to the individual patient and to hear the "patient's voice" (see The Patient's Voice 33.1). Smoking is an addictive behavior that for most patients has become intimately associated with daily reinforcing experiences, emotions, and coping mechanisms, despite the irrefutable evidence of its significant health risks. Assisting the patient in stopping smoking involves an empowerment process that enhances the patient's motivation and self-esteem. Providers can encourage patients to identify daily stressors and assist them to reframe situations and develop alternative coping strategies. Equally important is developing enhanced self-efficacy, which includes accepting and believing in one's own ability to succeed. Providers need to ask how the patient usually deals with stress and give simple and practical alternative coping strategies. A telephone hotline with recorded messages that empower and encourage the patient can be an effective way to manage and overcome the desire to smoke. Information about the rewards of smoking cessation, such as better health status with lower blood pressure and improved circulation and lung functioning, should also be provided

The Patient's Voice 33.1

BATTLEGROUND

"What is it with you and your cigarettes, anyway?" I angrily thought to myself after yet another heated debate with my father about smoking. As usual, he had been defending cigarettes as a source of pleasure, saying he always enjoyed smoking. He was against federal attempts to regulate levels of nicotine in cigarettes or restrict access. After smoking for 60 years, he quit last year, when the severity of his lung disease nearly took his life. Why couldn't I make him understand that cigarettes were killing people?

He must have sensed my frustration or read my mind, because as his O_2 concentrator clicked off and on, he looked at me and said softly, "You know, Snicklefritz, it was cigarettes that saved my life many times during the war." My father rarely talks about The War. He was a combat infantryman, a machine gunner—part of the Fifth Division known as "Roosevelt's Red Devils." He started slowly . . .

"At night we were the point. Machine gunners never got relieved. The cold was the worst. You couldn't imagine the cold. Raining—below freezing. We would take turns sleeping. You couldn't sleep for more than an hour. You had to rely on your buddies to wake you up. You had to keep moving to keep from freezing. Many only lasted one night and had to be sent back because their feet were frozen. I think we lost more men to cold that winter than from enemy fire."

"I remember standing up one night with tracers going by my head, yelling 'Go ahead and shoot me—put me out of my misery!' My buddy had to pull me down. He said. 'Have a cigarette—calm yourself!' We had to cover our heads with raingear to keep anyone from seeing me light up and give away our positions. You can't imagine the warmth and comfort in one cigarette. We were worried about living through the night."

"There were times the warmth of a cigarette was the only thing that kept us alive. We were short of supplies that winter, but they always kept us in cigarettes. Even our K-rations came with a pack—I'll give them that."

As he talked, I tried to imagine, to understand, the inhuman conditions he was describing and the meaning cigarettes held for him. As I listened to my father's story and watched him pull his arms to his chest and cup his hands to his face, as if he were holding something as precious as life itself, I finally heard what he had been saying for years. I began to feel my anger slipping away—anger with my father for smoking all those years and for nearly dying before my 3-year-old son had a chance to come to know him.

I felt my eyes fill with tears, not for the suffering my father had experienced during the war, but for the suffering he experienced because his daughter, the nurse, never understood.

—Shirley Countryman Gordon, from "Nightingale Songs." Publication of Florida Atlantic University College of Nursing.

(positive reinforcement). Individuals who cease smoking report more energy, enhanced taste and smell, monetary savings, freedom from addiction, feeling better about oneself, and better performance in sexual and sports activities. Smokers older than 55 years should be informed that despite many years of smoking, smoking cessation will improve their health. They will enjoy a better quality of life as ex-smokers and their risk for lung and other smoking-associated cancers will be reduced. Smokers die 5 to 8 years earlier than persons who have never smoked.

Additional rewards for older adults can be the satisfaction of being a positive role model for other family members and making a contribution to the improved health of their children, grandchildren, and others. To enhance recovery from nicotine addiction and prevent relapse, both individual and group cessation counseling and education should include a family focus with shared commitment and participation. The provider can facilitate this process by providing cessation information to both the patient and his or her family. In the absence of family, the clinician may focus on close friends or other social support network for the patient.

REFERENCES

American Academy of Otolaryngology—Head and Neck Surgery. Secondhand smoke exposure in children. https://www.childrenentdocs.com/docs/SecondHandSmokeExposure.pdf. Published 2017. Accessed June 2, 2017.

American Psychiatric Association. *Diagnostic and statistical manual of mental disorders.* 5th ed. Washington, DC: American Psychiatric Publishing; 2013.

Bornemann P, Eissa A, Strayer S. Smoking cessation: What should you recommend? *J Fam Pract.* 2016;26(2):22–29B.

Centers for Disease Control and Prevention. Best practices for comprehensive tobacco control programs. https://www.cdc.gov/tobacco/stateandcommunity/best_practices/index.htm. Published 2014. Accessed January 16, 2017.

Centers for Disease Control and Prevention. Burden of tobacco use in the U.S. https://www.cdc.gov/tobacco/campaign/tips/resources/data/cigarette-smoking-in-united-states.html. Published 2016. Accessed June 2, 2017.

Jameson JL, Fauci, Kasper, Hauser, Longo, Loscalzo, eds. *Harrison's principles of internal medicine.* 19th ed. New York, NY: McGraw-Hill; 2016.

Office of Disease Prevention and Health Promotion. Tobacco use. *Healthy People 2020.* https://www.healthypeople.gov/2020/topics-objectives/topic/tobacco-use.

Papadakis MA, McPhee SJ. *Current medical diagnosis and treatment.* New York, NY: Appleton-Lange/McGraw-Hill; 2017.

Peereboom D, Evers-Casey S, Leone F. Are you equipped to treat tobacco dependence? *Consultant.* 2014;54(12):903-907.

U.S. Department of Health and Human Services. *Ending the tobacco epidemic: A tobacco control strategic action plan for the U.S. Department of Health and Human Services.* Washington, DC: Office of the Assistant Secretary for Health; 2010.

U.S. Food and Drug Administration. FDA warns of health risks posed by e-cigarettes. https://www.fda.gov/ForConsumers/ConsumerUpdates/ucm173401.htm. Accessed June 2, 2017.

RESOURCES

Centers for Disease Control and Prevention: Smoking and Tobacco Use
https://www.cdc.gov/tobacco/

Smoking Cessation

1-800-QUIT-NOW.
https://www.cdc.gov/tobacco/quit_smoking/cessation/pdfs/1800quitnow_faq.pdf

American Cancer Society's Freshstart Program
https://www.cancer.org/healthy/stay-away-from-tobacco.html

American Lung Association's Freedom From Smoking
http://www.lung.org/stop-smoking/join-freedom-from-smoking

Centers for Disease Control and Prevention: Quit Smoking
https://www.cdc.gov/tobacco/quit_smoking/index.htm

Nicotine Anonymous
http://nicotine-anonymous.org

Quitnet.com
https://quitnet.meyouhealth.com/#/

Smokefree.gov
https://smokefree.gov/

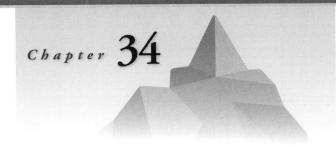

Chapter **34**

Common Cardiovascular Complaints

Kathryn B. Keller, PhD, RN, CNE

Jill E. Winland-Brown, EdD, APRN, FNP-BC

Brian Oscar Porter, MD, PhD, MPH, MBA

CHEST PAIN

Approximately 34% of individuals who experience a coronary event in any given year will die from it individuals will die of it (Mozaffarian, 2016). Although deaths from coronary heart disease have declined over the past 40 years, this decrease is mainly due to advances in medical and surgical treatment rather than lifestyle or behavioral changes. Several lifestyle changes can have a significant impact in reducing mortality risk, including smoking cessation (12%) and an increase in physical activity (5%) (Mozaffarian, 2016). *Healthy People 2020* continues to stress the need for lifestyle changes to reduce coronary heart disease–related deaths. The educational initiative over the past 25 years to inform women about the gender differences in heart attack characteristics has markedly increased women's awareness that cardiovascular deaths is their leading cause of mortality.

DIFFERENTIAL DIAGNOSIS

Although chest pain is often associated with cardiovascular problems, it may also have pulmonary, gastrointestinal, musculoskeletal, neurologic, psychogenic, or idiopathic causes. Obtaining a focused health history and physical examination are essential for accurate assessment and appropriate treatment of a patient with chest pain (see Fig. 34.1). Critical components of the history

include appraisal of the major symptoms of heart disease, including chest pain, dyspnea, syncope, and heart failure. The clinician should ask patients in all age groups about tolerance of exercise, especially whether exercise provokes any of the aforementioned complaints. The history of the present illness of the person with chest pain should focus on personal risk factors for cardiovascular disease.

The clinician should obtain a complete chest pain symptom analysis including location, quality, duration, aggravating or relieving factors, and associated symptoms or signs. In particular, localized, fleeting, and moving pain is rarely indicative of serious cardiac pathology. Anxiety and bereavement can cause diffuse chest pain lasting for hours. The pain of costochondritis (a type of chest wall syndrome [CWS]) is often described as localized, and it may be replicated with arm movement or pressing on the area of tenderness (point tenderness). CWS is largely a diagnosis of exclusion. Evidence-Based Nursing Practice 34.1 presents a study of a clinical prediction rule for CWS in the primary-care setting that could potentially prevent many tests and examinations used to rule out coronary related chest pain.

In contrast, the discomfort of angina pectoris is classically described as a diffuse, retrosternal sensation of pain, often with radiation, and a heavy, burning sensation, usually lasting more than 1 minute but less than 10 minutes. Exertional symptoms are usually more common in individuals with fixed atherosclerotic lesions. In assessing the person with known angina pectoris, it is critical to ascertain if there has been a change in the symptom pattern because this may indicate an alteration in vessel patency such as that found in accelerated atherosclerosis or vessel spasm. The word "pain" should be used with caution in taking the history of a person with suspected myocardial ischemia because the patient may deny that pain is present but may agree that tightness, burning, fullness, or other sensations more aptly describe the complaint.

The terms "unstable angina," "preinfarct angina," and "crescendo angina" are synonyms used to describe the new onset of cardiac ischemic chest pain at rest but without evidence of acute myocardial infarction (MI). Reports of symptoms at rest are more likely to be associated with coronary artery vasospasm, a condition usually seen in patients with coronary atherosclerosis. The combination of these two mechanisms of lumen narrowing places the patient at considerable risk for an acute coronary syndrome; in these cases, rapid and accurate assessment is vital to ensure appropriate disposition and treatment.

Diagnostic Reasoning Algorithm: Chest Pain

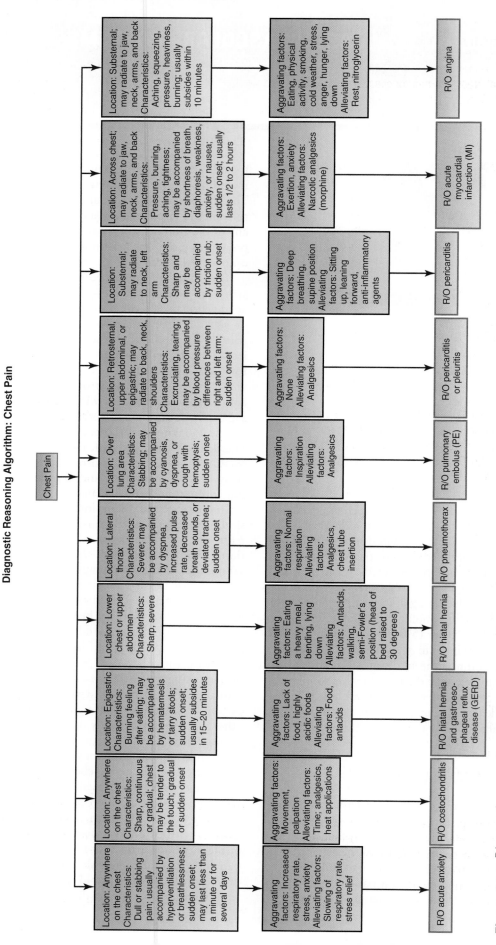

Figure 34.1 Diagnostic reasoning algorithm: chest pain.

Evidence-Based Nursing Practice 34.1

Ronga A, Vaucher P, Haasenritter J, et al. Development and validation of a clinical prediction rule for chest wall syndrome in primary care. *BMC Family Pract.* 2012;13:74.

ABSTRACT

Background: Chest wall syndrome (CWS), the main cause of chest pain in primary-care practice, is most often an exclusion diagnosis. We developed and evaluated a clinical prediction rule for CWS.

Methods: Data from a multicenter clinical cohort of consecutive primary-care patients with chest pain were used (59 general practitioners, 672 patients). A final diagnosis was determined after 12 months of follow-up. We used the literature and bivariate analyses to identify candidate predictors, and multivariate logistic regression was used to develop a clinical prediction rule for CWS. We used data from a German cohort (n = 1212) for external validation.

Results: From bivariate analyses, we identified six variables characterizing CWS: thoracic pain (neither retrosternal nor oppressive), stabbing, well localized pain, no history of coronary heart disease, absence of general practitioner's concern, and pain reproducible by palpation. This last variable accounted for 2 points in the clinical prediction rule and the others for 1 point each; the total score ranged from 0 to 7 points. The area under the receiver operating characteristic (ROC) curve was 0.80 (95% confidence interval 0.76–0.83) in the derivation cohort (specificity: 89%; sensitivity: 45%; cutoff set at 6 points). Among all patients presenting CWS (n = 284), 71% (n = 201) had pain reproducible by palpation and 45% (n = 127) were correctly diagnosed. For a subset (n = 43) of these correctly classified CWS patients, 65 additional investigations (30 electrocardiograms, 16 thoracic radiographies, 10 laboratory tests, eight specialist referrals, one thoracic computed tomography) had been performed to achieve diagnosis. False positives (n = 41) included three patients with stable angina (1.8% of all positives). External validation revealed the ROC curve to be 0.76 (95% confidence interval 0.73–0.79) with a sensitivity of 22% and a specificity of 93%.

Conclusions: This CWS score offers a useful complement to the usual CWS exclusion diagnosing process. Indeed, for the 127 patients presenting with CWS and correctly classified by our clinical prediction rule, 65 additional tests and examinations could have been avoided. However, the reproduction of chest pain by palpation, the most important characteristic to diagnose CWS, is not pathognomonic.

About one-third of patients with angina pectoris will have simultaneous dyspnea caused by a transient increase in pulmonary venous pressure that accompanies ventricular stiffening during an episode of myocardial ischemia. The presence of diaphoresis with chest pain is particularly worrisome, often indicating a significant drop in cardiac output during the episode of pain and subsequent decreased perfusion of the skin. In contrast to the patient who complains of anginal pain, the patient who is experiencing an acute MI often complains of anginal-like chest pain that lasts in excess of 20 minutes but occasionally waxes and wanes during that period. The pain is frequently accompanied by dyspnea, diaphoresis, nausea, and dizziness. The pain may radiate to the neck, jaw, shoulder, or arm (left side more than right). Patients show extreme variation in the amount of pain experienced with an MI, from complaining of a "vise around the heart" to apologizing for seeking assistance with "just a bit of indigestion that will not clear up." In particular, women, older adults, and people with diabetes mellitus are likely to have minimal or atypical symptoms with an acute MI. A more detailed discussion of the pain of angina and MI is provided in the sections on treatment of those conditions in Chapter 35.

PALPITATIONS

Palpitations are commonly reported by the individual who has or is at risk for heart disease. *Palpitations* are defined as the awareness of the beating of one's heart and may be benign or pathological in nature. When questioning the patient with palpitations, the clinician should obtain a detailed description of the sensation. If the patient reports a sensation of a strong but regular rhythmic beating of the heart after stress or exertion, this likely indicates a normal physiological response to increased catecholamine production. If there is a report of skipped or missed beats, particularly with the sensation that the heart "stopped" momentarily, this may indicate the presence of an atrial or ventricular ectopic beat.

DIFFERENTIAL DIAGNOSIS

Atrial ectopic beats are most often benign, occurring with excessive caffeine, alcohol, or tobacco use. On occasion, atrial ectopic beats occur with cardiac pathology, sometimes as a precursor to a supraventricular rhythm such as multifocal atrial tachycardia or atrial fibrillation. This is most likely in the patient with chronic obstructive pulmonary disease (COPD) or rheumatic heart disease and valvular dysfunction.

Ventricular ectopic beats are somewhat more likely to indicate cardiac pathology than atrial ectopy. If the patient is at high risk for or has known heart disease, the clinician must carefully assess the complaint of palpitations because ventricular ectopy may reflect an increased risk of sudden cardiac death.

Another variation on the presentation of palpitations is the patient who complains of a sudden onset of a very rapid heartbeat or fluttering of the heart. The etiology may be a supraventricular or ventricular tachycardia, often with equally rapid and unpredictable cessation of the rhythm, or a rhythmic paroxysm. Although this type of rhythmic sensation is usually regular, such as in paroxysmal supraventricular tachycardia or ventricular tachycardia, it may also be irregular, such as in intermittent atrial fibrillation. In any case, the clinician should query the patient carefully about accompanying symptoms, such as chest pain related to decreased coronary artery filling and increased myocardial oxygen demands, as well symptoms associated with low cardiac output.

Diagnostic testing should be directed by information obtained in the health history and physical examination. As with cardiac-related syncope, thyroid function (thyroid-stimulating hormone), blood chemistries, hemoglobin, and hematocrit should be evaluated to help rule out thyroid disorder, electrolyte imbalance, and anemia as possible, though less common, causes of palpitations. Ambulatory cardiac monitoring (Holter monitoring) until at least one event is recorded is most helpful in ascertaining the presence of a potentially lethal cardiac rhythm disturbance. Echocardiography may be necessary to assess cardiac outflow tract patency and to help rule out valvular stenosis or hypertrophic cardiomyopathy.

Intervention should be directed at the underlying cause of the palpitations. For example, if a rhythm disturbance such as recurrent supraventricular or ventricular tachycardia is the cause, treatment directed at eliminating this is warranted. In any event, the clinician should consult with a physician or cardiologist who has expertise in this area to ensure patient safety and optimal outcome.

A diagnostic algorithm for palpitations is presented in Figure 34.2.

SYNCOPE

Syncope is a loss of consciousness that occurs abruptly as a discrete episode and usually lasts for a short period of only a few minutes. The implied pathology is decreased cerebral blood flow caused by a marked decrease in cardiac output. Approximately one million people are affected by syncope in the United States every year. Whereas some of these episodes are explainable and of noncardiac origin (e.g., fluid loss, dehydration, emotional stress), the majority of these episodes are cardiovascular in origin, including the most common etiology of vasovagal or cardioneurogenic syncope.

Cardiac-related syncope is an ominous sign associated with high rates of mortality. A syncopal episode may be the only warning sign of impending sudden cardiac death. One of the most common cardiac causes of syncope is cardiac arrhythmias. A wide range of conduction disturbances can precede a syncopal event, including tachycardia-bradycardia syndrome (sick sinus syndrome), supraventricular and ventricular tachycardias, heart blocks, and bradycardia.

DIFFERENTIAL DIAGNOSIS

Cardiac outflow tract blockage, such as the obstruction that may occur in hypertrophic cardiomyopathy or aortic valve stenosis, can also produce syncope. This is most often seen in response to increased activity or stress when the outflow tract blockage impedes the increase in cardiac output needed to meet the increased demand for oxygen. This leads to syncope that typically lasts for a few seconds and ends when the "rest" period of the syncopal episode rebalances the supply of oxygenated blood with demand.

Presyncope, a state of light-headedness, feeling faint, and muscular weakness, is most often cardiovascular in origin. The etiology is usually the same as for syncope. In contrast, *vertigo* is the sensation of spinning that can often be reproduced by a change in head position. Vertigo is not usually caused by decreased cerebral blood flow; an inner ear disturbance is the most common cause.

Diagnostic testing for cardiac-related syncope should be directed by the information obtained in the health history and physical examination. Similar to the work-up for palpitations, blood chemistries, thyroid-stimulating hormone, hemoglobin, and hematocrit should be checked to help rule out electrolyte imbalance, thyroid disorder, and anemia as possible, though less common, causes of syncope. Ambulatory cardiac monitoring until at least one event is recorded is most helpful in ascertaining the presence of a potentially lethal cardiac rhythm disturbance. Echocardiography may be necessary to assess cardiac outflow tract patency and to rule out valvular stenosis or hypertrophic cardiomyopathy. A tilt-table test may be performed to assess for orthostatic syncope.

Intervention in cardiac-related syncope should be directed at the underlying cause. If a rhythm disturbance (as described previously) is the cause, treatment should be directed at eliminating the conduction disorder. Ablation, an internal cardiac defibrillator, and/or a permanent pacemaker may be indicated depending on the type of arrhythmia. In any event, the clinician should consult with a cardiologist to ensure patient safety and an optimal outcome.

DYSPNEA

Dyspnea, or shortness of breath, is a highly subjective complaint, yet it is one of the most common cardiac symptoms. The challenge to the clinician is to determine its etiology. As with any complaint, the patient with dyspnea should be asked about precipitating factors, quality, duration, alleviating factors, and the length of time needed to relieve the symptom after discontinuing the precipitating event. In addition, dyspnea may be an anginal equivalent, especially in older adults and individuals with diabetes.

Patients with a chief complaint of dyspnea vary markedly in presentation; however, because this is a subjective complaint, the patient's report should be placed into

Diagnostic Reasoning Algorithm: Palpitations

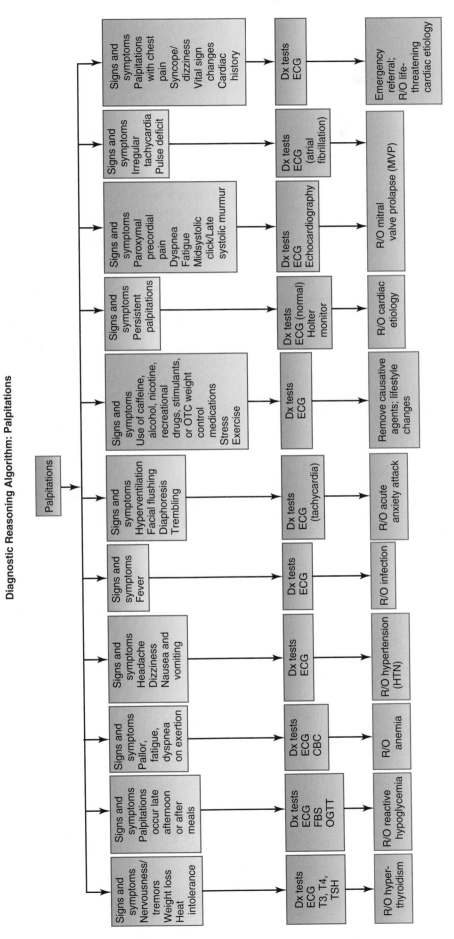

Figure 34.2 Diagnostic reasoning algorithm: palpitations.

context. As with the complaint of pain, the discomfort and degree of dyspnea represent the patient's reality; however, correlating the complaint with physical findings may help to establish the cause of the dyspnea, thus leading to an effective plan of intervention.

DIFFERENTIAL DIAGNOSIS

Dyspnea has a number of possible causes. With left-sided cardiac outflow tract blockage, such as in severe aortic stenosis or obstructive cardiomyopathy, dyspnea likely arises from the decrease in cardiac output. When dyspnea is associated with recurrent myocardial ischemia, as in angina pectoris, the shortness of breath is likely caused by an increase in pulmonary vascular pressure, coupled with a transient decrease in cardiac output. In right-sided cardiac problems, such as tricuspid and pulmonic valvular dysfunction, the complaint of dyspnea usually arises from increased pulmonary pressures and resistance to cardiac emptying of the right ventricle.

Another common cause of dyspnea is pulmonary disease, such as COPD, asthma, pleural effusion, pneumothorax, pulmonary embolus, or pulmonary hypertension secondary to interstitial lung disease or pulmonary fibrosis. Other noncardiac causes of dyspnea are severe anemia and metabolic acidosis (i.e., Kussmaul's respirations), obesity, physical deconditioning, and anxiety or emotional distress.

The patient's assessment of the severity of dyspnea may differ from the objective findings. For example, some patients who have been observed to have rather marked difficulty breathing have little complaint of breathlessness, whereas other patients who have few objective findings will describe marked difficulty breathing. In addition, when asked about difficulty breathing, one patient may admit to feelings of suffocation, in that getting sufficient air in and out of the lungs is a problem, whereas others will describe a need to take deep breaths.

Dyspnea is a poorly sensitive and nonspecific marker for cardiovascular disease. Factors contributing to the complaint of breathlessness in the absence of heart disease include poor conditioning and exercise intolerance related to inactivity and obesity. The patient usually reports that the onset of this type of dyspnea accompanies increased activity and resolves rapidly when the activity ceases. In cardiovascular disease, dyspnea is usually a result of increased stiffness in the lungs caused by increased pulmonary blood volume or pulmonary congestion. This is usually found in conditions that result in poor cardiac output, such as congestive heart failure (CHF), recurrent myocardial ischemia, poorly controlled hypertension, valvular dysfunction, and heart disease.

When dyspnea is the complaint, it is essential for the clinician to assess for any change in the patient's ability to perform typical daily activities. In particular, dyspnea is often first detected by the patient as the inability to talk during exertional activities. Pinpointing the onset of the symptoms and concurrent events may be helpful in determining its etiology. In addition, asking about cosymptoms such as wheezing and weight gain is crucial because dyspnea is the most common presenting complaint in CHF.

Orthopnea is shortness of breath that begins when the patient has been in a supine position, such as when lying face up in bed. The patient usually compensates for this sensation by sleeping on an increased number of pillows to elevate the upper body, hence the use of the qualifying term *three-pillow orthopnea*. If the person slides off the pillows while sleeping, shortness of breath reoccurs, causing the person to awaken. Orthopnea is usually caused by CHF as a result of increased right-sided heart pressure, which increases after the patient has been supine for a few hours, mobilizing fluid that pooled in the extremities during the more active awake hours.

Paroxysmal nocturnal dyspnea (PND) is shortness of breath that occurs 1 to 2 hours into sleep, concurrent with the redistribution of bodily fluids and a subsequent rise in left atrial pressure. The person awakens suddenly with significant difficulty breathing. He or she usually stands or sits up until symptoms are relieved in about 10 to 30 minutes. As with orthopnea, the diagnosis of CHF should be considered in patients with PND.

LEG ACHES

Leg aches associated with peripheral vascular disorders are caused by impaired blood flow to the extremities. Peripheral vascular disease (PVD) affects the arteries and veins. When the vascular disease is arterial, it is usually the result of atherosclerosis (accumulation of fatty streaks and fibrous plaques and high levels of low-density lipoproteins). Venous problems are related to venous incompetence secondary to valve obstruction, resulting in chronic venous insufficiency and varicose veins.

DIFFERENTIAL DIAGNOSIS

Patients presenting with leg aches may have a number of disorders other than PVD; therefore, a thorough history and physical examination must be performed to rule out thrombosis, phlebitis, polycythemia, anemia, Raynaud's disease, and Buerger's disease. Because some of the contributing factors to PVD may be smoking, high blood pressure, and diabetes, these problems must be addressed and underlying conditions managed. Both peripheral arterial disease and peripheral venous disease are discussed in more detail in Chapter 37.

PERIPHERAL EDEMA

Peripheral edema is the accumulation of tissue fluid within the interstitial spaces of the extremities. When the edema involves the lower extremities, it is a symptom of an

Diagnostic Reasoning Algorithm: Peripheral Edema

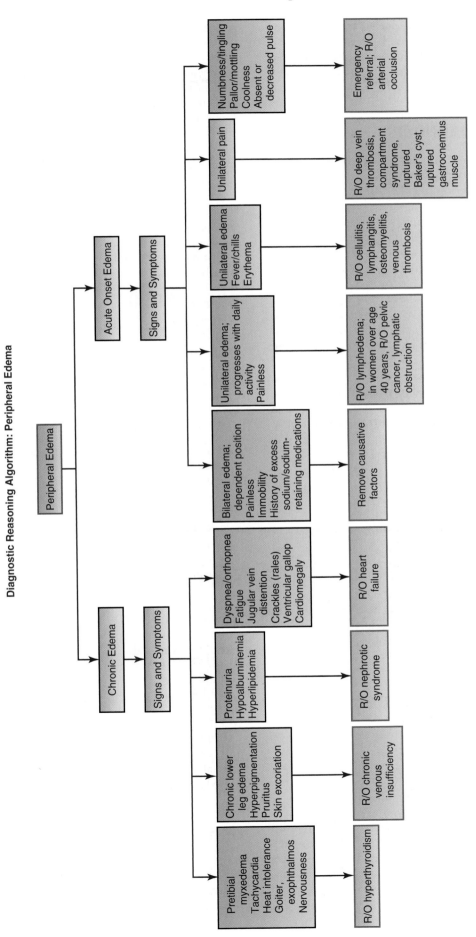

Figure 34.3 Diagnostic reasoning algorithm: peripheral edema.

underlying disorder and may be caused by cardiac conditions (e.g., heart failure, chronic venous insufficiency, or thrombophlebitis), renal or hepatic disease, trauma, tumors, or inflammation. Peripheral edema occurs equally in men and women.

DIFFERENTIAL DIAGNOSIS

Peripheral edema is usually diagnosed via the history and physical examination, although laboratory findings may also assist in determining the cause of the edema. It is essential that the underlying cause be identified and treated, or the peripheral edema will remain, possibly causing tissue ischemia from compressed and diminished arterial circulation. Specific diagnostic tests the clinician should order include a complete blood count, urinalysis, serum chemistries, and a thyroid profile. X-ray studies may be ordered if trauma or osteomyelitis is suspected, and a chest x-ray film should be ordered to assess the heart and lungs. A computed tomography scan may help to assess the distribution of edema and to pinpoint the extent of venous and lymphatic obstruction. An electrocardiogram is essential for assessing cardiac function, and Doppler studies may be ordered to evaluate for deep vein thrombosis.

A diagnostic algorithm for peripheral edema is presented in Figure 34.3.

REFERENCES

Goel R, Srivathsan K, Mookadam M. Supraventricular and ventricular arrhythmias. *Prim Care.* 2013;40(1):43–71.

Heart Rhythm Society. Syncope. http://www.hrsonline.org/PatientInfo/SymptomsDiagnosis/Fainting/index.cfm. Updated May 22, 2013.

Mozaffarian D, Benjamin EJ, Go AS, et al Heart disease and stroke statistics—2016 update: A report from the American Heart Assococation. *Circulation.* 2016;133(4):e38–e360.

Stochkendahl MJ, Christensen HW. Chest pain in focal musculoskeletal disorders. *Med Clin North Am.* 2010;94(2):259–273.

U.S. Department of Health and Human Services/Office of Disease Prevention and Health Promotion. Heart disease and stroke. *Healthy People 2020.* https://www.healthypeople.gov/2020/topics-objectives/topic/heart-disease-and-stroke/objectives. Accessed July 15, 2017.

RESOURCES

American College of Cardiology
    www.acc.org
American Heart Association (Contact AHA for local state affiliate)
    www.americanheart.org
American Medical Association (AMA)
    www.ama-assn.org
Healthy People 2020
    www.healthypeople.gov/hp2020/objectives/topicarea

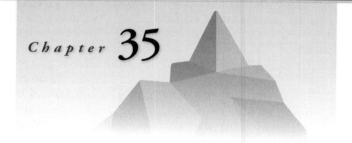

Chapter **35**

Cardiac and Associated Risk Disorders

Kathryn B. Keller, PhD, RN, CNE

Denese Sabatino, MSN, APRN, NP-C, CCRN

Jill E. Winland-Brown, EdD, APRN, FNP-BC

Brian Oscar Porter, MD, PhD, MPH, MBA

HYPERTENSION

Hypertension (HTN) is one of the most common chronic health problems seen in the primary-care setting, with nearly one-half of all American adults affected. The health implications of HTN are far reaching and widely recognized as a public health concern. *Healthy People 2020* includes 23 specific objectives for heart disease and stroke, six of which relate directly to HTN. The goals of these recommendations are improvement of cardiovascular health and quality of life through the prevention, detection, and treatment of risk factors, early identification and treatment of heart attacks and strokes, and the prevention of recurrent cardiovascular events.

EPIDEMIOLOGY AND CAUSES

HTN occurs in one of three Americans, or 34% of the U.S. population (approximately 85.7 million persons). It is projected that by 2030, 41.4% of the population will have HTN. Historically, HTN has been more prevalent in men, particularly in African American men. As of 2017, African American women surpassed African American men with a higher prevalence of HTN. However, this gender gap is narrowing and appears to be influenced by age. For persons younger than 45 years, men are affected more often than woman, whereas in persons 65 years of age and older, more woman than men have HTN. African Americans continue to experience HTN more often and at an earlier age than European Americans or Latinos.

The prevalence of HTN continues to increase with age. HTN is a common disorder that occurs with aging in industrialized societies. Data from the Framingham Heart Study suggest that even individuals who are normotensive at 55 years of age still have a 90% lifetime risk of developing HTN. There is a particular rise in systolic blood pressure (BP) that progresses throughout life, with a difference of 20 to 30 mm Hg between early and late adulthood.

More than 95% of patients with elevated BP have primary, or essential, HTN, with no single identifiable cause. Primary HTN results from multiple genetic and environmental factors, including lifestyle and behavioral influences. It is more common in individuals whose parents or other close family members have HTN, possibly due to a diminished ability to excrete excess sodium coupled with long-term high dietary sodium intake, which predisposes to increased peripheral vascular resistance and a rise in BP.

Less than 5% of patients have secondary HTN due to a specific and potentially reversible cause, such as an identifiable cardiac, renal, or endocrinological problem or the use of vasoconstricting medications. The onset of diastolic HTN, with or without systolic elevation after 60 years of age is unusual, and a diagnosis of new-onset secondary HTN should be considered in these individuals. In particular, renovascular disease is a common cause of new-onset diastolic HTN in this older age group.

HTN contributes to ischemic heart disease, heart failure (HF), diabetic complications, chronic kidney disease, and cerebrovascular disease. While recent 2017 data from the National Health and Nutrition Examination Survey (NHANES) demonstrated a 50% improvement in BP control among Americans with HTN, 45.6% of persons with HTN still had uncontrolled BP. Moreover, morbidity is worsened in the setting of overweight and obesity, the prevalence of which has increased over the last 15 years, with obesity rates growing from 30.5% to 37.7% in the United States. For example, a body mass index (BMI) of greater than 30 kg/m^2 raises the risk of high BP and cardiovascular disease, while doubling the lifetime risk of HF compared with persons with a BMI of less than 25 kg/m^2.

After decades of a steady reduction in rates of HTN-related diseases, researchers have reported a recent leveling off of coronary heart disease rates, coupled with a slight increase in end-stage renal failure and age-adjusted stroke rates. These changes are likely due to a number of factors,

including a growing elderly population; however, the role of undetected and untreated or inadequately controlled HTN contributes significantly. Thus, primary-care practitioners should be committed not only to the detection and treatment of HTN but also to its prevention.

PATHOPHYSIOLOGY

Essential Hypertension

The term "essential hypertension" describes high BP that has no identifiable etiology after a thorough clinical examination excludes possible secondary causes. The etiology and pathophysiology of essential HTN are incompletely understood. It is a complex, multifactorial disorder that involves genetic and environmental factors, diet and lifestyle practices, imbalances in vasoactive substances, and dysfunction of the arterial endothelium. Although the precise cause is unknown, endothelial dysfunction is thought to be the key pathophysiological process involved in essential HTN. The arterial endothelium is an important regulator of vascular tone, vascular structure, thrombosis, and inflammation. Endothelial dysfunction is central to many cardiovascular disorders, including HTN, atherosclerosis, and myocardial ischemia.

Vascular tone is maintained by endothelium-derived mediators such as nitric oxide, endothelin-1, and angiotensin II. Nitric oxide, a major vasodilator, counteracts the potent vasoconstrictors endothelin-1 and angiotensin II, which regulate normal vascular tone. In essential HTN, there is an imbalance in the vasodilator and vasoconstrictive substances secreted by the endothelium. Plasma levels of nitric oxide are diminished, whereas levels of endothelin-1 and angiotensin II are elevated. Reasons for this imbalance have not been elucidated, and it is not clear whether endothelial dysfunction precedes or is the result of HTN.

The role of altered sodium excretion by impaired epithelial cells in the kidney may also be a factor in the development of HTN. Renin levels are markedly abnormal in some hypertensive individuals, despite normal renal function. Individuals who secrete abnormally high levels of renin experience constant cycling of the renin-angiotensin-aldosterone cascade, which raises blood volume and BP. Low renin secretors, in general, are salt-sensitive hypertensive individuals. Ingestion of sodium increases water reabsorption into the bloodstream, which raises blood volume and BP. The cause of renin imbalance in some persons with essential HTN is unknown, but measuring plasma renin levels in patients with refractory HTN may assist in clinical diagnosis and treatment.

Other contributors include aging, sympathetic nervous system overactivity, toxins, and low numbers of nephrons. An often-overlooked cause of essential HTN is sleep apnea with its associated activation of the sympathetic and renin-angiotensin systems. More commonly, metabolic syndrome with its resultant insulin resistance and increased insulin levels also leads to increased sympathetic activity and hypertensive states (see Box 35.1). Worldwide epidemiological evidence demonstrates that age-related HTN is uncommon in societies where individuals maintain lower body weight, consume less sodium and more potassium, and engage in greater levels of physical activity. These findings indicate that high BP is influenced by environmental and modifiable lifestyle factors (e.g., smoking, obesity, stress) and is not an inevitable consequence of aging.

Genetic and ethnic influences also play a role in the development of HTN. Persons with a family history of HTN are four times more likely to have HTN than those with no family history of the condition. Studies show that the genetic contribution to essential HTN is complex, and multiple genes are likely involved. Most genetic effects involve gene–gene interactions and gene–environment interactions. Genes that encode components of the renin-angiotensin-aldosterone system are being extensively studied. Results of this line of investigation have implicated mutations in the angiotensinogen gene and angiotensin-converting enzyme gene.

Studies of HTN in African Americans demonstrate that ethnicity is related to HTN susceptibility and plays a role in the efficacy of specific types of drugs. Morbidity and mortality due to HTN and HTN-related disorders are more common in African Americans than in European Americans and non-Hispanic Americans. HTN also seems to follow a more malignant course in African Americans. Compared with European Americans with HTN, African Americans have an increased risk of left ventricular hypertrophy (LVH), HF, and renal failure.

HTN has localized and systemic adverse effects. Locally, high BP creates a shearing force against the arterial walls, which injures the endothelium and accelerates development of atherosclerosis. Endothelial injury initiates a detrimental localized reaction of vasoconstriction, inflammation, platelet aggregation, and fibrin and lipid deposition—the basis of arteriosclerotic plaque formation. In turn, target organs

that are damaged by HTN include the heart (LVH and coronary artery disease (CAD) resulting in angina or acute myocardial infarction [MI]), the kidneys (chronic renal insufficiency), the brain (transient ischemic attacks [TIAs], cerebrovascular accidents [CVAs], and increased risk of dementia), the eyes (retinal hemorrhages and hypertensive retinopathy), and the peripheral arteries (peripheral vascular disease).

Secondary Hypertension

Secondary HTN is elevated BP due to an identifiable, underlying condition. Detection of secondary HTN is critical to reverse the source of the pathological process and prevent hypertensive target organ damage (TOD). Much less common than essential HTN, secondary HTN has an overall frequency of 5% to 10% in primary-care practices. Secondary HTN is often distinguished from essential HTN by certain assessment findings, such as an age of onset younger than 30 years or older than 50 years, BP higher than 180/110 mm Hg at diagnosis, significant TOD at diagnosis, hemorrhages and exudates on funduscopic examination, renal insufficiency, LVH, accelerated or malignant HTN, and a poor response to therapy. Resistant HTN is often due to unexplored, reversible secondary causes.

Reversible causes of secondary HTN include obesity, obstructive sleep apnea, renovascular disease, chronic corticosteroid therapy, Cushing's syndrome, primary hyperaldosteronism, pheochromocytoma, coarctation of the aorta, hyperthyroid disease, parathyroid disease, and excess alcohol intake. Secondary HTN can also be drug induced, and a thorough history of the patient's medications, including herbal supplements, over-the-counter (OTC) agents, and any illicit drug use is essential. Common drugs that can cause HTN include NSAIDs, cyclooxygenase-2 (COX-2) inhibitors, sympathomimetics such as decongestants and anorectics (diet pills), oral contraceptives, erythropoietin,

---

Box 35.1 Lifestyle Modifications to Manage Hypertension

- **Weight reduction:** Maintain normal body weight (BMI, 18.5–24.9 kg/m²) (lowers BP by 5–20 mm Hg).
- **Adopt DASH (Dietary Approaches to Stop Hypertension) eating plan:** Consume a diet rich in fruits, vegetables, and low-fat dairy products, with a reduced content of saturated and total fat (lowers BP by 14–18 mm Hg).
- **Dietary sodium reduction:** Reduce dietary sodium intake to no more than 100 mmol (2.4 g sodium) per day (lowers BP by 2–8 mm Hg).
- **Physical activity:** Engage in regular aerobic physical activity such as brisk walking (at least 30 minutes/day on most days of the week) (lowers BP by 4–9 mm Hg).
- **Moderation of alcohol:** Limit consumption to no more than two drinks (1 oz or 30 mL of ethanol, e.g., 24 oz of beer, 10 oz of

wine, or 3 oz of 80-proof whiskey) per day for most men and to no more than one drink per day for women and lighter weight persons (lowers BP by 2–4 mm Hg).
- **Stop smoking and/or use of other tobacco products.**
- **Understand hot tub safety:** When combined with heat, antihypertensive drugs may cause vasodilation resulting in dizziness, light-headedness, fainting, and reduction of cerebral blood flow, with the potential for falling and risk of injury.
- **Maintain adherence to pharmacotherapeutic plan:** When medication regimen is not followed, BP will rise.
- **Monitor for drug-induced HTN:** Drugs that may induce HTN include NSAIDs, antidepressants, glucocorticoids, oral contraceptives, hormone replacement therapy, and OTC medications that contain decongestants.

cocaine, amphetamines, corticosteroids, tacrolimus, cyclosporine, and herbal ephedra supplements. Licorice, smoking, and chewing tobacco also increase BP.

"White Coat" Hypertension

"White coat" HTN, with a prevalence of 13%, is a transient rise in BP experienced by a patient when in the clinical or hospital setting, most likely due to anxiety. This condition of "pseudohypertension" is common in primary-care practice. The "white coat" effect can lead to an overestimation of BP and the prescribing of unnecessary antihypertensive treatment. In addition, the patient's transiently high BP can be misinterpreted as ineffectiveness of antihypertensive therapy. One review showed that 30% to 40% of patients who were diagnosed with HTN based on their BP readings in a clinical office had normal "out-of-office" BP readings according to ambulatory BP measurements (Cobos et al., 2015).

Care must be taken to use an appropriately sized BP cuff when assessing HTN in the clinic. Obese patients or those with large arms need to have a cuff that is large enough to measure BP accurately. If the cuff used is too small, an artificially high BP reading may result. Patients with white coat HTN are more accurately assessed through the use of ambulatory BP monitoring (ABPM), which provides an automated 24-hour recording of the patient's BP during normal daily activities that can be reviewed by the clinician. Alternatively, the patient may be instructed to measure and record intermittent BP readings over several weeks with reliable, consistent equipment for later review.

Masked Hypertension

Masked HTN is defined as HTN that is present during daily life and yet absent in clinical assessment. Studies conducted by the National Institutes of Health demonstrated that masked HTN may be present in as many as one in seven individuals with normal clinic-based BP readings. ABPM or home-based BP self-monitoring by the patient who is at high risk for masked HTN is a cornerstone of optimizing outcomes. Without active patient participation and education, however, this condition may go untreated. Risk factors identified for masked HTN include smoking, alcohol use, lack of physical activity, and work-related and physiological stressors. Patients with masked HTN have a higher incidence of cardiovascular events and subsequently a higher risk of mortality and morbidity due to missed opportunities to treat.

Malignant Hypertension

Malignant HTN (hypertensive urgency/emergency) has been noted in up to 1% of patients diagnosed with primary HTN. Malignant HTN is diagnosed when a patient presents with severely elevated BP in the range of 180/110 mm Hg or higher and evidence of acute TOD. Although these terms are often used interchangeably, *hypertensive emergency* or *hypertensive crisis* denotes this process acutely. If not treated with immediate parenteral antihypertensive therapy in an acute-care setting, a hypertensive emergency may prove fatal. In contrast, a significantly elevated BP alone with no evidence of TOD does not constitute an emergency and is classified as a *hypertensive urgency.*

Hypertensive urgencies may be treated with oral agents over a period of 24 to 48 hours to achieve stabilization. In a hypertensive emergency, a severely elevated BP can be reduced over the course of hours with oral and/or IV medications in an inpatient setting. Acute TOD most commonly involves the neurologic, cardiac, or renal systems, with evidence of TOD including the following:

- Cerebrovascular events
- Papilledema, hemorrhages, or exudates on funduscopic examination
- Acute myocardial ischemia or infarction
- HF
- Pulmonary edema
- Aortic dissection
- Acute renal failure or dysfunction evidenced by hematuria, proteinuria, or elevated serum creatinine
- States of catecholamine excess
- Epistaxis
- Preeclampsia or eclampsia
- Change in mental status or neurologic deficits on physical examination
- Dementia

CLINICAL PRESENTATION

Subjective

The history should include a thorough investigation of cardiovascular risk factors such as age, gender, menopausal status, diet, physical activity level, alcohol and caffeine use, smoking, dyslipidemia, diabetes mellitus, family history of heart disease, and current medications. Some medications, such as NSAIDs and sympathomimetic OTC cold remedies, may exacerbate BP elevation. Culture and ethnicity should be assessed within the history as well. As noted earlier, compared with European Americans, African Americans have a higher risk of HTN, diabetes mellitus, and renal impairment, which all requires aggressive management of BP and specific drug therapy.

Diagnosis of HTN is typically made after several routine outpatient visits with the patient complaining of no symptoms. Occasionally, if the BP is extremely elevated, the patient may present with a headache that occurs on awakening and is located in the occipital area. Hypertensive urgency or emergency may present with complaints related to the particular type of end-organ damage (e.g., chest pain from cardiac ischemia, blurred vision from papilledema, mental status changes from TIA).

Objective

A systematic approach should be used when assessing the person with or at risk of HTN.

A patient presenting with acute, severely elevated BP requires a thorough clinical examination that includes staging of the BP elevation and investigation for evidence of hypertensive TOD. This evaluation should include funduscopic examination, palpation of the chest for point of maximal impulse (PMI), auscultation of the heart, abdominal assessment for bruits or widened aortic diameter and enlarged kidneys, examination of the carotid arteries for bruits, palpation of peripheral pulses, and a neurologic examination, such as funduscopy, electrocardiogram (ECG), urinalysis, serum creatinine measurements, and a chest x-ray. A computed tomography (CT) scan of the head to rule out stroke may be necessary, if the patient presents with mental status changes.

Table 35.1 presents the most recent 2017 American Heart Association/American College of Cardiology (ACC/AHA) HTN classification guidelines. The assessment should include two measurements of BP in both arms, with the patient seated with both feet on a flat surface (crossing the legs may increase the systolic BP [SBP] by 2–8 mm Hg) and the back supported with the arm at heart level (diastolic BP [DBP] may be decreased by up to 6 mm Hg if the arm is below the level of the heart). The patient should remain quiet and not speak during the reading. As noted earlier, an appropriately sized cuff for the patient is critical because a cuff that is too large will provide a falsely low BP, whereas a cuff that is too small will provide a falsely elevated BP. When elevated BPs are detected, a bilateral assessment for confirmation should be obtained if not contraindicated (e.g., by the presence of an atrioventricular shunt or postmastectomy status). BP should be taken again after the patient has stood for at least 2 minutes, and the higher readings should be recorded.

In certain patient groups such as the elderly, the obese, and patients with arrhythmias, certain clinically meaningful findings should be noted. In the elderly, the clinician should note whether an auscultatory gap is common, as this may be associated with vascular disease and result in an underestimation of SBP. In addition, if severe vessel rigidity is present in the brachial artery, the BP cuff may be unable to adequately compress the calcified vessel, leading to a falsely elevated BP reading. This phenomenon is known as *pseudohypertension*. Although this may increase the BP reading by 30 mm Hg or more, it does not by itself represent a disease state.

The obese patient often has a short upper arm length relative to upper arm width; in this instance, a wrist cuff may be used with the wrist placed at heart level to obtain an accurate BP reading. In patients with highly irregular arrhythmias such as atrial fibrillation, the BP varies from beat to beat, so the clinician should measure the BP several times and average the readings. In patients with severe bradycardia, the provider should deflate the cuff more slowly to prevent underestimating SBP and overestimating DBP.

The United Kingdom's National Institute for Health and Clinical Excellence guidelines state that a diagnosis of primary HTN should be confirmed with 24-hour ABPM or sequential home BP readings. Twenty-four-hour ABPM is indicated to rule out "white coat" or "masked" HTN, to uncover apparent drug-resistant HTN, and to identify hypertensive symptoms while the patient is being treated with antihypertensive medication.

Advanced Assessment 35.1 lists common findings associated with HTN. Evidence of TOD includes retinopathy, which may appear as arteriolar narrowing, arteriovenous nicking, hemorrhages, or exudates. A bruit may be auscultated over either carotid artery, indicating stenosis. The chest may demonstrate a displaced PMI and/or an S_4 heart sound indicating left ventricular hypertrophy (LVH). Auscultation of an S_4 heart sound is associated with the decreased elasticity of the left ventricle (LV) that occurs in LVH. The patient should also be evaluated for the presence of HF, a known sequela of long-standing HTN. An S_3 gallop, pulmonary crackles, jugular venous distention, and peripheral edema are signs of HF. A bruit heard in the abdomen may indicate an aneurysm or renal artery stenosis. Palpation of a widened aortic pulsation is associated with abdominal aortic aneurysm. Diminished peripheral pulses and loss of sensation in the lower extremities can indicate peripheral arterial disease. Neurologic examination can reveal deficits associated with TIA or a CVA.

DIAGNOSTIC REASONING

Diagnostic Tests

Diagnostic testing of a patient who has or is suspected of having HTN should focus on the evaluation of target organs and related comorbidities, as well as on excluding certain causes of secondary HTN. Additional testing may

TABLE 35.1   Classification of Blood Pressure for Adults Aged 18 Years or Older

Blood Pressure (BP) Category	Systolic BP (mm Hg)	Diastolic BP (mm Hg)
Normal	<120 and	<80
Elevated	120–129	<80
Hypertension		
Stage 1	130–139 or	80–89
Stage 2	≥140 or	≥90

Source: Whelton PK, Carey RM, Aronow WS, et al. ACC/AHA/AAPA/ABC/ACPM/AGS/APhA/ASH/ASPC/NMA/ PCNA guideline for the prevention, detection, evaluation, and management of high blood pressure in adults: Executive summary: A report of the American College of Cardiology/American Heart Association task force on clinical practice guidelines. *J Am Soc Hypertens.* 2018;12:579.

✜ Advanced Assessment 35.1: Hypertension

Assessment	Common Findings
BLOOD PRESSURE MEASUREMENT	
Proper technique: • Cuff size has a bladder length of 80% and a width of at least 40% of arm circumference • Patient in a sitting position, arm resting at level of the heart with feet on flat surface and legs uncrossed. • Rest for 5 minutes before measurement. • Average two readings at least 2 minutes apart (if >5 mm Hg difference, obtain additional readings)	SBP >130 mm Hg DBP >80 mm Hg
PHYSICAL EXAMINATION	
Height, weight, BMI	Obesity (BMI >27 kg/m^2), especially with central or truncal pattern
Waist measurement	Men: >39 inches Women: >34 inches
Fundoscopy	Hypertensive retinopathy (arteriolar narrowing, arteriovenous nicking, hemorrhages, exudates, papilledema)
Carotid arteries	Bruits
Neck veins	Distention
Thyroid	Enlargement Nodules
Cardiac	Point of maximal impulse and apex displaced laterally; greater than one intercostal space S$_3$, S$_4$ heart sounds Murmur or mitral regurgitation
Lungs	Crackles Bronchospasm
Abdomen	Bruits, masses, abnormal aortic pulsations Enlarged kidneys
Extremities	Absence of peripheral arterial pulsations Bruits Edema
DIAGNOSTIC TESTS	
Urinalysis	Proteinuria
Blood urea nitrogen/creatinine	Increased
Complete blood count	May show anemia
Potassium	Increased or decreased
Blood glucose	May be increased
Lipids: triglycerides, high-density lipoprotein, low-density lipoprotein	Increased
12-lead ECG	May show target organ damage, e.g., LVH, left atrial enlargement
Brain natriuretic peptide	Hormone released by the ventricle indicative of increased myocardial demand

Abbreviations: BMI, body mass index; DBP, diastolic blood pressure; LVH, left ventricular hypertrophy; SBP, systolic blood pressure.

be indicated, particularly when concurrent diseases such as diabetes mellitus or hyperlipidemia are present.

The ECG is an important screening tool to assess for cardiac TOD in the hypertensive patient. It can be used to assess for the presence of left atrial enlargement (LAE), LVH, myocardial ischemia or infarction, premature ventricular contractions, and atrial fibrillation. LAE is one of the earliest ECG findings associated with HTN. An echocardiogram is useful to detect the presence of increased left ventricular wall thickness and hypertrophy.

Differential Diagnosis

The key to differential diagnosis is to determine the underlying etiology of the HTN, whether it is essential or secondary, for instance, and to assess the degree of HTN (and whether malignant or benign, etc.). A presumptive diagnosis is made if the average of at least two seated BP measurements on at least two or more visits exceeds either 80 mm Hg DBP or 130 mm Hg SBP in adults older than 18 years.

Some concurrent health problems, if inadequately treated, may also affect BP. For example, the normal pain response includes vasoconstriction and tachycardia; therefore, inadequate control of both acute and chronic pain can cause a rise in BP. In turn, adequate pain control may resolve the HTN. Certain clinical conditions may also necessitate the use of drugs that can cause or exacerbate HTN, such as cyclosporine, erythropoietin, and certain antidepressants (e.g., tricyclic antidepressants, selective serotonin-norepinephrine reuptake inhibitors). In this case, reducing the dose or stopping the causative agent of HTN should be explored, but if that is not possible, antihypertensive treatment must be chosen with care and an adequate dose prescribed, which may require referral to a HTN specialist.

MANAGEMENT

Approximately one in five adults will need medication to treat HTN. The key to HTN management is not only the reversal of HTN-related disease trends but also the prevention of TOD. The following recommendations are public health approaches to achieve a downward shift in BP distribution at the population level, thereby reducing morbidity, mortality, and the lifetime risk of an individual becoming hypertensive:

- Develop community health programs to stress reducing calories, saturated fat, and salt in processed foods.
- Encourage food manufacturers and restaurants to reduce the sodium in the food supply by 50% over the next decade.
- Increase community/school opportunities for physical activity.
- Address the diversity of racial, ethnic, cultural, linguistic, religious, and social factors in the delivery of community services to increase the community's receptiveness to use of public health services.
- Improve opportunities for treatment and control of HTN, as health-care providers help break down barriers to the diagnosis and treatment of HTN (e.g., nursing and work-site clinics that offer health services on evenings and weekends, thereby increasing the likelihood of access to care for those who work during weekday hours).

The use of lifestyle modifications (Box 35.2) should be a part of every patient's regimen to prevent or treat

elevated BP. The primary-care practitioner should work with the patient on a plan of lifestyle modification and medications as needed to lower the BP as much as is tolerated without symptoms. Patient-specific goals include the following:

- Increase awareness regarding the risks of prehypertension and the development of frank HTN. Teens and young adults with high-normal BP are at markedly increased risk of developing HTN in their fourth and fifth decades of life. Behavioral therapies such as a program of regular aerobic exercise and a diet that is low in fat and sodium and high in potassium should be initiated to help avoid HTN in otherwise healthy individuals.
- Know one's own BMI, which should serve as a guide to weight loss rather than just aiming for an ideal body weight, which may prove particularly daunting for some individuals.
- Improving HTN control in persons already diagnosed with HTN. Many patients diagnosed and started on treatment for HTN still have a BP greater than 130/80 mm Hg (see Table 35.1 for specific diagnostic thresholds), demonstrating inadequate control.
- Reduce cardiovascular risks, in addition to BP. Many patients with HTN will have additional modifiable cardiovascular disease risk factors such as diabetes mellitus, hyperlipidemia, tobacco use, and physical inactivity/sedentary lifestyle; therefore, a comprehensive plan to treat HTN must also address these issues.

In 2014, the panel appointed to the Eighth Joint National Committee (JNC 8) published new recommendations for HTN that raised BP treatment thresholds. The JNC 8 guidelines are presently guiding practice in many clinical settings and were supported by the Core Quality Measures Collaborative convened by the Centers for Medicare and Medicaid and America's Health Insurance Plans. Although they are a part of this collaborative, the AHA and ACC did not endorse the JNC 8 Guidelines, stating that the proposed relaxed BP targets could cause harm to millions of patients by placing patients at greater risk for stroke and heart disease. In November 2017, the ACC/AHA published stricter guidelines with lower BP treatment thresholds than those recommended by the JNC 8.

Patients with an elevated SBP up to 129 mm Hg and a DBP up to 80 mm Hg should adopt healthy lifestyle choices and have their BP reevaluated in 3 to 6 months. For patients with Stage 1 HTN, the 10-year cardiovascular risk of heart disease and stroke should be calculated. The AHA/American Stroke Association offers a calculator to determine the risk of heart disease and stroke that is based on a patient's age, lipid profile (total cholesterol [TC], as well as low-density lipoprotein [LDL], and high-density lipoprotein [HDL]), current BP, and related medical history, including whether the patient is being treated for HTN and whether the patient has a history of stroke,

Box 35.2　Metabolic Syndrome

Metabolic syndrome refers to a cluster of specific cardiovascular-related diseases and diabetes mellitus risk factors in which the underlying pathophysiology is thought to be related to insulin resistance. Because the term *metabolic syndrome* has been imprecisely defined, the primary-care practitioner should evaluate and treat all CVD risk factors without regard to whether a patient meets the criteria for diagnosis of metabolic syndrome. Nevertheless, clinicians need to be cognizant of new information pertaining to this syndrome, because definitions change rapidly.

Metabolic syndrome has been characterized as a combination of atherogenic and diabetogenic factors. Increased BMI, elevated SBP, hypertriglyceridemia, hyperglycemia, and low levels of protective HDL-C are found in affected persons. Any three of these conditions occurring together usually establish the diagnosis (see Table 35.2). The etiology of metabolic syndrome is unknown; however, environmental, genetic, and behavioral factors contribute to the development of metabolic syndrome, particularly physical inactivity and excess body fat. Elevated BMI is apparent as central obesity, with the affected individual demonstrating an "apple shape" or high waist circumference.

Metabolic syndrome is also a proinflammatory and prothrombotic disorder causing endothelial injury, as evidenced by elevations of the inflammatory marker C-reactive protein, increased platelet aggregation, and increased fibrinogen levels. In addition to hyperglycemia and deranged lipid metabolism, peripheral tissues are resistant to insulin. The pancreas over-secretes insulin to overcome tissue resistance, which results in hyperinsulinemia. Obesity enhances insulin resistance and predisposes the individual to type 2 diabetes mellitus.

Obesity is believed to contribute significantly to the development of metabolic syndrome. The National Cholesterol Education Program recommends obesity as the primary target for intervention. Abdominal obesity is defined as a high waist-to-hip ratio. Weight loss improves serum lipid profiles, reduces BP, decreases insulin resistance, and ameliorates glucose intolerance.

For further discussion of metabolic syndrome, see the section in Chapter 59.

TABLE 35.2　Components of Metabolic Syndrome

Risk Factor (three required for diagnosis)	Defining Level
Central (Abdominal) Obesity Men: Women:	*Waist Circumference* >40 inches >35 inches
Fasting Triglycerides	>150 mg/dL (or taking medication for high TGs)
HDL-C (cardioprotective form) Men: Women:	<40 mg/dL (or taking medication for low HDL-C) >50 mg/dL (or taking medication for low HDL-C)
Blood Pressure	≥130 / ≥85 mm Hg (or taking medication for HTN)
Fasting Glucose	>100 mg/dL (or taking medication for hyperglycemia)

Abbreviations: HDL-C, high-density lipoprotein-cholesterol; HTN, hypertension; TG, triglycerides.
Source: Adapted from http://www.heart.org/idc/groups/heart-public/@wcm/@hcm/documents/downloadable/ucm_300322.pdf.

In patients with diabetes mellitus, the American Diabetes Association continues to recommend a target SBP of less than 130 mm Hg and a target DBP of less than 80 mm Hg. For patients with chronic kidney disease and proteinuria, the therapeutic plan should be individualized with attention to balancing side effects of medications (e.g., hypotension or worsening renal disease) with recommended BP goals. Renal impairment should compel the clinician and patient to work together to maintain meticulous BP control in order to minimize the development of nephropathy. In addition to public health programs, community-affiliated programs, including parish-based, neighborhood, and work-site programs and health-promotion events, should be used to assist patients, as well as those with normal BP, to make healthy lifestyle choices.

Special Considerations for Older Adults

Nearly one-half of all adults aged 65 years and older develop isolated systolic HTN, defined as an SBP above 160 mm Hg with a normal DBP (80 mm Hg or below) as a consequence of atherosclerotic thickening of the vessels. More than two-thirds of persons older than 65 years develop HTN, and as the 2017 ACC/AHA guidelines are stricter than in the past, even more Americans are expected to meet the criteria for HTN and require treatment. Given its frequency, the development of isolated systolic HTN is often viewed as an unavoidable consequence of aging. However, primary-care practitioners should be aware that behaviorally based therapies used to prevent and

angina, diabetes mellitus, peripheral artery disease, MI, or atherosclerotic cardiovascular disease (ASCVD).

If their calculated cardiovascular risk is less than 10%, they should institute lifestyle changes and reassess their BP in 3 to 6 months. If their risk is more than 10%, they should institute lifestyle changes and start antihypertensive medication with monthly follow-up visits until their BP is controlled. If they have Stage 2 HTN, lifestyle changes should be instituted as well as antihypertensive medications from two pharmacologic classes, with monthly follow-up visits until the control of BP is achieved.

treat HTN can also help minimize age-associated increases in BP.

Historically, older adults with HTN have not received the emphasis on treatment that was merited. Present-day guidelines now stress the importance of treating HTN in older adults, which results in a significant reduction in congestive HF (CHF), cardiovascular, and cerebrovascular disease. Even in persons older than 50 years of age, SBP greater than 130 mm Hg is a much more important risk factor for cardiovascular disease than elevated DBP. Even patients with a normal BP at 55 years of age still have a 90% lifetime risk for developing HTN. In a patient with a BP of 115/75 mm Hg, the risk of cardiovascular disease doubles with each incremental increase of 20/10 mm Hg.

Pharmacologic Therapy

Antihypertensive drug therapy is not recommended if there is no compelling indication other than potential risk factors for HTN, for which lifestyle modifications should be instituted. In turn, monitoring for drug-induced HTN is essential before the initiation of pharmaceutical therapy, for example, iatrogenic HTN due to the use of NSAIDs, glucocorticoids, antidepressants, oral contraceptives, hormone replacement therapy, and OTC sympathomimetic decongestants (cold medications). The use of alcohol and tobacco must also be assessed, as well as the presence of sleep apnea.

For most patients with newly diagnosed HTN, therapeutic lifestyle changes should be instituted for 1 month and, if ineffective in lowering the BP after 1 month, pharmacotherapy should be added. In patients other than African Americans, including those with diabetes mellitus, initial antihypertensive treatment should include any one of four classes of oral medication, which improve cardiovascular outcomes: a thiazide-type diuretic, a calcium channel blocker (CCB), an angiotensin-converting enzyme inhibitor (ACEI), or an angiotensin receptor blocker (ARB). Initial therapy should consist of a low dose of the chosen agent, which may be increased in dose if it is well tolerated but BP control has not yet been achieved.

Thiazide-type diuretics are first-line antihypertensive drugs. These agents are useful in the presence of isolated systolic HTN. They are also helpful for patients with osteoporosis because they help preserve bone density. Use of thiazide-type diuretics has been shown to reduce stroke and cardiovascular-related mortality and morbidity. Chlorthalidone 12.5 to 25 mg per day is the recommended first-line thiazide diuretic drug. A second choice is hydrochlorothiazide initiated at a similar dose.

In African Americans, initial treatment may consist of either a CCB or a thiazide diuretic (ACEIs have been shown to be less effective in this population). In patients with chronic kidney disease, pharmacologic treatment should be initiated to lower SBP to less than 130 mm Hg

and DBP to less than 80 mm Hg. The initial agent of choice in patients with chronic kidney disease should be an ACEI or ARB.

The primary-care practitioner should choose an antihypertensive therapy with the patient's concurrent medical history and comorbid conditions in mind. Examples of antihypertensive drugs that can be used in patients with concurrent diseases include choices from the following pharmacologic classes:

- **Angiotensin-converting enzyme inhibitors** (ACEIs—drugs with generic names typically ending in -*pril,* such as captopril) are effective in the presence of HF and MI with systolic dysfunction to help limit the effects of myocardial remodeling. ACEIs should be used when certain comorbid conditions including renal insufficiency and diabetes mellitus are present, as these drugs may assist in preserving or enhancing renal function.
- **Angiotensin II receptor blockers** (ARBs) are helpful in antihypertensive individuals with comorbid conditions such as HF and type 2 diabetes mellitus. Because they have a higher cost than ACEIs and because long-term research is lacking, ARBs should be reserved for patients who develop a cough when taking ACEIs or are otherwise intolerant, although some clinicians consider there to be a risk of cross-reactivity to ARBs in patients who are anaphylactic to ACEIs and will consider both classes contraindicated in these patients. Given their related mechanisms of action, an ACEI and an ARB should not be used in combination.
- **Beta blockers** (drugs with generic names ending in -*lol,* such as metoprolol) are no longer commonly recommended for the primary management of HTN but may be used in the presence of angina, post-MI (to reduce cardiac workload and enhance rhythm stability), atrial tachycardia, migraine headache (as a nonselective agent for the reduction in frequency and severity of migraine headaches), and essential tremor (as a nonselective agent).
- Long-acting dihydropyridine **CCBs** (drugs with generic names ending in -*pine,* such as amlodipine) are suggested for black patients of African or Caribbean descent who are younger than 55 years, for patients with isolated systolic HTN, and for hypertensive patients with concurrent stable angina pectoris.
- **Alpha-adrenergic antagonists** (alpha blockers) are usually effective in patients with benign prostatic hyperplasia because they facilitate bladder emptying by decreasing prostate size.
- Additional drugs may include **combination therapies** with two drugs in one tablet, such as combinations of an ACEI and a CCB, an ACEI and a diuretic, an ARB and a diuretic, a centrally acting agent and a diuretic, or more than one diuretic (see Drugs Commonly Prescribed 35.1).

After the initiation of pharmacologic treatment, the BP should be reevaluated within a month. If the goal

Drugs Commonly Prescribed 35.1: Hypertension

MEDICATIONS PREFERRED WITH SPECIFIC COMORBID CONDITIONS (SEE DRUG CLASSIFICATIONS BELOW FOR ABBREVIATIONS)

Diabetes mellitus*	Angiotensin-converting enzyme inhibitor ACEI) or angiotensin II receptor blocker (ARB) For metabolic syndrome, ACEI or ARB or calcium channel blocker (CCB)
Chronic kidney disease	ACEI or ARB
Heart failure (HF)†	ACEI or ARB, mineralocorticoid receptor antagonist, beta blocker, diuretic (loop diuretic preferred) For left ventricular hypertrophy: ACEI or ARB, along with CCB
High-risk coronary artery disease (CAD)	Beta blocker or CCB for angina ACEI or CCB for asymptomatic atherosclerosis
Post–myocardial infarction (MI)	ACEI or ARB, beta blocker
Recurrent stroke prevention	Any effective antihypertensive

*To reduce risk for major cardiovascular events and slow progression of chronic kidney disease in adults with diabetes mellitus not on dialysis with urine albumin of <30 mg/24 hours, the blood pressure goal is <140/90 mm Hg. If urine albumin is >30 mg/24 hour, the goal is ≤130/80 mm Hg.
†Combined therapy should be used cautiously in those at risk for orthostatic hypotension.

DRUG CLASSIFICATION	INDICATION	ADVERSE REACTIONS AND PRESCRIBING CONSIDERATIONS
Diuretics		
Thiazide diuretics chlorthalidone (Hygroton) hydrochlorothiazide (HCTZ)	First-line diuretic to treat hypertension (HTN). Thiazide diuretics are indicated in the management of HTN, either as the sole therapeutic agent or to enhance the effect of other antihypertensive drugs in more severe forms of HTN.	Use with caution in severe renal disease, which may precipitate azotemia, and in patients with impaired hepatic function. Contraindicated in patients with anuria or known hypersensitivity to these products or other sulfonamide-derived drugs. Use with caution in patients with hepatic impairment, given the risk of hepatic coma. Hypokalemia, hyperuricemia, and rise in lipid levels may occur. May cause occasional urticaria and skin rash, postural hypotension, gastrointestinal (GI) distress, loss of appetite, impotence, and vertigo. Thiazide diuretics are less effective when creatinine is >1.8 mg/dL.
Loop diuretics bumetanide (Bumex) furosemide (Lasix)	Loop diuretics are more potent than thiazides in promoting diuresis; however, they are less effective than thiazides in blood pressure (BP) management. Indicated for the treatment of mild to moderate HTN and in the management of edema associated with congestive HF. Also beneficial in the management of HTN associated with hepatic and renal disease, including nephritic syndrome. Will likely remain effective in patients who have creatinine > 1.8.	May cause hypokalemia, hyponatremia, low magnesium, dehydration, postural hypotension, tinnitus, hyperuricemia leading to gout, increased sensitivity to sunlight. Hypertensive patients who cannot be adequately controlled with thiazides will probably also be inadequately controlled with furosemide alone.
Aldosterone receptor blockers spironolactone (Aldactone)	Weak antihypertensives. Potassium-sparing diuretics are indicated for the treatment of HTN or edema in patients who develop hypokalemia. Aldosterone antagonists block the effects of serum aldosterone and are effective at regulating Na+ and water homeostasis to maintain stable intravascular volume.	The use of potassium-sparing agents is often unnecessary in patients receiving diuretics for uncomplicated essential HTN, when such patients have a normal diet. May cause nervousness, skin rash, increased sensitivity to sunlight, confusion, irregular heart rhythm, shortness of breath, lethargy, and weakness. Hyperkalemia risk is increased with the use of ACEI or ARB. Use with caution in cases of renal impairment.

Continued

Drugs Commonly Prescribed 35.1: Hypertension—cont'd

DRUG CLASSIFICATION	INDICATION	ADVERSE REACTIONS AND PRESCRIBING CONSIDERATIONS
Beta-Adrenergic Receptor Blockers		
Carvedilol (Coreg) Metoprolol (Toprol) Propranolol (Inderal)	Not indicated as first-line management of HTN unless compelling indications such as acute coronary syndrome (ACS) or HF are present. May be used in combination with other antihypertensive agents, especially thiazide-type diuretics. Beta blockers are a component of core measures in patients with ACS.	May cause sinus bradycardia, atrioventricular block, hypotension, shortness of breath, depression, dizziness, fatigue, vivid dreams, diarrhea, nausea/vomiting, increased triglycerides, sexual dysfunction, pruritus, skin hyperpigmentation, alopecia, xerosis, and urticaria. Use with caution in patients with chronic obstructive pulmonary disease, asthma, and peripheral vascular disease. May increase the risk of developing type 2 diabetes mellitus.
Angiotensin-Converting Enzyme Inhibitors (ACEIs)		
Enalapril (Vasotec) Lisinopril (Zestril)	Use alone or in combination with thiazide diuretics. Effective for patients with HF, post-MI, left ventricular dysfunction, renal insufficiency, or glomerulosclerosis. Diabetes mellitus with nephropathy may likewise benefit. May be effective in the prevention of stroke. ACEIs are a component of core measures in patients with ACS.	May exacerbate hyperkalemia and carries the risk of severe angioedema of oral (e.g., tongue, lips) and upper respiratory tract structures. Avoid in pregnancy. May cause a chronic cough through effects on the bradykinin pathway. When given with an aldosterone receptor blocker, may cause orthostatic hypotension, sinus tachycardia, fatigue, dizziness, syncope, headache, or hyperkalemia. Renal adjustment is indicated in renal insufficiency. Do not dose in the presence of bilateral renal artery stenosis.
Angiotensin II Receptor Blockers (ARBs)		
Losartan (Cozaar) Olmesartan (Benicar) Valsartan (Diovan)	Use alone or in combination with other antihypertensive agents. ARBs are an alternative to ACEIs in patients who develop a chronic cough secondary to ACEI usage. Attention must be paid to the exact cause of the cough to rule out other etiologies, such as to identify possible worsening of HF.	Avoid use in pregnancy. May exacerbate hyperkalemia, hyponatremia, angioedema, renal impairment, orthostatic hypotension, syncope, dizziness, and insomnia.
Calcium Channel Blockers (CCBs)		
Nondihydropyridine CCBs Diltiazem (Cardizem) Verapamil (Calan) Dihydropyridine CCBs Amlodipine (Norvasc) Felodipine (Plendil)	Most potent antihypertensive agents routinely utilized. May be useful for the treatment of stable angina pectoris, especially dihydropyridines. CCBs may be effective in the management of angina from coronary artery vasospasm. Effective in reducing cardiac muscle burden and lessens myocardial demand for oxygen. Nondihydropyridines have antichronotropic effects on certain tachycardic arrhythmias (e.g., atrial fibrillation).	Use with caution in HF and second- and third-degree heart block (unless pacer is in place). Effects of CCBs are potentiated by grapefruit juice. May cause lower extremity edema. Avoid in patients with recent MI. May cause peripheral edema, headache, dizziness, flushing, palpitations, fatigue, nausea/vomiting, abdominal pain, and drowsiness. Caution in acute HF, renal, or hepatic impairment.

Drugs Commonly Prescribed 35.1: Hypertension—cont'd

DRUG CLASSIFICATION	INDICATION	ADVERSE REACTIONS AND PRESCRIBING CONSIDERATIONS
Alpha-Adrenergic Receptor Blockers		
Doxazosin (Cardura) Prazosin (Minipress) Terazosin (Hytrin)	Use with benign prostatic hyperplasia, prostatism, and dyslipidemia. May be used alone or in combination with diuretics, beta blockers, CCBs, or ACEIs.	Do not use as first-line or "solo" agents, as this is associated with higher rates of stroke and HF. Alters lipid metabolism by decreasing low-density lipoprotein and very low-density lipoprotein cholesterol. May cause mild sexual dysfunction, dizziness, light-headedness, headache, drowsiness, fatigue, nausea/vomiting, peripheral edema, nasal congestion, and palpitations. May cause complications years later during eye surgery (e.g., cataract removal) by leading to floppy iris syndrome.
Centrally Acting Agents		
Alpha-methyldopa (Aldomet) Clonidine (Catapres)	Effectively lower BP by decreasing central sympathetic outflow and peripheral resistance.	May cause drowsiness, impotence, dry mouth, increased respirations, increased GI motility, and miosis. Less common effects are depression and Coombs-positive anemia (with alpha-methyldopa). Abrupt withdrawal may lead to a rebound HTN.
Direct Vasodilators		
Hydralazine (Apresoline) Isosorbide dinitrate (Isordil) Isosorbide mononitrate (Imdur) Minoxidil (Loniten)	Good for HTN in pregnancy. Injectable hydralazine is used as a first-line agent in the treatment of hypertensive emergencies. Direct vasodilators play an important role in the treatment of severe HF.	May cause peripheral edema, headache, tachycardia, angina, hirsutism, mastalgia, and bullous rash, as well as orthostatic hypotension.
Combination Drug Therapy		
ACEI-CCB Benazepril-amlodipine (Lotrel) Enalapril-felodipine (Lexxel) Trandolapril-verapamil (Tarka)	Effective with atrial tachycardia or fibrillation (especially the nondihydropyridine CCBs) and diabetes mellitus types 1 and 2. CCBs may be useful in Raynaud's syndrome, as well as for isolated systolic HTN and those at high risk of CAD. The nondihydropyridine CCBs (e.g., verapamil and diltiazem) have been shown to reduce cardiovascular mortality, proteinuria, and progression of diabetic nephropathy independent of ACEI use.	See information under ACEIs and CCBs.
ACEI-Diuretic Benazepril-hydrochlorothiazide (Lotensin HCT) Captopril-hydrochlorothiazide (Capozide) Enalapril-hydrochlorothiazide (Vaseretic) Fosinopril-hydrochlorothiazide (Monopril HCT) Lisinopril-hydrochlorothiazide (Prinzide)	See information under ACEIs and Diuretics.	See information under ACEIs and Diuretics.

Continued

Drugs Commonly Prescribed 35.1: Hypertension—cont'd

DRUG CLASSIFICATION	INDICATION	ADVERSE REACTIONS AND PRESCRIBING CONSIDERATIONS
ARB-Diuretic Candesartan-hydrochlorothiazide (Atacand HCT) Eprosartan-hydrochlorothiazide (Teveten HCT) Irbesartan-hydrochlorothiazide (Avalide) Losartan-hydrochlorothiazide (Hyzaar) Olmesartan medoxomil-Hydrochlorothiazide (Benicar HCT) Telmisartan-Hydrochlorothiazide (Micardis) Valsartan-hydrochlorothiazide (Diovan HCT)	See information under ARBs and Diuretics.	See information under ARBs and Diuretics.
Diuretic Combination Spironolactone-hydrochlorothiazide (Aldactazide) HCTZ-triamterene (Dyazide)	Used to treat fluid retention and HTN. See information under Aldosterone receptor blockers and Diuretics.	May exacerbate hyperkalemia, metabolic acidosis, gynecomastia, gout, renal and hepatic impairment. May cause GI disturbances. Useful in patients with refractory HTN. Use in patients with need for potassium-sparing diuretic. Do not use potassium supplements or other diuretics. Advise patients to obtain emergency medical help if any signs of an allergic reaction occur, such as hives, difficulty breathing, swelling of face, lips, tongue, or throat, may cause numbness, muscle pain or weakness, uneven heartbeat, drowsiness, restless, light-headedness, change in urination pattern, shallow breathing, tremors, confusion, nausea, stomach pain, low fever, loss of appetite, dark urine, clay-colored stools, and jaundice.

BP is not attained, up-titration of the dose of the current pharmacologic agent may be required. Alternatively, the addition of a pharmacologic agent from another class may be added at a low starting dose. If BP goals are not obtained with the use of two BP agents, a third agent may be added, although the clinician must be aware of the risks of polypharmacy in such patients. Failure to respond to a triple-therapy regimen may require a referral to a cardiologist or HTN specialist. In addition, a more extensive evaluation for causes of secondary HTN may also be indicated in such patients.

Because small doses of two agents from different pharmacologic classes may have a synergistic effect in lowering BP while avoiding the problems of higher doses of either agent given alone (see Drugs Commonly Prescribed 35.1), these combination products may be appropriate as first-line antihypertensive therapy. In particular, a very low dose (12.5 mg) of chlorthalidone has the ability to potentiate the effect of other agents, without producing negative metabolic effects.

Choosing the Best Drug

Certain patient characteristics, including ethnicity, may influence the choice and efficacy of an antihypertensive agent. A common perception is that the best antihypertensive effect for African Americans and older adults with HTN can be achieved by using a combination of a diuretic and a CCB. This should not be viewed, however, as a contraindication to using ACEIs or ARBs in these populations, as these drugs may offer significant benefit in patients when certain concomitant diseases are present. For example, ACEIs or ARBs may be used in all groups with chronic kidney disease, although higher doses may be necessary in older adults and African Americans, and a longer period of time may elapse before improvement is seen.

An agent with once-daily dosing (i.e., 24-hour duration of action with at least 50% of activity in the past 12 hours) is recommended for chronic use to improve patient adherence and provide persistent, smooth control of HTN (see Drugs Commonly Prescribed 35.1). In addition, with longer-acting formulas, there is less risk of hypertensive rebound resulting from a missed dose, providing protection against risk of stroke, MI, or sudden death from cardiac arrest induced by a dramatic increase in BP.

In certain clinical situations, some medications should be used with caution or are contraindicated because they may have unfavorable effects on comorbid conditions (see Drugs Commonly Prescribed 35.1). The JNC 8 guidelines stress that if the patient's medications are effective, they should not necessarily be changed just because new guidelines have been published.

Age-Related Treatment Concerns

Certain age-related physical changes predispose older adults to difficulty with antihypertensive drug therapy. Because elderly patients benefit significantly from the control of HTN, the appropriate drug should be chosen in consideration of particular factors that increase the risk for postural hypotension, such as a decreased number of baroreceptors. As a result, BP should be measured with the patient in both standing and sitting positions. In addition, older adults should be instructed to change position slowly while on antihypertensive medication.

The force of myocardial contractility decreases with age, leaving older adults more sensitive to antihypertensive medications with negative inotropic effects, such as beta blockers. Because of lower circulating blood volume, diuretics, which are particularly effective antihypertensive agents for this age group, should be used in lower doses. In general, older adults usually have decreased renal excretory capacity; therefore, smaller doses of medications are required. In turn, the adage "Start low and go slow" should be followed, and the dose titration of antihypertensive medication should be monitored closely with every dose adjustment.

The Beers criteria is a clinical tool developed to assist clinicians in improving medication safety in older adults. The clinician should consult the Beers criteria for potentially inappropriate medication use in older adults (American Geriatrics Society 2015 Beers Criteria Update Expert Panel, 2015).

Concurrent Use of Select Concomitant Medications

NSAIDs can negate the BP-lowering effects of select antihypertensive medications such as ACEIs and diuretics by increasing sodium retention. In addition, use of vasoconstricting medications such as decongestants (e.g., pseudoephedrine, phenylpropanolamine, caffeine) and sympathomimetic drugs of abuse (e.g., cocaine, amphetamines) can cause persistently elevated BP readings, despite pharmacologic intervention. Excessive alcohol use may also prevent many antihypertensive medications from achieving their full therapeutic effect. In addition, one of the first manifestations of alcohol withdrawal is BP elevation. Nicotine and many of the chemically active, vasoconstricting substances patients are exposed to with cigarette smoke can also contribute to inadequate BP control.

FOLLOW-UP AND REFERRAL

For the patient undergoing lifestyle modification as initial treatment intervention for HTN, a follow-up visit should be scheduled every 3 to 6 months to determine effectiveness and adherence to the regimen of recommended behavioral changes. If lifestyle modifications are ineffective, pharmacologic therapy should be initiated. HTN can be controlled only if the patient is motivated, and using the *Circle of Caring* model to involve the patient in his or her own care may assist in increasing motivation.

After initiation of antihypertensive pharmacotherapy, a follow-up visit should be scheduled in 2 to 3 weeks for a BP check and possibly in 1 to 2 weeks for an electrolyte or side effect check in at-risk patients. Once the BP goal is reached, visits can be scheduled every 3 months. More frequent visits may be needed if comorbid conditions exist. Serum potassium and creatinine levels should be monitored several times per year.

Patients with refractory HTN, secondary HTN, or comorbid conditions known to increase BP (either by virtue of the condition itself or due to required concomitant medications) should be referred to a cardiologist or HTN specialist for further evaluation and management. In addition, the primary-care practitioner should refer patients with hypertensive emergency to an emergency department or an acute-care setting for appropriate diagnostic testing, monitoring, and treatment.

Patient Education: Hypertension

Lifestyle modifications need to be stressed at each visit, particularly with vigorous promotion of tobacco avoidance. Low-dose aspirin therapy should be initiated once BP control is achieved. If aspirin therapy is started when the patient is still hypertensive, there is a potential risk of hemorrhagic stroke. Because the majority of MIs occur in the morning, aspirin should be administered at night. If a patient is on two antihypertensive medications, one should be given in the morning and one in the evening.

A patient-directed interdisciplinary team approach is critical to successful HTN care. This team should include representatives from nursing, pharmacy, medicine, and nutrition for the continued education of the patient and family and therapeutic monitoring during antihypertensive therapy. Education is stressed to improve patient adherence to behavioral and pharmacologic therapy.

Numerous factors influence the efficacy of HTN therapy. Certain issues should be considered when HTN persists. Nonadherence to therapy is the most common reason for persistent HTN, and the most common reasons for nonadherence are (1) lack of perceived benefit of the intervention, (2) difficulty with provider follow-up, and (3) adverse effects of medication.

The clinician must work with the patient to develop a plan of care that will meet therapeutic goals and fit with the patient's needs. Choosing well-tolerated drugs for intervention and continually acting as the patient's advocate and coach for lifestyle changes are critical.

Using the *Circle of Caring* model, the patient will be involved with the clinician in addressing diet, exercise, tobacco use, and modifiable risk factors that may be positively changed. Family may be an important component of the *Circle of Caring* and should be present when patient teaching occurs. Often, a successful behavioral regimen is spearheaded by a conscientious family member.

The Clin Calc Pooled Cohort Risk Assessment equation can be used to predict the 10-year risk for a first ASCVD event. If a patient's assessed risk is greater than 7.5%, it is recommended that the clinician initiate lipid-lowering therapy in additional to antihypertensive treatment. The primary-care practitioner may choose to use this type of assessment tool with patients to reinforce the clinical impact of disease on their lives and to gain their commitment to make changes.

Oral contraceptives may increase BP, and the risk of HTN increases with the length of use. BP should be monitored regularly in women taking oral contraceptives. If a woman becomes hypertensive while taking oral contraceptives, the primary-care practitioner should advise the patient to consider other forms of birth control.

The frequency of erectile dysfunction (ED) is significantly higher in men who are hypertensive than in men who are normotensive. If ED occurs, the antihypertensive medication should be discontinued and treatment restarted with another agent. Male patients should be advised that there is a lower risk of ED in men who are physically active, nonobese, and nonsmokers. Therefore, pertinent lifestyle modifications should be encouraged in all men to prevent ED.

Because some older adults develop postural hypotension with antihypertensive drug therapy, the primary-care practitioner must educate these patients about avoiding abrupt positional changes while on antihypertensive medication and recommend that they sit on the edge of the bed for several minutes before arising in the morning. In addition, patients with postural hypotension should be urged to avoid volume depletion by drinking adequate quantities of water. In sum, lifestyle modifications cannot be stressed enough in the treatment and prevention of comorbidity due to HTN, and teaching at every visit should reinforce the suggestions listed in Box 35.2.

DYSLIPIDEMIA

Dyslipidemia, also referred to as *hyperlipidemia*, is a general term for elevated concentrations of any or all of the different types of lipids in the plasma. A major risk factor for CVD, increased lipid levels positively correlate with an increased risk of acute coronary syndrome (ACS). The ACC/AHA guidelines recommend considering statin therapy in individuals who do not currently have CVD but who have a 7.5% or greater risk for stroke or heart attack. This risk is calculated using an equation endorsed by the ACC/AHA that includes race, gender, age, TC, HDL, BP, use of BP meds, presence of diabetes mellitus, and smoking status.

The ACC/AHA recommend that the clinician begin a discussion to determine the best lipid-lowering therapy for each unique patient situation. These recommendations from the ACC/AHA are changing the way clinicians view traditional treatment guidelines, as the ACC/AHA stress that many patients are undertreated and not receiving maximal statin therapy. Additionally, the importance of high-intensity dosing of anticholesterol medication has been emphasized.

EPIDEMIOLOGY AND CAUSES

The correlation between dyslipidemia and coronary events is well documented. Elevated lipid levels present the greatest risk factor for the development of CAD. Table 35.3 shows normal and abnormal lipid values and classifications according to the Guidelines of the National Cholesterol Education Program (NCEP) of the National Heart, Lung, and Blood Institute (NHLBI) of the National Institutes of Health.

Dyslipidemia can arise as a result of rare genetic disorders, such as familial hypercholesterolemia. Behavioral factors and lifestyle choices, such as high dietary consumption of fats and a lack of physical activity, much more commonly play a role. Moreover, dyslipidemia can be part of a constellation of abnormalities known as metabolic syndrome characterized by abdominal obesity, glucose intolerance, insulin resistance, hyperinsulinemia, dyslipidemia, and HTN.

TABLE 35.3 Serum Lipid Levels	
Classification Level	*Laboratory Value*
Total Cholesterol (mg/dL)	
Desirable	<200 mg/dL
Borderline high	200–239 mg/dL
High	>240 mg/dL
Triglycerides (mg/dL)	
Normal	<150 mg/dL
Borderline high	150–199 md/dL
High	200–499 mg/dL
Very high	>500 mg/dL
HDL (mg/dL)	
Low	<40 mg/dL
High (optimal: cardioprotective)	>60 mg/dL

Adapted from the Guidelines of the National Cholesterol Education Program of the National Heart, Lung, and Blood Institute of the National Institutes of Health.

It is important to assess patients for secondary causes of dyslipidemia before instituting lipid-lowering treatment, as treatment of the primary disorder can improve or correct the dyslipidemia. Secondary causes of dyslipidemia include obesity, diabetes mellitus, hypothyroidism, nephrotic syndrome, end-stage renal disease, hepatic disorders, excessive alcohol consumption, estrogen administration, Cushing's syndrome, and glycogen storage disease. Certain drugs can cause lipid abnormalities such as thiazide diuretics, corticosteroids, beta blockers, anti-HIV protease inhibitors, isotretinoin, and growth hormone.

In the United States, CVD claims the lives of approximately 801,000 men and women each year. Approximately one in three deaths can be attributed to CVD. The Framingham Heart Study (the largest ongoing cohort study of heart disease in the United States) has documented that 40% of participants with an MI had a TC level between 200 and 250 mg/dL. A patient with a TC level greater than 259 mg/dL is three times more likely to develop CAD than a patient with a level of less than 200 mg/dL. It is important to recognize that dyslipidemia is only one of the many factors that increase the risk of developing CAD. The greater the number of risk factors present, the greater the probability of developing clinically significant CAD.

PATHOPHYSIOLOGY

Dyslipidemia is a heterogeneous metabolic disorder that involves abnormal levels of lipids and lipoproteins that increase the risk of atherosclerosis. Lipoproteins are molecules that carry cholesterol in the bloodstream. Lipoproteins differ in size, density, and atherogenicity and are divided into several classes: very low-density lipoprotein (VLDL), intermediate-density lipoprotein (IDL), LDL, lipoprotein (a) (Lp[a]), and HDL. Atherogenesis is mediated by the lower density lipoproteins: Lp(a), VLDL, IDL, and LDL. These small LDL particles migrate into the inflamed region of the blood vessel wall where they are oxidized and phagocytosed by macrophages to form foam cells, ultimately leading to the formation of fatty streaks and atherosclerotic plaques.

LDL cholesterol (LDL-C) is the specific type of cholesterol that constitutes the lipid core of arteriosclerotic plaque deposits. In clinical analyses, Lp(a), LDL, IDL, and VLDL are combined into the single fraction of LDL. Desirable levels of LDL are dependent on the existence of other CVD risk factors (see Table 35.3 for a classification of all lipid levels). Triglycerides (TGs) are large lipid molecules that also contribute to atherogenesis, which are formed from fats consumed directly in the diet or formed from sugars and alcohols. To prevent cardiovascular disease, the desirable TG level is less than 150 mg/dL.

Atherogenic forms of cholesterol–lipoprotein complexes include all types of non-HDL cholesterol (HDL-C) and triglyceride-transporting proteins: LDL, IDL, Lp(a), and

VLDL. TC in the blood arises both from ingested fats and from synthesis in the liver. The measurement of total blood cholesterol is based on LDL-C, TG, and HDL-C. The following equation is used to calculate TC: TC = LDL-C + TG/5 + HDL-C. The desirable level of TC in the blood without other cardiac risk factors is less than 200 mg/dL.

HDL-C is excreted from the body and, in contrast to LDL-C, is not deposited on arterial walls. HDL removes excess cholesterol from blood vessels and transports it back to the liver through reverse cholesterol transport. Once in the liver, cholesterol is excreted into the intestine as bile. HDL also plays a protective role by blocking the oxidation of LDL, which, in turn, inhibits atherogenesis. A low HDL level (40 mg/dL or less) is considered a cardiovascular risk factor, whereas a high level of HDL-C (60 mg/dL or more) is considered cardioprotective. Thus, an HDL-C level of more than or equal to 60 mg/dL is considered a "negative" or protective cardiovascular risk factor, allowing one to be subtracted from the total number of CVD risk factors, for the purpose of cardiovascular risk prediction.

CLINICAL PRESENTATION

Subjective

Typically, the patient may present without symptoms when diagnosed with dyslipidemia. Often, however, concurrent problems related to CVD, such as HTN or CAD, exist.

Objective

The clinician, on noting an abnormal lipid profile, may be the first to diagnose dyslipidemia in the unsuspecting patient. Physical examination may reveal a carotid bruit or corneal arcus. In some forms of dyslipidemia, yellowish skin deposits of cholesterol called xanthomas may develop. These deposits commonly occur around the eyelids (xanthelasma) and extensor tendons. Interestingly, even with effective lipid-lowering therapy, these deposits tend not to regress.

DIAGNOSTIC REASONING

Diagnostic Tests

The main goal of diagnostic testing for dyslipidemia is to adequately characterize the levels of various components of the plasma lipid compartment, as these levels are used to categorize disease and to set treatment goals. The fourth Adult Treatment Panel guidelines from the NCEP of the NHLBI were released in November 2013. Previous guidelines recommended specific LDL and non-HDL-C targets for patients with CVD, with some targeting LDL levels lower than 100 mg/dL and others proposing levels of less than 70 mg/dL. The latest ACC/AHA guidelines state that there is no evidence from trials to support treatment to a specific LDL target. These guidelines identify four groups of patients for whom to target primary and secondary prevention and concentrate efforts aimed at reducing CV events:

1. Patients with ASCVD
2. Patients with LDL levels greater than or equal to 190 mg/dL, such as those with familial hypercholesterolemia
3. Patients with diabetes mellitus aged 40 to 75 years with LDL between 70 and 189 mg/dL and without evidence of ASCVD
4. Patients without evidence of CVD or diabetes mellitus but who have LDL levels between 70 and 189 mg/dL along with a 10-year risk of ASCVD greater than or equal to 7.5% (as determined by a CV risk calculator)

Testing to assess these higher-risk groups of dyslipidemic patients is critical, as it is recommended that the first two groups use high-intensity statins and the last two groups use moderate-intensity statins.

Differential Diagnosis

Some potential causes of secondary dyslipidemia are listed in Table 35.4. Elevated TC levels may be present in CAD, type II familial hypercholesterolemia, idiopathic hypercholesterolemia, obstructive jaundice, biliary cirrhosis, hypothyroidism, von Gierke's disease (glycogen storage disease type I), pregnancy, uncontrolled diabetes mellitus, other pancreatic disease, chronic nephritis, glomerulosclerosis, and obesity. Although the primary clinical focus is on hyperlipidemia, given the implications for ASCVD, decreased TC levels may be present in malabsorption, starvation, anorexia nervosa, liver disease, severe cell damage, HTN, chronic anemia, and drug therapy with adrenal corticotrophic hormones.

Elevated TG levels may be present in liver disease, alcoholism, nephrotic syndrome, renal disease, hypothyroidism, uncontrolled diabetes mellitus, pancreatitis, gout, glycogen storage disease, post-MI (increased levels may last for 1 year), metabolic diseases related to endocrinopathies, von Gierke's disease, stress, high-carbohydrate diet, and HTN. In contrast, decreased TG levels may be

present in malnutrition, hyperthyroidism, exercise, and malabsorption syndrome.

An elevated HDL level may be associated with chronic liver disease or chronic alcohol abuse/intoxication, long-term aerobic exercise or other vigorous exercise, and elevated estrogen levels or birth control pills. A decreased HDL level may be caused by hypertriglyceridemia, hypothyroidism, end-stage liver disease, diabetes mellitus, obesity, chronic inactivity, uremia, and homozygous Tangier disease (familial alpha-lipoprotein deficiency).

An increased LDL level may be the result of familial hypercholesteremia or secondary causes such as a diet high in cholesterol and saturated fat, nephrotic syndrome, chronic renal failure, pregnancy, porphyria, diabetes mellitus, multiple myeloma, corticosteroid use, and estrogens. A decreased LDL level may be the result of malnutrition and malabsorption syndromes.

An increased VLDL level may be caused by familial hyperlipidemia or secondarily by alcoholism, obesity, diabetes mellitus, chronic renal disease, pancreatitis, pregnancy, estrogen, birth control pills, and progestins. A decreased VLDL level may be the result of malnutrition and malabsorption syndromes.

MANAGEMENT

The primary goals of dyslipidemia treatment are (1) lowering elevated LDL, (2) lowering elevated TG, and (3) raising suboptimal levels of HDL in order to prevent CVD.

Dietary Modification

A cholesterol-lowering diet is recommended for all Americans. Diets very low in total fat or in saturated fat, however, may lower protective HDL-C as much as they do LDL-C. Most nutritionists advocate reducing total fat to 25% to 30% of daily calories and saturated fat to less than 7% of daily calories. The Mediterranean diet has also been shown to decrease cholesterol levels in some patients. This diet is a heart-healthy eating plan that emphasizes fruits, vegetables, whole grains, beans, nuts and seeds, and healthy fats.

Pharmacologic Therapy

For years, diet has been the cornerstone of treatment for hyperlipidemia; however, recent studies have demonstrated that diet alone is often insufficient in lowering cholesterol. The 3-hydroxy-3-methylglutaryl coenzyme A (HMG-CoA) reductase inhibitors (medications with generic names ending in -*statin*) are the first-line drugs of choice in the majority of hyperlipidemic patients. Drugs Commonly Prescribed 35.2 presents information on the different levels of statin therapy along with specific dosages; statin therapies are categorized as either low, moderate, or high intensity. Although some practitioners recommend them, evidence is less consistent to support the use of fibrates, niacin, or fish oil to treat hyperlipidemia.

TABLE 35.4	Potential Causes of Secondary Hyperlipidemia
Causes	*Lipid Abnormalities*
Inactivity	HDL ↓
Alcohol abuse	TG ↑, HDL ↑, LDL ↑
Diabetes mellitus	TG ↑, HDL ↓, TC ↑
Hypothyroidism	TG ↑, TC ↑
Thiazide diuretic use (high dose)	TC ↑, LDL ↑, TG ↑
Beta blocker use (high dose)	LDL ↑, HDL ↓
Chronic renal insufficiency	TC ↑, TG ↑

Abbreviations: HDL, high-density lipoprotein; TC, total cholesterol; TG, triglycerides.

Drugs Commonly Prescribed 35.2: Statin Therapy for Hyperlipidemia

DRUG	EFFECT ON LIPIDS	ADVERSE REACTIONS AND PRESCRIBING CONSIDERATIONS
HMG-CoA Reductase Inhibitors (Statins)		
High-Intensity Atorvastatin (Lipitor) 40–80 mg Rosuvastatin (Crestor) 20–40 mg	Decreases LDL by up to 50% on average Increases HDL Decrease TGs	May cause myositis (especially in patients taking fibrates or niacin). Do not use with gemfibrozil. Take in the evening.
Moderate-Intensity Atorvastatin (Lipitor) 10–20 mg Lovastatin (Mevacor) 40 mg Pravastatin (Pravachol) 40–80 mg Rosuvastatin (Crestor) 5–10 mg Simvastatin (Zocor) 20–40 mg	Decreases LDL by 30%–50% on average	Do not give to patients with active or chronic liver disease. Monitor liver function tests before initiating therapy.
Low-Intensity Fluvastatin (Lescol) 20–40 mg Lovastatin (Mevacor) 20 mg Pravastatin (Pravachol) 10–20 mg Simvastatin (Zocor) 10 mg	Decreases LDL up to 30% on average	For patients who cannot tolerate a high- or moderate-dose statin
Combination Therapy		
Statin plus CCB Atorvastatin + amlodipine (Caduet)	Decreases LDL Increases HDL Decreases TGs	May cause edema, dizziness, palpitations, flushing, fatigue, constipation, dyspepsia, abdominal pain, drowsiness, myopathy, elevated liver enzymes, and rhabdomyolysis with renal dysfunction. Monitor liver function before the start of therapy. May increase serum levels of digitalis, hormone concentrations from birth control pills.
Statin plus cholesterol-absorption inhibitor	Decreases LDL Increases HDL Decreases TGs	Caution with moderate to severe liver disease.
Atorvastatin + ezetimibe (Liptruzet) Simvastatin + ezetimibe (Vytorin) Statin plus niacin Lovastatin + niacin (Advicor) Simvastatin + niacin (Simcor)	Atorvastatin + ezetimibe combination lowers LDL by approximately 10% more than atorvastatin alone, but this may not translate to better patient outcomes.	May cause headache, fatigue, myalgia, extremity pain, myopathy, rhabdomyolysis, and elevated serum transaminases. Avoid fibrates, alcohol, and grapefruit juice. May potentiate vasoactive drugs. Monitor warfarin and antidiabetics. Niacin-containing combinations may cause flushing, headache, pain, pruritus, and dyspepsia.

Abbreviations: CCBs, calcium channel blockers; HDL, high-density lipoprotein; LDL, low-density lipoprotein; TGs, triglycerides.

Once the initial dose of a statin medication is prescribed, the primary-care practitioner should consider whether to increase the dose or add another agent if the statin is ineffective or not fully effective at the initial dose. The clinician should caution patients about use of statins with hepatotoxic drugs or alcohol. Other adverse effects include muscle weakness and, in extreme cases, rhabdomyolysis with significant elevations in serum creatine phosphokinase (creatine kinase [CK]) and aldolase levels. GI complaints include dyspepsia and abdominal pain.

To determine if a patient should be on a statin, the primary-care practitioner should consider the following four questions; if any response is *yes*, the patient is a potential candidate:

1. Does the patient have a history of any of the following?
   a. ACS
   b. MI
   c. Stable or unstable angina
   d. Coronary or arterial revascularization
   e. Stroke, TIA
   f. Peripheral arterial disease of atherosclerotic origin
2. Does the patient have an LDL level of greater than or equal to 190 mg/dL (indicative of familial hypercholesterolemia)?

3. Is the patient 40 to 75 years of age with diabetes mellitus?
4. Is the patient 40 to 75 years of age with a 10-year cardiovascular risk of greater than or equal to 7.5%?

For patients with ASCVD who are younger than 75 years, high-intensity statin therapy should be used to reduce their LDL-C levels by 50%. For patients older than 75 years, moderate-intensity therapy should be instituted. Moderate-intensity statin therapy should be used for patients with diabetes mellitus aged 40 to 75 years because the goal is to reduce the LDL-C level by 30% to 49%. If these patients have a 10-year cardiovascular risk of greater than 7.5%, high-intensity therapy should be used. In addition, for patients aged 40 to 75 years without CVD or diabetes mellitus, but who have a cardiovascular risk score greater than 7.5% and an LDL level of 70 to 189 mg/dL, moderate-intensity therapy is also acceptable.

If patients do not fall into any of the previous categories, additional factors should be considered that suggest the need for statin therapy, such as family history of premature ASCVD in a first-degree relative, high-sensitivity C-reactive protein (hsCRP) greater than 2 mg/dL, presence of calcification on a coronary artery calcium scan, and an ankle-brachial index less than 0.9.

FOLLOW-UP AND REFERRAL

Because hyperlipidemia is so common, the primary-care practitioner must be prepared to treat patients with this condition. If treatment goals are not reached, consultation with a cardiologist may be indicated. Consultation with a nutritionist may be recommended if the patient cannot follow or understand how to adhere to a cholesterol-lowering diet. Endocrinological referral is indicated for familial hypercholesterolemia.

Patient Education: Dyslipidemia

Lifestyle counseling should occur at the initial and follow-up visits as the foundation for statin therapy and may lower the patient's overall risk of morbidity due to hyperlipidemia. It is important for the primary-care practitioner to provide ongoing support and reinforcement to patients undertaking both dietary modification and pharmacologic therapy for dyslipidemia. Many patients do not like to take medications and feel that dietary modification alone is sufficient to keep their cholesterol "under control." Showing patients their laboratory testing results and discussing what the numbers actually mean, especially the ratio of HDL to TC, in terms of the risk of having an MI, is an effective way to get the patient to focus on the potential benefits of combined dietary and pharmacotherapy.

Calculating the patient's 10-year cardiovascular risk score will facilitate the conversation about the possible need for statin therapy. In addition, discussing the patient's Framingham Heart Score to predict the risk of having an acute coronary event may help to motivate a patient in adhering to a comprehensive diet, exercise, and drug treatment program. The ACC/AHA urges clinicians to use shared decision-making models. The *Circle of Caring* model encourages shared decision making and supports patients in initiating long-term lifestyle and medication changes.

CORONARY HEART DISEASE

Coronary heart disease (CHD) is the leading cause of death in the United States, responsible for more than one in seven deaths per year. Mortality from CHD has declined in recent years because of patient education regarding risk factors, early recognition and treatment of CHD symptoms, management of comorbidities such as HTN, dyslipidemia, and diabetes mellitus, as well as therapeutic advances such as thrombolytic drugs.

EPIDEMIOLOGY AND CAUSES

Nearly 13 million Americans have CHD, the incidence of which increases with age. CHD is also a major killer of women, as more than 10 times the number of women die from ASCVD each year than from breast cancer.

The causes of CHD are reflected in a number of risk factors that are classified as nonmodifiable, modifiable, or contributing. These risk factors are ostensibly associated with the development of ASCVD, which is the primary etiology of CHD.

Risk Factors: Coronary Heart Disease

Nonmodifiable:

- Male gender
- Increasing age
- Family history of CAD
- African-American ethnicity

Modifiable:

- Hypertension (>140 mm Hg SBP and/or >90 mm Hg DBP, depending on age)
- Smoking
- Sedentary lifestyle
- Hyperlipidemia
- For women: natural or surgical menopause without estrogen replacement therapy; oral contraceptive use combined with cigarette smoking

Contributing:

- Diabetes mellitus
- Obesity
- Stress

PATHOPHYSIOLOGY

The coronary arteries provide arterial blood flow that supplies oxygen and nutrients to allow for optimal myocellular function of the heart. The coronary arteries dilate via the release of vasoactive substances that further augment oxygen delivery to keep pace with changing metabolic demands. In addition, the lumen of each coronary artery needs to be patent in order to maintain optimal tissue perfusion.

In CAD, arteriosclerotic plaque formation along the inner vessel walls hinders optimal blood flow and dilation of the coronary arteries. Coronary arteries become obstructed, stiffened, and incapable of vasodilation, which severely impedes perfusion of the myocardium. During physical exertion, when increased blood flow to the heart is required for greater myocardial contractility, coronary artery blood flow becomes insufficient for the oxygen demands of the myocardium.

This coronary insufficiency, in turn, leads to ischemia of heart muscle. Ischemia creates anaerobic conditions for the myocardium, particularly if acute occlusion of the coronary vessels results. Anaerobic metabolism yields inadequate energy (approximately 5% of normal) for myocardial demand, allowing for less than a 20-minute period of tissue viability after occlusion. Lactic acid is created as a waste product, leading to localized tissue acidosis. Because lactic acid is irritating to muscle tissue, lactic acid buildup is the source of chest pain in ischemic heart disease. Thus, if left untreated, CAD as a cause of CHD will progress to ischemia of the heart muscle, resulting in angina pectoris (i.e., chest pain due to cardiac ischemia), which can then lead to an MI if the ischemia is persistent.

Although it is the main cause of CHD, *atherosclerosis* (*arteriosclerosis*) is a systemic disease affecting all arteries of the body. *Arteriosclerosis* means "hardened arteries," which is an apt term for the rigid arteries resulting from long-term plaque formation along the vessel wall. Once CAD is diagnosed, it is likely that arteriosclerosis is present throughout all arterial systems, in addition to the heart. Likewise, if vascular disease is identified in target end-organs, CAD is likely to already be present. The process of arteriosclerosis begins with endothelial injury, which can be incited by a number of etiological agents.

Free radicals, HTN, hyperglycemia, and hyperlipidemia have all been found to be agents of injury to arterial endothelial cells that can precipitate atherosclerosis. Endothelial injury provokes an inflammatory reaction that attracts T cells, macrophages, monocytes, and platelets to the site. White blood cells (WBCs) secrete inflammatory cytokines, such as interleukins and tumor necrosis factor–α (TNF-α), as well as acute phase reactants like CRP, which perpetuate the inflammatory reaction. In turn, platelets aggregate and form microthrombi along the vessel wall. Inflammation is now thought to be the major force that drives atherosclerosis. This idea is supported by the prognostic utility of hsCRP levels as a predictor of cardiovascular risk in individuals with coronary arteriosclerosis.

Inflammation of the endothelium depletes nitric oxide, a major vasorelaxant of the arterial muscle wall. This depletion results in a net vasoconstrictive effect. Other proinflammatory mediators stimulate proliferation of vascular smooth muscle within the arterial wall, which further intensifies the vasoconstrictive effect. Concurrently, macrophages within the vessel wall engulf and ingest LDL, forming "foam cells." Disruptions of the arterial endothelium by inflammation, lipid-laden macrophages, platelets, and vasoconstricting mediators are the initiating events of arteriosclerosis and atherogenesis.

In the process of atherogenesis, an initial fatty streak on the arterial wall evolves over time, serving as a nidus for fibrin deposition to become a fibrous, calcified plaque. As they become lined by calcified arteriosclerotic plaque, arteries lose significant vasodilatory capacity. The lipid-rich, calcified plaque becomes brittle and unstable, easily rupturing with mechanical stress due to increased or turbulent blood flow, such as that seen with uncontrolled HTN. When disruption of the plaque occurs, this induces platelet aggregation and activation of the coagulation cascade. A thrombus forms at the site of endothelial injury that can ultimately break-free (embolize), lodge in, and obstruct the lumen of narrowed arteries.

In patients who die from unstable angina or MI, pathological studies find that death occurs as a result of a ruptured plaque with associated thrombosis. Obstruction due to thrombosis is the most common cause of ischemia in *any* arterially supplied region of the body. Ischemia-prone regions of the body include the myocardium, brain, and lower extremities. Common sites of arteriosclerosis are the coronary arteries (i.e., CAD potentially resulting in ACS, including MI), cerebral arteries (potentially resulting in stroke), and peripheral arteries of the lower extremities (potentially resulting in peripheral arterial insufficiency, a form of peripheral vascular disease).

CLINICAL PRESENTATION

Subjective

In most patients, CHD develops many years before the patient is aware of its existence. Because collateral circulation develops, the patient is usually unaware that anything is wrong unless other concomitant conditions are present, such as dyslipidemia or HTN. Thus, the medical history should include a detailed description of all risk factors that may be present, which will guide further assessment for resultant problems such as angina (pertinent questions related to angina are covered in the section on Acute Coronary Syndrome).

Typically, symptoms of CHD are not reported until 75% of a coronary artery is narrowed due to atherosclerosis. Eventually, if CHD is left untreated, the patient will usually present with exertional angina, which should lead the primary-care practitioner to suspect CHD. Angina is the presenting symptom in CHD in 38% of men and 61% of women. Middle-aged and older men and postmenopausal women are most prone to developing angina. Associated symptoms may include radiation of the discomfort to the left arm and jaw, nausea, shortness of breath, and light-headedness or syncopal episodes. It should be noted that not all patients present with these typical CHD symptoms (see Differential Diagnosis).

Objective

For the patient with known or suspected CHD, the primary-care practitioner should note all the peripheral pulses, auscultate for carotid bruits, note jugular venous distention, take the BP in sitting, lying, and standing positions, and examine the skin and nail beds for evidence of decreased perfusion (e.g., prolonged capillary refill time). Because atherosclerosis is a widespread problem, patients with CHD also have a much higher incidence of peripheral vascular disease and cerebrovascular disease than other individuals. In turn, the primary-care practitioner should assess for other symptoms that suggest vascular insufficiency, such as intermittent claudication or TIAs.

DIAGNOSTIC REASONING

Diagnostic Tests

An ECG, cardiac stress test, nuclear myocardial scanning, and coronary angiography may be ordered to determine the extent of CAD as an etiology of CHD and to identify which vessels are affected. Twelve-lead ECGs are discussed in detail later in this chapter in the section on Diagnostic Tests for ACS.

An exercise ECG or cardiac stress test may be ordered to detect and evaluate potential ischemia due to CAD. In these tests, carefully controlled and supervised exercise increases myocardial oxygen demand, which evaluates the coronary arteries' ability to meet this demand for increased myocardial perfusion successfully. When the patient is unable to achieve a vigorous level of exercise, a dipyridamole thallium-201 nuclear stress test may be used. These tests may produce false-positive readings, however, especially in women and in the presence of certain drugs such as beta blockers and CCBs that blunt the adrenergic response, as well as electrolyte imbalances. A stress test is contraindicated in the presence of known acute CVD (e.g., MI, unstable angina, or HF) because the heart cannot respond to the increased demand for oxygen.

Nuclear scanning of the heart (technetium-99m ventriculography) assesses the motion of the left ventricular wall and measures the ventricle's ability to eject blood, referred to as the ejection fraction (normally 55% to 75%). When ischemia is present because of a narrowed coronary artery, the segment of the myocardium served by that particular artery exhibits diminished wall motion (hypokinesis) or contractility that is represented as pooled blood within the ventricular and atrial chambers.

Contrast-enhanced CT scan imaging of the coronary arteries is a noninvasive imaging method of assessing overall "plaque burden" (i.e., the extent to which atheromatous plaque undermines the integrity of an arterial wall). Estimating plaque burden assesses the risk of atheromatous plaque rupturing from the vessel wall and causing ischemia. This type of CT scan, also termed *CT calcium scoring*, evaluates the overall burden of calcified atherosclerotic plaque in the coronary vessels.

A diagnostic cardiac catheterization with angiography for coronary artery visualization is commonly performed after stabilizing a patient in ACS or if there is a high suspicion of ACS. Visualization of the coronary arteries confirms the diagnosis of CAD and can evaluate the extent of coronary artery stenosis. Cardiac catheterization can also be used for interventional purposes to unblock clogged coronary arteries, as discussed in the section on Management of ACS.

Ultrasonography can be used with cardiac catheterization to add diagnostic information. Intravascular ultrasonography (IVUS) used during cardiac catheterization measures plaque burden through real-time intraluminal imaging of vessel walls. IVUS can also be used to assess plaque regression when the patient is on drug therapy for hyperlipidemia.

Because arteriosclerosis is a chronic inflammatory condition, the biomarker CRP is commonly elevated in individuals with CHD. CRP is an acute-phase inflammatory protein produced by the liver and the smooth muscle cells within arteriosclerotic coronary arteries. An elevated level of CRP, as detected by the hsCRP test with greater sensitivity (i.e., a lower limit of detection) than standard CRP testing, has been shown to be an independent predictor of the risk of MI, stroke, peripheral arterial disease, and sudden cardiac death. Measurement of hsCRP adds to the total cardiac risk assessment of the patient but should not be solely relied on as a confirmatory test given its lack of specificity, since CRP levels may be nonspecifically elevated in many different inflammatory conditions of a noncardiac etiology.

Epidemiological studies show that an elevated level of the amino acid homocysteine is an independent risk factor for arteriosclerosis and CHD. Homocysteine requires folic acid, vitamin B_6, and vitamin B_{12} for its metabolism. In turn, this amino acid accumulates in the blood and injures the endothelium when there are inadequate levels of the B complex vitamins and folate for its proper metabolism. Therefore, an elevated serum homocysteine level adds to the cardiac risk assessment of a patient. Of note, reducing homocysteine levels with vitamin supplements has not been shown to reduce the risk of heart disease.

Differential Diagnosis

The key clinical finding of CHD, angina pectoris, may be produced by many causes. A thrombus, coronary artery vasospasm, aortic stenosis, aortic insufficiency, severe HTN, or idiopathic subaortic hypertrophic stenosis can also lead to angina. In addition, the differential diagnosis for CHD also includes GI, pulmonary, and cardiac problems that are not related to ischemia. For example, gastroesophageal reflux disease, esophageal spasm, or biliary colic can present with angina and other symptoms similar to MI, and by the same token, patients with CHD or MI often present with epigastric pain that is misinterpreted as "heartburn" or related pain. This misinterpretation is often the reason for a patient's delay in obtaining prompt medical evaluation for ACS, including MI.

Patients with anxiety or panic attacks often present to the emergency department with symptoms that mimic angina or an MI. For example, extreme stress can precipitate chest pain, dizziness, dyspnea, and hyperventilation, all of which mimic the symptoms of angina or an MI. Costochondritis, a musculoskeletal problem due to nonspecific inflammation of the articular joints of the chest wall (e.g., rib cage, clavicle, sternum), can also present as chest pain that may be misinterpreted as CHD by patients. However, the pain of costochondritis is typically not constant and can usually be reproduced as point tenderness by pressing on the sternum and costochondral regions of the chest.

Persons with diabetes mellitus may experience angina or MI with minor symptoms or no symptoms at all (e.g., a silent MI), given the resultant nerve related damage that occurs with chronic hyperglycemia, which blunts cardiac-related pain. For example, some patients with CHD may experience nausea and vomiting, dyspnea, epigastric pain, diaphoresis, or dizziness with no complaint of chest pain. These symptoms are referred to as "anginal equivalents" and can be particularly common in elderly patients.

In addition, women experiencing angina or MI commonly present with anginal equivalents rather than with classic radiating chest pain. Historically, clinicians have underestimated the risk of CHD in women. Atypical presentations of ACS in women contributes to the lack of early recognition of cardiac symptoms by both patients and clinicians, including primary-care practitioners. Women classically delay seeking medical care for ischemic symptoms, which contributes to their overall higher morbidity and mortality rates with cardiac events (Arslanian-Engoren and Scott, 2017; Taghaddosi et al., 2010; Lefler and Bondy, 2004).

Because chest pain is often the impetus for the diagnosis of CHD, the pain characteristics that drive the differential diagnoses of CHD need to be carefully assessed. For example, in a young, otherwise healthy adult, reproducible point tenderness is likely musculoskeletal chest wall pain and not ischemic in nature. In addition, pneumothorax, pneumonia, pericarditis, pulmonary embolism, mitral valve prolapse, and aortic dissection are all less common causes of chest pain that may mimic ischemic angina due to CAD. Pleuritic chest pain worsens on inspiration and is likely due to lung pathology, such as pneumonia, especially if accompanied by fever and a productive cough. Thus, the primary-care practitioner needs to have a high level of suspicion and to complete a thorough cardiac risk assessment to rule out CHD, as well as frank MI, in all patients complaining of chest pain or "anginal equivalents."

MANAGEMENT

The principles of management of CHD include establishing the diagnosis, controlling symptoms, and preventing disease progression that may lead to MI or sudden death. During a cardiac catheterization, fibrinolytic agents may be infused directly into an occluded coronary artery in an attempt to restore coronary blood flow. Other therapeutic approaches include balloon angioplasty, stent placement, and coronary artery bypass graft. Presently there are two types of stents in use—bare-metal stents and drug-eluting stents impregnated with medication (e.g., everolimus, paclitaxel, sirolimus) designed to prevent re-stenosis of the stented lumen. With both types of stents, dual antiplatelet therapy (DAPT) should be started for its antithrombotic effects, consisting of aspirin and a $P2Y_{12}$ receptor inhibitor (e.g., clopidogrel [Plavix], prasugrel [Effient], ticagrelor [Brilinta], cangrelor [Kengreal]). Drug-eluting stents require a longer duration of DAPT anticoagulation therapy than bare-metal stents, i.e., at least 6 months versus 1 month, respectively.

Risk Factor Modification

Risk factor modification is essential to stop the progression of CHD. This involves aggressive lowering of lipid levels (as discussed in the section on Dyslipidemia), strict glycemic control in patients with diabetes mellitus (see Chapter 58), aggressive antihypertensive therapy (discussed in the section on Hypertension), smoking cessation (see Chapter 33) and cessation of all other tobacco use (chewing/dipping or nasal "snuff" tobacco), and modifying lifestyle behaviors to include regular exercise, stress reduction, and a heart-healthy diet (less than 300 mg of cholesterol per day and 7% or less of total calories from saturated fats).

Pharmacologic Therapy

Pharmacologic agents are used to control the anginal symptoms of CHD and to prevent subsequent cardiovascular events (see the section on Management of Acute Coronary Syndrome). Most clinicians recommend low-dose daily aspirin (81 to 325 mg) to decrease the incidence of a first MI in middle-aged men and women. Coated aspirin is recommended for individuals with gastric problems or GI intolerance. The dose should be decreased if the patient has a tendency to bruise or stopped if the patient has a bleeding diathesis. There is controversy over whether aspirin should be used concomitantly in patients on other anticoagulants and, if so, what dosage is recommended.

Complementary Therapy

Complementary Therapies 35.1 presents suggested vitamin, mineral, and herbal supplements for various cardiovascular disorders. Of note, the isolated effects of these agents have not been as rigorously tested for positive outcomes and an acceptable risk-benefit profile in

CHD or other cardiovascular conditions as the medications recommended in the Management sections of this chapter.

FOLLOW-UP AND REFERRAL

Patients need to understand the chronicity of CHD and be committed to frequent follow-ups for the control of cardiovascular risk factors. The primary-care practitioner should refer the patient to a cardiologist for a cardiac stress test and any further work-up indicated by the results.

Complementary Therapies 35.1: Cardiac Conditions

AGENT	INDICATION	ADVERSE REACTIONS AND CONSIDERATIONS*
Hawthorn	Angina, CHF, CHD, functional cardiovascular disorders, HTN (in diabetes mellitus), orthostatic hypotension	May cause abdominal discomfort, agitation, arrhythmia, diaphoresis, dizziness, dyspnea, fatigue, headache, palpitations, sleeplessness, or rash. Caution with the following: HTN medications (increased risk of hypotension), antilipemic agents (additive effects), CCBs (additive vasodilation), cardiac glycosides, and vasodilators (additive vasodilation). Monitor BP, coagulation panel, heart rate, and lipid profile.
Magnesium	Arrhythmia, acute MI, CHD, HTN, mitral valve prolapse	May cause areflexia, asthenia, cardiac arrhythmias, cardiac arrest, drowsiness, hypermagnesemia, hypotension, loss of tendon reflexes, polydipsia, or respiratory paralysis. Caution with the following: aminoglycosides (increased risk of muscular weakness and paralysis), antibiotics (decreased effects), antidiabetic agents (increased absorption), and antihypertensive agents (additive effects). Monitor alkaline phosphatase, blood glucose, BP, calcium levels, coagulation panel, cortisol, LFTs, ECG, and parathyroid hormone.
Beta-glucan	Antioxidant, CHD, cardioprotection during CABG, hyperlipidemia, HTN	May cause dizziness, flushing, headache, HTN or hypotension, inflammatory airway disease, keratoderma, nausea, polyuria, urticaria, or vomiting. Caution with the following: antidiabetic agents (additive effects), antihypertensive agents (additive effects), and antilipemic agents (additive effects). Monitor blood glucose, BP, lipid profile, and WBC count.
Selenium	Antioxidant, cardiomyopathy, CHD prevention, circulation	May cause digitalis dysfunction, garlic-like breath odor, hepatorenal dysfunction, irritability, loss or thickening of hair and nails, metallic taste, muscle tenderness, nausea/vomiting, nervous system abnormalities, skin lesions, thrombocytopenia, tremor, or weakness. Caution with the following: barbiturates (increased sedation), HMG-CoA reductase inhibitors (decreased efficacy), and niacin (decreased efficacy).
Vitamin B_6	Angioplasty, CHD, CHD risk reduction, coronary restenosis, reduction in homocysteine level	Prolonged excessive use may cause neuropathy. Monitor vitamin B_6 levels.
Vitamin B_{12}	Angioplasty, CHD, coronary restenosis, reduction in homocysteine level, orthostatic tremor (restless legs syndrome)	Monitor vitamin B_{12} levels.
Vitamin C	Atherosclerosis, circulation, ischemic heart disease, MI risk reduction	In large doses may cause abdominal cramps, diarrhea, nausea, or skin rashes. In diabetics, may cause falsely elevated blood glucose readings. Caution with iron (increased iron levels) and warfarin (in high doses, lowers prothrombin time). Monitor vitamin C levels, although excess is typically excreted in the urine.

Complementary Therapies 35.1: Cardiac Conditions—cont'd

AGENT	INDICATION	ADVERSE REACTIONS AND CONSIDERATIONS*
Vitamin E	Angina, arterial elasticity, atherosclerosis, CHD, HF, dyslipidemias, intermittent claudication, deep venous thrombosis	May cause abdominal pain, blurred vision, diarrhea, fatigue, or headache. Increased risk of mortality with high doses with history of severe CHD (stroke or MI). Caution with the following: anticoagulants/antiplatelet agents (increased risk of bleeding) and chemotherapy (interferes with effectiveness). Monitor coagulation panel (with high doses); monitor vitamin E levels. Discontinue use 2 weeks before dental or surgical procedures.
Flaxseed Oil	CHD, HTN, hyperlipidemia	May cause abdominal discomfort, anaphylaxis, bleeding, bowel obstruction, constipation, diarrhea, dyspnea, hypoglycemia, hypotension, mania, nausea/vomiting, increased risk of prostate cancer, pruritus, skin rash, sneezing, stuffy nose, seizures, or watery eyes. Contraindicated with hypertriglyceridemia. Caution with the following: anticoagulants/antiplatelet agents (increased risk of bleeding), antidiabetic agents (increased risk of hypoglycemia), antihypertensives (increased risk of hypotension), antilipemic agents (decreased effects on triglycerides), furosemide (decreased absorption of furosemide). Monitor alkaline phosphatase, blood glucose, coagulation panel, inflammatory markers, lipid profile, PSA, red blood cells, and triglycerides.
Garlic	Anticoagulant, atherosclerosis, familial hypercholesterolemia, hyperlipidemia, HTN, prevention of MI, peripheral vascular disease	May cause anorexia, bleeding, burning inside the mouth, chills, constipation, diarrhea, dizziness, diaphoresis, dyspepsia, dyspnea, fever, flatulence, halitosis, hyperglycemia or hypoglycemia.
Lycopene	CHD, HTN	May cause abdominal pain, cramps, anorexia, diarrhea, flatulence, or nausea/vomiting. Monitor androgen, lipid profile, and PSA.
Coenzyme Q10	Adjunct to statin therapy, angina, cardiomyopathy, cardioprotection during surgery, HF, CHD, hyperlipidemia, HTN, and MI	May cause bleeding, diarrhea, dizziness, dyspnea, fatigue, flu-like symptoms, GI upset, headache, heartburn, hyperglycemia or hypoglycemia, hypotension, insomnia, irritability, loss of appetite, nausea/vomiting, photosensitivity, pruritus, rash, thrombosis, or thyroid hormone alterations. Caution with antidiabetic agents (altered effects), antihypertensives (additive effects), antilipemic agents (additive effects), corticosteroids (decreased effects), and warfarin (decreased anticoagulant effects). Monitor blood glucose, BP, coagulation panel, LFTs, lipid profile, and CD4 lymphocyte T_4/T_8 ratio.
Calcium	HTN	May cause abdominal pain, arrhythmias, calcium deposits in heart and kidney, chalky taste in mouth, confusion, constipation, GI irritation, headache, irritability, MI, nausea/vomiting, nephrotoxicity, polydipsia, polyuria, renal calculi, skin reactions, or urinary incontinence. Caution with CCBs (decreased effects); levothyroxine (decreased effectiveness of levothyroxine). Monitor bone mineral density, calcium levels, and renal function tests.
Red yeast rice	CHD, hyperlipidemia	May cause bloating, dizziness, flatulence, GI discomfort, headache, or kidney damage. Caution with alcohol (increased risk of liver damage), gemfibrozil and niacin (increased risk of myopathy), HMG-CoA reductase inhibitors (increased risk of adverse effects), protease inhibitors (altered effects). Monitor LFTs and kidney function.

*For an extensive review and additional information on these agents, see Ulbricht, C. *Davis's pocket guide to herbs and supplements*. Philadelphia, PA: FA Davis; 2011.

Abbreviations: BP, blood pressure; CABG, coronary artery bypass graft; CCB, calcium channel blocker; CHD, coronary heart disease; ECG, electrocardiogram; HF, heart failure; HMG-CoA; 3-hydroxy-3-methylglutaryl coenzyme A; HTN, hypertension; GI, gastrointestinal; LFTs, liver function tests; MI, myocardial infarction; PSA, prostrate-specific antigen; WBC, white blood cell.

Patient Education: Coronary Heart Disease

At each visit, the primary-care practitioner should stress cardiac risk factor modification. The lifestyle modifications listed in Box 35.2 for managing HTN are good activities to stress in patient education for overall cardiovascular health.

ACUTE CORONARY SYNDROME

Acute coronary syndrome (ACS) is a term used for the disorders of myocardial ischemia—unstable angina, MI, and variant angina (Prinzmetal's angina). *Unstable angina* due to myocardial ischemia is newly diagnosed angina or previously diagnosed angina that has changed in pattern, frequency, or severity. Unstable angina is commonly a forerunner of acute *MI*, which is necrosis or death of the myocardium as a result of prolonged ischemia due to an insufficient supply of oxygenated blood. *Variant angina* may occur in patients with normal coronary arteries who have cyclically recurring angina at rest that is unrelated to effort.

Although ACS, by definition, refers to acute conditions, stable angina is also covered in this section. *Stable angina* (chronic exertional angina) is a diagnosed condition of myocardial ischemia that is predictable in pattern and frequency and controlled with medication.

EPIDEMIOLOGY AND CAUSES

Each year, an estimated 580,000 Americans have a new ACS attack and almost 210,000 have a recurrent attack. This amounts to a new coronary event approximately every 40 seconds. More men than women experience MIs; however, after menopause this gap dramatically closes. The average age for a first MI in men is 65.3 years and 71.8 years in women. MIs are more common in Western societies, and African Americans have a higher incidence of MI due to the greater incidence of HTN in that population. The mortality rate is approximately 30% for a severe MI.

The contributing causative factors for ACS (including MI) are the same as those for CHD discussed in the previous section. In addition, tachycardia, LVH, anemia, increased platelet aggregation, and the abuse of illegal substances (particularly sympathomimetics, such as cocaine and amphetamines) all may contribute to decreased perfusion of the coronary arteries.

PATHOPHYSIOLOGY

ACS is a broad term describing a continuum of disorders that arise from coronary artery occlusion. ACS denotes high-risk forms of angina pectoris (e.g., unstable or variant angina)

or an MI. In both angina and MI, decreased myocardial perfusion occurs because of coronary artery narrowing caused by thrombus formation subsequent to rupture of atherosclerotic plaque. In stable angina, which is not considered a form of ACS, coronary occlusion causes a brief episode of ischemia that is treatable and reversible. In contrast, in unstable angina, coronary occlusion causes ischemia with a high risk of MI, which can occur with prolonged ischemia. Variant angina, on the other hand, is an atypical form of angina pectoris that occurs as a result of vasospasm of otherwise normal coronary arteries.

Two types of MI are classified according to their electrocardiographic changes: non–ST-segment elevation MI (NSTEMI) and ST-segment elevation MI (STEMI). NSTEMI indicates an infarction caused by a *nonocclusive* thrombus that *partially* interrupts perfusion of the myocardium and results in an infarction affecting only part of the myocardial wall, rather than its full thickness. STEMI is caused by an *occlusive* thrombus that leads to a complete *transmural* MI—an infarction of the full thickness of the myocardial wall. The majority of MIs are NSTEMIs.

After myocardial ischemia occurs, anaerobic metabolism becomes the predominant form of energy production in the affected cardiac tissue. Anaerobic metabolism yields a low energy output that can sustain the heart tissue for a maximum of only 20 minutes. Death of myocardial tissue due to infarction occurs as energy requirements are not met, thus underscoring the importance of acute beta blocker therapy in the management of MI to decrease cardiac workload and myocardial oxygen demand. Moreover, lactic acid, a waste product of anaerobic metabolism, is noxious to surrounding cells, further disrupting cell function.

Necrosis in the infarcted region of the myocardial wall disrupts the conduction system and decreases the strength of the heart muscle as a mechanical pump. In turn, arrhythmias and HF are common sequelae of an MI. In particular, the more damage to the heart muscle, the greater the risk of HF. *Papillary muscle rupture* is also a common complication that may result from an MI. Heart valve leaflets are attached to papillary muscles via stringlike membranous attachments called chordae tendineae. Disrupted papillary muscles and ruptured chordae tendineae cause valvular dysfunction that manifests as a heart murmur due to turbulent blood flow. Specifically, MI of the LV with papillary muscle rupture can cause dysfunction of the mitral valve, and mitral regurgitation is a common complication of left ventricular MI.

CLINICAL PRESENTATION

Subjective

As a common symptom of ACS, the patient with angina pectoris typically complains of chest discomfort that may be described as pressure, tightness, burning, or heaviness. The patient should be asked to describe the pain in terms of its quality, location, radiation, precipitating factors, alleviating factors, and associated signs and symptoms during the acute episode. Although angina pectoris is classically described as chest discomfort, the pain may radiate elsewhere, including to the arms, chest, back, neck, jaw, or teeth. Patients frequently describe the discomfort as feelings of indigestion because angina pectoris may also be accompanied by nausea or vomiting. The patient may also complain of shortness of breath and sweating, with symptoms developing either at rest or with physical activity. The patient may also be anxious, light-headed, and tachycardic.

The pain of ACS may frequently occur after meals because of increased oxygen consumption during the meal and greater diversion of blood flow to the splanchnic circulation. Alternatively, ACS pain may be brought on by psychological stress. Rest and nitroglycerin, either via sublingual (SL) tablet or lingual spray, may relieve the symptoms of stable angina. In contrast, the pain of unstable angina tends to last longer and be of greater intensity than the pain of stable angina, while the pain of variant angina occurs at rest, due to spontaneous coronary vasospasm (see Table 35.5 for a description of the characteristics of the various forms of angina). Of note, patients may be in denial when experiencing angina pectoris and will often rationalize that the symptoms are caused by indigestion or overexertion.

In acute MI, the patient often complains of angina-like chest pain lasting more than 20 minutes, while occasionally waxing and waning during that period. Often,

TABLE 35.5 Forms of Angina

Type of Angina	Characteristics
Stable	Chest pain: transient episodes related to activities that increase myocardial oxygen demand Duration: typically lasts 3–15 minutes. Associated signs and symptoms: nausea, vomiting, shortness of breath Relief: rest and/or nitroglycerin tablets
Unstable	Chest pain: more severe and brought on with less exertion; may occur at rest Duration: prolonged Associated signs and symptoms: nausea, vomiting, shortness of breath, diaphoresis Relief: not relieved by rest and/or nitroglycerin tablets; relieved by morphine
Variant (Prinzmetal's)	Chest pain: episodes unrelated to activities that increase myocardial oxygen demand Duration: cyclical; often occurs during sleep (most common in early morning hours); pain intensifies quickly and lasts longer than that of stable angina Associated signs and symptoms: palpitation, syncope, bradycardia Relief: may subside with exercise

dyspnea, diaphoresis, nausea, and dizziness are also reported. Radiation of the pain to the neck, jaw, shoulder, or arm (left more often than right) is usually described. The degree of distress with these symptoms varies greatly, however, from the patient who complains of an "elephant standing on my chest" to the patient who is apologetic for seeking assistance with "just a bit of indigestion that will not clear up." In particular, women, older adults, and persons with diabetes mellitus are likely to have minimal or atypical symptoms with an acute MI.

About 15% of patients suffer a painless MI that may be detected only on a future ECG, on autopsy, or if the patient presents with other symptoms that prompt the clinician to more thoroughly evaluate for the possibility of an MI. This occurs more often in an older patient or a patient with diabetes mellitus or HTN. In these cases, patients may complain of dyspnea, general upper abdominal pain, exacerbation of HF, or acute confusion.

Objective

The cardiac examination in a patient suspected of having ACS should include inspection, palpation, and auscultation. As with any physical examination, the cardiac evaluation should begin with the general survey, as the primary-care practitioner or other clinician begins to develop a picture of the overall health status of the patient and continues to gather diagnostic clues.

In a patient with angina due to ACS, the clinician may auscultate a transient third (S_3) or fourth (S_4) heart sound, a transient mitral regurgitant murmur, and/or a carotid arterial bruit. In addition, the patient may appear dyspneic and be diaphoretic. In a patient specifically with an MI, the clinician may observe pallor, cool, and diaphoretic skin, crackles on auscultation, a third (S_3) or fourth (S_4) heart sound, cardiac murmurs, edema of the extremities, and possibly jugular venous distention. In addition, the patient may have a low-grade fever. The presence of diaphoresis with chest pain is particularly worrisome, often indicating a significant drop in cardiac output during the episode of pain and subsequent decreased perfusion of the skin.

DIAGNOSTIC REASONING

Diagnostic Tests

Although chest pain can be caused by a number of conditions, assessing for ACS in the patient with angina pectoris is critical. In particular, given the life-threatening implications of an MI, the diagnostic work-up of a patient with suspected ACS must always rule out infarction. The most specific laboratory tests to rule out MI are cardiac-specific troponin I (cTnI) and T (cTnT). These troponins are cardiac proteins released from dead heart muscle, and they are essentially undetectable in the blood of healthy individuals. Troponin levels rise within the first 2 to 4 hours after an MI and remain elevated for 7 to 10 days.

The muscle and brain isoforms of the creatine phosphokinase enzyme are also released from necrotic heart muscle after an MI. These isoenzymes are detected in the blood as a combined fraction of CK isoforms using the CK-MB test. CK-MB levels rise within 4 to 8 hours after an MI and generally return to normal by 48 to 72 hours. The rise in CK-MB fraction also correlates better with infarct size than does troponin level.

CK-MB remains elevated in the blood for a shorter period of time than the cardiac troponins. Therefore, episodes of recurrent ischemia with resultant MI are more readily diagnosed by a rise in cardiac troponins. However, the prolonged elevation of cardiac troponins does not allow for recognition of repeat episodes of acute MI within the first few days after the initial insult. If the diagnosis of an MI remains uncertain, serum cardiac biomarkers should be measured on admission, at 6 to 9 hours after admission, and again after 12 to 14 hours.

Myoglobin is a muscle protein that rises in the blood within only a few hours after an acute MI. It is one of the earliest serum cardiac markers to rise after an MI; however, it is nonspecific for cardiac muscle death and can rise with skeletal muscle injury as well. Blood levels return to normal within 24 hours of infarction and cannot be relied on for diagnosis of MI. Other cardiac enzymes, which are rarely used in diagnostic work-ups, include serum glutamic oxaloacetic transaminase and lactate dehydrogenase; they become elevated in the serum much later in the course of an MI and are, therefore, not sensitive as indicators of an acute MI.

Other laboratory tests that should be drawn as part of a full work-up of ACS include a complete blood count (CBC), erythrocyte sedimentation rate (ESR), serum electrolyte panel, blood urea nitrogen (BUN), and serum creatinine. Leukocytosis is a nonspecific indicator of myocardial injury, as WBC counts often reach levels of 12,000 to 15,000 cells/mcL. ESR, a general indicator of inflammation, also rises after MI and remains elevated for several days.

After the patient is stabilized, echocardiography and cardiac catheterization with angiography are procedures that provide significant prognostic information. Echocardiography can be done to detect cardiac wall motion abnormalities, right and left ventricular function, valvular or septal defects, and LV ejection fraction. Echocardiography is a noninvasive procedure that is easily performed in most emergency departments; however, it is not recommended as a reliable diagnostic test of MI. When the patient is assessed via angiography, coronary artery occlusion can be estimated using the thrombolysis in myocardial infarction (TIMI) grading system. The TIMI scale grades coronary artery occlusion from grade 0, indicating complete occlusion, to grade 3, indicating full perfusion of the coronary artery with normal blood flow.

In addition, radionuclide imaging can detect reversible ischemic regions or fixed infarcted areas of the heart. Injected radionuclide tracer substances are distributed in proportion to myocardial blood flow. This type of imaging reveals a "cold spot" with decreased myocardial perfusion during the first few hours after an MI. However, it cannot distinguish acute MI from the scarring of the myocardium due to an MI experienced in the past.

In the emergency department and urgent care settings, a 12-lead ECG is a critical tool to reveal myocardial ischemia, STEMI, NSTEMI, or cardiac arrhythmias, and should be performed promptly upon presentation of a patient with suspected ACS to a clinical setting. The 12-lead ECG presents 12 leads or "views" of the heart to detect and localize myocardial damage (Fig. 35.1) that shows the ECG wave configuration of a normal 12-lead ECG): leads I, II, and III are the three standard (bipolar) leads; leads aV_R, aV_L, and aV_F are the augmented or unipolar leads; V_1 through V_6 are the chest or precordial leads that view the heart in a horizontal plane. In ACS, ischemic and injured cells have an altered action potential and pathologic patterns of depolarization and repolarization that lead to deviations from the normal ECG pattern. By identifying the leads that contain these ECG changes, the location of myocardial damage and the corresponding coronary artery supply can be determined (Table 35.6).

Myocardial injury is demonstrated by ST-segment changes, and the ECG can delineate the location of myocardial ischemia and its corresponding coronary artery supply. With epicardial injury, injured cells depolarize normally but repolarize more rapidly than normal cells. This causes an elevation of the ST segment in the leads facing the areas of injury. In endocardial and subendocardial injury, the ST segment is more likely to be depressed (usually by 1 mm or more) in the leads facing the injury. With variant angina, an ECG taken during an acute attack will indicate ST-segment elevation rather than depression.

The decision to proceed with thrombolytic therapy in the setting of an acute MI is largely based on the presence of ST-segment elevation in two or more ECG leads. The presence of ST-segment elevation greater than 1 mm in contiguous leads (which evaluate the same anatomical area of the myocardium) usually indicates acute coronary artery occlusion, typically arising from thrombosis. In addition, clinically significant ST-segment elevation is observed during reperfusion therapy for coronary artery blockage.

The various waves of electrical activity on an ECG also show changes characteristic of myocardial ischemia and infarction. Myocardial ischemia is demonstrated by enlargement and inversion of T waves due to altered late repolarization. The ischemic area also remains depolarized when adjacent areas have returned to the resting, polarized electrical state, as infarcted cells have no action potential

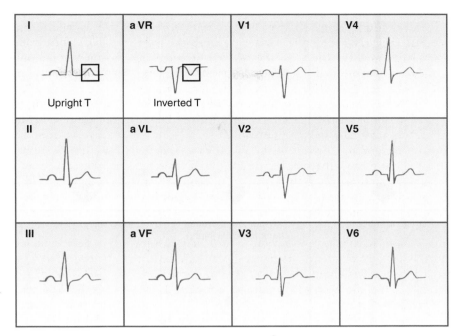

Figure 35.1 The normal 12-lead ECG. (Source: *Lipman B, Cascio T.* ECG assessment and intervention. Philadelphia, PA: FA Davis; 1994. Reprinted with permission.)

TABLE 35.6	Localizing Myocardial Infarction via ECG		
Location of MI	*Abnormal ECG Leads*	*Reciprocal ECG Changes*	*Coronary Arteries Affected*
Anterior	V_1–V_4	II, III, aV_F	Left anterior descending artery
Anteroseptal	V_1, V_2	None	Left anterior descending artery
Anterolateral	I, aV_L, V_4, V_6	II, III, aV_F	Left anterior descending artery Left circumflex artery
Inferior	II, III, aV_F	I, aV_L	Right coronary artery in 80%–90% Left coronary artery in 10%–20%
Posterior	V_1–V_3	R wave greater than S wave, depressed ST segment, elevated T wave	Right coronary artery Left circumflex artery
Lateral	I, aV_L, V_5, V_6	V_1, V_2	Left circumflex artery

and cannot conduct impulses through dead tissue. Thus, electrical impulses are deflected away, causing an abnormal Q wave. Because of the absence of depolarization of cells in the area of an acute MI, Q waves develop 1 to 3 days after the infarction. These abnormal Q waves are usually at least 0.04 seconds wide and 25% or greater in depth than the R wave is tall. Figure 35.2 shows the typical ECG changes seen with cardiac damage.

At times, myocardial perfusion halts temporarily and is then reestablished in a relatively short period of time. This may be the result of a coronary vessel spasm or a sudden drop in BP, such as with severe blood or fluid loss that is eventually compensated for by peripheral vasoconstriction. In this situation, a small portion of subendocardial tissue may be damaged, while adjacent myocardial tissue remains viable. As a result, ECG changes are present but differ significantly from those seen in a classic transmural MI. Q waves do not form because electrically active tissue backs up the area of infarction. Because tissue injury, ischemia, and infarction occur subendocardially, rather than being oriented toward the epicardium as in a transmural MI, the injury pattern is reflected in ST-segment depression.

Moreover, the ECG changes are transient—present only during the acute event and during tissue healing. Thus, if not found during the acute presentation, a non–Q wave MI may never be diagnosed. The terms Q–wave and non–Q wave MI are now referred to as STEMI and

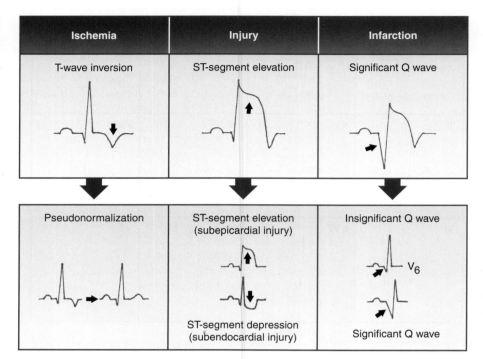

Figure 35.2 Typical ECG changes seen with cardiac damage. (Source: *Lipman B, Cascio T.* ECG assessment and intervention. Philadelphia, PA: FA Davis; 1994. Reprinted with permission.)

NSTEMI (as previously defined). There may be a temptation to consider a non–Q wave MI/NSTEMI as a "small heart attack" with limited long-term sequelae. However, these patients have well-demonstrated risk for future MI and other cardiac events, particularly during the next 3 to 6 months. The majority of patients with non–Q wave MIs are elderly adults (aged 70 years or older) with a history of prior MI and CHF. Figure 35.3 illustrates the difference between STEMI and NSTEMI ECG changes.

Systematic Approach to ECG Interpretation

The identification of the abnormal ECG patterns associated with an acute MI should not overshadow the wealth of information that can be obtained from a thorough and stepwise ECG reading. If the clinician is not systematic in her or his approach to ECG interpretation, the risk of error and oversight of critical findings increase. For example, if the presence of a left bundle branch block (LBBB) is not detected, these changes may be interpreted as Q waves in the inferior leads or ST elevations in the precordial leads.

An LBBB prevents a true evaluation of this area of the heart because the normal path of depolarization is blocked and does not travel directly down the typical electrical conduction pathway. This results in a distorted view, with the typical pattern of LBBB ECG changes. Therefore, after first determining the rate and rhythm on an ECG, observation for LBBB should be the next step. However, the clinician needs to keep in mind that an LBBB could also result from the acute ischemic process of an MI. Thus, if this is a new ECG finding, it should be noted and incorporated into the clinical picture to evaluate for possible MI.

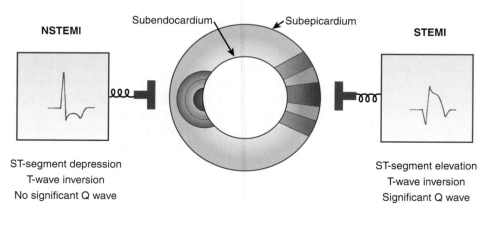

Figure 35.3 ST-segment versus non–ST-segment elevation myocardial infarction. (Source: *Lipman B, Cascio T.* ECG assessment and intervention. Philadelphia, PA: FA Davis; 1994. Reprinted with permission.)

The 12-lead ECG also provides information about cardiac electrical axis deviation, which is the third step in systematic interpretation, after rate/rhythm assessment and observation for LBBB. The cardiac electrical axis is, for all practical purposes, synonymous with the overall wave of myocardial depolarization. Healthy myocardial tissue depolarizes in a predictable pattern, thus recording on the ECG a predictable electrical axis. The normal wave of depolarization travels down the heart from the atria to the ventricles and from the right side to the left. This normal axis shows as a positive QRS complex in lead I and lead aV_F. This is because the net ventricular forces travel toward the pole of lead I and down toward the pole of lead aV_F.

With cardiac disease, the wave of depolarization swings away from areas of damage or necrosis, creating electrical axis deviation (a change from the norm). If the axis is shifted to the left, the QRS complex is positive in lead I and negative in lead aV_F. Left axis deviation is subdivided into normal left axis deviation (NLAD) and abnormal left axis deviation (ALAD). NLAD is often seen in the presence of LVH due to enlargement of the left-sided myocardium. ALAD is seen in a block of the anterosuperior division of the left bundle branch, often referred to as a left anterior fascicular block. ALAD is also seen in Q wave inferior wall MI and with a right apical pacemaker. Right axis deviation (RAD) is seen in a block of the posterior inferior division of the left bundle block, often referred to as a left posterior fascicular block. RAD can also be caused by an extensive Q-wave lateral wall MI and may be seen in hypertrophy of the right ventricle (RV).

Axis deviation is occasionally present in the absence of cardiac disease. In pregnancy, the heart is shifted in the cavity because of the height of the diaphragm. This may cause a left axis deviation. In addition, adults with abdominal obesity may demonstrate left axis deviation. In infants and children, as well as tall, thin adults, RAD is normal. Advanced Assessment 35.2 presents a rapid quadrant-based assessment method for determining ECG axis deviation.

The 12-lead ECG may also provide information about heart chamber enlargement. Chamber enlargement, or hypertrophy, is usually a consequence of obstruction of blood flow out of the affected area of the heart, given the need for greater contractility to increase cardiac outflow. For example, left atrial hypertrophy is a common consequence of mitral valve stenosis because the atrium must generate excessive pressure to compensate for the pathologically smaller valve opening, thereby becoming enlarged as a result of forcing open a stiff, diseased valve.

The following are typical ECG findings associated with chamber enlargement:

1. Right atrial hypertrophy, also known as P pulmonale
   - Peaked P wave in leads II, III, aV_F, and V_1

 Advanced Assessment 35.2: Assessing Axis Deviation

The quadrant method is a rapid and accurate system of assessing the ECG electrical axis. Although it does not yield an exact degree measurement, such as that obtained when using an ECG ruler, this method can be used without any special equipment. First, examine leads I and aVF for the presence of a positive or negative QRS complex. Then, apply following rules to characterize axis deviation:

- Normal axis: positive complexes (tall R wave) in leads I and aVF
- Left axis deviation: positive complex in lead I and negative complex in aVF
- Right axis deviation: negative complex in lead I and positive complex in aVF
- Extreme right axis deviation: negative complexes in leads I and aVF

   - P wave of more than 2.5 mm in leads II, III, and aV_F
2. LAE, also known as P mitrale
   - Notched P wave of more than 0.10 seconds in leads II, III, and aV_F
   - Prominent negative P terminus (latter portion) in V_1 (more than 1:1 size ratio)
3. Right ventricular hypertrophy (RVH)
   - Reversal of R wave progression in the precordial leads.
   - Although not routinely seen, RVH may be observed in patients with chronic obstructive pulmonary disease (COPD).
4. LVH, using the Estes Scoring System:
   - 3 points for any or all of the following: voltage (height) of 30 mm or more in the S wave in V_1 or V_2, 30 mm or more in the R wave in V_5 or V_6, or 20 mm or more in the R or S wave in lead I, II, III, aV_F, or aV_L
   - 1 point for secondary ST-segment/T-wave changes if the patient is taking digitalis
   - 3 points for secondary ST-segment/T-wave changes if the patient is not taking digitalis
   - 3 points for an abnormal P terminus in V_1, reflecting LAE
   - 2 points for LAD
   - 1 point for a QRS interval of more than 0.09 seconds
   - 1 point for an intrinsicoid deflection time (R wave peak time, i.e., the time from the beginning of the QRS complex to the peak of the R wave) in V_5 or V_6 of 0.05 seconds or more
   - *Total score interpretation*: 0 to 3 = LVH unlikely; 4 = LVH likely; 5 to 13 = LVH present

Although the pathologic ECG changes in ACS were discussed earlier in this section, given their relevance for the diagnosis of life-threatening conditions such as unstable angina and MI, identifying the leads that contain ECG changes to localize injury and assess for myocardial damage should actually be the *final* step in ECG interpretation. For example, if the determination of an LBBB has not been made prior to this last step, the ECG interpretation will be flawed. Moreover, focusing only on ischemic ECG changes in ACS may cause clinicians to overlook other important findings on this cornerstone diagnostic test, such as electrical axis deviation, conduction blocks, and underlying arrhythmias.

Importantly, even if the clinician is unable to fully interpret the 12-lead ECG due to an LBBB, the clinical context of the situation needs to be considered and further diagnostic and treatment interventions rapidly implemented. For example, if an acute STEMI is suspected, additional diagnostics should be obtained such as an echocardiogram and possibly left heart catheterization with angiography.

Differential Diagnosis

Differential diagnoses for ACS, whether presenting as angina pectoris or with further symptoms suspicious for an acute MI, include costochondritis, esophagitis, esophageal spasm, peptic ulcer, gastritis, cholecystitis, biliary tract disease, pericarditis, myocarditis, aortic dissection, pulmonary embolus (PE), pulmonary HTN, pneumothorax, anxiety, and panic disorders.

MANAGEMENT

In ACS, the goal is to promptly diagnose and appropriately treat the underlying etiology of myocardial ischemia. In the primary-care setting, the clinician can attempt to stabilize the patient with acetylsalicylic acid (aspirin, ASA) and nitroglycerin. However, the patient experiencing ACS must be transferred to a hospital-based emergency-care setting as soon as possible, preferably one with access to a cardiac catheterization laboratory.

Treatment of Angina

Although not included in the definition of ACS, it is important to distinguish stable angina from unstable angina, as the former is more readily treatable than unstable angina, which is a harbinger of more severe ischemia. If a patient presents with ischemic chest pain that is relieved by nitroglycerin and rest, this implies stable angina. Chronic anginal pain is typically of short duration, usually only for 3 to 5 minutes, but it may last up to 30 minutes or longer. For an acute attack of chronic stable angina, nitroglycerin may be given as an SL tablet or

lingual spray. One tablet or one spray should be administered under the tongue (the spray formulation may also be delivered directly onto the tongue) every 5 minutes for a maximum of three doses until the pain is relieved. If three doses are insufficient to relieve the pain, the local emergency medical services system should be activated to immediately transport the patient to the nearest emergency department.

After the patient's chest pain has been relieved, a beta blocker and/or long-acting nitrate agent may be prescribed. Beta blockers decrease myocardial oxygen demand by interfering with the effects of the sympathetic nervous system on beta-1 receptors of the heart. Long-acting nitrates, either in a topical or oral formulation, may be added to a beta blocker (e.g., atenolol, metoprolol, nadolol, propranolol) to increase myocardial oxygen supply through coronary artery vasodilation.

Long-acting topical nitrate formulations include the nitroglycerin transdermal patch or paste/gel, which are available in various strengths. The patch or paste must not be used continuously and should be applied for 12 to 14 hours and then removed for 12 hours to prevent the development of tolerance. The use of hydralazine is being evaluated as a way to inhibit tolerance to nitroglycerin paste. Isosorbide dinitrate is a long-acting oral nitrate agent, which may be taken daily as an alternative form of prophylaxis to prevent recurrent angina.

All patients with diagnosed angina should be placed on daily aspirin therapy to help prevent coronary thrombosis. ASA 81 to 325 mg may be taken daily (use enterically coated ASA in patients with concurrent gastric problems). Ticlopidine taken with food may be ordered for patients who are allergic to aspirin or those with a history of GI bleeding.

As unstable angina is defined as chest pain of new onset, a progressive nature, or a new pattern, if rest and nitroglycerin do not relieve the chest discomfort in typical fashion, the patient must be immediately transported by ambulance to the emergency department for further evaluation and to rule out an MI (Figure 35.4 presents a flowchart for the management of unstable angina). In variant angina, the ECG findings of ST-segment elevation will abate when the patient is treated with nitroglycerin and drugs that influence calcium metabolism, such as a CCB (e.g., verapamil HCl).

Treatment of Myocardial Infarction

The location and extent of infarcted myocardial tissue and the speed with which reperfusion is supplied to the "cutoff" areas of the myocardium determine prognosis following an MI. Because the use of early reperfusion therapy increases the likelihood of survival and improves left ventricular function, the patient with a suspected MI should be assessed rapidly in order to provide the most appropriate care. The Iceberg of Myocardial Infarction

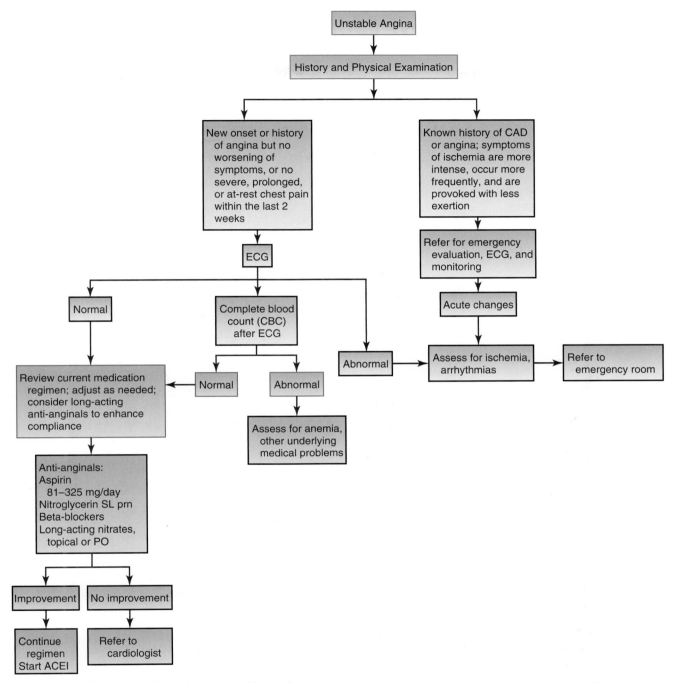

Figure 35.4 Treatment flowchart: unstable angina.

explores many facets involved in recognizing and treating a patient with an MI.

The pharmacologic treatment of ACS is directed primarily at dissolution of the intracoronary thrombus causing obstruction to blood flow by antiplatelet therapy (e.g., aspirin, glycoprotein IIb/IIIa receptor antagonists), anticoagulant therapy (e.g., heparin), and relief of symptoms by antianginal (e.g., nitroglycerin, beta blockers, supplemental oxygen therapy) and analgesic (morphine sulfate) medications. After an MI is confirmed, urgent

evaluation for salvage of viable myocardial tissue is initiated through reperfusion treatments based on coronary angiographic studies. Ultimately, the goal of management is to salvage the ischemic myocardium before it becomes necrotic by reperfusing the area as soon as possible. After that, the goal of ongoing treatment shifts to preventing future attacks.

Immediate interventions for a suspected MI mirror those of unstable angina, including rest, aspirin, and nitroglycerin to relief chest pain, in order to decrease

The Iceberg of Myocardial Infarction

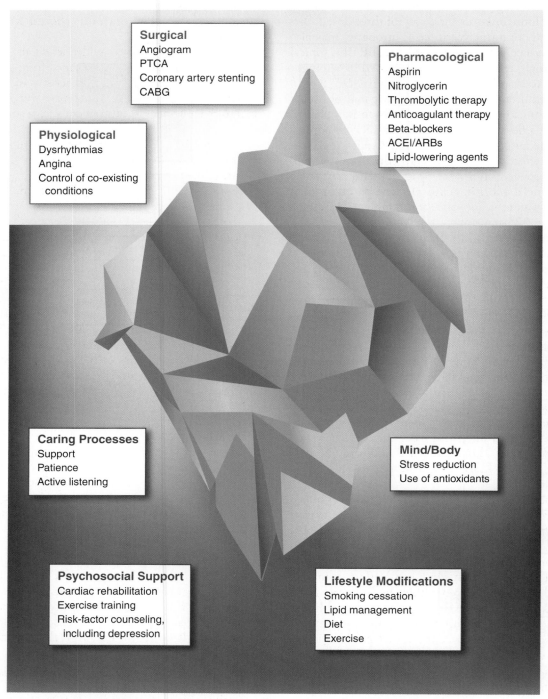

Surgical
Angiogram
PTCA
Coronary artery stenting
CABG

Pharmacological
Aspirin
Nitroglycerin
Thrombolytic therapy
Anticoagulant therapy
Beta-blockers
ACEI/ARBs
Lipid-lowering agents

Physiological
Dysrhythmias
Angina
Control of co-existing
  conditions

Caring Processes
Support
Patience
Active listening

Mind/Body
Stress reduction
Use of antioxidants

Psychosocial Support
Cardiac rehabilitation
Exercise training
Risk-factor counseling,
  including depression

Lifestyle Modifications
Smoking cessation
Lipid management
Diet
Exercise

PTCA - Percutaneous Transluminal Coronary Angioplasty
CABG - Coronary Artery Bypass Graft
ACEI - Angiotensin-Converting-Enzyme Inhibitor
ARB - Angiotensin Receptor Blocker

heart rate, BP, and myocardial oxygen demand. Nitroglycerin can be administered sublingually as a tablet or spray. If relief is not achieved within 2 to 3 minutes after the initial dose of nitroglycerin, a second or third dose can be given at 5-minute intervals for a total of three doses. One or more inches of nitroglycerin gel (Nitropaste) may also be used to induce vasodilation and lower BP. This topical form of nitroglycerin may be easily removed by wiping it off the skin to stop its effects. In more advanced clinical settings, an adjustable IV nitroglycerin drip may be used if appropriate nursing and medical supervision is available.

Aspirin at a dose of 162 to 325 mg can also be administered in the ambulatory care setting. Aspirin exerts an antiplatelet effect, whereas nitroglycerin decreases preload and coronary vasospasm, thus contributing to an overall beneficial effect in acute MI. The patient should initially chew and swallow one aspirin tablet. It is important that the 325-mg dosage not be exceeded, because that may negate the antiplatelet effect. This initiation of antiplatelet therapy given at the time of onset (within 70 minutes) of symptoms, before hospitalization, has been shown to lower the mortality rate in MI patients.

The patient should then be transferred to an emergency medical setting. The primary-care practitioner or first health-care provider to encounter the patient should place a large-bore IV if possible, provide supplemental oxygen via nasal cannula or face mask, and monitor the patient until the emergency medical services system can be activated. Once the patient is stabilized, emergency-care clinicians can determine if the patient is a candidate for emergent reperfusion treatment with intravenous thrombolytic agents or primary percutaneous coronary intervention (PCI). This approach should only be used for patients with a STEMI or with suspected acute MI in the setting of LBBB.

Thrombolytic agents, such as alteplase (recombinant tissue plasminogen activator), reteplase, or tenecteplase, are most effective when administered early in the course of an MI. The first thrombolytic agent, streptokinase, is not commonly used today because it is a non–fibrin-specific agent. For the best therapeutic effect, thrombolytics should be administered within the first three hours (ideally 30 minutes) of MI symptom onset, although studies have shown that thrombolytic therapy can be of benefit up to 12 hours after the initial presentation of symptoms of MI. Thrombolytic therapy can also be combined with the antiplatelet agents known as glycoprotein IIb/IIIa inhibitors, including abciximab (ReoPro), eptifibatide (Integrilin), and tirofiban (Aggrastat).

Cardiac catheterization with angiography can determine whether the patient is a candidate for reperfusion therapy, percutaneous transluminal coronary angioplasty (PTCA), coronary artery stenting, or coronary artery bypass grafting. Immediate coronary angiography and primary PCI, which includes stenting of the infarct-related artery, have been shown to be more effective than thrombolysis for STEMI if done within 90 minutes of

presentation to the clinical center. This 90-minute time frame is referred to as the "door to balloon time" and is managed only in specialized centers. Stenting may be done in conjunction with administrations of the platelet glycoprotein IIb/IIIa antagonist abciximab (ReoPro) in patients with acute MI.

The AHA has published guidelines for the management of patients with acute MI. Developed from the consensus opinion of nursing and medical experts, as well as evidence-based health-care practice outcomes, the AHA recommends the following for the patient with a suspected MI:

- Community systems, including primary-care practitioners, should work together to ensure prompt initial care of the patient with suspected MI. Once the patient enters care in the emergency department, initial evaluation should occur within 10 minutes.
- The following care should be provided immediately: administration of oxygen via nasal prongs; SL nitroglycerin, unless SBP is less than 90 mm Hg, heart rate is less than 50 or more than 100 beats per minute, or a phosphodiesterase-5-inhibitor (e.g., sildenafil, vardenafil, tadalafil) has been taken within the past 24 hours; adequate analgesia for angina pectoris with morphine sulfate or meperidine; ASA 162 to 325 mg taken orally (ASA should be administered regardless of whether thrombolytic therapy is being considered; chewable ASA has a more rapid effect and is preferred); in addition, some clinicians give a loading dose of clopidogrel (300 to 600 mg).
- Clinically significant ST-segment elevation largely dictates reperfusion therapy by use of thrombolytic therapy or PTCA. When thrombolysis is used, heparin is usually given for 48 hours to ensure continued vessel patency; an alternative to unfractionated heparin (if no renal or hepatic impairment is present) is a low-molecular-weight heparin such as enoxaparin sodium (Lovenox). If LBBB is present on an ECG and the clinical scenario is consistent with an acute MI, the same level of care should be offered; in contrast, patients with clinical presentations suggestive of an MI but without ST-segment changes should not receive thrombolysis until additional testing confirms the diagnosis of MI.
- The patient should be hospitalized and placed on continuous ECG monitoring for rhythm disturbances. Serial 12-lead ECGs should be obtained and the results correlated with laboratory measures of myocardial necrosis, such as CK-MB, cTnI, and cTnT levels.
- Daily aspirin therapy should be continued; the initial dosage should be 325 mg daily, with anywhere from 81 to 325 mg given daily after discharge indefinitely.
- The use of heparin should be considered in the presence of a large anterior MI or LV mural thrombus because of an increased risk of embolic stroke.
- If no contraindications are present, the Core Measures of the Joint Commission should be implemented, which include the following: aspirin on arrival and discharge,

ACEI or ARB therapy for left ventricular systolic dysfunction, beta blocker therapy as tolerated, and statin therapy on discharge. Beta blocker therapy and ACEI therapy should be initiated promptly because the use of these agents is associated with reduced mortality and morbidity after an MI. Beta blocker therapy should be continued indefinitely, with ACEIs being most appropriate for patients with LV dysfunction characterized by a systolic ejection fraction of less than 40% or the presence of HF. Beta blockers exert their beneficial effect in patients with an MI by reducing myocardial oxygen demand, decreasing myocardial wall stress, and antagonizing the arrhythmogenic effects of catecholamines. ACEIs reduce the progressive ventricular dilation and remodeling after an MI, and in some studies have been shown to reduce myocardial reinfarction, although by an unknown mechanism. ACEIs also decrease the incidence of HF, thereby reducing mortality in patients with large myocardial infarcts and those with LV dysfunction.

- Ongoing care includes the goal of reducing LDL-C to less than 100 mg/dL using diet, exercise, and, if necessary, drug therapy. This is in keeping with an overall plan to reduce or eliminate all cardiac risk factors in addition to dyslipidemia, including physical inactivity, tobacco use, and obesity.
- Coronary artery bypass surgery is not usually done during an evolving MI, unless the patient has a serious complication such as acute severe mitral regurgitation with or without papillary muscle rupture, acute septal rupture, or a free wall rupture that might be associated with a pseudoaneurysm, refractory cardiogenic shock, or recurrent severe postinfarction ischemia that cannot be managed with drugs or PTCA.

FOLLOW-UP AND REFERRAL

Stable patients whose cardiovascular risk profile has not yet been optimized should be followed every 3 months to determine their adherence to risk factor modification strategies and to monitor for the progression of comorbid factors related to ACS, for example, HTN, overweight, and obesity. Patients with stable angina may be managed by the primary-care practitioner with either beta blockers and short (e.g., SL tablets or lingual spray) and possibly long-acting (isosorbide) nitrates for as needed symptomatic relief and prophylactic use, respectively. However, given the potential for stable angina to evolve into unstable angina over time, it is appropriate to refer these patients to a cardiologist initially to confirm the nature of their angina and to ensure that more serious underlying cardiovascular pathology has not been missed.

In contrast, patients with unstable angina should be rapidly referred to an emergency department and a cardiologist for a complete evaluation. As unstable angina and an acute MI may only be distinguishable through a thorough diagnostic work-up, from the instant a clinician suspects a patient is experiencing an acute MI, the patient must be immediately transported to an emergency department for immediate treatment and rapid evaluation by a cardiologist.

The primary-care practitioner should follow the patient after hospitalization to coordinate ongoing care. This may include the cardiologist discharging the patient from his or her specialty care to long-term management by the primary-care practitioner, following an agreed upon plan of care. Ideally, the cardiologist should have already referred the patient to a cardiac rehabilitation program before discharge, and the primary-care practitioner should take on an active role in encouraging the patient to adhere to the prescribed program.

Upon discharge, a review of the core measures (Joint Commission) related to ACS should be completed. In addition to a beta blocker (and, if indicated, an ACEI), the patient should be prescribed nitroglycerin (SL tablet or spray) with instructions on when to take it and how to store it. The patient should also be taking a daily enteric-coated aspirin of at least 81 mg, as well as a cholesterol-lowering statin drug. For patients with residual myocardial ischemia or with significant left ventricular dysfunction, a longer-acting nitrate such as isosorbide (Isordil) should also be considered. Research has also shown that the addition of a diuretic for HTN provides a decrease in mortality.

Patient Education: Acute Coronary Syndrome

Patients should be taught about the purpose of their medications, proper usage, and adverse effects. For example, the primary-care practitioner should educate patients in how to take nitroglycerin to treat as well as prevent angina prophylactically. The clinician should stress that nitroglycerin tablets should remain in the light-resistant bottle in which they are packaged and not be put in another pill box or placed in areas that could become warm and humid. Once opened, the bottle must be dated and discarded after 6 months or the medication may decrease in effectiveness. Patients should also be taught to use nitroglycerin prophylactically before any stressful physical activity such as sexual intercourse.

Anxiety and fear often accompany anginal attacks because the patient may fear the onset of an MI. Patients and their families should be allowed to express their fears and concerns and should be collaborative partners in instituting necessary lifestyle changes. At every office visit, the primary-care practitioner should assist the patient in reducing the negative impact of all modifiable cardiovascular risk factors that may exacerbate angina and CHD, such as through smoking cessation, lipid management, stress reduction, and the use of antioxidants. In addition, coexisting medical conditions such as HTN, diabetes mellitus, anemia, hyperthyroidism, and HF should be managed aggressively.

In addition, the primary-care practitioner should encourage the patient to enter a cardiac rehabilitation program of safe exercise and risk factor modification, with activity limitations as determined by exercise tolerance testing. Patients with ACS should be placed on a low-fat diet that is calorie controlled if weight reduction is necessary. Caloric restrictions must take into account what is realistic for patients to adhere to, but weight loss generally occurs when daily caloric intake is less than 2,000 calories for women and 2,500 calories for men. However, these targets are affected by many factors, such as a patient's physical activity level.

As in all households of patients with cardiac conditions, family members should learn cardiopulmonary resuscitation and how to activate emergency medical services, as well as the immediate care they can provide in the case of a suspected MI. Education of the patient's family or immediate support network is critical, as most patients will be too anxious or confused to exhibit effective self-care practices during an acute MI (see The Patient's Voice 35.1 for an example of one person's experience of having an acute MI). It is also quite common for patients to minimize their symptoms during an acute MI and be in denial of their need for more aggressive clinical evaluation. Thus, patients and their families must understand the life-threatening consequences of failing to act on ACS symptoms early.

Patients and their families should be instructed not to exceed the 325-mg dose of ASA in the case of a suspected MI, as higher doses may negate the therapeutic effects of ASA during an acute MI. Therefore, if a patient takes ASA while waiting for emergency medical services, the patient or her or his family need to inform the providers as soon as they arrive that aspirin has already been taken. Additionally, for those patients taking daily ASA, the AHA recommends that it be taken at night for greater effectiveness, as more MIs occur in the early morning hours.

Patient education following an acute MI involves similar aggressive risk factor modification to prevent a recurrence, as listed in Box 35.2 for the prevention of HTN. This includes the need for an aggressive cardiac rehabilitation program, even if the patient has previously refused, in order to improve exercise tolerance, cardiac symptoms, lipid levels, and psychosocial well-being. The primary-care practitioner should explain that exercise training through cardiac rehabilitation increases arterial oxygen saturation and improves oxygen uptake by the peripheral tissues. This results in a decrease in the cardiac output required to perform exercises, allowing for more effective rehabilitation post-MI. The patient and her or his family also needs to understand that there is a markedly increased risk of clinical depression in the post-MI patient and that a comprehensive cardiac rehabilitation program that also addresses mental health and well-being can help prevent this serious sequela.

There are three phases of cardiac rehabilitation. Phase I begins in the early in-hospital postinfarct phase, with range-of-motion exercises progressing to an increase in activities of daily living. Phase II is a structured outpatient program of exercise training and risk factor counseling and education. Phase III establishes a lifelong pattern of regular aerobic exercise and further modification of risk factors and mental well-being; this third phase is usually undertaken in a community wellness center.

HEART FAILURE

Heart failure is a condition in which cardiac output is insufficient to meet the body's metabolic demands. Early identification of patients at risk for HF and effective patient education is key not only for the prevention of disease but also for the quality of life of these patients.

EPIDEMIOLOGY AND CAUSES

HF unlike other cardiac disorders, has been increasing in incidence and prevalence, especially in the older adult population. The AHA states that the number of adults living with HF increased from 5.7 to 6.5 million over a 5-year period from 2009 to 2012, according to longitudinal NHANES data. The incidence is increasing because of the use of newer medications and technologies that have increased survival at the expense of increased morbidity. The costs of this condition are high in the United States, as care and evaluation of HF patients exceed $30.7 billion in resources each year.

HF is the most common discharge diagnosis in patients older than 65 years and is diagnosed in 10% of the population by the time they reach the age of 75 years.

▲▲ The Patient's Voice 35.1

MYOCARDIAL INFARCTION

It was 4:30 A.M. … Damn, what a case of indigestion … Have to get to the golf course … It's the first day of the seniors' tournament, and employees will be there early. Driving to work, the indigestion seemed to be subsiding. Arrived at work and started getting things organized for the day's events. Started pulling kegs of beer to be placed around the course when the pain started coming back, and I got nauseated. Pain is getting worse now. Now it's starting to feel like someone is sitting on my chest. Someone called the paramedics…

I'm in the ambulance now. I'm sweating, feeling clammy … chest pain continues. We get to the hospital, and the people there ask if I'm allergic to anything. Pain is getting worse. They're sticking tubes and needles in me. A doctor tells me I'm having a heart attack … and not to worry, they have it all under control. *Not worry*—what does he think?! Then he tells me he's going to give me a clot-busting drug. I'm trying to listen, but I really don't understand what's going on. At least the chest pain is starting to go away.

But I'm only 40 … I can't be having a heart attack! This isn't happening to me!

Approximately 5.7 million adults in the United States have HF. About half of these people who have HF will die within 5 years of diagnosis.

HF may occur acutely, or it may occur after a cardiac abnormality has been present for years, when an increased demand is placed on a heart that is already in a long-term compensated state, resulting in further deterioration. It is critical for the primary-care practitioner to identify not only the underlying cause of heart disease but also the precipitating factors leading to HF, as prompt treatment and elimination of precipitating causes, if possible, may save the patient's life. Factors that increase the risk of HF include infectious disease, obesity, anemia, the physiologic stress of pregnancy, diabetes mellitus, chronic renal insufficiency, myocarditis, cardiomyopathies, valvular disorders, CAD, dysrhythmias, thyrotoxicosis, PE, sleep apnea, alcohol abuse, substance abuse, and chemotherapeutics. Table 35.7 summarizes many of the common causes of HF and their physiologic effects on the heart.

Because of the increasing incidence of HF, new theories are being generated to explain the elusiveness of this disease process to intervention and cure. Ongoing research is being conducted to explore the neurohormonal causal hypothesis of HF. This research began with the discovery that ACEIs and possibly beta blockers were more effective in reducing mortality in HF than potent afterload-reducing drugs. In the neurohormonal pathophysiologic model, active molecules that are released in HF are toxic to the myocardium. Noradrenaline, angiotensin, vasopressin, endothelin, and TNF-α have all been studied for their causal relationship to HF.

PATHOPHYSIOLOGY

HF is a constellation of clinical manifestations that result from the heart's inability to pump adequate amounts of blood to meet the oxygen demands of peripheral tissues. HF involves a number of complex pathophysiological changes that are progressive. It can result from a dysfunctional ventricle that is unable to eject an adequate amount of blood (*systolic dysfunction*) or from the inability of the ventricle to fill with a sufficient amount of blood (*diastolic dysfunction*). There are numerous etiologies of HF; however, ischemic heart disease and long-standing HTN are common underlying causes. Ischemic heart disease due to diminished coronary perfusion of the myocardium weakens the strength of contractility of the ventricles. HTN creates excess mechanical stress on the ventricles, resulting in the structural changes of myocardial hypertrophy and eventual left ventricular dilation.

Regardless of etiology, HF provokes hemodynamic changes, neurohormonal stimulation, vasoactive substance secretion, and cardiac structural alterations (myocardial remodeling)—all of which have systemic consequences. When cardiac muscle contraction is weakened, endothelin, a potent vasoconstrictor, is secreted

TABLE 35.7	**Precipitating Causes of Heart Failure**
Precipitating Causes	**Physiologic Effects on the Heart**
Infection	Increases demand on the heart secondary to fever, tachycardia, hypoxemia, and increased metabolic demands
Anemia	Increased heart rate to meet peripheral tissue oxygen demands leads to increased cardiac demand.
Pulmonary edema	Increased pulmonary arterial pressure leads to increased right ventricular afterload.
Pregnancy, thyrotoxicosis arrhythmias	Adequate tissue perfusion in these conditions requires increased cardiac output. Tachyarrhythmias decrease diastole and lead to cardiac ischemia. Loss of "atrial kick" leads to increased atrial pressures. Abnormal intraventricular conduction can lead to decreased cardiac output, which will lead to further attempts to compensate. Any arrhythmia that alters the formula (cardiac output = heart rate × stroke volume) has the potential to increase demand on an already decompensated heart.
Rheumatic heart disease and other forms of myocarditis	Alterations in cardiac output increase cardiac demand secondary to infectious or inflammatory processes.
Infective endocarditis; excesses in physical activity (overexertion), dietary intake, environmental conditions (e.g., excessive heat or humidity), or emotional states	Valvular damage, fever, inflammatory processes, and extreme conditions increase cardiac demand.
Systemic HTN	Sudden elevation of arterial pressure leads to increased systemic vascular resistance and increased cardiac workload.
MI	May lead to impaired ventricular function

by the arterial endothelium in response to a drop in BP. Although endothelin helps the body compensate by raising BP, chronic secretion increases afterload and resistance against the heart pump. The inflammatory cytokine TNF-α is also found in the circulation and heart muscle during HF. TNF-α is anorexigenic and increases wasting of lean body mass. Two other important vasodilator peptides are released with dilation of the atria and ventricles in HF: atrial natriuretic peptide (ANP) and brain natriuretic peptide (BNP). These are natural diuretic substances that stimulate the excretion of sodium and water to counteract the excess water reabsorption and fluid overload caused by activation of the renin-angiotensin-aldosterone cascade in response to decreased cardiac output.

HF can be described as *systolic* versus *diastolic dysfunction*, *right-sided* versus *left-sided HF*, *right ventricular* versus *left ventricular failure* (LVF), or *forward* versus *backward failure*. These complementary terms are descriptions that illustrate the different pathophysiological mechanisms of HF for academic purposes. However, clinically, most patients with HF exhibit a clinical presentation that is a combination of these processes. Given that HF typically presents with symptoms of vascular congestion (either primarily in the lungs or systemically in the venous return network to the heart) due to the reduced capacity of the heart to pump blood adequately into the peripheral circulation, HF is commonly referred to more specifically as "CHF" by most clinicians.

The terms *systolic dysfunction* or *forward failure* describe the same process in HF. In systolic dysfunction, the diminished ejection of blood from a weakened ventricle sets off a detrimental cascade of events. The weakened ventricle cannot pump sufficient blood volume forward into the arterial system, which results in decreased cardiac output and a hypoperfusion of end organs. Hypoperfusion of the arteries and kidneys stimulates a neurohormonal response, producing vasoactive substances and cytokines, which initially help the body adapt to changes from reduced cardiac output. However, in chronic HF, these substances cause further myocardial damage and impairment of cardiac function. As BP drops in the hypoperfused arteries, this is also detected by pressure sensors within arterial walls called baroreceptors, which stimulate the sympathetic nervous system to constrict the arteries in an effort to raise the BP.

Hypoperfusion of the kidneys stimulates renin production, which provokes the renin-angiotensin-aldosterone cascade. Renin circulates in the bloodstream, and when it reaches the liver, angiotensinogen is released. Angiotensinogen circulates, and when it reaches the lungs, this proenzyme is converted to angiotensin I. Within the lungs, a key reaction occurs, as angiotensin I is converted to angiotensin II by ACE. Angiotensin II acts in various ways to raise BP further and increase blood volume. Angiotensin II is a potent vasoconstrictor that directly incites peripheral arterial vasoconstriction. It also

stimulates the adrenal gland to secrete aldosterone, a hormone that acts at the nephron to increase sodium and water reabsorption into the bloodstream and to excrete potassium. Angiotensin II also directly provokes genetic changes within cardiac myocytes to promote hypertrophic remodeling. Increased BP and blood volume, increased peripheral vascular resistance, and myocardial hypertrophy are the net results of sympathetic stimulation and activation of the renin-angiotensin-aldosterone cascade.

Although compensatory, these effects increase blood volume and peripheral resistance, which increase workload on the weakened heart pump. Thus, as the ventricle endures greater workload, further systolic dysfunction occurs, and neurohormonal mechanisms are cyclically activated. This cycle increases blood volume and leads to fluid overload and further deterioration of systolic function, creating a vicious cycle of HF.

Diastolic dysfunction or *backward failure* describes an abnormality of filling, distensibility, or relaxation of the ventricles. There is elevated filling pressure in the left and/or RV, which causes backward buildup of hydrostatic pressure into the atria. In left ventricular diastolic dysfunction, there is a backup of hydrostatic pressure into the left atrium and, in turn, the pulmonary venous system, which results in the extravasation of fluid into the pulmonary interstitium. If this hydrostatic pressure builds to high levels, pulmonary capillary wedge pressure increases and high amounts of fluid buildup in the pulmonary interstitial spaces (*pulmonary edema*).

Left-sided HF or LVF is the most common type of HF. Most often the LV becomes dysfunctional due to long-standing HTN. Systemic HTN increases resistance against the LV, thereby increasing workload. This leads to LVH, and eventually the LV decompensates into failure. In addition, the LV is vulnerable to ischemic insults due to CAD and may endure an MI. One of the most common sites of arteriosclerosis is the left anterior descending artery, a branch of the left main coronary artery, a major supplier of blood flow to the LV. Repeated ischemic episodes can lead to weakening of the LV with eventual LVF.

LVF can occur as systolic dysfunction (forward failure) and/or diastolic dysfunction (backward failure) as described previously. The classic clinical presentation of LVF involves the pulmonary signs and symptoms of exertional dyspnea, cough, orthopnea (an inability to breathe comfortably while lying supine), paroxysmal nocturnal dyspnea (PND), crackles heard on auscultation, and the hemodynamic finding of elevated pulmonary capillary wedge pressure. These symptoms are a result of the buildup of hydrostatic pressure backward into the pulmonary vasculature due to a failing LV. Ejection fraction (EF) is decreased in LV systolic dysfunction to less than 50% of total ventricular volume (normal EF ranges from 55% to 70%). In contrast, in diastolic dysfunction, the EF may be normal or even increased to greater than 70%, representing the need for the LV to eject a larger proportion of its total blood volume during systole to compensate for reduced diastolic filling.

Right-sided HF or *right ventricular failure* (RVF) most commonly occurs as a result of LVF from a failure of forward cardiac output. The same cardiac muscle comprises both the right and left ventricles, which endures biochemical and hemodynamic stresses during HF. Therefore, in the clinical setting, manifestations of right- and left-sided HF often appear together. The RV can undergo systolic dysfunction (forward failure) and/or diastolic dysfunction (backward failure) in the same manner as the LV. In right-sided HF, the classic signs and symptoms are due to backup of hydrostatic pressure into the venous system. Venous congestion of the superior vena cava is reflected in the classic sign of jugular venous distention. Venous congestion of the inferior vena cava is reflected in the GI system as hepatomegaly, splenomegaly, and peritoneal edema *(ascites)*. Depending on the position of the patient, peripheral edema is apparent as either sacral edema or ankle edema.

Isolated RVF can also occur due to pulmonary disease. The term *cor pulmonale* is used to describe right-sided HF, which is a result of a pathological pulmonary process, such as pulmonary fibrosis, recurrent pulmonary emboli, or other phenomena leading to pulmonary HTN due to arterial vasoconstriction in the pulmonary vascular bed. Chronic hypoxia is a common cause of pulmonary arterial vasoconstriction. The high pulmonary arterial pressure leads to increased resistance against the RV. The RV hypertrophies in response to the increased workload initially. However, eventually the hypertrophic RV decompensates from the excess workload, leading to RVF.

HF severity has traditionally been described with the symptom-based New York Heart Association (NYHA) classification system. The ACC/AHA guidelines supplement this with a staging system that describes the progressive phases of HF. The two systems are complementary, with the NYHA system describing symptom severity and the ACC/AHA system providing a framework for a stage-based therapeutic approach. Patients who present with a past medical history of HTN, diabetes mellitus, CAD, previous exposure to cardiotoxic drugs, or a strong family history of cardiomyopathy may be screened using the following tools as put forth by the NYHA and ACC/AHA.

NYHA classification of HF severity:
  I. Patients with asymptomatic HF
  II. Patients with HF symptoms with significant exertion
  III. Patients with HF symptoms with minor exertion
  IV. Patients with HF symptoms at rest
ACC/AHA staging criteria of HF:
  A. Patients at risk for developing left ventricular dysfunction
  B. Patients with left ventricular dysfunction who have not developed symptoms
  C. Patients with left ventricular dysfunction with symptoms
  D. Patients with refractory end-stage HF

By assigning a combination of the NYHA HF class and the ACC/AHA HF stage to a patient, a more exact assessment and subsequent management plan can be implemented. The following are examples of combining the two systems:

- A patient with minimal or no symptoms but a large pressure gradient across the aortic valve or severe obstruction of the left main coronary artery is classified as function capacity I (NYHA class) and objective assessment D (ACC/AHA stage).
- A patient with severe anginal syndrome but angiographically normal coronary arteries is classified as functional capacity IV (NYHA class) and objective assessment A (ACC/AHA stage).

CLINICAL PRESENTATION

Subjective

The patient with HF may present with symptoms related to the pulmonary system, central nervous system (CNS), specific end organs such as the liver and spleen, and generalized systemic manifestations. Common complaints related to fluid in the pulmonary interstitium include cough, dyspnea at rest or on exertion, orthopnea (especially in the left lateral decubitus position), and PND. Some patients may even present with chest pain.

Patients report breathing easier with the head of the bed elevated because this position disperses fluid downward into the lung bases. Patients often report needing to be propped up on two or three pillows in bed to breathe comfortably at night, termed "two" or "three-pillow orthopnea." Patients with PND frequently report awakening in the middle of the night due to a "nightmare," feeling breathless, or with a dry cough from nighttime hypoxia due to fluid accumulation in the lungs. The clinician must have a high level of suspicion because the description of PND varies from patient to patient.

As HF progresses, the degree of dyspnea increases. However, if the progression is gradual, the patient may not be aware of the dyspnea or that she or he is hypoxic, although shortness of breath may be observed with activity. Some relief may be noted with sitting, standing, or inspiration of fresh outdoor air. When severe coughing and wheezing are associated with dyspnea, the condition is sometimes referred to as cardiac asthma.

Symptoms related to the CNS range from confusion, difficulty concentrating, impaired memory, delirium, insomnia, anxiety, and headache to hallucinations and unresponsiveness. Patients may report light-headedness, near-syncope, or frank syncopal episodes due to the impact of hypotension on the CNS.

Systemic complaints may include fatigue and generalized weakness, which are associated with low cardiac output and may occur at rest or upon exertion. These symptoms may also be caused by blood volume depletion and electrolyte imbalances secondary to overdiuresis in patients on diuretic therapy. Patients may also notice decreased urine output during the day due to decreased blood flow to the kidneys and renal filtration of sodium and water, which contrasts with the development of nocturia during sleeping hours that is the result of enhanced renal filtration secondary to recumbency. However, nocturia may not be reported if concurrent renal failure is present.

The patient may also complain of peripheral and dependent edema. Patients may present with ascites, feelings of abdominal fullness, nausea, vomiting, constipation, upper abdominal pain, anorexia, or symptoms related to congestion of the liver, spleen, or intestines.

Objective

A complete physical examination is necessary to diagnose HF, determine its etiology, and provide the clinician with enough information to optimize intervention strategies. On general inspection, the clinician may note breathlessness, dyspnea on exertion, peripheral cyanosis (as a result of low cardiac output), pallor in the extremities, and distended peripheral veins. There may be jugular venous distention along with abnormal pulsations. Skeletal or connective tissue deformities (as seen in Marfan's syndrome) may be noted. In addition, the patient may have dependent edema, jaundice (suggesting hepatic congestion), ascites, or anasarca (full-body edema).

Vital signs may show tachycardia, pulsus alternans (a weak pulse alternating with a strong pulse), atrial fibrillation (which may contribute to HF), rapid and shallow respirations at rest or with minimal exertion, and possibly Cheyne-Stokes respirations if the patient is asleep (a crescendo-decrescendo pattern of respiratory swings terminating in apnea) caused by a prolonged circulation time from the heart to the brain. Unless observed in an inpatient setting, verification of this type of sleep disturbance would need to be obtained from a family member or friend who has observed the patient during sleep.

On cardiac assessment, the clinician may note a lateral and downward shift in the PMI secondary to cardiac enlargement, the presence of a third heart sound (S_3) in adults older than 40 years (an increased likelihood by 11-fold), and the sudden development of the murmurs of mitral or tricuspid regurgitation. On lung assessment, the clinician may note dyspnea, wet crackles (rales), generally heard bilaterally in the bases or in the most dependent regions of the lungs on inspiration. The classic sign of pulmonary edema is pink, frothy sputum. Wheezing may also be present, as well as findings consistent with a pleural effusion, including stony dullness to percussion or shifting dullness with positional changes. In evaluating these symptoms, the clinician should also consider coronary arterial thromboembolism, which is present in 4% of patients with primary dilated cardiomyopathy.

DIAGNOSTIC REASONING

Diagnostic Tests

Several laboratory tests can assist in the initial diagnosis of HF. Cardiac myocytes and endothelial tissues secrete a family of structurally related peptide hormones termed natriuretic peptides, for example, ANP and BNP. ANP is secreted in response to the atrial stretch that occurs in HF due to increased hydrostatic pressure within the atria. BNP is abundant in the heart and rapidly rises in the bloodstream in the presence of HF. These peptides have diuretic, vasodilating, and kaliuretic (potassium-wasting) effects. In patients with dyspnea, the BNP blood test can be used to rule out HF, as it is highly sensitive and unlikely to be normal (negative) in the presence of HF. Thus, circulating serum BNP level is a useful indicator of the degree of HF, compared with a baseline value obtained in the absence of acute cardiac decompensation, but serum levels do not correlate well with clinical response and are not helpful when followed frequently during inpatient stays.

Of note, BNP is not specific for HF. BNP can be elevated in pulmonary edema, COPD, pulmonary embolism, renal disease, and other conditions. However, a BNP level that is greater than 500 pg/mL is highly indicative of HF. In the Breathing Not Properly study, a BNP cutoff of 100 pg/mL had a sensitivity of 90% and a specificity of 73% to diagnose HF in the emergency department setting and had a diagnostic accuracy of 81.2%, as compared with 74% for clinical judgment alone. There is also a pharmacologic form of BNP, nesiritide, that is used to treat HF. However, once nesiritide is initiated, BNP levels would not be of clinical use to assess the extent of HF.

A CBC may show severe anemia associated with high-output HF. A urinalysis that shows a high degree of proteinuria may indicate nephrotic syndrome, and RBCs or cellular casts may indicate glomerulonephritis. An ESR should be ordered because the ESR is typically decreased secondary to impaired fibrinogen synthesis and decreased fibrinogen concentration in patients with HF. A serum creatinine elevation may reflect volume overload caused by renal failure, with BUN similarly elevated secondary to decreased renal blood flow.

A serum electrolyte panel may show hyponatremia, which may be either genuine (secondary to prolonged sodium restriction and diuretic therapy) or dilutional (secondary to expansion of extracellular volume). Hyponatremia may also signal pronounced activation of the renin-angiotensin system. Hypokalemia may be secondary to diuretic therapy or activation of the renin-angiotensin-aldosterone axis. Hyperkalemia may be secondary to renal failure as a result of the HF, especially if ACEIs have been used. An arterial blood gas may also be ordered for further acid–base evaluation.

Liver function tests may show abnormalities as a result of hepatic congestion. There is also decreased hepatic blood flow; therefore, drugs metabolized by the liver should be appropriately dosed. Additionally, the thyroxine (T_4) and thyroid-stimulating hormone levels may indicate that the HF is aggravated by hypothyroidism or hyperthyroidism.

In addition to laboratory studies, several diagnostic tests and procedures are used to gather information in the diagnosis of HF. A chest x-ray may show an alteration in cardiac silhouette as evidenced by a change in cardiac size and shape, a change in the cardiothoracic (heart width to chest width) ratio (a ratio of more than 0.50 is considered cardiomegaly), and specific cardiac chamber enlargements. A chest x-ray may also show pulmonary venous congestion as evidenced by distention of the pulmonary veins upward from the hila. Normally in the upright position, larger vessels are seen in the bases; however, with increasing capillary pressures, there is compression of the vessels to the lower lobes and dilation of upper lobe vessels. This might present on x-ray studies as an equalization of upper and lower lobe vessel sizes, loss of definition of pulmonary vascular markings (which is usually caused by perivascular edema), haziness of hilar shadows, and thickness of interlobular septa (known as Kerley B lines). Kerley B lines usually result from distended lymphatic vessels. As pulmonary capillary wedge pressure exceeds 25 mm Hg, alveolar edema is indicated by diffuse haziness, usually extending downward toward both lung fields in a butterfly pattern.

Although there is no specific ECG pattern for HF, an ECG may help diagnose underlying causes of HF, such as dysrhythmias or an MI. An echocardiogram is the diagnostic test commonly used to confirm HF after noting a demonstrable elevation of BNP. Abnormalities of systolic and diastolic functions are easily visualized on cardiac ultrasound, and ejection fraction can be estimated. An echocardiogram can also visualize different etiologies of HF, such as diseases of the pericardium or myocardium (e.g., abnormal cardiac wall thickness), as well as heart valve defects. A radionuclide angiocardiography uses technetium-99m as a radioactive tracer to in a multigated acquisition scan to assess for blood pooling, in order to assess wall-motion abnormalities and to measure EF.

Right-heart catheterization is useful to measure of intracardiac pressures. Left-heart catheterization is not usually indicated in HF; however, once the condition is stabilized, catheterization can be useful in identifying the underlying causes of HF. Left-heart catheterization can be performed by a cardiologist if sudden murmurs are auscultated, including severe mitral regurgitation that may be caused by ruptured chordae tendineae, severe aortic regurgitation that may be caused by bacterial endocarditis, perforation of the interventricular septum, or papillary muscle rupture.

Differential Diagnosis

The symptoms of HF can be vague and progress slowly, or they can be sudden and overwhelming, which means HF may mirror several other diagnoses. In either presentation, the symptoms and findings of what appears to be HF may

have other causes such as anxiety, lung disease (e.g., COPD, asthma, pneumonia), venous insufficiency, nephrotic syndrome, hepatic cirrhosis, superior vena cava syndrome from a tumor or other obstruction, or pericardial effusion. In addition, as noted earlier, several pathologies affecting the heart and lungs and their membranous coverings (i.e., the pericardium and pleura) may be underlying causes of HF, including cardiomyopathy, myocarditis, constrictive pericarditis, and pleuritis with pleural effusion.

Takotsubo cardiomyopathy is a typically transient cardiomyopathy that presents as LV apical akinesis and mimics ACS. Its presentation may include chest pain, ST elevation on ECG, elevated cardiac troponins in 90% of cases, and frequently an increased BNP level. However, no coronary occlusions are observed during cardiac catheterization, which distinguishes it from ACS. The onset of Takotsubo cardiomyopathy has been noted in otherwise healthy patients after the occurrence of a particularly traumatic event, such as a sudden illness, a serious accident, or the loss of a loved one, which has resulted in its colloquial moniker of "broken-heart syndrome."

MANAGEMENT

The principles of HF management include identifying and treating precipitating or aggravating conditions, recognizing and treating underlying cardiac disease, and managing the cardiac failure. Prompt treatment of symptoms and underlying causes of HF is key; however, adequate treatment is often delayed for a number of reasons, particularly in elderly patients, as described in Evidence-Based Nursing Practice 35.1. Although HF is often a chronic

 Evidence-Based Nursing Practice 35.1

Jurgens CY, et al. Why do elders delay responding to HF symptoms? *Nurs Res.* 2009;58(4):274–282

Elderly individuals with heart failure (HF) are at risk for frequent hospitalizations for symptom management. Repeated admissions are partly related to delays in responding to HF symptoms. The purpose of this study was to describe contextual factors, such as prior illness experiences and social/emotional factors related to symptom recognition and response among elders hospitalized with decompensated HF. Seventy-seven patients completed several questionnaires in this study, revealing the median duration of early symptoms of HF decompensation was 5 to 7 days, but the duration of dyspnea ranged from 30 minutes to 90 days before action was taken. A longer dyspnea duration was associated with higher physical symptom distress. Sensing and attributing meaning to early symptoms of HF decompensation was problematic for the elderly patients in the study. The physical symptom experience and the cognitive and emotional response to HF symptoms were inadequate for timely care seeking for most of this older age sample.

condition that requires long-term treatment guided by the primary-care practitioner, in the past patients with an acute HF exacerbation were generally hospitalized; however, many may now be managed at home.

When managing HF, the primary-care practitioner must consider treatments that will decrease cardiac workload, decrease volume overload, optimize LV function, correct ventricular dyssynchrony, reduce mortality, and control the ventricular rate or convert atrial fibrillation to a sinus rhythm if present. To decrease the cardiac workload, the primary-care clinician should order rest for the patient until her or his "dry weight" (non–HF-exacerbated baseline weight) is achieved, order vasodilators, encourage weight loss if appropriate, and control HTN. Analysis of data acquired from the Systolic Hypertension in the Elderly Program indicates a marked effect in preventing the development of HF in older patients with isolated systolic HTN when diuretic therapy is initiated.

ACEIs are indicated for all patients with LV systolic dysfunction unless there are specific contraindications, such as a history of intolerance or adverse reactions to these agents, serum potassium greater than 5.5 mEq, or symptomatic hypotension. ACEIs may be the sole therapy for a HF patient with fatigue and mild dyspnea on exertion, and they are referred to as the "cornerstone of HF therapy." ACEIs have been shown to counteract many of the neurohumoral changes in HF and, therefore, decrease mortality.

For patients who cannot tolerate ACEIs, ARBs may be used, as ARBs have a lower risk of chronic cough and angioedema than ACEIs. However, given their related mechanisms, many clinicians reflexively choose to avoid ARBs in patients who have reacted badly to ACEIs. Both ACEIs and ARBs should be used with caution in patients with low systemic BPs, renal insufficiency, or elevated serum potassium levels. A recently approved combination therapy (Entresto) includes both an ARB (valsartan) and a neprilysin inhibitor (sacubitril) and has been shown to reduce mortality in HF. It should not be administered concomitantly or within 36 hours of taking an ACEI or with aliskiren in patients with diabetes mellitus. In addition, a previous history of hypersensitivity to either component of this combination drug or angioedema to an ACEI or ARB are contraindications to its use.

Vasodilators and nitrates can also be used in those who cannot tolerate ACEIs. Diuretics should be added to this regimen if symptoms persist or frank volume overload develops at the first signs of stage C overload, for example, orthopnea, PND. However, overdiuresis must be avoided, as this will lead to hypotension, renal insufficiency, and may interfere with other medications. For mild HF, thiazide diuretics are used, and for severe HF, loop diuretics such as furosemide (Lasix) or bumetanide (Bumex) are indicated. Dosages of these agents can be increased during acute HF exacerbations to counteract fluid overload. In addition, all patients should be on a sodium-restricted diet.

The sympathetic nervous system is stimulated as a compensatory mechanism in HF, causing arterial vasoconstriction and an increased heart rate, which have further detrimental effects on the weakened heart. For this reason, beta-adrenergic blockers, such as carvedilol, have been recommended as part of the drug treatment regimen in HF. Carvedilol is also an alpha-1 antagonist, and along with the beta-adrenergic blockade, will slow heart rate and limit peripheral arterial vasoconstriction, thereby decreasing the force of afterload against the ventricles and, in turn, the work of the heart. Bisoprolol and sustained-release metoprolol are other beta blockers that have been shown to reduce mortality. An additional category of HF drug is ivabradine (Corlanor), which is a sinoatrial node modulator that, when added to maximally tolerated doses of beta blockers, can assist in keeping the heart rate at 70 beats per minute or lower in symptomatic chronic HF.

Once HF has progressed to stage C, the aldosterone antagonist spironolactone has been shown to be of benefit in selected patients, as described in the latest AHA updates for stage C HF therapy. In addition, patients in stage C HF should be evaluated for biventricular pacing and an implantable defibrillator, as HF is often associated with ventricular remodeling and arrhythmias, such as LBBB. These conditions lead to unsynchronized ventricular contractions. Cardiac resynchronization therapy (CRT) is an option for patients who present with a left ventricular EF of less than or equal to 35%, a QRS greater than 120 milliseconds, NYHA class III of IV HF, or who are otherwise are not optimized on medical therapy. CRT involves implantation of a biventricular pacing device, and if necessary, an implantable cardioverter-defibrillator. CRT has been shown to improve cardiac mechanics by inducing concordant contraction of both ventricles.

Implantation of an internal cardiac automated defibrillator may be considered for primary prevention in chronic HF patients (NYHA functional class II or III and ACC/AHA stage C) with ischemic or nonischemic cardiomyopathy or with a patient with an EF of less than or equal to 35%, given the patient's increased risk of sudden cardiac death due to a greater risk of sustained ventricular tachycardia and ventricular fibrillation. As noted earlier, CRT may also be used for patients with NYHA class III or IV HF with persistent symptoms who are already receiving optimal medical therapy. Left ventricular assist devices as end-stage (destination) therapy or, alternatively, as a bridge to heart transplantation may be considered for patients who have exhausted all other treatment recommendations with poor efficacy (i.e., ACC/AHA stage D HF).

Historically, digoxin has been used to treat HF. However, with the establishment of ACEIs and ARBs along with beta blockers and diuretics as first-line treatment options in HF, the use of digoxin has declined. Digoxin may still be used in conjunction with other medications in patients with severe HF (ACC/AHA stage C), although it may not be necessary in patients who become asymptomatic after treatment with ACEIs and diuretics.

Intravenous inotropic agents that may be ordered in a monitored inpatient setting for end-stage cardiac failure (stage D) include dopamine (Intropin), dobutamine (Dobutrex), and milrinone (Primacor). When inotropic support is implemented in the inpatient setting and the patient is unable to be weaned from this therapy, the decision may be made with the patient, family, and care team to discharge the patient home with end-stage HF on home inotropic support.

Controlling the ventricular rate and, when possible, eliminating the arrhythmia of atrial fibrillation are essential in treating HF. Atrial fibrillation in patients with asymptomatic or symptomatic LV systolic dysfunction is associated with an increased risk of progression and death. Because of this, anticoagulation treatment is instituted in HF to decrease the formation of thrombi in the dysfunctional heart chambers, thus decreasing the risk of cerebral thromboembolism. Long-term oral anticoagulation with warfarin (Coumadin) is usually recommended, although newer anticoagulant agents (e.g., factor Xa inhibitors) that do not require frequent laboratory monitoring with PT/INR are being studied in HF.

In addition to optimal medical and electrophysiological therapy, other interventions for patients with HF include the following:

- Regular exercise should be encouraged for all patients with stable HF, because it improves functional status and decreases congestive symptoms, provided physical exertion does not exceed cardiac capacity and trigger a HF exacerbation.
- Cardiac rehabilitation programs, although not specifically indicated for patients with HF, might benefit patients who are anxious about exercising on their own or those who have low cardiac output.
- Dietary sodium should be restricted to 2 g per day or less.
- Limitation of fluid intake should be advised for each patient based on his or her HF status.
- Alcohol consumption should be discouraged. Patients should drink no more than one glass of beer or wine, or a mixed drink with no more than 1 ounce of alcohol per day.
- The patient should record his or her weight daily and notify the primary-care practitioner of a weight gain of 3 pounds in 24 hours or 5 pounds or more within 1 week, as this likely reflects significant fluid retention from a HF exacerbation.
- Immunization with influenza and pneumococcal vaccines reduces the risk of a respiratory infection, as per current Centers for Disease Control and Prevention recommendations.
- All barriers to medication adherence must be removed to assist the patient with management of the disease. Such barriers include the cost of medications, the complexity of the regimen (which typically includes multiple agents from different therapeutic classes), and adverse medication effects, including those related to polypharmacy.
- Psychological support is essential, and patient support groups have been shown to be effective in helping patients to cope with the lifestyle impacts of chronic HF and follow the prescribed treatment regimen.
- The patient must be counseled concerning the prognosis, so that he or she has the benefit of understanding the rationale for decisions made regarding the care plan and can effectively plan for the future. This must be done while maintaining hope, as the primary-care practitioner should explain that a good quality of life is still possible in cooperation with the recommended treatment regimen.
- The patient should be encouraged to complete an advance directive, given the risk of cardiac arrest with HF.

FOLLOW-UP AND REFERRAL

Patients in chronic cardiac failure may be treated on an outpatient basis, in which changes in cardiac status are assessed thoroughly, including questions regarding health-related quality of life (e.g., sleep quality, sexual function, mental health status, outlook on life, appetite, and social activities). After the patient, family, and caregiver have been educated on the condition, they should be encouraged to communicate all signs, symptoms, fears, and concerns related to HF, as patients are likely to experience changes in symptoms prior to developing evidence of deterioration on physical examination.

The frequency of follow-up of these patients generally depends on the underlying cause of their HF, although patients are typically seen by the primary-care practitioner at least every 3 months. Intensive home-care surveillance has been shown to decrease the need for hospitalization and to improve the functional status of older adult patients with HF.

Referral to a cardiologist is recommended with the onset of symptoms in HF; however, initial medical treatment should begin immediately as directed by the primary-care practitioner, followed by a phone referral to a cardiologist. Increasingly in the United States, dedicated HF clinics are becoming popular referral resources.

Patients in acute HF typically require hospitalization for aggressive medical intervention, unless mild in severity. The primary-care practitioner and cardiologist should work together to establish a plan of care with the patient for the long-term management of HF. The Joint Commission has mandated that specific core measures of care should be met before discharge. For example, there must be an assessment of LV function documenting an EF. If the EF is below 40%, the patient should be prescribed an ACEI or ARB. If the patient has had an allergic reaction to either of these drugs or otherwise cannot tolerate them, this must be documented in the medical record.

Additional core measures include advice and counseling on smoking cessation (as well as other tobacco use) and discharge instructions that include reconciliation of the prescribed medication regimen.

Patient Education: Heart Failure

Successful management of patients with HF requires an active partnership between the patient and all health-care providers in order to decrease the possibility of the patient becoming "crippled" by the disease process. This includes thorough patient education regarding the condition and encouragement for the patient to take responsibility for her or his own personal care. In turn, the primary-care practitioner should educate and facilitate the patient in achieving the following self-care goals:

- Keep a record of daily weights and notify the clinician of a 3-pound or greater weight gain in 24 hours or a 5-pound or greater weight gain in 1 week or less.
- Exercise regularly.
- Restrict dietary sodium to 2 g/day.
- Maintain an optimal body weight.
- Rest with elevation of the lower extremities and the upper body (i.e., head of the bed).
- Use elastic stockings to reduce the risk of venous thrombosis and PE.
- Ensure emotional rest and adequate relaxation.
- Advise the health-care provider of all symptoms or concerns related to HF.
- Discuss all changes the patient wants to make in self-care practices with the primary-care practitioner before taking action, as this will ensure the best possible outcome.

In working with the patient and her or his family to develop the patient's care plan, the primary-care practitioner should not lose sight of highly influential nature of her or his recommendations. The clinician should keep in mind that the family, who fears losing their loved one, will attempt to ensure the care plan is followed exactly. Therefore, the primary-care practitioner should remember to "build in"—and teach the patient and family how to "build in"—humane adaptations to the plan of care that allow for practical flexibility under certain circumstances.

For example, if the clinician stresses a diuretic must be taken every morning, she or he must realize that if the patient has an important family function one morning and chooses to take the diuretic later in the day, an inflexible mandate from the clinician may cause needless stress and guilt. The patient may be frightened of falling into distress if he or she does not follow the clinician's orders precisely, and the family may "harass" the patient for deliberately not following the plan of care. In turn, the patient may feel that participation in events that take place in the morning is forbidden and isolate him or herself to the detriment of the patient's social support system. Thus, it is critical that the primary-care practitioner ensures the patient and her or his family understand the rationale for the decisions about his or her care, as these perceived restrictions compromise the quality of the patient's life and are unnecessary.

With the rising incidence of HF, researchers are increasingly evaluating patient self-care practices and their impact on clinical outcomes. Exercise training is now being recommended for most individuals with moderate to severe HF, as activity intolerance associated with chronic HF leads to a decreased quality of life. Exercise training as therapy for chronic HF has shown to reduce morbidity and mortality (Van Craenenbroeck EM, 2017)

Coaching and encouraging a terminally ill patient in self-care may be time consuming and can be draining for the clinician and patient. However, the primary-care practitioner must maintain an authentic presence and respond to calls for assistance that are often not timed with the patient's regularly scheduled appointments, given the acute nature of HF exacerbations. To patients with chronic, progressive, and ultimately terminal illnesses, the significance of the effects of the illness on their lives is directly related to their perceptions of the attention and care being given by health-care providers.

REFERENCES

General

The American Geriatrics Society 2015 Beers Criteria Update Expert Panel. American Geriatrics Society 2015 Updated Beers Criteria for potentially inappropriate medication use in older adults. *J Am Geriatr Soc*. 2015;63(11):2227–2246.

Acute Coronary Syndrome

Benjamin EJ, Biaha MJ, Chiuve SE, et al. (2017). Heart disease and stroke statistics-2017 update: A report from the American Heart Association. *Circulation*. 2017;135(10):e146–e603.

Levine GN, Bates ER, Bittl JA, et al. 2016 ACC/AHA guideline focused update on duration of dual antiplatelet therapy in patients with coronary artery disease: A report of the American College of Cardiology/American Heart Association task force on clinical practice guidelines. *J Thorac Cardiovasc Surg*. 2016;152:1243–1275.

Coronary Heart Disease

Arslanian-Engoren C, Scott LD, (2017). Delays in treatment-seeking decisions among women with myocardial infarction. *Dimens criti care Nurs*. 2017;36(5):298–303.

Lefler LL, Bondy KN. Women's delay in seeking treatment with myocardial infarction: A meta-synthesis. *TJ Cardiovasc Nurs*. 2004;19(4):251–268.

Taghaddosi M, Dianati M, Fath Gharib Bidgoli J, Bahonaran J. Delay and its related factors in seeking treatment in patients with acute myocardial infarction. *ARYA Atheroscler*. 2010; Spring; 6(1): 35–41.

Dyslipidemia

Drozda JP, Ferguson B, Jneid H, et al. 2015 ACC/AHA focused update of secondary prevention lipid performance measures: A report of the American College of Cardiology/American Heart Association task force on performance measures. *Circ Cardiovasc Qual Outcomes.* 2016;9:68–95.

Heart Failure

National Center for Chronic Disease Prevention and Health Promotion, Division for Heart Disease and Stroke Prevention. 2016 heart failure fact sheet. **https://www.cdc.gov/dhdsp/data_statistics/fact_sheets/fs_heart_failure.htm.**

Van Craenenbroeck EM. Exercise training as therapy for chronic heart failure. European Society of Cardiology, vol 14. **https://www.escardio.org/Journals/E-Journal-of-Cardiology-Practice/Volume-14/Exercise-training-as-therapy-for-chronic-heart-failure.**

Yancy CQ, Jessup M, Bozkurt B, et al. 2017 ACC/AHA/HFSA focused update of the 2013 ACCF/AHA guideline for the management of heart failure: A report of the American College of Cardiology/American Heart Association task force on clinical practice guidelines and the HF Society of America. *Circulation.* 2017;136(10):e137–e161.

Zeitler EP, Eapen ZJ. Anticoagulation in heart failure: A review. *J Atr Fibrillation.* 2015;8(1):1250.

Hypertension

Chazal RA, Creager MA. New quality measure core sets provide continuity for measuring quality improvement: Concerns raised about conflicting blood pressure measures. *Hypertension.* 2016;67:1053–1054.

Cobos F, Haskard-Zolnierek K, Howard K. White coat hypertension: Improving the patient–health care practitioner relationship. *Psychol Res Behav Manag.* 2015;8:133–141.

James PA, Oparil S, Carter BL, et al. (2014). 2014 evidence-based guideline for the management of high blood pressure in adults: Report from the panel members appointed to the eighth joint national committee (JNC 8). *JAMA.* 2014;311(5):507–520.

Michigan Quality Improvement Consortium Guideline. Medical management of adults with hypertension. MQIC, 2017. **http://mqic.org/pdf/mqic_medical_management_of_adults_with_hypertension_cpg.pdf.**

Page MR. The JNC8 hypertension guidelines: An in-depth guide. www.ajmc.com/publications/evidence-based-diabetes-management/2014/jan-feb2014.

Shimbo D, Newman JD, Schwartz, JE, et al. Masked hypertension and prehypertension: Diagnostic overlap and interrelationships with left ventricular mass: The Masked Hypertension Study. *Am J Hypertens* 2012;25(6):664–671.

Whelton PK, Carey RM, Aronow WS, et al. ACC/AHA/AAPA/ABC/ACPM/AGS/APhA/ASH/ASPC/NMA/ PCNA guideline for the prevention, detection, evaluation, and management of high blood pressure in adults: Executive summary: A report of the American College of Cardiology/American Heart Association task force on clinical practice guidelines. *J Am Soc Hypertens.* 2018;12:579.

Metabolic Syndrome

Grundy SM, Cleeman JI, Daniels SR, et al. Diagnosis and management of the metabolic syndrome. *Circulation.* 2005;112(17):2735–2752.

McKinney L, Skolnik N, Chrush A. *Diagnosis and management of obesity.* Leawood, KS: American Academy of Family Physicians; 2013.

RESOURCES

American Heart Association/American Stroke Association Cardiovascular Risk Calculator
http://ccccalculator.ccctracker.com

Cardiovascular Risk Calculator
http://myamericanheart.org/cvriskcalculator

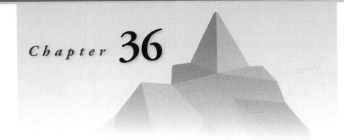

Chapter **36**

Dysrhythmias and Valvular Disorders

Kathryn B. Keller, PhD, RN, CNE

Denese Sabatino, MSN, APRN, NP-C, CCRN

Jill E. Winland-Brown, EdD, APRN, FNP-BC

Michael B. Keller, MD

Brian Oscar Porter, MD, PhD, MPH, MBA

ARRHYTHMIAS

Arrhythmias that the primary-care practitioner may encounter in the clinical setting include the atrial arrhythmias of atrial fibrillation, premature atrial contractions (PACs), atrial tachycardia, atrial flutter, and supraventricular tachycardia (SVT). Ventricular arrhythmias include premature ventricular contractions (PVCs) and ventricular tachycardia (VT). First-, second-, and third-degree heart blocks are other common arrhythmias. In the past, arrhythmias associated with digitalis toxicity were not uncommon, but they are seen less frequently today because of the decreased usage of digitalis preparations.

ATRIAL ARRHYTHMIAS

Atrial Fibrillation

Atrial fibrillation is one of the most common arrhythmias that clinicians will encounter in clinical practice. In most cases, atrial fibrillation initially will be associated with a rapid ventricular response, and most patients will have some type of underlying heart disease. In these patients, the loss of atrial contribution to left ventricular blood volume (atrial "kick"), along with a rapid ventricular rate, can have serious hemodynamic effects caused by diminished cardiac output. These effects may manifest as hypotension, diaphoresis, dizziness, and syncopal episodes.

The loss of mechanically effective atrial contractions in atrial fibrillation leads to stasis of blood in the left atrium that predisposes an individual to formation of embolic atrial thrombi. Thrombi that form in the left atrium tend to travel into the left ventricle and the aorta where they are propelled into the arterial circulation. A common route for a thrombus

from the aorta is to the brachiocephalic artery, carotid artery, and then into the cerebral circulation. This pathway makes atrial fibrillation a risk factor for ischemic stroke because an embolus may lodge in a branch of the middle cerebral artery.

All persons with atrial fibrillation should be evaluated for their risk of stroke and potential anticoagulant therapy using the most current version of the CHADS2 scoring tool. The CHADS2 risk score is calculated using 1 point each for CHADS, as shown in Table 36.1.

With a score of 2 or greater, oral anticoagulation is recommended. This CHADS score is the easiest one to use in the primary-care setting. The CHA2DS2-VASc score is recommended in patients with nonvalvular AF for assessment of stroke risk (January et al., 2014). This scoring includes the addition of having vascular disease and being a female.

Premature Atrial Contractions

PACs are common, yet in most cases, they have no clinical significance. PACs are usually a benign arrhythmia that does not require pharmacological intervention unless there are underlying causes that can be corrected. They are rarely symptomatic. This arrhythmia is commonly seen in young, healthy individuals. Cardiac stimulants such as caffeine, nicotine, alcohol, or over-the-counter medications sometimes induce PACs. They may also occur in patients with right atrial dilation caused by obstructive lung disease and heart failure.

Supraventricular Tachycardia

Supraventricular tachycardia is often used as a "catch-all" term that encompasses rapid arrhythmias originating just above the ventricles. There continues to be confusion over specific terminology with respect to different forms of SVT. This confusion originates from an inability to differentiate true atrial tachycardias or atrial flutter from paroxysmal supraventricular tachycardia (PSVT) that occurs because of electrical reentry circuits. The use of the term *paroxysmal atrial tachycardia* (PAT) further confounds the terminology issue. PAT describes a sudden onset of atrial tachycardia, yet this term is often incorrectly used for SVTs, such as atrial flutter or atrial fibrillation, whether they occur paroxysmally or not.

TABLE 36.1   CHADS2 Score for Stroke Risk Assessment in Atrial Fibrillation

	Condition	*Points*
C	Congestive heart failure	1
H	Hypertension (or treated hypertension)	1
A	Age >75 years	1
D	Diabetes	1
S	Prior stroke or transient ischemic attach	2

Adapted from de Jong, Jonas MD, PhD. CHA2DS2-VASc/HAS-BLED/EHRA atrial fibrillation risk score calculator. https://www.chadsvasc.org/

The two most common forms of PSVT are atrioventricular nodal reentrant tachycardia (AVNRT) and orthodromic circus movement tachycardia (CMT). For the purposes of this discussion, the condition SVT is subdivided into PSVT, which includes AVNRT and CMT, and non-PSVT, which includes atrial tachycardia of non-reentrant origin and atrial flutter. Although atrial fibrillation can also be classified as an SVT, this rhythm is discussed separately.

Current Advanced Cardiac Life Support treatment standards require that the clinician be able to differentiate tachycardias originating in the atrium that are included under the term *SVT.* The atrial rate differentiates atrial tachycardia from atrial flutter. This rate difference is particularly pertinent when the clinician is attempting to discern whether the arrhythmia is an atrial tachycardia with a heart block (as seen in digitalis toxicity) or an atrial flutter. Both rhythms can present with more than one observable P wave before the QRS. An atrial tachycardia rate (P-wave rate of 140–250 per minute) is slower than an atrial flutter rate (P-wave rate of 250–350 per minute). It is important for the clinician to remember that the P-wave rate needs to be counted separately from the QRS rate. Atrial flutter is less common than atrial fibrillation and most commonly occurs in older adults. Patients with atrial flutter typically have some form of organic heart disease. They must be referred to a cardiologist and may need to be managed in an acute care setting.

VENTRICULAR ARRHYTHMIAS

Premature ventricular contractions (PVCs) are usually a benign arrhythmia that does not require pharmacological intervention unless the rhythm progresses to VT, which may be associated with any form of heart disease. It may be sustained or nonsustained. In patients who have had a myocardial infarction (MI), nonsustained VT is a risk factor for sudden cardiac death.

HEART BLOCKS

Atrioventricular (AV) blocks are classified by the severity of disturbance in the impulse going through the electrical conduction system between the atria and ventricles. Heart blocks may be permanent or transient and are classified as first-, second-, or third-degree:

- A *first-degree AV block* is observed with a regular rhythm and only a prolonged P-R interval.
- *Second-degree AV block* may be classified further as type I (Mobitz I or Wenckebach) and type II (Mobitz II). Mobitz type I occurs in the AV nodal area with progressive lengthening of the P-R interval until a QRS complex (ventricular contraction) is dropped. Mobitz type II occurs within or below the bundle of His, with a normal or lengthened PR interval and a periodic drop of a QRS complex.

- A *third-degree AV block* or complete heart block occurs when the atria beat regularly and at a normal rate but no excitation is transmitted from the atria to the ventricles. In turn, the atria and ventricles contract independently at their own intrinsic rates. This complete lack of coordination between the chambers of the heart severely compromises cardiac output and can prove fatal. Third-degree heart block is further classified as third-degree at the junctional level or third-degree at the ventricular level, depending on where the block occurs anatomically.

Progression of heart block is an important clinical concept. A second-degree Mobitz type I block does not progress to Mobitz type II; rather, a Mobitz type I block typically progresses to a third-degree block with an idiojunctional response. In contrast, a second-degree Mobitz type II block progresses to a third-degree heart block with an idioventricular response that carries a more ominous prognosis. If a rhythm presents with two P waves for every QRS complex (referred to as 2:1 conduction) with a normal rate, the origin of nodal or subnodal pathology must be determined. This rhythm is often referred to as undifferentiated second-degree AV block. If the QRS complex is narrow (0.04–0.10 seconds), it can be deduced that the location of the block is from the junctional area and, therefore, Mobitz type I in origin. However, if the QRS complex is 0.12 seconds or wider, the block could be either from the junctional area (Mobitz I/Wenckebach area) with a preexisting bundle branch block or it could be a Mobitz II idioventricular response from the ventricular area.

ARRHYTHMIAS ASSOCIATED WITH DIGITALIS

Historically, one of the most common agents used in the treatment of heart failure and supraventricular tachyarrhythmias was digitalis. Although the use of digitalis is not as common today, it is still prescribed by many clinicians and merits discussion. It is a common cause of various degrees of AV block. There is a narrow therapeutic range for this drug, and signs of toxicity can occur before acute symptoms are recognized. Digitalis toxicity can cause almost any type of arrhythmia. Those arrhythmias most commonly seen in digitalis toxicity are atrial tachycardia with AV nodal block, accelerated junctional rhythms, atrial fibrillation with a slow or regular ventricular response, second-degree heart block—Mobitz type I (Wenckebach), and ventricular dysrhythmias. The serum digitalis level may not reflect the amount of digitalis bound to the myocardial membrane, where it cannot be measured. Thus, a normal digitalis level should not be the determining factor in assessing digitalis toxicity. The onset of atrial tachydysrhythmias, noncardiac subjective symptoms (particularly altered visual color perception), and a pertinent medication history should make the clinician highly suspicious of digitalis toxicity. Electrocardiograms (ECGs) representing these rhythms are shown in Figure 36.1.

Common Arrhythmias
ATRIAL ARRHYTHMIAS

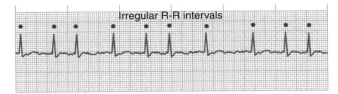

Figure 36.1a Atrial fibrillation. Fibrillatory waves distort the baseline, and the R-R interval is characteristically irregular. The ventricular rate is approximately 100 beats/min.

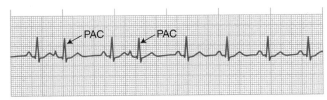

Figure 36.1b Premature atrial contraction (PACs) or atrial premature contractions (APCs). A single complex occurs earlier than the next expected sinus complex. After the PAC, sinus rhythm usually resumes.

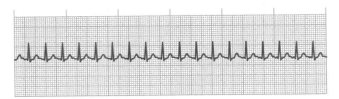

Figure 36.1c Atrial tachycardia with a rate of 180 beats/min.

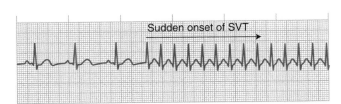

Figure 36.1d Paroxysmal supraventricular tachycardia (PSVT) or paroxysmal atrial tachycardia. (PAT). Sinus rhythm that changes into atrial tachycardia at a rate of 230 beats/min.

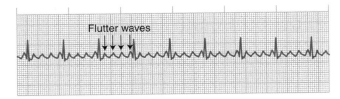

Figure 36.1e Atrial flutter. A characteristic sawtooth pattern at the baseline. Atrial flutter with a 4:1 conduction. The R-R interval is regular.

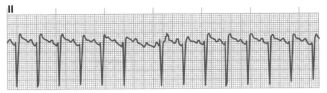

Figure 36.1f Atrial flutter with a 2:1 conduction. Initiation of carotid sinus massage temporarily slows the ventricular rate enough to unmask the flutter waves.

VENTRICULAR ARRHYTHMIAS

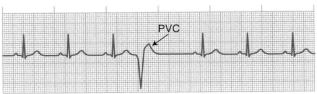

Figure 36.1g Premature ventricular contractions (PVCs). The ectopic QRS complex (the PVC) is wide, abnormally shaped, and appears earlier than expected. The length of the compensatory pause following a PVC indicates that sinus node discharge was undisturbed. A nonconducted sinus P wave distorts the T wave (the P wave appears on time).

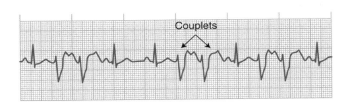

Figure 36.1h PVC couplets. Pairs of uniform PVCs originating from the same ectopic site.

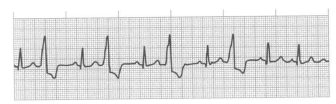

Figure 36.1i PVC bigeminy. A uniform PVC occurring from the same ectopic site; occurs every other beat.

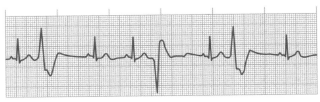

Figure 36.1j Multifocal PVCs. PVCs coming from two ectopic foci.

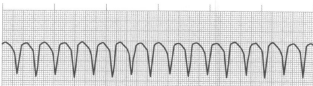

Figure 36.1k Ventricular tachycardia. The ventricular rate is approximately 160 beats/min. The QRS complexes are wide, they look alike, and the R-R interval is regular.

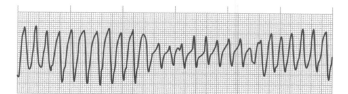

Figure 36.1l Torsade de pointes. Polymorphic ventricular tachycardia, congenital or drug-induced.

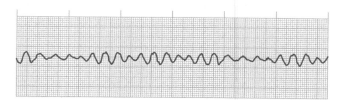

Figure 36.1m Ventricular fibrillation. Chaotic electrical activity with no ventricular contraction.

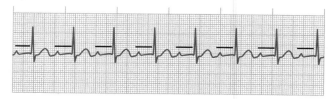

Figure 36.1n Atrioventricular (AV) heart blocks: First-degree AV block. The P-R interval is consistently prolonged at 0.20 second or longer, with an underlying sinus rhythm.

SECOND-DEGREE AV BLOCKS

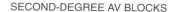

Blocked beat
X

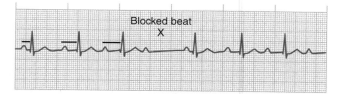

Figure 36.1o Type I (Mobitz I or Wenckebach). The P-R interval lengthens until a beat is dropped. The QRS complexes are narrow. The nonconducted P waves are easily visible.

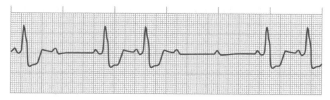

Figure 36.1p Type II (Mobitz II). The P-R interval remains fixed. The QRS complexes are wider than normal. The nonconducted P waves are visible. The conduction ratio (P waves to QRS complexes) is commonly 2:1, 3:1, or 4:1.

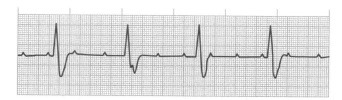

Figure 36.1q Third-degree AV block: There is no relationship between the P wave and the QRS complex. This is a third-degree AV block with a ventricular escape pacemaker.

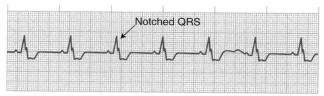

Notched QRS

Figure 36.1r Bundle branch block (BBB). Either the left or the right ventricle will depolarize late, creating a "notched" QRS complex. In this strip, we are unable to determine whether this is a right or left BBB. An RBBB is determined in lead VI and will show a notched pattern in a classic rsR (little r, s wave, larger R prime) upright qrs complex that is .12 or greater. If an LBBB is present, then V1 will retain the original formation (showing a small upright r wave with negative remaining complex) that is .12 or greater. This LBBB can be confirmed in either V5 or V6 also by a notched appearance but does not have a set pattern to the qrs as found in the rsR of a RBBB. It is necessary to be able to determine a LBBB in the setting of an acute MI because this will interfere with accurate 12-lead ECG interpretation of an acute injury pattern.

EPIDEMIOLOGY AND CAUSES

Atrial Arrhythmias

Most patients with atrial fibrillation have some form of heart disease. The most common form is coronary artery disease (CAD) associated with heart failure, followed by hypertension and rheumatic heart disease. Frequently, the precipitating event is an acute illness, electrolyte imbalance, or major cardiac surgery. Atrial fibrillation is seen in 60% of patients after valvular surgery and in 33% to 42% of patients with mitral valve stenosis. Other causes of atrial fibrillation include abrupt discontinuation of beta blockers, alcohol ingestion (sometimes called "holiday heart"), hyperthyroidism, acute MI, and cor pulmonale. A danger of untreated atrial fibrillation, with or without rapid ventricular response, is the significant increased risk of embolic stroke. The risk of stroke is increased in untreated atrial fibrillation after 48 to 72 hours; therefore, it is important to diagnose and treat this arrhythmia in an expeditious manner. A beta blocker or calcium channel blocker should be given to slow AV conduction and control the ventricular rate of atrial fibrillation.

PACs typically have no clinical significance. In a normal patient, tobacco, caffeine, alcohol, or emotional stress may cause PACs. They may also result from stretching of the myocardium, a sign associated with developing congestive heart failure. In patients with organic heart disease, common causes of PACs are mitral valve stenosis and cor pulmonale, which result in atrial enlargement. Occasionally in patients with organic heart disease, PACs may precipitate PSVT, atrial flutter, and atrial fibrillation. The most common cause of a pause on an ECG is a blocked PAC. Assessment of whether the P wave occurs early or is on time can help differentiate this diagnosis from heart block. If the P wave is early, it is a premature atrial ectopic beat. If the P wave is on time, heart block should be considered.

Ventricular Arrhythmias

Frequent PVCs are seen in patients with cardiomyopathies of differing etiologies and arteriosclerotic heart disease. These patients are rarely symptomatic and in general do not need to be treated specifically for the PVCs. In patients with frequent PVCs, however, it is worthwhile to rule out acute underlying causes of ventricular ectopy, such as hypokalemia, hypomagnesemia, hypoxia, myocardial ischemia, or digitalis toxicity. Other common causes are stress and stimulants, such as alcohol and nicotine. Sustained ventricular tachycardia is associated with a prior MI or CAD, electrolyte disturbances, and digitalis toxicity.

Heart Blocks

A first-degree heart block (P-R interval greater that 0.20 seconds) may occur as a result of drugs that slow AV conduction or in persons with CAD and digitalis toxicity. A transient second-degree AV heart block type I may be associated with an acute inferior MI. It may also be associated with heart failure or digitalis toxicity. A Mobitz type II AV block is a less common type of second-degree heart block; it is marked by an intermittent blocked impulse that can occur at the bundle of His or at the right or left bundle branches. This type of block may occur as the result of an anterior wall MI. As this block progresses, complete heart

block with an idioventricular response may follow. Insertion of a temporary pacemaker as soon as a Mobitz type II block is discovered is the standard of care. Other causes of AV block at this level are acute infections, valvular heart disease, and digitalis toxicity. This is not commonly a transient arrhythmia and can progress to third-degree AV heart block at the ventricular level; therefore, it must be monitored and treated appropriately.

PATHOPHYSIOLOGY

The mechanism of atrial fibrillation remains controversial. Cardiac disease associated with atrial enlargement is the primary cause of the rapid firing (400–700 beats per minute) of the ectopic foci throughout the atrium. Although electrical atrial activity is very rapid, only a small islet of myocardium is depolarized rather than the entire atrium. Because the atrium does not contract as a whole, there is no P wave. The chaotic atrial activity is seen as a wavy line between the QRS complex and is referred to as fibrillatory waves. These impulses are transmitted in variable fashion from the atria to the ventricles. The ventricular response rate to atrial fibrillation may be fast or slow, depending on the refractory nature of the AV node and the degree of AV nodal heart block or conduction delay within the AV node. In turn, therapy is usually geared toward rate control with AV nodal slowing agents, rather than toward complete resolution of the arrhythmia with antiarrhythmic medications.

Other pathological arrhythmias involve bypass tracks. Normally, electrical impulses from the sinoatrial node within the atria are conducted down the AV node to the His-Purkinje conduction system, disseminating throughout the two ventricles and leading to subsequent contraction. In addition to the AV node, some individuals have a fast-conducting accessory pathway between the atria and ventricles that bypasses the AV node. The tissue in these pathways depolarizes at a faster rate because of the presence of faster inward sodium transport channels. One of the most common and well-characterized examples of these bypass tracts is the bundle of Kent accessory tract, which is seen in individuals with Wolff-Parkinson-White (WPW) syndrome. Because conduction down this bypass pathway directly transmits a depolarizing impulse to the ventricles faster than impulses sent down the AV node, this has been termed a "preexcitation syndrome." ECG patterns in these patients demonstrate QRS fusion beats with a characteristic shape produced by the overlap of QRS complexes transmitted via each pathway in temporal proximity, hence creating a fusion complex. The first portion of the upswing in the R wave in this complex has a characteristic slanted appearance with a less steep angle than the remainder of the upward deflection, termed a "delta wave." Figure 36.2 shows a delta wave present in WPW syndrome.

The most common mechanisms of PSVT observed in symptomatic patients are CMT (40% of cases) and AVNRT

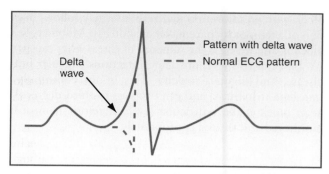

Figure 36.2 Delta wave present in Wolff-Parkinson-White syndrome.

(50% of cases). CMT is distinguished by the dependence of the circular, reentrant impulse on an accessory conduction pathway, separate from the AV node. Thus, the fast bypass tract found in WPW syndrome is an ideal setup for development of CMT. Normal physiology dictates that cardiac conducting tissue become refractory (i.e., resistant to depolarization and electrical conduction) for a brief period of time following transmission of an electrical impulse. Bypass pathways such as that seen in WPW syndrome typically have shorter refractory periods than the AV node. Once depolarizing impulses are transmitted down the AV node to the ventricles, the refractory nature of the AV node prevents retrograde conduction back up this pathway. However, the same impulse may be conducted in retrograde fashion from the ventricles back up the accessory bypass tract to the atria. In turn, this impulse may then be conducted back down the AV node, which will have recovered from its refractory state by this time, only to circle back around once again to the atria via the fast accessory pathway. This type of circular, orthodromic conduction accounts for 90% of CMT cases, with a P wave occurring immediately after the QRS complex, rather than before it. The remaining 10% of CMT cases are considered antidromic, with the depolarizing impulse initially conducted down the fast accessory tract, only to circle back up the slower AV nodal pathway to the atria to complete the circular movement.

In AVNRT, PSVT typically results from an interplay of two conducting pathways within the AV node itself—one fast and one slow. The key aspect of this type of PSVT is that reentry of the impulse is dependent on an AV nodal pathway, as opposed to an accessory bypass pathway. In AVNRT, the fast AV nodal conducting pathway has a refractory period that lasts longer than that of the slow AV nodal pathway. Thus, if an electrical impulse enters both pathways of the AV node simultaneously, the fast pathway will remain refractory longer. In turn, if an early PAC then enters the AV node while the fast accessory pathway is still refractory, it can depolarize the ventricles only via transmission down the slower AV nodal pathway. By the time the impulse has traveled down this open slow pathway, the fast pathway is no longer refractory, and the impulse may travel in retrograde fashion back up to the atria via the fast

pathway, and then back down again to the ventricles via the slow pathway. This mechanism activates the atria and the ventricles nearly simultaneously, which places the P wave within the QRS complex, distorting its terminal portion.

PVCs and VT may be the result of enhanced normal automaticity from catecholamines within the His-Purkinje system or abnormal automaticity anywhere in the ventricles from ischemia, injury, or electrolyte imbalances. Another mechanism for these arrhythmias is reentry through slowly conducting tissue within the His-Purkinje system or the ventricular myocardium related to catecholamines or digitalis excess.

Digitalis toxicity may cause delayed after-depolarizations that are oscillations in transmembrane potential that follow full repolarization of the membrane. These oscillations are caused by interference of the sodium-potassium pump by digitalis. Digitalis competes with potassium for a binding site on the cell membrane, which disables the sodium-potassium adenosine triphosphatase (ATPase) pump. The less potassium there is to bind to receptors, the greater the number of receptors available for digitalis; thus, hypokalemia potentiates digitalis toxicity. Triggered activity in which an abnormal action potential is triggered by a preceding action potential is another important mechanism in the pathophysiology of digitalis toxicity.

The mechanism of AV block is delayed conduction or nonconduction of an atrial impulse when the AV junction is not physiologically refractory. In first-degree AV block, there is not an actual block but rather a prolongation of conduction. In second-degree block, there is nonconduction of some of the atrial impulses. The pathology is either in the AV node itself or within or below the bundle of His. The QRS complex duration assists the clinician in localizing the level of the block. A narrow QRS complex is seen if the ventricular response is initiated at the level of AV node and conducted down both bundle branches simultaneously, as seen in Mobitz type I block. A wider QRS complex indicates that the block is located farther down the conduction system at the bundle of His or within the bundle branches. These criteria may not be helpful if the patient has a pre-existing right or left bundle branch block because such a patient could present with a prolonged P-R interval with a broad QRS complex. In turn, the pathology could be either in the AV node or within or below the bundle of His. The clinician would then need to assess the P-R interval carefully for varying lengths and Wenckebach conduction patterns. If the patient's ECG has a pattern of two P waves for every wide QRS complex (2:1 conduction), the origin of pathology is difficult to determine from the ECG.

CLINICAL PRESENTATION

Subjective

A patient presenting with atrial fibrillation may complain of shortness of breath, palpitations, angina, changing level of consciousness, and syncope. If the patient is aware of palpitations, the clinician should have him or her "tap" out the rhythm in the palm of the hand. Irregular tapping at irregular intervals (i.e., an irregularly irregular heart rhythm) can differentiate this rhythm from the regular patterns of other arrhythmias.

A patient experiencing SVT will complain of dizziness, shortness of breath, and chest pain. As part of the patient's history, the clinician should ask about polyuria that is associated with SVT. Polyuria may be present in patients with PSVT or atrial fibrillation. It is thought to be related to the cardiac secretion of atrial natriuretic factor due to changes in the heart rhythm and atrial pressure. Polyuria is particularly common in AVNRT with high atrial pressures.

A patient presenting with nonsustained VT may complain of palpitations or may present with symptoms similar to those of patients with sustained VT. Usually patients with sustained VT will demonstrate findings compatible with a loss of cardiac output, such as decreased levels of mentation and hypotension.

If the patient is taking digitalis, the clinician should question him or her about anorexia, nausea, and vomiting, which suggest toxicity. In addition, the patient should be asked about changes in the quality of color vision, especially red and green color distortions. These changes may be subtle, and patients often do not volunteer them unless asked. Visual disturbances such as scotomas and flickering halos, although advanced signs, may also be present. Neurological symptoms such as headache, malaise, memory lapses, and insomnia may also be reported.

A patient experiencing first-degree heart block will be asymptomatic. With third-degree AV heart block, the patient may exhibit signs of symptomatic bradycardia. The origin of the block may determine the degree of symptomatology. Patients with second-degree AV Mobitz type I block that progresses into a third-degree block with an idiojunctional response may or may not exhibit overt signs and symptoms of bradycardia. Hemodynamic symptoms will depend on the rate of the junctional response (anywhere from 40–60 beats per minute), the status of the patient's left ventricular ejection fraction, and the loss of atrial kick (up to 20%–30% of cardiac output). A patient whose Mobitz type II heart block progresses to third-degree heart block with a ventricular response of 20 to 40 beats per minute will almost always exhibit signs and symptoms of severe bradycardia, such as profound changes in level of consciousness and hypotension, which may preclude subjective symptom complaints.

Objective

Atrial Fibrillation

Physical examination of the patient with atrial fibrillation will yield an irregularly irregular heart rhythm. In most cases the rate is rapid (100–180 beats per minute). Some patients with a diseased AV node present with a slow or normal ventricular rate. Patients can be asymptomatic, although most present with symptoms such as palpitations, dizziness, a decrease in blood pressure (BP), or new-onset activity intolerance. In a few cases, a stroke can be the presenting manifestation of atrial fibrillation as a result of emboli traveling from a clot formed in the dysfunctional atrium into the cerebral vasculature.

Cannon waves, which are unpredictable expansions of the jugular pulse caused when the atria contract against closed AV valves resulting in a reflux of blood into the jugular vein, may be seen. When present in atrial fibrillation, cannon waves signify AV dissociation. The ECG strip will show fibrillatory waves representing an atrial rate of 350 to 600 beats per minute (although unmeasurable on an ECG), with a ventricular rate of 100 to 180 beats per minute. The rhythm is irregular, and there are no discernible P waves on the ECG, with a coarse or fine fibrillatory wave (f wave) present. This is the hallmark of this arrhythmia and represents chaotic atrial activity. Thus, the P-R interval cannot be measured, and the QRS wave is usually normal.

Premature Atrial Contractions

PACs may be found on a routine ECG. The rate is usually 60 to 100 beats per minute with a regular rhythm, except when premature beats are present. The premature beats have a different P-wave configuration because of origination outside the sinus node. The PAC P-R interval may be different from the sinus P-R interval, and the QRS complex may be normal, aberrant (e.g., wide QRS complex), or absent.

The most common cause of an electrical pause on an ECG rhythm strip is a blocked or nonconducted PAC. This occurs when the PAC comes so early that it falls in the T wave. If the AV node is still refractory, the early P wave does not conduct, and a pause is seen on the rhythm strip. If the clinician looks closely at the T wave and compares it with the patient's other T waves, the early nonconducted P wave may be seen distorting that specific T wave. If the nonconducted PACs present in a bigeminal pattern, the rhythm may be mistaken for profound sinus bradycardia or sinoatrial (SA) block. Thus, the clinician should always assess for nonconducted P waves within preceding T waves in any pauses observed on the ECG.

Observation of the neck veins may help the clinician rapidly distinguish between PSVT and VT. During PSVT, the atria contract against closed AV valves, resulting in a rapid, regular expansion of the neck veins (the same mechanism as cannon waves). This physical finding has been called the "frog sign" because the rapid, regular expansion of the neck veins resembles the puffing motion of a frog, which may be noted by the patient's family members.

Supraventricular Tachycardia

The ECG of a patient in SVT will show a regular rhythm with a rate of 150 to 250 beats per minute. The P waves are ectopic and distorted and may be initiated by a PAC. The P-R interval is shortened, and the QRS complex may be normal or distorted. If the patient is in atrial flutter, the atrial rate will be regular at 250 to 350 beats per minute, and the ventricular rate may be regular or slightly irregular. The P waves are discernible and "march out" (i.e., can be mapped out with a caliper) consistently throughout the strip. P-R intervals cannot be calculated, and the QRS complexes will have variable conduction.

Premature Ventricular Contractions

The ECG of a patient with PVCs will usually show a rate of 60 to 100 beats per minute. The rhythm will be irregular due to the premature ventricular beat. The PVC usually obscures the P wave; however, P waves may be visible if the PVC occurs late in diastole. These P waves are not related to the ectopic beat and occur at the same regular rate of the preceding sinus P waves. The P-R interval is not measurable on the PVC. The QRS complex for the PVC is wide and bizarre. It may be observed in patterns of ventricular bigeminy, trigeminy, or couplets. In the setting of an acute ischemic event, PVCs that occur close to the preceding T wave (R on T phenomenon) may precipitate ventricular fibrillation.

Ventricular Tachycardia

VT can be categorized as monomorphic or polymorphic. The ECG of a patient with monomorphic VT will show a rate greater than 100 beats per minute with a regular rhythm. The P wave will be buried in the QRS complex or may be discernible after the QRS complex because of retrograde conduction. The P-R interval is not measurable, and the QRS complex is wide and bizarre. The ECG of a patient with polymorphic VT will show a "flipping" of the ventricular axis. For example, torsades de pointe is a form of polymorphic VT in which the QT interval demonstrates prolongation before the onset of the dysrhythmia. It is essential to differentiate torsades de pointe from non–torsades polymorphic VT to optimize treatment (e.g., torsades de pointe may respond to magnesium treatment).

Heart Blocks

In first-degree AV block, the pulse will usually be 60 to 100 beats per minute. The ECG rhythm is usually regular, with a P wave preceding each QRS complex and a prolonged P-R interval longer than 0.20 seconds. QRS complexes follow every P wave and are usually a normal width.

A patient with second-degree AV block Mobitz type I will have a ventricular rate of 50 to 70 beats per minute, although it may vary. The atrial rate is regular, whereas the ventricular rate is irregular. P waves precede each QRS complex, and the P-R interval progressively lengthens. The QRS complex is usually normal in width, unless a preexisting bundle branch block is present. As the P-R interval progresses, eventually the QRS complex

disappears for a beat. In contrast, in a Mobitz type II AV block, the P-R interval may be prolonged or normal, but it remains constant, unlike the progressively lengthening P-R of a type I. The blocked P wave may occur in patterns of 2:1, 3:1, or 4:1. The width of the QRS complex indicates where the block is located. The wider the complex, the lower the block is located below the AV node. The P wave is regular and the P-R interval constant, with a wide QRS following every P wave until the QRS complex is not conducted.

With a third-degree block, the AV node (if the block is of a Mobitz I origin) or the ventricles (if the block is of a Mobitz II origin) generate an autonomous rhythm with a ventricular rate of 25 to 60 beats per minute. The atrial rate is 60 to 100 beats per minute. P waves are present and regular, but there is no relationship to the QRS complexes. The P-R interval cannot be calculated as it is variable, and the QRS complex is wider and longer than 0.12 seconds if the block is at the ventricles (Mobitz II origin), or it is normal if the block is at the nodal/junctional level (Mobitz I origin).

DIAGNOSTIC REASONING

Diagnostic Tests

An ECG is the routine diagnostic test to determine the type of arrhythmia so as to direct treatment appropriately. The most definitive diagnostics are confirmed by electrical physiology studies. Electrophysiological testing using intracardiac electrocardiographic recordings and programmed atrial and/or ventricular stimulation is used in the diagnosis and management of complex dysrhythmias. Electrophysiological testing can evaluate recurrent syncope of possible cardiac origin and differentiate supraventricular from ventricular dysrhythmias.

Tilt-table testing (autonomic testing) is useful in patients with arrhythmias when syncope may be due to a vasovagal response. The patient is tilted to approximately 70 degrees in conjunction with isoproterenol infusion. Syncope due to bradycardia and/or hypotension will occur in about one-third of patients with recurrent syncope.

Transesophageal echocardiography (TEE) is a diagnostic procedure used to visualize and rule out the presence of thrombi in the left atrium before cardioversion in atrial fibrillation. The presence of clots in the left atrium is a contraindication to cardioversion.

Differential Diagnosis

The differential diagnoses should consider conditions that could mimic the symptoms of dysrhythmia, such as a panic attack, anxiety, valvular disorders, and syncopal episodes either neurogenic or cardiac in origin.

MANAGEMENT

Management of these patients depends on the expertise of the clinician. If the clinician is at all unsure of the management of an arrhythmia, he or she should consult with a cardiovascular specialist.

Atrial Fibrillation

The initial goal of treatment in atrial fibrillation is to control the ventricular response and then convert the patient back to normal sinus rhythm (NSR) by using medications or electrical synchronized cardioversion.

Some patients with atrial fibrillation revert to NSR after cardioversion. However, many patients after cardioversion return to atrial fibrillation within a short period of time. This occurs particularly in patients with longstanding atrial fibrillation or in patients with advanced heart disease and a very large left atrium. Patients with new-onset atrial fibrillation or chronic atrial fibrillation with a very rapid ventricular response should be admitted to a unit where telemetry is available, so that the response to treatment can be carefully monitored. Drugs that may convert atrial fibrillation to sinus rhythm include amiodarone and disopyramide. Elective synchronized cardioversion is recommended if acute ischemic heart disease is present with a rapid ventricular rate (120–200 beats per minute) or if the patient is in clinical distress. All patients should be assessed for risk of atrial emboli before electrical shock.

Before cardioversion, the patient should undergo TEE to assess for the presence of mural thrombi. Successful cardioversion (in the absence of mural thrombi) and prevention of recurrence of atrial fibrillation depends on atrial size and the length of time in atrial fibrillation. In addition, valvular function should be assessed for further therapeutic interventions. Before electrical or pharmacological cardioversion is attempted, anticoagulants should be considered.

Anticoagulation therapy should be initiated in all patients who remain in atrial fibrillation for longer than 48 hours or who experience atrial fibrillation of unknown duration (see Drugs Commonly Prescribed 36.1). Patients may be placed on IV heparin for rapid anticoagulation and started on warfarin (Coumadin), which takes approximately 5 days to achieve its full anticoagulant effect. A prothrombin time (PT) with international normalized ratio (INR) is drawn and the patient is started on warfarin with the dose adjusted according to the patient's INR. The target INR in atrial fibrillation is between 2 and 3. The PT should be checked at regular intervals to ensure the INR remains within the appropriate range. Once a constant appropriate INR range has been achieved, the PT should be monitored monthly.

Alternatives to warfarin may include dabigatran (Pradaxa), rivaroxaban (Xarelto), or apixaban (Eliquis). These agents are for the management of the patient with nonvalvular atrial fibrillation. Commonalities of these agents are shorter half-lives, fewer drug–drug interactions, and earlier peak blood levels compared with warfarin. Additionally, these agents do not necessitate dose

---

Drugs Commonly Prescribed 36.1: Antithrombotic Treatment Options for Stroke Prevention in Nonvalvular Atrial Fibrillation

AGENT	DOSING	IMPLICATIONS FOR PRACTICE
warfarin* (Coumadin)	Starting dose: 2–5 mg daily in the evening	Goal INR 2.0–3.0; higher in mechanical valve patients. Antidote: vitamin K
dabigatran† (Pradaxa)	150 mg twice daily creatinine clearance (CrCl) >30 mg/mL 75 mg twice daily CrCl = 15–30 Contraindicated if CrCl <15	Requires no laboratory monitoring. Do not cut, crush, or open pill. Antidote: idarucizumab (Praxbind)
rivaroxaban† (Xarelto)	20 mg daily for CrCl >50 mg/mL 5 mg daily for CrCl = 15–49 mg/mL No dosing information for CrCl <15 mL/min	Requires no laboratory monitoring. If unable to swallow, pill may be crushed. No dosing if patient is on dialysis. Antidote: None (in development)
apixaban† (Eliquis)	5 mg twice daily 2.5 mg twice daily with at least two of the following: age >80 years, body weight <60 kg, or creatinine >1.5 Contraindicated if CrCl <25 mL/min	Requires no laboratory monitoring. Antidote: None

*Pregnant women (with the exception of those who have mechanical heart valves) should not receive warfarin.
†Should not be administered to patients with prosthetic heart valves, hemodynamically significant valvular heart disease, severe kidney failure, and/or advanced liver disease.

titration or laboratory monitoring. Comparative studies suggest that with these agents, there is a 10% reduction in mortality, fewer strokes, and fewer systemic emboli. However, a disadvantage for some of these drugs is that there is no established antidote for reversal. Dabigatran has an approved antidote; however, rivaroxaban and apixaban do not at this time. Patients in chronic atrial fibrillation who are difficult to convert with a controlled ventricular rate should be on anticoagulant therapy indefinitely. For patients refractory to these therapies, cardiac ablation therapy is an option.

A permanent implantable device is available for patients in nonvalvular atrial fibrillation. Placed via the femoral vein, the Watchman device closes the left atrial appendage of the heart and reduces the risk of stroke. After implantation for 6 weeks, patients discontinue warfarin but remain on clopidogrel (Plavix) for 4 months, which is then discontinued as well.

Premature Atrial Contractions

Treatment of PACs is not indicated unless the patient is symptomatic or an underlying cause can be corrected. Simple measures such as stopping tobacco use, reducing caffeine intake, and improving electrolyte imbalance may reduce the incidence of PACs. If symptoms persist, Holter monitoring may be indicated, and the patient should be instructed to maintain a diary of activities. The patient should be followed closely for the first 3 months to establish whether the condition is acute or chronic condition.

Supraventricular Tachycardia

The initial treatment for stable SVT consists of vagal maneuvers. Vagal maneuvers increase parasympathetic tone and slow conduction through the AV node. These techniques include coughing, lying on the floor while elevating legs against the wall, or squatting. If the clinician has experience with carotid sinus massage, this maneuver is usually effective. However, carotid massage is contraindicated in patients with carotid artery stenosis, bruits, or a history of transient ischemic attacks, or in patients older than 65 years of age who may have an exacerbated parasympathetic response to carotid pressure. Facial immersion in cold water (dive reflex) is another method that has been used. The clinician must never use eyeball pressure as a vagal maneuver because it may cause retinal detachment and is unpleasant for the patient.

In the case of PSVT, adenosine is the treatment of choice because it blocks electrical transmission through the AV node. If the patient has symptomatic atrial flutter, hypotension, ischemic pain, or severe heart failure, synchronized cardioversion is usually recommended. Pharmacological intervention may involve beta blockers and calcium channel blockers. Patients who have recurrent symptomatic and refractory PSVT will need to see an electrophysiologist for possible radiofrequency ablation of the accessory pathway. Ablation therapy is often chosen over a lifetime course of prophylactic drugs.

Premature Ventricular Contractions

Treatment for PVCs is not usually needed in healthy adults because many adults experience PVCs with no untoward effects. PVCs may be related to an MI, however, in which case it must be determined whether the PVCs are caused by a problem with oxygenation, hypotension, electrolyte disturbances, acid–base imbalance, other medications, or by an increased catecholamine state from unrelieved ischemic pain or anxiety. Typically, therapy in this case involves treating the underlying cause, such as the hypoxia, pain, electrolyte imbalance, or alterations in hemodynamics with nitroglycerin, oxygen, pain medications, and beta blockers.

Heart Blocks

Treatment for a first-degree AV block is not advised because it is an asymptomatic arrhythmia. However, the clinician should assess and take note of any drugs the patient is taking that may prolong AV conduction. For a Mobitz type I second-degree AV block, treatment may not be indicated unless symptomatic. Medications such as beta blockers, calcium channel blockers, and digitalis should be considered as a cause and decreasing or discontinuing dosages should be considered. Additionally, the patient should be evaluated for an inferior wall MI, which can also present with a Mobitz type I AV block. If symptomatic bradycardia develops, a temporary or transcutaneous pacemaker may be needed, whereas a permanent pacemaker may be required for a Mobitz type II AV block. For third-degree heart block, the underlying pathological site must be identified to prevent complications. The ability to determine whether the block has an idiojunctional response versus an idioventricular response is critical in determining the appropriate intervention, as third-degree heart block is considered an emergent and potentially life-threatening condition that would require a pacemaker.

Implantable Cardioverter-Defibrillators

Implantable cardioverter-defibrillator (ICD) devices are multiprogrammable antiarrhythmic devices capable of treating bradydysrhythmias, ventricular fibrillation, and ventricular tachycardia. These devices offer antitachycardia pacing, as well as low- and high-energy shocks in multiple ranges of tachycardic rates. These devices are placed under the skin of the left chest. Patients need close follow-up with a cardiologist and extensive patient education. Patients should carry a device identification card at all times. The American College of Cardiology/American Heart Association/North American Society of Pacing and Electrophysiology guidelines delineate indications for ICD therapy (Gregoratos et al., 2016).

FOLLOW-UP AND REFERRAL

A cardiologist should be consulted to establish the plan of care. The cardiologist may order a Holter monitor to assess the pattern of the arrhythmia. Electrophysiological studies may be indicated to evaluate the patient for cardioablation therapy for PSVTs, such as WPW syndrome.

Patient Education: Arrhythmias

The education of a patient for atrial fibrillation should include a list of foods and prescription and over-the-counter drugs that interfere with warfarin (see Table 36.2). A patient on warfarin is at risk for bleeding; therefore, the primary-care practitioner should provide literature on medical alert identification jewelry and instruct the patient how to assess for signs of bleeding, such as bruising and dark stools. These patients should also use electric razors and nightlights to avoid accidents. Patients should be taught to check their pulse rate. If the pulse rate is decreased (below 60 beats per minute) or the patient notices bursts in the heart rate, it should be reported to the primary-care practitioner.

For patients who have an ICD device implanted, if admitted to hospice care or on a treatment withdrawal protocol, the treating clinician should consider deactivating the ICD to avoid defibrillation in the case of cardiac arrest.

VALVULAR DISORDERS AND MURMURS

Heart valve disorders may be congenital or acquired and may be symptomatic or asymptomatic. Many are detected during cardiac auscultation when alterations in the normal heart rhythm, presence of extrasystole, murmurs, and abnormal heart sounds are heard. Mitral and aortic valve disorders are the most common of the heart valve disorders.

Heart murmurs are the sound of turbulent blood flow that typically result from specific valvular disorders. Blood traveling through the chambers and great vessels is normally a silent event. When turbulence exists along the wall of the heart or a great vessel, a murmur occurs. Murmurs may be benign, in that the clinician simply hears the blood flowing through the heart, but no cardiac or vascular structural abnormality exists. Certain cardiac structural problems, however, such as valvular or myocardial disorders, can contribute to the development of a murmur.

Types of Valvular Disorders

Table 36.3 describes the common valvular disorders, several of which are discussed in this section.

Aortic stenosis is the inability of the aortic valves to open to an optimal orifice. The aortic valve normally opens to

TABLE 36.2 Drugs and Foods That Interact With Warfarin

Increased Anticoagulant Effect	*Decreased Anticoagulant Effect*
Drugs	
acetaminophen (Tylenol)	carbamazepine (Tegretol)
allopurinol (Zyloprim)	cholestyramine (Questran)
amiodarone (Cordarone)	ethinylestradiol/
cephalexin (Keflex)	norethisterone (Loestrin)
ciprofloxacin (Cipro)	ethinylestradiol/norgestimate
cisapride (Propulsid)	(Ortho Tri-Cyclen)
disulfiram (Antabuse)	griseofulvin (Grifulvin)
erythromycin (E-Mycin)	rifampin (Rifadin)
famotidine (Pepcid)	spironolactone (Aldactone)
fluconazole (Diflucan)	sucralfate (Carafate)
fluoxetine (Prozac)	
gemfibrozil (Lopid)	
glimepiride (Amaryl)	
glipizide (Glucotrol)	
ibuprofen (Advil, Motrin)	
levofloxacin (Levaquin)	
metronidazole (Flagyl)	
penicillin V potassium (Pen VK)	
propranolol (Inderal)	
quinidine (Quinaglute)	
ranitidine (Zantac)	
sertraline (Zoloft)	
tetracycline (Achromycin)	
trimethoprim-sulfamethoxazole (Bactrim)	
valproate (Depakene)	
Foods and Nutrients	
cranberry juice	broccoli, brussels sprouts, chard, collard greens, kale, mustard greens, parsley, and spinach
excessive alcohol use	canola and soybean oils
vitamins A, E	green tea
	vitamin K

*Other drugs from the same class are likely to have similar effects.

3 cm^2; aortic stenosis usually does not cause significant symptoms until the valvular orifice is limited to 0.8 cm^2. The disease is characterized by a long symptom-free period, with rapid clinical deterioration at the onset of symptoms, including dyspnea, syncope, chest pain, and heart failure. The clinician should look for a narrow pulse pressure, which is a characteristic of severe aortic stenosis.

The murmur of *mitral regurgitation* (also referred to as mitral insufficiency) arises from mitral valve incompetency or the inability of the mitral valve to close properly. This allows for retrograde "regurgitant" flow from a high-pressure area (left ventricle) to an area of lower pressure (left atrium). Mitral regurgitation is most often caused by the degeneration of the mitral valve, most commonly by rheumatic fever, endocarditis, a calcific annulus, rheumatic heart disease, ruptured chordae tendineae, or papillary muscle

TABLE 36.3   Common Valvular Disorders

Disorder	Murmur Characteristics	Physical Exam	Diagnostic Findings
Aortic stenosis	Harsh systolic murmur usually crescendo-decrescendo pattern. Heard best: Second right intercostal space (RICS) near apex. Radiation: To carotids. Other: Softens with standing.	Cardiac: May have diminished S_2, slow-filling carotid pulse, narrow pulse pressure, loud S_4, heaving point of maximum impulse (PMI). Other: Anxiety, difficulty breathing, compromised mental status, cyanosis, peripheral edema, hair loss, shiny skin over shins, cool extremities, decreased systolic blood pressure, pulmonary edema.	Chest x-ray: Aortic valve calcification, left ventricle (LV) enlargement, prominent ascending aorta. ECG: Left ventricular hypertrophy (LVH), sinus tachycardia, atrial fibrillation, AV conduction delay, left or right bundle branch block (LBBB, RBBB). Echocardiogram: Limited aortic valve movement, thickened left ventricular wall. Cardiac catheterization: Increased pressure gradient in systole across aortic valve, decreased size of aortic orifice, increased left ventricular end-diastolic pressure (LVEDP).
Aortic regurgitation	High-pitched blowing diastolic murmur. Heard best: Third left intercostal space (LICS). Other: May be enhanced by forced expiration, leaning forward.	Cardiac: Usually with S_3, wide pulse pressure, sustained thrusting apical impulse, palpitations, dyspnea, orthopnea, paroxysmal nocturnal dyspnea (PND), syncope, signs of LV failure, peripheral edema, flushed skin, cardiomegaly. Other: More common in men, usually from rheumatic heart disease; fatigue, weakness, anxiety, compromised mental status.	Chest x-ray: Aortic valve calcification, LV enlargement, dilation of ascending aorta. ECG: LVH, sinus tachycardia, PVCs. Echocardiogram: Dilated and hyperdynamic LV, enlargement of aortic root and left atrium (LA), early closure of mitral valve, diastolic fluttering of aortic valve. Cardiac catheterization: Decreased aortic diastolic BP, increased LVEDP, reflux through aortic valve.
Aortic sclerosis	Soft systolic ejection "50 over 50" murmur (found in 50% of those over age 50 years). Heard best: Second RICS in aortic valve region. Other: Marker for increased risk of cardiovascular events; may precede aortic stenosis.	Cardiac: May also hear normal split of S2 heart sound.	Echocardiography: Best detected by two-dimensional echocardiogram. Benign thickening and/or calcification of aortic valve leaflets. Often accompanied by mitral annulus calcification.
Mitral stenosis	Mid-diastolic rumbling murmur. Accentuated S_1 in early disease.	Heard best at apex with the stethoscope bell with patient in left lateral decubiti position.	Echocardiography often reveals left atrial enlargement. ECG may show P mitrale, a broad notched P wave in several leads and/or a negative component to the P wave in V_1. Atrial fibrillation is often present. Chest x-ray may reveal pulmonary edema.
Mitral regurgitation	A holosystolic murmur.	Heard best at the apex and radiates to the axilla. Accentuated with clenching fists or lying supine. An S_3 may be present on auscultation. May palpate a laterally displaced PMI.	ECG may reveal left atrial abnormality, LVH. Chest x-ray may reveal pulmonary edema.
Mitral prolapse	A midsystolic click followed by a late systolic murmur.	Heard best at the apex. The click occurs later in systole with maneuvers that increase volume of left ventricle (i.e., squatting or lying supine).	Echocardiography will show protrusion of mitral valve into left atrium during systole.
Atrial septal defect (ASD)	A fixed splitting of S_2 during both inspiration and expiration.	May palpate right ventricular heave in advanced disease (e.g. Eisenmenger's syndrome)	Transthoracic echo may visualize ASD directly or visualize bubbles traversing ASD while performing a bubble study. ECG may present with first-degree AV block or right atrial abnormality.

dysfunction. In mitral regurgitation from rheumatic heart disease, there is usually also some degree of mitral stenosis. Once the person is symptomatic, the disease progresses in a downhill course of heart failure over the next 10 years.

Mitral valve prolapse (MVP) is the most common valvular heart problem, with an incidence of 2.4% in the general population based on two-dimensional echocardiographic criteria. In most cases, MVP is a benign condition. However, MVP with mitral regurgitation may predispose the individual to thrombi and endocarditis. In the past, the prevalence of MVP was overestimated, owing to lack of specific diagnostic procedures. Patients given this diagnosis more than 10 years earlier may not have the disorder at all and should be reevaluated with two-dimensional echocardiography.

Types of Murmurs

Benign systolic ejection murmurs (a type of physiological murmur) are found in the absence of cardiac pathology. The term implies that the reason for the murmur is something other than obstruction to flow and is present with a normal BP gradient across the valve. This murmur may be heard in up to 80% of thin adults or children if the cardiac examination is performed in a soundproof room; it is best heard at the left sternal border. It occurs in early to midsystole, leaving the two heart sounds intact. In addition, the patient with a benign systolic ejection murmur denies cardiac symptomatology and has an otherwise normal cardiac examination, including an appropriately located point of maximal impulse and full pulses. No cardiac pathology is present with a physiological murmur, so no endocarditis prophylaxis is needed.

A *hemic murmur* is heard in hyperkinetic or high-volume states such as anemia, fever, or in response to exercise. The murmur has a crescendo–decrescendo pattern and is harsh; both heart sounds are preserved. Because there is no cardiac pathology associated with this condition, it resolves when the underlying high-flow state normalizes. As with a physiological murmur, no structural cardiac abnormality is present, and no endocarditis prophylaxis is needed.

An *aortic sclerosis murmur* is also called the 50/50 murmur because it is present in about 50% of adults older than age 50 years. Its etiology is likely due to fibrotic and/or calcific changes in the aortic valve. The valve can open enough to prevent a significant pressure gradient but is restricted enough to cause the murmur. It differs from an aortic stenosis murmur in having an early peak and resolution, as well having no hemodynamic significance.

EPIDEMIOLOGY AND CAUSES

Bacterial endocarditis, rheumatic heart disease, and aortic calcification are common etiologies of valvular disorders that cause heart murmurs. Bacterial endocarditis is most often due to septicemia caused by *Staphylococcus aureus* or *Streptococcus viridans* (alpha-hemolytic) infection. Valvular deformities are among a spectrum of abnormalities associated with endocarditis. IV drug users and patients with indwelling IV catheters are at risk for bacterial septicemia that can lead to endocarditis. Patients with prosthetic heart valves, heart murmurs, or valvular damage require prophylactic antibiotics to prevent endocarditis before any invasive procedures such as dental or surgical interventions.

Rheumatic heart disease is another cause of heart valve injury. Rheumatic heart disease is a result of rheumatic fever, an infection caused by group A beta-hemolytic *Streptococcus* infection. The pathological mechanism involves antibodies developed by the body against the bacteria. Antistreptococcal antibodies are thought to cross-react with the body's own tissues and "mistakenly" attack the heart valves in susceptible individuals. Because of the wide availability of antibiotics, rheumatic fever has become a less common etiology of valvular disease.

Calcification of the aortic valve is a common finding in elderly patients who present with the systolic murmur of aortic stenosis. A calcified aortic valve is often the result of long-standing arteriosclerosis. This calcification causes narrowing of the aortic valve resulting in an audible disturbance in blood flow across the valve.

In children and younger adults, aortic stenosis may also be present; it is usually caused by a congenital bicuspid (rather than tricuspid) aortic valve or by a three-cusp valve with leaflet fusion. This defect is most often found in males and is commonly accompanied by a long-standing history of becoming excessively short of breath with increased activity, such as running. The physical examination is usually normal, except for the associated cardiac findings.

Mitral valve prolapse occurs in about 2% to 4% of the population and is usually detected in young adulthood. It is more common in women younger than 20 years, whereas the incidence is equal in men and women after age 20 years.

PATHOPHYSIOLOGY

Normal heart valves allow unidirectional, unimpeded forward blood flow through the heart. The entire stroke volume is able to pass freely during one phase of the cardiac cycle, and there is no backflow of blood. When a heart valve fails to open to its normal orifice size, it is considered stenotic. When it fails to close appropriately, the valve is incompetent, causing regurgitation of blood flow to the previous chamber or vessel. Both of these events place the patient at significant risk for embolic disease.

CLINICAL PRESENTATION
Subjective

Patients may or may not know whether they have a heart murmur because they may be asymptomatic or, depending on the specific problem, may complain of dyspnea, orthopnea, paroxysmal nocturnal dyspnea, fatigue, hoarseness, palpitations, weakness, chest pain, symptoms of heart failure, activity intolerance, vertigo, syncope, and peripheral edema.

Objective

Systolic murmurs are graded on a 1 to 6 scale, from barely audible to audible with the stethoscope held off the chest. Grade 4 to 6 murmurs have a palpable thrill. Diastolic murmurs are usually graded from 1 to 4 because these murmurs are not loud enough to reach grades 5 and 6. The bell of the stethoscope is most helpful for ausculting lower-pitched sounds, whereas the diaphragm is best used for hearing higher-pitched sounds. Advanced Assessment 36.1 gives more information about cardiac examination findings, including maneuvers to assess for heart murmurs. Advanced Assessment 36.1 lists the physical signs of common valvular disorders, which may underlie cardiac murmurs.

DIAGNOSTIC REASONING

Diagnostic Tests

Initially, the primary-care practitioner may be the first to discover a murmur on physical examination. Depending on the associated symptoms, the primary-care practitioner may refer the patient for subsequent testing or may refer the patient directly to a cardiologist for more invasive testing. Two-dimensional echocardiography is the definitive procedure to diagnose heart valve disorders. Additional diagnostic tests used to detect valvular lesions or structural heart changes include the ECG, chest x-ray, and cardiac catheterization. The primary-care practitioner usually orders an echocardiogram, ECG, and chest x-ray to confirm the definitive diagnosis of a murmur and then refers the patient to a cardiologist unless the primary-care practitioner and patient agree on an initial course of therapy as a trial, such as in MVP.

The ECG may reveal left ventricular hypertrophy or atrial enlargement. The chest x-ray may show an enlarged

✦ Advanced Assessment 36.1: Cardiac Examination and Assessment of Heart Murmurs

Focus of Examination	Factors to Assess	Potential Clinical Correlation
Skin temperature	Variations from normal	Cool, moist skin may indicate a decrease in cardiac output Cool, dry skin may reflect environmental temperature or use of vasoconstricting substances such as sympathomimetics (caffeine, nicotine)
Skin color	Central cyanosis Peripheral cyanosis Palmar erythema Pallor	Poor blood oxygenation Excessive removal of oxygen from the blood Suggests liver impairment May be present in severe anemia (hemoglobin [Hgb] <8 g/dL)
Pulse	Rate Rhythm Character and volume	Note presence of bradycardia or tachycardia Regular, irregular, regularly irregular (extrasystoles) or irregularly irregular (likely atrial fibrillation) Normally full and rapidly filling
Blood pressure	Pulse pressure (difference between the systolic and diastolic pressure readings)	Narrow pulse pressure may be found in volume depletion and aortic stenosis Wide pulse pressure may be found in aortic regurgitation
Point of maximum impulse (PMI)	Location	Normally located at fifth intercostal space (ICS) at midclavicular line With hypertrophy, PMI shifts laterally and may span more than one ICS
Apical impulse	Sensation and quality	Normally a gentle tapping sensation Forceful and thrusting with ventricular overload Diffuse and weak in cardiac hypertrophy Sustained in poorly controlled hypertension and aortic stenosis Double apical impulse in ventricular aneurysm
Heart sounds	S_1 (normal first heart sound)	Marks onset of systole Heard just before palpation of carotid artery pulse High-pitched, click-like sound

Advanced Assessment 36.1: Cardiac Examination and Assessment of Heart Murmurs—cont'd

Focus of Examination	Factors to Assess	Potential Clinical Correlation
	Variations from normal S_1	Unusually loud: mitral stenosis Unusually soft: In mitral stenosis, S_1 becomes softer as the valve calcifies and becomes more rigid and less mobile (mitral stenosis, mitral regurgitation) Abnormally wide split: delayed closure of tricuspid valve (as in right bundle branch block)
	S_2 (normal second heart sound)	Marks end of systole Vibration of aortic and pulmonic valves after closure
	Physiologically split S_2	Occurs at end of systole Widest split at peak inspiration May disappear with sitting or standing Normal finding in younger adult, which usually disappears by middle-age
	Fixed split S_2	Occurs at end of systole No closure of split with positional change Does not increase with inspiration Occurs with atrial septal defect and pulmonary stenosis
	Paradoxically split S_2	Splitting heard during expiration and disappears during inspiration Occurs with delayed closure of aortic valve (e.g., severe aortic stenosis, hypertrophic obstructive cardiomyopathy, left bundle branch block)
	S_3 (third heart sound, ventricular gallop, protodiastolic gallop)	Occurs in early diastole Likely produced by rapidly filling ventricles at a point when ventricular filling slows or by recoil of the heart as it is pushed against the chest Heard best by the diaphragm No change with respiration, although occasionally inspiration or expiration will increase sound Found with disorders of systolic emptying (e.g., heart failure, valvular heart disease, ischemic heart disease, hypertrophic cardiomyopathy)
	S_4 (fourth heart sound, atrial gallop, presystolic gallop, S_4 gallop)	May be caused by the tug of chordae tendineae and papillary muscles in the state of poor ventricular compliance Found with disorders of diastolic filling (e.g., poorly controlled hypertension, angina, ischemic heart disease)

cardiac silhouette, a left ventricular prominence, calcification of the aortic valve, and/or dilation and calcification of the ascending aorta. An echocardiogram is useful in demonstrating the underlying pathological process, whether the lesion involves the aortic root or if valvular disease is present. Cardiac catheterizations can provide an accurate assessment of regurgitation and stenosis, along with left ventricular function and pulmonary artery pressures. Coronary angiography is often indicated to determine the presence of coronary artery disease before valvular surgery.

Differential Diagnosis

The differential diagnoses for MVP include hypertrophic cardiomyopathies, papillary dysfunction, anxiety disorders, and congenital cardiac anomalies. The differential diagnoses for mitral stenosis include left atrial myxoma, vegetation caused by endocarditis, and calcium deposits. For mitral regurgitation, the differential diagnoses include calcified aortic stenosis, MVP, prosthetic mitral valve malfunction, and ventricular septal defect.

MANAGEMENT

Although asymptomatic patients typically require no treatment, the principle of management of valvular disorders is to help the patient maintain normal cardiac output, thus preventing the complications of heart failure, venous congestion, and inadequate tissue perfusion.

Proper management of certain valvular disorders involves preventive therapy to minimize the risk of developing infective endocarditis under certain circumstances, such as dental work or surgery, to which abnormal valves are prone. In recent years, the recommendations for antibiotic prophylaxis before dental work have undergone revision and are now more selective. For current guidelines pertaining to the use of prophylactic antibiotic therapy, the clinician is advised to refer to the American College of Cardiology/American Heart Association (ACC/AHA) guidelines for the prevention of infective endocarditis (see Treatment Standards/Guidelines).

Mitral Valve Disorders

Mitral Valve Prolapse

There is no medical treatment to correct MVP. Symptomatic management includes lifestyle changes, such as beginning a mild exercise program to reduce plasma catecholamines, lower the heart rate, decrease stress, and increase cardiac output and blood volume. Beta blockers may be prescribed for patients with MVP to help control heart palpitations. However, fatigue is a problem with this disorder, and it may be exacerbated by beta blockers.

The clinician should refer to the most current guidelines available from the ACC/AHA regarding the use of antibiotic prophylaxis. Antibiotics are no longer recommended for prophylaxis against infective endocarditis if patients are undergoing genitourinary or gastrointestinal tract procedures. Anticoagulation with aspirin (81–325 mg/day) is prescribed for some individuals with MVP who have also had a history of TIA, ischemic stroke, or atrial fibrillation.

Persons with MVP and severe mitral regurgitation should be followed periodically with stress echocardiography. Surgical intervention is indicated for MVP with severe mitral valve regurgitation.

Mitral Stenosis

For symptomatic mitral stenosis, diuretics and sodium restriction should be initiated to reduce blood volume and pulmonary and systemic venous pressures, along with anticoagulation therapy with warfarin if there is a history of systemic embolism, atrial fibrillation, or a

---

 ## Treatment Standards/Guidelines: Infective Endocarditis Prophylaxis

Source: Wilson W, Taubert KA, Gewitz M, et al. Prevention of infective endocarditis: guidelines from the American Heart Association: A guideline from the American Heart Association Rheumatic Fever, Endocarditis, and Kawasaki Disease Committee, Council on Cardiovascular Disease in the Young, and the Council on Clinical Cardiology, Council on Cardiovascular Surgery and Anesthesia, and the Quality of Care and Outcomes Research Interdisciplinary Working Group. *Circulation.* 2007;116(15): 1736–1754.

Only people at greatest risk for negative outcomes from infective endocarditis (IE) should receive preventive antibiotics. These include patients undergoing the following:

- Dental procedures involving the gingival tissues or periapical region of a tooth and for those procedures that perforate the oral mucosa
- Invasive respiratory tract procedures that involve incision or biopsy of the respiratory mucosa

Antibiotic prophylaxis is recommended for high-risk patients with any of the following:

- Prosthetic heart valves
- Previous history of IE
- Complex cyanotic congenital heart disease (surgically repaired or unrepaired)
- Cardiac valvulopathy in a transplanted heart

Antibiotic prophylaxis is not indicated for common valvular lesions; however, clinicians should exercise judgment in selecting the dose and duration of antibiotics in individual cases or under special circumstances.

Adequate oral hygiene is an important factor in preventing IE.

Endocarditis Prophylaxis (30–60 minutes before procedure)

If no penicillin allergy:

amoxicillin oral—adults 2 g; children 50 mg/kg
If no penicillin allergy and unable to take oral agents:
   ampicillin IM or IV—adults 2 g; children 50 mg/kg

If penicillin-allergic:

clindamycin oral—adults 600 mg; children 20 mg/kg
OR
cephalexin oral—adults 2 g; children 50 mg/kg
OR
azithromycin or clarithromycin oral—adults 500 mg; children 15 mg/kg
If penicillin-allergic and unable to take oral agents:
   clindamycin IV—adults 600 mg; children 20 mg/kg
   OR
   cefazolin or ceftriaxone IM or IV—adults 1 g; children 50 mg/kg

NOTE: Cephalosporins should not be used in persons with a history of serious penicillin allergy, such as anaphylaxis, angioedema, or widespread urticaria.

large left atrium. If the patient is in atrial fibrillation, the antiarrhythmic amiodarone or the calcium channel blocker diltiazem may be prescribed and are preferred to the use of digitalis. Surgical intervention may be required for some patients and may include mitral commissurotomy, balloon valvuloplasty, or mitral valve replacement.

Mitral Regurgitation

For a symptomatic patient with mitral regurgitation, vasodilators should be initiated to reduce ventricular filling volume and to decrease systemic vascular resistance. Diltiazem and anticoagulants should be prescribed to control the ventricular rate and decrease the risk of embolic complications if the patient has atrial fibrillation. Sodium restriction and diuretics will relieve symptoms of heart failure if they are present in patients with mitral regurgitation. A mitral valve replacement may be required.

Aortic Valve Disorders

Aortic Stenosis

Aortic valve replacement or aortic valve commissurotomy may be required for aortic stenosis.

Aortic Regurgitation

For the patient with symptomatic aortic regurgitation, digitalis and diuretics can be used to treat the symptoms of heart failure. Arterial vasodilators are used to reduce left ventricular afterload. Aortic valve replacement may be required.

FOLLOW-UP AND REFERRAL

The clinician should follow the patient at regular intervals for close monitoring, as well as whenever a new drug has been added or a dosage changed. The patient should be referred to a cardiologist if the diagnosis is unconfirmed or if symptoms are not well managed with medical therapy.

Patient Education: Valvular Disorders and Murmurs

Valvular heart disorders require lifelong management. Patients may benefit from maintaining a diary to monitor the effectiveness of lifestyle changes and compliance with specific drug therapy in controlling symptoms of the disorder. Patients with MVP should be instructed to begin a gradual program of exercise and to avoid caffeine, decongestants, and products containing ephedrine, alcohol, chocolate, or cheese. Provided MVP has not led to severe mitral regurgitation and subsequent congestive heart failure, patients should be encouraged to drink at least eight glasses of water a day to prevent dehydration. Patients with aortic stenosis often require activity restrictions. The patient should understand how to pace activity, note improvements in fatigue, and, ideally, accept activity restrictions. A

critical part of the evaluation of a person with a heart murmur is the decision to offer antimicrobial prophylaxis. No prophylaxis is needed with benign murmurs. Patients and their primary-care providers should follow current treatment guidelines for bacterial endocarditis prophylaxis.

REFERENCES

General

O'Gara PT, Kushner FG, Ascheim DD, et al. 2013 ACCF/AHA guideline for the management of ST-elevation myocardial infarction: A report of the American College of Cardiology Foundation/American Heart Association Task Force on Practice Guidelines. *Circulation.* 2013;127(4):e362–425.

Arrhythmias

Gregoratos G, Abrams J, Epstein AE, et al. ACC/AHA/NASPE 2002 guideline update for implantation of cardiac pacemakers and antiarrhythmia devices: summary article: a report of the American College of Cardiology/American Heart Association Task Force on Practice Guidelines (ACC/AHA/NASPE Committee to Update the 1998 Pacemaker Guidelines). *Circulation.* 2002;106(16):2145–2161.

Havard J. Why are we so bad in primary care at initiating warfarin in atrial fibrillation patients? *BJC Br J Cardiol.* 2009;16:237–240. https://bjcardio.co.uk/2009/09/why-are-we-so-bad-in-primary-care-at-initiating-warfarin-in-atrial-fibrillation-patients/. Accessed October 3, 2017.

January CT, Wann LS, Alpert JS, et al. 2014 AHA/ACC/HRS guideline for the management of patients with atrial fibrillation: A report of the American College of Cardiology/American Heart Association Task Force on practice guidelines and the Heart Rhythm Society. *Circulation.* 2014;130(23):e199–267. http://www.online jacc.org/content/64/21/e1. Accessed October 3, 2017.

Mobius-Winkler S, Sandri M, Mangner N, et al. The WATCHMAN left atrial appendage closure device for atrial fibrillation. *J Vis Exp.* 2012(60):3671. https://www.ncbi.nlm.nih.gov/pmc/articles/PMC3399494/. Accessed September 5, 2017.

Page RL, Joglar JA, Caldwell MA, et al. 2015 ACC/AHA/HRS Guideline for the Management of Adult Patients With Supraventricular Tachycardia: A Report of the American College of Cardiology/American Heart Association Task Force on Clinical Practice Guidelines and the Heart Rhythm Society. *Circulation.* 2016;133(14):e506–574.

Thompson D. Hospitalization rates soar for irregular heartbeat. *HealthDay.* http://consumer.healthday.com/senior-citizen-information-31/misc-aging-news-10/afib-hospitalization-rates-soaring-682259.html. Published November 18, 2013.

Valvular Disorders and Murmurs

Jneid H, Mack MJ, McLeod CJ, et al. 2017 AHA/ACC Focused Update of the 2014 AHA/ACC Guideline for the Management of Patients with Valvular Heart Disease. 2017 AHA/ACC Focused Update of the 2014 AHA/ACC Guideline for the Management of Patients With Valvular Heart Disease: A Report of the American College of Cardiology/American Heart Association Task Force on Clinical Practice Guidelines. Circulation. 2017;135(25):e1159–e1195.

Wilson W, Taubert KA, Gewitz M, et al. Prevention of infective endocarditis: Guidelines from the American Heart Association: a guideline from the American Heart Association Rheumatic Fever, Endocarditis, and Kawasaki Disease Committee, Council on Cardiovascular Disease in the Young, and the Council on Clinical Cardiology, Council on Cardiovascular Surgery and Anesthesia, and the Quality of Care and Outcomes Research Interdisciplinary Working Group. *Circulation.* 2007;116(15):1736–1754.

RESOURCES

CHA$_2$DS$_2$-VASc/HAS BLED/EHRA
Atrial fibrillation risk score calculator
www.chadsvasc.org

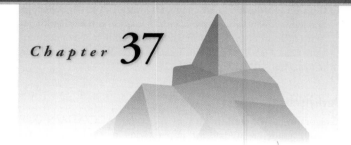

Chapter **37**

Disorders of the Vascular System

Kathryn B. Keller, PhD, RN, CNE

Denese Sabatino, MSN, APRN, NP-C, CCRN

Jill E. Winland-Brown, EdD, APRN, FNP-BC

Brian Oscar Porter, MD, PhD, MPH, MBA

Michael B. Keller, MD

PERIPHERAL ARTERY DISEASE

Peripheral artery disease (PAD) is an occlusive disorder of the arteries, which most commonly affects the lower extremities. PAD is most frequently the result of occlusive atherosclerotic plaques that impede blood flow to the peripheral vasculature. The resulting arterial insufficiency most commonly manifests itself in the form of lower extremity *claudication*—cramping pain triggered or exacerbated by exertion and relieved by rest. Although atherosclerosis is the most common etiology of arterial insufficiency, several other disorders may precipitate lower extremity ischemia, including vasculitis, radiation exposure, dissection, and aneurysm.

EPIDEMIOLOGY AND CAUSES

PAD is caused by atherosclerosis, blood clots, trauma, spasms of smooth muscle in the arterial walls, and congenital structural defects in the arteries. Approximately

8.5 million people in the United States have PAD, and its most common symptom is intermittent claudication. In patients older than age 60 years, 12% to 20% have PAD. The 5-year mortality rate for PAD approaches 30% as patients die from comorbid conditions of CAD and cerebrovascular disease. PAD is more common in men than women and nine times more common in smokers (see Risk Factors: Peripheral Artery Disease).

Risk Factors: Peripheral Vascular Disease (PVD)

Arterial Risk Factors:

- Smoking: Vasoconstriction/spasm-decreased circulation
- Obesity: Increased cardiac workload
- Inactivity: Decreased circulation
- Hypertension: Increased fibrous tissue, which decreases stretch of arterial walls and increases peripheral vascular resistance
- High cholesterol: Atherosclerotic plaque, which increases hyperlipidemia
- Diabetes mellitus: Increase in atherosclerosis of smaller vessels

Venous Risk Factors:

- Coagulation abnormalities
- Abdominal/pelvic surgery: Venous pooling/stasis
- Estrogen/oral contraceptives
- Pregnancy: Venous congestion
- Obesity: Increased cardiac workload, venous pooling
- Heart disease: Venous stasis
- Advanced neoplasm: Coagulation abnormalities, interference with venous blood flow

PATHOPHYSIOLOGY

Atherosclerosis is the most common cause of arterial insufficiency of the lower extremity, also referred to as PAD. Arteriosclerotic plaque obstructs optimal arterial blood flow to the muscles of the lower extremity. With increased muscle activity, there is an increased need for arterial blood flow. For this reason, during ambulation or exercise, limitations of arterial blood flow cause muscle pain due to ischemia. This cramping muscle pain is referred to as *intermittent claudication* because in the initial stages of PAD, ischemia occurs periodically. Muscle activity of the lower extremity requires increased circulation and arterial vasodilation. PAD causes lack of arterial vasodilatory ability. Thus, as PAD worsens, arterial circulation diminishes, and less muscle activity causes pain due to worsening ischemia. Eventually pain at rest occurs, which is a sign of severe PAD.

In general, the clinical manifestations of PAD are extremity pain (claudication), weak pulse, pallor, paresthesias, and palpable coolness of the lower extremity. Long-standing PAD causes muscle atrophy, diminished hair growth, and discolored, hardened toenails of the extremity. All of these signs and symptoms are due to lack of arterial blood supply to the lower extremities. Early recognition of the signs of PAD and treatment are critical because severe ischemia can lead to the need for amputation.

Arteriosclerotic plaque formation within the lower extremities is accelerated by the presence of diabetes mellitus; therefore, PAD is more common in persons with diabetes. Hyperglycemia in diabetes causes endothelial injury, damaging arterial vessels. Clinical manifestations of arterial insufficiency are apparent in the lower extremities of individuals with diabetes. Many suffer the complications of diminished circulation of the legs, which include poor wound healing and peripheral neuropathy. The smaller caliber arterial vessels of the most distal regions of the lower extremity are initially affected. Therefore, careful periodic physical assessment of the feet and lower extremities is recommended in persons with diabetes, inspecting for poor wound healing and diminished peripheral pulses.

Aneurysms, another manifestation of PAD, result from weakening in arterial walls, which renders them susceptible to rupture. The most common cause of this weakening is arteriosclerosis. Aneurysms appear as bulges in the arterial wall and are classified according to location. The aorta and cerebral arteries are the most common sites of aneurysms. In the aorta, a dissecting aneurysm, which is an incomplete tear in the vascular wall, may occur when elevated blood pressure leads to separation of the layers of aortic tissue.

Arteritis, a form of vasculitis, involves inflammation of arterial blood vessels. Inflammation decreases the vasodilatory capacity of arteries and may cause spasm of the arteries. This condition is often associated with autoimmune disease. *Raynaud's phenomenon* is a result of cold-induced vasospasm of the small blood vessels in the fingers and toes, causing a characteristic blanching that sometimes extends to the hands or feet. A tricolor change may also be stimulated, which appears first as blanching of the finger tips and toes, followed by cyanosis and rubor (redness).

CLINICAL PRESENTATION

Subjective

The patient with PAD will usually present with intermittent leg pain (intermittent claudication) that increases in severity with exertion, including normal walking. The location of the lower extremity pain depends on where the occlusion is located. Aorto-iliac occlusions typically produce claudication of the thigh and buttock, whereas occlusions of the femoral artery produce pain in the upper calf. The pain is described as severe, "grabbing," and cramp-like. The pain lasts minutes (at most), is relieved by rest, and does not reoccur until the patient walks the same distance again. Pain at rest frequently signifies severe PAD. The patient usually denies swelling, pain at night, or color or temperature changes. The patient may also complain of thick toenails with corn-like (dead skin callus) material under the nails. Eventually, the lower legs and ankles may assume a purple-black color, characteristic of cyanosis and gangrene.

Objective

A thorough history distinguishes the cause of leg pain in more than 90% of patients. Assessing risk factors assists in the diagnosis. The next step should be to determine the rapidity of onset of symptoms. PAD must be differentiated from a limb-threatened state that may need immediate treatment. If the onset of claudication is gradual, this is more consistent with the progressive obliteration of the lower extremity vessels and the formation of collateral circulation, as seen with PAD, rather than an acute event such as an embolus from the heart or a proximal abdominal aortic aneurysm.

The clinician should evaluate the cervical, radial, ulnar, brachial, femoral, popliteal, dorsalis pedis, and posterior tibial pulses bilaterally. A consistent grading system should be used. Usually 0 refers to an absent pulse, 1+ a diminished pulse, 2+ normal, and 3+ bounding. The clinician should keep in mind that about 10% of the population has absent pedal pulses. Because a bruit indicates turbulence and possible atherosclerotic narrowing, the following pulse sites should be assessed using the diaphragm of a stethoscope: cervical, supraclavicular, abdominal, flank, and inguinal areas.

To differentiate chronic venous insufficiency from PAD, the clinician should raise the patient's legs for several minutes. When the legs are dependent again, the patient with PAD will have pale, dusky red (rubor) extremities, while the patient with chronic venous insufficiency will have improved color in the extremities. The six P's of PAD—pain, pulselessness, paresthesia, paralysis, poikilothermia (coolness), and pallor—should be assessed to evaluate the presence of acute arterial ischemia. The clinician should do a sensory examination to rule out peripheral neuropathy associated with ischemia in patients with diabetes.

With PAD, the clinician may observe decreased or absent peripheral extremity pulses. The affected leg may be smaller in size as a result of muscular atrophy. The clinician may note thinning of the skin, loss of hair over the affected area, and possible leg ulcers. The extremity may be cool and pale, and the toenails will be thickened. The patient will have a history of delayed wound healing.

When the extremity is dependent, it will appear reddish-blue in color.

DIAGNOSTIC REASONING

Diagnostic Tests

If arterial insufficiency is suspected and the pulses are absent, a Doppler ultrasound flow study should be performed, which can quantify the degree of the ischemia. The ankle-brachial index (ABI), a comparison of arm blood pressure to the ankle pressures, should be calculated during the Doppler flow study using a blood pressure cuff. The normal ratio of ankle to brachial pressure is more than 0.9. An ABI reading of 0.6 to 0.9 indicates a moderate level of disease, and levels less than 0.5 indicate severe ischemia. Although an arteriogram is not usually ordered as a diagnostic tool, it should be obtained preoperatively, if the patient requires assessment by a vascular surgeon.

Additional assessment tools and diagnostic procedures for PAD include a walking impairment questionnaire (WIQ), treadmill exercise testing, lipid profile, and magnetic resonance angiogram (MRA). The WIQ is used to assess the ability of patients to walk defined distances at certain speeds and to climb stairs.

Differential Diagnosis

Differential diagnoses for PAD include chronic venous insufficiency, thrombosis, phlebitis, polycythemia, anemia, Raynaud's disease, vasculitis such as Buerger's disease, aneurysms, and peripheral neuropathy.

MANAGEMENT

Treatment for PAD is aimed at improving blood flow by removing or lessening the cause of impaired circulation. Because the condition is usually chronic and irreversible, treatment involves education and lifestyle changes. Patients with PAD should be counseled about modification of risk factors, and hypertension and diabetes should be aggressively managed. The clinician should encourage the patient to walk at least 30 minutes three to four times per week. Any ulcers or traumatic lesions to the extremities will need immediate care. The patient should be encouraged to keep the legs dependent to improve blood flow and, therefore, oxygenation in the extremities. Tight bandages and stockings should be avoided.

Although drug therapy is not a substitute for exercise, some medications have been helpful in extending ambulation distances for more than 25% of patients. Patients with PAD should be started on antiplatelet therapy with aspirin, or if they cannot tolerate aspirin, clopidogrel. These antiplatelet agents do not provide a measurable improvement in symptoms of claudication but are prescribed to reduce the risk of concomitant atherosclerotic disease such myocardial infarction and stroke. A statin should also be added to this regimen.

Current American College of Cardiology (ACC) and American Heart Association (AHA) guidelines recommend cilostazol (Pletal) for the treatment of claudication. Cilostazol is a phosphodiesterase-3 inhibitor that causes vasodilation and inhibits platelet aggregation. Cilostazol may be ordered specifically to treat leg pain and cramping due to the blockages from atherosclerosis in the leg arteries. Cilostazol should not be prescribed in the presence of any degree of heart failure.

Most patients with moderate PAD can be effectively managed with medical therapy and risk modification alone. Surgical intervention and angioplasty are used selectively in patients with severe PAD. Indications for surgical or percutaneous revascularization include profound functional and occupational limitation due to claudication, disease refractory to pharmacological therapy, and limb-threatening critical ischemia. Patients must be able to demonstrate improvement in their symptoms on revascularization and not be severely disabled by other comorbid conditions (e.g., severe pulmonary disease, heart failure, coronary artery disease) that may render revascularization futile.

FOLLOW-UP AND REFERRAL

All patients with PAD should be followed at least every 3 months to assess the effectiveness of lifestyle changes, skin care, and management of ulcers. If ulcers are present, the patient may need to be seen on a weekly basis. Patients with PAD may be referred to a vascular surgeon for evaluation and potential surgery, including a balloon angioplasty in the distal extremity or an arterial graft using a section of the great saphenous vein or a synthetic graft.

Patient Education: Peripheral Artery Disease

Patients who have been diagnosed with PAD should be counseled about the modification of risk factors. They should totally abstain from nicotine. It is essential to control hypertension and diabetes if present. Dietary control must include limitation of fat and salt intake. Patients must be taught to do meticulous daily foot care that includes inspecting feet daily for sores, ulcers, and abrasions, including the use of a mirror to check the soles of the feet. Patients should not walk barefoot and should wear well-fitting supportive shoes. They should not soak their feet and should be careful trimming their nails. All patients should be taught to watch for the signs and symptoms that might indicate progressive ischemia, such as increased pain, increased pallor or cyanosis, and rest pain.

Patients with PAD should be encouraged to perform Buerger-Allen exercises three to four times per day. The clinician should teach the patient to raise and lower the extremities, with each of five repetitions taking about 2 minutes. The legs should be raised to a 45-degree angle, and then lowered again to the supine position. The changes in position cause the veins of the legs to refill by gravity.

Additionally, exercise therapy is recommended for PAD because it stimulates collateral vessel growth in the lower extremities. Patients should be encouraged to walk distances until moderate pain occurs, stop until pain subsides, and then resume walking. A supervised treadmill walking program three times a week over a 6-month period is part of cardiovascular rehabilitation. Treadmill grade and speed are gradually increased over time as the patient improves.

DEEP VEIN THROMBOSIS/ CHRONIC VENOUS INSUFFICIENCY

Deep vein thrombosis (DVT) is a disorder of the venous system characterized by clot formation in the deep vessels of the venous vasculature. DVT primarily results as a complication associated with Virchow's triad—venous stasis, endothelial injury, and hypercoagulable state. The resulting thrombus formation may lead to a variety of complications including chronic venous insufficiency and, most notably, pulmonary embolism (PE). Pulmonary embolism is a potentially life-threatening complication of DVT in which venous thrombi propagate to the pulmonary vasculature resulting in respiratory compromise. It is estimated that 10% to 30% of patients will die within 1 month of diagnosis of DVT/PE and that sudden death is the first symptom in about 25% of people who have a PE. About one-third of patients who have a DVT/PE will have a recurrence within 10 years.

Chronic venous insufficiency is a disorder characterized by valvular incompetence, which manifests as lower extremity edema, skin discoloration, and ulceration as a result of poor antegrade venous flow. Although the condition is commonly a complication of DVT, it may be the result of inflammatory conditions such as phlebitis or anatomical disturbances.

EPIDEMIOLOGY AND CAUSES

DVT and PE are often complications encountered during the treatment of medical and surgical patients. Approximately 300,000 to 600,000 hospitalizations can be associated with DVT and PE each year. Up to 50,000 deaths occur annually because of PE. It is estimated that there are more than 2 million cases per year of DVT. The actual number of cases is often underdiagnosed due to the silent nature of the problem. Risk factors are listed below.

Risk Factors: Deep Vein Thrombosis (DVT)—Virchow's Triad

Venous Stasis

- Possible causes include immobility, venous insufficiency, prolonged sedentary position, poststroke, post–myocardial infarction, and heart failure

Vessel Injury

- Possible causes include trauma, surgery (especially orthopedic), and indwelling IV catheters.

Hypercoagulability

- Possible causes include high estrogen states (oral contraceptives or hormone replacement therapy), pregnancy/postpartum period, cancer, and inherited coagulation abnormalities

Source: Teri Capriotti, DO, MSN, CRNP.

Patients undergoing various types of surgical procedures, such as orthopedic, gynecological-obstetric, urological, neurosurgical, and general surgical procedures, are at high risk for developing DVT and PE. Of these groups, orthopedic patients appear to be especially prone to thrombosis, particularly patients with hip fracture. All elective orthopedic surgical patients undergoing lower extremity surgery are at risk for DVT. The risk is greatest for patients undergoing hip surgery and knee reconstruction, for which DVT rates range from 45% to 70%.

Patients with various types of medical diseases, usually chronic, are also at a high risk for venous thrombotic events. The risk of DVT in pregnancy has been reported to be five times higher than in nonpregnant patients in the same age-group and may be increased postpartum. A silent DVT may cause a postphlebitic syndrome. Postphlebitic syndrome is characterized by swelling and pain in an extremity that was previously affected by thrombophlebitis.

A frequent complication of DVT is PE, which can obstruct blood flow to the lungs and cause significant morbidity. The mortality of PE is estimated to be approximately 30%, although with the availability of newer diagnostic tools such as computed tomography angiogram, which can detect smaller peripheral emboli, it is estimated that the actual mortality rate of PE is about 10%. More than 80% of patients who died from PE showed DVT on autopsy.

Chronic venous insufficiency usually results from venous incompetence secondary to valvular dysfunction. More than 20% of the population is affected with chronic venous insufficiency; the incidence increases with age with no evident ethnic predisposition. Chronic venous insufficiency is more common in women than men.

PATHOPHYSIOLOGY

Blood clots can originate anywhere in the venous system, but the majority begin in the deep veins of the pelvis and lower extremities, with a significant number at or above the popliteal vein. Clots that originate in the proximal veins are potentially more dangerous because they are larger in size and result in more clinically significant thromboembolic events.

The causative factors in the formation of blood clots are referred to as *Virchow's triad* (see earlier discussion). Clots are likely to form when two of the three factors in the triad—stasis, vessel wall damage, and coagulation changes—are altered. Stasis of blood may result from immobility, edema, or anesthesia; blood tends to coagulate in and around the valve cusps of the veins, thus increasing the likelihood of clot formation. Vessel wall damage may result from trauma, surgical incision, laceration, venous wall distention from immobility or anesthesia, or a previous DVT. Coagulation changes leading to activated coagulation factors as a result of damaged endothelium may be the result of surgery, trauma, injury, disease states (such as sepsis, infection, or cancer), pregnancy, or foreign substance invasion via IV lines or catheters. The damaged endothelium causes the local activation of coagulation factors as platelets come in contact with the exposed collagen found in connective tissue, including skin, bone, ligaments, and cartilage. In turn, the platelets release substances that cause vasoconstriction and accelerate clotting.

Once formed, a DVT can propagate, embolize, or lyse. When the clot propagates, it extends proximally and becomes larger and thus more dangerous, by obstructing blood flow, which causes the vein to dilate and the vessel wall to be damaged. When a clot embolizes, it travels; it may lodge itself in the arteries of the lungs, resulting in PE. When a clot lyses, it breaks down. Even if a clot lyses, it can still cause irreversible valve damage by allowing blood to reflux in the veins. The damage sets up a cycle of pooling and hypertension known as the postphlebitic syndrome. Patients with this syndrome experience chronic pain, swelling, and venous ulcers.

Deep venous thrombophlebitis and thromboembolism is a critical disorder of the veins of the lower extremity. The presence of a thrombus within a deep vein with an accompanying inflammatory response is termed *deep venous thrombophlebitis* or *deep venous thrombosis*. If the thrombus breaks away from the wall of the vein and travels upward toward the heart, it is termed a *venous thromboembolism*. Common causes of hypercoagulability are estrogen use, pregnancy, and neoplasms. Venous stasis occurs most often as a result of immobility. Vascular injury can be due to surgery or trauma. Orthopedic surgery is a major risk factor for DVT, and there is a high incidence of concurrent DVT in persons with cancer of the pancreas, lungs, breast, genitourinary tract, and stomach. PE is a potential complication of DVT. The venous thrombus may break free from the venous wall and travel from the lower extremity to the inferior vena cava and up to the right atrium, right ventricle, and into the pulmonary arterial circulation. This may cut off blood flow to an entire lung segment, resulting in potentially fatal ventilation/perfusion (V/Q) mismatch. In addition, any abnormal communication between the right and left chambers of the heart (e.g., atrial septal defect, patent foramen ovale, ventricular septal defect) creates the potential for cerebral thromboembolism and a subsequent cerebrovascular accident (stroke).

It is critical to diagnose DVT early because the complication of PE can be life-threatening. A PE is a thrombus that obstructs circulation within the lungs, causing lack of oxygenation of blood. Signs of pulmonary embolism can be subtle or severe depending on the size of the embolus. Sudden death can result from pulmonary embolism and may not be heralded by clearly observable signs of DVT.

Chronic venous insufficiency is a disorder of the valves within the deep veins of the lower extremities. Valves within veins assist venous blood to flow upward toward the heart, regulating unidirectional flow by preventing retrograde flow of venous blood away from the heart. Weakened venous valves do not form tight closures, failing to prevent retrograde blood flow.

The appearance of superficial varicose veins may be associated with chronic venous insufficiency. Superficial varicose veins are benign in most cases and are treatable with conservative measures. However, under more severe circumstances, venous stasis results, as excess pressure builds up in the legs, causing distention of the veins, thinning and scaling of the skin with dusky discoloration (stasis dermatitis), and eventually large venous ulcers. In addition, dependent edema and poor wound healing result.

CLINICAL PRESENTATION

Subjective

Although many lower extremity thrombi are silent, the patient may present with a complaint of pain in the calf muscle, slight swelling of the calf or asymmetry, or muscle tenderness when massaging the affected area.

The patient with chronic venous insufficiency will complain of dependent edema, venous engorgement (varicose veins), and localized pain. The patient may complain of a darkened color in the lower extremities, along with dryness and scaling of the skin.

Objective

The signs of DVT may be subtle. Overt signs of DVT may include tenderness and a palpable cord along the course of a vein, although more often than not, the only sign is a unilateral swelling of an extremity with or without signs of inflammation. The most common complaint is calf pain. Although used in the past, a positive *Homans's sign* (pain on dorsiflexion of the foot) is now considered an unreliable diagnostic indicator, given its lack of specificity. The clinician may assess for warmth or heat of the affected extremity and note distention of the superficial veins. A slight fever and tachycardia may also be present. An acute DVT in the femoral or iliac veins may show symptoms of tenderness over the veins, swelling, and a slightly bluish skin color.

In patients with chronic venous insufficiency, the clinician may note a brownish hyperpigmentation of the extremities, edema, subcutaneous fibrosis, and possibly leg ulcers. When the clinician elevates the extremity, the sharp, deep muscle pain may be lessened. The peripheral pulses may be normal or diminished. There may be superficial ulcers around the medial malleolus.

DIAGNOSTIC REASONING

Diagnostic Tests

If DVT is suspected, the clinician should first assess for the probability of thrombosis. This may be done using a clinical probability assessment model, which estimates the probability of DVT, such as the Well's criteria that consist of 10 yes/no questions. Further diagnostic work-up is contingent on the patient's clinical likelihood of DVT. If the patient is determined to have a low clinical probability of DVT, a D-dimer level may be ordered, which has become increasingly available in primary-care practices. A low Well's score and a negative D-dimer test result would indicate the absence of DVT. However, if a high or intermediate Well's score is calculated, then no screening D-dimer is needed and further investigation is required.

The D-dimer assay can be helpful in ruling out but not definitively confirming the diagnosis of DVT. D-dimer is a breakdown product of fibrin and is positive in venous thrombosis and PE. However, the D-dimer assay has low specificity and cannot be solely relied on for diagnosis. If a D-dimer is present, it does not prove a DVT exists because many conditions (e.g., advanced age, malignancy, recent surgery, pregnancy, infection) may cause a positive result. However, given its high sensitivity for venous thrombosis, if the D-dimer is negative, it effectively rules out the presence of DVT. A false-negative result can occur if the sample is drawn too early after thrombus formation or if testing is not done in an acute time period.

In patients with an intermediate or high clinical probability of DVT, compression ultrasonography of the femoral and popliteal regions has become the diagnostic standard.

The ascending venogram was long considered the "gold standard" for the diagnosis of venous thromboembolism; however, it is rarely used today. If pulmonary embolus is suspected, a V/Q scan or a spiral (helical) computed tomography scan of the lungs and pulmonary arterial system would be indicated.

To confirm venous insufficiency if the history and physical examination are inconclusive, a venogram may be performed. This is a radiological test in which the suspected vein is injected with a radiopaque dye. Sequential films will show the engorged and tortuous veins if venous insufficiency is present. In addition, plethysmography may be done to determine the changes in fluid volume of the extremities. The air-cuff plethysmography measures the changes in the circumference of a limb by recording the changes in pressure in an air-filled cuff surrounding the extremity. However, this test is rarely done because the history, physical examination, and other tests are usually adequate to confirm the diagnosis.

Differential Diagnosis

Patients with chronic venous insufficiency may exhibit some of the symptoms of DVT. Patients who suffer from chronic venous insufficiency have swelling and dilated superficial veins. They may also complain of aching or fatigue in the legs while standing or walking. Other differential diagnoses for DVT include cellulitis, lymphedema, and muscle strain.

MANAGEMENT

Chronic Venous Insufficiency

For the patient with chronic venous insufficiency, conservative treatment is effective in alleviating symptoms in 85% of patients. The degree of dependent edema can be a guide to the effectiveness of therapy. The clinician should order light exercise, support or compression stockings, weight loss, and elevation of the legs several times each day for approximately 30 minutes. Subsequent management involves aggressively treating any ulcers and reducing factors that cause atherosclerosis.

Deep Vein Thrombosis

Pharmaceutical modalities prevent coagulation changes in the blood that result in clot formation or prevent extension of the clot. In the past, the initial treatment of DVT involved the use of subcutaneous low molecular weight fractionated heparin or IV unfractionated heparin. However, with newer oral anticoagulants (dabigatran [Pradaxa], rivaroxaban [Xarelto], and apixaban [Eliquis]), approaches to the treatment of DVT are expanding, as laboratory monitoring with PT/INR (prothrombin time and international normalized ratio) test to judge the level of anticoagulation is not required, given their standardized dosing regimens.

Traditionally patients with DVT were admitted to the hospital for anticoagulant treatment. Current guidelines suggest outpatient treatment for selected patients in the primary-care outpatient setting for an otherwise healthy patient with no significant comorbidities. Candidates for outpatient heparin therapy must have a supportive home environment, be hemodynamically stable, and not have renal failure or a high risk for bleeding. If the patient exhibits a massive DVT, symptoms suggestive of PE, is at high risk for bleeding on anticoagulant therapy, or has significant comorbid conditions—the patient needs to be admitted to an acute care facility.

In the hospital, patients have traditionally been treated aggressively with anticoagulant therapy, IV unfractionated heparin, or subcutaneously injected low molecular weight heparin (LMWH) and monitored for signs of further thrombosis or iatrogenic bleeding. The dosage of heparin should be adjusted according to the partial thromboplastin time (PTT). The goal is to achieve a PTT of two times the control value. Alternatively, LMWH can be used as inpatient or outpatient management of DVT until warfarin is at a therapeutic level.

Enoxaparin (Lovenox), dalteparin (Fragmin), and tinzaparin (Innohep) are examples of types of LMWH, which can be administered subcutaneously once or twice daily. Inpatient Lovenox may be used at a dose of 1 mg/kg injected subcutaneously every 12 hours or in an outpatient setting at 1.5 mg/kg SC daily. The side effect of heparin-induced thrombocytopenia is less likely with LMWH, and less laboratory testing is required, as monitoring PTT need not be done. Simultaneous initiation of warfarin and LMWH has not shown any adverse effects.

Only unfractionated heparin is readily reversible after several hours, once the IV drip is turned off. Subcutaneously injected LMWHs, on the other hand, will exert their effect for at least 12 hours after each dose. In the past, warfarin therapy would be initiated after the patient had been on heparin for 1 to 5 days; however, the current practice is to start warfarin and heparin simultaneously, in order to achieve adequate levels of anticoagulation faster with oral therapy.

Dosing recommendations for warfarin are highly individualized, with starting doses recommended from 2 to 5 mg daily for the first 2 days, before checking the first follow-up PT/INR result. Provided anticoagulation with a parenteral agent (e.g., IV unfractionated heparin) has already been started, some clinicians choose to start warfarin cautiously at a lower daily dose to minimize the risk of bleeding from over-anticoagulation. However, in otherwise healthy adults, some clinicians start with doses as high as 7.5 to 10 mg daily for the first 2 days. Regardless, the warfarin dose is adjusted as needed every 2 to 3 days, based on PT/INR results to achieve the desired level of anticoagulation.

Warfarin therapy should not be started in the absence of a parenteral (IV or SC) anticoagulant to minimize the risk of warfarin-induced skin necrosis. Given the differing half-lives of the vitamin k-dependent clotting proteins inhibited by warfarin (i.e., protein C and factor VII having shorter half-lives than factors II, IX, and X), warfarin may induce relative deficiencies in protein C and factor VII during the first several days of therapy, especially at high initial doses. This imbalance in clotting factors can lead paradoxically to a hypercoagulable state and the formation of intravascular thromboses that can block blood flow to the skin and lead to marked skin necrosis. Thus, starting parenteral anticoagulant therapy with unfractionated heparin or LMWH (which work via a different mechanism than warfarin) concurrently with warfarin for at least 5 days (i.e., "bridging") until the target PT/INR level is reached will help prevent paradoxical warfarin-induced thrombosis and its sequelae.

For selected patients who are being treated as outpatients by a primary-care practitioner, several approaches may be utilized: LMWH overlapped with warfarin, pretreatment with LMWH followed by the oral anticoagulant dabigatran [Pradaxa], or anticoagulation with rivaroxaban [Xarelto] or apixaban [Eliquis] only (with no heparin used). Approaches to anticoagulant therapy should be individualized based on patient comorbidities, risk of bleeding, access to follow-up care and monitoring, patient preferences, and costs.

If anticoagulant therapy is contraindicated, filtering devices such as a vena cava filter may be used to trap emboli before they reach the lungs and cause a PE. Vena caval filters are mechanical barriers that are inserted in the inferior vena cava under percutaneous radiological guidance. Although they do not prevent clot formation, they prevent potentially fatal clot migration from the legs to the lungs.

High-risk patients without active lower limb thrombosis within the last 6 months should receive nonpharmacological prophylaxis with intermittent pneumatic compression of the lower legs in the postsurgical setting or during other episodes of significant immobilization. External pneumatic compression and gradient compression stockings are effective alternatives for decreasing lower leg thrombosis, if lower extremity trauma does not preclude their use. However, use of pneumatic compression devices on limbs with a known DVT is not recommend. Rather, patients should elevate the affected limb, apply heat, and limit activity as anticoagulant therapy is initiated.

Thrombolysis is not indicated for DVT except in cases of massive ileofemoral thrombus. Thrombolytic agents are indicated for patients with massive PE and associated hemodynamic instability. The role of thrombolysis in patients with lesser sized PEs is controversial, given the significant associated bleeding risk.

FOLLOW-UP AND REFERRAL

Most patients with acute DVT are hospitalized for about 1 week. Follow-up treatment for these patients includes anticoagulant therapy for 6 months after an initial episode of DVT and for 1 year after each subsequent episode. The clinician will follow the patient after he or she is released from the hospital. The patient on warfarin must be seen daily, with PT/INR typically checked every

2 to 3 days for potential dose adjustments, until the target INR range is achieved (usually in the hospital), then on a monthly basis thereafter.

Patient Education: Deep Vein Thrombosis

Patients should be educated about DVT prevention and treated prophylactically, depending on the number of risk factors exhibited and the resulting need for hospitalization or surgery. To prevent DVT, prophylactic methods should be used for all patients at risk, including pharmacological treatments, physical or mechanical modalities, or some combination of the two.

Physical modalities that prevent DVT by reducing venous stasis include leg elevation, passive leg exercises, and early ambulation. Although these techniques are somewhat effective, each has some drawbacks and should be combined with other physical measures, such as graduated elastic compression or external pneumatic compression devices. Graduated compression stockings provide safe, simple, and inexpensive prophylaxis. Besides preventing stasis, they also prevent venous distention, which can initiate vessel wall damage. Pneumatic compression devices are more effective at emptying the veins, sustaining femoral blood flow velocity, and expelling the blood from behind the valve cusps in the femoral vein, thus stimulating fibrinolysis.

Education for patients recovering from DVT includes teaching about the need to avoid trauma to the affected veins. The clinician should be educated regarding potential adverse effects of anticoagulant medications, including signs and symptoms of bleeding, anticoagulant-induced skin necrosis, and when to seek medical care. The patient must avoid food fads and crash diets and should not drink alcohol or take vitamin E, cold medicines, antibiotics, aspirin, cimetidine (Tagamet), thyroid hormones, or NSAIDs without first consulting the clinician. Immobility should be discouraged. Patients must know when to return for a follow-up PT if they are on warfarin.

 For additional resources please visit **https://davisedge.fadavis.com/**

REFERENCES

Deep Vein Thrombosis/Chronic Venous Insufficiency

Ali M, Young V. Shifting DVT identification into primary care. *Br J Healthc Manage.* 2012;18(4):211–214.

Centers for Disease Control and Statistics. *Venous thromboembolism—data & statistics.* Division of Blood Disorders, National Center on Birth Defects and Developmental Disabilities, Centers for Disease Control and Prevention. **https://www.cdc.gov/ncbddd/dvt/data.html.** Published 2017. Accessed 9/8/17.

Lip GYP, Hull RD. Overview of the treatment of lower extremity deep vein thrombosis (DVT). *UpToDate.* http://www.uptodate.com. Published 2017.

Michielss JJ, Maasland H, Moossdorff W, Lao M, Gadiseur A, Schroyens W. Safe exclusion of deep vein thrombosis by a rapid sensitive ELISA D-dimer and compression ultrasonography in 1330 outpatients with suspected DVT. *Angiology.* 2016;67(8):781–787.

Peripheral Artery Disease

Centers for Disease Control and Statistics. Peripheral Arterial Disease (PAD) Fact Sheet. Division for Heart Disease and Stroke Prevention. CDC. **https://www.cdc.gov/dhdsp/data_statistics/fact_sheets/fs_pad.htm.** Published 2016. Accessed September 8, 2017.

Gerhaard-Herman MD, Gornik HL, Barrett C, et al. 2016 AHA/ACC Guideline on the Management of Patients With Lower Extremity Peripheral Artery Disease: A Report of the American College of Cardiology/American Heart Association Task Force on Clinical Practice Guidelines. *Circulation.* 2017;135;e726–e779.

RESOURCES

Well's Criteria: DVT Risk Assessment Calculator
https://www.mdcalc.com/wells-criteria-dvt

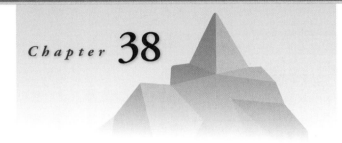

Chapter 38

Common Abdominal Complaints

Debera J. Thomas, DNS, RN, FNP/ANP

ABDOMINAL PAIN

Abdominal pain is one of the most common complaints for which people seek medical attention. According to the 2013 National Ambulatory Medical Care Survey, abdominal pain is one of the top 20 leading principal reasons for office visits. The causes of abdominal pain are numerous; a few are serious enough to require surgical intervention. Conditions associated with an acute abdomen can be inflammatory, metabolic, or structural; therefore, any acute abdominal pain must be evaluated quickly and precisely. Abdominal pain that occurs without any other signs or symptoms is rarely a serious problem. In instances when the exact cause of pain is not immediately evident, an empiric trial of therapy or test selection may help suggest the underlying pathophysiology, narrow the differential diagnoses, and guide further assessment and treatment. It is important to keep in mind that nongastrointestinal etiologies such as ovarian cancer, ectopic pregnancy (see Chapter 48), or myocardial ischemia (see Chapter 35) may present as abdominal pain.

Half of patients who complain of abdominal pain do not receive an accurate diagnosis. The source of the abdominal pain may be from one of a triad of vascular emergencies: mesenteric ischemia, abdominal aortic aneurysm, or myocardial infarction. Conditions in this triad can cause severe pain and should not be excluded from the differential diagnosis.

DIFFERENTIAL DIAGNOSIS

Total patient presentation and a careful history is the key when evaluating abdominal pain and determining the severity of the condition. The onset, location, duration, characteristics, any associated/aggravating factors, relieving factors, temporal factors, and severity, as well as what the pain means to the patient, are useful in the diagnostic reasoning. The presence or absence of bowel sounds is also an important diagnostic factor. Tachycardia, tachypnea, and hypertension often indicate the intensity of the pain. Many nonsurgical conditions can present with classic acute "surgical" abdomen symptoms such as intense pain, rebound tenderness, and guarding. All patients with abdominal pain should undergo rectal, genital, and pelvic evaluations. Blood found in the stool or intense pain on examination may indicate more serious conditions.

Abdominal pain can be caused by mechanical, inflammatory, and ischemic factors. The characteristics of a patient's abdominal pain often give clues as to the specific factors involved. For example, abdominal organs are sensitive to stretching and distention but not as sensitive to cutting, crushing, or tearing. *Visceral pain* is caused by distention or spasm of a hollow viscus and is usually generalized and dull. Distention of an organ capsule, such as Glisson's capsule around the liver; vascular compromise; and mucosal irritations cause pain that is visceral in nature. Conversely, *parietal pain,* described as sharp and well localized, is caused by irritation of the peritoneum. Appendicitis often causes this type of pain as the peritoneum becomes involved. Abdominal pain described as *colicky,* which means that it comes and goes, may result from gallstones or renal stones. *Burning pain,* caused by irritation of the gastric mucosa by gastric contents, is associated with peptic ulcers and esophagitis.

A thorough history and physical examination are essential to narrow the list of differential diagnoses of patients with abdominal pain. First, the nature of the pain is assessed to provide clues to the mechanism of the pain. Although location of the pain is valuable information, it is important to remember that abdominal pain can be referred from other areas. Timing of the pain (onset, duration, frequency, and relationship to associated symptoms) can help eliminate some causes. The palliative and provocative aspects of the pain can give clues about the cause of the pain. For example, does moving, eating certain foods, assuming different positions, or taking medications make the pain better or worse? Associated symptoms will further narrow the list of diagnostic possibilities. Some causes of abdominal pain will necessitate a surgical referral. Any time the pain is very severe and associated with a rigid abdomen, referral to a physician is essential. Abdominal pain can be the presenting symptom of many pathophysiological processes, ranging from very mild gastritis to more serious forms of abdominal pain associated with bowel obstruction or appendicitis.

A complete blood count, serum chemistries, liver function tests, urinalysis, pregnancy test, and abdominal films will help determine the acuity of the problem. Figure 38.1 presents diagnostic algorithms for abdominal pain. Treatment of abdominal pain depends on the cause.

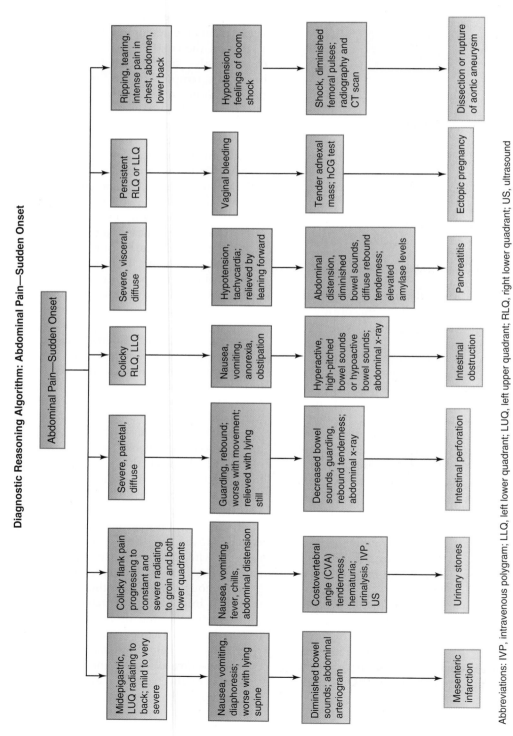

Diagnostic Reasoning Algorithm: Abdominal Pain—Sudden Onset

Abbreviations: IVP, intravenous polygram; LLQ, left lower quadrant; LUQ, left upper quadrant; RLQ, right lower quadrant; US, ultrasound

Figure 38.1a Diagnostic reasoning algorithm: abdominal pain–sudden onset.

Diagnostic Reasoning Algorithm: Abdominal Pain—Burning

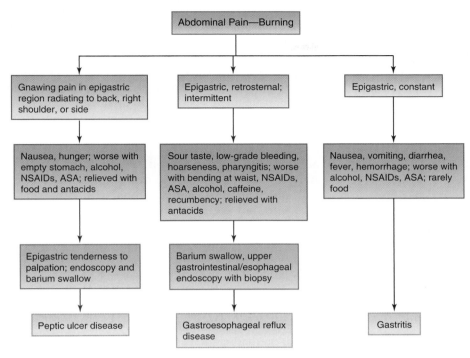

Abbreviations: ASA, acetylsalicylic acid; NSAIDs, nonsteroidal anti-inflammatory drugs; RLQ, right lower quadrant

Figure 38.1b Diagnostic reasoning algorithm: abdominal pain–burning.

Diagnostic Reasoning Algorithm: Abdominal Pain—Cramping

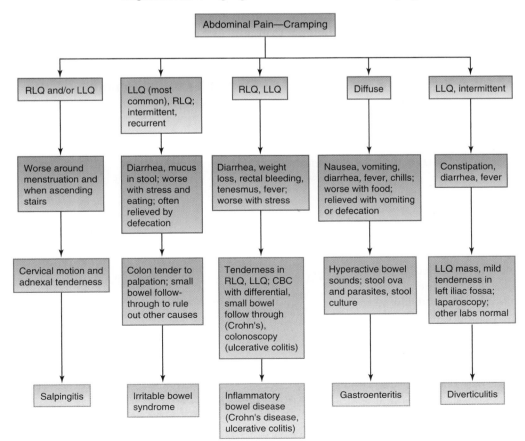

Abbreviations: CBC, complete blood count; LLQ, left lower quadrant; RLQ, right lower quadrant

Figure 38.1c Diagnostic reasoning algorithm: abdominal pain–cramping.

Diagnostic Reasoning Algorithm: Abdominal Pain—Visceral

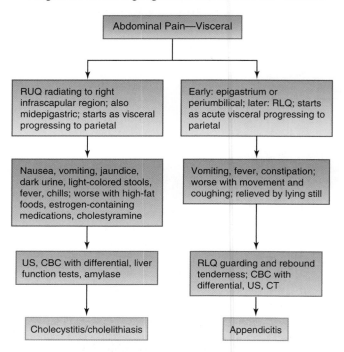

Abbreviations: CBC, complete blood count; CT, computerized tomography; LLQ, left lower quadrant; RLQ, right lower quadrant; RUQ, right upper quadrant; US, ultrasonography

Figure 38.1d Diagnostic reasoning algorithm: abdominal pain–visceral.

CONSTIPATION

Constipation, or difficult or infrequent defecation, is a common symptom in Western society and is the most common gastrointestinal (GI) disorder in the United States, particularly in older adults and sedentary individuals. The clinician and the patient must have a similar operational definition of constipation and what a normal bowel pattern is for that patient.

The most common cause of constipation in the United States is a lack of dietary fiber; the recommended amount is 30 grams daily for optimal bowel health. The average American consumes only about 10 grams per day. Other common causes of constipation are habitual use of laxatives, irritable bowel syndrome (IBS), decreased physical activity, a change in environment or travel, use of medications with constipating potential, suppression of the urge to defecate, and painful defecation caused by anorectal problems. Other less common but serious causes of constipation include bowel tumors and metabolic disorders such as hypothyroidism, diabetes, hypercalcemia, and depression.

Generally, there are three categories of constipation:

- *Functional constipation* generally results from a diet that is low in fiber. A sedentary lifestyle contributes

as well. In addition, some people have difficulty defecating in an environment other than their own home and suppress the urge to defecate, thereby promoting functional constipation.

- *Disordered motility* is most often seen in older adults and is caused by slowed transit time. Megacolon and megarectum are also common disorders of motility, but they most frequently occur in children with conditions such as Hirschsprung disease. Other conditions that cause disordered motility and constipation include IBS and diverticular disease.

- *Secondary constipation* often is a result of medications such as opioids, analgesics, calcium channel blockers, antidepressants, antiparkinsonian drugs, cough medicine, and aluminum antacids. Box 38.1 presents a list of constipating drugs. Other common causes of secondary constipation are chronic laxative use, prolonged immobilization, and organic diseases of the lower GI system, such as colorectal cancer.

Chronic constipation rarely results from a serious condition, and the patient can usually be treated symptomatically by increasing dietary fiber. Patients who have constipation that has developed with a recent disability, a change in diet, recent depressive illness, or the ingestion of a constipating medication can also be treated symptomatically. Patients who develop constipation that cannot be explained, have abdominal pain, report blood or mucus in their stool, or require a substantial increase in their laxative use require more investigation. Constipation occurs in fewer than 30% of patients with colon cancer.

Box 38.1 Medications That Commonly Cause Constipation

Aluminum-containing antacids	Antiparkinsonian drugs
Anticholinergics	Antipsychotics
Anticonvulsants	Bismuth-containing products
• Phenobarbital	
• Phenytoin	• bismuth subsalicylate (Pepto-Bismol)
• Carbamazepine	
	Iron preparations
Antidepressants	NSAIDs
	Opiates
• Amitriptyline	
• Doxepin	• Codeine
• Imipramine	• Morphine
• Nortriptyline	• Heroin
• Protriptyline	• Fentanyl
	• Methadone
Antihistamines	• Propoxyphene
Antihypertensives	• Tramadol
• Calcium channel blockers	
• Clonidine	Sympathomimetics

DIFFERENTIAL DIAGNOSIS

An accurate description of the feces can give clues to the cause of the constipation. For example, ribbon-like stools often indicate a motility disorder but can also be caused by an organic narrowing of the distal or sigmoid colon. If the patient complains of a progressive decrease in the diameter of the stools, this suggests an organic lesion. If steatorrhea and greenish-yellow stools are associated with the constipation, the practitioner should look for a small bowel or pancreatic lesion. Constipation alternating with diarrhea is often a result of IBS.

The cause of constipation is multifactorial, which can make the differential diagnosis difficult. Figure 38.2 presents various causes of constipation.

MANAGEMENT

The management of simple constipation is straightforward. Most patients respond well to education about bowel habits, activity, and dietary intervention. Some patients may require pharmacological intervention as well. Patients should be instructed to slowly increase the amount of dietary fiber to 25 to 35 grams per day, with at least 12 to 15 grams at breakfast. Mild exercise after the morning meal is often helpful in stimulating peristalsis and promoting defecation. Uninterrupted toilet time in the morning is also helpful. Adequate hydration is essential, and patients should be encouraged to drink at least 64 ounces of fluids daily.

Treatment with a pharmacologic agent may be needed for patients who do not respond to increases in fiber, fluids, and exercise. Most drugs should be used for a short time only, and most are available without a prescription. Because these agents are available without a prescription, patients may have self-medicated for some time; by the time they seek medical attention, they may either have overused laxatives or may have a more serious underlying pathology. The only agents that are appropriate for long-term use are bulking agents. The different agents used in the treatment of constipation are listed in Drugs Commonly Prescribed 38.1. Complementary Therapies 38.1 lists the uses of vitamins, minerals, and herbs for constipation as well as other GI problems.

DIARRHEA

As with constipation, there is no single definition of diarrhea, but it is generally defined as an increase in the frequency, volume, or fluid content of bowel movements over what is normal for the individual. Because dietary intake of fiber in the United States is low, the average daily stool for each individual weighs about 200 grams. For most individuals, if the daily stool is more than 200 grams or the frequency of bowel movements is more than three times a day, the patient's condition is diarrhea.

There are several types of diarrhea that include the following:

- *Osmotic diarrhea* results when the osmotic gap between the stool and the serum is over 50 mOsm/kg. Normally, the fecal osmolality is equal to the serum osmolality. An increasing osmotic gap implies either ingestion or malabsorption of a substance that is osmotically active. Carbohydrate malabsorption is the most common cause and includes lactose, fructose and sorbitol. Other causes include laxative abuse and other malabsorption syndromes. Osmotic diarrhea usually responds to fasting. Celiac disease is a malabsorption syndrome related to an immune reaction to gluten in the diet. It is most common in women, and the peak incidence is in women aged 40 to 50 years. Gluten is found in food products that contain wheat, barley, and rye. The effects on the intestinal mucosa cause the villi to become flat, the crypts to hypertrophy, and an increased number of intraepithelial lymphocytes and plasma cells to appear. Complications such as collagenous sprue and intestinal ulcers, nutritional complications, and malignancy are possible. The patient will have a history of chronic diarrhea, foul-smelling stools, abdominal bloating, weakness, and fatigue. A presumptive diagnosis is based on a combination of clinical presentation and positive serology. Distal duodenal biopsy is needed to confirm the diagnosis. Treatment includes a lifelong gluten-free diet and treatment of nutritional deficiencies such as iron, folate, and vitamin B_{12}.
- *Secretory diarrhea* produces voluminous, watery stools but is unresponsive to fasting. Most cases of acute and chronic diarrhea are secretory in nature. Secretory diarrhea results from bacterial toxins (most notably from cholera and strains of *Escherichia coli*) and viruses (norovirus). However, it can also be caused by laxative abuse; bile salt malabsorption, which stimulates colonic secretion; and endocrine tumors that stimulate pancreatic or intestinal secretion.
- Diarrhea is associated with *morphological changes* within the mucosa of the intestinal wall that occur with inflammatory conditions of the intestines, and these changes can result in acute or chronic diarrhea. Both Crohn's disease and ulcerative colitis cause inflammation of the mucosa of the intestinal lumen, resulting in diarrhea.
- *Altered intestinal motility* secondary to diabetic neuropathy, dumping syndrome, or IBS can also cause diarrhea. Chronic parasitic infections with organisms such as giardia, *Entamoeba histolytica*, and Cyclospora can cause diarrhea. Some medications, such as antibiotics, can induce diarrhea by disrupting the normal balance of bacteria. Probiotics have been studied in the treatment of diarrhea. A systematic review of 30 randomized clinical trials of the use of probiotics in adults at risk for antibiotic-associated diarrhea (AAD) revealed that the

Diagnostic Reasoning Algorithm: Constipation

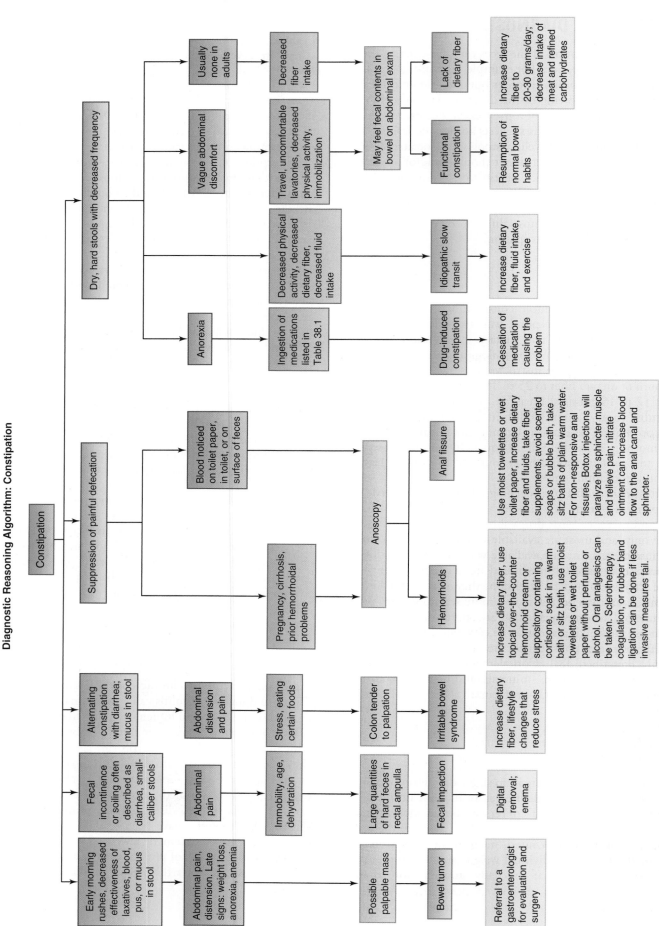

Figure 38.2 Diagnostic reasoning algorithm: constipation.

Drugs Commonly Prescribed 38.1: Constipation

DRUG	INDICATION	ADVERSE REACTIONS AND PRESCRIBING CONSIDERATIONS
Bulking agents Psyllium preparations Methylcellulose preparations	Irritable bowel syndrome Chronic constipation Diverticulitis	Causes flatulence, bloating and requires adequate fluid intake.
Stool softeners Docusate sodium	Frequently used for prevention of constipation but not effective	Hepatotoxic if combined with irritant laxatives.
Saline laxatives Magnesium hydroxide	Intermittent use in chronic constipation and bowel prep	Can cause dehydration and electrolyte imbalance.
Stimulant/irritant laxatives Bisacodyl Senna cascara	Acute constipation; should not be used for chronic constipation	Patient can become dependent. Also causes dehydration and electrolyte imbalance.
Lubricants Mineral oil	Intermittent use in chronic constipation	Can cause lipid pneumonia if aspirated.

Complementary Therapies 38.1: Complementary Therapies for Gastrointestinal Problems

AGENT	INDICATION	ADVERSE REACTIONS AND PRESCRIBING CONSIDERATIONS
Senna *(Cassia senna)*	Constipation	1–2 tsp dried leaves per 8 oz water taken as a tea once daily (not to be taken for longer than a few days)
Acupuncture	Heartburn	8–12 treatments
Ginger	Nausea and motion sickness	250 mg daily

risk of AAD was reduced in adults but not in the elderly (Jafarmejad, Shab-Bidar, Speakman, et al., 2016). In another systematic review that included five studies on the effectiveness of probiotics in reducing *Clostridium difficile*–associated diarrhea in the elderly, results were mixed and showed no difference compared with placebo in elderly hospitalized patients (Vernaya, McAdam, & Hampton, 2017). Probiotic use for travelers' diarrhea, *C. difficile,* and inflammatory bowel disease (IBD) has not proved efficacious. Pathogenic bacteria also cause increases in GI motility and intestinal secretions. There have been promising results with the use of fecal microbiota transplantation (stool transplant) for the treatment of *C. difficile* diarrhea. This procedure involves taking fecal bacteria from a healthy person and infusing this via enema into the person with the *C. difficile* infection.

DIFFERENTIAL DIAGNOSIS

Differential diagnosis of diarrhea is aided by separating acute diarrhea from chronic diarrhea. *Acute diarrhea* usually has an abrupt onset and lasts for less than 1 week. Nausea, vomiting, or fever may be associated with acute types of diarrhea. *Chronic diarrhea* lasts for more than

2 weeks or recurs over months or years. When diarrhea occurs suddenly in an otherwise healthy patient without signs or symptoms of other organ involvement, the most likely cause is an infectious agent, most often viral. The most frequent causes of chronic diarrhea are IBS, medications, dietary factors, IBD, and colon cancer.

A thorough history and comprehensive review of systems can elicit information that the patient may not think is important but that can facilitate diagnosis. For example, recent travel is particularly important because viral, bacterial, and protozoan causes are endemic in many areas. Hikers and campers in the United States who drink unfiltered water are at a high risk for giardiasis. Focus on History: Diarrhea presents important information to obtain from the patient's history.

Focus on History: Diarrhea

Characteristics of Feces

- Frequency
- Amount and fluidity
- Color and characteristics: bloody, tarry, black, steatorrheic, mucus

Other History

- Diet history: intolerance to lactose or certain foods
- Recent travel
- Source of drinking water: well or city water supply
- Medication use: magnesium-containing antacids (or supplements), antibiotics, chemotherapy, immunosuppressive agents
- Medical/surgical history: diabetes mellitus, hyperthyroid, HIV, organ transplant, GI surgery
- Sexual practices: frequency of anal intercourse, number and sex of partners
- Social history: living conditions
- Family history: colon cancer, IBD

Other Factors

- Associated symptoms: abdominal pain, fever, vomiting, neurological symptoms, headache, malaise, myalgia, muscle weakness
- Exacerbating or alleviating factors

Acute viral gastroenteritis is the most common cause of diarrhea. (Gastroenteritis is discussed in detail later in Chapter 39.) Other common causes of diarrhea the practitioner should consider are IBS, IBD, ingestion of magnesium-containing antacids, lactose intolerance, antibiotic therapy, laxative abuse, and AIDS. Figure 38.3 presents a diagnostic algorithm for diarrhea.

Diagnostic Reasoning Algorithm: Diarrhea

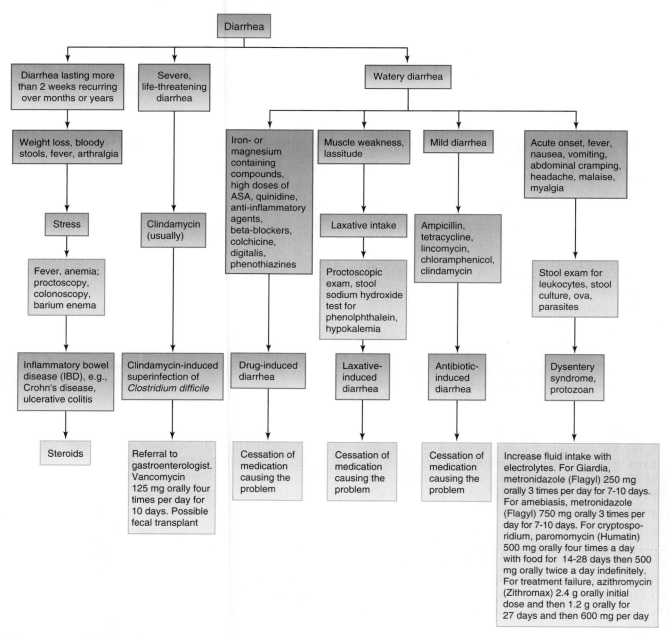

Figure 38.3 Diagnostic reasoning algorithm: diarrhea.

Diagnostic Reasoning Algorithm: Diarrhea (Continued)

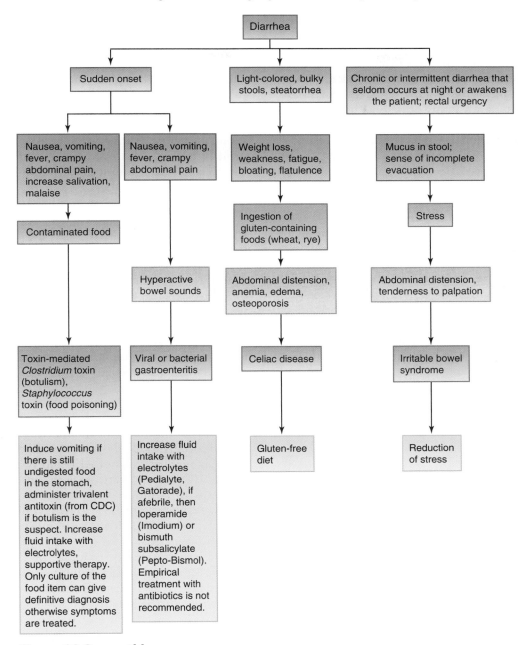

Figure 38.3—cont'd

DYSPEPSIA AND HEARTBURN

The frequency with which patients present with dyspepsia and heartburn as their chief complaint has been diminishing, probably because of the availability of over-the-counter histamine-2 receptor blockers and proton pump inhibitors. Aggressive advertising of these products by pharmaceutical companies over the past decade has led to increased self-medication for what could be a serious illness that the individual mistakes as simple heartburn.

DIFFERENTIAL DIAGNOSIS

Dyspepsia and heartburn are two different entities. *Heartburn* is occasionally described as extreme pain, and this makes it difficult to distinguish heartburn pain from that of angina pectoris or myocardial infarction. Patients with heartburn sometimes describe the pain as radiating to the back, arms, or jaw, which further complicates the diagnosis. Symptoms of *dyspepsia* include epigastric discomfort, postprandial fullness, early satiety, anorexia, belching, nausea, heartburn, vomiting, bloating, borborygmi, dysphagia, and abdominal burning.

These symptoms most often have functional or organic causes. The possibility of an organic cause for dyspepsia increases as a person ages. Patients who ingest alcohol in significant amounts or take drugs such as salicylates, corticosteroids, NSAIDs, erythromycin (E-Mycin), or theophylline (Theo-Dur, Theo-24) often have dyspepsia as a result of medication-induced gastritis. Giardiasis can cause dyspepsia with only occasional bouts of diarrhea. Nonulcer dyspepsia caused by *Helicobacter pylori* causes vague abdominal pain, a sense of fullness, nausea, and bloating, which are worse after eating. If the symptoms of dyspepsia are continuous and associated with anorexia and weight loss, gastric cancer may be the cause.

Heartburn, a retrosternal burning sensation, is common in the general population, with 7% complaining of daily symptoms, 14% having weekly episodes, and 36% experiencing heartburn at least once in their lives. The most common cause of heartburn is gastroesophageal reflux disease. Pregnant women have a high incidence of esophagitis, most often later in the pregnancy because of increased intra-abdominal pressure. Heartburn is commonly relieved by the ingestion of alkali (antacids) and is precipitated and aggravated by recumbency. Figure 38.4 provides a diagnostic algorithm for heartburn and dyspepsia.

JAUNDICE

Jaundice (icterus) is a yellow coloration of the skin, mucous membranes, and sclera resulting from an accumulation of bilirubin in the blood. Patients who develop jaundice usually seek medical attention promptly because it is so dramatic, frightening, and difficult to ignore.

The hyperbilirubinemia that causes the jaundice can be a result of increased production, decreased uptake, decreased conjugation, or decreased excretion of bilirubin. The etiology of hyperbilirubinemia is shown in Box 38.2. Hyperbilirubinemia and jaundice in most patients result from cholestasis, either because of impaired bile formation and/or bile flow, which can be the result of extrahepatic biliary tract obstruction or hepatic parenchymal disease.

DIFFERENTIAL DIAGNOSIS

Understanding laboratory values reported for typical liver function tests is essential in determining the cause of hyperbilirubinemia and establishing a diagnosis. Icterus is not usually evident until the serum bilirubin level exceeds 2.5 to 3.0 mg/dL. The normal serum bilirubin level is 0.3 to 1.0 mg/dL. Most bilirubin is formed from the heme portion of the breakdown of red blood cells. This initial bilirubin is unconjugated and therefore not soluble in water. When measured in the serum, it is reported as indirect bilirubin. This form of bilirubin is reversibly bound to albumin and transported to the liver, where it is taken up by hepatocytes and conjugated with glucuronic acid. Conjugated bilirubin, which is water soluble, is transported from the hepatocyte into the bile. It is measured in the serum as the direct fraction of bilirubin. Only conjugated bilirubin, by nature of its water solubility, is found in the urine of patients with hyperbilirubinemia. Problems in the metabolism of bilirubin can occur at any point of the cycle.

Serum levels of the transaminases–aspartate aminotransferase (AST) and alanine aminotransferase (ALT)–are good indicators of hepatocyte damage from a variety of causes. Elevated transaminase levels reflect the activity of the disease process, but actual serum levels do not necessarily correlate with the overall severity of the liver disease, nor with the prognosis. AST is found in hepatocyte mitochondria and cytoplasm and in nonhepatic tissues such as skeletal muscle, the heart, and the brain. ALT is found primarily in hepatocyte cytoplasm, making it a much more specific marker for hepatocyte damage. Levels of AST and ALT that are below 300 U/L are nonspecific; however, some extreme elevations can be diagnostic. For example, it is uncommon for the AST to be elevated 15 times the normal value in biliary obstruction except when it occurs suddenly or is associated with cholangitis. Striking elevations of ALT and AST (greater than 1,000 U/L) occur in patients with acute viral hepatitis, toxin- or drug-induced hepatitis, and ischemic liver injury. If the ratio of AST to ALT is high, it generally indicates severe hepatic necrosis, most often caused by alcoholic hepatitis.

Alkaline phosphatase is found in the biliary canalicular membranes and is useful in assessing cholestasis. Cholestasis is also characteristically accompanied by an increase in the serum gamma-glutamyl transpeptidase (GGT) and 5(-nucleotidase. Extreme elevations in alkaline phosphatase (greater than three times normal) in conjunction with elevation of the GGT indicate a mechanical obstruction of the biliary system by a tumor, stricture, or stone. Because alkaline phosphatase is also found in bone, an isolated elevation of that enzyme without elevation of the GGT is indicative of a bone disorder rather than a cholestatic process.

A patient who presents with jaundice often has complaints of pruritis, anorexia, nausea, vomiting, fever, light-colored stools, weight loss, and fatigue. Examination may reveal right upper quadrant pain and tenderness, dark urine, and abdominal distention. Pruritus, dark urine, and light-colored stools in conjunction with the jaundice are indicative of cholestasis, either intrahepatic or extrahepatic, such as cholelithiasis, cirrhosis, or other biliary obstruction.

Diagnostic Reasoning Algorithm: Heartburn and Dyspepsia

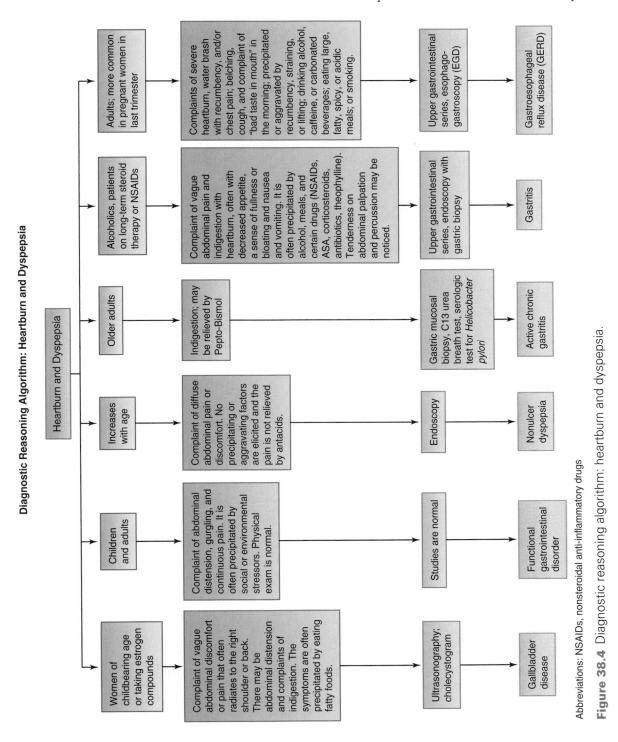

Abbreviations: NSAIDs, nonsteroidal anti-inflammatory drugs

Figure 38.4 Diagnostic reasoning algorithm: heartburn and dyspepsia.

MELENA

Melena is defined as black, tarry stools that test positive for occult blood. The most common cause of melena is upper gastrointestinal (GI) bleeding, but bleeding in the small bowel or the right colon can also produce melena. It is the action of gastric acid and intestinal secretions that reduces bright red blood to black, tarry stools. To produce melena, about 100 to 200 mL of blood must be present. Because

of GI transit time, it is possible for melena to continue for several days after the acute bleeding has stopped.

DIFFERENTIAL DIAGNOSIS

Some patients may present with black, tarry stools that do not test positive for blood. The most common causes for this are iron supplements, bismuth subsalicylate (Pepto-Bismol), and a variety of foods. Box 38.3 lists common

---

Box 38.2   Causes of Hyperbilirubinemia

Increased Production

Hemolysis, resorption of hematomas, ineffective erythropoiesis

- Megaloblastic anemia, iron-deficiency anemia, sideroblastic anemia
- Thalassemia minor
- Polycythemia vera
- Lead poisoning

Decreased Clearance

Inherited disorder of bilirubin metabolism

- Gilbert's syndrome, Crigler-Najjar syndrome, Dubin-Johnson syndrome, Rotor's syndrome

Cholestasis

- Hepatocellular disease: viral, drug-induced, or alcoholic hepatitis
- Biliary tract obstruction: choledocholithiasis, tumor, sclerosing cholangitis, chronic pancreatitis, pancreatic cancer, primary biliary cirrhosis

Drugs

- Antibiotics (erythromycin, trimethoprim/sulfamethoxazole, amoxicillin/clavulanic acid, nitrofurantoin, griseofulvin)
- Analgesics (propoxyphene, sulindac, diflunisal)
- Allopurinol
- Warfarin
- Steroids (contraceptive and anabolic)
- Phenytoin
- Thiazide diuretics
- Phenothiazines
- Tricyclic antidepressants
- Haloperidol
- Parenteral gold
- Oral hypoglycemics (chlorpropamide, tolbutamide)

Box 38.3   Common Causes of Gastrointestinal Bleeding

Upper Gastrointestinal Tract

Peptic ulcer

- Gastric ulcer
- Duodenal ulcer

Gastric erosions
Erosive esophagitis
Esophageal varices

Lower Gastrointestinal Tract

Diverticular disease
Colon cancer
Intestinal polyps
Inflammatory bowel disease
Ulcerative colitis
Crohn's disease
Infectious colitis
Meckel's diverticulum
Small bowel neoplasm

---

causes of GI bleeding. Signs and symptoms associated with GI bleeding depend on the source, rate of bleeding, and coexistent diseases. GI bleeding from a peptic ulcer is common and accounts for roughly half of all episodes of upper GI hemorrhage. A complete blood count can give clues about the severity and duration of the bleeding. Endoscopy is useful in diagnosing the upper GI tract as the source of the bleeding.

NAUSEA AND VOMITING

Nausea is an unpleasant sensation in the stomach that is difficult to define because it is a sensory experience. It is often accompanied by diaphoresis, increased salivation, and the vasovagal signs of hypotension and bradycardia.

Nausea can occur alone or precede vomiting. Vomiting is the forceful expulsion of gastric contents; it is a reflex response to stimulation of receptor sites in the mucosa of the upper gastrointestinal (GI) tract, the labyrinthine apparatus in the inner ear, higher cortical centers in response to emotional stimuli, or the chemoreceptor trigger zone of the medulla oblongata. Afferent nerve fibers carry these impulses to the vomiting center, where efferent fibers then send impulses to relax the gastric fundus and the gastroesophageal sphincter, contract the pylorus, and cause reverse peristalsis in the esophagus. The abdominal muscles and diaphragm contract, increasing the intra-abdominal pressure, which forces the gastric contents out through the mouth.

DIFFERENTIAL DIAGNOSIS

Gastroenteritis is the most common cause of nausea and vomiting in adults and children. Contaminated food should be considered in cases of acute nausea and vomiting, especially when more than one person is affected. Gastritis, usually associated with alcohol consumption or drugs (aspirin, NSAIDs, antibiotics, and illicit drugs), is also a common cause of acute nausea and vomiting in adults. Nausea and vomiting are listed as adverse effects of many medications; they are also common presenting symptoms for many disease entities such as hepatitis, myocardial infarction, and peptic ulcer. Box 38.4 provides common causes of nausea and vomiting.

A careful history and documentation of signs and symptoms are often necessary to determine the cause of

Box 38.4 Common Causes of Nausea and Vomiting

Gastrointestinal Disorders and Problems

Gastroenteritis
Acute gastrointestinal infections
Food poisoning
Gastritis, including alcoholic
Peptic ulcer disease
Hepatitis
Food intolerance
Celiac disease (Celiac sprue)
Lactase deficiency
Ingestion of fatty foods
Intestinal obstruction
Appendicitis
Cholecystitis
Peritonitis
Diabetic gastric atony

Central Nervous System Disorders and Problems

Increased intracranial pressure
Migraine headache
Meningitis
Acute labyrinthitis
Ménière's disease
Altitude sickness

Other Disorders and Problems

Motion sickness
Uremia
Bulimia nervosa
Diabetic ketoacidosis
Adrenal insufficiency
Acute myocardial infarction
Congestive heart failure
Gastroparesis
Postinfectious gastroparesis

Acute Systemic Infections Accompanied by Fever

Pregnancy
Adverse Effect of Drugs and Chemicals
Antibiotics (erythromycin, metronidazole)
Opiates
Estrogen
Ipecac
Digitalis
Chemotherapy
Theophylline

the nausea and vomiting. The circumstances surrounding the episode or episodes give clues to the cause. Vomiting following a meal can occur with gastritis and in digitalis toxicity. If the vomiting occurs 1 to 2 hours after eating, diseases of the biliary tract or pancreas should be suspected. Projectile vomiting without nausea is classically a sign of a neurological source, such as increased intracranial pressure. If the nausea and vomiting occur in the early morning, the cause may be uremia, pregnancy, or chronic alcohol ingestion. The duration of the nausea and vomiting depends on the cause. Infectious agents in the GI tract usually cause nausea and vomiting only for 24 hours or less. Nausea as a result of pregnancy can last for weeks.

The characteristics of the vomitus are important in determining the cause. For example, repeated vomiting without bile staining is indicative of pyloric obstruction, which can be caused by scars from an ulcer or a tumor, whereas vomiting of undigested food could indicate an esophageal obstruction. The odor of the vomitus is important information to elicit from the patient in determining the cause. Odorless vomitus indicates a lack of gastric acid, possibly from esophageal stricture or achalasia. Fecal odor, on the other hand, indicates a bowel obstruction or gastrocolic fistula.

Associated symptoms can further narrow the field of possibilities. Ménière's disease or middle ear disturbances should be suspected if the patient complains of vertigo, tinnitus, or hearing loss. Nausea and vomiting often accompany migraine headaches, which are usually unilateral. Nausea and vomiting with diarrhea and abdominal pain are often caused by gastroenteritis. Figure 38.5 provides a diagnostic algorithm for nausea and vomiting.

MANAGEMENT

Management of nausea and vomiting is aimed at the underlying cause, which is covered in detail in specific chapters in this section and in other chapters of this book. Symptomatic relief, however, is useful for the comfort of the patient and in preventing complications such as dehydration and electrolyte imbalance. Drugs Commonly Prescribed 38.2 presents a list of medications commonly used for the control of nausea and vomiting

DYSPHAGIA

Dysphagia is defined as difficulty swallowing that may or may not have a component of *odynophagia,* or painful swallowing. Although dysphagia may accompany odynophagia, classic dysphagia is not usually painful. The prevalence increases with age and is common in older adults.

The process of swallowing is complex and involves 50 pairs of muscles and many nerves. Swallowing has three phases: (1) The *oral phase* involves movement of the tongue and jaw allowing for mastication and preparation of food into a bolus and making it ready for swallowing; (2) the *pharyngeal phase* includes the reflexive passage of the bolus from the oral cavity through the pharynx and

Diagnostic Reasoning Algorithm: Nausea and Vomiting

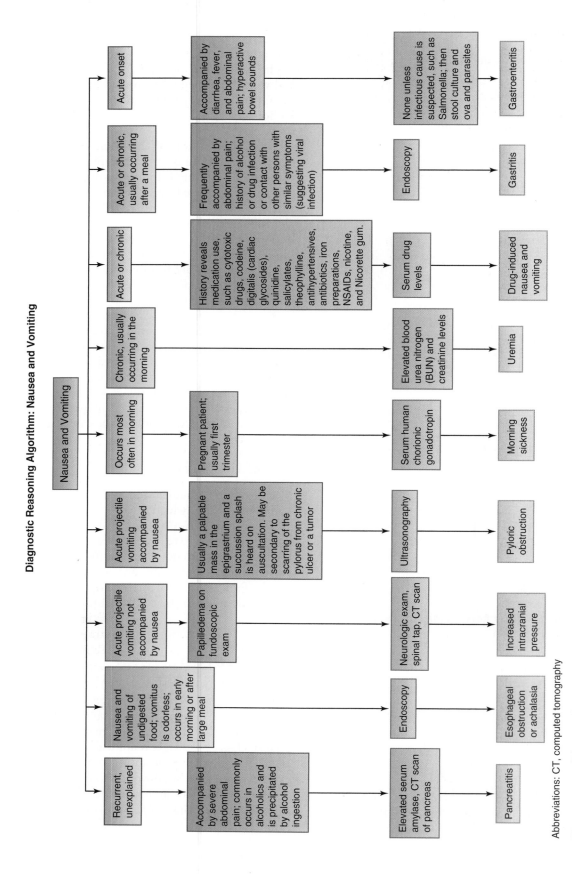

Abbreviations: CT, computed tomography

Figure 38.5 Diagnostic reasoning algorithm: nausea and vomiting.

Drugs Commonly Prescribed 38.2: Nausea and Vomiting

DRUG	INDICATION	ADVERSE REACTIONS AND PRESCRIBING CONSIDERATIONS
Antihistamines (dimenhydrinate, promethazine, hydroxyzine, meclizine)	Motion sickness Drug-induced nausea Postoperative During labor	Sedation, dry mouth, blurred vision, headache
Antidopaminergics (prochlorperazine)	Chemotherapy- and radiation-induced nausea and vomiting Postoperative	Sedation, dry mouth, urinary retention, constipation, extrapyramidal effects
Antidopaminergics and cholinergics (metoclopramide)	Postoperative Diabetic gastroparesis	Restlessness, drowsiness, fatigue, extrapyramidal effects
Cholinergic antagonists (scopolamine)	Motion sickness	Dry mouth, blurred vision, tachycardia, constipation, sedation
Serotonin receptor antagonists (ondansetron, granisetron)	Chemotherapy- and radiation-induced nausea and vomiting	Anxiety, euphoria, depression, headache, insomnia, restlessness, weakness

into the upper esophagus; and (3) the *esophageal phase* is the reflexive passage of the bolus through the esophagus and into the stomach. There is often a combination of underlying factors that cause dysphagia.

DIFFERENTIAL DIAGNOSIS

Dysphagia can be caused by mechanical obstruction or a functional problem that impairs motility. Mechanical obstruction can be either intrinsic (strictures, tumors, diverticular outpouchings) or extrinsic (a tumor or other growth outside the esophagus that presses inward to compress the esophageal wall). Functional dysphagia can have a neurological or muscular cause. Neurological conditions that interfere with voluntary swallowing or peristalsis are cerebrovascular accidents, Parkinson's disease, multiple sclerosis, amyotrophic lateral sclerosis, and achalasia. Eighty percent of oral phase and pharyngeal phase abnormalities have a neurologic origin. Dermatomyositis is a muscular disease that causes functional problems in the upper esophagus leading to dysphagia. Dysphagia may be the first sign of such an underlying disorder. Psychological conditions may also cause the symptoms; the term *globus hystericus* refers to a manifestation of acute anxiety disorders and panic attacks. Dysphagia may also be associated with an underlying depressive disorder.

Alterations of the swallowing process may manifest differently depending on the underlying pathology. For example, if there is a problem in the oral phase, dribbling, spillage, pocketing of food in the mouth, or aspiration may be present. The pharyngeal phase is the first reflexive, or involuntary, phase; problems during this phase are characterized by nasal regurgitation, aspiration, and/or altered voice. This is the phase where aspiration most commonly occurs during swallowing. Esophageal phase problems are characterized by neck pain, heartburn, and the sensation of food becoming "stuck" below the sternum.

An upper endoscopy is the first choice to evaluate chronic dysphagia and has the benefit of direct visualization and the ability to obtain a biopsy if an abnormality is found. A videofluoroscopic swallow study is useful in evaluating swallowing. This imaging technique videotapes the entire swallowing process and shows an outline of the structures from the oral cavity to the stomach, as well as assessing the velocity and movement of oral and hypopharyngeal structures and their temporal relationship to each other. Through observation of the ingestion of various food consistencies, such as thin liquids, thick liquids, semisolids, and solids, the safest plan for oral intake can be determined.

MANAGEMENT

There are a number of approaches to treating dysphagia depending on the cause. One approach involves muscle strengthening exercises of the facial muscles to improve the coordination of swallowing. Most approaches involve instructing the patient and family members in ways to improve safe food intake, including positioning (usually sitting upright, with the head tilted slightly forward and downward) and food-consistency modification (no thin liquids, mechanical soft diet) during food intake. However, if the risk of aspiration is severe, the clinician may have to consider elimination of oral intake. For these patients, enteral feeding is the next choice.

REFERENCES

Bascom A. *Incorporating herbal medicine into clinical practice.* Philadelphia: FA Davis; ; 2002.

Domino FJ, Baldor RA, Golding J, Stephens MB, eds. *The 5-minute clinical consult,* 26th ed. Philadelphia: Wolters Kluwer; 2018.

Edmunds MW, Mayhew MS. *Pharmacology for the primary care provider,* 4th ed. St. Louis: Mosby/Elsevier; 2013.

Goldberg EJ, Bhalodia S, Jacob S, et al. *Clostridium difficile* infection: A brief update on emerging therapies. *Am J Health Syst Pharmacol.* 2015;72:1007–1012.

Huether SE. Alterations in digestive function. In McCance KL, Huether SE (eds.), *Pathophysiology: The biologic basis for disease in adults and children,* 7th ed. St. Louis, MO: Mosby; 2014:1423–1485.

Jafarnejad S, Shab-Bidar S, Speakman JR, et al. Probiotics reduce the risk of antibiotic-associated diarrhea in adults (18–64 years) but not the elderly (>65 years): A meta-analysis. *Nutrition in Clinical Practice,* 2016;31:502–513.

Vernaya M, McAdam J, Hampton MD. Effectiveness of probiotics in reducing the incidence of *Clostridium difficile*–associated diarrhea in elderly patients: A systematic review. *JBI Database System Rev Implement Rep.* 2017;15:140–164.

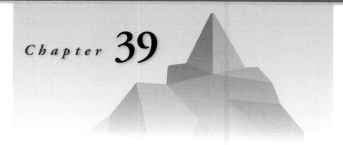

Chapter **39**

Infectious Gastrointestinal Disorders

Debera J. Thomas, DNS, RN, FNP/ANP

GASTROENTERITIS

Gastroenteritis is an inflammation of the stomach and intestine that manifests as anorexia, nausea, vomiting, and diarrhea. Gastroenteritis can be acute or chronic and can be caused by bacteria, viruses, parasites, injury to the bowel mucosa, inorganic poisons (sodium nitrate), organic poisons (mushrooms or shellfish), and drugs. Chronic causes include food allergies and intolerance, stress, and lactase deficiency. Gastroenteritis caused by bacterial toxins in food is often referred to as food poisoning; it should be suspected when groups of individuals present with the same symptoms.

The symptoms and subsequent electrolyte imbalances are usually self-limiting in the healthy adult but can have serious consequences for older adults and immunocompromised or pediatric patients. The severity of the illness is indicated by the presence of dehydration secondary to profuse watery diarrhea, fever greater than 101°F (38.3°C), vomiting, or dysentery (frequent small stools containing blood and mucus). A careful history and physical exam provides clues about the causative agent and the suspected vector of transmission. Travel, dining locations, and antibiotic history should be included as part of the assessment.

EPIDEMIOLOGY AND CAUSES

Acute gastroenteritis results most often from an infectious agent. Although it is one of the most frequent diagnoses in primary-care practice (about 30% of patients seen each year), the exact number of individuals affected is not known because acute gastroenteritis presents with a group of nonspecific symptoms that often go unreported or the etiology cannot be determined. Estimates are that the annual rate for gastroenteritis is approximately one episode per adult per year in the United States and Western Europe. Food- and waterborne outbreaks are of particular importance and gain the attention of the news media in an effort to identify and treat all the individuals who were exposed to the harmful pathogen.

The most common mode of transmission for acute infectious gastroenteritis is the fecal–oral route from contaminated food or water. Person-to-person transfer of the disease is more common within the hospital setting and within day-care centers where there are larger groups of people capable of transmitting the disease. Groups considered at high risk for developing gastroenteritis include anyone traveling to a developing country, immunocompromised patients, anyone engaging in anal intercourse, residents of institutions or nursing homes, infants and children attending day-care centers, and individuals consuming raw shellfish and seafood.

Bacterial pathogens account for 30% to 80% of acute gastroenteritis cases and are an important cause of morbidity in tropical areas and in travelers to areas of high risk for the pathogens (traveler's diarrhea). Areas considered high risk for developing traveler's diarrhea include Africa, Southeast Asia, and developing countries in the Middle East or Latin America. Table 39.1 presents the most common bacterial, viral, and parasitic causes of gastroenteritis.

TABLE 39.1 Organisms Causing Gastroenteritis

Pathogen	Pathogenesis	Duration/Onset	Clinical Findings	Diagnosis and Treatment
Bacterial Pathogens *Bacillus cereus*	Type of food poisoning from formation of enterotoxins within food or gut; two forms, differing in duration of illness.	Duration is normally less than 24 hours. Onset is within 1–8 hours after exposure.	Illness begins with vomiting and proceeds to diarrhea; no fever. Commonly occurs in rice dishes; the spores are heat resistant and not affected by cooking.	No antibiotic treatment is required; oral hydration and supportive care.
Campylobacter jejuni	Found primarily in eggs and poultry but may be found in domestic animals. Organism invades the intestinal mucosa and produces a cholera-like toxin. Organism grows within ileum and jejunum.	Duration of illness is 2–6 days. Onset of symptoms approximately 48 hours after ingestion of pathogen.	Common cause of traveler's diarrhea from ingestion of contaminated water. Symptoms include fever, bloody diarrhea, and abdominal pain. Stool is positive for polymorphonuclear neutrophils.	Normally self-limiting. Erythromycin ethylsuccinate can be used in severe cases. Rapid antibiotic resistance is common. Stool culture requires special media. Quinoline antibiotics have been effective in increasing recovery.
Clostridium botulinum	Anaerobic gram-positive bacillus that produces seven distinct toxins. In the foodborne type the toxin is ingested with contaminated food. Once absorbed, the toxin blocks the release of acetylcholine from peripheral nerve endings. Canned foods are the primary source.	Duration of illness depends on diagnosis and treatment. Mortality rate is high. Onset is abrupt, although incubation can be as long as 4–8 days.	GI symptoms often precede neurological findings, which are bilateral, are symmetrical, and occur in a descending fashion. Initial neurological symptoms include dry mouth, diplopia, and loss of pupillary reflex. Dysphagia and dysarthria can lead to aspiration pneumonia. Progression of neurological insult leads to paralysis of the diaphragm and death if mechanical ventilation is not employed.	Diagnosis is made by isolation of organism in suspected food, the serum, or feces. Symptoms are often confused with Guillain-Barré. Treatment is to first eliminate any unabsorbed food (toxin) by inducing vomiting or by gastric lavage, then administration of trivalent antitoxin (A, B, or E) from the Centers for Disease Control and Prevention. The antitoxin does not reverse the existing neurological symptoms but prevents progression. Little benefit if given after 72 hours. Toxin may cause serum sickness or anaphylaxis. Mechanical ventilation must be considered in an emergency.

Continued

TABLE 39.1 Organisms Causing Gastroenteritis—cont'd

Pathogen	Pathogenesis	Duration/Onset	Clinical Findings	Diagnosis and Treatment
Clostridium difficile	Gram-positive anaerobe maintained in spore form. It colonizes bowel when normal bowel flora are suppressed by antibiotics. It produces two toxins: toxin A, an enterotoxin, and toxin B, a cytotoxin causing pseudomembranous colitis and necrosis.	Duration and intensity of disease vary. Onset normally is in a hospitalized patient who has had recent antibiotic treatment.	Symptoms range from none to acute abdomen secondary to toxic megacolon with perforation; symptoms usually begin after initiation of antibiotics. Profuse, watery, or mucoid diarrhea, which may be blood tinged, accompanied by fever, abdominal cramping and distention, white blood cells (WBCs) greater than 20,000, and ascites. Metabolic acidosis indicates severe colitis or toxic megacolon. Common cause of nosocomial infections in hospitals.	Diagnosis is confirmed with isolation of toxin A or B in the stool. Culture alone is no longer diagnostic because of the number of patients who are asymptomatic carriers. Flexible sigmoidoscopy may reveal pseudomembranous colitis. It is associated with recent abdominal surgery. It is treated with oral metronidazole (Flagyl) 250 mg four times daily for 10 days, vancomycin (Vancocin) 125 mg four times daily for 10 days. Relapse (20%) is treated with second course of above. Patients with multiple relapses may require 30 days of antibiotic treatment. Avoid antimotility agents.
Clostridium perfringens	Found in soil, feces, air, water. Outbreaks caused most often by contaminated meat. Type A enterotoxin causes mild to moderate gastroenteritis. Type C enterotoxin can be fatal.	Duration of illness is similar to mild gastritis, lasting 1–4 days without medical intervention. Fatal cases are less common. Onset is usually within 12 hours of ingestion of contaminated food.	Abrupt onset of diarrhea without fever. If fatal, cases have severe diarrhea with abdominal pain and distention.	Diagnosis is made by isolating organism in food or feces. Cultures usually show many clostridia in food or feces. No treatment is necessary for mild forms other than supportive care. Penicillin may be useful in severe cases.
Escherichia coli	Five identified strains classified by pathogenesis of diarrhea. All are gram-negative rods.	Dependent on strain; epidemics are due to ingestion of contaminated meat or dairy products.		
	Enterohemorrhagic *E. coli* (EHEC). Most serious; produces a hemorrhagic infection; O157:H7 strain produces two toxins, which inhibit protein synthesis in intestinal cells.	Duration typically 1–8 days. Onset is 24 hours after ingestion of contaminated food.	Acute onset of dysentery with 12–24 hours of abdominal cramps, watery diarrhea, and fever is followed by bloody stools. Can cause hemorrhagic infection of colon and can be fatal. Complications include hemolytic-uremic syndrome or thrombolytic thrombocytopenic purpura. WBCs are greater than 20,000; azotemia; dehydration. Infants and older adults are most prone to adverse effects.	Diagnosis is by isolation of *E. coli* O157:H7 in stools. Look for the source of undercooked meat. It can be transmitted in feces and dirty diapers. Treatment is supportive. Antibiotics have not proved effective.

TABLE 39.1 **Organisms Causing Gastroenteritis—cont'd**

Pathogen	Pathogenesis	Duration/Onset	Clinical Findings	Diagnosis and Treatment
	Enterotoxigenic *E. coli* (ETEC). Adheres to the mucosa of small bowel releasing toxins, which cause diarrhea.	Duration 2–4 days. Incubation period is 24–36 hours.	Most common cause of traveler's diarrhea from contaminated food or water. Mild fever, abdominal cramps, watery stool, nausea, and vomiting are common.	Usually self-limiting, requiring no treatment other than supportive care. It is common in developing countries.
	Enteropathogenic *E. coli* (EPEC).	Duration is 1–3 days; 12- to 36-hour incubation period.	Profuse, watery, foul-smelling diarrhea. It is of special concern to infants and older adults who are prone to dehydration.	Usually self-limiting. Infants and older adults may require hospitalization. It is rare in the United States.
	Enteroinvasive *E. coli* (EIEC) causes invasion and proliferation within enterocytes, much like *Shigella* infection.	Duration is 4–10 days; 12- to 72-hour incubation period.	It is an uncommon cause of food-borne dysentery in the United States. Patients have fever, anorexia, cramps, and watery diarrhea. Stools may be mucoid or bloody. Clinical presentation is much like that of *Shigella* infection.	May isolate leukocytes in stool. Diarrhea is self-limiting. Food poisoning of this kind is rare in the United States.
	Enteroadherent *E. coli* (EAEC) is rare and adheres to liver cells.		Mild, nonbloody diarrhea; strain is uncommon.	No leukocytes in stool.
Vibrio cholerae	Commonly found in areas with poor sanitation; food and water contaminated with feces. Enterotoxin causes hypersecretion in small intestine. Rarely found in the United States but may be endemic along the Gulf Coast.	Incubation is 1–3 days. Duration is 1–2 weeks.	Most cases in the United States are hemolytic and are transported here from contaminated foods. Diarrhea can be severe, causing septicemia, especially in immunocompromised patients, children, or older adults. Diarrhea is profuse, "rice water" and can be life-threatening. There is no abdominal cramping or fever. Patients may stool at the rate of 1 L/hr.	To diagnose *V cholerae* a special *Vibrio*-selective medium must be used in the stool culture. Diarrhea requires prompt replacement of fluids and electrolytes. Antibiotic: tetracycline 500 mg by mouth (PO) every 6 hours for 2 days or Bactrim DS every 12 hours for 2 days.
Vibrio parahaemolyticus	Pathogen found in seafood. Produces toxins in the gut or invades intestinal mucosa. Outbreaks frequent in summer; usually associated with improperly cooked seafood.	Incubation period 8–24 hours. Duration is 1–3 days.	Patient presents with abdominal cramping, headache, fever. Usually associated with explosive, noninflammatory, watery diarrhea, which may be bloody depending on the degree of mucosal destruction.	Stool is positive for *Vibrio*. Often diagnosed when a group of people become sick after consuming seafood. Food cultures are positive.

Continued

TABLE 39.1	**Organisms Causing Gastroenteritis—cont'd**			
Pathogen	*Pathogenesis*	*Duration/Onset*	*Clinical Findings*	*Diagnosis and Treatment*
Yersinia enterocolitica	Primarily transmitted via fecal-oral route; food borne. It is rare in the United States; more common in northern Europe and Canada. Organism forms an enterotoxin and invades the intestinal epithelium.	Onset and incubation are unknown. Duration usually resolves in 1–3 weeks.	Symptoms include fever, abdominal pain, and bloody diarrhea. Older children may develop mesenteric adenitis, which presents with fever, right lower quadrant pain, and leukocytosis; similar to symptoms of appendicitis. Adults may present with polyarthritis, Reiter's syndrome, and erythema nodosum. *Yersinia* can cause bacteremia.	Diagnosis is made by isolation of organism in the stool. Stool also tests positive for fecal leukocytes. Treatment for severe cases is tetracycline 250–500 mg every 6 hours for 7–10 days; ciprofloxacin 500 mg PO twice daily; tobramycin 3–5 mg/kg per day every 8 hours.
Salmonella	One of the major causes of diarrhea worldwide. Three species: *S. typhi, S. choleraesuis, and S. enteritidis.* Found primarily in chicken, eggs, and livestock, causing 85% of community-acquired *Salmonella* outbreaks. Individuals must ingest 10,000–1 million organisms to become infected.	Duration is 2–5 days; onset is 8–48 hours after ingestion. Patients may become "chronic carriers," defined as individuals with positive stool cultures 1 year after initial disease.	Peak incidence is in summer and fall. Symptoms begin with nausea and vomiting, followed by colicky abdominal pain and bloody or mucoid diarrhea. Enteric fever results from organisms entering the bloodstream via the bowel lymphatics, causing bacteremia, headache, and myalgias. Tissue abscesses may develop. Stools may be foul smelling.	Diagnosis is made by isolation of organism in stool. No treatment is necessary unless associated with fever and systemic disease. Treatment includes trimethoprim-sulfamethoxazole (Bactrim DS) or a quinoline, norfloxacin 400 mg or ofloxacin 400 mg PO twice daily for 7–10 days. Stress proper handling of food, thorough cooking, and good hand washing.
Shigella	One of the most common causes of bacillary dysentery. Several species: *S. sonnei* is isolated in 75% of cases in the United States. Because of poor hygiene and overcrowding, it is spread via the fecal–oral route and requires only a small number of organisms to produce disease. Organism causes epithelial invasion of intestinal mucosa.	Duration usually 4–7 days and is self-limiting. Incubation period of 1–2 days after exposure or ingestion of pathogen.	Initially patients present with watery diarrhea and high fever. Later colitis-type symptoms develop: Abdominal cramps, tenesmus, urgency, frequent small stools with blood and mucus. Low-grade fever may persist for 2–20 days. Complications can include hemolytic-uremic syndrome and colitis.	Diagnosis is made by isolation of organism in stool or rectal swab. In severe cases sigmoidoscopy shows mucosal hyperemia, friability, and ulceration. Treat with Bactrim DS twice daily for 3 days if infection was acquired in the United States.
Staphylococcus	Common cause of food poisoning. Caused by ingestion of enterotoxin found in improperly handled or stored foods. Enterotoxins produced by *Staphylococcus* act on receptors in the gut, which then transmit impulses to medullary centers.	Abrupt onset 1–8 hours after ingestion of contaminated food. Duration is usually less than 24 hours.	Abrupt onset of nausea, vomiting, colicky abdominal cramps, profuse watery diarrhea.	Definitive diagnosis is made only if contaminated food source is tested; otherwise, diagnosis is made based on short incubation and duration of symptoms.

TABLE 39.1 Organisms Causing Gastroenteritis—cont'd

Pathogen	Pathogenesis	Duration/Onset	Clinical Findings	Diagnosis and Treatment
Viral Pathogens Rotavirus	Very common cause of gastroenteritis in industrialized areas. Organism most often implicated in deaths from diarrhea. Frequently involves small bowel. A disaccharidase deficiency is common after rotavirus infections. Rotavirus is an RNA virus with four antigenic serotypes.	Incubation period 24–36 hours. Duration is 4–6 days.	Common in children younger than age 3. Peak incidence at age 6–24 months. Uncommon in adults because most have developed immunity. Symptoms include low-grade fever and copious watery diarrhea. Outbreaks are more common in winter months.	Diagnosis is made by electron microscopy. Serological enzyme-linked immunosorbent assay tests are available. No leukocytes found in stool.
Norwalk virus	Cube-shaped virus with seven known antigenic variants. It can cause large epidemics when spread by contaminated water. It is transmitted by the fecal–oral route. It is a common cause of absenteeism due to "viral gastroenteritis."	Incubation is 18–48 hours. Duration is 48–72 hours.	Illness can be very debilitating to some patients. Symptoms are mild and brief and include vomiting, frequent watery diarrhea, diffuse myalgias, chills, and sometimes fever. Often causes family outbreaks.	No known antiviral therapy is available. Fluid and electrolyte replacement is the treatment of choice. Virus can be isolated with electron microscopy but is costly and the disease is self-limiting.
Protozoal Pathogens *Giardia lamblia*	Approximately 4% of healthy U.S. citizens harbor *G. lamblia* in their intestines and are asymptomatic. *G. lamblia* is a protozoon that attaches to the mucosa of the small bowel. Patients with hypogammaglobulinemia and achlorhydria are predisposed to giardiasis. It is transmitted via oral–anal intercourse and is a common cause of traveler's diarrhea and diarrhea in children who attend day-care centers.	Incubation is 1–4 weeks. Duration usually 1–6 weeks.	Symptoms range from nonspecific complaints of bloating, flatulence, nausea, and watery, noninflammatory diarrhea to chronic diarrhea with weight loss, anorexia, and malabsorption.	Diagnosis can be made by examination of stool but is most often made by duodenal aspirate or small bowel biopsy. Stool exam is positive for trophozoites in about 50% of confirmed cases. Treatment with quinacrine hydrochloride (Atabrine) 100 mg three times daily after meals for 5–7 days or metronidazole (Flagyl) 250 mg three times daily for 5–7 days.

Continued

TABLE 39.1 Organisms Causing Gastroenteritis—cont'd

Pathogen	Pathogenesis	Duration/Onset	Clinical Findings	Diagnosis and Treatment
Entamoeba histolytica (amebiasis)	Transmitted via contaminated food and water, primarily in tropical areas with poor sanitation. Common in Mexican migrant workers and military personnel returning from the Far East. Human host becomes a reservoir after ingesting cysts from source and can transmit disease via fecal–oral route. Sexual transmission is men who have sex with men.	Most common clinical variant is the asymptomatic cyst carrier who can be a reservoir for an undetermined length of time. Duration can be weeks to months.	Symptoms include abdominal cramps, abdominal pain, and weight loss. Diarrhea contains blood and mucus. Patients may have hepatomegaly and pain over the cecum and ascending colon. Some patients may have fever, tenesmus, and acute dysentery illness. Complications can include peritonitis, toxic megacolon, and hepatic abscess. The encysted ameba is passed into the environment, where it can survive for up to 10 days.	Diagnosis is important to distinguish amebiasis from ulcerative colitis because treatment with glucocorticoids can accelerate amebic colitis and enhance systemic invasion. Sigmoidoscopy reveals discrete rectosigmoid ulcers with normal intervening mucosa. Indirect hemagglutination test is effective in detecting invasive amebic disease but remains positive long after treatment. Treat with metronidazole (Flagyl) 750 mg three times daily for 7–10 days.
Cryptosporidium	Enteric protozoan parasite that invades the small bowel located just below the basement membrane. Causes two distinct syndromes— one in immunocompetent and one in immunosuppressed individuals. Common cause of waterborne outbreaks from inadequate filtration. Parasite produces an exotoxin.	Incubation is 1–3 weeks. Usually self-limiting but can last 1–2 weeks in immunocompromised patients.	Outbreaks can occur after ingestion of water contaminated with livestock waste. Also common in day-care centers and patients with AIDS. Immunocompromised patients develop severe cholera-like diarrhea, which can last for months and cause daily fluid losses of 5–10 L/day.	Diagnosis by isolation of parasite in stool. Commercially available immunofluorescent antibody test can also assist diagnosis. Leukocytes not present in stool. Intestinal mucosa not inflamed but with ulcerations. Suggested treatment includes paromomycin (Humatin) 500 mg PO four times daily with food for 14–28 days, then 500 mg twice daily indefinitely. If treatment fails: azithromycin (Zithromax) 2.4 g PO on day 1, 1.2 g PO for 27 days, and then 600 mg/day for maintenance indefinitely.

Gastroenteritis can also be caused by dietary factors such as coffee, tea, and sodas containing caffeine, medications (primarily antacids and antibiotics), and metabolic factors, including diabetes mellitus, hyperthyroidism, and adrenal insufficiency.

PATHOPHYSIOLOGY

Pathophysiological causes of gastroenteritis are numerous; however, bacterial, viral, and parasitic infections are among the most common. Almost all forms of enteric infection manifest with diarrhea. Diarrheal diseases cause an increase in the frequency of stools, less well-formed feces, and an increase in the fecal water content. The definition of diarrhea is dependent on each patient's normal bowel habits. Diarrhea is not considered a medical emergency unless it affects children or older adults who are less able to regulate their fluid intake. Diarrhea is a major cause of infant mortality in developing nations.

The gastrointestinal (GI) tract has several defenses against the development of infection. When bacterial or viral pathogens can overcome these barriers, they proliferate, causing varying degrees of gastroenteritis. The acidity of the stomach is normally maintained at a pH of 2, which creates a hostile environment for most microorganisms. This acidic barrier protects the small bowel and colon from ingested pathogens. If the organism is resistant to the acid environment or the patient has taken medications that alter the pH, the organism may thrive and cause illness.

Another host defense mechanism is the constant peristalsis of the small bowel, which prevents the colonization of pathogens within the lumen. Patients who have small bowel stasis as a result of obstruction, diverticula, or blind loop syndrome frequently develop an overgrowth of bacteria within the stagnant segment, causing gastroenteritis resulting from the increased number of bacteria in the small bowel. In contrast, the colon is relatively stagnant; it typically harbors about 1 billion bacteria per gram of intestinal contents. Normal feces are composed primarily of water and bacteria. These beneficial bacteria protect against potential pathogens by consuming available nutrients and producing by-products that create a hostile environment to the invading pathogens.

The GI tract also produces specific immunoglobulins that protect against invading organisms. After exposure to certain organisms, immunoglobulins may even protect against future invasions by the same organism, much like an antigen–antibody response. IgA, a secretory immunoglobulin, may help defend against many of the bacteria that cause gastroenteritis by invading the intestinal mucosa.

Ingestion of contaminated food can result in clinical symptoms of gastroenteritis, depending on the number and virulence of the organisms in the food. Almost all bacteria are capable of producing mild diarrhea if ingested in large enough quantities. Other organisms (e.g., *Shigella, Salmonella, Campylobacter, Cryptosporidium*) have such a high virulence that only a small inoculum can produce symptoms.

Often, the incubation time of the pathogen, coupled with the presenting symptoms, will give specific clues for establishing a diagnosis. Infectious processes of the small intestine often result in watery, secretory, or a malabsorptive type of diarrhea; infections of the large intestine tend to produce bloody diarrhea and abdominal pain. Gastroenteritis with an onset of nausea and vomiting within 6 hours after exposure to the pathogen suggests food poisoning resulting from the ingestion of a preformed toxin such as that of *Bacillus cereus*. Incubation periods greater than 14 hours and the initial symptom of vomiting are highly suggestive of viral infections.

CLINICAL PRESENTATION

Subjective

Patients with gastroenteritis present with varying degrees of nausea, vomiting, diarrhea, fever, and abdominal pain and cramping. Symptoms depend on the underlying cause but can also include fatigue, malaise, anorexia, tenesmus, and borborygmus. Individuals with profuse diarrhea may complain of rectal burning and hematochezia from rectal abrasion and bleeding. Patients may complain of symptoms that suggest dysentery, including passage of numerous small-volume stools containing blood and mucus. Reports of voluminous stools are suggestive of a source in the small bowel or proximal colon; small stools accompanied by a sense of urgency suggest a source in the left colon or rectum. Bloody stools suggest mucosal damage and an inflammatory process secondary to invasive pathogens. Frothy stools and flatus suggest a malabsorption problem.

Objective

The physical exam is usually normal except for the aforementioned GI problems. Depending on the degree of dehydration, the skin turgor may be poor, and mucous membranes may be dry. Vital signs may reflect dehydration, such as a fever with an increased heart rate. Older and very young patients with gastroenteritis may show signs of severe dehydration such as orthostatic hypotension and dizziness. Patients who have had prolonged illness and are malnourished may present with edema resulting from hypoalbuminemia.

DIAGNOSTIC REASONING

Diagnostic Tests

Evaluation of the history is paramount to the appropriate diagnosis and management of the patient with gastroenteritis. The patient must be questioned thoroughly about the temporal association of symptoms with the suspected pathogen. Patient history should include a thorough drug history, including over-the-counter drugs and supplements, antibiotics, antacids, laxatives, alcohol, and sugar substitutes. It is important to know the patient's travel history, surgical history, and sexual orientation and practices. The duration of the illness is important in the differential diagnosis because acute diarrhea is usually caused by infectious agents or toxins, whereas chronic diarrhea usually has a noninfectious etiology.

Laboratory diagnosis of acute gastroenteritis is not always necessary in patients with nonbloody diarrhea and no evidence of systemic toxicity. In the average, otherwise healthy adult, the disease will normally run its course without incident, and there is no need for costly evaluation. Selection of the most appropriate tests is based on information received from the history and physical exam. In patients with severe diarrhea and dehydration, stools should be examined for consistency, blood, and fecal leukocytes. Numerous fecal leukocytes in patients with acute diarrhea is indicative of diffuse colonic inflammation and is highly suggestive of an invasive pathogen such as *Shigella, Salmonella,* or *Campylobacter*. Other causes of leukocyte-positive stools include *Clostridium difficile, Yersinia, Vibrio parahaemolyticus,* and *Escherichia coli*. In patients with chronic diarrhea, fecal leukocytes suggest inflammatory bowel disease (IBD) or ischemia.

A stool culture should be done on any patient who has severe diarrhea, a fever of 101.3°F (38.5°C) or higher, the presence of bloody stools, or stools that test positive for leukocytes, lactoferrin, or occult blood because these findings are indications of a bacterial pathogen. Routine stool culture will identify the presence of *Shigella, Salmonella, Campylobacter, Aeromonas,* and *Yersinia.* In diarrheal illnesses that are suspected to be caused by eating contaminated hamburger meat, stools can be cultured for *E. coli.*

Blood cultures should be obtained from patients who show clinical signs of typhoid or enteric fever or from any hospitalized patient who has an intestinal illness with high fever. It is essential that the blood cultures be obtained before initiation of antibiotic therapy.

Stools should be examined for ova and parasites in cases of persistent diarrhea, especially if the symptoms began after travel to Russia, Nepal, the Rocky Mountains, or other mountainous regions, or after exposure to infants in a day-care center. Parasites should also be considered in men who have sex with men or any patient with HIV/AIDS who presents with diarrhea, as well as in a patient with diarrhea who lives in a community where a waterborne outbreak has occurred. If a patient has diarrhea that has lasted longer than 2 weeks and the stool is negative for fecal leukocytes, a stool exam for parasites should be considered. Patients with intestinal amoebiasis usually have no leukocytes in their stool because of the noninflamed areas of intestinal mucosa between the areas of ulceration, as well as the lytic effects of the exotoxins produced by the parasite. If parasitic infection is highly suspected but the stool culture is negative, a small bowel biopsy is indicated to identify the causative agent. Immunofluorescent antibody tests and diagnostic enzyme-linked immunosorbent assay (ELISA) tests are more sensitive than microscopic studies for identifying *Giardia* and *Cryptosporidium.*

In patients with epidemiological evidence, stool samples should be sent to the laboratory for specific enteropathogen studies that are not normally detected with routine stool culture, such as enterohemorrhagic colitis (*E. coli* O157:H7), *Vibrio cholerae,* other noncholera vibrios, and other Shiga toxin–producing *E. coli.* Routine stool culture identifies certain strains of *Yersinia* and *E. coli* O157:H7; however, some strains can be detected only by research laboratories. Any patient who develops diarrhea after initiation or completion of antibiotic therapy should have tissue culture assay or an ELISA test for *C. difficile* toxin.

Viral gastroenteritis should be suspected in patients who present with vomiting as the major symptom and in cases where food- or waterborne contamination is suspected and the incubation period is greater than 12 hours. Although there are commercially available test kits that identify rotaviruses, their application is limited because there is no known treatment for viral causes of illness.

Flexible sigmoidoscopy is usually reserved for patients with colitis that is unresponsive to antibiotic therapy and for patients with persistent diarrhea undiagnosed by laboratory evaluation. Tissue biopsy can help identify the offending pathogen, as well as differentiate infection from chronic inflammatory changes consistent with IBD or celiac disease.

Differential Diagnosis

The differential diagnosis of gastroenteritis, particularly in patients with persistent or chronic diarrhea and severe abdominal pain, should include irritable bowel syndrome, IBD, ischemic bowel disease (especially in patients with peripheral vascular disease), partial bowel obstruction, and pelvic abscess. Other considerations for diagnosis should include ruling out complications from diabetes mellitus, small bowel diverticulosis, Whipple's disease, chronic pancreatitis, and any surgical alteration of the GI tract that might interfere with normal absorption.

MANAGEMENT

All patients who present with diarrhea require fluid and electrolyte management, particularly children, older adults, and the immunosuppressed. Patients who are dehydrated and able to tolerate oral fluid replacement need to drink fluids with a sodium content of 45 to 75 mEq/L (Pedialyte or Gatorade) or be provided with oral rehydration salts. In patients who are severely dehydrated or those who have chronic diseases and are hypotensive, hospitalization for IV hydration may be indicated. In otherwise healthy adult patients who are not dehydrated, sports drinks, diluted fruit juices, and broths or soups are usually adequate for fluid and sodium replacement.

Patients with diarrhea require a diet that includes calories that come from boiled starches and cereals (potatoes, pasta, rice, wheat, and oats), which will facilitate enterocyte renewal, with the addition of salt for the duration of illness. Once stools have started to become formed, the diet can be advanced as tolerated. Some authors advise avoiding dairy products; however, this is not necessary unless there is clinical evidence of lactose intolerance.

Nonspecific symptomatic treatment of acute diarrhea can decrease the occurrence by 50% and is most effective against secretory diarrhea. Antimotility drugs are the most frequently prescribed and most effective drugs for the treatment of symptomatic gastroenteritis. These agents work by slowing intraluminal peristalsis, thereby slowing the passage of fluids through the lumen, which facilitates absorption. Patients with febrile dysentery should not receive antimotility medications because slowing the intraluminal time may prolong the duration of the disease. Drugs Commonly Prescribed 39.1: Symptomatic Treatment of Acute Diarrhea lists medications commonly recommended for the symptomatic treatment of acute diarrhea.

Drugs Commonly Prescribed 39.1: Symptomatic Treatment of Acute Diarrhea

DRUG	INDICATION	ADVERSE REACTIONS AND PRESCRIBING CONSIDERATIONS
bismuth subsalicylate (Pepto-Bismol)	Acute diarrhea	Not as effective as loperamide in acute diarrhea. May potentiate the effects of antidiabetic medications. Do not use with antibiotics in patients with HIV infection.
loperamide (Imodium)	Acute diarrhea	Drug of choice for afebrile, nondysentery cases of acute diarrhea. Minimal central opiate effect.
diphenoxylate with atropine (Lomotil)	Acute diarrhea	Prescription only. For use in afebrile, nondysentery cases of acute diarrhea. Has central opiate effects. Overdose possible. Atropine has adverse effects that may limit use.

Empiric antimicrobial therapy is recommended for patients with severe diarrhea, especially those with fever or stool positive for leukocytes. Empirical treatment for traveler's diarrhea is dependent on the location of the travel because of the different organisms prevalent in different areas. For example, *E. coli* is found in most locations, but *Salmonella* is found in South and Southeast Asia, *Campylobacter* is prevalent in Southeast Asia, and *Shigella* is prevalent in South Asia and Africa. On July 26, 2016, the U.S. Food and Drug Administration (FDA) issued an enhanced black box warning for fluoroquinolones stating their association with disabling and potentially permanent side effects and that they should be reserved only for conditions where there are no other options available. In light of this recent warning, the antibiotic of choice for traveler's diarrhea is azithromycin (Zithromax) 1,000 mg orally once a day for 1 to 3 days. Nonantibiotic preventive therapy includes bismuth subsalicylate (Pepto-Bismol), two tablets before each meal and at bedtime for a total of eight tablets/day for the entire trip. This remedy has an approximately 60% effectiveness rate.

FOLLOW-UP AND REFERRAL

Follow-up is not usually required except in those patients with the chronic forms of infectious diarrhea such as from *C. difficile*. Often, patients with serious infectious diarrhea will require home administration of IV antibiotics. Patients who require sigmoidoscopy for biopsy of intestinal mucosa for identification of the pathogen should be referred to a gastroenterologist.

Patient Education: Gastroenteritis

The aim of patient education is prevention of the spread of disease from patients with infectious diarrhea to other individuals. Teaching includes good hand washing and safe disposal of waste products. Any infant or child with infectious diarrhea should not attend day care until the diarrhea has stopped or the child has completed the prescribed course of antibiotics. Good hand washing technique is imperative to prevent household outbreaks of the disease.

Patients traveling in high-risk areas should be instructed to consume only safe foods and beverages there and on the airplane leaving the area. "Safe" foods include acidic foods such as unpeeled citrus fruits; dry foods such as breads and cereals; steamed foods and beverages such as coffee, tea, and cooked vegetables; foods containing high amounts of sugar such as syrups, jellies, and jams; and bottled carbonated drinks such as soda and beer. It is generally not considered safe to drink bottled water (unless bottled from a safe source) or to eat raw, uncooked vegetables, including salad. Patients with known HIV infection and any other individuals with a known debilitating illness who may not tolerate any degree of gastroenteritis should be encouraged to take antibiotic prophylaxis.

HEPATITIS

Hepatitis is a common problem throughout the world and has many causes, including infectious, drug, vascular, and metabolic etiologies. Many cases of hepatitis are subclinical. Symptoms may be "flu-like" and go unreported so that the true incidence of the disease may be underestimated. Table 39.2 lists some of the causes of acute hepatitis.

Acute viral hepatitis is a systemic infection that predominantly affects the liver and can lead to liver inflammation and necrosis. There are many viral agents that cause hepatitis, but the most common, and the ones that have public health concerns, are hepatitis A virus (HAV), hepatitis B virus (HBV), hepatitis C virus (HCV), hepatitis D virus (HDV), and hepatitis E virus (HEV). All are endemic to the United States except HEV, which is most common in Asia, the Middle East, Africa, and

TABLE 39.2	Causes of Acute Hepatitis
Viral	Cytomegalovirus; Epstein-Barr virus; hepatitis A, B, C, D, and E viruses; herpes virus; rubella; varicella-zoster virus; yellow-fever virus
Nonviral	Amebic abscess, bacterial abscess, Lyme disease, syphilis
Metabolic disorders	Alpha-1-antitrypsin deficiency, Wilson's disease
Vascular	Budd-Chiari syndrome, congestive heart disorders failure, ischemia (hypotension, shock)
Drugs	Acetaminophen, allopurinol, ASA (high doses), captopril, carbamazepine, isoniazid, ketoconazole, methyldopa, NSAIDs, procainamide, sulfonamides
Toxins	Alcohol (ethanol), carbon tetrachloride, herbs, mushrooms

Central America. However, although there seems to be a high prevalence of antibodies to HEV in the general population in the United States, there are few cases of acute illness reported and those that are can usually be attributed to travel to an area where HEV is endemic.

EPIDEMIOLOGY AND CAUSES

Hepatitis A

HAV is a small, single-stranded RNA virus of the picornavirus family. HAV is endemic in the United States, with periodic outbreaks. Because the symptoms of HAV are often mild and nonspecific, many cases remain undetected. Many other cases are asymptomatic, making it almost impossible to quantify the number of infections annually. The Centers for Disease Control and Prevention (CDC) estimated a total of 2,800 new cases of HAV infection in 2015. Risk factors include crowded conditions, such as prisons, nursing homes, and day-care centers, and poor sanitation. Contaminated food or water is a common source of HAV. HAV can cause fulminant liver failure on rare occasions, usually in combination with an underlying liver disease. The HAV vaccine became available in 1995, and since that time, the rate of infection in the United States has decreased by 95%.

Transmission is by the fecal–oral route, but there have been rare cases of HAV being transmitted via transfusion. People contract HAV by consuming contaminated water or ice; raw shellfish harvested from sewage-contaminated water; and fruits, vegetables, or other foods eaten uncooked that may have become contaminated in handling. The virus is killed by heating at 185°F for 1 minute. Adequate chlorination of water also kills the virus. The incubation period is 30 days but can be as long as 6 weeks. Excretion of HAV in feces occurs up to

2 weeks before clinical illness. It is rarely found in feces after the first week of illness. Blood and stools are infectious throughout the incubation period and early illness until the aminotransferase levels peak. A person is most infectious about 2 weeks before and during the first week that symptoms appear.

Chronic HAV does not occur. There is no carrier state, and HAV usually causes no long-term damage. HAV may persist for up to 1 year with relapses before full recovery. The mortality rate is about 0.02 deaths per 100,000 cases, which has stayed the same since 2011.

Hepatitis B

HBV is a DNA hepadnavirus with eight genotypes and replicates in the liver. The CDC estimated a total of 21,900 new cases of acute HBV infection in 2015. The overall rate has decreased by about 82% since 1991 when a national strategy was implement and vaccination was first recommended for infants and children. The risk for chronic infection decreases with increasing age, for example, 90% of infants, 25% to 50% of children aged 1 to 5 years and 5% of adults become chronically infected. The CDC estimates that there are 850,000 individuals living with chronic HBV (CHB) in the United States. Some studies cited by the CDC estimate the number of people living with CHB infection to be more like 2.2 million.

High-risk groups include men who have sex with men, injection drug users, first-generation immigrants from endemic regions (Southeast Asia, China, and the Middle East), and people with multiple sex partners. Other high-risk groups include nurses, physicians, dentists, and personnel working in clinical and pathology labs and blood banks where direct needle-stick contamination may occur. The risk of infection from a contaminated needle is 10% to 30%. Patients and staff at hemodialysis centers are also at high risk. The risk of contracting HBV from a blood transfusion is now rare in the United States.

Transmission is usually by direct contact with infected blood or blood products or by sexual contact. The highest concentrations of HBV are found in the blood; however, other body fluids such as semen, cervical secretions, saliva, and wound exudates contain lower concentrations of hepatitis B surface antigen (HBsAg). Parenteral exposure is the most efficient route of transmission, most often occurring in IV drug abusers sharing or using contaminated needles and in health-care workers by accidental needle sticks. HBV can be transmitted from contact with contaminated inanimate objects because the virus is capable of living in the open environment for approximately 1 week. HBV is not transmitted via the fecal–oral route. The incidence of HBV is highest in the 30- to 39-year-old age-group, with more men becoming infected than women. Pregnant women who are HBsAg-positive may transmit HBV to their babies during childbirth. HBV is not spread through food, water, or casual contact. The average incubation period for HBV is 12 to 14 weeks but can be anywhere from 6 weeks to 6 months.

The mortality rate for acute HBV infection is 0.4% to 1% but is higher when hepatitis D is superimposed. Patients with chronic hepatitis are at an increased risk for cirrhosis and hepatocellular cancer. Infection with HBV is also associated with arthritis, glomerulonephritis, and polyarteritis nodosa.

Hepatitis C

HCV was first identified in 1989 and was previously known as hepatitis non-A non-B. It is a single-stranded RNA virus with 6 genotypes and more than 50 subtypes. Genotype 1 is the most common type in the United States and accounts for 74% of cases. The clinical significance of the genotype is unclear, but different genotypes and subtypes have different responses to treatment. The incubation period of HCV is 6 to 7 weeks. Transmission of HCV is primarily by percutaneous exposure to blood and blood products and include the following:

- Injection drug use (most common): injection drug use accounts for about 60% of HCV cases today
- Recipient of donated blood, blood products, or organ before 1992 (Screening for HCV became available in 1992.)
- Health-care workers (needlestick injury)
- Transmission from HCV-infected pregnant women to newborns

Infrequent routes of transmission include sex with an HCV infected person, sharing razor or toothbrush with infected person and invasive health-care procedures.

Forty-one states reported 2,436 cases of hepatitis C in 2015. The CDC estimates that the overall incidence is 0.8 cases per 100,000 of the population and that after adjusting for underreporting, the actual number of cases is about 33,900, an increase from 2012.

About 3.2 million Americans have chronic hepatitis C infection. The prevalence of this infection is greatest in those individuals born between 1945 and 1965. They were most likely infected in the 1970s and 1980s. Injection drug use is the strongest risk factor. Having sex with an injection drug user is also a risk factor, although less robust. There is a 5% risk of maternal–neonate transmission at the time of birth, which some studies suggest is greatest in patients with high circulating levels of HCV RNA. Anti-HCV antibodies are more common in non-Hispanic black and Mexican American people. Low family income and a lifetime history of more than 20 sexual partners are also risk factors. Rates of HCV infection are higher for men than for women, possibly due to more risky behavior. Other possible transmission can be through body piercing and tattooing, although there is little evidence to date. For many patients infected with HCV, the source is never determined.

Fewer than 25% of people with HCV infection are symptomatic, making diagnosis and treatment difficult in the 75% who are HCV RNA positive. Most acute cases go undetected until they present with symptoms of chronic liver disease. Seventy-five percent to 85% of patients with HCV develop chronic hepatitis. Sixty percent to 70% progress to chronic liver disease and 5% to 20% will develop cirrhosis over 20 to 30 years. The consequences of chronic infection are liver cancer and cirrhosis. Alcohol consumption appears to increase the chances of chronic disease and serious complications. The U.S. Preventive Services Task Force recommends screening for HCV in persons who are at high risk for the infection. They also recommend that all people born between 1945 and 1965 be offered a one-time screening for HCV infection.

Hepatitis D

HDV is an RNA virus that requires HBsAg for its replication. Only individuals with HBV are at risk for HDV. The major risk factor for HDV is injection drug use. Transmission is by the parenteral route and should be suspected in any HBsAg-positive person with acute or chronic hepatitis. New cases of HDV are uncommon in the United States today, probably because of widespread vaccination for HBV. Incubation is 1 to 6 months, and the mortality rate is 3%.

Hepatitis E

HEV is a single-stranded RNA virus that is usually transmitted via the fecal–oral route. It is similar to HAV but not as easily transmitted. It is transmitted through fecally contaminated water and is responsible for waterborne hepatitis outbreaks; it is endemic in Asia, the Middle East, Africa, and Central America. Contaminated shellfish was responsible for an outbreak on a cruise ship, and there have been foodborne transmission outbreaks in China, Taiwan, and Japan. Large outbreaks have occurred in refugee camps in Sudan and Chad. There have been relatively few cases in the United States, and most have been associated with global travel. There are documented cases in Germany and Japan of HEV infection with consumption of meat from animals that are infected with the virus. The illness is usually self-limiting, but chronic HEV is possible in immunocompromised patients. The incubation period is from 15 to 60 days. The mortality rate is low except in pregnant women, in whom the mortality rate is 10% to 20%. Table 39.3 lists the features of hepatitis A, B, C, D, and E.

Chronic Hepatitis

Chronic hepatitis, characterized by elevated aminotransferase (aspartate aminotransferase [AST] and alanine aminotransferase [ALT]) levels for more than 6 months, occurs in 1% to 2% of immunocompromised adults with

TABLE 39.3   Key Features of Hepatitis A, B, C, D, and E

Features	Hepatitis A Virus (HAV)	Hepatitis B Virus (HBV)	Hepatitis C Virus (HCV)	Hepatitis D Virus (HDV)	Hepatitis E Virus (HEV)
Transmission	Fecal–oral through sewage-contaminated water and shellfish; possibly through blood	Percutaneous and permucosal through infected blood and body fluids; sexual transmission	Percutaneous through infected blood and body fluids; community, many infected individuals have no known risk factors	Percutaneous, but must have co-infection with HBV	Fecal–oral
Incubation period (days)	15–50 (average 20–37)	25–160 (average 60–110)	42–49	Same as for HBV	10–56
Laboratory tests	Anti-HAV IgM (acute); anti-HAV IgG (resolving)	HBsAg (confirms), IgM anti-HBs (acute phase), IgG anti-HBs (resolving/immunity), HBeAg, anti-HBe, anti-HBc (persists in carriers)	Anti-HCV appears in 6–37 weeks	Anti-HDV appears late	Anti-HEV IgM detected within 26 days of jaundice; IgG antibody persists
Immunity/immunization	45% of United States population has antibodies against HAV; HAV vaccine available	5%–15% of U.S. population has anti-HBs; HBV vaccine available	Unknown; no vaccine available	People immune to HBV are also protected against HDV	Unknown
Prevalence	Increasing in adults	Decreasing in the United States	4% of post-transfusion hepatitis; 50% IV drug users	Common in IV drug abusers	Rare in United States; endemic in Southeast Asia, India, North Africa, Mexico
Course/mortality	Does not progress to chronic state; mortality is 0–0.2% with fulminant hepatitis	Chronic liver disease occurs in 1%–5% of adults and 80%–90% in children; mortality rate is 0.3%–1.5%	Chronic active hepatitis develops in 70%–90% of cases; 20% develop chronic liver disease; mortality rate is the same as for HBV	Chronic liver disease develops if present in chronic HBV; mortality rate is 2%–20% for acute icteric hepatitis	Does not progress to chronic liver disease; mortality rate is 1%–2% but as high as 10%–15% in pregnant women

IgG = immunoglobulin G; IgM = immunoglobulin M.

HBV and in as many as 90% of neonates and infants with HBV. Chronic hepatitis occurs in up to 85% of the people infected with HCV. Cirrhosis develops in 40% of patients with chronic HBV, and 20% of those with chronic HCV are at high risk for developing hepatocellular carcinoma as well.

PATHOPHYSIOLOGY

Hepatitis is an inflammation of the liver. It can result from a variety of causes. Viral hepatitis usually presents in one of three clinical manifestations: anicteric, icteric,

or cholestatic. Despite the presentation, the progression of the disease follows the same pattern, differing only in severity, enzymatic abnormality, and possible outcomes. The pathological lesions of hepatitis are similar to those caused by other viral infections. Regardless of the type of hepatitis causing the infection, all the liver acini cells are affected by patchy cell dropout, acidophilic hepatocellular necrosis, scarring, Kupffer cell hyperplasia, and mononuclear inflammatory infiltrate. The degree of cellular change is proportional to the severity of infection. Hepatocellular injury is mediated by cell-mediated immune response. Cytotoxic T cells and natural killer cells play an important part by killing the infected cells and releasing inflammatory cytokines. An intense immune response can decrease the chance of chronic infection; however, it does foster development of hepatocellular necrosis. Histological examination of tissue from livers infected with hepatitis demonstrates that even early in the disease process, liver regeneration has already started.

Normally, in patients infected with hepatitis, the underlying reticulin network is preserved, allowing for complete histological recovery. If extensive necrosis of the bridging acini occurs, however, the inflammatory process can damage and obstruct the bile canaliculi, causing cholestasis and obstructive jaundice. In most mild cases of hepatitis, the liver parenchyma is not damaged; HBV and HCV tend to be the more severe forms of hepatitis, with histological evidence of parenchymal inflammation and necrosis. Although the histological changes in the liver tissue are the same for each type of hepatitis, occasionally HBV can be diagnosed from the presence of "ground-glass" hepatocytes caused by HBsAg-infiltrated cytoplasm and by using special staining techniques that detect certain viral components. These findings are most often associated with chronic HBV infection. The long-term, asymptomatic chronic-carrier state is thought to result from an immunological tolerance to the hepatitis virus. The virus is not totally cleared by the immune system, and the hepatocellular injury is minimal, leading to a lifelong asymptomatic carrier state. This carrier state is most common in infants, whose immune system is immature and may be unable to overcome the virus. This chronic-carrier state is associated with a 10- to 100-fold risk of hepatocellular carcinoma.

HCV causes hepatocellular injury through direct cytopathic invasion by the virus. The viral load is directly proportional to the histological inflammation seen on liver biopsy. HCV is capable of rapid mutation, which allows it to elude immunity by development of resistant strains to the existing antibodies. Autoimmune hepatitis is most commonly associated with HCV, lending itself to the multiple extrahepatic manifestations of the disease. These patients develop autoimmune responses leading to membranous glomerulonephritis, vasculitis, dermatitis, pulmonary fibrosis, and rheumatoid arthritis. Chronic HCV occurs in approximately 60% to 70% of cases, with inflammatory changes leading to cirrhosis within 20 to 30 years.

Different drugs can cause different histopathological abnormalities in the liver. For example, acetaminophen damages hepatocytes by producing toxic metabolites that damage the cellular and subcellular structures of the liver. Hepatic injury resulting from sepsis is caused by direct bacterial invasion of the parenchyma, circulating endotoxins, and hypoxia. Cytotoxic lymphocytes attack hepatocyte membrane antigens in autoimmune chronic active hepatitis. All of these agents result in varying degrees of hepatocyte injury.

CLINICAL PRESENTATION

Subjective

The clinical presentation of viral hepatitis is extremely variable; it can range from asymptomatic infection without jaundice to a sudden severe infection and death in a few days. Table 39.4 displays the clinical findings and corresponding laboratory values for the different phases of viral hepatitis.

TABLE 39.4 Clinical Findings: Viral Hepatitis		
Stage	*Subjective and Objective Complaints*	*Laboratory Tests*
Incubation	None	HBsAg late in the stage HBeAg
Prodromal	Onset abrupt or insidious Anorexia, nausea, vomiting, malaise, upper respiratory infection (nasal discharge, pharyngitis), myalgia, arthralgia, easy fatigability, fever (HAV), abdominal pain	HBsAg in HBV
Icteric	Jaundice, dark urine, light-colored stools Continued prodromal complaints with gradual improvement	Anti-HBc Anti-HAV (IgG and IgM) Anti-HCV HBsAg becomes negative High urine bilirubin Markedly elevated ALT and AST Elevated LDH, bilirubin, alkaline phosphatase Markedly increased PT indicates increased mortality
Convalescent	Increased sense of well-being Appetite returns Jaundice, abdominal pain, and fatigability abate	Anti-HAV IgG Anti-HBs Decreased liver enzymes

ALT = alanine aminotransferase; AST = aspartate aminotransferase; IgG = immunoglobulin G; IgM = immunoglobulin M; LDH = lactate dehydrogenase; PT = prothrombin time.

Prodromal Phase

During the prodromal phase, the onset may be abrupt or insidious with anorexia, nausea, vomiting, malaise, upper respiratory infection, or flu-like symptoms. The patient may also complain of myalgia, arthralgia, and easy fatigability. Many patients report an aversion for smoking if they are smokers. Nausea and vomiting occur frequently. Diarrhea or constipation may be reported. In the early stage of acute HBV, skin rashes and arthritis may be seen.

Fever is usually present but rarely exceeds 103°F (39.4°C), except in HAV, in which it may go higher. Chills may mark an acute onset. A decrease in fever often coincides with the onset of jaundice.

Abdominal pain is usually mild and constant in the right upper quadrant or epigastrium. The pain can be aggravated by jarring or exertion. It is occasionally severe enough to simulate cholecystitis or cholelithiasis.

Icteric Phase

During the icteric phase, jaundice and dark urine appear, usually 5 to 10 days after the initial symptoms, although some patients do not experience jaundice. With the onset of jaundice, the prodromal symptoms worsen and are followed by progressive clinical improvement.

Convalescent Phase

The convalescent phase is marked by an increased sense of well-being. The jaundice, abdominal pain and tenderness, and fatigability disappear and the appetite returns. Chronic HBV begins at this point in the case of chronic disease.

The acute illness usually subsides over 2 to 3 weeks. Complete clinical and laboratory recovery occurs by the ninth week in HAV and after 16 weeks in HBV. Five percent to 10% of the cases may last longer, and fewer than 1% have an acute fulminant course. Hepatitis B and C may become chronic.

Hepatomegaly is present in 50% of patients with viral hepatitis, and splenomegaly is seen in 15% of cases. Lymphadenopathy, especially in the cervical and epitrochlear areas, is commonly present. Signs of general toxemia may vary from minimal to severe. The clinical features of all the types of viral hepatitis are similar, with the exception of onset. Hepatitis A and E usually have an abrupt onset, whereas hepatitis B, C, and D have a more insidious onset, and the liver enzyme levels are higher. HVC is often asymptomatic.

DIAGNOSTIC REASONING

Diagnostic Tests

Laboratory tests are used to diagnose, identify the serological type, and determine the current status of the disease.

Hepatitis A

Two types of antibodies to HAV can be detected by radioimmunoassay and ELISA. The first type of antibody to HAV is the immunoglobulin M (IgM) antibody (IgM anti-HAV), which appears about 4 weeks after exposure, or just before hepatocellular enzyme elevation occurs, and disappears in 3 to 6 months. Detection of IgM is the diagnostic gold standard for acute hepatitis A. The second type of antibody, immunoglobulin G (IgG) anti-HAV, appears about 2 weeks after the IgM anti-HAV begins to increase and peaks after about 1 month of disease. The IgG antibody persists for more than 10 years and provides immunity. If the IgM is elevated in the absence of IgG, acute hepatitis is suspected. If IgG is elevated in the absence of IgM, this indicates previous exposure to HAV, noninfectivity, and immunity to recurring HAV infection.

Hepatitis B

Acute and chronic HBV can be differentiated from other forms of viral hepatitis by serological markers representing the body's immunological response. The HBV is made up of an inner core surrounded by an outer capsule. The outer capsule contains HBsAg (hepatitis B *surface* antigen). The inner core contains the HBV *core* antigen (HBcAg). HBeAg (the *extracellular* form of HBcAg) is also found within the core. Antibodies to these antigens are called anti-HBs, anti-HBc, and anti-HBe.

Detection of HBsAg is diagnostic for HBV and is the first test to order when HBV is suspected. It will appear 1 to 10 weeks after exposure to the hepatitis B virus and will remain positive throughout the acute phase of the illness. If HBsAg persists longer, this may indicate chronic hepatitis. HBsAg rises before the onset of clinical symptoms, peaks during the first week of symptoms, and returns to normal by the time the jaundice subsides. HBsAg indicates acute infection and infectivity. Anti-HBs appears about 4 weeks after the disappearance of the surface antigen and signifies recovery from the infection and noninfectivity, as well as immunity.

There are no tests available to detect the HBV core antigen (HBcAg), but the IgM anti-HBc appears shortly after HBsAg is detected and can persist for 3 to 6 months. The anti-HBc level is elevated during the time lag between the disappearance of HBsAg and the appearance of anti-HBs; this interval is called the *core window*. During this window, anti-HBc is the only detectable marker of a recent hepatitis infection. Anti-HBs is composed of IgG and IgM antibodies. The IgM titer is diagnostic for acute hepatitis, whereas the IgG antibody is usually positive for life after infection.

HBeAg is generally not used for diagnostic purposes but rather as an index of viral replication and infectivity. The presence of HBeAg correlates with early and active disease and with high infectivity in patients with acute

HBV infection. HBeAg appears during the incubation period shortly after the detection of HBsAg. The continued presence of HBeAg predicts the development of CHB infection. Table 39.5 displays the serology testing and results for HBV infection.

Hepatitis C

The diagnosis of HCV is based on enzyme immunoassays or chemiluminescence immunoassay (CIA) that detect antibodies to HCV (anti-HCV). Limitations of these tests include moderate sensitivity for the diagnosis of acute HCV (false-negative result) and low specificity (50%) in healthy blood donors and some people with elevated gamma-globulin levels (false-positive result). The diagnosis of HCV may be confirmed by use of a polymerase chain reaction (PCR) to detect HCV RNA. The risk of transfusion-associated HCV has decreased from 10% in the early 1990s to less than 0.1% today as a result of the testing of donated blood for HCV.

Hepatitis D

Diagnosis of HDV is via detection of anti-HDV or HDV RNA in the presence of hepatitis B markers. Rising titers of anti-HDV indicate acute infection and are detectable early in the disease.

Hepatitis E

In a patient with acute hepatitis where other causes have been ruled out, serology can be performed especially in those patients who have traveled to an area where HEV is common. Immunoassay tests for IgM anti-HEV and IgG anti-HEV are available but not FDA approved. Tests for HEV RNA are only performed in research labs. IgM anti-HEV is detected 3 to 4 weeks after exposure and peaks at about 7 weeks then quickly decreases and is undetectable in about 13 weeks. IgG anti-HEV is detected 3 to 4 weeks after exposure and persists.

Additional Testing

In any patient in whom hepatitis is suspected, liver enzyme levels should be checked for signs of injury. Elevated aminotransferase levels are the hallmark of all forms of acute hepatitis. AST is usually markedly elevated early in hepatitis. ALT is often very elevated early in hepatitis,

as is lactate dehydrogenase. All of these hepatocellular enzymes are elevated during the acute and chronic active phases of hepatitis. AST and ALT levels fluctuate during the course of the disease for unknown reasons. Bilirubin and alkaline phosphatase are usually elevated and may remain elevated after the AST and ALT have normalized.

The white blood cell count is normal or low, especially in the preicteric phase. Large atypical lymphocytes may occasionally be seen and are similar to those found in infectious mononucleosis. Mild proteinuria is common, and there is bilirubinuria just preceding and during the icteric phase. The prothrombin time may be prolonged in severe hepatitis and signifies increased mortality risk. Liver biopsy is rarely indicated unless there is evidence of liver damage from a chronic state of hepatitis.

Differential Diagnosis

Differential diagnosis for hepatitis includes other viral diseases that affect the liver, such as infectious mononucleosis, cytomegalovirus infection, and herpes simplex virus. Drug- or toxin-induced liver damage should also be included in the differential diagnosis list, as well as conditions that cause jaundice.

MANAGEMENT

The principle of hepatitis management includes prevention of transmission and symptomatic relief. Vaccinations are available to prevent HAV and HBV. HAV vaccination is recommended for all children at 1 year. HAV vaccine is also recommended for person traveling to countries with high to moderate rates of hepatitis A, men who have sex with men, injectable drug uses, persons who have chronic liver disease, and those who have occupational risk for infection.

HBV vaccine is recommended for:

- all children under age 19 who have not been previously vaccinated
- people with high-risk factors, such as health-care workers and day-care workers
- injection drug users
- men who have sex with men

TABLE 39.5 Serologic Testing for Hepatitis B					
Interpretation	*HBsAg*	*Anti-HBs*	*HBeAg*	*Anti-HBe*	*Anti-HBc*
Acute hepatitis (confirms diagnosis)	+	−	+	−	IgM
Acute hepatitis	−	−	+ or −	−	IgM
Recovery from hepatitis (immunity)	−	+	−	+ or −	IgG
Vaccination (immunity)	−	+	−	−	−
Chronic HBV with active viral replication	+	−	+	−	IgG
Chronic HBV with low viral replication	−	−	−	+	IgG

- anyone with multiple sex partners
- household contacts of HBsAg positive persons
- residents and staff of facilities for developmentally disabled persons
- persons with chronic liver disease or HIV infection
- travelers to endemic areas of HBV infection

Treatment for hepatitis, no matter what the cause, is largely supportive. Patients rarely require hospitalization. Balanced nutrition with adequate calories and fluids is recommended, and avoidance of alcohol is stressed. Activity is generally restricted during the acute phase and during a relapse with gradual resumption of activity.

The American Association for the Study of Liver Diseases has developed guidelines for the treatment of CHB infection. For treatment decisions, they list four phases of CHB:

1. Immune-tolerate phase, in which the virus is replicating rapidly but there is a low inflammatory response.
2. HBeAg-positive immune-active phase, in which there are elevated ALT and HBV DNA levels and evidence of liver injury.
3. Inactive CHB phase, in which HBV DNA level are low or undetectable, ALT is normal, and there is anti-HBe present.
4. HBeAg-negative immune reactivation phase, in which those who are anti-HBe positive continue to have elevated ALT and high HBV DNA levels.

Patients with CHB should be referred to a hepatologist for treatment. The phase of CHB dictates what treatment options are most effective. Currently there are six agents approved for treating CHB (see Drugs Commonly Prescribed 39.2). They are used alone or in combination depending on factors such as the phase of CHB, level of viral replication, ALT levels, and seroconversion to anti-HBe. The goal of therapy is to reduce HBV DNA levels to the lowest possible and normalizing ALT levels and preventing liver cell damage. Nucleotide and nucleotide analogs (NUC/A) are the preferred treatment because they can be taken orally and have a better side effect profile. Pegylated interferon alfa-2a (Peg-IFN-2a) intramuscularly

is still used alone or in combination with a NUC/A. All of the agents used have serious side effects.

HCV causes chronic hepatitis and liver damage. The goal of treatment is to eradicate HCV RNA. With newer treatment regimens using direct-acting antiviral (DAA) medications, a cure is now possible for most patients. Treatment is dependent on the genotype, subtype, and presence or absence of cirrhosis. Patients should be referred to a hepatologist for evaluation and treatment. Drugs Commonly Prescribed 39.3 lists the medications commonly recommended in the treatment of HCV.

Response to therapy is judged by an ALT returning to normal by 12 weeks and negative viral markers (HCV RNA). After the ALT has returned to normal, treatment is slowly discontinued. Consuming alcohol increases the risk of these patients progressing to cirrhosis and liver failure, so abstinence from all forms of alcohol (including in medications) is especially important.

Hepatic transplantation is indicated for patients with advanced liver disease as a result of chronic HCV, and in fact it is the most common reason for liver transplantation in the United States.

FOLLOW-UP AND REFERRAL

Any patient diagnosed with HCV should be referred to a hepatologist for follow-up because of the high risk of chronic infection. Patients with HAV usually do not require follow-up. Patients with HBV should be seen in 1 month and should have blood drawn for HBsAg after 6 months. Persistent elevation of HBsAg indicates a chronic state, and these patients should be referred to a hepatologist.

Patient Education: Hepatitis

Patients and their intimate contacts should be given careful instructions about the cause of hepatitis, the mode of transmission, and measures to prevent the transmission. It is

---

Drugs Commonly Prescribed 39.2: Chronic Hepatitis B Infection

DRUG	DOSAGES	ADVERSE REACTIONS AND PRESCRIBING CONSIDERATIONS
Peg-INF-2a	180 g intramuscularly weekly	Fatigue, flu-like symptoms, mood disturbances, autoimmune disorders
Entecavir	0.5 or 1.0 mg orally once a day on an empty stomach	Lactic acidosis
Tenofovir	300 mg orally once a day	Nephropathy, osteomalacia, lactic acidosis
Adefovir	10 mg once a day orally	Acute renal failure, lactic acidosis, diarrhea
Lamivudine	100 mg once a day orally	Lactic acidosis, diarrhea, headache, fatigue, muscle pain, depression, fever
Telbivudine	600 mg once a day orally	Peripheral neuropathy, lactic acidosis, creatine kinase elevations and myopathy, diarrhea

Drugs Commonly Prescribed 39.3: Treatment for HCV

DRUG	GENOTYPE	CONSIDERATIONS	ADVERSE REACTIONS
NS3/4A Protease Inhibitors			
Simeprevir	1 and 4	Combined with Peg-INF-2a, ribavirin or sofosbuvir	Liver toxicity Fatigue, nausea, pruritus, weakness
Paritaprevir	1 and 4	Combined with ombitasvir and das-abuvir and ritonavir*	Liver toxicity Fatigue, nausea, pruritus, weakness
Grazoprevir	1, 4, 5, 6	Used in combination with elbasvir.	Liver injury Fatigue, weakness, nausea, insomnia, pruritus.
NS5A Inhibitors			
Ledipasvir	1, 4, 5, 6	Used in combination with sofosbuvir	Liver injury Fatigue, weakness, nausea, insomnia, pruritus.
Ombitasvir	1 and 4	Used in combination with paritaprevir and ritonavir*	Liver injury Fatigue, weakness, nausea, insomnia, pruritus.
Elbasvir	1-6	Used in combination with grazoprevir	Liver injury Fatigue, weakness, nausea, insomnia, pruritus.
Velpatasvir	1-6	Used in combination with sofosbuvir	Liver injury Fatigue, weakness, nausea, insomnia, pruritus.
NS5B Nucleos(t)ide Polymerase Inhibitor			
Sofosbuvir	1-6	Used in combination with Peg-INF-2a and ribavirin or with simeprevir or daclatasvir or ledipasvir or velpatasvir depending on the genotype	Liver injury Fatigue, weakness, nausea, insomnia, pruritus.
NS5B Non-nucleos(t)ide Polymerase Inhibitor			
Dasabuvir	1 and 4	Used in combination with Paritaprevir, ritonavir*, and ombitasvir.	Liver injury Fatigue, weakness, nausea, insomnia, pruritus.
Combination drugs			
Epclusa (sofosbuvir/velpatasvir)	1-6	Used in combination with ribavirin. No need to use Peg-INF-2a	Headache, fatigue Symptomatic bradycardia
Technivie (ombitasvir, paritaprevir and ritonavir*)	4	Used in combination with ribavirin. (No need to be used with Peg-INF-2a)	Liver injury in those with advanced liver disease. Fatigue, weakness, nausea, insomnia, pruritus.
Zepatier (elbasvir and grazoprevir)	1 and 4	Can be used in combination with ribavirin.	Diarrhea, headache, insomnia, weakness, anemia, fatigue, pruritus Liver injury
Viekira Pak (ombitasvir-paritaprevir-ritonavir and dasabuvir)	1a and 1b		Liver injury Fatigue, weakness, nausea, insomnia, pruritus.

*Ritonavir has no activity against HCV but is a pharmacologic booster.

recommended that household contacts and sexual contacts be given passive immunity (immunoglobulin) for HAV and HBV, as well as active immunization. Hand washing and personal hygiene can help prevent the spread of the disease. Patients should also be taught not to share personal items such as toothbrushes, razors, and eating utensils during the period of infectivity. Patients with chronic hepatitis or a carrier state should be instructed to practice safe sex.

Patients who develop chronic liver disease as a result of hepatitis can contact the American Liver Foundation for information about treatment.

APPENDICITIS

The appendix is a fingerlike projection located at the apex of the cecum just below the ileocecal valve. It has no known function in humans; however, it is thought to have some immunological function, based on the amount of lymphoid tissue it contains. The appendix fills with food, just as the cecum does, but because the lumen of the appendix is smaller, it has a tendency to become obstructed. Appendicitis is the inflammation of the vermiform appendix caused by an obstruction and/or infection. It is the most common cause of acute right lower quadrant (RLQ) abdominal pain requiring surgical intervention. Acute appendicitis results in more than 250,000 appendectomies annually in the United States and represents 1 million hospital day stays.

EPIDEMIOLOGY AND CAUSES

Appendicitis can occur at any age; however, it is most common between ages 10 and 30 years. It is rare in infants and in older adults and is often associated with higher morbidity within these age-groups because of delayed diagnosis and intervention. During the peak incidence years, men are twice as likely to be diagnosed with appendicitis as are women, but the occurrence in both genders tends to equalize over the life span. It is estimated that appendicitis will affect 10 in 100,000 people in the United States, with an incidence of 1.1 cases per 1,000 people per year.

Appendicitis is more common in Western countries, where people have diets that are low in fiber, high in fat, and high in refined sugars and other carbohydrates. Obstruction of the appendix by a variety of pathological processes is the cause of the majority of appendicitis. Other contributing factors include intra-abdominal tumors and positive family history. Recent roundworm infestation or viral infection of the GI tract have also been implicated.

PATHOPHYSIOLOGY

Appendicitis typically begins with dilation of the appendix, followed by obstruction and subsequent bacterial infection. When the lumen of the appendix is obstructed by hardened feces (fecalith), inflammatory processes (including parasites, viruses, or bacteria), strictures, neoplasms, or foreign bodies (including vegetable or fruit seeds or barium), the mucosa of the appendix continues to secrete fluid, which further distends the lumen, impairing the venous blood flow and leading to tissue necrosis. Left untreated, this increased distention impedes arterial inflow. Bacteria continue to proliferate and, in the absence of treatment, perforation of the appendix occurs. The incidence of perforation in patients with appendicitis is between 17% and 40%, with rates as high as 60% to 70% in older adults because of the nonspecific presenting symptoms. Gynecological disorders and gastroenteritis are the most common causes of misdiagnosis.

CLINICAL PRESENTATION

Subjective

The diagnosis of acute appendicitis is made clinically and is based primarily on the patient's history and physical exam. The historical presentations of signs and symptoms are important keys to prompt diagnosis and treatment; therefore, it is important to obtain a thorough and accurate account of the events. The classic presentation of appendicitis begins with the acute onset of mild to severe colicky, epigastric, or periumbilical pain. The pain is often vague at first, but within 24 hours usually it shifts and localizes over the RLQ and is exacerbated by walking or coughing. In male patients, the pain may radiate into the testicles; pain (rigidity) also may be associated with abdominal muscle spasm in male or female patients. Most patients complain of nausea and anorexia after the onset of pain, which may or may not be associated with vomiting. If vomiting is present, the patient usually reports that abdominal pain was present before vomiting began. The sensation of constipation is typical, although diarrhea is present in some patients.

A mildly elevated temperature of 99°F to 100°F is common. If the patient with RLQ pain presents with shaking chills (rigors), perforation of the appendix should be suspected. An important point to remember is that the very young and older adults may have an atypical presentation, which can mimic other less acute disease processes. For example, older adults with appendicitis may present with weakness, anorexia, abdominal distention, and mild complaints of pain. A delay in the diagnosis in this age-group has led to an associated increase in morbidity and mortality.

Objective

On physical examination, the patient may or may not look sick depending on the degree of pain and other symptoms. The patient may have hypertension and tachycardia proportionate to the degree of fever and pain. When the patient is lying recumbent, he or she may flex the right knee upward to relieve the tension on the iliopsoas muscle, which overlies the appendix. Palpation of the abdomen early in the process may reveal diffuse tenderness over the umbilicus and midepigastric areas. As the process progresses, the tenderness localizes over the RLQ and may be accompanied by guarding. *Guarding* is defined as "the voluntary contraction of the abdominal muscles in anticipation of examination," as opposed to *rigidity*, which is caused by "the involuntary reflexive spasm of the muscles of the abdominal wall." Rebound tenderness is tested by placing the palmar aspect of the hand on the abdomen and pressing hard enough to depress the peritoneum. This may cause the patient pain, but the clinician should keep the abdomen depressed with constant pressure until the patient becomes accustomed to the pressure, and the pain decreases. Then, without warning, the clinician should remove the hand suddenly, preferably when the patient's attention is directed elsewhere. If positive for rebound tenderness, the patient will grimace in pain, which is a more reliable sign than a subjective complaint of pain. Asking the patient to cough helps to localize exactly the site from which the pain is coming. Advanced Assessment 39.1 outlines exam maneuvers that aid in the diagnosis of appendicitis.

A rectal exam can be performed, but it is open to greater subjective interpretation. Patients with appendicitis will normally perceive greater tenderness and fullness on the right than on the left during the rectal exam. The provider must keep in mind that both the bowel and the appendix are mobile organs; they can shift posteriorly or suprapubically, causing altered exam findings. Bowel sounds are a nonspecific finding—they may be present, absent, or decreased in patients with appendicitis.

Other physical exam findings can include alterations in vital signs consistent with increased pain, such as tachycardia or elevated blood pressure. Patients may be reluctant to take a deep breath for fear they will cause themselves pain.

If there is perforation of the appendix, there may be a sudden cessation of the pain, which is considered an emergency. Findings consistent with peritonitis include diffuse abdominal tenderness with rigidity. The patient may exhibit signs of septic shock, with marked leukocytosis, fever, and hemodynamic instability.

DIAGNOSTIC REASONING

Diagnostic Tests

Laboratory findings are not diagnostic and are nonspecific, so they must be used in combination with data from the history and physical exam. A complete blood count usually reveals a mild to moderate leukocytosis

Advanced Assessment 39.1: Physical Exam Maneuvers for Diagnosing Appendicitis		
Maneuver	**Examination**	**Comments**
Rovsing's sign	Deep palpation over the left lower quadrant with sudden, unexpected release of pressure.	This causes tenderness over the right lower quadrant (RLQ) and is considered a positive finding.
Psoas sign	The patient is instructed to try to lift the right leg against gentle pressure applied by the examiner or by placing the patient in the left lateral decubitus position and extending the patient's right leg at the hip.	An increase in pain is considered positive and is an indication of the inflamed appendix irritating the psoas muscle.
Obturator sign	With the right hip and knee flexed, the examiner slowly rotates the right leg internally, which stretches the obturator muscle.	Pain over the RLQ is considered a positive sign and indicates irritation of the muscle by the inflamed appendix.
McBurney's sign	Pressure is applied to McBurney's point, which is located halfway between the umbilicus and the anterior spine of the ilium.	Pain when pressure is applied to this area is considered a positive response.

(white blood cell count 10,000–20,000 mcg/L) with a left shift. Urinalysis shows microscopic hematuria or pyuria in 25% of patients. Women should have a urine human chorionic gonadotrophin test completed to rule out (ectopic) pregnancy. The lack of laboratory findings should not preclude the diagnosis of appendicitis.

No radiological exam is of diagnostic importance early in appendicitis, but x-ray studies become more important as appendicitis progresses. A chest x-ray film rules out pneumonia as a source of abdominal pain and is necessary as part of the preoperative procedure in most hospitals. Plain x-ray films of the abdomen may show evidence of a fecalith, a gas-filled appendix, small bowel ileus, a deviation in the bowel gas pattern, or a loss of the right iliopsoas shadow. Any of these findings is suggestive of appendicitis when combined with a suspect history and physical exam.

A computed tomography scan of the abdomen is helpful in ruling out other diagnostic possibilities, as well as determining whether there has been perforation of the appendix or development of a periappendiceal abscess. An abdominal ultrasound helps to visualize the inflamed appendix and is also useful in ruling out other potential diagnoses. Diagnostic laparoscopy may be considered in female patients to rule out ectopic pregnancy, tuboovarian processes, or pelvic inflammatory disease (PID).

Differential Diagnosis

The differential diagnoses of appendicitis comprise a host of problems, which include, but are not limited to, urinary tract infection, ectopic pregnancy, ovarian cyst, pneumonia, gastroenteritis, Crohn's disease, diverticulitis, mesenteric adenitis, pancreatitis, PID, and cholelithiasis. If the diagnosis of appendicitis remains questionable after the history and physical exam have been completed and initial lab work has been obtained, radiographic studies are helpful in ruling out many of the processes found within the differential diagnoses. For women of childbearing age, the clinician should always obtain a pregnancy test before ordering any radiographic studies. In some cases, laparotomy or laparoscopy may be required to assist in definitive diagnosis.

Careful attention must be given to the sexual and menstrual history of all female patients because of the myriad of potential gynecological problems that present with the same signs and symptoms as appendicitis. A pelvic exam and a diagnostic laparotomy are often necessary for differential diagnosis.

Many GI disorders have symptoms that mimic those of appendicitis, and watchful waiting may be indicated in some cases. If appendicitis is at all a suspicion, however, the prudent practitioner will follow these patients closely until a diagnosis has been reached.

MANAGEMENT

The treatment of appendicitis is surgical; therefore, once a definitive diagnosis is made, prompt referral to a surgeon should follow. The incidence of appendiceal perforation ranges from 17% to 40% in patients with appendicitis; it is as high as 60% to 70% in older adults. With effective and timely treatment, the mortality rate is less than 1%; however, in the older adult population, mortality remains at 5% to 15%.

Preoperative management includes correction of fluid and electrolyte imbalances; bedrest; nothing by mouth, with placement of a nasogastric tube if indicated; and IV antibiotics. Narcotics should be avoided if possible because they mask any developing symptoms that might indicate a complication such as perforation. Laxatives are contraindicated in patients with appendicitis because they may cause the appendix to rupture. Stool softeners may be given if the patient is complaining about constipation and diarrhea is not present.

Third-generation cephalosporins are the antibiotics of choice. If there has been perforation and peritonitis is suspected, antibiotic coverage for both gram-negative aerobic and anaerobic organisms is recommended. Some of the choices include ampicillin, gentamicin, clindamycin, metronidazole (Flagyl), ampicillin-sulbactam (Unasyn), and ticarcillin/clavulanate (Timentin).

Patients are normally discharged the same day as surgery unless there are complications. Early ambulation is encouraged, with progression to full activity as soon as possible. Diet is advanced when bowel sounds return. The patient is given standard postoperative guidelines for individuals who have had abdominal surgery.

FOLLOW-UP AND REFERRAL

The patient is normally followed by the surgeon, who will see the patient 5 to 7 days postoperatively to remove the sutures. If there was perforation of the appendix and the patient must remain hospitalized, the surgeon will follow the patient until discharge.

Patient Education

The patient will be given standard postoperative instructions from the surgeon, which should include advice to return to the hospital if anorexia, nausea, vomiting, abdominal pain, fever, or chills develop. Patients should be instructed to avoid heavy lifting for at least 2 weeks.

REFERENCES

Appendicitis

Guibentif L, Ris F, Scheffler M, Reny J, Prendki V. Acute appendicitis in elderly adults: A difficult diagnosis. *J Am Geriatr Soc.* 2016;64(6):1377–1379.

Huston JM, Kao LS, Chang PK, Sanders JM, Buckman S, Adams CA, et al. Antibiotics vs. appendectomy for acute uncomplicated appendicitis in adults: Review of the evidence and future directions. *Surg Infect.* 2017;18(5):527–535.

Kim HK, Kim YS, Lee HH. Impact of a delayed laparoscopic appendectomy on the risk of complications in acute appendicitis: A retrospective study of 4,065 patients. *Dig Surg.* 2017;34(1):25–29.

Gastroenteritis

Barnes D, Yeh AM. Bugs and guts. *Nutr Clin Pract.* 2015;30(6):747–759.

Freeland AL, Vaughan GH, Banerjee SN. Acute gastroenteritis on cruise ships—United States, 2008–2014. *MMWR Morb Mortal Wkly Rep.* 2016;65(1):1–4.

Nair D. Travelers' diarrhea: Prevention, treatment, and post-trip evaluation. *J Fam Pract.* 2013;62(7):356–361.

White MB, Rajagopalan S, Yoshikawa TT. Infectious diarrhea: Norovirus and *Clostridium difficile* in older adults. *Clin Geriatr Med.* 2016;32(3):509–522.

Wikswo ME, Kambhampati A, Kayoko S, Walsh KA, Bowen A, Hall AJ. Outbreaks of acute gastroenteritis transmitted by person-to-person contact, environmental contamination, and unknown modes of transmission—United States, 2009–2013. *MMWR Morb Mortal Wkly Rep.* 2015;64(12):1–16.

Hepatitis

American Association for the Study of Liver Diseases. *HCV guidance: Recommendations for testing, managing, and treating Hepatitis C.* http://www.hcvguidelines.org. Published 2017.

Centers for Disease Control and Prevention. *Viral hepatitis surveillance, United States, 2015.* https://www.cdc.gov/hepatitis/statistics/2015surveillance/pdfs/2015HepSurveillanceRpt.pdf. Published 2017.

Centers for Disease Control and Prevention. *Viral hepatitis.* https://www.cdc.gov/hepatitis/hbv/index.htm. Published 2015.

Cordeiro da Silva SG. A rare case of transfusion transmission of hepatitis A virus to two patients with haematological disease. *Transfus Med Hemother.* 2016;43(2):137–141.

National Library of Medicine. *LiverTox: Clinical and research information on drug-induced liver injury, Simeprevir.* https://livertox.nih.gov/Simeprevir.htm. Published 2017.

Terrault NA, Lok ASF, McMahon BJ, Chang K-M, Hwang JP, Jonas MM, et al. AASLD guidelines for treatment of chronic hepatitis B. *Hepatology.* 2015;63(1):261–283.

Tseng TC, Kao JH. Treating immune-tolerant Hepatitis B. *J Viral Hepat.* 2015;22(2):77–84.

U.S. Food & Drug Administration. FDA approves Technivie for treatment of chronic hepatitis C genotype 4. https://www.fda.gov/newsevents/newsroom/pressannouncements/ucm455857.htm. Published 2015.

U.S. Food & Drug Administration. FDA approves Epclusa for treatment of chronic Hepatitis C virus infection. https://www.fda.gov/newsevents/newsroom/pressannouncements/ucm508915.htm. Published. 2016.

RESOURCES

American Association for the Study of Liver Diseases (AASLD)
https://www.aasld.org/publications/practice-guidelines-0
American Liver Foundation
http://hepc.liverfoundation.org/
Centers for Disease Control and Prevention (CDC)
https://www.cdc.gov/nchs/pressroom/sosmap/liver_disease_mortality/liver_disease.htm

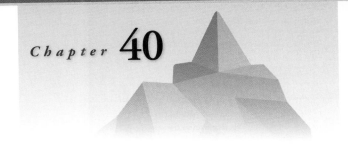

Chapter **40**

Gastric and Intestinal Disorders

Debera J. Thomas, DNS, RN, FNP/ANP

GASTROESOPHAGEAL REFLUX DISEASE

Esophageal reflux is the backward flow of stomach or duodenal contents into the esophagus without associated retching or vomiting. It can occur in otherwise healthy people. If symptoms become severe or frequent or are associated with esophageal mucosal damage, the potential for serious clinical consequences becomes more likely, and the esophageal reflux is considered a disease.

Gastroesophageal reflux disease (GERD) is a syndrome that results from esophageal reflux; the characteristic symptoms are caused by repeated exposure of the esophageal mucosa to the deleterious effects of gastrointestinal (GI) contents and the gradual breakdown of the mucosal barrier (see the Iceberg of GERD).

EPIDEMIOLOGY AND CAUSES

GERD can occur at any age. Some research indicates that it increases with age and then decreases after age 69. The prevalence of GERD is equal across gender, ethnic, and cultural groups in the United States; it is a common condition. Higher rates of GERD occur in individuals who are overweight or obese and have a body mass index over 25. The prevalence rate for GERD (those experiencing symptoms at least once a week) in the United States is approximately 20%. The prevalence rates in other countries are less, ranging from 0.1% to 5% in China to 10% to 15% in the United Kingdom. In the United States, 35% to 45% of the adult population complain of heartburn at least once a month, and 10% of the adult population complain of symptoms daily. These figures may be significantly underestimated because many people with mild symptoms use over-the-counter (OTC) medications (histamine 2 blockers or proton pump inhibitors [PPI]) or antacids. Many individuals also believe that it is

The Iceberg of GERD

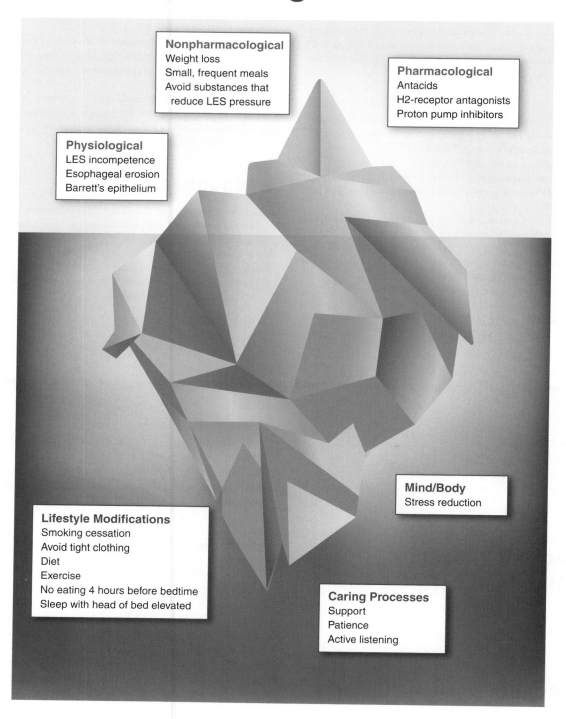

Nonpharmacological
Weight loss
Small, frequent meals
Avoid substances that
    reduce LES pressure

Pharmacological
Antacids
H2-receptor antagonists
Proton pump inhibitors

Physiological
LES incompetence
Esophageal erosion
Barrett's epithelium

Lifestyle Modifications
Smoking cessation
Avoid tight clothing
Diet
Exercise
No eating 4 hours before bedtime
Sleep with head of bed elevated

Mind/Body
Stress reduction

Caring Processes
Support
Patience
Active listening

normal to have symptoms from time to time and attribute them to stress or dietary indiscretion.

The primary cause of GERD is the inappropriate, spontaneous, transient relaxation of the lower esophageal sphincter (LES) to an unknown stimulus. In most patients, the normal resting or baseline LES pressure is 10 to 30 mm Hg. In patients who have severe disease,

the LES is incompetent, with a resting pressure of less than 10 mm Hg. An incompetent LES results in free reflux during abdominal straining, lifting, bending, and recumbency. Gastric contents are acidic, and it is this low pH (less than 3.9) that causes injury to the esophageal mucosa in most patients with GERD. Normally, refluxate is neutralized by swallowing salivary bicarbonate and

---

Box 40.1   Substances That Reduce Lower Esophageal Sphincter Pressure or Irritate the Gastric Mucosa

Food Substances

Alcohol
Caffeinated beverages (cola, tea, coffee)
Chocolate
Citrus fruits
Decaffeinated coffee
Fatty foods, fats (butter, margarine, shortening), and oils
Onions
Peppermint and spearmint
Tomatoes and tomato-based products (ketchup, cocktail sauce, tomato sauce, tomato paste)

Nonfood Substances

Anticholinergic drugs
Beta-adrenergic blocking agents
Calcium channel blockers
Diazepam
Estrogen and progesterone
Nicotine, including secondhand smoke
Theophylline

---

cleared by esophageal peristalsis. The decreased rate of swallowing (by two-thirds) during sleep, coupled with recumbency, significantly increase the duration of exposure of the mucosa to acid at night.

Hiatal hernia, which displaces the LES into the thorax, is found in 75% of patients with severe erosive gastritis and 90% of patients with Barrett's esophagus but in only 25% of patients with nonerosive GERD. Delayed gastric emptying, which often worsens as people age, causes increased intra-abdominal pressure and may contribute to reflux. Obesity is also a risk factor for GERD. Several foods and pharmacological agents are known to lower LES pressure. Box 40.1 lists the common substances that reduce LES pressure or cause direct gastric mucosal irritation.

PATHOPHYSIOLOGY

Physiologically, gastric acid is prevented from reflux into the esophagus by the presence of two areas of high pressure in the distal esophagus. The upper esophageal sphincter is a 3-cm segment at the proximal end of the esophagus. The LES is a 2- to 4-cm segment of the esophagus just proximal to the gastroesophageal junction that prevents the reflux of gastric contents. These areas of the esophagus are under muscular, hormonal, and neural control. The anatomical placement of the LES within the abdomen supports its function, as does the acute angle

(angle of His) that is formed as the esophagus enters the stomach.

Esophageal reflux occurs when the gastric volume (e.g., a large meal) or the intra-abdominal pressure is elevated (e.g., in pregnancy). It can also occur when the sphincter tone of the LES is decreased (e.g., by caffeine) or when the LES undergoes inappropriate relaxation. Gravity, saliva, and peristalsis combine to return refluxed contents to the stomach. As the esophagus becomes inflamed with repeated exposure to gastric acid, it cannot eliminate the refluxed material as quickly or efficiently, prolonging the duration of the contact with each subsequent exposure.

Because gastric contents are so irritating to the esophageal mucosa, an inflammatory response is established. With repeated exposure, the inflammation becomes chronic. In response to chronic inflammation, blood flow to the area increases, and erosion occurs. Frank bleeding is unusual, but minor capillary bleeding is common. As the erosion heals, the body replaces the normal squamous epithelium with metaplastic columnar epithelium (Barrett's epithelium) containing goblet and columnar cells. This new epithelium is more resistant to acid and, therefore, supports esophageal healing. Barrett's epithelium is a premalignant tissue, however, and confers a 40-fold increased risk for the development of esophageal adenocarcinoma. Fibrosis and scarring also accompany the healing process, leading to esophageal strictures.

CLINICAL PRESENTATION

Subjective

The most typical symptom of GERD is heartburn, ranging in degree from mild to severe. It is usually associated with other symptoms, including regurgitation, water brash (reflex salivation), dysphagia, sour taste in the mouth in the morning, odynophagia, belching, coughing, hoarseness, or wheezing, usually at night. Substernal or retrosternal chest pain may also be present, but additional questioning can determine if the pain is activity induced, leading to the conclusion that the pain may be cardiac in origin. Factors that precipitate or make the symptoms worse, such as reclining after eating; eating a large meal; ingesting alcohol, chocolate, caffeine, fatty or spicy foods, or nicotine; wearing constrictive clothing; or working in an occupation in which heavy lifting, straining, or working in a bent-over position is involved also help establish the diagnosis of GERD. It is equally important to ask what the patient does that makes the symptoms better, such as taking antacids, sitting upright after a meal, or eating small meals.

Patients with chronic GERD may present with dysphagia as their chief complaint. The dysphagia is usually present only with the first swallow of every meal and is not progressive. Should the patient complain of progressive or persistent dysphagia, adenocarcinoma, or the development of a stricture should be suspected.

Objective

The physical exam of the patient with GERD is usually normal. The only physical sign may be a stool positive for occult blood on rectal exam resulting from microhemorrhages in the irritated esophageal epithelium.

DIAGNOSTIC REASONING

Diagnostic Tests

Diagnosis of GERD is usually made by history alone and has a sensitivity of 80%. The severity of the symptoms does not correlate well with the severity of the disease; some patients with the most severe disease have virtually no symptoms. GERD may also manifest with atypical symptoms such as adult-onset asthma, chronic cough, chronic laryngitis, sore throat, or noncardiac chest pain.

When the diagnosis of GERD is unclear or when the patient fails to respond to 4-8 weeks of empiric once daily PPI therapy, the test of choice is esophagogastroduodenoscopy (EGD, also called an upper endoscopy). The benefit of EGD is direct visualization of the mucosa to determine the extent of tissue damage. The EGD can also detect complications of GERD such as Barret epithelium, esophageal stricture and cancer. The American College of Gastroenterology (ACG) guidance for EGD in adults with GERD symptoms recommends EGD for patients with heartburn and dysphagia, bleeding, anemia, weight loss, or recurrent vomiting rather than initial empiric therapy and those who have persistent symptoms despite 8 weeks of PPI therapy. Upper endoscopy is recommended for surveillance evaluation in anyone with Barrett's esophagus every 3 to 5 years and more frequently if there is Barrett's esophagus with dysplasia.

Differential Diagnosis

The symptoms of GERD are similar to those of peptic ulcer disease (PUD), and the two conditions often coexist. Unlike GERD, however, PUD usually produces epigastric pain and tenderness on palpation. One pattern that can help differentiate GERD from PUD is that heartburn from PUD is usually relieved by food. This is not the case in GERD; instead, the symptoms are worse shortly after eating. Another possible differential diagnosis is gallbladder disease, which usually presents with epigastric or right subcostal pain. Nausea and possibly vomiting are usually associated with cholelithiasis and cholecystitis; this is not the case in gastric reflux. There may be a strong association between the ingestion of a high-fat meal and the development of the symptoms of cholelithiasis. Occasionally, GERD may present with chest pain. In these patients, the clinician must differentiate between symptoms of cardiac origin and those of GERD. If the pain is of cardiac origin (e.g., angina), the patient's history usually reveals that the pain is associated with exercise and is relieved by rest and nitrates. Patients with angina are often treated with medications (calcium channel blockers, beta-adrenergic blockers, nitrates) that decrease the LES pressure and produce a coexistent esophageal reflux, which complicates the differential diagnosis further.

MANAGEMENT

Initial Treatment

The goal of the management of GERD is to rapidly eliminate or reduce symptoms; prevent meal- or exercise-related symptoms; and prevent the complications of esophageal stricture, esophageal ulcer, Barrett esophagus's, pulmonary aspiration, and esophageal hemorrhage all in the most cost-effective way. The focus of management is patient education coupled with pharmacological intervention. The ACG conditionally recommends lifestyle modifications that include weight loss (moderate level of evidence); elevating the head of the bed 6 to 8 inches and avoidance of meals 2 to 3 hours before bedtime (low level of evidence); and avoidance of certain foods known to trigger reflux (chocolate, alcohol, caffeine, acidic or spicy foods)[low level of evidence].

The ACG recommends an 8-week trial of PPIs based on a high level of evidence. It found no difference in the effectiveness of different PPIs. A moderate level of evidence suggests that traditional PPIs should be taken 30 to 60 minutes before a meal for the best pH control. The newer PPIs can be taken on a more relaxed schedule, a conditional recommendation based on a moderate level of evidence.

For patients with mild, intermittent symptoms, lifestyle changes may relieve symptoms. For patients with mild to moderate symptoms without esophageal erosion, an 8-week course of PPI once daily before the first meal of the day is the treatment of choice (strong recommendation, moderate level of evidence). In those patients with a partial response to this therapy, tailoring the dose and timing especially for those patients with symptoms at night, or with sleep disturbance (strong recommendation, low level of evidence) is indicated. If the patient has a partial response, changing to a twice a day dosing schedule or switching to a different PPI may be effective (conditional recommendation, low level of evidence).

Troublesome Symptoms or Symptoms Unresponsive to 8 Weeks of PPI Therapy

Patients who have severe symptoms and have endoscopically documented erosive esophagitis or Barrett's esophagus should be treated with PPIs such as omeprazole, rabeprazole, pantoprazole, or lansoprazole once a day 30 minutes before breakfast. An 8-week course of once-daily treatment usually provides adequate control of heartburn in 80% to 90% of the cases and healing of erosive esophagitis in 80%, whereas twice-daily dosing heals 95% of cases. If twice-daily dosing provides inadequate symptom relief, the patient should be evaluated with upper endoscopy. Chronic maintenance therapy with PPIs may be necessary for severe erosive esophagitis.

Patients with severe erosive esophagitis, Barrett's esophagus, peptic stricture, or who required twice-daily PPI therapy for initial symptom control should be maintained on long-term therapy. More than 80% of patients who achieved good symptom control with initial therapy and discontinue treatment will relapse. These patients may require intermittent 2- to 4-week courses of PPI therapy.

Evidence suggests that PPIs are more effective than H_2-receptor antagonists (H_2RAs) in all cases of GERD. These agents should not be used in combination, especially with older adults. The PPIs should be taken 30 to 60 minutes before breakfast to maximize effectiveness. If the patient requires twice-daily dosing, the second dose should be taken 30 to 60 minutes before dinner as well. Patients on long-term therapy should have their symptoms reevaluated every 6 months in an effort to avoid potential adverse effects such as PPI-associated pneumonia, *Clostridium difficile*, osteoporosis, and vitamin B_{12} deficiency.

Unresponsive Disease

The 5% of patients who do not respond to any of the above treatments may require surgical intervention. However, for patients that do not respond to PPI therapy, surgical intervention is generally not recommended (strong recommendation, high level of evidence). For those patients who do require surgery, preoperative ambulatory pH monitory is mandatory if they do not have evidence of erosive esophagitis (strong recommendation, moderate level of evidence). Before referring a patient for surgical intervention, other causes of refractory GERD, such as gastrinoma, proton pump resistance, pill-induced esophagitis, scleroderma-like esophagus, or patient noncompliance, should be investigated. Under investigation for future treatments include transient lower esophageal sphincter relaxation (TLESR) inhibitors, such as metabotropic glutamate receptor 5 antagonists (e.g., AZD2066) and cannabinoid receptor agonists. Drugs Commonly Prescribed 40.1 outlines the PPIs and other medication used to treat GERD.

FOLLOW-UP AND REFERRAL

GERD is a lifelong condition, and patients must be reevaluated on a regular basis to minimize the development of severe complications. Patients with mild-to-moderate symptoms should be instructed in the appropriate lifestyle modifications and treated with PPIs for 4 to 8 weeks. Antacids or OTC H_2-RAs may be effective for some patients, but the treatment of choice is a PPI. If on the 8-week follow-up visit there is no improvement in the symptoms, the patient can be advanced to twice daily dosing. If this regimen is ineffective, the patient should be referred to a gastroenterologist. Patients who have self-medicated for a length of time may have developed erosive esophagitis or Barrett's esophagus and need aggressive treatment.

Patient Education: GERD

Education for patients with GERD includes instructing them on appropriate lifestyle modifications. Patients who are obese should be referred to a dietitian for counseling about weight loss. Dietary modifications may improve symptoms and include reducing the ingestion of foods that are irritating to the gastric mucosa and those that reduce LES pressure. Factors that increase intra-abdominal pressure should be avoided, such as large meals, tight or restrictive clothing, and bending or straining. It is most helpful for patients to eat small, frequent meals, with the main meal at midday. Eating less than 4 hours before bedtime, including snacks, should be avoided because this increases the chance of reflux during the night. Although the clinical evidence is not robust, sleeping with the head of the bed elevated, which can be accomplished by placing blocks or bricks under the legs of the head of the bed, may improve symptoms. Patients should be given assistance in smoking cessation, but the use of supplemental nicotine should be avoided because it reduces LES pressure. Programs for stress management have not been found to be helpful in reducing the symptoms of GERD.

PEPTIC ULCER DISEASE

PUD is a generic name for both gastric ulcers and duodenal ulcers. A peptic ulcer is a break in the surface mucosa of the stomach or duodenum, which results when there is disruption of the normal mucosal defenses and the tissue is exposed to the damaging effects of acid and pepsin. By definition, a peptic ulcer penetrates the muscularis mucosa and is usually larger than 5 mm in diameter. Peptic ulcers occur when there is an imbalance between the protective factors of the mucosa and aggressive factors as acid and pepsin. The initial damage to the mucosa is usually a result of infection by *Helicobacter pylori* or medications, particularly NSAIDs.

EPIDEMIOLOGY AND CAUSES

The actual incidence of PUD in unknown, but the estimate is about 10% to 17% of the population. An individual has a 10% lifetime risk of developing a peptic ulcer. Approximately 500,000 new cases are diagnosed each year in the United States. Most duodenal ulcers occur in patients between ages 30 and 55, but gastric

Drugs Commonly Prescribed 40.1: Treatment for GERD

DRUG	INDICATION	ADVERSE REACTIONS AND PRESCRIBING CONSIDERATIONS
Proton pump inhibitors: Omeprazole 20 mg orally Rabeprazole 20 mg orally Lansoprazole 30 mg orally Dexlansoprazole 60 mg orally Esomeprazole 40 mg orally Pantoprazole 40 mg orally *H2-receptor antagonists may be effective in some patients and are less expensive	Mild, intermittent symptoms	Trial for 4–8 weeks Take 30 minutes before breakfast PPIs are generally well tolerated. Common side effects include headache, diarrhea, constipation, abdominal pain, flatulence, fever, vomiting, nausea or rash. Serious side effects: increased risk of *Clostridium difficile* infection, serious allergic reactions, Stevens-Johnson syndrome, toxic epidermal necrolysis, reduced kidney function, pancreatitis, reduced liver function, erythema multiforme.
Proton pump inhibitors (PPIs): Omeprazole 20 mg orally Rabeprazole 20 mg orally Lansoprazole 30 mg orally Dexlansoprazole 60 mg orally Esomeprazole 40 mg orally Pantoprazole 40 mg orally	Moderate symptoms or partial response to once daily dosing	Twice dialing dosing or switch to a different PPI (conditional recommendation, low level of evidence) Long term use of PPIs can cause vitamin B_{12} deficiency and risk for osteoporosis
Optimize PPI therapy (strong recommendation, low level of evidence) Future treatment: Research is being done on transient lower esophageal sphincter inhibitors and cannabinoid receptor agonists.	Troublesome symptoms or refractory gastroesophageal reflux disease	Upper endoscopy Explore other etiologies; possible referral to pulmonary and allergy specialists (strong recommendation, low level of evidence) Refractory patients with ongoing evidence of reflux should be considered for surgery or increasing the dose of PPI

ulcers are more prevalent between ages 55 and 70 years. Because of the eradication of *H. pylori*, the actual incidence of duodenal ulcers has declined dramatically over the past 30 years. However, because of the widespread use of NSAIDs and low-dose aspirin, the incidence of gastric ulcers has increased.

A variety of conditions are considered to be risk factors for the development of PUD, but the two major causes are infection with *H. pylori* and chronic ingestion of aspirin and other NSAIDs. Less than 5% to 10% of ulcers are attributed to other causes such as acid hypersecretion syndromes (Zollinger-Ellison syndrome, systemic mastocytosis). Genetics, blood type, personality type, and cigarette smoking may also play a role in the development of PUD. Patients with chronic obstructive pulmonary disease, cirrhosis, renal failure, and renal transplant have a higher incidence of PUD than the general population, but the mechanism is not known. Dietary factors such as caffeine, alcohol, and spicy foods, as well as stress do not cause ulcers.

PATHOPHYSIOLOGY

Most ulcers are located in the duodenum and approximately 95% occur within 3 cm of the pylorus. Almost all patients with gastric ulcers have normal or subnormal amounts of gastric acid secretion. Only about 35% of patients with duodenal ulcers have demonstrated above-average rates of acid secretion but have impaired duodenal bicarbonate secretion that is *H. pylori* dependent. The breakdown of the local mucosal defenses appears to play a larger role in the pathogenesis of ulcer formation. Mucosal defense is supported by surface mucus and bicarbonate, which form a thin alkaline gel coating mucosal cells, and by prostaglandin-enhanced mucosal blood flow and cell renewal.

A variety of factors can affect the development of ulcers. Cigarette smoking facilitates ulcer formation, which is proportional to the amount smoked. The mechanism by which cigarette smoking causes ulcer formation is unclear. Aspirin and other NSAIDs decrease the mucosal defense mechanisms by inhibiting prostaglandin synthesis, leaving the area vulnerable to the effects of gastric hydrochloric acid and pepsin. Many infectious agents have been detected in patients with ulcer disease, but *H. pylori* is the most important. As many as 70% to 90% of patients with duodenal ulcers are infected with *H. pylori*, and the bacterium is present in most gastric ulcer patients although the association with gastric ulcers is less. Not everyone with *H. pylori* infection, however, develops PUD.

CLINICAL PRESENTATION

Subjective

The hallmark of PUD is a complaint of a burning or gnawing (hunger) sensation or pain (dyspepsia) in the epigastrium, which is often relieved by food or antacids. These complaints, however, are not specific or sensitive enough to be diagnostic of ulcer disease. Patients with PUD usually describe an episodic pattern of complaints in which the pain tends to cluster and last for minutes, with the episodes separated by periods of no symptoms. It is this alternating pattern that is more predictive of ulcer disease than the nature of the symptoms themselves. Almost half the patients with NSAID-induced ulcers are asymptomatic.

Nocturnal pain is present in two-thirds of patients with duodenal ulcers and one-third of those with gastric ulcers. This corresponds to the circadian stimulation of acid secretion. Nausea and anorexia sometimes occur in patients with gastric ulcer, whereas vomiting and weight loss are indications of more serious complications such as gastric malignancy or pyloric obstruction. Patients with duodenal ulcers may report a reduction in pain after eating; patients with gastric ulcers tend to experience more intense pain after eating, which is a result of secretion of gastric acids.

Objective

The physical exam is not useful in differentiating PUD from other types of upper GI disorders. Patients with duodenal ulcers often demonstrate epigastric tenderness 2.5 cm to the right of the midline, but this may also be present with cholecystitis, pancreatitis, nonulcer dyspepsia, and other GI disorders. Reports of melena or coffee-ground–like emesis usually indicate a bleeding ulcer, and a perforated ulcer may present with abdominal rigidity.

DIAGNOSTIC REASONING

Diagnostic Tests

Most routine laboratory tests are normal in patients with ulcer disease unless there is significant bleeding or vomiting, in which case the results show anemia and fluid and electrolyte disturbances. When a patient is actively bleeding, a complete blood count (CBC) to evaluate hemoglobin levels is paramount. If the patient has leukocytosis, then the clinician should suspect perforation. The diagnostic standard for PUD is EGD. It provides direct visualization and the opportunity to obtain a biopsy. Although duodenal ulcers are usually benign, 3% to 5% of benign appearing gastric ulcers prove to be cancer.

Research has implicated *H. pylori* gastritis in 90% to 95% of both duodenal and gastric ulcers that are not associated with NSAIDs. *H. pylori* infection increases with age, and in the United States more than 50% of asymptomatic persons older than 60 years show evidence of active or past infection. Worldwide, at least 30% to 50% of the population is colonized with this bacterium, but the rate is declining. The mode of transmission is unknown. In response to *H. pylori,* the stomach produces more gastrin, which in turn leads to an increase in the amount of acid secreted by the parietal cells. The excess acid and pepsin on the stomach lining can cause the lining to erode and leads to the development of an ulcer. There are four tests used to detect *H. pylori*: (1) fecal antigen assay, (2) urea breath test, (3) biopsy with histological examination, and (4) serological antibody (enzyme-linked immunosorbent assay) test (not as sensitive or specific as the three other tests).

In patients for whom an increase in gastric acid secretion is suspected, a fasting serum gastrin level should be obtained. Levels higher than 200 pg/mL should be confirmed on repeat testing and followed by basal and peak acid-output measurements. Zollinger-Ellison syndrome should be suspected in patients whose fasting serum gastrin level is greater than 600 pg/mL and who have a basal acid output of more than 15 mmol/hr.

Differential Diagnosis

PUD must be distinguished from other causes of epigastric distress. A variety of thoracic and upper abdominal disorders can cause similar pain such as nonulcer dyspepsia, cholecystitis, pancreatitis, irritable bowel syndrome (IBS), GERD, gastric cancer, myocardial ischemia, gastritis, and gastroenteritis. If the pain does not respond to food or antacids and there is severe pain and rebound tenderness, the cause is not likely to be an uncomplicated peptic ulcer. If the patient presents with weight loss, anemia, or exacerbation of the pain when eating, gastric cancer should be suspected.

MANAGEMENT

The principal aim of management for patients with PUD is to relieve pain, heal the ulcer, and prevent complications or recurrences. Pharmacological therapy is the foundation of management for PUD, but nonpharmacological measures, such as smoking cessation, should be used as well. Cigarette smoking increases the risk for PUD; in patients with documented ulcers, smoking impairs healing, promotes recurrence, and increases the morbidity and mortality. There are no firm dietary measures for patients with PUD other than instructions to avoid foods that precipitate dyspepsia. Pharmacological intervention for PUD consists of H_2-RAs, PPIs, and agents that enhance the mucosal defenses, such as antacids, sucralfate (Carafate), bismuth subsalicylate (Pepto-Bismol), and prostaglandin analogs (misoprostol), as well as antibiotics.

Proton Pump Inhibitors

The PPIs are the drugs of choice for treating PUD. The duration of action of the PPIs is more than 24 hours and a once-a-day dosing schedule. The usual dosage is either omeprazole 20 mg, rabeprazole 20 mg, lansoprazole 30 mg, esomeprazole 40 mg, dexlansoprazole 30 mg, or pantoprazole 40 mg. All PPIs inhibit parietal cell hydrogen-potassium adenosine triphosphatase (ATPase), which mediates hydrogen ion secretion. PPIs heal 90% of duodenal ulcers in 4 weeks of therapy and 90% of gastric ulcers after 8 weeks. Long-term use of these drugs is associated with slightly decreased absorption of vitamin B_{12} and iron.

H₂-Receptor Antagonists

If a patient has mild symptoms and no indicators of complications or a more serious disease, empiric therapy with an H_2-RA should be instituted for 2 weeks. After the initial treatment period, if symptoms persist or worsen, EGD should be considered for a more definitive diagnosis. When H_2-RAs are used for peptic ulcer treatment, the standard treatment is to administer an H_2-RA once a day at bedtime or half the daily dose twice a day for 8 weeks. More than 80% of ulcers are healed by the completion of this regimen. H_2-RAs effectively reduce basal and food-stimulated secretion of gastric acid and thus facilitate healing; they are generally well tolerated. Cimetidine (Tagamet), however, inhibits the hepatic cytochrome P-450 system and can increase levels of other medications that are metabolized by these enzymes, including warfarin (Coumadin), theophylline (Theo-Dur), and phenytoin (Dilantin). The other H_2-RAs have fewer adverse effects.

Other Pharmacological Agents

Antacids were traditionally the mainstay of ulcer treatment for decades and are still useful today. They neutralize acid rapidly, are generally well tolerated, and are inexpensive. One of the major disadvantages is that they require frequent (1- to 3-hour) dosing, which can contribute to patient nonadherence. They should be used with caution in patients with renal failure because of the risk of aluminum and magnesium toxicity. Antacids that contain calcium should not be used in patients with PUD because calcium causes rebound acid secretion.

Sucralfate is an aluminum hydroxide salt of sucrose that enhances the mucosal defenses and is used in healing duodenal ulcers and in the long-term treatment to prevent recurrence. Sucralfate works by forming a protective barrier to the action of acid and pepsin in the ulcer base. It also stimulates mucus, bicarbonate secretion, and prostaglandin production and binds fibroblast growth factor. Studies have shown that sucralfate 1 g four times daily heals duodenal ulcers as well as H_2-RAs do.

Bismuth preparations promote ulcer healing by stimulating mucosal bicarbonate and prostaglandin production. Bismuth also has antimicrobial action against *H. pylori* and has been shown to eradicate the organism in up to 33% of cases. The two types of bismuth preparation available in the United States are bismuth subsalicylate and ranitidine bismuth citrate. Bismuth causes feces to darken or turn black. Patients should be warned of this effect to lessen their anxiety when it occurs. Bismuth subsalicylate also potentiates the effects of antidiabetic medications, so patients should be warned about the possibility of hypoglycemia.

Misoprostol (Cytotec), a prostaglandin analog, stimulates ulcer healing by promoting mucus and bicarbonate secretion. It is indicated for use only as a prophylactic measure to prevent gastric ulcer formation in patients who require treatment with NSAIDs for other conditions. It is ineffective in preventing duodenal ulcers caused by NSAID use. Misoprostol should not be used in pregnancy because it can cause abortion, premature birth, or birth defects.

Several regimens are used to eradicate *H. pylori,* enhance ulcer healing, and prevent ulcer recurrence. Most regimens use a combination of several drugs, including bismuth, antibiotics, and PPIs for 2 weeks. The standard triple-drug therapy is the combination of two antibiotics (clarithromycin and either amoxicillin or metronidazole) with a PPI all twice a day for 14 days and has been shown to be very effective in the eradication of *H. pylori* (75%–90%). Amoxicillin is preferred over metronidazole because there are resistant strains of *H. pylori,* and the adverse effects of metronidazole hamper patient adherence. Eradication of *H. pylori* has also been demonstrated by combining bismuth subsalicylate and two antibiotics, but the dosing schedule is four times daily and has a higher incidence of adverse effects. The standard quadruple therapy consists of 14 days of a PPI twice a day, bismuth subsalicylate two tabs four times a day, tetracycline four times a day and metronidazole three times a day. Drugs Commonly Prescribed 40.2 presents the drugs used for PUD.

FOLLOW-UP AND REFERRAL

Successful eradication of *H. pylori* should be confirmed 4 weeks after the completion of therapy. In patients with non–*H. pylori* associated ulcer disease, follow-up is necessary only if symptoms recur. If after 2 weeks the patient has seen no improvement or symptoms have progressed, referral to a gastroenterologist for upper endoscopy is indicated. Any time a gastric ulcer is suspected rather than a duodenal ulcer, the patient should be referred to a gastroenterologist because the incidence of gastric cancer in these patients is increased. Follow-up is necessary for any patient who does not respond to therapy or who experiences worsening symptoms.

Drugs Commonly Prescribed 40.2: Peptic Ulcer Disease

DRUG	INDICATION	ADVERSE REACTIONS AND PRESCRIBING CONSIDERATIONS
First-Line Therapy		
Antacids only for symptom relief Mylanta II 2–4 tsp between meals and at bedtime Sucralfate 1 g four times per day for 4–8 weeks H2-receptor antagonists: Cimetidine 800 mg Ranitidine 300 mg Nizatidine 300 mg Famotidine 40 mg OR Proton pump inhibitors (PPIs)—all should be administered orally 30 minutes before breakfast Omeprazole 20 mg Lansoprazole 30 mg Esomeprazole 40 mg Rabeprazole 20 mg Pantoprazole 40 mg	Peptic ulcer disease (non–*H. pylori* related) Uncomplicated ulcer	These medications should be used only as long as the patient is symptomatic and as needed. Uncomplicated duodenal ulcer treatment is once a day for 6 weeks. Uncomplicated gastric ulcer treatment is half the dose twice a day for 8 weeks Uncomplicated duodenal ulcer treatment is 4 weeks. Uncomplicated gastric ulcer treatment is 8 weeks
Standard Triple Therapy (14 days)		
PPIs as above twice daily PLUS Clarithromycin 500 mg orally twice a day PLUS Amoxicillin 1 g orally twice a day (OR metronidazole 500 mg orally twice a day if penicillin allergic) PPI as above PLUS Tetracycline 500 mg orally 4 times per day PLUS Metronidazole 500 mg orally 3 times a day PLUS Bismuth subsalicylate two tablets 4 times a day	Ulcer disease associated with *H. pylori*	These medication may inhibit absorption of digoxin, tetracycline antibiotics, and quinolone antibiotics and should be used for 14 days. PPIs should be continued once daily for an additional 4–6 weeks if the ulcer is large. Long-term use of PPIs is not advised.

Patient Education: Peptic Ulcer Disease (PUD)

The most important aspect of patient education is to stress the importance of following the treatment regimen prescribed. The patient's anxiety can be eased by informing him or her of possible bothersome side effects of any medications, such as a change in fecal color when taking bismuth preparations. If the patient is taking sucralfate in conjunction with an antacid, PPI, or H$_2$-RA, it should be stressed that the sucralfate cannot be taken at the same time as the other medications or at the same time as digoxin, ciprofloxacin, or phenytoin because sucralfate binds to all of these medications. Dispelling myths about ulcers is also an important part of patient education.

HEMORRHOIDS

Hemorrhoids are defined as a mass of dilated and tortuous veins that represent prolapsed submucosal tissue. Hemorrhoids are classified as either internal or external, depending on their location. The primary cause of hemorrhoids is believed to be straining during defecation, which is further complicated by constipation, prolonged sitting, pregnancy, and anal infection. Some hemorrhoids are asymptomatic, require no treatment, and typically resolve on their own within 3 weeks; others can result in profuse bleeding, requiring emergency ligation.

EPIDEMIOLOGY AND CAUSES

Every year approximately 1 million people, or 5% of the U.S. population, visit their medical provider for symptoms of hemorrhoids. Although hemorrhoids can occur at any age, their incidence increases with age.

Although the cause of hemorrhoids is not completely known or understood, they are common in countries where there is a known deficiency of dietary fiber. Thus, increased straining during defecation has been recognized as an important predisposing factor in the development of hemorrhoids. Heredity may also be a factor because 10% of the patients with hemorrhoids have a family history of the disease. Patients with illnesses characterized by chronic diarrhea, such as inflammatory bowel disease (IBD), are also more likely to develop hemorrhoids.

PATHOPHYSIOLOGY

External hemorrhoids are dilated varicose veins originating from the inferior hemorrhoidal plexus and are located below the anal-rectal line. Internal hemorrhoids are a dilation of the veins within the superior hemorrhoidal plexus and are located within the distal rectum and the anal canal. Internal hemorrhoids are classified by the degree of prolapse present (Table 40.1).

The inferior hemorrhoidal plexus is prone to increased distention during defecation, which can result in rupture of a vessel and subsequent development of a perianal hematoma or thrombus within one of the vessels of the plexus. Patients who have a thrombosed hemorrhoid may present with a painful perianal lump.

CLINICAL PRESENTATION

Subjective

External hemorrhoids may present with an abrupt onset of pain that is associated with the development of a perianal lump. Many patients complain of more intense pain after defecation or other straining maneuvers, which result in further inflammation and engorgement. Mucus discharge from the anus can lead to poor hygiene and complaints of pruritus. The natural history of a resolved hemorrhoid is the formation of external skin tags, which are asymptomatic but may be irritating and interfere with daily hygiene.

Objective

On physical examination, external hemorrhoids may not be visible at rest but usually protrude on standing or with the Valsalva maneuver. Thrombosed hemorrhoids may appear as shiny, blue masses located at the anus. Evidence of hemorrhoidal skin tags may appear at the site of resolved hemorrhoids; these skin tags are fibrotic and painless.

TABLE 40.1	Classification of Internal Hemorrhoids
Severity	*Description of the Process*
First degree	Protrude into the lumen of the anal canal, usually without the sensation of protrusion.
Second degree	Protrude beyond the anal canal during defecation but spontaneously reduce when defecation is completed.
Third degree	Protrude beyond the anal canal during defecation but must be manually reduced after the completion of the bowel movement.
Fourth degree	Protrude beyond the anal canal and are permanently prolapsed despite attempts at manual reduction.

Internal hemorrhoids most often present with rectal bleeding described as bright red streaks on the toilet paper. Patients may report that blood drips into the toilet after a bowel movement. Occasionally the bleeding is sufficient enough to cause anemia, which in any case merits further investigation.

DIAGNOSTIC REASONING

Diagnostic Tests

Initial diagnosis is made by visual inspection of the anal area. Digital rectal examination is not considered an accurate means of diagnosis because most internal hemorrhoids are soft swellings that usually are not palpable, nor are they painful unless they have thrombosed or become infected, or unless a fissure has developed. External hemorrhoids can usually be diagnosed at physical exam, whereas internal hemorrhoids are visible on physical examination only if they have prolapsed.

Definitive diagnosis of internal hemorrhoids requires anoscopy for a proper inspection of the anal canal. With the anoscope in place, the patient is asked to strain as he or she would while having a bowel movement so that the degree of prolapse can be assessed. Patients may undergo proctosigmoidoscopy to effectively rule out any precipitating or coexisting diseases of the colon or rectum.

Differential Diagnosis

The differential diagnosis of hemorrhoids includes polyps, carcinoma of the anus, anorectal fistula, cryptitis, papillitis, or rectal prolapse. Proctosigmoidoscopy is an effective means of establishing the appropriate diagnosis.

MANAGEMENT

Initial treatment for symptomatic external hemorrhoids is focused on adequate pain relief with oral analgesia and sitz baths. If the hemorrhoids do not spontaneously regress, care is directed at decreasing straining with defecation and modification of toilet habits. Patients are encouraged to avoid sitting on the toilet for long periods of time, to use some form of bulk-forming laxative, and to increase their daily fiber intake slowly to 25 to 35 g to establish regular, formed stools. Patients who suffer from diarrhea should be treated accordingly to control frequent loose stools. Individuals who suffer from pruritus should be instructed to maintain anal hygiene. Sitz baths, witch hazel, and application of topical hydrocortisone creams are all effective in controlling pruritus. If the external hemorrhoids continue to be painful or bothersome despite treatment, referral for surgical excision should be made.

Medical treatment of internal hemorrhoids follows the same principles previously outlined, with attention toward avoiding straining during defecation, modification of diet with the addition of fiber, increasing fluids, and the addition of bulking agents. If medical treatment is not effective, other nonsurgical treatments may be employed. First-degree hemorrhoids can be treated by injection sclerotherapy or infrared coagulation. Infrared coagulation, much like electrocoagulation, uses high-intensity light to shrink the swelling. Second- and third-degree hemorrhoids are normally treated with rubber-band ligation, in which a rubber-banded ring is placed around the base of the hemorrhoid. This band acts a tourniquet, strangulating the tissue while fixing the mucosa proximal to the ligation into the muscularis. All of the nonsurgical techniques used to treat internal hemorrhoids are associated with some degree of pain and bleeding.

Large, advanced-degree hemorrhoids will most often require referral to a surgeon for a formal hemorrhoidectomy. Again, proper anal hygiene and correction of chronic constipation and diarrhea are essential to prevent the recurrence of hemorrhoids.

FOLLOW-UP AND REFERRAL

Excision of a single external hemorrhoid, evacuation of a thrombosed external hemorrhoid, and injection sclerotherapy of simple internal hemorrhoids can all be performed in the office by a trained provider. Band ligation and other specialized treatment of hemorrhoids will require referral to a gastroenterologist more familiar with these procedures. Follow-up will be based on the patient's postprocedure course. Most patients will require no further care except for instruction on proper anal hygiene and diet. The addition of a nonirritating laxative after the procedure will usually prevent the development of constipation and the associated fear of defecation.

Patient Education: Hemorrhoids

Patient education for hemorrhoids is aimed at preventing the problem through increasing fiber in the diet. Fiber should be increased to 25 to 35 g/day, but this should be done slowly to

prevent bloating and gas formation. Teaching patients to read food labels can help them gain control over their nutrition. Often, patients associate salad and cereal with very high levels of fiber. This is not accurate information in many cases; for example, most breakfast cereals have only 1 to 3 g of fiber per serving, and iceberg lettuce has very little fiber as well. OTC bulking agents, such as psyllium (Metamucil), can be suggested to help eliminate constipation. It is important to teach patients the necessity of drinking 64 ounces of water a day.

ABDOMINAL HERNIAS

An abdominal hernia is the protrusion of a peritoneally lined sac through some defect or weakened area in the abdominal wall. A history of heavy physical labor or heavy lifting can elicit a hernia. There are several types of hernias, which are usually classified by the anatomical location of the protrusion.

EPIDEMIOLOGY AND CAUSES

It is estimated that up to 10% of the population has some form of hernia. *Groin hernias* are the most common type and are classified as *indirect inguinal hernias,* which are responsible for 50% of hernias treated; *direct inguinal hernias,* which represent 25% of hernias seen; and *femoral hernias,* which represent 10% of hernias. Hernias occurring through the anterior abdominal wall are called *ventral hernias;* these account for only 15% of all hernias. Ventral hernias are further broken down into epigastric hernias (5%), incisional hernias (5%), and umbilical hernias (3%).

Groin hernias are by far the most common type of hernia and occur in both men and women. Indirect inguinal hernias are the most common and occur in both genders, although they are frequently seen in young men. Direct inguinal hernias are more common in men older than age 40 and are caused by a congenital abnormality. Femoral hernias occur more often in women than in men and are rare in children.

The recurrence rate of hernias in general is about 10%, with direct and indirect hernias having a recurrence rate that is approximately equal. The subsequent recurrence rate of recurrent hernias is much higher, at 35%.

Ventral hernias include all other hernias of the anterior abdominal wall. Epigastric hernias are much more common in men than in women and are multiple in 25% of the cases. The peak age of incidence is between ages 20 and 50 years. Umbilical hernias are considered a normal occurrence in newborn infants, with about 20% of infants being affected. These hernias are more common in males of all ages and in African Americans of either gender. The presence of an umbilical hernia is considered normal until the child reaches age 2. Incisional hernias are considered the only iatrogenic type of herniation.

Approximately 2% to 11% of all patients undergoing abdominal surgery develop incisional hernias. Women are affected twice as often as men.

Hernias occur because there is sufficient pressure to force tissue out through a defect in the abdominal wall, as well as a potential space for that protrusion. The etiology of hernias is multifactorial, with biological, congenital, and environmental influences contributing to their development.

PATHOPHYSIOLOGY

In general, for any type of groin hernia to occur, two of the body's protective mechanisms must be overcome. The first is called the *shutter mechanism,* whereby the internal oblique muscle and the transversus abdominis muscles contract to overlap, strengthening the posterior wall of the inguinal canal. Second, a *closure* or *sphincter-type mechanism* causes contraction of the musculature, displacing the transversalis fascia, which in effect decreases the diameter of the deep inguinal ring.

Indirect Inguinal Hernias

Indirect inguinal hernias result when tissue herniates through the internal inguinal ring, which in men extends the length of the spermatic cord. With continued pressure, the sac can reach the scrotum, where it is then palpable just proximal to Hesselbach's triangle. The pathophysiology of indirect inguinal hernias in most cases begins with the herniation of tissue through a still-patent vaginal process that remains after the descent of the testes. In women, the vaginal process exists within the canal of Nuck. Indirect inguinal herniation is caused by a combination of this congenital defect and a disruption in the functioning of the sphincter mechanism as a result of a variety of environmental conditions, including increased abdominal pressure and trauma to the area.

Direct Inguinal Hernias

Direct inguinal hernias occur when the transversus abdominis and internal oblique muscles are attached, forming a high arch on the inferior border that results in a faulty shutter mechanism. Any environmental factors that increase abdominal pressure enhance the chance of herniation. As with indirect inguinal hernias, the presence of this congenital defect does not explain why herniation is more common later in life.

Femoral Hernias

Femoral herniation occurs at the fossa ovalis where the femoral artery exits from the abdomen. It is presumed to be attributable to women's larger femoral canal and smaller iliopsoas muscles. Other factors that contribute to femoral herniation are femoral engorgement during pregnancy and the size of the female pelvis.

Epigastric Hernias

Epigastric hernias occur along the midline between the xiphoid process and the umbilicus. The fibers along the linea alba are brought together in a patchwork-type closure; the defect exists within this decussation. As these fibers weaken, the contents can herniate through the abdomen. Epigastric hernias are three times more likely to occur in men than in women. Peritoneal fat, bowel, and omentum are the most common abdominal contents to protrude through the wall.

Umbilical Hernias

Umbilical hernias that develop in adulthood occur through a weakening in the abdominal wall around the umbilical ring. The herniation of abdominal contents through this defect is also dependent on environmental factors that increase intra-abdominal pressure. Of particular importance when diagnosing an umbilical hernia is to look for underlying ascites secondary to liver disease.

Incisional Hernias

Incisional hernias can occur anywhere along a surgical incision into the abdomen. They are classified into those that cannot be controlled by surgical technique and those that can be controlled by surgical technique. Controllable factors include the type of incision chosen and choice of suture and surgical techniques. Factors that are considered uncontrollable include the prior medical history of the patient, age, steroid use, nutritional status, obesity, and complications of the surgery, especially wound sepsis.

CLINICAL PRESENTATION

Subjective

In any patient presenting with an abdominal hernia, the provider must determine whether there is an abnormal increase in intra-abdominal pressure that has contributed to the herniation. A thorough history and physical exam, with special attention to the genitourinary, respiratory, and GI systems, will provide clues. All male patients who present with an abdominal hernia, regardless of age, require a prostate exam to determine if there is any obstructive process inhibiting urinary output, which in effect increases intra-abdominal pressure. Patients should be evaluated for ascites, which also increases intra-abdominal pressure.

Patients who have respiratory difficulty, such as obstructive pulmonary disease, have an increased risk of hernia because of the increased abdominal pressure associated with coughing and the downward expansion of the diaphragm found with hyperinflated lungs.

Objective

The presentation of inguinal hernias is not always obvious and is quite often an incidental finding on routine exam. Patients may present with complaints of pain while straining or lifting heavy objects or a swelling in the groin area. In general, the physical exam for all groin hernias begins with visual inspection of both groins and the genitalia. With the male patient standing, the spermatic cord is located on both sides and is palpated for any swelling into the scrotum. Once the inguinal canal has been palpated, three additional areas must be examined. After invaginating the scrotal sac, the examining finger follows the spermatic cord up to the external inguinal ring and the fascia of the external oblique muscle. The posterior wall is inspected for weakness or bulging, and the inguinal ring is also palpated for structural soundness. Once these areas have been examined, the provider then withdraws the finger slightly and the patient is asked to cough, which increases the intra-abdominal pressure. If the provider feels the presence of a tissue-like sac tapping against the finger, hernia is present. Other findings indicative of herniation are feeling a rush of fluid (peritoneal) under the examining finger or a patient's report of pain. In a female patient, the femoral areas are palpated while the patient increases intra-abdominal pressure by performing the Valsalva maneuver. Any bulging in the area is considered a positive finding.

Once a groin hernia has been diagnosed, the practitioner must determine whether the hernia is incarcerated or strangulated, both of which require immediate surgical attention, or whether a more chronic situation is present, which can be cared for electively. Most often this can be determined by patient history, as well as the physical ability to reduce the hernia on examination. A strangulated hernia is a nonreducible herniation in which the blood supply to the herniated tissue is compromised. An incarcerated hernia is a hernia that has caused a bowel obstruction as a result of the protrusion.

An indirect inguinal hernia presents as a soft swelling within the internal ring, when either provoked or unprovoked, and often descends into the scrotum. A direct inguinal hernia presents as a bulge around Hesselbach's triangle (Fig. 40.1). Direct inguinal hernias are usually painless and easily reducible. The hernia bulges anteriorly, pushing against the side of the examining finger. Femoral hernias are more common on the right side and may be accompanied by severe pain. There is a palpable bulge through the femoral ring, and the inguinal canal is empty. Normally, it is the intestine that has herniated through the abdominal wall.

Epigastric hernias are normally asymptomatic and present as a small bump or bulge along the midline

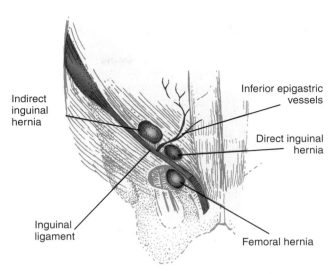

Figure 40.1 Locations of indirect and direct inguinal and femoral hernias. Anterior view of the groin, showing locations of indirect inguinal hernia, direct inguinal hernia, and femoral hernia, based on anatomical landmarks. Source: Kozol AK, Fromm D, Konen JC. *When to call the surgeon: Decision making for primary care providers.* Philadelphia: FA Davis; 1999:170. Reprinted with permission.

above the umbilicus. There may be variation in size with increasing intra-abdominal pressure. Peritoneal fat, omentum, and bowel are usually the tissues that herniate through the abdomen. The smaller hernias tend to be more painful because they involve the herniation of the preperitoneal fat, which is irritating. Larger hernias must be examined for incarceration and obstruction.

Incisional hernias manifest along the incision line of a previous abdominal operation and can be painful. Patients with incisional hernias may also have signs and symptoms of bowel obstruction, which are discussed under Bowel Obstruction later in this chapter.

DIAGNOSTIC REASONING

Diagnostic Tests

Hernias are diagnosed almost exclusively by physical exam findings, as described in the preceding text. On occasion, a radiographic study is necessary to determine if an obstructive process is taking place. Other studies, such as pulmonary function testing or evaluation of a mass or lesion within the abdomen, may be indicated to assess the cause and/or extent of increased intra-abdominal pressure.

Differential Diagnosis

The differential diagnosis list for hernia is limited. It includes hydrocele, psoas abscess, femoral adenopathy or inguinal adenopathy, and ectopic testis.

MANAGEMENT

When a hernia is detected, the patient should be referred to a surgeon. Despite the evolution of hernia repair over the last century, the underlying principles remain the same: reinforce the two natural defense mechanisms discussed previously; decrease the size of the inguinal ring; and strengthen the posterior wall of the canal. Repair of femoral hernias is accomplished by reducing the size of the canal, whereas repair of indirect hernia is accomplished by dissecting the hernial sac and reduction of the repaired tissue. Frequently, there is not sufficient tissue to reconstruct and strengthen the posterior wall of the canal and synthetic mesh materials are used. Laparoscopic surgery has decreased the recovery time and allowed for a single intervention for bilateral hernia repair. All ventral hernias should be repaired to decrease the possibility for incarceration.

Postoperatively, the patient may experience incisional pain, which is relieved by oral analgesics. Pain that persists for more than a few days suggests impending wound infection. Normally, there is slight postoperative swelling, ecchymosis, and erythema of the skin, up to the scrotal area in male patients. Hernia repair with significant scrotal involvement may result in increased scrotal edema, which can be relieved with ice packs, elevation, and wearing a scrotal support. In female patients, swelling is usually limited to the surgical site but may extend to the labia and vulva.

FOLLOW-UP AND REFERRAL

All patients with abdominal hernias require surgical consultation, whether emergently or electively, and appropriate referral should be made. The patient is usually seen in the surgeon's office 3 to 7 days after surgery.

Patient Education: Abdominal Hernias

After typical groin surgery, the patient can return to normal activities, including work, after about 1 week but is instructed to avoid heavy lifting or contact sports for at least 4 to 6 weeks. Patients who have undergone laparoscopic repair of groin hernias can resume regular activities, including heavy lifting, as soon as 2 days postprocedure. Patients who have had a ventral hernia repair should follow routine postoperative instruction as directed by the surgeon.

IRRITABLE BOWEL SYNDROME

IBS is a functional GI disorder characterized by abdominal pain or discomfort and a change in bowel habits. To be considered IBS, two of the following features must be present: abdominal pain or discomfort that is relieved by defecation; change in frequency in stool; and a change in the appearance of the stool. Patients usually have other symptoms such as frequent stools (more than three per day) or fewer stools (less than three per week); passing mucus; feelings of straining, urgency, or incomplete evacuation; flatulence, and abdominal distention. IBS is a common GI problem encountered in primary care. When patients present for medical attention, they have usually had the complex of symptoms for several weeks to several months.

EPIDEMIOLOGY

Traditionally, women have been affected more often than were men, at a rate of 3:1. Recent epidemiological studies, however, suggest that men and women are affected equally, but that men are underdiagnosed based on the current IBS diagnostic criteria. It is estimated that up to 10% of the general population is affected by symptoms that can be classified within the diagnosis of IBS, but fewer than one-third of those individuals seek medical attention. Typically, the symptoms first present in late adolescence and early adulthood but rarely in patients older than age 50 years.

PATHOPHYSIOLOGY

The exact cause of IBS is unknown. IBS was once considered to have no organic cause, but several mechanisms have been identified. Normal bowel function is regulated by segmental contractions that limit the movement of bowel contents through the colon. An increase in these contractions causes constipation, and a decrease in the contractions results in frequent stooling or diarrhea. Myoelectric studies of colonic movement in individuals with IBS were inconclusive for diagnostic criteria, but the studies did demonstrate patterns of hypermotility, including high-amplitude pressure waves in patients, with pain as the predominant symptom during an acute IBS attack. Likewise, patients with diarrhea-predominant IBS had decreased and lower-amplitude pressure waves. Studies have confirmed alterations in colonic activity during periods of emotional stress, in which motility is decreased or inhibited with depression and increased with feelings of hostility and anger.

Another major investigative focus of IBS has centered on visceral hypersensitivity. Approximately 50% of the patients with IBS have perceptual abnormalities including heightened gut sensitivity, leading to a lower tolerance for abdominal pain and distention of the colon with gas and feces. Studies in which the rectums of IBS patients were distended by balloon dilation resulted in spastic contractions, leading to the characteristic symptoms seen with IBS. Patients with IBS are acutely aware of the intraluminal activities occurring with the digestive process. Sensations range from mild discomfort and tugging to frank pain. In summary, IBS patients do show evidence of abnormal colonic smooth muscle activity; however, the level at which the lesion originates is yet unknown.

Up to 10% of patients with IBS develop the disorder after bacterial gastroenteritis. It appears that patients with increased life stressors are more prone to developing IBS postinfection. Although the importance is unknown at this time, increased inflammatory cells have been found in all layers of the bowel in some patients with IBS.

In those patients who seek medical care for symptoms of IBS, about 50% have underlying depression, anxiety, or somatization. These psychological abnormalities my affect how a person reacts to visceral sensations and to changes in bowel habits. Chronic stress may also affect the nervous system processing of visceral sensations and may alter GI motility.

The correlation between the symptoms of IBS and food intolerance is high. Careful diet history is necessary to distinguish between the two. The most common dietary triggers are lactose, fructose, sorbitol, and glutens.

CLINICAL PRESENTATION

Subjective

Individuals with IBS typically present with symptoms that fall into two broad categories—those with abdominal pain and altered bowel habits, consisting of both diarrhea and constipation, and those with painless diarrhea.

Most patients with abdominal pain describe their pain as originating over some area of the colon, with the left lower quadrant (LLQ) being most often affected. The pain can be sharp and burning with cramping or a diffuse, dull ache. The description of the pain usually remains constant for the individual but can vary greatly among the patient population. Pain is often precipitated by eating or stress and can be relieved with a bowel movement or passing of flatus. The pain associated with IBS is usually not significant enough to interfere with sleeping, nor is it great enough to wake the patient from sleep.

More than 50% of patients with IBS describe an overly acute sensory ability with regard to the GI tract and the digestive process. This visceral hypersensitivity is manifested by frequent complaints of abdominal distention, gas, and belching. Many of these symptoms occur 2 hours after having a meal and are often thought to be food intolerances. Patients typically complain of urgency to defecate, abdominal pain, bloating, and gas. Some patients with IBS have upper GI complaints, including dyspepsia, pyrosis, nausea, and vomiting.

Patients who present with painless diarrhea usually report an urgent need to defecate immediately on awakening or after eating. Although diarrhea rarely occurs nocturnally, urgency is so great that it may cause incontinence.

Alteration in bowel habits is the most consistently reported symptom. The typical presentation is diarrhea alternating with constipation. Patients report that constipation that was once responsive to laxatives has become continuous and that the stool has become harder and is decreased in caliber. Many patients complain of a sense of incomplete evacuation and thus repeated attempts at defecation are necessary within a short period of time. Periods of predominant constipation can last for months, interrupted by periods of diarrhea and then back to constipation. Patients who have diarrhea as their predominant symptom complain of frequent, low-volume (less than 200 mL), loose stools. Diarrhea does not normally occur at night; however, it can be exacerbated by eating or stress. Many patients report the passage of large volumes of mucus within the stool. This differs from the mucus occurring with colitis because there is no associated inflammatory process nor is there any blood in the stool, other than if there is an incidental finding of hemorrhoids.

Patients diagnosed with IBS frequently have an associated psychiatric diagnosis, which presents in the form of anxiety, depression, and somatoform disorders. A recent stressful life event often precipitates IBS symptoms such as marital discord, death, or abuse.

Objective

As with any illness, a thorough and detailed patient history is the key to definitive diagnosis. The physical exam is usually normal except for tenderness in some area of the colon, most often the LLQ and over the umbilicus or epigastric area in those with small bowel involvement. Digital rectal exam is normal but may reveal tenderness and exacerbate symptoms in some individuals.

There is usually no associated weight loss or deterioration in health. History of psychosocial stressors can often be correlated with the onset of symptoms. Key to diagnosis is the lack of other systemic symptoms such as fever, leukocytosis, or bloody stools, which might suggest an organic cause for symptoms.

DIAGNOSTIC REASONING

Diagnostic Tests

IBS is diagnosed based on a careful history and physical that reveals the characteristic increase in bowel symptoms with the onset of pain, relief of pain with defecation, heightened sensation of bowel activity, or sense of incomplete defecation. The criteria used for diagnosing IBS are provided in Advanced Assessment 40.1.

Initial laboratory testing should include CBC, erythrocyte sedimentation rate (ESR), chemistry panel including electrolytes and serum amylase, urinalysis, and stools for occult blood, ova and parasites, and cultures. Any abnormal lab value should prompt further investigation in the direction of the abnormal finding because most laboratory studies in the patient with IBS are normal and any diagnostic clue as to the cause is helpful. If white blood cells (WBCs) are found in the stool, it suggests an infectious or inflammatory process and not IBS.

Advanced Assessment 40.1: Criteria for Diagnosing Irritable Bowel Syndrome

Abdominal pain or discomfort that is consistently relieved by defecation or has been associated with a change in the frequency or a change in the consistency of the stool for a period of 3 months either continuously or recurrently within that time frame
AND
Defecation with varying patterns of constipation and diarrhea 25% of the time
AND
Two or more of the following:

Altered stool frequency
Altered stool form including hard, loose, watery, mucoid
Altered sensory act of defecation including straining, urgency, tenesmus
Passage of mucus
Varied degrees of bloating and abdominal distention

 Differential Diagnosis 40.1: Irritable Bowel Syndrome

Food intolerance

- Lactase deficiencies
- Caffeine
- Fermentable carbohydrates
- Artificial sweeteners

Fat or bile acid intolerances
Pathogen-precipitated processes

- Intestinal parasites
- Bacterial overgrowth

Medication-induced alterations in bowel motility

- Laxative abuse
- Magnesium-based antacids
- Antibiotics
- Opiate analgesics

Fuctional upper gastrointestinal (GI) disorders

- Dyspepsia
- Pyrosis
- Gastroesophageal reflux disease
- Peptic ulcer disease
- Cholelithiasis
- Biliary pain
- GI malignancy

Functional lower GI disorders

- Inflammatory bowel disease
- Crohn's disease
- Ulcerative colitis
- Diverticulitis
- Intestinal obstruction
- Hemorrhoids
- Lower GI malignancy
- Ascites

Endocrine disorders

- Hypothyroidism
- Hyperthyroidism
- Autonomic diabetic neuropathy

Psychological disorders

- Depression
- Anxiety

Flexible proctosigmoidoscopy enables the provider to see up to 60 cm of the colon. No abnormalities are seen with IBS with the possible exception of an increased volume of mucus; however, increased tenderness and spasm may inhibit passage of the scope beyond 15 cm. Patients who present for initial treatment at age 40 or older should also be given a colonoscopy.

Food intolerances should be ruled out, especially in patients who present with diarrhea and gas as predominant symptoms. Lactase deficiency can be identified with a hydrogen breath test or lactose tolerance test. Other intolerances are identified by removing the most common causative agents from the diet for 3 weeks and then slowly reintroducing them to the diet one at a time.

IBS is no longer a diagnosis of exclusion; thus, the practitioner must direct diagnostic testing as information is received and lends itself toward an organic cause of the symptoms. Patients should not be subjected to endless batteries of expensive and uncomfortable tests in search of an organic disease. Laboratory findings that support a cause other than IBS include elevated ESR, anemia, leukocytosis, blood or WBCs in the stool, or stool volumes greater than 300 mL.

Differential Diagnosis

The differential diagnosis of IBS can include any of the processes in Differential Diagnosis 40.1, with emphasis on the organic GI disorders. Most of the disease processes can be ruled out with careful history and physical exam. Patients presenting with diarrhea as the dominant symptom should have thyroid function tests, 24-hour stool check for fecal fat, and stool weight and stool testing for laxative content. Patients who present with constipation as their predominant symptom may require referral to a specialist who can measure colonic transit time. A careful medication history is necessary for either presentation.

Patients with epigastric pain must have the pain differentiated from that produced by biliary tract pain, ulcerative disease, or malignancies of the stomach and pancreas.

MANAGEMENT

The initial step to successful management of IBS is making the diagnosis and then identifying the symptom pattern for each individual patient. Based on the symptom pattern of each patient, therapy may include diet, education, and pharmacological and supportive interventions. The patient with IBS requires reassurance and guidance throughout the course of the disease and a therapeutic relationship between the provider and the patient can reduce symptomatology. Patients must understand that there is no proven treatment and that the therapy is often symptomatic. Much of the recent literature suggests that there is a high degree of placebo effect with varying treatments.

A careful diet history is important in identifying foods that may precipitate symptoms. IBS is often confused with lactose intolerance and can be evaluated by removing lactose from the diet for 2 weeks and monitoring the symptoms. Other foods that are frequently identified in producing IBS syndromes include caffeine, legumes (and other fermentable carbohydrates), and artificial sweeteners. If any foods are identified that provoke symptoms, they should be eliminated from the diet. Patients who seem to suffer from postprandial discomfort may alleviate symptoms by eating a lower-fat diet that contains more protein. Dietary consultation can be helpful in assisting patients in developing a diet program that is palatable to them.

Diets high in fiber are beneficial regardless of predominant bowel habit. Patients are encouraged to increase their fiber intake to 20 to 30 grams per day. The hydrophilic properties of fiber or bulk-producing agents help to prevent excessive hydration or dehydration of stool; thus, fiber is indicated for both diarrhea and constipation symptom presentations. Foods high in fiber include whole grains, cereals, fruits, and vegetables; however, they must be introduced slowly for IBS patients to avoid the sensation of bloating. Bulk-producing agents can be substituted for individuals who choose not to change their diet. Commercially prepared bulk-producing agents are started once a day and increased gradually to three to four times daily. Patients are encouraged to continue treatment for at least 2 months before termination to allow the bowel to adjust to the bulking agents. All patients should try to drink at least eight 8-ounce glasses of water per day. Individuals with constipation as their predominant symptom should be aware that fiber-bulking agents are not overnight laxatives, and they should not abandon this therapy because they did not get overnight results.

There is a moderate level of evidence indicating the use of probiotics is effective for patients with IBS. There are several mechanisms of probiotics in IBS proposed. Probiotics increase the mass of beneficial bacteria in the gut. Some research has shown that some lactobacilli strains may induce the expression of μ-opioid and cannabinoid receptors in the intestinal mucosal barrier thereby modulating intestinal pain. Probiotics may also reduce intestinal permeability and bacterial translocation. The probiotic that seems to have the best results in multiple clinical trials is VSL#3, one packet orally twice a day and *Bifidobacterium infantis*, one tablet orally twice a day.

Pharmacological treatment is reserved for patients with moderate to severe symptoms and is directed at specific symptoms. Antidiarrheal medications are used only as a temporary measure. When the diarrhea is severe, episodic use of loperamide (Imodium) 2 mg or diphenoxylate (Lomotil) 2.5–5.0 mg every 6 hours can be used as needed. Patients who anticipate stressful situations can use antidiarrhea medications prophylactically.

Patients with constipation who have not responded to a high-fiber diet, hydration, exercise, and bulking agents may benefit from intermittent use of stimulant laxatives such as lactulose or magnesium hydroxide. Long-term use of laxatives is discouraged.

Antispasmodic agents have been used successfully in controlling abdominal pain caused by intestinal spasm. Patients who suffer with postprandial pain not responsive to diet therapy can benefit from dicyclomine 10 to 20 mg three to four times a day by mouth or hyoscyamine 0.125 to 0.75 mg twice a day. Anticholinergics should be avoided in patients with glaucoma and benign prostatic hypertrophy because of the adverse effects and used with caution in the elderly.

Tricyclic antidepressants and selective serotonin reuptake inhibitors have been shown to relieve symptoms in some individuals. Individuals with IBS need reassurance and understanding that their disease is chronic. They often benefit from support groups and counseling. Psychiatric interventions that teach behavior modification and biofeedback or that can provide psychotherapy or hypnosis are helpful alternative measures for patients with refractory IBS.

FOLLOW-UP AND REFERRAL

The emotional support provided by regular follow-up appointments is important in the management of patients with IBS. A strong, honest relationship with the patient is necessary to allay fears and prevent unrealistic expectations of the patient regarding his or her disease. Follow-up is important to encourage preventive behaviors including high-fiber diet, regular exercise, and avoidance of foods that precipitate symptoms. Patients who are not responding to treatment should be referred to a gastroenterologist.

Patients who have IBS are often dissatisfied with treatment because no organic cause of their symptoms can be found. A second opinion is helpful in the management of these individuals; however, they must also be discouraged from continuing to search for organic causes for their symptoms. Referral for psychological intervention tends to be more helpful in patients with intermittent symptoms; those with chronic pain or intractable symptoms usually respond poorly.

Patient Education: Irritable Bowel Syndrome

Care of patients with IBS requires a positive and honest practitioner–patient relationship. Education is important in reducing the number of return visits for symptoms common to patients with IBS. The patients should understand that they have a real intestinal disorder, which is characterized by hypersensitivity to certain foods, hormonal changes, and stressors. Patients should be taught how to recognize these triggers and how to avoid or diminish their effects. Patients should understand that they have a chronic disease but that they do not have a shorter life expectancy because of it. A thorough understanding of the treatment regimen and setting realistic goals regarding treatment is the key to building a positive relationship with the patient. Patients must understand that the goal of treatment is to improve their symptoms, not cure the disease, and that improvement in symptoms can be a time-consuming process.

Dietary education is paramount to relief of the symptoms. Increasing fiber and water intake is an important component of the treatment. Teaching patients how to read nutrition labels will help them to quantify the amount of fiber they are consuming daily. Patients must be encouraged to take an active role in their treatment program and to understand that elimination of foods that trigger symptoms can be time consuming and requires their careful attention.

Establishing good bowel habits is also important in the treatment of IBS. A high-fiber diet and increasing water intake to eight 8-ounce glasses per day can help in maintaining a regular bowel program. Patients who suffer with constipation should avoid laxatives and instead practice bowel training. Allowing adequate time after breakfast to sit on the toilet without straining can help establish a daily schedule.

Helping patients recognize and understand environmental stressors that trigger symptoms should be included in patient education. Involving the patient's family is important in establishing a support system. A resource available to patients for both education and support is the International Foundation for Bowel Dysfunction (see Resources).

CELIAC DISEASE

Celiac disease, also known as gluten-sensitive enteropathy or celiac sprue, is a gluten-sensitive autoimmune disorder that affects the small intestinal villous epithelium in individuals with a genetic predisposition and exposure to the cereal protein gluten (gliadin) in wheat, rye, and barley.

EPIDEMIOLOGY AND CAUSES

Celiac disease is a multisystem autoimmune disease caused by an immunologic response to gluten. Once thought of as a disease in children, the majority of cases are diagnosed in adulthood. The estimated prevalence in adults is between 0.40% to 0.95%. Serologic testing indicates that 1:100 whites of Northern European descent have the disease but only 10% have had the diagnosis made. It is likely that the incidence and prevalence is much higher. Risk factors for celiac disease include a family history of celiac disease, Down's syndrome, HLA-DQ2 or HLA-DQ8, Turner's syndrome, or other genetic based autoimmune disease such as type 1 diabetes mellitus and thyroiditis.

PATHOPHYSIOLOGY

Celiac disease is a disorder involving the complex interaction of genetic, immune, and environmental factors. The immune reaction is mainly T-cell-mediated, although a humoral immune reaction occurs as well. Celiac disease only develops in people with the haplotype HLA-DQ2 (95%) or HLA-DQ8 (5%). The pathogenesis remains unclear, since 40% of the population has HLA-DQ2 or -DQ8. In susceptible individuals, there is an environmental trigger (gluten) that causes T-cell-mediated autoimmune injury to the intestinal epithelial cells. Anti-gliadin, anti-endomysium, and anti-tTG IgA antibodies develop in the presence of gluten. T-cells destroy the mucosal cells causing inflammation, atrophy, and flattening of the small intestinal villi, usually in the duodenum and jejunum; however, the ileum can be involved as well. The brush border disappears and there is a decrease in the surface area for nutrient absorption. It should be noted that patients with celiac disease have a threefold increased risk of developing non-Hodgkin's lymphoma.

CLINICAL PRESENTATION

Subjective

Many patients are asymptomatic. Patients may complain of diarrhea, weight loss, dyspepsia, and flatulence. Atypical complaints may be fatigue (resulting from anemia), joint pain, and depressed mood; in women, amenorrhea, difficulty getting pregnant, and early menopause may occur.

Objective

The physical exam may be normal. In severe cases, there may be signs of malabsorption such as muscle wasting, pallor (anemia), reduced subcutaneous fat, ataxia, and peripheral neuropathy (vitamin B_{12} deficiency). Dermatitis herpetiformis occurs as a cutaneous variant of celiac disease in less than 10% of patients. Patients presenting with dermatitis herpetiformis almost always have signs of celiac disease on intestinal biopsy.

DIAGNOSTIC REASONING

Diagnostic Tests

When a patient is suspected of having celiac disease, serologic testing for anti-tTG IgA antibodies should be done. This test is inexpensive and has a high sensitivity and specificity. A total IgA should be done as well because 2% of patients with celiac disease also have an IgA deficiency and will test falsely negative. The only way to assess the extent of damage to the intestinal mucosa is through upper GI endoscopic small bowel biopsy and histologic examination. This may show partial or complete villous atrophy and intraepithelial lymphocytes.

In lieu of definitive testing and in those with very mild symptoms, patients may try a gluten-free diet and evaluate for symptom improvement. For those already on a gluten-free diet, serology may be normal. In these cases, a gluten challenge can be attempted and the appearance of symptoms evaluated as well as serologic markers determined.

The clinician should consider testing for nutritional deficiencies associated with the malabsorption related to celiac disease. These include hemoglobin, iron, folate, vitamin B_{12}, calcium, and vitamin D.

Differential Diagnosis

Patients with chronic diarrhea, abdominal bloating, and flatulence are often misdiagnosed with IBS. Other diseases that can cause malabsorption of nutrients should be excluded such as IBDs (Crohn's disease, ulcerative colitis, and microscopic colitis). Symptoms of celiac disease mimic lactose intolerance and should be considered.

MANAGEMENT

The treatment of choice for patients with celiac disease is a strict gluten-free diet. A referral to a dietician or nutritionist who specializes in celiac disease is helpful. The risk of developing non-Hodgkin's lymphoma is reduced if the patient can maintain the strict gluten-free diet for more than 5 years. A gluten-free diet usually reduces symptoms and eliminates mucosal damage. For patients who do not have a robust response to a gluten-free diet, other sources of gluten intake should be investigated, such as medications. A dietician specializing in celiac disease can assist the patient to be sure of complete removal of gluten. Some patients may require more aggressive treatment with immunomodulating agents.

FOLLOW-UP AND REFERRAL

Patients suspected of having celiac disease should be referred to a gastroenterologist for definitive diagnosis and once that is made, they should see a dietitian specializing in celiac disease. Patients should be monitored for the development of complications or other diseases associated with celiac disease including Addison's disease, Graves's disease, type 1 diabetes mellitus, myasthenia gravis, scleroderma, atrophic gastritis, and pancreatic insufficiency.

Patient Education: Celiac Disease

Patient education about gluten-free diets is essential to preventing the cellular changes that lead to malabsorption of nutrients. This is best done by a dietitian who specializes in celiac disease. With the expansion of gluten-free products on the market, there is concern about contamination with gluten in processing, and minimizing the use of highly processed, convenience foods should be encouraged.

BOWEL OBSTRUCTION

Bowel obstruction is the consequence of any condition that inhibits the normal flow of chyme through the intestinal lumen. It can be complete or partial and can involve any segment of the large or small bowel. Bowel obstruction is considered simple when it results from a mechanical blockage or functional (paralytic ileus) when there is a disruption in motility.

EPIDEMIOLOGY AND CAUSES

Intestinal obstruction can be classified according to the onset. Acute obstruction is sudden and can be caused by torsion, herniation, or intussusception (the slipping of a proximal piece of intestine into the part below it). Chronic obstruction usually indicates a slow, gradual process, often from tumor growth or strictures. Obstructions are also classified according to the degree of obstruction, either complete or partial, and the location of the obstructing lesion. Obstructions can develop within the lumen, as in the case of foreign bodies, tumors, or intraluminal fibrosis. This type of obstruction is considered intrinsic. Conversely, they can be extrinsic or from obstruction that arises outside the intestine. For example, intussusception, torsion (volvulus), fibrosis, and hernia can all cause intestinal obstructions from outside the bowel. Another aspect in the classification of intestinal obstruction is the effect it has on the intestinal wall. A simple obstruction indicates that there is no impairment of the blood supply to that portion of the intestine. A strangulated obstruction means that the lumen is obstructed and the blood supply is compromised. Bowel obstruction can be a complication of adhesions, which are fibrous bands of tissue that develop after a surgical procedure.

PATHOPHYSIOLOGY

There are numerous physiological alterations resulting from an intestinal obstruction related to the onset, location of the obstruction, and the amount of intestine proximal to the obstruction. Immediately after the obstruction begins, there is distention of the intestine with sequestration of fluid and gas proximal to the obstruction. The gas is a result of bacterial fermentation and swallowed air. When the intestine begins to distend, its ability to absorb water and electrolytes decreases and more is left in the lumen, adding to the distention. Sources of water and electrolytes include saliva, gastric juice, bile, and pancreatic juice, as well as intestinal secretions. Within 24 hours, as much as 8 L can accumulate in the intestinal lumen, leading to vomiting. Because of the vomiting and sequestration of fluid and electrolytes in the intestinal lumen, profound fluid and electrolyte imbalances result, leading to dehydration, hemoconcentration, and ultimately hypovolemic shock. The increasing distention causes pressure on the diaphragm, thereby reducing the respiratory volume leading to atelectasis and pneumonia.

Depending on the location and stage of the intestinal obstruction, alkalosis or acidosis is possible. Alkalosis occurs early in intestinal obstruction or if the obstruction is in the proximal portion of the small bowel. This occurs because gastric juice, which is high in hydrogen ions, does not get absorbed through the intestinal lumen, resulting in loss of the ion. However, later in the course of obstruction, or if the obstruction is more distal, acidosis occurs because alkaline pancreatic secretions and bile cannot be reabsorbed. Potassium is sequestered in the intraluminal fluid, causing hypokalemia, which promotes acidosis and atony of the intestinal wall.

As pressure within the intestinal lumen increases, arterial blood flow may be compromised leading to ischemia, necrosis, perforation, and peritonitis. Metabolic acidosis is compounded by the buildup of lactic acid that results from the decreased arterial blood flow. Venous return is reduced leading to edema within the bowel wall. As the edema progresses, there is an increase in capillary permeability causing fluid to be lost into the peritoneum, contributing to the hypovolemia already present.

CLINICAL PRESENTATION

Subjective

In general, patients with obstruction generally complain of a sudden onset of colicky abdominal pain accompanied by nausea and vomiting. The pain is usually intermittent and corresponds to peristaltic waves. Patients with obstruction at the jejunum or below may have emesis that has changed to a brownish, feculent type material. They may complain of initial bouts of diarrhea, but this is soon followed by constipation.

In the later stages of obstruction, patients may have constipation and lack of flatulence. It is important to obtain information regarding previous abdominal operations, which may help in the diagnosis of intestinal obstruction. The abdominal pain of small bowel obstruction is usually centered about the umbilicus or in the epigastric area, and vomiting usually occurs early in the disease process. If the arterial circulation to the bowel is compromised, the pain becomes more constant and severe. Perforation produces severe generalized abdominal pain, as well as the classic signs of peritonitis.

Objective

The physical exam should include careful inspection for abdominal scars and the presence of hernias. The patient may show signs of dehydration including poor skin turgor, dry mucous membranes, sunken eyeballs, and tachycardia. Blood pressure may be elevated depending on the degree of pain and if there is evidence of strangulation and subsequent ischemia. The degree of abdominal distention depends on the level of obstruction. The more distal the obstruction, the greater the length of proximal intestine producing greater distention. Also, if the obstruction is in the distal portion of the intestine, vomiting may occur only late in the course of the disease. The abdomen may be tender to palpation if strangulation is present. Bowel sounds are high pitched and hyperactive; they may be accompanied by rushes, which coincide with the colicky abdominal pain. Patients with strangulation tend to have increased distention, abdominal tenderness, tympany to percussion, and hypoactive or absent bowel sounds. Sometimes a mass is palpable. If perforation has occurred, there may be a short period of pain relief, which is soon followed by increased pain, rebound tenderness, and fever, all suggestive of peritonitis.

Patients presenting with large bowel obstruction usually have a more gradual onset of symptoms, beginning with increasing constipation and abdominal distention. Large bowel obstruction is rare in patients younger than age 50. Lower abdominal cramps are unproductive of feces and are painful. Patients report a several-day history of no stools or flatus production. Vomiting occurs if there is an incompetent ileocecal valve or if there is a resultant superimposed, small bowel obstruction. The most common cause of large bowel obstruction is carcinoma of the sigmoid colon or diverticulosis.

Physical exam findings include a distended abdomen, particularly over the transverse and descending colon, with the presence of borborygmi. Patients are normally afebrile unless diverticulitis is suspected. There is usually no abdominal tenderness or guarding unless there are areas of ischemic bowel or associated small bowel obstruction with impending cecal perforation. A mass may be palpable over the area of obstruction. Rectal exam reveals an empty vault without tenderness unless there are obstructing rectal carcinomas. The systemic manifestations of large bowel obstructions are much less serious than those caused by small bowel obstruction.

DIAGNOSTIC REASONING

Diagnostic Tests

Before diagnostic testing, patients must be thoroughly examined for any type of hernia that may be precipitating the obstruction. Diagnosis of small bowel obstruction is usually confirmed by supine and upright abdominal x-ray films that reveal a ladder-like distention of the small bowel. Upright films show multiple air-fluid levels within the loops of small bowel, which are the hallmark of small bowel obstruction. Findings indicative of other causes of small bowel obstruction are evidence of a foreign body or an actual mass suggestive of infarcted bowel. Oral contrast with small bowel follow-through can identify areas of partial obstruction. Oral barium studies are contraindicated and must be avoided unless large bowel obstruction has been ruled out.

Laboratory studies include CBC and chemistry profile but are rarely useful for the diagnosis. Leukocytosis can indicate impending ischemia or strangulation of the bowel but is not diagnostic of such. Chemistry evaluation can help with proper fluid and electrolyte replacement. Serum amylase may be elevated and can lead to the erroneous diagnosis of pancreatitis. A finding of metabolic acidosis or an elevated lactic acid is highly suggestive of intestinal infarction.

Abdominal x-ray films of patients with large bowel obstruction usually show distention of the intestine down to the level of the obstruction. It is important to note the size of the cecum because as the diameter approaches 14 cm, the danger of perforation is imminent. If air is noted under the diaphragm, it is likely that perforation of the cecum or sigmoid colon has occurred.

Differential Diagnosis

The differential diagnosis of small and large bowel obstruction is presented in Differential Diagnosis 40.2. Volvulus, a twisting of the bowel on itself, can happen suddenly, with loss of blood supply to the area and subsequent ischemia. Cecal volvulus presents as a large gas bubble within the midabdomen or left upper quadrant on abdominal x-ray film. A volvulus of the sigmoid colon usually occurs only in older adults. It typically appears as a "coffee bean" dilation arising from the pelvis. For both cecal and sigmoidal volvulus, a barium enema is done to reveal the precise location of the obstruction.

Colonoscopy and endoscopy are contraindicated in patients suspected of mechanical bowel obstruction because to visualize the intestine, air must be introduced into the colon and can increase the chance of perforation.

MANAGEMENT

All patients with suspected intestinal obstruction should be hospitalized and immediately referred to a surgeon. Therapy must be administered as definitive diagnosis is

 Differential Diagnosis 40.2: Bowel Obstruction

Pseudo-obstruction
Toxic megacolon
Twisting of a loop of bowel

- Cecal volvulus
- Sigmoid volvulus

Incarcerated or strangulated hernias

- Abdominal
- Femoral
- Inguinal

Kinking of a loop of bowel

- Adhesions secondary to previous abdominal surgery

Concentric narrowing of the lumen of the intestine

- Neoplasms
- Diverticulitis
- Crohn's disease

Foreign body

- Gallstones
- Ingested objects

Intussusception
Paralytic ileus

being obtained. Most patients with a bowel obstruction will require placement of a nasogastric tube to decrease passage of secretions, aid in decompression, and ameliorate vomiting if present. Rehydration with IV fluids and replacement of electrolytes should be done as indicated by laboratory studies. Placement of an indwelling urinary catheter is necessary to monitor urine output accurately, which is recorded on a daily intake and output sheet.

Treatment of small bowel obstruction proceeds after the aforementioned therapies have been instituted and the patient is medically stabilized. Patients with upper small bowel obstruction are prone to alkalosis and hypokalemia caused by emesis; they must be monitored carefully and given IV fluid and electrolyte replacement as necessary. All medications that can decrease intestinal motility, including anticholinergics, narcotics, and calcium channel blockers, should be discontinued. If strangulation is suspected, the patient should be started on broad-spectrum antibiotic therapy, which provides coverage for anaerobic and gram-negative organisms. Laparotomy is indicated for all patients with complete bowel obstruction.

Patients with a large bowel obstruction are rehydrated and stabilized as previously described. If the patient has evidence suggestive of sigmoidal volvulus, an initial attempt to reduce the volvulus can be made with sigmoidoscopy, but surgery is required if that attempt is unsuccessful. Patients with Crohn's disease, intestinal lymphoma, or diverticulitis with subsequent concentric narrowing of the intestinal lumen may be given a trial of medical therapy specific to the disease process in an attempt to relieve the obstruction before surgical intervention.

Obstructing carcinomas can be treated with surgical resection and anastomosis. (Colon cancer is discussed later in this chapter.) If fecal impaction has been identified as the cause, it can often be removed digitally. If the impaction is barium and is located within the sigmoid colon, open laparotomy is required for removal. Adhesions can be relieved by surgical intervention; however, the chances are great that they will recur. Hernia reduction is indicated if this is the determined cause of obstruction. All patients who have undergone surgical intervention as definitive therapy must be monitored for paralytic ileus postoperatively.

FOLLOW-UP AND REFERRAL

All patients with suspected bowel obstruction must be referred to a surgeon, who will manage the patient's hospitalization and postoperative care. The prognosis of appropriately treated simple intestinal obstruction is good, with a mortality rate of less than 2%. If strangulation is suspected and intervention is delayed, the mortality rate can be as high as 25%.

Because patients are usually acutely ill, postoperative teaching should be delayed until the patient is more receptive to instruction. Initial follow-up visits should be with the consulting surgeon, who will direct the patient's care until the patient is released to his or her primary-care provider.

Patient Education: Bowel Obstruction

Follow-up of patients with bowel obstruction will be guided by the surgeon. Instructions on care of the incision, including dressing changes and signs and symptoms of infection, are provided before discharge from the hospital. Once the patient has been cleared by the collaborating surgeon, he or she will return to the primary-care setting. Patients should be instructed to report any recurrent abdominal pain with or without vomiting, fever, or problems regarding bowel function. Laxatives should not be taken without consulting the primary-care provider first. Stool softeners are prescribed as needed, and patients are encouraged to avoid foods that cause constipation. Patients should refrain from strenuous activity for at least 6–8 weeks.

DIVERTICULAR DISEASE

Diverticular disease is the term used to describe the inflammatory changes that occur within the diverticular mucosa of the intestine (diverticulitis), as well as the asymptomatic, uninflamed outpouchings called diverticulosis. Diverticula are pouchlike protrusions of the intestinal mucosa that occur most often within the descending and sigmoid segments of the colon. They decrease in frequency in the cecum and rarely are found in the rectum. Diverticula occur infrequently in the small bowel. There are two types, congenital and acquired. Congenital diverticula are situated on the antimesenteric margin of the bowel and consist of the intestinal wall layers. Acquired diverticula occur on the mesenteric margin of the bowel, where the blood vessels enter the bowel wall. A diverticulosis of the small bowel may cause malabsorption and steatorrhea. Diverticula tend to form at weakened areas of the intestinal wall, usually where arterial vessels perforate the colon. The inner layer of these pouchlike protrusions forms a narrow neck, which is continuous with the inner layer of the colon, and the sac herniates through the muscle wall. Most diverticula are asymptomatic and pose a problem only when they become inflamed or bleed. Most diverticula are found incidentally with endoscopy or barium enema (BE). Diverticula vary in size from 3 mm to 3 cm in diameter.

EPIDEMIOLOGY AND CAUSES

Diverticula are uncommon (less than 20%) in individuals younger than age 40, with the prevalence increasing steadily after that. The prevalence increases to 60% by age 60 years. Diverticular disease is more common in developed nations than in less-developed countries, with estimates of 5% to 45% in Western populations. The incidence is 2,200 to 3,000 per 100,000 people, occurring equally among men and woman. Diverticula are a rare finding in pediatric patients.

Although there is no known cause for diverticular disease, a low-fiber diet has been implicated because it causes increased intraluminal pressures within the colon, which lead to mucosal herniation through the weaker areas in the bowel wall. Dietary fiber and eating a vegetarian diet reduce the incidence of symptomatic disease. In a large study (47,000 men), diverticular disease was significantly increased in those with a diet that is low in fiber and high in total fat or red meat. Obesity is associated with a higher risk for diverticular disease as well as increased risk for diverticular bleeding. Other factors believed to contribute to the formation of diverticula include hypertrophy of the segments of the circular muscle of the colon, chronic constipation and straining, irregular and uncoordinated bowel contractions, and weakness of the bowel muscle brought on by aging. Risk factors are directly related to the suspected causes of the disease: age older than 40 years, low-fiber diet, previous diverticulitis, and the number of diverticula present within the colon. Diverticula occur most often in the sigmoid colon; a right lower quadrant presentation is a rare condition, with a higher incidence in Asian populations.

PATHOPHYSIOLOGY

The exact cause of diverticulosis is unknown; therefore, the pathophysiology is based on the speculative findings already mentioned. As a consequence of increased ingestion of refined foods and decreased fiber intake, the stool bulk is decreased and the colon transit time is increased, leading to the development of diverticula. Diverticula are thought to result from the increased pressure produced with the segmental contraction of the muscular portion of the wall of the colon. This increased pressure causes the herniation of the bowel wall through the weaker points in the muscle layer of the colon, normally occurring along the teniae at the penetration site of the colonic vasculature. Inflammation occurring around the diverticular sac is often caused by the retention of undigested food and bacteria, which when formed into a hardened mass is called a *fecalith.* This mass in turn can disrupt the blood flow and lead to abscess formation. When the opening of this saclike projection becomes occluded and inflammation ensues, it can progress to the point of rupture. Acute diverticulitis is the result of this localized inflammation within the wall of the colon or peritoneum, causing the characteristic LLQ abdominal pain and tenderness. If the perforation is not localized, the patient can develop acute peritonitis and septic shock.

Fistula formation following acute diverticulitis is the result of a tract forming between the colon and other structures within the abdomen. These fistulas include colovesicular fistulas (urinary bladder), colovaginal fistulas (vagina), entero-enteric fistulas (loop of bowel), and colocutaneous fistulas (peritoneal tissue). Pericolitis is inflammation around the colon, which can result in fibrous strictures and obstruction.

Bleeding is a common complication of diverticulosis and is the most common cause of substantial lower GI bleeding. Postbleeding examinations have discovered that most bleeding occurs from uninflamed rather than inflamed diverticula.

CLINICAL PRESENTATION

Subjective

Approximately 25% of patients with diverticular disease develop symptoms. Patients with diverticulosis characteristically present with pain in the LLQ of the abdomen. Some patients report that the pain is worse after eating, which may be a result of colonic distention, and that the pain is sometimes relieved with a bowel movement or passing flatus. Elimination patterns may alternate between diarrhea and constipation, and there may be associated abdominal distention and tenderness. Diverticulitis may present with bleeding, which can be massive and is not associated with pain or discomfort.

When the diverticula become inflamed, there are the usual signs and symptoms of infection—fever, chills, and tachycardia. Patients typically present with localized pain and tenderness in the LLQ of the abdomen with associated anorexia, nausea, and vomiting. If there is fistula formation, there are symptoms associated with the particular organ involved. Patients may complain of dysuria, pneumaturia (passage of air in the urine), and/or fecaluria (passage of fecal matter in the urine) if there is fistula formation involving the bladder. Patients may be concerned about the development of hematochezia or frank bleeding from the rectum.

Objective

A physical exam reveals tenderness in the LLQ of the abdomen, and—if the patient can tolerate more vigorous examination—a firm, fixed mass may be identified in the area of the diverticula. Patients may have rebound tenderness with involuntary guarding and rigidity. Bowel sounds may initially be hypoactive or can be hyperactive if an obstructive process has developed. Examination of the rectum may reveal tenderness, and the stool is usually positive for occult blood.

DIAGNOSTIC REASONING

Diagnostic Tests

Initial laboratory testing can show mild to moderate leukocytosis, depending on whether the patient presents with diverticulitis or with a more advanced inflammatory process such as peritoneal abscess. The WBC count is usually normal in patients with diverticulosis. Hemoglobin and hematocrit may be low if there is associated rectal bleeding. If there is fistula formation between the diverticula and the bladder, urinalysis may show elevated levels of both WBCs and red blood cells, and urine culture may be positive. Patients with signs suggestive of peritonitis should have a blood culture to assess for bacteremia.

Abdominal x-ray films should be obtained on all patients with suspected diverticulitis, especially if there are signs of perforation or peritonitis. Plain films of the abdomen can reveal free air (indicating perforation), ileus, or obstruction (small or large bowel). A BE outlines the lumen of the bowel clearly defining diverticula and is thus most helpful in the diagnosis of the disease process. If perforation is suspected, the study can be performed with diatrizoate meglumine and diatrizoate sodium (Gastrografin, a water-soluble contrast medium). Barium studies help to identify sinus tracts, fistula formation, or obstructive processes. Diverticula are often an incidental finding on colonoscopy; however, colonoscopy is much less sensitive for the diagnosis of diverticular disease than barium studies. Colonoscopy may be helpful in ruling out cancer as the source of the symptomatology, as is cystoscopy in evaluation of colovesicular fistula.

Although diverticulitis can often be diagnosed clinically, a computed tomography (CT) scan with oral contrast is a much more sensitive and accurate test for cases in which confirmatory testing is necessary. CT scan can also determine if there is clinical deterioration by measuring the thickness of the bowel wall and assessing for the development of phlegmon over time using serial exams.

Patients who present with lower GI bleeding may require radioisotope scanning to locate the site of bleeding. Angiography is often nondiagnostic because the rate of bleeding is too slow or because bleeding has stopped.

Differential Diagnosis

The differential diagnosis of diverticular disease includes IBS, carcinoma of the colon, IBD, lactose intolerance, pelvic inflammatory disease, ovarian cyst, colitis (infectious or ischemic), appendicitis, and pyelonephritis. Most often the diagnosis can be made using the clinical findings and initial noninvasive ultrasonography. Colonoscopy is helpful for definitive diagnosis of diverticulitis and colon surveillance for other colonic disease processes but the AGA suggests it should not be used until after the resolution of the episode of acute diverticulitis.

MANAGEMENT

With early detection and treatment of diverticulitis and the associated complications, the prognosis is good. An incidental finding of uncomplicated diverticulosis requires no further intervention and can be managed with a high-fiber diet or daily fiber supplementation with psyllium. Treatment of a patient presenting with mild symptoms can often be managed on an outpatient basis with rest and a clear liquid diet. The American Gastroenterological Association (Stollman, Smalley, Hirano, & AGA Institute Clinical Guidelines Committee, 2015) suggests that antibiotics should not be routinely used because acute diverticulitis is more of an inflammatory process rather than an infectious one, as well as concerns about overuse of antibiotics. When antibiotics are deemed necessary, amoxicillin and clavulanate potassium 875/125 mg orally twice a day or metronidazole (Flagyl) 500 mg orally three times a day with trimethoprim/sulfamethoxazole (Bactrim DS) 160/800 mg orally twice a day for 7 to 10 days or until the patient is afebrile for 3 to 5 days. The symptoms usually subside quickly; then the diet can be advanced to soft, low roughage and next to high fiber as tolerated. Pain due to spasms can be managed with antispasmodics such as hyoscyamine (Levsin) 0.125 mg every 4 hours, dicyclomine (Bentyl) 20 to 40 mg four times daily, buspirone (BuSpar) 15 to 30 mg/day.

Patients with more acute illness require hospitalization for intravenous antibiotics and hydration, analgesia, bowel rest, and possible nasogastric (NG) tube placement. If the patient requires analgesia, morphine sulfate should be avoided because it increases intraluminal pressures within the colon and causes or exacerbates the presenting symptoms or perforation. An NG tube should be placed if there is evidence of ileus or if there is intractable nausea and vomiting.

The choice of antibiotics will depend on the severity of the disease process and should cover both gram-negative bacteria and anaerobic organisms. If cultures are obtained from the diverticular abscess, antibiotic coverage can be altered according to the results of the culture. Use and dosage of aminoglycosides should depend on renal function as indicated by the creatine clearance. Patients who are immunocompromised will require broader antibiotic coverage, including an anti-*Pseudomonas* agent. IV antibiotic therapy is normally continued for 7 to 10 days and may be continued orally for an additional 7 to 10 days after discharge, depending on the severity of the illness.

Patients will usually experience relief in symptoms after 72 hours of antibiotic therapy and may resume oral intake as tolerated. Once patients are able to maintain adequate nutrition and hydration, they can be discharged. A colonoscopy should be scheduled to evaluate treatment once the acute phase is resolved.

Patients whose cases are complicated by bleeding that does not subside will require angiography to locate the site of bleeding; they may also require infusion of vasopressin (Pitressin) 0.2 to 0.3 units/min via an intra-arterial catheter placed during the radiographic procedure. If the patient shows signs and symptoms of acute blood loss, transfusion may be indicated. Twenty percent of patients who have experienced diverticular bleeding bleed again within a year.

If there is no improvement or if there is clinical deterioration after 72 hours of medical treatment, surgical intervention may be indicated. Approximately 20% to 30% of patients with the diagnosis of diverticulitis require surgical management. Surgery is usually required for patients who have had several episodes of diverticulitis within 2 years or for those who have had a single episode of diverticulitis with complications. Findings such as generalized peritonitis and large abscesses that do not respond to medical treatment are indications for emergent surgical intervention. The surgical procedure of choice is colon resection. Patients who have undergone the surgical procedure will require routine postoperative care, with emphasis on pain management, pulmonary hygiene, hydration, nutrition, and wound assessment.

Localized abscesses can be drained percutaneously with the assistance of an interventional radiologist. Despite medical treatment, it is estimated that up to 40% of patients with diverticulitis continue to experience symptoms, and approximately one-half of these patients will need surgical intervention.

FOLLOW-UP AND REFERRAL

To evaluate or diagnose diverticular disease, all patients will require colonoscopy at some point during their disease process; therefore, referral to a gastroenterologist is indicated for symptoms that do not respond to treatment after 6 months. Early in the disease process, patients with diverticulitis should consult with a surgeon who can follow them and determine the necessity for emergent surgical intervention if complications should develop. Any patient who has had an acute attack of diverticulitis before age 40 will usually require surgical intervention and should be referred accordingly.

Patient Education: Diverticular Disease

Patients diagnosed with diverticular disease will need to make modifications in their diets with an emphasis on increasing the amount of dietary fiber. Diet changes should be made slowly to avoid bloating, gas, and other GI problems that may discourage compliance. Fiber can be increased by eating bran, fresh fruits, vegetables, and whole grains. The goal of diet therapy is to avoid constipation and straining during bowel movements, which can further increase intraluminal pressures and cause complications.

Patients should also be instructed to drink at least eight 8-ounce glasses of water a day to have regular, soft bowel movements. If patients continue to have constipation despite increasing their fiber and fluid intake, a bulk-forming laxative such as psyllium (FiberCon, Metamucil) can be added.

Symptoms recur in approximately one-third of all patients with diverticulitis who were initially treated with medical management. Therefore, all patients with diverticular disease should be instructed to return for follow-up if they develop signs and symptoms of infection or other associated complications of diverticulitis. Patients should understand that despite adherence to diet and medication, they may have another attack.

INFLAMMATORY BOWEL DISEASE

Inflammatory bowel disease is the term used to describe a chronic immunological disease that manifests in intestinal inflammation. The two most common IBDs are ulcerative colitis (UC) and Crohn's disease (CD), but microscopic colitis (MC) is increasing in prevalence and includes collagenous colitis (CC) and lymphocytic colitis (LC). IBD is characterized by exacerbations and remissions that are experienced throughout an individual's lifetime and therefore result in significant disruption in the quality of life. The Patient's Voice 40.1 describes the impact of CD on a 39-year-old woman with a 20-year history of the disease.

The Patient's Voice 40.1: Crohn's Disease

As a 39-year-old woman with a 20-year history of severe Crohn's disease (CD), I remain undecided as to which has been most difficult to deal with: the symptoms of the disease—uncontrolled diarrhea, bowel incontinence, malnutrition, pain, bloating, and flatulence, to name a few; the results of the symptoms—fatigue, malaise, anemia, anorexia, anxiety, embarrassment, guilt, fear, and shame; or the constant discipline necessary to incorporate lifestyle changes instrumental to the adaptation and management of this debilitating disorder—diet, stress elimination, exercise, rest, vitamin supplementation, and prescription compliance. Experience with CD has taught me that health and wellness is a personal choice and that whatever intestinal ailments or conditions one struggles with, incorporating the dietary changes necessary to promote wellness through nutrition, particularly raw, fresh fruit and vegetable juices, should be part of a comprehensive approach to achieving optimal health.

UC and CD are both IBDs that share similar characteristics and causes but are two separate diseases, however, the same pharmacologic agents are used for both. UC involves only the mucosal surface of the colon, which ultimately results in friability, erosions, and bleeding. It occurs most often in the rectosigmoid area but can involve the entire colon but not the small bowel. CD is characterized by segmental or patchy transmural inflammation of the bowel wall involving any portion of the GI tract from the mouth to the anus. Disease of the terminal ileus is present in about 80% of patients with CD, and in 20% of the cases only the colon is involved. The incidence of both CD and UC is increasing globally and ranges from 3 to 300 per 100,000 persons.

EPIDEMIOLOGY AND CAUSES

The incidence and prevalence of these diseases vary widely, which supports a multifactorial theory in the development of the disease. Research supports a genetic predisposition for IBD, even though less than 15% of cases are familial. A gene on chromosome 16 that encodes the protein nucleotide-binding oligomerization domain 2 *(NOD2)* has variants that are found in about 62% of patients with CD. Genes associated with IBD have also been found on chromosomes 10 and 7 that encode for proteins that mediate epithelial cell–cell interactions and the transport of molecules into and out of cells. Another factor is the ability of bacteria in the gut to cause inflammation related to abnormal T-cell reactions to commensal microflora and other luminal antigens. The intestinal epithelium plays an important role in the immune response, interacting with microbes and antigens and communicating with immune cells triggering the production and secretion of cytokines and chemokines.

The incidence of IBD is about equal in men and women. The age at onset for UC and CD is frequently in early adulthood but can be anywhere from age 10 to 40, whereas microscopic colitis is more common in people over 40 years of age. LC affects men and women equally, but CC is 20 time more common in women. Table 40.2 compares UC and CD.

PATHOPHYSIOLOGY

Ulcerative Colitis

The inflammatory process of UC is confined to the mucosa of the colon and rectum and begins with neutrophil infiltration at the base of the crypt of Lieberkühn. The disease most often occurs in the rectum and sigmoid colon. The mucosa in this area is thinner and has a dark red and velvety appearance in susceptible individuals. The cytokines released from the macrophages and neutrophils during the

inflammatory response are responsible for tissue damage. Ulcers form in the eroded tissue, and abscesses form in the crypts. These abscesses become necrotic and ulcerate. The muscularis mucosa becomes edematous and thickened, narrowing the lumen of the colon. Bleeding, cramping pain, and the urge to defecate result from the mucosal destruction. The characteristic stool is diarrhea that contains blood and purulent mucus. There is also a loss of the absorptive surface leading to large volumes of watery diarrhea. Fecal leukocytes are always present with active colitis. Absence of these inflammatory changes within the deeper layers of the intestinal mucosa helps to differentiate UC from other inflammatory processes. Patients diagnosed with severe UC are at risk for a perforated colon. They require close observation and should have consultation with a surgeon.

Crohn's Disease

CD is an inflammatory process that begins in the submucosa of the intestine and gradually spreads to involve the mucosa and serosa. Any portion of the GI tract can be

TABLE 40.2 Comparison of Ulcerative Colitis and Crohn's Disease		
Feature	*Ulcerative Colitis*	*Crohn's Disease*
History		
Age at onset	Age 10–40	Age 15–25; age 50–80
Etiology	Unknown	Unknown
Genetic tendency	Familial tendency	Familial tendency
Nicotine use	Nonsmoker	Smoker
Assessment Findings		
Serological	+ (positive) for antineutrophil cytoplasmic antibodies (pANCA)	– pANCA
Fever/malaise	With severe disease	Common
Weight loss	Uncommon	Common
Rectal bleeding	Common	Dependent on location of lesion; occurs in about 50% of cases
Abdominal pain	Usually mild	Can be moderate to severe
Abdominal mass	Negative	May be present
Perianal lesions	Absent	May develop fissures, abscesses
Fistulas	Absent	Common
Strictures	Uncommon	Common
Common		
Rectal involvement	Always	50% of the cases
Distribution	Confined to colon; continuous	Any portion of gastrointestinal tract; discontinuous, skipped lesions
Mucosa	Friable, granular	Cobblestone appearance
Ulceration	Crypt abscess development	Aphthous or linear ulcers
Inflammation	Surface involvement	Transmural involvement

affected, but 80% of patients have small bowel involvement. There are abnormalities in the intestinal immune response where proinflammatory cytokines, interleukins, and tissue necrosis factor produce areas of tissue damage. Typically, some haustra segments are affected while others are not, creating a pattern called skip lesions. The ulcerations form longitudinal and transverse fissures, extending inflammation into Peyer's patches and the lymphoid tissue. The typical lesion is granulomatous with projections of inflamed tissue surrounded by scar tissue. It is described as a "cobblestone" appearance. With progression of the disease, fibrosis thickens the bowel wall, narrowing the lumen. Serosal inflammation causes bowel loops to adhere to one another, contributing to transmural inflammation, ulceration, and fibrosis, which can lead to obstruction, fistulas, and shortening of the bowel.

Individuals with IBD are at greater risk for developing colorectal cancer than the general population. Clinical findings suggest that carcinoma is less common in patients with CD than with UC and is attributed to the treatment of CD with colectomy.

Microscopic Colitis

Some research indicates that LC and CC may be different phases of the same disease. In LC, lymphocytes infiltrate the colonic epithelium by. Lymphocyte infiltration also occurs in CC along with a thickening of the subepithelial collagen band or table (a band of collagen below the epithelial cells). Patients with CC have increased levels of immunoreactive prostaglandin E2 and nitric oxide (NO) in the colonic epithelium, which is believed to contribute to secretory diarrhea. Other processes have been implicated, such as increased mucosal secretion of transforming growth factor-1 and endothelial growth factor. Although a definitive cause for microscopic colitis has not been found, there is a strong correlation between consumption of nonsteroidal anti-inflammatory agents and the risk of CC. Other drugs, including aspirin, ranitidine, PPIs, and ticlopidine, are associated with microscopic colitis.

CLINICAL PRESENTATION

Subjective

Individuals with mild forms of UC commonly report four or fewer loose bowel movements per day associated with abdominal cramps that are relieved with defecation, small amounts of blood and mucus in the stool, and sometimes tenesmus. Usually there are no associated systemic symptoms. With moderate disease, patients have four to six loose stools a day containing more blood and mucus. They also have systemic symptoms such as tachycardia, mild fever, and weight loss and may have mild edema depending on the serum albumin level. Severe disease manifests with more frequent bloody bowel movements (6–10) per day; abdominal pain and tenderness;

and symptoms of anemia, hypovolemia, and impaired nutrition.

The most common presenting symptoms of CD are abdominal cramping and tenderness, fever, anorexia, weight loss, spasm, flatulence, and right lower quadrant (RLQ) pain or mass. Individuals may report an increase in symptomatology during periods of stress or emotional upset or after meals consisting of poorly tolerated foods such as fatty or spicy foods or milk. Stools are soft or semiliquid. Observable blood is found in the stool intermittently; when present, it occurs in a larger amount than with UC. Because of the loss of healthy bowel mucosa, there may be insufficient resorption of bile salts, causing steatorrhea (foul-smelling, fatty stools). CD can involve the entire thickness of the bowel wall, causing microperforations and symptoms of acute localized peritonitis, which can mimic appendicitis or diverticulitis. If there is fistula formation, these symptoms may dominate the clinical picture.

The most common presenting symptom for MC is protracted, nonbloody diarrhea that has been present from several months to 2 to 3 years. Forty percent of patients with CC complain of weight loss. Abdominal cramping and fecal incontinence are reported less often than diarrhea.

Several patterns of symptom onset for UC and CD are recognized: gradual, with vague abdominal discomfort, malaise, cramping, and bloody, mucopurulent stools; abrupt, with frequent periods of bloody diarrhea, anorexia, fever, and weight loss; and abrupt and fulminating, with sudden, violent diarrhea occurring nocturnally, high fever, intense abdominal cramping, signs of peritonitis, weight loss, and anorexia. Stools may contain blood, mucus, and/or pus. Typically, CD has a more insidious and gradual onset. Individuals often experience intermittent symptoms long before presenting for medical attention. The disease is characterized by periods of acute exacerbation alternating with complete remission.

If the UC is confined to the rectal or sigmoid area, the stools can be normal or hard and dry; however, the rectum will continue to dispel mucus containing both red and white blood cells. As the disease process moves proximally, the stools become looser. Patients may report eating less to decrease the frequency of bowel movements, which leads to more pronounced nutritional deficiencies.

Objective

On physical exam, there may be tenderness in the left lower quadrant or across the entire abdomen, often accompanied by guarding and abdominal distention. A digital rectal exam should be performed to assess for anal and perianal inflammation, rectal tenderness, and blood in the stool. Depending on the severity of the disease and the extent of potential complications, signs and symptoms of ileus and peritonitis may be found. Perirectal abscesses and fistulas are not associated with UC.

The physical exam may reveal abdominal tenderness with a tubular, tender mass in the RLQ. Fifty percent of individuals with CD have perianal involvement, including anal fissures, perianal fissures, and edematous, pale skin tags, which are often misdiagnosed as prolapsed hemorrhoids. Extra-intestinal findings include episcleritis, erythema nodosum, nondeforming peripheral arthritis, and axial arthropathy, which may be more apparent than bowel symptoms and should prompt the practitioner to look for a diagnosis of CD.

CD tends to present in one of four patterns: (1) inflammation, RLQ abdominal pain, and tenderness, often presenting as appendicitis; (2) obstruction, fibrosis, and stenotic changes within the bowel, causing recurrent obstruction associated with severe colic, abdominal distention, constipation, and vomiting; (3) diffuse jejunoileitis involving the jejunum and ileum and characterized by both inflammation and obstruction, which can result in malnutrition and chronic debility; and (4) abdominal fistulas and abscesses, normally occurring late in the disease process and causing fever, generalized wasting, and abdominal masses. Although CD is uncommon among children, those with CD often present with extra-intestinal symptoms, especially growth retardation, fever of unknown origin, and anemia.

Generally, patients with MC have no abnormalities on physical exam. Patients with severe and prolonged disease may have signs of dehydration, malnutrition, and weight loss.

DIAGNOSTIC REASONING

Diagnostic Tests

Definitive diagnosis is made by correlating the symptoms with the history and physical exam. Results of diagnostic testing help to differentiate UC from CD. Stool analysis and cultures are obtained to rule out bacterial, fungal, or parasitic infection as the cause for diarrhea. The stool is also examined for mucus and blood, which are normally present with UC.

Patients with CD who have small intestine involvement may also require evaluation for additional conditions caused by malabsorption and vitamin and mineral deficiencies, including anemia secondary to bleeding and iron deficiency and macrocytic anemia, which results from inflammation of the terminal ileum and poor absorption of folate. In addition, patients should be evaluated for hypocalcemia and vitamin D deficiency, hypoalbuminemia, and steatorrhea resulting from bile salt deficiency. Liver function tests may be helpful in screening for primary sclerosing cholangitis and other liver problems associated with IBD. Fluid and electrolyte disturbances are common in both diseases because of the extracellular fluid loss. CD may also present with an elevated WBC count and sedimentation rate, as well as a prolonged prothrombin time.

Diagnosis of acute UC is best made by sigmoidoscopy. Barium enema should not be performed because of the risk of precipitating toxic megacolon. Early in the disease, the mucous membrane is granular, friable, and edematous, with loss of the normal vascular pattern. In many patients, there may be scattered areas of hemorrhage that bleed with minor trauma. The resulting ulcerations develop after the mucosa breaks down, leaving the mucous membranes dotted with numerous bleeding and pus-oozing ulcers. Severe disease is characterized by copious amounts of purulent exudate. Colonoscopy should be avoided in individuals with severe colitis or deep ulcerations because of the risk of perforation. Although there are periods of remission, sigmoidoscopy shows some degree of friability and granulation in patients with UC. Biopsy results reveal chronic inflammation.

Plain films of the abdomen can help estimate the severity and proximal extent of the disease by demonstrating loss of haustration and the absence of formed stool within the diseased sections of bowel.

Every patient with UC requires a colonoscopy to determine the extent of the disease, but in order to avoid perforation, this is reserved for patients who have shown improvement on treatment. Ulcers suggestive of UC are shallow and confluent; they are erythematous, edematous, and friable, causing them to bleed easily. Individuals with UC usually have disease that begins in the rectum and extends proximally, without "skipped areas."

Definitive diagnosis of CD is normally made based on clinical manifestations and supporting endoscopic, pathologic, and radiographic evidence. The earliest manifestations of CD are aphthous and linear ulcers, which are best visualized with barium upper GI series with small bowel follow-through, depending on the location of the lesions. The ileum is stiff and nodular, and the lumen shows signs of thickening and narrowing. In advanced disease, the upper GI tract with small bowel follow-through may show the characteristic "string sign"—ileal strictures and evidence of bowel loop separation resulting from marked circumferential inflammation and fibrosis.

Colonoscopy reveals ulcers that are either minor erosions or deep longitudinal fissures. Segmental transverse fissuring creates the characteristic cobblestone appearance and is usually found above the rectum and rectosigmoid areas. Biopsies may be obtained to rule out pseudopolyposis, adenomatosis, or cancer. CT is often used in the evaluation of CD to identify bowel wall thickening or abscess formation. If an abscess is found, CT may be useful for guided drainage of the abscess.

MC is confirmed on colonoscopy with biopsy. In most patients with MC, the mucosa appears normal on colonoscopy. Biopsy in individuals with CC reveals a thick subepithelial collagenous deposit; in those with LC, there is a pronounced intraepithelial lymphocytic inflammation. An infiltrate of plasma cells, lymphocytes, and eosinophils in the lamina propria caused by chronic inflammatory may be seen on histologic examination.

There may be epithelial cell flattening, subepithelial blebs, and denuded epithelium. CC has the same histologic features of LC, along with a thickened subepithelial collagen layer in the lamina propria.

Differential Diagnosis

Differential diagnosis of UC must begin with the exclusion of an infectious cause for the colitis before treatment is initiated. Enteric infection is ruled out through fresh stool culture for ova and parasites. Infectious colitis caused by *Entamoeba histolytica, Campylobacter enteritidis,* and *Shigella* species and *Chlamydia* species can cause acute colitis, which is difficult to differentiate from UC both clinically and endoscopically. The distinction must be made because treatment with corticosteroids can be catastrophic. Obtaining a thorough travel, sexual, and antibiotic history is imperative. If the individual has had antibiotic exposure within the last 30 days, a stool sample to test for *Clostridium difficile* should be obtained. Homosexual men practicing anal intercourse should be screened for infectious proctitis as a cause of colitis. Individuals with HIV are susceptible to many opportunistic infections, which must also be considered as part of the differential diagnosis and treatment.

Older adults, patients with a history of coagulation disorders, and young women using oral contraceptives should be examined for ischemic colitis. Radiographic findings of "thumbprinting" and segmental distribution of lesions are typical of ischemic colitis. Although colon cancer rarely presents with fever and purulent diarrhea, it should be ruled out as a cause for bloody diarrhea.

As with UC, evaluation of CD must begin with ruling out infectious enteritis as the source of colitis. Enteric tuberculosis and fungal disease must also be considered in the differential diagnosis of CD. *Yersinia enterocolitica* enteritis, although a self-limiting infection, may require a 3-month follow-up examination because the initial clinical presentation is so similar to that of CD.

Although only 20% of patients with CD have disease that is limited to the colon, differentiation from UC must be made. CD is the more likely diagnosis when there is evidence of perianal disease and rectal bleeding. RLQ pain without a history of chronic bowel symptomatology may mimic appendicitis, pelvic inflammatory disease, ectopic pregnancy, ovarian cysts, or tumors; all of these must be ruled out in the differential diagnosis of CD. Both diverticular disease and ischemic colitis can present with the segmental involvement and luminal stricturing characteristic of CD.

Many drugs have been implicated in drug-induced colitis, the most common being NSAIDs and antibiotics. Many individuals who routinely take NSAIDs may have damage to the GI tract characterized by bloody diarrhea and weight loss. Some antibiotics alter the bowel flora, allowing overgrowth of pathogens such as *C. difficile,* which produces a toxin that is damaging to the bowel

mucosa and can cause bloody diarrhea, abdominal pain, and weight loss. Although initial radiographic studies may be similar to those for CD, endoscopic examination reveals a more segmental distribution of lesions, and biopsy results are not supportive of inflammatory disease.

Colon cancers can cause bloody diarrhea; however, they usually do not have the associated fevers, leukocytosis, and purulent discharge. Diverticulitis can cause abdominal pain, fever, leukocytosis, obstruction, and diarrhea; however, endoscopic evaluation reveals the characteristic mucosal herniations in the bowel wall.

Patients with MC are often misdiagnosed with diarrhea-predominant IBS. Other differential diagnoses include celiac disease, ischemic colitis, infectious colitis, hyperthyroidism CD, UC, and laxative abuse.

MANAGEMENT

There is no cure or definitive treatment for IBD. The initial therapy should depend on the severity of the presenting symptoms and must be individualized. Medical therapy is directed at reducing inflammation, correcting or maintaining fluid and electrolyte balance, and relieving the signs and symptoms of the disease.

Ulcerative Colitis

Initial treatment of UC includes nutrition counseling. Patients should avoid caffeine, raw fruits, vegetables, and other foods high in fiber, which can cause trauma to the already inflamed mucosal surface. Some patients may benefit from a lactose-free diet, but this is not recommended unless a trial produces symptomatic relief. A bland diet that is high in calories and protein yet low in fat can help to control diarrhea and flatulence and maintain nutrition and weight. Parenteral nutrition may be necessary in individuals with severe anorexia or uncontrollable diarrhea.

Antidiarrheal medications should be avoided in the acute phase but can be helpful for patients with mild symptoms. Patients with mild to moderate diarrhea may benefit from diphenoxylate with atropine (Lomotil) 2.5 to 5.0 mg orally twice a day and up to four times per day, loperamide (Imodium) 2 mg after each bowel movement, or codeine 15 to 30 mg orally every 4 to 6 hours.

Disease that is limited to the rectosigmoid area can often be successfully treated with topical mesalamine (see Drugs Commonly Prescribed 40.3). Steroid enemas and foams (e.g., hydrocortisone [Cortifoam] 100 mg) should be administered nightly for 2 weeks. If effective, this treatment will bring about remission in 70% of initial episodes of idiopathic UC. Patients may then taper the dose over the next week to prevent the side effects associated with rapid steroid withdrawal. Mesalamine (Rowasa), a form of 5-aminosalicylate (5-ASA), is more expensive; it is sometimes more effective than hydrocortisone for patients with refractory or left-sided colitis and is available in enema and suppository forms. Oral preparations of 5-ASA medications (e.g., Asacol, Azulfidine) help to maintain remission after the enemas have been discontinued. Sulfasalazine (Azulfidine) contains 5-ASA and sulfapyridine. It is the sulfapyridine that is responsible for many of the side effects of sulfasalazine. Other formulations of 5-ASA preparations (mesalamine) lack the sulfapyridine and have fewer adverse effects, and are better tolerated for prolonged courses of treatment. Subsequent exacerbations of

UC tend to show increasing resistance to therapy, requiring longer treatment regimens. Budesonide (Entocort) is an oral corticosteroid with a high first-pass loss in the liver, facilitating less systemic activity and more topical anti-inflammatory activity. An enteric-coated preparation of budesonide (Uceris) has delayed release and delivery throughout the colon.

Advanced disease usually requires the addition of a systemic glucocorticoid in combination with sulfasalazine or other 5-ASA therapy. Glucocorticoids are especially

Drugs Commonly Prescribed 40.3: Inflammatory Bowel Disease

DRUG	INDICATION	ADVERSE REACTIONS AND PRESCRIBING CONSIDERATIONS
5-Aminosalicylic Acid Agents		
mesalamine (Asacol) sulfasalazine (Azulfidine)	Ulcerative colitis (UC)	Research indicates that these drugs are of little value in Crohn's disease (CD). Continue to be used for ulcerative colitis. Headache, malaise, cramping and flatulence Rare: pneumonitis, pericarditis, pancreatitis, interstitial nephritis
Antidiarrheals		
loperamide (Imodium) diphenoxylate with atropine (Lomotil)	Diarrhea First- line treatment for microscopic colitis (MC)	Do not use in acute ulcerative colitis. Constipation may occur. Do not use if toxic megacolon occurs.
Corticosteroids		
prednisone budesonide (Entocort) or (Uceris)	Moderate to severe disease In severe cases of MC	Drastically suppresses clinical symptoms. This preparation is released in the ileum and induces remission in 50%–70% of cases of CD. Treatment is for 8–16 weeks followed by a 2–4 week taper in 3-mg increments.
hydrocortisone (Cortifoam, Anucort, Rectocort)	Initial treatment	Topical rectal application in suppository, foam or enema. Can be very irritating to the rectal mucosa. Cost is about $800 for a 4-week supply.
Immunomodulating Drugs		
Azathioprine (Imuran) Mercaptopurine (Purinethol) Methotrexate (MTX)	Moderate to severe disease that does not respond to corticosteroid therapy (CD, UC, MC)	This class of drugs can cause bone marrow suppression, and patients are at risk for life-threatening infections.
Anti-TNF Therapies		
Infliximab (Remicade) adalimumab (Humira) golimumab (Simponi) certolizumab (Cimzia)	Moderate to severe disease	This class of drugs causes bone marrow suppression and increases the risk for life-threatening infections.
Anti-Integrins Monoclonal Antibodies		
Natalizumab (Tysabri) Vedolizumab (Entyvio)	CD patients who do not respond do anti-tumor necrosis factor therapies CD and UC patients who do not respond to other treatments	Natalizumab can cause progressive multifocal leukoencephalopathy in immunocompromised patients. Should not be used with concomitant immunosuppressants. Vedolizumab does not have this adverse effect. Common side effects include fatigue and allergic reactions.

helpful in controlling the extracolonic manifestations of UC, which include peripheral arthritis, ankylosing spondylitis, erythema nodosum, anterior uveitis, and pyoderma gangrenosum. Peripheral arthritis and the skin lesions often parallel the course of the disease. Oral prednisone (Prelone), up to 40 to 60 mg in single or divided doses, must be tapered and not discontinued abruptly.

Severe or fulminant UC is manifested by 10 or more bloody stools per day, abdominal tenderness, fever, colon dilation, and tachycardia. Patients often require hospitalization for these symptoms. Patients with severe disease must be monitored closely for the development of toxic megacolon and colonic perforation. Any patient who does not show improvement after 7 to 10 days of maximized therapy should be considered for surgical intervention. Subtotal or total colectomy is often required to prevent perforation of the bowel and its complications. Some individuals may require restoration of their fluid volume and electrolytes, as well as blood transfusions, depending on the severity of the diarrhea and bleeding.

Immunosuppressive agents—azathioprine (Imuran), cyclosporine, and metabolite 6-mercaptopurine (6MP)— are used in cases of UC that are unresponsive to other medical treatment and in patients who are not surgical candidates. The long-term use of immunosuppressive agents for relapse prevention must be balanced with the increased risk of developing a malignancy. Most commonly, these agents are used to allow patients to reduce the maintenance dosage of glucocorticoids. For disease that is unresponsive to other therapies, anti–tumor necrosis factor (TNF) agents can be used. These include infliximab (Remicade) 5 mg/kg and adalimumab (Humira) administered subcutaneously 160 mg at week 1, 80 mg at week 2, and then maintenance of 40 mg every other week beginning at week 4. Anti-integrins are monoclonal antibodies that have been shown to be effective for inducing and maintain remission in patients with UC. These include natalizumab (Tysabri) 300 mg IV over 1 hour once every 4 weeks and vedolizumab (Entyvio) 300 mg IV at weeks 0, 2, and 6 for induction then a maintenance dose of 300 mg IV every 8 weeks.

Individuals who progress to fulminant disease are at risk for developing toxic megacolon—an atonic and distended, thin-walled colon. Approximately 1% to 2% of patients with UC develop this complication, which is characterized by fever, sepsis, electrolyte imbalances, hypoalbuminemia, and dehydration. Definitive diagnosis is made when radiographic measurement of the midtransverse colon shows it to be dilated to greater than 6 cm. The patient is at risk for perforation until the dilation is reduced. If medical reversal is not accomplished within 48 hours, surgical intervention is indicated and consultation should be made early.

Patients with toxic megacolon should receive nothing by mouth, a nasogastric tube should be placed for intermittent suction, and all antidiarrheal medications should be discontinued. Fluid and electrolyte disturbances,

particularly hypokalemia, should be corrected, and total parenteral nutrition may be required until the patient is able to tolerate oral food and fluids. Broad-spectrum antibiotics for peritonitis prophylaxis and parenteral administration of glucocorticoids are indicated. Patients must be monitored closely for signs and symptoms of perforation, which may be blunted because of the large doses of glucocorticoids. Loss of hepatic dullness on percussion may be the first sign of perforation. Daily abdominal x-ray films are necessary to assess colon distention and the presence of free air within the abdomen.

Over the long term, 25% of those with UC will require surgery. Emergent total colectomy is indicated for patients who do not respond to intensive medical therapy within 48 hours or who have massive hemorrhage or perforation. Surgical intervention is sometimes done in stages for patients who are severely ill. The most common procedure is the proctocolectomy with a Brooke ileostomy; it is a curative and functional procedure. Surgical intervention is also considered in patients who require large maintenance doses of glucocorticoids, are experiencing quality of life issues caused by severe diarrhea, or in children who are manifesting signs of growth retardation.

Crohn's Disease

Treatment of CD parallels that of UC including sulfasalazine (Azulfidine); however, 5-ASA medications have not been shown through research to be of any benefit. Glucocorticoids are used when initial treatment fails and for patients with moderate to severe disease. There is no curative therapy for CD; therefore, treatment is aimed at suppressing the inflammatory process and symptomatic relief of complications. The patient with CD has a much greater incidence of relapse once medications are discontinued; 70% of patients started on steroid therapy must remain on the therapy to prevent relapse. Oral prednisone 40 to 60 mg/day is used as initial outpatient treatment. Once maximal response has been achieved, the dose can be tapered over 2 to 4 months. Some patients may require a daily maintenance dose of 5 to 10 mg/day. As with UC, steroids are often helpful in managing the extra-intestinal manifestations of the disease. Patients with disease within the rectum may benefit from enema preparations as well.

Sulfasalazine (Azulfidine) remains a common treatment for CD; however, new research is showing that it may have little value. There is a high incidence of intolerance, including nausea, anorexia, rash, and headache. When it is used, the initial dose of sulfasalazine for treatment of mild to moderate disease of the colon or ileocolon is 500 mg twice daily; the dose can be increased to 3 to 4 g/day. Clinical improvement is usually noted in 3 to 4 weeks, at which time the medication can be tapered to 2 to 3 g/day for 3 to 6 months. Sulfasalazine interferes with folic acid absorption, so patients should receive folic acid 1 mg/day while taking this medication.

The use of metronidazole has been effective in patients who are intolerant of sulfasalazine, although metronidazole's use is also limited by adverse effects, including nausea, anorexia, metallic taste, furry tongue, and paresthesias. Although the mechanism of action is not clear, metronidazole has been effective in the treatment of perianal disease and in controlling Crohn's colitis. There is a high rate of relapse, however, once the drug has been discontinued. Other antibiotics such as ciprofloxacin, ampicillin, and tetracycline have been effective in controlling CD ileitis and ileocolitis.

The use of immunosuppressive medications has been shown to be effective in patients with CD that is unresponsive to other treatments, in individuals dependent on high-dose steroids, or in those with nonhealing fistulas. The clinical benefit of 6MP (the active metabolite of azathioprine [Imuran]) can take up to 3 months before being realized. These drugs can cause bone marrow suppression and pancreatitis; therefore, patients must be monitored frequently for leukopenia. The risk for developing malignancy is low but still must be considered. Patients remain on treatment for up to 2 years; in extremely refractory cases, treatment is continued indefinitely. Cyclosporine (Neoral, Sandimmune), an immunosuppressant drug typically used to prevent organ transplant rejection, is helpful in patients with steroid-resistant CD. Its use remains experimental, and it should be administered by practitioners who are experienced in caring for patients with complicated CD.

Other immunomodulating agents called TNF-alpha blockers such as infliximab (Remicade), adalimumab (Humira), and certolizumab are proving helpful in patients with moderate to severe CD. Rapid improvement is seen when infliximab is used initially. The regimen includes an initial dose of infliximab 5 mg/kg followed by repeat doses again at 2 weeks and 6 weeks, with maximal response seen in the first 2 weeks. Adalimumab (Humira) by subcutaneous injection is prescribed at 160 mg at week 1, 80 mg at week 2, and then maintenance of 40 mg every other week beginning at week 4. The side effects include infusion-related reactions and hypersensitivity reactions as a result of the development of antinuclear antibodies. This can be reduced by concomitant administration of other immunosuppressive medications. Serious infections may develop while patients are being treated with this medication. Anti-integrins are monoclonal antibodies that have been shown to be efficacious for inducing and maintain remission in patients with CD. These include natalizumab (Tysabri) 300 mg IV over 1 hour once every 4 weeks and vedolizumab (Entyvio) 300 mg IV at weeks 0, 2, and 6 for induction then a maintenance dose of 300 mg IV every 8 weeks.

Surgical intervention for CD is normally not indicated except for complications including intestinal obstruction, fistulas and abscess drainage, or perforation. Over the long term, up to 75% of patients with CD will require surgery. Patients with fistula formation (which may be enterocutaneous, enterovaginal, or enterovesicular) should be managed with bowel rest, parenteral nutrition, and antibiotic therapy before surgery is considered. Surgery is not curative and must be reserved for complications that are resistant to medical therapy. Intestinal obstruction caused by stricture formation is often successfully treated with strictureplasty, thus avoiding multiple colon resections and the risk of short bowel syndrome. Patients with symptoms of obstruction should avoid foods that contain nuts or seeds.

As with UC, the use of anticholinergic and antidiarrheal medications should be avoided in patients with severe disease because the drugs may precipitate toxic megacolon or ileus. Loperamide (Imodium), diphenoxylate (Lomotil), and codeine may be helpful in controlling chronic diarrhea in patients with mild CD colitis.

FOLLOW-UP AND REFERRAL

UC and CD are both complex illnesses with periods of exacerbation and remission requiring lifelong intervention and follow-up. Adjustment of therapy is based on symptom analysis and examination. Confirmation of the diagnosis and uncontrolled exacerbations should be referred to the physician. Referral to a gastroenterologist is often necessary for endoscopic evaluation and tissue biopsy. Long-term use of steroids and immunosuppressive drugs dictates ongoing patient follow-up. Repeat evaluation may be indicated if symptoms of a major complication have developed. Routine colonoscopy for colon cancer surveillance is necessary in any patient with long-standing disease. Stool analysis for occult blood is not an effective means of surveillance. Individuals whose disease is not controlled with established medical therapy of low-dose prednisone should be referred to a gastroenterologist who is knowledgeable in the treatment of these chronic disease processes.

Patient Education: Inflammatory Bowel Disease

All patients need to be informed about the disease process, the treatment options, and the expected outcome of the treatment regimens. Patients must be a part of the treatment plan and must have the knowledge necessary to make informed decisions. Education about the disease, diagnostic and laboratory tests, and diet and lifestyle changes should be included in the education. Open, honest information is important in helping patients to develop realistic expectations regarding treatment and outcomes.

The importance of adequate rest and stress reduction to decrease bowel motility and promote healing is essential. Stress management techniques, such as guided imagery, should be taught, and patients can be referred for counseling if necessary. Patients should be provided with the information and addresses for national organizations such as the Crohn's and Colitis Foundation of America that have up-to-date information and local support groups.

Dietary concerns for patients with CD include a low-residue diet when obstructive symptoms are present. Patients on a low-residue diet should avoid all foods high in fiber, including whole grain breads and cereals, all fresh fruits and vegetables, and seeds and nuts. Patients can have canned fruits and vegetables and should have only white breads. If the patient is unresponsive to medical treatment or is exhibiting signs of growth retardation, oral elemental or parenteral nutrition may be necessary. Patients who are intolerant of lactose should be taught to avoid dairy foods. When patients are not in the middle of an acute attack, they can eat whatever they can tolerate.

Dietary instruction for patients with UC is the same as that for CD. If they are not having symptoms of an acute attack, patients may eat whatever they can tolerate. During an acute exacerbation, parenteral nutrition or oral supplementation for malnutrition may be necessary. Some patients will ask questions about the use of diet as a treatment. Studies to date show that diet is ineffective as a treatment or therapy for UC. Foods that can cause diarrhea and gas-producing foods should be avoided during acute attacks.

Female patients with IBD require special guidance and counseling before they attempt pregnancy. Pregnant patients must be followed closely by a gastroenterologist throughout their pregnancy.

COLORECTAL CANCER

The majority of cases of colorectal cancer are both curable and preventable if detected early. Colorectal tumor presentation can be either symptomatic or asymptomatic and is dependent on the location of the tumor. Polyps, the most benign form of tumors, are classified as hyperplastic (nonneoplastic), adenomatous (neoplastic), or submucosal (lipomas). Adenomatous polyps are believed to be the precursors to the malignant adenocarcinomas, which comprise more than 95% of all malignant tumors of the colon. Over the past 20 years, there has been a decline in the mortality rate associated with colorectal carcinoma, which has been attributed to improvement in screening, diagnosis, and treatment. Cure rates of colorectal carcinoma are estimated to be as high as 50%.

EPIDEMIOLOGY AND CAUSES

Of cancers affecting both men and women, colorectal cancer is the second leading cancer killer in the United States. The estimated number of new colon cancer cases in 2017 is 135,430 with an estimated number of deaths at 50,260. It is estimated that 4.3% of the population will develop colorectal cancer in their lifetime. Since 1985, the number of new cases of colorectal cancer has decreased and the 5-year survival rate has increased.

Age is the most important risk factor for developing colorectal cancer in the United States. The risk increases steadily with age, especially after age 45, and is rare in individuals younger than age 35 unless they have genetic risk factors. The older adult population is at the greatest risk of developing colorectal carcinoma, with the median age at the time of diagnosis of 71 years. Colon cancer affects men and women equally; however, rectal cancers are more common in men. The overall survival rate of patients with colorectal cancer is approximately 66% and is attributed to early detection and treatment. African American males and members of low-income minority groups have, for unknown reasons, lower survival rates in comparison to national data for other groups. It is presumed—although not proved—that the lower survival rates among minorities are in part a result of inequalities in access to health care, including screening and treatment.

Seventh Day Adventists are a religious group that subscribes to a vegetarian diet, and they also have a lower incidence of colorectal cancer. In the past, studies have shown that the Japanese have had a lower incidence of colorectal cancer; however, Japanese Americans who have adopted a diet high in fat, refined carbohydrates, and red meat have a higher incidence of this type of cancer. In general, groups that migrate from areas of low to high incidence of colorectal cancer experience a change in cancer incidence that parallels that of the new region.

Other risk factors for colorectal cancer include a family history and a personal history of adenomatous polyps (multiple polyps or individual polyps greater than 1 cm in size) or colon cancer. Twenty-five percent of patients diagnosed with colon cancer have a family history of colon cancer. The risk of developing colon cancer is directly proportional to the number of first-degree relatives affected: For patients who have one first-degree relative with colon cancer, the risk increases twofold to threefold. Disorders involving increased colon mucosal cell turnover (such as IBD and UC) have been implicated in greater risk for colon cancer. Familial adenomatous polyposis is an autosomal dominant condition that results in the development of thousands of adenomas within the colon but accounts for less than 1% of colon cancers. Other hereditary conditions that increase the chance of developing colorectal cancer include Peutz-Jeghers syndrome, Gardner's syndrome, and Turcot's syndrome. Patients with a family history or personal history of gynecological (breast, ovarian, endometrial) cancers and individuals diagnosed with Barrett's esophagus also have an increased risk of developing colon carcinoma.

Although the etiology of colorectal cancer (adenomas) is unknown, both environmental and genetic factors have been implicated. Geographic variances and a positive correlation in the incidence of disease among migrant workers both suggest that environmental factors play a role. Diets high in fat, red meat, and refined carbohydrates and low in plant fiber have been correlated with the areas of highest incidence of colorectal cancer, whereas areas with the lowest incidence of colorectal cancer have diets high in fiber and rich in vegetables and fruits. It has been theorized that the excess fat interacts with colonic bacteria to form deconjugated bile acids, which have been associated with tumor-producing activity, increased deposition of fatty acids within the cell membranes, and increased synthesis of prostaglandins, which further stimulates cell proliferation. Ketosteroids are thought to be metabolic by-products of cholesterol that induce genetic damage and have been found in higher concentrations among high-risk populations. Products of pyrolysis—decomposition of organic matter secondary to increases in temperature such as those resulting from charbroiling and frying—have also been implicated in carcinoma of the colon. Diets high in processed meats also increase the risk of colorectal cancer. Geographic areas with low levels of selenium also have higher incidence of colorectal cancer.

Conversely, diets high in fiber tend to reduce the transit time within the colon, thus decreasing exposure to potentially carcinogenic substances and altering the gut flora and decreasing fecal pH. (Populations with the highest incidence of colorectal cancer have an associated higher fecal pH.) When fecal contents take longer to transit the bowel, the deionized bile acids and free fatty acids stay in contact with the intestinal mucosa, which has been associated with development of colorectal cancer.

Other risk factors include being overweight or obese. Physical inactivity is associated with a greater risk of developing colorectal cancer. Long-term smoking and heavy use of alcohol are also risk factors. However, moderate alcohol use, defined as no more than 2 drinks per day for men or 1 drink a day for women, may lower the risk for colorectal cancer.

PATHOPHYSIOLOGY

Most colorectal cancers are adenocarcinomas. The evolution from adenoma to invasive carcinoma can take up to 10 years. *Adenomas* are benign neoplasms composed of granular epithelium that are not capable of metastasis or invasion of the muscularis mucosa. They are either sessile (attached by a broad base) or pedunculated (attached by a stalk). Most smaller adenomas (less than 1 cm in diameter) are of the tubular type, and less than 1% contain carcinoma. As the polyps increase in size (greater than 2 cm in diameter), they begin to show villous changes with increasing dysplasia; the chance of one of these polyps containing cancer is about 50%.

Most adenocarcinomas of the colon form hard, nodular areas that grow irregularly. Colon cancers are staged

or classified according to histological changes in the infiltrative character of the tumor. The most common classification system used today is the tumor-node-metastasis system (TNM) (Table 40.3). Histologically, colon cancers vary from well-differentiated cells that appear normal (grade 1) to highly anaplastic, poorly differentiated cells (grade 4). The accuracy of specimen collection is crucial. The most accurate method of evaluating a polyp is by removing the entire lesion for cytological examination. If the polyp is less than 7 mm in diameter, tissue for biopsy can be obtained while the polyp is destroyed through "hot" (fulguration) biopsy.

Metastatic progression of colon cancer usually involves spread by local invasion, lymphatic extension with spread to the mesenteric lymph nodes first, and then hematogenous spread through the portal system to the liver. In

TABLE 40.3 Staging Classifications of Colorectal Cancer (TNM)				
Stages	*Tumor*	*Node*	*Metastasis*	*Description*
Stage 0	Tis	N0	M0	Carcinoma in situ
Stage 1	T1	N0	M0	Tumor invades submucosa; greater than 80% 5-year survival
	T2	N0	M0	Tumor invades muscularis
Stage II	T3	N0	M0	Tumor penetrates through bowel wall; 60%–80% 5-year survival
	T4	N0	M0	Tumor invades adjacent organ; no regional lymph node involvement
Stage III	T1, T2	N1 or N2	M0	Any bowel wall perforation with lymph node involvement; 20%–50% 5-year survival
	T3, T4	N1 or N2	M0	One to three pericolic or perirectal lymph nodes.
Stage IV	Any T	Any N	M1	Distant metastasis; less than 25% 5-year survival

Source: used with permission of the American College of Surgeons, Chicago, Illinois. Original source for this information is the AJCC Cancer Staging Manual, Eighth Edition (2017) published by Springer International Publishing.

some patients, the cancer metastasizes throughout the peritoneal cavity and to the lungs. Rectal carcinoma spreads by direct extension through the perirectal fat to the lymph nodes and less often to the lungs and distant organs through hemorrhoidal circulation. Prognosis of colorectal carcinoma is a function of several factors, including poorly differentiated tissue histology, mucin production, aneuploidy (DNA abnormalities), tumor invasion to other organs, perforation, and venous involvement. The prognosis is not influenced by tumor size.

Colon cancers can develop as polyps within the lumen of the intestine or as a mass on the wall of the colon. Bulky polypoid tumors are more common within the right colon, whereas tumors that encircle the bowel, causing obstruction, are more common on the left side of the colon. Tumor growth is normally slow and, in most cases, is asymptomatic until the tumor becomes large. Diagnosis is usually made late in the course of the disease, often after metastasis, thereby making a surgical cure difficult. Colon cancers that produce intracellular mucin are called signet ring–type carcinomas; these tumors tend to be more aggressive in their spread.

Several types of colon cancers have been linked to specific genetic defects. Hereditary nonpolyposis colorectal cancers include two autosomal dominant conditions that have been associated with a markedly increased risk for developing colon cancer. Although these patients have few or no adenomatous polyps, individuals diagnosed with Lynch syndrome I are at increased risk of developing colon cancer at an early age. This cancer has a propensity for the right side of the colon. Lynch syndrome II includes the features of Lynch syndrome I as well as an increased risk of developing tumors within the ovary, uterus, urinary tract, and stomach.

CLINICAL PRESENTATION

Subjective

Signs and symptoms in patients with colorectal cancer will vary, depending on the tumor size, anatomical location, and associated complications, if any. There are few early warning signs of colorectal carcinoma; in fact, most individuals are asymptomatic. Frequently, the cancer is found incidentally during abdominal surgery or during screening sigmoidoscopy.

Patients may present with melena or bright red bleeding from the rectum, depending on the location of the tumor. A change in bowel habits, including constipation alternating with diarrhea or a change in stool caliber (described as narrowed or ribbonlike), can be signs of colon cancer. Stools streaked with blood may be mistakenly dismissed as a sign of hemorrhoidal irritation. Abdominal pain is a rare presenting symptom but may indicate obstruction resulting from tumors on the left side of the colon, which has a smaller diameter lumen, or from invasion of the bowel wall by a tumor. Patients rarely report colicky pain as a result of a right-sided colon cancer because of the larger diameter of the colon and the liquid consistency of the stool. Patients with rectal cancer may complain of tenesmus (spasm of the anal sphincter), urgency, and/or hematochezia. Patients with chronic occult blood loss from an undiagnosed tumor may experience weakness and fatigue caused by iron-deficiency anemia. Weight loss and anorexia are common with any malignant process but are usually manifested late in the disease process.

Objective

Physical exam may reveal a mass within the abdomen or an enlarged liver, which may be suggestive of metastasis. A digital rectal exam should be done even though most tumors are not palpable. The stool should be tested for occult blood, which, if positive, is pathognomonic for right-sided colon cancer. Approximately 50% of patients with a positive fecal occult blood test have either an adenoma (38%) or a neoplasm (12%). Conversely, fecal occult blood testing is positive in only 60% to 70% of patients with known large intestinal cancers; however, annual screening can reduce colorectal mortality rates by 33%.

DIAGNOSTIC REASONING

Diagnostic Tests

Although there are no definitive laboratory tests for diagnosis of colorectal cancer, a CBC should be obtained to assess for iron-deficiency anemia or anemia of chronic blood loss, either of which can be a common finding in patients with colorectal cancer. Liver function tests may reveal an elevation of the liver enzymes, especially of alkaline phosphatase if there has been metastasis to the liver and/or bone. Usually, when there is liver metastasis, the bilirubin level tends to remain normal until late in the disease process.

The serum immune assay for carcinoembryonic antigen (CEA) was developed with the intent of providing an early means of detection for colon cancer; however, the test is too insensitive and nonspecific for screening. CEA levels have been poorly correlated with the stage of cancer; however, this test is useful for monitoring a patient's response to therapy, whether surgical or chemotherapeutic. CEA levels usually normalize after colon resection, and levels that remain elevated are associated with poor prognosis. A secondary spike in the CEA level after surgery is highly suggestive of recurrence and must be evaluated.

Colonoscopy establishes the diagnosis of colon cancer with almost 100% accuracy and is thus the diagnostic procedure of choice. Flexible sigmoidoscopy can be used for confirming lesions within the rectosigmoid area; however, full colon examination with colonoscopy is preferred. Computed tomography (CT) scan is used for evaluation of distant metastasis. Endoscopic ultrasound has been used to stage regional rectal cancers and is more accurate than CT scan in this area.

Patients with colonic polyps will require histological examination of the polyp. Polyps larger than 7 mm should be totally removed. Polyps that are less than 7 mm in size are usually not malignant and can be removed by "hot" biopsy, which destroys the polyp while obtaining the necessary tissue for cytological exam.

Differential Diagnosis

The symptoms of colorectal cancer are nonspecific; therefore, many disease processes can mimic the presenting symptoms of colon carcinoma and must be differentiated from it. Most of the inflammatory and IBD processes can be confused with colon carcinoma. Ischemic colitis, diverticular disease, IBS, IBD, or infectious colitis can form strictures within the bowel that are indistinguishable from colon carcinoma. Colonoscopy with biopsy of the lesion is the diagnostic procedure of choice. Any patient older than age 50 who presents with iron-deficiency anemia, stool positive for occult blood, change in bowel habits, or hematochezia should have a thorough evaluation to rule out the possibility of neoplasm.

MANAGEMENT

The first step in the treatment of colon cancer is the staging of the disease. The staging of the cancer is of critical importance not only for the determination of the patient's long-term survival but also for determining which patients should receive adjuvant therapy. Staging of a neoplasm first involves understanding the characteristics used to describe the histological findings: tissue of origin (adenocarcinoma, sarcoma, carcinoid), origin of specimen (colon, breast), and the degree of tissue differentiation. Staging of the carcinoma includes both the primary site and the metastatic sites and allows for the development of the most optimal treatment plan based on those findings. More than half of all cancers are not curable using approved treatments available today. Many of the treatment regimens involve some form of experimental drugs or procedures; therefore, accurate staging is necessary to determine the efficacy of the treatment.

The only known cure for colon cancer is surgical resection. This is the treatment of choice for all patients who can tolerate the surgery. Even patients who have known metastasis can benefit from surgical intervention to reduce the chance of developing an intestinal obstruction or rectal hemorrhage later in the disease process. Most patients with colorectal cancer present with penetration of the mass through the bowel wall and with associated lymph node involvement. The surgeon will decide, based on the staging, what type of surgical resection is appropriate. The anatomical location of the tumor—left or right side of the colon—will dictate whether left or right hemicolectomy is performed. A wide margin of intestine (with careful ligation of the total arterial blood supply) will be resected to ensure that mesenteric and associated lymph node drainage is removed.

Lesions located within the rectosigmoid area are usually treated with anterior resection, which protects the rectal sphincter. (The rectum is the distal 8–11 cm of large bowel.) If the rectal lesions are small and are discovered early, they can sometimes be treated by local incision, laser photoablation, or cryosurgery. Larger lesions located within this lower portion of the large bowel usually require a combination of abdominal-perineal resection with a colostomy. Nonresectable rectal cancers can be palliated with a diverting colostomy, or, if the patient is a poor surgical candidate, laser fulguration of the tumor mass can minimize the bleeding and maintain the patency of the rectum.

Adjuvant chemotherapy for colon cancer is based on the stage of the disease (see Table 40.3). Treatment of Stage III cancer includes 6 months of chemotherapy. A combination of 5-fluorouracil (5-FU), leucovorin, and oxaliplatin is the treatment of choice for the best 5-year survival rate (73.3%) compared with 5-FU and leucovorin alone (67.4%). Stage IV metastatic cancer is treated with the same chemotherapy combination as Stage III but with the addition of a biologic agent such as bevacizumab (monoclonal antibody), which improves survival but only for a mean of 2 to 5 months.

Rectal carcinomas have a lower long-term survival rate than colon cancers and are typically treated with chemoradiation of 5-FU or capecitabine. When given preoperatively, the chemotherapy sensitizes the cancer cells to the effects of the radiation therapy, leading to better outcomes. After surgery, chemotherapy with 5-FU, leucovorin, and oxaliplatin is used along with 6 months of radiation.

Twenty percent of patients with colorectal cancer have known metastases at the time of diagnosis. Patients with known metastases to the liver may have improved survival rates with resection. Some patients with liver metastases have opted for infusions of 5-FU into the hepatic artery or portal vein, which has proved superior in the treatment of hepatic disease; however, this treatment has little effect on the overall survival rate for colorectal cancer and can be extremely toxic to the patient.

Although the oncologist will manage the patient's chemoradiation therapy, the primary-care practitioner will continue to work closely with the patient to treat any of the numerous adverse effects caused by the chemotherapy and the radiation therapy. The potential toxic effects of adjuvant therapy for colorectal cancer are numerous and can range from nausea, vomiting, and weight loss to cystitis and radiation proctitis.

Radiation therapy to the pelvic area can cause severe GI disorders, including intractable diarrhea and even malabsorption syndromes.

FOLLOW-UP AND REFERRAL

Initial assessment and screening for colorectal carcinoma is the responsibility of every primary-care provider. Patients who are known to be at higher risk for the development of colorectal cancer, such as those who have a first-degree relative with the disease, a family history of adenomas, a personal history of adenomas or colorectal cancer, or a long-standing history of IBD, require a more in-depth screening by a practitioner who is well trained in this area. Screening for high-risk patients should include colonoscopy, which is best done by an experienced gastroenterologist. The recommended screening for average- and high-risk individuals is provided in the accompanying feature.

✛ Screening Recommendations/Guidelines: Colon Cancer Screening American College Gastroenterology (ACG) 2009

Risk	Screening Recommendations
Average risk: Beginning at age 50 through age 75 years; for African Americans, begin screening at age 45 years	Colonoscopy every 10 years For those who decline colonoscopy: annual fecal immunochemical test (FIT) Alternatives: Flexible sigmoidoscopy every 5–10 years Computed tomography colonography every 5 years (replaces the double contrast barium enema) Annual Hemoccult Sensa or fecal DNA testing every 3 years
Higher risk • Family history of colorectal cancer or polyps before age 60 years • Family history of a hereditary colorectal cancer syndrome	Colonoscopy every 5 years starting at age 40 or 10 years younger than the age at diagnosis of the youngest affected relative.

Follow-up is vitally important in the treatment of colorectal cancer. To prevent recurrence, scheduled colon surveillance is required. Early detection and removal of adenomas can improve survival rates. Close surveillance is necessary for patients who have undergone "curative resection" surgery. Recommendations include office visits every 3 months, which should include a CEA level, an annual CT of the abdomen and pelvis, and a chest x-ray film for the first 3 years postoperatively. A colonoscopy should be completed postoperatively; but, if the exam was not completed at that time, a colonoscopy should be scheduled for 3 months postoperatively and then again at 1 year, with special attention to anastomotic recurrences. If the results of the exam are within normal limits, patients may continue with follow-up exams every 3 years. Patients whose CEA levels normalize or stabilize after surgery and then spike suddenly require a thorough examination.

Patients who have undergone surgical resection for colon cancer and have a temporary or permanent colostomy may benefit from assistance from an enterostomal therapist. Consultation with a urologist for urological or sexual dysfunction resulting from surgical or radiation therapy may provide medical and social support. Patients with metastatic disease can be referred to hospice service personnel, who are trained in providing comfort and support to both the family and the patient.

Patient Education: Colon Cancer

Patient education should focus first on the prevention of colon cancer, stressing a diet that is low in fat and refined carbohydrates and high in fiber, fruits, vegetables, and complex carbohydrates. Since obesity and sedentary lifestyle are risk factors, patients should be assisted in pursuing weight loss and exercise. The risk/benefit/cost ratio makes these preventive measures worth suggesting.

REFERENCES

Lower Gastrointestinal Diseases

Bascunan KA, Vespa MC, Araya M. Celiac disease: Understanding the gluten-free diet. *Eur J Nutr.* 2017;56:449–459.

Ben-Horin S, Kopylov U, Chowers Y. Optimizing anti-TNF treatments in inflammatory bowel disease. *Autoimmun Rev.* 2014;13(1):24–30.

Cornett PA, Dea TO. Cancer. In Papadakis M, McPhee S, eds. *Current medical diagnosis & treatment.* New York: McGraw Hill; 2017:1636–1644.

Dai C, Zheng CQ, Jiang M, Ma X-Y, Jiang LJ. Probiotic and irritable bowel syndrome. *World J Gastroenterol.* 2013;19(36):5973–5980.

Kahi CJ, Boland R, Doinitz JA, et al. Colonoscopy surveillance after colorectal cancer resection: Recommendations of the US multi-society task force on colorectal cancer. *Am J Gastroenterol.* 2016;150(3):758–768.

Kroser JA. Collagenous and lymphocytic colitis. http://emedicine.medscape.com/article/180664-overview. Published 2017.

Lin JS, Piper MA, Perdue LA, Rutter CM, Webber EM, O'Connor E, et al. US Preventive Task Force: Evidence report. Screening for colorectal cancer: updated evidence report and systematic review for the US Preventive Services Task Force. *JAMA.* 2016;315(23):2576-2594.

Luthy KE, Larimer SG, Freeborn DS. Differentiating between lactose intolerance, celiac disease and irritable bowel syndrome-diarrhea. *J Nurse Pract.* 2017;13(5):348–353.

McQuaid KR. Gastrointestinal disorders. In Papadakis M, McPhee S, eds. *Current medical diagnosis & treatment.* New York: McGraw Hill; 2017:578–673.

Nalley C. Celiac disease update. *Nurse Pract Persp.* 2015;2(3):24–30.

National Cancer Institute. Colon cancer treatment (PDQ)—health professional version. https://www.cancer.gov/types/colorectal/hp/colon-treatment-pdq. Updated 2017.

Rex DK, Johnson DA, Anderson JC, Schoenfeld PS, Burke CA, Inadomi JM. Colorectal screening. *Am J Gastroenterol.* 2009;104:739–750.

Richman E, Rhodes JM. Review article: Evidence-based dietary advice for patients with inflammatory bowel disease. *Aliment Pharmacol Ther.* 2013;38(10):1156–1171.

Salazar CA. Crohn disease: Diagnosis and treatment. *Clin Advisor.* 2016;19(3):28–33.

Siegel RL, Miller KD, Jemal A. Cancer statistics, 2017. *Cancer J Clin.* 2017;67(1):7–30.

Stollman N, Smalley W, Hirano I, AGA Institute Clinical Guidelines Committee. American Gastroenterological Association Institute Guideline on Management of Acute Diverticulitis. *Gastroenterology.* 2015;149(7):1944–1949.

U.S. Preventive Services Task Force. Screening for celiac disease: US Preventive Services Task Force Recommendation Statement. *JAMA.* 2017;317(12):1252–1257.

Upper Gastrointestinal Diseases

Bashashati M, Hejazi RA, Andrews CN, Storr MA. Gastroesophageal reflux symptoms not responding to proton pump inhibitor: GERD, NERD, NARD, esophageal hypersensitivity or dyspepsia? *Can J Gastroenterol Hepatol.* 2014;28(6):335–341.

Chan FK, Ching JYL, Suen BY, Tse YK, Wu JCY, Sung JJY. Effects of *Helicobacter pylori* infection on long-term risk of peptic ulcer bleeding in low-dose aspirin users. *Gastroenterology.* 2013;144(3):528–535.

Cohen E, Bolus R, Khanna D, Hays RD, Chang L, Melmed GY, et al. GERD symptoms in the general population: Prevalence and severity versus care-seeking patients. *Dig Dis Sci.* 2014;59(10):2488–2496.

Fu W, Song Z, Zhou L, Xue Y, Suo B, Tian X, Want L. Randomized clinical trial: Esomeprazole, bismuth, levofloxacin, and amoxicillin or cefuroxime as first-line eradication regimens for Helicobacter pylori infection. *Dig Dis Sci.* 2017;62:1580–1589.

Graham DY. *Helicobacter pylori* update: Gastric cancer, reliable therapy, and possible benefits. *Gastroenterology.* 2015;148(4):719–731.

Helgadottir H, Metz DC, Bjornsson ES. Study of gender differences in proton pump inhibitor dose requirements for GERD: A double-blind randomized trial. *J Clin Gastroenterol.* 2015;51(6):486–493.

Katz PO, Gerson LB, Vela MF, et al. Guidelines for the diagnosis and management of gastroesophageal reflux disease. *Am J Gastroenterol.* 2013;108(3):308–328.

Maradey-Romero C, Fass R. New and future drug development for gastroesophageal reflux disease. *J Neurogastroenterol Motil.* 2014;20(1):6–16.

RESOURCES

Crohn and Colitis Foundation of America
www.ccfa.org
Celiac Disease Foundation
https://celiac.org
International Foundation for Bowel Dysfunction
https://www.iffgd.org/
National Cancer Institute—Health Professional Version
https://www.cancer.gov/types/colorectal/hp

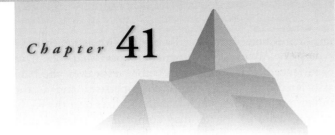

Chapter **41**

Gallbladder and Pancreatic Disorders

Debera J. Thomas, DNS, RN, FNP/ANP

CHOLECYSTITIS

Cholecystitis is an acute inflammation of the gallbladder wall, which is usually the result of an impacted calculus within the cystic duct, causing inflammation proximal to the obstruction. Cholelithiasis is found in more than 90% of patients presenting with cholecystitis. Cholecystitis without gallstones, acalculous cholecystitis, is a very serious disease with high morbidity and mortality rates. It usually occurs in patients who are already critically ill because of trauma, burns, surgery, or sepsis and who have had no oral intake or have been supplemented with hyperalimentation. Patients present with severe pain and tenderness in the epigastrium or right upper quadrant (RUQ) of the abdomen accompanied by nausea, vomiting, fever, and leukocytosis.

EPIDEMIOLOGY AND CAUSES

Cholecystitis/cholelithiasis is prevalent in Western societies. Researchers estimate that the disease affects approximately 20 million Americans, the majority of whom are not aware they have cholelithiasis. About 50% of these asymptomatic patients never require treatment. Gallstones form in people as early as their 30s. In fact, 75% of American Indian women over age 25 have gallstones. The risk of requiring a cholecystectomy increases with age as a consequence of complications secondary to the lithiasis. By age 65, about 20% of women and 10% of men have symptoms related to gallstones that require medical attention. As many as 5,000 to 6,000 deaths each year are attributed to gallstone-related disease.

Cholesterol stones are the most common form and account for 75% of all gallstones. The remaining 25% are pigmented stones, which are categorized as black or brown depending on their chemical composition. Cholesterol stones contain between 50% and 90% cholesterol; the remainder of the stone is made of calcium salts from bilirubin pigment, carbonate, bile acids, phospholipids,

fatty acids, and proteins. Risk factors for cholelithiasis are listed below.

Risk Factors Associated with Cholelithiasis

Cholesterol Stones:

- Female gender
- Obesity
- Pregnancy
- Increased age
- Drug-induced (oral contraceptives, clofibrates)
- Cystic fibrosis
- Rapid weight loss
- Spinal cord injury
- Ileal disease with extensive resection
- Diabetes mellitus
- Sickle cell anemia

Pigmented Stones:

- Hemolytic diseases
- Increasing age
- Hyperalimentation
- Cirrhosis
- Biliary stasis
- Chronic biliary infections

The well-known mnemonic regarding the typical cholelithiasis patient is the "six Fs": fat, female, forty (age 40 years), flatulent, fertile, and fat-intolerant. After age 50, the gender distribution of cholelithiasis is equal. Pregnancy also predisposes women to cholelithiasis, presumably because of the increased abdominal pressure and increased cholesterol levels during the third trimester. Any condition that increases the development of cholelithiasis increases the chance of developing cholecystitis.

PATHOPHYSIOLOGY

More than 90% of cholecystitis cases are associated with cholelithiasis. Cholesterol stones are the most common form of gallstones. Cholesterol is insoluble in water; it is made soluble though interaction with bile salts and phospholipids, allowing it to be carried within the bile. There are two known transport systems for cholesterol within the bile, vesicular and micellar; both are needed le to maintain equilibrium of the various bile components. When this equilibrium is disturbed and the bile contains more cholesterol than can be maintained, crystallization of the cholesterol, referred to as nucleation, occurs. Gradual deposition of cholesterol on these crystals leads to the development of a cholesterol gallstone. Although this process seems to contribute to the formation of gallstones, not all people with cholesterol-saturated bile form stones. Thus, there is more to the process of lithogenesis than is known.

The gallbladder is of primary importance in the development of gallstones because it provides an arena for bile stasis and allows time for the slow crystallization of cholesterol, which may also be enhanced by yet unknown proteins or other materials within the bile. Biliary cholesterol is increased by ingestion of estrogen and oral contraceptives, multiparity, and inflammatory terminal ileal disease, which decreases the bile acid pool. Bile stasis, which can contribute to gallstone formation, is increased by strictures within the ductal system, parenteral hyperalimentation, fasting, and mechanical obstruction secondary to tumor or cyst formation.

The pathogenesis of pigmented stones is less well understood but seems to be directly related to elevation in levels of unconjugated bilirubin. Any disease state that increases the amount of bilirubin increases the risk for pigmented lithogenesis. Black-pigmented stones are formed within the gallbladder and are commonly associated with hemolytic diseases, cirrhosis, long-term parenteral hyperalimentation. Black-pigmented stones are more fragile and seem to crush more easily than cholesterol stones.

Brown pigmented stones are composed of alternating layers of calcium bilirubinate and calcium fatty acids. Chronic bacterial infections are believed to be partly responsible for the formation of brown pigmented stones because the enzymes the bacteria produce predispose the patient to this type of stone formation. Brown stones are typically found within the intrahepatic ducts and are rarely found within the gallbladder.

The pathophysiological changes occurring within the gallbladder before the diagnosis of acute cholecystitis are directly related to the amount of time the duct has been obstructed and the degree of inflammation that has taken place. The earliest pathological findings are erythema, edema, and a fibrinosuppurative exudate. Tissue examination reveals inflammatory infiltration, hemorrhage, and edema resulting in ulceration of the mucosa within a short period of time. The result is the development of gangrene with abscess formation. As the acute process resolves, collagen deposits develop, usually within 1 to 2 weeks. The gallbladder eventually contracts and becomes scarred, causing thickening of the wall. Often the gallbladder becomes filled with pus preceding the development of gangrene. Perforation may occur, most often at the fundus, but it can occur anywhere there is erosion of an impacted stone. Perforation of the gallbladder allows bile to spill into the peritoneal cavity, causing bile peritonitis, abscess, and fistula formation.

CLINICAL PRESENTATION

Subjective

Acute cholecystitis causes various symptoms, ranging from generalized gastrointestinal complaints to intractable pain. Most patients complain of indigestion, nausea, and vomiting, especially after consuming a meal high in fat. Acute cholecystitis usually begins with acute, colicky-type pain. About 80% of patients report that they have experienced this type of pain before. However, the pain associated with acute cholecystitis persists, and as the inflammation progresses, the pain localizes over the RUQ or epigastrium. Patients may complain of referred pain that radiates to the middle of the back, infrascapular area, or right shoulder. The pain is increased by any movement, including respiration. If the inflammation extends to the peritoneal area, the pain worsens, the abdominal muscles become rigid, and a fever is usually evident.

Objective

Physical findings reflect the degree of inflammation present. As the pain over the RUQ becomes severe, there is often involuntary guarding of the abdominal muscles over the right side. A positive Murphy's sign is elicited when the right subcostal region is so tender that there is painful splinting with deep inspiration or when palpation over the RUQ area causes transient inspiratory arrest. The gallbladder is palpable in fewer than 50% of the patients. Fever is usually low grade, 99° to 101°F (38.3°C); high fever suggests sepsis. Patients may develop mild jaundice from edema of the common bile duct. Hyperbilirubinemia should raise the suspicion of choledocholithiasis. Bowel sounds may be diminished.

In most cases, acute cholecystitis subsides spontaneously, with improvement in the first few days and resolution of symptoms after about 4 days. If symptoms persist or become more severe, the potential for perforation, gangrene, empyema, and septic shock increases. Rebound tenderness, shaking chills, or increased fever should raise suspicion that perforation has occurred. Surgical referral is indicated early in the disease process.

DIAGNOSTIC REASONING

Diagnostic Testing

During the acute presentation of cholecystitis, there is usually mild elevation of the white blood cell count, to 15,000/mL. Serum transaminases can be elevated up to four times the normal amount; aspartate aminotransferase and alanine aminotransferase can be elevated to 300 U/L. Alkaline phosphatase is elevated two to four times above normal levels, and bilirubin can be as high as 4 mg/dL. Profound elevation of alkaline phosphatase and bilirubin is highly suggestive of choledocholithiasis. An elevation in amylase can be the result of passage of a stone through the common bile duct but may also indicate gallstone pancreatitis.

Abdominal x-ray films may reveal gallstones, enlarged gallbladder, or air within the biliary system or peritoneal cavity. The gold standard for diagnosis of acute cholecystitis is abdominal ultrasound; it is a quick, noninvasive, reliable, and cost-effective means of identifying the presence of cholelithiasis. An obstructed cystic duct is the cause of acute cholecystitis in the most patients and is best seen with hepatobiliary imaging (cholescintigraphy) using a radiographic tracer (sometimes referred to as a HIDA scan). A computed tomography (CT) scan is useful if gangrene or perforation of the gallbladder is suspected.

Differential Diagnosis

The differential diagnosis of acute cholecystitis in the presence of RUQ pain, nausea, vomiting, and fever includes pancreatitis, myocardial infarction, appendicitis, peptic ulcer, pneumonia, and hepatitis. Most of these potential diagnoses can be effectively ruled out via standard laboratory tests and ultrasound. Electrocardiogram can rule out myocardial infarction and is necessary as part of preoperative studies.

MANAGEMENT

Treatment of cholelithiasis depends on many variables, including age; presenting symptoms; past medical history; and size, type, and number of gallstones involved. Patients with symptomatic cholelithiasis can often be safely managed on an outpatient basis. Patients must be advised to avoid foods high in fat, which can provoke an attack. Nonsurgical options for the treatment of gallstones include dissolution of the stone by oral ingestion of ursodeoxycholic acid (ursodiol) or direct dissolution by percutaneous instillation of methyl-tertiary-butyl ether. Both types of dissolution therapies are of limited value and can be used only with cholesterol stones. Recurrence rates with these treatments are almost 100%, and duration of treatment may be as long as 2 years.

Patients who are deemed poor surgical risks can also undergo extracorporeal shock wave lithotripsy along with chemical dissolution in an attempt to reduce the size of the stones. Patients who continue to have biliary colic or who have developed other complications should be hospitalized for further treatment, with prompt referral to a gastroenterologist and/or a surgeon.

Initial Management

Initial treatment begins with definitive diagnosis. For many, the diagnosis of gallstones is made as an incidental finding during medical treatment for another problem. These patients are often asymptomatic and require no further treatment except awareness of the signs and symptoms of a "gallbladder attack." Patients who are considered a poor surgical risk can be treated nonsurgically with dissolution therapy or lithotripsy. However, the recurrence rate is high and in the elderly, the complication rate and mortality are high. Those who remain symptomatic despite treatment or have developed other complications

should be hospitalized in an attempt to reduce the risk of a life-threatening event such as gangrene, perforation, or septic shock.

Management of acute cholecystitis includes rehydration with IV fluids, antibiotics, analgesics, and GI rest. If vomiting is persistent, a nasogastric tube is inserted. A second or third generation cephalosporin is started once the diagnosis is made. If sepsis is suspected, an aminoglycoside is added to the antibiotic coverage.

The treatment of choice for acute cholecystitis is early surgical intervention. Patients in the acute phase of the disease are usually stabilized before a cholecystectomy is scheduled; however, early surgical intervention is associated with a decreased length of stay, lower cost, and patient satisfaction. Patients who are considered a poor surgical risk may benefit from cholecystotomy, either operatively or percutaneously. Emergency decompression with cholecystotomy may be necessary to remove stones and purulent material before a cholecystectomy, which should be deferred for 6 to 8 weeks.

The mortality rate associated with acute cholecystitis is 5% to 10% and is usually associated with patients older than age 60 with comorbid conditions and those with septic complications. The mortality rate for cholecystectomy is less than 0.2%. Approximately 50% of patients who do choose not to undergo cholecystectomy have a recurrence within 5 years, and complications are common.

Subsequent Management

The most common complications of acute cholecystitis are empyema and perforation. Perforation into the abdominal cavity can occur early in the disease process and is associated with a 30% mortality rate. Perforation may also occur into another hollow viscus or into the colon, causing draining fistulas, which may relieve the symptoms associated with cholecystitis. Surgical removal of the gallbladder with fistula repair is indicated when the patient is medically stable for surgery.

FOLLOW-UP AND REFERRAL

Patients with acute cholecystitis require referral to a general surgeon for removal of the gallbladder. Referral should be made after diagnosis of acute cholecystitis. Follow-up includes routine postoperative visits according to the surgeon. Patients who have persistent symptoms after removal of the gallbladder (postcholecystectomy syndrome) may have a mistaken diagnosis, a functional bowel disorder, retained or recurrent common bile duct stones, or spasm of the sphincter of Oddi. Patients with incidental findings of asymptomatic gallstones should be referred to a surgeon and given the option for elective surgery, medical dissolution therapy, lithotripsy, or contact solvent dissolution.

Patient Education: Gallbladder Disease

Patient education for individuals declining surgical intervention should include the risks and benefits of each therapy. Dietary counseling should include weight loss for those patients who are obese and the avoidance of fatty foods that provoke attacks. Patients taking oral contraceptives should be given information about alternative forms of birth control, and menopausal women taking estrogen should be counseled about alternative sources of phytoestrogens, such as soy products.

ACUTE PANCREATITIS

Acute pancreatitis is defined as acute inflammation of the pancreas and the surrounding tissues resulting from the release of pancreatic enzymes. These enzymes cause a chemical burn in the retroperitoneal spaces, which leads to systemic toxicity. The degree to which the microcirculation within the pancreas is preserved determines the histological classification of pancreatitis. If the microcirculation remains intact, the process is defined as acute interstitial pancreatitis. If the microcirculation is disrupted, it is defined as necrotizing pancreatitis. Acute pancreatitis normally resolves both clinically and histologically.

EPIDEMIOLOGY AND CAUSES

Although there are many causes of acute pancreatitis, approximately 80% of all hospital admissions for acute pancreatitis are the result of biliary tract disease (passing of a gallstone) or alcoholism. See Box 41.1 for all the causes of pancreatitis. Up to 25% of patients will experience recurrence in the first several years after the initial diagnosis. More than 300,000 hospital admissions and a cost of more than $2 billion is attributed to acute pancreatitis annually.

Acute pancreatitis is usually the result of some other process, such as passing of a gallstone, excessive alcohol

---

Box 41.1 Causes of Pancreatitis

- Infection (mumps)
- Hyperlipidemia (particularly types I, IV, and V)
- Metabolic disorders (hyperparathyroidism, hypercalcemia)
- Drugs (furosemide, valproic acid, sulfonamides, thiazides)
- Endoscopic retrograde cholangiopancreatography (ERCP)
- Structural abnormalities of the pancreatic duct (stricture, carcinoma, pancreas divisum)
- Structural abnormalities of the common bile duct and ampullary region
- Surgery (particularly of the stomach and biliary tract)
- Vascular disease (atherosclerosis, severe hypotension)
- Trauma

---

intake, or other type of biliary tract disease. Clinical pancreatitis is seen in up to 9.5% of alcoholic patients, and histological evidence is found in 17% to 45% of this group. Cholelithiasis is present in 60% of nonalcoholic patients with pancreatitis.

PATHOPHYSIOLOGY

Pathological changes associated with pancreatitis range from acute edema and cellular infiltration to necrosis and hemorrhage. Although the exact pathogenesis is not known, temporary impaction of the sphincter of Oddi by a gallstone before its passage into the duodenum may cause edema or obstruction of the ampulla of Vater, with subsequent reflux of bile into the pancreatic ducts and injury to the acinar cells. This cascade of events causes an autodigestive process within the pancreas that can progress to shock and death without appropriate intervention. Inflammation is confined to the pancreas in edematous pancreatitis, and the mortality rate is less than 5%.

When inflammation and tissue necrosis extends beyond the pancreas, the associated mortality rate is 10% to 50%. Pancreatic exudate containing toxins and activated enzymes permeates the retroperitoneum and causes a chemical burn that increases the permeability of the blood vessels within the peritoneal cavity. As a result, large amounts of protein-rich fluid from the circulation are sequestered in these third spaces, producing hypovolemia and shock. As these toxins and enzymes enter the systemic circulation, they can further reduce vascular tone and thus the ability to correct the hypotension and shock.

Acute pancreatitis can be classified as either mild or severe. Mild acute pancreatitis normally improves within 48 to 72 hours and does not involve other organ systems. There is minimal interstitial edema, with only occasional microscopic acinar cell necrosis. Severe, acute pancreatitis is often associated with complications and multisystem organ failure. It can be a life-threatening condition, and the patient may require monitoring in the intensive care unit (ICU).

Complications during the first few days of diagnosis are associated with hemodynamic instability: shock, renal failure, respiratory compromise secondary to adult respiratory distress syndrome (ARDS), and hypoxemia. Pancreatic necrosis with secondary gram-negative sepsis has an associated 100% mortality rate unless there is extensive surgical debridement of the infected tissue. Up to 25% of patients diagnosed with acute pancreatitis develop some degree of fluid collection within a few days of diagnosis that resolves spontaneously half of the time. Patients in whom fluid collection does not resolve may form pseudocysts, abscesses, and other necrotic collections.

Pancreatic pseudocysts take at least 4 weeks to form and resolve spontaneously after about 6 weeks in 40% of cases. If the pseudocyst does not resolve within 12 weeks after acute pancreatitis, the risk of complications in symptomatic patients (infection, bleeding, rupture) is as high as 60%, but there is little associated risk in asymptomatic patients. The decision for invasive intervention depends on the progression of symptoms and cyst size.

CLINICAL PRESENTATION

Subjective

The patient with acute pancreatitis usually presents with abrupt onset of deep epigastric pain that persists for hours to days and may radiate straight through to the back. The pain is intense and often refractory to large doses of parenteral narcotics. It is aggravated by any vigorous activity, such as coughing, and by lying supine; it improves when the patient is seated and leaning forward. The patient appears acutely ill, often with intractable nausea and vomiting. In some cases, depending on the severity, the patient may experience sweating, weakness, and anxiety. The patient may report a history of ingestion of alcohol or a big meal before onset of symptoms or mild biliary colic preceding the episode.

Objective

On physical exam, there is severe abdominal tenderness, particularly over the epigastric area, which may be accompanied by guarding but without rigidity or rebound tenderness, and there may be milder pain in the lower abdomen without guarding or rigidity. Abdominal distention is present in approximately 20% of the patients. Bowel sounds can be hypoactive or absent if associated with paralytic ileus. The rectal exam is normal, and the stool is usually negative for occult blood.

The patient is tachycardic (100–140 beats/min) with rapid, shallow respiration. Inspiratory effort is poor because deep inspiration causes pain. Blood pressure may be high secondary to pain or low if shock is imminent. The patient's temperature may initially be normal or subnormal but increases to 100.4° to 102.2°F (38°–39°C) within a few hours. Mild jaundice and scleral icterus may be present. The patient's skin may be pale, cool, and clammy if shock is present.

Uncommon findings that can result from the pancreatic inflammatory process include left-sided pleural effusion, bluish discoloration over the flanks (Grey Turner's sign) or around the umbilicus (Cullen's sign), jaundice caused by impingement on the common bile duct, and epigastric mass secondary to pseudocyst development.

DIAGNOSTIC REASONING

Diagnostic Tests

The diagnosis of pancreatitis is made on the basis of the presence of abdominal pain, elevated serum amylase and/or lipase levels, and imaging findings consistent with acute pancreatitis. The gold standard for diagnosis is an elevated serum amylase level (up to three times the normal value); however, in one-third of patients with alcoholic pancreatitis, the serum amylase level may be normal. The diagnosis of pancreatitis is supported by a concurrent elevation of serum lipase. Serum amylase and lipase levels are increased on the first day of acute symptoms and return to normal in 3 to 7 days. Levels remain normal if there has been repeated prior damage to acinar cells, which renders them incapable of further enzyme secretion. The level of elevation of amylase and lipase is not indicative of the severity of the disease.

The white blood cell (WBC) count is usually between 12,000 and 20,000 cells/mL. The hematocrit can be as high as 50% to 55% because of hemoconcentration resulting from sequestered fluids in the third spaces.

A decrease in serum calcium may indicate saponification and is indicative of the severity of the pancreatitis. Calcium levels below 7 mg/dL (with normal serum albumin) can cause tetany and are associated with poor prognosis. Elevated C-reactive protein is correlated with pancreatic necrosis. The risk of infection is positively correlated with pancreatic necrosis and accounts for most of the deaths. Pancreatic necrosis requires surgical intervention; computed tomography (CT)–guided aspiration of the necrotic tissue for gram stain and culture is indicated.

Patients presenting with biliary pancreatitis have an elevation of the liver enzymes. When alanine aminotransferase is up to three times the normal limit, the positive predictive value is 95% that the pancreatitis is caused by biliary disease (gallstones). Concomitant increases in the aspartate aminotransferase, alkaline phosphatase, and bilirubin suggest gallbladder disease.

Diagnostic imaging, especially CT of the abdomen, can provide fast and accurate information for the definitive diagnosis of acute pancreatitis. Although the CT scan can be normal in 15% to 30% of patients with mild acute pancreatitis, it is the most efficient means of discerning acute pancreatitis from other potentially fatal intra-abdominal processes. CT is also helpful in monitoring the progression or resolution of pancreatic pseudocysts.

Patients with acute pancreatitis and no obvious alternative causes should undergo abdominal ultrasonography (US) to detect the possible causes such as cholelithiasis or neoplasms. US can also detect dilation of the common bile duct, indicating obstruction. Endoscopic retrograde cholangiopancreatography (ERCP) with sphincterotomy and stone extraction can be performed and has been proved to decrease morbidity and mortality.

If there is evidence that the pancreatitis is severe, additional testing with IV contrast is recommended; the necrotic pancreas has damage to its microcirculation and thus is not enhanced with IV contrast. If the microcirculation remains intact, there is uniform enhancement of the pancreas. Pancreatic necrosis is associated with much higher morbidity, mortality, and infection rates.

TABLE 41.1   Ranson's Criteria for Assessing the Severity of Pancreatitis

At admission or at time of diagnosis:

1. Age older than 55 years
2. White blood cell count greater than 16,000/mcL
3. Blood glucose greater than 200 mg/dL
4. Base deficit greater than 4 mEq/L
5. Serum lactate dehydrogenase (LDH) greater than 350 IU/L
6. Aspartate transamine (AST) greater than 250 U/L

During the initial 48 hours:

1. Hematocrit (Hct) drop of more than 10 percentage points
2. Blood urea nitrogen (BUN) rise of greater than 5 mg/dL
3. Arterial PO_2 of less than 60
4. Serum calcium (Ca) of less than 8 mg/dL
5. Estimated fluid sequestration of greater than 6 L

Number of Diagnostic Criteria	Mortality Rate (%)
0–2	1
3–4	16
5–6	40
7–8	100

Adapted from Ranson JH, Rifkind KM, Roses DF, Fink SD, Eng K, Spencer FC. Prognostic signs and the role of operative management in acute pancreatitis. *Surg Gynecol Obstet.* 1974;139(1):69–81,.

Pancreatic infection is a complication that requires immediate diagnosis and intervention. Infection should be suspected when the patient has persistently elevated WBC counts and fever. The patient normally looks very sick. Positive blood cultures and visualization of gas bubbles within the retroperitoneum on CT support the diagnosis.

Ranson's criteria are useful for assessing the severity of acute pancreatitis. Identification of early prognostic signs may provide the best indication of a serious outcome and can alert the practitioner that the patient may require transfer to the ICU. Table 41.1 lists the 11 objective signs used to classify the severity of pancreatitis. Mortality rates correlate directly with the number of diagnostic criteria present. Pancreatitis is classified as severe when three or more of Ranson's criteria are met.

Differential Diagnosis

Differential diagnosis of acute pancreatitis is made by history and physical exam and supported by laboratory data and imaging studies. CT scan is useful in differentiating other intra-abdominal processes from acute pancreatitis. However, it is less helpful in identifying gallstones as a potential cause. Laboratory data are helpful in differentiating other causes of acute abdominal pain with associated hyperamylasemia. Box 41.2 differentiates hyperamylasemia resulting from pancreatic and nonpancreatic causes.

Box 41.2   Hyperamylasemia: Pancreatic and Nonpancreatic Causes

Pancreatic Hyperamylasemia	Nonpancreatic Hyperamylasemia
Pancreatic pseudocyst	Salivary adenitis (secondary to mumps)
Perforated duodenal ulcer	Ruptured ectopic pregnancy
Small bowel perforation	Postabdominal surgery
Mesenteric infarction	Lactic acidosis
Mesenteric vascular thrombus	
Opiate administration	Leaking aortic aneurysm
Post–endoscopic retrograde cholangiopancreatography	Renal insufficiency

MANAGEMENT

Treatment of acute pancreatitis is aimed at limiting the severity of pancreatic inflammation, preventing further complications by interrupting the pathological processes, and managing symptoms. Mild acute pancreatitis usually resolves spontaneously in a few days; these patients can be managed conservatively as outpatients. Fasting is necessary until the symptoms of acute inflammation have subsided.

Treatment includes maintaining fluid status with parenteral fluids to prevent hypovolemia and hypotension. Pain has traditionally been controlled with meperidine (Demerol) rather than with other opiates to prevent increased pressure within the sphincter of Oddi. However, research indicates that morphine causes no more spasms in the sphincter of Oddi than meperidine. The patient is allowed nothing by mouth, and nasogastric (NG) tube insertion should be considered when there is persistent nausea, vomiting, or evidence of ileus. The use of empiric antibiotics, H_2-receptor antagonists, and pancreatic enzyme inhibitors have not been proved effective and are not recommended.

Judicious introduction of clear liquids can be instituted once the patient is pain free, amylase and lipase levels have returned to normal range, and bowel sounds have returned. A low-fat diet may be instituted as the patient tolerates.

Patients with more severe pancreatitis tend to have sequestered larger amounts of fluid as a result of the "chemical burn" sustained by the tissues within the retroperitoneal space. These patients are usually transferred to the ICU under the care of a gastroenterologist or surgeon. Aggressive volume replacement is necessary and may require invasive hemodynamic monitoring to maintain appropriate fluid balance. Fluid resuscitation is an important part of therapy and 6 to 8 L/day may be required. Some patients may require infusion of fresh frozen plasma or serum albumin or blood transfusions, which can increase the risk of the development of ARDS. Cardiac function and fluid status can be monitored with a central line or pulmonary artery catheter. Measurement of hourly urine output is also necessary. If hemodynamic stability is not achieved through volume replacement, vasopressors may be necessary.

Daily monitoring of serum calcium, magnesium, glucose, electrolytes, total protein, albumin, amylase, lipase, and complete blood count with subsequent correction of abnormalities is required. In febrile patients, cultures of blood, urine, and sputum should be obtained, as well as CT-guided needle aspiration of necrotic areas of the pancreas with initiation of appropriate broad-spectrum antibiotic coverage as necessary to prevent increased morbidity and mortality. Arterial blood gas readings should be obtained daily, and hypoxemia treated accordingly. The patient may require assisted ventilation if hypoxemia persists or ARDS develops.

Correction of serum glucose is done with caution and should not begin until levels are greater than 250 mg/dL. Hypocalcemia is often corrected with the administration of albumin-containing fluids. Neuromuscular irritability, if present, can be corrected with a 10% solution of calcium gluconate. If there is a coexisting hypomagnesemia, correction of the magnesium level will often restore the calcium to its normal level. In patients with renal impairment, magnesium must be replaced cautiously.

Patients with severe pancreatitis must be maintained in a fasting state for prolonged periods of time, often for 2 to 4 weeks. Administration of antacids through an NG tube can help to prevent stress ulceration. The nutritional needs of the patient can be maintained with total parenteral nutrition until the gut becomes functional; enteral feedings can then be started, using the distal jejunum to reduce pancreatic stimulation. Oral feedings should not be started until all complications have been treated, the patient is free from nausea and vomiting, and amylase and lipase levels have returned to normal.

Surgical intervention is normally reserved for a pancreatic pseudocyst that has persisted for more than 6 weeks with ongoing symptomatology, necrotizing pancreatitis, pancreatic abscess, or severe hemorrhagic pancreatitis. Despite surgical intervention, the mortality rate for necrotizing pancreatitis remains high.

For pancreatitis caused by cholelithiasis, surgical intervention is determined by the presenting course of events. If biliary decompression is necessary, it can often be accomplished with ERCP. If the pancreatitis is mild, a cholecystectomy can be performed at a later time.

FOLLOW-UP AND REFERRAL

Patients with severe acute pancreatitis or those who do not respond to conservative treatment should be referred to a gastroenterologist for management. Surgical referral should be made once the diagnosis of pancreatitis is made. The patient who develops a pseudocyst requires long-term follow-up with serial CT scans to observe the resolution or growth of the cyst, which may require

surgical intervention. The patient who has gallstone disease should have a cholecystectomy.

The prognosis of the patient with pancreatitis correlates directly with the severity of the inflammatory process. Patients with interstitial, or edematous, pancreatitis even with systemic complications have a mortality rate of 1% to 2%; however, patients with necrotizing pancreatitis have a mortality rate of 10% with sterile necrosis and up to 30% with infected necrosis.

In patients for whom no cause has been found, studies have suggested that half of these patients have occult gallstone disease (biliary sludge) or sphincter of Oddi dysfunction. These patients require repeated abdominal US exams to detect the development of biliary sludge. Patients with hereditary hypercholesterolemia are often missed because serum triglycerides are not obtained until after several days of fasting, at which time the triglyceride level may have fallen to within normal limits.

Patient Education: Acute Pancreatitis

Patients with biliary disease as the cause of the pancreatitis should be informed of the need for a cholecystectomy, as well as the benefit of reducing their dietary intake of fat. If the etiology of pancreatitis is alcohol abuse, the patient should be encouraged to abstain. Patients with genetic hyperlipidemia require diet instruction and information on avoidance of precipitating factors such as alcohol, estrogens, and certain drugs. These patients may benefit from lipid-lowering medications and must be taught to control their diabetes if present. If a drug is the suspected cause of the pancreatitis, it should not be restarted.

CHRONIC PANCREATITIS

Chronic pancreatitis is defined as a slowly progressive inflammatory process that results in irreversible fibrosis of the pancreas with destruction and atrophy of the exocrine and endocrine glandular tissue. There are varying degrees of ductal dilation and fibrosis. There can be intraductal formation of protein plugs, which calcify and cause further dilation and obstruction. *Chronic relapsing pancreatitis* is defined as acute attacks that occur in the setting of chronic pancreatitis and are usually precipitated by a specific event such as binge drinking or the passage of a stone.

EPIDEMIOLOGY AND CAUSES

There is little reliable information on the prevalence or incidence of chronic pancreatitis. Alcoholism may account for between 70% and 80% of the cases in industrialized countries. Although there is no threshold for alcohol consumption and the development of chronic pancreatitis, there is a statistically significant increase in individuals who consume 120 g of ethanol per day (eight 12-ounce beers, 8 ounces of 100-proof whiskey, or 30 ounces of wine). Diets high in protein in combination with either high or low fat can further predispose patients to pancreatic injury from alcohol.

Other causes of chronic pancreatitis include autoimmune disease, genetic mutations, hereditary predisposition, hypertriglyceridemia, severe malnutrition (especially protein-calorie deficiency in developing countries), tropical pancreatitis, and obstruction of the main pancreatic duct caused by stenosis, stones, tumor, or cystic fibrosis. In 10% to 30% of persons with chronic pancreatitis, the cause is unknown, but patients are divided into two groups: (1) those who present with abdominal pain (usually between ages 15 and 30) and (2) older individuals (ages 50–70) who present, often without pain, with pancreatic calcifications, glandular insufficiency, and diabetes.

The tropical, or nutritional, form of chronic pancreatitis is almost exclusively found in tropical countries. In these countries, the disease begins in early childhood and results in death in early adulthood because of complications. This type of pancreatitis also involves large intraductal calculi and a high susceptibility to pancreatic cancer. Malnutrition has a significant role, but it is not the sole cause because many areas with comparable malnutrition do not have equal prevalence of the disease. Key features of tropical pancreatitis include abdominal pain, maldigestion leading to steatorrhea, and diabetes.

PATHOPHYSIOLOGY

The pathogenesis of chronic pancreatitis is unclear. Two characteristic findings in chronic pancreatitis are hypersecretion of protein without a subsequent increase in ductal bicarbonate secretion and inflammation. Chronic pancreatitis results in irreversible structural damage with permanent functional impairment of the pancreatic gland. For individuals who have alcohol-related disease, ductal obstruction is thought to be caused by changes in the chemical composition of the pancreatic juice, leading to protein plugging, calcification, and subsequent pancreatic damage. Another theory postulates that continuous injury to the acinar cells causes inflammation, necrosis, and fibrosis. Analysis of pancreatic juice obtained from alcoholic patients revealed protein plugs but not always chronic pancreatitis. Proponents of the theory favoring repeated damage to the pancreatic acinar cells believe that ductal obstruction is a result of changes in the pancreatic juice that cause increased viscosity and damage to the gland itself. These changes in the enzymatic properties result in chronic inflammation and fibrosis of the gland. Biliary disease has not been identified as a causative factor in the development of chronic pancreatitis.

With the progressive inflammatory changes occurring with chronic pancreatitis, it is not uncommon to find a fibrotic common bile duct and jaundice secondary to the obstructed common bile duct. Upper gastrointestinal bleeding can result from the formation of gastric varices

or the development of a pseudoaneurysm in an artery within the pancreatic area. Steatorrhea and diabetes mellitus result from destruction of the pancreatic gland with subsequent endocrine and exocrine insufficiency. Steatorrhea develops as lipase and protease secretion drops below 10% of normal. Islet cell destruction reduces insulin secretion, causing glucose intolerance and diabetes.

CLINICAL PRESENTATION
Subjective

The most frequent presenting symptoms are intractable abdominal pain, weight loss, and diarrhea, but symptoms can be as mild as dyspepsia, nausea, and vomiting. Abdominal pain is usually epigastric or located in the left upper quadrant, may radiate to the back or left lumbar region, and is described as dull and constant. Pain may be absent in 5% to 10% of the cases or may represent an exacerbation of acute or relapsing pancreatitis. Pain may precede the development of other symptoms of chronic pancreatitis by years. The pain is often precipitated or aggravated by food or alcohol intake. In some patients, the pain diminishes over time (5–15 years) and is associated with failure or calcification of the gland. Between 10% and 20% of older adults with idiopathic chronic pancreatitis have no pain with the disease.

Weight loss may result from anorexia caused by pain and nausea, malabsorption secondary to pancreatic exocrine insufficiency, or poorly controlled diabetes mellitus. Diabetes mellitus is present in approximately 50% of patients and is often the presenting sign in individuals who have no pain associated with pancreatitis. Steatorrhea develops after the pancreas loses the ability to secrete digestive enzymes, which results in bulky, foul-smelling, fatty stools. Patients often complain of "oil leakage" from the rectum or an "oil slick" in the toilet bowl, which is indicative of pancreatic insufficiency.

Objective

Abdominal assessment in patients presenting with pain reveals mild to moderate epigastric tenderness with no rebound tenderness or guarding. A palpable abdominal mass is suggestive of a pancreatic pseudocyst. Bowel sounds may be absent in patients with paralytic ileus. Lung sounds may be diminished in the bases, which is indicative of pleural effusion.

DIAGNOSTIC REASONING
Diagnostic Tests

Diagnosis of chronic pancreatitis is normally made through evaluation of pancreatic function and radiographic visualization of structural abnormalities such as pancreatic calcification or abnormalities in the size or consistency of the pancreatic tissue. The patient usually presents with chronic abdominal pain, weight loss, exocrine insufficiency (malabsorption), and diabetes mellitus.

Tests for pancreatic function include assessment of endocrine and exocrine function. A 2-hour postprandial blood sugar level greater than 200 mg/dL or fasting glucose greater than 120 mg/dL on two occasions is diagnostic for diabetes mellitus. Glucosuria may also be present. The serum amylase level may remain within normal limits because the pancreas has lost the ability to mount a response due to the chronicity of the disease. Malabsorption is documented by a 72-hour stool analysis for fecal fat content. Although helpful for diagnosis of exocrine function, steatorrhea is not diagnostic of chronic pancreatitis because patients do not develop steatorrhea until lipase falls below 10% of normal.

Pancreatic insufficiency can be confirmed by the bentiromide (nitroblue tetrazolium–*para*-aminobenzoic acid [NBT-PABA]) test, which measures urinary excretion of pancreatic chymotrypsin, or a secretin stimulation test, which is more sensitive but is unavailable in many places. The test involves placing a tube within the duodenum and collecting pancreatic secretions after IV stimulation with secretin. Collections of normal volume and low in bicarbonate (HCO_3^-) suggest chronic pancreatitis; collections low in volume and normal HCO_3^- suggest pancreatic cancer. The detection of decreased fecal chymotrypsin or elastase helps to diagnose pancreatic insufficiency, but these tests do not have widespread availability.

Imaging studies include plain films of the abdomen, which may show intraductal stones or a calcified pancreas caused by pancreatolithiasis and mild ileus. CT and/or US of the abdomen may show an abnormal size or consistency of the pancreas, a pancreatic pseudocyst, or dilated pancreatic ducts. Magnetic resonance cholangiopancreatography is a noninvasive procedure that is considered safer procedure than ERCP. ERCP is associated with an increased risk of acute pancreatitis from dye injection into the pancreas. Endoscopic ultrasound can be used to visualize the pancreatic and bile ducts.

Differential Diagnosis

Differential diagnosis includes diseases that present with persistent abdominal pain such as peptic ulcer disease or mesenteric ischemia; diseases that result in weight loss and abdominal pain, including abdominal malignancies, especially cancer of the pancreas; and intestinal disorders that may present with steatorrhea. The diagnosis of chronic pancreatitis can be confirmed by visualization of the calcified pancreas on x-ray films, which will also rule out most other disease processes.

MANAGEMENT

The treatment of chronic pancreatitis is aimed at preventing further pancreatic damage, managing pain, and supplementing exocrine and endocrine function. The major cause of chronic pancreatitis is alcohol abuse; therefore, complete abstinence is imperative. Pancreatic enzyme supplementation may relieve pain in some patients. Generally, narcotics are necessary to manage pain. Patients whose pain is not managed by analgesics or pancreatic enzyme therapy should be considered for operative treatment.

Malabsorption is managed with a low-fat diet (less than 50 g/day) and oral pancreatic enzyme supplementation. Oral supplementation should be administered 20 to 30 minutes before meals and snacks. The usual dose is 30,000 units of lipase. Non–enteric-coated pancrelipase formulations (Viokase or Cotazym) should be given with H_2-receptor antagonists to prevent degradation by gastric acids. Enteric-coated preparations of pancrelipase (Pancrease or Creon) or pancreatin (Donnazyme) are stable at an acid pH and should not be given with acid neutralizers because this will promote enzyme release within the stomach. Fat-soluble vitamin (A, D, E, and K) replacement may be required. Favorable outcomes are weight gain, decreased number of stools per day, decrease in oil seepage from the rectum, and subjective improvement in well-being.

Endocrine insufficiency is controlled with insulin supplementation. Extreme caution must be used with insulin supplementation because there is a deficiency of glucagon secretion, which can lead to prolonged hypoglycemia. Serum glucose levels of 200 to 250 mg/dL are considered acceptable and do not require treatment. The principal step in the management of diabetes associated with chronic pancreatitis is the correction of poor nutritional habits, malabsorption and malnutrition, and the elimination of alcohol. Normal insulin requirements range from 5 to 15 units per day but may fluctuate up to 40 units per day. It is best to maintain these patients at a higher than normal glucose level to avoid hypoglycemia while avoiding significant glucosuria.

Surgical intervention may be required to drain persistent pseudocysts, for relief of pain, or to treat other complications associated with chronic pancreatitis. The goal of surgical intervention is to alleviate biliary tract disease, establish the free flow of bile into the duodenum, and remove obstruction of the pancreatic duct. Distal pancreatectomy may be necessary if the disease is located at the tail of the pancreas, and the Whipple procedure is performed when the disease is most extensive at the head of the pancreas. These procedures relieve the pain for 60% to 80% of patients.

In patients with alcoholic pancreatitis, ERCP examination often reveals alternating stricture and dilation ("chain of lakes") of the pancreatic duct. Treatment is a modified Puestow procedure (lateral pancreaticojejunostomy), which relieves pain in 70% to 80% of patients.

FOLLOW-UP AND REFERRAL

Follow-up of the patient with chronic pancreatitis depends on the complications resulting from the disease and the medical and surgical interventions employed to remedy the disease. Patients who have developed pseudocysts that have not resolved spontaneously will require periodic CT scans to monitor resolution or evolution of the cysts. Cysts that are consistently larger than 6 cm and are expanding should be referred for invasive treatment.

A nutritionist may be helpful in managing protein-calorie malnutrition. The pancreas is very nutrition sensitive, and an improper diet can lead to atrophy and fibrosis. Follow-up with the nutritionist is often necessary for control of diabetes mellitus as well.

Patient Education: Chronic Pancreatitis

Patients should be taught about the pathophysiology of this chronic disease, common complications, and the long-term outlook. Patients with chronic pancreatitis can expect that after 5 to 10 years, the episodes of pancreatic pain diminish in frequency and may disappear. Patients should understand their medicine regimen, including appropriate timing of medication doses and adverse effects. Patients tend to be more compliant when they understand that the goal of treatment is to control diarrhea and gain body weight. Patients can be provided with written instructions to assist with adherence.

Patients should be cautioned against long-term narcotic analgesic use because it can result in drug dependence. If long-term narcotic use is necessary, patients may benefit from referral to a pain control clinic to learn how to relieve pain using nonpharmacotherapeutic measures.

REFERENCES

Abraham S, Rivero HG, Erlikh IV, Griffith LF, Kondamudi VK. Surgical and nonsurgical management of gallstones. *Am Fam Physician.* 2014;89(10):795–802.

Afdhal NZ. Epidemiology of and risk factors for gallstones. *UpToDate.* http://www.uptodate.com./online/content/topic.do?topicKey= biliaryt/5497&selectedTitle=4%7E150&source=search_result. Published November 28, 2016.

Bergman S, Al-Bader M, Sourial N, et al. Recurrence of biliary disease following non-operative management in elderly patients. *Surg Endosc.* 2015;29(12):3485–3490.

Bollen TL. Acute pancreatitis: International classification and nomenclature. *Clin Radiol.* 2016;71(2):121–133.

Cucher D, Kulvatunyou N, Green DJ, Jie T, Ong ES. Gallstone pancreatitis: A review. *Surg Clin North Am.* 2014;94(2):257–280.

Ranson JH, Rifkind KM, Roses DF, Fink SD, Eng K, Spencer FC. Prognostic signs and the role of operative management in acute pancreatitis. *Surg Gynecol Obstet.* 1974;139(1):69–81.

Tenner S, Baillie J, DeWitt J, Vege SS. American College of Gastroenterology Guideline: Management of acute pancreatitis. *Am J Gastroenterol.* 2013;108:1400–1415.

RESOURCES

The National Pancreas Foundation
About acute pancreatitis
   https://pancreasfoundation.org/patient-information/acute-pancreatitis/acute-pancreatitis-diagnosis-and-treatment/

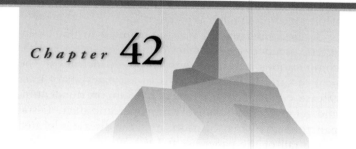

Chapter **42**

Cirrhosis and Liver Failure

Debera J. Thomas, DNS, RN, FNP/ANP

Cirrhosis is result of hepatocellular injury involving the entire liver, resulting in fibrosis, nodular regeneration, and distorted hepatic architecture. Cirrhosis is considered permanent and irreversible. Fibrous bands are formed during nodular regeneration in an attempt by the liver to repair itself, and these bands give the liver

a hobnailed appearance. The fibrotic changes that occur within the liver parenchyma cause disruption and compression of the vascular, biliary, and lymphatic vessels and result in many of the characteristic findings common to liver failure.

EPIDEMIOLOGY AND CAUSES

In the Western Hemisphere, cirrhosis is a leading cause of death in individuals older than age 40. The prevalence of cirrhosis in the United States is approximately 0.27% (633,323 people) and may be higher. Although there are many causes of cirrhosis (Box 42.1), chronic alcohol abuse and viral hepatitis remain the leading pathological insults in the United States.

There are three consequences of alcohol abuse: fatty liver, alcoholic hepatitis, and alcoholic cirrhosis. Fatty liver is a reversible condition where large vacuoles of triglycerides accumulate in the hepatocytes. The accumulation of fat in the liver causes an inflammatory reaction in the liver called steatohepatitis and is

Box 42.1   Causes of Cirrhosis

Alcohol

Direct hepatotoxins

- Carbon tetrachloride
- Phosphorus

Indirect hepatotoxins

- Tetracycline
- Methotrexate
- Acetaminophen
- Mushroom toxin—*Amanita phalloides*
- Alkylated anabolic steroids
- 6-Mercaptopurine

Hepatitis B and hepatitis C virus infection

Autoimmune chronic active hepatitis

Diabetes mellitus and insipidus

Thyroiditis

Ulcerative colitis

Glomerulonephritis

Biliary cirrhosis

Primary biliary cirrhosis

Primary sclerosing cholangitis

Chronic pancreatitis

Sclerosing cholangitis

Vasculitis

Cholelithiasis

Cystic fibrosis

Genetic diseases

- Wilson's disease
- Hemochromatosis
- Galactosemia

Vascular/congestive disorders of the liver

- Budd-Chiari syndrome
- Ischemic hepatitis/shock liver
- Right-sided heart failure (chronic)

a precursor of cirrhosis. Alcoholic hepatitis results from moderate to severe alcohol abuse for years and can lead to alcoholic cirrhosis quickly even with abstinence, but it is not an obligatory phase in the development of cirrhosis.

Alcoholic cirrhosis is the most common type of cirrhosis in the United States. The incidence of alcohol use disorder (AUD) is increasing in the United States; an estimated 18 million people in the United States abuse alcohol. However, only 35% of individuals with AUD develop cirrhosis.

The toxic effects of alcohol metabolism on the liver, immunologic alterations, oxidative stress, and malnutrition cause alcoholic cirrhosis. Although alcoholic cirrhosis is often associated with nutritional and vitamin deficiencies, it can occur in well-nourished individuals. Studies have found no safe amount of alcohol that can be ingested daily without causing cirrhosis, which supports the theory that there are additional factors (genetic, environmental, nutritional) that may influence the development of alcoholic liver disease. Women tend to develop cirrhosis more quickly with less alcohol intake than men, which suggests that a smaller, leaner body mass and enhanced absorption are both factors in the development of alcoholic cirrhosis.

Primary biliary cirrhosis (PBC) is a disease that almost exclusively affects women aged 40 to 60. It is an autoimmune disease that causes destruction of the intrahepatic bile ducts, resulting in cholestasis. Autoimmune disorders such as scleroderma, Raynaud's syndrome, autoimmune thyroid disease, celiac disease, and Sjögren's syndrome have been linked to the development of PBC.

Primary sclerosing cholangitis (PSC) is most common in men aged 20 to 40 and is associated with inflammatory bowel disease (75%), as well as with the histocompatibility antigens HLA-B8, HLA-DR3, and HLA-DR4, suggesting a genetic link. It is characterized by diffuse inflammation and fibrosis throughout the biliary tree. Factors contributing to the development of PSC are anything that obstructs or inhibits the flow of bile through both the extrahepatic and intrahepatic bile ducts. Smoking is associated with a *decreased* risk of PSC.

Budd-Chiari syndrome (BCS) is a disorder resulting from hepatic vein thrombosis and outflow obstruction, which can occur anywhere from the hepatic veins to the inferior vena cava (IVC) or the right atrium. Other disease processes associated with this form of cirrhosis are coagulopathies, lymphoreticular malignancies, ischemic hepatitis resulting from profound hypotension associated with shock, and liver arteriovenous malformations characteristic of hemorrhagic telangiectasia. There are numerous causes for BCS, and definitive diagnosis is found in only approximately 65% to 75% of cases. In the Western Hemisphere, thrombosis of the hepatic veins is most often associated with myeloproliferative and coagulation disorders, as well as oral contraceptive use. Venous thrombosis is also an associated risk factor in the third trimester of pregnancy. Malignant tumors arising from within the liver or metastatic renal carcinoma can result in mechanical obstruction of the IVC, causing thrombosis within the hepatic veins and resulting in cirrhosis.

Wilson's disease and *hemochromatosis* are both autosomal recessive metabolic disorders that often present with hepatocellular dysfunction and can lead to cirrhosis if left untreated. The liver is the primary organ involved in the metabolism of both iron (hemochromatosis) and copper (Wilson's disease); overload of either metal can cause cirrhosis. Hemochromatosis is diagnosed primarily in middle-aged whites, whereas Wilson's disease is a disease of adolescents and young adults of all ethnicities.

PATHOPHYSIOLOGY

Cirrhosis is the irreversible, end stage of liver injury caused by a variety of insults. Fibrotic scarring and hepatocellular changes result from chronic inflammation; obstruction; and toxic, metabolic, and congestive injuries. The morphological changes resulting from the injury are often classified according to the size of the regenerative nodules: Patients may have micronodular, macronodular, and mixed forms of cirrhosis. Cirrhosis also may result from severe acute injury, as is seen with hepatitis caused by HBV, HCV and chemical injury; subsequent to moderate damage sustained over months, as seen with obstructive biliary diseases; or from chronic continuous abuse, as seen in alcoholic cirrhosis.

Liver Changes in Cirrhosis

In individuals with cirrhosis, the normal lobular liver architecture is replaced by diffuse disorganization, resulting in proliferation of bands of fibrous tissue and nodular regeneration of the surviving hepatocytes. The extent to which this occurs depends on the degree of injury, the length of exposure to the injury, and the liver's reaction to the insult. The end result is a decrease in the total liver cell mass because of collagen formation or fibrosis. During the repair process, there is distortion of the microcirculation resulting in an increased resistance to blood flow, thereby causing portal venous hypertension. As the liver attempts to repair itself, it develops a series of collateral vessels from the newly regenerated nodules to the existing portal vein and hepatic artery. These vessels, which are much less efficient than those of the normal circulation, cause portal hypertension.

Histological Classification

Histological classification of cirrhosis is useful for describing the major anatomical changes that result from the various insults. This type of classification gives no etiological information other than narrowing the scope to the injurious agents resulting in this specific histological category of injury. Moreover, it is important to remember that at any point in the disease process, a patient may exhibit varying degrees of histological change.

Micronodular (Laennec's) cirrhosis is characterized by regenerative nodules that are 1 cm in diameter or less, no bigger than normal liver lobules. Histological examination fails to identify portal tracts and hepatic venules. Alcohol abuse often results in this type of cirrhosis; the theory is that continuous damage to the liver caused by alcohol exposure prevents it from regenerating. Initially the liver becomes enlarged and fatty as changes in lipid metabolism lead to fatty infiltrates. As disease progresses, the liver atrophies and hardens. Fibrous tissue forms in thin, regularly spaced bands throughout the liver, which in time result in a decreased liver mass.

Macronodular cirrhosis is characterized by larger nodules (diameters of 5 cm), which may be multinodular with varying size nodules and may contain central veins. These nodules are surrounded by broad fibrous bands of varying thickness, which correspond to the postnecrotic type of cirrhosis associated with chronic hepatitis. As the normal liver architecture collapses, the portal tracts converge between the fibrous scars, which is a key histological finding. *Mixed cirrhosis* has characteristics of both micronodular and macronodular cirrhosis.

Causes of Cirrhosis

Drug-induced liver disease can be the result of a toxicity from a single drug for from a combination of the toxic effects from multiple drugs. The resultant liver toxicity may be caused by metabolism that is enhanced, altered, or the result of idiosyncratic processes, such as hypersensitivity or a genetic predisposition to liver damage. Intrinsic hepatic injury is drug-dose dependent and is influenced by environmental and genetic factors, whereas idiosyncratic drug reactions are more frequent and are not dose dependent. Patients who have hypersensitivity reactions to a drug develop hepatotoxicity secondary to the formation of drug metabolites, which are harmful to the liver.

Both chronic active hepatitis B (HBV) and hepatitis C (HCV) can cause severe liver injury leading to cirrhosis and liver failure. About one-third of those diagnosed with HCV will progress to cirrhosis, and 15% of those with chronic HCV go on to develop cirrhosis. The chronic hepatitis causes repeated inflammation resulting in fibrosis and structural change of the liver.

PBC and PSC are both chronic cholestatic liver diseases that affect adults. There is an immunological component to both diseases that causes inflammation and fibrosis, which ultimately results in bile duct destruction. Liver biopsy in patients with PBC is of limited value because the disease varies from portal tract to portal tract; biopsy is, however, helpful to validate cirrhotic changes. The beginning stages of PSC are characterized by portal infiltration of lymphocytes, plasma cells, macrophages, and eosinophils. These inflammatory changes are followed by "ductular proliferation," which is characterized by the replacement of mature bile ducts with small, ineffective ones. The inflammatory changes lead to fibrosis, and as fibrotic changes ensue, increased signs of cholestasis appear. The result of these changes is cirrhosis.

Primary sclerosing cholangitis can involve any part of the biliary tract from the ampulla of Vater to the small bile ducts within the liver. The lumens of these ductal systems can be narrowed or completely obstructed by fibrous scar tissue, resulting in cholestasis the key functional abnormality seen in this disease. Biopsy results show fibrosis with inflammatory changes similar to those described for PSC. Bacterial infections that often occur in the area above the strictures and in the presence of long-standing disease lead to biliary cirrhosis.

The pathophysiology of liver disease caused by hereditary factors is essentially the same for both Wilson's disease and hereditary hemochromatosis. Wilson's disease results from decreased hepatic excretion of copper and excessive absorption of copper from the small intestine. There is a gradual accumulation of copper within the tissues, resulting in hepatotoxicity. Initial presentation of Wilson's disease may vary from acute hepatitis or chronic hepatitis, neuropsychiatric disease, cirrhosis, or fulminant hepatic failure in young adults. Histological examination of the initial lesions reveals hepatic steatosis, with increased glycogen deposits. These lesions eventually progress to fibrosis and finally cirrhosis.

Hereditary hemochromatosis is characterized by increased intestinal absorption of iron. Liver biopsy reveals increased iron deposition, predominantly within the hepatocytes. When levels of iron exceed 20,000 mcg/g of liver tissue, fibrosis and cirrhosis usually ensue.

Vascular disorders of the liver, which include BCS and congestive hepatopathy, cause cirrhosis as the end result of necrosis. Liver biopsies show centrilobular congestion, hemorrhage, necrosis, and dilation. The resultant disruption of the hepatic circulation causes portal hypertension, fibrosis of the surrounding tissues, and ultimately cirrhosis.

CLINICAL PRESENTATION

Cirrhosis is often an incidental finding, revealed either by an asymptomatically enlarged liver or an elevation of the liver enzymes. The clinical manifestations of cirrhosis are the result of hepatocellular damage and portal hypertension. The cumulative effect of these signs and symptoms is often referred to as the "stigmata of liver disease." The onset of symptoms is usually gradual, and patients with cirrhosis may appear well and remain asymptomatic for years.

Subjective

Initial complaints generally include weakness, anorexia, weight loss, and fatigue. Malnutrition is usually evident and can be the result of anorexia or the effect of reduced bile salt excretion, resulting in fat malabsorption and deficiency of fat-soluble vitamins.

As cirrhosis advances, patients may present with upper gastrointestinal (GI) bleeding from esophageal varices, which develop secondary to portal hypertension. As the liver continues to fail, patients may present with ascites and/or encephalopathy. Patients with cirrhosis may complain of abdominal pain that is caused by the enlargement of the liver and stretching of Glisson's capsule or by the ascites itself.

Menstrual abnormalities, loss of libido, impotence, sterility, and gynecomastia are manifestations of increased levels of estrogen that result from the liver's inability

to inactivate hormones. These symptoms may prompt individuals to seek medical attention.

Objective

Physical exam findings depend on the stage and severity of the disease process. Initial exam findings may reveal an enlarged, firm liver edge (the left lobe) that is palpable below the right costal margin; however, in patients with advanced disease, the liver may be small and difficult to palpate. Often, a firm smooth mass is palpable over the epigastric area, which is the right lobe of the liver (Riedel's lobe). Occasionally, nodular deformities may be palpable along the liver's edge. These areas of liver enlargement are dull to percussion, which can aid in measuring the expanse of the liver.

Manifestations of cirrhosis that are nonspecific but suggestive of chronic liver disease include spider nevi, which are normally found over the anterior chest; pectoral alopecia; generalized muscle wasting; Dupuytren's (palmar) contractions; parotid gland enlargement; palmar erythema; hair loss; and testicular atrophy. Patients may have dilated cutaneous veins called *caput medusae* (Medusa's head) radiating from around the umbilical area. These varicose veins are a result of the shunting of blood to the paraumbilical veins and are a manifestation of portal hypertension. Signs of vitamin and mineral disturbances are glossitis, cheilitis, and peripheral neuropathies. Fever may indicate complications such as peritonitis, cholangitis, or hepatitis.

Jaundiced sclera, skin, and mucous membranes usually develop in the later stages of cirrhosis. Hyperbilirubinemia is a consequence of the liver's inability to conjugate and excrete bilirubin. Patients with hereditary hemochromatosis may have bronze-colored skin from increased levels of iron and melanin stored in the tissue. Pruritus, although nonspecific, is often the presenting symptom in several forms of cirrhosis and can develop as a result of bile salts accumulating in the skin. Disruption in the liver's ability to synthesize clotting factors may manifest with bruising and complaints of a tendency to bleed. Peripheral edema results because of the decreased plasma osmotic pressure caused by hypoalbuminemia.

Ascites is a direct result of portal hypertension, which is a consequence of increased portal vein pressure. As liver function fails and healthy hepatic cells are replaced with fibrous nodules, blood flow through the liver is impaired, causing increased resistance and back pressure that result in the accumulation of serous fluid within the abdomen. An abdominal exam reveals a positive fluid wave and shifting dullness on percussion. Splenomegaly results from splenic vein congestion. Esophageal varices, another consequence of portal hypertension, may be discovered if bleeding causes hematemesis, hematochezia, and/or melena. Hemorrhoids, which result from portal hypertension, are also present and cause bright red bleeding from the rectum.

Hepatic encephalopathy can range from mild confusion to coma and is the result of increasing blood ammonia, which is toxic to the brain. Characteristics of encephalopathy include asterixis (liver flap), reversal of sleep–wake patterns, tremors, hyperactive deep-tendon reflexes, dysarthria, delirium, and drowsiness.

Patients who present with Wilson's disease may have golden brown rings of color—called Kayser-Fleischer rings—located within Descemet's membrane of the cornea. These rings are usually found in patients with central nervous system (CNS) involvement and are seen with a slit lamp.

DIAGNOSTIC REASONING

Diagnostic Tests

Results of initial laboratory testing vary depending on the stage of the disease process. In many patients with early-stage cirrhosis, laboratory results may be normal; however, in some patients, elevation of liver enzymes may be the only indicator of liver disease. Laboratory testing may reveal abnormalities, but these results are nonspecific unless correlated with the history and physical exam.

Alcoholic cirrhosis may manifest in different ways depending on other coexisting processes, such as malnutrition or hepatitis. A complete blood count commonly shows macrocytic anemia and, depending on the severity of the disease, pancytopenia from the overall suppression of the bone marrow. The mean corpuscular volume does not correct quickly with abstinence from alcohol and may be the only key to occult alcohol use. Anemia can represent suppression of erythropoiesis from folic acid deficiency, occult losses from the GI tract, or a combination of the two. The white blood cell and platelet counts can vary depending on whether there is infection or splenic sequestration. As the liver continues to fail and liver cell mass decreases, the prothrombin time (PT) increases as the liver loses the ability to synthesize the proteins necessary to produce clotting factors.

Blood chemistry test results may show mild to moderate increases in alanine aminotransferase (ALT) and aspartate aminotransferase (AST) levels; however, if the patient has a superimposed alcoholic hepatitis, the classic enzyme elevation of ALT/AST may be reversed, with an AST/ALT ratio ranging from 2:1 to 3:1. The levels of AST/ALT do not reflect the severity of the disease process. The gamma-glutamyl transpeptidase level is a good measurement of recent alcohol ingestion and declines rapidly with abstinence. Alkaline phosphatase levels may be markedly elevated when there is biliary obstruction; in this scenario, serum bilirubin levels can be as high as 30 mg/dL. Hypoalbuminemia is common and contributes to the development of edema.

The diagnosis of alcoholic cirrhosis may be difficult to differentiate from alcoholic hepatitis, which is a reversible process, unless a liver biopsy is obtained. Histological examination reveals hepatocellular necrosis and evidence of Mallory bodies within the damaged cells. Depending on the stage of the disease, there is fatty infiltration and fibrosis. In early disease, there are micronodular changes, which over time develop into macronodular cirrhosis.

Abdominal ultrasound (US) is helpful in determining the size of the liver and any ascites or nodule formation. Doppler studies, in combination with US, are used to evaluate patency of the venous system that, if disrupted, can lead to portal hypertension. Computed tomography (CT) and magnetic resonance imaging of the liver can further characterize nodules. Any nodular findings that are suspicious for malignancy should be biopsied. If a patient presents with melena or hematemesis, an esophagogastroscopy should be performed to assess for esophageal varices or ulcerative processes.

Diagnosis of cholestatic liver disease, specifically PBC and PSC, may be made in conjunction with various autoimmune disease processes. The initial hepatic blood work-up usually shows an alkaline phosphatase level that is three to four times normal, with mild to moderate increases in the transaminases. Cholestatic liver disease can lead to prolonged PT.

Patients with PBC may also present with mild elevation of serum bilirubin and more often hypercholesterolemia. Serum immunoglobulin M levels are elevated in 50% of cases. Antimitochondrial antibodies (AMAs) are found in 95% of the patients with PBC; titers can exceed 1:500. Definitive diagnosis is made via liver biopsy, which reveals granulomatous bile duct destruction and accumulation of inflammatory cells within the portal tracts with resultant segmental necrosis of the interlobular and septal bile ducts (chronic nonsuppurative destructive cholangitis). US evaluation of the biliary tree is negative for biliary obstruction.

Laboratory studies of patients with PSC show the typical cholestatic profile; however, unlike with patients with PBC, the AMA titer is negative. Total cholesterol levels increase as the disease progresses. Endoscopic or transhepatic cholangiography reveals characteristic beading and stricture of the intrahepatic and extrahepatic bile ducts. Liver biopsy is diagnostic for fibrous obliterative cholangitis, in which the hepatic ductal system being replaced with fibrous cords of connective tissue. The end result for both PBC and PSC is biliary cirrhosis.

Diagnosis of cirrhosis caused by vascular disorders such as BCS and other veno-occlusive diseases is normally made through imaging studies because laboratory findings are nonspecific. Serum bilirubin, transaminases, and alkaline phosphatase can be elevated as much as four times normal. A CT scan demonstrates failure of the hepatic veins to opacify, indicating an occlusive process. Pulsed Doppler studies illustrate absent hepatic flow; a normal pulsed Doppler effectively rules out BCS. Venographic studies also demonstrate narrowing and obstruction of the hepatic venous system. Histological exam reveals centrilobular congestion with associated hemorrhage and necrosis.

Wilson's disease and hemochromatosis are inherited metabolic liver diseases that result in cirrhosis if diagnosis and treatment are not made early. Diagnosis of Wilson's disease is suggested by elevated serum copper levels in conjunction with low serum ceruloplasmin levels. Once an abnormal ceruloplasmin level has been documented, a 24-hour urine check for copper should be completed. Definitive diagnosis is made through quantitative copper levels in the liver on biopsy. Most patients with Wilson's disease have histological findings consistent with hepatic steatosis, which in time progresses to fibrosis and cirrhosis.

Iron metabolism studies are used to diagnose hereditary hemochromatosis and should be collected with the patient in the fasting state. The presence of an elevated transferrin saturation level in combination with an elevated ferritin level is suggestive of hereditary hemochromatosis. Liver biopsy is necessary for definitive diagnosis. Histological studies with quantitative iron levels greater than 20,000 mcg/g are consistent with advanced disease and cirrhosis.

Differential Diagnosis

The patient who presents with cirrhosis can be a diagnostic challenge. The differential diagnosis of cirrhosis varies little between the different etiologies; therefore, the challenge is determining the cause to prevent further liver damage. The differential diagnosis of alcohol-induced liver disease includes biliary tract disease, idiopathic hemochromatosis, nonalcoholic fatty liver disease, drug toxicity, and/or viral hepatitis. US exam of the liver can often rule out an obstructive process. Patients with AUD and chronic pancreatitis frequently develop jaundice secondary to stricture of the common bile duct, which is differentiated through endoscopic retrograde cholangiopancreatography. A liver biopsy is often the only definitive test for differentiating many of the hepatobiliary diseases from each other. Thorough history and physical exam can suggest a diagnosis, but histological study is necessary to distinguish one process from another.

Patients who abuse alcohol also have a high incidence of co-infection with hepatitis, the cause of which is often unclear; the presence of this infection can alter the typical serological findings. A hepatitis panel can reveal active or prior infection. Drug toxicity, specifically with acetaminophen, even in low doses, can alter transaminase levels and necessitates obtaining a careful drug history from each patient. Because of preexisting liver injury, patients who abuse alcohol who present with acetaminophen toxicity have significantly higher morbidity and mortality with relatively low doses of acetaminophen.

The differential diagnosis of cholestatic liver disease must include all other causes of chronic cholestasis, such as tumors, strictures, or obstructions resulting from stone formation. Autoimmune chronic active hepatitis can mimic the signs and symptoms of PBC; however, laboratory studies will show a low or negative titer for AMA. US exam may reveal biliary duct dilation, a process consistent with both PBC and PSC, thus making cholangiography the diagnostic test of choice.

MANAGEMENT

Treatment of cirrhosis is aimed at identifying and removing the causative agent, treating the symptoms, and preventing complications.

Alcohol-Induced Liver Disease

In a patient with alcohol-induced liver disease, the most effective treatment remains abstinence. Patients who continue to ingest alcohol and present with ascites can increase their 2-year survival rate to 95% if they can completely abstain from alcohol. Those who continue to drink have a 2-year survival rate of less than 25%. The liver has a remarkable regenerative potential; despite slow progress, the patient can become functional if he or she is motivated to remain abstinent. Nutritional assessment with dietary supplementation to ensure adequate caloric intake (25–35 kcal/kg body weight per day) is imperative because many patients with alcohol-induced liver disease are also malnourished. Protein intake should be increased to 1 to 1.5 grams per kilogram of body weight per day unless there is evidence of hepatic encephalopathy, which necessitates a reduction in protein intake. Daily vitamin and mineral supplementation is also indicated. Specifically, patients should receive a multivitamin, additional vitamin B$_{12}$, folate, thiamine, magnesium, and zinc supplementation if 100% of the daily requirement of these minerals is not contained in the multivitamin. Patients who continue to show clinical deterioration despite abstinence can be considered for liver transplantation, provided they have remained alcohol free for more than 6 months.

Treatment of Complications

Many of the complications of alcohol-induced liver disease are the direct result of the development of portal hypertension and include ascites, hepatic encephalopathy, anemia, hemorrhage, spontaneous bacterial peritonitis, hepatorenal syndrome, hepatopulmonary syndrome, and hepatocellular carcinoma. Box 42.2 presents the treatment of these complications.

Irreversible, Chronic Liver Disease

Liver transplantation is the treatment of choice for irreversible chronic liver disease. Cirrhosis, hepatitis C, PBC, primary sclerosing cholangitis, alcoholic liver disease, autoimmune hepatitis, and genetic disorders of the liver are diseases for which transplantation has been successful. Five-year survival rates are documented as high as 80% with advancements in surgical techniques and immunosuppressive agents such as T-cell depleting monoclonal antibodies (muromonab-CD3, Alemtuzumab), calcineurin inhibitors

---

Box 42.2 Complications of Alcohol-Induced Liver Disease

Portal Hypertension and Variceal Hemorrhage

Portal hypertension is the result of disruption of the hepatocellular circulation, causing an increase in portal venous pressure. As the liver becomes progressively more cirrhotic, collateral venous circulation develops between the portal and systemic circulation to overcome the increased resistance to blood flow. The collateral circulation that forms, specifically the azygos vein, is a much weaker system and results in dilated, tortuous vessels commonly known as varices. Development of varices within the esophagus and submucosa of the gastric fundus predisposes patients to hemorrhage when the portal pressure gradient is greater than 12 mm Hg.

Management of this complication is as follows:

- A combination of band ligation or sclerotherapy and octreotide, which results in reduced splanchnic and hepatic blood flow to decrease portal pressure, is the most effective treatment for bleeding varices.
- Patients who have failed both endoscopic and pharmacological intervention require emergent insertion of a Sengstaken-Blakemore tube for balloon tamponade of the bleeding variceal site. The risk for aspiration, esophageal rupture, or rebleed is great, and patients normally require intensive care monitoring.
- Some patients may benefit from surgical placement of a portacaval shunt or placement of a transjugular intrahepatic portosystemic shunt. Both procedures are performed to decrease portal hypertension but are associated with a high operative mortality rate, especially if performed on an urgent basis. Prevention of future bleeding also may be accomplished using these procedures.

Ascites

Ascites, the excess accumulation of serous fluid within the peritoneal cavity, is associated with unfavorable outcomes. Ascites results from a combination of increased hydrostatic pressure (portal hypertension), decreased oncotic pressure (hypoalbuminemia), peripheral vasodilation probably mediated by nitric oxide released from the splanchnic vasculature, volume expansion resulting from a disturbance in the renin-angiotensin system with subsequent sodium and water retention, and impaired activation of aldosterone by the liver.

Ascites can be clinically observed on physical exam when 1,000 mL or more of fluid has accumulated within the abdominal/peritoneal cavities; smaller amounts are detectable with the use of ultrasound. Shifting dullness to percussion and a positive fluid wave are two findings consistent with the diagnosis of ascites.

Management of ascites includes the following:

- Initial treatment is sodium restriction of 400 to 800 mg/day with daily monitoring of weight, serum electrolytes, and renal function. The goal of treatment for the patient with ascites and peripheral edema is a daily weight loss of approximately 1 pound. For patients with hyponatremia (serum levels less than 125 mEq/L), fluid restriction of 800 to 1,000 mL/day, is recommended.

- Diuretic therapy is usually required in addition to sodium and water restriction. Initial therapy is with spironolactone (Aldactone), a potassium-sparing, aldosterone antagonist. Furosemide (Lasix), a loop diuretic, is added if effective diuresis has not been achieved.
- In the 10% of patients who do not respond to either of the above treatments, large-volume paracentesis is performed. Up to 4 to 6 L of fluid can be removed per procedure. Intravascular volume expanders can be infused simultaneously to prevent hemodynamic instability secondary to removal of large volumes of ascitic fluid. The procedure can be performed daily until ascites is resolved, and then the patient can be maintained on diuretic therapy.

Spontaneous Bacterial Peritonitis

Spontaneous bacterial peritonitis (SBP) is a common complication of cirrhosis that can be fatal. Patients may present with abdominal pain, increasing ascites, fever, and progressive encephalopathy. Definitive diagnosis is made by paracentesis. The gold standard for the diagnosis of SBP is a total white cell count of greater than 300 cell/mcL with a polymorphonuclear neutrophil cell count of greater than 250/mcL. The protein concentration is usually less than 1 g/dL. Gram-negative bacilli are the causative pathogen in 70% of patients with SBP, with *Escherichia coli* being isolated in 50% of the cases. Gram-positive organisms are isolated in approximately 25% of the cases, and infection with anaerobic organisms is rare due to the high oxygen content of the ascitic fluid. The mortality rate for untreated SBP is 50%.

Management of SBP includes empiric treatment with cefotaxime (Claforan), a broad-spectrum, third-generation cephalosporin. Post-SBP prophylaxis can be accomplished with norfloxacin.

Hepatorenal Syndrome

Hepatorenal syndrome is a terminal complication frequently associated with advanced liver damage and is almost always found in patients with advanced ascites. The syndrome is characterized by oliguria, hyponatremia, azotemia, low urine sodium (less than 10 mEq/L), and hypotension. The hallmark to diagnosis is a disproportionate rise in creatinine with respect to the blood urea nitrogen. Histologically, the kidneys are normal, and diagnosis is often one of exclusion. Patients are often misdiagnosed with prerenal failure, and the only way to differentiate between the two is through insertion of a central venous catheter and assessment of venous pressures. Large-volume paracentesis, aggressive diuresis aimed at decreasing ascites, or sepsis can precipitate hepatorenal syndrome in individuals with decompensated cirrhosis and ascites.

Management of hepatorenal syndrome includes restoring the intravascular volume and avoiding any procedures that will dramatically disturb the patient's volume status, such as large-volume paracentesis and aggressive diuresis. The definitive treatment of patients with hepatorenal syndrome is liver transplantation.

Box 42.2 Complications of Alcohol-Induced Liver Disease—cont'd

Hepatic Encephalopathy

Hepatic encephalopathy, also known as portosystemic encephalopathy, is a complex process involving a change in mental status resulting from the failure of the liver to detoxify elements of gut origin and shunting of this blood from the portal to the systemic circulation and then to the brain. Nitrogenous agents such as ammonia are believed to enter the central nervous system by way of shunted blood resulting in disturbances in neurological function. Although ammonia is thought to be the sole toxin responsible for hepatic encephalopathy, the serum levels do not correlate with the degree or presence of encephalopathy.

The diagnosis of hepatic encephalopathy is made clinically and often follows an event such as increased dietary protein, GI bleeding, constipation, infection, deterioration in hepatic function, hypokalemia, azotemia, alkalosis, and hypovolemia. Physical exam findings include an altered mental status such as personality (mood) changes, decreased reaction time, and intellectual deterioration, as well as neuromuscular dysfunctions such as asterixis or metabolic flap, absence of fixed sensory or motor deficits, and hyperreflexia. Other findings include fetor hepaticus (garlic odor of the breath caused by exhalation of sulfur-containing mercaptans), hyperthermia, and hyperventilation. Obtaining a fasting arterial blood ammonia level or a spinal fluid glutamine level can be helpful in confirming the diagnosis of hepatic encephalopathy although they are not necessary.

Management of hepatic encephalopathy involves identification and treatment of factors that cause encephalopathy in patients with liver disease. For instance, gastrointestinal bleeding and diets high in protein lead to the formation of ammonia and other nitrogenous compounds from the action of bacteria in the gut, which can induce or aggravate the symptoms of encephalopathy. The goal of treatment is to reduce formation of ammonia and other nitrogenous compounds. This is achieved by decreasing the numbers of colonic bacteria with the antibiotic neomycin and inducing acidification of the colon contents with lactulose (Cephulac, Heptalac), a nonabsorbable synthetic disaccharide that is fermented by intestinal bacteria. The lower stool pH binds the ammonia in the colon, rendering it nonabsorbable. Lactulose also changes the bowel flora so that there are fewer ammonia-forming bacteria.

Iron-Deficiency Anemia

Iron-deficiency anemia is a common finding in individuals with AUD. It can be treated with ferrous sulfate taken three times daily after meals. To avoid the constipating effect of iron, a stool softener can be given as well. If there is evidence of a macrocytic anemia, the patient may benefit from 1 mg of folic acid daily.

Hepatopulmonary Syndrome

Hepatopulmonary syndrome is a recently recognized pulmonary complication of cirrhosis and portal hypertension, which manifests as abnormal arterial oxygenation. The diagnosis is made when intrapulmonary dilation occurs in the absence of other morphological pathology. This syndrome is reversible with liver transplantation.

(tacrolimus, cyclosporine), mammalian target of rapamycin inhibitors (sirolimus, everolimus), and interleukin-2 receptor antagonists (daclizumab, basiliximab). Contraindications to transplantation include malignant hepatobiliary processes, sepsis, and advanced cardiopulmonary disease. In cases of hepatitis B and C, the virus can infect the new liver.

Primary Biliary Cirrhosis

Treatment of PBC is symptomatic. Pruritus is often the most aggravating manifestation of PBC. Cholestyramine (Questran) or colestipol relieves itching in patients with cholestasis by lowering serum bile acids and increasing the intestinal secretion of bile by preventing its resorption. The usual dose is 4 or 5 g, respectively, in water or juice three times daily until the pruritus has been controlled, and then the dosage is decreased to that which maintains control of the symptom. Rifampin (Rifadin) 150 to 300 mg twice daily has been beneficial in relieving pruritus in some cases; ondansetron, a 5-HT$_3$ serotonin receptor antagonist, shows promise as well.

Fat-soluble vitamin deficiency occurs with the onset of steatorrhea and can be made worse with the administration of cholestyramine (a bile acid sequestrant). Vitamins A, D, E, and K can be replaced orally. Laboratory studies will reveal vitamin K deficiency as a prolonged PT. The deficiency can be treated with 5 to 10 mg daily of vitamin K by mouth; subsequent monitoring of the PT will indicate whether therapy is adequate. Because overdose of vitamin A can cause hepatotoxicity, the dosage must be individualized based on serum levels and response to treatment.

Patients with PBC often have associated osteoporosis because of an imbalance in bone remodeling. If patients have been diagnosed with PBC and have osteomalacia or osteoporosis, bisphosphonates (Fosamax, Boniva, Aclasta, Actonel) have been shown to be affective. Anyone with cirrhosis from any cause should receive calcium supplementation with 1 g per day and vitamin D$_3$ 800 IU/day in an effort to prevent osteomalacia or osteoporosis. Patients should be instructed to eat foods rich in calcium and phosphorus and to increase their exposure to sunlight.

Several immunosuppressive agents including corticosteroids, methotrexate, and azathioprine and the antifibrinogenic colchicine have been effective in reducing elevated serum alkaline phosphatase and bilirubin levels. Ursodeoxycholic acid (ursodiol), a choleretic, acts by stimulating excretion of bile by the liver, is much less toxic than the other drugs mentioned and has been effective in reducing symptoms and improving long-term survival.

Surgical reconstruction of the biliary tract, choledochoduodenostomy, and choledochojejunostomy are palliative treatments that alleviate the symptoms of PBC. If there is notable stricture within the biliary tree, patients often do well with stenting. Liver transplantation for advanced PBC is the treatment of choice.

Hemochromatosis and Wilson's Disease

Two important but treatable inherited metabolic causes of cirrhosis are hemochromatosis and Wilson's disease. Early diagnosis and treatment are key to the management of hereditary hemochromatosis (HHC) and begin with liver biopsy for definitive diagnosis. If treatment is initiated before cirrhosis ensues, the disease can be controlled with weekly phlebotomies of 1 unit (500 mL) of blood, which contains approximately 250 mg of iron. This process is continued until there is depletion of the iron stores (which can be 2 years or more). Every 2 to 3 months, iron metabolism studies monitor the patient's progress. Once the iron stores are depleted—when serum ferritin levels fall below 50 ng/mL and transferrin saturation is less than 50%— patients can be maintained with periodic phlebotomies. Patients who are exhibiting cardiac symptoms may require the use of iron-chelating agents such as deferoxamine. Administered intramuscularly, it increases the urinary excretion of iron up to 5 to 18 g annually. Phlebotomy decreases the cardiac conduction defects and lowers insulin requirements. Patients should be instructed to consume a low-iron diet that eliminates foods such as red meat, and they should avoid alcohol, vitamin C, raw shellfish, and any supplement containing iron. Patients may require specific treatment of diabetes mellitus, heart disease, arthropathy, hypopituitarism, and portal hypertension, all complications due to HHC. Patients whose disease has progressed to cirrhosis must be monitored for hepatocellular carcinoma either by liver US or measurement of alpha-fetoprotein levels. Because the disease is inherited, screening of all first-degree relatives is necessary.

Wilson's disease is also an inherited disease the early diagnosis and treatment of which can prevent the development of neurological or hepatic damage. Treatment includes both dietary and medicinal components. Limiting dietary intake of copper (legumes, animal organs, and shellfish) should become a lifelong habit. The administration of oral penicillamine (Depen) 0.75 to 2 g/day in divided doses induces the urinary excretion of chelated copper. If GI upset or hypersensitivity prohibits the use of penicillamine, trientine (Syprine) 250 to 500 mg three times daily can be substituted. Oral administration of zinc 50 mg three times daily as maintenance therapy also promotes excretion of copper in the feces. Patients who are receiving penicillamine, an antimetabolite of vitamin B_6, should receive pyridoxine (supplemental vitamin B_6) 50 mg/week. Liver transplant is the treatment of choice for patients with cirrhosis or fulminant hepatitis. Siblings and family members should be screened for the disease.

Vascular or Congestive Liver Disorders

Management of patients who present with vascular or congestive liver disorders, such as those with BCS and other hepatic occlusive diseases, is essential. Because of the many causes of BCS, initial treatment must begin with finding and treating the cause of the hepatic congestion. Hepatic vein thrombus is difficult to manage and requires a multidisciplinary approach including a hematologist, surgeon, hepatologist, and gastroenterologist. Ascites is initially managed with sodium restriction and diuretics; however, over time this is usually ineffective, and most patients will require large-volume paracentesis or shunting for symptomatic relief.

If diagnosis of acute thrombus is made early, thrombolytic therapy can be instituted and long-term anticoagulation with warfarin (Coumadin) can help prevent further thrombus formation. Surgical decompression shunting for refractive ascites can delay development of hepatic failure or cirrhosis but often results in graft thrombus. Patients with associated myeloproliferative diseases and hypercoagulopathies may benefit from low-dose aspirin therapy and chemotherapy as directed by a hematologist.

FOLLOW-UP AND REFERRAL

Any patient with advanced liver disease should be referred to a hepatologist or gastroenterologist trained to treat the disease and its complications. All patients require referral for liver biopsy to establish a definitive diagnosis. The primary-care provider should be able to recognize the onset of liver disease, obtain the necessary tests, and provide results of all diagnostic testing performed to the consulting physician. Patients with end-stage liver disease should be referred to a liver transplant facility. Patient follow-up can be shared between the primary-care practitioner and the consulting physician. Patients with chronic or advanced liver disease will require indefinite monitoring of their liver function tests, as well as their fluid and electrolyte status. Maintaining good nutrition is an important component of treatment of any disease process. Patients with advanced liver disease may benefit from consultation with a registered dietitian, who can review dietary restrictions and help patients understand how to achieve a balanced diet.

Patient Education: Cirrhosis

Patients with hepatic failure should be instructed to check their weight daily as a way to monitor increasing fluid retention and ascites, which may indicate a developing complication. Patients with cirrhosis have a life-threatening terminal disease; therefore, attention must be given to promoting psychological well-being. Patients should be provided with education regarding medications to prevent further hepatotoxicity, such as acetaminophen (Tylenol), vitamin A, cocaine, tetracycline (Sumycin), phenytoin (Dilantin), and ethyl alcohol. Patients with liver failure should always ask their health-care provider about the potential liver toxicity of each of their medications. Patients with hepatic encephalopathy should avoid CNS depressants, which might intensify their lethargy or fatigue. These patients may also require education about the need for self-administering enemas if they become constipated to decrease the time for bowel absorption of nitrogen-based compounds. All patients with ascites must be informed of the signs and symptoms of infection, which may indicate developing spontaneous bacterial peritonitis.

 For additional resources please visit
https://davisedge.fadavis.com/

REFERENCES

Grant BF, Chou SP, Saha TD, et al. Prevalence of 12- month alcohol use, high-risk drinking, and *DSM-IV* alcohol use disorder in the United States, 2001–2002 to 2012–2013. Results from the National Epidemiologic Survey on Alcohol and Related Conditions. *JAMA Psychiatry.* 2017;74(9):911–923.

Guirguis J, Chhatwal J, Dasarathy J, et al. Clinical impact of alcohol-related cirrhosis in the next decade: Estimates based on current epidemiological trends in the United States. *Clin Exp Res.* 2015;39(11):2085–2094.

Moni M, Schilsky ML, Tichy EM. Review on immunosuppression in liver transplantation. *World J Hepatol.* 2015;7(10):1355–1368.

Murali AR, Attar BM, Katz A, et al. Utility of platelet count for predicting cirrhosis in alcoholic liver disease: Model for identifying cirrhosis in a US population. *J Gen Int Med.* 2015;30(8):111201117.

Scaqlione S, Kliethermes S, Cao G, et al. The epidemiology of cirrhosis in the United States: A population-based study. *J Clin Gastroenterol.* 2015;49(8):690–696.

Volk ML, Kanwal F. Quality of care in the cirrhotic patient. *Clin Transl Gastroenterol.* 2015;7(4):e166. doi:10.1038/ctg.2016.25; published online April 21, 2016

RESOURCES

American Liver Foundation
www.liverfoundation.org

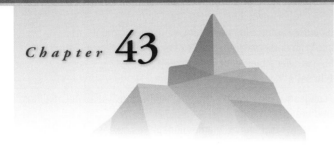

Chapter **43**

Common Urinary Complaints

Debbie Nogueras Conner, PhD, ANP/FNP-BC, FAANP

Debera J. Thomas, DNS, RN, FNP/ANP

Brian Oscar Porter, MD, PhD, MPH, MBA

DYSURIA

Dysuria is the subjective experience of pain or a burning sensation on urination and can also be accompanied by urinary frequency, hesitancy, urgency, and strangury (slow, painful urination). Symptoms of dysuria can be secondary to several medical conditions or certain medications. For example, a light burning sensation or discomfort can be normal when associated with concentrated acidic urine. However, dysuria is most commonly associated with lower urinary tract infection. Selective serotonin reuptake inhibitors, such as citalopram (Celexa), escitalopram (Lexapro), paroxetine (Paxil), fluoxetine (Prozac), and sertraline (Zoloft), may also cause dysuria. Other prescribed medications such as opiates and those used to prevent motion sickness (e.g., scopolamine) may also cause dysuria, given their anticholinergic effects on the renal system.

DIFFERENTIAL DIAGNOSIS

Dysuria is most often associated with a bladder problem and rarely with renal disease. Inflammatory lesions of the prostate, bladder, and urethra—including prostatitis in men, urethrotrigonitis in women, and bladder and urethral infections in both men and women—are the most common causes of dysuria. When caused by bladder problems, urinary frequency usually occurs secondary to diminished bladder capacity or with pain when the bladder becomes distended. Urinary frequency may be a manifestation of urinary incontinence and can occur with prostatic hypertrophy or neurogenic bladder disorders and in women with pelvic organ prolapse.

Other conditions associated with dysuria are bladder tumors, chronic renal failure, nephrolithiasis, and occasionally diseases of the upper urinary tract. Dysuria may also be associated with diseases outside the renal system, such as sexually transmitted diseases, vaginitis, or prostatitis. For example, female patients may present with symptoms of dysuria or external irritation from urine passing over irritated vulvar tissues. Any woman who presents with dysuria should be questioned about an associated vaginal discharge or irritation. Symptoms of dysuria may lead to other diagnoses, such as urethral strictures, pelvic organ prolapse, pelvic peritonitis, cancer of the cervix or prostate, dysmenorrhea, and disorders of the prostate.

Urinalysis is the easiest, least invasive, and most economical way to identify urinary tract infections and other renal problems (see Advanced Assessment 43.1). Once the underlying problem has been identified, appropriate treatment can be instituted.

Conditions associated with dysuria, such as bladder tumors, chronic renal failure, nephrolithiasis, and infections of the lower and upper urinary tracts are discussed in Chapters 44 and 45. Problems associated with dysmenorrhea are discussed in Chapter 48, and conditions associated with the prostate in Chapter 49.

HEMATURIA

Hematuria is defined as blood in the urine and can be visible (gross) or occult (microscopic). Asymptomatic microhematuria has many benign causes such as infection, menstruation, vigorous exercise, viral illness, and trauma. In the primary-care setting, the dipstick method to detect hematuria has a sensitivity of 95% and a specificity of 75%. Positive results should be confirmed with a microscopic examination because of the possibility of a false-positive test result. On microscopic examination, hematuria is characterized by more than three red blood cells (RBCs) per high-power microscopic field (hpf). Normal urinary excretion of RBCs is 2,000,000 cells per day, which corresponds to two

⁘ Advanced Assessment 43.1: Urinalysis

Urinalysis Result	Finding/Abnormal Value	Common Differential Diagnosis
Appearance	Colorless	Diabetes insipidus, diuretic agents, fluid overload
	Dark	Hematuria, malignancy, stones, acidic urine
	Cloudy	Urinary tract infection, hematuria, bilirubin, mucus
	Pink/red	Hematuria, hemoglobin, myoglobin, beets, food coloring
	Orange/yellow	Phenazopyridine (Pyridium), rifampin (rifampicin), bile pigments
	Brown/black	Myoglobin, bile pigments, melanin, cascara (laxative), iron preparation
	Green	Bile pigments, methylene blue, indigo carmine (food dye)
	Foamy	Proteinuria, bile salts
Specific gravity	Increased	Dehydration, congestive heart failure, adrenal insufficiency, diabetes mellitus, nephrosis, antidiuretic hormone
	Decreased	Diabetes insipidus, pyelonephritis, glomerulonephritis, excess fluid intake
pH	Acidic	Diet, medications, acidosis, ketoacidosis, chronic obstructive pulmonary disease
	Alkaline	Diet, sodium bicarbonate, vomiting, metabolic alkalosis, urinary tract infection
Bilirubin	Positive	Jaundice, hepatitis
Blood	Positive	Kidney stones, tumors, kidney disease, trauma, infection, injury from instrumentation, coagulation problems, menses
Glucose	Positive	Diabetes mellitus, pancreatitis, Cushing's disease, shock, burns, corticosteroids, renal disease, hyperthyroidism, cancer
Ketones	Positive	Starvation, diet, ketoacidosis, vomiting, diarrhea, pregnancy
Nitrate	Positive	Infection
Protein	Positive	Kidney disease, pregnancy, congestive heart failure, diabetes mellitus, cancer, benign cause
Leukocyte esterase	Positive	Infection
Reducing substance	Positive	Signifies the presence of glucose, fructose, or galactose, lactose, pentose May also signify certain medications (e.g., salicylates, levodopa, ascorbic acid, nalidixic acid, tetracyclines) Liver disease, hyperthyroidism

or three RBCs per hpf. It takes only a small amount of blood to make the urine appear red, as urine will appear pink with between 20 and 30 RBCs per hpf and will become red at about 100 RBCs per hpf. There is a direct relationship between the quantity of blood found in the urine and the likelihood of pathology.

Transient hematuria occurs on a single occasion whereas *persistent hematuria* occurs on two or more consecutive occasions. Both transient and persistent hematuria can be a sign of serious underlying disease. Urine color can vary widely from light pink to dark red and is sometimes characterized as "smoky." The color of urine depends on the amount of blood present, as well as on dietary intake, the use of medications, and the dilution and pH of the urine. For example, the ingestion of beets can color the urine red to pink, and medications such as rifampin (rifampicin) and phenazopyridine (Pyridium) can give urine a reddish-orange color. The presence of porphyrins, hemoglobin, or myoglobin can color the

urine reddish-brown. Pus in the urine is indicative of bacterial infection somewhere along the urinary tract, such as cystitis, urethritis, or prostatitis.

Rates of hematuria in the general population are usually less than 1% but can be as high as 15%. The age, gender, and activity level of the patient with hematuria should be considered during the assessment. For example, long-distance runners and other athletes can have rates of hematuria as high as 18%. However, even transient hematuria in men older than 50 years may be an indication of serious disease, with up to 2.4% of this population having urinary tract malignancies, typically transitional cell carcinoma. In men older than 60 years, the incidence of urinary tract malignancy increases to 9%. In older men with gross hematuria, the rate of associated malignancy is as high as 20%. In general, there is a higher correlation between underlying malignancy and gross hematuria, as opposed to microscopic hematuria, especially in patients with a history of cigarette smoking.

DIFFERENTIAL DIAGNOSIS

The causes of hematuria are grouped according to anatomical site of the blood source. For example, *isolated hematuria* (i.e., with no other abnormal urine components) may be due to bleeding anywhere from the renal pelvis to the urethra but is rarely caused by a systemic disease. RBC casts usually indicate injury to the nephron and are diagnostic of hematuria of renal origin. However, intact uniform RBCs with no casts suggests hematuria originating in the lower urinary tract. The presence of bacteria in the urine is diagnostic of an infectious origin, as is also suggested by fever. Acute cystitis and urethritis produce gross hematuria and are more common in women. The presence of both proteinuria and hematuria is suggestive of glomerular or interstitial nephritis. A drug history is important because many drugs can cause hematuria. In addition, dietary substances such as caffeine, spices, tomatoes, chocolate, aged cheeses, citrus fruits, and soy sauce may act as bladder irritants. Alcohol and cigarettes are also bladder irritants. Thus, the patient's drug and food intake history should be assessed to rule out these substances as causative agents. The drugs involved may be prescribed, over the counter, herbal, supplemental vitamins, or recreational in nature. β-Lactam antibiotics (e.g., amoxicillin with clavulanic acid [Augmentin]), sulfonamides (e.g., sulfamethoxazole/trimethoprim [Bactrim]), NSAIDs, rifampin (rifampicin), ciprofloxacin (Cipro), allopurinol (Zyloprim), cimetidine (Tagamet), and phenytoin (Dilantin) can all cause *nephritis*, typically allergic interstitial nephritis, which can result in destruction of nephrons and subsequently lead to impaired renal function and hematuria. Papillary necrosis can result from the use of anticoagulants such as warfarin (Coumadin), heparin, aspirin, and NSAIDs. Glomerulonephritis can be caused by the use of hydralazine, hydrocarbons (including glue and paint sniffing), gold, penicillamine (Cuprimine), amphetamines, NSAIDs, allopurinol (Zyloprim), and Paraquat (a type of weed killer). Urolithiasis (discussed in Chapter 44), which often presents with hematuria, can occur with the use of carbonic anhydrase inhibitors, the diuretic triamterene (Dyazide, Maxzide), sulfonamides, and vitamin D metabolites.

Menstrual history is always important in a female patient with hematuria. Patients should be asked about recent strenuous exercise, streptococcal infection (which suggests poststreptococcal glomerulonephritis), a history of nephrolithiasis, pertinent family history (e.g., polycystic kidney disease), and recent travel to tropical areas (which suggests potential exposure to parasitic infections). Gross painless hematuria is a cardinal sign of certain malignancies such as bladder cancer.

Physical examination may reveal costovertebral angle tenderness, which could indicate pyelonephritis, tumor, or glomerulonephritis. An abdominal mass may indicate a neoplasm (e.g., renal cell cancer) or polycystic kidney disease. Suprapubic tenderness is indicative of a bladder etiology, whereas urethral discharge indicates urethritis. An enlarged prostate could indicate benign prostatic hypertrophy, whereas a tender prostate would more likely be suggestive of prostatitis, and a prostate nodule may indicate a prostatic neoplasm. Ecchymosis (large superficial bruising) of the skin may indicate an underlying coagulopathy or vasculitis.

Hematuria accompanied by colicky flank pain suggests a ureteral stone. When bleeding occurs only at the beginning or end of urination, a prostatic or urethral source is likely. Hematuria accompanied by hypertension, edema, and a sore throat or a skin infection may be indicative of poststreptococcal glomerulonephritis. Thirty percent of patients with gross hematuria are diagnosed with a malignancy of the prostate, urethra, bladder, kidney, or ureter. Differential Diagnosis 43.1 lists possible differential diagnoses of hematuria.

The most important diagnostic tool in cases of hematuria is urinalysis. One drawback of the common urine dipstick test is that it detects the presence of heme (an iron-containing nonprotein portion of the hemoglobin molecule) in the urine but not actual RBCs. If the dipstick is positive for heme, but the number of RBCs on the microscopic examination is within normal limits, myoglobinuria and hemoglobinuria should be suspected.

When hematuria of renal origin is suspected, laboratory tests should include an antinuclear antibody test, immunoglobulins, cryoglobulins, antiglomerular basement membrane antibodies, a full serum chemistry panel including creatinine clearance and blood urea nitrogen, a complete blood count and platelet count, an antistreptolysin O titer, serum protein electrophoresis, and a Venereal Disease Research Laboratory test (to rule out syphilis). If these studies indicate a renal problem, the patient should be referred to a nephrologist. A urine culture and sensitivity should be done on all patients with hematuria, and if bacterial infection is found, treatment with appropriate antibiotics should be instituted with reevaluation for persistent hematuria 2 weeks after the completion of treatment.

Isolated asymptomatic hematuria is often found on a routine screening urinalysis with no apparent source determined by history or physical examination. The possibility of occult malignancy or other potentially serious etiology in this setting increases with age, and if the patient is older than 35 years, he or she should be evaluated for urological tumors. Patients younger than 35 years should be monitored at least monthly for 3 months, and if the hematuria persists, a more aggressive work-up is indicated.

Examination of the morphology of RBCs present in the urine using phase-contrast microscopy can provide clues as to the etiology of hematuria. Dysmorphic RBCs may indicate glomerular disease. A fresh urine sample is essential because changes in morphology occur if the urine is allowed to sit for a prolonged time after collection. If the hematuria persists without evidence of infection, an IV pyelogram or renal ultrasound should be done to assess kidney structure. The American Urological

⊞ Differential Diagnosis 43.1: Hematuria

Origin of Pathology	Differential Diagnoses
Urethra	Urethritis (gonococcal, nongonococcal) Stricture Calculus Trauma
Prostate/male genitourinary tract	Infection (prostatitis, epididymitis) Benign prostatic hypertrophy Tumor
Kidney	Infection (pyelonephritis) Nephrolithiasis Renal cell cancer Trauma Glomerular disease (vasculitic, idiopathic) Ischemia (embolism, thrombosis, papillary necrosis) Allergic interstitial nephritis (drug-induced)
Ureters	Nephrolithiasis Tumor Endometriosis
Bladder	Infection (bacterial, parasitic) Calculus Tumor Endometriosis Drugs (hemorrhagic cystitis)
Pseudohematuria	Menstrual contamination Phenothiazines Red food dye Beet consumption Quinine Rifampin (rifampicin) Hemoglobinuria
Systemic illness	Pyelonephritis Coagulopathies (thrombocytopenia, hemoglobinopathy, sickle cell)
Functional causes	Intense exercise

Association recommends cystoscopy for all patients who present with risk factors for urinary tract malignancies, such as irritative voiding symptoms, current or past cigarette smoking, and certain chemical exposures, regardless of age (AUA, 2016).

PROTEINURIA

The primary proteins found in urine are globulin and albumin. *Proteinuria* is usually indicative of renal pathology, most often of glomerular origin. Proteinuria can be functional as a result of acute illness, emotional stress, or excessive exercise, in which case it is a benign process or simply a resultant sign of a transient condition. However, proteinuria can also reflect more serious disease. Abnormalities in the glomerular basement membrane produce glomerular proteinuria, and damage to the proximal tubule where filterable proteins are reabsorbed can result in tubular proteinuria. Proteinuria may also develop due to the overproduction of filterable plasma proteins, such as Bence Jones proteins associated with multiple myeloma. Bence Jones proteinuria (characterized by free monoclonal light chain components of immunoglobulin proteins) may also be associated with lymphosarcoma, Hodgkin's disease, and leukemia.

Intermittent proteinuria is most often asymptomatic, associated with functional disorders, and discovered incidentally through urine dipstick testing. Continuous proteinuria is associated with renal pathology. Importantly, the standard dipstick proteinuria test does not detect Bence Jones proteins or other light chain immunoglobulins, as it is most sensitive to larger proteins such as albumin. A false-negative reading can occur because of a diluted urine sample, alkaline pH (normal pH = 4.5 to 8 [usually range = 5.5 to 6.5]), or with Bence Jones proteinuria. Thus, the most accurate way to quantify the amount of protein in the urine is with a 24-hour urine collection; however, a spot urine albumin to urine creatinine ratio can be measured as a close approximation of the 24-hour urine measurement. A 24-hour urine collection with more than 150 mg of protein is considered abnormal, and a specimen with more than 3.5 g is indicative of a nephrotic process. A urine albumin to urine creatinine ratio of less than 0.2 is normal and corresponds to an excretion of less than 200 mg/dL of protein.

DIFFERENTIAL DIAGNOSIS

Proteinuria may occur from benign or functional causes, in which it is a resultant sign of an acute or transient condition. Such causes include orthostatic proteinuria, vigorous exercise, environmental conditions, fever, and acute illnesses. Orthostatic proteinuria occurs when the urinary protein level is elevated only when the patient has been standing for a prolonged time, but not while he or she has been reclining. Exercise-induced proteinuria may occur in athletes such as runners or boxers, and it may be accompanied by elevated catecholamines, hemoglobinuria, or hematuria. Proteinuria caused by environmental conditions such as emotional stress, exposure to cold, prolonged lordotic posture, and excess norepinephrine levels will resolve spontaneously when the precipitating element is eliminated and subsequently avoided. Mild, transient proteinuria may result from an albumin infusion or acute illnesses such as infection with fever (given the release of inflammatory cytokines), congestive heart failure, acute pulmonary edema, head injury, or

TABLE 43.1   Proteinuria

Type of Proteinuria	Major Mechanism	Associated Disease Process
Bence Jones proteinuria	Elevated plasma concentration	Multiple myeloma (also lymphosarcoma, leukemia, Hodgkin's disease)
Tamm-Horsfall proteinuria	Increased tubular cell secretion	Normal mucoprotein in urine
Tubulointerstitial area involvement	Decreased tubular reabsorption of normal filtered protein	Pyelonephritis
Altered glomerular capillary permeability	Increase of filtered proteins	Glomerulonephritis, nephrotic syndrome
pH >8.0	High-alkaline urine	False positive

cerebrovascular accident. This type of proteinuria typically resolves as the medical condition improves.

When proteinuria is identified in a low-risk (nondiabetic or nonpregnant) patient, the urine should be tested for Bence Jones proteins, the presence of which suggests multiple myeloma. In addition, a full serum chemistry panel should be done, including a fasting blood sugar, a lipid profile, urine culture and sensitivity, and a complete blood count with differential. If the patient's urine is positive for Bence Jones proteins, a serum protein electrophoresis should be done.

Persistent proteinuria that is not classified as functional proteinuria requires a further work-up, beginning with a 24-hour measurement of urine protein and creatinine levels. If the excretion rate is above 3.0 to 3.5 g per day, the patient, by definition, has nephrotic syndrome and must be referred to a nephrologist. Nephrotic syndrome can lead to acute renal failure, hypertension, and end-stage renal failure. If the excretion rate of protein is more than 2 g in 24 hours, a glomerular cause is most likely and further evaluation is warranted.

If renal function is normal in a patient with elevated urinary protein, the patient should be evaluated for orthostatic proteinuria. This involves having the patient collect a urine specimen upon awakening but before assuming an upright position for longer than 1 minute. After the patient has been standing or walking for 2 hours, a second specimen is collected. If the patient has orthostatic proteinuria, the first specimen will be free of protein and the second will be positive for protein, and referral to a nephrologist is necessary. Although this condition is largely benign and self-limited, orthostatic proteinuria is not well understood. Patients with nonorthostatic proteinuria and normal renal function in whom no Bence Jones proteins have been detected

should also be referred to a renal specialist for renal biopsy. Descriptions of proteinuria associated with specific disease processes involving the renal system is presented in Table 43.1.

Management of proteinuria depends on the underlying cause. Angiotensin-converting enzyme agents have been found to reduce proteinuria by decreasing interglomerular pressure. If hyperlipidemia and/or hypertension is present, these conditions should be aggressively treated. Patients found to have chronic renal failure should also be aggressively managed by a nephrologist to prevent or delay the onset of end-stage renal disease.

REFERENCES

Davis R, Jones JS, Barocas DA, et al. Diagnosis, evaluation and follow-up of asymptomatic microhematuris (AMH) in adults. American Urological Association. https://www.auanet.org/guidelines/asymptomatic-microhematuria-(2012-reviewed-and-validity-confirmed-2016). Published 2012, Accessed July 26, 2017.

Lerma EV. Proteinuria. Medscape. http://emedicine.medscape.com/article/238158-overview. Published 2016. Accessed August 26, 2017.

Michels TC, Sands JE. Dysuria: Evaluation and differential diagnosis in adults. *Am Fam Physician.* 2015;92(9):778–786.

RESOURCES

American Urological Association
    www.auanet.org
National Bladder Foundation
    www.bladder.org
National Kidney Foundation
    www.kidney.org

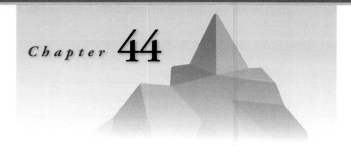

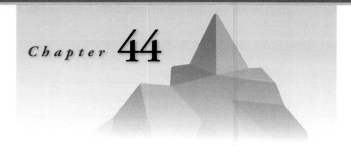

Chapter 44

Urinary Tract Disorders

Debbie Nogueras Conner, PhD, ANP/FNP-BC, FAANP

Debera J. Thomas, DNS, RN, FNP/ANP

Brian Oscar Porter, MD, PhD, MPH, MBA

URINARY INCONTINENCE

Urinary incontinence (UI) is the involuntary loss of urine from the bladder. Incontinence is so frequent in women that many patients mistakenly believe that it is an unavoidable consequence of aging. Incontinence is also common in older men as a result of an enlarging prostate. Incontinence can affect a person's quality of life and may be psychologically devastating. Ignoring incontinence, or inadequate treatment of this condition, can lead to social isolation, body image problems, anxiety, or depression; therefore, prompt treatment is essential (see The Iceberg of Incontinence).

EPIDEMIOLOGY AND CAUSES

UI affects more than 25 million Americans. The direct cost of treating and managing UI is reported to be more than $26 billion per year and includes costs associated with diagnostic testing, medication, and adult incontinence products such as disposable pads and undergarments. One study estimates that more than 40% of American women are affected, and there seems to be a strong association between UI and major depression. The prevalence of UI in the community population varies from 5% to 15%, depending on age and sex; more than 50% of patients in long-term care facilities have incontinence. Women are more likely than men to have incontinence, and the incidence increases with age; in fact, the risk of UI increases 14% with each decade of life.

Transient UI is characterized by sudden onset and can have several causes, including delirium, infection, pharmacologic agents, or underlying systemic illnesses such as diabetes, fecal impaction, and restricted mobility. Most new-onset incontinence that occurs in the

hospital resolves with appropriate treatment, but this acute transient phase can become a chronic problem if left untreated. The basic types of persistent UI are categorized as stress, urge, overflow, and functional UI. A patient may present with mixed symptoms of urge and stress incontinence. Table 44.1 provides an overview of the types of UI.

PATHOPHYSIOLOGY

The physiology of micturition involves three major components of urine storage and release: the central nervous system (CNS), the bladder, and the bladder outlet (urethral sphincters). Within the CNS, micturition is controlled by both the cortical (central) and brainstem (pontine) micturition centers. The cortical micturition center coordinates inhibitory stimuli from the frontal lobes and basal ganglia, permitting bladder relaxation and filling, as well as urethral sphincter closure to prevent urinary leakage, as the bladder increases in size. These efferent signals originate in spinal levels T11 to L2 and are mediated by alpha-adrenergic receptors and cholinergic somatic stimulation. This maintains urethral pressure along the bladder outlet by both internal and external sphincters. Alpha-adrenergic stimulation causes muscle contraction of the internal sphincter, whereas the external sphincter is under voluntary control of striated muscle tissue (allowing patients to "hold their urine" for purposes of social appropriateness).

In contrast, bladder emptying is mediated by the parietal lobes and the thalamus, which modulate afferent proprioceptive stimuli from the distended bladder wall detrusor muscle, sensing an increase in bladder pressure that is interpreted as bladder fullness. Once the patient has the urge to void, the inhibition by the cortical micturition center ceases. In turn, the brainstem micturition center sends impulses from the pons down the spinal cord to the sacral micturition center at S2 to S4, subsequently triggering the bladder detrusor muscle to contract via cholinergic stimulation of parasympathetic M2 and M3 type muscarinic receptors found within the smooth muscle of the bladder walls. (This latter action is simulated by the pharmacologic agent bethanechol [Urecholine], which is used to treat urinary retention caused by an atonic or poorly responsive bladder.) In addition, preganglionic sympathetic inhibition relaxes the urethral sphincter, allowing for the egress of urine.

Age-related changes that may affect urological functioning are decreased bladder capacity, increased postvoid residual urine volume (greater than 50 mL), increased disinhibition of bladder contractions (i.e., overactive bladder [OAB]), increased nocturnal sodium and fluid

The Iceberg of Incontinence

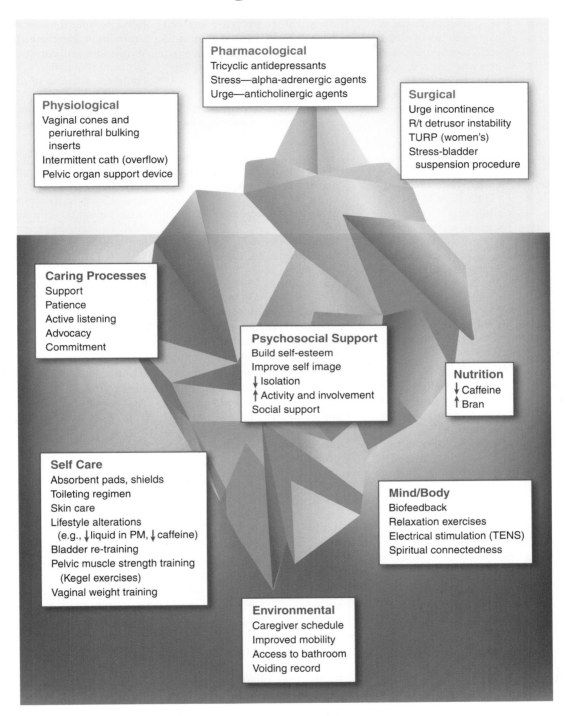

Pharmacological
Tricyclic antidepressants
Stress—alpha-adrenergic agents
Urge—anticholinergic agents

Physiological
Vaginal cones and
  periurethral bulking
  inserts
Intermittent cath (overflow)
Pelvic organ support device

Surgical
Urge incontinence
R/t detrusor instability
TURP (women's)
Stress-bladder
  suspension procedure

Caring Processes
Support
Patience
Active listening
Advocacy
Commitment

Psychosocial Support
Build self-esteem
Improve self image
↓ Isolation
↑ Activity and involvement
Social support

Nutrition
↓ Caffeine
↑ Bran

Self Care
Absorbent pads, shields
Toileting regimen
Skin care
Lifestyle alterations
  (e.g., ↓ liquid in PM, ↓ caffeine)
Bladder re-training
Pelvic muscle strength training
  (Kegel exercises)
Vaginal weight training

Mind/Body
Biofeedback
Relaxation exercises
Electrical stimulation (TENS)
Spiritual connectedness

Environmental
Caregiver schedule
Improved mobility
Access to bathroom
Voiding record

excretion (nocturia), urinary overflow phenomena resulting from increased urethral resistance in men related to benign prostatic hypertrophy, and weakness of the pelvic floor in women. Postmenopausal estrogen deficiency in women can result in decreased competence of the internal and external sphincters via atrophy of the urethral mucosal epithelium resulting in atrophic urethritis, loss of compliance, and a diminished urethral mucosal seal. It is important to note, however, that normal aging does not cause UI.

TABLE 44.1 Types of Urinary Incontinence

Type	Cause	Assessment	Management
Stress incontinence	Leakage of urine due to hypermobility of bladder neck, intrinsic sphincter deficiency, or neurogenic sphincter deficiency Medications: sedatives, hypnotics, antispasmodics	History of vaginal deliveries, urine leakage with cough or sneeze Evidence of urine loss Pelvic examination, pad test, stress test, urinalysis with culture and sensitivity, video-urodynamics, cystometrogram	Pelvic floor re-education with biofeedback (Kegel exercises) Weight loss, if obese Electrical stimulation Hormone replacement therapy (estrogen) Alpha-adrenergic agonist Surgical correction of hypermobile bladder neck Periurethral bulking injections
Urge incontinence	Leakage of urine due to urinary tract infection; vaginitis; bladder stones and tumors; cortical, sub-cortical, and suprasacral lesions; cerebrovascular accident; dementia; multiple sclerosis; Parkinson's disease; spinal cord transection Medications: diuretics, narcotics	History of dysuria, frequency, urgency, hematuria, or nocturia Evidence of a large amount of urine loss Evidence of unstable detrusor function with decreased capacity Assess perineal hygiene Pelvic examination, smear, neurologic examination, urinalysis with culture and sensitivity, cystometrogram, video-urodynamics	Antimicrobial agents, antiseptics, topical estrogen, anticholinergics, smooth muscle relaxants, tricyclic antidepressants (imipramine) Pelvic floor re-education with biofeedback (Kegel exercises) Prompted voiding and scheduled voiding Fluid intake management Removal of bladder stones Tumor resection and/or treatment
Overflow incontinence	Failure to empty bladder due to underactive detrusor activity, outlet obstruction, or diabetes mellitus Medications: anticholinergics, disopyramide, antihistamines, calcium channel blockers	History of hesitancy, dribbling, decreased stream, feeling of incomplete bladder emptying, constipation Neurologic examination, prostate examination (for men), prostate-specific antigen (for men), urinalysis with culture and sensitivity, serum creatinine, voiding cystometrogram, video-urodynamics	Scheduled toileting Credé's maneuver Treatment of underlying conditions Urinary collection devices (intermittent or suprapubic) Alpha blockers Resection of prostate, balloon dilation
Functional incontinence	Delirium, fecal impaction, lack of manual dexterity, or decreased mobility Medications: diuretics, hypnotics, alcohol, narcotics, decongestants	Fecal impaction Assess sleep patterns, mental state, hearing, vision, functional ability, intake and output, toilet accessibility, infection, neurologic function	Remove barriers to rapid toileting Provide barrier-free environment Bowel and bladder program Urinary collection devices Physical therapy Habit training

CLINICAL PRESENTATION

Subjective

Assessments of the urinary system should begin with a detailed medical and surgical history, including the patient's voiding history. A voiding history includes the date of incontinence onset, the number of times per day or night the patient voids, the amount of urine voided each time, the fluid-intake history including types of fluids consumed, and the characteristics of the patient's UI (e.g., "occurs when sneezing," nocturia,

frequency, urgency, dysuria). Information regarding underlying medical conditions that act as risk factors such as diabetes, cancer, acute illness, and neurologic disease should also be elicited.

Objective

The aim of the physical examination is to identify the underlying pathophysiological causes of incontinence, which can be multiple. The neurologic assessment is important in differentiating diagnoses such as cerebrovascular accident (stroke) and Parkinson's disease and should include an assessment of functional and cognitive ability. This provides information about limitations in mobility, self-care ability, mental status, and communication deficits, such as aphasia or language barriers.

An abdominal examination may rule out constipation, fecal impaction, masses, distended bladder, or cystitis, which can lead to incontinence. A pelvic examination will reveal the degree of pelvic floor strength, conditions such as uterine prolapse, and any problems associated with perineal structures. A rectal examination should be done to determine the sphincter tone and the presence or absence of feces that may suggest causative complications such as fecal impaction. In men, a prostate examination is crucial in evaluating urinary tract complaints. Inspection of the skin around the pelvic area is important. For example, in women there may be atrophic vaginitis, and in men there may be abnormalities of the foreskin, penis, or perineum. In addition, the patient's skin should be evaluated for breakdown or pressure areas during the pelvic examination. Incontinence can cause skin breakdown in the perineal area and buttocks, which may lead to decubitus ulcers. In female patients, particularly postmenopausal women, the perineum should be assessed for dryness and atrophy of the vaginal mucosa as a result of decreased estrogen.

During the physical examination, signs of congestive heart failure (CHF) should be assessed because 50% of people with CHF experience incontinence. A cough stress test (which will allow direct observation of urine loss with a full bladder), bladder scan (ultrasound), or catheterization (if necessary) to determine postvoid residual volume should be done as well. The patient or caretaker should be instructed to keep a voiding record for 3 to 7 days. The voiding record includes the time of the incontinence episode, the amount of urine, whether there was an urge to void, and the patient's activity at the time of the voiding. This record also includes an hourly record of fluid intake. For patients with a questionable history of UI, a "pad test" can be done. This involves having the patient take oral phenazopyridine (Pyridium), which will color the urine orange, and then wear a sanitary pad that can be checked at intervals for staining.

DIAGNOSTIC REASONING

Diagnostic Tests

A urinalysis and urine culture and sensitivity should be done, as well as measurements of serum electrolytes, blood urea nitrogen, creatinine, calcium (for polyuria in the absence of diuretics), and glucose. Catheterization to assess postvoiding residual volume is important even on initial evaluation of the patient, unless a reliable measurement can be obtained by bladder scan. Further testing depends on whether the onset of incontinence is acute, in which case testing related to other concurrent conditions may be warranted. Urinalysis results are often normal but may show glycosuria (in patients with diabetes), proteinuria (in patients with glomerular disease), white blood cells (WBCs; in patients with a bacterial infection), red blood cells (RBCs) (which may indicate the presence of a tumor), or bacteria (another sign of infection). A urine culture that is positive for a predominant bacterial species (i.e., other than mixed or normal flora) also indicates infection, and specific findings can be used to guide antibiotic therapy.

Other diagnostic options include urodynamic testing and cystometry, cystometrogram, video-urodynamics, and a postvoid residual catheterization to indicate the amount of retained urine and patients requiring these tests are usually referred to a urologist. Reviewing the patient's use of medications for possible drug interactions, obtaining an accurate record of intake and output, and evaluating for other risk factors contributing to UI are also important. Patients who have indwelling catheters should be urodynamically evaluated for possible bladder retraining. Renal ultrasound may show renal pathology; a transrectal ultrasound can provide evidence of prostatic disease; and a pelvic ultrasound may demonstrate pelvic pathology. A cystogram may show abnormal sphincter pressure or bladder pathology.

Differential Diagnosis

Many older patients may normally compensate for their incontinence, but any marked alteration in status either physiologically or psychologically—such as a hospitalization—can precipitate the acute onset of incontinence. For example, the administration of IV hydration in an acutely ill or older adult may be sufficient to precipitate incontinence. Although the end point is the same for all types of incontinence (involuntary bladder emptying), the context in which this occurs may vary markedly. Thus, the primary goal of differential diagnosis is for the clinician to correctly identify the type and etiology of incontinence, which in turn drives management and treatment decisions. Normal micturition requires a complex interplay of neurologic, structural, and functional components of the urinary system:

- The cerebral cortex exerts an overall inhibitory influence on the sacral spinal cord reflex. Delirium, dementia, parkinsonism, and stroke may all lead to urge incontinence without the patient's awareness. Conversely, the brainstem and suprasacral spinal cord exert a predominantly facilitating and coordinating influence that may be overcome in disorders such as stroke and multiple sclerosis, leading to overflow incontinence without awareness. This type of incontinence is referred to as neurogenic or detrusor-sphincter dyssynergy. Injuries to the sacral spinal cord, which controls reflex bladder filling and emptying, may lead to an acontractile bladder and overflow incontinence. This type of incontinence also results from the sacral nerve damage that can occur in uncontrolled diabetes mellitus.

- Local irritation and bladder or outflow obstructions may lead to urge incontinence because the smooth muscle in the obstructed bladder can have enhanced spontaneous contractile activity. Increased outflow obstruction may be caused by anatomical obstruction by the prostate, pelvic stricture, or cystocele, resulting in chronic urinary retention and overflow incontinence and without the patient being aware that they are incontinent.

- The bladder and lower genitourinary tract must be able to store urine and empty properly for normal micturition to occur. Failure to store urine may be a result of a hyperactive or poorly compliant bladder (e.g., secondary to cystitis, stones, tumor, or diverticula), leading to urge incontinence. OAB is an overarching term used to describe urine storage symptoms such as urgency, frequency, and nocturia and may or may not be accompanied by urge incontinence.

- Laxity of pelvic floor muscles and bladder outlet or sphincter weakness, and in women, hypermobility of the urethra may cause diminished outflow tract resistance, leading to stress incontinence. Increased intra-abdominal pressure (pregnancy, obesity, tumors, sneezing, coughing) can precipitate stress incontinence.

Mixed types of incontinence are common. In a patient with mixed signs and symptoms, multiple etiological factors must be considered, and a variety of interventions must be made available. The assessment and management of a patient with incontinence are best approached through the *Circle of Caring* (see discussion of this model in Chapter 1).

MANAGEMENT

Effective treatment of UI is largely driven by the pathophysiologic basis of its etiology, as well as specific causative factors in individual patients. Understanding the mechanics of the various causes of incontinence helps clarify management.

Stress Incontinence

Stress incontinence is the involuntary loss of urine resulting from increased intra-abdominal pressure, such as that caused by coughing, sneezing, and laughing. In this condition, the bladder is unable to retain urine because of hypermobility of the bladder neck, intrinsic sphincter deficiency, neurogenic sphincter deficiency, or use of certain medications, such as sedatives, hypnotics, alpha-blockers, and/or antispasmodics that relax smooth muscle and increase urine flow. Patients who present with stress incontinence report urinary leakage with coughing or sneezing and typically have a history of vaginal deliveries and/or hysterectomy. A detailed history guides the diagnostic work-up, which should include a pelvic examination, a pad test to determine the amount and

frequency of urinary leakage, a cough stress test, urinalysis with culture and sensitivity, video-urodynamic testing, and/or a cystometrogram.

Once the diagnosis of stress incontinence has been made, treatment should be individualized and instituted to meet the patient's needs. Noninvasive treatments include pelvic floor re-education (e.g., Kegel exercises) with biofeedback, electrical stimulation (an advanced form of biofeedback), weight loss (if the patient is obese), anti-incontinence devices or pessaries, and medications such as alpha-adrenergic agonists, which improve the muscle tone of the urinary tract. Eliminating diuretics will also improve symptoms. Surgical options include correction of the hypermobile bladder neck and periurethral bulking injections. See Drugs Commonly Prescribed 44.1 for a list of medications used for UI.

For cases in which uterine malpositioning is putting undue pressure on the bladder (e.g., as may be seen with uterine prolapse), vaginal cones or rings may be used to retain the uterus in a less problematic (and more physiologic) position. Thus, vaginal cones can reduce the pressure on the bladder of prolapsed uterine musculature and subsequent UI. Vaginal pessaries are divided into two categories: support and space filling. Pessaries are an effective option, particularly for older women or in those who do not tolerate the medications well or in whom medications are contraindicated.

Surgical intervention may be appropriate if all other measures have failed or if used in conjunction with the previously discussed conservative treatment approaches. Surgery may be indicated to correct anatomical abnormalities such as a prolapsed uterus, hypermobile bladder neck, or obstructions such as an enlarged prostate or urinary tract and bladder tumors. Surgery should be used as the last treatment option unless the causative agent is diagnosed as a tumor or severe urinary tract obstruction.

Urge Incontinence

Urge incontinence, also known as detrusor instability, is the involuntary leakage of urine resulting from an inability to delay voiding. The patient has the sensation of a full bladder but is not able to store the urine long enough to reach the toilet. This failure can be caused by urinary tract infection (UTI); vaginitis; bladder stones; bladder tumors; cortical, subcortical, or suprasacral CNS lesions; stroke; dementia; multiple sclerosis; Parkinson's disease; prostate problems; spinal cord transection; and medications such as diuretics and narcotics. The patient's history and physical examination may reveal evidence of dysuria, increased frequency or urgency, hematuria, large amounts of urine loss, and unstable detrusor muscle activity with decreased urinary capacity, or nocturia. Assessment should include perineal hygiene, pelvic examination with vaginal discharge smear, and a neurologic examination including an assessment of mental status; a urinalysis with a culture and sensitivity

Drugs Commonly Prescribed 44.1: Urinary Incontinence

DRUG	INDICATION	ADVERSE REACTIONS AND PRESCRIBING CONSIDERATIONS
Anticholinergic/Antispasmodic Agents		

Tolterodine (Detrol LA)
Oxybutynin (Ditropan XL, Urotrol)
Solifenacin (VESIcare)
Darifenacin (Enablex)
Trospium chloride (Sanctura XR)
Transdermal oxybutynin (Gelnique)
Fesoterodine (Toviaz)
	Urge incontinence
	Overactive bladder (OAB)
	Stress incontinence
		Contraindications:
		  Closed-angle glaucoma
		  Myasthenia gravis
		  Partial or complete gastric obstruction
		  Severe colitis
		  Urinary retention
		  Gastric retention
		Side effects:
		  Dry mouth
		  Drowsiness
		  Blurred vision
		  Urinary hesitance
		  Urinary retention
		  Decreased gastrointestinal motility
		  Headache
		  Constipation
		  Vertigo/dizziness
		  Abdominal pain

Alpha-1-Adrenergic Blocking Agents (used predominantly in men)		

Tamsulosin hydrochloride (Flomax)
Terazosin hydrochloride (Hytrin)
Doxazosin mesylate (Cardura)
	Benign prostatic hypertrophy and related urinary symptoms	Contraindications:
		  Hypersensitivity to tamsulosin terazosin, or doxazosin
		Side effects:
		  Orthostatic hypotension
		  Palpitations
		  Dizziness
		  Impotence
		  Gastrointestinal upset
		  Headache

Tricyclic Antidepressants		

Imipramine (Tofranil)
Amitriptyline (Elavil)
	OAB
	Urge incontinence
		Contraindications:
		  Hypersensitivity to tricyclic antidepressants
		  Use of monoamine oxidase inhibitors
		Side effects:
		  Dry mouth
		  Urinary retention
		  Blurred vision
		  Orthostatic hypotension
		  Sedation
		  Confusion in the elderly
		  Tachycardia
		  Anxiety and nervousness
		  Sexual dysfunction
		  Constipation

Continued

Drugs Commonly Prescribed 44.1: Urinary Incontinence—cont'd

DRUG	INDICATION	ADVERSE REACTIONS AND PRESCRIBING CONSIDERATIONS
Other		
Botulinum toxin (Botox) injection	OAB from neurogenic conditions OAB that does not respond to anticholinergic drugs	Side effects: Urinary tract infection Need for transient self-catheterization

should also be ordered. Invasive procedures that may be needed include cystometrogram and video-urodynamics.

Treatment begins conservatively, with pelvic floor re-education and biofeedback, if the patient is capable. Scheduled or prompted voiding by a caregiver, with management of the patient's fluid intake, may be useful for patients who have cognitive impairments or are forgetful. Medications such as antimicrobial agents may be necessary to treat underlying conditions. Other medications may include anticholinergics, smooth muscle relaxants, and tricyclic antidepressants to improve the neuromuscular function of the bladder and urethral sphincter (see Drugs Commonly Prescribed 44.1). Surgical treatment may be indicated for the removal of bladder stones or tumors.

Overactive Bladder

The term *overactive bladder* is often used interchangeably with the term *urge incontinence*; however, they are different conditions. OAB is a syndrome of symptoms that include urgency, frequency, and nocturia, all of which are associated with involuntary contractions of the detrusor muscle. Urge incontinence (the sudden intense urge to urinate and an involuntary loss of urine) may or may not be a feature of this syndrome, as about one-third of patients with OAB have urge incontinence.

OAB may also occur as a component of other types of UI, such as stress incontinence. OAB is caused by many factors, including disorders of the lower urinary tract, ingestion of alcohol and caffeine, use of a variety of prescribed drugs, or neurologic conditions. This condition is most common in women and often results in anxiety and depression because of restricted daily functioning. Sexual dysfunction can occur because of the fear of urine loss during sexual intercourse. It is estimated that only about 6% to 27% of women with this condition seek treatment.

Pharmacotherapy plays an important role in management of OAB. Antimuscarinic agents are commonly used drugs for OAB and are effective because they inhibit the muscarinic action of acetylcholine and prevent unwanted contractions of the detrusor muscle. Botulinum toxin A injection in the detrusor muscle is effective for patients with refractory OAB. See Drugs Commonly Prescribed 44.1 for a complete list of medications used for OAB.

Overflow Incontinence

Overflow incontinence is the involuntary leakage of small amounts of urine. This is caused by an overdistended bladder in a patient who does not feel the need to void because of an atonic detrusor muscle, outlet obstruction, benign prostatic hypertrophy, diabetes mellitus, or the use of medications such as anticholinergics, disopyramide (Norpace), antihistamines, diuretics, or calcium channel blockers. The history and physical examination may indicate hesitancy, dribbling, nocturia, decreased stream, feeling of not emptying the bladder, and/or constipation. A neurologic examination, prostate examination, urinalysis with culture and sensitivity, serum creatinine, voiding cystometrogram, and/or video-urodynamic testing should be done.

Management of overflow incontinence consists of treating the underlying condition, teaching scheduled toileting and Credé's maneuver, and the prescribing of medications such as alpha blockers (see Drugs Commonly Prescribed 44.1). Credé's maneuver involves applying pressure over the symphysis pubis and slowly pressing down. This is particularly helpful in patients who have a spinal cord injury or other neurologic problems. It may be necessary to discontinue certain medications or to alter dosages to reduce the adverse effects causing overflow incontinence. Alternative collection devices may also be indicated, including the use of external catheters; pads; and indwelling, intermittent, or suprapubic catheterization. In the case of urinary outlet obstruction in men, resection of the prostate may be necessary.

Functional Urinary Incontinence

Functional UI is incontinence that occurs with a normal functioning urinary system. The leakage of urine is caused by factors outside the lower urinary tract and can be transient in nature. The causes of functional incontinence may vary from delirium or fecal impaction to lack of manual dexterity and immobility problems. Medications such as diuretics, hypnotics, narcotics, and decongestants, as well as alcohol, may also play a role. Assessment for fecal impaction, sleep pattern disturbances, mental status, hearing and vision, functional ability, fluid intake, infection (especially of the urinary tract), and neurologic function is essential.

Treatment for functional UI may consist of some combination of removing barriers to effective toileting, providing education regarding a scheduled bowel and bladder program, the use of urinary collection devices, referring patients for physical or occupational therapy, and toileting habit training. Barriers to elimination may be identified when the patient cannot remove clothing or reach the toilet in sufficient time to avoid leakage. By identifying the barrier(s), interventions to resolve the problem can be developed. Some solutions include the use of hook-and-loop (Velcro) closures (which are easily managed by arthritic hands and fingers) instead of buttons and zippers, bedside commodes for nighttime use to eliminate the amount of time needed to get to the bathroom, or monitors for obtaining immediate assistance in getting out of bed and to the toilet.

A caregiver may be necessary to assist the patient in toileting; therefore, it is imperative to assess the caregiver's ability to provide care and determine his or her level of competency. Nursing research shows that caregivers want to give "good" care; however, the caregiver must be physically capable of providing this care with sufficient manual dexterity, strength, and mental cognition. Furthermore, the caregiver must be able to comprehend and follow through with instructions that may be complex and require problem-solving ability.

Identifying patients who need physical or occupational therapy to improve their functional skills may be required. Initiation of a bowel and bladder program can decrease the incidence of constipation and fecal impaction. Patients should also be encouraged to retrain the bladder to empty completely on a regular basis. For patients who cannot avoid UI, alternatives are available to keep them clean and dry. Condom catheters are effective in keeping male patients dry, and pads of various types are available for both men and women. Indwelling catheters, suprapubic catheters, and intermittent catheterization are options for urine collection in patients who cannot maintain bladder function or who have frequent or regular UI.

Medications used to treat incontinence are effective for patients who are unable to store urine. Pharmacologic agents should be used in conjunction with other treatment modalities such as toileting and behavioral modification. Scheduled toileting along with regulation of fluid intake can have a positive effect on bladder control. Behavioral modification treatment such as pelvic floor re-education is designed to increase pelvic floor muscular strength and endurance. Re-education is accomplished through Kegel exercises of the targeted muscle group using biofeedback for a period of 4 to 6 weeks. Kegel exercises are the tightening and releasing of the pubococcygeal and levator ani muscles, accomplished by tightening the muscle group used to avoid defecation or urination. The patient may experience results within 2 weeks to several months of initiating the program. This treatment is noninvasive and, when appropriate, should be attempted before surgical intervention (Box 44.1).

FOLLOW-UP AND REFERRAL

Close follow-up is essential for patients with UI. This may be done biweekly at first, while the patient is being taught therapeutic exercises (e.g., Kegel exercises) or medication dosages are being adjusted. Quarterly follow-up visits may be sufficient once incontinence is under control and medication doses have been stabilized. The patient should be monitored for adverse effects of medications and orthostatic hypotension. Periodic urinalysis should be done to detect any UTIs early. Women should have regular pelvic examinations to detect pelvic abnormalities early, and men should have regular rectal examinations to detect prostatic abnormalities.

Patient Education: Urinary Incontinence

Patient and family education is crucial in the treatment of UI. Medical side effects as contributing factors to UI cannot be overemphasized. Particularly in elderly patients, polypharmacy is a key contributor to iatrogenic UI and may be further exacerbated by the reactionary additional of new anti-incontinence medications. Environmental assessment should include recommendations about proximity of toilet facilities. An individualized toileting schedule should be geared to each patient's pattern of incontinence. Bladder training in the form of timed voiding, working up to 3-hour intervals, is an important intervention. Good general nutritional and exercise practices are important to the upkeep of overall health. Support and encouragement are essential. Interventions geared toward preventing social isolation, setting up necessary support services, and optimism in dealing with the problem are important interventions in the primary-care setting.

Box 44.1 Kegel Exercises: Patient Instructions

- Locate the correct muscle. To do so, try stopping your urine flow by contracting the muscle. When the urine slows or stops, you are using the pubococcygeus muscle.
- Squeeze the muscle for 2 seconds (do not hold your breath or contract your abdomen, buttocks, or thighs), then relax for 10 seconds. This is one repetition. Do 10 repetitions twice a day.
- After you have mastered the technique, begin to lengthen the time you contract the muscle. Increase the time by 1 second every few days until you are able to contract the muscle for 10 seconds at a time (and relax for 10 seconds). Continue to do 10 repetitions twice a day.

LOWER URINARY TRACT INFECTIONS

A lower UTI occurs when the normally sterile environment of the urinary tract system is invaded by pathogenic bacteria. Infections of the lower urinary tract can occur in the urethra, bladder, and, in men, the prostate. Infection of the urethra (*urethritis*) and infection of the urinary bladder (*cystitis*) usually occur together. Women may be diagnosed with chronic inflammation of the bladder wall (*interstitial cystitis* [*IC*]). *Prostatitis* is infection of the prostate gland.

Infections can be acute, chronic, recurrent, complicated, or uncomplicated. *Acute infections* are characterized by the onset of UTI in a previously symptom-free individual. Infections can become *chronic* when unresolved after standard treatment is rendered. UTIs become chronic because of obstructions, antibiotic-resistant bacteria, or the presence of multiple strains of bacteria that are not susceptible to the antibiotic therapy prescribed. A UTI is considered *recurrent* when it occurs again within 2 weeks of the original infection. A *complicated* UTI is either an acute or chronic infection that is accompanied by factors that predispose a patient to the infection or make treatment more difficult, such as instrumentation (e.g., indwelling, suprapubic, or intermittent catheterization), underlying chronic disease, systemic symptoms, or pregnancy. An *uncomplicated* UTI is one that can be resolved without addressing such factors and is localized to the lower urinary tract.

EPIDEMIOLOGY AND CAUSES

Lower UTI is a common problem that affects approximately 20% of women and 1% of men each year. This condition accounts for more than 6 million visits to primary-care practitioners annually. Although common in women of all ages, UTI rarely occurs in men younger than 50 years and is usually caused by urinary catheters, anatomical abnormalities of the urinary tract, unprotected anal intercourse, or vaginal intercourse with a woman who has a bacterial infection. UTI may occur at any age, but it is more prevalent in sexually active adults, very young children, or frail older adults. Other populations at risk include individuals with predisposing conditions such as a suppressed immune system, pregnancy, urinary obstruction, catheter dependency, neurogenic bladder, or diabetes mellitus.

Lower UTI may be the result of other conditions within the renal system. A urethral obstruction can create stasis of urine, providing a medium for bacterial growth. Other conditions that can contribute to UTI are a descending infection from the kidney, an anatomically short urethra (in female patients), and acute infections elsewhere in the body. UTI may also occur as a result

of poor or nonsterile catheterization technique or reuse of disposable catheters, poor hygiene, unprotected anal intercourse, or simply from a normal indwelling catheter, which, as a foreign body, serves as a nidus of infection.

IC is found primarily in women. An estimated 3 to 8 million women and 1 to 4 million men seeking treatment for bladder pain are diagnosed with IC, also known as painful bladder disease. The cause of this condition is unknown, but some researchers theorize that an abnormality in the bladder surface allows potassium and urea to leak into the bladder interstitium. Other etiologies being investigated include lymphatic, infectious, neurological, neurologic, autoimmune, and vasculitic mechanisms. Notably, IC does not respond to antibiotics.

PATHOPHYSIOLOGY

Lower UTIs usually occur as a result of contamination from the patient's own gastrointestinal tract. Bacteria may be introduced into the urinary tract from fecal contamination secondary to poor perineal hygiene, unprotected sexual (particularly anal) intercourse, and/or an anatomically shortened urethra in women. The use of a spermicide during intercourse (especially with diaphragm forms of contraception) alters the vaginal microenvironment, predisposing to bacterial colonization. Immunosuppressed or medically compromised patients may have difficulty in suppressing bacterial growth as bacteria ascend the urethra. Patients who are dependent on catheters are at risk for introduction of bacteria into the urinary tract through contamination of the catheter.

Alkaline urine is a common complication of diabetes mellitus. The elevated pH of the urine creates a medium in which bacteria can more readily grow and proliferate. Renal stones can also create an environment that promotes bacterial growth, as the blockage causes stasis of urine or reflux. In turn, contamination can occur in the kidney when urine "backs up" due to vesicoureteral reflux, in which urine flows back freely into one or both ureters, resulting in urinary stasis.

In women, approximately 80% to 90% of cases of uncomplicated UTI are a result of the gram-negative rod bacterium *Escherichia coli*. The second most common cause (5% to 20% of cases) of uncomplicated bacterial infection is the gram-positive coccus *Staphylococcus saprophyticus*, although this agent is rare in complicated UTI. Other gram-negative rods identified as causative pathogens in a smaller number of cases, but particularly in complicated UTI, include *Proteus mirabilis*, *Klebsiella*, *Enterobacter*, *Serratia*, and *Pseudomonas*. In addition, the gram-positive coccus *Enterococcus* has been identified. *Staphylococcus aureus* is a gram-positive coccus that can be introduced into the urinary tract through instrumentation or as a complication of renal stones.

Fungi, particularly *Candida* species, may also be causative agents in complicated UTI that fails to respond to antibiotic therapy, especially in the presence of an indwelling catheter. Candiduria may be asymptomatic, and fungal structures should be sought on urine microscopy because fungal colonies may be more difficult to elaborate under standard urine culture conditions, in turn leading to delays in treatment.

In up to 50% of all bacterial species associated with cystitis, genetic virulence determinants may be identified that contribute to the uropathogenicity of these organisms, such as adherence factors that allow for greater binding affinity to the uroepithelium. Another is the urease gene, expressed by certain gram-negative bacteria such as *Proteus*, *Klebsiella*, *Ureaplasma*, *Providencia*, and *Pseudomonas* species. This enzyme splits urea molecules within the urinary tract, creating ammonium and hydroxyl ions that produce an alkaline microenvironment. This higher pH facilitates survival of these bacteria, particularly when housed within triple phosphate (magnesium ammonium phosphate) stones, also known as struvite stones.

Cystitis is rare in men because the increased length and drier environment around the urethra contribute to less frequent bacterial colonization. In addition, prostatic fluid has inherent antibacterial properties. Thus, when UTI does occur, it is often associated with abnormal urethral anatomy or inadequate treatment of prostatitis. Most antibiotics do not penetrate the prostatic tissue and therefore do not eliminate prostatic infection. As a result, the bladder is reinfected from contaminated prostatic fluid, even if a lower UTI initially clears upon treatment.

Two well-documented phenomena related to classic UTI are asymptomatic bacteriuria and dysuria–pyuria syndrome. In asymptomatic bacteriuria, patients experience no obvious clinical symptoms or signs of UTI (including altered mental status in the elderly), yet urinalysis and culture yield findings consistent with bacteriuria. In contrast, dysuria–pyuria syndrome (also called "acute urethral syndrome") is characterized by painful urination with WBCs on microscopic urinalysis in the absence of a positive bacterial culture. This condition may be due to organisms such as *Chlamydia* that do not grow well under standard urinary culture conditions. Dysuria–pyuria syndrome may, however, be difficult to distinguish clinically from vaginitis due to sexually transmitted infection (STI).

CLINICAL PRESENTATION

Subjective

The presenting signs and symptoms of UTIs vary widely in intensity and occurrence. Women may present with urethritis and cystitis simultaneously. The most frequently reported symptoms in both men and women are dysuria, urinary frequency or urgency, nocturia, hematuria, low back or suprapubic pain, UI, and cloudy, foul-smelling urine. These symptoms can occur in any combination. In elderly patients, altered mental status may be the sole manifestation of UTI and should create a high level of suspicion.

Urethritis in men is rare; if left untreated or treated inadequately, it can lead to complications such as urethral strictures, periurethral abscess, urethral diverticula, and fissures. Vaginal discharge in women and urethral discharge in men may suggest (STI). Purulent urethral discharge (*Neisseria gonorrhoeae*) or whitish-mucoid discharge (*Chlamydia trachomatis*) should be treated aggressively with the appropriate antibiotic therapy (see Chapter 51 for a full discussion of STIs).

Objective

Physical examination in the outpatient setting should include a "clean catch" midstream urine sample for urinalysis. Urinalysis findings that are associated with an infectious process in the urinary tract system include cloudy appearance, alkaline pH, hematuria, elevated levels of nitrites, leukocyte esterase (detecting pyuria of greater than 10 leukocytes per high power field [hpf]), and urinary sediments of RBCs, WBCs, mucus, and bacterial overgrowth.

Of note, *Enterobacteriaceae* convert urinary nitrates to nitrites, producing positive results on urine dipstick analysis if present in adequate numbers (greater than 100,000 organisms/mL). In contrast, however, *Staphylococcus* does not convert this substrate and is not detectable by this test. Moreover, false-positive urinary nitrite tests may result in the presence of the urinary tract analgesic phenazopyridine. A urine culture with antibiotic sensitivities may be ordered to speciate and determine the sensitivity of the causative organism to specific antibiotic therapy.

Patients with IC may present with the need to urinate frequently because of reduced bladder capacity. This may occur up to 60 times per day in extreme cases. Other symptoms include pain or discomfort in the abdominal area that holds the bladder.

DIAGNOSTIC REASONING

Diagnostic Tests

Diagnosis of lower UTI is made based on the subjective complaints of the patient and a clean-catch midstream urine sample showing the presence of bacteria, especially if more than 100,000 organisms/mL of the same morphology are present in a sample from a female patient. Traditionally, a bacterial concentration of at least 100,000 colony-forming units (CFUs)/mL on urine culture has been used to define UTI, but UTI may result from far lower bacterial loads. UTI is currently defined as a urine sample with greater than 100 organisms/mL in the presence of characteristic clinical symptoms.

The method of urine collection also influences interpretation of the urine culture because the sterility of commonly performed "clean catch" techniques is heavily dependent on the patient's ability to self-clean around the urethra before voiding. Sterile wipes containing iodine, chlorhexidine, or other acceptable cleaning agent must be used to wipe the urethral opening at least two to three times consecutively in a direction away from the perineum to minimize contamination by anorectal flora (e.g., normal skin flora or bacteria from vaginal discharge or fecal matter). Alcohol swabs are unacceptable cleaning agents. Straight catheterization samples obtained with sterile technique are the most reliable, whereas samples obtained from receptacles connected to indwelling catheters may prove unreliable owing to repeated manipulation of the collecting bag.

Although urine culture is considered the gold standard with the greatest sensitivity for laboratory confirmation of UTI, urinalysis with microscopy is also helpful and provides rapid results. Urinalysis typically indicates pyuria (greater than 10 neutrophils per hpf on microscopic examination) and often the presence of RBCs. Hematuria is common in UTI but not with urethritis or vaginitis; however, blood in the urine is not a marker of complicated infection.

UTIs may be treated with empiric antibiotic therapy based on knowledge of the most common bacterial etiologies. However, urine culture and antibiotic sensitivity testing will aid in definitively identifying the infecting microorganism and the appropriate antibiotic therapy. Although the diagnosis of UTI is made both clinically and by urinalysis, generally urine culture and antibiotic sensitivities are indicated if complicated infection is suspected, atypical symptoms are present, or symptoms persist or recur within 1 month of the patient receiving a prior empirical course of antibiotic therapy or a new treatment regimen is desired.

IC is primarily a diagnosis of exclusion. Although somewhat controversial due to low sensitivity and specificity in some settings, a diagnostic tool for this condition is the potassium sensitivity test. This test involves slow instillation of 40 mL of sterile water into the bladder via catheterization and left for 5 minutes, after which the patient is asked to grade any discomfort on a 0 (none) to 5 scale, with 5 being the most severe. This establishes a baseline comparison. The water is then emptied and a 0.4 M potassium chloride solution is instilled into the bladder and left for 5 minutes, with any discomfort again graded by the patient. IC is suggested when there is a at least a two-point increase in pain or urgency, indicating abnormal epithelial dysfunction.

Differential Diagnosis

The differential diagnosis of tumors, upper UTI (pyelonephritis), vaginitis, and STIs must be explored in cases of suspected lower UTI. Tumors of the renal system and upper UTI are discussed in Chapter 45. Vaginitis and

STIs are discussed in Chapters 46 and 51. Patients with upper UTI usually show signs of sepsis such as fever and chills, have WBC casts in the urine (reflecting the passage of neutrophils through the renal tubules), or experience flank and costovertebral angle tenderness on examination, as in pyelonephritis.

MANAGEMENT

Pharmacologic antimicrobial management is the mainstay of treatment. Drugs Commonly Prescribed 44.2 presents the oral agents typically used for the treatment of lower UTI. Uncomplicated lower UTI may often be treated effectively with a short (3-days) course of trimethoprim-sulfamethoxazole (TMP-SMX) or a longer 10-day course of ampicillin. However, epidemiological surveillance has revealed increasing rates of resistance in *E. coli* isolates to ampicillin and sulfonamides, whereas only a small percentage of these isolates were resistant to nitrofurantoin (Macrodantin, Macrobid), which is known to concentrate in the urine. Thus, a 7-day course of nitrofurantoin should be used as an alternative in patients with documented sulfa drug allergy or in patients with previous antibiotic use within the past 3 months.

Nitrofurantoin is also effective against many gram-positive cocci such as *Enterococcus faecalis*, whereas other key uropathogens such as *Proteus*, *Enterobacter*, and *Klebsiella* may be highly resistant. Thus, both TMP-SMX (Bactrim) and nitrofurantoin should be used as empirical therapy for uncomplicated UTI only, as they may prove inadequate. Indeed, one of the strongest risk factors predicting microbial resistance to TMP-SMX is the previous use of this or any other antimicrobial agent for any infection within the past 3 months. However, selecting an alternative antibiotic regimen entails important considerations, such as local antibiotic resistance patterns, typically available from local health authorities or hospital systems. In addition, ciprofloxacin (Cipro) and other fluoroquinolones should be reserved as an alternative antibiotic class only in cases when no other antibiotic agents are appropriate, given concerns over the development of resistant uropathogens, the risk of tendon rupture and other connective tissue abnormalities, and the potential for severe, permanent, and disabling peripheral neuropathy.

The cost-effective 3-day treatment regimen for uncomplicated lower UTI reduces the risk of nonadherence and the development of *Candida* vaginitis due to clearance of normal urogenital flora. It is recommended for TMP-SMX, but not for nitrofurantoin, which requires a longer 7-day course of therapy for maximum efficacy. Complicated UTI, on the other hand, requires at least 10 to 14 days of antibiotic therapy.

The antimicrobial effects of these medications persist for several days after the final dose is administered. In particularly severe cases of UTI (especially in high-risk groups

Drugs Commonly Prescribed 44.2: Urinary Tract Infection (UTI)

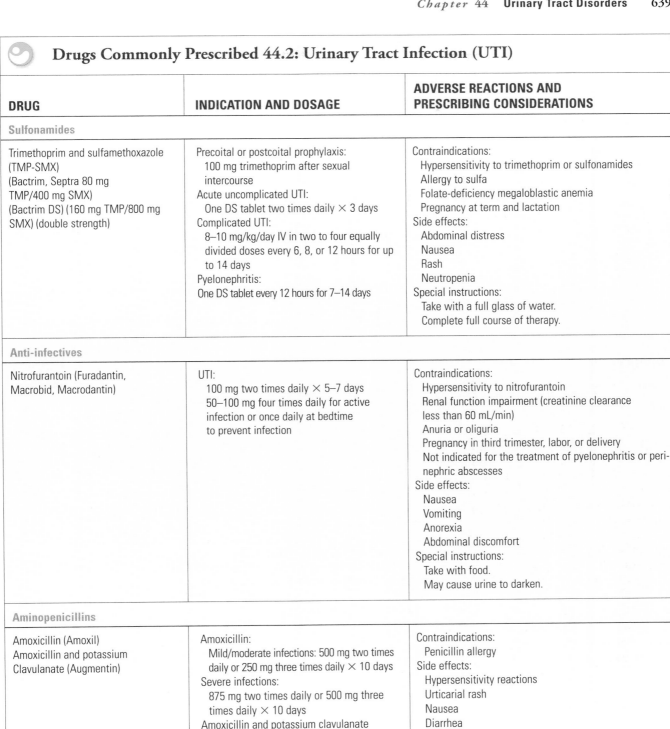

DRUG	INDICATION AND DOSAGE	ADVERSE REACTIONS AND PRESCRIBING CONSIDERATIONS
Sulfonamides		
Trimethoprim and sulfamethoxazole (TMP-SMX) (Bactrim, Septra 80 mg TMP/400 mg SMX) (Bactrim DS) (160 mg TMP/800 mg SMX) (double strength)	Precoital or postcoital prophylaxis: 100 mg trimethoprim after sexual intercourse Acute uncomplicated UTI: One DS tablet two times daily × 3 days Complicated UTI: 8–10 mg/kg/day IV in two to four equally divided doses every 6, 8, or 12 hours for up to 14 days Pyelonephritis: One DS tablet every 12 hours for 7–14 days	Contraindications: Hypersensitivity to trimethoprim or sulfonamides Allergy to sulfa Folate-deficiency megaloblastic anemia Pregnancy at term and lactation Side effects: Abdominal distress Nausea Rash Neutropenia Special instructions: Take with a full glass of water. Complete full course of therapy.
Anti-infectives		
Nitrofurantoin (Furadantin, Macrobid, Macrodantin)	UTI: 100 mg two times daily × 5–7 days 50–100 mg four times daily for active infection or once daily at bedtime to prevent infection	Contraindications: Hypersensitivity to nitrofurantoin Renal function impairment (creatinine clearance less than 60 mL/min) Anuria or oliguria Pregnancy in third trimester, labor, or delivery Not indicated for the treatment of pyelonephritis or perinephric abscesses Side effects: Nausea Vomiting Anorexia Abdominal discomfort Special instructions: Take with food. May cause urine to darken.
Aminopenicillins		
Amoxicillin (Amoxil) Amoxicillin and potassium Clavulanate (Augmentin)	Amoxicillin: Mild/moderate infections: 500 mg two times daily or 250 mg three times daily × 10 days Severe infections: 875 mg two times daily or 500 mg three times daily × 10 days Amoxicillin and potassium clavulanate Mild/moderate infections: 500 mg/125 mg two times daily or 250 mg/ 125 mg three times daily × 10 days Severe infections: 875 mg/125 mg two times daily or 500 mg/ 125 mg three times daily × 10 days	Contraindications: Penicillin allergy Side effects: Hypersensitivity reactions Urticarial rash Nausea Diarrhea Superinfections Special instructions: Complete full course of therapy. May decrease effectiveness of oral contraceptives. Augmentin should be given with food to decrease nausea.

Continued

Drugs Commonly Prescribed 44.2: Urinary Tract Infection (UTI)—cont'd

DRUG	INDICATION AND DOSAGE	ADVERSE REACTIONS AND PRESCRIBING CONSIDERATIONS
Cephalosporins—Second Generation		

Cefaclor (Ceclor)
Cefuroxime (Ceftin)
	Cefaclor:
	  500 mg three times daily × 7 days
	Cefuroxime uncomplicated UTI:
	  250 mg two times daily × 7–10 days
		Contraindications:
		  Allergy to cephalosporins
		Side effects:
		  Pruritus
		  Urticaria
		  Erythema multiforme
		  Rashes
		  Arthritis/arthralgia (with or without fever)
		  Diarrhea
		  Nausea
		Special instructions:
		  Renal dysfunction prolongs half-life.
		  May be taken without regard to meals.
		  Complete full course of therapy.

Cephalosporins—Third Generation		

Cefpodoxime (Vantin)	Cefpodoxime 100 mg two times daily
	× 7 days
		Contraindications:
		  Allergy to cephalosporins
		Side effects:
		  Diarrhea
		  Abdominal pain
		  Nausea
		  Dyspepsia
		  Flatulence
		Special instructions:
		  Avoid antacids 2 hours before and after dose.
		  Complete full course of therapy.

Urinary Analgesics		

Phenazopyridine (Pyridium)	Relief of pain, burning, urgency, and frequency from UTI:
	  200 mg three times daily after meals;
	  maximum 2 days
		Contraindications:
		  Hypersensitivity to phenazopyridine
		Side effects:
		  Headache
		  Rash
		  Itching
		Special instructions:
		  Take after meals.
		  May turn urine reddish-orange color and stain fabric.

Antispasmodics		

Flavoxate (Urispas)	Relief of dysuria, urgency, frequency, and incontinence of the urinary system:
	  100–200 mg three to four times a day
		Contraindications:
		  Use with caution in patients with glaucoma and older adults.
		Side effects:
		  Nausea
		  Vomiting
		  Dry mouth
		  Headache
		  Drowsiness
		  Blurred vision
		  Vertigo

such as elderly or bed-bound patients) or in cases involving urinary tract instrumentation, hospitalization and broad-spectrum IV antibiotic coverage (e.g., ceftriaxone, piperacillin-tazobactam, or ampicillin plus gentamicin) may be required until symptoms wane and urine culture and antibiotic sensitivities confirm the most appropriate narrow-spectrum antibiotic choice. The same approach may be required for upper UTI (i.e., pyelonephritis).

Empirical treatment of UTI in men (by definition, a complicated UTI) should be extended to at least 7 days. Nitrofurantoin and beta-lactams should be avoided.

Treatment of UTI during pregnancy is especially important because an established link exists between premature delivery and UTI (especially pyelonephritis). Empirical therapy may include ampicillin 500 mg by mouth four times daily, nitrofurantoin (Macrobid, Macrodantin) 100 mg orally two times daily, cephalexin (Keflex) 500 mg orally two times daily, or sulfisoxazole 1 g orally four times daily. Broader-spectrum regimens may include amoxicillin-clavulanate (Augmentin) 500 mg/125 mg orally two times daily or cefpodoxime (Vantin) 100 mg orally two times daily. Most clinicians will choose to treat UTI during pregnancy for 1 full week. Fluoroquinolones should be avoided, given concern for their effects on bone and cartilage formation in the developing fetus, and TMP-SMX should be avoided in the first and third trimesters of pregnancy.

Fungal UTI due to *Candida* infection is typically associated with an indwelling urinary catheter, and nearly half of all cases resolve simply with removal of the catheter. However, reinsertion of a new catheter is associated with a high rate of relapse. Antifungal treatment is typically not required for asymptomatic colonization, but if indicated in the presence of dysuria, an appropriate regimen would be fluconazole (Diflucan) 200 mg orally daily for 7 to 14 days.

The management of asymptomatic bacteriuria deserves special mention. This condition should be treated with antibiotics in pregnant women because it increases the risk of premature delivery. Although some studies suggest that treatment in girls beyond preschool age is not warranted, given the high rate of recurrent asymptomatic infection without obvious sequelae, general practice also calls for treating asymptomatic bacteriuria in young children. Treatment is also indicated in patients before they undergo a urological procedure to avoid operating on a contaminated field, after removal of a bladder catheter in place for less than 1 week, and in any patient with an underlying structural abnormality of the urinary tract, vesicoureteral reflux, or struvite stones. In contrast, treatment of this condition in adult men, nonpregnant women, the elderly, diabetic persons, and spinal cord patients with indwelling urinary catheters is not warranted. Although asymptomatic bacteriuria may be a harbinger of future UTI, antibiotic therapy has not been shown to persistently eradicate bacteriuria or urinary tract colonization in these populations.

After completion of antibiotic treatment, follow-up cultures may be obtained to ensure complete eradication of the pathogen in patients with a history of recurrent infection, during pregnancy, or in those prone to complicated UTI. Chronic or recurrent UTI may be prevented through prophylactic treatment either on a daily basis or after sexual intercourse, but this should be done only after all options to eliminate the causative factors of UTI have been explored. In women with a prior history of recurrent UTI, postcoital prophylaxis with a single oral dose of nitrofurantoin 50 mg or cephalexin 250 mg has been shown to be highly effective. Strategies should be emphasized to decrease the incidence of infection through the guidelines outlined under Patient Education: Lower Urinary Tract Infections.

Although appropriate antibiotic treatment is often adequate to relieve dysuria, certain medications may also be prescribed for the first few days to decrease the pain and discomfort of UTI. Use of these agents should not be prolonged, however, given their significant side effect profile. Effective treatment may involve anticholinergics, which produce an antispasmodic effect, including atropine (Donnatal), hyoscyamine (Levsin, Cystospaz), propantheline (Pro-Banthine), or oxybutynin (Ditropan). However, anticholinergics may also contribute to urinary retention (especially in the elderly), which is a clear risk factor for UTI, and should thus be used with caution. Analgesics may be prescribed such as phenazopyridine (Pyridium), but this alters the color of urine to orange and may cause urinary leakage secondary to anesthetization of the urethra and sphincter.

IC does not respond to antibiotics. However, this condition may be treated with pentosan polysulfate sodium (Elmiron), which tends to reduce the bladder wall inflammation. This drug has been shown to improve symptoms in 38% of patients with IC. Of note, IC is not curable, but it is controllable. If IC is untreated, it becomes more difficult to treat and in severe cases can progress to the development of a fibrotic contracted bladder.

FOLLOW-UP AND REFERRAL

Patients with complicated or repeated UTI, those who have pyelonephritis or are pregnant should have a follow-up urinalysis or culture to assess for effectiveness of treatment. UTI that is secondary to other pathological conditions will not resolve until the primary causative factor is addressed. Thus, indwelling urinary catheters should be changed every 4 to 6 weeks with new equipment, using sterile technique.

It is important to maintain adequate hydration and to monitor the urine output for signs of obstruction or renal failure. Urinary tract obstructions must be identified and removed to reduce the chances of chronic infection and renal damage that can lead to renal insufficiency and failure. It may be necessary to prescribe analgesics for the patient to reduce the pain associated with UTI.

Pain-relieving medications such as phenazopyridine (Pyridium) can be effective but should be prescribed for no more than 3 days.

Self-medication is usually adequate for female patients who have relatively few recurrences of UTI. If a diagnosis of recurrent bacterial UTI is confirmed, the patient should be given a supply of an antibiotic (preferably TMP-SMX or nitrofurantoin) and instructed to take it for 3 to 7 days whenever the symptoms recur. The patient should keep a diary of her infections and response to treatment and review it annually with a health professional so as to track medication-associated problems. The patient should also be advised to notify the clinician if symptoms such as flank pain, fever, hematuria, or lack of response to treatment occur.

If UTI recurs frequently (e.g., monthly), prophylactic therapy should be prescribed. After a course of 10 to 14 days of a suitable antibiotic for recurrent infection, the patient should begin low-dose antimicrobial prophylaxis every other day at bedtime over a 4- to 6-month period, which has proved as effective as daily dosing. Nighttime therapy is recommended because the patient generally does not void for a prolonged period, thus giving the bacteria the opportunity to adhere to the bladder wall. If this period of prophylaxis has been effective, the patient may switch to self-medication. If the frequency of recurrence increases at this point, however, prophylaxis should be extended to every other night indefinitely. However, all lifestyle issues should be investigated first. Given inconsistencies in the literature, there remains a need for well-designed studies to evaluate whether cranberry products may reduce the frequency of UTI recurrence as another prophylactic strategy.

Patient Education: Lower Urinary Tract Infections

Patient education should focus on teaching the patient to prevent the recurrence of UTI by advising the patient to follow these guidelines:

- Complete the full course of antibiotic therapy even if all symptoms subside early on in the course of treatment (prescribed treatment courses may be anywhere from 3 to 14 days in duration).
- Increase fluid intake to eight to ten 8-ounce glasses of water per day; this is most important to continue flushing out bacteria.
- Consider taking cranberry supplements (300–400 mg twice daily) or drink cranberry juice because this may decrease the bacteria's ability to adhere to the epithelial cells that line the bladder.
- Wear cotton underclothes rather than nylon to avoid moisture buildup and avoid wearing "thong" underpants.
- Avoid the use of harsh soaps or feminine hygiene products that can irritate the urethra.

- Use condoms to provide a barrier to infection from intercourse.
- Use proper techniques for self-catheterization (if indicated) to reduce the incidence of introducing bacteria.
- Empty the bladder frequently to avoid stasis of urine.
- Void after sexual intercourse.
- Take showers instead of tub baths or bubble baths to avoid chemical irritation of the urethra.
- Keep a diary of urinary symptoms and review it annually if recurrent infections are a problem.
- Empty the bladder completely, possibly by double-voiding (i.e., completely emptying the bladder two times in 5 minutes), especially if recurrent infections are a problem.

The patient should also be educated regarding any potential adverse effects of medications, including urinary leakage associated with phenazopyridine (Pyridium) treatment or the subsequent development of vaginal yeast infections following antibiotic treatment.

UPPER URINARY TRACT INFECTION: PYELONEPHRITIS

Pyelonephritis is an infection of the kidney that is characterized by infection within the renal pelvis, tubules, or interstitial tissue that may be unilateral or bilateral. The condition may be classified as either acute or chronic. The chronic condition leads to changes in the kidney that create atrophy and scarring of the kidney and calyceal deformity that may eventually lead to renal failure.

EPIDEMIOLOGY AND CAUSES

Pyelonephritis occurs in both men and women, but it is more common in women. The incidence is higher in older adults (especially if institutionalized or hospitalized), children, and immunocompromised patients. At least 250,000 cases are diagnosed annually with a treatment cost of $2.14 billion per year in the United States. The incidence and risk of developing this disease are increased in patients with predisposing factors including anatomical abnormalities such as ureterovesical reflux, urinary obstruction, stress incontinence, multiple or recurrent UTIs, renal disease, kidney trauma, pregnancy, and metabolic disorders such as diabetes mellitus. Having an indwelling urinary catheter is always a prominent risk factor for pyelonephritis, especially in hospitalized elderly women. An episode of acute pyelonephritis within the prior year also puts the patient at increased risk. Most of these risk factors alter the vaginal microenvironment and predispose individuals to lower UTI, as well.

In acute pyelonephritis, the actual infectious insult to the kidney may be from hematogenous seeding or urinary tract reflux, but most commonly it is an ascending infection from the bladder. Thus, it can often be attributed to an untreated lower UTI that spreads to the upper urinary system or is introduced through instrumentation. Chronic pyelonephritis usually has no specific pathological explanation if anatomical abnormalities have been ruled out.

PATHOPHYSIOLOGY

Pyelonephritis is typically caused by fecal flora that colonize the vaginal introitus and subsequently ascend along the urinary tract to the kidneys. It is unclear whether lower UTI always precedes pyelonephritis, because many patients present without clinical evidence of prior cystitis. However, bacteria are believed to enter through the urethral meatus and ascend upward from the lower urinary tract (urethra and bladder) to one or both kidneys via the ureters, the bloodstream (hematogenous spread), or the lymphatic system.

E. coli (75% to 95% of cases), *P. mirabilis*, *Klebsiella*, and *Pseudomonas* are the most common gram-negative causative agents. From 5% to 10% of cases are caused by gram-positive organisms, including *Enterococcus*, *S. saprophyticus*, and *S. aureus* (particularly in severe infection). *Ureaplasma urealyticum* and *Mycoplasma hominis* are rarer causative agents. In patients with normal urogenital systems, nearly all bacterial agents of pyelonephritis express virulence factors that contribute to their uropathogenicity (e.g., the *pap* and *sfa* operons and pathogenicity islands found in virulent *E. coli* strains).

In acute pyelonephritis, swelling of the renal parenchyma occurs as a result of the patchy distribution of the acute infectious process throughout the kidney. In rare instances, scarring of the renal parenchyma leading to kidney atrophy, renal hypertension, and renal failure may occur if left untreated. When the infection is severe, abscesses may develop in the renal medulla, leading to necrosis of the renal papillae. This infection can be potentially life-threatening in the elderly, children, or immunocompromised patients. In addition, diagnosis and treatment in pregnant women are particularly critical because upper UTI has a clear association with premature delivery.

Chronic pyelonephritis is usually caused by a recurrent or chronic bacterial infection of the kidney, often related to the presence of instrumentation such as an indwelling catheter that serves as a nidus of infection. Patients often have other urological problems such as vesicoureteral reflux, neurogenic bladder, or urinary obstruction caused by renal tumors, stones, or prostatic hypertrophy. The persistent unresolved infection and inflammation cause fibrosis (scarring) of the tubulointerstitium, which may lead to hypertension as the body senses decreased renal blood flow or eventually chronic renal insufficiency.

CLINICAL PRESENTATION

Subjective

Acute pyelonephritis presents with a classic triad of fever, costovertebral angle pain, and nausea and/or vomiting. The fever may persist over a few hours or days and range up to 103°F (39.5°C). The patient may present with shaking, chills, nausea, and vomiting, as well as unilateral flank or localized back pain over the affected kidney, fatigue, diarrhea, or other symptoms resembling those of gram-negative sepsis. Signs of urinary urgency or frequency and suprapubic discomfort may be present. In some cases, the presentation may mimic pelvic inflammatory disease. Otherwise, the patient may be largely asymptomatic and then progress to full-blown sepsis (i.e., urosepsis). In the elderly patient, altered mental status may be the initial manifestation of pyelonephritis.

Chronic pyelonephritis may present with the patient complaining of fatigue, nausea, decreased appetite with weight loss, nocturia, and/or polyuria. Patients may present with symptoms of renal failure resulting from asymptomatic chronic pyelonephritis that has persisted for several years. Symptoms of renal failure are discussed in detail in Chapter 45.

Objective

The physical examination will elicit marked tenderness on deep abdominal palpation and/or percussion of the affected flank and back overlying the affected kidney (costovertebral angle tenderness). Patients usually do not have a severely toxic appearance but may appear ill due to discomfort. Patients with underlying hypertension may present with blood pressure above their baseline. With severe pyelonephritis, patients may remain symptomatic for several days, even if appropriate antibiotic therapy is administered.

Patients with chronic pyelonephritis may show minimal symptoms or symptoms similar to those of acute pyelonephritis. Early signs and symptoms may be vague, and chronic pyelonephritis is usually first diagnosed when the patient presents with impaired renal function caused by damage to the kidneys.

DIAGNOSTIC REASONING

Diagnostic Tests

Diagnosis of pyelonephritis is confirmed through urinalysis, which is positive for bacteria, proteinuria, leukocyte esterase, urinary nitrites, hematuria, pyuria, and specifically WBC casts (reflecting the passage of neutrophils through the renal tubules), as well as urine culture, which typically demonstrates greater than 100,000 CFU/mL, allowing for identification of the causative organism. Any of these findings may be altered, however, if the patient is already on antibiotic therapy, and colony counts may be as low as 10,000 CFU/mL in some cases. Blood cultures may also be positive in 10% to 20% of mild to moderate pyelonephritis cases, reflecting urosepsis.

Cystoscopy with ureteral catheterization, renal ultrasound (to reveal hydroureter and/or hydronephrosis), or an intravenous pyelogram (IVP) may be indicated. However, the nuclear medicine–based dimercaptosuccinic acid (DMSA) scan is most sensitive for detecting pyelonephritis and renal scarring. Although rarely used, renal biopsy in acute pyelonephritis may reveal abscess formation with neutrophilic invasion. The area of the infection is wedge shaped, pointing toward the medulla, and the glomeruli are spared. Findings in chronic pyelonephritis include fibrosis, scarring, and reduction of renal tissue, with calyceal clubbing, dilation, and distortion. A voiding cystourethrogram may reveal vesicoureteral reflux, which predisposes to both lower and upper UTIs.

Differential Diagnosis

It can be difficult to differentiate pyelonephritis from cystitis; however, the presence of WBC casts is diagnostic for pyelonephritis. In women, a pelvic examination should be performed to rule out an alternative or additional diagnosis. Hematuria is also often present in lower and upper UTIs, but not in vaginitis or urethritis. Chronic pyelonephritis can sometimes be diagnosed through IVP, DMSA scan, or renal ultrasound, which may identify atrophied kidneys with "clubbing" of the affected calyces. A definitive diagnosis of chronic disease is made by identifying persistent pyuria and positive urine cultures. Sometimes chronic pyelonephritis is diagnosed only via kidney biopsy.

MANAGEMENT

Aggressive therapy is necessary to prevent permanent damage to the kidneys, a potential complication of upper versus lower UTI. Tissue penetration of antibiotics into the renal medulla appears more important than serum or urine drug levels. Oral antibiotics may be prescribed in mild cases of acute pyelonephritis, characterized by the absence of nausea and vomiting or signs of sepsis. Antibiotic choice should consider the local antibiogram and drug-resistance rates for the community and patient population in which the infection was likely acquired. Drugs Commonly Prescribed 44.2 presents the oral agents commonly given for lower UTI and mild to moderate pyelonephritis (not requiring hospitalization or IV therapy).

Hospitalization may be indicated, depending on the patient's ability to maintain adequate fluid intake and to tolerate oral antibiotics, along with the severity of the symptoms and evidence of bacteremia. Hospitalization of patients who are pregnant, vomiting, or dehydrated should be strongly considered. Likewise, the patient's degree of systemic illness (bacteremia or urosepsis), age, history of chronic disease, or nonadherence to therapy

may lead to the assessment that hospitalization is necessary. Ninety-five percent of patients demonstrate a positive therapeutic response to IV antibiotic treatment within 48 hours and may be discharged on appropriate oral medication, once urine culture and antibiotic sensitivity results are available and subsequent antimicrobial therapy may be narrowed in spectrum. Treatment courses should typically last for 7 to 10 days for mild to moderate cases, 14 days for severe cases, or 21 days in particularly slow responders. Ample evidence has demonstrated that once common 6-week regimens lead to increased adverse effects without improved treatment effectiveness. Selection of a regimen should be based on local antibiotic resistance and susceptibility results.

Second-line therapy includes ceftriaxone (Rocephin) 1 g IV daily, as well as other extended-spectrum cephalosporins or penicillins, carbapenems, monobactams (in penicillin allergy), and aminoglycosides (except in pregnant patients) such as gentamicin or tobramycin.

If the patient does not respond adequately within 48 hours, he or she should be reevaluated, the cultures reviewed, and an ultrasound, IVP, or DMSA scan performed. IV antibiotics may need to be administered for up to 7 to 10 days in severe cases. During treatment, the patient must increase fluid intake, and an accurate intake and output record must be maintained for appropriate fluid management. Surgery may be indicated to remove or correct secondary causes of UTI such as urinary obstruction or anatomical abnormalities and neuropathic genitourinary tract lesions. Diagnostic studies requiring the insertion of instruments should be delayed until the urine is sterile or free of bacteria and/or pus, to avoid the complications of bacteremia or septic shock. A urological anatomical evaluation should be performed for all men with pyelonephritis and women with recurrent pyelonephritis to detect any structural abnormalities that may be contributing to or causing the condition.

FOLLOW-UP AND REFERRAL

If undergoing outpatient treatment, the patient should be seen 48 hours later to assess responsiveness to therapy. Similarly, patients in the hospital should be evaluated in 48 hours for response to therapy and consideration of discharge. Follow-up urine cultures are not routinely recommended in asymptomatic patients. However, for those with recurrent pyelonephritis, reculturing at 2, 6, and 12 weeks after antibiotic therapy is initiated that may be done to ensure complete and lasting eradication of infection.

Further treatment decisions are based on clinical findings such as fever, pain, and the culture of causative bacteria. When a diagnosis of chronic pyelonephritis is determined, the patient should be referred to a nephrologist because of the severe damage that can occur to the kidney. As discussed previously, a renal ultrasound, renal colic CT scan, or voiding cystourethrogram may detect structural abnormalities, renal stones, or vesicoureteral reflux—all of which predispose the patient to infection. Patients should also be monitored and treated for other conditions secondary to the pyelonephritis such as hypertension, chronic infection, renal insufficiency, or renal failure.

Patient Education: Upper Urinary Tract Infections

The focus should be on teaching the patient to prevent recurrence of lower UTI and pyelonephritis by following these instructions:

- Complete the full course of antibiotic therapy even if symptoms subside early on in the course of treatment.
- Prevent or reduce the incidence of lower UTIs by following the guidelines under Patient Education in the previous section.
- Increase fluid intake to eight to ten 8-ounce glasses of water per day.
- Report any recurrence of UTI symptoms immediately.
- Consider taking cranberry supplements (300–400 mg twice daily) or drink cranberry juice because this may decrease the bacteria's ability to adhere to the epithelial cells that line the bladder.
- Control hypertension with medications, dietary regimen, and lifestyle changes, as detailed in Chapter 35.

NEPHROLITHIASIS

Nephrolithiasis is a condition in which stones (renal calculi) originate in the kidney. The stones form from calcium salts (approximately 75% to 85%), struvite (approximately 10% to 15%), uric acid (approximately 7%), and cystine (1% to 2%). These stones often cause acute episodes of urinary tract obstruction, infection, and severe pain in adults.

EPIDEMIOLOGY AND CAUSES

Renal calculi may occur in people aged 20 to 60 years, but the incidence peaks in those aged 20 to 30 years. It affects approximately 2% to 5% of individuals at some point during their lifetime, or about 70 to 210 per 100,000 of the population. Formation of renal calculi is more prevalent in the Southeast, West, and Midwest United States.

The typical patient may report a sedentary lifestyle or occupation that exposes him or her to high environmental temperatures. Calcium oxalate stones occur more often in men, whereas struvite stones are more common in women. Renal stones can occur because of obstruction, urinary stasis, infection, dehydration and urine concentration, increased consumption of calcium or vitamin D, excessive excretion of uric acid, or vitamin A deficiency. Hereditary factors can also predispose the patient to kidney stone formation.

Calcium oxalate and calcium phosphate stones account for 65% to 85% of all cases of renal calculi. These types of stones are found predominantly in men and in individuals whose diet is high in salt, animal fat, animal protein, and oxalate from green leafy vegetables. Interestingly, a low-calcium diet is also a risk factor, as it leads to increased oxaluria because less oxalate is bound to calcium in the gastrointestinal tract. Vasectomy is a risk factor as well, and hypertension doubles the risk of stone formation for reasons that are as yet unclear.

Patients with calcium oxalate or calcium phosphate stones typically do not have hypercalcemia except with certain disorders such as hyperparathyroidism, sarcoidosis, and hyperuricemia, which may lead to hypercalciuria or hyperuricosuria. Loop diuretics such as furosemide (Lasix) also promote calciuria. Similarly, hypocitraturia and hyperoxaluria similarly predispose to calcium stone formation because an increased amount of calcium is available for complexing with oxalate or phosphate within the urinary tract. Inflammatory bowel disease is associated with marked hyperoxaluria. Medullary sponge kidney disease is found in 10% to 30% of persons with calcium stones.

Several other forms of renal calculi have been noted. Struvite stones are found predominantly in women; these stones are associated with UTIs. They occur when the urine is alkaline (pH greater than 7.0) and a urea-splitting organism, such as *Proteus* or *Klebsiella*, is present. Uric acid stones are formed from an increase in uric acid production or ineffective elimination of uric acid, as found in gout. This may result from dietary intake of foods high in uric acid, acidic urinary pH (e.g., type I renal tubular acidosis, significant bicarbonate loss associated with severe diarrhea), regional enteritis, hereditary factors (including a predisposition to gout), or ulcerative colitis. Uric acid stones account for approximately 15% to 20% of all cases of nephrolithiasis. Cystine stones are created because of a rare autosomal recessive disorder called cystinuria. These stones are formed when there is a metabolic error that causes a decrease in tubular reabsorption in the kidney, leading to urinary cystine concentrations greater than 250 mg/L. Cystine stones account for approximately 1% to 3% of all cases of renal stones.

PATHOPHYSIOLOGY

Renal stone formation occurs when normally soluble mineral substances supersaturate the urine and deposit out of solution as crystals, which serve as nuclei for stone-forming substances such as calcium oxalate, calcium phosphate, triple-phosphate struvite (magnesium ammonium phosphate), uric acid, or cystine. Stone formation may also be facilitated by extremes in urinary pH (alkaline or acidic). This crystal combination becomes trapped within the renal system, where it continues to attract other crystals, causing the stone to increase in size.

Stones are typically anchored at the ends of collecting ducts at sites of epithelial injury. The calculi vary in size and composition and typically grow within the renal tubules, calyces, renal pelvis, ureters, or bladder. Large stones are called staghorn calculi if they span more than one of the renal calyces. Although over the span of years their presence in the kidneys may lead to chronic renal failure, unless they fragment and pass through the urinary system, they are generally asymptomatic.

The four major types of stones and their characteristics, causes, etiology, diagnosis, and treatment are listed in Table 44.2. These forms are not mutually exclusive and share certain risk factors. Many patients have renal stones of mixed etiology. Calcium stones are light in color; their crystals characteristically resemble RBCs in shape and size or may be a larger "dumbbell" form. Formation of these stones may be secondary to hypercalcemia or they may be idiopathic. Hyperoxaluria and hyperuricosuria are more associated with calcium oxalate stones, whereas calcium phosphate stones are more associated with primary hyperparathyroidism.

Struvite stones are flat and consist of hexagonally shaped crystals that are radiopaque. They often form secondary to UTI caused by *P. mirabilis*. Staghorn calculi are more likely to be struvite stones. Uric acid stones are radiolucent and red-orange in color, with a teardrop or flat square shape. Formation of these stones may be associated with a hereditary etiology of gout or with idiopathic causes. Uric acid crystals may also serve as a nidus for calcium stone formation. Cystine stone crystals are lemon yellow, hexagonal, and sparkle under light microscopy. Certain medications promote crystalluria and predispose the patient to renal stones, including topiramate,

triamterene, and sulfadiazine. The protease inhibitor indinavir (Crixivan) used to treat HIV-positive patients may actually precipitate within the renal collecting system, causing direct stone formation.

The incidence of recurrence of certain stones is approximately 40% to 50% within 5 years, with an estimated one-third of patients eventually losing a kidney if the condition is untreated or inadequately treated. Complications can occur when the stone obstructs the flow of urine. This can lead to urinary retention, accumulation of uremic wastes, end-stage renal failure, and/or electrolyte imbalances. Stones can also predispose the patient to UTI and hematuria.

CLINICAL PRESENTATION

Subjective

The patient with an acute episode of nephrolithiasis may present with a variety of signs and symptoms, depending on the location, size, and type of stone. Onset is usually sudden with renal colic, which is a type of flank pain that is not relieved by changes in position or other measures. The pain may present with a referral pattern that originates in the flank or kidney area and radiates across the abdomen down into the groin, perineal area, and inner thigh. This colicky pain occasionally progresses to constant pain at a level that can be excruciating and intractable. Other symptoms of renal calculi may include nausea, urinary frequency, vomiting, diaphoresis, dysuria, hematuria, and weakness. The patient may report a history of a recent or chronic UTI, previous diagnosis with nephrolithiasis, a dietary history consistent with stone formation, or alterations in voiding patterns.

TABLE 44.2 Renal Calculi			
Type of Stone (Percentage of all Stones)	**Characteristics**	**Causes**	**Management**
Calcium (75%–80%)	Resemble RBCs in shape and size or large dumbbell form Light color	Idiopathic, hypercalcemia, or increased levels of uric acid	Thiazide diuretics Diet Cholestyramine Surgery
Struvite (15%)	Flat, hexagonal shape Radiopaque	Alkaline urine, infection with urea-splitting organisms such as *Pseudomonas*	Antibiotic therapy Surgery
Uric acid (7%)	Teardrop-shaped or flat square plates Red-orange color	Increased uric acid production, high intake of uric acid, acidic urine, regional enteritis, ulcerative colitis, or idiopathic	Allopurinol Fluid replacement Diet Surgery
Cystine (<1%)	Lemon yellow, sparkling	Hereditary (autosomal recessive cystinuria)	Force fluids D-Penicillamine Tiopronin

Objective

The patient may present with abdominal distention and guarding on palpation, flank tenderness on percussion, and decreased or absent bowel sounds on auscultation. Fever may be present if there is acute infection related to obstruction. Blood pressure (as well as pulse rate and respiratory rate) may be elevated because of pain.

DIAGNOSTIC REASONING

Diagnostic Tests

The diagnostic work-up should begin with a routine urinalysis, complete blood count, and blood chemistry profile. Urinalysis may be normal or it may show RBCs, WBCs, crystals, mineral casts, bacteria, pus, and an alkaline or acidic pH. Table 44.3 identifies the tests and expected results that would lead to the suspicion of renal calculi. Either gross or microscopic hematuria is observed in the majority of cases but may be absent in up to 30% of cases, depending on the time of presentation. Identification of the type of stone formation is important for the appropriate treatment to be instituted. The results of these tests should lead the clinician to continue the diagnostic work-up with noninvasive tests to identify obstructions, masses, or anatomical abnormalities.

TABLE 44.3 Tests for Renal Calculi

Test	Rationale
Urinalysis	Shows RBCs, WBCs, crystals, casts, minerals, bacteria, pus, abnormal pH
24-hour urine	May show increased levels of creatinine, uric acid, calcium, phosphorus, oxalate, or cystine
Serum chemistry	May show increased levels of magnesium, calcium, uric acid, phosphorus, protein, and electrolytes
Serum blood urea nitrogen (BUN) and creatinine	Shows BUN elevated secondary to urinary tract obstruction; creatinine elevated secondary to damage to the kidney
Complete blood count	May show infection or septicemia
Kidney and upper bladder ultrasound	Shows calculi and/or anatomical changes
Intravenous pyelogram	Shows calculi and any abnormality in anatomic structures
Cystourethroscopy	May show calculi and/or abnormal structural defects
Computed tomography scan	Identifies calculi and other masses in the renal system

These further diagnostic tests may include x-ray studies of the kidney, ureters, and bladder, abdominal or transvaginal ultrasonography (used for pregnant women and those of childbearing age in whom radiation must be avoided), or noncontrast helical computed tomography scan (IV contrast dye is avoided due to potential renal toxicity). Invasive procedures may be necessary to visualize or assist in removing the stone through IVP, cystourethroscopy, or other surgical procedures.

Differential Diagnosis

The differential diagnosis for renal calculi includes a variety of diseases, including appendicitis, diverticulitis, mesenteric adenitis, pancreatitis, ileus, peptic ulcer disease, abnormalities of the fallopian tubes and ovaries including ovarian cysts, ectopic pregnancy, gallbladder disease, and abdominal aneurysms. A tentative diagnosis of renal calculi is made from the history and findings on physical examination showing increased intensity of renal colic with flank pain or a pattern of referred pain coupled with flank tenderness. Because hematuria may be the only presenting sign of stone formation, malignancy (renal cell carcinoma), which is typically painless, must also be considered. The diagnosis of renal stones is confirmed by urinalysis that is positive for blood and visualization of the renal system by radiography or ultrasound.

MANAGEMENT

Treatment goals are to decrease the symptoms and complications arising from existing renal stones and to prevent subsequent recurrence. It is important, therefore, to decrease the concentration of stone-forming substances in the urine. An intake of six to eight 8-ounce glasses of water a day is essential, unless prevented by cardiac complications, such as CHF. This high fluid intake must continue indefinitely. Most stones smaller than 5 mm pass spontaneously. Rates of spontaneous passage steadily decrease for stones larger than this, and spontaneous passage is highly unlikely for renal stones larger than 10 mm.

Initially, pain management is the priority. Oral NSAIDs in dosages of 600 to 800 mg three times daily or oral narcotics such as hydrocodone-acetaminophen (Vicodin, Lortab), acetaminophen-codeine (Tylenol #3), or oxycodone-acetaminophen (Percocet) are often necessary. In some cases, intramuscular or IV narcotic analgesics may be necessary, but most studies have demonstrated that NSAIDs are as effective as oral opiates, although they are slower acting. In addition, they have also been shown to relax ureteral smooth muscle, which may facilitate stone passage. Antispasmodics such as flavoxate or oxybutynin may also provide temporary relief, but the anticholinergic effects of these medications must be taken into account because they may lead to urinary retention. Warm compresses to the lower back, focused breathing, imagery, and diversional activities may provide minimal relief.

Certain drugs help to reduce urinary excretion of stone-forming substances. Thiazide diuretics (e.g., hydrochlorothiazide) reduce calcium excretion; allopurinol reduces uric acid production by inhibiting xanthine oxidase; and D-penicillamine affects the excretion of cystine. Importantly, loop diuretics such as furosemide (Lasix) and triamterene increase calciuria and typically worsen renal stone formation.

Noninvasive or invasive surgical interventions may be necessary if the stone does not pass spontaneously; these are presented in Table 44.4. Noninvasive procedures to treat renal calculi are aggressive and carry many of the same risks as surgery. Extracorporeal shock-wave lithotripsy (ESWL) is the least invasive technique, sending shock waves throughout the outside of the body to disrupt proximal and midurethral calculi and is preferred for stones smaller than 10 mm. NSAIDs should be avoided at least 3 days before this therapy to minimize the risk of bleeding. The percutaneous ultrasonic lithotriptor applies therapeutic ultrasound waves to the outside of the body to achieve the same results. A lithotriptic agent may also be used to dissolve the renal calculus.

Invasive procedures may be necessary to remove the stone because of its location or the failure of noninvasive procedures to destroy the stone. The procedure chosen is dependent on the location, size, and type of stone (e.g., struvite stones typically require ESWL or surgical intervention). First and second generation lithotripters originally visualized stones via fluoroscopy or ultrasonography. However, advances in urethroscopy with flexible fiber-optic systems now allow for the direct visualization of stones virtually anywhere along the urinary tract from the urethra to the renal pelvis. Stones may be crushed via electrohydraulic or laser lithotripsy in conjunction with these visualization techniques. Flexible ureteroscopy combined with laser lithotripsy is now the preferred treatment for proximal ureteral stones larger than 10 mm. The patient is then able to eliminate the stones naturally after they are crushed into smaller pieces.

Lithotomy is an incision into the bladder or ureter to remove calculi or to place a ureteral stent, whereas *lithotony* specifically denotes arthroscopic extraction of a renal stone from the bladder. Ureteral stents may be placed within the ureters to facilitate the passage of stones through natural elimination. *Lithonephrotomy* is an incision into the kidney to remove a stone.

Preventive measures should be taken to reduce the incidence of recurrence. The incidence of calcium-based stones may be reduced by increasing fluid intake (greater than 2 L/day) and taking thiazide diuretics or allopurinol. In addition, an acidic diet higher in meat content promotes calcium excretion. Hypocitraturia and hyperuricosuria may both be treated with potassium citrate supplementation. However, this may alkalinize the urine, creating another risk factor for stone formation, and care must be taken to stop this drug if urine pH is greater than 6.0. In similar fashion, appropriate treatment of UTI must be initiated to avoid recurrence of struvite stones, and the urease inhibitor acetohydroxamic acid (Lithostat) 250 mg orally three to four times daily may be given as adjunctive therapy to prevent urinary alkalinization, if infection with urease-producing organisms is confirmed.

Oxalate-containing stones may be prevented with a low-oxalate diet (see Patient Education: Nephrolithiasis). Struvite stone production may be decreased by preventing UTIs through patient education and self-care as previously discussed, maintenance of antibiotic therapy, or acidifying the urine with methenamine mandelate. Uric acid stones may be decreased through diet modification

TABLE 44.4 Surgical and Other Procedures for Renal Calculi Management			
Procedure	*Type of Procedure*	*Location of Calculi*	*Description*
Lithotripsy	Invasive	Bladder or urethra	Crushing of the calculi under direct visualization using a lithotriptoscope
Lithotony	Invasive	Renal system	Arthroscopic removal of the calculi
Lithonephrotomy	Invasive	Kidney	Incision of the kidney to remove the calculi
Lithotomy	Invasive	Bladder or urethra	Incision of the bladder or ureter to remove the calculi
Ureteral stent	Invasive	Kidney or ureter	Stent is placed in front of the calculi to facilitate elimination
Lithotrophic	Noninvasive	Renal system	Agent used to dissolve calculi
Percutaneous ultrasonic lithotriptor	Noninvasive	Renal system	Ultrasound waves are applied to the outside of the body to crush the calculi
Extracorporeal shock-wave lithotripsy	Noninvasive	Renal system	Shock waves are applied to the outside of the body to crush the calculi

(see Patient Education) or medications that facilitate uric acid excretion, such as allopurinol. Recurrence of cystine stones may be reduced through maintenance doses of D-penicillamine, tiopronin, or captopril, which binds cystine via sulfhydryl moieties.

FOLLOW-UP AND REFERRAL

Most patients with renal calculi are treated and followed on an outpatient basis. The patient may need hospitalization for secondary complications that can occur, such as severe nausea and vomiting leading to dehydration, urinary obstruction, decreased renal function, severe bleeding, intractable pain, and significant infection. The patient should be referred to a urologist and/or nephrologist for stone removal under these circumstances or if stone formation is thought to be secondary to a metabolic abnormality.

Patient Education: Nephrolithiasis

The patient should be instructed to increase fluid intake to six to eight 8-ounce glasses per day unless contraindicated (e.g., presence of cardiac complications, such as congestive heart failure). Increasing fluids will assist in the elimination of the stones. The patient should monitor intake and output and strain the urine for passed stones. Over-the-counter drugs that contain phosphorus or calcium, such as many antacids (e.g., Tums), and most vitamin supplements, especially vitamin D_3, should be avoided. The role of vitamin C supplementation is controversial. Although some research suggests that high-dose vitamin C supplementation helps to acidify the urine and facilitates stone dissolution (especially the calcium phosphate type), excess vitamin C (1 g/day) is known to undergo chemical conversion to oxalate, which may promote oxaluria and calcium oxalate stone formation. In contrast, vitamin B_6 and magnesium are both known to decrease oxaluria by facilitating oxalate metabolism. Magnesium further competes with calcium, reducing calcium-containing stone formation. In turn, supplementation of vitamin B_6 and magnesium has been shown to reduce the incidence of oxalate stones, although the ideal doses have not been established.

The patient should be encouraged to increase his or her activity level as tolerated because inactivity contributes to stone formation secondary to calcium shifts and urinary stasis. Dietary modification is also important. In general, caffeine, beer, and wine should be avoided. A low-oxalate diet is recommended to prevent calcium oxalate stones, in which oxalate-rich foods including beets, black tea, chocolate and cocoa, lamb, nuts, rhubarb, and spinach are excluded. A low-phosphorus diet for calcium phosphate or struvite stones should eliminate milk products and cola drinks. A low-purine diet is often effective in reducing stones formed from excess uric acid.

This diet limits the intake of purine-rich foods, such as organ meats, red meats, seafood (especially sardines, anchovies, and scallops), poultry, legumes, whole grains, and alcohol (which decreases uric acid clearance).

REFERENCES

Nephrolithiasis

National Kidney and Urologic Diseases Information Clearinghouse. Kidney and urologic diseases statistics for the United States. http://kidney.niddk.nih.gov/kudiseases/pubs/kustats/#urologic. Updated December 2016. Accessed September 9, 2017.

Urinary Incontinence

Amundsen CL, Richter HE, Menefee SA, et al. OnabotulinumtoxinA vs sacral neuromodulation on refractory urgency urinary incontinence in women: A randomized clinical trial. *JAMA.* 2016;316(13):1366–1374.

Coyne KS, Wein A, Nicholson S, Kvasz M, Chen CI, Milsom I. Economic burden of urgency urinary incontinence in the United States: A systematic review. *J Manag Care Pharm.* 2014;20(2): 130–140.

Dumoulin C, Hunter KF, Moore K, et al. Conservative management for female urinary incontinence and pelvic organ prolapse review 2013: Summary of the 5th International Consultation on Incontinence. *Neurourol Urodyn.* 2016;35(1):15–20.

Hsieh P, Chiu H, Chen K, Chang C, Chou E. Botulinum toxin A for the treatment of overactive bladder. *Toxins.* 2016;8(3). https://www.ncbi.nlm.nih.gov/pmc/articles/PMC4810204/. Accessed October 8, 2017.

Sukhu T, Kennelly MJ, Kurpad R. Sacral neuromodulation in overactive bladder: A review and current perspectives. *Res Rep Urol.* 2016;8:193–199.

Urinary Tract Infections

Fulop T. Acute pyelonephritis medication. http://emedicine.medscape.com/article/245559-medication#2. Published 2016. Accessed August 10, 2017.

Kazemier BM, Koningstein FN, Schneeberger C, et al. Maternal and neonatal consequences of treated and untreated asymptomatic bacteriuria in pregnancy: A prospective cohort study with an embedded randomised controlled trial. *Lancet Infect Dis.* 2015;15(11):1324–1333.

Nicolle LE. Management of asymptomatic bacteriuria in pregnant women. *Lancet Infect Dis.* 2015;15(11):1252–1254.

RESOURCES

American Urogynecologic Society (AUGS)
https://www.augs.org/
National Association for Continence
www.nafc.org
National Institutes of Diabetes and Digestive and Kidney Diseases (NIDDK)
https://www.niddk.nih.gov/

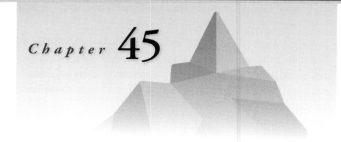

Chapter 45

Kidney and Bladder Disorders

Debbie Nogueras Conner, PhD, ANP/FNP-BC, FAANP
Debera J. Thomas, DNS, RN, FNP/ANP
Brian Oscar Porter, MD, PhD, MPH, MBA

ACUTE KIDNEY INJURY

Acute kidney injury (AKI), also known as *acute renal failure*, is the sudden and rapid deterioration of renal function resulting in an inability to maintain acid-base, fluid, and electrolyte balance and the accumulation of nitrogenous wastes. AKI now has a universal definition and staging system to allow for earlier detection and the management of disease. AKI is defined when one of the following criteria is met: serum creatinine rises to 26 mol/L or more within 48 hours or 1.5-fold or greater from the reference value, which is known or presumed to have occurred within 1 week, or urine output is less than 0.5 mL/kg/h for more than 6 consecutive hours. The reference serum creatinine should be the lowest creatinine value recorded within 3 months of the event.

AKI is commonly caused by intrarenal injury associated with renal hypoperfusion or nephrotoxins. The signs and symptoms vary with each patient and are most often attributed to uremia or its underlying cause. Persons with AKI usually do not experience the profound neurologic and musculoskeletal disorders seen in patients with chronic renal failure (CRF). Although recovery from AKI may be rapid and complete, this disorder nonetheless has a high, albeit wide-ranging, mortality rate, estimated at anywhere between 5% and 80%, depending on the patient's age, the cause of AKI, and the extent of multiorgan involvement.

EPIDEMIOLOGY AND CAUSES

It is estimated that 1% of patients admitted to hospitals have AKI at the time of admission. Between 2% and 5% of all hospitalized patients develop AKI; for patients in intensive care units, the rate is as high as 15%. Two percent to 7% of all open-heart surgery patients are estimated to develop AKI postoperatively. Fifty percent of AKI that develops in hospitalized patients is considered iatrogenic. AKI affects all ages and both sexes equally.

A major risk factor for AKI is surgery, especially for older patients or patients of any age with elevated creatinine levels. Community-based AKI occurs more frequently among vulnerable populations such as individuals with underlying renal disease, multiple myeloma, or diabetes mellitus. AKI is also one of the potential risks related to open-heart surgery and other cardiac procedures (e.g., cardiac catheterization) and use of IV contrast dyes. Any problem that causes decreased blood flow to the kidneys can lead to AKI: anaphylactic shock caused by drug or transfusion reactions, ingestion of nephrotoxic substances (aminoglycosides, angiotensin-converting enzyme [ACE] inhibitors in renal artery stenosis), malignancy, sepsis, cardiac problems, aneurysm, liver cirrhosis, trauma, dehydration, or shock.

AKI is classified into three major groups based on the anatomical nature of the lesion: prerenal azotemia, intrarenal azotemia, or postrenal azotemia. *Prerenal azotemia* is any condition that leads to an overall decrease in renal perfusion; etiologies in this group include hypovolemia, renovascular disease, decreased cardiac output, systemic vasodilation, renal vasoconstriction, and impairment of renal autoregulation of blood flow, which is often associated with drugs such as ACE inhibitors or NSAIDs. *Intrarenal* azotemia refers to disorders that affect the renal parenchyma itself, such as glomerulonephritis, acute tubular necrosis (ATN) (often caused by ischemic insult or nephrotoxic drugs such as aminoglycosides), interstitial nephritis (often an allergic reaction to various drugs or transfusion reactions), and tubular obstruction. Immune-mediated phenomena may lead to AKI following acute bacterial infection, for example, thrombotic thrombocytopenic purpura (TTP) or hemolytic uremic syndrome (HUS) following *Escherichia coli* gastroenteritis. *Postrenal* azotemia refers to any etiology that might lead to an obstruction of urine flow from the kidneys, including ureteral obstruction, bladder neck obstruction, or urethral obstruction. Major causes include benign prostatic hyperplasia/hypertrophy (BPH), prostate or bladder cancer, and metastatic disease affecting the urinary tract. An important consideration in the male patient with preexisting BPH is the use of over-the-counter sympathomimetic decongestants and other cold remedies with alpha-agonist properties, which may lead to acute worsening of prostatic hypertrophy with resultant anuria.

Box 45.1 presents the major causes of AKI. *Prerenal, intrarenal,* and *postrenal* mechanisms of AKI are not mutually exclusive; however, many patients present with a combination of these pathologies. Complications commonly seen as a result of AKI include intravascular volume overload, metabolic acidosis, anemia, hyperkalemia, and uremic syndrome, which is characterized by nausea, vomiting, anorexia, pericarditis, and central and peripheral nervous system abnormalities, including altered mental status, seizures, or coma.

Box 45.1 Major Causes of Acute Kidney Injury

Prerenal Acute Kidney Injury

- Fluid and electrolyte depletion
- Hemorrhage
- Septicemia
- Cardiac failure
- Liver failure
- Heat stroke
- Burns

Intrarenal Acute Kidney Injury

- Ischemia
- Toxins
- Radiocontrast agents
- Hemoglobinuria
- Myoglobinuria

- Acute glomerulonephritis
- Arterial or venous obstruction
- Tubulointerstitial nephritis
- Pyelonephritis
- Papillary necrosis
- Precipitation from hypercalcemia
- Urates
- Myeloma protein

Postrenal Acute Kidney Injury

- Prostatism (hypertrophy or malignancy)
- Bladder tumor
- Pelvic tumor
- Retroperitoneal tumor
- Renal calculi

PATHOPHYSIOLOGY

Prerenal Azotemia

Prerenal azotemia is caused by decreased blood flow to the kidneys, usually associated with poor systemic perfusion. Etiologies includes hypovolemia; altered peripheral vascular resistance; diminished cardiac output; congestive heart failure; renal artery disorders such as vasculitis and, to a lesser extent, thromboembolic disease. Chronic liver diseases, such as cirrhosis and the hepatorenal syndrome, are also recognized causes of prerenal azotemia.

The kidney's compensatory responses to hypoperfusion are autoregulation and activation of the renin-angiotensin-aldosterone axis via the release of renin. In response to renal tissue damage, these mechanisms attempt to shunt blood to undamaged nephrons in a process called adaptive hyperfiltration. Autoregulation depends on the body's ability to control afferent arteriole dilation and efferent arteriole constriction in order to maintain normal glomerular filtration rate (GFR) and creatinine clearance.

The release of renin activates the conversion of proenzyme angiotensinogen to the biologically inactive angiotensin I. In turn, ACE converts angiotensin I into angiotensin II, one of the most potent vasoconstricting agents in the body. Its production results in peripheral vasoconstriction and increased sodium reabsorption via increased aldosterone production. Antidiuretic hormone (ADH) is released in response to the increased plasma sodium concentration. ADH further enhances vasoconstriction and increases water reabsorption, thereby decreasing urinary output and increasing blood volume.

These mechanisms attempt to maintain systemic and renal perfusion. However, if the adaptive mechanisms of the kidneys fail, AKI develops because of hypoperfusion. As a result, glomerular filtration and the excretion of urea decrease, along with increased sodium and water reabsorption, resulting in an overall increase in blood urea nitrogen (BUN). Thus, although adaptive hyperfiltration is initially beneficial, allowing normal serum creatinine to be maintained in the face of mild renal insufficiency, prolonged activation of this compensatory mechanism leads to progressive renal failure.

Intrarenal (Parenchymal) Azotemia

Intrarenal azotemia results from injury to renal tissue; it is usually associated with intrarenal ischemia, toxins, or both. Accounting for up to 50% of all cases, intrinsic dysfunction is considered after prerenal and postrenal causes have been excluded. The sites of injury are the glomeruli, vasculature, interstitium, and tubules.

ATN is the most common cause of intrarenal azotemia and AKI in general. In ischemic ATN, the ischemic event is prolonged hypoperfusion and ischemia of the kidneys, with a sustained mean arterial pressure (MAP) in adults of less than 75 mm Hg. When renal autoregulation fails, the sympathetic nervous system (SNS) responds by initiating the renin-angiotensin system as the kidney attempts to redirect blood flow to the remaining healthy nephrons (adaptive hyperfiltration, as explained in the preceding paragraph). Again, however, this initial compensatory mechanism can eventually lead to progressive renal failure, because the SNS response and possible endothelin production may lead to severe afferent renal arteriole constriction. As a result, overall glomerular hydrostatic pressure, glomerular blood flow, and GFR are decreased.

The duration of the ischemic episode determines the amount and degree of renal cellular damage, which may continue after MAP and renal reperfusion are restored. Studies in animal models have demonstrated that a number of immunological mechanisms contribute to renal tubular injury. These include early complement activation, intracellular adhesion molecule–1 expression (which may promote neutrophilic damage to the endothelium), T-cell–mediated cytotoxicity, macrophage activation, and proinflammatory cytokine expression (e.g., tumor necrosis factor–α, interleukin [IL]-6, IL-7, chemokines).

Renal blood flow can be reduced by 50% after an ischemic episode; this is termed the *no-reflow phenomenon*. The kidneys are unable to synthesize vasodilating prostaglandins, which usually exacerbates the ischemic injury. Blood flow is redistributed from the cortex to the medulla as a result of SNS stimulation and angiotensin II production. This further decreases glomerular capillary flow and worsens tubular ischemia because these structures are located primarily in the cortex.

With renal ischemia, the availability of nutrients and oxygen for basic cellular metabolism and the tubular transport system is diminished. There is a significant decrease in the production of adenosine triphosphate (ATP) by the mitochondria, and, with insufficient oxygen and ATP, metabolism shifts from aerobic to anaerobic. This shift corresponds with extracellular and intracellular acidosis that alters kidney function. Ischemia also causes a decrease in renal cellular potassium, magnesium, and inorganic phosphate and an increase in intracellular sodium, chloride, calcium, and reactive oxygen species. Sodium and calcium (Ca) exchange is abnormal because of low ATP, altered Ca-ATPase activity, and increased intracellular sodium. This results in an increase in intracellular calcium, which seems to increase cell injury. The formation of free radical reactive oxygen species further exacerbates cellular damage and apoptosis (programmed cell death) during reperfusion after a prolonged renal ischemic event, an event termed *reperfusion injury*.

The glomerular basement membrane is altered by tubular cellular edema and becomes necrotic because of prolonged tubular ischemia. Tubular obstruction occurs from sloughed necrotic cells and renal cast formation, which seem to be facilitated by a translocation of basement membrane cellular adhesion proteins called integrins to the luminal membrane. Tubular hydrostatic pressure and Bowman's capsule hydrostatic pressure (which opposes glomerular hydrostatic pressure) increase as a result of tubular obstruction. This decreases GFR. Injury to the basement membrane increases tubular permeability, allowing tubular filtrate to leak back into the interstitium and peritubular capillaries, further decreasing tubular filtration.

Ischemic ATN is usually associated with oliguria (urine production of less than 500 mL/day in adults) because of extensive nephronal injury. Other clinical indications of ATN include decreased urea excretion and elevated BUN, decreased creatinine clearance and elevated serum creatinine, abnormal renal handling of sodium, and an inability to concentrate urine. Urinary osmolality may approximate plasma osmolality of 300 to 350 mOsm/L, a condition called *isosthenuria*.

Toxic ATN involves exposure to toxic by-products of microorganisms or to nephrotoxic agents. Renal toxic drugs often cause allergic interstitial nephritis, characterized by eosinophilic damage. Toxic ATN begins with an event that causes injury to tubular cells. Subsequent pathophysiology is similar to that of ischemic ATN because there is tubular cell necrosis, cast formation, tubular obstruction, and altered GFR. Unlike in ischemic ATN, however, the basement membrane is usually intact and the injured necrotic areas are more localized. Other differences include improved urine production, in that nonoliguria occurs more often with toxic ATN than with ischemic ATN, as well as the extent of injury with toxic ATN, which may be less than with ischemic ATN. The healing process, therefore, can be more rapid in patients with toxic ATN.

There are several reasons why the kidney is susceptible to toxic damage. Blood continuously circulates through the kidney, repeatedly exposing the tissues to all substances carried by the blood. Also, the kidney is the major excretory organ for toxic substances, and, as these substances await transport within renal cells, they disrupt cellular function. If liver disease is present, substances that are usually detoxified by the liver can overload the kidney. The kidney also transforms many substances into metabolites that can be toxic to the kidney, and the countercurrent mechanism concentrates metabolic and urinary waste by-products and other substances that, in increased concentrations, can be toxic to the kidney.

Postrenal Azotemia

Bilateral (ureteral) or distal (bladder outlet or urethral) postrenal obstruction impedes urine flow and results in oliguria or frank anuria. Urine congestion increases pressure retrograde through the urinary collecting system and the nephrons, slowing the tubular fluid flow rate and GFR. Increased reabsorption of sodium, water, and urea results in decreased urine sodium, increased urine osmolality, and increased BUN. The decreased GFR results in decreased creatinine clearance and, therefore, in an increased serum creatinine level. If postrenal obstruction is prolonged, the collecting system dilates and compresses parenchymal tissue. Nephrons are injured, which results in dysfunction of the urinary concentrating and diluting mechanism, increasing urine osmolality and urinary sodium level to approximate those of plasma. In contrast, if postrenal obstruction is temporary, there is little dilation of the collecting system or loss of renal tissue.

CLINICAL PRESENTATION

Subjective

Symptoms of AKI are not usually present until the GFR falls to approximately 10% to 15% of normal. The most common symptoms, which are secondary to the accumulation of toxic metabolites such as urea, are fatigue, malaise, nausea, vomiting, pruritus, and mental status changes. Of note, the development of uremic syndrome symptoms bears no direct correlation to the increases in BUN or serum creatinine, despite the critical role of hemodialysis in clearing the body of both identified and unidentified uremic toxins. Oliguria or even anuria may also be a presenting symptom of AKI but is not present in every case, as urine output depends largely on the stage of AKI and the precipitating cause. In some cases, fluid overload may be present, resulting in dyspnea and orthopnea.

A detailed history can give clues as to the etiology of AKI. The patient should be questioned about any history of illicit or prescription drug use, herbal preparations, surgery, trauma, or infection as possible sources of renal insult. However, the actual diagnosis of AKI is often made by routine laboratory assessment.

There are multiple signs and symptoms of AKI and four identified stages: initiating, oliguric, diuretic, and recovery. The *initiating stage* begins when the kidney is injured; this stage is variable in length, from minutes to several days (e.g., renal damage caused by contrast dye may occur within 2 minutes). Decreased urine volume and other signs and symptoms of renal impairment may then become evident. These may include anorexia, lethargy, nausea, headache, muscle cramps, and fatigue. If AKI is recognized at this stage, its cause should be determined and the plan of treatment should be established in consultation with a nephrologist.

The *oliguric stage* usually lasts from 5 to 15 days but can persist for weeks, depending on the nature of renal damage. Renal repair begins as tubular cells regenerate. The destroyed basement membrane is replaced with fibrous scar tissue, and nephrons become obstructed with a build-up of inflammatory products. Decreases in glomerular filtration, tubular transport of substances, urine formation, and renal clearance occur. When AKI persists for weeks or longer, renal endocrine functions, such as the secretion of erythropoietin, are altered. The longer this stage persists, the poorer the prognosis.

The next phase is the *diuretic stage*, defined as beginning when urine output increases to greater than 400 mL per day and BUN begins to fall. This stage is considered to last until the BUN level stabilizes or is in the normal range and may take from 1 to 2 weeks.

The fourth and final stage of AKI, referred to as the *recovery phase*, extends from the time BUN stabilizes and urine output returns to normal to the day the patient returns to normal activity. This recovery process may take up to 10 months or more, and some patients never recover but instead progress to CRF.

Objective

The objective manifestations of AKI depend on the stage of the disorder and may be extremely variable; however,

these signs can provide an assessment of the degree of renal failure and provide clues as to the underlying etiology. Orthostatic vital signs, skin turgor, and distention of jugular veins should be assessed to obtain information about the patient's fluid balance. Signs of fluid depletion can point to a prerenal etiology, whereas signs of fluid overload suggest a greater degree of renal impairment. Severe proteinuria from renal losses may lead to generalized edema (anasarca) due to the lack of intravascular oncotic pressure from hypoalbuminemia. Abdominal bruits can suggest renovascular disease. In cases of polycystic kidney disease or hydronephrosis, the kidneys may be palpable. A pelvic or renal examination may reveal causes of outflow obstruction such as an enlarged prostate or pelvic mass.

DIAGNOSTIC REASONING

Diagnostic Tests

Elevated BUN and serum creatinine levels assist in establishing the diagnosis of AKI. GFR is difficult to measure directly and is most commonly estimated using a simplified formula for creatinine clearance (see the Diagnostic Tests section under Chronic Renal Failure for a complete discussion). However, because acute trends are most important in the diagnosis and follow-up of AKI, direct serum creatinine levels are often used as an estimate of renal function. It is important to note that these absolute values are heavily influenced by a patient's muscle mass, age, and sex, as well as the presence of any underlying renal disease. Thus, serum creatinine levels may overestimate or underestimate renal function in certain populations (e.g., elderly or obese patients).

Serum electrolyte levels (sodium, potassium, chloride, bicarbonate, calcium, phosphate) should be monitored for potentially life-threatening abnormalities that may develop secondary to impaired renal function. The presence of red blood cells (RBCs), either intact or as cellular casts, may suggest a vascular or glomerular lesion, whereas white blood cells (WBCs) and WBC casts are seen in cases associated with infection and interstitial nephritis. Eosinophiluria, in particular, is characteristic of allergic interstitial nephritis due to renal toxic drugs. "Muddy-brown" granular casts and epithelial cell casts are strongly associated with ATN but are not considered specific. Moreover, their absence does not exclude intrinsic renal disease.

Urinary sodium tends to be less than 20 mEq/L in prerenal disease, whereas in ATN, the kidneys "leak" or "spill" sodium due to failure to reabsorb this electrolyte. This results in urinary sodium values typically greater than 40 mEq/L. However, variations in water reabsorption also affect urinary sodium concentration. Thus, the fractional excretion of sodium (FENa) is easily calculated as the urinary clearance of sodium divided by the GFR, using the following simplified formula:

$$FENa = 100\% \times \frac{\text{Sodium (urinary)} \times \text{creatinine (plasma)}}{\text{Sodium (plasma)} \times \text{creatinine (urinary)}}$$

The FENa is helpful in distinguishing prerenal azotemia from ATN. The FENa is generally less than 1% in prerenal disease related to hypoperfusion because the kidneys try to preserve intravascular volume by maximally conserving sodium. A FENa of greater than 2% reflects ATN, as the kidney loses its ability to resorb sodium effectively, but values between 1% and 2% are considered inconclusive. Of note, FENa has little or no predictive value in the presence of diuretic therapy, because natriuresis is a mechanistic outcome of both thiazide and loop diuretics. Thus, increased urinary sodium may not exclude a prerenal etiology or implicate ATN. In addition, FENa is less helpful when ATN is superimposed on a chronic intravascularly depleted state, such as in hypoalbuminemic cirrhotic liver disease.

ATN is also characterized by the inability to concentrate urine; in turn, urine osmolality is typically lower than 450 mOsm/L and in many cases, it can be lower than 350 mOsm/L. In contrast, the urine is highly concentrated in prerenal azotemia due to the secretion of ADH and intensified water reabsorption, producing urine osmolalities of greater than 500 mOsm/L. As renal tubular function worsens under prerenal conditions, however, this distinction tends to blur, and concentrating ability may wane as ischemic damage sets in.

If a glomerular process is suspected, measurement of antinuclear antibodies, antineutrophil cytoplasmic antibodies (ANCA, as seen in Wegener's granulomatosis), antiglomerular basement membrane (anti-GBM) antibodies, complement levels, and cryoglobulins can help the clinician determine whether immune-mediated disease is present.

A 24-hour urine collection is the most accurate way to measure proteinuria. A protein loss of more than 3.0 to 3.5 g every 24 hours indicates a glomerular lesion, whereas lesser amounts in the urine are more indicative of an interstitial disorder. Given the unwieldy nature of this test, however, and its practical challenges in the outpatient (home-based) setting, spot-urine checks for proteinuria are often used as a surrogate.

Renal ultrasound is commonly used to assess kidney size and rule out hydronephrosis. Ultrasound is used instead of an intravenous pyelogram (IVP) to avoid the risk of radiocontrast nephrotoxicity. If hydronephrosis indicative of renal obstruction is detected, the patient should be referred to a urologist. Computed tomography (CT) scan, a retrograde pyelogram, and cystoscopy may all be useful in determining the exact location of the obstruction. A nuclear renal scan may be helpful in detecting unilateral renal artery stenosis but is less sensitive in detecting bilateral renal artery disease. Renal artery stenosis is better diagnosed via CT scan or magnetic resonance imaging/magnetic resonance angiography (MRI/MRA), although direct renal angiography is still considered the (albeit invasive) gold standard for diagnosis.

If a noninvasive work-up proves inconclusive, renal biopsy may be indicated in some cases. Most notably, biopsy is performed in cases of isolated glomerular hematuria with proteinuria to confirm acute nephritic syndrome, to better characterize nephrotic syndrome or suspected vasculitis, and to aid in the diagnosis of acute or subacute renal failure of unknown etiology. Percutaneous versus open biopsy techniques are chosen based on the propensity for bleeding diatheses and the difficulty in reaching the affected kidney as determined by renal imaging.

Differential Diagnosis

The main diagnostic challenge in AKI is to determine the underlying cause. This is often complicated by fluid and electrolyte alterations. Assessment of the patient involves a thorough history, physical examination, and appropriate laboratory studies. When determining whether or not prerenal azotemia exists, the patient's history can provide information reflecting episodes of poor renal and/or systemic perfusion. This may include surgery, high fever, alterations in diet or fluid status (such as a patient receiving nothing by mouth and undergoing bowel preparation repeatedly for diagnostic tests), a low-sodium diet with fluid restriction, use of diuretics and antihypertensives, anaphylactic drug or transfusion reactions, penetrating or nonpenetrating abdominal trauma, hemorrhage, burns, shock, excessive sweating and dehydration, peritonitis, malignancies, sepsis, neurogenic shock, drug overdose, acute myocardial infarction, congestive heart failure, cardiac tamponade, cardiac dysrhythmias, cardiac arrest survival, renal artery emboli, thrombi, stenosis, aneurysm, occlusion, trauma, and liver cirrhosis.

Physical assessment findings may vary depending on the etiology of AKI and should be correlated with the patient's history and laboratory findings, such as fluid volume depletion or oliguria. Findings on physical examination consistent with a prerenal etiology may include dry mucous membranes, poor skin turgor, reduced jugular venous pressure, hypotension, oliguria, or weight loss. Significant laboratory findings in prerenal AKI include increased urine osmolality and specific gravity, decreased urine sodium and urea concentration, increased BUN, increased BUN to plasma creatinine ratio (especially a ratio greater than 20:1, because plasma creatinine is usually normal), a normal urinary sediment (seen in most cases), and oliguria. In turn, prolonged azotemia caused by a prerenal condition often leads to intrarenal failure.

Nephrotoxic agents that can cause damage to the kidneys include certain drugs (e.g., antineoplastics, anesthetics, antimicrobials, and anti-inflammatory agents), imaging contrast media, biological substances (e.g., metabolic toxins, tumor products, and heme pigments from hemoglobin or myoglobin), environmental agents (e.g., pesticides and organic solvents), heavy metals (e.g., lead, mercury, and gold), and certain plant and animal substances (e.g., toxic mushrooms and snake venoms).

Other conditions that may injure renal (parenchymal) tissue include inflammatory processes related to bacterial or viral infections; preeclampsia; immune processes such as autoimmunity, hypersensitivity, and tissue or organ transplant rejection; trauma or radiation to the kidney; and urinary tract obstruction (e.g., caused by neoplasm, stones, or scar tissue). Intravascular hemolysis related to blood transfusion reactions or microangiopathic hemolytic anemia as seen in TTP and HUS also causes damage to renal tissue. In addition, systemic and vascular disorders, such as renal vein thrombosis, nephrotic syndrome, Wilson's disease, malaria, multiple myeloma (due to direct proteinaceous deposition of immunoglobulin light chains into the renal parenchyma), sickle cell disease, malignant hypertension, diabetes mellitus, and systemic lupus erythematosus, can all cause intrarenal injury. Pregnancy-related disorders, such as septic abortion, preeclampsia, abruptio placentae, intrauterine fetal death, and idiopathic postpartum renal failure, can also cause damage to the kidneys.

Data that identify events or agents that may have caused renal injury, especially those related to ischemia or exposure to toxins, should be collected during the history. These may include exposure to nephrotoxins; radiological tests that require administration of contrast dye; hypersensitivity reactions to a drug or dye; recent infections; trauma; sepsis; use of antineoplastic medications with or without radiation therapy; multiple myeloma; pregnancy; or a history of cardiac, renal, or liver disease.

There is no one specific finding that pinpoints the cause of intrarenal azotemia during a physical assessment. Findings on examination must be correlated with history and laboratory findings. Differentiating prerenal problems from actual ATN is a challenge. Because prerenal problems often correspond with the onset phase of ATN and because this is a reversible phase, it is essential for diagnosis and aggressive management to begin early.

Serum laboratory tests, urinalysis, and microscopic examination of the urine provide important data that can help to differentiate prerenal azotemia from ATN. Prerenal problems are indicated by high urinary specific gravity and osmolality, low urinary sodium caused by decreased renal blood flow, avid tubular sodium reabsorption, and decreased GFR. The kidneys interpret these changes as a state of dehydration and respond via the actions of aldosterone and ADH to maximize sodium and water reabsorption from the distal tubule and collecting duct into the peritubular capillary plasma. This results in a small amount of very concentrated urine with a high specific gravity and high osmolality. Despite maximal sodium reabsorption, the urine is concentrated because of urea or other solutes. Urinary and serum creatinine levels often

show wide variation in prerenal etiologies of AKI, with a slower rate of rise than in ATN and periodic decreases in serum creatinine.

ATN is characterized by altered renal ability to conserve sodium. Clinically, ATN is seen as a urinary sodium level greater than 20 mEq/L. However, depending on the state of hydration, the serum sodium levels vary in ATN. Oliguria is usually associated with postischemic ATN, whereas either oliguria or nonoliguria may be associated with nephrotoxic ATN. Creatinine clearance is severely decreased, and plasma creatinine rises approximately 0.5 to 1 mg/dL per day in ATN. The BUN to serum creatinine ratio does not typically exceed 10:1 to 15:1 in ATN.

Response to therapy is another factor that distinguishes ATN from prerenal etiologies. The kidneys typically respond very quickly to therapy aimed at correcting an underlying prerenal problem in which no actual damage to nephrons has occurred; however, in ATN, the response to treatment of the underlying cause may be minimal depending on the degree of nephron damage. Additional therapy for ATN should be aimed at correcting alterations related to the inability of the kidneys to maintain functionality.

Postrenal azotemia results from interference with the flow of urine from the kidneys and is associated with obstruction or disruption of the urinary tract. Ureteral, bladder, bladder neck, or urethral obstruction may be the result of calculi, urinary tract or bladder neoplasms, sloughed renal papillary tissue, strictures, trauma, blood clots, congenital or developmental abnormalities, foreign objects, surgical ligation, prostatic hypertrophy, retroperitoneal fibrosis, abdominal and pelvic neoplasms, pregnancy, a neurogenic bladder, bladder rupture, or the use of drugs such as antihistamines and tricyclic antidepressants with significant anticholinergic effects or ganglionic blocking agents. The history should focus on collecting data that reflect obstruction or disruption of the urinary tract. Significant findings include a change (decrease) in urine volume; a history of prostatic disease, abdominal neoplasms, urinary tract stones, or nephralgia; pregnancy; recent abdominal surgery; and paralysis (e.g., quadriplegia).

Postrenal azotemia physical assessment findings also vary with etiology and need to be correlated with laboratory and history findings (e.g., nephralgia associated with moving urinary tract stones or rapidly developing hydronephrosis; bladder distention associated with prostate, bladder neck, or urethral disorders). Laboratory findings include variations in urine volume such as oliguria, polyuria, or abrupt anuria, urine osmolality (may be increased or similar to plasma osmolality), urine specific gravity, or a decrease in urinary concentration of sodium or urea, as well as a BUN to serum creatinine ratio that is normal to slightly increased. Microscopy of the urinary sediment is usually normal unless urinary tract infection (UTI) is present.

MANAGEMENT

Approximately 50% of patients with AKI are nonoliguric and have less severe signs and symptoms than oliguric patients. Frequent causes of death in the setting of severe AKI and renal failure include cardiac arrest resulting from hyperkalemia, gastrointestinal bleeding, and severe infection; thus, patients should be monitored very closely and treated appropriately on a day-to-day basis. The main goal is to keep the patient alive and to determine the underlying cause of the renal failure. The etiology of AKI will determine long-term management strategies.

Prerenal azotemia secondary to absolute hypovolemia necessitates the restoration of intravascular volume. Replacement of fluids depends on the mechanism of loss. Gastrointestinal fluid loss is generally hypotonic and should be replaced accordingly; fluid loss as a result of hemorrhage usually indicates the need for administration of both saline and transfused packed RBCs. In addition, electrolyte imbalances must be managed. Hyperkalemia in AKI can be life-threatening; emergent management is required in patients with extreme elevation of potassium levels (more than 6.5 mmol/L) or in any patient with electrocardiogram (ECG) abnormalities.

Certain diseases, such as glomerulonephritis or Wegener's granulomatosis, require immunosuppressive treatment with prednisone and cyclophosphamide to prevent irreversible renal damage. In cases of ATN caused by nephrotoxic agents, the removal of the offending agent will allow renal function to return gradually to normal. In the meantime, supportive measures may be provided to hasten the removal of toxins, such as peritoneal or hemodialysis.

Several indications exist for temporary hemodialysis, including fluid overload unresponsive to diuretic therapy, hyperkalemia with symptoms or ECG changes, uremic encephalopathy, severe metabolic acidosis, cardiorespiratory failure, pleuritis, pericarditis, and other forms of inflammatory serositis. Forms of dialysis include traditional intermittent hemodialysis via large-bore venous and arterial catheters; peritoneal dialysis, which operates by osmotic diffusion via an indwelling dialysate within the peritoneal cavity; and continuous renal replacement therapy, which is a prolonged form of low-flow arteriovenous or venovenous hemofiltration that is indicated for hemodynamically unstable patients.

Postrenal azotemia involves identification of the level of obstruction followed by treatment to relieve the obstruction. If the obstruction is higher in the urinary tract, such as at the vesicoureteral junction or in the ureter or renal pelvis, percutaneous nephrotomy or ureteral stent placement by a urologist is necessary. For urethral obstruction, bladder catheterization or placement of a suprapubic tube may be sufficient to relieve the obstruction. Intermittent bladder catheterization four to five times a day poses less risk of UTI than an indwelling urinary catheter and is the preferred method for urinary outflow in cases of bladder atony and neuromuscular compromise such as with spinal cord injury. However, the presence of a bladder outlet or urethral obstruction, which is more likely to cause AKI, may necessitate placement of a long-term catheterization device until surgical intervention is possible.

FOLLOW-UP AND REFERRAL

After hospitalization, patient follow-up is necessary in about 1 week as an outpatient, and then at 1 month, 3 months, 6 months, and annually thereafter, provided there are no further complications. Serum chemistries (basic metabolic profile) and a complete blood count (CBC) should be checked at each follow-up visit. The patient should be assessed for signs and symptoms of fluid overload, such as crackles on lung auscultation, elevated blood pressure (BP), shortness of breath, weight gain, jugular vein distention, or edema.

Patient Education: Acute Kidney Injury

During the recovery stage there is no special form of treatment other than general healthy living. However, lack of knowledge about the causative factors is a major problem with regard to acute episodes of renal failure and may contribute to repeat episodes. Thus, patients benefit from continual education throughout their clinical pathway of treatment and recovery from AKI. Follow-up care, emotional support, and prevention of another episode should be the teaching focus.

CHRONIC KIDNEY DISEASE

Chronic kidney disease (CKD) is characterized by a progressive loss of functional nephrons, eventually leading to end-stage renal disease (ESRD). As the functional reserve of the kidneys is lost, signs and symptoms of renal failure appear. These signs may arise as sequelae of AKI, but most often CKD arises as a complication of chronic systemic disease, such as diabetes or hypertension. The time frame for the development of CKD typically ranges from months to years, whereas AKI usually occurs over days to weeks (see previous section).

EPIDEMIOLOGY AND CAUSES

According to the National Health and Nutrition Examination Survey (NHANES), a large population-based representative health survey of the United States done every 2 years, CKD affects approximately 13% of the U.S. population. The number of people with a chronic elevation of creatinine greater than 2.0 mg/dL is estimated to be 2.8 per 100,000 persons. There are approximately 485,000 people in the United States with ESRD, of whom 341,000 are on chronic dialysis. Men are 1.3 to 1.4 times more likely than women to have ESRD. The peak age of onset of ESRD is between 65 and 75 years, with older adults representing 33.8% of new patients. Geriatric patients have both the highest incidence rates of ESRD and the highest morbidity and mortality rates.

Compared with the general population, African Americans are 3.9 times more likely to have ESRD and 6.7 times more likely to have hypertensive ESRD. It is estimated that HIV-associated nephropathy may soon be the third leading cause of ESRD (after diabetes mellitus and hypertension) in African Americans aged 20 to 64 years.

Renal disease can result from many age-related illnesses. The major underlying conditions leading to ESRD are diabetes mellitus and primary hypertension seen in approximately 70% of cases, with glomerulonephritis, cystic disease, and other urological diseases accounting for another 15% of cases. Renal artery stenosis and chronic ischemic renovascular disease may cause up to 20% of CKD cases in persons older than 50 years. Analgesic overuse (e.g., NSAIDs), cigarette smoking, collagen vascular diseases, AIDS-related nephropathies, cirrhosis, and multiple myeloma are examples of other risk factors for the development of CKD. Several hereditary renal diseases (e.g., polycystic kidney disease and Alport syndrome, which also causes congenital deafness) can lead to CKD in children and some adults.

Overall, hypertension is present in at least 85% of patients with CKD. Hypertensive and diabetes-related CKD are forms of microvascular end-organ damage caused by these cardiovascular risk factors. Thus, these patients must also be evaluated for other forms of end-organ damage related to atherosclerotic disease, as a significant correlation exists between microvascular CKD, peripheral vascular disease, coronary artery disease, and cerebrovascular disease.

PATHOPHYSIOLOGY

The pathophysiology of renal failure varies depending on the underlying cause, although the end result is the same—a nonfunctional kidney. The most common causes of CKD are diabetic nephropathy, hypertensive nephropathy, and glomerulonephritis.

Diabetic Nephropathy

Diabetic nephropathy is the most common cause of ESRD and involves several mechanisms, including hyperglycemia, hormonal imbalances, and renal hemodynamic changes. Hyperglycemia leads to alterations in tubuloglomerular feedback, abnormalities in polyol (e.g., sorbitol) metabolism, and the formation of advanced glycosylation end products (AGEs) in tissues. Increases in circulating AGE peptides parallel the severity of renal dysfunction in diabetic nephropathy. Ultimately, defects

in glomerular cellular metabolism lead to hemodynamic changes in the kidney.

Renal hemodynamic changes implicated in diabetes mellitus and ESRD include both glomerular hyperfiltration and glomerular hypertension. Hormonal imbalances associated with diabetes mellitus and ESRD include decreased insulin secretion, increased growth hormone and glucagon production (both of which have been shown to produce glomerular hyperfiltration in laboratory studies), and altered concentrations or responsiveness to vasoactive hormones (e.g., angiotensin II, catecholamines, and prostaglandins), which can also result in hyperfiltration. Regardless of the inciting event, factors such as hyperglycemia-induced increases in extracellular fluid volume, renal hypertrophy, and/or altered glycoregulatory or vasoregulatory hormonal actions contribute to increased pressure and flow across the glomerular membrane, resulting in glomerular hypertension.

These factors, along with associated renal vasodilation and hyperfiltration, increase transglomerular protein filtration, which leads to proteinuria and mesangial deposition of circulating proteins. As a result, mesangial expansion and glomerulosclerosis cause the destruction of nephrons, as the glomerulus eventually becomes a fibrinous scar that can no longer function. In addition, a positive feedback stimulus for compensatory hyperfiltration is initiated, with further increases in GFR and progressive renal injury. Ultimately, it is glomerular hypertension that mediates progressive nephronal destruction. Based on this glomerular hypertension–hyperfiltration hypothesis, therapies directed at lowering glomerular hypertension would be expected to protect the kidney from further progression of nephropathy.

Hypertensive Nephropathy

Following diabetes mellitus, hypertensive nephropathy is the second most common cause of renal failure. The kidney is one of the major organs injured by hypertension, which results in *nephrosclerosis*. Benign nephrosclerosis is associated with chronic, mild, or moderate hypertension in which renal insufficiency develops slowly. The renal arterial vessels become thickened while their lumens narrow, resulting in decreased renal blood flow and autoregulation. Renal tubular changes correlate with the degree of reduction in renal blood flow. Signs and symptoms vary with the severity of renal injury and may include proteinuria, nocturia, urinary casts, and azotemia. Patients with benign nephrosclerosis are susceptible to AKI when a situation occurs that decreases blood flow to the kidney. Treatment is focused on control of hypertension.

Malignant nephrosclerosis is associated with marked hypertension, headache, congestive heart failure, and blurred vision. Unlike the progression of benign nephrosclerosis, renal failure develops rapidly in malignant nephrosclerosis. Renal arterioles and glomerular capillaries become thickened and necrotic, and renal tubules atrophy. Signs include hematuria with red cell casts, proteinuria, and azotemia. Treatment involves the immediate reduction of BP, which is necessary to prevent permanent loss of renal function and damage to other organs.

Renal artery stenosis occurs when the renal artery and its branches become thickened, stiff, and narrow due to atheromatous plaques (two-thirds of cases) or fibromuscular dysplasia (one-third of cases). As the body perceives the decreased blood flow (i.e., hypoperfusion) via the stenotic renal arteries as hypovolemia, the renin-angiotensin-aldosterone axis is activated and mild to severe hypertension results from the resulting retention of sodium and water. This condition becomes critical if both renal arteries are affected or if blood flow is compromised in patients with only a single kidney, either due to a congenital defect or after live organ donation of the other kidney. Other signs include a bruit auscultated in the flank or midabdominal region over the affected renal artery and an elevated blood renin level from the ipsilateral renal vein. The incidence of fibromuscular dysplasia is higher in women than in men, especially from 20 to 40 years of age. The treatment required is angioplasty or surgical repair to stent or reconstruct the stenotic vessels, along with medical therapy consisting of antihypertensives and diuretics.

Glomerulonephritis

Glomerulonephritis (GN) is the third most common cause of renal failure. GN is an inflammatory process that primarily affects the glomerular capillaries. It is also a major cause of ESRD. Approximately 25% of GN cases result from nonimmune mechanisms, whereas 60% to 75% stem from autoimmune mechanisms. Glomerular injury can be divided into two major categories based on pathology: *nephritis*, which is characterized by glomerular inflammation and/or necrosis; and *nephrosis*, which is characterized by abnormal permeability of the glomerular membrane. Both allow macromolecules such as albumin to pass into the urine, although more so in nephrosis. Of note, these two forms of glomerular injury are not mutually exclusive, and a single etiology can produce both forms of kidney injury.

The immunological injury that characterizes glomerulonephritis may occur by several different mechanisms. Anti-GBM disease is the result of direct glomerular injury occurring as a result of inflammation triggered by antibodies directed against components of the glomerular basement membrane. Linear deposits of immunoglobulin are seen via immunofluorescence (IF) microscopy of renal tissue and may reveal granular immunoglobulin deposits. Part of the inflammatory response that occurs is secondary to the glomerular deposition of immune complexes composed of antibodies bound to a variety of circulating antigens. The presence of these immune complexes is referred to as *immune complex disease*. Finally, pauci-immune ANCA-positive disease is characterized by the presence of serum antibodies against neutrophilic cytoplasm that are associated with the multisystem disease. Minimal or no immunoglobulin is seen by IF, however, hence the name "pauci-immune." Nonetheless, the glomerular injury is still believed to be immune mediated in nature.

The hallmark of nephrosis is increased permeability of the glomerular capillary wall to macromolecules, including serum proteins. Inflammatory changes are generally not seen but may be present. In classic forms of glomerulonephrosis, nephrotic syndrome develops, and various degrees of proteinuria may be present. In addition to hypertension, other characteristic findings include hypercholesterolemia with lipiduria and central edema from hypoalbuminemia due to albuminuria. In more than two-thirds of cases of glomerulonephrosis in adults, the cause is idiopathic; in the remainder, nephrosis is secondary to systemic disease such as diabetes, lupus, or amyloidosis.

CLINICAL PRESENTATION

Subjective

Because of the significant functional reserve of the kidneys, symptoms do not generally appear until renal function (as measured by the GFR) declines to 10% to 15% of normal. At about 30% to 40% of normal GFR, biochemical evidence of renal failure may be apparent, but patients typically remain asymptomatic. Early prominent symptoms in renal failure include anorexia, lassitude, fatigability, and weakness.

The inability of the kidneys to perform their normal excretory, metabolic, and endocrine functions results in *uremia*, a complex syndrome that includes a variety of physiological and clinical abnormalities. Dermatological abnormalities may result in the patient with complaints of pruritus and dry skin, and gastrointestinal alterations may manifest as complaints of anorexia, nausea, vomiting, and hiccoughing. Neurologic complaints may include emotional lability or depression, insomnia, fatigue (especially on exertion), confusion, headache, seizures, and coma. There may be an odor of urine to the breath and perspiration, complaints of shortness of breath, a metallic taste in the mouth, impotence, nocturia, and muscle cramps. The patient may present with foot drop, infection, bleeding, or gout. Often the patient is being treated for a major systemic disease such as diabetes mellitus. The primary-care provider should be alert to the potential for the onset of CKD in patients who present with these signs and symptoms who have a major systemic disease

Objective

The patient may appear pale, with a characteristic uremic frost appearance to the skin, or, conversely, hyperpigmentation may be apparent. There may be bruising and asterixis (i.e., hand-flapping on hyperextension of the wrists with complete forward extension of the upper extremities). Peripheral neuropathy and altered mental status may be present, along with peripheral edema and ascites from severe proteinuria and the resulting hypoalbuminemia, as well as auscultatory crackles in the lungs and a pericardial rub. There may be an elevated BP and a hard, rapid pulse. Some abnormalities are the result of the accumulation of toxic metabolites; others are caused by underproduction (e.g., vitamin D and erythropoietin) or overproduction (e.g., renin) of biochemically active substances produced by the kidney.

DIAGNOSTIC REASONING

Diagnostic Tests

If a patient has a condition known to predispose the individual to the development of CKD, especially if that patient is in a high-risk population, biochemical monitoring (BUN, creatinine, and creatinine clearance) should be done to detect renal failure before it becomes clinically apparent. Serum creatinine can track the progression of CKD. However, the GFR, which is normally well above 90 mL/min (with values as high as 130 mL/min in healthy adults), can decrease to 40% to 50% of normal with only small changes noted in serum creatinine levels. Accurate measurement of the GFR is based on experimental calculations of renal inulin clearance. Inulin is a polymer of fructose secreted from the blood exclusively via renal glomeruli with no tubular reabsorption. Measurement of inulin clearance, however, requires a complex assay too cumbersome for regular clinical use and tends to be reserved for research purposes. Alternatively, GFR can be estimated in milliliters per minute using the Cockcroft-Gault formula for creatinine clearance (see Box 45.2).

It is important to realize that trends in GFR (as estimated by creatinine clearance or serum creatinine levels) are far more important in assessing renal function and stability of CKD than are the absolute values of these indices. A meta-analysis of 13 studies found that a lower GFR and a higher albuminuria independently predict mortality and ESRD in patients with CKD. This is especially true of direct serum creatinine measurements, whose interpretation must take into account a patient's muscle mass, age, and gender. Thus, creatinine clearance is a far more informative diagnostic tool as a measure of renal function.

Although no universally agreed upon definition of CKD exists, GFR and proteinuria are often used to stratify CKD patients by disease severity. The third NHANES Survey defined the stages as follows:

- **Stage 1** disease is characterized by persistent albuminuria with a normal GFR greater than 90 mL/min per 1.73 m² of BSA.
- **Stage 2** disease is characterized by albuminuria with a GFR between 60 and 89 mL/min per 1.73 m² of BSA.
- **Stage 3** disease is defined as a GFR between 30 and 59 mL/min per 1.73 m² of BSA.
- **Stage 4** disease is defined as a GFR between 15 and 29 mL/min/1.73 m² of BSA.
- **Stage 5** disease is ESRD, defined as a GFR less than 15 mL/min/1.73 m² of BSA.

Routine monitoring of the CBC can detect anemia secondary to erythropoietin deficiency. Monitoring of urinalysis can detect increasing proteinuria. When renal function declines further, closer monitoring of routine laboratory tests to detect dangerous electrolyte imbalances (e.g., hyperkalemia) and acidosis is required.

Numerous laboratory alterations occur in patients who develop ESRD. A CBC will usually reveal a normochromic and normocytic anemia, decreased hematocrit, increased bleeding time, capillary fragility, thrombocytopenia, and a decreased immune responsiveness. Blood chemistries typically reveal some of the following abnormalities: decreased active vitamin D, elevated ammonia, BUN, serum creatinine, uric acid, sulfate, potassium, phosphate, parathyroid hormone, and glucose levels, along with insulin resistance and hyperlipidemia (particularly hypertriglyceridemia). Urinalysis may reveal proteinuria (the greater the proteinuria, the more rapid the progression of CKD) and coarse granular casts. Ketosis may artificially raise creatinine levels, and certain drugs (e.g., cimetidine, trimethoprim, cefazolin) may also alter diagnostic test results.

Twenty-four-hour urine studies (e.g., urinary protein level, creatinine clearance) may be collected although samples often are difficult to obtain in ambulatory patients and have been largely replaced by spot urine checks. Complement levels, antinuclear

---

> **Box 45.2** **Glomerular Filtration Rate Using the Cockcroft-Gault Formula for Creatinine Clearance**
>
> - (140 minus age × lean body weight in kilograms) divided by (72 × stable serum creatinine in mg/dL)
> - This value is multiplied by 0.85 (i.e., reduced by 15%) for women.
> - Creatinine clearance values are normalized per 1.73 m² of body surface area (BSA) in order to adjust for very heavy (obese) or very thin patients by multiplying the estimated creatinine clearance value by 1.73 m² and then dividing the product by the total body surface area of the patient in m²*.

*Most adults have a BSA that falls within 1.6 to 1.9 m² (hence, the value of 1.73 m² representing the average adult BSA). This correction factor is sometimes not applied in clinical practice, with creatinine clearance reported in units of mL/min, rather than mL/min per 1.73 m² of BSA.

antibody, and serum and urine protein electrophoresis may all provide data as to the underlying pathophysiology of CKD.

Renal ultrasound performed at least at baseline when impaired renal function is first noted is indicated in all cases of CKD. Among other pathologies, sonography may reveal decreased kidney size (less than 11 cm), polycystic kidney disease, or an obstructed ureter or bladder outlet with hydroureter and/or hydronephrosis. Renal CT scan/CT angiography or MRI/MRA may detect and localize harder to visualize structural abnormalities, renal parenchymal disease, or renal artery stenosis. Duplex Doppler ultrasonography to assess renal vascular flow has a high sensitivity and specificity for renal artery stenosis if conducted by an experienced ultrasonographer, but renal angiography remains the diagnostic gold standard for this condition. However, unilaterally decreased kidney size on renal imaging is highly suggestive of vascular occlusive disease and may be helpful as a screening method. Renal biopsy is not utilized for CKD as much as for AKI, unless noninvasive diagnostic testing is unable to suggest a likely etiology.

Differential Diagnosis

The differential diagnosis of CKD is aimed at identifying the underlying etiology of renal failure, as discussed earlier. Although the terms *chronic kidney disease* and *chronic renal insufficiency* (CRI) are often used interchangeably, some authorities reserve the use of CKD to imply a dialysis-dependent state, whereas CRI denotes an earlier form of the condition not yet requiring dialysis or kidney transplantation, but that may clearly progress to CKD. The signs and symptoms and diagnostic test results commonly seen in the three stages of CKD (decreased renal reserve, renal insufficiency, and ESRD) are presented in Table 45.1.

MANAGEMENT

General principles of CKD management include (1) the determination and control of the underlying causative etiology, (2) monitoring changes in renal function, (3) conservative treatment of the physiological effects of CKD, and (4) instituting more aggressive treatment (dialysis and/or renal transplantation) as appropriate in later stages of treatment-refractory disease.

TABLE 45.1   Differentiating the Stages of Chronic Kidney Disease

Stage	Glomerular Filtration Rate	Signs and Symptoms	Management
1. Decreased renal reserve	Normal kidney function: Greater than 90 mL/min per 1.73 m² of BSA	• Asymptomatic • Hypertension (mild)	Control blood pressure and observation.
2. Kidney damage	Mildly reduced kidney function: 60–89 mL/min per 1.73 m² of BSA	• Hypertension (mild) • ↑ PTH • Early bone disease • ↑ BUN and serum creatinine	Control blood pressure and observation.
3. Renal insufficiency 3a. 3b.	Moderately reduced kidney function: 45–59 mL/min per 1.73 m² of BSA 30–44 mL/min per 1.73 m² of BSA	• Hypertension • Anemia due to ↓ erythropoietin • ↑ BUN and serum creatinine • Risk of cardiovascular events	• Refer to specialist. • Evaluate serum creatinine, potassium, hemoglobin, and urinary protein every 6 months. • Control blood pressure.
4. Severe renal insufficiency	Severely reduced kidney function: 15–29 mL/min per 1.73 m² of BSA	• Moderate hypertension • Anemia • Hyperphosphatemia • ↑ Triglycerides • Metabolic acidosis • Hyperkalemia • Water/salt retention • ↑ BUN and serum creatinine	• Refer to specialist. • Control hypertension. • Oral phosphate binders. • Cholesterol-lowering therapy. • Administration of erythropoietin (epoetin-alpha) for anemia.
5. End-stage kidney disease or kidney failure	<15 mL/min per 1.73 m² of BSA or on dialysis	• Severe hypertension • Anemia • Hyperphosphatemia • Uremia	• Refer to specialist. • Dialysis. • Renal transplant. • Same management as for Stage 4.

Abbreviations: BSA, body surface area; BUN, blood urea nitrogen; PTH, parathyroid hormone
Adapted from www.renal.org/whatwedo/InformationResources/CKDeGUIDE/CKDstages.aspx and www.kidney.org/PROFESSIONALS/kdoqi/guidelines_ckd/toc.htm.

Management of Hypertension

Glucose levels and hypertension must be strictly controlled in diabetic patients, with a target hemoglobin A1c of less than 7%. For any patient with proteinuria of more than 1 g per day, the target BP is 125/75 mm Hg; for a patient with proteinuria of less than 1 g per day, the goal is a BP of no more than 130/80 mm Hg. Given the importance of maintaining renal perfusion, systolic BPs lower than 110 mm Hg should be avoided. ACE inhibitors or the newer class of angiotensin II receptor blockers (ARBs) should be used for BP control in patients with diabetes mellitus, given their renoprotective effects. If monotherapy with one of these agents is insufficient to control BP, a diuretic should be added, followed by a calcium channel blocker (diltiazem or verapamil) or a beta blocker, as needed. If combination therapy using agents from these additional classes proves ineffective, an ACE inhibitor or ARB should be added (whichever class was not used initially).

For patient with renal artery stenosis, pharmacologic BP management is equally as important. However, ACE inhibitors and ARBs are usually avoided in patients with bilateral renal artery stenosis, because their vasodilatory effect on the efferent renal arterioles effectively decreases GFR due to reduced afferent blood flow from stenotic the renal arteries. In turn, this may precipitate potentially devastating acute or CRF. Percutaneous angioplasty or surgical revascularization with arterial stenting should be considered for patients with severe hypertension refractory to pharmacotherapy, recurrent episodes of flash pulmonary edema due to CKD-related fluid overload, and progressive renal insufficiency that fails to improve despite effective BP control. Individuals with particularly severe CKD (serum creatinine greater than 4 mg/dL) or chronically atrophied kidneys (less than 7 cm) are unlikely to respond to such interventions, however. Revascularization is more likely to be effective in patients whose renal function rapidly declines, particularly after beginning ACE inhibitor or ARB therapy.

Management of Fluids and Electrolytes

Dietary therapy is a cornerstone of conservative management of CKD. Restriction of fluid intake (to maintain a serum sodium concentration of 135 to 145 mEq/L) and sodium intake (especially if volume expanded) may decrease secondary hypertension or congestive heart failure, although volume depletion must be avoided given the potential for acute worsening due to renal hypoperfusion. A restricted goal of 2 g per day of sodium intake and 2 L per day of fluid intake may be needed if the patient is volume overloaded. Restricted protein intake is recommended (0.6 to 0.8 g/kg/day), although an adequate caloric intake (40 to 50 cal/kg/day) should be maintained, because malnutrition is a common complication of CKD. Consultation by a skilled nutritionist is recommended at the time of diagnosis and periodically as the disease progresses and the patient's nutritional needs change. Foods rich in essential amino acids are the most effectively utilized source of nitrogen. Restriction of dietary phosphate (800 mg/day) and potassium may be necessary because of reduced excretion and the potential for hyperphosphatemia and hyperkalemia. Strict dietary restrictions may be unnecessary in older patients because they often have low protein and sodium intake, but treatment regimens must be individualized. Low-dose sodium polystyrene sulfonate (Kayexalate) 5 mg PO one to three times daily with meals may be used as a potassium binder for hyperkalemia. Oral phosphate binders such as calcium carbonate (2.5 to 20 g/day), calcium acetate (Phos-Lo; 1334 mg three times daily), or sevelamer (Renagel; 800 mg three times daily) are typically taken with meals when GFR falls below 30 mL/min. Sevelamer is used when CKD is complicated by iatrogenic hypercalcemia. Aluminum- and magnesium-containing salts should be avoided, owing to cumulative toxicity.

Given the kidneys' reduced ability to synthesize activated vitamin D in CKD and the propensity for subsequent hypocalcemia and renal osteodystrophy, oral 1,25-dihydroxyvitamin D (calcitriol 0.25 mg daily) and calcium carbonate (600 mg two times daily) supplements should be given, along with a renal-specific multivitamin (Nephrocaps). Importantly, however, this chronic treatment may result in hypercalcemia and worsen coronary artery calcification. Thus, close monitoring of serum calcium levels is critical.

If diuretic therapy is instituted for edema, dehydration must be avoided. Thiazide diuretics may be tried first, but they are far less effective at a GFR of less than 20 to 30 mL/min per 1.73 m^2 of BSA (approximated by serum creatinine levels of greater than 2.5 mg/dL); however, they provide an additive effect when used with a loop diuretic initiated for refractory edema. Potassium-sparing diuretics should be avoided, owing to the kidneys' reduced ability to excrete potassium.

Treatment of Anemia

Anemia should be treated with erythropoietin (80 to 120 units/kg subcutaneously per week), taking care not to induce polycythemia (goal Hgb = 11 to 12 g/dL) with its attendant risk of stroke. Dosing usually begins around 10,000 units per week but may be adjusted upward in frequency or dose as needed. Darbepoetin alfa is an alternative erythropoietic agent with a longer half-life, allowing for less frequent dosing (0.45 mcg/kg subcutaneously per week). Patients with iron-deficiency anemia should take ferrous sulfate 325 mg by mouth one to three times daily with meals, with lower doses being less likely to induce constipation in elderly patients. Gentle transfusion with packed RBCs may be required in cases of extreme or acutely worsened anemia, but care must be taken not to induce high-output heart failure or fluid overload, because the heart typically adapts to the chronic anemia of CKD.

Bleeding diatheses due to uremic platelet dysfunction are not uncommon in both AKI and CKD. Active bleeding in these patients should be treated with desmopressin, cryoprecipitate, estrogen, or dialysis to remove uremic toxins believed to be qualitatively inhibiting platelet function.

Management of Hypercholesteremia

Because CKD is considered a coronary artery disease risk equivalent, hypercholesterolemia should be treated with a statin drug, with a low-density lipoprotein goal of less than 100 mg/dL. Recent evidence suggests this goal should be even lower to minimize the rate of disease progression due to atherosclerotic renovascular disease. Dietary modification to restrict cholesterol and saturated fats is also critical to adequately address hyperlipidemia, especially hypertriglyceridemia.

Ongoing Management of Symptoms

Both hypovolemia (renal hypoperfusion) and renal toxic drugs may exacerbate CKD and must always be considered when acute or CRF is observed. A judicious trial of isotonic fluid repletion may be appropriate in patients displaying the physical stigmata of dehydration, and careful attention must be paid to the dosing of all chronic and newly started medications. All nephrotoxic agents (e.g., NSAIDs, radiocontrast dye) should be avoided.

Other measures to relieve symptoms include skin moisturizers for dry skin; menthol or phenol lotion, a trial of capsaicin cream, or the antihistamine diphenhydramine (Benadryl) may all be useful in treating pruritus. Vitamin E may also be helpful in treating muscle cramps.

Management of Progressive CKD

As CKD progresses, the patient will have increased difficulties with fluid balance and may experience episodes of hyperkalemia, hypertension, acidosis, and severe uremia with altered mental status and qualitative platelet dysfunction with a tendency for bleeding diatheses. Metabolic acidosis should be treated initially with sodium bicarbonate 600 mg two times daily, in order to titrate serum bicarbonate to the 16 to 20 mEq/L range. However, patients must display adequate respiratory function to avoid the accumulation of metabolized carbon dioxide and respiratory acidosis. The potassium and calcium levels should be monitored during treatment of acidosis, because both might fall. Hospitalization may be required for the control of fluid overload, hypertension, hyperkalemia, or infection.

A GFR of less than 10 mL/min, a serum creatinine level approaching 12 mg/dL, or a BUN of greater than 100 mg/dL all typically require more aggressive therapies to avoid life-threatening sequelae, including peritoneal or hemodialysis. Continuous venovenous or arteriovenous hemofiltration may be used in hemodynamically unstable patients, as an alternative to classic hemodialysis. Such therapies must be done only under the supervision of a nephrologist, however. Life-threatening indications for dialysis include pericarditis, diuretic-refractory fluid overload (e.g., pulmonary edema), medication-resistant or rapidly worsening hypertension, uremic syndrome with an attendant bleeding diathesis or neurologic symptomatology, and persistent nausea and vomiting. In addition, protein malnutrition in the face of a creatinine clearance of less than 20 mL/min is considered an indication for early dialysis.

FOLLOW-UP AND REFERRAL

The course of CKD is typically punctuated by periods of rapid deterioration, often precipitated by dehydration or infection. The rate of progression to kidney failure will depend in part on the underlying renal disease. It is usually more rapid in patients with diabetic nephropathy or severe hypertension and slower in patients with polycystic kidney disease.

Patients with CKD should be referred to a nephrologist, given the progressive nature of the disease. In patients with advanced renal failure (creatinine levels greater than 10 mg/dL), mean survival time without intervention (e.g., dialysis or transplantation) is only 100 to 150 days. Vascular access for hemodialysis (arteriovenous grafts or fistulae) must be obtained 2 to 3 months in advance to permit maturation of the fistulae and allow for potential revisions. Decisions regarding dialysis and transplantation require a team approach with the primary-care practitioner, nephrologist, patient, and family. Comprehensive evaluation of the patient's medical, psychological, and social contexts is necessary for successful planning and follow-up.

In general, the multiplicity of metabolic demands on the patient with CKD will require careful and close follow-up and constant adjustments in treatment. The most important cornerstone of care is the monitoring and treatment of all underlying disorders known to lead to CRF. Depending on the course of disease, at some point during follow-up, the patient may need to be hospitalized to control fluid overload, hypertension, hyperkalemia, or infection. Successful therapy depends in good part on the maintenance of a strong relationship between the health-care provider and the patient and family.

Nowhere is the *Circle of Caring* approach more important than in a chronic, progressive disorder such as CKD. Interventions should be geared toward maximizing the patient's independence and reducing social isolation. Given the fact that CKD may be rapidly progressive depending on its etiology and reach its end-stage in relatively young patients, clinicians and their patients may be faced with emotionally challenging situations related to the death and dying process, which necessitate a range of approaches.

Patient Education

For care to be effective, the patient and family must have a thorough understanding of the chronic and progressive nature of CKD, of the importance of treating all underlying systemic diseases such as diabetes and hypertension, and of the specifics of the treatment plan. Avoidance of infection is critical, as is maintaining a healthy, renally adjusted diet as recommended. Patients should know when and how to report bleeding, fever, decreases in urine output, or episodes of nausea and vomiting.

RENAL TUMORS

Renal tumors (*neoplasms*) are characterized by abnormal tissue formations on or around the kidney that may cause or contribute to renal disease. They may be primary or secondary (resulting from malignant spread), although the latter are rarely clinically relevant and are typically found during postmortem examination. *Renal adenomas* (benign tumors) and *adenocarcinomas* (malignant tumors) are rare; these tumors usually create complications requiring surgical removal.

EPIDEMIOLOGY AND CAUSES

Renal tumors are responsible for approximately 3.8% of all new cancer cases in 2017. The incidence is higher in men (although the difference in incidence has been decreasing over time). Kidney cancer is the sixth most common cancer in men and the tenth most common in women. Age of onset is typically between 55 and 70 years, while rarely occurring in people younger than 45 years. The average age of diagnosis is 64 years.

Renal cell carcinomas originating in the renal cortex are the most common (85%) type of malignant renal tumors. These tumors occur most often in the parenchyma of the kidney, with ureteral and urethral tumors occurring only rarely. Histologically, renal cell carcinomas are classified as clear cell (75% to 85%), chromophilic or papillary (15%), chromophobic (5%). Rare forms include oncocytic and collecting duct tumors. Transitional cell carcinomas are the next most common type of renal carcinoma, comprising 5% to 8% of all tumors; these typically affect the bladder and are discussed extensively in the next section (see Bladder Tumors).

Renal cell carcinomas are curable in more than 90% of patients if they are superficial and/or localized in the renal pelvis or ureter. Tumors that are invasive, however, have only a 10% to 15% chance of being cured. In children, nephroblastoma (Wilms' tumor) is common, comprising 5% of primary tumors, whereas sickle cell disease has a known, albeit rare, association with carcinoma of the renal medulla.

Risk factors for renal cell carcinoma include obesity; exposure to asbestos, cadmium, and/or gasoline; the use of phenacetin- and aspirin-containing analgesics and chronic hemodialysis for acquired polycystic kidney disease. In addition, cigarette smoking has a 25% to 30% correlation with the development of renal cell carcinoma.

PATHOPHYSIOLOGY

The urinary system is lined with transitional cell epithelium where tumors may form. The tumors often are asymptomatic and grow undetected until complications from the tumor present clinically. The tumors are usually encapsulated and located near the cortex unilaterally. Renal neoplasms may be diagnosed as benign or malignant, and they may be identified as either primary (originating in the kidney) or secondary (originating or spread from another source). Primary malignancies usually spread through the lymph nodes and blood vessels to the lungs, liver, and bone. Metastatic disease that spreads to the kidney, usually from the lung as the primary source, is more common than primary renal neoplasms. Metastatic lesions to the ureter typically originate via hematogenous spread from the breast or colorectal primary lesions. Direct extension into the ureter may also occur from cervical or colonic neoplasms, as well as pelvic retroperitoneal lymphoma. Benign renal neoplasms are rare but should be removed because of complications that may develop such as pain, bleeding, and urinary obstruction.

Carcinogen exposure has been associated with specific gene mutations that appear to underlie the development of various forms of hereditary renal cell carcinoma. However, definitive causal relationships between various mutational hot spots and renal cancer have not been proven.

Clear cell carcinomas consistently display mutations spanning the 3p14 to 3p26 chromosomal region. In contrast, chromophilic carcinomas lack these mutations but have been associated with various trisomies, including those of chromosomes 12, 16, and 20. Chromophobic carcinomas, which arise from the intercalated cells of the collecting duct system, typically display hypodiploidy, with a wide variety of whole chromosomal deletions. The much less common oncocytic carcinomas have been associated with deletions in chromosome 11q13, but as with collecting duct tumors, no consistent chromosomal abnormalities have been identified.

CLINICAL PRESENTATION

Subjective

Symptoms vary depending on the size of the tumor. Early signs of tumor growth are silent. Approximately 60% of the time, asymptomatic patients present with gross hematuria as the only outward sign. However, 30% of patients complain of dull, achy flank pain or an abdominal mass. In 10% to 15% of patients, the triad of flank pain, hematuria, and an abdominal mass is observed, which is often a sign of advanced disease.

Objective

Examination of the patient may reveal other signs that may present alone or in combination with hematuria. General signs of advanced disease include weight loss and fatigue. More specific signs and symptoms of renal tumors include intermittent fever not associated with infection and palpable abdominal mass, which may be associated with the complaint of nephralgia. The spread of primary renal tumors typically involves the lungs, lymph nodes, liver, bones, and contralateral kidney, with metastasis of renal cancer indicating a poor prognosis.

DIAGNOSTIC REASONING

Diagnostic Tests

The diagnosis of a renal mass is initially confirmed by IVP with nephrotomography; however, it is often impossible to determine if the mass is solid or cystic with these diagnostic imaging tests. Generally speaking, a cancerous tumor splays, distorts, or occludes the visualization of the collecting system and prevents normal filling and draining of the renal system. Although hematuria is common, urine cytology is not consistently reliable for diagnosing these tumors. Ureteroscopy or ultrasonography with IVP can be used to differentiate potentially neoplastic tissue from renal cyst formation by direct or indirect visualization of the entire renal system. Once tissue biopsy samples are obtained, flow cytometric analysis is used to determine the ploidy (DNA content) of the tumor, and histological analysis determines morphology and tumor grade (degree of cellular differentiation). Urine cytology samples often provide inadequate tissue for such analyses, however, and the mass must be biopsied directly. Figure 45.1 presents a flowchart for the evaluation and treatment of a renal mass.

MRI and CT scan are useful in the preoperative work-up and staging of metastatic lesions. It is necessary to stage the advancement of the tumor and potential for survival in order to initiate appropriate treatment. Staging of the neoplasm is confirmed through surgical intervention. The tumor-node-metastasis (TNM) staging of renal cell carcinoma is as follows:

- Stage I is defined as a tumor confined within the kidney capsule; it is treated by nephrectomy. The 5-year survival rate is 60% to 75%.
- Stage II is defined as the invasion of the renal capsule that is confined within the Gerota's fascia; it is treated by nephrectomy. The 5-year survival rate is 47% to 65%.

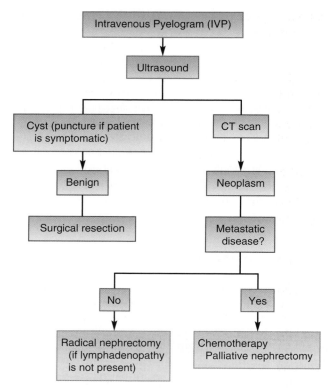

Figure 45.1 Flowchart for the treatment and evaluation of renal tumors.

- Stage III is defined as involvement of the regional lymph nodes ipsilaterally, the renal vein, or the vena cava. The 5-year survival rate is 5% to 15%.
- Stage IV is defined as distant metastasis, with a 5-year survival rate of less than 5%.

Approximately 30% of patients with renal tumors have metastatic disease at diagnosis. The most common sites of metastasis are the lung (50% to 60%), bone (30% to 40%), regional lymph nodes (15% to 30%), brain (10%), and adjacent organs.

Differential Diagnosis

A renal cyst is differentiated from a renal tumor by biopsy. Renal calculi and renal infarction must also be ruled out, as well as (rarely) renal tuberculosis. In addition, polycystic kidney disease and hydronephrosis must be considered and may be ruled out via imaging such as renal CT scan or on biopsy.

MANAGEMENT

As with any cancer, treatment of renal cancer requires immediate specialist referral to a urologist or surgical oncologist, often with additional consultation by a medical oncologist or nephrologist, depending on the patient's renal function. Treatment for a renal neoplasm is primarily surgical with a partial or total nephrectomy, with or without regional lymphadenectomy if no metastatic disease is present. Less radical surgical interventions have been suggested by a minority of urologists, who stress the poor prognosis of advanced renal tumors, regardless of surgical intervention, as well as the increased morbidity and mortality associated with radical surgery.

No universal standards have been accepted for adjunctive treatment after nephrectomy. Chemotherapy is not effective with this type of cancer; however, immunotherapy using lymphokine-activated killer cells, with or without IL-2 treatment, may be helpful for selected patients. Radiation therapy is controversial but may be used in combination with nephrectomy or for palliative effects in patients with bone metastases.

FOLLOW-UP AND REFERRAL

For follow-up of patients with a total nephrectomy, a CT scan of the abdomen and renal fossa should be done in 3 to 6 months. The patient may then be followed with renal ultrasound every 6 months for 3 years and annually thereafter, unless symptoms occur. Chest x-rays are done quarterly for a year to monitor for pulmonary metastasis.

At the time of diagnosis of the neoplasm, the patient should be referred to a urologist for a surgical evaluation and to an oncologist for potential cancer treatment. The patient should be seen by a primary-care practitioner for problems not related to the cancer and to assist the patient with counseling and support regarding grief, death and dying issues, body image changes, and alterations in quality of life.

Patient Education: Renal Tumors

Patients typically require preparation for surgical intervention. Postoperatively, the focus is on pain management and promoting comfort through the use of moist heat, analgesics or opioids, or positioning the patient on their side with pillows and back support. Additional interventions include preventing pneumonia and atelectasis by encouraging the patient to do coughing and deep breathing exercises, incisional care, and monitoring bowel and bladder function.

BLADDER TUMORS

Bladder tumors are abnormal tissue masses that occur in the bladder wall lining, which is composed of transitional cell epithelium (urothelium). These tumors commonly recur despite aggressive treatment.

EPIDEMIOLOGY AND CAUSES

Bladder tumors are the most common cancer of the urinary system; they represented approximately 4.7% of all new cancer cases in 2017 and result in 3% of cancer deaths per year. Bladder cancer is the fifth most common neoplasm in the United States; it occurs in men three times more often than in women and most often in adults aged 60 to 70 years. It is also more common among non-Hispanic white men than in other ethnic or racial groups.

There is a significant correlation between bladder tumors and risk factors including cigarette smoking; the presence of renal tumors; exposure to aromatic amine dyes known as arylamines (e.g., beta-naphthylamines, xenylamine, 4-nitrobiphenyl, and benzidine) and arsenic; chronic use of phenacetin-containing analgesics; use of saccharin (in rodent studies); chronic lower UTI; schistosomiasis; and recurrent nephrolithiasis. Other predisposing factors for bladder tumors include previous radiation treatment for cervical, ovarian, or prostate cancer and prior cyclophosphamide chemotherapy.

PATHOPHYSIOLOGY

Bladder tumors are primarily transitional cell carcinomas, which arise from the transitional cell uroepithelium (urothelium). Transitional cell carcinomas, in general, are the second most common form of renal carcinomas, arising from the urothelia that lines the mucosal surfaces of the collecting tubules, renal calyces, renal pelvis, ureters, bladder, and urethra. Specifically, transitional cell carcinomas account for 90% of all tumors of renal pelvic or ureteral origin. Bladder tumors may also be squamous cell carcinomas or adenocarcinomas. Transitional cell carcinomas of the bladder have the most favorable prognosis.

Bladder tumors are described as papillary (90%) or nonpapillary (10%). Papillary bladder lesions form as a small protuberance attached to a stalk. Nonpapillary lesions are more invasive and have a poorer prognosis. Primary bladder cancer tends to metastasize to the lymph nodes, liver, bones, and lungs. However, bladder cancer may also develop secondary to local extension and/or metastatic disease from adjacent organs, such as the cervix in women and the prostate in men.

Genetic analyses of transitional cell carcinomas demonstrate a loss of heterozygosity at any one of multiple chromosomal locations, including 9q (most common), 5p, 8p, 10q, 11p, and 17p—all of which may represent sites of tumor suppressor genes. Genetic predisposition also appears to be based on allelic variants of the p450 cytochrome enzyme complex. For instance, smokers with bladder cancer express p450 enzyme variants that lead to increased activation of arylamine metabolites, a required step in their contribution to bladder carcinogenesis. Along this same line, allelic variants exist for the *N*-acetyltransferase gene *NAT2*, which (along with *NAT1*) serves as the primary pathway for the metabolism and detoxification of arylamines via *N*-acetylation. Individuals with *NAT2* variants conferring a "slow-acetylation" phenotype are up to 17 times more likely to develop bladder cancer than those with a "fast-acetylation" phenotype. A similar phenomenon exists regarding the glutathione-*S*-transferase Mu 1 gene (*GSTM1*), which contributes to detoxification and secretion of carcinogenic compounds via their conjugation to glutathione. In the United States, nearly 50% of white men display deletions in both alleles of this gene, effectively eliminating any enzymatic activity from the *GSTM1* gene product.

Transitional cell carcinomas often present multifocally along the urinary tract, spreading via intraluminal seeding or intraepithelial migration via a process known as "field cancerization." Such multifocal tumors display monoclonality along their entire distribution. Squamous cell carcinoma, a less common form of bladder cancer that also accounts for 7% of renal pelvis tumors, is typically associated with an underlying inflammatory process, such as chronic UTI and renal calculi. These tumors tend to be deeply invasive and have a poor prognosis.

CLINICAL PRESENTATION

Subjective

The patient with a bladder tumor is frequently asymptomatic until he or she has an episode of hematuria that varies in severity from microscopic to gross amounts and may be intermittent or continuous. Other presenting symptoms may include dysuria, urinary frequency, chills, low-grade fever, weight loss, and urinary urgency. Patients with advanced disease may complain of pelvic pain and other symptoms associated with urethral obstruction.

Objective

The physical examination may be positive for a palpable mass and/or metastatic manifestations. The urinalysis shows trace to gross hematuria, possibly with abnormalities in protein level, RBCs, or WBCs. The serum CBC may indicate the presence of anemia.

DIAGNOSTIC REASONING

Diagnostic Tests

The diagnosis of a bladder tumor is confirmed by visualization of the lesion through transurethral resection of the bladder tumor. Urine cytology that is positive for transitional cell cancer can confirm the diagnosis; however, negative results do not rule out the possibility of bladder cancer. Cystoscopic evaluation can be used to confirm the suspected diagnosis, determine the location of the tumor, and aid in staging of the tumor. The cystoscopy should include a bladder washing for cytology and a mucosal biopsy. An abdominal or pelvic CT scan,

with or without IVP, may be useful for determining the metastatic progress of the disease.

According to the TNM system of the American Joint Committee on Cancer, the stages of transitional cell carcinoma are as follows:

- Stage 0 tumors are confined to the mucosa.
- Stage I tumors invade the lamina propria.
- Stage II tumors invade the muscular layer.
- Stage III tumors extend to the peripelvic fat or renal parenchyma.
- Stage IV indicates metastatic disease.

Urine tumor marker tests can detect recurrent bladder tumors. The *N*-benzoyl-L-tyrosyl-*p*-aminobenzoic acid and nucleoside 5′-monophosphate tests are more sensitive in detecting recurrent tumors than urine cytology.

Differential Diagnosis

Because this disease most often presents as painless hematuria, differential diagnoses to be ruled out include renal stones, infection, trauma, other tumors such as renal cell carcinoma, arteriovenous malformations, and glomerulonephropathies. The differential diagnosis for bladder irritability includes inflammation, the passage of renal stones, neurologic dysfunction, and foreign bodies in the bladder or urinary system. Visualization and biopsy may be necessary for a definitive diagnosis.

MANAGEMENT

Treatment depends on the type, size, and degree of invasion of the bladder tumor, which is classified as superficial, invasive, or metastatic. *Superficial tumors* (Stages 0 and I) involve the bladder mucosa and submucosa; they are treated by endoscopic resection or laser resection. These tumors tend to recur, and the patient must be reexamined every 6 months. *Invasive tumors* (Stages II and III) involve the muscle and/or perivesical fat around the bladder. These tumors are treated with radical cystectomy or with radiation and chemotherapy. Neoadjuvant chemotherapy can improve the survival rate in cases of advanced urothelial cancer. *Metastatic tumors* (Stage IV) from the bladder involve spread to the lymph nodes, bone, or other viscera and are treated with radiation and/or chemotherapy. Treatment by TMN stage is outlined in Table 45.2.

For the majority of bladder tumors, surgical resection is the treatment of choice. Immediate referral to a urologist or surgical oncologist is critical, as well as follow-up with a medical oncologist and/or nephrologist, depending on functional renal status. Intravesical chemotherapy instilled directly into the bladder may prevent recurrence, but radiation therapy for bladder tumors is less effective than the other interventions.

TABLE 45.2 Bladder Tumor Treatment Based on TNM Staging

Stage	Description	Treatment Options	Characteristics
Stage 0	Noninvasive papillary carcinoma (Ta). Cancer has grown from urothelium toward hollow center of bladder but not into connective tissue or muscle of bladder wall. Has not spread to lymph nodes or distant sites.	Transurethral resection (TURBT) followed by close follow-up or immunotherapy with Bacillus Calmette-Guerin	Recurrence is common; follow-up every 6 months 5-year survival rate of 98%
Stage I	Cancer has grown into the layer of connective tissue under the urothelial lining layer but has not reached the muscular layer of the bladder wall. Has not spread to lymph nodes or distant sites.	• TURBT • For high-grade or large tumors, a radical cystectomy is recommended. • If the patient is a poor surgical risk, radiation and chemotherapy are recommended.	5-year survival rate of 88%
Stage II	Cancer has grown into thick muscular layer of bladder wall, but has not passed through the muscle to reach the fatty tissue surrounding the bladder. Has not spread to lymph nodes or distant sites.	Radical or partial cystectomy with lymph node resection. Radiation and chemotherapy may be done pre-operatively to shrink the tumor.	5-year survival rate of 63%
Stage III	Cancer has grown into the fatty tissue surrounding the bladder. May have spread to prostate, uterus, or vagina, but not growing into pelvic or abdominal wall. Has not spread to lymph nodes or distant sites.	• Neoadjuvant chemotherapy to shrink tumor preoperatively. • Radical cystectomy and lymph node resection. • Chemotherapy is usually indicated.	5-year survival rate of 46%
Stage IV	Cancer has grown through the bladder wall and into pelvic or abdominal wall. May have spread to nearby or distant lymph nodes or to sites such as the bones, liver, or lungs.	• Treatment is palliative only. • Systemic chemotherapy and/or radical cystectomy or external beam radiation therapy.	5-year survival rate of 12%-15%

FOLLOW-UP AND REFERRAL

All patients diagnosed with bladder cancer should be referred to a urologist or surgical oncologist for evaluation and treatment. A urinalysis and cystoscopy should be performed every 3 to 6 months because of the significant risk of recurrence of bladder tumors. Patients with invasive or metastatic disease or should be referred to a medical oncologist and possibly a radiation oncologist as well, given that treatment typically involves chemotherapy and/or radiation therapy.

Home health or hospice care may be appropriate for patients who need skilled care and ongoing patient teaching, although less advanced forms of bladder cancer tend to have high cure rates. An ostomy nurse may be necessary for patients who have undergone an ileostomy or urostomy, as a result of surgical resection.

Patient Education: Bladder Tumors

It is critical for clinicians to teach the importance of ongoing follow-up care, given the potential for bladder cancer recurrence and infection of the urinary tract. This includes stressing the preventive measures of not smoking and avoiding chemical carcinogens. The possible development of associated signs and symptoms should also be discussed with patients, including nausea and vomiting, weight loss, anorexia, impotence, sterility, pain, and fatigue. Teaching ileostomy and urostomy care is indicated for patients whose bladders have been surgically removed.

Although many forms of bladder cancer have high cure rates, for terminal patients with advanced disease, death and dying issues need to be addressed and education to improve quality of life is important for both patients and their caregivers. Key emotional and mental states to be addressed include fear, anxiety, grieving, and anticipation, as well as self-image issues (including the potential loss of hair from chemotherapy or skin changes from radiation therapy). The potential loss of one's job is a critical issue for patients, while coping with the possible loss of a loved one is an important consideration for the patient's family.

For additional resources please visit
https://davisedge.fadavis.com/

REFERENCES

Acute Kidney Injury

Durand F, Graupera I, Ginès P, Olson JC, Nadim MK. Pathogenesis of hepatorenal syndrome: Implications for therapy. *Am J Kidney Dis.* 2016;67(2):318–328.

8. RENAL PROBLEMS

Hobson C, Ozrazgat-Baslanti T, Kuxhausen A et al. Cost and mortality associated with postoperative acute kidney injury. *Ann Surg,* 2015;261(6):1207–1214.

Holmes J, Rainer T, Geen J, et al. (2016). Acute kidney injury in the era of the AKI E-Alert. *Clin J Am Soc Nephrol.* 2016;11(12):2123–2131.

Panek R, Tennankore KK, Kiberd BA. Incidence, etiology and significance of acute kidney injury in the early post kidney transplant period. *Clin Transplant.* 2016;30(1):66–70.

Wang AY, Bellomo R, Cass A, et al. Health-related quality of life in survivors of acute kidney injury: The Prolonged Outcomes Study of the Randomized Evaluation of Normal versus Augmented Level Replacement Therapy study outcomes. *Nephrology.* 2015;20(7):492–498.

Bladder Tumors

Baris D, Waddell R, Beane Freeman LE, et al. (2016). Elevated bladder cancer in northern New England: The role of drinking water and arsenic. *J Natl Cancer Inst.* 2016;108(9).

Cumberbatch MG, Cox A, Teare D, et al. Contemporary occupational carcinogen exposure and bladder cancer: A systematic review and meta-analysis. *JAMA Oncol.* 2015;1(9):1282–1290.

National Cancer Institute: Surveillance, Epidemiology, and End Results Program. Cancer stat facts: Bladder cancer. https://seer.cancer.gov/statfacts/html/urinb.html. Accessed October 6, 2017.

National Comprehensive Cancer Network. NCCN Clinical Practice Guidelines in Oncology. Bladder cancer, version 2. http://www.nccn.org/professionals/physician_gls/pdf/bladder.pdf. Published 2016. Accessed October 17, 2017.

Chronic Kidney Disease

Hill NR, Fatoba ST, Oke JL, et al. Global prevalence of chronic kidney disease - A systematic review and meta-analysis. *PLoS One.* 2016;11(7):e0158765.

Ketteler M, Elder GJ, Evenepoel P, et al. Revisiting KDIGO clinical practice guideline on chronic kidney disease—mineral and bone disorder: A commentary from a kidney disease: Improving global outcomes controversies conference. *Kidney Int.* 2015;87(3):502–508.

Levey AS, Becker C, Inker LA. Glomerular filtration rate and albuminuria for detection and staging of acute and chronic kidney disease in adults: A systematic review. *JAMA.* 2015;313(8):837–846.

United States Renal Data System. Chapter 1: CKD in the general population. USRDS annual data report: Epidemiology of kidney disease in the United States. Bethesda, MD: National Institutes of Health, National Institute of Diabetes and Digestive and Kidney Diseases. https://www.usrds.org/2015/view/v1_01.aspx. Published 2015. Accessed October 17, 2017.

Renal Tumors

American Cancer Society. Cancer facts & figures 2017. https://old.cancer.org/acs/groups/content/@editorial/documents/document/acspc-048738.pdf. Accessed October 17, 2017.

Hanske J, Sanchez A, Schmid M, et al. A comparison of 30-day perioperative outcomes in open versus minimally invasive nephroureterectomy for upper tract urothelial carcinoma: Analysis of 896 patients from the American College of Surgeons-National Surgical Quality Improvement Program Database. *J Endourol.* 2015;29 (9):1052–1058

Siefker Radtke AO, Dinney CP, Shen Y, et al. A phase 2 clinical trial of sequential neoadjuvant chemotherapy with ifosfamide, doxorubicin, and gemcitabine followed by cisplatin, gemcitabine, and ifosfamide in locally advanced urothelial cancer. *Cancer.* 2013;119(3):540–547.

RESOURCES

American Cancer Society

Bladder Cancer
    https://www.cancer.org/cancer/bladder-cancer.html
Kidney Cancer
    https://www.cancer.org/cancer/kidney-cancer.html

National Institute of Diabetes and Digestive and Kidney Diseases

Acute Kidney Injury
    https://www.niddk.nih.gov/research-funding/research-programs/acute-kidney-injury
Chronic Kidney Disease
    https://www.niddk.nih.gov/health-information/kidney-disease/chronic-kidney-disease-ckd
Kidney Failure
    https://www.niddk.nih.gov/health-information/kidney-disease/kidney-failure

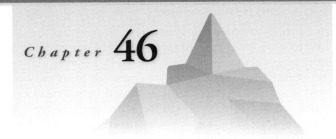

Chapter **46**

Common Reproductive System Complaints

Susan Bulfin, DNP, APRN, FNP-BC

Debera J. Thomas, DNS, RN, FNP/ANP

Brian Oscar Porter, MD, PhD, MPH, MBA

Many patient complaints or issues raised in the primary-care setting relate to the male and female reproductive system. These common complaints associated with a patient's reproductive organs (related to the interplay of genetic and hormonal developmental factors) may be separate and distinct from a patient's gender identity (psychosexual self-identification as male or female) or sexual orientation (sexual attraction to men, women, or both). Thus, the following issues and complaints commonly raised in the primary-care setting may occur in patients regardless of their gender identity or sexual orientation. In addition, transgender individuals may experience these disorders as related to their underlying sexual anatomy, either pre- or postsurgically, if in the process of gender reassignment.

FAMILY PLANNING

Although not necessarily considered a patient complaint in the primary setting, one of women's primary health concerns from menarche to menopause is prevention of unintended pregnancy, otherwise known as *family planning*. The rate of unintended pregnancy in the United States is around 45% of all pregnancies (Centers for Disease Control [CDC], 2016). The decision to pursue pregnancy and regulate its timing is related to one's values; professional goals; personal, cultural, and religious beliefs; self-perception; health status; economics; social and family support; sexual lifestyle; accessible reproductive options; and partner status. Ideally, birth control options should be affordable, easy to use, easy to obtain, safe and effective, and acceptable for users and their partners. Women who want to have children in the future also need to consider whether the method is reversible. Popular birth control methods include intrauterine devices, oral contraceptive pills (OCPs), Depo-Provera injections, barrier methods such as the diaphragm and condoms, and sterilization.

Although preventing pregnancy is a major concern with sexual activity, some sexual practices also increase the risk of acquiring a sexually transmitted infection (STI). To control both pregnancy and disease, routine health care is important, and a thorough gynecological history and physical evaluation are essential to address both issues.

The gynecological history reviews risks for STIs, as well as any past and current use of birth control methods, and identifies needs for health promotion. A thorough history also identifies sexual dysfunction or sexual concerns. Reviewing anatomy and physiology with the patient may help her understand her body and result in healthier lifestyle choices. Other items important in history taking include menstrual cycle information (including the date of the last menstrual period), age at menarche, change in menses, number of sexual partners in the past year and lifetime, age at first sexual encounter, presence of dyspareunia, history of STIs, medications used, results of previous cervical cancer screening tests and resolution of any cervical abnormalities, as well as cigarette, drug, and/or alcohol use or abuse. It is important to obtain a basic health history as well to identify potential contraindications to new or previous birth control methods. A helpful guide for this determination is the U.S. medical eligibility criteria (U.S. MEC) for contraceptive use, 2016. The U.S. MEC uses categories 1 to 4 to classify hormonal contraceptives and IUDs for use in women with particular conditions.

- Category 1: There are no restrictions for the use of the contraceptive method.
- Category 2: The advantages of using the method outweigh the possible risks.
- Category 3: The risks of using the method outweigh the advantages.
- Category 4: Use of the contraceptive method is unacceptable.

The charts and tables available from the CDC are easy to use and invaluable to the clinician.

Wording questions during history taking in a nonjudgmental, supportive, accepting manner enables the patient to be open and honest in an area of great sensitivity and possible emotional pain. The clinician should address areas of concern, such as poor body image, depression, poor nutrition, emotional or physical problems, myths, domestic violence or sexual abuse, smoking, obesity, alcohol or drug abuse, and family problems.

A well-woman assessment includes a physical examination, blood pressure measurement, weight, and height. Breast examination, bimanual pelvic examination, and cervical cancer screening may be performed according to current recommendations for the patient's age and pertinent risk factors. The American College of Obstetrics and Gynecology in its Women's Preventive Services Initiative recommends the following schedule for routine cervical cancer screening in average-risk women:

- Ages of 21 and 29 years: Every 3 years using cervical cytology (papanicolaou [Pap] test). The use of human papillomavirus (HPV) testing in women younger than 30 years is not currently recommended.
- Ages 30 to 65 years: A Pap test and cervical HPV testing should be done every 5 years in women or Pap test alone every 3 years.
- Older than 65 years who have had three consecutive negative Pap test results: No screening.

These recommendations do not apply to women at higher risk for cervical cancer such as those infected with HIV or who are immunocompromised, women exposed to diethylstilbestrol in utero, or women treated in the past 20 years for cervical intraepithelial neoplasia Grade 2 or higher. Testing for STIs and other infections may also be indicated based on the patient's risk factors and presenting information.

Some health-care facilities require signed consent forms for the birth control method selected to ensure the patient has been given, in writing, full information on the use, risks, benefits, and follow-up needs of the particular method. Other facilities educate the patient at the time of the visit and give her the product insert and educational material to read at home. Ideally, the patient and her sexual partner(s), if possible, need comprehensive information on birth control methods so that the choice is an educated decision based on their lifestyle and needs. The success or failure of a birth control method depends on the woman's motivation, adherence, partner support, consistency, and comfort of use with the form of contraception. The most common contraceptive methods are listed in Figure 46.1 and are discussed in detail in the following sections.

INTRAUTERINE DEVICE

The *intrauterine device* (IUD) is a highly effective (greater than 99%), reversible contraceptive method. An IUD may be inserted by a clinician trained in the procedure at any time during the menstrual cycle in a nonpregnant woman. The contraceptive mechanism of action of an IUD is not completely understood, but it is believed to act either as a spermicide or to have inhibitory effects on sperm capacitation and transport. However, an IUD is not an abortifacient, and contrary to previous thought, nulliparity is not a contraindication to IUD use.

Several IUDs are available in the United States that slowly release levonorgestrel (e.g., Mirena, Skyla, Liletta, Kyleena). The Copper T-380A IUD is also available. A 6- to 8-week wait is customary postpartum before insertion of an IUD, although an IUD may be safely inserted immediately postpartum. An IUD has two long, off-white monofilament tails that project from the cervix into the vagina. The patient should be instructed to check for this string after each menstrual period to ensure the IUD is still in place. A visual inspection of the cervix and bimanual pelvic examination are performed before insertion to check for abnormalities. STI testing may be done in women who have risk factors.

If a levonorgestrel-releasing IUD is inserted within 7 days of the start of the menstrual period, no backup contraceptive method is needed; for insertions after day 7 of the start of menses, a backup method should be used for a minimum of 7 days. In contrast, the copper IUD requires no form of backup contraception. Mirena and Kyleena are effective for about 5 years, whereas Skyla and Liletta for about 3 years and the Copper T-380A for up to 10 years. The CDC's U.S. selected practice recommendations for contraceptive use, 2016 provides excellent guidance for the use of IUDs and all forms of contraception.

Side Effects

Adverse effects of the copper IUD include heavier menstrual periods, bleeding between periods, and increased menstrual pain. These side effects often lessen or go away completely within 1 year. With the levonorgestrel IUDs, bleeding may be unpredictable for the first few months of use. One-third of patients using Mirena and Kyleena and a small number of patients using the other levonorgestrel IUDs will have amenorrhea after the first year of use. Spontaneous expulsion of the IUD occurs in 2% to 10% of patients during the first year of use, but the expulsion rate is higher when the IUD is inserted immediately after childbirth (10% to 25%). There is a slightly increased risk of pelvic infection in the first month after insertion of an IUD, although there does not appear to be any greater risk of infection other than that of acquiring a new STI. If a patient wants to become pregnant while using an IUD, the device can be removed with no effect on fertility.

Contraindications

There are few absolute contraindications for the use of an IUD. They include pregnancy, a distorted uterine cavity, unexplained vaginal bleeding, pelvic tuberculosis, cervical or endometrial cancer, malignant trophoblastic disease, acute pelvic inflammatory disease (PID), post septic abortion, postpartum sepsis, and purulent cervicitis. In

Effectiveness of Family Planning Methods

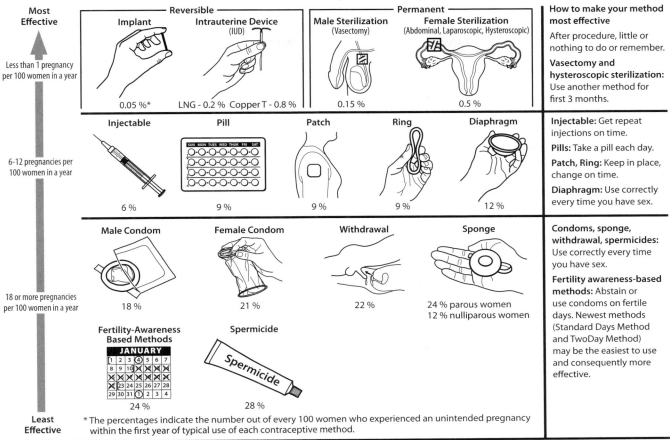

	Reversible		Permanent		How to make your method most effective

Most Effective

Less than 1 pregnancy per 100 women in a year

Implant 0.05 %*

Intrauterine Device (IUD) LNG - 0.2 % Copper T - 0.8 %

Male Sterilization (Vasectomy) 0.15 %

Female Sterilization (Abdominal, Laparoscopic, Hysteroscopic) 0.5 %

How to make your method most effective

After procedure, little or nothing to do or remember.

Vasectomy and hysteroscopic sterilization: Use another method for first 3 months.

6-12 pregnancies per 100 women in a year

Injectable 6 %

Pill 9 %

Patch 9 %

Ring 9 %

Diaphragm 12 %

Injectable: Get repeat injections on time.

Pills: Take a pill each day.

Patch, Ring: Keep in place, change on time.

Diaphragm: Use correctly every time you have sex.

18 or more pregnancies per 100 women in a year

Male Condom 18 %

Female Condom 21 %

Withdrawal 22 %

Sponge 24 % parous women / 12 % nulliparous women

Condoms, sponge, withdrawal, spermicides: Use correctly every time you have sex.

Fertility awareness-based methods: Abstain or use condoms on fertile days. Newest methods (Standard Days Method and TwoDay Method) may be the easiest to use and consequently more effective.

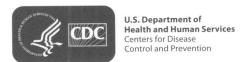

Fertility-Awareness Based Methods 24 %

Spermicide 28 %

Least Effective

* The percentages indicate the number out of every 100 women who experienced an unintended pregnancy within the first year of typical use of each contraceptive method.

CS 242797

U.S. Department of Health and Human Services
Centers for Disease Control and Prevention

CONDOMS SHOULD ALWAYS BE USED TO REDUCE THE RISK OF SEXUALLY TRANSMITTED INFECTIONS.
Other Methods of Contraception

Lactational Amenorrhea Method: LAM is a highly effective, temporary method of contraception.
Emergency Contraception: Emergency contraceptive pills or a copper IUD after unprotected intercourse substantially reduces risk of pregnancy.

Adapted from World Health Organization (WHO) Department of Reproductive Health and Research, Johns Hopkins Bloomberg School of Public Health/Center for Communication Programs (CCP). Knowledge for health project. Family planning: a global handbook for providers (2011 update). Baltimore, MD; Geneva, Switzerland: CCP and WHO; 2011; and Trussell J. Contraceptive failure in the United States. Contraception 2011;83:397–404.

Figure 46.1 Methods of birth control. Source: *Centers for Disease Control and Prevention. Adapted from World Health Organization (WHO) Department of Reproductive Health and Research, Johns Hopkins Bloomberg. School of Public Health/Center for Communication Programs (CCP). Knowledge for health project. Family planning: A global handbook for providers (2011 update). Baltimore, MD; Geneva, Switzerland: CCP and WHO; 2011; Trussell J. Contraceptive failure in the United States. Contraception. 2011;83:397–404.*

addition, women with breast cancer should not use a levonorgestrel-releasing IUD.

ETONOGESTREL IMPLANT

The progestin-only etonogestrel (ENG) implant (Implanon) is a highly effective (greater than 99%), flexible, 4-cm single rod inserted subdermally in the upper arm. The implant releases 60 to 70 mcg per day in weeks 5 to 6 postimplantation and gradually decreases to approximately 25 to 30 mcg per day at the end of the third year. The implant can be inserted at any time if the woman is not pregnant. Backup contraception should be used if insertion occurs after day 5 of the start of menses. Risks

outweigh benefits for women with the following conditions: cirrhosis, liver tumors, systemic lupus erythematosus, and unexplained vaginal bleeding. Use of the implant is contraindicated in women with breast cancer.

COMBINED ORAL CONTRACEPTIVE PILLS

OCPs contain either a combination of estrogen and progestin or progestin only (commonly called the "mini-pill"; discussed subsequently). The most popular OCPs are the 4-week cycle combination pills. Combination OCPs have a failure rate of 0.3% when used correctly, while the failure rate is 8% typical use, due to some degree of nonadherence to prescribed usage instructions.

The combination OCPs are taken each day for 3 weeks, with inert (placebo) pills taken during the fourth week. During the nonhormonal (fourth) week, withdrawal uterine bleeding occurs. Combination extended cycle OCPs contain 84 active and 7 inert pills (Seasonale, Seasonique, LoSeasonique) and result in menses only every 3 months (four times a year). Ethinyl estradiol (EE) and levonorgestrel (Amethyst, Aviane, Falmina, Levlen, Orsythia, Vienva) is a combination OCP that is taken 365 days a year and results in no menstruation.

Combination estrogen-progestin OCPs are classed as monophasic, biphasic, triphasic, and quadraphasic and contain different doses of hormones during the month and all suppress ovulation, thereby preventing pregnancy. Estrogen in the pill inhibits implantation of the egg by altering normal maturation of the uterine lining, while the progestins in the pill slow ovum transport and uterine motility. Progestins also cause the cervical mucus to become thick and scanty, slowing sperm transport and capacitation. In addition, the pH of the genital tract is altered, and the cervical and uterine environment becomes hostile to sperm.

EE is currently the most popular estrogen used in OCPs in the United States. The progestins currently used include desogestrel (in Mircette, Cyclessa, Ortho-Cept, Desogen), levonorgestrel (in Alesse, Nordette, Seasonale, Trivora, Triphasil), norethindrone (in Estrostep, Norinyl 1/35, Ortho-Novum 1/35 and 7/7/7, Necon 1/35, Modicon, Ovcon 35, Loestrin 1.5/30, Tri-Norinyl), norgestimate (in Ortho-Cyclen, Ortho-TriCyclen), drospirenone (in Yasmin), and *dl*-norgestrel (in Lo-Ovral, Low-Ogestrel).

All progestins, even in low doses, offer excellent cycle control and minimal metabolic changes. Progestins have variable estrogenic, androgenic, and progestational effects. The third generation progestins (desogestrel, drospirenone, norgestimate) are the least androgenic and are preferred for women with acne or hirsutism. However, there have been studies with conflicting results that suggest that women taking a contraceptive containing drospirenone are at a 1.5-fold increased risk for developing blood clots.

The amounts of estrogen and progestin in combined OCPs have been greatly reduced since their inception. The lower the effective dose, the lower the rate of adverse effects; the lowest acceptable dose is guided by the ability of the pill to prevent breakthrough bleeding, which is an undesirable adverse event. Estrogen content is usually 20 to 35 mcg of EE per tablet, with no more than 50 mcg in formulations available in the United States. Progestin content ranges from 0.1 to 3 mg. Both the estrogen and progestin doses may either be constant in a cycle pack (with monophasic contraceptives) or variable (with multiphasic contraceptives). The ratio of estrogen to progestin in combination pills can range from 1:5 or 1:50; most commonly, the ratio is 1:10 to 1:30. In a normal menstrual cycle, the ratio is 1:10 (early follicular phase), 1:5 (preovulation phase), or 1:30 (luteal phase). Multiphasic OCPs are used to replicate these hormonal ratios; however, they may be associated with a higher incidence of breakthrough bleeding than monophasic pills.

Eligibility Criteria for Combined Oral Contraception

In the presence of certain medical conditions, the risks associated with combined oral contraception are considered unacceptable or outweigh it benefits. These conditions include current breast cancer, being less than 21 days postpartum, severe cirrhosis of the liver, current or past history of deep vein thrombosis (DVT), major surgery with prolonged immobilization, vascular disease, having diabetes mellitus for more than 20 years, diabetic retinopathy, and a history of migraine with aura. Other conditions in which risks typically outweigh the advantages of the use of OCPs include a history of breast cancer with no disease for 5 years, a low risk for DVT, or OCP-related cholestasis.

Instructions for use of OCPs

OCPs should be started either with the onset of menses (same-day start) or on the first Sunday of the week in which menses starts (Sunday start). With a Sunday start, a backup contraceptive method (e.g., condom or abstinence) should be used for at least 7 days, unless Sunday is the first day of menses.

The effectiveness of OCPs is dependent on patient adherence. Each pill must be taken at the same hour every day. Once the start date is established and the pack is started, there is no waiting needed or menstrual impact in starting the subsequent pack. As soon as the initial pack is completed, the next pack is started on the next day. Patients may need suggestions as to how to take the pill on time and every day, whether it is when brushing teeth, at mealtime, or at bedtime—as long as it is at the same hour, every day. For women who experience nausea when taking OCPs, taking them at bedtime can minimize this adverse effect.

Combination OCPs are provided in 28-day pill packs, color coded by dose and time, which include 21 active and 7 inert tablets. Some manufacturers include iron supplements in the 7 inert (placebo) pills, while some eliminate the 7 inert pills and provide simply a 21-day pack. To keep a patient adherent and on time, it is usually best to recommend the habit of taking one pill a day, without stopping for the last 7 days, to prevent forgetting when to restart again.

Missed doses of OCPs

If the patient forgets to take one or more doses of OCPs, the following guidelines are recommended:

- One dose late (less than 24 hours) or one missed (24 to 48 hours): Take the missed dose as soon as remembered and then the next dose at the usual time. No additional contraception is needed.

- Two or more doses (more than 48 hours): Take the missed dose as soon as possible and discard any other missed pills and continue taking the remaining pills at the regular time. Use a backup form of birth control or avoid sexual intercourse until the remaining pills have been taken for 7 consecutive days. If the OCP was missed in the last week of the hormone containing pills (days 15 to 21), then omit the hormone-free interval and begin the next new cycle. If unable to start a new pack, then backup contraception should be used until the new pack has been taken for 7 consecutive days. Emergency contraception should be considered if the dose was missed in the first week of the cycle and unprotected sex occurred in the 5 days prior.

Some patients experience breakthrough bleeding with missed pills or the doubling of pills. Some practitioners do not advocate using the methods outlined here but instead tell their patients to discontinue the pack, use a barrier method, and restart with a new pack when regular menses begins. If menses does not occur as usual, a pregnancy test must be performed.

Special Considerations With OCPs

Patients need special instructions when starting OCPs if they had a recent full-term delivery, are nursing, had a recent abortion or miscarriage, have infrequent or irregular menses, or are using other medications. Many patients inquire about starting or restarting OCPs postpartum. The U.S. Food and Drug Administration (FDA) package insert indicates that because the postpartum period lends itself to a higher risk of thromboembolism, OCPs should be started no earlier than 4 to 6 weeks after delivery in nonnursing mothers. Ovulation rarely takes place before 4 weeks postpartum of a full-term pregnancy; however, if a patient is using drugs (e.g., bromocriptine [Parlodel]) to suppress lactation, ovulation may occur earlier, so she will need an additional form of contraception before initiating OCPs.

Similarly, many patients who are breastfeeding inquire about starting on OCPs. Because estrogen decreases the amount and quality of breast milk, OCPs are not recommended for lactating women. Conversely, progestins promote breast milk production, so progestin-only OCPs may be used in women who are breastfeeding and desire contraception. However, combination estrogen and progestin oral contraceptives should not be prescribed until at least 6 weeks postpartum.

Because ovulation is a possibility within 14 days after either a recent abortion or miscarriage, OCPs should be started either immediately or no later than 7 days after a first-trimester (5 to 13 weeks) abortion. After a midtrimester abortion, OCPs should be started in the same manner as after a full-term pregnancy. If a patient is not pregnant (as confirmed by a pregnancy test), OCPs may be started at any time, with backup contraception used throughout the first cycle of pills. If OCPs are started within 5 days of normal menses, no backup contraceptive method is necessary. In women with amenorrhea or infrequent menstrual cycles, discontinuation of OCPs may cause anovulatory or fully amenorrheic if their history includes secondary amenorrhea, oligomenorrhea, or irregular menstrual cycles. These patients should therefore consider another method of birth control.

Noncontraceptive Benefits of OCPs

The combination OCPs are an effective reversible form of birth control, relatively inexpensive, and the least invasive method of correcting painful and irregular menstrual cycles. Additional benefits include reduced blood loss resulting in a lower incidence of anemia, less risk of ectopic pregnancy and salpingitis, fewer ovarian cysts, reduction in dysmenorrhea, reduction in risk of ovarian and endometrial cancer, improvement in acne, decreased risk of developing myomas in long-term (greater than 4 years) users, and a beneficial effect on bone mass. These benefits reduce the need for costly hospitalizations. In addition, excessive facial and body hair is often reduced in OCP users, although hair loss is not usually related to OCP use and should be referred to a dermatologist for evaluation.

Adverse Effects of OCPs

If a woman taking OCPs complains of any of the adverse effects typically associated with OCPs (e.g., nausea, abdominal bloating, hair changes, weight gain, leg pain, cramps, swelling), switching the patient to a pill with a lower estrogen dose or one with a less androgenic progestin formulation will often relieve the problem. Although switching to a lower estrogen dose or different progestin component may relieve abdominal bloating, bowel irregularity can also cause bloating and should be evaluated. If a patient complains of nausea, she should be instructed to take the pill with food or at bedtime. If the nausea or bloating persists or worsens, the patient may need to consult a gastroenterologist.

The benefits and safety of OCPs are dependent on adherence but are also affected by other factors such as smoking. There is an increased risk of cardiovascular disease and thromboembolic disease in women who are older than 35 years and who smoke more than 15 cigarettes a day while taking OCPs. Women older than 40 years who are nonsmokers may safely continue low-dose OCPs. The use of OCPs is safest throughout the menstrual lifetime of women who are of normal weight, are nonsmokers, have normal blood pressure and cholesterol levels, do not have diabetes mellitus, and have no family history of heart disease.

The Nurses' Health Study, Nurses' Health Study II, and the Women's Health Initiative are long-term prospective studies examining the effects of OCPs and menopausal hormone therapy on cardiovascular risk, thromboembolic risk, and cancer risk. These studies generated safety data demonstrating that OCPs have a wide range of adverse effects. Overall, the constant presence of low-level hormones creates a pregnancy-like environment in the female body. Thyroid hormone and cortisol levels may be elevated, progestins may alter the lipid profile, and estrogens can decrease glucose tolerance (thus, women with diabetes mellitus should be monitored closely if using OCPs). Estrogen-related increases in clotting factors result in an increased risk of thromboembolism; thus, women who will be undergoing surgery and postoperative bed confinement should discontinue OCPs at least 4 weeks before surgery.

The risk of developing hypertension in OCP users increases with the duration of use and in older women. If a woman develops hypertension while taking OCPs, the pills should be stopped and another form of contraception adopted. However, if a woman is younger than 40 years, does not smoke, and has mild hypertension that is controlled with medication, OCPs may be used as long as blood pressure is closely monitored. The use of OCPs is not recommended in women with a history of migraines with aura because OCPs can precipitate migraine or vascular headaches or make existing migraines worse. Another form of contraception should be used if headaches increase in severity or frequency.

Women taking OCPs (particularly pills with 50 mcg or more of estrogen) are at a higher risk of myocardial infarction. The risk is further increased in women who smoke, are obese, have hypertension, diabetes mellitus, or hyperlipidemia. Similarly, the risk of thromboembolic disease is increased in women taking OCPs, particularly formulations that are higher in estrogen. Leg pain, cramps, and swelling usually disappear after three cycle packs, but severe extremity pain, especially if unilateral, can indicate a thrombosis and requires immediate discontinuation of the OCP and rapid medical evaluation.

Other adverse effects of OCP use are an increased risk of cervical dysplasia and cancer in long-term (greater than 5 years) users who have also had persistent cervical HPV infection. There is some evidence that there is a higher incidence of benign liver tumors or gallstones conferred by OCPs, which is usually associated with higher hormonal dosages, longer-term use, and older patient ages. It is unclear whether OCPs contribute to breast cancer. FDA packaging inserts imply an association related to duration of use and medical history. Fibrocystic breast discomfort has been found to be less frequent in OCP users. Breast swelling and tenderness are common premenstrual complaints, and low-dose OCPs seem to decrease this complaint, as does reducing caffeine intake, avoiding smoking, and reducing sodium intake.

Because the cervical mucus is affected by the progestin component in OCPs and estrogen can cause cervical mucorrhea, it is not uncommon for OCP users to experience mucus-generating irritations of the genital tract, including *Candida* infections of the vagina and vulva. Antibiotic therapy may also cause this condition.

Patients who use OCPs may have increased pigmentation of the face and forehead. Combination pill users find this in the areola and perineum as well. Weight gain may or may not be an OCP effect; it may be simply overeating, lack of exercise, fluid retention, thyroid problems, or poor nutrition, but a gain of 2 to 5 pounds is not uncommon. To metabolize OCPs properly, certain vitamins are needed as micronutrients, which may not be effectively stored in the body. Thus, women should be instructed to take a daily multivitamin and vitamin C supplements while taking OCPs to prevent deficiency of these nutrients.

Discontinuing Use of OCPs

When combination OCPs are discontinued, 90% of women resume ovulation and menses within 3 months. A pregnancy test should be done to ensure the patient is not pregnant if normal cycles are not established after 3 months. If a woman does not wish to become pregnant, another form of contraception should be used when OCPs are discontinued. If a woman becomes pregnant while using OCPs, most studies show no increased incidence of congenital birth defects. However, it is best not to use OCPs if a patient suspects she is pregnant but rather use another method of birth control until a state of pregnancy is established or not.

CONTRACEPTIVE PATCH

The *transdermal contraceptive patch* (Xulane) is a highly effective form of combined hormonal contraception and has potential advantages over OCPs. Because the transdermal delivery bypasses the liver, there is no first-pass hepatic metabolism and lower doses of hormones are possible. With the patch, hormone levels are constant without peaks and troughs. In addition, because the patch is applied once every 7 days, compliance is enhanced.

The patch contains EE and norelgestromin and is applied weekly. About 20 to 35 mcg of EE and 150 mcg of norelgestromin are released from the patch on a daily basis. Since it is a combined hormonal contraceptive, the mechanism of action is the same as that of OCPs. The effectiveness is 99% if used perfectly and 91% in typical use, although obesity decreases the effectiveness of the patch.

Eligibility and Contraindications for Use

Because the patch is a combined hormonal contraceptive, the eligibility criteria for its use are the same as that for OCPs. The contraindications to the contraceptive patch are also the same as those for combined OCPs: history of thromboembolism, an estrogen-dependant tumor, or abnormal liver function. In addition, if a woman has sensitive skin or exfoliative dermatitis, she may not be a candidate for the patch. Some women may experience skin sensitivity to any component of the transdermal system and should not use the patch.

Instructions for Use of the Patch

The patch should be initiated on either the first day of menses or the Sunday following the start of menses; however, if the Sunday start is 5 days after the beginning of menses, then an additional form of contraception (condom) is suggested for the first 7 days.

The patient should be instructed to apply the patch to the buttock, abdomen, upper arm, or upper torso, but avoiding the breast. The patch should be changed in 7 days and at the same time and the old patch removed and the new patch applied to a different site. It is important to inform the patient that lotions should not be used at the site of the patch and an occlusive dressing cannot be used at the patch site. The patch is changed every 7 days for 3 weeks and then is followed by a patch-free week.

If there is a delay in removing and replacing the patch during the second or third patch cycle, the woman should apply a new patch as soon as possible. If the new patch is applied within 48 hours of the patch day, there is an adequate release of hormones and the patch change day can remain the same. If it is after this 48-hour time period, the day that she remembers and applies a new patch becomes the new patch day, and either avoid intercourse or use a backup contraceptive method for 7 days following the application. If a patch becomes detached for less than 24 hours, it can be reapplied to the same location; however, if it has lost its stickiness, it cannot be used. If it is less than 24 hours, a new patch can be applied in the event that the original patch is no longer adhesive. If the patch is detached for longer than 24 hours, then a new patch should be applied and this then becomes the new patch change day and an additional form of contraception should be used for the next 7 days.

Adverse Effects of the Patch

As with OCPs, the transdermal patch has similar adverse effects particularly on coagulation factors. Although both OCPs and the patch have an increased risk of venous thromboembolitic events (VTE), patch users have a higher risk over OCP users. In particular, women with diabetes have a VTE risk greater with the patch than with OCPs. This is attributed to the higher overall EE concentrations with the patch because it is not metabolized by the liver on the first pass.

Side Effects of the Patch

There may be breakthrough bleeding in the first two cycles after initiating the patch. This is very common. The most commonly reported side effects were breast tenderness, headache, application site reactions, nausea, and dysmenorrhea but less than 2% discontinued use of the patch because of these side effects.

CONTRACEPTIVE VAGINAL RING

The *contraceptive vaginal ring* (NuvaRing) is a combined hormonal contraceptive containing both estrogen and progestin and has the same benefits as OCPs and the transdermal patch but has the advantage that it is left in place for 3 weeks. Like the patch, it also has the advantage of consistent hormone release without peaks and troughs but rather peaks immediately after insertion and has a slow decrease over the 3-week cycle. Also, there is not first-pass loss in the liver because it is absorbed vaginally so the EE concentration is lower than with OCPs.

The contraceptive vaginal ring is a flexible ring measuring 54 mm in diameter and 4 mm in cross section.

The ring releases 15 mcg of EE and 120 mcg of ENG per day. The mechanism of action is the same as the other combined hormonal contraceptives with the addition of thickening the cervical mucus and preventing the penetration of sperm. The ring has the same effectiveness rating at the patch, 99% if used perfectly and 91% in typical use. Several medication decrease the effectiveness of the ring: Rifampin, Rifampicin and Rifamate, Griseofulvin, certain HIV medications, and the herb St. John's wort.

Eligibility and Contraindications for Use

Because the ring is a combined hormonal contraceptive, the eligibility criteria for its use are the same as that for OCPs and the transdermal patch and outlined by the CDC.

Instructions for Use of the Ring

The patient should be instructed to insert the ring on the first day of menses, but some women will not like the idea of insertion while they have their period. Alternatively, the ring can be inserted at any point during their cycle provided there is no possibility they could be pregnant. This is referred to as the quick start method. Backup contraception should be used for the first 7 days if the ring is not inserted within the first 5 days of menses.

Insertion of the ring is similar to insertion of a diaphragm. The woman should be in a comfortable position and have the sides of the ring pressed together and insert it into the vagina as high as possible. The higher the insertion, the less likely of discomfort or the ring falling out. The ring is left in position for 3 weeks and then removed. During the 3 weeks, the woman should be instructed to periodically check to be sure the ring is still in place. After one ring-free week, a new ring is inserted on the same day of the week and time that the old ring was removed. If the ring is left in place for more than 3 weeks but less than 5 weeks, it should be removed and a new one inserted after a week ring-free interval to allow for withdrawal bleeding. If the ring is left in place for longer than 5 weeks, then backup contraception should be used until the new ring has been in place for 7 days.

If the ring is removed or falls out, it can be rinsed in cool water and reinserted within 3 hours. If the ring is out of the vagina for more than 3 hours and it is during the first 2 weeks of the cycle, the ring can be reinserted as soon as possible, and backup contraception should be used until it has been in place for 7 days. If the removal occurs during week 3 of the cycle, it should be discarded and instruct the patient either to insert a new ring and begin the 3-week cycle with backup contraception for 7 days or wait 7 days and insert a new ring, using backup contraception during the ring-free week and for 7 days after the insertion of the new ring. Fertility is restored rapidly with the median time to ovulation at 19 days.

Adverse Effects of the Ring

The adverse effects of the ring are the same as those for OCPs. There may be a slight increase in VTE risk in ring users, but there is little evidence.

Side Effects of the Ring

The side effects of the ring are the same as the other forms of hormonal contraception with the addition of local vaginal symptoms such as vaginitis, increased wetness and leukorrhea.

PROGESTIN-ONLY PILL

The progestin-only pill (or "mini-pill") contains progestin exclusively and has a reported failure rate of 1% to 4%—slightly higher than that of combined OCPs. Progestin-only pills contain either 0.35 mg of norethindrone (Ortho Micronor, Nor-QD) or 0.075 mg of *dl*-norgestrel (Ovrette) and are taken continuously, beginning on the first day of the menstrual cycle. The progestin inhibits ovulation inconsistently but causes thickening of the cervical mucus (creating a hostile environment for sperm), alters ovum transport (leading to a higher risk of ectopic pregnancy), and inhibits implantation. The advantages of the mini-pill are that it is safe during lactation and may increase the flow of milk; it can be used in women older than 35 years; it can be used in women with sickle cell disease; and it can be used in women with myomas. The progestin-only pill is less likely than combination OCPs to cause headaches, high blood pressure, depression, cramps, premenstrual syndrome, or elevations in glucose.

Disadvantages of the mini-pill include contraceptive failure and ectopic pregnancy. Irregular menstrual bleeding (e.g., amenorrhea, breakthrough bleeding, prolonged flow) is common in progestin-only users and may necessitate frequent pregnancy tests. Absolute contraindications include pregnancy and breast cancer. Conditions in which the risks of progestin-only OCPs typically outweigh their benefits include having cirrhosis of the liver, diabetes mellitus for more than 20 years, diabetic retinopathy, nephropathy, neuropathy, vascular or cardiovascular disease, a history of stroke, and unexplained vaginal bleeding.

MEDROXYPROGESTERONE ACETATE INJECTIONS

Depot medroxyprogesterone acetate (DMPA) is available in several long-acting forms of contraception. Depo-Provera injectable consists of deep intramuscular (IM) injections of 150 mg, whereas Depo-SubQ Provera 104 consists of subcutaneous injections of 104 mg. Each type of injection is given every 3 months. These injections have efficacy rates of 94% to 99.7%. The initial injection is typically given on day 5 of menses but may be given at any time if the woman is not pregnant (including immediately postpartum). If the injection is given after day 7 of the start of menses, the woman needs to abstain from intercourse or use a backup method of birth control for 7 days following the injection. If a woman wishes to become pregnant, she should be counseled that it may take an average of 9 to 10 months for fertility to return after stopping the injections.

Use of DMPA is contraindicated if the woman is pregnant or has breast cancer. Risks outweigh advantages for use of DMPA for the following conditions: undiagnosed vaginal bleeding, current breast cancer, thromboembolic disorders, cerebrovascular disease, hepatic tumors (benign or malignant), active hepatic disease, papilledema, retinal vascular lesions, and sudden onset vision loss. Risks outweigh benefits in patients with a history of breast cancer; diabetic nephropathy, retinopathy, or neuropathy; ischemic heart disease; liver tumors; multiple risk factors for atherosclerotic cardiovascular disease; severe hypertension (persistent values of 160/100 mm Hg or more); diabetes mellitus with vascular involvement; and systemic lupus erythematosus with positive antiphospholipid antibodies or severe thrombocytopenia. The use of DMPA is associated with an increase in weight and percent body fat over that of OCP. In 2004, the FDA issued a "Black Box" warning on the long-term use of DMPA because of the possibility of loss of bone mineral density. However, there is no research to indicate any increase in fracture risk later in life, and the World Health Organization concluded that there is no reason for restriction of use in women aged 18 to 45 years.

BARRIER METHODS

Barrier methods include male and female condoms, the diaphragm, and cervical cap. Some barrier methods have the dual advantage of preventing pregnancy and STIs. The most common STIs are caused by herpes simplex virus, HPV, HIV, *Neisseria gonorrhoeae*, and *Chlamydia*. Preventing HPV infection also reduces the risk of cervical cancer. Adverse effects and challenges with the use of barrier methods include messiness, handling of the genitalia, precoital interruption of spontaneity, and allergy or contact dermatitis to component materials or lubricants. In turn, the use of barrier methods requires motivation on the part of both partners. Condom use is promoted based more on the general principles of preventing sexually transmitted infections rather than on epidemiological data because protection against HPV transmission is not 100% effective. HPV can be found in many genital areas (e.g., genital tract skin and mucous membranes). Hence, condoms do not protect the vulva from microscopic HPV particles on the skin.

Male Condom

The *male condom* is the most common barrier method of contraception and is most effective at preventing pregnancy when combined with a spermicide such as non-oxynol-9. However, condoms containing nonoxynol-9 have not been shown to reduce the rate of STI transmission, and some studies have demonstrated higher rates of HIV transmission associated with nonoxynol-9 use in condoms, which is associated with an increased risk of vaginal lesions. Thus, the World Health Organization currently recommends that nonoxynol-9 not be used by women at high risk of HIV infection.

Condoms are available in various sizes, colors, flavors, strengths, and states of lubrication. The tip should extend one-half inch beyond the penis to collect the ejaculate. Care must be taken during withdrawal of the penis to prevent the condom from coming off and spilling the semen. Other adverse effects include irritation, allergic reactions, unfavorable oral sex, and accidental breakage of the condom. With typical use, failure rates for condoms used without spermicide are approximately 18%, and when used with a spermicide, the contraceptive failure rate is equivalent to that of OCPs. However, condoms may not be the best contraceptive choice for people younger than 25 years because of noncompliance, inconsistent use, and low motivation in this age-group. Note, however, that these considerations regarding contraceptive effectiveness are separate from requirements for STI prevention because barrier methods are the most effective means of preventing transmission of sexually acquired infections.

Female Condom

The *female condom* is a device that is disposable and made of seamless polyurethane. It fits loosely inside the vagina and covers the perineum. There are flexible rims on both ends. The inner rim sits on the closed end and is compressed for placement into the vagina over the cervix, which prevents direct contact with bodily secretions. The condom is soft, lubricated by spermicide, relatively inexpensive, and may be purchased over the counter. However, many patients state that it is difficult to use. Adverse effects include irritation and allergic reactions. The failure rate of the female condom is 5% (perfect use) to 21% (typical use) and comparable to the efficacy of the diaphragm. Perfect use refers to the use prescribed for research subjects, and typical use is everyday use by regular people.

Diaphragm

A *diaphragm* is a latex hemisphere with a flexible rim that fits over the cervix. The failure rate is 6% (perfect use) to 12% (typical use) when used with spermicidal jelly. This method allows the woman control over contraceptive decision making and has no systemic side effects. The largest size that covers the cervix comfortably is best. Once the device has been fitted, the patient should insert and remove the diaphragm, and then return for a recheck after 1 week of practice while using a backup contraceptive method. Before insertion, one teaspoon of spermicide is placed in the cup and a small amount is spread around the rim. The diaphragm must be left in place for 6 hours after intercourse; if additional intercourse is desired, additional spermicide must be inserted into the vagina. The diaphragm should not be left in place for more than 24 hours. There is a new single size contoured diaphragm (Caya) now available in the United States. Instead of the metal rim typically found in diaphragms, the Caya uses a nylon rim that is more comfortable and flexible. Although Caya fits most women who have used 65- to 80-mm diaphragms, a test fit should be done for women who have never been fitted for a diaphragm.

Once removed, the diaphragm is washed with a mild soap, dried, and stored. Before the diaphragm is used again, it should be held up to the light to check for holes, tears, and breaks. The patient should be instructed to urinate before inserting and after removing the diaphragm to reduce the risk of urinary tract infections (UTIs). Under normal circumstances, the diaphragm is fitted during the annual gynecological visit; however, if the patient has pelvic surgery, pregnancy, or a weight change of 10 to 20 pounds, the diaphragm must be refitted. This may not be necessary for the Caya diaphragm.

Cervical Cap

The *cervical cap* is a cup-shaped plastic or rubber device that fits snugly around the cervix, with a failure rate of 23% (typical use) and 8% (perfect use) but is less effective in multiparous women. Like the diaphragm, the cap is used with a spermicide. Because the cap is smaller than the diaphragm, it may be more difficult to insert and remove. The advantage of the cervical cap is that it can be used in women who are unable to use a diaphragm because of a relaxed anterior vaginal wall or in those who have recurrent UTIs with the use of a diaphragm. The cervical cap should not be left in place for at least 6 and up to 48 hours after intercourse. The cervical cap should not be used by women with a history of PID, abnormal Pap tests, severe cervicitis, or an abnormally shaped cervix. Adverse effects of the cervical cap are similar to those associated with the diaphragm: allergic reactions, irritation, and displacement.

Vaginal Contraceptive Sponge

A *vaginal contraceptive* sponge is a one-size-fits-all disposable sponge of polyurethane treated with a spermicide, which protects against pregnancy but not against STIs. The sponge available in the United States must be thoroughly wet with two tablespoons of water before being inserted into the vagina. The failure rate for the sponge is approximately 12% for nulliparous women and up to 24% for parous women. Adverse effects include displacement, irritation, and a slight risk of TSS (1 per 2 million sponges). It should be left in place for 6 hours after intercourse, but not more than 30 hours. It is not recommended for use during menses or the puerperium (up to 6 weeks after childbirth).

Contraceptive Foam, Cream, Film, Jelly, and Suppository

Nonoxynol-9 is the most common spermicide contained in contraceptive foam, cream, film, jelly, and suppositories. These products have an overall failure rate of 2% to 30% when used correctly. The advantages to these forms of contraception are that they are available without a prescription, easy to use, readily available, and relatively inexpensive. Nonoxynol-9 may have some virucidal and bactericidal activity but does not offer any protection against HIV and has not been shown to reduce rates of STIs. Other disadvantages of these products are that they can cause irritation and allergic reactions.

FERTILITY AWARENESS METHODS

Fertility awareness methods are techniques that can be used for both preventing and achieving pregnancy. Abstaining from sexual intercourse during the days of the menstrual cycle when the ovum is most vulnerable to fertilization is one way of avoiding pregnancy. Likewise, if achieving pregnancy is the desired outcome, engaging in sexual intercourse at this time is desirable.

There are several fertility awareness methods that can be used to predict the best time for abstinence. The *calendar method* is based on the assumptions that the ovum is viable for 24 hours after ovulation, spermatozoa are viable for 48 hours after coitus, and ovulation occurs 12 to 16 days before menses. The woman records the length of her cycle for several months and establishes her fertile period by deducting 18 days from her shortest cycle and 11 days from her previous longest cycle to determine the ovulation period of each cycle. During each subsequent menstrual cycle, abstinence should occur during this calculated fertile period. The patient must have regular menstrual cycles to use this method effectively.

Other fertility awareness methods include the basal body temperature method, the cervical mucus method, and the symptothermal method. When several techniques are used in combination, the period of abstinence can be reduced and the effectiveness increased for both preventing pregnancy or achieving pregnancy (if this is the goal).

In the *basal body temperature method*, the patient measures basal body temperature daily. Abstinence is observed from menses to 3 days of elevated temperature. Although this method does not predict ovulation effectively, it can be used to learn the pattern of temperature changes over time. The lengthy abstinence period required plus abstinence in anovulatory cycles make this a less favorable method for many. In the *cervical mucus method*, a woman learns to recognize and interpret changes in the amount and consistency of cervical that occur in response to changes in estrogen and progesterone levels associated with the menstrual cycle. Abstinence begins in menses (and every day thereafter to reduce the risk of confusing mucus with semen) until the first day of slippery,

copious cervical mucus is detected. Abstinence is observed every day thereafter until 4 days after the last day mucus is present or the peak mucus day, since ovulation typically occurs within 2 days of the peak day of mucus production. In the *symptothermal method*, the fertile period is determined by calendar calculation and cervical mucus changes to predict the fertile period; changes in mucus and basal temperature are used to pinpoint the end of this period. This method is difficult to learn but is the most effective natural method to prevent pregnancy.

The greatest obstacle to acceptance of these techniques is the need to avoid sexual relations for many days in each cycle. Some couples use a barrier method during fertile times for greater acceptance and to reduce the failure rate. Self-administered ovulation prediction kits are also available for the detection of hormonal changes in urine, which reduce the required abstinence period to just several days per cycle.

POSTCOITAL CONTROLS

Postcoital controls are another method of birth control. There are three types: withdrawal, postcoitus douche, and emergency contraception. The simplest, most effective, and most practical method of preventing implantation after unprotected sex is the administration of emergency contraception. Emergency contraception is available over-the-counter and is known as "Plan B One-Step." Plan B One-Step is levonorgestrel 1.5 mg and is a one-tablet regimen to be taken as soon as possible after unprotected sex but must be within 72 hours. Available only by prescription is Ulipristal (Ella). The emergency contraceptive contains 30 mg of ulipristal and prevents pregnancy by blocking progesterone receptor sites. It should be taken as soon as possible but can be taken up to 5 days after unprotected intercourse.

STERILIZATION

Sterilization is a permanent method of birth control. After risks and benefits of sterilization are reviewed with the patient, informed consent is obtained. Up to 10% of patients who undergo sterilization procedures later request reversal of sterilization particularly for those women younger than 30 years.

Male sterilization consists of vasectomy performed on an outpatient basis; the procedure typically takes 20 minutes under local anesthesia. Complications include hematoma (5%), sperm granuloma, and spontaneous reanastomosis. After vasectomy, the man is not considered sterile until two sperm-free ejaculates have been produced. Semen analysis should be performed 8 to 16 weeks after the procedure. About 15 to 20 ejaculations are required postvasectomy for absolute sterility.

Female sterilization can be performed in several ways. A minilaparotomy is usually performed postpartum, where the fallopian tubes are brought up through a small incision. Usually a small section of each tube is removed, but the entire tube can be removed. The procedure can be performed laparoscopically through a small incision. Both of these require general anesthesia. Another option is hysteroscopic sterilization. In this procedure, the hysteroscope is introduced into the opening of each fallopian tube where an inner coil of stainless steel and polyethylene terephthalate fibers and an outer coil of nickel-titanium. This causes scar tissue to form and block the opening. This is done under local anesthesia in the provider's office. A hysterosalpingography must be done 3 months after the procedure to be sure that the tubes are blocked. The failure rate is roughly 1 per 1,000 cases for all forms.

ABORTION

An elective abortion is one of the most common gynecological procedures in the United States and has been legal since 1973. In accordance with the landmark *Roe v. Wade* Supreme Court decision, the state may not interfere with the practice of abortion in the first trimester. To protect the health of the mother, a second-trimester abortion may be performed, and limiting restrictions have been declared unconstitutional. Since abortion was legalized in the United States, the maternal mortality rate has fallen significantly.

The primary method used for elective abortion in the first trimester is vacuum aspiration under local anesthesia and involves dilation of the cervix and vacuum aspiration of the products of conception. Second-trimester abortion (after 13 weeks) can be done with dilation of the cervix and evacuation of the pregnancy (D&E) or with medication (medical abortion). A D&E is most often used because it has fewer complications than medical abortion. A D&E is a surgical procedure that can be performed either under local or general anesthesia. Because the fetus may be too large to remove by suction alone, forceps are inserted through the cervix, and the fetus is removed. Methods of medical abortion include hypertonic saline solution that is instilled into the amniotic cavity, or prostaglandins may also be used to induce labor. The prostaglandins used most often are PGE_2 as a vaginal suppository and 15-methyl $PGF_{2\alpha}$ as an IM injection. They are given at 2- to 3-hour intervals until evacuation of the fetus. Both instillation of hypertonic saline and prostaglandin administration are difficult for the patient. Abortions are rarely performed after 20 weeks, because the lower limit of fetal viability is considered to be 24 weeks of gestational age but are performed for medical reasons such as severe defects in the fetus.

Complications from abortions increase as gestational age increases and include retained products of conception and unrecognized ectopic pregnancy. Currently, most abortions (90%) are performed before 12 weeks of gestation, and there is an overall mortality rate of 1 in 100,000 cases. Patients should be counseled to obtain an abortion as early as possible in the pregnancy if this is their choice to minimize complications.

In September 2000, the FDA-approved mifepristone (RU486), a synthetic antiprogestational-antiglucocorticoid pill, as an oral abortifacient. RU486 is used to induce an abortion during the first 9 weeks of pregnancy. RU486 is given as a single dose of 200 mg and has a success rate of 85%, but if it is followed in 36 to 48 hours with a prostaglandin vaginal suppository, the success rate in terminating pregnancy is 95%. Adverse effects include nausea, vomiting, bleeding, and abdominal pain.

Patient Education: Contraception

Contraception is not just a method; it is a life decision and part of a family planning process. With regard to female contraception, there is no ideal method for every woman, but because so many options are available today, contraception can be tailored for each person's lifestyle, motivation, and partner's participation. Research in reproductive biology may provide less invasive and more effective contraceptive methods in the future. However, at present, maximum effectiveness still depends on consistent and accurate use; thus, the human element is the primary source of error.

Every heterosexual woman should consider contraception as part of her overall personal health maintenance, regardless of her desired form (including the choice of abstinence), just as every woman should include the following in her health regimen: an annual gynecological examination, balanced nutrition, smoking and alcohol cessation, weight control, mental health, exercise, and risk reduction. Fertility control and health and wellness work hand in hand for the female patient and her future life plans.

BREAST MASS

A breast mass is a lump in the breast, and discovering such a mass is one of the most anxiety-producing events a woman may encounter in her lifetime. Seventy percent of patients with breast cancer present with a lump in the breast; 90% of these breast masses are discovered by the woman herself. Benign breast disorders (e.g., fibroadenoma) are referred to as *fibrocystic changes* or *fibrocystic disease* and are the most common breast lesions. Fibrocystic changes are extremely common and are considered a normal variant of breast tissue. In benign breast disorders, the breast masses or lumps are tender and usually bilateral. There may be a rapid fluctuation in the size of benign masses compared with breast malignancies, which slowly increase in size. In premenopausal women, masses should be reassessed in 2 to 3 weeks during a different phase of the monthly cycle. Typically, the tenderness and size of the mass may increase before menses. Fibrocystic breast disease is most common in women aged 30 to 50 years or in postmenopausal women on hormone replacement therapy. If accompanied by significant pain, nipple discharge, or palpable lump on physical examination, the patient should be evaluated for possible breast cancer.

DIFFERENTIAL DIAGNOSIS

The characteristics that differentiate a breast cyst from breast cancer are tenderness, fluctuations in size, and multiplicity of lesions. It is difficult to distinguish a breast cyst from cancer based on clinical findings alone; therefore, testing is warranted. The first step is to rule out benign causes of a breast mass such as infection (e.g., mastitis or cellulitis). A mammogram is usually the first test performed; however, the breast tissue in patients with fibrocystic breast disease may be too radiodense to provide a conclusive diagnosis. Digital breast tomosynthesis, another diagnostic screening tool, generates a three-dimensional radiographic image, which has demonstrated higher cancer detection rates than traditional mammography and fewer patient recalls for additional testing (American College of Radiology, *2014 Position Statement on Breast Tomosynthesis*). If a mass is present, a breast ultrasound will differentiate a cystic mass from a solid mass, although a definitive diagnosis is made via breast biopsy. Aspiration of a cystic lesion will relieve the breast pain and assist in the diagnosis.

MANAGEMENT

Treatment of fibrocystic breast disease consists of avoiding trauma, wearing a firm bra throughout the day and night, eliminating coffee, tea, and chocolate from the diet, and taking 400 IU of vitamin E daily. Patients may be prescribed diuretics, oral contraceptives, NSAIDs, and supplemental progestin. For patients with severe pain, danazol (Danocrine) 100 to 200 mg twice daily is helpful. Danazol is an androgen derivative that suppresses pituitary gonadotropins. With its androgenic side effects such as acne, edema, and hirsutism, most women find that the treatment is more troublesome than the condition itself and prefer to try milder forms of pain relief.

ABNORMAL UTERINE BLEEDING

A change in the pattern or volume of menstrual bleeding is a common health concern of women from puberty to menopause. The literature suggests that during their reproductive years, 10% to 20% of women have abnormal uterine bleeding (AUB) at least once. Women may describe abnormal bleeding episodes as infrequent, occurring between regular menstrual periods, prolonged in duration, and/or excessive in volume. Acute AUB is defined as an episode of bleeding in a nonpregnant woman of reproductive age that, in the opinion of the provider, requires immediate intervention to prevent further blood loss. Chronic AUB is uterine bleeding that is abnormal in duration, volume, and/or frequency and has been present for the majority of the past 6 months. Chronic AUB is associated with a reduction in work productivity by approximately 30% (Frick, 2009).

Traditionally, genital bleeding in women has been vaguely defined, with inconsistent and confusing terminology. Heavy menstrual bleeding describes a woman's perception of excessive menstrual blood loss without regard to regularity, duration, or frequency of menses. In an effort to develop consistency, consensus, and clear terminology, the International Federation of Obstetrics and Gynecology Menstrual Disorders Committee developed a flexible classification system in 2011. This system, known as PALM-COEIN, classifies causes of AUB in the reproductive years. The normal frequency of menses is 24 to 38 days, with an average duration of 4.5 to 8 days and approximately 5 to 80 mL of blood loss per month. Determination of abnormal bleeding involves recognizing variations in frequency, regularity, duration, and volume of flow. Causes of AUB are categorized by the PALM-COEIN acronym, which stands for the following possible causes: polyp, adenomyosis, leiomyoma, malignancy and hyperplasia, coagulopathy, ovulatory dysfunction, endometrial, iatrogenic, and not yet classified. Factors of the "PALM" group are considered structural causes, while the "COEIN" group entities are not defined by imaging or histopathology.

DIFFERENTIAL DIAGNOSIS

Initial evaluation of bleeding from the vagina involves determining its source. Structural causes due to a polyp, leiomyoma, or adenomyosis can be identified via ultrasound. Anovulatory bleeding is the cause of AUB in approximately 95% of women younger than 20 years and in 90% of perimenopausal women who experience AUB for 2 to 3 years before the onset of menopause. In contrast, ovulatory cycles are associated with certain features such as midcycle pain, specific vaginal mucus changes, dysmenorrhea, and premenstrual breast tenderness. Approximately one-half of ovulating women experience midcycle spotting that is self-limited. Irregular endometrial shedding may occur with the prolonged production of progesterone with a persistent corpus luteum resulting in AUB.

A thorough history, physical examination, pelvic examination, and selected laboratory tests will usually yield the appropriate diagnosis. The history should include the woman's age, date of last menstrual period, birth control method, frequency of menses, amount of menstrual blood flow (e.g., the estimated number of pads or tampons used daily), duration of menses, and if there is a menstrual pattern change. In women who report profuse acute bleeding episodes, the diagnosis of pregnancy or miscarriage (e.g., passing tissue, nausea, vomiting, breast tenderness) must be excluded. In an ectopic pregnancy, the woman may complain of abdominal pain. Complaints of fainting spells may be indicative of a ruptured ectopic pregnancy. If the woman describes bleeding only with urination or defecation, or when wiping with toilet tissue, bladder or GI disorders should be explored.

Up to 10% of women who use OCPs and other forms of hormonal contraception report irregular bleeding episodes. Any woman who presents with AUB and is 35 years of age or older should be evaluated for cervical and uterine cancer. Endometrial sampling is an office procedure to rule out unchecked proliferation of the endometrium that can lead to hyperplasia and potentially endometrial adenocarcinoma. Similarly, a colposcopy, cervical biopsy, and endocervical curettage are used to diagnose cervical cancer. Women older than 30 years who are HPV-positive and have an atypical squamous cells of undetermined significance (ASC-US) or other abnormal Pap test results should be referred for colposcopy. In women aged 25 years and older with low-grade squamous intraepithelial lesion should be referred for colposcopy, and any woman with ASC-H (H indicates that high-grade squamous intraepithelial lesion cannot be excluded) should be referred for colposcopy. Trauma and foreign bodies as a cause of bleeding from the vagina are seen more commonly in children. A less common cause of uterine bleeding is a blood dyscrasia creating a tendency to bleed, such as von Willebrand's disease or thrombocytopenic purpura. This is particularly true if the patient is an adolescent and presents with heavy menstrual bleeding.

Physical examination should focus on findings pointing to possible sources of bleeding, such as an anal fissure, cervical laceration, an enlarged, irregular, or boggy uterus, blood clots in the vaginal vault, uterine tenderness, copious blood flow, or adnexal masses or tenderness. Laboratory work-up is directed by the history and physical examination findings and usually consists of hematocrit, hemoglobin, platelet count, peripheral smear with differential, pregnancy evaluation, and Pap test. In severe bleeding, tests for partial thromboplastin time, prothrombin time, and bleeding time are indicated. Hysteroscopy may be performed immediately before a cervical dilation and curettage of the uterus to assist in the diagnosis of polyps, exophytic endometrial cancer, or fibroids (leiomyomata). Prolactin level and thyroid function tests are ordered to rule out hyperprolactinemia and hypothyroidism, respectively.

MANAGEMENT

Management of AUB is directed toward controlling bleeding and preventing a recurrence. For teenagers, management includes observation for those with mild cases and no anemia and prescribing medroxyprogesterone or an OCP. For women of reproductive age, treatment is based on the woman's desire for fertility or contraception. For women who cannot take OCPs, medroxyprogesterone is offered. OCPs containing EE are used in acute bleeding episodes. For women with severe acute bleeding but who remain hemodynamically stable, conjugated estrogen is used until bleeding stops.

DYSPAREUNIA

Dyspareunia is painful sexual intercourse that can occur as a result of either introduction of the penis (natural or artificial) into the vagina or deep penile penetration. Dyspareunia can also be experienced by same-sex lesbian partners with the introduction into the vagina of multiple fingers or sex toys (e.g., vibrators, artificial penises or "dildos"). The pain a woman experiences can be a consequence of vaginal inflammation, structural (anatomical) abnormalities, vaginal atrophy, insufficient vaginal lubrication, pelvic pathology, or psychological issues.

Because patients tend not to report painful sexual intercourse, it is difficult to determine the incidence of dyspareunia. A review of studies reporting the prevalence of chronic pelvic pain indicates that the rates of dyspareunia ranged from 1.3% to 45.7% in more than 154 studies that included over 35,973 women. One study of 313 patients documented that more than 60% had experienced dyspareunia at some point in their lives. Risk factors include a history of sexual trauma, history of STIs, recurrent candidiasis infection, poor hygiene, menopause, psychological issues, and difficulties in intimate personal relationships.

DIFFERENTIAL DIAGNOSIS

Obtaining a thorough history requires creating a comfortable and nonjudgmental environment that normalizes the topic of sexuality, which is essential in ascertaining the cause of dyspareunia. As noted earlier, pain may occur with initial or deep vaginal penetration and may occur with the first episode of intercourse or after a long time of pain-free sexual experiences. The patient may complain of vaginal discharge or irritation. There may be a history of unrelated pelvic pain, recent pregnancy or childbirth, pelvic or abdominal trauma, chemotherapy, radiation, or surgery. The patient may, upon questioning, reveal difficulty in using tampons or difficulty tolerating prior pelvic examinations.

On physical examination, the patient may present with signs of vulvar or vaginal mucosal irritation, inflammation, lesions, discharge, atrophy, hymenal remnants, Bartholin's cyst or abscess, or vestibulitis. *Vaginismus*, the involuntary contraction of perineal muscles, may occur during the speculum examination, impeding full visualization and examination of the vaginal vault and cervix. The clinician must proceed with sensitivity, allowing the patient control over the pelvic examination. The bimanual examination may reveal a pelvic mass, cervical motion tenderness, uterine prolapse, a rectocele, or a cystocele.

The laboratory work-up is directed by findings from the history and physical examination and usually consists of a urinalysis, a wet mount of vaginal discharge, and cervical cultures. Urinalysis is useful in identifying any urinary tract conditions that may be a contributing factor to the source of the pain. The presence of white blood cells (WBCs), red blood cells, or bacteria may indicate a UTI. Wet mount examination of vaginal discharge can reveal the presence of bacterial vaginosis (*Gardnerella vaginalis*), trichomoniasis, or candidiasis. Cervical cultures are useful in determining the presence of *Chlamydia* and gonorrhea.

MANAGEMENT

Management of dyspareunia depends on the patient's symptoms and etiology. If the cause is atrophic vaginitis, estrogens (especially vaginal estrogens) may be helpful for postmenopausal women. A water-soluble lubricant (Astroglide, K-Y Jelly) can be used for vaginal lubrication and comfort. STIs are treated with appropriate antibiotic therapy. Progressive dilation and muscle awareness exercises such as Kegel exercises are recommended for treatment of vaginismus, hymenal strands, an anatomically narrow introitus, and scar tissue. If psychological factors, such as sexual trauma, relationship conflicts, stress, and a restrictive sexual attitude, appear to be the cause, referral to a psychotherapist is indicated.

NOCTURIA IN MEN

Nocturia is currently defined by the International Continence Society as having to wake at night one or more times to void, each time being preceded and followed by sleep. Recording the number of times a patient urinates at night and making a reasonable estimate of the amount voided is extremely important. The frequency of urination may vary from large volumes of urine (polyuria) voided infrequently to small quantities passed at frequent intervals. Adult men normally void five to six times during the day and once or not at all during the night. As men age, nocturia is usually a sign of a prostatic problem, most often benign prostatic hyperplasia (BPH). Typically, 50% of men older than 50 years have BPH, and the rate increases by 10% for every 10 years of age (i.e., to 60% of men older than 60 years, to 70% of men older than 70 years, and so on). BPH is discussed in more detail in Chapter 49.

The occurrence of nocturia without discomfort may be due to diminished bladder capacity, overflow incontinence, or habit. In men with a normal bladder, the absence of nocturia while suffering from increased frequency of urination during the day suggests a psychogenic origin. A rare finding might be a polyp or irritative lesion in the posterior urethra that is relieved by recumbence, so nocturia is not present.

Detrusor muscle instability may cause urinary incontinence as well as nocturia. Fifty percent of male patients in nursing homes are incontinent, whereas 15% to 30% of elderly men in the community have urinary incontinence, which may be caused by decreased bladder capacity,

increased residual urine (from an inability to empty the bladder), or involuntary bladder contractions. Moderate dribbling of urine may indicate overflow from a partially incompetent outlet and can be a congenital or an acquired anomaly. Less common causes of incontinence are spinal cord disease, multiple sclerosis, tumors, trauma, syphilis, and diabetic neuropathy. Microorganisms that can cause nocturia and incontinence include *Klebsiella pneumoniae*, *Proteus mirabilis*, *Enterobacter*, *Staphylococcus*, enterococci (*Streptococcus* bacteria associated with the intestines), or *Pseudomonas*.

Medications, such as methyldopa, phenothiazines, diazepam, excessive vitamin D, and diuretics, may also cause nocturia, as well as precipitate or aggravate incontinence. Drugs that cause urinary retention include alpha-adrenergic agents, androgens, and sympathomimetic agents, such as ephedrine and pseudoephedrine. In turn, urinary retention can lead to nocturia and incontinence.

DIFFERENTIAL DIAGNOSIS

Nocturia may occur as a result of primary disease of the urinary tract or from metabolic diseases such as diabetes mellitus or diabetes insipidus; it may also be associated with cardiovascular disorders, fluid shifts into the lower limbs, polypharmacy, and emotional tension. Documentation of the pattern of urination during a 24-hour period is vital to a diagnosis of nocturia. Although a patient may complain if he or she awakens frequently to urinate, the precipitating events and activities of the day may also give a hint as to the cause. For example, alcohol intake before sleep may increase the number of times the patient urinates at night and may also increase urine volume.

Urgency, a desire to urinate, can be constant or intermittent. Urgency and frequency of urination often occur together. Urgency is frequently the result of prostatic disease or bladder infection. *Stress incontinence* is involuntary loss of urine during physical activity or upon exertion, such as due to a cough, laughing, lifting a heavy object, changing positions, or with exercise. Incontinence is further discussed in Chapter 44. *Hesitancy* refers to difficulty in initiating a urine stream. *Oliguria* is a decrease in urinary output and can be caused by a decrease in the production of urine secondary to acute glomerulonephritis or other renal disease, as well as conditions that drastically decrease cardiac output. *Dribbling* can be symptomatic of disease; it may occur at night or during the day and usually indicates the presence of a urethral stricture, prostatic obstruction, or less commonly, a neurologic disorder.

MANAGEMENT

Treatment of nocturia depends on identifying the cause. A simple urinalysis is performed to rule out UTI. A prostate-specific antigen blood test and a digital rectal examination are done to rule out a prostatic problem in men. The results may indicate a need for further diagnostic testing. Specific aspects of patient education are discussed under the particular disease causing the nocturia.

CHRONIC PELVIC PAIN SYNDROME IN WOMEN

Pelvic pain is seen in 1% to 2% of female patients in primary-care practice. Pelvic pain is categorized as acute, chronic, or recurrent and may present as pelvic and/or lower abdominal pain. Common causes of pelvic pain include genitourinary (e.g., pelvic adhesions, endometriosis, interstitial cystis), gastrointestinal (e.g., irritable bowel syndrome), or musculoskeletal system diseases or dysfunction that may cause sudden, acute pain in both areas. Chronic or recurrent pelvic pain is typically less urgent than acute pain. Recurrent pain may or may not be associated with menstruation, whereas chronic pain can be related to benign or malignant neoplasms or characterized as psychogenic.

DIFFERENTIAL DIAGNOSIS

Acute onset of pelvic pain may be the result of pelvic disorders including PID, ruptured ovarian cyst, torsion of an ovarian cyst, ovary, or fallopian tube, or ectopic pregnancy with rupture. PID accounts for approximately 20% of acute pelvic pain in women, ovarian cysts for up to 40%, and adnexal torsion for about 16%. Ten percent of women

who report acute pelvic pain may have extrapelvic disease such as appendicitis.

Women reporting recurrent pain with menstruation may have primary or secondary dysmenorrhea, endometriosis, adenomyosis, chronic PID, and/or pain related to IUDs. Endometriosis is seen in up to 50% of women with chronic pelvic pain. Recurrent pain that is not associated with menses may have many causes, including Mittelschmerz (a pain syndrome caused by the release of a mature ovum from the ovary), leaking ovarian cysts, incompletely treated or recurrent pelvic infections, or UTI. Physical findings may include vaginismus, uterine or adnexal masses, enlargements or tenderness, or pelvic floor muscle relaxation. Nongynecological etiologies include adhesions, inflammatory bowel disease, and irritable bowel syndrome. Imaging tests are important to complete the assessment process. However, for as many as 37% of women with chronic or recurrent pelvic pain, no physiological cause of the pain can be determined.

MANAGEMENT

Treatment for pelvic pain depends on the underlying cause. Differential Diagnosis 46.1 outlines the differential diagnosis for pelvic pain and possible treatments. If short-term medical management is ineffective or the work-up is inconclusive, a laparoscopy may be indicated.

Resources are available for providers and patients through the International Pelvic Pain Society (IPPS).

⊞ Differential Diagnosis 46.1: Pelvic Pain

Clinical Findings	Diagnosis	Treatment
Lower abdominal tenderness Cervical motion tenderness Adnexal tenderness Oral temperature above 101°F (38.3°C) ↑ Erythrocyte sedimentation rate Abnormal cervical/vaginal discharge abscess Evidence of *Chlamydia trachomatis* or *Neisseria gonorrhoeae* ↑ WBCs	Pelvic inflammatory disease	Antibiotics (see CDC guidelines for sexually transmitted infections*). Hospitalization may be required with an uncertain diagnosis, pelvic abscess, or pregnancy.
Smooth mobile adnexal mass Percussive dullness on affected side Diffuse pain/pressure (if ruptured)	Ovarian cyst	Monitor cysts <10 cm with repeat imagining. Cysts >10 cm in size require evaluation via laparoscopy and possible surgical removal.
Localized or diffuse colicky or dull pain Shoulder pain with hemoperitoneum Rebound tenderness/guarding (if ruptured) Abnormal vaginal bleeding Amenorrhea Quantitative serum human chorionic gonadotropin immunoassay positive (1 week after conception)	Ectopic pregnancy	Surgery

Continued

⁜ Differential Diagnosis 46.1: Pelvic Pain—cont'd

Clinical Findings	Diagnosis	Treatment
Dysmenorrhea Dyspareunia Pain on defecation Infertility	Endometriosis	Continuous combined hormonal contraceptive may offer some benefit because of the elimination of menses. Depot medroxyprogesterone acetate and progestin contraceptive implant reduce the pain from endometriosis. Gonadotropin-releasing hormonal agents NSAIDs Possible laparoscopy to rule out pelvic pathology
Flank pain and/or suprapubic pain Dysuria and/or urinary frequency Fever, nausea and/or vomiting	Urinary tract infection (UTI), including pyelonephritis	Antibiotics (see Chapter 44 for specific treatment for lower and upper UTI)
Acute, progressively severe pain Mass/tenderness on affected side on palpation Symptoms more impressive than physical examination	Adnexal torsion	Hospitalization/surgery
Initially: epigastric to midabdominal pain and anorexia Later: lower quadrant to suprapubic to flank pain and vomiting Rebound tenderness/guarding: tenderness over McBurney's point Psoas/obturator sign Low-grade fever	Appendicitis	Hospitalization and surgery
Palpable mass on uterus Back pain/pressure Dysmenorrhea/menorrhagia Anemia Frequency/constipation	Uterine fibroid (leiomyomata)	Hysterectomy Uterine artery embolectomy
Variable in intensity of pain lasting up to several hours	Mittelschmerz	No treatment for mild cases over-the-counter analgesics, such as acetaminophen or NSAIDs Combined hormonal contraception may be offered to inhibit ovulation

*Centers for Disease Control and Prevention. Sexually Transmitted Diseases Treatment Guidelines, 2015. *MMWR Recomm Rep.* 2015;64(No. RR-3):1–140.

CHRONIC PELVIC PAIN SYNDROME IN MEN

The term *prostatodynia* is often used as a designation for unexplained chronic pelvic pain in men, which may be mistaken for inflammatory prostatitis. However, the nomenclature and conceptualization of prostatodynia have been expanded in modern clinical practice into a broader disorder called *chronic pelvic pain syndrome* (CPPS), which is defined by the absence of a causative bacterial infection (e.g., prostatitis, as detailed in Chapter 49). This is considered predominantly a non-inflammatory disorder that has many causes, including voiding dysfunction and pelvic floor dysfunction, but the prostate is normal.

The term *prostatodynia* is not considered accurate nomenclature for CPPS because it suggests that the condition stems from the prostate itself, despite the term being used historically to describe nonspecific groin pain of unclear etiology. No unifying cause of CPPS is known. CPPS affects mostly young and middle-aged men and is characterized by pain in the groin that may extend to the genitalia and perineum. In the United States, for men older than 50 years, chronic prostatitis is the most common diagnosis for urologists and ranks third as the most frequent diagnosis in men younger than 50 years, with the majority characterized as suffering from CPPS (Watson, 2017).

CPPS is considered by some clinicians to be equivalent to chronic nonbacterial prostatitis, although several lines of evidence point to nonprostatic causes. It may be considered an umbrella disorder of male patients with an array of chronic pelvic symptoms, consisting predominantly of groin pain that relates largely to anatomical structures in proximity to the prostate gland. Importantly, the symptoms of CPPS have no adequate treatment, cure, or objective explanation, although the disorder appears to relate to a combination of dysfunctional immune, endocrine, neurologic, and psychological factors.

DIFFERENTIAL DIAGNOSIS

CPPS is often mistaken for chronic prostatitis because many of the symptoms and signs of these disorders are the same. The patient with prostatodynia may present with low back and perineal pain, urinary hesitancy, and interruption of urine flow. Unlike in chronic prostatitis, there is no history of UTIs with CPPS. On physical examination (including digital rectal examination), the prostate is normal, but there may be increased anal sphincter tone and periprostatic tenderness. The primary value of physical assessment is in ruling out identifiable diagnoses, such as prostatitis, urethritis, and prostate cancer.

There are no tests that specifically diagnose CPPS. Elevated prostate-specific antigen is not typically associated with classic prostatodynia and is more consistent with prostatitis. Urinalysis is normal without bacteriuria or pyuria, as are expressed prostatic secretions in most patients. Of note, some patients with CPPS have evidence of WBCs in prostatic secretions, suggesting an inflammatory component, although this finding is not classically associated with prostatodynia. Moreover, significantly elevated WBCs in prostatic secretions should trigger the suspicion of acute or chronic infectious prostatitis.

There may be detrusor contraction without urethral relaxation, high urethral pressures, and spasms of the urinary sphincter on urodynamic testing. However, these tests are not performed unless the patient has no response after a trial of alpha blocker or anticholinergic medication, as described in the following section on management.

The differential diagnoses for prostatodynia include acute and chronic prostatitis and nonbacterial prostatitis. Because the urinalysis is normal, acute infection can be ruled out. The normal expressed prostatic secretions distinguish prostatodynia from nonbacterial prostatitis. Of note, however, some clinicians may diagnose CPPS in patients, despite evidence of an inflammatory component to their condition, as reflected by WBCs in expressed prostatic secretions, suggesting heterogeneity of the diagnosis.

MANAGEMENT

The patient with CPPS is usually treated with alpha blocker medications to reduce bladder neck and urethral spasms. The most commonly used drugs are terazosin (Hytrin) 1 to 10 mg PO daily, doxazosin (Cardura) 1 to 8 mg PO daily, and tamsulosin (Flomax) 0.4 to 0.8 mg PO daily. Some patients benefit from myofascial release therapy and warm sitz baths, whereas others may experience relief using the muscle relaxant diazepam and biofeedback to relieve tension myalgia associated with pelvic floor muscle dysfunction. Psychotherapy is appropriate if sexual dysfunction accompanies CPPS. Antibiotics have no established role, given that CPPS is not infectious in origin, yet patients may be inappropriately prescribed antibiotics for prolonged periods of time, given the lack of a clear etiology.

Given that CPPS should only be diagnosed after thorough evaluation that rules out chronic prostatitis and other identifiable causes for persistent symptoms, referral to a urological specialist may be required for patients with intransigent symptoms. Several patient education resources are available for patients with CPPS, including the chronic prostatitis/CPPS network, the Prostatitis Foundation, and the International Association for the Study of Pain interest group on pain of urogenital origin.

TESTICULAR PAIN

Testicular pain is one of the most urgent complaints in male patients. Testicular pain as an isolated symptom is a fullness or heaviness of the scrotum, ranging from a dull ache to a stabbing pain, and may occur in a wide variety of patients with no differentiation based on culture, ethnicity, or socioeconomic status.

Testicular pain is often directly related to anatomical causes. During development, the processus vaginalis gives rise to the tunica vaginalis anterior and lateral to each testis, which represents the detached portion of the peritoneal cavity within the scrotum. The processus vaginalis normally closes and obliterates over time; however, a patent processus vaginalis can predispose the patient to an indirect or congenital hernia. A painful hernia can also occur when an evagination of the peritoneal cavity is occluded by the adult spermatic cord. Partial occlusion of a patent processus vaginalis can result in a fluid accumulation, or hydrocele, that cannot be distinguished from a hernia or an incompletely descended testicle until surgery is performed.

DIFFERENTIAL DIAGNOSIS

A cause of testicular pain may be swelling of the testis, the epididymis, or the spermatic cord or torsion of the testicle (the testicle may become twisted around the spermatic cord, causing acute pain; this condition is a urological emergency). Differential diagnoses for testicular pain include hydrocele, varicocele, epididymitis, and prostatitis. Pain from prostatitis usually occurs in the lower back, radiates to the testicles, and is typically accompanied by fever. Cultures usually show *Escherichia coli*, with or without fistula formation. Hernias, hydroceles, and hematomas must all be excluded. A detailed history and physical examination will direct the assessment to exclude other diagnoses. A spermatocele may also cause testicular pain, although most spermatoceles are painless. A syphilitic gumma is a possibility, as is a varicocele; however, these conditions are usually not painful.

Because of multiple potential diagnoses, specialized tests are performed to differentiate the etiology of testicular pain. A scrotal ultrasound can identify a mass originating in the testicles and is noninvasive. An echo-texture pattern reveals the presence of a hypoechoic mass that is distinct from surrounding normal testicular tissue, a spermatocele, hydrocele, or varicocele. The specific cause of testicular pain determines the appropriate treatment, as described in the specific sections for each of these disorders (see Chapter 50).

TESTOSTERONE DEFICIENCY

Testosterone levels peak during adolescence and early adulthood and then gradually decline about 1% per year after age 30 years. As men age, there is a rise in the level of follicle-stimulating hormone, which controls sperm production, as well as luteinizing hormone, which controls testosterone production. Simultaneous to this is a decline in testosterone levels. Normal testosterone levels are less than 300 ng/dL and are best assessed in the morning between 7:00 and 10:00 a.m. Testosterone decline may be a function of normal aging or may be due to hypogonadism. Other factors suppressing testosterone levels include stress, obesity, tobacco and alcohol use, obstructive sleep apnea, diabetes mellitus, and illness. Medications such as suramin (Germanin), ketoconazole (Nizoral), glucocorticoids, alkylating agents, and opiates may cause a decrease in serum testosterone if used chronically.

Low testosterone (low T) affects multiple bodily systems. Cardiovascular effects include dyslipidemia and hypertension. Metabolic syndrome consists of these disorders, in addition to obesity and glucose intolerance, which collectively increase the risk of cardiovascular disease. Low T is associated with diabetes mellitus type 2, and men with the lowest levels of free testosterone are four times more likely to have diabetes mellitus. Osteopenia, osteoporosis, and fracture prevalence rates are greater in hypogonadal men, with 30% of fractures occurring in men with low T. Erectile dysfunction and decreased libido correspond with a decline in testosterone, which regulates nerve structure and function in areas of the spinal cord that are involved in erections. In addition, a decline in mental functioning has also been associated with low T.

MANAGEMENT

First-line treatment for symptomatic men with low testosterone levels is testosterone replacement therapy. Testosterone gels and patches are the most prevalent hormone replacement formulations and can be found in the Drugs Commonly Prescribed 50.1 for erectile dysfunction in Chapter 50. Testosterone therapy is contraindicated in men with breast or prostate cancer, palpable prostate nodules or induration, untreated obstructive sleep apnea, severe lower urinary tract symptoms with an International Prostate Symptom Score of greater than 19, and New York Heart Association Class III or IV heart failure.

VULVOVAGINITIS

Vulvovaginitis is defined as the simultaneous inflammation of the vulva and vagina. The patient typically complains of vaginal itching, burning, and discharge, which comprise the triad of vulvovaginitis symptoms and account for some of the most common reasons women seek health care from primary-care practitioners. Although frequently the result of infection, vulvovaginitis may also have noninfectious causes including allergic reactions, foreign body irritation, atrophic vaginitis, traumatic vaginitis, vulvar disease, or collagen vascular disease.

DIFFERENTIAL DIAGNOSIS

The delicate vaginal environment can be altered by numerous intrinsic and extrinsic influences. In addition to the effects of normal changes in the body's hormonal condition, such as ovulatory midcycle mucus production, menstruation, or the atrophic mucosal changes that occur after menopause, the use of antibiotics, presence of diabetes mellitus or glycosuria, and stress can all cause symptoms of vulvovaginitis.

A thorough history should include time of symptom onset and a full description of the vaginal discharge and the relationship of symptoms to the menstrual cycle, coitus, and use of medications (especially antibiotics). A detailed sexual history helps to identify whether the patient is at increased risk for the development of an STI. It is important to determine whether the patient's partner has symptoms of infection (e.g., penile discharge or lesions in a male partner) and if the woman has used spermicidal preparations, douches, bubble baths, feminine hygiene deodorants, sex toys, and if she has administered any type of self-treatment to the vagina.

The most common cause of abnormal vaginal discharge, itching, and burning is infection from bacteria, yeast, parasites, or vulvovaginal atrophy. Bacterial vaginosis caused primarily by *Gardnerella* accounts for almost 50% of all vaginal infections, followed closely by candidiasis (approximately 25%) and trichomoniasis (approximately 20%). Each infection is diagnosed based on the clinical presentation, which includes the type, amount, color, odor, and pH of the discharge. Atrophic vaginitis is common in peri- and postmenopausal women and is characterized by burning, itching, vaginal dryness, and dyspareunia. Vulvar conditions such as lichen sclerosis can be debilitating if left untreated.

Physical examination to distinguish these causes includes visualization of the vulva and vagina for the presence of lesions, discharge, erythema, or atrophy. The cervix is also examined for the presence of lesions, erosions, friability, or erythema. During the bimanual examination, the clinician should pay particular attention to the presence of cervical motion tenderness or the presence of adnexal and uterine tenderness or masses.

Laboratory work-up is directed by findings from the history and physical examination and usually consists of a saline wet mount of vaginal discharge to determine the presence of *Gardnerella*, *Trichomonas*, or atrophic vaginitis and a potassium hydroxide wet mount to determine the presence of *Candida*. A Gram stain of vaginal discharge can reveal the presence of gonorrhea. In addition, a urinalysis and urine culture should be performed to rule out UTI.

MANAGEMENT

Differential Diagnosis 46.2 presents the differential diagnoses for vulvovaginitis. Treatment for vulvovaginitis depends on the cause. Drugs Commonly Prescribed 46.1 lists the treatments for the different causes of vulvovaginitis.

✠ Differential Diagnosis 46.2: Vulvovaginitis

Clinical Findings	Diagnosis
Vaginal discharge, mild or none Vaginal pH: <4.5 No amine odor KOH examination: negative	Physiological leukorrhea
Pruritus Dyspareunia Vulvar erythema and edema Thick, white, floccular, nonadherent vaginal discharge Vaginal pH: <4.5 No amine odor KOH examination: pseudohyphae Saline microscopy: pseudohyphae	Candidiasis
Malodorous, gray-yellow-green, watery or thick adherent vaginal discharge Burning with urination No dyspareunia Vaginal pH: >4.5 Amine odor present KOH examination: positive Saline microscopy: clue cells	Bacterial vaginosis (*Gardnerella*)
Homogeneous, malodorous, purulent, green-yellow, thick, frothy vaginal discharge "Strawberry" cervix Vulvovaginal erythema Itching Burning on urination Dyspareunia Vaginal pH: 5–6 No amine odor KOH examination: negative Saline microscopy: motile trichomonads	Trichomoniasis

Continued

▓ Differential Diagnosis 46.2: Vulvovaginitis—cont'd

Clinical Findings	Diagnosis
Dyspareunia Vaginal dryness Thinning of vestibular and vaginal tissue Vulvar and vaginal burning Bleeding Itching Vaginal pH: >6 Amine odor present KOH examination: negative	Atrophic vaginitis
Dyspareunia Itching Thinning and progressive atrophy of the epidermis Hyperkeratosis White streak or shiny plaque on vulva Wrinkled, parchmentlike appearance of vaginal skin and tissue Disappearance of the vulvar sulci Biopsy to confirm diagnosis	Vulvar lichen sclerosus

◉ Drugs Commonly Prescribed 46.1: Vulvovaginitis

DRUG	INDICATION	ADVERSE REACTIONS AND PRESCRIBING CONSIDERATIONS
Butoconazole 2% (Gynazole-1, Mycelex-3) cream 5 g intravaginally once at bedtime OR Miconazole 2% cream (Monistat) 5 g intravaginally (1,200 mg at bedtime for 1 day or 200 mg at bedtime for 3 days or 100 mg at bedtime for 7 days) OR Clotrimazole 1% (Lotrimin) cream 5 g intravaginally for 7–14 days OR Clotrimazole 2% cream intravaginally for 3 days OR Clotrimazole 100 mg vaginal tablet for 7 days OR Tioconazole 6.5% (Vagistat-1) ointment 5 g intravaginally in a single application OR Terconazole 0.4% cream 5 g intravaginally for 7 days Terconazole 0.8% cream 5 g intravaginally for 3 days OR Fluconazole (Diflucan) 150 mg PO × one dose for uncomplicated cases; if severe, 150 mg every 72 hours × two doses; for recurrent cases, 150 mg weekly for 6 months	Candidiasis	Adverse reactions include vulvovaginal burning, itching, irritation, swelling, cramping, abdominal pain, and headache. Do not use contraceptive diaphragm or condoms within 3 days. Do not use tampons, douches, or spermicides within 7 days. Adverse reactions include headache, nausea, abdominal pain, gastrointestinal upset, dizziness, taste perversion, and hepatotoxicity. Use with caution in the elderly. High-dose fluconazole in early pregnancy may cause birth defects but the evidence is minimal.

Drugs Commonly Prescribed 46.1: Vulvovaginitis—cont'd

DRUG	INDICATION	ADVERSE REACTIONS AND PRESCRIBING CONSIDERATIONS
Metronidazole 500 mg PO twice daily for 7 days OR Metronidazole gel 0.75% one full applicator (5 g) intravaginally daily for 5 days OR Clindamycin cream 2% One full applicator (5 g) intravaginally at bedtime for 3–7 days	Bacterial vaginosis	Avoid ingestion of alcohol with metronidazole and for 24 hours after treatment is complete. Adverse reactions include gastrointestinal upset, metallic taste, dysuria, cystitis, incontinence, *Candida* overgrowth, seizures, peripheral neuropathy, and neutropenia. OK in pregnancy. It is unlikely to cause preterm birth, low birth weight or congenital anomalies. Do not use in patients with a history of enteritis or colitis. Do not use contraceptive diaphragm or condom for 72 hours after treatment.
Metronidazole 2 g PO single dose OR Metronidazole 500 mg PO twice daily for 7 days for recurrent infection	Trichomoniasis	Must treat partner. Avoid alcohol for 24 hours after treatment is completed.
Estrogen cream (Premarin vaginal cream) 0.5 g twice weekly continuously or as 21 days of continuous therapy followed by 7 days off therapy	Atrophic vaginitis	Decrease dose or stop completely based on symptom improvement.
High-potency topical corticosteroids (e.g., clobetasol propionate) daily for 1–3 months	Vulvar lichen sclerosus	Early detection and treatment are important in halting progression of disease.

REFERENCES

Abnormal Uterine Bleeding

Whitaker L, Critchley HOD. Abnormal uterine bleeding. *Best Pract Res Clin Obstet Gynecol.* 2016;34:54–65.

Breast Mass

American College of Radiaology, 2014 Position Statement on Breast Tomosynthesis. https://www.acr.org/Advocacy-and-Economics/ACR-Position-Statements/Breast-Tomosynthesis. November 24, 2014. Accessed 9/28/2018.

Chronic Pelvic Pain Syndrome

Centers for Disease Control and Prevention. Sexually transmitted diseases treatment guidelines. *MMWR Recomm Rep.* 2015;64 (No. RR -3):1–140.

Magistro G, Wagenlehner FME, Grabe M, et al. Contemporary management of chronic prostatitis/chronic pelvic pain syndrome. *Eur Urol.* 2016;69(2):286–297.

Watson RA. Chronic pelvic pain in men treatment & management. Emedicine. http://emedicine.medscape.com/article/437745-treatment. Updated May 22, 2017. Accessed September 14, 2017.

Family Planning

Berenson AB, Rahman M. Changes in weight, total fat, percent body fat, and central-to-peripheral fat ratio associated with injectable and oral contraceptive use. *Am J Obstet Gynecol.* 2009;200(3):329.e1–8.

Buckman RT. Transdermal contraceptive patch. Up-To-Date. https://www.uptodate.com/contents/transdermal-contraceptive-patch. Accessed January 13, 2018.

Caya. For providers. How Caya works. http://caya.us.com/services/for-providers/. Accessed January 3, 2018.

Curtis KM, Tepper NK, Jatlaoui TC, et al. U.S. medical eligibility criteria for contraceptive use, 2016. *MMWR Recomm Rep.* 2016;65(No. RR-3):1–104. Accessed September 14, 2017.

Curtis KM, Jatlaoui TC, Tepper NK, et al. U.S. selected practice recommendation for contraceptive use, 2016. *MMWR Recomm Rep.* 2016;65(4):1–66. Accessed January 3, 2018.

Evans G, Sutton EL. Oral contraception. *Med Clin North Am.* 2015;99(3):479–503. Accessed January 3, 2018.

Golobof A, Kiley J. The current status of oral contraceptives: Progress and recent innovations. *Semin Reprod Med.* 2016;34(3):145–151. Accessed January 3, 2018.

Jackson AV, Karasek D, Dehlendorf C, Foster DG. Racial and ethnic differences in women's preferences for features of contraceptive methods. *Contraception.* 2016;93(5):406–411.

Kerns J, Darney PD. Contraceptive vaginal ring. Up-To-Date. https://www.uptodate.com/contents/contraceptive-vaginal-ring. Published 2017. Accessed January 13, 2018.

Lopez LM, Grimes DA, Schulz KF, Curtis KM, Chen M. Steroidal contraceptives: Effect on bone fractures in women. Cochrane Library. http://onlinelibrary.wiley.com/doi/10.1002/14651858.CD006033.pub5/full. Published 2014. Accessed January 3, 2018.

Phillips SJ, Tepper NK, Kapp N, et al. Progestogen-only contraceptive use among breastfeeding women: A systematic review. *Contraception.* 2016;94:226–252.

Women's Preventive Services Initiative. Recommendations for preventive services for women final report to the U.S. Department of Health and Human Services, Health Resources & Services Administration, December 2016. The American College of Obstetricians and Gynecologists. http://www.womenspreventivehealth.org/wp-content/uploads/2017/08/WPSI_2016FullReport.pdf. Published 2017.

Nocturia in Men

Hofmeester I, Kollen BJ, Steffens MG, et al. Impact of the International Continence Society (ICS) report on the standardization of terminology in nocturia on the quality of reports on nocturia and nocturnal polyuria: a systematic review. *BJU Int.* 2015;115(4):520–536.

Testicular Pain

Wright S, Hoffmann B. Emergency ultrasound of acute scrotal pain. *Emerg Med.* 2015;22(1):2–9.

Testosterone Deficiency

Cunningham GR, Stephens-Shields AJ, Rosen RC, et al. Testosterone treatment and sexual function in older men with low testosterone levels. *J Clin Endocrinol Metab.* 2016;101(8):3096–3104.

Vulvovaginitis

Lee A, Bradford J, Fischer G. Long-term management of adult vulvar lichen sclerosus: A prospective cohort study of 507 women. *JAMA Dermatol.* 2015;151(10):1061–1067.

RESOURCES

American College of Obstetricians and Gynecologists
    https://www.acog.org
U.S. Medical Eligibility Criteria (US MEC) for Contraceptive Use
    https://www.cdc.gov/reproductivehealth/contraception/mmwr/mec/summary.html
Centers for Disease Control and Prevention
    https://www.cdc.gov/reproductivehealth/contraception/pdf/summary-chart-us-medical-eligibility-criteria_508tagged.pdf
Centers for Disease Control and Prevention: 2015 Sexually Transmitted Diseases Treatment Guidelines
    https://www.cdc.gov/std/tg2015/default.htm

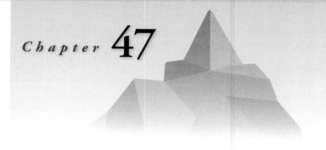

Chapter **47**

Breast Disorders

Debera J. Thomas, DNS, RN, FNP/ANP
Brian Oscar Porter, MD, PhD, MPH, MBA

MASTITIS

Mastitis is a general term that refers to inflammation of the breast. The terminology for the various types of mastitis can be confusing because there are overlapping definitions and contradictions in the literature. For this discussion, there are three general categories: puerperal mastitis, nonpuerperal mastitis, and periductal mastitis. Each category is defined further by an explanation of the cause of the mastitis.

Puerperal mastitis is a cellulitis that develops in the lactating or nonlactating breast after childbirth. Epidemic puerperal mastitis was a hospital-acquired infection most commonly seen in the preantibiotic era. The most common contagion for epidemic puerperal mastitis is *Staphylococcus aureus*. *S. aureus* is spread by cross-transmission from neonate to mother, as well as cross-transmission in the nursery. There is multiple duct involvement, which results in inflammation of several nonadjacent lobes of the breast. With the progression of rooming-in and the introduction of antibiotics, epidemic puerperal mastitis has become a rare occurrence. Sporadic puerperal mastitis is an acute process that is far more common in women who breastfeed rather than in those who bottle-feed their children. It usually occurs in the second to sixth week postpartum; however, it has been reported in patients even after breastfeeding for 1 year. It is hypothesized that the higher occurrence of mastitis in the earlier postpartum period is due to the prevalence of nipple and feeding problems at this time, a risk factor for the disease. Feeding problems are more likely to occur in first-time breastfeeding mothers.

Nonpuerperal mastitis is a rare disease found in patients who are immunocompromised, have undergone radiation therapy, or have had an autoimmune disorder. It can also occur in neonates. It is common in late adolescence or early adulthood. Nonpuerperal mastitis is a ductal abnormality or a local manifestation of a systemic problem. Several pathological pathways may be involved, including squamous metaplasia of the lactational ducts (the most common cause in nonpuerperal mastitis), periareolar abscesses, and cellulitis. Mastitis can also be caused by several obscure pathogens or by a substance in the breast such as silicone. This disease usually presents as a palpable mass and a known infectious process such as tuberculosis (TB) or syphilis. Nonpuerperal mastitis must always be evaluated for the presence of underlying carcinoma.

Periductal mastitis has been referred to and cross-referenced under several other names, such as mammary duct ectasia, mastitis obliterans, plasma cell mastitis, comedomastitis, and secretory disease of the breast. *Duct ectasia* is a condition in which dilated lactiferous ducts of the breast are filled with keratin and secretions. Periductal mastitis is the inflammatory process that occurs around these ducts. Some degree of duct dilation normally occurs with aging. Some researchers have suggested that periductal mastitis seen in younger patients represents a different disease from the more chronic clinical presentation seen in older women. The primary event of periductal mastitis is controversial. Some hypothesize that duct ectasia precedes the inflammatory process and vice versa. The disease is characterized by dilation of the subareolar ducts. The ducts become thick walled and surrounded by plasma cells. Inside the ducts there is a pasty, lipid-rich, yellow-brown secretion. The periductal regions become fibrotic and inflamed. This may be caused by rupture and leaking of the ducts themselves. Fat necrosis is often evident.

EPIDEMIOLOGY AND CAUSES

The incidence of mastitis in breastfeeding women has been reported to be between 2% and 10%. Studies done in other countries report an incidence between 18% and 24%, with the majority of cases occurring in the first 6 weeks postpartum.

There are a multitude of factors that contribute to puerperal mastitis. Cracked, abraded, or otherwise damaged nipples provide a portal of entry for infecting microorganisms. Patients who are having latch-on and positioning difficulty during feeding also increase their risk for both nipple skin disruption and milk stasis, which can lead to mastitis. A slow milk ejection reflex, breast engorgement, failure to empty the breast adequately, waiting too long between feedings, supplemental feedings, the use of pacifiers, wearing a tight and restrictive bra, sleeping positions that constrict the breast, and weaning also contribute to a woman's risk of developing mastitis. Each of these situations can lead to blocked ducts and milk stasis. Unresolved milk stasis provides a medium for bacterial overgrowth.

The causative organism of sporadic puerperal mastitis is *S. aureus* in at least 50% of reported cases. *S. aureus* is frequently found on skin and cultured from the neonate's mouth. Other organisms implicated in the infection are *Escherichia coli*, group A and group B *Streptococcus*, and *Mycobacterium tuberculosis*. Tuberculosis mastitis occurs in populations in which TB is endemic. Physiological and psychological stress are both significant risk factors that increase the likelihood of puerperal mastitis. Fatigue, improper nutrition, and life stress are predictors for breast infections. These situations lead to lower maternal immune defenses and an increased likelihood of the illness.

Periductal mastitis/mammary duct ectasia is seen primarily in perimenopausal and postmenopausal women. The peak incidence is between 40 and 49 years of age, but it can occur at any time after menarche. The inflammatory process has been observed on microscopic examination in 30% to 40% of women older than 50 years; however, clinical disease occurs much less frequently. The actual incidence of the disease is unknown. Duct ectasia has a reported incidence of 5.5% to 25%, as demonstrated on postmortem examinations. An important (and modifiable) risk factor for periductal mastitis is cigarette smoking. The mechanism by which smoking increases the incidence of this disease is unknown, but there is a clear statistical link. Inverted nipples have been suggested to be a source of duct obstruction, which could lead to ectasia, but they have not been shown to be a risk factor.

The cause of periductal mastitis and duct ectasia is unknown. There may be an autoimmune explanation, but this has not been clarified. Infection by anaerobes and other bacteria may play a role, but this has not been verified either. Some patients with this type of mastitis do have bacteria in their nipple discharge.

PATHOPHYSIOLOGY

The causative mechanism of the various forms of mastitis (puerperal, nonpuerperal, and periductal) has been discussed in the preceding text. However, the pathophysiology of the infectious process in the most common form, puerperal mastitis, is a classic example of a breakdown in the body's protective outer epithelial barrier. This results in entry of bacteria from the infant's mouth or the mother's skin into her breast through cracked nipple skin or the nipple pores. With one or more lobes of the breast seeded, infection develops. Moreover, the symptoms of the disease, which include pain, tenderness, and maternal fatigue, contribute to further decreases in effective feeding practices and adequate emptying of the breast, thus worsening the infection. Milk of a mastitic breast has a higher than normal sodium and chloride content, and it is not unusual for an infant to refuse to nurse from that breast.

Because the infection of puerperal mastitis is located primarily in the extraductal tissue, breastfeeding generally poses no harm to the infant, provided skin breakdown has not resulted in frank bleeding from the nipples and there is no evidence of purulent nipple discharge. Purulent material may be present within the ducts, however. In addition, although bilateral infection is possible, mastitis is usually unilateral and localized to the upper outer quadrant of the affected breast. The incidence of mastitis progressing to a subareolar breast abscess has been reported to be as high as 4% to 11% in patients treated for the disease. It is much higher for those who do not seek treatment for mastitis.

CLINICAL PRESENTATION

Subjective

The clinical presentation is acute in nature. The patient's first complaint is fatigue followed by the onset of flu-like symptoms and breast tenderness. The involved breast segments may be red and warm. Patients describe the affected area as being tender to painful. A fever of at least 100.0°F (37.8°C) can be expected with myalgia, malaise, and chills. Nausea and vomiting can accompany these symptoms.

Many patients with periductal mastitis are asymptomatic. Others present with breast tenderness or pain, a breast mass, nipple discharge, nipple retraction, a nonpuerperal breast abscess, or a mammary fistula. The pain is usually subareolar and noncyclical. The nipple discharge varies in color and may contain occult blood. It is most frequently green and sticky and occurs spontaneously. The mastitis can be unilateral or bilateral. Nipple retraction and noninflammatory masses occur more commonly in older women. Pain and abscesses tend to occur in younger women. Periductal mastitis and duct ectasia account for 3% to 12% of benign breast lumps. The pain is usually focused behind the areola and tends to be more severe in younger patients.

Objective

On examination, varying degrees of erythema and edema of the affected breast may be noted. The erythema is most commonly in a V-shaped distribution and may or may not feel hard. Sometimes there is purulent nipple discharge. There may or may not be a palpable blocked duct.

DIAGNOSTIC REASONING

Diagnostic Tests

Milk cultures are rarely done in first-occurrence cases of mastitis because they are costly and may delay treatment. They are warranted with a recurrence or failure of initial treatment. A breast milk culture can be obtained by manual expression of a midstream, clean-catch specimen. Washing the nipple with water and sterile gauze preps the breast. The first 2 to 3 mL of milk expressed should

be discarded. The specimen needs to be fresh when sent to the laboratory. Breast milk is rarely found to be sterile and normally contains leukocytes. A normal leukocyte count is 1,000 to 4,000 white blood cells (WBCs) per milliliter.

With patients symptomatic for mastitis, there are three diagnostic categories when cytology and cultures are performed on breast milk samples. Milk stasis is present with a WBC count of less than 10^6 cells/mL and a bacterial count of less than 10^3 colony-forming units (CFUs)/mL. Noninfectious breast inflammation is present with a WBC count of more than 10^6 cells/mL and a bacterial count of less than 10^3 CFU/mL. A WBC count of more than 110^6 cells/mL with a bacterial count of more than 10^3 CFU/mL is indicative of infectious mastitis. With the help of a milk culture and antibiotic sensitivities, appropriate antibiotic treatment can be initiated. There are occasionally situations in which a patient develops chronic puerperal mastitis. These patients may have anatomical strictures of some lactiferous ducts, which lead to chronic plugged ducts. Long-term antibiotic therapy and attentive breastfeeding management can improve the outcome.

Ultrasound examination of the breast or mammogram may be helpful in making the diagnosis of periductal mastitis. The mammogram shows tubular dilated ducts. Calcification may be present in the lumen and walls of the affected ducts. Intense periductal mastitis may simulate carcinoma on the mammogram. Because carcinoma and mastitis can coexist, a biopsy may be warranted with such findings. In older patients, the mass from the duct ectasia can be difficult to differentiate from carcinoma. Both masses can be hard, irregular, and either fixed or not fixed to the surrounding tissue, with skin or nipple retraction potentially seen with the former. When the nipple discharge is bilateral and multiple ducts are involved, the likelihood of malignancy is reported to be remote. Another diagnostic tool is needle aspiration and the culture of areas of inflammation. Fine-needle aspiration (FNA) may show polymorphs, plasma cells, lymphocytes, and giant cells.

Differential Diagnosis

The first point to consider when presented with a patient symptomatic for puerperal mastitis is to identify whether milk stasis or plugged ducts have led to an infectious process versus a potentially more serious pathophysiologic mechanism, such as breast cancer. The clinical presentation is invaluable in this judgment. There have been several cases of breast cancer in patients who are lactating or pregnant, and reports differ on infants rejecting a breast later diagnosed with cancerous disease. Inflammatory breast cancer is a rare disease, but it can present with some of the same symptoms as classic puerperal mastitis. The patient with inflammatory breast cancer may have a red, swollen breast and sometimes (but rarely) a fever.

The patient commonly has no palpable breast mass and may or may not have *peau d'orange* (breast skin resembling an orange peel in texture). When inflammatory cancer is present, symptoms do not respond to antibiotic treatment as mastitis generally does. With any suspicion of a cancerous process, the patient must be referred for biopsy and a definitive diagnosis.

Breast engorgement is often mistaken for mastitis but does not have the accompanying systemic symptoms of infection (e.g., fever, erythema, myalgia). If the infant has signs of poor "latch-on" during feeding (infant showing sunken cheeks, clicking sounds signifying breaking of suction, contact between the upper and lower lips at the corners of the mouth while feeding, etc.), this can also predispose the mother to mastitis. Galactoceles (milk retention cysts), which may result from plugged ducts, appear hard and red and may be quite painful with breast soreness, as opposed to the shooting pains of mastitis; however, galactoceles lack the systemic signs of mastitis. Interestingly, hard, tender breasts with shooting pains but without redness or fever may be more associated with fungal infection.

MANAGEMENT

The basic principle of management in puerperal mastitis is to decrease contributing factors to the inflammation and infection while generally improving breastfeeding management. Flu-like symptoms should always be treated as mastitis in postpartum patients unless proven otherwise. With a first occurrence, the diagnosis can be made by clinical symptoms alone. If there is no response to antibiotic treatment, or if there is recurrent mastitis, further diagnostics are indicated.

It is vital that the infant continue to breastfeed to avoid milk stasis. Because the infection is extraductal, there is no risk to the infant in continuing to breastfeed, except in HIV-infected mothers due to the potential for viral transmission. Massage of the breasts during feeding helps to better drain the breast, and additional pumping may be needed, particularly if the infant is not nursing effectively on the affected side. Pumping in addition to frequent infant feeding decreases the duration of symptoms (it is recommended to feed or pump every 6 hours) and sequelae of disease, notably the development of breast abscess. Breastfeeding management should include correction of any latch-on or positioning difficulties and aggressive discovery and care of cracked or sore nipples.

Bedrest is imperative during the acute phase of the illness. The mother should be assisted with her household duties and rest in bed with her infant. Moist heat to the affected breast can be useful before feeding and pumping to increase milk expression. A cold compress to the affected breast may provide comfort between feedings. Pain and other uncomfortable symptoms can be treated with nonsteroidal analgesics such as acetaminophen. Stress management techniques should be implemented.

Empirical antibiotic therapy is recommended to treat the infection. Without treatment, only 15% of patients recover without recurrent infection or breast abscess. Approximately 50% improve with breast pumping alone as treatment, and more than 95% recover completely with combination therapy of breast pumping and antibiotics. The patient must be instructed to continue her pharmacologic therapy for the duration of the prescription to avoid partially treated disease and the development of antibiotic-resistant organisms.

The best response is expected is when antibiotics are started within the first 24 hours of symptom onset. Broad-spectrum antibiotics such as dicloxacillin 500 mg or cephalexin (Keflex) 500 mg orally four times daily or amoxicillin-clavulanate (Augmentin) 500 gm orally three times daily is recommended for 10 to 14 days. In addition, antibiotic sensitivities should be obtained from the milk culture in recurrent or nonresponsive cases to help focus therapy. For patients with a beta-lactam allergy, clarithromycin 500 mg orally twice daily for 10 to 14 days is recommended. If community acquired methicillin-resistant *S. aureus* (CA-MRSA) is suspected, then clindamycin 300 mg orally three times daily or trimethoprim-sulfamethoxazole one DS tablet twice daily may be given for 10 to 14 days. Doxycycline 100 mg orally twice daily for 10 to 14 days can be used if the woman is not breastfeeding or pregnant.

In the management of periductal mastitis, broad-spectrum antibiotics have been successful. They treat the periareolar inflammation associated with this condition and reduce pain. If a mass is present, it must be biopsied to rule out carcinoma. In the presence of a suspicious nipple discharge, a ductal excision is necessary to confirm the diagnosis. The wound infection rate after breast biopsies where periductal mastitis and/or duct ectasia is present is high. The infection rate is 2% after biopsies with no evidence of this disease but 10.2% when it is present. This appears to be unrelated to trends in culture results. Symptomatic treatment includes nipple and areolar hygiene; some clinicians recommended no oral nipple stimulation.

Notable sequelae of this type of mastitis are breast abscesses and fistulas. Nonpuerperal breast abscesses are seen more frequently than those associated with lactation. The incidence of periareolar abscess is 10% in patients with symptomatic duct ectasia. The bacteria cultured are usually *S. aureus* and anaerobes. Surgical excision and broad-spectrum antibiotic coverage is the treatment of choice. Needle aspiration may be performed if the risk of malignancy is low, but this treatment frequently needs to be done repetitively.

Abscess is one of the more common sequelae of puerperal mastitis. It can occur when the disease progresses either with or without treatment. The patient presents with worsening local symptoms and may or may not have systemic manifestations. A breast ultrasound can be useful to confirm the diagnosis. Most abscesses are surgically incised and drained under anesthesia. Biopsy of the cavity has been recommended to check for the presence of carcinoma. A drain is put in place, and broad-spectrum parenteral antibiotics should be started with anaerobic coverage pending culture results. A polymicrobial infection is common. The drain can be covered with sterile gauze. It is not unusual for breast milk to leak around the drain because of severed lactiferous ducts. There are occasions when a breast abscess is treated with recurrent needle aspiration, but this is not the treatment of choice.

A recurrence of mastitis may occur for several reasons, including inadequate antibiotic therapy. When a recurrence is evident, a breast milk culture is indicated, as well as further exploration of the patient's breastfeeding management. Chronic mastitis is treated with an antibiotic to cover MRSA as noted earlier.

After antibiotic therapy, infection of the nipples with *Candida albicans* is not unusual. Topical treatment for the patient and concomitant oral nystatin for the infant is necessary. Fungal (*Candida*) mastitis may develop, which is characterized by fiery pain shooting up the duct system; oral antimycotic treatment is indicated in this setting.

FOLLOW-UP AND REFERRAL

The patient may benefit by referral to a board-certified lactation consultant for professional evaluation and assistance with infant feeding. The lactation consultant evaluates and corrects problems related to the infant's feeding, which may be causing or contributing to the occurrence of infection. If a patient's symptoms are not resolved after reasonable treatment attempts, or if there is no change in the size or condition of a breast lump presumed to be a plugged duct after 48 hours of care and treatment, the patient must be referred for further diagnostic evaluation.

Patient Education: Mastitis

Appropriate patient teaching and breastfeeding management in the early postpartum period can be the best prevention tool for puerperal mastitis. Early and frequent infant feedings with correct infant latching and positioning is necessary. No harsh substances such as soaps and lotions should be put on the nipples, and correct bra sizing, rest, and dietary instruction can all help with disease prevention.

Patients with periductal mastitis and duct ectasia need significant support because it can simulate breast cancer. The fear of carcinoma in this age-group (perimenopause and menopausal) is high, and the patient must be reassured that a cancer diagnosis has been considered and ruled out. Because of the connection between periductal mastitis and cigarette smoking, smoking cessation should be discussed at each visit.

BREAST CANCER

Cancer of the breast is the most common cancer in American women and accounts for approximately 30% of all cancers in women in the United States. The Centers for Disease Control and Prevention statistics indicate that 236,968 women were diagnosed with breast cancer in 2014 (most recent data available) and that 41,211 women and 465 men died from breast cancer. Breast cancer is second only to lung cancer as the leading cause of cancer death among women and is the main cause of death in women aged 40 to 44 years. During the 1980s, there were yearly increases in breast cancer incidence rates, probably as a result of an increase in screening; however, this rise has slowed over the past few years. Mortality rates have been decreasing since 1990, most likely because of earlier detection and advances in breast cancer treatment.

EPIDEMIOLOGY AND CAUSES

In general, the lifetime risk of a woman getting breast cancer is one in eight, and the lifetime risk of dying from breast cancer is 1 in 28. In North America, the lifetime odds of a woman getting breast cancer are 1 in 6 for non-Hispanic white women, 1 in 14 for African American women, 1 in 21 for New Mexican Hispanics, and 1 in 40 for New Mexican American Indians. Risk increases with age; it is low in women in their second and third decades of life but rises with each subsequent decade, with the median age for breast cancer diagnosis being 64 years. Increasing age and other risk factors (see Risk Factors: Breast Cancer) have been associated with the development of breast cancer, but these factors explain only 50% of cases. All women have the potential for the development of breast cancer. Screening recommendations and guidelines are presented in Screening Recommendations/Guidelines: Breast Cancer.

 Screening Recommendations/ Guidelines: Breast Cancer

The American Cancer Society (ACS) (2015) recommends the following:

For women of average risk:

- Screening mammogram beginning at age 45 years and performed annually in women 45 to 54 years. Women should have the opportunity to begin screening at age 40 years.
- Biennial screening for women 55 years and older with the opportunity to screen annually.
- Continue screening as long as overall health is good and life expectancy is at least 10 years.

The U.S. Preventive Services Task Force (USPSTF) (2016) recommends the following:

For women of average risk:

- Biennial screening mammography for women 50 to 74 years of age.
- Screening mammography before age 50 should be an individual choice.
- No recommendation for women over age 75.

Note: The ACS does not recommend clinical or self-breast examination for women at average risk.
Note: The USPSTF does not recommend clinical or self-breast examination for women at average risk.

Risk Factors: Breast Cancer

- Female gender
- Increasing age (>50 years)
- Personal history of breast cancer (in situ or invasive)
- Family history of breast cancer in a first-degree relative (parent, sibling, or child)
- Residing in North America or Northern Europe
- Biopsy-confirmed atypical hyperplasia
- Early menarche (before age 12 years)
- Late menopause (after age 55 years)
- Nulliparity or first live birth at a late age (after age 30 years)
- Long-term use of postmenopausal hormone therapy, especially combined hormonal therapy
- Exposure to high-dose radiation
- History of ovarian or uterine fundus cancer
- Higher education and socioeconomic status
- High-fat diet, being overweight, and obesity
- Alcohol consumption (two or more drinks per day)
- Physical inactivity
- Cigarette smoking, especially during adolescence
- Exposure to pesticides and other chemicals

PATHOPHYSIOLOGY

Breast cancer is a disease of various cell populations, with different growth rates, cell surface markers, and tendencies to metastasize. It is often considered a systemic disease at the time of first diagnosis because many patients with "early" breast cancer already have established but clinically occult micrometastases, reflecting the importance of adjuvant hormonal therapy (e.g., tamoxifen, anastrozole). Invasive breast cancer is often preceded by carcinoma in situ lesions of either ductal or lobular distribution. However, a malignant breast mass may be present for many years before the initial diagnosis, and it is not uncommon for invasive disease to be identified at the time of diagnosis, rather than a premalignant lesion. Breast cancers spread by contiguous, lymphatic, and/or vascular channels. The most common areas of metastasis are the regional lymph nodes, lung, skin, bone, liver, and brain.

The development of frank breast cancer may also be preceded by a variety of benign breast conditions characterized by multicentric proliferation of breast tissue. Several genetic mutations have been recognized in both precancerous and cancerous lesions, including genes affecting cellular proliferation, DNA mismatch repair, and the conversion of procarcinogens to carcinogenic compounds. Two of the most widely publicized breast cancer susceptibility genes are the tumor suppressor genes *BRCA1* and *BRCA2*, first cloned in the mid-1990s. These gene products are involved in the repair of double-stranded DNA breaks and mutations in women; they increase susceptibility not only to breast cancer but also to cancers of the ovary, pancreas, and prostate. However, *BRCA1/BRCA2* mutations are rare, accounting for one-fifth of familial breast cancer cases.

The Knudsen hypothesis of malignant transformation is often credited with explaining the pathogenesis of breast cancer. In this model, at least two sequential genetic "hits" or mutations that interfere with DNA repair are thought to underlie malignant transformation of normal breast tissue, which ultimately loses its capacity for programmed cell death (apoptosis). In familial cancers, the first of these hits is thought to be the inherited germline mutation, and the second mutation may be induced by an environmental carcinogen or related to one of many other predisposing risk factors.

CLINICAL PRESENTATION

Subjective

History and risk assessment should include age, ethnicity, education, and socioeconomic status. The clinician should assess for a breast lump or area that feels denser (with or without pain), tenderness, dimpling, nipple retraction, nipple ulceration, erythema or *peau d'orange* ("orange peel"); change in breast shape, breast enlargement, and/or an alteration in the vein pattern of the breast tissue; nipple discharge; or one or more palpable enlarged axillary lymph nodes. The date of onset, location, and duration of any change in the patient's breast and if trauma occurred should also be elicited.

Assessment should also include any systemic symptoms, especially those that may indicate metastases to the skeleton (bone pain, fracture), spinal cord (localized and radicular back pain, lower extremity weakness, paresthesias, paralysis, bladder/bowel dysfunction), brain (headache, seizure, mental status changes, vision and speech defects, sensory loss/muscle weakness, ataxia, persistent nausea/vomiting), bladder or bowel (incontinence), lungs (chest pain, dyspnea on exertion, shortness of breath, cough), and liver (abdominal pain or distention, jaundice, weakness, fatigue, nausea, vomiting, appetite, weight loss, lower extremity edema).

The medical history should include illnesses, especially a previous breast cancer, a benign or preinvasive breast condition, another cancer such as ovarian cancer, prior radiation exposure, medications, allergies, dietary and other health habits (fat intake, alcohol consumption, cigarettes, weight gain, exercise), and past surgical history, especially breast biopsy and/or surgery. Questions should be asked regarding gynecological and obstetric history: age at menarche, age at menopause, last menstrual period, pregnancy history (age when first full-term pregnancy occurred, abortions, miscarriages), and any use of hormone therapy. Frequency of mammograms and date of last mammogram, results of previous mammograms (noting any abnormalities), and other related diagnostic tests and results must also be sought. Family history questions should include information regarding a first-degree relative with a history of breast cancer (note age at diagnosis and bilaterality of disease) and a family history of ovarian cancer associated with breast cancer.

Objective

A thorough physical examination with a focus on the breasts and axillary and supraclavicular lymph nodes should be performed. Inspection should include contour, asymmetry, skin changes, and nipple changes. In premenopausal women, this assessment should be done during the follicular phase of the menstrual cycle, when hormone levels are low and less likely to affect the breast tissue. Examination of the breasts includes inspection and palpation in the upright and supine positions. The size, location, mobility, and consistency of any palpable breast mass or dense area, as well as the lymph nodes should be documented. Any breast changes noted on inspection and the characteristics of any nipple discharge are also recorded.

Clinical manifestations of breast cancer include those already stated, but some patients may present only with an abnormality detected on a mammogram, as pain and tenderness are present in fewer than 10% of patients with cancer. The Patient's Voice 47.1 illustrates the individuality of symptoms and their impact on different patients' life experiences.

DIAGNOSTIC REASONING

Diagnostic Tests

A diagnostic mammogram is necessary in any woman with a palpable breast mass, suspicious nipple discharge, or a suspicious area on a screening mammogram. A spot compression flattens and isolates a lesion. A diagnostic mammogram determines the needs for subsequent testing, and it determines whether other suspicious nonpalpable areas are present in one or both breasts.

Suspicious areas on a mammogram include (1) asymmetry with definitive borders or discernible masses; (2) architectural distortion (a "pulling in" of breast structures) not resulting from previous surgery; (3) a nodule that is more radiodense, irregularly shaped, and has unclear margins; (4) calcifications that are irregularly shaped, clustered, and of varying sizes; (5) skin changes such as thickening or retraction; (6) spiculations (needlelike); and (7) axillary and/or intramammary lymph nodes more than 2 cm in diameter.

Additional studies that may be scheduled to further delineate the abnormality are ultrasound, ductal lavage, and galactography or ductography. An ultrasound, which differentiates solid from fluid-filled masses, may distinguish between benign and malignant diseases. It may better visualize abnormalities in patients with dense breast tissue (women younger than 30 to 35 years) and is used in place of mammography in pregnant patients. Genetic testing for the *BRCA1* and *BRCA2* gene is expensive and done only in women with a high suspicion of a familial breast–ovary cancer syndrome who have undergone extensive pretest (and posttest) counseling.

Mammography views with the Eklund technique are used in a patient with a breast implant to provide additional views behind the implant. Galactography or ductography is used in the presence of serous or bloody nipple discharge without a palpable mass to visualize an intraductal lesion; however, it cannot distinguish between benign and malignant diseases.

A biopsy is performed next. Suspicious areas noted on a mammogram or ultrasound must be submitted for

---

 The Patient's Voice 47.1

A BREAST MASS

It was on my 48th birthday that I noticed a slightly tender enlargement in my left breast. I had consistently checked my breasts for years during my period. I had no family history for breast cancer and never experienced breast tenderness or lumps on a regular basis. Even before my one pregnancy at age 34, I had never experienced significant breast soreness. My nurse practitioner saw me the next day and stated that she could feel something. She sent me for a mammogram. I had one 2 years earlier, so I was sent to the same place. Two days later, I was told there are "changes," and I was referred to a surgeon. I did not know what that meant, except I knew it could be serious. I wanted to do everything they told me to do. I wanted to get better. I had a biopsy and then shortly after, a "lumpectomy." I was told I was very lucky because although the biopsy was positive for cancer, they said my "nodes" were cancer free. I was told I would need radiation therapy since I only had the lump removed. I experienced too much stress and fear at that time in my life. My yoga classes were very important to me then because they helped me relax and heal. I have been going for 7 years since the surgery and now teach yoga too. I know I was lucky and grateful that my nurse practitioner could see me the day after I felt the lump. Waiting is so stressful.

ANOTHER PATIENT'S VOICE

I went for my annual mammogram and later got the call; I was referred to a breast specialist and had a biopsy. On my 45th birthday, I got the news that I had bilateral breast cancer. I have had a bilateral mastectomy, and almost a year of treatment, first chemo and now radiation. I have a young son and husband. This will be the first Christmas since my diagnosis, and I am grateful to be here. Having this diagnosis made me rethink the important things in life. I have slowed down and appreciate all the people in my life. I know people say this, but the diagnosis of breast cancer has really been a gift. I appreciate the small things, like a beautiful sunset, the gentle breeze in my face, and the love of family and friends. I don't take life for granted any more!

biopsy for a definitive tissue diagnosis. A mammogram may not always result in a visible lesion; therefore, all clinically suspicious palpable masses must be submitted for biopsy whether or not they are seen with mammography. The patient should be referred to a surgeon for further evaluation at this point. One or more of the following biopsy techniques may be done in the outpatient setting, usually under local anesthesia:

- *FNA.* FNA may be performed by a primary-care practitioner experienced in the procedure. A 21- or 22-gauge needle is used to aspirate a cyst or extract cells from a palpable solid lesion for analysis. It is easy to perform and provides rapid results with little trauma to the tissue. It is highly reliable when used as an adjunct to the clinical examination and mammogram. On the negative side, FNA requires an experienced cytopathologist, may yield false-negative results, and does not differentiate in situ from invasive cancer. A stereotactic or ultrasound-guided biopsy can be performed on nonpalpable lesions.
- *Core-needle biopsy.* A large-gauge cutting needle is used to provide a large core of tissue from the lesion for histological examination. The results of a core-needle biopsy are as accurate as those of a surgical biopsy, but the procedure is less invasive with better cosmetic results. A stereotactic or ultrasound-guided biopsy can be performed on nonpalpable lesions.
- *Incisional biopsy.* This procedure may be done when a mass is very large and cannot be removed without major surgery. A wedge of tissue is removed for histological examination.
- *Open surgical excisional biopsy (lumpectomy).* This procedure involves the entire removal of a palpable mass or a nonpalpable lesion (after stereotactic or ultrasound-guided biopsy or mammographic needle localization). To qualify as a lumpectomy, lesions suggestive of cancer should be removed with a margin of at least 1 cm of normal tissue. X-ray films of needle-localization specimens are obtained to confirm removal of the mammographically detected abnormality. A postexcision mammogram should confirm complete excision. The open surgical excisional biopsy provides complete pathological assessment but may result in poor cosmesis.

If there is suspicion of inflammatory breast cancer or Paget's disease, a skin biopsy or nipple biopsy should be done at the time of the breast mass biopsy.

Prognosis

Preinvasive breast cancers include ductal carcinoma in situ (DCIS) and lobular carcinoma in situ (LCIS). DCIS has malignant potential but infrequently disseminates; therefore, approximately 98% of patients are cured with local–regional therapy (total mastectomy or breast-conserving surgery and radiation therapy). The addition of tamoxifen (Nolvadex) decreases the incidence of subsequent invasive disease. LCIS has a propensity for

bilaterality, multicentricity, and a 25% to 40% risk for the development of a subsequent invasive cancer. It is managed with close surveillance, a bilateral mastectomy, or chemoprevention (tamoxifen).

Invasive breast cancers have the potential to disseminate through lymphatic and vascular channels to other organs. Most of these cancers are adenocarcinomas. Approximately 80% are infiltrating ductal carcinomas, and 10% are invasive lobular carcinomas. Their prognosis is identical. Invasive lobular carcinoma differs in its slightly greater tendency toward bilaterality and metastasis to meningeal and serosal surfaces. Other histological subtypes are pure mucinous, tubular, medullary, and papillary carcinomas. These subtypes have a slight to somewhat better prognosis resulting from a smaller risk of dissemination. Paget's disease of the breast and inflammatory breast carcinoma are rare. Paget's disease of the breast, unilateral eczema of the nipple, is always associated with DCIS or invasive ductal carcinoma. Inflammatory breast carcinoma has the poorest prognosis of all breast cancers.

Prognostic factors, or tumor-related features, are biological measures done on the breast tissue specimen. They serve as guides for the oncologist in determining systemic adjuvant therapy for the breast cancer patient. In addition to the histological types of invasive breast cancer, lymph node status (0, 1–3, 4–9, or 10 or more [range of good to poor prognosis]), tumor size (1 cm or less in diameter [good prognosis]), and histological differentiation (range of well differentiated [low grade] to poorly differentiated [high grade]) are the standard predictors of risk of recurrence and survival. High-grade tumors are poorly differentiated and carry a worse prognosis, whereas lower grade, well-differentiated tumors carry a more favorable prognosis. With reference to these factors, patients with breast cancer have an excellent prognosis if they have the following features: DCIS, negative lymph nodes with an invasive tumor size less than 1 cm in diameter, and special histological subtypes of breast cancer (e.g., pure tubular) less than 3 cm in diameter.

Patients who have potentially high recurrence rates and who would, therefore, greatly benefit from systemic therapy have the following features: positive regional lymph node(s) or invasive tumors more than 2 cm in diameter even with negative lymph nodes. Breast cancer patients who have a tumor that is poorly differentiated have an increased risk of recurrent disease, but they may also have a greater response to chemotherapy.

Hormone receptor status—for example, the presence or absence of estrogen (ER) and progesterone receptors (PR)—is another important prognostic factor, especially in guiding the oncologist in the selection of hormonal therapy. More patients with breast cancer respond favorably if ER levels are high and if both ERs and PRs are present. Also, a positive status of the pS2 protein (an ER-regulated secretory protein expressed mainly by ER-positive tumors) is indicative of a better prognosis in women with both negative and positive lymph nodes.

Other prognostic factors such as those indicative of the proliferative capacity of the tumor (mitotic index, thymidine labeling index, S-phase fraction, ploidy, and Ki-67), nuclear grade, tumor necrosis, tumor microvessel density, peritumoral lymphatic vessel invasion, the protease cathepsin D, and expression of proto-oncogenes (*ERBB2* [*HER-2/neu*, c-*erbB-2*] and c-*myc*), and the *p53* tumor-suppressor gene may be helpful in predicting response to treatment. For example, the overexpression of c-*erB-2* may predict that a breast cancer patient will be resistant to certain chemotherapy agents and possibly to hormonal therapy. It may also predict a shorter disease-free interval.

Reference to these additional prognostic factors, along with the standard ones, may be valuable in determining the need for systemic therapy in women who have an intermediate prognosis, such as node-negative patients with invasive tumors 1 to 2 cm in diameter.

Staging

After the diagnosis of breast cancer is confirmed, the stage of the disease is evaluated (Table 47.1). Certain laboratory tests may reflect distant metastasis. A complete blood count may show an abnormality of WBCs and platelets, and a low hematocrit may indicate bone marrow infiltration and occult metastatic disease. Liver enzymes and calcium and phosphorus abnormalities may indicate occult liver metastasis and/or bone metastasis. Abnormalities in tumor markers (e.g., CEA, Ca 27.29) may indicate occult metastatic disease. If the tumor marker is abnormal, it will be useful in assessing response to treatment, disease progression or recurrence. Radiological examinations can also assist in detecting distant metastasis. A chest x-ray abnormality may indicate lung metastasis, and abnormal findings on a bone scan/skeletal survey or liver scan (if warranted by signs, symptoms, or laboratory tests) may reflect specific metastasis.

Differential Diagnoses

Several differential diagnoses should be considered. With breast cancer, a palpable mass is usually persistent, unilateral, solitary, discrete, firm, irregularly shaped, nontender, and may or may not be fixed to the skin or underlying

---

TABLE 47.1   Tumor/Node/Metastasis (TNM) Staging of Primary Breast Cancer

Stage	TNM Staging	Description
	TX, NX, MX	Primary tumor (T), regional lymph nodes (N), or distant metastasis (M) respectively cannot be assessed (X)
0	Tis, N0, M0	Carcinoma in situ or Paget's disease of nipple with no tumor
I	T1, N0, M0	Tumor ≤2 cm; no regional lymph node metastasis; no distant metastasis
IIA	T0, N1, M0	No evidence of tumor; metastasis to moveable ipsilateral axillary lymph node(s); no distant metastasis
	T1, N1, M0	Tumor ≤2 cm; metastasis to moveable ipsilateral axillary lymph node(s); no distant metastasis
	T2, N0, M0	Tumor >2 to ≤5 cm; no regional lymph node metastasis; no distant metastasis
IIB	T2, N1, M0	Tumor >2 to ≤5 cm; metastasis to moveable ipsilateral axillary lymph node(s); no distant metastasis
	T3, N0, M0	Tumor >5 cm; no regional lymph node metastasis; no distant metastasis
IIIA	T0, N2, M0	No evidence of tumor; metastasis to ipsilateral axillary lymph node(s) fixed to one another or to other structure; no distant metastasis
	T1, N2, M0	Tumor ≤2 cm; metastasis to ipsilateral axillary lymph node(s) fixed to one another or to other structure; no distant metastasis
	T2, N2, M0	Tumor >2 to ≤5 cm; metastasis to ipsilateral axillary lymph node(s) fixed to one another or to other structure; no distant metastasis
	T3, N1 or N2, M0	Tumor >5 cm; metastasis to ipsilateral axillary lymph node(s) fixed to one another or to other structure; no distant metastasis
IIIB	T4, any N, M0	Tumor of any size with direct extension to chest wall (excluding pectoral muscle) and/or edema (including *peau d'orange*) or ulceration of the skin or satellite skin nodules confined to the same breast, or inflammatory carcinoma; any nodal status as described above; no distant metastasis
IV	Any T, N3, M0	Any tumor status as described above; metastasis to ipsilateral internal mammary node(s); no distant metastasis
	Any T, any N, M1	Any tumor or nodal status as described above; distant metastasis, including metastasis to ipsilateral supraclavicular lymph nodes

Source: used with permission of the American College of Surgeons, Original source for this information is the AJCC Cancer Staging Manual, Eighth Edition (2017) published by Springer International Publishing.

tissue. Breast distortion and skin changes such as diffuse erythema, edema, *peau d'orange*, dimpling, nipple retraction, or nipple ulceration are also indicative of cancer. If present, nipple discharge is spontaneous, persistent, unilateral, localized to a single duct, watery or sticky, and clear, sanguineous, serosanguineous, or serous in color. Lymph nodes suggestive of a malignancy are typically large, firm, and fixed (matted).

Fibrocystic changes (cystic breast disease, chronic cystic mastitis, or mammary dysplasia) may be difficult to distinguish from breast cancer by palpation alone. Fibrocystic changes are so common that they are considered a normal variant of breast tissue. However, if accompanied by significant pain, nipple discharge, or palpable physical examination findings that raise suspicion for breast cancer, the condition is termed *fibrocystic disease*. Cystic areas are unilateral or bilateral, somewhat more diffuse, 1 mm to many centimeters in diameter, soft, and mobile; they may also be tender and painful due to stromal edema, dilation of ducts, and accompanying inflammation. These cysts are hormonally regulated and may be worse premenstrually; this variation with menses usually distinguishes fibrocystic changes from fibroadenomas and breast cancer. Aspiration of clear fluid with complete disappearance of the cyst on follow-up examination or the appearance of a fluid-filled cavity on ultrasound confirms the diagnosis. These changes are most common in patients aged 30 to 55 years.

Fibroadenomas are benign, solid masses of fibrous and glandular tissue that are often confused with breast cancer. These masses may be isolated or multiple and are typically firm, nodular, well-defined, freely mobile, and possibly tender. Growth of the tumor is hormonally stimulated; thus, it may grow rapidly during pregnancy, lactation, or hormonal manipulation. These are most common in younger patients and are not associated with an increased risk of breast cancer if in their simple form. However, *complex fibroadenomas* (i.e., with cysts greater than 3 mm in size, calcification on mammography, or histological evidence of sclerosing adenosis or papillary apocrine changes) have been associated with a greater risk of breast cancer when accompanied by proliferation of surrounding glandular tissue.

Hamartomas composed of stromal and epithelial tissue and *tubular adenomas* consisting of ductal tissue are less common benign tumors of the breast that may present similarly on physical examination but are not considered cancerous. Fat necrosis or *panniculitis* is another benign condition and is typically trauma induced. The mass associated with panniculitis is firm and possibly tender, often with calcification seen on mammography. *Diabetic mastopathy* results in a breast lump with a dense mammographic appearance but benign histology consisting of keloidal scar tissue and lobular, lymphocytic inflammation. This is most often seen in women with type 1 diabetes mellitus who also suffer from other end-organ microvascular damage such as retinopathy or neuropathy. *Intraductal papilloma* is a benign condition with a small, usually solitary and nonpalpable mass in one mammary

duct, with an associated spontaneous sanguineous or serosanguineous nipple discharge. If large enough to palpate, the mass is most often close to or beneath the areola, soft, mobile, 1 to 3 cm in size, poorly delineated, nontender, and sometimes associated with skin dimpling. It is most common in patients aged 35 to 55 years. Solitary papillomas are not considered premalignant; however, diffuse papillomatosis characterized by the formation of multiple papillomas carries with it a greater risk of eventual breast cancer.

Duct ectasia is a benign condition involving inflammation of a subareolar duct, which may produce subareolar erythema and swelling, a mass with nipple retraction and/or skin dimpling, dull nipple pain, tenderness, burning, and itching. Nipple discharge is pasty and straw colored, cream colored, green, or brown. It is most common in perimenopausal or postmenopausal patients who have had children and have nursed.

Ductal hyperplasia without atypia is distinguished from ectasia, in that it is the most common benign breast lesion clearly associated with an increased risk of breast cancer. Epithelial cell proliferation along the basement membranes of the ducts, although benign histologically, varies in size and shape. *Atypical ductal hyperplasia* is associated with an even greater risk of breast cancer (up to sixfold in women with a strong family history of breast cancer), especially in premenopausal women. It is characterized by a loss of apical-basal cellular organization within ductal tissue. *Atypical lobular hyperplasia* is even more concerning because it is qualitatively (albeit not quantitatively) equivalent to LCIS, which is considered a precursor lesion to invasive breast cancer.

Sclerosing adenosis, most common in patients aged 35 to 45 years, is a benign proliferation of the breast epithelium with increased fibrous and glandular tissue, with hard, pea-sized nodules throughout the affected area. There is mild to moderate pain and swelling premenstrually. The presence of this condition has also been associated with an increased risk of breast cancer. *Radial scars* are another benign histological finding consisting of a fibroelastic core from which ducts and lobules radiate outward. If large, these lesions may appear similar to a spiculated carcinoma on mammography and are indeed associated with an increased risk of breast cancer.

Mastitis, a typically benign infectious condition of the breast that may or may not include formation of an abscess, presents with redness, induration, pain, possible purulent nipple discharge, fever, chills, and myalgia. It is more common during lactation.

MANAGEMENT

The patient diagnosed with breast cancer is referred to oncology specialists, such as a surgeon, medical oncologist, and/or radiation oncologist for treatment of the disease (Table 47.2). The choice of treatment is influenced by such factors as tumor stage, ER and PR levels

TABLE 47.2	Management of Invasive Breast Cancer	
Stage	*Surgery/Radiation Therapy*	*Adjuvant Therapy*
I	Breast-conserving surgery with separate axillary node dissection and radiation therapy (RT) to the breast *or* modified radical mastectomy (MRM)	Suitable estrogen receptor (ER)-negative patients: adjuvant chemotherapy ER-positive patients: adjuvant chemotherapy or tamoxifen 20 mg daily
II	Breast-conserving surgery with separate axillary node dissection and RT to the breast. or MRM Consider RT to the chest wall and regional nodes for patients at high risk of local-regional recurrence, including those with known residual disease or four or more involved nodes.	*Node-positive patients:* Premenopausal and postmenopausal (ER-negative) patients: adjuvant combination chemotherapy with or without tamoxifen Postmenopausal patients with positive hormone receptors: tamoxifen alone *Node-negative patients:* ER-negative or ER-positive patients with large tumors: adjuvant chemotherapy ER-positive patients: adjuvant chemotherapy or tamoxifen 20 mg daily
IIIA	*In operable cases:* MRM with or without RT or radical mastectomy (removal of breast tissue, all axillary lymph nodes, and underlying chest muscle) with or without RT. RT may be given because of the high risk of local recurrence; postoperative external beam RT to chest wall with or without boost as necessary for positive or close margins.	Combination chemotherapy with or without hormones Neoadjuvant therapy: chemotherapy may be given preoperatively if primary resection is not feasible or technically difficult.
IIIB	Biopsy for diagnosis and estrogen receptors/progesterone receptors (ER/PR) If good response to chemotherapy or hormonal therapy: local therapy with surgery and/or RT If poor response to chemotherapy or hormonal therapy: palliative RT	Chemotherapy/hormonal therapy: combination chemotherapy with or without hormonal therapy *or* tamoxifen (if ER/PR-positive)
IV	Biopsy for diagnosis and ER/PR receptors External beam RT or palliative mastectomy to control local disease	If visceral disease is minimal or absent and ER/PR-positive: hormonal therapy (as initial therapy) For premenopausal patients: tamoxifen or oophorectomy For patients who relapse after a period of response or prolonged stability on initial hormone therapy: megestrol 40 mg four times daily or anastrozole 1 mg daily or letrozole 2.5 mg daily If visceral disease present or ER/PR-negative: combination chemotherapy
Inflammatory Breast Cancer	Refer to options for Stage IIIB or IV	Refer to options for Stage IIIB or IV

and other prognostic factors, patient age, menopausal status, and the patient's general health. When detected in early stages, invasive breast cancer that is treatable with surgery, radiation therapy, chemotherapy, and/or hormonal therapy may be highly curable.

Surgical Management

The initial surgical management of Stage I and Stage II breast cancer includes one of several types of surgery. Breast-conserving surgery may include a partial mastectomy, lumpectomy, wide excision, segmental mastectomy, or quadrantectomy with a separate axillary node dissection and radiation therapy to the breast. A modified radical mastectomy is a total mastectomy with axillary node dissection. Breast-conserving surgery removes a portion of the breast tissue, whereas a total mastectomy removes all but approximately 2% to 3% of the breast tissue. The survival rates for these two surgical treatment options, breast-conserving or radical mastectomy, are equivalent.

The type of initial surgery for a particular patient usually depends on the location and size of the tumor, breast size, characteristics of the disease on mammography, patient age, and the patient's feelings regarding breast preservation. Breast-conserving surgery may not be an option if there is a tumor beneath the nipple, a large tumor-size-to-breast-size ratio, multicentricity, extensive intraductal carcinoma, diffuse malignant-appearing calcifications on the mammogram, or contraindications to radiation therapy such as pregnancy, collagen-vascular disease, or prior radiation therapy to the breast or chest wall.

After a mastectomy, the patient may choose immediate or delayed breast reconstruction with a submuscular saline implant or expander, a transverse rectus abdominis myocutaneous flap, or a latissimus dorsi flap. Depending on the type of breast surgery, the adverse effects may be wound infection, seroma, bleeding or hematoma, phantom breast syndrome (pain, numbness, or nipple pruritus), paresthesias, muscle atrophy, arm or shoulder weakness or stiffness, lymphedema, phlebitis, or a winged scapula (protruding scapula resulting from intraoperative injury to the long thoracic nerve). A new technique under investigation, lymphatic mapping and sentinel lymph node biopsy, may eliminate the need for an axillary lymph node dissection in some patients and thus avoid some of these adverse effects. The sentinel node (the first lymph node along a lymphatic drainage pathway) is identified after peritumoral injection with a radioisotope or vital blue dye. If the sentinel node is negative for metastatic disease, a complete axillary lymph node dissection is not indicated.

Radiation Therapy

Radiation therapy is indicated for local–regional control of the primary breast cancer or palliation of metastatic disease. After breast-conserving surgery, primary treatment includes external-beam radiation to the entire breast with or without a boost (interstitial radioactive implant or external-beam radiation) to the primary site. After a modified radical mastectomy, radiation therapy to the chest wall and regional lymph nodes is considered in women at high risk of local or regional recurrence, including those with known residual disease or four or more involved lymph nodes. Patients undergoing an axillary lymph node dissection generally do not require radiation therapy to the axilla. Internal mammary lymph nodes may be treated, and patients with four or more positive lymph nodes may require supraclavicular radiation therapy to reduce the risk of supraclavicular lymph node recurrence. A pregnant patient with breast cancer can begin radiation therapy after delivery. Potential adverse effects of radiation therapy include fatigue, edema, breast pain or tenderness, skin reactions, brachial plexopathy, radiation pneumonitis, and myocardial damage if the left breast is treated. Secondary malignancies, such as sarcomas, leukemias, and lung cancer, are rare, although smokers have an increased risk of lung cancer in the ipsilateral lung.

Breast surgery or radiation therapy may make subsequent mammograms difficult to interpret. Masses (postoperative fluid collections and scarring), edema, skin thickening, and calcifications may be seen on these mammograms, especially during the first 6 months after treatment. During the next 6 to 12 months, slow resolution of these changes takes place and stability occurs within 2 years.

Chemotherapy

Neoadjuvant therapy is increasingly being used. It refers to the systematic treatment of breast cancer preoperatively. Neoadjuvant therapy can be chemotherapy, but it can also include endocrine therapy in certain patients. Neoadjuvant chemotherapy is associated with better clinical response rates and increases the likelihood for breast conservation surgery; however, it has not been shown to improve overall survival rates.

Antineoplastic chemotherapy as adjuvant therapy is indicated for the eradication of micrometastatic disease that may be present at the time of the original diagnosis. It should be initiated within 6 weeks (preferably less) of surgery (radiation therapy would follow the chemotherapy). Combination chemotherapy is the standard of care for the treatment of primary breast cancer because it most likely would overcome the potential for drug resistance.

The most widely used regimens include the following:

- CMF (cyclophosphamide [Cytoxan], methotrexate [amethopterin], and fluorouracil [Adrucil])
- CAF (FAC) (cyclophosphamide, doxorubicin [Adriamycin], and fluorouracil)
- AC (doxorubicin and cyclophosphamide) with or without sequential paclitaxel (Taxol)

Alternative regimens include the following:

- CMFVP (CMF and vincristine [Oncovin] and prednisone [Deltasone])
- CFM (CNF, FNC) (cyclophosphamide, fluorouracil, mitoxantrone [Novantrone])
- NFL (mitoxantrone, fluorouracil, leucovorin [Wellcovorin])
- Sequential Dox-CMF (doxorubicin followed by CMF)
- VATH (vinblastine, doxorubicin, thiotepa [Thioplex], and fluoxymesterone [Halotestin])
- Vinorelbine (Navelbine) plus doxorubicin
- Second-line or later therapy, in the event of disease progression or recurrent disease, includes agents such as vinorelbine, paclitaxel, docetaxel (Taxotere), or gemcitabine (Gemzar)

Some of the more common potential adverse effects of chemotherapy include myelosuppression, nausea and vomiting, anorexia, mucositis, alopecia, fatigue, and neurotoxicity. Less common toxicities include hemorrhagic cystitis (alkylating agents), cardiomyopathy (anthracyclines), thromboembolic events, and early menopause (in premenopausal patients). Paclitaxel and docetaxel may also produce myalgia and rare allergic reactions; docetaxel may cause cumulative fluid retention and symptomatic pleural effusions. A rare complication of antineoplastic chemotherapy may be the development of secondary leukemia.

Hematopoietic growth factors (erythropoietin, granulocyte colony-stimulating factor [Neupogen], granulocyte-macrophage colony-stimulating factor [Leukine], and oprelvekin [Neumega]) and cytoprotective agents such as amifostine (Ethyol) and dexrazoxane (Zinecard) may help to prevent or reduce some chemotherapy-related complications related to myelosuppression. Pamidronate (Aredia), a second generation aminobisphosphonate, is used in cases of osteolytic bone metastases to prevent pathological fractures, cord compression, the need for radiation therapy or surgery to the bone, and hypercalcemia, and it significantly reduces bone pain. Pregnant breast cancer patients may receive antineoplastic chemotherapy during their third trimester or after delivery.

Monoclonal Antibodies

The newest treatment for metastatic breast cancer, trastuzumab (Herceptin), a recombinant DNA–derived humanized monoclonal antibody, is used as a single agent in second-line or later therapy for those patients with metastatic breast cancer whose tumors overexpress the HER2 protein. The combination regimen of trastuzumab and paclitaxel is used for the same patient populations who have not previously received chemotherapy for their metastatic disease. Potential adverse effects include cardiomyopathy, anemia, leukopenia, diarrhea, and infection.

Hormonal Therapy

Hormonal therapy includes the use of antiestrogens (tamoxifen), progestins (e.g., megestrol acetate), luteinizing hormone–releasing hormone (LHRH) agonists (e.g., leuprolide), or aromatase inhibitors (anastrozole and letrozole). Tamoxifen is the most commonly prescribed of these agents, and the treatment period is 5 years. Because of its antiestrogenic effect, it is beneficial in breast cancer patients whose tumors have positive hormone receptors, with its greatest effect in those who have both ER-positive and PR-positive tumors. However, tamoxifen also exhibits an estrogenic effect on the endometrium; therefore, it may increase the incidence of endometrial cancer. Potential adverse effects include mild nausea, hot flashes, menstrual irregularities, vaginal discharge, vaginal dryness and irritation, benign ovarian cysts, thromboembolic events, and ophthalmological toxicities.

Local Recurrent Disease

Local recurrent disease is usually indicative of widespread recurrence, especially in postmastectomy patients. Some patients initially treated with breast-conserving surgery

and radiation therapy who later develop a local recurrence in the ipsilateral breast may be cured with surgery and/or radiation therapy. Prolonged survival is more likely if there is a chest wall recurrence less than 3 cm in diameter, axillary and internal mammary (not supraclavicular) lymph node recurrence, and a disease-free interval of more than 2 years after initial therapy. Treatment options for recurrent disease include surgery, radiation therapy, chemotherapy, and/or hormonal therapy. Surgery and/or radiation may be used for a local or visceral recurrence.

In asymptomatic patients with a positive or unknown ER/PR status, and with absent or minimal visceral disease in only one organ, tamoxifen in premenopausal and postmenopausal patients or oophorectomy (or LHRH agonists) in premenopausal patients is a treatment option. In the event that a patient had an initial response to hormonal therapy but had a subsequent relapse, another type of hormonal therapy may be prescribed, such as tamoxifen, anastrozole, letrozole, Megace, androgens, LHRH agonists (for premenopausal patients), or aminoglutethimide. A subset of patients may respond to hormonal therapy withdrawal for approximately 10 months before switching to another form of hormonal therapy.

Patients with positive visceral disease and a negative ER/PR status should receive chemotherapy. If a patient relapses a year or more after receiving adjuvant treatment with CMF, this same regimen may be readministered. If the patient relapses after treatment with an anthracycline-containing regimen, she may be retreated with other agents mentioned earlier. Recurrent breast cancer treatment may be palliative in nature, such as the use of radiation therapy to relieve the pain of bone metastases.

FOLLOW-UP AND REFERRAL

Depending on the breast cancer patient's risk for both local and distant recurrence, a history and physical examination may be done according to the following schedule: every 3 to 6 months during the first 3 years (more frequently during adjuvant therapy), every 6 months for the next 2 years, and annually after the fifth year (more frequently for patients at very high risk for recurrence).

A baseline mammogram should be done 3 to 9 months after tumor excision and at the completion of all treatment. Thereafter, it should be done at least annually to detect a recurrence in the ipsilateral breast of patients who had breast-conserving surgery or to detect a second primary in the contralateral breast of most breast cancer patients. Further testing such as bone scans, chest x-ray films, computed tomography scans, and liver function tests are ordered for symptomatic patients as indicated. Patients treated with tamoxifen should have routine pelvic examinations. If abnormal uterine bleeding occurs, further evaluation is warranted.

The 5-year relative survival rate for patients with localized breast cancer is 98.4%, with regional spread it is 84.6%, and with distant metastases, it declines to 24.3%. The 10-year survival rate for localized breast cancer declines to 82% and 15-year survival declines to 75%.

Patient Education: Breast Cancer

The primary-care practitioner may be involved at various phases of the patient's care, for example, at prediagnosis, diagnosis, treatment, and posttreatment. Therefore, the clinician is in a valuable position to teach the patient and significant others regarding breast cancer prevention and detection and to reinforce information about a breast cancer diagnosis and treatment options (including both benefits and potential complications). For example, primary and secondary breast cancer screening recommendations should be reviewed and discussed with the patient, since if diagnosed at an early stage, breast cancer may be curable with standard treatment (see Evidence-Based Nursing Practice 47.1).

The breast cancer patient needs to learn how to prevent potential postsurgical and/or radiation therapy complications such as lymphedema. In this situation, the patient should be taught range-of-motion exercises for the involved arm and shoulder. The need to avoid infections, injuries, strains, and constriction of the arm is stressed. Antineoplastic chemotherapy and other forms of breast cancer treatment can be teratogenic; therefore, the patient must be advised to use effective contraception during treatment.

The breast cancer patient should be taught about the pharmacologic and nonpharmacologic management of the adverse effects of potential chemotherapy, radiation therapy, or hormonal therapy. For example, the patient may be instructed to take medications such as ondansetron (Zofran) and dexamethasone (Decadron) to prevent delayed chemotherapy-induced nausea and vomiting and to perform techniques such as relaxation with guided imagery to prevent or minimize these symptoms. The patient may also be directed in the purchase of a breast prosthesis, mastectomy bra, or wig.

The patient diagnosed with breast cancer may face many physical and psychosocial issues, such as an alteration in body image and sexuality, a role change, anxiety, denial, anger, and depression. The primary-care practitioner is in a prime position to counsel and support the patient and significant others and to direct them to the many breast cancer resources available to the public that offer individual and group counseling, among other services.

> ### ◢◣ Evidence-Based Nursing Practice 47.1
>
> Kenison TC, Silverman P, Sustin M, Thompson CL. Differences between nurse practitioner and physician care providers on rates of secondary cancer screening and discussion of lifestyle changes among breast cancer survivors. *J Cancer Surviv.* 2015;9:223–229.
>
> This study examined the frequency of cancer screening and discussion of healthy lifestyles between provider types: surgical and medical oncologists, primary-care physicians, and nurse practitioner (NP) survivorship specialists. The researchers surveyed breast cancer survivors regarding the type of provider they saw most, lifestyle changes since cancer diagnosis, cancer screening, and discussion. The response rate was 78.7% with 759 breast cancer survivors completing the survey. There was no difference across providers in the rates of cancer screening. However, a larger proportion of patients seeing an NP reported they discussed physical activity (78.6%; $p < 0.001$) than with any of the other provider. Discussion of nutrition and weight management showed a similar pattern (NP 70.0%, oncologist 36.5%, surgeon 25.7%, radiation oncologist 48.7%, and primary-care physicians 35.5%). Self-reported lifestyle change was basically the same across groups of patients working with different types of providers. The researchers suggest using providers specializing in lifestyle modification to achieve better outcomes in this area.

REFERENCES

Breast Cancer

Cancer stat facts: Female breast cancer. National Institutes of Health, National Cancer Institute: Surveillance, Epidemiology, and End Results Program. https://seer.cancer.gov/statfacts/html/breast.html. Accessed December 17, 2017.

Ciatto S, Houssami N, Bernardi D, et al. Integration of 3D digital mammography with tomosynthesis for population breast-cancer screening (STORM): A prospective comparison study. *Lancet Oncol.* 2013;14(7):583–589.

Elmore JG, Aronson MD, Melin JA. Screening for breast cancer: strategies and recommendations. UpToDate. https://www.uptodate.com/contents/screening-for-breast-cancer-strategies-and-recommendations. Published 2017. Accessed September 8, 2017.

Kenison TC, Silverman P, Sustin M, Thompson CL. Differences between nurse practitioner and physician care providers on rates of secondary cancer screening and discussion of lifestyle changes among breast cancer survivors. *J Cancer Surviv.* 2015;9:223–229.

National Cancer Institute. Breast cancer treatment (PDQ)—Health professional version. https://www.cancer.gov/types/breast/hp/breast-treatment-pdq#link/_551_toc. Updated August, 23, 2017. Accessed September 8, 2017.

Oeffinger KC, Fontham ETH, Etzioni R, et al. Breast cancer screening for women at average risk: 2015 guideline update from the American Cancer Society. *JAMA.* 2015;314(15):1599–1614. http://jamanetwork.com/journals/jama/fullarticle/2463262. Accessed September 8, 2017.

U.S. Preventive Services Task Force. Breast cancer: Screening. https://www.uspreventiveservicestaskforce.org/Page/Document/UpdateSummaryFinal/breast-cancer-screening1. Published 2016. Accessed September 11, 2017.

Mastitis

Dixon JM. Lactational mastitis. UpToDate. https://www.uptodate.com/contents/lactational-mastitis. Updated July 21, 2017. Accessed September 8, 2017.

Khanal V, Scott JA, Lee AH, Binns CW. Incidence of mastitis in the neonatal period in a traditional breastfeeding society: Results of a cohort study. *Breastfeed Med.* 2015;10(10):481–487.

Miller AC. Mastitis empiric therapy. Medscape. http://emedicine.medscape.com/article/2028354-overview. Published 2017. Accessed September 8, 2017.

RESOURCES

Breastcancer.org
　　www.breastcancer.org
National Breast Cancer Foundation
　　www.nationalbreastcancer.org/breast-cancer-facts
National Cancer Institute
　　https://www.cancer.gov/
The Susan G. Komen Breast Cancer Foundation
　　https://ww5.komen.org/

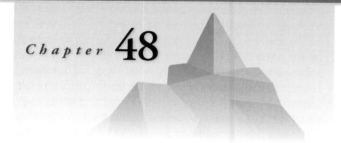

Chapter **48**

Vaginal, Uterine, and Ovarian Disorders

Kimberly Rae Gould, DNP, RN, FNP-C

Debera J. Thomas, DNS, RN, FNP/ANP

Brian Oscar Porter, MD, PhD, MPH, MBA

FERTILITY PROBLEMS

Fertility is the quality of producing ova, fertilized ova being able to implant, and implantation being sustained. Although the medical techniques that facilitate fertility continue to advance, chance continues to play a large role in achieving pregnancy. *Infertility* is defined as the failure to achieve pregnancy despite regular unprotected sexual intercourse for at least 12 months. Over a 12-month period, studies have shown an 85% cumulative probability of achieving pregnancy in normal fertile couples who are not using contraception. Infertility occurs in 10% to 15% of reproductive-aged couples in the United States. A woman younger than 35 years is considered infertile if pregnancy does not occur after 1 year of unprotected intercourse. This time frame is shortened to 6 months in women aged 35 years and older. A man is considered infertile if he does not produce and deliver enough quality sperm to initiate a pregnancy. Given that infertility may arise from causes in both men and women, the full spectrum of causes in both sexes is discussed in this section.

Infertility is divided into two categories. *Primary infertility* refers to a woman who is unable to bear a child, either due to failure to become pregnant or to carry a pregnancy to a live birth. *Secondary infertility* applies to a woman who has delivered at least one child, but subsequently fails to become pregnant or to carry a pregnancy to a live birth. *Sterility* is a term applied when there is an irreversible factor preventing reproduction. Cycle fecundability is the probability of a successful pregnancy occurring in a single menstrual cycle, and cycle fecundity is the probability that a live birth will occur in a single cycle.

EPIDEMIOLOGY AND CAUSES

On average, 30% of fertile couples will achieve pregnancy within 1 month of unprotected intercourse, 80% within 6 months, and 85% within 12 months. At age 25 years, the age at which couples are the most fertile, the average length of time needed to achieve pregnancy is 5.3 months. The average 20- to 30-year-old American couple has intercourse one to three times a week, a frequency that should be sufficient to achieve pregnancy if all other factors are satisfactory. Primary infertility occurs in about 1 of 12 couples (8.3%).

The American Society for Reproductive Medicine (ASRM) estimates there are more than 6 million women between the ages of 15 and 44 years with infertility problems in the United States. However, fertility is determined by factors affecting both partners, including age, underlying disease, and exposure to toxins, drugs, and radiation. A major difference between male and female reproductive potential is that women have a finite reproductive life span (approximately 35 years), whereas men, after puberty, have the capacity to reproduce for the rest of their lives. Nevertheless, aging does affect fertility and sexual function in both men and women.

One in seven couples aged 30 to 34 years is infertile, which increases with age to one in five couples aged 35 to 39 years, and one in four couples aged 40 to 44 years. These declines reflect the natural aging process and emphasize the need for rapid evaluation and treatment of infertility, especially in a female patient older than 35 years. Infertility can be multifactorial and may result from factors affecting the male or female patient, or a combination of both. Although not well defined, infertility is thought to result from male factors in 20% of cases, female factors in 38%, and a combination of factors in both in 27%, whereas the cause of infertility may be unidentified in up to 15% of couples.

Male fertility involves pretesticular, testicular, and/or post-testicular factors. Pretesticular conditions account for 2% to 5% of infertility and include diseases of the pituitary gland and hypothalamus, or factors that affect the hypothalamic-pituitary axis. Testicular defects in spermatogenesis account for up to 80% of male infertility cases, and post-testicular causes include sperm transport disorders, which account for 5% of cases. Ten percent to 20% of cases in men are idiopathic. Female causes of infertility include ovulatory disorders (25%), endometriosis (15%), pelvic adhesions (12%), tubal obstruction or related abnormalities (22%), and hyperprolactinemia (7%). An important factor that affects fertility in women is delaying pregnancy until after age 35 years. With increasing age, the risk that one or more physiological processes are necessary to achieve pregnancy will be inadequate. By age 40, only about 5% of women are able to achieve pregnancy without reproductive assistance.

In general, infertility is caused by one of four conditions: the inability to produce healthy gametes (sperm or eggs); the failure of healthy gametes to come into close physical proximity, thus preventing fertilization; the inability of the fertilized egg to attach to the uterine lining successfully; and the inability of a woman to carry a pregnancy to term postimplantation. Couples should be referred for an infertility evaluation if they have been unable to achieve pregnancy after 1 year of regular unprotected intercourse. If the woman is between 35 and 40 years of age, the couple should be referred for evaluation after 6 months of unprotected intercourse, and immediate evaluation is encouraged in women older than 40 years, given the rapid increase in follicular atresia that occurs after age 37 years.

PATHOPHYSIOLOGY

Numerous processes are essential to normal fertility in women. One of the ovaries must produce a mature follicle and release a mature ovum. There must be no obstruction between the ovary and fallopian tube, and the movements of the fimbria must facilitate transfer of the ovum to the fallopian tube. The quality of the cervical mucus must be favorable to ensure survival of the spermatozoa and its transport to the uterus and fallopian tube. Fertilization usually takes place in the fallopian tube, and the tube must be patent to allow the fertilized ovum to travel to the uterus. The follicle that released the ovum will become a corpus luteum and must produce a large amount of progesterone, an adequate amount

of estrogen, and inhibin A to prepare the endometrium for implantation of the blastocyst and to sustain normal growth and development.

In men, normal fertility requires that the testes must produce an adequate number of morphologically normal, motile sperm. Genital tract secretions from the seminal vesicles and prostate gland must be normal, and because sperm travels from the testis through the epididymis and vas deferens to the urethra, the male genital tract must not be obstructed. In addition, the ejaculated spermatozoa must be deposited in the female genital tract in such a manner that they reach the cervix and enter the uterus where they may contact oocytes either within the uterus, or more commonly within the fallopian tubes.

Fertility can be affected by structural problems in the fallopian tubes, uterus, endometrium, and cervix, and by systemic and genetic factors. Tubal infertility refers to conditions originating in the fallopian tubes. The most common cause of tubal infertility is uterine infection that extends into the fallopian tubes. Pelvic inflammatory disease (PID), most commonly caused by infection with *Neisseria gonorrhoeae* and *Chlamydia trachomatis*, can lead to the formation of scar tissue that can inhibit transport of the sperm to the ovum and/or the ovum to the uterus. Obstruction can then lead to development of hydrosalpinxes, which are collections of fluid within the fallopian tubes. These significantly interfere with the success of in vitro fertilization (IVF), possibly because components in the hydrosalpinx fluid are toxic to developing embryos.

In addition, obstruction may result from tubal endometriosis, pelvic tuberculosis, and adhesions from previous pelvic surgery.

Uterine anatomical abnormalities have not been consistently identified as causal sources of infertility because many women with abnormal uteri are able to become pregnant and carry pregnancies to term. However, septate uteri, synechiae (severe endometrial scarring), and polyps are more common in infertile women. Similarly, uterine leiomyomata or fibroids (benign smooth muscle monoclonal tumors) are the most common form of pelvic tumors in women and have been observed in greater frequency in infertile women. This may be due to lower oocyte implantation that may occur with intracavitary or submucosal leiomyomata.

Other factors also exist that can affect fertilization and pregnancy. Endometriosis occurs when endometrial tissue is found outside the uterus. These tissue implants can occur in multiple areas, including the abdomen, bowel, bladder, fallopian tubes, ovaries, the outer surface of the uterus, the cervix, and more rarely in distant organs such as the lungs. Endometriosis is more common in infertile women and may compromise fertility in a number of ways. The endometrial tissue can irritate surrounding organs and cause the development of adhesions and scar tissue. In addition, direct damage to ovarian tissue by endometrial implants or subsequent surgical removal can occur. Cytokines and cellular growth factors produced by endometrial implants can also interfere with ovulation, fertilization, or oocyte implantation.

Fertility may also be affected by cervical stenosis, which can be a congenital condition or may occur following trauma or infection, with subsequent scarring. Cervical stenosis and alterations in cervical mucus may impair the entry of sperm into the uterus. Problems can also occur after implantation of the fertilized oocyte. If development of the corpus luteum is impaired, inadequate progesterone production can occur and delay endometrial maturation. Likewise, despite the presence of adequate progesterone, the endometrium may not be adequately responsive to this hormone. However, the significance of luteal phase defects as a direct cause of infertility is not well understood.

Systemic factors also exist that affect the ability to initiate or maintain pregnancy. Hypercoagulable states such as antiphospholipid antibody syndrome, systemic lupus erythematosus, and other autoimmune and connective tissue disorders are known to be associated with early, first-trimester miscarriages, which are most likely due to immunological rejection of the developing embryo or microthrombosis of placental vessels leading to placental insufficiency. Genetic defects have been associated with infertility in men and women, the most common being Turner's syndrome (karyotype: 45 chromosomes, XO) in women and Klinefelter's syndrome (karyotype: 47 chromosomes, XXY) in men. Other genes and gene products capable of affecting fertility if mutated include *KAL1* (Kallmann's syndrome) which leads to congenital hypothalamic hypopituitary hypogonadism, fragile X mental retardation 1 (fragile X syndrome), gonadotropin-releasing hormone (GnRH) receptor, follicular-stimulating hormone (FSH) receptor, *DAX1*, *FGFR1*, and *GPR54*.

In men, primary hypogonadism is the most common identifiable cause of infertility. Infertility may be a result of congenital disorders (including chromosomal disorders such as Klinefelter's syndrome and fragile X syndrome), azoospermia from cryptorchidism (failure of testicular descent from the abdominal cavity during in utero development), defects in androgen production (e.g., 5-α-reductase deficiency) or receptor activity, as well as Y chromosome deletions, especially in the long arm at the Yq6 region. Acquired disorders such as testicular infection (e.g., viral orchitis from the mumps paramyxovirus, echovirus, or arbovirus), drugs toxic to sperm (e.g., alkylating immunosuppressants such as cyclophosphamide, antiandrogens such as spironolactone, ketoconazole), radiation exposure, tobacco smoking, and hyperthermia have all been associated with decreased male fertility, as well as underlying systemic disease such as chronic renal insufficiency and cirrhosis. Antisperm antibodies have also been identified in some infertile men that presumably affect fertility, but it is not clear whether these antibodies form spontaneously or as a result of testicular injury that compromises the testicular–blood barrier.

Disorders affecting the hypothalamic-pituitary-gonadal axis may also affect fertility. A failure of hypothalamic

GnRH secretion and/or pituitary gonadotropin production may result from congenital defects (e.g., Kallmann's syndrome) or acquired conditions, such as secreting or nonsecreting pituitary macroadenomas, prolactinomas, craniopharyngiomas, or infiltrative processes such as sarcoidosis, histiocytosis, or tuberculosis.

Sperm transport may be inhibited anywhere along the male reproductive tract. Intrauterine estrogen exposure may lead to epididimal defects, and infection (e.g., epididymitis caused by *Neisseria gonorrhoeae*, *Chlamydia trachomatis*, or tuberculosis) and certain chemical toxins (e.g., chlorohydrin) may affect spermatozoa function within the epididymis. The vas deferens may similarly be affected by infection, intentional ligation (surgical vasectomy), inspissation of mucoid secretions (Young's syndrome), or congenital absence due to defects in cAMP-regulated chloride ion channels (cystic fibrosis).

Erectile dysfunction and ineffective ejaculation may result from spinal cord damage, neurologic disease, or defects in autonomic function caused by diabetes mellitus. Although secretions from the prostate and seminal vesicles contain several components (e.g., fructose) that contribute to sperm viability and motility, defects in glandular secretion have not been causally related to infertility. Varicoceles (venous dilation of the pampiniform plexus proximal to the testicle) are also more common in infertile men, but they may also be present in men with normal fertility. Although no definitive evidence exists, varicoceles are thought to impair spermatogenesis via increased testicular temperature, hypoxia, or vascular stasis with delayed clearance of serum metabolites that are toxic to sperm.

CLINICAL PRESENTATION

Subjective

The typical presentation of infertility involves a couple who presents to the primary-care specialist with the complaint of an inability to become pregnant, despite the desire to have a child. An assessment of persons seeking evaluation and treatment of infertility should begin with a comprehensive history. A detailed medical, social, and family history should be obtained from both partners, as well as a thorough review of systems. In some cases, the history alone will reveal the etiology. The history of both partners should include information about diet; exercise; occupation; presence of stress or depression; allergies; past illnesses, injuries, and surgeries; current medications; use of illicit drugs; and exposure to radiation, chemotherapy, or toxic environmental substances such pesticides, lead, iron, zinc, or copper.

The duration of infertility and whether it is primary or secondary should be determined in both partners. In females, the onset of menses and characteristics of the menstrual cycle; presence of premenstrual symptoms; prior use of contraception; frequency and timing of sexual intercourse; sexual history; characteristics of any vaginal discharge; and history of cervicitis, pelvic infections, surgery, and trauma should be obtained. Relevant information to obtain from men includes a history of mumps, orchitis, trauma, diabetes mellitus, herniorrhaphy, use of anabolic steroids, and problems with urination or libido. Men should also be questioned about exposure to heat (e.g., from ambient temperatures or tight clothing). Finally, although diethylstilbestrol (DES) has not been used in the United States since 1978, couples should still be queried about maternal use during pregnancy, because intrauterine exposure can affect fertility in men and women.

Objective

Both partners should have a complete physical examination that includes body habitus, body mass index (BMI), fat distribution, and identification of characteristics that may suggest developmental delays, genetic abnormalities, or androgen excess. Women should have a pelvic examination that includes inspection of the external genitalia, vagina, and cervix and palpation of the uterus and adnexa. The male examination should include inspection of the external genitalia, evaluation of the scrotum for varicocele or hernia, and measurement of testicular size to determine decreased volume (less than 15 mL is considered abnormal) and testicular length (less than 3.6 cm is considered abnormal).

DIAGNOSTIC REASONING

Diagnostic Tests

Infertility testing can be costly, time-consuming, and emotionally distressing. Testing should always follow a comprehensive history and physical examination. In addition, data should be obtained to confirm the timing of intercourse and the length of time a couple has been having unprotected intercourse. The couple should understand when ovulation occurs, the signs of ovulation, and the most effective times for intercourse.

Diagnostic testing ranges from simple to complex. In women, a basic test of ovulatory function can be done by serial measurements of basal body temperature (BBT), which can aid in identifying follicular, ovulatory, and luteal phase abnormalities. With additional documentation of coitus, serial BBT charts can help identify when ovulation is likely to occur and if intercourse is occurring at the ideal time to achieve pregnancy. One proposed schedule for intercourse based on serial BBT charts is every other day beginning 3 to 4 days before and continuing for 2 to 3 days after the expected time of ovulation.

In men, semen analysis is the single most important diagnostic study and should be done early in the couple's evaluation and always before invasive testing of the female partner. The most important parameters in semen analysis are sperm concentration (count), motility, and morphology. A normal sperm count is between 40 and 300 million/mL of semen, and according to the ASRM, a sperm count below 15 million indicates infertility. The

normal range for total motility is 40%, and at least 25% must demonstrate progressive forward mobility. Morphology refers to the size and shape of sperm, and between 4% and 14% of sperm must have a normal appearance to be considered adequate. Low sperm counts, decreased mobility, and low normal morphology may all adversely impact fertility. Semen pH is also important, as low pH is correlated with decreased fertility.

Cellular debris and agglutination are of concern for antibody-mediated autoimmune destruction of sperm. Antibodies may be detected and are considered concerning if they coat more than 50% of spermatozoa. The presence of immature germ cells may represent a maturation defect, and the presence of sperm leukocytes (greater than 1 million/mL) reflects infection within the reproductive tract. Although a semen culture is often performed, it is usually not diagnostically useful.

It is important to note that an absence of sperm may be due to spermatic duct obstruction, rather than a lack of sperm production by the testes. Patients lacking sperm in the semen should be referred to urology to rule out retrograde ejaculation, congenital absence of the vas deferens, or other forms of obstruction. A postejaculatory urine specimen will reflect retrograde ejaculation if sperm is present, whereas an absence of sperm may reflect obstruction or impaired spermatogenesis. Evaluation of the male partner may include at least two semen analyses to confirm or rule out a seminal deficiency.

The female evaluation includes assessing the hypothalamic-pituitary axis to determine ovulatory function. Progesterone levels are measured at different points along the luteal phase to confirm ovulation. Elevated levels of progesterone are noted when ovulation has occurred. In addition, luteinizing hormone (LH) levels can be measured in the serum and with home urine tests to help predict ovulation. A normal surge should occur 1 to 2 days before ovulation, which can help determine the optimal timing of intercourse. Home urine tests have an 85% sensitivity rate but are not as sensitive as serum testing that is done during a formal fertility evaluation. Due to variations in renal clearance of LH, urine testing may not detect the LH surge.

Examination of vaginal discharge for increased volume and clear, slippery mucus that stretches into strings (Spinnbarkeit) is a strong indicator of preovulatory estrogen effect. The progesterone challenge test, in which medroxyprogesterone acetate 10 mg is given daily for 5 days and the induction of uterine bleeding is monitored in the week after treatment, confirms adequate production of estradiol (estrogen). An FSH level should be drawn on day 3 of the cycle to check for adequate ovarian reserve; a value less than 15 IU/mL is suggestive of adequate reserve. A prolactin level should also be checked in all women with amenorrhea and/or galactorrhea to rule out hyperprolactinemia or the presence of a prolactinoma. Hyperprolactinemia can be treated with a dopamine agonist, such as bromocriptine, pergolide, or cabergoline.

Endocrine evaluation of men includes serum LH, FSH, and testosterone levels. Elevated LH and FSH levels and a low testosterone level are consistent with primary hypogonadism, whereas normal to low LH and FSH reflect secondary hypogonadism. In men with low testosterone and normal to low LH levels, prolactin should be measured to rule out prolactinomas.

If the results of both the male and female infertility workups are negative, further evaluation may be necessary. Magnetic resonance imaging (MRI) and a hysterosalpingogram (fluoroscopic radiographic imaging) are done to evaluate the structure and function of the cervix, uterus, fallopian tubes, and ovaries. Laparoscopy is more sensitive for detecting tubal abnormalities than hysterosalpingogram alone and may be unnecessary if the findings from the hysterosalpingogram are normal. Also, the performance of the hysterosalpingogram itself (flushing the tubes with oil-based contrast medium) increases the likelihood of pregnancy.

Table 48.1 outlines fertility tests and results that suggest a couple is capable of achieving pregnancy.

TABLE 48.1   Fertility Tests and Favorable Clinical Findings

Gender	Test	How Obtained	Favorable Clinical Findings
Male	Semen analysis	48–72 hours after abstinence from ejaculation	Normal amount of ejaculate (3–5 mL; range 1–7 mL) No agglutination of sperm (agglutination suggests infection or autoimmunity) Normal seminal fluid Sperm count greater than 20,000,000 cells/mL with at least 50% motility 2 hours after ejaculation and more than 60% normal-appearing cells
	Karyotyping (in men with severe oligospermia or azoospermia)	Blood/bone marrow sample	Chromosomal abnormalities not detected
Female	Basal body temperature measurement	Oral temperature taken daily before arising, throughout several menstrual cycles	Biphasic pattern with persistent temperature elevation for 12–14 days before menses
	Post coital test	Vaginal examination within 8 hours after unprotected intercourse, during time of presumed ovulation	Cervical mucus suggestive of ovulation. Microscopic ferning pattern present. Watery, slippery, abundant mucus. Spinnbarkeit is present, suggesting normal mucosal consistency (the act of pulling out a string of cervical mucus and measuring how far it can be stretched before breaking). Presence of normal live and motile sperm in cervical mucus.
	Serum progesterone measurement	Blood sample	3–4 ng/mL in early luteal phase 10 ng/mL at midluteal phase
	Serum luteinizing hormone (to predict ovulation)	Blood sample	6.17–17.2 IU/L at ovulation
	Karyotyping (in women with ovarian failure or repeated spontaneous abortions)	Blood sample/bone marrow	Chromosomal abnormalities not detected. Evidence of normal pelvic anatomy and tubal functioning
	Immunoassay tests	Semen and male/female serum	Absence of antibody reaction
	Hysterosalpingogram	Dye injected through cervix into uterus, followed by fluoroscopic visualization of the spread of dye through fallopian tubes; done during first half of menstrual cycle before ovulation	Patency of fallopian tubes and absence of abnormalities in uterine cavities and fallopian tubes
	Laparoscopy	Direct visualization of pelvic structures via insertion of fiber-optic cameras through a small abdominal incision	Normal pelvic structures and absence of signs of infection, adhesions, endometriosis, or lesions

MANAGEMENT

The goal of management is to assist the couple in achieving pregnancy before or during the natural age-related decline in female fertility. Several lifestyle changes can increase the chances that a couple will become pregnant. Women should limit caffeine intake to no more than 250 mg (e.g., two cups of coffee) per day. Studies show that consumption of more than 300 mg caffeine daily can delay pregnancy and increase the risk for miscarriage and preterm labor. Caffeine intake in men does not seem to affect fertility. Likewise, alcohol affects fertility in women, and intake should be limited to no more than four drinks per week. Increasing sexual intercourse to two to three times a week is also advisable. These measures should be recommended before any other interventions.

If the woman's BMI is less than 20 or greater than 27, attempts should be made to achieve ideal body weight. Loss of 5% to 10% of body weight in obese, anovulatory women with polycystic ovary disease (PCOS) can restore ovulation within 6 months and should be a first-line intervention. For women with PCOS, in addition to weight loss, insulin-sensitizing drugs such as metformin have been shown to improve fertility. A low percentage of body fat resulting from eating disorders (e.g., anorexia nervosa, bulimia) or from extreme exercise can lead to anovulation through GnRH or gonadotropin suppression and must be addressed. Pulsatile GnRH therapy may restore ovulation in these women.

If an ovulatory defect has been identified during fertility testing, treatment depends on the specific cause of the problem. In 70% to 85% of cases, the ovaries and prolactin level are normal and the pituitary gland is intact. This type of anovulation is called normogonadotropic, normoestrogenic anovulation (i.e., World Health Organization class 2 anovulation). In these women, clomiphene citrate (Clomid), a selective estrogen receptor modulator (SERM) with both agonist and antagonist effects on the estrogen receptor, may effectively induce ovulation. Ovulation occurs in up to 80% of properly selected women, and pregnancy rates approach 40%. The risk of multiple gestation with clomiphene is 5% and occurs almost exclusively with twins.

Dosing includes a 50-mg dose of clomiphene daily on days 5 through 9 of a woman's cycle. Ovulation can be expected to occur 5 to 10 days after the last dose. If ovulation is not achieved during the first cycle of therapy, the dose may be increased in 50 mg increments to a maximum of 200 to 250 mg daily for 5 days. After the first treatment cycle, a pelvic examination should be done to rule out ovarian enlargement or hyperstimulation. Ovarian enlargement and abdominal discomfort may result from follicular growth and the formation of multiple corpus lutea. Other adverse effects include hot flashes, nausea and vomiting, vision problems, headache, and dryness or loss of hair. Clomiphene citrate should not be used for more than six cycles because it is unlikely to work after that many attempts.

Tamoxifen is another SERM that works with fewer antiestrogen effects, but it has no added fertility benefit over clomiphene citrate. Aromatase inhibitors such as letrozole (Femara) and anastrozole (Arimidex) have a shorter half-life than the SERMs and fewer antiestrogen effects, producing fewer follicles and lower estradiol levels, reducing the risk of multiple gestation and miscarriage. These agents may be used for patients who do not respond to clomiphene.

Women who have not had success with SERMs or aromatase inhibitors may respond to ovarian stimulation with injectable gonadotropins. This treatment requires much closer monitoring, has a higher cost, and a higher risk of multiple gestation; it is, however, considered the most effective medication to use with intrauterine insemination. Intrauterine insemination (IUI) just before ovulation (based on LH measurements) is often effective when other methods have failed. IUI may be tried before IVF because it is often effective and less expensive than IVF. IUI done high in the uterus is more effective than intracervical injection, which approximates normal intercourse. With high IUI, the probability of pregnancy is improved through concurrent treatment with clomiphene for three to six cycles, and if this fails, IUI with gonadotropin injections for at least three cycles can be tried.

The final option infertile couples is assisted reproductive technologies (ART), which includes IVF and embryo transfer or, if the fallopian tubes are patent and normal, gamete intrafallopian transfer (GIFT) or zygote intrafallopian transfer (ZIFT). GIFT and ZIFT are done in less than 1% of cases. In some cases of tubal occlusion (e.g., women with a low success rate of tubal repair of less than 30%), IVF appears to be preferable to surgery because of the more rapid pregnancy rate. IVF has the highest pregnancy rate in the shortest amount of time, but it is also the costliest intervention at $50,000 to $100,000 per attempt. Some studies show an improvement in success rates with intratubal transfer of embryos over transcervical transfer, although this finding is inconsistent. The Society for Assisted Reproductive Technology has valuable information for both provider and patients on their website.

The pregnancy rate with IVF varies significantly between fertility clinics due to the complexity of the techniques required, whereas the pregnancy rate with GIFT is more consistent. The mean live delivery rates per egg retrieval cycle with IVF and GIFT are approximately 21% and 28%, respectively. Ectopic pregnancy occurs in about 4% to 5% of these pregnancies, whereas the rate of fetal abnormalities is slightly increased with a relative risk of 1.32 (95% confidence interval).

It is also possible to achieve pregnancy with IVF, donor sperm and embryo transfer using donor eggs, with a higher success rate than with regular IVF and embryo transfer (47% per retrieval). The eggs generally come from young fertile women (e.g., sisters or anonymous volunteers). The recipient's uterus can be prepared for optimal uterine receptivity by replacement doses of estradiol and progesterone. There are many ethical considerations associated with ART, some of which are presented in Box 48.1.

Less frequently used is a procedure done during a laparoscopy called ovarian drilling. The procedure is performed in women who have PCOS and have failed to ovulate with metformin or clomiphene. During laparoscopy, a laser or electrosurgical needle is used to puncture the ovary several times. This procedure may help women respond better to clomiphene. Cervical stenosis can be treated with catheter dilation of the cervix for several days and concurrent antibiotic prophylaxis (doxycycline 100 mg by mouth [PO] twice daily). Women with systemic clotting disorders may also benefit from aspirin and heparin anticoagulation therapy to improve the likelihood of pregnancy and decrease the chance of pregnancy loss.

Male infertility from hypogonadotropic hypogonadism may be treated with human chorionic gonadotropin (hCG) injections 1,500 to 2,000 IU administered subcutaneously or intramuscularly (IM) three times per week for at least 6 months. hCG acts similarly to LH. If this treatment does not work, human menopausal gonadotropin 37.5 to 75 IU three times per week is added that contains FSH. Thus, this treatment can last more than a year. This combination therapy is typically needed for Kallmann's syndrome (congenital hypogonadotropic hypogonadism). Recombinant LH/FSH is also available. Pulsatile GnRH treatment delivered via IV pump is also available for hypothalamic hypogonadotropic hypogonadism.

Sperm autoimmunity may be treated in the male partner with high-dose steroids (prednisone 40 to 80 mg PO daily) for up to 6 months, but this regimen may be poorly tolerated. Thus, intracytoplasmic sperm injection (ICSI) is an important IVF alternative with a clinical pregnancy rate of up to 20%. Retrograde ejaculation may be treated with IUI, traditional IVF, or ICSI as well. Repair of varicoceles to increase fertility is controversial and is usually recommended only with large defects or in younger men, because prolonged damage to the testes—indicated by testicular atrophy, epithelial damage, and severe oligospermia or azoospermia—is unlikely to be reversed by surgical ligation of the varicocele. Reversal of male vasectomy can result in successful pregnancy in a female partner in up to 50% of cases. In cases of obstruction along the reproductive tract, sperm may be retrieved for ICSI via direct microsurgical aspiration from the epididymis or the seminiferous tubules of the testes. In all cases of congenital reproductive tract defects, such as an absent vas deferens, genetic counseling is required before microsurgical aspiration and ICSI, given the risk of passing genetic defects, such as the cystic fibrosis gene, Klinefelter's syndrome (an extra X chromosome in males), or deletions in the Y chromosome, onto these men's offspring.

FOLLOW-UP AND REFERRAL

Following a thorough examination and counseling regarding the frequency and timing of intercourse, couples who wish to proceed with testing and/or treatment need to be

---

Box 48.1   Ethical Considerations of Assisted Reproductive Technologies

In vitro fertilization (IVF) has been a welcome solution for many couples who have been unable to achieve pregnancy. Recently, advances in the application of IVF technology have spurred the emergence of even more new avenues of achieving pregnancy and parenting. With hormone therapy and donor egg embryos, women past menopause can achieve pregnancy. Other options include cryopreservation, fertilization of donor gametes (donor eggs, sperm, or both), IVF with the use of a gestational carrier, embryo adoption, and the use of surrogacy. All of these options are complicated by the introduction of a third party into the reproductive process and by ethical considerations. Some of the issues raised in connection with these techniques include the following:

1. Is it a constitutional right for individuals or couples to be able to use donor gametes or to contract with a woman to carry their embryo to treat their infertility?

2. With a multiple pregnancy rate approaching 20% in couples undergoing IVF procedures, the potential (<3%) of having a grand multiple gestation forces, some couples to consider embryo reduction (selective abortion) to avoid an adverse obstetric and/or fetal outcome.

3. If excess embryos are frozen for storage, how long can and should they be stored? What should be done in cases of death

of one or both partners, divorce, or when couples choose not to claim their embryos?

4. Do providers have the right to decide who can participate in using donor gametes, embryos, gestational carriers, and surrogates? What about single women, lesbian couples, or when donor arrangements cross-generational lines (e.g., a daughter being a donor for a mother)?

5. Does the use of assisted reproductive technologies take into consideration the best interests of all parties involved, including those of the resultant offspring? For example, what are the effects on a child of knowing or not knowing the identity of one or more gamete donors?

6. How can the potential for consanguinity (having a close ancestor in common) be controlled in the case of gamete and/or embryo donation?

7. Does the existence of new technologies make it more difficult to accept childlessness by increasing pressure on women to follow every avenue in an attempt to become pregnant?

8. To what extent should health insurance policies cover these modes of treating infertility at a time of growing health-care costs?

referred to a reproductive endocrinologist or clinic that specializes in infertility, and this is usually done after a year of unprotected intercourse. Infertile couples need a great deal of support and advocacy, as well as education and assistance in decision making. The options must be presented in a nonjudgmental way to facilitate the couple's own decision making. Providing anticipatory guidance for the battery of diagnostic tests to which patients are subjected during infertility evaluation is critical. Providing referral to other sources of assistance is another way in which the clinician supports the infertile person or couple. One important source of information is RESOLVE, a national organization composed of self-help groups that provide support and information about infertility.

Patient Education: Infertility

An important component of care for infertile persons is emphasizing and teaching self-care. Couples who experience infertility often describe feeling a loss of control over their lives. Identifying and using successful coping strategies help the patient regain this sense of control. Stress-reduction techniques, such as exercise, relaxation techniques, and meditation, may be especially useful both for those with general concerns about fertility and for those concerned over specific diagnostic or treatment procedures. Infertility can become an all-encompassing concern, resulting in alterations in health and recreation patterns and a loss of interest in other aspects of life. It should be emphasized that one can be creative, productive, and successful in other areas of life even if unable to produce children. In addition, other options such as adoption can also be discussed as viable options for raising children and expanding one's family. The emotional problems surrounding infertility illustrate the need for emphasis on family-centered care because infertility is a highly emotional issue that has far-reaching implications for many family members.

PREMENSTRUAL SYNDROME AND PREMENSTRUAL DYSPHORIC DISORDER

Premenstrual syndrome (PMS) and *premenstrual dysphoric disorder* (PMDD) occur during the luteal phase of the menstrual cycle. Symptoms may be mild and cause little disruption in daily life; moderate, causing interference in some aspects of life; or severe, resulting in symptoms that significantly impair a patient's ability for daily activities and impact her life, work, and relationships.

PMS is defined as a cyclic recurrence of a constellation of physical and psychological symptoms that arise during the second, or luteal, phase of the menstrual cycle and resolve 1 to 3 days after the onset of menses. The most common symptoms of mild PMS are headache, bloating, breast tenderness, and irritability. Both somatic symptoms (e.g., depression, angry outbursts) and physical symptoms (e.g., breast pain, bloating) are present in patients with PMS. Although the severity may vary each month, the symptoms are generally mild, of short duration, and manageable. If symptoms related to the luteal phase lead to economic or social dysfunction (e.g., work absenteeism, decreased work productivity, relationship problems) and have occurred for at least three consecutive cycles, a diagnosis of PMS can be made.

In contrast, PMDD is a severe mood disorder that is recognized in the *Diagnostic and Statistical Manual of Mental Disorders, Fifth Edition* (*DSM-5*). To meet *DSM-5* criteria for PMDD, women must have experienced symptoms during most of the menstrual cycles that occurred in the preceding year, and the symptoms must have caused significant distress and interfered with usual activities and quality of life. In addition, at least one of the core symptoms described in the *DSM-5* criteria, and an overall total of five symptoms must be present to meet criteria for the diagnosis. Core symptoms include mood swings, sudden sadness, anger, irritability, depressed mood, tension, and anxiety. Other symptoms include difficulty concentrating, food cravings, loss of interest in usual activities, low energy, feeling overwhelmed, breast tenderness, bloating, weight gain, joint pain, and alterations in sleep (see Box 48.2).

EPIDEMIOLOGY AND CAUSES

PMS is a common problem. During the reproductive years, up to 75% of women will experience minor physical and emotional symptoms for 1 to 2 days before the onset of menses. Between 20% and 40% of women will experience clinically significant PMS, and 5% to 8% of women will experience symptoms that severely disrupt their daily lives and meet criteria for a diagnosis of PMDD. PMS and PMDD can affect women across the full range of reproductive years, and there do not appear

---

Box 48.2 Common Symptoms of Premenstrual Syndrome

Core Symptoms

- Irritability, anger
- Tension, anxiety
- Dysphoria, depression
- Labile mood, mood swings

Other Symptoms

- Headache
- Food craving
- Anger
- Backaches
- Tender breasts
- Clumsiness
- Crying
- Dizziness
- Feeling faint
- Fatigue
- Fluid retention
- Forgetfulness
- Bloating
- Hostility
- Joint swelling
- Confusion
- Migraine

to be significant geographic, ethnic, or cultural differences or predispositions. Family history appears to be a risk factor for the development of PMS, and social and environmental factors such as low education and smoking are also implicated.

Lifestyle habits, including nutrition and stress, are related to PMS as the possibility of physical influence. Although no association between cyclic hormone changes and PMS has been found, it has been suggested that some women may have an abnormal response to normal cyclical hormonal changes. Cyclical changes in levels of estrogen and progesterone appear to impact levels of the neurotransmitter serotonin, and treatment with selective serotonin reuptake inhibitors (SSRIs) has been an effective treatment option. In addition, women with a personal history of anxiety or depression also appear to have an increased risk of developing PMDD.

PATHOPHYSIOLOGY

The influence of cyclical ovarian hormones on various neurotransmitters has been documented, including β endorphins and γ-aminobutyric acid (GABA). In fact, there is a lower concentration of the progesterone metabolite allopregnanolone, which potentiates GABA receptor function, in women experiencing PMS. However, the majority of evidence supports a deficiency in the tryptophan-derived neurotransmitter serotonin as the primary factor in the pathogenesis of PMS. Serum serotonin levels and serotonin uptake by platelets are both reduced during the luteal phase of the menstrual cycle in women with PMS. Moreover, the serotonin agonist fenfluramine and SSRIs both improve PMS symptoms, whereas tryptophan depletion and the serotonin antagonist metergoline both worsen the syndrome.

Fluctuations in ovarian steroids are believed to underlie these abnormalities in neurotransmitter levels, as demonstrated by the efficacy of GnRH treatments (e.g., leuprolide) that suppress ovarian hormones and relieve the symptoms of PMS. Interestingly, the concentrations of serum estrogen and progesterone do not differ between women experiencing PMS and controls; thus, it is the cyclical nature of the sex hormones and the individual response to hormonal changes that appear to be key. Several subcategories of PMS have been suggested, which are synonymously termed categories of premenstrual tension (PMT). PMT-A is categorized by the symptoms of anxiety, irritability, and nervous tension. PMT-B is categorized by fluid retention, abdominal bloating, mastalgia, and weight gain. PMT-C is categorized by premenstrual cravings for sweets, increased appetite, and food binges. PMT-D is categorized by depression, withdrawal, insomnia, forgetfulness, and confusion. Although these categories have some overlap, they may be helpful in differentiating severity of PMS and focusing on where to target interventions.

CLINICAL PRESENTATION

Subjective

A thorough medical, social, sexual, reproductive, and family history should be completed for all patients presenting with PMS symptoms. It is important to ask about family history of PMS or PMDD, personal history of depression or anxiety, and current symptoms including duration and severity. Patients should also be asked about dietary habits, drug and alcohol consumption, exercise, and social and occupational history.

Premenstrual cognitive symptoms that may be reported include crying spells, depression, hostility, anxiety, irritability, relationship conflicts, feelings of inadequacy, increased or decreased libido, and an inability to cope with ever-recurring symptoms. These symptoms often persist for years, and women tend to delay seeking help from a health-care professional until adverse events are linked with these alterations in mood. This delay in seeking help could come from a fear of being labeled as a hypochondriac or mentally unstable. A recent crisis, threat, or ultimatum from a significant other may precipitate a perceived need for professional help, and often women seek help out of a sense of desperation.

Multiple physical symptoms may be reported that range from mild to severe and may vary from month to month. The following is a list of reported symptoms organized by body system:

- Gastrointestinal (GI): abdominal bloating (occurring in 90% of women), nausea, vomiting, constipation, increased thirst
- Respiratory: colds, hoarseness, rhinitis, asthma, sinusitis, sore throat
- Urological: oliguria, urethritis, cystitis
- Ophthalmological: conjunctivitis, vision changes, glaucoma, eye infection
- Mammalogical: breast tenderness (in more than 50% of women), swelling, heaviness
- Dermatological: acne, boils, urticaria, spot bruising, recurrence of herpes
- Neurologic: headaches/migraines (in more than 50% of women), aggravation of epilepsy, vertigo, syncope, fainting, paresthesia of the hands or feet
- Musculoskeletal: backache, joint pain, edema of extremities
- Constitutional: fatigue (affecting more than 90%), weight gain
- Miscellaneous: palpitations, pelvic or low abdominal pain, cold sweats, hot flashes, food cravings, compulsive eating

Other changes perceived as "positive" have been reported by patients during the premenstrual period, including increased libido, more energy, more creative ideas, and increased ability to accomplish tasks. Although women most often initially present with physical symptoms, mood alterations are the most incapacitating and distressing.

Premenstrual symptoms occur in one of four cyclic patterns:

1. Symptoms appear at midcycle, disappear, and reappear the week before menstruation.
2. Symptoms begin at midcycle, with subtle changes that gradually escalate until menses.
3. Symptoms appear the week before menses and intensify until menstruation ensues.
4. Symptoms appear in the first or second luteal weeks and do not disappear until the end of menstruation.

Objective

Increased age and parity may increase the possibility of PMS and are, therefore, important indicators to consider when assessing symptoms are their association with PMS. A 3-month symptom diary that includes the severity and timing of symptoms in relation to menses should be completed by the patient. The diary should also include treatments the patient has tried and the effect of these treatments on symptoms. In addition, notation should be made of the effects the patient's PMS symptoms have had on family members and colleagues. The patient may find this diary a useful tool when exploring her expectations concerning evaluation and therapy. The examination of a patient presenting with PMS symptoms should also include a neurologic examination and screenings for depression and anxiety.

DIAGNOSTIC REASONING

Diagnostic Tests

The most commonly accepted method to diagnose PMS uses a diary during at least two menstrual cycles (three is preferred). If the intensity of symptoms increases at least 30% in the 6 days before onset of menses (compared with days 5 to 10 of the cycle), and if the symptoms occur in two consecutive months, the patient is likely experiencing PMS. This is a rather subjective method of diagnosis because women are asked to assess the percentage of increase in symptoms subjectively, and there is no objective means of comparison with other patients. Once symptoms are determined to be associated with the luteal phase of the menstrual cycle and abatement of symptoms are noted to occur during other parts of the cycle, a presumptive diagnosis of PMS can be made.

A complete physical examination, including a gynecological examination, is necessary to assess the health of women with PMS symptoms. This will enable the provider to rule out other possible causes of the symptoms. Diagnostic tests that may be useful in eliminating other illnesses as possible etiologies include a thyroid-stimulating hormone, complete blood count, urinalysis, FSH, blood sugar, and prolactin level. Depression and anxiety scales are also an important assessment tool and should be used routinely when evaluating a patient for PMS. These assist the practitioner to rule out depression

during the follicular stage of the menstrual cycle versus objectively associating mood and depressive symptoms to the luteal phase of the menstrual cycle.

Differential Diagnosis

One of the most important assessment parameters in making a diagnosis of PMS is that symptoms occur only during the luteal phase of the menstrual cycle. If symptoms appear during the follicular phase, this may reflect a mood or anxiety disorder. It is important to note that there is a lifetime incidence of psychiatric disorders, especially depression, in nearly 80% in women diagnosed with PMS. Differential diagnoses should include cyclothymic disorder, a dysfunctional marital/intimate partner situation, depression, bipolar disorder, menopause transition, poor diet, endocrine abnormalities (e.g., hypoglycemia, diabetes mellitus, hypothyroidism, hyperprolactinemia, hyperandrogenism), alcoholism and drug abuse, and tumors of the brain, breast, and ovaries. The possibility of these conditions should be clinically correlated and ruled out prior to making a definitive diagnosis of PMS. To avoid missing a diagnosis or providing the wrong diagnosis, the primary-care practitioner should be wary of diagnosing PMS without sufficient evaluation.

MANAGEMENT

The main principle of management is to assist the patient in developing strategies to gain control over her symptoms, alleviate symptoms as much as possible, and normalize the patient's life experience. Once an accurate diagnosis of PMS is made, appropriate interventions can be individualized. There are two principles to consider when developing a plan of care. First, PMS is a chronic disorder that may last until menopause. Second, patients have different symptoms and symptom severity and will respond differently to various treatments. Treatment plans should address the chronicity of the problem and provide management options that can be modified as needed. In addition, cognitive behavior therapy should be included for patients with mood disorders, depression, and negative thoughts about self and circumstances.

Lifestyle Changes

Lifestyle changes are considered a first-line treatment for PMS and PMDD and include dietary changes, regular aerobic exercise (shown to decrease depression), and relaxation. Dietary interventions that have been identified as effective include a reduction in salt, sugar, alcohol, and caffeine intake, as well as an increase in complex carbohydrates. It is hypothesized that carbohydrates are involved in the serotonergic pathway, and an increase in serotonergic activity caused by increased complex carbohydrate consumption may help to relieve symptoms. In one trial, a cohort of patients was given a carbohydrate-rich beverage during the late luteal phase of the menstrual cycle, and a control group was given an isocaloric control beverage. The patients who drank the carbohydrate-rich beverage reported lower adverse mood symptom scores, whereas the control group reported no effect on mood.

Aerobic exercise can cause an increase in endorphin levels and, thereby, improve mood. Epidemiological studies comparing the severity of premenstrual symptoms in patients who exercise to those who do not have suggested that those who exercise have fewer symptoms. This is especially true for premenstrual depression. Moreover, it appears that the benefits are independent of the intensity of exercise; therefore, low levels of exercise intensity may be beneficial. An activity as simple as sitting quietly for 20 minutes twice a day and deep breathing while listening to relaxing music has been shown to reduce mood symptoms of PMS twice as effectively as no active therapy

Calcium and magnesium supplements have been shown to help control the emotional and physical symptoms of PMS. In several large clinical trials, 1,000 mg of calcium per day decreased all PMS symptoms as well as any other medication or treatment. Women taking magnesium also experienced a reduction in total symptoms. This effect is thought to be due to the reversal of lower than average mononuclear blood cell magnesium concentrations in patients with PMS. Other dietary supplements including vitamin B_6, folic acid, and vitamin E have been explored, but studies are limited or results are inconclusive. However, adverse effects of most vitamins used at recommended doses are minimal, and a daily supplement may be helpful in some women.

Medications

In addition to lifestyle changes, selective serotonin reuptake inhibitors (SSRIs) such as fluoxetine, sertraline, paroxetine, and citalopram are considered first-line treatment options and have demonstrated effectiveness in relieving tension, irritability, and dysphoria. The recommended starting daily doses of SSRIs are as follows: fluoxetine 20 mg, sertraline 25 to 150 mg, escitalopram 10 to 20 mg, paroxetine 10 to 20 mg, and citalopram 20 to 30 mg. These medications are relatively inexpensive and have minimal adverse effects overall. The most common adverse effects include nausea, headache, jitteriness, and a decrease in libido. Lowering the dose of the SSRI may eliminate some of the adverse effects. If a therapeutic response is not reached within several cycles, the dose may be increased. Although SSRIs are generally administered daily, these drugs have been shown to be effective when administered only during the luteal phase, which has the advantage of lower treatment costs and minimizing adverse effects. Other antidepressants including clomipramine (a tricyclic antidepressant) and venlafaxine (a serotonin-norepinephrine reuptake inhibitor or SNRI) have also been used. However, these medications

have more adverse effects and are not recommended over SSRIs, as their effectiveness has not been well established.

Benzodiazepines such as low-dose alprazolam have been used during the luteal phase in women who fit the strict diagnostic criteria of PMDD and have not had symptom relief from SSRIs. However, the risk of drug dependence is high with benzodiazepines, and the International Society for Premenstrual Disorders does not consider benzodiazepines to be an evidence-based treatment for PMDD.

Combination estrogen-progesterone oral contraception is second-line treatment and should be considered prior to initiating treatment with GnRH agonists. When used continuously, ovulation is suppressed, which suppresses symptoms. Although it is commonly believed that combination oral contraception pills (OCPs) help relieve PMS symptoms, research has shown that there is little difference in symptomatology in users and not users. The only regimen that has been shown to improve both physical and psychologic symptoms of PMS and PMDD in randomized controlled trials is a combined OCP containing ethinyl estradiol 30 mcg with drospirenone. Patients should be screened for the risk of deep vein thrombosis (DVT) before initiation of therapy.

Patients who do not respond to the preceding measures are candidates for a trial of ovulatory suppression therapy with danazol 200 to 800 mg daily. Danazol is a GnRH agonist and a nortestosterone hormone derivative with progestin-like effects that induces ovarian suppression. It works by continuously suppressing pituitary gonadotropin secretion of LH and FSH. It must be given continuously because pulsatile administration leads to LH and FSH secretion. When this therapy is used, "add back" treatment is also used to provide some of the hormones suppressed by the GnRH agonist, with estrogen and progestin given in low doses. Danazol has several undesirable adverse effects, such as weight gain, increased facial hair, and acne. For patients on GnRH agonist therapy, long-term alendronate is given to help prevent bone mineral density loss.

Fluid retention is commonly reported during the luteal phase of the menstrual cycle and accounts for some of the physical symptoms of PMS. Spironolactone 100 mg daily dosed during the luteal phase has been shown to significantly reduce physical and psychological symptoms of PMS versus placebo. With the use of spironolactone, participants reported improvement in irritability, depression, swelling, breast tenderness, and food cravings. Other classes of diuretics, such as thiazides, do not demonstrate effective reduction of PMS symptoms.

NSAIDs administered during the luteal phase significantly reduce the physical symptoms of PMS. Naproxen sodium 500 mg twice daily, started 1 week before the onset of menses and continued through the first few days of bleeding, is effective for both PMS symptoms and dysmenorrhea. This treatment is not recommended for patients with renal impairment, GI disorders, or inflammatory bowel disease. As with any NSAID, GI distress and bleeding may occur. Although they are not first-line therapy for patients with PMDD, NSAIDs may be beneficial for patients with moderate symptoms, especially if associated with dysmenorrhea, headaches, or other musculoskeletal symptoms. NSAIDs are a relatively inexpensive and safe form of therapy for younger patients and may provide the help they need to function normally during this period of the menstrual cycle.

Surgical oophorectomy is an option for women who have failed to improve on GnRH agonist therapy for at least 6 months. This option is limited to women who no longer desire pregnancy and would likely need therapy for several more years.

Many folk remedies and complementary therapies have been used by women for centuries with varying degrees of success. Complementary Therapies 48.1 presents some of these therapies for women's health issues.

FOLLOW-UP AND REFERRAL

The first follow-up visit should be in 2 months to evaluate the data collected by the patient between visits to assess symptom patterns, enabling the diagnosis of PMS to be made and to begin treatment. Frequent visits may be required after that time to evaluate the effectiveness of treatments and to encourage patients to continue to examine and develop treatment plans. Eventually, once symptoms have been controlled, yearly visits should be sufficient.

Complementary Therapies 48.1: Women's Health Problems

PROBLEM	THERAPY	DOSAGE	COMMENTS
Premenstrual syndrome	Evening primrose oil	250 mg orally up to three times daily 2–3 days before menses	May decrease breast tenderness. Common side effects include headache and gastrointestinal (GI) symptoms.
	Calcium	1,200–1,600 mg orally daily	May reduce luteal phase symptoms. Should be taken in divided doses and with recommended daily dose of vitamin D (400 IU daily).
	Vitamin B$_6$	40–100 mg orally daily	Common side effects include numbness, paresthesia, and unsteady gait. Patients with Parkinson's disease or taking levodopa should consult their provider before starting.
	Vitamin C	1,500–3,000 mg orally daily	Take in divided doses for better absorption and to avoid diarrhea.
	Essential oils: chamomile, basil, lavender, marjoram	Use as directed on label	Aromatherapy
Menopausal symptoms	Black cohosh	40–200 mg orally daily	Not recommended for more than 6 months
	Chaste tree berry	Extracts or tinctures to provide 20 mg of crude fruit or 30–40 mg of fruit decoction	Possible adverse GI effects; contraindicated in pregnancy
	Vitamin B complex	50 mg orally daily	High levels of estrogen related to hormone fluctuations can deplete vitamin B$_6$, resulting in anxiety, irritability, and depression.
	Vitamin C	1,500–3,000 mg orally daily	Take in divided doses for better absorption and to avoid diarrhea.
	Vitamin E	400–800 IU orally daily	Can interfere with anticoagulant therapy; avoid if taking anticoagulants; consult with provider before starting.
Breast tenderness	Chaste tree berry Evening primrose oil	As above As above	
Candidiasis (yeast infection)	Vitamin C	3,000–6,000 mg orally daily	Take in divided doses for better absorption and to avoid diarrhea.
Decreased sexual desire	Essential oils: jasmine, neroli (bitter orange tree), rose, sandalwood, ylang-ylang, clary sage, patchouli	Use as directed on label	Aromatherapy; aphrodisiac

Referrals to a specialist may be required, depending on findings from diagnostic tests and the physical examination. The use of certain treatments for severe PMS, such as GnRH agents, is managed by a gynecologist. The diagnosis of PMDD requires referral to a psychiatrist for treatment.

Patient Education: Premenstrual Syndrome

It is important to listen to and evaluate the concerns of patients when they present with symptoms typically associated with PMS. PMS must not be identified with weakness on the part of the patient, but rather recognized as a disease entity that must be investigated and treated. It may take time and energy to manage symptoms and help the patient maintain a good quality of life. When a woman is able to reduce the symptoms of PMS, whether severe or mild, it helps her to function at a higher level.

MENOPAUSE

According to the North American Menopause Society (NAMS), menopause is the permanent cessation of menses resulting from loss of ovarian follicular function. It is defined as the final menstrual period (FMP) and is reached when there have been 12 consecutive months of amenorrhea. Menopause most often occurs due to aging and represents the permanent decline of sex hormone levels. In addition to aging, menopause can also be induced surgically (i.e., bilateral oophorectomy) or medically (e.g., due to chemotherapy or pelvic irradiation) at any age.

The average age of menopause is 51.5 years, and 95% of women will experience their FMP between the ages of 48 and 55 years. Perimenopause refers to the time period before menopause when hormonal, physical, and emotional changes occur and fertility begins to decline. The menopause transition begins with the onset of changes in the menstrual cycle. This is known as the early menopause transition and can precede menopause by several years. The late menopause transition is recognized by the onset of vasomotor symptoms and a greater than 60-day interval between periods. The menopause transition ends with the FMP. The postmenopausal period refers to the period of time after menopause.

Menopause is not a disease state, but it does signal permanent changes in the hormonal, emotional, and reproductive lives of women. Some women may experience an increased awareness of the significance of menopause. They may have philosophical and personal beliefs about managing menopause and treating their symptoms, and because, on average, 30 years of a woman's life will be lived after menopause, they may need help to understand menopause and age-related changes, so that they can make informed decisions about how best to manage this stage of their lives. The management of menopause has received a great deal of attention in recent years. As the average life span for women lengthens—currently at 84 years—it is evident that menopause does not signal the end but rather the beginning of another phase of life recognized by its own issues, challenges, and opportunities.

EPIDEMIOLOGY AND CAUSES

Perimenopause includes three phases in a woman's reproductive life span; the early and late menopausal transition; menopause (FMP); and the postmenopausal period (12 months after the FMP). The menopausal transition signals the nearing of menopause and can begin up to 10 years before the FMP, usually between the ages of 38 and 42 years. The onset may be abrupt or insidious. During this time, ovulation becomes less frequent, and the number of ovarian follicles is decreased as they become less likely to mature. There may be a small increase in the level of FSH. Women note the beginning of this phase with persistent changes in the menstrual cycle, usually with shorter cycle length and/or increased menstrual bleeding. Immediately before menopause, in the late menopause transition, menses may occur after a short luteal phase or after an estradiol peak without ovulation. In approximately 70% of patients, menses will then become lighter and occur less often until ceasing completely. Ten percent of patients will simply stop menstruating suddenly with few or no symptoms, and 20% will experience heavier and often unpredictable bleeding. FSH levels measured at this time will be greater than 25 IU/L. All women who experience cessation of menses before age 40 years should be assessed for primary ovarian insufficiency. If the FSH level is above 40 IU/L, the patient should be referred to an endocrinologist for further evaluation.

In patients with heavy bleeding, there is risk for anemia and other causes should be considered. In addition to menopause, abnormal uterine bleeding (AUB) in this age-group can be caused by endometrial hyperplasia, cancer or polyps, uterine leiomyomata, or systemic clotting disorders.

PATHOPHYSIOLOGY

Menopause is the permanent cessation of menses and ovarian function in a woman. To fully understand menopause, knowledge of normal ovarian development is required. Oocyte development is characterized by germ cell differentiation and the formation of primordial ovarian follicles. This process begins during embryonic development, and at 20 weeks' gestation the fetus will have as many as 6 to 7 million oocytes. FSH drives this process by stimulating granulosa cell formation in ovarian follicles and inducing LH receptor formation, which will eventually allow for ovulation to occur later in life in response to surges in LH at the time of menarche. In a sexually mature ovulatory female, follicular release of an oocyte leads to transformation of the follicle into a corpus luteum cyst, which produces less estrogen and increasing amounts of progesterone that will subsequently support the uterine lining and facilitate implantation of the oocyte and maintenance of pregnancy.

Follicular atresia and oocyte destruction begin during late fetal development and are normal, continuous processes that occur until menopause. At birth, the number of oocytes will have decreased from its peak of 6 to 7 million to 1 to 2 million, and to approximately 300,000 at the onset of puberty. Animal and human studies have shown reduction in oocyte number may be driven by reductions in FSH, decreased androgen production by ovarian thecal cells (reducing substrate for estrogen production via androgen aromatization), the upregulation of proapoptotic genes such as *Bax*, and the downregulation of antiapoptotic genes such as *bcl-2* in both oocytes (primarily a fetal process) and follicular granulosa cells (primarily in adults). Although follicular atresia occurs continuously throughout a woman's reproductive lifetime, it increases rapidly after 37 years of age.

The perimenopause period, which is 2 to 8 years before and 1 year after the FMP, is characterized by waxing and waning of ovarian function, as reflected in both ovulatory and anovulatory (estrogen-only) menstrual cycles of unpredictable duration and intensity, extended periods of estrogen deficiency, and heightened FSH and LH secretion with occasional follicular development and estradiol production. Over time, estrogen feedback to the hypothalamic-pituitary axis declines. In some women, estrogen positive feedback no longer leads to an LH surge capable of triggering ovulation, whereas in others, estrogen negative feedback fails to suppress LH production during the follicular phase. Moreover, the failure of the corpus luteum cysts after ovulation leads to a decrease in progesterone and increased exposure to unopposed estrogen, which accounts for the increase in AUB and endometrial hyperplasia observed during this period.

Factors that influence the timing of menopause have been the subject of much research. Whereas age at menarche has steadily declined over recent decades (having been linked to nutritional status, environmental factors, and general health), the average age at menopause has remained remarkably constant since ancient times. Today, several factors are known to lower the age at menopause, including smoking (which decreases the age of onset of menopause by 2 years on average), nulliparity, menstrual regularity and a shorter cycle length, a family history of early menopause, increased galactose (a monosaccharide component of lactose) intake, concurrent type 1 diabetes mellitus, and certain genetic variants in the estrogen receptor and galactose-1-phosphate uridyl transferase gene. Menopause occurring past age 55 years is defined as late menopause.

With the depletion of ovarian follicles that are able to respond to gonadotropins, both follicular development and cyclical estrogen production cease during menopause. FSH levels rise as the body tries unsuccessfully to stimulate follicular production of estrogen. FSH levels above 40 IU/mL signal the approach of menopause, even though a woman may still experience occasional menstrual bleeding. LH concentration is also elevated, but menopausal levels are difficult to distinguish from LH elevations seen during preovulatory gonadotropin surges in the normal menstrual cycle. Persistently high LH levels lead to continued androgen production by ovarian thecal cells, namely androstenedione, contributing to some of the undesirable physical changes experienced by postmenopausal women such as increased facial hair. Biochemical studies have revealed that the gonadotropins in older women have a longer half-life (contributing to their increased serum levels) and also contain higher levels of carbohydrate that tend to render them less biologically active. Moreover, although residual oocytes and differentiating follicles have been identified in postmenopausal women, the follicles are typically atretic and eventually become cystic in the absence of viable oocytes.

Without a follicular source, circulating levels of estrogen fall significantly during menopause—particularly the active form estradiol, produced from the aromatization of testosterone. High gonadotropin levels stimulate the ovarian stroma to produce the less potent hormone estrone, rather than estradiol, while androstenedione produced by the adrenal glands is converted to estrone by aromatization in the periphery, particularly within adipose tissue, which contains significant levels of the aromatase enzyme. In addition, serum levels of the hormone inhibin B also decline, closely correlating to the rise in FSH, implying an inhibitory action of inhibin B on FSH. Estrone and androstenedione levels remain relatively constant as the patient ages, whereas testosterone levels decline.

Obese women, with larger amounts of adipose tissue, typically display higher levels of circulating estrogens; however, they are still subject to vasomotor symptoms triggered by estrogen deficiency. Patients who are thin tend to experience vaginal dryness and other symptoms associated with low estrogen levels, whereas obese patients are at greater risk of experiencing symptoms associated with unopposed estrogen, such as AUB, endometrial hyperplasia, and endometrial neoplasms. In turn, women who do not experience the vasomotor symptoms of estrogen deficiency during menopause, such as hot flashes, should be monitored yearly for endometrial pathology with vaginal ultrasound and biopsy as appropriate.

CLINICAL PRESENTATION

Subjective

Most women go through menopause without experiencing symptoms debilitating enough to seek medical attention, but may report them during their annual gynecological examination. Information gathered during the examination should include a medical, social, sexual, surgical, and family history. Several factors may influence the timing of menopause and should be noted in the health history: genetic abnormalities, family history, surgical removal of the ovaries or uterus, smoking, and history of chemotherapy or radiation treatments. While removal of the ovaries results in immediate surgical menopause, sparing the ovaries during a hysterectomy may hasten the cessation of follicle stimulation and ovulation by 1 to 2 years. Family history is significant as there is a similarity in menopausal age between mothers and daughters. Women who smoke and those with chronic disease may experience earlier menopause, and menopause can be induced during and following chemotherapy and radiation treatment by virtue of their impact on ovarian function.

About 20% of patients will seek health-care attention for one or more symptoms related to menopause. The most common symptom of menopause is hot flashes (vasomotor symptoms), and up to 80% of women will experience them to varying degrees. Vasomotor symptoms are caused by thermoregulatory dysfunction in which inappropriate peripheral vasodilation, cutaneous blood flow, and perspiration lead to a rapid loss of heat and a fall in core body temperature, causing an involuntary reaction of chills or shivering. Hot flashes can occur during the day and at night, causing night sweats that interrupt sleep. Sleep disturbances and insomnia are reported in 32% to 45% of all menopausal women, and nighttime hot flashes and night sweats can make sleep disturbances significantly worse. Sleep disturbance has been linked to mood disorders including depression, irritability, anxiety, and fatigue. It is important to note that during the menopause transition, women are at increased risk for developing depression, and women with a history of depression may experience worsening of symptoms at the onset of menopause.

Other symptoms of menopause include vaginal dryness, joint pain, diminished libido, and cognitive changes. Estrogen is essential to the health of vaginal tissue, and menopause can cause changes in the epithelium that lead to dryness and atrophy. Lack of estrogen leads to decreased blood flow to the vaginal mucosa and vulva, leading to thinning of the vaginal epithelial lining, decreased vaginal rugae (transverse ridges in vaginal mucous membranes), loss of elasticity, and decreased vaginal mucus. Vaginal dryness is progressive, affecting 21% of women in the late menopause transition, and up to 45% of women 3 years after the FMP. The severity of symptoms will vary, some women may experience mild symptoms such as itching, and others may experience severe dryness that can lead to bleeding. Vaginal dryness and atrophy can also result in sexual dysfunction. A decrease in estrogen influences peripheral blood flow responses to sensory stimulation, affecting the timing and degree of the vasocongestive response during sexual activity. Symptoms may include diminished sexual responsiveness, dyspareunia, decreased sexual activity, a decline in sexual desire, and relationship changes.

Vaginal atrophy may contribute to the symptoms of both stress and urge incontinence in the menopausal woman, particularly atrophy of the urethral epithelium with atrophic urethritis, loss of compliance, and irritation interfering with adequate seal of the urethral meatus. Atrophy of the bladder trigone (outlet tract) and decreased responsiveness of alpha-adrenergic receptors at the bladder neck and urethral sphincter may also contribute to incontinence symptoms

Objective

Estrogen receptors are found throughout the body, and a thorough physical examination may demonstrate signs of estrogen deficiency in the menopausal patient. The physical examination of women in any stage of menopause should include measurement of height and weight and inspection of skin, hair, and vaginal tissue. Many women gain weight during the menopause transition and may have a more difficult time shedding visceral fat. Although weight gain during this time is most likely due to aging, there is some evidence that menopause may change body composition and fat distribution.

Estrogen also helps maintain bone health, and because there is an escalation of bone loss during the menopause transition, a decrease in height can be an early indicator of low bone mass. Because low bone mass can also affect the teeth, an examination should be done to assess oral health. It is significant that during the climacteric, women may lose 2% to 5% of bone mass per year. Skin function is also impacted by falling estrogenic activity, and during menopause there is a rapid decline in skin collagen and skin thickness. These changes lead to dry skin, wrinkling, and atrophy of the vaginal tissue. Menopause can also cause development of facial hair that has the appearance of peach fuzz, as well as abnormal hair growth on the chin.

DIAGNOSTIC REASONING

A diagnosis of menopause can be made based on a history of amenorrhea and the presence of menopause-associated symptoms in age-appropriate women. If these symptoms are present within this context, laboratory testing is not necessary. If the age of the patient and history are not consistent with age-related estrogen deficiency, however, other causes of amenorrhea and menopause symptoms must be considered.

Diagnostic Tests

Several tests are appropriate for women presenting with amenorrhea. Initially, a quantitative beta–hCG test should be done. An elevated level could reflect intrauterine pregnancy, molar pregnancy, ectopic pregnancy, or even certain germ cell tumors. Serum FSH and LH levels may be checked and will be elevated in menopause. FSH levels between 10 to 25 IU/mL suggest relative ovarian resistance consistent with menopausal transition. FSH levels of greater than 40 IU/mL are consistent with complete cessation of ovarian function. LH levels are a less sensitive indicator of hormonal and ovarian function. While they do rise during the menopausal transition, they may also be elevated during the midcycle surge and in cases of chronic anovulation.

Women younger than 40 years presenting with amenorrhea and menopausal symptoms may be given a progesterone challenge test, in which medroxyprogesterone acetate 10 mg is given daily for 5 days and the induction of uterine bleeding is monitored in the week after treatment. If no bleeding occurs, a measurement of a serum estradiol may be helpful. Normal estradiol levels range between 40 and 300 pg/mL. A level greater than 30 pg/mL may indicate some degree of residual ovarian function. Levels less than 30 pg/mL indicate cessation of ovarian function. All women experiencing menopause earlier than 40 years will require additional testing to assess cause.

Women on combined oral contraceptive pills should have hormone levels drawn between cycle days 5 and 7 of the placebo-pill week to assess accurate FSH and estradiol levels. This would be appropriate for menopause-aged women who are taking the pill for contraception and want to know when it is safe to discontinue. Those on progestin-only contraceptive pills can have levels drawn at any time because progesterone does not affect FSH and estradiol levels.

Women who present with amenorrhea and have no vasomotor symptoms may have overproduction of estrogen and should be assessed via pelvic ultrasound to rule out endometrial hyperplasia. Menopausal status can also be determined by vaginal cytological examination. On microscopic examination, parabasal cells will predominate, indicating a lack of epithelial maturing resulting from low estrogen levels.

Differential Diagnosis

The differential diagnoses for patients presenting with menopausal symptoms include pregnancy, spontaneous abortion, anovulation, endometrial hyperplasia, carcinoma, infection, abnormalities of the uterus such as fibroids or polyps, endometriosis, adenomyosis, or injury, and abnormalities of the ovaries such as tumors or cysts. Absence of menses can also be caused by endocrine abnormalities such as hyperprolactinemia and hypothyroidism, as well as excessive stress or exercise.

MANAGEMENT

Treatment of menopause focuses on symptom management and will vary depending on degree of symptom intensity, medical history, type of menopausal symptoms, and personal preference.

Vasomotor Symptoms

Lifestyle modifications are often sufficient to manage mild hot flashes. Simple interventions that can be helpful include using fans, lowering room temperature, dressing in layers, and avoiding triggers such as stress, caffeine, and alcohol. Women with high BMIs experience more hot flashes, and weight loss and regular exercise can be helpful. Physically active women have 50% fewer hot flashes than their sedentary counterparts, and NAMS recommends regular aerobic exercise. Although exercise may initially precipitate perspiration and hot flashes, these symptoms will ease as physical conditioning improves. Insomnia often accompanies vasomotor symptoms and may be relieved with exercise as well. Implementing a diet that is high in complex carbohydrates and fiber (25 to 30 g daily), low in fat (less than 30% of calories from fat) and animal fat in particular, and high in antioxidants (e.g., fresh fruits and vegetables) may also be beneficial.

Several pharmacologic therapies are available for vasomotor symptoms. Women with moderate vasomotor symptoms may benefit from treatment with SSRIs and SNRIs, as both can be effective in reducing the frequency of hot flushes. Menopausal hormone therapy (HT) is appropriate for women with moderate to severe symptoms who have no contraindications such as breast cancer, as well as a low risk of coronary artery disease, DVT, and stroke. The antihypertensive medication clonidine 100 to 150 mcg daily can be given orally or transdermally to relieve hot flashes, but the adverse effects of dry mouth, drowsiness, and hypotension make it less desirable. A new classification of drugs called tissue selective estrogen complexes also provide an option for treatment of vasomotor symptoms and osteoporosis. One such drug combination (Duavee) combines an SERM (bazedoxifene 20 mg) with conjugated estrogen 0.45 mg. The primary advantage of this medication is that the estrogen antagonistic effect of bazedoxifene on the uterus allow patients to obtain the benefits of estrogen without needing to take a progestin.

In women who desire alternative options to prescribed medications, cognitive behavioral therapy, hypnosis, acupuncture, and oral supplements may be tried. A wide variety of herbal and other plant-derived preparations have been developed, such as isoflavonoid phytoestrogens that come from plant fiber and are functionally similar to estradiol. Phytoestrogens are found in soy products such as tofu and soy milk and have estrogenic effects that may reduce vasomotor symptoms. It should be noted, however, that use of soy-based products is controversial because of their unknown effects on estrogen receptors located in breast tissue. Because the safety and efficacy of these supplements is not well established, they should be avoided by women with breast, ovarian, or uterine cancer, endometriosis, and uterine fibroids.

Black cohosh (*Cimicifuga racemose* or *Actaea racemose*) has been used for many years to treat menopausal symptoms. Although the safety and efficacy of this supplement have not been established, there is some evidence that it may reduce hot flashes in some women, and the incidence of adverse reactions is relatively low.

Genitourinary Symptoms of Menopause

Genitourinary symptoms in menopause include genital symptoms (e.g., dryness, burning, and irritation), sexual symptoms (e.g., dryness, discomfort, pain with intercourse), and urinary symptoms (e.g., urgency, dysuria, recurring urinary tract infections). For patients who complain of genital symptoms, a physical examination, cervical cytology, vaginal culture and pH measurement, and urinalysis should be done to assess whether the symptoms are related to estrogen deficiency and not to abnormal cellular changes or infection. If infection or cellular abnormalities (other than parabasal cells) are found, these must be addressed and then the patient reassessed.

The most effective treatment for vulvovaginal atrophy is intravaginal estrogen, which is available as a tablet, vaginal ring, or cream. These products, at low doses, have very little systemic absorption and are suitable for long-term use. At low doses, progesterone therapy is not necessary because there is little systemic absorption. If used at higher doses, adding a progesterone is recommended because of the increased risk of endometrial hyperplasia and cancer with unopposed estrogen. Ospemifene (Osphena), a relatively new SERM, is an oral non-estrogen drug that targets vaginal epithelial tissue and has shown improvement in vaginal dryness and dyspareunia.

Water-soluble or silicone-based vaginal lubricants can be used as an alternative to intravaginal estrogen or as an adjunctive therapy. Lubricants (e.g., Astroglide, K-Y Jelly) used before intercourse to decrease dyspareunia do not alleviate the symptoms of vaginal atrophy but may decrease discomfort. In addition, regular intercourse may improve the health of the vaginal tissue and reduce distressing symptoms.

Estrogen deficiency in menopause affects the lower urinary tract and can lead to symptoms of dysuria, urgency, frequency, nocturia, urinary incontinence, and recurring UTIs. Low dose vaginal estrogen is the primary recommendation for treating urinary symptoms associated with menopause. Kegel exercises continue to be recommended for treatment of urinary frequency and incontinence. These exercises are a safe, nonpharmacologic therapy that may improve the tone of the pelvic floor muscles and urethral sphincter in patients with stress incontinence.

Emotional Symptoms

Many women experience emotional problems with menopause including depression, irritability, and anxiety. Depression associated with menopause occurs more often in women who experienced depression at other times in their lives. In addition to relieving symptoms of depression, many antidepressants also have a favorable effect

on other symptoms of menopause, such as hot flushes. For example, in addition to their effects on mood, SSRIs (e.g., paroxetine 12.5 to 25 mg or venlafaxine 37.5 to 75 mg given once daily) may relieve hot flashes as well as hormonal therapy.

In additional to pharmacologic therapies, regular aerobic exercise improves cognitive function, enhances mood, and promotes daytime alertness and nocturnal sleepiness. Recent studies have shown that a brisk daily walk enhances wellness and promotes a sense of well-being.

Hormone Therapy

Menopausal HT has been approved by the U.S. Food and Drug Administration (FDA) for the prevention of osteoporosis, relief of vasomotor symptoms, and the treatment of vulvovaginal atrophy associated with menopause. The NAMS position statement on HT recognizes HT as the most effective treatment for vasomotor symptoms and genitourinary symptoms of menopause. HT can also aid in the prevention of bone loss. For healthy menopausal women younger than 60 years and who are within 10 years of menopause, HT is a reasonable option for menopause symptom management. In healthy, young postmenopausal women taking combination HT for 5 years, the risk of adverse effects is low. Women without a uterus do not need to take progestin, and the risk of adverse effects remains low for 10 years.

Treatment guidelines for menopause symptom management and HT were revised after findings from the Women's Health Initiative (WHI) study demonstrated an increased risk of heart disease, stroke, venous thromboembolism, and breast cancer with HT. Although the intervention aspect of the study was halted prematurely, data continue to be collected on the health effects of HT, dietary modifications, memory, and calcium and vitamin D supplementation. Also, an observational study is ongoing examining multiple cardiovascular, bone health, and cancer-related outcomes. This study was considered groundbreaking and continues to inform treatment recommendations and guidelines. Today, HT is considered appropriate to treat menopausal symptoms in selected women, but it is not appropriate for the prevention of chronic disease. Specifically, it is not considered cardioprotective, and there is no evidence to suggest it prevents dementia.

HT is contraindicated in patients with hormone-dependent cancers, such as breast, endometrial, and ovarian cancer, and undiagnosed vaginal bleeding. Patients with liver disease, active thrombosis, or history of stroke should not take estrogen, and progestin should be used with caution. Pregnancy is an absolute contraindication for HT. Migraine headache is a relative contraindication for the use of estrogen because of the vasoactive properties of estrogen in some patients. Estrogen use has also been associated with a small increased risk of gallbladder disease, and recent studies have demonstrated an association between estrogen therapy (ET) and adult-onset asthma. An increased risk for the development of systemic lupus erythematosus exists when taking estrogen; however, the incidence is low.

The primary-care practitioner should thoroughly review all risks and benefits of HT and work with the patient to identify the most appropriate type, dose, and method of delivery. HT should be individualized to manage specific symptoms, and consideration should be given to patient preference, cost, and convenience of use. See Drugs Commonly Prescribed 48.1 for a description of HT options available in the United States. When prescribing HT, it is important to understand basic prescribing terminology and guidelines:

- ET: In most cases, estrogen-only therapy is used in women who do not have a uterus or are treating genitourinary symptoms with low-dose topical preparations
- Estrogen plus progestin therapy (EPT): Combination therapy is used in women who have a uterus to prevent endometrial hyperplasia. EPT can be taken continuously (taking both estrogen and progestin daily) or cycled to mimic a menstrual cycle using a continuous-sequential

(CS-EPT) or continuous-combined (CC-EPT) method. When using the CS-EPT method, estrogen is given on cycle days 1 to 21 of each month, and a progestin is given on cycle days 7 to 21. HT is withheld on cycle days 22 to 30, causing endometrial sloughing and bleeding. When using the CC-EPT method, estrogen and a progestin are taken daily. Patients may experience intermittent spotting for a few months, but this should subside once the endometrium thins in response to the HT.

Estrogen products originate from different sources. For example, 17-beta estradiol products are derived from plants (in particular soy) and are considered bioidentical (structurally identical to the human form of estrogen). Conjugated equine estrogen is a synthetic hormone derived from the urine of pregnant horses. It contains naturally occurring estrogens, such as estradiol and estrone, as well as products not native to humans. This product is similar to the human form of estrogen, but not bioidentical.

Androgens also play a role in HT. Levels of androgens, primarily testosterone and androstenedione, but also dihydrotestosterone (DHT), dehydroepiandrosterone

---

🌀 Drugs Commonly Prescribed 48.1: Hormone Therapy for the Treatment of Menopause Symptoms

ORAL ESTROGEN*	DOSING OPTIONS
Conjugated estrogen (Premarin)	0.3, 0.625, 0.9, 1.25 mg; can be given cyclically or continuously
Synthetic conjugated estrogen (Menest, Enjuvia)	0.3, 0.625, 0.9, 1.25 mg; can be given cyclically or continuously
Estradiol products (Estrace)	0.5, 1.0, 2.0 mg; can be given cyclically
Esterified estrogens (Menest)	0.3, 0.625, 1.25, 2.5 mg
Estropipate (Ogen)	0.75, 1.5, 3 mg (may give up to 6 mg per day)
TRANSDERMAL ESTROGEN	**DOSING OPTIONS (RELEASED IN MG/DAY)**
Alora patch	0.025, 0.05, 0.075, 0.1 mg (twice weekly)
Climara patch	0.025, 0.0375, 0.05, 0.06, 0.075, 0.1 mg (once weekly)
Minivelle patch	0.25, 0.0375, 0.05, 0.075, 0.1 mg (twice weekly)
Menostar patch	14 mcg/24 hours (once weekly)
Vivelle-Dot patch	0.25, 0.0375, 0.05, 0.075, 0.1 mg (twice weekly)
Divigel gel	0.1% estradiol: 0.25 g/packet (0.25 mg estradiol/day); 0.5 g/packet (0.5 mg estradiol/day); 1 g/packet (1 mg estradiol/day)
Elestrin gel	0.06% estradiol: 0.0125 mg per day
Evamist spray	Estradiol 1.53 mg/spray (once daily)
VAGINAL ESTROGEN	**DOSING OPTIONS**
Estrace cream	0.01% estradiol: 0.01 mg/g
Estring ring	0.0075 mg/24 hours (one every 3 months)
Vagifem tablet	10 mcg estradiol (twice weekly)
Premarin cream	0.625 mg/g cream; given cyclically—3 weeks on/1 week off

Continued

Drugs Commonly Prescribed 48.1: Hormone Therapy for the Treatment of Menopause Symptoms—cont'd

ORAL ESTROGEN PLUS PROGESTIN	DOSAGE AVAILABLE
Angeliq	0.5 mg estradiol/0.25 drospirenone; 1 mg estradiol/0.5 mg drospirenone
Femhrt	2.5 mcg ethinyl estradiol/0.5 mg norethindrone; 5 mcg ethinyl estradiol/1 mg norethindrone
Activella	0.5 mg estradiol/0.1 mg norethindrone; 1 mg estradiol/0.5 mg norethindrone
Prefest	1 mg estradiol and 1 mg estradiol/0.09 mg norgestimate (3 days of 1 mg estradiol followed by 3 days of estradiol and norgestimate)
Premphase cycle	0.625 mg conjugated estrogens/10 mg medroxyprogesterone
Prempro	0.3 mg conjugated estrogens/1.5 mg medroxyprogesterone 0.45 mg conjugated estrogens/1.5 mg medroxyprogesterone 0.625 mg conjugated estrogens/2.5 mg medroxyprogesterone 0.625 mg conjugated estrogens/5 mg medroxyprogesterone
ORAL ESTROGEN PLUS TESTOSTERONE	**DOSING OPTIONS**
Covaryx	0.625 mg esterified estrogens/2.5 mg methyltestosterone
Covaryx HS	0.625 mg esterified estrogens/1.25 mg methyltestosterone
TRANSDERMAL ESTROGEN PLUS PROGESTIN	**DOSING OPTIONS**
Climara Pro	0.045 mg estradiol/0015 mg levonorgestrel (once weekly)
CombiPatch	0.05 mg estradiol/0.14 mg norethindrone; 0.05 mg estradiol/0.25 mg norethindrone (twice weekly)
ORAL PROGESTINS	**DOSING OPTIONS**
Medroxyprogesterone acetate (Provera)	2.5, 5.0, 10.0 mg (continuously or taken on cycle days 14–25)
Norethindrone acetate (Aygestin)	5 mg (continuously or taken on cycle days 14–25)
Micronized progesterone (Prometrium)	100, 200 mg (continuously or taken on cycle days 14–25)

*Estradiol, 17-β-estradiol.

(DHEA) and dehydroepiandrosterone sulfate (DHEA-S). Androgen levels decrease slowly in patients who experience natural menopause and more rapidly in patients who have undergone oophorectomy because the majority of androgens are produced in the ovary. Androgens are also produced in skin, muscle, and bone tissue. Androgens are available in synthetic form, either alone as methyltestosterone, or combined with estrogen. A natural micronized testosterone may be procured from a compounding pharmacy.

A positive correlation may exist between reduced androgen production and decreased libido in postmenopausal patients. Because the effects of androgen depletion on libido occur only in patients with testosterone levels of less than 20 to 60 ng/dL, a testosterone blood level is indicated before initiation of therapy. Long-term effects of testosterone and its effect on breast tissue in postmenopausal patients is unknown. Androgens have been shown to decrease high-density lipoprotein levels, an undesirable effect; however, they have also been shown to decrease triglyceride levels.

Postmenopausal Osteoporosis

Bone loss is a concern for all aging and postmenopausal women. In the WHI study, combination of estrogen and progestin was found to reduce the risk of vertebral and hip fractures by 34% and other osteoporotic related fractures by 23%. However, when HT is being considered in postmenopausal women of typical age solely for the prevention of osteoporosis, the recommendation is to initially consider nonestrogen options. However, ET is appropriate to use for osteoporosis prevention in women younger than 50 years who experienced early menopause.

Bone density should be assessed in all women older than 65 years and in younger postmenopausal women with risk factors (e.g., small body build, tobacco smoker, corticosteroid use, hypothyroidism, fracture following minimal trauma, family history of fracture). Bisphosphonates are considered first-line therapy for the prevention and treatment of postmenopausal osteoporosis and include both oral preparations [alendronate (Fosamax), ibandronate (Boniva), and risedronate (Actonel)] and intravenous administration of zoledronic acid (Reclast, Aclasta). These drugs have been shown to increase spine and hip bone mineral density and decrease the risk of postmenopausal fracture. The patient should be instructed to take these drugs on an empty stomach in the morning and wait at least 30 minutes before eating or drinking. The patient must remain upright for 30 minutes after taking the medication. If heartburn or difficulty swallowing occurs, the patient should be instructed to stop the medication and seek medical attention, given the risk of pill esophagitis with these medications.

Raloxifene HCl (Evista) is an SERM that may be used as a first-line therapy for the prevention and treatment of postmenopausal osteoporosis. It protects patients from bone loss associated with decreased levels of estrogen. It has an agonistic effect on bone and an antagonistic effect on breast and uterine tissue. Breast tenderness, spotting, and other symptoms that can occur with the initiation of ET do not occur with raloxifene. To date, raloxifene has not demonstrated an increased risk of breast or uterine cancer. A common adverse reaction to raloxifene is hot flashes that may improve over time.

A newer classification of drugs used to prevent bone loss are receptor activator of nuclear factor-kappa B ligand antagonists. The first FDA-approved drug in this category is the monoclonal antibody denosumab (Prolia), which is appropriate for patients with a previous fracture and/or multiple risk factors for osteoporotic fractures. Appropriate patients also include those who have failed to respond to other options, cannot tolerate bisphosphonates, have hypocalcemia, are receiving aromatase inhibitor treatment for breast cancer, or have renal insufficiency. Denosumab is administered subcutaneously two times per year.

Calcitonin nasal spray can also be used to decrease bone resorption in postmenopausal women and can be used alone or in conjunction with hormonal therapy. It is the drug of choice for women who cannot take HT, bisphosphonates, or raloxifene (Evista). The dose of calcitonin is 100 IU/day subcutaneously or 200 IU intranasally daily.

Bone mineral density can also be increased with administration of daily subcutaneous injections of teriparatide (Forteo, Parathar), a parathyroid hormone (parathormone) analog. It is administered subcutaneously in 20 mcg per day doses. A serious adverse effect is an increased risk of osteosarcoma when teriparatide is administered in high doses (based on studies in rats).

Vitamin D and calcium should be taken as supplements by most women. The recommendation is 1,200 to 1,600 mg of daily calcium and 400 to 1,000 IU of vitamin D (ergocalciferol, vitamin D_2) to maintain bone health. Calcium supplements can be either calcium citrate or calcium carbonate. Some sources indicate that calcium citrate is better absorbed from the GI tract.

Bioflavonoids are thought to have estrogenic activity. One study showed that grapefruit juice increased the bioavailability of administered estradiol and estrone. Black cohosh, blue cohosh, ginseng, and wild yam have all demonstrated estrogenic effects. These compounds may result in endometrial hyperplasia, however, if unopposed with progesterone in patients with intact uteri.

FOLLOW-UP AND REFERRAL

When therapies recommended for the treatment of menopause symptoms do not offer adequate relief, a referral to a gynecologist is recommended. In addition, a referral should be initiated for all patients with abnormal bleeding or suspected abnormalities, especially carcinoma. Abnormal bleeding in perimenopausal or postmenopausal periods requires further evaluation with pelvic vaginal ultrasound to check for endometrial hyperplasia and endometrial biopsy to rule out abnormal pathology. A normal postmenopausal endometrium should be less than 4 mm in thickness. Measurements over 4 mm require further work-up.

Estrogen-progestin therapy usually treats AUB, but intermittent ovulation may require low-dose OCPs. In smokers or women with contraindications to OCPs (e.g., history of thromboembolism, breast, or uterine cancer) and no significant symptoms of estrogen deficiency, progestin therapy with medroxyprogesterone acetate 5 to 10 mg daily for 2 weeks per month can induce withdrawal bleeding and prevent endometrial hyperplasia. A depressed menopausal patient who does not respond to lifestyle changes and medications should be referred to a mental health specialist for counseling. Patients who are not responsive to therapy for insomnia may be referred to a sleep disorder clinic.

Patient Education: Menopause

Educating women about menopause is challenging. Because menopause is an event that occurs with normal aging, it is important to educate women about generally expected age-related changes versus changes that are specific to menopause. Patients should be steered toward evidence-based sources of education, such as NAMS. Patients in perimenopause should be reminded that it is still possible to get pregnant, and a pregnancy test should be done for all perimenopausal women presenting with amenorrhea. Patients should receive counseling about safe methods of birth control until menopause has been achieved.

The patient plays a key role in menopause treatment decisions, and adequate education about risks and benefits of various therapies is necessary. Before initiating HT, patients should be screened for cervical, breast, and colon cancer as appropriate. In addition, a serum chemistry panel, lipid panel, blood pressure, FSH, and thyroid hormone levels should be checked. All patients experiencing abnormal vaginal bleeding should have an endometrial biopsy prior to starting HT.

Patients undergoing menopause may have deep feelings and significant emotional investment about what is happening to their bodies. The primary-care practitioner must assess and evaluate these feelings to understand better how to assist the patient. Studies show that fear, lack of knowledge about menopause, and the lack of an informed decision-making process are some of the factors underlying a woman's reluctance to seek treatment for menopausal symptoms. There is considerable conflicting information in the media and among clinicians about HT, and patients will benefit from clarification of the risks and benefits of all the treatments for menopausal symptom relief.

AMENORRHEA

Menarche usually occurs between ages 11 and 14 years, and the average age in the United States today is 12.4 years. Absence of menstruation is considered amenorrhea and can be primary or secondary. *Primary amenorrhea* is the failure to menstruate by age 15 in girls with secondary sex characteristics (breast development) or within 3 years of thelarche (breast budding). *Secondary amenorrhea* is the absence of menstruation for 3 or more consecutive months in a woman who has achieved menarche.

EPIDEMIOLOGY AND CAUSES

Primary amenorrhea occurs in about 0.3% of women and may result from hypothalamic or pituitary failure, ovarian failure, or chromosomal or enzymatic abnormalities. Amenorrhea is a manifestation of a pathological process and is not a diagnosis itself. Causes of primary amenorrhea include congenital defects of gonadotropin production; genetic disorders (Turner's syndrome); congenital central nervous system (CNS) defects such as hydrocephalus; congenital anatomical malformations of the reproductive system (absence of vagina or uterus); abnormal outflow tract (vaginal aplasia or imperforate hymen); and acquired CNS lesions, including trauma, infection, and tumors. Females without a uterus or vagina usually have normal ovarian function in which skeletal growth and secondary sex characteristics develop in the proper sequence, but menses does not occur. In cases of uterine hypoplasia, the uterus does not respond to hormonal stimulation during puberty.

If a woman is not pregnant (the most common cause of amenorrhea), secondary amenorrhea is likely and usually associated with anovulation caused by neuroendocrine dysfunction. Secondary amenorrhea occurs in approximately 1% to 3% of women, with a higher incidence among college students (3% to 5%) and athletes (5% to 50%). Amenorrhea reflects a disruption in the normal physiological or anatomical function of the hypothalamus, pituitary gland, and ovary or outflow tract. Hormones produced by these structures play major roles

in ovulation; any slight change in production may result in anovulation and absence of menstruation. Women taking anabolic steroids (weightlifters, bodybuilders), elite athletes with low body fat, and those with anorexia nervosa may present with secondary amenorrhea.

PATHOPHYSIOLOGY

The hypothalamic-pituitary-ovarian-uterine axis needs to function in a coordinated manner for menstruation to occur. The most frequent cause of primary amenorrhea is dysfunction of the ovaries resulting from gonadal dysgenesis. This may be caused by various chromosomal abnormalities that result in a depletion of oocytes and ovarian follicles, subsequently impairing the regulated cycle of menses. Turner syndrome, characterized by an XO (single X-chromosome) genotype, is one of the most common chromosomal disorders. In this condition, the ovaries are replaced by fibrous tissue (known as streak ovaries), which has a very limited or absent capacity for estrogen production.

In addition, primary ovarian insufficiency (i.e., menopause occurring before age 40 years), PCOS (characterized by concurrent hyperandrogenism), and estrogen or androgen-secreting tumors may all cause amenorrhea. Secondary amenorrhea is nearly universally a hormonal problem because, by definition, normal female sexual development has already occurred. By far, the most common cause of secondary amenorrhea is the normal hormonal changes associated with pregnancy, that is, increased progesterone production needed to maintain the pregnant uterus.

Under normal conditions, the hypothalamus produces GnRH in a pulsatile fashion. In response to GnRH, the anterior pituitary gland produces the gonadotropins FSH and LH. In response to FSH and LH, the ovaries produce estrogen and progesterone, which subsequently drive secondary sexual development and cyclic menstruation. Factors such as stress, weight changes, nutritional deficiencies, strenuous exercise, or infiltrative CNS lesions including hypothalamic tumors (e.g., lymphoma, histiocytosis) or sarcoidosis may all disrupt the normal pulsatile release of GnRH. Pulsatile production of GnRH may also be affected by rare pituitary tumors including macroadenomas and microadenomas, which cause hyperprolactinemia and account for 20% of secondary amenorrhea cases. Amenorrhea may occur before or after the treatment (e.g., surgical resection) of such tumors, depending on the underlying production of pituitary gonadotropins. Functional hypothalamic amenorrhea (which may be primary or secondary) is characterized by an absence of histological CNS pathology, despite an underproduction or overproduction of GnRH that leads to a decrease in gonadotropin surges and results in amenorrhea. In contrast, a complete absence of hypothalamic GnRH production may occur congenitally, inherited in an autosomal dominant, autosomal recessive, or X-linked fashion.

Whereas acquired endometrial scarring known as Asherman's syndrome is essentially the only anatomical uterine etiology of secondary amenorrhea, nearly 25% of primary amenorrhea cases are due to structural abnormalities that prevent menstrual outflow, including imperforate hymen, vaginal agenesis, absent or abnormal uterus, or the presence of a transvaginal septum between the hymen and the cervix. Such conditions may not be connected to any specific event or environmental exposure. However, some conditions may result from biochemical abnormalities in hormone receptor functioning, manifested on either an XX or XY genetic background. Thus, an advanced work-up of patients with primary amenorrhea should also include karyotyping to confirm that the patient is an XX genetic female.

Primary amenorrhea often is the presenting symptom in patients with complete androgen insensitivity syndrome (testicular feminization syndrome). This syndrome occurs when the external genitalia of an XY fetus is unable to respond to testosterone because of a receptor defect and thus fails to undergo differentiation into a phenotypically male form. Internally, however, the testes produce functional Müllerian inhibiting factor, causing the regression of all internal female reproductive organs, thus leading to primary amenorrhea. Individuals with this syndrome have a male genotype (XY) but appear outwardly female on clinical examination. A congenital lack of 5-α-reductase enzymatic activity causes a similar phenomenon of external sexual ambiguity in which XY males do not undergo full secondary sexual development at puberty, because testosterone cannot be converted into its more potent metabolite DHT.

CLINICAL PRESENTATION

Subjective

Amenorrhea is a symptom and is usually the reason the patient seeks health care. Other subjective data from the patient usually are obtained during the history. The detailed history must include a complete menstrual history including age at menarche, date of last menstrual period and last normal menses, cycle regularity, and flow, as well as obstetrical history, including number of pregnancies, lactation, and birth control methods. Other components include developmental data to evaluate for short stature or growth hormone or thyroid deficiency, nutritional history including anorexia, diet, stress factors, sports activities, family history, (especially mother's onset of menopause), symptoms that may arise from systemic disorders (e.g., diabetes, thyroid disorders), the presence or absence of secondary sex characteristics, and any medications being taken, such as antihypertensive medications or OCPs. Cyclic pelvic pain in a young teen or preteen could indicate Müllerian outflow tract obstruction.

Objective

The physical examination should include a neurologic examination to assess for headaches and visual field abnormalities to rule out a pituitary tumor, olfactory testing to screen for Kallmann's syndrome (hypothalamic or pituitary tumor), a pelvic and rectal examination to assess for the presence of a vagina, condition of the hymen, and presence of a uterus, the existence of skin lesions, acne, needle marks, and skin darkening to rule out adrenal insufficiency, and a breast examination to check for galactorrhea, which may be a sign of hyperprolactinemia.

DIAGNOSTIC REASONING

Diagnostic Tests

A urine pregnancy test should be the first test performed in the patient with amenorrhea. It is inexpensive, easy to perform, and should be done despite what the patient indicates about her sexual history. If the test is positive, a serum beta–hCG level for approximate staging of pregnancy should be drawn. Other tests include baseline blood chemistry profiles to evaluate for renal or hepatic disease, thyroid function tests, and tests for estrogen, FSH, LH, and prolactin levels.

Tests for secondary amenorrhea include androgen studies of total testosterone and DHEA-S, which are specifically done in women who have clinical signs of hyperandrogenism such as acne and hirsutism, a progesterone challenge test, and prolactin and FSH levels, which evaluate the hypothalamic-pituitary-ovarian axis. A progestin (or progesterone) challenge test indirectly provides information regarding outflow tract patency. This test, only administered once a negative pregnancy test result is obtained, consists of giving medroxyprogesterone acetate 10 mg PO for 5 to 10 days or 200 mg IM once to induce withdrawal bleeding or spotting, which should occur within 14 days after the last dose. If withdrawal bleeding occurs, this indicates intact pituitary-gonadal function, and amenorrhea is probably the result of anovulation. The test is negative if no withdrawal bleeding occurs and suggests low levels of estrogen (premature ovarian failure or hypothalamic pituitary failure) or a nonpatent outflow tract.

Differential Diagnosis

Differential diagnoses for amenorrhea include pregnancy (intrauterine or ectopic), menopause, premature ovarian failure, genetic and chromosome-related problems, and hyperprolactinemia related to tumor, stress, or thyroid dysfunction. Outflow-tract abnormalities include Asherman's syndrome, which is characterized by endometrial adhesions and scarring as a result of aggressive dilation and curettage (D&C), uterovaginal malignancies, cervical stenosis, or imperforate hymen.

MANAGEMENT

The goal of management for amenorrhea is to initiate or restore menses while determining the cause. Treatment of amenorrhea is dependent on its etiology and the patient's wishes. For primary amenorrhea, ET is indicated for patients to develop secondary sex characteristics and to prevent osteoporosis.

For a patient with secondary amenorrhea whose progestin challenge test is negative, treatment consists of oral estrogen 1.25 to 2.5 mg daily for 21 to 25 days, along with oral progesterone 10 mg daily during the last 5 to 10 days of the estrogen doses. The patient should experience bleeding if the endometrium is normally responsive to estrogen and the outflow tract is patent.

For a patient with secondary amenorrhea who is anovulatory and has adequate endogenous estrogen, the common practice is to administer periodic or cyclic progesterone 10 mg PO daily for 10 days each month. These patients must experience withdrawal bleeding for at least 3 months to prevent endometrial hyperplasia or endometrial carcinoma related to unopposed estrogen. If the patient is anovulatory and wants to become pregnant, ovulation may be induced with clomiphene citrate (Clomid) 50 mg PO on days 5 to 9 of the cycle after induction of bleeding with progesterone.

If the patient requires contraception, hormonal contraceptives are beneficial for monthly cycle regulation. For patients with hyperprolactinemia, bromocriptine (Parlodel) is the drug of choice. Once hypothalamic failure is established, GnRH may be given in a pulsatile fashion. GnRH is given as a combination with estrogen and calcium because these patients are hypoestrogenic and at high risk for osteoporosis. In patients with thyroid dysfunction, replacement therapy should be initiated, and amenorrhea should be corrected.

Surgical intervention is possible for women with endometrial scarring (Asherman's syndrome) from endometritis. Diagnosis and treatment are accomplished in the same way, through hysteroscopic inspection and the lysis of adhesions. After this procedure, antibiotics are given and a small Foley catheter is placed in the uterus to be left in for 1 week. When the catheter is removed, an intrauterine device is inserted and left in place for 2 months while the patient receives cyclic estrogen and progesterone to build the endometrial lining. This treatment usually restores normal menses and fertility, but complications of pregnancy are common, including spontaneous abortion.

FOLLOW-UP AND REFERRAL

A gynecologist and an endocrinologist should be consulted for further testing. If a CNS problem is detected, computed tomography (CT) scanning or MRI should be performed to rule out pathology. The gynecologist may also consider an endometrial biopsy for patients who are at high risk (those with diabetes, hypertension, and obesity) for endometrial hyperplasia and adenocarcinoma before prescribing medications. Pelvic ultrasound may also be used to measure endometrial thickness and rule out ovarian masses. Once the work-up is completed, the patient should be evaluated annually. Patients with primary amenorrhea should be referred to a gynecologist. Patients with secondary amenorrhea may need to be referred if their initial treatment is unsuccessful.

Patient Education: Amenorrhea

Frequently, teenagers and their parents are apprehensive when menses does not start "on schedule," but reassurance and watchful waiting may be all that is needed but the girl should be evaluated if menstruation does not occur by age 15 years or 3 years after breast budding. Patients should be taught about their medication regimen and the importance of taking medications exactly as prescribed. Patients must be aware of the need to notify their health-care provider if they take any new medications, given the potential for drug–drug interactions with many hormonal therapies. Patients should be encouraged to maintain a healthy diet and exercise regimen, because having inadequate body fat from excessive exercise or calorie restriction can result in amenorrhea.

DYSMENORRHEA

Dysmenorrhea is painful menses. It may be primary with no pelvic pathology or secondary and usually accompanied by pelvic pathology.

EPIDEMIOLOGY AND CAUSES

Primary dysmenorrhea usually begins 1 to 2 years after the onset of menstruation, is associated with ovulatory cycles, and lasts for 1 or 2 days each month. There is no associated pathology in this condition, which 50% to 75% of women experience at some point in their lives. The menstrual pain associated with primary dysmenorrhea may lessen for some women as they age or after the birth of children, or it can last until menopause.

Secondary dysmenorrhea is caused by a physical condition. Women who experience this type of dysmenorrhea tend to be older than those who have primary dysmenorrhea, sometimes beginning when a woman is in her third and fourth decades of life. Menstrual pain is the predominant symptom, as in primary dysmenorrhea. Possible conditions responsible for secondary dysmenorrhea include endometriosis, PID, fibroids (uterine leiomyomas), adenomyosis, and endometrial polyps. Secondary dysmenorrhea is most common in women aged 40 to 50 years.

It is estimated that more than 140 million who lost work hours are a result of dysmenorrhea. It is the most common gynecological complaint of women and the main cause of missed work, school, or other activities. An estimated 42 million women in the United States experience painful menstrual symptoms each month. Risk factors for primary dysmenorrhea include obesity, low BMI, long menstrual cycles, menarche occurring before 12 years of age, nulliparity, cigarette smoking, and a positive family history for dysmenorrhea. Risk factors for secondary dysmenorrhea include endometriosis, pelvic infection, and sexually transmitted infections.

PATHOPHYSIOLOGY

Dysmenorrhea is caused by the production of prostaglandins and leukotrienes, chemical substances that are released when uterine tissue breaks up and is sloughed off during menstruation. Prostaglandin F_2 (PGF_2) and PGE_2 are two of the most important players. Elevated uterine levels of these arachidonic acid metabolites, and more specifically an increased ratio of PGF_2 to PGE_2, have been directly correlated with increases in subjective pain. Increased prostaglandin levels found in uterine tissue, but not in plasma, cause dysrhythmic uterine contractions and increased resting tone by stimulating smooth muscle tissue to contract, which compromises blood supply and oxygenation to uterine muscle, thus causing severe pelvic pain known as "cramps."

These uterine contractions may last for several minutes at a time, producing maximal pressures of up to 400 mm Hg, with resting pressures as high as 80 mm Hg. In turn, if uterine muscle tone is consistently higher than systemic arterial pressure, uterine ischemia ensues, resulting in the production of anaerobic metabolites that stimulate small type C pain fibers. In turn, pain relief has been directly correlated with decreases in uterine contraction pressure.

Because smooth muscle is found in the stomach, intestines, and blood vessels, as well as in the uterus, excessive stimulation accounts for nausea, diarrhea, and headache that often accompany dysmenorrhea. Cramps facilitate the release of menstrual tissue, and because the cervical opening is usually widened after childbirth or years of menstruation, cramps may lessen in the older patient. In contrast, intensified cramps are associated with anovulatory menstrual cycles—a common phenomenon in young women, affecting up to half of adolescents within 2 to 4 years after the start of menses.

CLINICAL PRESENTATION

Subjective

Description of the pain is an important factor. The type, severity, and duration of pain should be noted. A patient with dysmenorrhea may present with sharp stabbing pain and cramping, low back pain, nausea and possible vomiting, bowel changes, and fatigue. The pain with primary dysmenorrhea usually starts within 24 hours of menses and may last for 48 to 72 hours. Secondary dysmenorrhea may have the onset of pain a week or more before the onset of menses and continue after cessation of flow for a few days. The patient may state that she is immobilized by her period every month for the first day. Her pain may be so severe that at times she cannot do anything except stay in bed with a heating pad on her abdomen. The patient may lose her appetite and eat very little during this time. Patients may also complain of pain during intercourse.

DIAGNOSTIC REASONING

Diagnostic Tests

A physical examination that reveals no signs of pathology and a history of consistent symptoms for 1 or 2 days each month will usually substantiate the diagnosis of primary dysmenorrhea, because the symptoms are fairly typical. Patients with secondary dysmenorrhea may have slightly varying description of symptoms; some menses are more painful than others, and the level of discomfort may be progressive. If the complaint of painful intercourse is present, a diagnosis of secondary dysmenorrhea, possibly related to endometriosis, should be explored.

Laboratory studies in the evaluation of dysmenorrhea are ordered to rule out potential causes of pelvic pain. They include a quantitative beta-hCG, a complete blood count, urinalysis, an erythrocyte sedimentation rate, and stool for occult blood. Serum cancer antigen-125 (CA-125) levels are known to be elevated in women with endometriosis (a common cause of dysmenorrhea), as well as ovarian pathology; however, this test is not sufficiently sensitive to serve as a reliable screening tool.

Imaging studies are the choice for the initial evaluation of suspected pelvic disease. Gynecological consultation with visualization of pelvic organs via ultrasound is the initial procedure for the evaluation of pelvic pathology. If such testing does not produce a definitive diagnosis, it should be followed up by laparoscopic exploration to directly visualize pathological conditions such as endometriosis.

Differential Diagnosis

The ultimate goal of the differential diagnosis of dysmenorrhea is to exclude underlying pelvic pathology to differentiate between primary and secondary dysmenorrhea. This includes diagnosing conditions that may produce or mimic dysmenorrhea such as endometriosis, ovarian cysts, ectopic pregnancy, urinary tract infection, vaginitis, AUB, uterine leiomyomas, appendicitis, lower back pain, trauma from sexual assault, and PID. Endometriosis is the most common cause of secondary dysmenorrhea.

MANAGEMENT

The principle of management for primary dysmenorrhea is to relieve the menstrual pain as much as possible. For secondary dysmenorrhea, the goal is to find a diagnosis. For pain relief, NSAIDs or aspirin every four hours, started 1 or 2 days before menstruation, are helpful because of their antiprostaglandin activity. Dietary changes such as the avoidance of caffeine during the first few days of menstruation have been shown to be helpful. Exercise may be of some benefit because it raises levels of beta-endorphins—neurotransmitters in the brain associated with pain relief. Cigarette smoking has also been linked to increasing the duration of dysmenorrhea.

Interestingly, in clinical studies, placebo treatments have been shown to improve symptoms of dysmenorrhea, albeit often only transiently. However, the NSAID ibuprofen (Advil, Motrin) 400 to 800 mg PO three to four times daily as needed remains the mainstay of dysmenorrhea therapy and is considered the most effective over-the-counter pain reliever for cramps. Several studies have demonstrated that if ibuprofen fails to relieve a patient's symptoms, it is appropriate to try an alternative NSAID agent such as naproxen sodium (Naprosyn 500 mg or Aleve 220 mg ¥ two tablets PO two times daily as needed), indomethacin (Indocin), fenoprofen (Nalfon 300 to 600 mg PO two to three times daily as needed), or mefenamic acid (500 mg PO initially, followed by 250 mg four times daily for up to 3 days). The latter agent not only inhibits new prostaglandin formation but also inhibits the activity of preformed prostaglandins. In contrast, acetaminophen (Tylenol) appears to be less effective because it does not inhibit prostaglandin formation and is not an anti-inflammatory agent.

Application of a hot-water bottle or heating pad to the abdomen or hot baths may help relieve discomfort and in some studies has been shown to be as effective as NSAID therapy. However, interestingly, the combination of heat therapy and NSAIDs together has been shown to be counterproductive. Acupuncture, transcutaneous electrical nerve stimulation therapy, and specific herbal teas (e.g., mint tea, certain ayurvedic preparations) have all been shown to decrease uterine spasms in small clinical trials. Relaxation or yoga-type exercises may also help to relieve pain. Dietary restriction of both caffeine and salt is also recommended, and vitamin E, vitamin B_1, vitamin B_6, magnesium, and vitamin D were found to reduce symptoms. There is some evidence that vitamin E therapy 400 IU/day beginning 2 days before the onset of menstruation and for 5 days total for two cycles decreases dysmenorrhea. Other research indicates that ingestion of a single high oral dose of vitamin D has a favorable effect on dysmenorrhea.

For some women, even prescribed prostaglandin inhibitors are ineffective. Combined estrogen-progestin oral contraceptive agents may be considered for these patients because they relieve cramping by inhibiting arachidonic acid production and ovulation, in turn hindering high levels of prostaglandin production. These therapies may be given daily as 21-, 63-, or 105-day continuous courses, each followed by 7 days off medication, before repeating the cycle. Longer cycles of OCPs and other hormonal agents decrease the frequency of menstruation occurring during the off-therapy week.

If no relief is achieved after NSAIDs and OCPs, ultrasonography and exploratory laparoscopy may be appropriate to rule out pelvic pathology. If endometriosis (the most common cause of secondary dysmenorrhea) is found, a GnRH analog may be prescribed in continuous fashion to inhibit menses (see the section "Management" under "Endometriosis").

FOLLOW-UP AND REFERRAL

Patients with dysmenorrhea should have follow-up care since treatment is ongoing and requires further evaluation for persistent relief of symptoms or additional diagnostic evaluation for continued symptoms. The prognosis for primary dysmenorrhea is good with the use of antiprostaglandins, with 70% to 80% relief of symptoms in some cases.

Patient Education: Dysmenorrhea

Patients should be educated that aspirin and other NSAIDs can significantly reduce prostaglandin levels associated with painful menstruation if started 1 to 2 days before menstruation begins. Education about changes in exercise and diet may also be useful. Dietary supplementation with omega-3 fatty acids has been shown to help provide relief in adolescents. Patients should be encouraged to stop smoking and decrease alcohol intake. Patients can also be told that symptomatic treatment with a warm bath or locally applied heat may be helpful.

ENDOMETRIOSIS

Endometriosis is a painful, chronic disease characterized by the presence and proliferation of abnormally located endometrial tissue, which responds to hormonal changes in the woman's body. Abnormally located endometrial tissue has been found outside the uterus, usually in the abdomen, on the ovaries, fallopian tubes, and the ligaments that support the uterus, as well as in the area between the vagina and rectum, on the outer surface of the uterus, and in the lining of the pelvic cavity. Other sites for these endometrial growths may include the bladder, bowel, vagina, cervix, vulva, and in abdominal surgical scars. Rarely, endometrial tissue may be located in the lung, arm, thigh, brain, or other non–reproductive tract locations.

This tissue reacts to hormonal changes in the same way as uterine endometrial tissue during the menstrual cycle. The bloody discharge produced by such tissue typically has no outlet, and the presence of such discharge may cause severe pain with each menstrual cycle, either during ovulation, menstruation, or both. The accumulation of the discharge may form dense fibrous tissue, leading to adhesions, infertility, and the destruction of ovarian tissue.

The Iceberg of Endometriosis

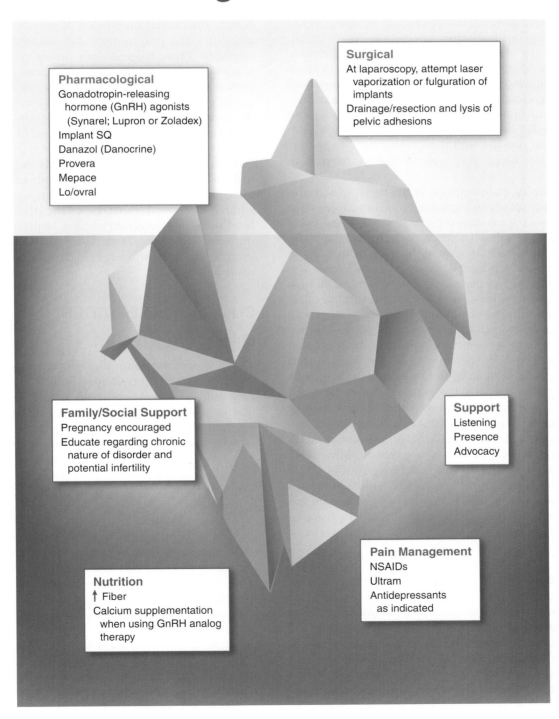

Pharmacological
Gonadotropin-releasing
   hormone (GnRH) agonists
      (Synarel; Lupron or Zoladex)
Implant SQ
Danazol (Danocrine)
Provera
Mepace
Lo/ovral

Surgical
At laparoscopy, attempt laser
   vaporization or fulguration of
   implants
Drainage/resection and lysis of
   pelvic adhesions

Family/Social Support
Pregnancy encouraged
Educate regarding chronic
   nature of disorder and
   potential infertility

Support
Listening
Presence
Advocacy

Nutrition
↑ Fiber
Calcium supplementation
   when using GnRH analog
   therapy

Pain Management
NSAIDs
Ultram
Antidepressants
   as indicated

EPIDEMIOLOGY AND CAUSES

Endometriosis affects an estimated 5.5 million women in the United States and Canada. A study of 3,684 premenopausal women undergoing laparoscopy or laparotomy found a prevalence of endometriosis varying from 12% to 45%, depending on the indication for surgery. Women at all levels of society and of all races may be affected, although Japanese women are twice as likely to have endometriosis as Caucasian women. The highest level of occurrence is reported in women 25 to 29 years of age, and the lowest incidence is found in women older than 44 years; however, the disease can be found at any age, including in adolescents.

A delay in diagnosing endometriosis is common. Research conducted by the Endometriosis Association found that the recognition and diagnosis of endometriosis still take a combined average of 9 years (a 4.7-year delay in seeking medical help and a 4.6-year delay in obtaining a physician diagnosis). From the sample of 4,000 respondents, almost one-half said they had to see a doctor five times or more before they were diagnosed, referred, or treated.

The cause of endometriosis is unknown. The retrograde menstruation and implantation theory suggests that during menses some amount of menstrual tissue backs up through the fallopian tubes, implants in the abdomen, and proliferates in response to ovarian steroids. In turn, conditions that lead to genital tract obstruction and impede menstrual outflow contribute to reflux through the fallopian tubes. However, this theory does not explain all of the possible sites of endometriosis, and some experts believe that all women experience some degree of menstrual tissue backup. Direct transplantation may account for endometriosis that develops in uterine surgical scars after a cesarean section or episiotomy. Another theory suggests that endometrial tissue is distributed from the uterus to other parts of the body through either the lymphatic or hematological circulatory systems. The coelomic (peritoneal) metaplasia theory suggests that undifferentiated cells lining the peritoneal cavity are triggered to differentiate into endometrial tissue by hormonal irregularities. There may also be a genetic predisposition to endometriosis. In addition, research by the Endometriosis Association has recently linked dioxin exposure to the development of endometriosis.

PATHOPHYSIOLOGY

In addition to the etiological theories discussed in the preceding text, a link to immune system dysfunction and the pathogenesis of endometriosis have also been suggested. Reduced T-cell and natural killer cell function are thought to impair the ability of the body to recognize and destroy abnormally implanted endometrial tissue via immunosurveillance. Interestingly, however, an increased number of peritoneal leukocytes and macrophages has been identified within ectopic endometrium. Increased levels of cytokines and chemokines produced by these cells have been identified, including interleukin-1 (IL-1), IL-6, IL-8, tumor necrosis factor, and RANTES (regulated upon activation normal t cell expressed and presumably secreted). These mediators act as growth factors for ectopic endometrium, and vascular endothelial growth factor stimulates capillary proliferation into this tissue. Women with endometriosis are also more likely than controls to suffer from autoimmune inflammatory diseases.

Any pelvic organ may be a possible site of endometriosis. The cyclical production of ovarian sex hormones allows for the proliferation and maintenance of these implants. Thus, endometriosis occurs primarily during a woman's active reproductive phase, rather than during premenstrual, immediately postmenarchal, or postmenopausal phases. This bleeding may cause severe pelvic pain, dyspareunia, infertility, and debilitation. In addition, inflammation of pelvic tissues may lead to adhesions and cyst development.

Endometriosis may be progressively staged from minimal (Stage I: isolated implants without adhesions), mild (Stage II: superficial implants less than 5 cm in aggregate without adhesions), moderate (Stage III: multiple superficial and invasive implants with or without tubo-ovarian implants), to severe (Stage IV: multiple superficial and invasive implants with large ovarian endometriomas and dense adhesions).

CLINICAL PRESENTATION

Subjective

The primary symptom of endometriosis is recurrent abdominal and/or pelvic pain, which may range from very mild to completely incapacitating. Some patients may complain only of premenstrual spotting. However, for those with pain, it may be associated with menstruation (dysmenorrhea) or may occur slightly before the menstrual period begins. Pain may be experienced as generalized abdominal or pelvic pain or pain associated with sexual intercourse (dyspareunia), urination, or defecation. Fatigue, diarrhea, constipation, or nausea may accompany the pain.

A careful history of menstruation should be taken, with significant attention to any complaints of pain. A history of allergies, chemical sensitivities, and recurrent yeast *(Candida)* infections may be present. Complaints of infertility should be noted, as infertility is associated with endometriosis in 30% to 40% of cases.

Objective

On physical examination, tenderness in the posterior fornix is the most common symptom. Lateral deviation of the cervix may be due to internal scarring, and bimanual examination may reveal palpable nodules on supporting ligaments and affected ovaries. However, a definitive diagnosis cannot be made via history and physical examination alone.

DIAGNOSTIC REASONING

Diagnostic Tests

Direct visualization and pathological testing of endometrial implants through laparoscopy is the preferred diagnostic method, because most implants are located on the pelvic organs. A complete blood count may be done to diagnose anemia associated with blood loss resulting from endometriosis, and an elevated white blood cell count may also show evidence of an infection. This would tend to make endometriosis less likely, although it would not exclude the presence of abnormally located endometrial tissue. Serum CA-125 levels are more likely to be elevated with advanced (Stages III–IV) endometriosis, but this serum marker is not particularly sensitive and not an adequate screening tool.

Differential Diagnosis

The clinical manifestations of endometriosis are associated with many genitourinary disorders. The pain experienced is often discounted by the patient or clinician because pain is a frequent (and presumed normal) accompaniment to menstruation. Pelvic and abdominal pain can be caused by gastroenteritis, appendicitis, ovarian cysts, fibroids, or ectopic pregnancy, and these diagnoses must be ruled out. Specific differential diagnoses that must be considered also include adenomyosis and endometrial polyps.

Adenomyosis is the presence of ectopic endometrial glands and stroma within the musculature of the uterus, which induces hypertrophy and hyperplasia of the myometrium in response to estrogen (and possibly progesterone). It may be microscopic or nodular on gross inspection, but endometrial biopsy is typically negative because changes are primarily in the myometrium. Adenomyosis seems to be more associated with childbearing, but the pathogenesis is unknown. Although a third of women are asymptomatic, adenomyosis may present with AUB, dysmenorrhea, and menorrhagia—just as with endometriosis. Abdominal ultrasound may be able to distinguish this diagnosis, but laparoscopy is necessary to diagnose endometriosis.

Endometrial polyps are hyperplastic pedunculated or sessile growths of endometrial glands and stroma at the endometrial surface (millimeters to centimeters in size). They are common in middle-aged women, and metrorrhagia (irregular uterine bleeding) occurs in 50% of cases. Less frequently, menorrhagia (abnormally heavy uterine bleeding), postmenopausal bleeding, uterine prolapse through the cervical os, and breakthrough bleeding on hormonal treatments can occur as symptoms. A definitive diagnosis is made on microscopy (after D&C, biopsy, or hysterectomy), and sonohysterography (instillation of saline into the uterus before ultrasound) is preferred to transvaginal ultrasound (TVUS) for noninvasive evaluation (although it is not diagnostic). Curettage guided by hysteroscopy, rather than done blindly, is preferred for detecting polyps.

MANAGEMENT

Currently, there is no cure for endometriosis. Management is linked to relieving or reducing pain, shrinking or slowing endometrial growths, preserving or restoring fertility, and preventing or delaying the recurrence of the disease. In women with mild disease or those who are perimenopausal and will soon stop ovarian cycling and the hormonal fluctuations that trigger bleeding endometriosis, expectant management (observation) is an important option.

Medication administration should begin with the onset of menstruation to avoid the possible influence of medications on pregnancy. With consistent reevaluation of symptom reduction, the risks associated with medications can be minimized. Prescription pain medications may be necessary to control symptoms, although conservative management is to use the least powerful medications first.

Pain relief is often achieved with NSAIDs and other prostaglandin inhibitors, although NSAIDs are usually sufficient only for disease with minimal pain. Typical medications include ibuprofen (400 to 600 mg four times daily), naproxen sodium (220 mg four times daily), indomethacin, and mefenamic acid (Ponstel; 250 mg four times daily to 500 mg three times daily). Oral contraceptives may also provide adequate relief for women with mild disease. Studies indicate that low-dose drospirenone/ethinyl estradiol 3 mg/20 mcg OCPs used either continuously or cyclically are effective in reducing pelvic pain resulting from endometriosis, although any of the combination OCPs and other hormonal contraceptives discussed in Chapter 46 can be used. Breakthrough bleeding may occur and is treated with conjugated estrogen 1.25 mg daily for 1 week or estradiol 2 mg daily for 1 week. Adverse effects are discussed in Chapter 46.

For women with moderate to severe disease, other hormonal therapies may help relieve symptoms. Drugs such as nafarelin nasal spray (0.2 to 0.4 mg twice daily), long-acting leuprolide acetate (3.75 mg IM once a month), or goserelin (3.6 mg subcutaneously once a month) are GnRH analogs that suppress ovulation by suppressing pituitary gonadotropin secretion and, thus, ovarian estrogen secretion. These drugs are used for 3 to 6 months, although the optimum length of therapy is unclear. Adverse effects of these medications are vasomotor symptoms (e.g., hot flashes), vaginal dryness, dyspareunia, decreased libido, insomnia, breast tenderness, headache, depression, and bone demineralization, which can be mediated by "add back" therapy with norethindrone 5 to 15 mg daily.

Another hormonal treatment is danazol (200 to 400 mg twice daily), which is used for 6 to 9 months. Danazol is a testosterone derivative that acts like progesterone and suppresses menstruation. Adverse effects are androgenic and include weight gain, acne, hirsutism, muscle cramps, lower HDL levels, and decreased breast size.

Progesterone alone, in the form of medroxyprogesterone acetate 100 mg IM administered every 2 weeks for four doses and then every 4 weeks, can be given to inhibit endometrial tissue growth and initiate decidualization and atrophy of the endometrium. Oral therapy with medroxyprogesterone 10 mg three times daily or norethindrone 5 mg daily can also be used for 6 to 9 months. These treatments provide 80% of women with complete or partial symptom relief. Oral estrogen can be added to control breakthrough bleeding. Aromatase inhibitors that decrease estrogen production are still investigational. Regimens may be developed that combine these drugs with progestins or GnRH analogs.

Laparoscopy is used to ablate endometrial implants, which greatly reduce pain. Some women require removal of ovarian endometriomas along with ablation of implants, and this procedure improves fertility. For women who no longer desire to have children, a total abdominal hysterectomy and bilateral salpingo-oophorectomy (TAH-BSO) will treat endometriosis definitively, but in women with deep implants, TAH-BSO may not be sufficient.

Medical treatment alone is inappropriate for moderate to severe disease, and in addition, it does not improve fertility in these women. Only surgical interventions are shown to improve fertility. For example, some reviews have shown that with observation alone, pregnancy rates with mild, moderate, and severe endometriosis are 50%, less than 25%, and only 5%, respectively. With surgery, pregnancy rates rise to 50% and 39% in patients with moderate and severe disease, respectively. However, IVF is usually needed postoperatively for women with severe disease in whom hysterectomy can be avoided. Infertile women who are trying to improve their chance of pregnancy typically benefit from laparoscopic ablation of endometrial implants.

Alternative therapies are gaining acceptance in the treatment of endometriosis. Visualization techniques, patterned breathing, and massage therapy may each have their place in the treatment of this disorder. Dietary therapy and therapy to maximize function of the immune system may also be useful. Treatment must be evaluated for an appropriate match between patient and therapeutic choice. Financial issues may also be of concern, as hormonal therapies are significantly more expensive than dietary changes or massage therapy (see Complementary Therapies 48.1).

FOLLOW-UP AND REFERRAL

The signs and symptoms of endometriosis are related to the menstrual cycle. Follow-up visits should be timed to allow prescribed treatments to have already affected the symptoms associated with the next menstrual cycle. The patient should be referred to a gynecologist experienced in laparoscopic diagnosis and the treatment of endometriosis if the most conservative medical treatments are not sufficient to ameliorate symptoms.

Patient Education: Endometriosis

Each patient must receive appropriately formulated educational materials about endometriosis, including its signs and symptoms and the effects they may produce, because this is usually a lifelong condition (see The Patient's Voice 48.1).

LEIOMYOMAS (UTERINE FIBROIDS)

Leiomyomas (leiomyomata) are commonly called *uterine fibroids*. Fibroids are the most common benign tumor of the uterus and arise from smooth muscle cells in the myometrium. Most are small and asymptomatic.

EPIDEMIOLOGY AND CAUSES

Leiomyomas are extremely common. Their prevalence increases in women between 30 and 50 years of age and decreases with menopause. By age 50 years, 50%

 The Patient's Voice 48.1

ENDOMETRIOSIS

I had a very painful menstruation from day 1. As long as I can remember, every month I was in bed doubled over in pain. Nothing seemed to relieve the intensity of the pain . . . even taking birth control pills. My periods were not heavy, but I always had pain and even a little spotting, especially after my period every month. About 1 year after the delivery of my third child, I began experiencing great discomfort with intercourse. My gynecologist suggested that since I was almost 40 years old, a surgical intervention was needed. He explained that laparoscopy or laparotomy and eventual hysterectomy was the usual treatment for women with severe pain. My first surgery did reveal that I had endometriosis . . . a small amount . . . but my surgeon said that some of the locations of the endometriosis made it even more painful. I had a difficult time with the hysterectomy . . . a lot of pain. But, since they removed my uterus, the pain I had for almost 27 years is finally gone. Why did it take so long for someone to give me relief?

of African American and Asian American women have leiomyomas and about 30% of white women have them.

The cause of leiomyomas is unknown, but clearly there is a hormonal link. Girls before menarche do not have leiomyomas, and they shrink after menopause, implicating estrogen. If a pregnant woman has a fibroid, it dramatically increases in size during pregnancy, but decreases after delivery. Risk factors for the development of leiomyomas include nulliparity, age between 30 and 50 years, obesity, and a sedentary lifestyle. Interestingly, smoking seems to decrease the risk for developing fibroids.

PATHOPHYSIOLOGY

Leiomyomas develop from a single neoplastic smooth muscle cell with abnormal chromosomal patterns. Leiomyomas are classified by their location within the uterine wall and can be subserosal, submucosal, and/or intramural. Pedunculated fibroids may also grow out from the surface of the uterus or into the cavity of the uterus. Rarely, a leiomyoma can be intraligamentous, cervical, or parasitic (deriving its blood supply from an organ to which it becomes attached). Most uterine fibroids are surrounded by compressed but otherwise normal myometrium. When leiomyomas outgrow their blood supply, they can become necrotic and ulcerate.

CLINICAL PRESENTATION

Subjective

Most leiomyomas are asymptomatic. When symptoms are present, AUB is the most common symptom. The woman may also complain of pain, particularly with intercourse. If the fibroid is large enough, it can cause pressure on the bladder, resulting in urinary frequency, urgency, and possibly dysuria. The complaint of abdominal or genital heaviness is also common with large fibroids.

Objective

Pelvic examination will reveal one or more uterine masses. Leiomyomas are usually firm and nontender. If there are multiple fibroids (which occurs in most cases), the uterus will feel irregular and nodular in shape.

DIAGNOSTIC REASONING

Diagnostic Tests

Because most women with leiomyomas have AUB, a complete blood count is ordered. Hemoglobin is decreased because of the increased amount and frequency of menstrual bleeding. Occasionally, polycythemia may be present. A pregnancy test should be done to rule out intrauterine pregnancy. An endometrial biopsy may be done and will be normal, which helps rule out other diagnoses. Pelvic ultrasound or MRI will confirm the diagnosis of a leiomyoma, but TVUS is used most often. Occasionally, hysterography or hysteroscopy is used to confirm cervical or submucosal myomas.

Differential Diagnosis

Differential diagnoses should include other disorders that cause uterine enlargement and AUB, including pregnancy, adenomyosis (presence of endometrial glands and stroma in the myometrium), endometriosis, an ovarian neoplasm, a tubo-ovarian inflammatory mass, uterine cancer, and possibly diverticulitis.

MANAGEMENT

No treatment is necessary for women with asymptomatic or very small leiomyomas. If the patient is severely anemic, measures should be undertaken to stop the prolonged, heavy menstrual periods and boost her hemoglobin. Medroxyprogesterone acetate 150 mg IM given every 28 days or Danazol 400 to 800 mg PO daily will usually slow or stop the bleeding. Patients should be instructed to take OTC iron preparations (ferrous sulfate, ferrous gluconate, or ferrous fumarate 300 mg) daily. Folic acid 400 mcg PO daily will help boost red blood cell production as well.

The goal of conservative medical management is to shrink the leiomyomas. Oral contraceptives may be effective for some women, but for others, the estrogen in OCPs causes enlargement of leiomyomas, so frequent monitoring is important. GnRH agonists are given to decrease LH and FSH levels, thereby producing a hypoestrogenic effect that usually causes leiomyomas to shrink. This is frequently used before surgery, because the risk of surgical complications is increased with large tumors. The GnRH agents that are used are leuprorelin (Lupron) depot injection of 3.75 mg every 28 days for 3 months or a single dose of 11.25 mg IM. Treatment lasts 8 to 12 weeks and is very costly. Because these drugs induce a menopausal state, the adverse effects reflect those of menopause (see previous section on Menopause). These medications are contraindicated in women with undiagnosed AUB and in women who are breastfeeding. Insertion of a levonorgestrel-containing intrauterine contraceptive device (e.g., Mirena) has been shown to significantly decrease bleeding with fibroids that are associated with menorrhagia. This device is removed after 5 years.

There are several surgical approaches for problematic leiomyomas. Myomectomy is surgical removal of the myoma and is done when preservation of fertility is desired and the tumor is larger than 12-week gestational size. Hysterectomy (with or without removal of the ovaries) is the definitive treatment for very large fibroids, particularly when bleeding is very heavy and the patient is markedly anemic. Few adverse effects occur as a result of hysterectomy, although infection, bleeding, and damage to surrounding organs are always a possibility with any surgical procedure. Other possible consequences of hysterectomy and oophorectomy include depression, sexual dysfunction, and severe menopausal symptoms.

Uterine artery embolization is a relatively new alternative to surgery. The uterine arteries are embolized, producing end-organ ischemia, necrosis, and subsequent shrinkage of the uterus. This procedure is effective in reducing menorrhagia, pain, and uterine volume in 80% of patients. However, a large number of women report severe pelvic pain, fever, malaise, and nausea and vomiting resulting from the infarcted uterine tissue.

FOLLOW-UP AND REFERRAL

Any woman with severe bleeding, marked anemia, and palpable leiomyomas should be referred to a gynecologist for evaluation and treatment. Women with small uterine myomas should be reexamined at 3- to 6-month intervals or more often if symptoms increase. If menorrhagia is present, hemoglobin and hematocrit should be monitored frequently.

Patient Education: Leiomyomas

Women with leiomyomas should be reassured that this does not increase their chances of developing uterine cancer. If increased bleeding is a problem, the woman should be instructed to take an iron supplement daily and to increase iron-rich foods in her diet. She should report any shortness of breath, palpitations, or increase in fatigue or pain immediately.

PRECANCEROUS LESIONS AND CANCER OF THE CERVIX

As a precursor of cervical cancer, cervical intraepithelial neoplasia (CIN) has been explored and studied more than any other premalignant lesion of the genital tract. The accessible anatomical location of the upper vagina and cervix facilitates investigation and the early detection of premalignancy and cancerous lesions of the cervix. In addition, the development and use of colposcopy to identify sites of potential dysplasia and assist in directing biopsy have positively affected patient outcomes in the management of CIN and cervical cancer.

EPIDEMIOLOGY AND CAUSES

Several terms have been used to describe premalignant lesions of the cervix. These changes are described on a continuum from mildly atypical to the potential to progress to invasive carcinoma. The grades of severity of premalignant lesions are CIN 1 (mild dysplasia), CIN 2 (moderate dysplasia), and CIN 3 (severe dysplasia to carcinoma in situ). With regard to the degree of dysplasia, mild involvement includes one-third of the cervical epithelium, moderate involvement includes two-thirds of the epithelium, and severe involvement includes the full thickness of the epithelium. Carcinoma in situ is considered the most advanced premalignant change.

Cervical cancer is the 14th most common cancer in women in the United States and the most common cancer in women worldwide. With the prevalence of Papanicolaou (Pap) test screening in the United States, mortality rates due to cervical cancer have fallen by more than 45% since the 1970s. The American Cancer Society (ACS) estimates that there will be 12,820 new cases of invasive cervical cancer and that more than 4,210 women will die of the disease in 2017. Most cases of cervical cancer are found in women younger than 50 years, but 15% of cases are found in women older than 65 years. Hispanic women in the United States have the highest incidence of cervical cancer, followed by African American women. American Indians and Alaskan native women have the lowest risk.

Precancerous dysplasia, or CIN, occurs more often in younger women, with the incidence peaking in the early third decade of life. About 12% of women will have cervical dysplasia by 20 years of age. However, the American College of Obstetricians and Gynecologists (ACOG) has issued new recommendations for cervical cancer screening, which should begin at age 21 years in all women, regardless of sexual history, and is recommended every 3 years.

The cause of CIN and cervical cancer remains unknown; however, studies implicate several factors. In particular, the sexually transmitted human papillomavirus virus (HPV) is believed to support the development of premalignant and malignant cervical lesions. There are more than 150 genotypes of the HPV virus and 13 have been associated with various anal/genital lesions (e.g., condylomata or genital warts), and two specific genotypes, HPV-16 and HPV-18, have been most frequently (66%) associated with neoplasia (i.e., higher grades of dysplasia and cervical cancer). HPV-31 and HPV-45, and to a lesser extent HPV-33, HPV-52, and HPV-58 account for another 15% of cases of cervical cancer. Condom use is promoted based more on the general principles of preventing sexually transmitted infections rather than on epidemiological data because protection against HPV transmission is not 100% effective. HPV can be found in many genital areas (e.g., genital tract skin and mucous membranes). Hence, condoms do not protect the vulva from microscopic HPV particles on the skin.

Although flat HPV cervical lesions are strongly associated with cellular transformation to CIN, most HPV infections are subclinical. Women may be unaware of their HPV status. In addition, women who have a history of early intercourse (age 14 or 15 years), begin to have children at an early age, and/or have a history of multiple sexual partners are at greater risk for developing carcinoma of the cervix.

Risk Factors: Cervical Neoplasia

History

- Early intercourse
- Multiple sex partners (more than two)
- Early childbearing
- Prostitution
- Immunosuppression
- Prior exposure to radiation
- Intrauterine DES exposure
- OCP use
- Cigarette smoking
- Vitamins A, B, and C and folic acid deficiencies

Male Partner

- History of genital cancer, especially penile carcinoma; sexually transmitted infections (STIs), especially penile or urethral condylomas; CIN or cervical cancer in a previous partner; low socioeconomic status; multiple sex partners

Infections

- SITs
- HPV infection (serotypes 16 and 18)
- Herpes simplex infection
- HIV infection
- *Chlamydia trachomatis*
- Cytomegalovirus infection

PATHOPHYSIOLOGY

The normal cervical transformation zone includes columnar epithelium and squamous metaplasia. The squamocolumnar junction (SCJ) of the cervix is viewed via a colposcope, which magnifies the epithelium of the transformation zone. Colposcopic examination of this landmark site is important because this area is most vulnerable to neoplastic changes.

Examination of the exocervix reveals where the cervical glandular, columnar epithelium (which is grapelike in appearance) meets the native squamous epithelium distal to the external os in young adult women. After childbirth, this area may enlarge and move farther away from the cervical os. The junction usually recedes after menopause into the endocervical canal. Throughout a woman's reproductive life, squamous metaplasia, a physiological process involving squamous tissue replacing columnar tissue, occurs. This process is most active during fetal development, adolescence, and pregnancy.

The SCJ is first delineated in utero; however, metaplasia is an estrogen-dependent process that accelerates during puberty and pregnancy. SCJ cells are more vulnerable and especially prone to damage at these times in a woman's reproductive life. An abnormal transformation zone in the SCJ is caused by neoplastic squamous epithelium, thus explaining why exophytic tumors are the most common presentation of cervical cancer.

HPV infection may alter the morphology of the cervical epithelium, leading to nuclear enlargement and multinucleation, hyperchromasia, and perinuclear cytoplasmic halos. Cellular findings of HPV infection on biopsy can be histologically similar to dysplasia, and misdiagnosis can occur. However, the diagnosis of HPV does not imply clinical disease. Thus, treatment is limited only to symptomatic patients (e.g., those with condylomas) or those with evidence of neoplasia (e.g., positive colposcopy findings). Vaccines (e.g., Cervarix, Gardasil) have been developed to prevent HPV infection and, therefore, reduce the risk of developing HPV-associated cancers in both females and males, including cervical cancer in women and penile cancer in men. Gardasil also protects against genital warts and cancer of the anus, vagina, and vulva that are also associated with HPV infection. Girls should be vaccinated at 11 years of age but can be vaccinated up to the age of 26 years. Boys should be vaccinated at 11 years of age but can be vaccinated through the age of 21 years.

In worldwide studies, epitheliotropic HPV infection has been identified in greater than 99% of cervical neoplasias. Certain viral serotypes that undergo episomal replication (i.e., independent replication of viral genetic material without integration into the host genome) typically lead to condylomata acuminata or histologically low-grade squamous intraepithelial lesion (LSIL in The Bethesda system [TBS]), which correlates to CIN 1 (e.g., HPV-6, HPV-11), whereas oncogenic forms of the virus (e.g., HPV-16, HPV-18, HPV-58, HPV-52, HPV-31, HPV-45) that integrate into the host DNA are more likely to contribute to malignant transformation, including high-grade squamous intraepithelial lesion (HSIL), which usually corresponds to CIN 2 or CIN 3, invasive squamous cell carcinoma, and adenocarcinoma. Infection alone is not sufficient for the development of squamous cervical neoplasia or most cervical cancers. Most women infected with HPV do not develop high-grade cervical abnormalities and cancer. Research indicates that women with a persistent infection with HPV (1 to 2 years) are likely to develop high-grade CIN or CIN 3+.

The HPV E6 protein degrades the cell cycle inhibitory protein p53, and the HPV E7 protein interacts with the retinoblastoma protein Rb, which leads to dysregulated cell cycle progression. E7 protein also leads to upregulation of the inflammatory cytokines IL-6 and IL-8, both of which contribute to cervical cancer progression. The HPV serotypes HPV-16 and HPV-18 most strongly correlate with invasive squamous cell carcinoma, with HPV-18 portending a worse prognosis. It is clear, however, that HPV infection alone is insufficient to cause cervical neoplasia, and further insult by cigarette smoking, immunosuppression, or other risk factors appears necessary.

Although squamous cell carcinoma comprises 80% of all cervical cancers, at least 15% are attributed to adenocarcinomas, with another 3% to 5% being of a mixed adenosquamous phenotype. The incidence of adenocarcinoma of the cervix has steadily increased in women younger than 35 years since the 1970s, but this may be due to improved screening detection and early treatment of squamous cell disease. However, a greater association of adenocarcinoma with oral contraceptive use seems to imply the importance of underlying hormonal mechanisms in its pathogenesis. Far rarer forms of cervical cancer include neuroendocrine tumors, small cell carcinomas, and rhabdomyosarcomas.

CLINICAL PRESENTATION

Subjective

Patients with premalignant cervical lesions may present with one or more of the following: a history of one or more epidemiological risk factors associated with the development of cervical cancer, a concurrent vaginal infection with symptoms, no recent gynecological care, and no cervical cytology screening for a prolonged time.

Women with invasive carcinoma may describe a brownish discharge or a history of abnormal vaginal bleeding occurring spontaneously or after intercourse. Women with a history of postcoital bleeding or irregular vaginal bleeding that cannot be explained should be referred to a gynecologist for further evaluation. Typically, only with extensive disease spread will other symptoms manifest (e.g., weight loss, decreased appetite, back pain).

Objective

Women with abnormal cervical cytology are usually asymptomatic with normal cervical, vaginal, and abdominal findings on physical examination. Even if cervical cytology findings are normal, any cervical or vaginal lesion that appears abnormal, friable, raised, or has the appearance of condyloma requires a referral for colposcopy. The location of the dysplasia directs the treatment.

The cervical cytology report should include a statement on the adequacy of the specimen for examination, a general categorization, and a descriptive diagnosis. Results are described as follows:

- Satisfactory but limited (less than optimal; may be secondary to partially obscuring inflammation)
- Unsatisfactory (not acceptable for diagnostic evaluation and may require repeat testing or follow-up)
- Within normal limits
- Other (may require follow-up care; the report will have an additional notation if further action is required)

A protocol for the triage and referral of patients with abnormal cervical cytology results is presented in Table 48.2.

TABLE 48.2 Advanced Practice Nursing Interventions: Pap Test Results and Treatment Protocols	
The Bethesda System Category	*Treatment Protocol*
Normal cytology	Repeat Pap test as recommended in current guidelines (ages 21–29 every 3 years; 30–65 every 3 years or every 5 years with HIV cotesting).
Unsatisfactory for evaluation	Repeat Pap test in 2–4 months. If HPV positive and older than 30 years, colposcopy is acceptable.
Infection • *Trichomonas vaginalis* • Fungal organisms morphologically consistent with *Candida* spp. • Shift in flora suggestive of bacterial vaginosis • Bacteria morphologically consistent with *Actinomyces* spp. • Cellular changes consistent with herpes simplex virus • Cellular changes consistent with cytomegalovirus	Treat infections that present with symptoms or identified with cytology results, or test to confirm organism.
SQUAMOUS CELL ABNORMALITIES	
Low-grade squamous intraepithelial lesion indicates mild dysplasia (CIN 1). High-grade squamous intraepithelial lesion indicates moderate or severe cervical intraepithelial neoplasia (CIN 2 or CIN 3) but does not necessarily mean the presences of cervical cancer. Squamous cell carcinoma	Refer to gynecologist Colposcopic examination likely

TABLE 48.2	Advanced Practice Nursing Interventions: Pap Test Results and Treatment Protocols—cont'd	
The Bethesda System Category	**Treatment Protocol**
GLANDULAR CELL ABNORMALITIES	REFER TO GYNECOLOGIST
Atypical glandular cells	Refer to gynecologist
AGC—not otherwise specified	Refer to gynecologist
AGC—favor neoplasia	Refer to gynecologist
AIS (adenocarcinoma in situ)	Refer to gynecologist
Adenocarcinoma	Refer to gynecologist

DIAGNOSTIC REASONING

Diagnostic Tests

The ACS has developed cervical cancer screening guidelines that are supported by the American Medical Association, National Cancer Institute, American Nurses Association, ACOG, and American Academy of Family Physicians. However, an issue that is the subject of ongoing debate is the mandated frequency for performing cervical cytology screening. Currently, the ACS recommends the following:

- Screening should begin at age 21 years.
- Women aged 21 to 29 years should have a Pap test every 3 years. HPV cotesting is not necessary for this group but may be done after an abnormal Pap test.
- Starting at 30 years of age, screening includes a Pap test and an HPV test every 5 years until age 65 years. An alternative option is screening with a Pap test alone every 3 years.
- Women with suppressed immune systems have a higher risk of cervical cancer. Any woman with HIV infection, organ transplant, or long-term cortical steroid use or with an in utero exposure to DES may need to be screened more often.
- For women 65 years and older who have had regular screening for the 10 years prior and with and with no serious precancers (CIN 2 or CIN 3) in the past 20 years can discontinue screening.
- Screening is no long necessary for a woman after total hysterectomy with removal of the cervix unless the surgery was performed as treatment for cervical cancer or precancer. Women who have had a hysterectomy but have an intact cervix should continue with screening as just outlined.

Differential Diagnosis

Differential diagnosis should include evaluation for cervical and endocervical infections that can cause inflammation of the cervix as well as testing for HPV since the majority of lesions are a result of persistent HPV infection. Postcoital bleeding can be a result of cervical polyps, cervical myoma, endometriosis, and cervical precancer and cancer.

It is important that the cytology laboratory complies with state and national regulations, utilizes a sufficient number of reputable cytologists, maintains a quality assurance program, and supports open, clear communication between health-care professionals and the testing laboratory. Historically, several reporting systems have been developed to enhance communication between the cytopathologist and the clinician performing the Pap test. The oldest system was the class system that provided limited information and did not reflect newer risk factors such as HPV infection. See Therapeutic Procedure 48.1 for specific techniques for obtaining cervical cytology specimens for testing.

Therapeutic Procedure 48.1: Smear and Liquid-Based Cervical Cell Collection (Pap Test)

TECHNIQUE FOR OBTAINING ROUTINE PAP TEST

1. Complete the cytology request form with all pertinent data.
2. Label the slide.
3. Insert the dry or water-lubricated speculum. Direct the speculum in a downward and posterior direction.
4. Expose the cervix.
   - Avoid sampling if a vaginal infection is present.
   - Take the Pap test sample before any other cervical sample.
5. Insert the cytobrush or cotton-tipped applicator in the cervical os.
6. Use a vigorous rotary endocervical technique in clockwise fashion.
7. Use a paintbrush motion to place the sample on the glass slide.
8. Scrape the external os area with the cytology spatula.
9. Note the individual topography of the squamocolumnar juncture.
10. Obtain a vaginal specimen if needed (e.g., DES exposure, hormone evaluation, history of hysterectomy).
11. Smear the slide and fix immediately.

Continued

Therapeutic Procedure 48.1: Smear and Liquid-Based Cervical Cell Collection (Pap Test)—cont'd

TECHNIQUE FOR OBTAINING LIQUID-BASED CERVICAL CELL COLLECTION

1. Complete the cytology request form with all pertinent data.
2. Label the container.
3. Insert the dry or water-lubricated speculum. Direct the speculum in a downward and posterior direction.
4. Expose the cervix.
5. Insert cervical broom with central portion into the cervical os.
6. Rotate one-quarter turn only.
7. Place broom in fixative container and vigorously move about to dispel all particles into solution.

TBS currently uses only two terms to describe the wide spectrum of squamous cell precursors: *LSIL* and *HSIL*. TBS has also established a category called *atypical squamous cells* (ASC), and this is further qualified into two categories: *atypical squamous cells of undetermined significance* (ASC-US) and *atypical squamous cells; cannot exclude high-grade SIL* (ASC-H). *Atypical glandular cells* (AGC) may be endocervical, endometrial, or glandular cells. *Atypical glandular cells not otherwise specified* in origin (AGC-NOS), and these women are at lower risk for neoplasia than women with AGC.

Per TBS, if the Pap test shows AGC, this favors neoplasia. More worrisome is endocervical adenocarcinoma in situ or true adenocarcinoma. These glandular findings are associated with a high rate of premalignancy or true neoplasia, and these women should be referred for colposcopy. Women older than 35 years and those with significant unexplained anovulatory bleeding should also get an endometrial biopsy. If all cells are endometrial in origin only, colposcopy may be avoided in favor of an initial endometrial biopsy.

LSIL is a combination of cytological changes consistent with HPV, without evidence of dysplasia or changes consistent with mild dysplasia (CIN I). ASC-US is limited to epithelial abnormalities of uncertain significance and usually represents about 5% of the tests in most populations screened. When cells are described as atypical, further evaluation is necessary.

Obtaining endocervical cells becomes more difficult as the patient ages and the SCJ migrates inwardly. An optimal smear contains squamous cells, endocervical cells, and potentially metaplastic cells. Absence of endocervical cells on cytology may indicate an inadequate sample and requires the sample to be repeated. Box 48.3 presents factors affecting Pap test results.

MANAGEMENT

The principle of management varies depending on the degree and extent of the CIN. The patient with an abnormal cytology should be referred to a gynecologist for the proper treatment. Small lesions that are visible and do not extend to the endocervix may be handled with cryosurgery (by a gynecologist). A laser can be used on large visible lesions and vaporizes the transformation zone and 5 to 7 mm of the endocervical canal. This procedure is done under colposcopy with special training. Loop

---

Box 48.3   Factors Affecting Cervical Cytology Results

Patient History

- Previous treatment and/or surgery of reproductive tract
- Previous abnormal Pap test
- Diethylstilbestrol (DES) exposure in utero
- Current or recent vaginal or cervical infection
- Pelvic inflammatory disease
- Any medications, especially hormones
- Bleeding abnormalities
- History of any malignancy
- Pregnancy, suspected or current
- Partner history of genital or urological problems (e.g., discharge, infection, bumps/warts/rash on male or female genitalia)

Patient Factors

- Intercourse
- Douching

- Birth control methods
- Menses
- Infection
- Obtaining inadequate or inaccurate gynecologic, obstetric, or sexual history

False Negatives

- Rate for properly performed cytology smears is 1% to 80%, suggesting false or less than optimal reports are caused by clinician, patient, or cytopathologist factors.
- Rate of sampling error (i.e., diagnostic cells not on the slide) is 60%.
- Rate of screening error (cells present on slide but missed by cytotechnologist) is 40%.

False Positives

- Rate is <1%.

electrosurgical excision procedure excision can also be used on clearly visible lesions. In this procedure, a wire loop is used to excise the lesion and the tissue is sent to pathology. Conization of the cervix is surgical removal of the entire transformation zone and endocervical canal and is reserved for CIN 3 or carcinoma in situ and can be achieved with any of the methods mentioned above.

Cancer of the cervix is treated with hysterectomy. If the cancer is considered carcinoma in situ, and the woman desires to preserve fertility, then conization is the treatment of choice. For invasive carcinoma, hysterectomy is done usually with radiation and chemotherapy. If maintaining fertility is desired, radiation and chemotherapy can be done without hysterectomy.

FOLLOW-UP AND REFERRAL

The follow-up and referral depend on the specific diagnosis, extent of the cervical dysplasia or presence of cancer, and the management, but patients with abnormal cytology should be referred to a gynecologist. Patients who have undergone treatment need close follow-up in the first 2 years and women who have CIN 2 or CIN 3 and been treated with the methods outlined earlier (not hysterectomy) should have cytology repeated every 4 to 6 months for 2 years.

Patient Education: Precancerous Lesions and Cancer of the Cervix

Since the majority of cervical cancer is related to HPV infection, education about HPV prevention should begin in adolescence. Women should be educated on the guidelines for cervical cancer screening. The American College of Obstetricians and Gynecologists has prepared a patient education fact sheet with the most current guidelines as outlined earlier. The National Cervical Cancer Coalition offers educational material for patients in English and Spanish.

ENDOMETRIAL CANCER

Endometrial cancer arises from the lining of the uterus, known as the endometrium. The majority of these cancers are pure adenocarcinomas. Endometrial cancer accounts for at least 20% of cases of postmenopausal uterine bleeding.

EPIDEMIOLOGY AND CAUSES

Cancer of the endometrium is the most common of all gynecological cancers, accounting for 50% of all cases. The National Cancer Institute estimates there will be approximately 61,380 new cases of endometrial cancer in 2017, with 10,920 deaths in the United States. The overall 5-year survival rate is 80% to 85%, but is as high as 98% if the cancer is detected early and the depth of invasion is less than 66% of total endometrial thickness. The 5-year survival rate decreases to 78% if the depth of invasion is more than 66%.

The average age at diagnosis is 60 years, and about 25% of all cases occur before menopause. African American women are at greater risk for most forms of endometrial cancer than the general population, and their stage-for-stage survival rates are worse compared with those for Caucasian women. OCPs have been shown to have a protective effect against ovarian and endometrial cancer. Women who use combination estrogen-progestogen OCPs have half the risk of developing these cancers as women who do not, and women who use OCPs for at least 1 year experience this protective effect even after the OCPs are discontinued.

Risk factors for endometrial cancer include exposure to unopposed estrogen, early menarche, advanced age, a high-fat diet, nulliparity, obesity, hypertension, and diabetes mellitus. Routine screening for endometrial cancer is neither cost-effective nor warranted, except in extremely high-risk women (40% to 60% risk) with certain familial malignancy syndromes, such as Lynch syndrome II (i.e., endometrial, ovarian, and colorectal cancers) who are also at risk for hereditary nonpolyposis colorectal cancer. However, endometrial cancer screening has rarely been shown to be justified in asymptomatic women, even those on unopposed estrogen hormone replacement or the SERM tamoxifen, which is known to have estrogen agonist effects on the endometrium that increase the risk of endometrial cancer.

PATHOPHYSIOLOGY

The precursor of endometrial cancer is a hyperplastic state that may progress to invasive carcinoma. Endometrial hyperplasia of glandular tissue occurs when estrogen does not have progesterone as a counterbalance, resulting in a greater gland-to-stroma ratio. The mitogenic effect of estrogen on endometrial tissue appears to result from upregulation of the cell cycle protein cyclin D, as well as various proto-oncogenes and cellular growth factors and their receptors. These findings are also consistent with the protective effects of progestin-containing OCPs or continuous progestin therapies.

An unopposed estrogenic state, which increases the risk of endometrial cancer, may occur from multiple etiologies, including chronic anovulation such as in polycystic ovary syndrome, an estrogen-secreting ovarian tumor, obesity that causes increased aromatization of androstenedione to estrone and testosterone to estradiol in peripheral adipose tissue with decreased levels of sex hormone–binding globulin, iatrogenic estrogen exposure from older HT regimens of estrogen monotherapy (10-fold increase in risk) or the SERM tamoxifen (two- to three-fold increase in risk), which is used as adjuvant therapy for breast cancer. The potential for cytological atypia increases with chronic unopposed estrogen stimulation, creating a persistent proliferative phase within the endometrium, rather than the normal cycling of proliferative and progesterone-induced secretory phases.

The premalignant condition of endometrial hyperplasia is characterized by either a simple (i.e., cystic dilation of the glands with occasional outpouching) or complex (more abundant and adjacent glands with outpouching and minimal stroma) architectural pattern of the endometrium, as well as the presence or absence of nuclear atypia and glandular mitoses. Simple hyperplasia without atypia is unlikely to develop into endometrial carcinoma (in just 1% of cases), whereas complex architecture with atypia is most likely to progress to malignancy (in 30% of cases). Atypia is the key negative prognostic factor, because 25% of women with atypia on biopsy have coexistent malignancy on further evaluation. In fact, some pathologists group complex architecture with atypia together with differentiated adenocarcinoma under the common heading of endometrioid neoplasia. Indeed, 75% to 80% of all endometrial cancers are estrogen-dependent (type I) endometrioid carcinomas.

Not all endometrial malignancy arises from hyperplastic tissue, however. For example, papillary serous endometrial tumors (5% to 10% of cases) arise from atrophic rather than hyperplastic tissue. As with clear cell (1% to 5% of cases), mucinous, and squamous cell (fewer than 2% of cases) endometrial cancers, these tumors are estrogen independent (type II). These rarer forms of endometrial cancer tend to be more poorly differentiated (higher nuclear grade) than type I cancers, are highly aggressive with lymphatic invasion, and portend a worse prognosis.

Uterine sarcoma is a rare form of cancer (5% of uterine malignancies), which may be completely nonepithelial in origin or of a mixed epithelial-nonepithelial phenotype. Most commonly arising from the uterine myometrium (e.g., mixed Müllerian carcinosarcoma of fibrous, vascular, or lymphatic tissue; leiomyosarcoma), uterine sarcoma may also arise from the endometrium and invade the myometrium (e.g., endometrial stromal sarcoma). These cancers are more aggressive than more common hyperplastic endometrial forms, are prone to metastasis to the retroperitoneal and intra-abdominal lymph nodes and via the bloodstream to the lungs, and carry a poorer prognosis (50% 5-year survival rate for Stage I disease vs. 90% for more common forms of endometrial cancer). They are more common in African American women (except the endometrial stromal form) and in women aged 40 to 60 years. There appears to be a correlation with prior pelvic irradiation and, possibly, tamoxifen use.

Endometrial cancers may be mediated by mutations in a host of genes, such as the *p53* tumor suppressor gene, which is a late mutation in 20% of endometrioid carcinomas, an early mutation in 90% of serous adenocarcinomas, but is rarely mutated in endometrial hyperplasia. Estrogen-dependent cancers also demonstrate mutations in *PTEN* (an early mutation seen in 80% of cases), microsatellite DNA (20% to 30% of cases), and K-*ras* (a late mutation seen in 20% of cases). The cancerous cells lining the endometrium may extend directly into the cervix and through the uterine serosa. Both the pelvic (paravaginal) and para-aortic lymph nodes may become involved. Although endometrial cancer metastasizes slowly, malignant cells can be found in the peritoneal cavity.

CLINICAL PRESENTATION

Subjective

The patient, usually postmenopausal, presents with abnormal bleeding in 80% of cases. Typically, this is the only patient complaint. Patients who are perimenopausal tend to have irregular periods of bleeding; however, irregular uterine bleeding must not be discounted in these women without further exploration.

Objective

The patient usually does not demonstrate any pain on examination unless metastasis has already occurred and the pelvic organs are affected.

DIAGNOSTIC REASONING

Diagnostic Tests

Any postmenopausal patient with AUB should be referred for endometrial biopsy. Eighty percent of cases of abnormal bleeding are from benign causes. A Pap test is not a reliable diagnostic indicator for endometrial cancer. Any AGC reported on the Pap test should be followed up by endometrial biopsy to rule out hyperplasia or carcinoma; the same may be done for women older than 40 years with normal endometrial cells on Pap test, but this is more controversial.

If endometrial biopsy reveals hyperplasia with atypia, a more extensive hysteroscopy with curettage should be done to rule out coexistent endometrial cancer. If abnormal bleeding persists after an otherwise normal endometrial biopsy (i.e., showing only atrophy, proliferative or secretory endometrium, or disordered/dyssynchronous endometrium reflecting irregular endometrial shedding seen with unopposed estrogen exposure or endometritis), further assessment should be done with TVUS, hysteroscopy, and directed biopsy/curettage. TVUS is helpful in ruling out carcinoma in women not on HT. A biopsy is done if the endometrial thickness is greater than 4 mm or in any woman with persistent uterine bleeding, regardless of endometrial thickness. However, TVUS cannot replace biopsy as a definitive means of ruling out cancer. Depending on the results of the endometrial biopsy, the patient should be referred to a surgeon, and CA-125 should be checked to predict the extent of extrauterine spread, if cancer is suspected.

Differential Diagnoses

Differential diagnoses may include benign tumor (leiomyomas [fibroids]), ectopic pregnancy, intrauterine pregnancy, GI masses, endometriosis, adenomyosis, and pelvic abscess or adhesions. Endometrial polyps should also be considered because they present mostly in middle-aged women but account for 25% of cases of abnormal bleeding in premenopausal and postmenopausal women. They are hyperplastic pedunculated or sessile growths of endometrial glands and stroma at the endometrial surface (millimeters to centimeters in size) and are only rarely neoplastic (benign in 70% of cases, hyperplasia without atypia in 25%, atypia in fewer than 5%, and cancer in fewer than 1%). Metrorrhagia (irregular uterine bleeding) occurs in 50% of cases of endometrial polyps; less frequently, menorrhagia, postmenopausal bleeding, prolapse through the cervical os, and breakthrough bleeding on hormonal treatments occur as symptoms. The only definitive diagnosis for endometrial polyps is via microscopy (after D&C, biopsy, or hysterectomy), but sonohysterography (instillation of saline into the uterus before ultrasound) is preferred to TVUS for noninvasive evaluation (although it is not considered diagnostic). Curettage guided via hysteroscopy, rather than done blindly, is preferred for detecting polyps.

Adenomyosis is the presence of ectopic endometrial glands and stroma within the musculature of the uterus, which induces hypertrophy and hyperplasia of the myometrium in response to estrogen (and possibly progesterone). It may be microscopic or nodular on gross inspection, but endometrial biopsy is typically negative because changes are limited to the myometrium. It seems to be more associated with childbearing, but the pathogenesis is unknown (it is perhaps related to invagination of the endometrium or it may arise de novo from Müllerian remnants). The uterus is large and boggy (as opposed to firm with uterine fibroids). Adenomyosis is not related to endometriosis, although it is another form of ectopic endometrium. Although a third of women are asymptomatic, adenomyosis may present with AUB, dysmenorrhea, and menorrhagia.

MANAGEMENT

The primary principle of management is to obtain a correct diagnosis as early as possible, because the cure rate for endometrial cancer is very high if treated early. Because primary prevention is the best management, women with chronic anovulation may benefit from the protective effects of progestin or progesterone-containing regimens against hyperplasia and carcinoma, with doses decreased from standard recommendations in women with significant side effects. Women with hyperplasia without atypia can be given medroxyprogesterone acetate 10 mg daily for 12 to 14 days each month for 3 to 6 months, whereas women with atypia (premalignancy) need hysteroscopy with D&C and preferably a hysterectomy, if childbearing is no longer desired. If no cancer is found, women can receive megestrol acetate 10 to 80 mg four times daily on a continuous basis to suppress hyperplasia or undergo a hysterectomy if fertility is no longer desired and the patient can tolerate the surgery. Any ET should be stopped in these cases.

In postmenopausal women not on HT who have hyperplasia without atypia, a hysteroscopy and D&C are done to determine the source of estrogen (e.g., tumor, obesity). Women can be given medroxyprogesterone acetate 10 mg daily for 3 months and then reevaluated by biopsy as a guide for further management. If the woman is taking HT, it should be stopped immediately and a similar assessment done. In postmenopausal women with atypia, a hysteroscopy with D&C is done to rule out carcinoma, and a hysterectomy (preferred) is considered. As an alternative, megestrol acetate 40 mg two to four times daily can be given with a repeat biopsy in 3 months and hysterectomy done if atypia persists. Otherwise, if the atypia regresses, megestrol can be given and repeat biopsies done every 6 to 12 months for the rest of the woman's life.

Treatment of endometrial cancer is based on International Federation of Gynecology and Obstetrics (FIGO) staging. Stage I is confined to the uterine corpus, Stage II involves the cervix, Stage III is regional spread to the pelvis, and Stage IV is spread outside the pelvis (20% to 25% 5-year survival). Lymph node biopsy (lymphadenectomy) is done for clinically suspicious nodes and for cases beyond Stage I disease—a tumor greater than 2 cm, type II endometrial cancer, or myometrial invasion of greater than 50%—because all of these indicate an increased risk of metastasis. Peritoneal cytology is also sent as a part of surgical staging, because a positive result with nonendometrioid tumors may indicate the need for postsurgical adjuvant chemotherapy. Bilateral salpingo-oophorectomy is done to check for adnexal micrometastases and to eliminate endogenous estrogen production.

In contrast to the treatment of early Stage type I endometrial cancer, uterine sarcoma is treated with TAH-BSO with adjuvant radiotherapy (either external beam or brachytherapy). Although adjuvant chemotherapy has not been shown to be effective for uterine sarcoma, recurrent disease is treated with chemotherapy. Uterine adenocarcinoma of Stage II or higher is also treated with TAH-BSO, if the patient can tolerate surgery. Pelvic irradiation is an alternative to hysterectomy but entails significant comorbidities from fibrotic tissue damage that is progressive and nonreversible.

Adjuvant postsurgical radiation may be used for women at intermediate to high risk of recurrent disease (Stage I or II disease extending greater than 50% beyond the myometrium [Stage IC] or Stage II to IV disease) or reserved as salvage treatment for recurrent disease. Disease at high risk of recurrence (Stage II disease extending to the cervix with greater than 50% myometrial involvement, Stage III disease, involvement of the lymphatic or vascular system or other metastases) should be treated with surgery and adjuvant chemotherapy or pelvic irradiation; the choice is individualized depending on potential side effects and patient tolerance. Recurrent or highly advanced disease is treated with a combination of chemotherapy and hormonal therapy, although the choice of regimen is controversial. Localized relapse may be treated with salvage surgery or pelvic irradiation.

FOLLOW-UP AND REFERRAL

If endometrial cancer is suspected in a postmenopausal patient with AUB, an immediate referral should be made to a gynecologist or oncologist for an endometrial biopsy. Follow-up will be guided by the type of intervention chosen, as the only definitive cure for endometrial cancer is hysterectomy, with complete removal of all endometrial tissue.

Patient Education: Uterine Cancer

Healthy postmenopausal patients should be encouraged to seek care at the first sign of any abnormal bleeding. In addition, obese women should be encouraged to lose weight because it may be protective and possibly therapeutic for women with chronic anovulation. The use of HT for any indication is controversial in women with prior endometrial cancer. All women should be encouraged to follow treatment regimens for any concurrent diseases, such as hypertension and diabetes mellitus.

OVARIAN CANCER

Tumors of the ovary are common, and most are benign. However, malignant ovarian tumors are the leading cause of reproductive system cancer deaths. There are three primary types of *ovarian cancer*, which are classified according to their cell type of origin: surface epithelial tumors, ovarian germ cell tumors, and ovarian stromal tumors.

EPIDEMIOLOGY AND CAUSES

The causes of ovarian cancer are largely unknown. However, known risk factors for developing ovarian cancer include advanced age (more than half of patients are older than 65 years), family history of a grandmother, mother, or sister with ovarian, breast, or colon cancer or a father or brother with colon cancer (5% to 10% of cases are familial), nulliparity, early menarche, and late menopause ("incessant ovulation" increases the risk of ovarian epithelial damage and inactivation of tumor suppressor genes), lifestyle factors (e.g., high-fat diet, positive smoking history, lack of exercise), and a history of prolonged use of fertility drugs.

Ovarian cancer is quantitatively the rarest but most deadly of the gynecological cancers. In the United States, more than 25,000 cases of ovarian cancer are diagnosed annually, with approximately 14,500 deaths. It is the seventh most common cancer in women worldwide, with the greatest incidence occurring in industrialized countries. It is most commonly diagnosed in light-skinned women of northern European ancestry who have a strong family history. This familial predisposition may be strictly genetic or multifactorial in etiology, including environmental causes.

The highest incidence of ovarian cancer occurs in the postmenopausal years, with a gradually rising incidence after the age of 45 years. Ovarian cancers have been associated with the number of ovulations in a woman's lifetime; nulliparity increases the number of ovulations that occur and, therefore, the risk of cell mutations occurring. Likewise, infertility drugs, which are known to hyperstimulate the ovaries, increase the risk of a cancerous mutation.

Despite public awareness that early detection is crucial for cancer prevention and effective treatment in general, no mass screening test has proven effective enough for ovarian cancer to be recommended at this time. However, for women who have risk factors for ovarian cancer, a pelvic examination, CA-125 level, and a transvaginal pelvic ultrasound can be done annually to increase the chance of early detection. However, surveillance has not been shown statistically to increase early diagnosis.

PATHOPHYSIOLOGY

There are several distinct types of ovarian malignancies: epithelial cell, germ cell, and sex cord stromal cell. By far the most prevalent and life-threatening tumors arise from the surface epithelial cells that cover the ovary and are continuous with the peritoneal mesothelium. Tumors arising from epithelial cells account for 80% to 90% of all ovarian cancer diagnoses. Epithelial cell tumors are further subdivided into papillary serous cystadenocarcinomas, which resemble the cells lining the fallopian tubes (75%), mucinous cystadenocarcinomas, which simulate the endocervical epithelium (10%), endometrioid tumors (10%), which are similar to endometrial cancers, and the much rarer clear cell, Brenner transitional cell, undifferentiated, and mixed cell–type tumors.

Germ cell tumors comprise 20% to 25% of ovarian tumors, with fewer than 5% of these being malignant. Dysgerminomas are the most common (30% to 50%), followed by yolk sac (endodermal sinus) tumors and immature/mature teratomas—each of which accounts for approximately 20% of germ cell tumors. Much rarer forms of germ cell tumors include embryonal carcinoma, polyembryoma, choriocarcinoma, and carcinoid tumors.

Stromal cell tumors are less common, comprising only 5% to 8% of primary ovarian neoplasms. Neoplasms of stromal cells originate from the cells of the supporting structure of the ovary. These can be divided into gonadal support structures, which are the cells that support the ova or egg, and nongonadal stromal cells that are the nonspecialized support structures of the ovary. The gonadal cells are further divided into two specialized subgroups called the granulosa-theca and the Sertoli-Leydig cells. Granulosa-theca cells surround the site on the ovary where the ovum is released and produce female sex hormones. The second subgroup, the Sertoli-Leydig cells, is responsible for producing male sex hormones. The nongonadal stromal cell tumors are derived from the smooth muscle and ligaments that give the ovary its basic structure and form.

Various germline mutations have been associated with epithelial ovarian tumors, such as *BRCA1*, *BRCA2*, and the hereditary nonpolyposis colorectal cancer gene, but only in a small minority of cases, with serous ovarian adenocarcinomas predominating. These cancers, which appear to run in families, have an earlier age of onset than those in the general population. Mutations in well-characterized oncogenes including *HER-2/neu*, c-*myc*, *Akt*, and the tumor suppressor genes *p53*, *p16*, and *PTEN* have also been associated with noninherited forms of ovarian cancer. However, the precise pathogenetic mechanisms implicating these mutations, as well as most ovarian cancer risk factors, have yet to be determined.

A likely mechanism appears to be the increased frequency of genetic mutations associated with repeated injury and repair to the ovarian epithelium that occurs with cycled ovulation, thus explaining the correlation of ovarian cancer with nulliparity and early menses and the protective effect of oral contraceptives that suppress ovulation. Hormonal stimulation of ovarian tissue by high estrogen levels and possibly also androgens has also been cited as a factor in malignant transformation, whereas progesterone has been shown to have protective effects. Interestingly, some case-controlled studies have demonstrated a connection between ovarian carcinogenesis and environmental agents believed to enter through the genitourinary tract that travel retrograde to the ovaries (e.g., perineal talc, although a causative role is unclear).

CLINICAL PRESENTATION

Subjective

Symptoms can be vague or nonexistent in the early stages of the disease or seemingly unrelated to the ovaries. Such early symptoms include pelvic or abdominal pain, bloating, inability to eat or feeling full quickly, and urinary urgency or frequency. As the tumor enlarges and the disease progresses, commonly expressed symptoms include a sense of pelvic pressure or discomfort; urinary frequency, pressure, and urgency; abdominal swelling and gassy bloating; nausea and vomiting; indigestion; rectal pressure; painful intercourse; diarrhea or constipation; abnormal vaginal bleeding; unexplained weight loss; and jaundice.

Objective

During the pelvic examination, a pelvic mass, decreased mobility of the cervix and uterus, fullness in the adnexal areas of cul-de-sac, and pain on palpation of the ovaries may be detected. A rectal examination may confirm a pelvic mass as well.

DIAGNOSTIC REASONING

Diagnostic Tests

A comprehensive diagnostic work-up begins with a complete history and must include questions and discussions regarding the woman's current complaints, past health experiences, obstetric history, family history, and dietary habits. Further information that could be useful would be bowel and bladder habits and menstrual history. If an ovarian neoplasm is suspected, a bimanual pelvic examination is the first step in the diagnostic work-up. Malignant ovarian tumors are usually large with irregular contour and decreased mobility, unlike benign tumors and cysts, which usually have smooth borders, are relatively small (less than 5 cm), and are mobile.

When a mass is palpated and suspicious for malignancy, subsequent diagnostic testing should include a pelvic ultrasound to evaluate the size, shape, and consistency of the mass, as well as a serum CA-125 level. If the CA-125 level is greater than 35 U/mL, there is a greater likelihood that the ovarian mass is malignant, but the level may also be elevated in postmenopausal women with benign disease (e.g., endometriosis). CA-125 is most helpful for following the response to therapy and to help determine prognosis, but it is not an effective or sensitive screening tool.

A TVUS can help differentiate malignant ovarian masses from those that are benign. An intravenous pyelogram will demonstrate if the mass is impinging on the ureters or bladder. A barium enema determines involvement of the rectum or colon. In some cases, a diagnostic laparoscopy can be used for direct visualization of the mass. Abdominal/pelvic CT and MRI are not useful to establish the diagnosis for pelvic masses, but these imaging tests are helpful in establishing the presence or degree of metastases from ovarian cancer or determining whether a primary cancer site exists outside the ovaries. A biopsy is not routinely recommended when an ovarian mass is present because this may cause the tumor cells to disseminate into the peritoneal cavity.

As part of a preoperative evaluation to rule out non-ovarian primary cancer sites, a colonoscopy or barium enema should be done if a stool occult blood test is positive or if the patient has GI obstruction. An upper GI x-ray series is done if an upper GI site of pathology is suspected, bilateral mammography if any breast mass is present, and endometrial biopsy with curettage if AUB is present.

Differential Diagnosis

Differential diagnoses include ovarian cysts, benign ovarian tumors, ectopic pregnancy, hydrosalpinx, GI masses, pelvic kidney, endometriosis, tubo-ovarian abscess or adhesions, and intrauterine pregnancy. Also included in the differential diagnosis are metastases to the ovaries from other primary sites of cancer, such as the breast, uterus, or GI tract.

MANAGEMENT

The main principle of management of ovarian cancer is early diagnosis and referral for treatment (surgical and/or medical). Ovarian cancer is surgically staged, and the staging determines the specific treatment approach. Staging is done using FIGO staging, which guides treatment. Stage I disease is confined to the ovaries. In Stage II, there is extension to the pelvis, and Stage III indicates spread beyond the pelvis to the peritoneal cavity or para-aortic/inguinal lymph nodes (but within the abdomen). Stage IV disease denotes distant metastasis. Seventy-five percent of women with epithelial disease present in Stages III to IV, and 25% present in Stages I and II. The 5-year survival rate for Stage I ovarian cancer is 90%, but only 25% of all cases are diagnosed at this early Stage. The 5-year survival rate declines rapidly as the stage of disease increases: 40% to 60% for Stage II disease, 15% to 20% for Stage III, and less than 5% for Stage IV.

Unlike other cancers, surgical resection for optimal cytoreduction is the standard of care for both early and advanced ovarian cancer. Therapy is based on appropriate surgical staging, unless there are clear contraindications to surgery. Surgery improves disease-related symptoms, improves response to chemotherapy (if cytoreduction leaves a tumor of less than 2 cm in the widest dimension), and decreases tumor-produced immunosuppressive cytokines. Surgical staging is done via laparotomy, checking for fluid in the cul-de-sac, as well as exploring the entire abdomen for disease. The para-aortic and pelvic lymph nodes are dissected as well to evaluate for microscopic extension into the nodes (Stage III disease), which can occur in up to a third of cases that initially appear to be Stage I.

Surgical removal usually includes hysterectomy and bilateral oophorectomy (because there is a large risk of contralateral disease) with appendectomy (which may be a site of isolated metastasis), along with additional resection of pelvic/abdominal structures as needed (especially the omentum). In very early stage disease, unilateral oophorectomy may be performed only if future fertility is desired, but endometrial biopsy should be done.

After surgical treatment, the patient is usually given a course of chemotherapy, with or without radiation. The amount and type of chemotherapy are based on the surgical findings, staging, and subsequent pathological diagnosis and grading of the tumor. Carboplatin plus paclitaxel is the standard of care for Stage III to IV epithelial cancers. This same chemotherapy regimen may also be used for Stage I to II epithelial cancers after surgery. It may suffice to just observe low-grade Stage I disease after surgical resection, rather than treat with chemotherapy, as long as higher Grade 2 or 3 disease is not noted. Chemotherapy is started 4 to 6 weeks after surgery and continues for three to six cycles, depending on extent of disease and response to therapy (the patient is followed with physical examination, interim history, CA-125 levels, imaging via CT scan, etc.).

Most patients respond to postsurgical first-line chemotherapy, but chemotherapy may also be used for palliative care in the case of recurrence. Patients with bulky residual disease survive a median of 26 months, whereas for those with small-volume residual disease, median survival is 60 months. Neither maintenance chemotherapy (longer regimens of single or combination chemotherapeutic agents) nor intraperitoneal (IP) chemotherapy are current standards of care and are under investigation. IP chemotherapy has the advantage of direct contact with cancer cells, less systemic adverse effects, and less collateral damage to nonmalignant tissue. At present, for Stage III and IV disease, surgery followed by systemic chemotherapy is indicated, but studies are ongoing to evaluate neoadjuvant (preoperative) chemotherapy. Currently, neoadjuvant chemotherapy is used for patients with poor performance status who would not tolerate surgery before treatment. Secondary cytoreduction after initial surgery and first-line systemic chemotherapy may be beneficial, however.

The diagnosis and treatment of ovarian cancer (and other gynecological cancers) may be devastating for the patient and her family. Several phenomenological studies have identified the themes of uncertainty, perceived lack of control, feelings of isolation, and hopelessness as prominent in the patient experience. These feelings can impact recovery and may manifest in physical symptoms. Researchers at the Yale University School of Nursing conducted a single-blinded randomized clinical trial to determine if a specialized nursing intervention designed to help patients develop and maintain self-management skills and participate in decisions affecting their treatment would improve quality of life scores over women who did not have the intervention. The women in the intervention group experienced less uncertainty, less symptom distress, and better scores on the quality of life instrument than the control group (McCorkle et al., 2009).

FOLLOW-UP AND REFERRAL

When an adnexal mass is detected, the patient should be referred to a gynecologist and possibly a surgeon for prompt treatment. Patients who have been diagnosed with ovarian cancer and have undergone surgical and chemical treatment will have CT scans repeated at 6-month intervals for 2 years and may be encouraged to have a second-look surgical procedure to assess the results of the prior treatments, both surgical and medical. Follow-up will be determined by the type of intervention.

Patient Education: Ovarian Cancer

As mentioned previously, the number of ovulations in a patient's lifetime increases the risk of ovarian cancer; therefore, both pregnancy and use of hormonal contraception lower the risk of ovarian cancer. Patients should be aware of early signs and symptoms and screening modalities and guidelines, especially if they have any risk factors. Annual gynecological examinations should be encouraged, and the importance of a low-fat diet and weight control should be stressed.

VULVODYNIA

Vulvodynia is a complex, multifactorial chronic vulvar pain syndrome. The most recent definitions and descriptions of vulvar pain were developed in 2015 at the Vulvar Pain and Vulvodynia Consensus Conference. At this conference, The International Society for the Study of Vulvovaginal Diseases, the International Society for the Study of Women's Sexual Health, and the International Pelvic Pain Society collaborated to develop consistent nomenclature for the disease. The 2015 classification lists two main categories: chronic vulvar pain related to specific disorders (inflammatory, neoplastic, traumatic) and vulvodynia. Vulvodynia in this classification is defined as idiopathic vulvar pain lasting at least 3 months. Vulvodynia is classified based on the location of the pain (generalized or localized), whether the pain is provoked or unprovoked (upon contact, spontaneous), whether the pain is intermittent or constant, and the type of onset.

EPIDEMIOLOGY AND CAUSES

Vulvodynia is believed to affect as many as 10% to 28% of reproductive-aged women. The exact cause is unknown and until recently, the problem was not recognized as a distinct and diagnosable pain syndrome. It is estimated that the costs of vulvodynia in the United States are between $31 and $72 billion each year. This figure includes both direct health-care costs and indirect costs (e.g., lost work productivity). It does not, however, consider the significant psychological costs to the women affected and their partners. Sexual and physical abuse can be a risk factor for developing vulvodynia. In fact, women with vulvodynia reported severe sexual and physical abuse three times more often than women without vulvodynia.

PATHOPHYSIOLOGY

To date, no definitive cause of vulvodynia is known. Studies have confirmed an increased number and density of nociceptor nerve endings in the vulvar vestibular tissue of some women with vulvodynia. Some researchers have found serotonin receptor gene (5HT-2A) polymorphisms in women with provoked vulvodynia (PVD), indicating a possible link to the serotonergic system. There is some evidence that women with PVD have augmented CNS neural activity in response to painful vestibular stimulation.

There is some question of a genetic predisposition to developing PVD, and studies have focused on polymorphisms that increase the risk of *Candida* infections and the possibility that genetic factors permit an exaggerated inflammatory reaction to such infections in the vestibule. In turn, a large portion of the research into vulvodynia is focused on inflammation. Women with vulvodynia are also more likely to report having hives before the onset of vulvar pain, leading researchers to consider mast cells as a trigger for nerve sensitization in vulvodynia.

CLINICAL PRESENTATION

Subjective

The most common symptom of vulvodynia is burning, stinging pain. It is sometimes described as irritation or sharp pain in the vulvar vestibule area. The pain can be intermittent, constant, or occur when the area is touched (provoked). The woman may relate that it occurs only during sexual activity, insertion of a tampon, or during periods of prolonged sitting, bike riding, or other activity that places pressure on the vulvar area.

Objective

Pain can be elicited in many cases by touching the vulvar vestibule, but no other objective signs are typically noted.

DIAGNOSTIC REASONING

Diagnostic Tests

The diagnosis of vulvodynia is made largely on history. A pelvic examination is done to rule out infectious processes. In addition, the patient should be checked for specific localized areas of pain. This is usually done with a cotton swab gently applied to the vulvar tissue to elicit a pain response.

Differential Diagnosis

Given the idiopathic nature of vulvodynia, differential diagnoses include vaginitis (due to yeast or bacterial infection), lichen planus, vulvar cancer, vaginal atrophy, and a Bartholin gland cyst. These diagnoses are ruled out by visual inspection, vaginal culture, and biopsy if needed.

MANAGEMENT

Because the cause of vulvodynia is unknown, treatment can be difficult. The most important step in the management of vulvodynia is validating that the pain the woman is feeling is genuine. The clinician should explore the patient's psychological health and sexual health. Depression is common in anyone with chronic pain and should be assessed. If depression is present, antidepressant medication may be indicated. Psychotherapy and cognitive behavioral therapy can also be helpful for women experiencing sexual pain secondary to vulvodynia.

Pelvic floor physical therapy has been shown to be effective for some women with vulvodynia. Performing Kegel maneuvers coupled with superficial perineal massage can help the woman increase her awareness of the contraction and relaxation of her pelvic floor muscles. The Valsalva maneuver can help by increasing the capacity of the introitus, which perineal massage can also help to gradually desensitize the area.

No research has documented convincing efficacy of any therapeutic intervention. Oral adjuvant analgesic therapy, antidepressants (tricyclic agents), and anticonvulsants (e.g., gabapentin, pregabalin, lamotrigine) have all been studied, with widely varying success rates from 27% to 100%, which leads some researchers to believe these results may be due largely to placebo effects. Surgical intervention has been researched as a treatment for PVD; however, it is considered a last resort, given the lack of an identifiable cause. The typical procedure is a modified vestibulectomy, after which women have reported an improvement in their pain.

FOLLOW-UP AND REFERRAL

Because vulvodynia is a chronic pain syndrome that may involves a combination of biological, psychological, and social factors that contribute to the condition, a multidisciplinary approach is preferred. Acknowledging vulvodynia as a chronic pain condition is the first step toward patient recovery, as follow-up may be prolonged, as the woman learns to adapt to this condition if her symptoms cannot be eliminated completely. Referral to a gynecologist for a thorough assessment of the reproductive tract is indicated, and referral to a physical therapist who specializes in pelvic floor exercises and sexual health may also be beneficial, as may be a referral for sexual and cognitive therapy.

Patient Education: Vulvodynia

Vulvodynia is a complex condition that requires an individualized and holistic approach to the management plan. Women should be reassured that this is a genuine condition, and the clinician should reinforce the teaching of Kegel exercises and all aspects of the treatment plan. Results from any treatment may take up to 2 years to be effective and the primary-care practitioner can support the patient through reassurance and active listening.

REFERENCES

Amenorrhea

Genazzani AD, Podfigurna-Stopa A, Czyzyk A, et al. Short-term estriol administration modulates hypothalamo-pituitary function in patients with functional hypothalamic amenorrhea (FHA). *Gynecol Endocrinol.* 2016;32(3):253–257.

Kowanci E, Schutt AK. Premature ovarian failure. *Obstet Gynecol Clin North Am.* 2015;42(1):153–161.

Dysmenorrhea

Abaraogu UO, Tabansi-Ochuogu CS. As acupressure decreases pain, acupuncture may improve some aspects of quality of life for women with primary dysmenorrhea: A systematic review with meta-analysis. *J Acupunct Meridian Stud.* 2015;8(5):220–228.

Iacovides S, Avidon I, Baker FC. What we know about primary dysmenorrhea today: A critical review. *Hum Reprod Update.* 2015;21(6):762–778.

Endometrial Cancer

Howlader N, Noone AM, Krapcho M, et al., eds. SEER cancer statistics review, 1975–2014. Bethesda, MD: National Cancer Institute. **https://seer.cancer.gov/csr/1975_2014.** April 2017.

Endometriosis

Brown J, Farquhar C. An overview of treatments for endometriosis. *JAMA.* 2015;313(3):296–297.

Dunselman GAJ, Vermeulen N, Becker C, et al. ESHRE guideline: Management of women with endometriosis. *Hum Reprod.* 2014;29(3):400–412.

Prescott J, Farland LV, Tobias DK, et al. A prospective cohort study of endometriosis and subsequent risk of infertility. *Hum Reprod.* 2016;31(7):1475–1482.

Fertility Problems

Brunham RC, Gottlieb SL, Paavonen J. Pelvic inflammatory disease. *N Engl J Med.* 2015;372(21):2039–2048.

Crawford NM, Steiner AZ. Age-related infertility. *Obstet Gynecol Clin North Am*. 2015;42(1):15–25.

Kovanci E, Schutt AK. Premature ovarian failure: Clinical presentation and treatment. *Obstet Gynecol Clin North Am*. 2015;42(1):153–161.

Leiomyomas (Uterine Fibroids)

Stewart EA. Uterine fibroids. *N Engl J Med*. 2015;372(17): 1646–1655.

Menopause

Cauley JA. Estrogen and bone health in men and women. *Steroids*. 2015;99:11–15.

Collins P, Webb CM, DeVilliers TJ, et al. Cardiovascular risk assessment in women-an update. *Climacteric*. 2016;19(4):329–336.

Kim HK, Kang SY, Chung YJ, Kim JH, Kim MR. The recent review of genitourinary syndrome of menopause. *J Menopausal Med*. 2015;21(2):65–71.

Ovarian Cancer

McCorkle R, Dowd M, Ercolano E, et al. Effects of a nursing intervention on quality of life outcomes in post-surgical women with gynecological cancer. *Psychooncology*. 2009;18(1):62–70.

Nezhat FR, Apostol R, Nezhat C, Pejovic T. New insights in the pathophysiology of ovarian cancer and implications for screening and prevention. *Am J Obstet Gynecol*. 2015;213(3):262–267.

Oza AM, Cook AD, Pfisterer J, et al. Standard chemotherapy with or without bevacizumab for women with newly diagnosed ovarian cancer (ICON7): Overall survival results of a phase 3 randomised trial. *Lancet Oncol*. 2015;16(8):928–936.

Precancerous Lesions and Cancer of the Cervix

Sawaya GF, Smith-McCune K. Cervical cancer screening. *Obstet Gynecol*. 2016;127(3):459–467.

Up-To-Date. Patient education: Follow-up of high grade abnormal Pap tests (beyond the basics). **https://www.uptodate.com/contents/follow-up-of-high-grade-abnormal-pap-tests-beyond-the-basics.** Accessed January 10, 2018.

Waxman AG, Chelmow D, Darragh TM, Lawson H, Moscicki AB. Revised terminology for cervical histopathology and its implications for management of high-grade squamous inteaepithelial lesions of the cervix. *Obstet Gynecol*. 2012;120(6):1465–1471.

Premenstrual Syndrome and Premenstrual Dysphoric Disorder

Hantsoo L, Epperson CN. Premenstrual dysphoric disorder: Epidemiology and treatment. *Curr Psychiatry Rep*. 2015;17:87. **https://link.springer.com/content/pdf/10.1007%2Fs11920-015-0628-3.pdf.**

Yonkers KA, Casper RF. Clinical manifestations and diagnosis of premenstrual syndrome and premenstrual dysphoric disorder. UpToDate. **https://www.uptodate.com/contents/clinical-manifestations-and-diagnosis-of-premenstrual-syndrome-and-premenstrual-dysphoric-disorder?source=search_result&search=clinical%20manifestations%20and%20diagnosis%20of%20premenstrual%20syndrome&selectedTitle=1~150.** Updated 2016. Accessed September 19, 2017.

Vulvodynia

DeAndres J, Sanchis-Lopez N, Asensio-Sampler JM, et al. Vulvodynia—an evidence-based literature review and proposed treatment algorithm. *Pain Pract*. 2016;16(2):204–236.

Pukall CF, et al. Vulvodynia: Definition, prevalence, impact, and pathophysiological factors. *J Sex Med*. 2016;13(3):291–304.

Sadownik LA. Etiology, diagnosis, and clinical management of vulvodynia. *Int J Womens Health*. 2014;6:437–449.

Stockdale CK, Lawson HW. 2013 Vulvodynia Guideline update. *J Low Genit Tract Dis*. 2014;18(2):93–100.

RESOURCES

American Society for Reproductive Medicine
http://www.asrm.org

Fertilitext
http://www.fertilitext.org

International Council on Infertility Information Dissemination
http://www.inciid.org

Internet Health Resources: Infertility Resources
http://www.ihr.com/infertility

National Cancer Institute Resources
For patients: https://www.cancer.gov/resources-for/patients
For providers: https://www.cancer.gov/resources-for/hp

National Cervical Cancer Coalition
http://www.nccc-online.org/resources/educational-materials

The American College of Obstetricians and Gynecologists, Patient Education Fact Sheet
https://www.acog.org/-/media/For-Patients/pfs004.pdf?dmc=1&ts=20180113T1931084368

The American Society for Colposcopy and Cervical Pathology (ASCCP): The Society for Lower Genital Tract Disorders Guidelines
http://www.asccp.org/asccp-guidelines

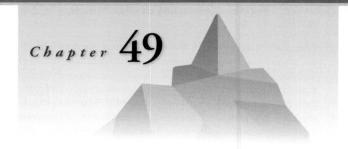

Chapter 49

Prostate Disorders

Debbie Nogueras Conner, PhD, ANP/FNP-BC, FAANP

Debera J. Thomas, DNS, RN, FNP/ANP

Brian Oscar Porter, MD, PhD, MPH, MBA

BENIGN PROSTATIC HYPERPLASIA

Benign prostatic hyperplasia (also called benign prostatic hypertrophy or BPH) is the common name for nodular hyperplasia of the prostate and is one of the most common conditions affecting men older than 40 years. The prostate gland is a walnut-size gland positioned at the base of the bladder and in front of the rectum. The prostate gland, which starts enlarging in puberty and stops growing at around 20 years, begins to enlarge again after 50 years.

The prostate is composed of acinar glands and their ducts, which are arranged in a radial fashion, with the stroma containing blood vessels, lymph vessels, and nerves. The prostate gland secretes 0.5 to 2 mL of fluid a day, which constitutes 10% to 20% of the seminal fluid of the ejaculate. The prostatic fluid contains citric acid, prostaglandins, and fibrinogen. The epithelial cells of the prostate gland are the only source of the glycoprotein prostate-specific antigen (PSA).

The prostate lies between the base of the urinary bladder and the upper surface of the levator ani and deep transverse peritoneal muscles. The anterior surface is adjacent to the retropubic space; the posterior surface lies adjacent to the seminal vesicles and recto-vesicular (rectum–bladder) septum. Given this location, the prostate is palpable per rectum. The normal prostate gland is 2 to 3 cm across; at its midpoint, it is typically twice the breadth of the examining finger and weighs approximately 20 g (i.e., walnut sized).

A slightly enlarged gland is documented as +1 and is considered three finger-breadths across, with +2 being twice the normal breadth or four finger-breadths across. Occasionally a +3 or +4 classification will be noted, which involves the anterior pelvic outlet with marked encroachment of the posterior lobe on the rectal wall, reducing the caliber of the rectal passage. A normal prostate posterior area can be palpated without moving the hand, but the clinician may need to move the hand side to side to palpate an enlarged prostate or nodular area.

The prostate gland is subdivided into five lobes, which include the left and right lateral lobes (which are extensive and make up what was formerly termed the anterior lobe), the left and right posterior lobes (which also include the apex of the gland), and the median lobe. Prostatic cancer is known to have a propensity for the gland's posterior and apical peripheral zone (thus accounting for the ability to palpate many cases of prostatic cancer through the rectal wall), whereas BPH tends to affect the transition zone that surrounds the urethra.

The prostate has three distinct zones: the central zone, the peripheral zone, and the transition zone, which lies adjacent to the urethra. BPH develops primarily in the transition zone, whereas carcinoma of the prostate usually develops in the peripheral zone. Symptoms of BPH are reported earlier than when clinical evidence becomes apparent, with 25% of men at age 55 years describing a change in voiding patterns (see Pathophysiology).

EPIDEMIOLOGY AND CAUSES

The cause of BPH is not fully understood, but androgens play a key role. Aging is a primary risk factor, and BPH occurs in more than 50% of men older than 50 years and 90% of men older than 80 years. Of these, 20% of men older than 60 years have obstructive and irritative symptoms that are severe enough to require treatment. Genetic susceptibility to the disorder is also underscored by twin concordance and family history studies, with inherited forms predominating in men younger than 60 years.

Epidemiological studies of BPH have been hampered by inconsistencies in the definition and clinical criteria of this disorder. Most authorities consider not only prostate size (greater than 30 mL) but also decreased urinary flow rates (less than 15 mL/s) and significant postvoid residual (PVR) bladder volumes (greater than 50 mL).

BPH arises from a systemic hormonal alteration, which may or may not act in combination with growth factors that stimulate stromal or glandular hyperplasia. One risk factor for BPH is intact testes—more specifically, functioning Leydig cells. Castrated men or those with untreated hypogonadism before age 40 years rarely develop BPH. There has been no concrete evidence that dietary, environmental, or sexual practices are implicated in BPH, although obesity substantially increases the risk of BPH.

PATHOPHYSIOLOGY

The prostate consists of two main sections based on secretory function. The inner section of the gland produces secretions needed to keep the lining of the urethra moist.

The outer section contributes to seminal secretions. Prostatic secretions form part of the seminal fluid during ejaculation. The ejaculatory ducts from the seminal vesicles pass through the prostate gland and enter the urethra.

The importance of dihydrotestosterone (DHT) as a key androgenic hormone in the pathogenesis of BPH is well supported. Although concentrations of this prohormone (which is subsequently converted into testosterone) do not differ in men with or without BPH, prostatic receptors for this hormone have a much more heterogenous distribution in men with BPH, whereas in normal controls, these receptors predominate within the epithelia. Thus, although necessary for the pathogenesis of BPH, androgen exposure alone is not sufficient to cause the disorder. Similarly, estrogen has been implicated as a necessary factor to maintain BPH in older men, but it is not sufficient to cause its pathogenesis alone. The data are conflicting, however. For instance, the concentration of estrogen receptors is actually lower in hyperplastic prostatic tissue, whereas the concentration of progesterone receptors does not differ in BPH versus the normal prostate.

The earliest histological signs of BPH usually appear in men in their third and fourth decades of life. The development of pathological BPH is similar in most cases. BPH usually presents as a predominance of stromal nodules (up to a fourfold increase), consisting primarily of smooth muscle and connective tissue, in the periurethral area of the transition zone. This may be followed by glandular hyperplasia (up to a twofold increase) with an increase in epithelial cells. Key growth factors include fibroblast growth factor, insulin-like growth factor–2, and transforming growth factor–β. In vitro data demonstrate a wider array of growth factors that stimulate prostatic epithelial cell growth. Antiapoptotic factors such as bcl-2 are also upregulated in BPH tissue, and animal studies have implicated higher numbers of stem cells in hyperplastic prostatic tissue.

There are two documented mechanisms of obstruction— static and dynamic. *Static constriction* is caused by the buildup of prostatic tissue, with direct obstruction of the bladder neck. *Dynamic constriction* is an increase in prostatic muscle tone through adrenergic stimulation, leading to constriction of the bladder neck. A predominance of alpha-adrenergic receptors in the sympathetic nervous system controls stromal hyperplasia. If middle lobe enlargement of the prostate predominates, the symptoms produced are similar to those of a ball-valve obstruction at the bladder neck.

Obstruction of the bladder outlet forces the bladder to generate higher pressures than normal to achieve micturition. Increased muscle mass in the bladder leads to reduced bladder elasticity and compliance, which manifests as a reduction in bladder capacity. If the bladder neck obstruction is not relieved, the bladder's smooth muscle begins to be replaced by connective tissue, leading to bladder failure.

CLINICAL PRESENTATION

Subjective

Use of a standardized questionnaire such as the American Urological Association Symptom Index (AUASI) (shown in Table 49.1), also known as the International Prostatic Symptom Score, is important in assessing the impact of BPH on the patient. This questionnaire is designed to uncover the degree of symptomatology in each patient and should be calculated before starting therapy. There are seven items on the questionnaire that determine the severity of obstructive or irritative symptoms. Symptom scores are helpful to quantify the patient's symptoms. A score of 7 or higher on the AUASI, for example, can reinforce the need for further investigation of the cause of the symptoms. Although the scores alone are not diagnostic, they help to support the diagnosis, as well as being useful in following a patient after initiating therapy to track the decrease in symptoms. In addition, however, a detailed urinary history should be obtained to rule out other possible causes of the symptoms.

The symptoms of BPH vary and are dependent on the type of obstruction, but usually include a combination of obstructive and irritative voiding symptoms. Because the symptoms are not specific to BPH and may have other causes, a complete work-up is necessary. BPH is non–life-threatening, but it is a lifestyle-changing diagnosis.

Symptoms of obstructive BPH include decreased force of stream, hesitancy, postvoid dribbling, sensation of incomplete bladder emptying, overflow incontinence, inability to voluntarily stop the urinary stream, urinary retention, double voiding (voiding a second time within 2 hours), and straining. Irritative symptoms of BPH include nocturia, urinary frequency, urgency, dysuria, and urge incontinence.

Objective

A digital rectal examination (DRE) is done to determine enlargement of the prostate gland. The prostate in BPH is usually diffusely smooth and enlarged. If the prostate is nodular and unusually firm, prostate cancer may be present. The size of the prostate does not correlate with the severity of the symptoms in men with BPH. Many men with palpably enlarged prostates are asymptomatic, whereas some patients with small prostates have irritative or obstructive symptoms. A focused neurologic examination should also be performed on these patients to help determine if dysfunctional urinary symptoms are related to a neurologic disorder.

Objective findings can include gross hematuria (especially in men older than 60 years), observation of a weak urinary stream, bladder distention to greater than 150 mL as detected by percussion, an increased PVR volume to more than 100 mL, and prostatic enlargement to more than the normal "walnut" size of 20 g or less.

TABLE 49.1 American Urological Association (AUA) Symptom Score Index

Directions: Circle one number on each line.

Question to be Answered	Not at All	Less Than 1 Time in 5	Less Than Half the Time	About Half the Time	More Than Half the Time	Almost Always
1. Over the past month, how often have you had a sensation of not emptying your bladder completely after you finished urinating?	0	1	2	3	4	5
2. Over the past month, how often have you had to urinate again less than 2 hours after you finished urinating?	0	1	2	3	4	5
3. Over the past month, how often have you found you stopped and started again several times when you urinated?	0	1	2	3	4	5
4. Over the past month, how often have you found it difficult to postpone urination?	0	1	2	3	4	5
5. Over the past month, how often have you had a weak urinary stream?	0	1	2	3	4	5
6. Over the past month, how often have you had to push or strain to begin urination?	0	1	2	3	4	5
7. Over the past month, how many times did you most typically get up to urinate from the time you went to bed at night until the time you got up in the morning?	0	1 time	2 times	3 times	4 times	5 times

Total sum of the 7 circled answers (AUA Symptom Score): _____

AUA Symptom Score Index

Score	Severity
0–7	Mild
8–19	Moderate
20–35	Severe

Source: Barry MJ, et al. The American Urological Association symptom index for benign prostatic hyperplasia. *J Urol.* 1992;148(2):1549–1557.

DIAGNOSTIC REASONING

Diagnostic Tests

Urinalysis should be done to exclude infection or hematuria. The AUA no longer recommends serum creatinine as part of the initial evaluation. A PSA test is optional, but is usually done if the patient's life expectancy is greater than 10 years. PSA is a glycoprotein that aids in the liquefaction of the seminal coagulum. The PSA in BPH is usually less than 10 ng/mL. Its use in screening is controversial, however, because there may be an elevation of the PSA in either prostate cancer or BPH. Acute lower urinary retention or prostatitis will also elevate the PSA. Therefore, the PSA value alone is not diagnostic of cancer or BPH.

An elevated urinary pH results from the chronic residual urine retained in the bladder. If an obstructive uropathy is present, the serum creatinine level will be elevated.

Urine cultures are sometimes positive for bacteria because of the chronic residual urine. Urine cytology should be done to rule out carcinoma, particularly when hematuria is present. An intravenous pyelogram can identify an increased PVR volume of urine, a large prostatic impression on the bladder, a trabeculated bladder, bladder diverticula, upper tract dilation, and/or bladder stones.

Subsequent testing should be done by a urologist if initial treatment does not relieve symptoms or if prostate cancer is suspected. Uroflow, for example, measures the amount of urine voided per unit of time. Flow of less than 10 mL/s is indicative of obstruction. This test is accurate when the voided volume is greater than 200 mL. A cystometrogram measures bladder compliance and is usually reserved for patients with suspected neurologic disease or whose prostate surgery was unsuccessful in relieving symptoms. A cystoscopy is usually done only to determine the best surgical approach for BPH.

Differential Diagnosis

The differential diagnoses that must be considered when evaluating a patient with suspected BPH are numerous and fall into three distinct categories: bladder outlet obstruction, nonobstructive etiologies, and irritative symptoms. Differential Diagnosis 49.1 presents the differential diagnosis for BPH.

When BPH is the presumptive diagnosis, other obstructive etiologies of the lower urinary tract (bladder calculi, bladder neck contracture, urethral stricture, and prostate cancer) should be explored. Careful history may reveal previous urethral instrumentation, urethritis, or trauma as the source of the obstruction. Bladder calculi may present with pain and hematuria. Irritative etiologies (bladder cancer, lower urinary tract infection [UTI], prostatitis, or urethritis) may present with hematuria, urgency, and frequency. A history of diabetes mellitus, stroke, neurologic diseases, or spinal cord injury can contribute to a neurogenic bladder, which has many of the same symptoms as BPH. Likewise, cancer of the prostate and BPH have many of the same symptoms.

Differential Diagnosis 49.1: Benign Prostatic Hyperplasia

Bladder Outlet Obstruction

- Prostate cancer
- Urethral stricture due to trauma or sexually transmitted disease
- Bladder neck contracture (acquired or congenital)
- Anterior or posterior urethral valve failure
- Müllerian duct cysts
- Inability of bladder neck or external sphincter to relax during voiding

Nonobstructive Etiologies

- Neurogenic bladder (detrusor denervation)
- Myogenic cause (detrusor muscle failure)
- Diabetes mellitus
- Parkinson's disease
- Cerebrovascular accident
- Medications (parasympatholytics, sympathomimetics)
- Psychogenic stress–induced performance anxiety

Irritative Symptoms

- Neurogenic bladder (detrusor denervation)
- Neoplasm
- Bladder cancer
- Bladder calculi
- Prostatitis
- Urinary tract infection
- Urethritis

MANAGEMENT

Medical Management

Most patients with BPH can be treated as outpatients; the goal is to relieve the symptoms of dysfunctional urination, specifically nocturia. The Patient's Voice 49.1 illustrates the patient's desire for symptom relief. Inpatient treatment is required to manage fluid and electrolyte abnormalities of obstructive uropathy.

Most urologists and primary-care providers have adopted a "watchful waiting" approach for patients with BPH who have only mild symptoms. A patient with mild to moderate symptoms, minimal PVR, and no objective changes in the urinary tract may only require monitoring; thus, watchful waiting is considered the most conservative and the most appropriate management approach for BPH, as long as more serious conditions have been ruled out. Watchful waiting is also the recommended treatment when BPH has little or no impact on quality of life. As lifestyle changes do occur, however, or as the AUA score increases, several options may be offered to the patient. Avoidance of caffeine, alcohol, and highly seasoned foods, known to be bladder irritants, is recommended. A patient with a high AUA symptom score, urinary retention, or complications of BPH, including a high PVR, renal insufficiency, hematuria, bladder stones, or anatomical urinary tract abnormalities, should not be observed with only watchful waiting because these conditions require more vigorous treatment.

Once prostatic cancer has been ruled out, medications may be tried initially to treat the symptoms of BPH. Medical management is used when there is no strong indication for surgery, when a patient refuses surgery, or if the patient is a poor surgical candidate. Because the prostate and bladder contain alpha$_1$-adrenergic receptors that cause the prostate and bladder neck to contract when bound, alpha-adrenergic blockade decreases this effect and results in objective and subjective improvement in the manifestations of

---

The Patient's Voice 49.1

NOCTURIA

I had been getting up three or four times a night to urinate. It was getting to be a nuisance. At my annual examination, I was told I had mild BPH and that my PSA was normal. I told my primary-care provider that I was tired of getting up so often at night and that it made me tired the next day. The primary-care provider told me that if getting up several times a night was bothering me, then there were some lifestyle changes I could make (decrease evening fluids, completely emptying my bladder when I void) and medications I could use, so I decided to give it a try. What relief! Some simple changes and a daily pill, and now I can sleep all night and wake up in the morning refreshed. I feel great, and I am grateful that my primary-care provider took time to listen to me.

BPH. Most of the alpha-adrenergic used in the treatment of BPH are selective alpha$_1$-adrenergic antagonists. These include silodosin (Rapaflo) 4 or 8 mg daily, terazosin (Hytrin) 1 to 10 mg daily, and doxazosin (Cardura) 1 to 8 mg daily. Silodosin should be taken with a meal. No dosage adjustment is required with mild to moderate hepatic impairment or mild renal impairment. However, with moderate renal impairment, the dose should be reduced to 4 mg daily. For those with severe hepatic or renal impairment, silodosin is contraindicated. These long-acting alpha$_1$-adrenergic blockers have the advantage of once-daily dosing but still require a gradual dose titration. For example, terazosin is started at 1 mg nightly for 7 days, then 2 mg nightly for 7 days, then 5 mg nightly for 7 days, and finally up to 10 mg nightly for adequate symptom relief. Similarly, doxazosin is usually started at 1 mg daily and then doubled in dose every 1 to 2 weeks up to a maximum dose of 8 mg daily (taken in the morning or evening).

The subtype of alpha$_{1A}$-adrenergic receptors have been identified in the bladder neck and prostate, as compared to alpha$_{1B}$-adrenergic receptors found on blood vessels. This has led to the development of medications for BPH that selectively target the alpha$_{1A}$ subtype of receptors in the prostate and, therefore, have less adverse effects related to hypotension than earlier generation alpha$_1$-antagonists. These include tamsulosin (Flomax) 0.4 or 0.8 mg daily and alfuzosin (UroXatral) 10 to 15 mg daily (immediately after the same meal each day). The alpha$_{1A}$-adrenergic blockers (tamsulosin and alfuzosin) do not need to be titrated, but should be started at the lowest dose and then increased if necessary.

Another class of medications used to treat BPH are the 5-alpha-reductase inhibitors, which include finasteride (Proscar) and dutasteride (Avodart). These medications block the conversion of testosterone to DHT by inhibiting the enzyme 5-alpha-reductase. The action of DHT is primarily responsible for the enlargement of the prostate gland. The maximum reduction in prostate size (20% reduction) may take up to 6 months of therapy. However, improvement in symptoms is seen only in men with very enlarged prostates (greater than 40 g).

Finasteride is well tolerated in most patients, but adverse effects include decreased ejaculate volume, reduced libido, and erectile dysfunction in 3% to 5% of all patients. The adverse effects may decrease with time, however, and are reversible with the cessation of treatment. Dutasteride (a second generation 5-alpha-reductase inhibitor) produces a more rapid reduction in DHT. For example, dutasteride 0.5 mg daily for 2 weeks reduced serum DHT concentrations by 90% and resulted in significant improvement in symptoms after 3 to 13 months of treatment. The side effects of dutasteride were similar to those of finasteride but decreased over time and were only slightly higher than in men receiving placebo. Finasteride and dutasteride also decrease the PSA concentration by almost 50%, which can complicate prostate cancer detection and may increase the risk of patients being diagnosed with more advanced, high-grade prostate cancer; thus, the U.S. Food and Drug Administration (FDA) has included this risk in the labels of all 5-alpha-reductase inhibitors.

There is some evidence that combination therapy of terazosin and finasteride is superior to single-medication therapy (with either an alpha-adrenergic-blocker or 5-alpha-reductase inhibitor) in long-term but not in short-term treatment. If a patient has reached the maximum dose of the alpha blocker and symptoms continue to progress, finasteride can be added at that point to improve prostate size and symptoms.

Complementary therapies may also be used to treat BPH. Complementary Therapies 49.1 presents herbal therapies, along with vitamin and mineral therapies, that may be used in the treatment of the symptoms of BPH.

Invasive and Surgical Management

Urological surgery is another treatment option for BPH and is the second most common surgery in men (second only to cataract surgery). Prostate surgery is indicated when there is urinary retention or when other symptoms are intractable because of prostatic obstruction, as gauged by the AUA index in patients with a score of greater than 8. Obstructive uropathy, recurrent and persistent UTIs due to prostatic obstruction, or recurrent gross hematuria caused by an enlarged prostate is also an indication for surgical resection.

Transurethral resection of the prostate (TURP) is the surgical treatment of choice for BPH. Candidates for surgical intervention include patients with severe symptoms,

Complementary Therapies 49.1: Benign Prostatic Hyperplasia

THERAPY	COMMENTS
Saw palmetto	Available in tablet, liquid, or tea form: 320 mg by mouth daily. Inhibits 5-α-reductase activity and mimics the effects of finasteride; combination of saw palmetto, lycopene, and selenium is thought to be more effective. PSA levels may be artificially lowered by saw palmetto.
African wild potato (*Hypoxis hemerocallidea*)	Sixty to 130 mg of β-sitosterol (a constituent of African wild potato) divided into two or three doses daily. It acts by decreasing inflammation.

high PVRs, complications, upper urinary tract changes, and those who fail medical therapy. TURP is performed through a cystoscope, using a diathermy loop for the resection of prostatic tissue. It is usually performed under spinal or general anesthesia, with a urethral catheter maintained in place for 36 to 48 hours postoperatively. Some patients may also need to be discharged from the hospital with a urinary catheter in place for up to 2 weeks after surgery. Symptomatic improvement following a TURP occurs in 90% of the patients. Flow-stream rates are increased as much as 15 mL/s. Unfortunately, complications of TURP include retrograde ejaculation, which occurs in 65% of patients, and erectile dysfunction, which occurs in up to 15% of patients. Less frequent problems include bleeding, UTI, and urethral stricture.

A transurethral incision of the prostate (TUIP) is limited to patients with moderate to severe symptoms and a small prostate who have an elevated bladder neck or posterior commissure hyperplasia. In this procedure, an instrument is passed through the urethra to make one or two cuts in the prostate and the prostatic capsule, reducing the urethral stricture in order to relieve symptoms. This procedure can be performed on an outpatient basis under local anesthesia and sedation or during a 24-hour hospital stay. TUIP has a lower complication rate than TURP.

Open prostatectomy is a surgical option reserved for prostate glands weighing more than 40 to 100 g. An open prostatectomy is the surgical removal of the inner portion of the prostate via a suprapubic or retropubic incision in the abdominal area. This procedure requires longer hospitalizations than the other two options and has far more complications. Nonetheless, this may be the only alternative for a patient who has failed medical treatment or when carcinoma of the prostate is suspected.

Robotic simple prostatectomy is used for patients with very large prostates. During the procedure, the inner part of the prostate that is causing the obstruction is removed. This is a substitute for open prostatectomy and has drastically reduced blood loss, postoperative pain, and hospital length of stay. Although robotic prostatectomy has better outcomes with regard to sexual and urinary function than open prostatectomy, most patients will experience some sexual dysfunction and urinary incontinence.

There are several minimally invasive procedures for BPH. Transurethral laser–induced prostatectomy (TULIP) is a type of coagulation necrosis and is done under transrectal ultrasound guidance. Other types of laser surgery (coagulation necrosis) are performed under direct visualization. In laser procedures, the ablated tissue sloughs off in 3 weeks to 3 months. The main advantage of laser surgery is that it is minimally invasive and can be done in the outpatient setting. There is also minimal blood loss, and the occurrence of retrograde ejaculation and erectile dysfunction is reduced. Also, this procedure can be performed in patients who are taking anticoagulants.

Another procedure is transurethral electrovaporization of the prostate. This seems to provide results equivalent to those of laser ablation. In transurethral electrovaporization, a grooved roller-blade electrode administers diathermic energy to the prostate, vaporizing the prostatic tissue. The procedure provides a patient with improved urinary flow through the urethra. This may be the procedure of choice for patients who require anticoagulation because the anticoagulation does not need to be interrupted, further decreasing the risk of procedural complications. Because this is a recent innovation, long-term studies are not yet available.

Transurethral microwave thermotherapy (TUMT) is another procedure that results in the ablation of prostatic tissue. In TUMT, microwave energy is applied to the prostate through a microwave antenna in a urethral catheter; temperature monitoring of the rectum and urethra is essential. Prostate tissue is heated to 55°C, resulting in necrosis of the tissue, causing obstruction. Urethral cooling prevents urethral necrosis and limits postoperative irritative symptoms. One of the adverse effects of TUMT postoperatively is urinary retention, requiring catheterization. Although symptom score and urine flow rates are improved, long-term studies are needed to assess its efficacy.

In transurethral needle ablation (TUNA), two radiofrequency energy waves are administered to prostatic tissue via needle electrodes applied through a cystoscope. Temperatures up to 120°F (48.9°C) destroy the prostatic tissue that had caused the urinary retention or obstruction while preserving the prostatic urethral mucosa.

Another means of thermal tissue ablation is high-intensity focused ultrasound. A rectal probe delivers a short burst of high-intensity focused ultrasound energy that heats the prostate tissue, resulting in coagulative necrosis. Clinical trials are ongoing and demonstrate symptom improvement, but long-term efficacy is not yet known.

Stents have been placed cystoscopically and may be effective in relieving severe urinary obstruction or retention without further surgical intervention. Within 4 to 6 weeks after placement, the stents become covered in urothelium. Stent placement is reserved for patients who are poor surgical risks or who have a limited life expectancy. Stent placement is being used less since the development of minimally invasive procedures such as the TUNA and TULIP.

Transurethral (balloon) dilation of the prostate involves the insertion of a catheter with a balloon at the end through the urethra and into the prostatic urethra. The balloon is then inflated to stretch the urethra at the stricture where it has been narrowed. Although this treatment has been associated with fewer complications, dilation is less effective than other methods. It may provide only a temporary solution, with symptoms recurring within 2 years, and is thus rarely used today.

Selective prostatic artery embolization (PAE) is a promising alternative treatment for those with prostates greater than 80 mL in size who failed medical treatment and are unsuited for surgery. PAE is still considered experimental while studies are ongoing to establish it as a standard of care treatment.

FOLLOW-UP AND REFERRAL

Patient monitoring includes the use of the AUA symptom index, which should be monitored every 1 to 6 months; urodynamic testing, which should be done every 3 to 6 months; and yearly DRE. The American Cancer Society does not recommend routine PSA screening because of overdiagnosis and the severe side effects of inappropriate cancer treatment. If a man makes an informed decision to be screened for prostate cancer, then a PSA blood test may be obtained. If the PSA is less than 2.5 ng/mL, the patient should be retested every 2 years versus yearly if the results are greater than 2.5 ng/mL. Urodynamic studies should be done every 3 to 6 months to evaluate flow rates and voiding pressures. Any patient with BPH who is suspected to have prostatic carcinoma or develops urinary retention should be referred to a urologist.

Patient Education: Benign Prostatic Hypertrophy

It is extremely important to stress to the patient with BPH that taking over-the-counter medications containing alpha-adrenergic agonists or anticholinergic agents can cause acute urinary retention that can result in acute renal failure. These patients may require an indwelling urinary catheter until the acute urinary retention is resolved. The most common offending medications are various cold and flu preparations. Patients should also be advised to avoid bladder irritants such as coffee, spicy foods, and alcohol. Patients should be instructed to void at least every 2 hours to help reduce the possibility of UTI.

PROSTATITIS

Prostatitis is one of several inflammatory and/or painful conditions affecting the prostate gland. Prostatitis accounts for about 25% of all office visits by men, and 50% of men will experience prostatitis in their lifetime. The classification of the type of prostatitis is important for both diagnostic and treatment purposes. Patients may present with acute bacterial prostatitis, chronic bacterial prostatitis, nonbacterial prostatitis, or prostatodynia. Chronic nonbacterial prostatitis is the most common type; it is eight times more frequent than bacterial prostatitis.

In an effort to standardize this classification schema, the National Institutes of Health suggested that nonbacterial prostatitis and prostatodynia be grouped together as chronic prostatitis/chronic pelvic pain syndrome, which may be inflammatory or noninflammatory in nature. In addition, a final category of asymptomatic inflammatory prostatitis is used to denote persons with a significant inflammatory infiltrate in prostatic secretions, but without overt pain or difficulty with urination.

EPIDEMIOLOGY AND CAUSES

Acute prostatitis occurs predominantly in sexually active men aged 30 to 50 years, whereas chronic bacterial prostatitis is more common in patients older than 50 years. Acute bacterial prostatitis is always associated with a UTI and has a characteristically abrupt onset. Chronic bacterial prostatitis is a major cause of recurrent bacteriuria and is associated with a history of recurrent UTI, presumably due to repeated seeding of the urinary tract by an infected prostate. Thus, risk factors for prostatitis include advanced age (older than 50 years), a history of a previously diagnosed UTI, and a history of prostatic calculi.

Nonbacterial prostatitis has findings similar to those associated with chronic bacterial prostatitis, but no evidence of bacterial infection will be present in a urine culture. Prostatodynia presents with signs and symptoms of prostatitis but without evidence of inflammation. Athletes who run long distances—including cross-country runners and athletes who have vigorous exercise regimens—may be predisposed to prostatitis, although the etiology is not well documented at present. Some sources have suggested noninfectious prostatitis may be the most common form of prostatitis, although the lack of a clear etiologic agent in most of these cases makes epidemiologic tracking difficult.

Acute and chronic bacterial prostatitis are both caused by an infection that originates from the ascending urethral flexion or from the reflux of urine into the prostatic ducts. Infection may also spread directly to the prostatic ducts from the rectum. Infection may spread via the lymphatic system or bloodstream, with prostatic calculi serving as a nidus for infection. The most common aerobic gram-negative bacteria involved in prostatitis include *Klebsiella*, *Pseudomonas*, *Enterobacter*, *Escherichia coli*, *Proteus mirabilis*, and *Neisseria gonorrhoeae*. The most common gram-positive bacteria are *Streptococcus faecalis* and *Staphylococcus aureus*. Some organisms suspected as causative agents but as yet unproven are *Staphylococcus epidermidis*, *Micrococcus*, non–group D *Streptococcus*, and diphtheroids. Rarely, fungi and *Mycobacteria tuberculosis* have been implicated in chronic prostatitis. The cause of nonbacterial prostatitis is currently under scrutiny; however, *Ureaplasma*, *Trichomonas vaginalis*, and *Chlamydia trachomatis* may be involved.

PATHOPHYSIOLOGY

The infectious processes resulting in acute or chronic bacterial prostatitis are a result of the organisms mentioned previously. Purulent prostatic discharge may or may not be evident in the absence of prostatic massage. Among patients who fall into the chronic prostatitis/chronic pelvic pain category, prostatic massage will effectively double the number of cases that are considered inflammatory, due to the presence of white blood cells (WBCs) in postmassage urine or seminal fluid.

The pathophysiology of nonbacterial prostatitis is less clear, but it may be related to a voiding dysfunction such as spasm of the bladder neck or urethra. The cause of prostatodynia is unclear, although it may be related to internal urethral sphincter problems or to abnormal tension of the pelvic floor musculature. Prostatodynia may also be related to stress, anxiety, and depression.

CLINICAL PRESENTATION

Subjective

The patient may present complaining of *tenesmus* (a spasmodic contraction of the anal sphincter), with pain and a persistent desire to empty the bowel or bladder, accompanied by involuntary and ineffective straining efforts. "Focus on History: Prostatitis" presents common signs and symptoms of the different types of prostatitis. Obstructive symptoms, including weak urine stream, incomplete bladder emptying, and terminal dribbling, are common in both acute bacterial prostatitis and prostatodynia. Irritative symptoms are present in all of the classifications but are more common in chronic bacterial prostatitis and prostatodynia. In addition, the patient with prostatodynia typically does not have a history of recurrent UTIs.

Objective

The practitioner should assess the patient for the signs and symptoms listed in "Focus on History." The rectal examination should be performed gently with care because vigorous manipulation of the prostate can result in septicemia. In chronic prostatitis, the rectal examination may reveal a tender prostate, but it is usually not swollen or boggy.

Focus on History: Signs and Symptoms of Prostatitis

Acute bacterial prostatitis

- General complaints: fever, chills, low back pain, malaise, arthralgia, myalgia
- Urinary complaints: frequency, urgency, dysuria, nocturia, bladder-outlet obstruction
- Physical examination: warm, tense, boggy, very tender prostate

Chronic bacterial prostatitis

- General complaints: symptoms often absent, perineal pain, low back pain, lower abdominal pain, scrotal pain, penile pain, pain on ejaculation
- Urinary complaints: dysuria, irritative voiding
- Physical examination: normal, boggy, or focally indurated prostate

Nonbacterial prostatitis and prostatodynia

- General complaints: pelvic pain
- Urinary complaints: irritative voiding, abnormal flow
- Physical examination: similar to chronic bacterial prostatitis, tender on palpation

---

DIAGNOSTIC REASONING

Diagnostic Tests

A complete blood count will show leukocytosis and a shift to the left if the patient has acute bacterial prostatitis. In acute prostatitis, a urinalysis will show bacteriuria, pyuria, and possibly hematuria. In chronic prostatitis, it is necessary to culture the expressed prostatic secretions in order to confirm diagnosis. Prostatic massage is controversial and some clinicians feel that vigorous prostatic massage can lead to bacteremia. Referral to a urologist is advised. A urine sample from a patient with nonbacterial prostatitis will show the presence of WBCs, but the urine culture will be negative. There are no abnormal laboratory findings associated with prostatodynia.

If a malignancy or abscess is suspected, computed tomography scanning or transrectal ultrasonography is indicated. A needle biopsy of the mass or aspiration of the abscess for culture may be done by the urologist.

Differential Diagnosis

The differential diagnosis for prostatitis includes cystitis, urethritis, pyelonephritis, epididymitis, prostatic abscess, malignancy, obstructive calculi, foreign bodies, and acute urinary retention. Prostatic abscesses are more common in men who are HIV positive. The manifestations of acute prostatitis can mimic those of acute diverticulitis, but history and laboratory tests usually differentiate between the two conditions. In the case of nonbacterial chronic prostatitis or chronic pelvic pain syndrome, the diagnosis is one of exclusion; other sources of perineal pain (hernias, testicular masses, and hemorrhoids) should be ruled out first. Asymptomatic inflammatory prostatitis is not yet fully understood, and guidelines as to its natural history and need for treatment are not yet established.

MANAGEMENT

The main principle of management for prostatitis is to treat the patient on an outpatient basis if he does not have a fever. However, an extremely ill patient with bacterial prostatitis should be treated in the hospital, as hospitalization may be necessary if the patient is toxic, is immunocompromised, has a proven or suspected abscess, or has signs of urosepsis. It is extremely important that the patient with acute bacterial prostatitis be kept well hydrated, and percutaneous suprapubic catheterization may be required if urinary retention develops because urethral catheterization is contraindicated in patients with acute bacterial prostatitis to avoid trauma to the inflamed prostate and possible seeding of bacteria.

Most men with acute bacterial prostatitis may be treated on an outpatient basis for 5 days with levofloxacin (Levaquin) 750 mg by mouth (PO) daily or ciprofloxacin (Cipro) 750 mg PO every 12 hours. However, given increasing concerns regarding antibiotic resistance and significant adverse effects, such as tendinitis and tendon rupture, the fluoroquinolone antibiotics as a class should only be used when no other treatment options exists, as reflected in their labeling that includes an FDA-mandated black-box warning. Alternatives to fluoroquinolones are trimethoprim/sulfamethoxazole (TMP/SMX [160 mg/800 mg]: Bactrim, Septra, Cotrim) one double-strength (DS) tablet every 12 hours for 10 to 14 days. Treatment may be extended an additional 2 weeks if the patient remains symptomatic after the first course.

For chronic bacterial prostatitis, the best cure rates are associated with treatment with levofloxacin (75% eradication rate), although other antibiotics such as ofloxacin, moxifloxacin, TMP-SMX, azithromycin, and fosfomycin are effective as well. As with acute bacterial prostatitis, however, the fluoroquinolones should only be used if there are no other effective alternative antibiotic choices. The patient with chronic infection is usually treated for 4 to 6 weeks, with an additional 4 to 6 weeks if the first course results in only a partial symptomatic response.

The etiology of nonbacterial prostatitis is uncertain, and treatment may be primarily supportive. The irritative voiding symptoms associated with nonbacterial prostatitis may be treated with NSAIDs, muscle relaxants, anticholinergic agents, warm sitz baths, nontraumatic sexual activity with regular ejaculation, and regular mild exercise. Avoidance of spicy foods, caffeine, and alcohol may help some patients to alleviate the irritative voiding symptoms as well. For patients with severe urinary retention, insertion of a suprapubic catheter may be necessary. Surgical resection for intractable chronic disease or to drain an abscess may also be performed.

The effective use of antibiotic agents has also been reported for nonbacterial prostatitis, although their mechanism of action in noninfectious cases is unclear. Their use is restricted to cases in which expressed prostatic secretions are noted to be inflammatory (10 or more WBCs/high-power field), possibly suggesting the presence of occult infection. These patients may benefit from erythromycin 250 mg four times daily, TMP-SMX DS one tablet daily, or one of these agents in combination with a fluoroquinolone. Other patients with nonbacterial prostatitis have responded to treatment with nitrofurantoin (Furadantin, Furalan, Furanite, Macrodantin, Nitrofan, Nitrofurantoin) 100 mg daily.

FOLLOW-UP AND REFERRAL

Depending on the acute nature of the illness and the patient's response to treatment, referral to a urologist may be warranted. The patient with hematuria or significantly elevated prostate PSA should prompt immediate urological referral. Patient monitoring for acute bacterial prostatitis should include a follow-up urinalysis and culture 30 days after beginning treatment. Chronic bacterial

prostatitis requires urinalysis and culture every 30 days. Monitoring should continue until the patient no longer shows signs of infection. Suppression therapy with prophylactic antibiotics may also been used if recurrent symptomatic infections occur.

Patient Education: Prostatitis

The patient should be told that the prognosis for recovery from prostatitis is good, with a 55% to 97% cure rate. The cure rate depends on the population and the medications used. Prostatitis can, however, be difficult to cure and can persist for a prolonged time. The National Kidney and Urologic Diseases Information Clearinghouse has printed information available for patient education.

PROSTATE CANCER

Timely clinical recognition and treatment of prostate cancer is informed by an understanding of the prostatic anatomy and function as reviewed earlier. The epithelial cells of the prostate gland are the only source of the glycoprotein PSA. Prostatic cancer is known to have a propensity for the gland's posterior and apical peripheral zone (thus accounting for the ability to palpate many cases of prostatic cancer through the rectal wall).

EPIDEMIOLOGY AND CAUSES

Carcinoma of the prostate is the most common cancer found in American men and ranks third in the number of cancer deaths (lung cancer and colorectal cancer ranked first and second). About one in seven men will be diagnosed with prostate cancer during his lifetime. Prostate cancer is rare before age 40 years, and the average age at the time of diagnosis is approximately 66 years with 60% of men diagnosed at that age or older. Most men diagnosed with prostate cancer do not die from it; more than 2.9 million men with prostate cancer are living today. Although approximately 67% of men 80 years of age have prostate cancer, only about 3% are expected to die from it.

The clinical incidence of prostatic carcinoma is highest in North America and Europe and lowest in the Far East, suggesting that there may be genetic, dietary, or environmental factors that increase prostatic growth. Genetic susceptibility foci for prostate cancer have been identified on several chromosomes through genome-wide studies, and consistent with a genetic predisposition, a man with a first-degree relative (i.e., a father or a brother) with prostate cancer is twice as likely to develop the disease and to do so at an earlier age. In the United States, those at highest risk for prostate cancer are African Americans, men with a family history of prostate cancer, and men with a diet high in fat, particularly animal fat. In addition, occupational and environmental risks for the development of prostate cancer include exposure to cadmium nitrates and heavy metals. As an occupational group, farmers are at the highest risk for development of prostate cancer. Smoking has also been identified as an important risk factor for prostate cancer, and the risk appears to be proportional to the number of cigarettes smoked, which may be related to their cadmium content. A patient's endogenous hormonal influences, namely, increased levels of testosterone, have also been shown to increase risk.

PATHOPHYSIOLOGY

Prostate cancer is believed to result from a sequential accumulation of genetic abnormalities affecting the androgen receptors on prostatic tissue. These defects have been characterized as either genetic predispositions to disease that run in families (e.g., deletions in chromosome 1q); somatic mutations that activate prostatic oncogenes such as c-*myc*, *MKP-1*, *bcl-2*, and telomerase (e.g., mutations in the 7p and 8q regions); or somatic mutations that inactivate tumor suppressor genes such as *PTEN/MMAC-1*, *Mxi1*, *GSTP1*, *TGF-1*, and *Rb* (e.g., mutations in the 8p, 10q, 12q, 13q, and 17p regions). Such mutations accumulate over time, thus accounting for the strong correlation between advanced age and disease prevalence.

The degree of malignancy may be graded according to several scales. One method (the Jewett system) uses the following stages:

- A1–A2 and B1–B2 neoplasms are confined within the capsule.
- C1 has extension of the carcinoma beyond the capsule.
- C2 has malignancy that involves the seminal vesicles.
- D1 involves metastatic disease in the regional lymph nodes.
- D2 involves metastatic disease in the bone or other organs.

The left and right posterior lobes of the prostate are most predisposed to malignant transformation. Extensive carcinoma may involve the capsule and the periprostatic tissues. Carcinomas of the prostate usually extend to the base of the bladder and the region of the seminal vesicles to form a shelf or a plateau. Usually, the periprostatic spread is limited by Denonvilliers' fascia, but once this area has been invaded, circumferential extension about the rectum occurs.

The lethality of malignant prostate cancers is a direct function of the heterogeneity in their cellular composition, which consists of both androgen-sensitive and androgen-insensitive cells. Antitestosterone therapies work by suppressing androgen, which itself represses proapoptotic genes in cancer cells that would otherwise lead to cellular death. However, the apoptosis (nonnecrotic or programmed cell death) of androgen-insensitive cancer cells is not induced by antiandrogen therapies. Through progressive genetic mutations, the androgen receptors on cancerous prostatic tissue are increased in number, level of androgen-independent activity, and resistance to apoptotic death signals from tumor suppressor genes. This accounts for the progressive and inevitably increased androgen insensitivity of malignant prostatic tissue and, in turn, the persistent spread of disease.

CLINICAL PRESENTATION

Subjective

Men with prostate cancer are usually asymptomatic early in the disease process and may even be asymptomatic in late stages of disease. Latent symptoms include bone pain, weight loss, anemia, shortness of breath, lymphedema, and lymphadenopathy. Neurologic symptoms (e.g., an inability to perceive touch, pain, and temperature in the perineal or scrotal areas and a lack of sensation of bladder distention) occur with epidural metastasis and cord compression. Patient complaints can also include bladder-outlet symptoms or acute urinary retention with very large or locally extensive tumors, although these symptoms are most often due to BPH.

Objective

Rectal examination reveals a palpable hard prostate that may be localized or diffuse. Several hard areas may be noted or the nodules may be limited to one hardened area. Induration of the prostate may also be noted. Hematuria and hemospermia are signs that appear late in the course of the disease and are only rarely detected in early prostate cancer. Evaluation of contraction of the rectal sphincter in response to the bulbospongiosus (bulbocavernosus, Osinski) reflex in which the glans penis is squeezed should direct attention to a possible lesion at the level of the conus medullaris of the spinal cord.

DIAGNOSTIC REASONING

Diagnostic Tests

PSA is prostate specific but not cancer specific because it is found only in the cytoplasm of both benign and malignant prostatic cells. The effectiveness of using PSA in screening programs for prostate cancer has been questioned because of the lack of evidence that routine screening for PSA can improve the quality and quantity of life for the overall population. The predominant age range for the onset of prostate cancer is 50 to 60 years, which influences the recommendations for screening.

The American Cancer Society (ACS) recommends that men with no symptoms of prostate cancer, who are in relatively good health and can expect to live at least 10 more years, should start screening at age 50 years. ACS recommends that African American men and men who have a father, brother, or son diagnosed with prostate cancer before the age of 65 years begin conversations about initiating prostate cancer screening at age 45 years. Men at higher risk should be screened beginning at age 40 years. The American Urological Association (AUA) recommends the use of PSA-based screening programs in conjunction with DRE to detect prostate cancer in men aged 55 to 69 years who are at average risk and asymptomatic. The AUA guidelines state that PSA screening is not recommended for men younger than 40 years, for men 40 to 54 years who are at average risk, for men 70 years and older, or for men with a life expectancy of less than 10 to 15 years.

Research continues on PSA levels as a means of identifying true prostate cancer, and the goal is to increase the specificity of the test. The strongest evidence of benefit for PSA screening is in men aged 55 to 69 years. In younger, higher-risk men, screening should be individualized based on the uncertainty of benefit and associated harms of screening (e.g., anxiety, false positives, unnecessary biopsies, postsurgical complications). Recent guidelines recommend 2-year PSA testing intervals, and for men older than 60 years with PSA levels below 1.0 ng/mL, PSA screening intervals may be even longer, up to 4 years.

There is no PSA level below which prostate cancer can be definitively ruled out; rather, the risk of prostate cancer increases as the PSA level increases. As mentioned previously, PSA levels may be elevated in individuals with BPH, but with regard to cancer screening, traditionally a PSA level greater than 4.0 ng/mL is considered positive and a level of 4.1 ng/mL has been considered a threshold for performing prostatic biopsy. Serial PSAs are thought to be more accurate than a single test for prostate cancer screening because persistent elevations increase risk. Age-specific PSA norms have also been suggested as a method to increase the accuracy of the PSA test for the diagnosis of prostate cancer. However, the use of age-specific norms as a biopsy decision point is controversial, given that they may potentially delay detection of prostate cancer in some patients.

Most clinical experts agree that considering the complexity of current guidelines for PSA screening and the possible risks of biopsy (e.g., bleeding, infection, nerve damage), individualized informed decision making with the patient's active involvement is the best practice with regard to PSA testing and subsequent interventional diagnostic procedures. The ACS, the AUA, and the American College of Physicians all recommend that health-care providers have an open discussion with patients about the benefits and risks of prostate cancer screening and decide on a mutually agreeable course of action based on the patient's individual risk of developing prostate cancer and the implications of such a diagnosis (i.e., the morbidity and mortality of both prostate cancer and its

surgical or medical treatment). If screening is agreed to, it should begin at age 55 to 69 years for most men and at age 40 years for African American men or those with a family history of prostate cancer, especially in a father or brother. Screening may stop by age 75 years or in those with severe health problems because prostate cancer is unlikely to be the cause of death for the large majority of these patients.

If prostate cancer is suspected (e.g., PSA greater than 10 ng/mL or laboratory-specific threshold), the patient should be referred to a urologist for a TRUS and transrectal biopsy of the prostate. The identification of malignancy using TRUS-guided biopsy is not only a conclusive diagnostic finding; this procedure provides information that is helpful in staging the disease and in planning subsequent treatment, which may include radiation therapy and/or chemotherapy. Prostate screening using a combination of DRE, TRUS, and PSA with age-related values provides the greatest positive predictive value for diagnosing prostate cancer.

Potential complications of the TRUS-guided biopsy include hematospermia, hematuria, fever, hematochezia, or rectal bleeding. Biopsy may be repeated if initial results are negative and cancer is highly suspected. Free PSA levels in the bloodstream have also been tested as a screening tool and criteria for patients to have a follow-up TRUS. Free PSA occurs in greater concentrations in men without prostate cancer. In turn, the ratio of complex (protein-bound) PSA to total PSA is higher in individuals with prostate cancer. Complex PSA is PSA bound to the protease inhibitor alpha-1-antichymotrypsin, which is the form of PSA that is most elevated in prostate cancer. The predicted value of the complex PSA/total PSA ratio in prostate cancer is approximately 25%, based on patients who underwent biopsies after having had a free PSA test.

Prostate-specific antigen density (PSAD) has also been investigated as a screen for prostate cancer. PSAD may help differentiate BPH from prostate cancer, as it is calculated by dividing the PSA value by the volume of the prostate as estimated by TRUS. In addition, molecular diagnostic testing of urine collected postprostatic massage (i.e., with expressed prostatic sections) is also in development to detect highly specific genetic markers of prostate cancer, such as DNA hypermethylation of the genetic promoter for the tumor suppressor gene glutathione *S*-transferase (*GSTP1*), which downregulates its transcriptional activity and thereby reduces its protective anticancer effects.

Diagnostic testing may also be used to detect complications of more advanced disease, such as metastases. Serum alkaline phosphatase is typically elevated in patients with metastases (due to bone invasion), but this finding is not specific for cancer of the prostate. Additional studies done in patients with prostate cancer to detect metastases may include a bone scan, computed tomography of the pelvic lymph nodes, lymphoscintigraphy, and magnetic resonance imaging.

Differential Diagnosis

BPH is the first differential diagnosis the clinician must consider in an individual with suspected prostate cancer because the urinary outlet symptoms of nocturia, frequency, hesitancy, and weak urinary stream can be seen in both conditions but are far more commonly due to BPH. New-onset erectile dysfunction, hematuria, and hematospermia are less common presentations of prostate cancer. Other differential diagnoses for prostate cancer include a benign nodule, prostate stones, nodular whorls, and seminal vesicle enlargement.

MANAGEMENT

Neither chemotherapy nor immunotherapy can definitively cure prostate cancer once it has spread beyond the gland, although duration and quality of life may be preserved, depending on the individual patient's circumstance. Thus, if findings are positive on both DRE and PSA, the patient should be referred to a urologist for a definitive diagnosis (biopsy) and staging.

Staging

Prostate tumors are classified according to the Gleason system in which an initial grade (score) is applied to the architectural pattern of the cancer in the largest segment of the specimen and then a second grade is given to the next largest area. The pathologist adds the two scores together to produce the Gleason score, which is on a scale from 1 to 10. Accurate staging provides an indication of the best treatment options.

- Gleason score 1 to 4: indicates a well-differentiated cancer that is likely to be slow growing
- Gleason score 5 to 7: indicates a moderately differentiated cancer
- Gleason score 8 to 10: indicates a poorly differentiated cancer that is likely to be aggressive and rapidly growing

Prostate cancer is further staged according to the extent of the tumor, based on additional diagnostic studies or findings at the time of surgery. The most commonly used staging system is the American Joint Committee on Cancer tumor-node-metastasis system, which grades tumors numerically within more detailed subcategories: "T" describes *tumors* according to their degree of differentiation; "N" describes the extent of *nodal* involvement; and "M" describes the degree of *metastasis*. For example, T1 tumors are microscopic, nonpalpable, and not visible by TRUS. Tumors classified as T2 are palpable but not beyond the prostate itself, and T3 tumors extend beyond the capsule or into the seminal vesicles. T4 tumors are fixed and extend far beyond the prostate. Prostate cancer extending beyond the prostate itself is often fatal, and treatment is typically only palliative; however, localized disease is often curable by surgery, radiation therapy, and/or chemotherapy.

Patients Older Than 70 Years

Patients older than 70 years are usually offered conservative treatment as an alternative to surgery. Radiation external beam therapy or brachytherapy with implants and total androgen ablation are the general measures used to treat prostate cancer in older men.

Patients Younger Than 70 Years

If the patient is younger than 70 years, surgery is often recommended for a prostate cancer cure. Surgical interventions may be used for Jewett stages A and B and selected C stages. If the patient agrees, an orchiectomy may be warranted to ablate endogenous hormonal effects.

The standard treatment options for prostate cancer include radical prostatectomy, radiation therapy, and watchful waiting. Treatment decisions are based more often on the adverse effects, long-term risks, and financial and emotional costs of different therapies, depending on the individual patient. Younger, otherwise healthy patients are often encouraged to undergo the most radical treatment, whereas older patients are often directed to watchful waiting (observation) or radiotherapy.

Currently, surgery is usually performed with robotic assistance. In this technique, a few small incisions are made to access the prostate, rather than the typical large abdominal incision, and numerous ports are made for the insertion of a magnified, three-dimensional, high-definition vision apparatus. Mechanical wristed instruments allow the surgeon to operate with enhanced vision, precision, dexterity, and control. The benefit of this surgical approach is more precise removal of the prostate that leads to less nerve injury, thereby preserving sexual function and decreasing the risk of postsurgical urinary incontinence. In addition, there is less blood loss during surgery and fewer postoperative complications; however, surgical time may be longer.

Other treatments for prostate cancer include hormonal therapy to inhibit cancer growth by testosterone deprivation or administration of endogenous estrogen to block the release of luteinizing hormone from the hypothalamus. Adverse effects of estrogen therapy include hypercoagulopathy, cardiomegaly, and gynecomastia. Alternative hormonal preparations include leuprolide (Lupron), goserelin acetate (Zoladex), triptorelin (Trelstar), and histrelin (Vantas), which block the release of follicle-stimulating hormone and luteinizing hormone. Luteinizing hormone–releasing hormone antagonists such as degarelix (Firmagon) reduce testosterone levels more quickly and are used to treat advanced prostate cancer. These agents are typically administered monthly. Adverse effects include loss of libido, erectile dysfunction, gynecomastia, hot flashes, and anemia (rarely).

Oral antiandrogens are also available, including bicalutamide (Casodex), flutamide (Eulexin), and nilutamide (Nilandron), which inhibit the binding of testosterone to cancer cells. Finasteride (Proscar) is used to block the enzyme 5-alpha-reductase, which converts testosterone into DHT. Other antiandrogen treatments include enzalutamide (Xtandi), which blocks signaling from the androgen receptor to the prostate cancer cell, and abiraterone (Zytiga), which blocks the CYP17A1 enzyme in the testosterone synthetic pathway and, in turn, reduces androgen production.

Cryosurgical ablation of the prostate is used to destroy cancer cells through freezing in patients who have had negative bone scans for metastatic prostate cancer. The major adverse effects of this ablation technique include possible destruction of nerves and/or circulation, which can cause urinary incontinence and erectile dysfunction.

Importantly, aggressive surgical interventions, radiation therapy, and chemotherapeutic or hormonal treatments may not be appropriate options in patients for whom the morbidity and mortality risk of the cancer itself are outweighed by the potential adverse effects of therapy (e.g., elderly men for whom prostate cancer is unlikely to be their cause of death). Thus, some research has been directed toward the strategy of watchful waiting (i.e., observation and monitoring for progressive complications of disease in the absence of immediate intervention).

FOLLOW-UP AND REFERRAL

Patient follow-up is determined by the urologist or radiation oncologist, depending on the type of treatment utilized. Without fail, the patient should have a clinical examination every 3 months for the first year. Chest x-ray studies and bone scans should be done every 6 months for a year and then yearly thereafter. Potential complications of treatment may include cardiac failure, phlebitis, and pathological fractures secondary to the hormonal changes (testosterone suppression), as well as those mentioned in the Management section. With early diagnosis and treatment, the expected prognosis is good, and lesions should be curable, especially in young, otherwise healthy men.

Once prostate cancer has been diagnosed and the treatment regimen has been implemented, the patient should be followed by the specialist and also seen by the primary-care practitioner regularly for health maintenance, emotional reassurance, reinforcement of a positive outlook, and follow-up laboratory testing.

Patient Education: Prostate Cancer

Support groups and other advocacy organizations for prostate cancer patients are available, along with books on the subject, including reports and personal testimonies from prostate cancer survivors. Churches are also being used as a forum for patient education, particularly those with older congregations. Given the widespread impact of prostate cancer, it is important for the clinician to be knowledgeable regarding the latest diagnostic and treatment options, as well as to remain attuned to patients' desires and fears regarding this diagnosis.

REFERENCES

General

Ulbricht C. *Davis's pocket guide to herbs and supplements.* Philadelphia, PA: F.A. Davis; 2011.

Benign Prostatic Hypertrophy

American Urological Association. Clinical guidelines: Management of BPH. http://www.auanet.org/benign-prostatic-hyperplasia-(2010-reviewed-and-validity-confirmed-2014). Published 2010.

Barry MD, Fowler FJ, O'Leary MP, Bruskewitz RC, Holtgrewe HL, Mebust WK. American Urological Association symptom index for benign prostatic hyperplasia. *J Urol.* 1992;148:1549–1557.

Parsons JK, et al. Obesity and benign prostatic hyperplasia: Clinical connections, emerging etiological paradigms and future directions. *J Urol.* 2013;189(1):S102–S106.

Suskind AM, Walter LC, Zhao S, Finlayson E. Functional outcomes after transurethral resection of the prostate in nursing home residents. *J Am Geriatr Soc.* 2017;65(4):699–703.

Wang MQ, Guo LP, Zhang GD, et al. Prostatic arterial embolization for the treatment of lower urinary tract symptoms due to large (>80 mL) benign prostatic hyperplasia: Results of midterm follow-up from Chinese population. *BMC Urol.* 2015;15(33).

Wang XY, Zong HT, Zhang Y. Efficacy and safety of prostate artery embolization on lower urinary tract symptoms related to benign prostatic hyperplasia: A systematic review and meta-analysis. *Clin Interv Aging,* 2016;11:1600–1622.

Prostate Cancer

American Cancer Society. Key statistics for prostate cancer. https://www.cancer.org/cancer/prostate-cancer/about/key-statistics.html. Published 2017. Accessed August 17, 2017.

American Urological Association. PSA testing for the pretreatment staging and posttreatment management of prostate cancer. http://www.auanet.org/guidelines/prostate-specific-antigen-(2009-amended-2013). Published 2009.

Jemal A, Fedewa SA, Ma J. (2015). Prostate cancer incidence and PAS testing patterns in relation to USPSTF screening recommendations. *JAMA,* 314(19):2054–2061.

Ladjevardi S, Berglund A, Varenhorst E, Bratt O, Widmark A, Sandblom G. Treatment with curative intent and survival in men with high-risk prostate cancer. A population-based study of 11,380 men with serum PSA level 20-100 ng/mL. *BJU Int.* 2013;111(3):381–388.

National Comprehensive Cancer Network. NCCN clinical guidelines in oncology: Prostate cancer. http://www.nccn.org/professionals/physician_gls/f_guidelines.asp.

Parsons JK, Sarma AV, McVary K, Wei JT. American Urological Association. Early detection of prostate cancer. https://www.auanet.org/guidelines/prostate-cancer-early-detection-(2013-reviewed-for-currency-2018). Published 2013.

Prostatitis

Kraemer SD, Shetty S. Chronic bacterial prostatitis treatment and management. Medscape. http://emedicine.medscape.com/article/458391-treatment#d9. Published July 2, 2017.

Nickel CJ. Inflammatory and pain conditions of the male genitourinary tract: Prostatitis and related pain conditions, orchitis, and epididymitis. In: McDougal WS, Wein AJ, Kavoussi LR, et al, eds. *Campbell-Walsh urolog*. 11th ed. Philadelphia, PA: Elsevier; 2016.

Polackwich AS, Soskes DA. (2016). Chronic prostatitis/chronic pelvic pain syndrome: a review of evaluation and therapy. *Prostate Cancer and Prostatic Diseases*, 19:132–138.

RESOURCES

National Cancer Institute
    https://www.cancer.gov/types/prostate
Prostate Cancer Foundation
    https://www.pcf.org/
Prostate Diseases
    https://medlineplus.gov/prostatediseases.html

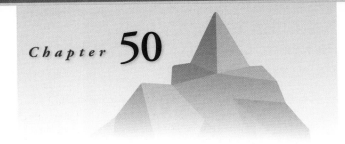

Chapter **50**

Penile and Testicular Disorders

Debera J. Thomas, DNS, RN, FNP/ANP

Debbie Nogueras Conner, PhD, ANP/FNP-BC, FAANP

Brian Oscar Porter, MD, PhD, MPH, MBA

ERECTILE DYSFUNCTION

Erectile dysfunction (ED) is the inability to achieve or maintain an erection that is sufficient for satisfactory sexual performance. ED can also manifest as a lack of sexual desire or an inability to ejaculate. ED can result from many causes, including physiological, psychological, endocrinological, vascular, and neurologic etiologies.

EPIDEMIOLOGY AND CAUSES

Fifty percent of men older than 40 years have some degree of ED. ED is classified as mild if the patient fails to achieve a satisfactory erection in 2 out of 10 attempts. If all attempts at satisfactory erection fail, ED is classed as severe, while moderate ED falls somewhere between mild and severe. It is difficult to estimate the number of men with ED because the definition is broad and some men may be reluctant to seek medical attention for the problem. Transient and limited episodes of impotence occur in about half of all adult men at some point in their lives and are not pathological. Aging affects sexual functioning, and more than 25% of men older than 65 years have ED. Most cases of ED have an identifiable physical as opposed to psychogenic cause.

Although the focus of this section is on the physiological causes of ED, it is critical for the primary-care practitioner to assess both physical and mental health aspects in the patient with ED and make appropriate specialist referrals if needed. In some cases, ED may result from a combination of both physical and psychological or emotional (psychogenic) causes because such etiologies are not mutually exclusive. In turn, it is critical to determine whether the patient with ED still experiences sexual arousal, despite the inability to achieve or maintain an erection.

Several categories of ED should be considered when determining the cause of the problem. A failure to generate the nerve impulse required to initiate an erection may be caused by a number of endocrinological or neurologic conditions, or it can be psychogenic in origin. ED can also be the result of a failure to adequately fill penile blood vessels, most often arteriogenic in origin. Another category is the failure to retain blood in the penis, which is usually veno-occlusive in origin.

A loss of libido may indicate androgen deficiency arising from either pituitary or testicular disease, resulting in a failure to initiate the nerve impulse needed to initiate an erection. Plasma levels of testosterone and gonadotropins are measured to rule out this possibility. Endocrine factors are unlikely if the patient has a normal semen volume. Some of the physical, nonpsychogenic causes of ED are listed in Box 50.1.

The Iceberg of Erectile Dysfunction

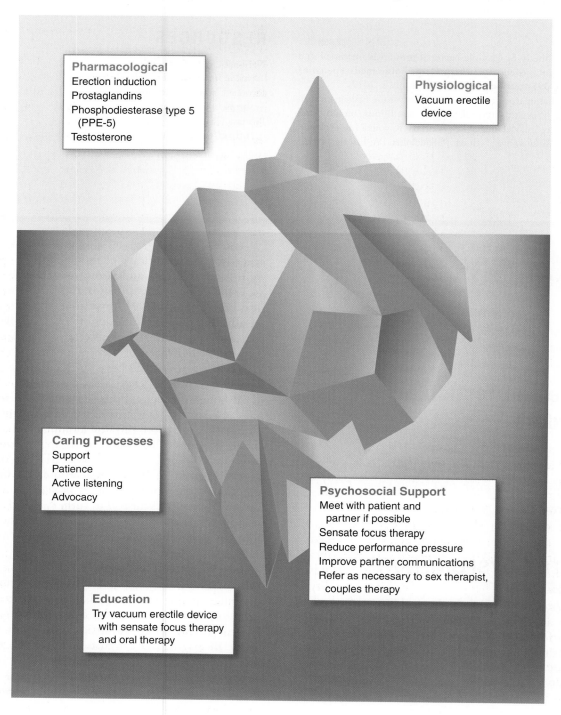

Pharmacological
Erection induction
Prostaglandins
Phosphodiesterase type 5
   (PPE-5)
Testosterone

Physiological
Vacuum erectile
device

Caring Processes
Support
Patience
Active listening
Advocacy

Psychosocial Support
Meet with patient and
   partner if possible
Sensate focus therapy
Reduce performance pressure
Improve partner communications
Refer as necessary to sex therapist,
   couples therapy

Education
Try vacuum erectile device
   with sensate focus therapy
   and oral therapy

Medications are a common cause of ED, either directly or by adverse effects. Loss of erection can be caused by central sympatholytic agents such as methyldopa, clonidine, and reserpine, whereas alpha blockers cause few problems with erection. However, beta-adrenergic blocking agents and spironolactone can cause a loss of libido. Certain drugs, such as calcium channel blockers, can increase prolactin secretion and thereby cause ED. Some drugs of addiction can decrease testosterone levels and lead to ED. In addition, zinc deficiency seen in malabsorption or malnourishment syndromes may also cause ED.

Box 50.1 Nonpsychogenic Causes of Erectile Dysfunction

Neurologic Diseases

- Anterior temporal lobe lesions
- Disease of the spinal cord
- Loss of sensory input (secondary to diabetes mellitus, polyneuropathies), tabes dorsales (disease of dorsal root ganglia)
- Disease of nervi erigentes (secondary to complete prostatectomy, retrosigmoid operations, aortic bypass)

Vascular Disease

- Leriche syndrome

Endocrine Disorders

- Testicular failure (primary or secondary)
- Hyperprolactinemia

Penile Disorders

- Failure of detumescence
- Priapism
- Penile trauma
- Peyronie's disease

Medications

- Phenothiazines
- Thioridazine
- Imipramine
- Methyldopa
- Guanethidine
- Reserpine
- Spironolactone
- Alcohol
- Heroin
- Methadone
- Estrogen
- Beta blockers
- Thiazide diuretics
- Antihypertensives

PATHOPHYSIOLOGY

To understand ED, knowledge of normal erectile physiology is necessary. Normal sexual function in men has five phases: libido, erection, ejaculation, orgasm, and detumescence. For an erection to occur, there must be an intact autonomic and somatic nerve supply to the penis and the pudendal arteries. Erection begins with neurologic and vascular stimulation and is maintained by increased arterial blood flow, increased venous resistance, and relaxation of the smooth muscle of the sinusoids in the corporal bodies of the penis. Additional rigidity of the penis is accomplished by contraction of the bulbospongiosus and ischiocavernosus muscles. The process is initiated by neurotransmitters, vasoactive intestinal peptide, acetylcholine, prostaglandins, and possibly nitric oxide, although the exact mechanism is unknown.

In addition to the increase in arterial blood flow, efflux of blood is reduced. As erectile tissue expands, the peripheral veins are compressed against the enveloping tunica albuginea, which effectively impedes drainage of blood from the cavernous sinuses. The less turgid corpus spongiosum allows the urethra to dilate during ejaculation.

With continued sexual stimulation, the urethral meatus dilates and sperm move to the ejaculatory duct. Seminal fluid is added to the sperm cells by the seminal vesicles and prostate gland. At the time of vaginal penetration, the male secretions produced by the bulbourethral glands and the glands of the penile urethra combine with female cervical secretions. The bulbourethral fluid serves to neutralize the acidity of any urine residue in the urethra and helps to neutralize the acidity of the vagina. In addition, this fluid provides some lubrication for the tip of the penis, thereby promoting the survival of sperm. The sperm cells move by emission into the prostatic urethra, where they become activated by seminal fluid and are motile. In the male, orgasm is concomitant with ejaculation, which is brought about by sympathetic activity transmitted along the hypogastric nerve and lateral pelvic plexus, and then through the prostatic and cavernous plexuses. Ejaculation is the strong rhythmic contraction of the vas deferens, seminal vesicles, epididymis, prostate, urethra, and penis. Retrograde ejaculation is prevented by partial bladder neck closure, mediated by sympathetic nerves. Orgasm is a sensory phenomenon in which rhythmic muscular contractions are perceived as pleasurable.

Postcoital resolution, or detumescence, results from sympathetic outflow to the genital area. The periarterial muscle increases its tone, thereby reducing the blood flow to the erectile tissues of the penis. A refractory period of variable duration follows, during which time another erection cannot occur.

An understanding of vascular disease as a cause of ED is essential, as continual high blood flow into the vascular system of the penis is necessary to maintain an erect state. Atherosclerosis can cause a failure of the vascular system to fill; therefore, risk factors for this type of ED include heart disease, cigarette smoking, diabetes mellitus, aging, dyslipidemia, and hypertension. Trauma can also damage the pudendal and cavernous arteries from, for example, prolonged bicycling, and thereby cause a failure to fill. Leriche's syndrome, with impedance of blood flow into the penis, occurs as the result of obstruction of the distal aorta at the bifurcation of the common iliac arteries. Presenting symptoms of this syndrome are claudication and ED, either separately or in combination.

Because resistance to the efflux of blood from the penis is necessary to maintain an erection, anything that impairs this ability is considered a failure-to-store defect. It can result from insufficient relaxation or fibrosis of the corporeal smooth muscle. Adrenergic agonists and/or psychological stress can cause insufficient relaxation of the corporeal smooth muscle, whereas atherosclerosis and penile trauma can result in fibrosis. *Priapism*, persistent painful erection, is usually idiopathic but can be associated with sickle cell anemia, chronic granulocytic leukemia, or spinal cord injury. The persistent erection disrupts this vascular network and can lead to fibrosis and subsequent failure to store.

In addition to the inability to achieve or maintain an erection, ED may also involve abnormal functioning of several other sexual processes. Premature ejaculation seldom has an organic cause. It is usually related to anxiety about the sexual situation, performance-related fears, or an emotional disorder. Psychological disorders such as depression, bipolar disorder, anxiety disorders, and relationship dysfunction may all cause ED.

The absence of emission may be caused by three organic disorders: retrograde ejaculation, sympathetic denervation, or androgen deficiency. Retrograde ejaculation may occur after surgery on the bladder neck, or it may develop spontaneously in a male patient with diabetes. A postcoital urine sample can be analyzed to confirm the diagnosis. Smooth muscle contractions may not occur at the time of ejaculation as a result of the loss of autonomic innervation of the prostate and seminal vesicles after sympathectomy. An androgen deficiency may lead to an absence of secretions from the prostate and seminal vesicles. If libido and erectile function are normal, the absence of orgasm is almost always due to a psychiatric disorder.

Various penile diseases and anatomical abnormalities may also cause ED. Structural causes of ED include micropenis, Peyronie's disease, scarring of the corpora cavernosa, phimosis, hypospadias, and postsurgical sequelae. Peyronie's disease results from localized fibrotic thickening of the tissue around the corpora cavernosa. Plaque may be palpated along the penile shaft, usually on the dorsum, but plaque is sometimes present on any part of the corpora cavernosa. Inelasticity produces a curvature of the penile shaft on erection that may be very painful. There is a high correlation between Peyronie's disease and Dupuytren's contracture of the palmar fascia.

CLINICAL PRESENTATION

Subjective

Because male sexual dysfunction can manifest in many ways and because the causes are numerous, a careful history is essential for the correct diagnosis of ED and subsequent treatment. Impotence is a very personal complaint, and discussion requires a trusting relationship between patient and clinician and sufficient time during the visit for the patient to voice his concerns. He may complain of a loss of sexual desire, an inability to obtain or maintain an erection, premature ejaculation, an absence of emission, or an inability to achieve orgasm. Frequently, the patient has a combination of these symptoms. It is essential to determine whether the patient has normal erections, particularly during sleep or early in the morning. If an erection does occur, an organic cause is most likely not the cause of the ED. In 25% of cases, medication use may be the cause of ED. The use of alcohol, tobacco, and recreational drugs increases the risk of sexual dysfunction.

A physical examination, including a thorough genital examination to rule out any abnormalities of the penis itself, is critical. The testes should be palpated for size or abnormal masses. If their length is less than 4 cm, hypogonadism should be considered. Evidence of feminization such as gynecomastia and abnormal body hair distribution should be assessed. All pulses should be palpated, including the penile pulse, which can be felt by pressing both corpora between the thumb and forefinger and palpating

to either side of the midline. If there is an indication of a vascular etiology from either the patient's history or physical examination, an aortogram may be indicated.

A neurologic examination to evaluate the erectile reflex, including anal sphincter tone, perineal sensation, and the bulbospongiosus reflex, should be part of the physical examination. The reflex can be evaluated by squeezing the glans penis and noting the degree of anal sphincter constriction. An examination for signs of peripheral neuropathy, including distal muscle weakness and loss of tendon reflexes in the legs, is important, along with tests that will reveal any impairment of vibratory, position, tactile, or pain sensation.

DIAGNOSTIC REASONING

Diagnostic Tests

Initially, laboratory tests that rule out the various causes of ED should be done. These tests include a fasting blood sugar to rule out diabetes mellitus, a lipid profile to rule out dyslipidemia, thyroid-stimulating hormone (TSH), and a testosterone level. If the testosterone level is below 300 ng/dL, a serum prolactin level is warranted. Laboratory tests for patients with established ED should include a complete blood count, a blood chemistry profile (including fasting glucose or glycosylated hemoglobin levels), a TSH level, and prostate-specific antigen (PSA) in men as young as 40 years if they have a family history of prostate cancer. Most men older than 55 years will have some abnormal laboratory findings or risk factors, but these may not necessarily be the cause of the ED.

Several specialized tests can be done but usually only if the cause of the ED is not apparent following the standard testing regimen. The most useful of these additional tests are the nocturnal penile tumescence and rigidity (NPTR) test and color Doppler sonography of the penis. NPTR testing is useful to assess the patient's physical ability to achieve an erection. Sensors are placed at the base and tip of the penis and record the circumference and rigidity of the penis during sleep. Typically, the test is done from one to three nights. Men usually have erections during rapid eye movement sleep. A physiological cause of ED is indicated if there is an absence or impairment of erections during sleep. This test is self-administered in the patient's home; however, it can be used in the clinical setting to determine erectile response to sexual stimuli.

There are, however, two medical conditions that cause ED in sexual situations yet still allow normal erectile activity during NPTR. The first is disruption of the afferent nerves that amplify the erectile response to external sexual stimuli but are bypassed in nocturnal erectile activity. The second is called *pelvic steal syndrome*, which may occur in physiological states when the patient is awake, but not when he is asleep. This condition involves partial blockage of the iliac vessels and causes all erections to occur when the patient is at rest. Loss of erection ensues, however, with gluteal muscle activity during thrusting.

Color Doppler sonography is used to assess vascular causes of ED. It measures the integrity of arterial influx in the cavernous artery during erection by measuring the peak systolic blood flow velocity in this artery.

Differential Diagnosis

Differential diagnosis of ED requires consideration of fibrosis secondary to trauma, severe urethritis, late-stage syphilitic lesions, penile infiltration with lymphogranuloma venereum, benign and malignant tumors, and congenital penile curvature. Urethral strictures produce an indurated area that may be identified by careful palpation along the penile urethra. A stricture can be identified more easily by the passage of a small urethral probe or catheter (urethral sound). Occasionally, strictures may be recognized by the presence of an indolent, firm, tender mass that may involve the skin over the penile shaft. Restricted erection may cause ventral curvature of the penis, periurethral inflammation, and, in severe cases, purulent urethrocutaneous fistula.

MANAGEMENT

A number of options are available for the treatment of ED. If an organic cause cannot be found, these men will most likely benefit from behaviorally based sex therapy. Pharmacologic treatments including hormone therapy are presented in Drugs Commonly Prescribed 50.1. Nonpharmacologic interventions including vacuum constriction devices, vasoactive therapy, penile prostheses, and penile revascularization are discussed in the sections that follow.

Hormone Therapy

For men with documented testosterone deficiency who do not have prostate cancer or benign prostatic hypertrophy (BPH), breast cancer, or cardiovascular disease, testosterone therapy is the treatment of choice. However, testosterone therapy should not be used in men with high blood pressure, clotting disorders, and may increase the severity of sleep apnea. Testosterone therapy can be accomplished

Drugs Commonly Prescribed 50.1: Erectile Dysfunction

DRUG	ADVERSE REACTIONS	PRESCRIBING CONSIDERATIONS
Hormone Therapy		
Parenteral agents: Testosterone cypionate (Depo-Testosterone) Testosterone enanthate (Delatestryl)	Sodium retention with dependent edema, increased risk of bleeding, pain at injection site, mild gynecomastia, mood swings, lipid abnormalities	Do not use in patients with serious liver, kidney, or cardiac disease, prostate or breast cancer, or in those with mercury allergy. Peak and trough effects may lead to aggression, feelings of well-being, energy, and increased libido within 72 hours of injection. As peak level falls, patient may experience depressed mood and loss of libido.
Oral agents: Fluoxymesterone (Halotestin) Methyltestosterone (Android, Methitest, Testred, Virilon)	Same as for parenteral agents Not used as much as transdermal or parenteral formulations because of difficulty in achieving adequate blood levels due to high first-pass metabolism in the liver	Oral agents are not generally recommended because of hepatotoxicity and unreliable androgenic effects.
Transdermal testosterone patch (Androderm, Testoderm)	Local irritation; burn-like blistering or irritation of skin where transdermal patch is applied	NOT to be applied to the scrotum. Should be applied to the arm, back, abdomen, or thigh. May cause local irritation.
Transdermal testosterone topical gel or solution (AndroGel 1%, 2.5–5 g packets) (Testim 1% Gel, 5–10 g packets) (Axiron solution, 60–120 mg)	Burn-like blistering or irritation of skin where gel is applied Problems with urination	Apply to the axilla, upper arm, or shoulder, but NOT the scrotum. May transfer to partner during intimate skin-to-skin contact.
Testosterone implantable pellets (Testopel, 150–450 mg)	Infection at implantation site and pellet extrusion	Produces steady blood levels; must be implanted in subcutaneous tissue every 3–4 months Less flexibility in dose adjustment
Testosterone buccal system (Striant, 30 mg)	Mouth or gum irritation Allergic reactions Swelling of ankles or legs Breathing disturbances, including those associated with sleep Liver damage	Insertion twice daily in the morning and evening provides continuous systemic delivery of testosterone

Continued

Drugs Commonly Prescribed 50.1: Erectile Dysfunction—cont'd

DRUG	ADVERSE REACTIONS	PRESCRIBING CONSIDERATIONS
Vasoactive Therapy		
Oral agents: Sildenafil (Viagra) Vardenafil (Levitra) Tadalafil (Cialis) Avanafil (Stendra)	Headache, flushing, dyspepsia, nasal congestion, and visual color changes Back and lower limb pain for all PDE$_5$ inhibitors	None of these agents should be used in patients taking nitrates or alpha blockers. Must wait 24 hours before giving nitrate medication after sildenafil or vardenafil and 48 hours for tadalafil.
Injectables: Alprostadil (Caverject, Edex)	Penile pain, prolonged erection, penile fibrosis, injection site hematoma, numbness, yeast infection, and priapism May also cause upper respiratory infection, headache, dizziness, and hypotension	Taking along with anticoagulants or heparin may increase risk of bleeding. Should not be used in patients with sickle cell anemia, penile fibrosis, coagulopathy, severe cardiovascular disease, myeloma, leukemia, penile deformity, morbid obesity, or penile implants. Can be used only once every 24 hours and a maximum of three times a week. Patient should be instructed to choose injection site along side of proximal one-third of penis, alternate injection sites, and avoid visible veins.
Transurethral suppositories: Alprostadil (Muse)	May cause urethral irritation	As above. Should not be used if partner is pregnant unless a condom is used. Suppository is inserted in penis to approximately 1 inch, after the patient urinates. Button on top of applicator is pushed to release suppository; gentle rocking motion will separate suppository from applicator. After applicator is removed, patient should massage penis firmly for approximately 10 seconds while standing. Erection will begin in 5–10 minutes.

by several delivery methods that include injections, oral medication, topical patches, or topical gels.

Vacuum Constriction Devices

Most vacuum devices work in similar ways, using a process that takes about 2 minutes. The patient inserts his penis into the cylinder, then uses the pump to create a partial vacuum. This causes venous blood to enter the corpora cavernosa, initiating tumescence and rigidity. Once a sufficient erection is achieved, a latex constriction ring is placed around the base of the penis to help maintain the erection. This is a noninvasive procedure and complications are rare. Vacuum constriction devices are now available over the counter and cost between $300 and $500.

Vasoactive Therapy

The development of drugs that decrease the breakdown of 5-cyclic guanosine monophosphate (cGMP) has revolutionized ED treatment. cGMP is the intracellular second messenger of nitric oxide, which is the primary vasodilator and neurotransmitter involved in the erectile response. The first of these drugs was sildenafil citrate (Viagra). Sildenafil is an orally active cGMP-specific phosphodiesterase inhibitor. It results in increased blood flow necessary for successful penile erection. The standard dose is sildenafil 50 mg taken orally at least 1 hour before sexual activity. Contraindications that can cause severe hypotensive effects with sildenafil are listed in Drugs Commonly Prescribed 50.1. Other medications in this class include vardenafil (Levitra), avanafil (Stendra), and tadalafil (Cialis). Phosphodiesterase-5 (PDE$_5$) inhibitors do not affect libido and do not initiate an erection without sexual stimulation.

Vasoactive prostaglandins have been shown to be an effective treatment for ED. Alprostadil (Caverject) 5 to 40 mcg is injected directly into the base and lateral aspect of the penis using a tuberculin syringe. Erection occurs within 20 minutes and lasts for approximately 30 to 60 minutes. Prolonged erection (priapism) occurs rarely, but the patient should be instructed to seek medical attention if this does occur. Alprostadil is also available in a transurethral suppository in dosages of 125, 250, 500, or 1,000 mcg. Suppositories produce an erection in about 5 to 10 minutes (see Drugs Commonly Prescribed 50.1 for instructions for use).

Penile Prostheses

Several prosthetic devices that can be surgically implanted into the penis are available in a variety of sizes and diameters. They are placed directly in the corporal bodies. Penile prostheses may be rigid, semifirm, hinged, or inflatable. The inflatable devices are more natural appearing; however, there is more opportunity for mechanical failure. Implantation of a prosthesis, which is a highly reliable but invasive form of therapy, may help men who have failed therapy with other methods. It is very expensive and not without the risks that accompany surgery. Implantation may be covered by some insurance plans. Most patients desiring implants prefer spontaneity and therefore choose this invasive treatment. Significant problems associated with implants are infection, erosion, and occasional mechanical failure (in less than 5% of patients). The most common types of implants are nonhydraulic (using semirigid rods) and hydraulic (using inflatables). Both types of implants involve surgical placement of two cylinders inside the corpus cavernosum. Healing takes 4 to 6 weeks, after which the patient may have intercourse.

Penile Revascularization

The experience with penile revascularization is limited, and some patients fail to have a sufficient erection even after the procedure. Patients with arterial disorders may be candidates for the various procedures, which include endarterectomy and balloon dilation, or arterial bypass. For patients with venous disorders, ligation of the deep dorsal vein or emissary vein or ligation of the crura of the corpora cavernosus may be effective.

In younger men, several conditions may warrant penile revascularization surgery. Men younger than 45 years whose impotence is caused by severe pelvic trauma are the best candidates for this surgery. In patients with impotence of sudden onset, the possibility that trauma to the peritoneum or pelvis may have led to vascular injury should be considered. A congenital shunt should be ruled out in any patient who reports that he has never had a full erection.

Low-Intensity Shock Wave Therapy

Low-intensity shock wave therapy (LIST) has met with success in Europe in patients with severe ED who are unresponsive to treatment with PDE$_5$ inhibitors such as sildenafil (Viagra), tadalafil (Cialis), and vardenafil (Levitra). It is not yet approved in the United States, but research is ongoing. It is believed that LIST promotes the release of angiogenic factors that lead to revascularization of the penis.

FOLLOW-UP AND REFERRAL

Hormonal therapy should be guided by a clinician experienced in the evaluation and monitoring of patients on hormonal therapy. For example, patients on testosterone therapy should undergo monitoring prostate examinations and PSA screening tests, given the theoretical risks of BPH and prostate cancer associated with testosterone exposure. Blood levels of the hormone being supplemented (e.g., serum testosterone) and other regulatory hormones along the hypothalamic-pituitary-gonadal axis (e.g., luteinizing hormone, which stimulates testosterone secretion) should also be followed to prevent the sequelae of medication overexposure. However, interpretation of these levels requires expert knowledge of reproductive endocrinology and is influenced by the timing of both the hormonal treatments and the monitoring blood draws.

Common psychogenic causes of ED include performance anxiety and relationship problems. Thus, referrals to sex therapy and/or marriage and couples counseling may be particularly helpful for some patients, especially in combination with other therapies. In addition, all of the invasive surgical interventions already described require appropriate referrals to a qualified urologist or pelvic surgeon.

Patient Education: Erectile Dysfunction

The primary role of the provider in educating the patient with ED is to stress the importance of management of chronic conditions such as hypertension, diabetes mellitus, and stress. Guided imagery, regular exercise, and yoga may be recommended as modalities to reduce stress. Tight control of blood pressure and blood sugar should be encouraged as a way to limit further deterioration of erectile function. In addition, counseling for the psychogenic causes of ED is essential.

Instructions regarding topical hormone formulations should include warnings regarding the possibility of transfer to sexual partners during intimate contact, as well as the general risk to women and children from unintended exposure to medications affecting the hormonal axis. The risks of hormonal overexposure (e.g., cardiac events) should also be reviewed, including BPH, an increased risk of obstructive sleep apnea, polycythemia, peripheral edema, and both cardiac and hepatic dysfunction.

EPIDIDYMITIS

Epididymitis is an inflammation of the epididymis, the coiled structure connecting the sperm-producing rete testis to the vas deferens that allows for maturation and immunosurveillance of the sperm. This inflammation results in scrotal pain, swelling, and induration of the posterior-lying epididymis, with eventual scrotal wall edema and involvement of the adjacent testicle, possibly with reactive hydrocele formation. The inflammation of the testicle results in a unilateral painful testicle known as *epididymo-orchitis*.

EPIDEMIOLOGY AND CAUSES

There is a predisposition to epididymitis when the patient has a history of unprotected intercourse, a new sexual partner, a history of UTI with dysuria, or urethral discharge. Symptoms may also occur following heavy lifting or straining. Younger sexually active men or older men with UTI are the patients who most commonly present with epididymitis. It may also (but rarely) occur in prepubertal boys, which likely heralds a structural abnormality in the genitourinary tract.

The causes of epididymitis in males younger than 35 years are usually sexually transmitted diseases such as *Chlamydia* or *Neisseria gonorrhoeae* infections. There is usually a difference in the type of discharge. *Chlamydia* infection produces a serous urethral discharge, whereas gonorrhea produces a purulent discharge.

Causes of epididymitis in men 35 years and older include coliform bacteria (such as *Escherichia coli*, which is most common) and sometimes *Pseudomonas aeruginosa* or *Staphylococcus aureus*. Epididymitis is often associated with a distal urinary tract obstruction in men older than 35 years or with coliform infections in men engaging in insertive anal intercourse. Tuberculous epididymitis will present with sterile pyuria and nodularity of the vas deferens, as well as pain. Another cause of epididymitis is sterile urinary reflux following transurethral prostatectomy. A granulomatous reaction following bacille Calmette-Guérin intravesical therapy for superficial bladder cancer may also cause epididymitis.

Rare causes of epididymitis include syphilis, brucellosis, blastomycosis, coccidioidomycosis, and cryptococcosis. When nonbacterial epididymitis and epididymo-orchitis occur, the cause is not clear but may be secondary to retrograde extravasation of urine.

PATHOPHYSIOLOGY

UTI and prostatitis, in particular, predispose a patient to the development of epididymitis. Other risk factors include transmission of pathogens via indwelling urethral catheters or urinary instrumentation, or as a consequence of transurethral prostate surgery. A urethral stricture of any type may also be a risk factor. Epididymitis caused by STDs is transmitted through the urethra and may be accompanied by symptomatic or asymptomatic urethritis.

Other causes include immunosuppression, trauma, or reflux of urine from the urethra through the vas deferens, causing chemical inflammation and edema within the epididymis that leads to ductal obstruction. Predisposing factors for subacute presentations of epididymitis in otherwise healthy postpubertal male patients include heavy physical activity, prolonged bicycle or motorcycle riding, and sexual activity. These patients may have negative urinalyses and often do not experience dysuria.

CLINICAL PRESENTATION
Subjective

The major complaint of patients with epididymitis is scrotal pain that often radiates along the spermatic cord or to the flank. The pain may appear relatively acute over several hours. Many men experience pain at the tip of the penis and complain of urethral discharge or other symptoms of UTI, such as frequency of urination, dysuria, cloudy urine, or hematuria. Initially, only the lowermost tail section of the posterior-lying epididymis will be painful, tender, and indurated. Elevation of the testes and the epididymis will relieve the discomfort. Patients with sensory neuropathy as a result of diabetes mellitus may have only minimal pain despite severe infections or abscesses; older adult patients may also present without significant pain. Fever and chills occur with severe infection or abscess formation.

Objective

Physical examination reveals scrotal swelling, and the testis may be indistinguishable from the epididymis. The scrotum wall will be thick and indurated, and a reactive hydrocele may occur. In addition to nodularity of the vas deferens and tenderness of the epididymis, patients with the nonsexually transmitted variety of epididymitis will have pyuria. Rectal examination reveals a tender prostate.

DIAGNOSTIC REASONING
Diagnostic Tests

Initially, a urinalysis will show pyuria and leukocytosis. A Gram stain of the urethral discharge may reveal gram-negative intracellular diplococci that are diagnostic of *Neisseria gonorrhoeae*. Culture of the penile discharge may be consistent with *Chlamydia* or gonorrheal infection. If no organisms are visible on the urethral smear but WBCs are evident, the diagnosis is usually nongonococcal urethritis, in which *Chlamydia* is the most likely pathogen. A complete blood count shows increased WBCs with a left shift to more immature forms. Interstitial congestion and fibrotic scarring may be present. An ultrasound of the scrotum can confirm the diagnosis of epididymitis.

Differential Diagnosis

The differential diagnoses for epididymitis include epididymal congestion following a vasectomy, testicular torsion, torsion of the appendix testis, mumps, orchitis, testicular tumor, and testicular trauma. An epididymal cyst, spermatocele, hydrocele, or varicocele should also be ruled out as part of the differential diagnosis. In epididymitis, the pain often improves when the scrotum is elevated above the level of the pubic symphysis (Prehn's sign).

MANAGEMENT

Initial treatment includes bedrest with scrotal elevation and ice packs, along with appropriate antibiotics; in severe cases, a spermatic cord block with local anesthetics may be necessary to relieve the pain. In men younger than 35 years with sexually transmitted epididymitis, treatment is a one-time dose of ceftriaxone (Rocephin) 250 mg intramuscular (IM) in addition to doxycycline (Vibramycin) 100 mg twice daily for 10 days. If the patient is allergic to cephalosporins or tetracyclines, a fluoroquinolone such as ofloxacin 300 mg PO twice daily or levofloxacin 500 mg PO daily can be given for 10 days. It is important to treat the sexual partner as well. Patients with nonsexually transmitted forms of epididymitis may be treated with ciprofloxacin 750 mg PO twice daily, ofloxacin 200 to 300 mg PO twice daily, or TMP-SMX (Bactrim, Septra) one DS tablet PO twice daily for 2 to 3 weeks. For the septic or toxic hospitalized patient, ceftriaxone 1 to 2 g IV or IM given every 24 hours is the preferred treatment. An aminoglycoside (gentamicin) 1 mg/kg IV or IM given every 8 hours (adjusted to the patient's renal function, after a loading dose of 2 mg/kg) may also be administered.

For patients with noninfectious epididymitis, treatment consists of NSAIDs, rest, and scrotal support. Antibiotic therapy is reserved for patients who are refractory to conservative treatment, in order to treat possible occult infection or fastidious organisms that are difficult to culture from urethral swabs or penile discharge. Tylenol with codeine may be used for moderate to severe pain.

Surgical procedures may be needed, depending on the severity of the case. An aspiration of the hydrocele may assist in examination of the scrotal contents and relieve discomfort. A vasostomy to drain the infected material may be done as well. Scrotal exploration should be done if there is uncertainty in differentiating epididymitis from testicular torsion. Drainage of abscesses, epididymectomy, or orchiectomy may be considered in severe cases that do not respond to antibiotics. The activity of the patient after these procedures is limited to bedrest for a minimum of 1 to 2 days.

FOLLOW-UP AND REFERRAL

Patient monitoring with office visits should continue until there are no signs of infection. Early treatment of prostatitis may prevent the development of epididymitis. Vigorous rectal examination of patients experiencing acute prostatitis should be avoided because this can lead to epididymitis. The prognosis is good if epididymitis is treated promptly. Pain improves in 1 to 3 days, but induration may last several weeks and take several months to resolve completely.

Complications of epididymitis include infertility or decreased fertility, recurrent epididymitis, abscess formation, or Fournier's gangrene (fulminant necrotizing fasciitis of the perineum and/or genitalia, due to synergistic polymicrobial infection)—all of which are possible if treatment is delayed or inadequate.

Patient Education: Epididymitis

The patient should be instructed to limit activity and immobilize the scrotal contents, which will relieve the pain and aid in treating the infection. The patient will need to wear an athletic supporter and avoid sexual contact and physical activity as long as pain persists. Patient education includes stressing the need to complete the full course of all antibiotics, even after the patient becomes asymptomatic.

TESTICULAR TORSION

Testicular torsion is the twisting or rotation of the testes, resulting in acute ischemia. It is a urological emergency. The torsion may vary from 90 to 360 degrees about the spermatic cord. An even more common phenomenon is torsion of the testicular appendix or appendiceal torsion, in which a small vestigial remnant of the Müllerian duct located on the anterosuperior portion of the testis twists about its base.

The average-sized testis is approximately $4.5 \times 3 \times 2.7$ cm. Within the scrotum, each testis is surrounded by the tunica albuginea, a tough layer of connective tissue, as well as the tunica vaginalis, which is a potential space formed by a membranous sac covering the anterior two-thirds of the testicle. A cryptorchid testis that fails to descend into the scrotal sac is most prone to undergoing torsion.

EPIDEMIOLOGY AND CAUSES

Testicular torsion can occur at any age, from in a newborn to age 80 years; however, two-thirds of cases occur between the ages of 10 and 20 years, with the peak incidence at age 14 years. Testicular torsion is possible but rare in older men. Torsion of the appendix testis is more common in children aged 7 to 14 years.

Testicular torsion is usually an idiopathic and spontaneous occurrence. There is a history of trauma in 20% of cases, with one-third of patients having had prior episodic testicular pain. One initiating factor of torsion appears to be the contraction of the cremaster muscle, which may occur during sleep in approximately 50% of patients. The contraction of the cremaster muscle may also be stimulated by trauma, exercise (most frequently in runners), extreme cold (torsion is more common in winter months), and sexual stimulation. Paraplegics are also at high risk for developing testicular torsion, probably as a result of constant pressure while sitting. Other factors contributing to testicular torsion are alterations in testosterone levels and cremasteric contractions during the nocturnal sex response cycle, as well as congenital abnormalities of the tunica vaginalis or the spermatic cord.

PATHOPHYSIOLOGY

If the base of the testis is inadequately fixed to the tunica vaginalis via the gubernaculum, the testis may twist around the spermatic cord under several of the conditions listed in the preceding paragraphs. Arterial inflow becomes compromised and venous outflow is obstructed, resulting in ischemia of the testis. This is exquisitely painful and may lead to necrosis if it is not treated emergently. Irreversible cellular damage may result in as little as 6 to 12 hours. Even if the testis is salvaged, fertility may be permanently compromised owing to a disruption of the blood–testis immunological barrier. This exposes germ cell antigens to the systemic circulation, resulting in sperm-specific antibodies that lead to permanent destruction of spermatozoa.

CLINICAL PRESENTATION

Subjective

The most common symptom of testicular torsion is acute onset of pain accompanied by swelling. Torsion of the appendix testis also presents with pain, but it may be more gradual in onset. The patient may have pain for several days before seeking medical attention.

Objective

The most common clinical sign of testicular torsion is the absence of the cremasteric reflex. The testicle may also be high in the scrotum, with a transverse, rather than longitudinal, lie known as a "bell-clapper" deformity. Elevation of the testis does not relieve testicular pain, as is sometimes observed in epididymitis (Prehn's sign). However, this physical finding is insufficiently specific to distinguish between these two disorders. Occasionally with torsion of the appendix testis there may be a small lump that is palpable on the superior pole of the testis. If the skin is pulled tautly over it, the lump may appear blue ("blue dot sign"). This "blue dot" results from infarction and necrosis of the appendix testis and is present in about one-fifth of cases.

DIAGNOSTIC REASONING

Diagnostic Tests

Testicular torsion is diagnosed by history and presenting manifestations. The only initial assessment required is a physical examination. Color Doppler ultrasonography or radionuclide scanning can be used to diagnose both testicular torsion and appendiceal torsion. Doppler ultrasound can detect an absent or reduced pulse with torsion and an increased flow with an inflammatory process,

although Doppler ultrasound is reliable only in the first 12 hours following torsion. A radionuclide testicular scintigraphy with technetium 99-m (99m-Tc) pertechnetate will show absent or decreased vascularity in patients with torsion; increased vascularity will be evident in patients with an inflammatory process, including torsion of the appendix testis.

Differential Diagnosis

Differential diagnoses for testicular torsion include epididymo-orchitis, an incarcerated or strangulated inguinal hernia, an acute hydrocele, a traumatic hematoma, idiopathic scrotal edema, a torsion appendix testis, an acute varicocele, a testicular tumor, or Henoch-Schönlein purpura. Scrotal abscesses and leukemic infiltrates are also important considerations in the differential diagnosis and must be ruled out. Some pathological findings associated with testicular torsion include venous thrombosis, tissue edema, necrosis, and arterial thrombosis.

MANAGEMENT

Compression of the testicular vessels leads to ischemic necrosis of the testes within 6 hours. Failure to recognize the torsion and intervene immediately results in the loss of the testicle in 80% of cases, with subsequent atrophy of the testis in 10% or more. Fertile resolution occurs in only 10% of patients.

Upon diagnosis, immediate referral of the patient to the emergency department is indicated, as testicular torsion is a urological emergency. In the emergency department, manual reduction may be successful. Manual reduction of the testis is classically done with gentle external rotation of the testis toward the thigh, because most cases of torsion occur with medial rotation away from the thigh. However, retrospective studies have demonstrated lateral testicular torsion in up to one-third of cases. Relief of pain, resolution of the "bell-clapper" deformity, and a restoration of arterial blood flow are used as the primary indications of effective reduction of testicular torsion. Reduction is followed by surgical exploration. Any testis that is not clearly viable is removed. Surgical exploration via scrotal approach—with detorsion, evaluation of testicular viability, orchidopexy (permanent anchoring of the testis in the scrotum) of the viable testicle, and orchidectomy (removal) of the nonviable testicle—is the preferred surgical intervention. Surgery should be done within 4 hours after the onset of symptoms to preserve the testicle; after 12 hours the viability of the testicle is diminished.

For a patient with torsion of the appendix testis, surgery may also be performed, but recovery is quicker than that for testicular torsion. Conservative medical treatment may be initiated with rest, ice, and NSAIDs, but recovery is much slower, and pain may persist for weeks to months. The dead appendiceal tissue is usually reabsorbed, however, and fertility is preserved.

FOLLOW-UP AND REFERRAL

Testicular salvage is directly related to the duration of torsion; the salvage rate is 85% to 90% if torsion has persisted for less than 6 hours. The salvage rate becomes less than 10% if the duration of the torsion is greater than 24 hours. Depressed spermatogenesis occurs in 80% to 94% of individuals and may be related to the duration of ischemic injury.

Patient Education: Testicular Torsion

As many as two-thirds of testes salvaged may atrophy in the first 2 to 3 years posttorsion. The possibility of testicular atrophy in a salvaged testis, along with depressed sperm counts, necessitates patient education and understanding of these potential sequelae. Patients should be taught to seek immediate care when experiencing testicular pain to prevent permanent sequelae.

HYDROCELE

A *hydrocele* is a collection of peritoneal fluid within the scrotum around the testes, between the parietal and visceral (adjacent to the testis) layers of the tunica vaginalis—the two-layered sac that surrounds the testis and spermatic cord. A hydrocele forms when secretion of fluid into this potential space outweighs its reabsorption. These collections may range from only a few milliliters of fluid to enormous volumes measured in liters.

EPIDEMIOLOGY AND CAUSES

The incidence rate of hydrocele is about 1% in adult men. Most hydroceles occur in men older than 40 years. Causes of an acute hydrocele include nonspecific acute epididymitis, tuberculous epididymitis, trauma to the testes, tumor of the testes, or sequelae as complications of radiation therapy. Exstrophy of the bladder (protrusion of the bladder through the abdominal wall) may increase the risk for hydrocele formation. Patients with Ehlers-Danlos syndrome have an increased risk for hydrocele, as do patients with a ventricular peritoneal shunt for dialysis or peritoneal dialysis.

PATHOPHYSIOLOGY

A basic knowledge of scrotal anatomy is required to understand the pathogenesis of a hydrocele. The processus vaginalis originates as a diverticulum of the peritoneal sac that lines the abdomen, just inferior to the testis. During development, as the testis descends into the scrotum, it brings this diverticulum down with it, eventually becoming engulfed by it. The sac surrounding the testis (now called the tunica vaginalis) remains connected to the peritoneal sac via the processus vaginalis. Typically, throughout infancy and childhood, the connecting portion of the sac between the tunica vaginalis and the processus vaginalis gradually closes, breaking communication with the peritoneal sac.

Hydroceles in infants typically result from a patent processus vaginalis that fails to close during in utero development, allowing for the free flow of fluid between the peritoneal sac and the tunica vaginalis. These hydroceles have been directly correlated with the risk of indirect inguinal herniation in which gut contents bulge through a patent processus vaginalis. A noncommunicating hydrocele results from complete closure of the processus vaginalis, trapping peritoneal fluid within the tunica vaginalis. This type of hydrocele may be self-limited in adults. A hydrocele of the spermatic cord forms when the distal processus vaginalis closes but the midportion surrounding the cord remains patent and filled with fluid. The proximal portion may be opened or closed.

Rapidly forming hydroceles may result from reactive inflammatory processes within the scrotum such as testicular or appendiceal testicular torsion, epididymitis, and even testicular cancer. A chronic hydrocele may result from gradual fluid accumulation within the tunica vaginalis in young boys or men, caused by an imbalance in fluid secretion, conduction, and reabsorption.

CLINICAL PRESENTATION

Subjective

Patients with a hydrocele typically present with swelling in the scrotum or inguinal canal. If the size of the scrotum fluctuates, a communicating hydrocele could exist. Hydroceles are usually painless, although patients report a sense of heaviness in the scrotum. If pain is present, it may radiate to the lower back.

Objective

The scrotum is transilluminated with a penlight in a darkened room during the physical examination. The trapped fluid appears light pink, yellow, or red. The hydrocele can be illuminated to show the full size and shape, which assist in the diagnosis. The testes themselves do not transilluminate, nor do hematomas. Swelling may be noted in the groin or in the upper scrotum.

DIAGNOSTIC REASONING

Diagnostic Tests

A detailed description of the events that precipitated finding the hydrocele should be obtained. Details of any trauma incurred will assist in the evaluation. If a hydrocele cannot be confirmed, the patient should be referred for an inguinoscrotal ultrasound, which can distinguish the presence or absence of bowel within the inguinal ring. A testicular nuclear scan is used to distinguish testicular torsion. Abdominal x-ray studies may be useful in distinguishing an incarcerated hernia from a hydrocele but are rarely needed.

Differential Diagnosis

The differential diagnoses for hydrocele include indirect inguinal hernias (because of the location of the hydrocele), orchitis (inflammation or infection of the testes), epididymitis (an inflammatory process that can produce symptoms that mimic those of a hydrocele), or a varicocele (a mass of varicose veins in the spermatic cord within the scrotum). Pain is more likely to be present with epididymitis. Traumatic injury to the testes must be ruled out by history and physical examination. Torsion of the testicle or torsion of the appendix of the testes must also be ruled out. Exploratory surgery is indicated for the definitive diagnosis of a patent processus vaginalis in a communicating hydrocele. A scrotal mass of any type requires further evaluation for testicular or scrotal cancer.

MANAGEMENT

For adults, no treatment of a hydrocele is required unless complications are present or the clinician suspects a significant underlying cause, such as a tumor. If the hydrocele is painful, large, unsightly, or uncomfortable, however, several treatments are available. For example, a variety of outpatient surgical procedures are used to treat hydroceles. The Jaboulay-Winkelmann surgical procedure is for thick hydrocele sacs that form when the hydrocele has wrapped itself posteriorly around the cord structures. The Lord procedure is used for a thin hydrocele sac; a radial suture is used to gather the hydrocele sac posterior to the testis and the epididymis. The hydrocele can be surgically drained and the tunica vaginalis resected. Sclerotherapy (injection of a sclerotic irritant into the tunica vaginalis to induce scarring and adhesions between the adjacent layer of the tunica) and endoscopic procedures can also be performed to alleviate hydroceles. Aspiration of hydroceles is usually not done because the fluid rapidly reaccumulates; however, it may be done for a postoperative hydrocele.

FOLLOW-UP AND REFERRAL

Patient monitoring for a hydrocele should be at 3-month intervals until the decision is made for or against surgery. Postoperatively, patient monitoring should be at 2- to 3-week intervals, followed by 2- to 3-month intervals until there is resolution.

Postoperative traumatic hydroceles are common and usually resolve spontaneously. Other possible complications may be injury to the vas deferens spermatic vessels,

a suture granuloma, a hematoma secondary to the surgery, or a wound infection.

Patient Education: Hydrocele

For patients with a hydrocele, education regarding an explanation of the disease process and management plan is appropriate, along with reassurance of the overall benign nature of the condition (depending on the underlying cause).

VARICOCELE

A *varicocele* is an abnormal degree of venous dilation of the pampiniform plexus in the spermatic cord above the testes, which usually results in pain and engorgement of the testis.

EPIDEMIOLOGY AND CAUSES

There is no ethnic predisposition or age differentiation among patients with varicoceles. The overall rate of incidence is 8% to 20%. In men evaluated for infertility, however, the rate of varicocele increases to 25% to 40%. A weak wall in the spermatic vein or excessive pressure is the leading cause of varicoceles.

PATHOPHYSIOLOGY

The pathophysiology of a varicocele results from vascular engorgement of the internal spermatic vein. A varicocele almost always appears on the left or bilaterally, because the left spermatic (gonadal) vein empties into the left renal vein, whereas the right spermatic vein empties into the inferior vena cava. One of the longest veins in the body, the left spermatic vein, empties into the left renal vein at a perpendicular angle. Compared with the right renal vein, the left renal vein has a higher intravascular pressure owing to its anatomical positioning between the aorta inferiorly and the superior mesenteric artery. In turn, if the valves of the left renal vein become incompetent because of this increased pressure, retrograde blood flow causes back pressure to be transmitted to the pampiniform venous plexus, which overlies the testis. In contrast, a unilateral right-sided varicocele may result from serious pathology, causing increased pressure within the inferior vena cava, such as a tumor or thrombus.

CLINICAL PRESENTATION

Subjective

The patient may present with pain and engorgement of the testes. The recognition of a varicocele is usually secondary to a problem with fertility, however. A patient with a varicocele often describes the sensation of palpating the affected portion of the scrotum as feeling like a "bag of worms."

Objective

On physical examination, with the patient in an upright position, tortuous veins located posterior to and above the testis can be assessed. The engorged veins may extend up into the external inguinal ring. Venous dilation can be increased by having the patient perform the Valsalva maneuver in a recumbent position. The reverse is also true; in the recumbent position, the venous distention will abate. Testicular atrophy with impaired circulation may be present.

DIAGNOSTIC REASONING

Diagnostic Tests

A system of grading has been established to better define varicocele. A *Grade 1* varicocele is one that is palpable only when the patient performs the Valsalva maneuver. A *Grade 2* varicocele is palpable when the patient is standing. A *Grade 3* varicocele may be assessed with light palpation and visual inspection.

Sperm count and motility of the sperm are significantly decreased in patients with a varicocele approximately 65% to 75% of the time. There is evidence of a progressive decline in fertility in men with varicocele. Scrotal ultrasound, venography (showing testicular venous reflux from a varicocele), and thermography (shows increase in temperature at the varicocele) all help to confirm the diagnosis.

Differential Diagnosis

The differential diagnosis for varicocele includes hydrocele, spermatocele, testicular tumor, epididymal cyst, and renal tumors. A diagnostic priority is questioning the patient thoroughly for any contributing factors and the time course of the finding. It is essential to note whether the onset of the testicular abnormality has been rapid or has resulted from a gradual increase in the varices or other structures surrounding the testicles, as this will point the clinician in a particular diagnostic direction. Of note, in an elderly patient, the development of a varicocele may be a late sign of a renal tumor.

MANAGEMENT

After a varicocele has been diagnosed, referral to a surgeon is indicated, although most patients do not require surgery because most varicoceles are minor. Surgical treatment of a varicocele involves ligation of the internal spermatic vein, which usually results in decompression of the varicocele and improvement in the quality of semen, as well as a decrease in pain. The surgery can be laparoscopic, anteriorly via an inguinal or subinguinal approach, posteriorly via a lumbar approach, or even microsurgical. Embolization with coils is a second-line approach but appears to have a higher complication rate owing to possible migration of the coils. Testicular atrophy is a definite indication for treatment. Conservative treatment in older men with only minor pain or for whom fertility is no longer an issue or for men with normal fertility may consist of NSAIDs and scrotal support. Treatment has not consistently improved sperm count or fertility in controlled trials.

FOLLOW-UP AND REFERRAL

Complications of a varicocele (if not corrected) include infertility and testicular atrophy. A referral to a urologist is recommended for affirmation of the diagnosis and further explanation of treatment options. Any patient with a recent onset of varicocele, infertility, pain, or testicular atrophy should have a urology consultation to rule out more serious pathology and to optimize the treatment plan.

Patient Education: Varicocele

Education for the patient should include an explanation of the disease process, signs, symptoms, and implications. The patient should be taught how to monitor growth and symptoms of the varicocele, especially if it is right sided. To relieve pain, the patient should be encouraged to wear a scrotal support; for some patients, wearing more supportive jockey shorts (briefs) rather than loose boxer shorts is sufficient to relieve discomfort.

TESTICULAR CANCER

Primary testicular neoplasms may arise from any testicular or adnexal cell component. Each testis is covered externally by two layers of fascia: the outer layer called the tunica vaginalis and the deeper albuginea layer, which extends internally and divides the testis into 250 to 300 lobules. Each lobule contains seminiferous tubules (the site of spermatogenesis) and the interstitial cells that produce androgens, including testosterone. The epididymis lies along the external surface of each testis and is the site of sperm maturation and storage. Tumors of the germ cells and the seminiferous tubules are the most common testicular carcinomas.

EPIDEMIOLOGY AND CAUSES

Although testicular malignancies comprise only 1% to 2% of all neoplasms in men (1 out of every 263 men will develop testicular cancer), the psychological and physically debilitating effects of testicular cancer affecting young men aged 15 to 35 years deserve mention because testicular cancer is the most common solid malignancy in this age-group. Fortunately, it is also one of the most curable of the solid cancers.

In the United States, there are 5.7 per 100,000 new cases of testicular cancer diagnosed per year in men. It is less common in African Americans than in the overall population, at 0.9 cases per 100,000 males. In adult men, germ cell cancers comprise 90% to 95% of testicular cancers, and in boys they represent 60% to 75%. The peak age at onset is between age 20 and 40 years, with an average age at diagnosis of 33 years. Although testicular cancer is mainly a disease of younger men, 7% of cases occur in men aged 55 years and older.

No clear cause-and-effect relationships are identified for testicular cancer. Prior cryptorchidism is the only undisputed risk factor for this type of cancer, with 10% of testicular tumors associated with this condition. Importantly, a fourth of these tumors occur in the contralateral, descended testis. In addition to cryptorchidism, a family history of testicular cancer and a personal history of previous testicular cancer also appear to confer a greater risk.

Other possible risk factors that have been identified for testicular cancer include higher social status, being unmarried, or living in a rural area. Weak associations demonstrate that hormonal imbalances associated with in utero exposure to estrogen may increase the risk for testicular cancer later in life. One study of mothers who used diethylstilbestrol during the first trimester found a 2.5- to 5-fold increase of testicular cancer in the sons of exposed mothers.

PATHOPHYSIOLOGY

Primary testicular neoplasm may arise from any testicular adnexal cell component. These are divided into germinal (90% to 95%) and nongerminal (sex cord–stromal) tumors. For treatment purposes, the germinal tumors are further divided based on histology into seminomas and nonseminomas (e.g., embryonal carcinomas, teratomas, choriocarcinomas, and yolk sac tumors), which are epithelial in nature. In contrast, far rarer are the sex cord–stromal tumors, which consist primarily of Leydig cell variants that produce estrogen due to increased aromatase activity and Sertoli cell tumors, which may also present with estrogenic overload.

Only a small number of molecular markers have been consistently associated with testicular cancers, for example, an isochromosome of chromosome 12p, activating mutations in c-*kit*, increased p53, and telomerase expression. Abnormal DNA ploidy is also common in germ cell tumors. Although certain genetic alterations differ in germ cell tumors found in prepubertal males, all germ cell tumors are believed to arise from pluripotential primordial germ cells. One exception to this is the relatively rare spermatocytic seminoma, the pathogenesis of which appears to be fundamentally different based on unique molecular markers.

Except for spermatocytic seminomas, all germ cell tumors may be preceded by a premalignant condition known as intratubular germ cell neoplasia of unclassified type (ITGCNU) or testicular carcinoma in situ. It is found adjacent to 90% of germ cell tumors, implying that genetic mutations lead to gonadal dysfunction and subsequent malignancy over a large area of tissue—a phenomenon known as a field defect. At least half the cases of untreated ITGCNU will progress to invasive malignant disease within 5 years, predictably spreading to the retroperitoneal draining lymph nodes. Men with a history of cryptorchidism are recommended to have empiric testicular biopsy between the ages of 18 and 20 years to evaluate for ITGCNU.

CLINICAL PRESENTATION

Subjective

Typically, the patient with testicular cancer presents with a hard lump or nodule on his testis that he felt while performing a testicular self-examination. Generally, testicular cancer presents as a painless enlargement of the testis. The patient may also note scrotal swelling, heaviness in the scrotum that may be interpreted as pain, a sensation of fullness, or a previously small testis that has enlarged to the size of a normal testis or the contralateral testis.

Objective

During routine physical examinations (e.g., a sports physical), a scrotal nodule or swelling is most commonly detected in men with testicular cancer. A firm, nontender mass within the confines of the tunica albuginea is typically palpable and distinct from the spermatic cord structures. Acute or chronic epididymitis or epididymoorchitis may result in a delay in the diagnosis of testicular cancer in about 10% of cases. Gynecomastia may be present in 5% of patients with testicular malignancies. Hydroceles (seen in 5% to 10% of patients) may develop secondary to testicular cancer.

As many as 10% of patients with testicular cancer will be asymptomatic, and another 10% will present with manifestations of metastasis. Symptoms of metastases may include respiratory symptoms (cough) due to lung metastases, low back pain and nerve root or psoas muscle irritation due to retroperitoneal metastasis, or lower extremity swelling from obstruction of the vena cava.

DIAGNOSTIC REASONING

Diagnostic Tests

Several biochemical markers can aid in the diagnosis of testicular carcinoma, but their main use is in following disease progression or remission after treatment by monitoring for trends in blood levels. These tests include human chorionic gonadotropin (hCG) and alpha-fetoprotein (AFP).

AFP levels are elevated by the pure embryonal carcinoma, teratocarcinoma, yolk sac tumor, or combinations of these three malignancies, but not by pure choriocarcinoma or seminoma. However, AFP may also be elevated in benign liver disease, telangiectasis, tyrosinemia, and malignancies of the liver, pancreas, stomach, and lung. Heavy marijuana smoking can also elevate levels of AFP.

hCG levels are elevated by all choriocarcinomas and occasionally with seminomas; however, hCG is also elevated in liver, lung, pancreatic, and stomach malignancies, as well as with kidney, breast, and bladder tumors. Forty percent to 60% of patients with an embryonal carcinoma and 5% to 10% of patients with seminomas have detectable levels of hCG (usually under 500 ng/mL). In general, elevated AFP, hCG, or lactate dehydrogenase is a poor prognostic sign in testicular cancer, and prognosis worsens with the degree of elevation. Elevated placental alkaline phosphatase (PLAP) may be the marker of choice for seminomas in 70% to 90% of patients. Patients with recurrent or disseminated seminomas have elevated PLAP levels. However, PLAP is not entirely specific because it may also be elevated by heavy tobacco smoking.

Scrotal ultrasound is also a useful diagnostic tool for testicular cancer because the mass can usually be seen clearly originating within the testis. Using an echotexture (hypoechoic) pattern, the mass will appear distinct from the surrounding normal testicular tissue on ultrasound. Uniformly cystic or fluid-filled masses are not likely to be testicular cancer, which is a solid tumor. However, ultrasound is not accurate for staging and should not replace orchiectomy as the procedure of choice. Magnetic resonance imaging is not usually more informative than scrotal ultrasound or pelvic/abdominal computed tomography (CT) for staging and identifying enlarged retroperitoneal lymph nodes that signify the need for lymph node dissection. Positron emission tomography scanning is usually used only to identify residual masses after treatment.

Chest x-ray studies, with both posterior-anterior and lateral views, are important for the identification of metastasis and to rule out the spread of malignancy above the diaphragm. A CT scan is able to define pelvic retroperitoneal and mediastinal lymphadenopathy, as well as to detect metastases to the abdominal viscera.

Differential Diagnosis

A definitive diagnosis of testicular cancer may be made with a transinguinal scrotal exploration and biopsy and/or radical orchiectomy (excision of the testicle and spermatic cord). Transscrotal open or cutaneous biopsy and transscrotal orchiectomy are contraindicated because of the potential for anatomical trespassing into the various lymphatic drainage systems. Testicular cancer is typically a painless mass in the testis, but the differential diagnosis includes epididymitis, hernia, hydrocele, hematoma, spermatocele, syphilitic gumma, and varicocele.

MANAGEMENT

The main principle of management for testicular cancer is a radical orchiectomy, which is also the major diagnostic tool because the whole testis is removed for biopsy. Testicular cancer is very treatable, with fewer than 400 deaths per year in the United States at present. Treatment does, however, leave the patient with a high possibility of being infertile. Sperm-banking (semen cryopreservation) should be done before radiographic diagnostic studies, if desired. Many of these men have gonadal dysgenesis with a low baseline sperm count and morphology problems, but banking works well in general, and future children fathered by this banked sperm do not have higher rates of congenital defects.

Testicular carcinoma is divided into two main categories when considering treatment. The first category, nonseminomas, includes embryonal cell carcinomas (20%), teratomas (5%), choriocarcinomas (less than 1%), and mixed cell types (40%). The second category is seminomas (35%). Staging depends on the type of tumor (seminoma vs. nonseminoma). In addition, the American Joint Committee on Cancer classifies tumors using the TNM(S) system. The size of the tumor (T), the spread to nearby lymph nodes (N), any metastasis (M), and serum markers (S) are considered in this system of staging (see Table 50.1 for testicular tumor staging criteria).

The TNM classification of the American Joint Cancer Committee is also used for testicular cancer. The primary tumor (T) is classed from T0 (no evidence of primary tumor) to T4 (invades scrotum). Lymph node assessment (N) is from N0 (no regional lymph node metastasis) to N3 (metastasis in lymph node greater than 5 cm). Distant metastasis (M) is classified from M0 (no distant metastasis) to M1b (distant metastasis to sites other than nonregional lymph nodes or lungs).

Seventy-five percent of nonseminomas can be cured with orchiectomy alone, usually with a modified retroperitoneal lymph node dissection. This is done to preserve the sympathetic innervation so the patient will still have ejaculatory function. The serum markers are monitored postorchiectomy, and those patients whose levels return to normal have an excellent prognosis. For patients with nonseminomas that have metastasized or who have significant lymph node involvement (greater than 3 cm), combination chemotherapy is used following orchiectomy. Commonly used chemotherapeutic agents include cisplatin (Platinol), etoposide (VePesid), and bleomycin (Blenoxane) or paclitaxel (Taxol). If the serum tumor markers do not normalize after chemotherapy, salvage chemotherapy is needed. Salvage chemotherapy includes cyclophosphamide (Cytoxan) or ifosfamide (Ifex)–based protocols, with mesna (Mesnex) to protect against hemorrhagic cystitis.

The 5-year survival rate for patients with Stage A nonseminomas is 96% to 100% after treatment. Patients with Stage B nonseminomas have an almost 90% 5-year survival rate after treatment. For patients with Stage C

TABLE 50.1 Staging and Classification for Testicular Carcinoma

Nonseminoma Germ Cell Tumor Staging

Stage A		Lesion confined to testis
Stage B		Regional lymph node involvement in the retroperitoneum
Stage C		Distant metastasis

MD Anderson System for Seminomas

Stage I		Lesion confined to testis
Stage II		Spread to retroperitoneal lymph nodes
Stage III		Supradiaphragmatic nodal or visceral involvement

American Joint Committee on Cancer (AJCC) TNM staging system
T = tumor, N = lymph node involvement, M = metastasis, S = serum tumor marker

Stage 0	pTis N0 M0 S0	Cancer only in the seminiferous tubules with no other part of the testicle involved (pTis). No lymph node involvement; no metastasis and tumor marker levels are normal.
Stage I	pT1–pT4 N0 M0 SX	Local spread beyond seminiferous tubules and possibly outside the testicle (pT1–pT4). No lymph nodes; no metastasis and tumor marker not done or not available.
Stage IA	pT1 N0 M0 S0	Tumor beyond the seminiferous tubules but within the testicle (pT1). No lymph nodes; no metastasis and tumor marker are normal.
Stage IB	pT2–pT4 N0 M0 S0	Tumor beyond the testicle and into nearby structures (pT2–pT4). No lymph nodes; no metastasis and tumor marker within normal limits.
Stage IS	Any pT N0 M0 S1–S3	Tumor may have spread outside the testicle (any pT). No lymph nodes; no metastasis but at least one tumor marker is higher than normal (S1–S3).
Stage II	Any pT N1–N3 M0 SX	Tumor may or may not have spread beyond testicle. One or more nearby lymph nodes (N1–N3). No metastasis; tumor marker results not done or not available.
Stage IIA	Any pT N1 M0 S0 or S1	Tumor may or may not have spread beyond testicle. At least one nearby lymph not involved (but less than 5) and no lymph node greater than 2 cm. No metastasis; tumor markers normal (S0) or one tumor marker slightly elevated (S1).
Stage IIB	Any pT N2 M0 S0 or S1	Tumor may or may not have spread beyond testicle. At least one lymph node greater than 2 cm but less than 5 cm OR spread outside the lymph node OR more than 5 positive lymph nodes. No metastasis; tumor markers normal (S0) or one tumor marker slightly elevated (S1).
Stage IIC	Any pT N3 M0 S0 or S1	Tumor may or may not have spread beyond testicle. At least one lymph node greater than 5 cm (N3). No metastasis; tumor markers normal (S0) or one tumor marker slightly elevated (S1).
Stage III	Any pT Any N M1 SX	Tumor may or may not have spread beyond testicle. May or may not have positive lymph nodes. Spread to distant parts of the body. Tumor marker results not done or not available.
Stage IIIA	Any pT Any N M1a S0 or S1	Tumor may or may not have spread beyond testicle. May or may not have positive lymph nodes. Spread to distant lymph nodes or the lungs (M1a). Tumor markers normal (S0) or one tumor marker slightly elevated (S1).

TABLE 50.1	Staging and Classification for Testicular Carcinoma—cont'd	
American Joint Committee on Cancer (AJCC) TNM staging system		
T = tumor, N = lymph node involvement, M = metastasis, S = serum tumor marker		
Stage IIIB	Any pT N1–N3 M0 S2	Tumor may or may not have spread beyond testicle. One or more positive lymph nodes but no metastasis. At least one tumor marker significantly elevated (S2).
	OR	
Stage IIIB	Any pT Any N M1a S2	Tumor may or may not have spread beyond testicle. May or may not have positive lymph nodes. Spread to distant lymph nodes or the lungs (M1a). At least one tumor marker significantly elevated (S2).
Stage IIIC	Any pT N1–N3 M0 S3	Tumor may or may not have spread beyond testicle. One or more positive lymph nodes but no metastasis. At least one tumor marker is extremely elevated (S3).
	OR	
Stage IIIC	Any pT Any N M1a S3	Tumor may or may not have spread beyond testicle. May or may not have positive lymph nodes. Spread to distant lymph nodes or the lungs (M1a). At least one tumor marker is extremely elevated (S3).
	OR	
Stage IIIC	Any pT Any N M1b Any S	Tumor may or may not have spread beyond testicle. May or may not have positive lymph nodes. Metastasis to other locations outside of lymph nodes or to the lungs (M1b). Tumor marker level may or may not be elevated.

Source: American Joint Committee on Cancer (AJCC) TNM staging system used with permission of the American College of Surgeons. Original source for this information is the AJCC Cancer Staging Manual, Eighth Edition (2017) published by Springer International Publishing.

nonseminomas, the 5-year survival rate is between 55% and 80%.

Seminomas are chemosensitive and have a good chemotherapeutic response. They are also extremely sensitive to radiation therapy. All patients with seminomas should have radical orchiectomy surgery. Then, depending on the stage of the cancer, irradiation and chemotherapy will be used. For patients with Stages I and IIa (retroperitoneal disease less than 10 cm), surgery and radiation are the treatments of choice and are associated with a 5-year survival of 98% and 92% to 94%, respectively.

More advanced Stage II (retroperitoneal disease greater than 10 cm) and Stage III seminomas receive primary chemotherapy either with etoposide and cisplatin or a combination of cisplatin, etoposide, and bleomycin. If enlarged lymph nodes (more than 3 cm in diameter) persist after chemotherapy, a retroperitoneal lymph-node resection is done. In 40% of cases, there is residual carcinoma in these lymph nodes. Ninety-five percent of patients with Stage III seminoma have a complete response to orchiectomy and chemotherapy.

As with all chemotherapeutic agents, the precautions are specific for each type of agent. Cisplatin causes ototoxicity, nephrotoxicity, and neurotoxicity. Etoposide may cause thrombocytopenia. Cyclophosphamide and ifosfamide may cause hemorrhagic cystitis, and patients must be well hydrated to flush the bladder and minimize the risk of hemorrhagic cystitis. Patients receiving ifosfamide should also receive mesna to reduce the risk of hemorrhagic cystitis. Bleomycin causes pulmonary fibrosis, while the alternative drug carboplatin (Paraplatin) can cause ototoxicity. Ondansetron (Zofran), dronabinol (Marinol), metoclopramide (Reglan), and similar medications may be used to control nausea.

FOLLOW-UP AND REFERRAL

Follow-up is extremely important for patients with testicular malignancies. In the first year after orchiectomy for testicular cancer, the National Comprehensive Cancer Network recommends a history and physical examination every 3 to 6 months with an abdominal/pelvic CT scan at 3, 6, and 12 months. In years 2 to 3, a history and physical examination and CT scan should be done every 6 to 12 months, and in years 4 to 5, the history and physical examination should be done annually with a CT scan done every 1 to 2 years.

If the patient had adjuvant chemotherapy or radiation therapy after orchiectomy, a history and physical examination should be done every 6 to 12 months with an abdominal/pelvic CT scan done annually. A history and physical examination should be done annually thereafter with an annual CT scan starting in year 3.

This level of monitoring is critical, as nonseminomatous tumors are more likely (50% to 70%) to metastasize than seminomas (25%). Men who have been cured of testicular cancer in one testicle have a 2% to 4% chance of developing cancer in the remaining testicle. If cancer develops in the other testicle, it is almost always a new cancer, however, and not a metastasis from the first episode. Men with HIV are also at a much higher risk of developing cancer in the remaining testicle.

Patient Education: Testicular Cancer

Although testicular cancer patients may be reassured of the high rate of cure associated with this disease, patients should also be fully informed of the risks of chemotherapy, radiation therapy, and surgical interventions. For example, adverse effects of chemotherapy include hair loss, immunosuppression, loss of appetite, nausea, and vomiting. Radiation therapy can cause extreme fatigue and interfere with sperm production; it can also cause diarrhea, vomiting, and skin reactions at the treatment site, as well as nephritis or enteritis. Complications from retroperitoneal lymph node dissection include loss of seminal emission and/or hypoalbuminemia.

Open discussions and reassurance are extremely important in patients diagnosed with testicular cancer. Concerns over quality of life after testicular cancer are extremely important to most patients. The patient must be able to cope with the way testicular cancer affects his self-image. Patients who are concerned about their appearance after losing a testis can be educated about the availability of prostheses that simulate the weight and feel of a testicle. A low sperm count may also occur after the loss of a testis, so patients (and, if given permission, their partners) should also be educated about the risk of infertility associated with the primary disease and its treatments, as well as options such as sperm banking. Although surgery to remove lymph nodes does not compromise a man's ability to have an erection or reach orgasm, it can interfere with ejaculation. Some men naturally regain the ability to ejaculate, while others require medication. Thus, patients should also be educated about sterility and hormone supplements.

REFERENCES

Erectile Dysfunction

Abu-Ghanem Y, Kitrey ND, Gruenwals I, Appel B, Vardi Y. Penile low-intensity shock wave therapy: A promising novel modality for erectile dysfunction. *Korean J Urol.* 2014;55(5):295–299.

Evens JD, Hill SR. A comparison of the available phosphodiesterase-5 inhibitors in the treatment of erectile dysfunction: a focus on avanafil. *Patient Preference and Adherence.* https://www.ncbi.nlm.nih.gov/pmc/articles/PMC4542406/pdf/ppa-9-1159.pdf. Published 2015. Accessed September 9, 2017.

Kim, E. D. *Erectile dysfunction treatment & management.* http://emedicine.medscape.com/article/444220-treatment. Updated October 11, 2016. Accessed September 9, 2017.

Lu Z, Lin G, Reed-Maldonado A, Wang C, Lee Y, Lue TF. Low-intensity extracorporeal shock wave treatment improves erectile function: A systematic review and meta-analysis. *Eur Urol.* 2017;71(2):223–233.

Epididymitis

Taylor SN. Epididymitis. *Clin Infect Dis.* 2015;61(Suppl. 8):S770–S773. https://academic.oup.com/cid/article/61/suppl_8/S770/345636/Epididymitis. Accessed September 14, 2017.

Hydrocele/Varicocele

Kolon TF. Evaluation and management of the adolescent varicocele. *J Urol.* 2015;194(5):1194–1201.

Kuhn AL, Scortegagna E, Nowitzki KM, Kim YH. Ultrasonography of the scrotum in adults. *Ultrasonography.* 2016;35(3):180–197.

Testicular Cancer

NIH, National Cancer Institute. Testicular cancer treatment (PDQ)—health professional version. https://www.cancer.gov/types/testicular/hp/testicular-treatment-pdq#link/_713_toc. Updated January 26, 2017. Accessed September 9, 2017.

Osterberg EC, Bernie AM, Ramasamy R. Risks of testosterone replacement therapy in men. *Indian J Urol.* 2014;30(1):2–7.

Sachdeva K. Testicular cancer follow-up. http://emedicine.medscape.com/article/279007-followup. Updated July 5, 2017. Accessed September 9, 2017.

U.S. Preventive Services Task Force. Final recommendation statement: Testicular cancer screening. https://www.uspreventiveservicestaskforce.org/Page/Document/RecommendationStatementFinal/testicular-cancer-screening. Accessed September 9, 2017.

Testicular Torsion

Sheth K, Keays M, Grimsby GM, et al. Diagnosing testicular torsion before urological consultation and imaging: Validation of the TWIST score. *J Urol.* 2016;195(6):1870–1876.

Ta A, D'Arcy FT, Hoag N, D'Arcy JP, Lawrentschuk N. Testicular torsion and the acute scrotum: Current emergency management. *Eur J Emerg Med.* 2016;23(3):160–165.

RESOURCES

American Cancer Society—Testicular Cancer
    https://www.cancer.org/cancer/testicular-cancer.html
Erectile Dysfunction—WebMD
    https://www.webmd.com/erectile-dysfunction/default.htm

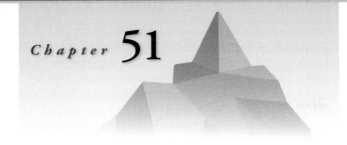

Chapter 51

Sexually Transmitted Infections

Kimberly Rae Gould, DNP, RN, FNP-BC

Debera J. Thomas, DNS, RN, FNP/ANP

Brian Oscar Porter, MD, PhD, MPH, MBA

Sexually transmitted infections (STIs) in men and women are caused by viruses, bacteria, and parasites and can occur in the throat, eyes, anal and perianal areas, external genitalia, vestibular glands, vagina, cervix, uterus, or adnexa. Sexually transmitted infections are spread through sexual intercourse or intimate person-to-person contact. An STI typically occurs when the mucous membranes of these areas are exposed to specific pathogens. Common STIs include herpes simplex virus (HSV), human immunodeficiency virus (HIV), human papillomavirus (HPV), *Chlamydia trachomatis*, *Neisseria gonorrhoeae*, *Trichomonas vaginalis*, and *Treponema pallidum* (the causative agent of syphilis). Less common STIs include chancroid (*Haemophilus ducreyi*), donovanosis or granuloma inguinale (*Klebsiella granulomatis*), mycoplasma genitalium, and lymphogranuloma venereum. In addition, hepatitis B virus (HBV), hepatitis C virus (HCV), molluscum contagiosum, pediculosis pubis, scabies, and methicillin-resistant *Staphylococcus aureus* are known to be transmitted through sexual contact. Some common vaginal infections, such as Candida infections and bacterial vaginosis (BV), may be related to sexual activity by causing a change in the vaginal pH. However, they are not considered sexually transmitted infections (STIs). Table 51.1 presents the causative pathogens for common STIs.

EPIDEMIOLOGY AND CAUSES

STIs are the most prevalent communicable diseases in the United States after upper respiratory infections, and the number of STI cases continues to increase. The Centers for Disease Control and Prevention (CDC) estimates the number of STI cases in the United States at 110 million, with 20 million new infections each year and an annual cost burden exceeding $16 billion. The most common STI is genital HPV, which infects approximately 45% of men and 39% of women between the ages of 18 and 59 years. Chlamydia is the most commonly reported STI, followed by gonorrhea and syphilis. Annually, there are an estimated 1.5 million new cases of chlamydia, 400,000 new cases of gonorrhea, and 24,000 new cases of syphilis.

STIs disproportionally affect adolescents and young adults between the ages of 15 and 24 years, primarily because of increased sexual encounters and risk-taking behaviors. This age-group accounts for 25% of the sexually active population and 50% of all new STIs. High-risk groups also include men who have sex with men and racial minorities. Overall, it is estimated that one in five Americans is infected with an STI other than HIV, indicating the risk is high in all age-groups. Perhaps even more alarming is that the United States has the highest STI rate of any nation in the industrialized world, despite being one of the most educated populations and having the highest standard of living.

Four common STIs (chlamydia, gonorrhea, syphilis, and trichomonas) can be treated with antibiotics and cured. Viral STIs (e.g., HSV, HPV, HIV), although chronic, can be treated and managed. Untreated or inadequately treated STIs can cause serious health issues in men and women. In women, mucopurulent cervicitis can result from infection with multiple organisms, including chlamydia, gonorrhea, syphilis, and genital herpes. Untreated, this condition can lead to ascending infection and affect the uterus, fallopian tubes, and ovaries. This more advanced infection, called pelvic inflammatory disease (PID), causes inflammation and formation of scar tissue in the genitourinary tract, which can result in a higher risk of miscarriage, ectopic pregnancy, and infertility. BV and trichomoniasis are also risk factors for preterm delivery of low-birth-weight infants. In men, untreated chlamydia, gonorrhea, and trichomoniasis can cause asymptomatic urethritis, epididymitis, and prostatitis and lead to disseminated gonococcal infection. Chronic inflammation of the prostate can also occur, leading to an increased risk of prostate cancer. In both men and women, untreated syphilis may lead to a tertiary form of infection that can cause serious injury to the central nervous system (CNS), aortitis, and nodular granulomatous lesions on the skin, bone, and solid organs known as gummas.

HPV is the most common virus-caused STI. There are more than 100 serotypes of HPV and 40 of them can infect the genitalia. Of these 40, 13 serotypes are considered high risk for further disease complications. High-risk HPV serotypes can be oncogenic, and persistent infection can progress to cancers of the genital tract, such as cervical, vaginal, and penile cancer. Infection with low-risk HPV serotypes causes genital warts on male and female genitalia, but although unsightly, they generally do not pose a serious health risk, unless bulky growth in immunocompromised hosts is complicated by significant bleeding.

The most serious viral STI is HIV. Left untreated, HIV will progress to AIDS over a period of 2 to 10 years, destroying the immune system and leading to increasing numbers of opportunistic fatal infections of the lungs, skin, genitourinary tract, and CNS. Both HIV and AIDS are discussed further in Chapter 63.

PATHOPHYSIOLOGY

Given the length of the male urethra and relatively small area of exposed mucosa at the urethral meatus, men have traditionally been thought to be less susceptible to STIs. However, microabrasions in the outer skin of the penile shaft sustained during sexual activity serve as entry points for sexually transmitted organisms to penetrate the skin barrier. The female reproductive tract is naturally protected from infection by several mechanisms, including a low acidic pH resulting from vaginal secretions and the presence of commensal nonpathogenic microbial flora, namely hydrogen peroxide–producing *Lactobacillus*. The normal flora of the vagina environmentally competes and provides protection against the overgrowth of potentially pathogenic anaerobic and gram-negative bacteria. Alterations of the vaginal pH can occur from hormonal influences, aging, douching, antibiotic use, exposure to semen, existing infections, and underlying diseases such as diabetes. These pH changes disrupt the natural balance

(Text continued on page 785)

TABLE 51.1 Sexually Transmitted Infections

Pathogen	Clinical Presentation	Diagnostic Reasoning	CDC Treatment Recommendations (2015)
Chancroid *Haemophilus ducreyi*	Painful, irregularly shaped, deep red ulcer with red halo and undermined edges. Found on the penis, labia, fourchette, and vaginal walls. Painful inguinal adenopathy with buboes. Females may have multiple lesions and may be asymptomatic.	Risk factors: coinfection with HIV, HSV, or syphilis. Test patients for HIV at time of diagnosis. Definitive diagnosis is obtained with culture (no FDA-approved PCR test available in United States).	Azithromycin 1 g orally single dose OR Ceftriaxone 250-mg intramuscular injection single dose OR Ciprofloxacin 500 mg orally twice a day for 3 days OR Erythromycin base 500 mg orally four times a day for 7 days
LGV *Chlamydia trachomatis*	Primary lesion: small painless erosion that heals quickly Inguinal stage: inguinal lymphadenopathy; may have headache, fever, and polymyalgia Late stage: anorectal swelling, perirectal abscesses, fistulae, swelling and ulcerations on labia	Risk factors: history of travel and sexual contact in endemically infected area. Diagnosis is confirmed with serological LGV complement fixation test; suspect if titer above 1:16 and diagnostic if titer above 1:64.	Doxycycline 100 mg orally twice a day for 21 days OR Erythromycin base 500 mg orally four times a day for 21 days.
Granuloma inguinale (donovanosis) *Klebsiella granulomatis*	Initial papule progresses into a painless, broad, superficial ulcer with clean, sharp rolled edges; may spread to inguinal folds. Lesion may be friable. Genital edema may occur. Late development of perianal fistulae and abscesses.	Risk factors: history of travel and sexual contact in endemically infected area. Diagnosis: Cannot be cultured; most reliable diagnostic method is direct visualization of Donovan bodies (i.e., rod-shaped, oval bacteria in the cytoplasm of mononuclear phagocytes or histiocytes) on stained tissue samples.	Azithromycin 1 g orally weekly for 3 weeks or 500 mg daily for 3 weeks OR Doxycycline 100 mg orally twice a day for 3 weeks OR Ciprofloxacin 750 mg orally twice a day for 3 weeks OR Trimethoprim-sulfamethoxazole 160 mg/800 mg one tablet orally twice a day for 3 weeks OR Erythromycin base 500 mg orally twice a day for 4 weeks

TABLE 51.1 Sexually Transmitted Infections—cont'd

Pathogen	Clinical Presentation	Diagnostic Reasoning	CDC Treatment Recommendations (2015)
Genital HSV	Multiple painful vesicular or ulcerated lesions that may last 12 days in the initial outbreak or 4–5 days in recurrent outbreaks. Flu-like symptoms (common with first outbreak), adenopathy, and tingling at the site before outbreak.	NAAT (PCR assays for HSV DNA) Type-specific serology testing is available and useful when developing plan of care.	First episode: Acyclovir 400 mg orally three times a day for 7–10 days OR Acyclovir 200 mg orally five times per day for 7–10 days OR Valacyclovir 1 g orally twice a day for 7–10 days OR Famciclovir 250 mg orally three times a day for 7–10 days Recurrent episodes: Acyclovir regimens 400 mg orally three time a day for 5 days 800 mg orally twice a day for 5 days 800 mg orally three times a day for 2 days OR Valacyclovir regimens 500 mg orally twice a day for 3 days 1 g orally once a day for 5 days OR Famciclovir regimens 125 mg orally twice a day for 5 days 1 g orally twice a day for 1 day 500 mg orally once and then 250 mg orally twice a day for × 2 days Suppression therapy: Acyclovir 400 mg orally twice a day OR Valacyclovir 500 mg orally once a day OR Valacyclovir 1 g orally once a day OR Famciclovir 250 mg orally twice a day Evaluate after 1 year for recurrent episodes.
Molluscum contagiosum *Poxvirus*	Usually asymptomatic Pearly, raised, painless, flesh-colored lesions (mollusca) with umbilicated (dimpled) centers; may be diffuse or singular; may be self-limited	Diagnosis is based on visual inspection of characteristic lesions.	No treatment; lesions may last months to years and often heal spontaneously. Once healed, the patient has lifetime immunity to the virus. Physical treatments to remove lesions, such as cryotherapy or curettage, may be considered in extreme cases or for lesions in unsightly areas, but these methods may lead to scarring.

Continued

TABLE 51.1 Sexually Transmitted Infections—cont'd

Pathogen	*Clinical Presentation*	*Diagnostic Reasoning*	*CDC Treatment Recommendations (2015)*
Syphilis *Treponema pallidum*	Primary: painless ulcer at initial site of contact (chancre), adenopathy Secondary: maculopapular rash on the palms and soles, flu-like symptoms, mucocutaneous lesions, lymphadenopathy Tertiary/late: cardiac, neurologic, ophthalmic, auditory, and gummatous lesions	Risk factors: test all patients for HIV and other common STIs. Definitive diagnosis: dark-field microscopy positive for spirochetes. Presumptive diagnosis: 1. Nontreponemal test (VDRL or RPR) 2. Confirmation with treponemal test (e.g., FTA-ABS, TP-PA)	Treatment is driven by staging. Primary and secondary or early latent (<1 year since infection): Benzathine PCN G 2.4 million units intramuscularly one time If PCN allergy: Doxycycline 100 mg orally twice a day for 14 days OR Tetracycline 500 mg orally four times a day for 14 days OR Ceftriaxone 1 g intramuscularly or intravenously daily for 8–10 days Late latent, latent of unknown duration, or tertiary with normal cerebrovascular fluid examination: Benzathine penicillin B 2.4 units intramuscularly once a week for 3 doses If PCN allergy: Tetracycline 400 mg orally four times a day for 4 weeks OR Doxycycline 100 mg orally twice a day for 4 weeks Neurosyphilis and ocular syphilis: Aqueous crystalline penicillin G 3–4 million units intravenously every 4 hours for 10–14 days (or continuous infusion). Alternate therapy if compliance is assured: Procaine penicillin 2.4 million units intramuscularly daily PLUS Probenecid 500 mg orally four times a day for 10-14 days If PCN allergy: Desensitize and treat with penicillin as above OR Ceftriaxone 2 g intramuscularly/intravenously once a day for 10–14 days
Trichomoniasis *Trichomonas vaginalis*	Most infected persons have minimal or no symptoms. Some infected women may have diffuse, frothy, malodorous, or yellow-green discharge and vulvar irritation. Infected men may have symptoms of urethritis, epididymitis, or prostatitis.	Vaginal pH >5; cervical smear wet mount shows motile protozoa and WBCs. Strawberry cervix may rarely be noted on examination. NAAT is highly sensitive: APTIMA *T. vaginalis* assay, amplified DNA Assay. In men, obtain penile-meatal swab. Rapid testing is available.	Metronidazole 2 g orally for one dose OR Tinidazole 2 g orally for one dose OR Metronidazole 500 mg orally twice a day for 7 days Avoid alcohol consumption during treatment with metronidazole.

TABLE 51.1 Sexually Transmitted Infections—cont'd

Pathogen	Clinical Presentation	Diagnostic Reasoning	CDC Treatment Recommendations (2015)
Urethritis *Neisseria gonorrhoeae* (most common) Nongonococcal Urethritis (NGU) *Chlamydia trachomatis,* *Mycoplasma genitalium*	May be asymptomatic Dysuria, urethral pruritus, mucoid or purulent discharge	Microscopic examination of urethral secretions will show WBCs and GNID or MB/GV purple intracellular diplococci. Test all patients for *C. trachomatis*; test men with NGU for HIV and syphilis. In men, complications of NGU include epididymitis, prostatitis, and reactive arthritis. No FDA-approved test for *M. genitalium.*	Treat with drug regimens recommended for *N. gonorrhoeae* and *C. trachomatis.* *M. genitalium* responds better to azithromycin than doxycycline.
Gonorrhea *Neisseria gonorrhoeae*	Usually asymptomatic. Partner may have an infection, requiring treatment. Women may report purulent, yellow, or green vaginal discharge; bleeding or pain with intercourse; and pelvic pain; may have inflammation of Skene's and Bartholin's glands. Men may report inflammation of the urethra, discharge, and dysuria.	Gonococcal culture and NAAT Women: endocervical swab Men: urethral swab	Primary therapy: Ceftriaxone 250 mg intramuscularly for one dose PLUS Azithromycin 1 g orally for one dose Alternative therapy (less effective): Cefixime 400 mg orally for one dose PLUS Azithromycin 1 g orally for one dose If azithromycin allergy: Doxycycline 100 mg orally twice a day for 7 days AND test of cure in 1 week. Follow CDC guidelines for complicated or refractory gonorrhea; consider EPT.
Chlamydia *Chlamydia trachomatis*	Asymptomatic infection is common in men and women. Women may report dysuria and mucopurulent vaginal discharge. Men may report purulent urethral discharge, dysuria, or pain/swelling of testicle(s).	NAAT Women: vaginal swab Men: urethral or rectal swab or first-catch urine specimen	Primary therapy: Azithromycin 1 g orally in a single dose OR Doxycycline 100 mg orally twice a day for 7 days Alternate therapy: Erythromycin base 500 mg orally four times a day for 7 days OR Ofloxacin 300 mg orally twice a day for 7 days OR Levofloxacin 500 mg orally once a day for 7 days

Continued

TABLE 51.1 Sexually Transmitted Infections—cont'd

Pathogen	Clinical Presentation	Diagnostic Reasoning	CDC Treatment Recommendations (2015)
HPV May infect the urethra, penis, groin, scrotum, vulva, perineum, external anus, and perianal area, including anogenital warts	Lesions are usually asymptomatic. Men and women may report itching or pain, depending on location. External warts are flat, papular or pedunculated lesions, single or multiple, and of varying sizes.	Risk factors: Early sexual debut, multiple sex partners. Diagnosis by visual inspection is based on characteristics of lesion. Cervical and intravaginal lesions are identified during colposcopy following an abnormal Pap test or a normal Pap test in the presence of high-risk HPV serotype infection.	Preventive: Gardasil, Gardasil 9, or Cervarix HPV vaccine times three doses Patient-applied: Podofilox 0.5% solution or gel applied twice daily three times per week for weeks OR Imiquimod 3.75% or 5% cream applied at bedtime three times per week for 16 weeks OR Sinecatechins 15% ointment applied three times a day for 16 weeks Provider-administered: Cryotherapy with liquid nitrogen or cryoprobe, repeated every 1–2 weeks OR Surgical removal by excision, curettage, laser, or electrosurgery OR TCA or BCA 80%–90% solution applied weekly Alternate therapy for external genital warts: Podophyllin resin 10%–25% in compound tincture of benzoin applied to each wart; may repeat weekly; strict application guidelines for provider-administered therapy must be followed.
HIV	Initial presentation of acute retroviral syndrome with fever, malaise, adenopathy, and maculopapular rash may occur. HIV: Malaise, headache, lymphadenopathy, gastritis, weight losws, bloody diarrhea, vaginal infections, thrush. AIDS: Encephalitis, meningitis, blindness, *Pneumocystis* pneumonia, tuberculosis, skin cancer.	Positive enzyme-linked immunosorbent assay is confirmed by positive Western blot.	Treat concurrent STIs and opportunistic infections as recommended by CDC; refer to specialist. Offer long-term counseling and management. HAART is key for the treatment of HIV; initiation of therapy is a function of T-cell count, viral load, and concurrent symptoms. Treatment is heavily influenced by the ability to comply with treatment regimens.

Abbreviations: AIDS, acquired immunodeficiency syndrome; BCA, bichloracetic acid; BV, bacterial vaginosis; CDC, Centers for Disease Control and Prevention; EPT, expedited partner therapy; FDA, U.S. Food and Drug Administration; FTA-ABS, fluorescent treponemal antibody absorption; GNID, gram-negative intracellular diplococci; HAART, highly active antiretroviral therapy; HIV, human immunodeficiency virus; HSV, herpes simplex virus; LGV, lymphogranuloma venereum; MB/GV, methylene blue/gentian violet; NAAT, nuclear antigen amplification test; NGU, nongonococcal urethritis; PCN, penicillin; PCR, polymerase chain reaction; PCT, polymerase chain reaction; RPR, rapid plasma reagin; STI, sexually transmitted infection; TP-PA, *Treponema pallidum* passive particle agglutination assay; TCA, trichloroacetic acid; VDRL, Venereal Disease Research Laboratory; WBCs, white blood cells.

of microbial flora and predispose the reproductive track to infection. Susceptibility is also influenced by aging and the presence of an existing infection. The incidence of chlamydia and HPV infections is higher in young women because the squamocolumnar junction, a vulnerable area for infection, is prominent on the ectocervix. In contrast, older women are more prone to infection secondary to drying and thinning of the vaginal and vulvar tissue.

In both sexes, the presence of one STI increases the risk of becoming infected with another—especially HIV. This is likely due to compromise of mucosal and outer skin barriers, as well as cellular and immune responses. The infectious organisms themselves may also express virulence factors that allow growth and colonization of opportunistic pathogens.

STIs also affect other areas of the body and may occur through nonsexual contact as well. Gonococcal pharyngitis can occur following receptive oral intercourse, and chlamydial conjunctivitis can be contracted by newborns during birth by passage through the birth canal. Women with HIV, HSV, and syphilis can transmit these diseases to a fetus during pregnancy and to infants via breastfeeding. HSV can also be transmitted to a newborn during birth. Less frequent modes of transmission include exposure to contaminated needles, surgical instruments, blood transfusions, and organ donation.

CLINICAL PRESENTATION

Subjective

According to the World Health Organization, most STIs have no symptoms or have symptoms that are so mild that they are not recognized as an STI. Genital warts caused by HPV infection and the chancre that occurs in the initial stage of syphilis are both painless lesions that usually resolve on their own but are, nevertheless, still infectious. The failure to recognize and treat infections early may worsen the course of the disease in men and women. In women, symptoms of chlamydia and gonorrhea may not present until PID develops, and men may develop prostatitis after an asymptomatic infection. Men and women who experience symptoms may report either a painful or painless lesion on the penis or vulva that is vesicular or ulcerated. Lymph node swelling, abnormal vaginal or penile discharge, abdominal or pelvic pain, dysuria, itching, and dyspareunia may also be noted. Women may also report abnormal vaginal bleeding. In advanced infections, fever, chills, and back pain can be present.

Objective

Examination of the female patient includes inspection of the external genitalia, anal and perianal areas,

urethra, and vestibular glands (Skene's glands and Bartholin's glands). In the male patient, the penis, glans, urethra, scrotum, and anal area are inspected. A finding of erythema, inflammation, or a lesion may indicate the presence of a STI. A primary syphilitic lesion, called a chancre, may manifest as a red bump that eventually indurates and ulcerates. A HPV lesion may appear warty, and HSV lesions may be vesicular.

A speculum examination should be done to inspect the vaginal tissue and cervix and to look for the presence of discharge or bleeding. Normal vaginal discharge is clear or white. Odorous, purulent, and colored discharge is found in BV, chlamydia, gonorrhea, and trichomonas. A finding of pain when the cervix is moved with a gloved finger (cervical motion tenderness) may indicate PID. A bimanual examination should be done to assess uterine size, mobility, and tenderness, as well as to assess for adnexal masses or tenderness.

In men, the testes, epididymis, and lower abdomen should be palpated, and if prostatitis is suspected, a digital rectal examination should be done to assess the prostate. The presence of urethral discharge or swelling and tenderness of the testes may indicate infection caused by chlamydia and gonorrhea. In either sex, the presence of pink or red maculopapular, pustular, or nodular skin lesions should raise suspicion for syphilis. Table 51.1 presents the clinical presentation for common STIs.

DIAGNOSTIC REASONING

Diagnostic Tests

Testing for STIs may be done to obtain a diagnosis or for screening purposes. Choosing the correct screening tests is based on the patient's age, sexual behavior, symptomatology, physical examination findings, and prevalence of infection in the community. Co-infections are common, and it may be necessary to test for more than one infection in some patients. High-risk sexual behaviors that result in syphilis, gonorrhea, or herpes also put the patient at risk for infection with HIV. Similarly, patients with HIV are at risk for acquiring all other STIs.

Screening for STIs is recommended for specific conditions and age-groups. The U.S. Preventive Services Task Force (USPSTF) recommends annual screening for chlamydia, gonorrhea, HIV, and syphilis in all nonpregnant women with high-risk sexual behaviors, as well as screening for chlamydia and gonorrhea in all sexually active women younger than 25 years. All pregnant women should be screened for HBV, HIV, and syphilis. In addition, pregnant women younger than 25 years or those engaged in high-risk behaviors should also be screened for chlamydia and gonorrhea. Screening for cervical cancer should begin at age 21 years, and specific screening for high-risk HPV serotypes begins at age 30 years.

Men engaging in high-risk behaviors should be screened for HIV and syphilis, and all persons diagnosed with syphilis, chancroid, or HSV should be screened for HIV because these infections increase the risk of acquiring and transmitting HIV. The USPSTF recommends HIV screening for everyone aged 15 to 65 years of age.

Methods available to test for STIs include microscopy, culture, and nucleic acid amplification testing (NAAT). Testing may be laboratory based or done at the point of care (POC). The choice of testing method will depend on the availability of equipment, cost, and the training and experience of available personnel. Currently, NAAT testing is U.S. Food and Drug Administration–approved for the detection of chlamydia, trichomonas, HSV, HBV, HCV, HPV, HIV, and gonorrhea, with some exceptions. If gonorrhea is suspected in the oropharynx, conjunctiva, or rectum, a culture should be done. Not all laboratory-based or POC tests offer optimal specificity, and some tests (e.g., for HIV and syphilis) require supplemental testing for confirmation. Practitioners should be familiar with the specificity and sensitivity of each test used in their practice, and treatment decisions should always be clinically correlated with findings on history and physical examination. Table 51.1 presents diagnostic reasoning and treatment for common STIs and vulvovaginal infections.

Differential Diagnosis

Following a comprehensive assessment, all subjective and objective findings are considered when developing differential diagnoses for the patient presenting with a suspected STI. A differential list may include contact dermatitis, psoriasis, lichen sclerosis, vulvodynia, urinary tract infection, renal calculi, PID, endometriosis, pregnancy, pelvic abscess, ovarian torsion, ectopic pregnancy, appendicitis, toxic shock syndrome, atrophic vaginitis, trauma, and presence of a foreign body in the genitourinary tract.

MANAGEMENT

Management goals include making a correct diagnosis, prescribing appropriate treatment, and providing education that focuses on prevention of reinfection and implementation of risk-reducing behaviors. Treatment should follow the guidelines issued by the CDC in 2015.

Prevention of reinfection largely depends on the concurrent treatment of intimate partners and the use of barrier protection during sexual contact. Patients with chlamydia and gonorrhea must be queried about

the sexual partners they have had in the preceding 60 days, and all efforts should be made to ensure treatment of these partner(s). The timeline for partner assessment of those with syphilis depends on the duration of symptoms and the stage at diagnosis (primary, secondary, or tertiary). Partners in the preceding 3 to 12 months will typically require notification and treatment.

Although limited to heterosexual individuals in current CDC guidance, expedited partner therapy (EPT) is considered a useful option to prevent reinfection. EPT is legal in most states and allows the practitioner to treat partners of patients with chlamydia and gonorrhea by giving the partner's prescription to the patient, if the practitioner cannot be reasonably sure the partner(s) will seek treatment. Data on the effectiveness of EPT with same-sex partners are limited, and concern about untreated concurrent infections (such as HIV) has prevented EPT from being extended to same-sex partners. In some states, EPT can also be used to treat partners of patients with trichomoniasis. Of note, because the recommended treatment for gonorrhea is intramuscularly injected ceftriaxone plus oral azithromycin, EPT cannot be ideally applied because partner prescriptions can only be given for oral medications. However, as of 2016, the CDC endorses EPT for gonorrhea in heterosexual partners because the risk of untreated partner infection is greater than the risk associated with suboptimal oral cephalosporin treatment. Table 51.1 presents current treatment recommendations for common STIs and vulvovaginal infections.

FOLLOW-UP AND REFERRAL

Routinely testing for cure is not recommended for most patients with chlamydia and gonorrhea when approved protocols are used. However, it is advisable to test for cure if symptoms persist, treatment compliance is a concern, there is risk of reinfection, or an alternative and less effective treatment regimen was used (e.g., an oral cephalosporin for gonorrhea). If compliance is a concern, treating the patient during the office visit should be considered. Because of high reinfection rates with trichomoniasis, testing for reinfection is recommended at 3 months.

Practitioners are required to report certain STIs to their state health department. Although state guidelines differ, the following currently require reporting in all states: HIV, AIDS, syphilis, gonorrhea, chancroid, and chlamydia. In some states, the testing laboratory and practitioner are responsible for completion of the reporting documentation. The practitioner is responsible for reporting the date of diagnosis, type of treatment, pregnancy status, and partner treatment and notification.

Patient Education: Sexually Transmitted Infections

Educating patients about risk-reducing behavior is paramount in decreasing overall morbidity and mortality associated with STIs. Effective education should emphasize prevention and result in behavioral changes that reduce the risk of contracting and spreading STIs. Primary prevention behaviors include HBV and HPV vaccination, using condoms 100% of the time, delaying sexual debut, and limiting the number of sexual partners. Secondary prevention measures include cervical cancer screening beginning at 21 years of age and STI screening in patients with high-risk behaviors, in women younger than 25 years, and during pregnancy. Teaching patients the importance of medication compliance, reinforcing the need for partner treatment, and discussing the risk of reinfection are examples of tertiary prevention. Patients should be assessed for such risks at each visit.

Due to the chronicity of viral STIs (e.g., HPV, HSV, HBV, HCV, and HIV), affected patients need education, counseling, and compassionate care. Discussing the expected course of the illness, remission and progression potential, management of outbreaks, and prevention of transmission are topics that should be presented and reinforced over the course of multiple visits. Patients may benefit from individual or group counseling, involvement in support groups, more frequent office visits, media-based educational interventions, and age-appropriate literature.

For additional resources please visit
https://davisedge.fadavis.com/

REFERENCES

Bowen VB, Torrone EA, Peterman TA. Verifying treatment of reported cases of gonorrhea. *Sex Transm Dis.* 2016;43(2):130–133.

Caini S, Gandini S, Dudas M, Bremer V, Severi E, Gherasim A. Sexually transmitted infections and prostate cancer risk: Systematic review and meta-analysis. *Cancer Epidemiol.* 2014;38(4):329–338.

Centers for Disease Control and Prevention. Recommendations for the laboratory-based detection of *Chlamydia trachomatis* and *Neisseria gonorrheae*. *MMWR Morb Mortal Wkly Rep.* 2014;63(2):1–16.

Centers for Disease Control and Prevention. Sexually transmitted diseases treatment guidelines. *MMWR Morb Mortal Wkly Rep.* 2015;64(3):1–137.

Clement ME, Okeke NL, Hicks CB. Treatment of syphilis: A systematic review. *JAMA.* 2014;312(18):1905–1917.

Fleming E, Hogben M. Assessing different partner notification methods for assuring partner treatment for gonorrhea: Looking for the best mix of options. *J Public Health Manag Pract.* 2017;23(3):247–254.

Klein J, McLaud M, Rogers D. Syphilis on the rise: diagnosis, treatment, and prevention. *J Nurse Pract.* 2015;11(1):49–55.

Lamont RF, Keelan JA, Larsson PG, Jorgensen JS. The treatment of bacterial vaginosis in pregnancy with clindamycin to reduce the risk of infection-related preterm birth: A response to the Danish Society of Obstetrics and Gynecology guideline group's clinical recommendations. *Acta Obstet Gynecol Scand.* 2017;96(2):139–143.

Peterman TA, Newman RR, Maddox L, Schmitt K, Shiver S. Risk of HIV following a diagnosis of syphilis, gonorrhea or chlamydia: 328,456 women in Florida, 2000–2011. *Int J STD AIDS.* 2015;26(2):113–119.

Phillippi JC, Latendresse GA. Sexually transmitted infections. In: McCance KL, Huether, SE eds. *Pathophysiology: The Biologic Basis for Disease in Adults and Children.* 7th ed. St. Louis, MO: Mosby/Elsevier; 2014:918–944.

Tan H, Fu Y, Yang C, Ma, J. Effects of metronidazole combined probiotics over metronidazole alone for the treatment of bacterial vaginosis: A meta-analysis of randomized clinical trials. *Arch Gynecol Obstet.* 2017;295(6):1331–1339.

Unemo M. Editor in chief. Ballard, R, Ison C, Lewis D, Ndowa F, Peeling R. Laboratory diagnosis of sexually transmitted infections, including human immunodeficiency virus. Geneva, Switzerland: World Health Organization, Department of Reproductive Health and Research; 2013.

RESOURCES

Centers for Disease Control and Prevention (Expedited Partner Therapy Guidance)
https://www.cdc.gov/std/ept/default.htm

U.S. Preventive Services Task Force
https://www.uspreventiveservicestaskforce.org/

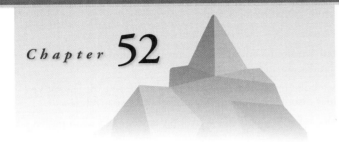

Chapter **52**

Common Musculoskeletal Complaints

Patricia Vanhook, PhD, MSN, APRN, FNP-BC, FAAN, FAANP

Lynne M. Dunphy, PhD, APRN, FNP-BC, FAAN, FAANP

Brian Oscar Porter, MD, PhD, MPH, MBA

Lori Martin-Plank, PhD, APRN, FNP-BC, GNP-BC, FAANP

Conor Luskin, PA-C

OVERVIEW

Musculoskeletal pain and dysfunction are some of the most common reasons for visits to a primary-care provider. Because of the complex nature of these problems and the variable differential diagnoses involved, the actual number of people affected is difficult to ascertain with true accuracy. Musculoskeletal problems in general are the most frequent cause of disability in workers, and population surveys show a greater than 50% prevalence of musculoskeletal disorders among older Americans.

Acute musculoskeletal complaints are generally self-limiting. However, some conditions, if left untreated, can lead to a cycle of progressive joint instability and a higher risk of subsequent injury if recovery is not complete. It is essential to rule out any musculoskeletal emergencies (see Table 52.1; see Chapter 73 for assessment of musculoskeletal emergencies). Delayed recognition of certain diagnoses may lead to permanent disability or death. Once these diagnoses have been excluded, proceed with an orderly evaluation of other diagnostic possibilities.

Musculoskeletal complaints can be a diagnostic challenge for the primary-care provider. There are no routine tests that can be employed in clinical practice to determine the presence of inflammation or muscle spasm. Much of the diagnosis is dependent on patient's self-reporting of symptoms. An accurate patient history and clinician knowledge of underlying anatomy and physiology of the musculoskeletal system are essential keys to a correct diagnosis. A useful approach to the initial patient encounter is to determine whether the musculoskeletal complaint is:

- Acute or chronic in duration.
- Articular or nonarticular in origin.
- Inflammatory or noninflammatory in nature.
- Localized or systemic in distribution.

Many musculoskeletal disorders resemble each other at onset, and some may take time to evolve into an identifiable diagnosis. Differential diagnoses of musculoskeletal problems include trauma, infection, metabolic or circulatory disorders, tumors, synovial conditions, congenital or developmental problems, or degenerative disorders.

Identifying the anatomical location of the musculoskeletal complaint is important. The primary-care provider should first distinguish between articular and nonarticular structures (see Box 52.1). Articular structures include the synovium, synovial fluid, articular cartilage, intra-articular ligaments, joint capsule, and juxta-articular bone. Disorders of these structures are characterized by deep or diffuse pain, limited range of motion (ROM) on active and passive movement, swelling (caused by synovial proliferation, effusion, or bony enlargement), crepitation, instability, "locking," or deformity. Nonarticular (or periarticular) structures are identified as supportive extra-articular ligaments, tendons, bursae, muscle, fascia, bone, nerve, and overlying skin. Nonarticular disorders are characterized by painful and active but not passive ROM, point or focal tenderness in regions distinct from articular structures, and physical findings far from the joint capsule. Crepitus, instability, or deformity is not likely to be associated with these disorders.

Inflammatory disorders may be infectious or idiopathic. These are identified by the presence of all or some of the four cardinal signs of inflammation (erythema, warmth, pain, or swelling); systemic symptoms (fatigue, weight loss, morning stiffness, fever); or laboratory evidence of inflammation (elevated erythrocyte sedimentation rate [ESR] or C-reactive protein [CRP], anemia of chronic disease, hypoalbuminemia, or thrombocytosis). Noninflammatory disorders tend to be related to trauma (meniscus tear), ineffective repair (osteoarthritis [OA]), neoplasm, or pain amplification (fibromyalgia).

TABLE 52.1 Musculoskeletal Emergencies

Clinical Manifestations	Musculoskeletal Emergencies: Differential Diagnoses
History	
Significant trauma	Soft-tissue injury, internal derangement, fracture
Constitutional signs and symptoms (fever, weight loss, malaise)	Infection, sepsis, systemic rheumatic disease
Hot, swollen, painful joint	Infection, systemic rheumatic disease, gout, pseudogout
Physical Examination	
Weakness	
Focal	Compartment syndrome, entrapment neuropathy, mononeuritis, motor neuron disease, radiculopathy
Diffuse	Myositis, metabolic myopathy, paraneoplastic syndrome, degenerative neuromuscular disorder, toxin, myelopathy, transverse myelitis
Neurogenic pain (burning, numbness, paresthesia) Asymmetrical	Radiculopathy, reflex sympathetic dystrophy, entrapment neuropathy
Symmetrical	Myelopathy, peripheral neuropathy
Claudication pain pattern	Peripheral vascular disease, giant cell arteritis (with jaw pain), lumbar spinal stenosis

---

Box 52.1 Comparison of Articular and Nonarticular Structures

Articular Structures	Nonarticular Structures
Synovium and synovial fluid	Supportive extra-articular ligaments
Articular cartilage, intra-articular ligaments	Bone
Joint capsule	Nerve, overlying skin
Juxta-articular bone	Muscle, tendons, fascia

Box 52.2 Examples of Disorders of Inflammation Versus Noninflammation

Inflammatory Musculoskeletal Disorders	Noninflammatory Musculoskeletal Disorders
Infectious	Ineffective repair (osteoarthritis)
Crystal induced	Pain amplification (fibromyalgia)
Immune related (rheumatoid arthritis, systemic lupus erythematosus)	Trauma
Idiopathic	Neoplasm

There may be pain without swelling or warmth, absence of inflammatory or systemic features, minimal or absent morning stiffness, and normal (for age) laboratory testing (see Box 52.2).

The differential diagnoses may be narrowed by the identification of the underlying pathological process and the exact site of the complaint. These help to determine whether there is need for immediate diagnostic or therapeutic intervention or for continued observation.

The clinical history should contain the patient profile, including age, sex, race, family history, occupational history, medications, and activities. The chronology of the complaint gives important diagnostic clues and may be divided into onset (e.g., abrupt), evolution (chronic, intermittent, migratory), and duration. The number and distribution of involved articulations should be noted. Articular disorders are classified based on the number of involved joints: monoarticular (one joint), periarticular (two to four joints), or polyarticular (more than four joints). Nonarticular disorders are classified as either focal or widespread. Precipitating events such as trauma or drug ingestion must be documented, as well as antecedent or current illnesses that may contribute to the patient's complaint. If the problem is chronic, ask the patient why he or she is addressing it now. A review of

systems may provide useful diagnostic information, eliciting systemic features of diseases such as fever (systemic lupus erythematosus [SLE], infection). Musculoskeletal complaints may be associated with other organ systems, for example, such as the nervous system (Lyme disease, vasculitis), eye (sarcoidosis, Reiter's syndrome), and gastrointestinal tract (scleroderma, inflammatory bowel disease) (see Focus on History: Musculoskeletal Problems).

Guided by the history, the physical examination helps to distinguish between mechanical problems, soft-tissue disease, and noninflammatory and inflammatory joint diseases. A major goal of the physical examination is to detect warmth over a joint, joint effusion, and pain on joint motion. These are hallmarks of synovitis. Limitations in movement and instability are also important to assess and are of concern in knee and ankle pain. The medial and lateral collateral ligaments (MCL and LCL) of the knee can be assessed by valgus and varus stress of the joint. Excess laxity of the knee on anterior drawer test or Lachman test may indicate an anterior cruciate ligament (ACL) tear.

Focus on History: Musculoskeletal Problems

Questions to ask:

1. Have you injured yourself?
2. Describe exactly how your injury occurred:
   - When the injury occurred, did it make a noise or sound? If so, describe the sound.
3. Where does it hurt? Does the pain radiate, or is it localized, or diffuse?
4. Do you have numbness or tingling?
5. Is there loss of function?
6. Is there swelling?
7. When did the pain first occur?
   - What relieves it?
   - What makes it worse?
   - What time of day does it occur?
   - Does the pain awaken you at night?
8. Is there joint stiffness?
   - Does activity make it worse or better?
9. Do you have any other symptoms (or systemic processes)?
   - Do you have a fever?
   - Do you have a rash?
   - Do you have general fatigue?
   - Have you recently been traveling or camping?
   - Have you recently been immunized?
   - Have you recently been treated with antibiotics?
   - Do you have a history of upper respiratory infection? Sexually transmitted disease? Chronic disease?
   - Were you ever treated with steroids?
10. Describe your daily activities—work, hobbies, home.

The Physical Examination

A general guide to the physical examination is provided in Advanced Assessment 52.1. The examiner should begin by inspecting the affected part, observing for side-to-side symmetry. The patient must be undressed and draped so that visual inspection can be done. The examiner should look for signs of trauma, ecchymosis, erythema, skin lesions, abrasions, lacerations, symmetry, and edema. The uninvolved side should be examined initially and compared with the involved side. The painful part should be examined last.

If the patient complains about a specific anatomical area, that area should be examined. Certain pain patterns often suggest specific diagnoses. For example, pain over the greater trochanter suggests hip trochanteric bursitis. A history of hand numbness that awakens the patient at night suggests carpal tunnel syndrome, even with no physical findings. Foot pain that begins the first thing in the morning when the patient puts his or her foot out of bed is suggestive of plantar fasciitis or early rheumatoid arthritis (RA). Crepitus (joint noises or palpable grinding during joint motion) may be due to articular surface abnormalities, meniscus tear, and arthritis. Crepitus not associated with pain or limitation of motion is generally of no clinical significance.

After the target area, if any, has been visually inspected, or if the patient reports diffuse generalized musculoskeletal pain, the next step in the physical examination is palpation. Bony enlargements of the distal interphalangeal joints or Heberden's nodes are indicative of OA, whereas soft-tissue swelling may indicate RA; inflammation may also be indicated by swelling of the metacarpophalangeal joints. Evidence of tender points and trigger points, as well as the absence of inflammation or swollen joints, increases the likelihood of a soft-tissue problem.

ROM testing is an important part of the physical examination. ROM testing measures the degree of movement of a joint or body part. Performance of ROM testing can be passive, active-assistive, or active. In passive ROM testing, the examiner moves the joint or body part; the patient does not actively participate in the movement. In active-assistive ROM testing, the examiner assists the patient in movement of the joint or body part; the patient participates in the movement but not significantly.

Two general assessments that should be included in all evaluations are to ask the patient to rise from a chair without holding on. If the patient cannot do this, there is an abnormality of the joints, nerves, or muscles, which requires further examination, usually by a specialist. The patient's gait also should be assessed by asking the patient to walk a few steps across the room.

All maneuvers described should take less than 2 minutes and should be included in the "general" physical examination. Note any endocrinopathies (irregular heart rhythms, weight gain, and thyromegaly) and possible malignancy (severe pain, weight loss, or palpable masses). Extra-articular abnormalities, such as oral/nasal ulcers; iritis; rash; nodules; pericardial or pulmonary rub; enlargement of liver, spleen, or lymph nodes; or neurologic abnormalities, suggest a systemic disease.

Diagnostic Tests

Laboratory Tests

Laboratory tests may be of limited use in true orthopedic complaints. These tests can be misleading and produce false-positive and false-negative results. For example, many people with RA have normal blood tests and x-ray findings, particularly early in the disease, when aggressive treatment might be most effective. Some tests are useful to research laboratories in the identification and understanding of pathogenic mechanisms, but do not add anything to the meaningful diagnosis and management of the patient. A review of associated laboratory tests is presented here.

- Complete blood count—the presence of anemia may be a clue to inflammation, and leukopenia is seen in active
- ESR and CRP—elevated ESR or CRP values are nonspecific indicators of inflammation. A highly elevated value indicates an increased likelihood of inflammatory rheumatic disease, infection, or malignancy. ESR

Advanced Assessment 52.1: Physical Examination for Musculoskeletal Disorders

1. Visual examination
   Does the effected extremity have any erythema, ecchymosis, overlying skin lesions, previous scars from surgery, deformities?
2. Palpation of the effected joint above and below
   Crepitus of the joint, crepitus at a fracture sight, joint effusion present, is the patient tender to palpation of the joint, soft tissues?
3. Range of motion (ROM)
   Active ROM: How the patient can move their extremity without assistance?
   Passive ROM: How you can move the patient's extremity.
   Is there a discrepancy?
4. Strength examination
   a. 0/5: no muscle twitching or movement (paralyzed limb)
   b. 1/5: muscle twitching but no movement
   c. 2/5 pt can actively move the extremity but cannot move it above gravity
   d. 3/5 pt can move the extremity against gravity
   e. 4/5 pt has weakness of the extremity but can move it against gravity
   f. 5/5 pt has full strength of their extremity
5. Joint stability
   a. Stress testing: Evaluate for increased pain and/or increased or decreased laxity relative to opposite side.
   b. Joint play: Evaluate for increased pain and/or increased or decreased mobility relative to opposite side.

6. Special tests
   Special tests are specific for certain pathologies. Examples include the following:
   a. Shoulder-Empty can test (rotator cuff), Neer/Hawkins impingement tests
   b. Knee-McMurray test (meniscus), Lachman test (anterior cruciate ligament)
   c. Cervical spine—Spurling's test (radiculopathy)
   d. Lumbar spine—straight leg/reverse straight leg raise (herniated disc)
   e. Achilles rupture—Thompson test
7. Neurovascular examination
   a. Test sensation of the extremity. Is it normal or limited?
   b. Check peripheral pulses.
      i. Upper extremity: radial pulse
      ii. Lower extremity: dorsalis pedis, posterior tibialis pulse
   c. Assess capillary refill for hand and toe injuries.
   d. Note peripheral edema.
      Grade on a scale of 0–4.
   e. Assess motor function.
      Can the patient move all their fingers and toes?
   f. Perform extremity reflex testing at the following locations to check specific spinal nerves:
      i. L4: knee
      ii. S1: Achilles tendon
      iii. C5–C6: biceps
      iv. C7: triceps

---

increases with age, as does CRP, and some people (as many as 5% to 10% of the general population) have elevated values with no explanation. Up to 40% of patients who present with RA have normal ESRs and CRPs. In patients with giant cell arteritis and polymyalgia rheumatica, the ESR is almost always markedly elevated and is therefore diagnostically useful.

- Rheumatoid factor (RF)—25% of patients with RA never have an elevated RF. This value may also be elevated with other inflammatory conditions (e.g., SLE, subacute bacterial endocarditis, vasculitis, viral infection).
- Fluorescent antinuclear antibody (ANA) test—this test is positive in 99% of patients with SLE; however, it is also positive in 5% to 10% of normal blood donors, meaning that only 1 in 100 people with a positive ANA has SLE. A positive ANA can also occur with certain drugs (procainamide, hydralazine); it may be transiently positive in people with a severe infection; and it is positive in a high percentage of people with other inflammatory rheumatic conditions, including RA (30% to 50%), scleroderma (20% to 50%), polymyositis (10% to 30%), and idiopathic pulmonary fibrosis (10% to 20%). Other antibody tests are more specific for certain inflammatory disorders.
- Lyme borreliosis antibodies—Lyme disease is identified serologically by antibodies to the Lyme *Borrelia* organism. From 5% to 10% of normal individuals

have a positive Lyme borreliosis titer, even in the best laboratories. A test for Lyme disease is not appropriate in patients with unexplained arthritis unless there are other risk factors such as living in an endemic area and frequent outdoor activities.

- Uric acid—uric acid measurement is often included in evaluation of patients with musculoskeletal symptoms because elevated uric acid is seen in more than 90% of people with gout, a condition that affects the musculoskeletal system and is often a part of the differential diagnosis. A definitive diagnosis of gout, however, requires identification of uric acid crystals in synovial fluid (see Chapter 59 for a detailed discussion of gout). Alcohol and diuretics may cause moderately elevated uric acid levels.
- Screening panels—these tests are available from all national laboratories and are marketed as "rheumatology screening panels" to rule out an inflammatory rheumatic disease. The simplest include RF, ANA, and uric acid, although more elaborate tests are available. These screens tend to be a major source of potential false-positive information in patient evaluations and are not advised for use by the general practitioner.

Imaging Tests

Imaging studies are indicated (1) when examination cannot localize the anatomical structure that is causing symptoms, (2) after a significant trauma, (3) when there is a loss of joint function (e.g., unable to bear weight), (4) when pain continues despite conservative management, (5) when a fracture or bone infection is suspected, or (6) when there is a history of malignancy. Clinicians who are unfamiliar with what views to order should contact the radiologist for guidance. The following lists common imaging studies used in the diagnosis of musculoskeletal disorders:

- *Radiography* (plain x-ray films) will be unrevealing (and are therefore not indicated) for most patients with acute and new symptoms of mechanical back pain and/ or soft-tissue disorders. For patients with typical acute mechanical low back pain, a plain radiograph adds little to the management decisions. Radiographs may confirm the diagnosis of OA and assess its severity, but normal findings on radiographs do not rule out the presence of OA. In addition, radiography can reveal the following:
  - Erosions
  - Calcifications and cysts
  - Osteopenia
  - Narrowing of joint spaces
  - Deformity of bones
  - Separations (fractures, dislocations)
- *Ultrasonography* may be useful in the detection of soft-tissue abnormalities but has limited clinical value. The foremost application of ultrasound is in the diagnosis of synovial (Baker's) cysts and other superficially prominent lesions, such as lipomas.
- *Computed tomography* (*CT*) has proved most useful in the evaluation of the axial skeleton because of its ability to visualize in the axial plane. CT is useful in the diagnosis of low back pain syndromes (herniated intervertebral disc, spinal stenosis, spinal trauma) and advanced osteonecrosis. Helical or spiral CT can be useful in the detection of obscure fractures.
- *Magnetic resonance imaging* (*MRI*) is most useful for the diagnosis of soft-tissue disorders such as muscle and tendon tears and intra-articular disorders such as labrum tears and meniscus tears, as well as spine disorders.

A bone scan may be useful when osteomyelitis, stress fractures, or bony metastases are a concern. In general, MRI is useful for assessing soft-tissue and spinal cord elements, whereas nuclear medicine studies are best for assessing bone turnover. Bone scans should not be ordered routinely in family practice. MRI should be reserved for patients who have failed conservative management of a soft-tissue disease after approximately 6 weeks.

- *Nerve conduction studies* (*EMG*) may be indicated when neurologic abnormalities or paresthesias are present in disorders such as carpel tunnel and a herniated disc.

Differential Diagnosis

Differential diagnoses of musculoskeletal problems include the following:

- Trauma
- Infection
- Metabolic or circulatory disorders
- Tumors
- Synovial conditions
- Congenital or developmental problems
- Degenerative disorders

Joint symptoms of one and up to a several joints may be due to trauma, infection, crystal-induced inflammation (gout, pseudogout), or primary inflammatory arthritis (including spondyloarthropathies and atypical presentation of RA). If both active and passive ROM are limited, soft-tissue contracture, synovitis, or a structural abnormality of the joint is possible. In acute monoarthritis, it is essential that infection of a joint be diagnosed or excluded, and this can be done only via joint aspiration and synovial fluid analysis and culture (see Advanced Assessment 52.2). Joint aspiration is usually performed by an orthopedic specialist, but this can include physician assistants and nurse practitioners with education and training. Chronic monoarticular symptoms with little or no effusion are usually from OA.

The combination of point tenderness, reduced active ROM, and preserved passive ROM suggests soft-tissue

Advanced Assessment 52.2: Synovial Fluid Analysis

	Normal	Grade I: Noninflammatory	Grade II: Inflammatory	Grade III: Infectious
Visual analysis	Clear, straw-colored	Clear or slightly bloody and turbid	Turbid	Turbid, gray, or yellow
Viscosity	Normal	Decreased	Decreased	Decreased
WBCs per mm³	30–150	<2,500	2,500–25,000	>50,000
PMNs (%)	<20	20–50	50–70	70–90
Protein (g/dL)	1–4	1–5	3–6	3–7
Examples		OA, SLE, mechanical derangement	RA, gonococcal arthritis, rheumatic fever, gout, pseudogout, Reiter's syndrome	Septic arthritis, tuberculosis

Abbreviations: OA, osteoarthritis; PMNs, polymorphonuclear leukocytes; RA, rheumatoid arthritis; SLE, systemic lupus erythematosus; WBC, white blood cell.

disorders, including bursitis, tendinitis, or muscle injury. Tendinitis and bursitis generally involve one joint region, and physical examination is usually diagnostic. Common syndromes include de Quervain's tenosynovitis, olecranon bursitis, medial and lateral epicondylitis, bicipital and rotator cuff tendinitis, rotator cuff tear, trochanteric bursitis, patellar bursitis and prepatellar bursitis, anserine bursitis, plantar fasciitis, posterior tibial tendinitis, and Achilles tendinitis.

Polyarthritis has an extensive differential diagnosis. The presence of prolonged morning stiffness, systemic symptoms, Raynaud's phenomenon, rash, or sicca symptoms and manifestations of other organ involvement suggest a rheumatic disease. The specific evaluation is guided by the clinical manifestations and should screen organ symptoms that can be involved without overt signs, such as the lung, heart, liver, kidney, and bowel, for potential involvement. Precise diagnosis and management usually requires referral.

Generalized arthralgias and/or myalgias without physical findings have an extensive differential diagnosis. Often, no definitive diagnosis is possible at the initial presentation. Common causes include fibromyalgia or polymyalgia rheumatica; viral and bacterial infections such as mononucleosis, Rocky Mountain spotted fever, and Lyme disease; an overuse syndrome (tendon strain associated with repetitive motion injuries or muscle fatigue); neuropathy; hypothyroidism; or psychogenic causes. More than one syndrome may occur concomitantly. For example, bursitis may coexist with pain from fibromyalgia. If the inflammation from the bursitis is overlooked, the patient may not receive the treatment indicated for the acute disorder. In addition, certain medications (e.g., some diuretics, some of the statin drugs, ciprofloxacin, and clofibrate [Atromid-S]) also may cause myalgia (Fig. 52.1). If the history and physical examination do not provide a diagnosis, symptomatic management and reassessment over several weeks are more productive initially than is laboratory testing or diagnostic imaging.

ACUTE MUSCULOSKELETAL INJURY

Acute muscle injury encompasses many common conditions and is characterized by acute pain of less than 6 weeks' duration. These injuries include damage to muscles, tendons, ligaments, nerves, and bursae. The most common types of injuries are as follows:

- Spasm—persistent, painful, and reversible contracture of striated muscle
- Strain—muscle injury caused by excessive tensile stress placed on a muscle that results in stiffness and decreased function

- Sprain—stretching or tearing of ligaments that occurs when a joint is forced beyond its normal anatomical range

DIFFERENTIAL DIAGNOSIS

Sprains and strains may occur in the context of a specific syndrome, such as low back pain and ankle sprain (see Differential Diagnosis 52.1). Sometimes a traumatic injury, such as from a car accident, or other significant precipitating factor, such as lifting a heavy object, may be identified as the initiating factor. In some cases, a trivial movement, such as bending over to tie a shoe or coughing, may precipitate the injury.

Differentiating between a strain and a sprain involves a careful patient history and physical examination. Patients who present with a sprain usually have some degree of swelling, pain, and disability. In severe sprains, deformity of the joint may be noted. Sprains can be classified as follows:

- A *first-degree sprain* involves stretching of ligamentous fibers.
- A *second-degree sprain* involves a tear of part of the ligament, with pain and swelling.
- A *third-degree sprain* results in complete ligamentous separation.

The patient with a sprain often has a history that includes a sudden injury or fall that resulted in acute pain and swelling that worsen over the next few hours and an inability to move the joint. Redness and bruising over the affected joint are usually noted, and both active and passive ROM of the joint are decreased, with pain usually elicited upon moving the joint. Radiographs to rule out fracture are warranted when there is an obvious deformity, bone tenderness, and inability to put weight on a joint.

In contrast, strains affect the muscles or tendons that connect a muscle to a bone. Minor strains usually do not cause swelling or redness. Patients may complain of a "pulled muscle" and are usually able to use the affected limb, although ROM may be limited.

In severe strains, the entire muscle or tendon may be torn, causing inflammation, swelling, weakness, and loss of function. Surgery may be needed to repair a torn muscle or tendon.

The primary-care provider should also be alert to the possibility of muscle strains and sprains that mimic potentially serious conditions. For example, *costochondritis*, also called *anterior chest wall syndrome*, is an inflammation of one or more costochondral junctions that manifest with chest wall pain. The pain may be sharp and acute or dull and persistent in nature. It is the most frequently occurring nontraumatic type of chest pain in adolescents and young adults. Pain is located over the costochondral and costosternal areas of the anterior chest and is caused by inflammation of the costochondral junctions manifesting

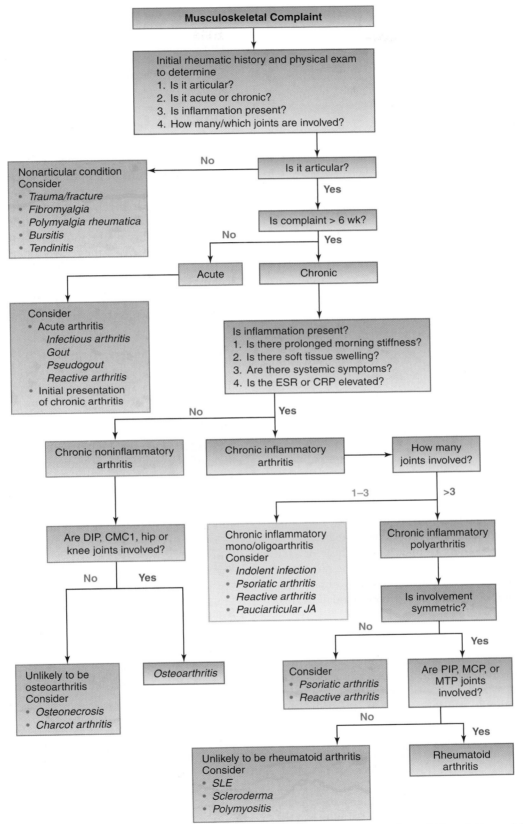

Figure 52.1 Diagnostic reasoning algorithm: articular and musculoskeletal disorders. Abbreviations: MCP, metacarpophalangeal joint; MTP, metatarsophalangeal joint; PIP, proximal interphalangeal joint; SLE, systemic lupus erythematosus. Source: *Kasper DL, et al., eds.* Harrison's principles of internal medicine. *16th ed. New York, NY: McGraw-Hill; 2005.*

✺ Differential Diagnosis 52.1: Classification of Sprains

Grade	Degree of Injury	Treatment
Grade I	Partial tear; no instability or opening of the joint on stress maneuvers	Symptomatic only
Grade II	Partial tear with some instability indicated by partial opening of the joint on stress maneuvers	Immobilization to protect injured part, but full healing expected
Grade III	Complete tear with complete opening of joint on stress	Immobilization; possible repair

only with pain in the absence of erythema, heat, or swelling. Repetitive minor trauma is currently believed to be the most likely etiology.

The following are management principles in acute musculoskeletal pain/injury not requiring emergent treatment (see Chapter 73 for emergency care and Chapter 54 for discussion of specific joint sprains):

- The acronym PRICE is commonly employed: *Pro*tect and *R*est the affected part, apply *I*ce for 48 hours, *C*ompression (Ace bandage wrap), and *E*levation.
- Reassurance—most injuries are self-limiting, and improvement should occur within approximately 2 weeks.
- Limitation of activity—immobilization of the injured area is appropriate during the diagnostic phase; if appropriate, bedrest should be limited to the most acute period (2 days or less) to control spasm and promote healing.
- Physical therapy—therapy may include heat or cold application with the goal of returning the patient to full function as soon as possible with minimal limitation. Commonly cold/ice is recommended for 48 hours, and then heat.
- Pain relief—NSAIDS are the first-line choice for pain relief. NSAIDs can be continued until symptoms have resolved. However, long-term use of NSAIDs can lead to serious gastrointestinal disease, such as ulcers, gastritis, and hemorrhage. Thus, patients with gastrointestinal histories should use these drugs cautiously. Using the lowest possible effective dose can help to prevent this problem. It is particularly important to use caution in recommending dosages for elderly patients who are more sensitive to the adverse effects of NSAIDs. This class of medicines affects renal and gastrointestinal prostaglandins and may cause fluid retention, edema, and increases in blood pressure; thus, patients should be monitored for weight gain. These problems may be significant in elderly patients and in people with congestive heart failure. *Opioids are not indicated for acute muscle injury and should be avoided.*

- Referral—the patient should be referred to an orthopedic specialist if there is no relief with conventional methods.
- Imaging studies—radiography, CT, and MRI are usually *not* indicated for acute musculoskeletal injuries.

MUSCLE CRAMPS

Muscle cramps may be described as sudden, involuntary, painful contractions of a muscle or muscle part that last from seconds to several minutes. Cramps may occur spontaneously while at rest or may be precipitated by a brief muscle contraction. The cause is usually related to hyperexcitability of the motor neurons supplying the muscles. In many cases, the reason for episodic, recurrent muscle cramps may remain unclear, even after complete diagnostic evaluation. Muscle cramps may also occur related to vigorous exercise and during sporting events and may be caused by dehydration.

DIFFERENTIAL DIAGNOSIS

The initial history should elicit whether the cramps occur with exercise or at rest. In pregnant women and children, leg cramps tend to occur at rest and are most often benign, requiring no treatment (see Differential Diagnosis 52.2). Certain medications (e.g., some diuretics, some of the statin drugs, and clofibrate [Atromid-S]) may cause muscle cramping. Leg pain and cramps in adults that are precipitated by exercise and relieved by rest are usually caused by peripheral vascular disease. Blood chemistry tests may be necessary, including serum

✺ Differential Diagnosis 52.2: Muscle Cramps

Symptom	Possible Diagnosis
Cramplike symptoms	Intermittent claudication related to ischemia; drug induced (such as statin-induced myopathy)
Contracture	Thyroid disease, McArdle's disease
Tetany	Hypoglycemia, hypomagnesemia, respiratory alkalosis, hypokalemia
Dystonia	Occupational (such as writer's cramp) Drug-induced (antipsychotics, antiparkinsonian) metabolic/neurologic
True cramps	Ordinary (nocturnal), dehydration, drug-induced (nifedipine, beta agonists), lower motor neuron, hemodialysis (volume and electrolyte shifts), heat induced (volume depletion, hyponatremia)

Source: McGee SK. Muscle cramp. *Arch Intern Med.* 1990;150:571.

enzymes, to rule out causes such as dehydration (from diarrhea or sweating).

PARESTHESIAS

Paresthesia is the sensation of numbness, prickling, or tingling experienced in central and peripheral nerve lesions. Frequently, the patient's understanding and use of the terms will differ from the clinician's; therefore, it is necessary to clearly establish the character of the patient's complaint. During the history, the provider should differentiate between the lack of use of a limb from the sensation of tingling and numbness and the total loss of sensation. It is also important to ascertain whether the loss or altered sensation ascends onto the abdomen or thorax.

The location of the paresthesia may be focal or generalized. It may also be nonspecific, as in multiple sclerosis, in which the initial presentation may be bilateral diminution of sensation or paresthesia in the upper or lower extremities, or unilateral, as in stroke or transient ischemic attack, in which unilateral extremity or face paresthesias may occur.

Paresthesias may be the result of anatomical or mechanical peripheral nerve injury, such as entrapment and compression neuropathies. These are most likely to occur at sites that are more susceptible to damage due to an increase in pressure and mechanical forces, such as entrapment or compression of the medial nerve at the wrist (carpal tunnel syndrome), radial nerve of the forearm, ulnar nerve at the elbow, and peroneal nerve at the knee.

A characteristic set of signs and symptoms known as radiculopathy is caused by compression or injury of spinal nerve roots due to spondylosis (degeneration of the vertebrae) or disc herniation. Radiculopathy includes weakness, numbness, and tingling that typically occur along the distribution of the affected nerve root. Commonly affected nerves are cervical nerve roots C5 to C8, lumbar nerves L3 to L5; and sacral nerve S1 (see Advanced Assessment 52.3). Patients who present with paresthesias should undergo a detailed neurologic assessment to determine whether sensory or motor deficits are present. MRI is indicated when paresthesia is accompanied by motor or sensory deficit or hyporeflexia to rule out spinal cord compression. Any change in bowel or bladder function (cauda equina syndrome) constitutes an emergency and needs immediate assessment by a specialist.

Other causes of paresthesias include chlorinated hydrocarbon exposure, respiratory alkalosis, and the use of certain drugs, such as carbonic anhydrase inhibitors (which are used in the treatment of glaucoma).

DIFFERENTIAL DIAGNOSIS

In addition to the causes described in the previous section, other causes of paresthesias include brachial plexus injury, thoracic outlet syndrome, and peripheral polyneuropathy.

Advanced Assessment 52.3: Paresthesias and Affected Nerve Roots

Nerve Root	Paresthesia
C6 (sixth cervical)	Thumb: dorsal and lateral aspects
C7 (seventh cervical)	Fingers: index and middle
C8 (eighth cervical)	Fingers: fifth and ulnar half of fourth Hand: ulnar side
L4 (fourth lumbar)	Thigh: anterior, just above knee
L5 (fifth lumbar)	Foot: dorsal aspect Great toe: dorsal aspect
S1 (first sacral)	Foot: lateral aspect Small toe: lateral aspect

Brachial plexus injuries include a broad array of neurologic dysfunction ranging from momentary paresthesias to completely flail extremities. The mechanism of injury is equally diverse, from high-energy motor vehicle crashes, falls from a height, and gunshot wounds to lower-energy injuries such as most athletic injuries. The symptoms are severe—burning upper arm and shoulder pain that radiates down the arm, followed by weakness affecting C5 and T1 (thoracic) nerve root distributions. The patient is often seen holding the arm on the affected side, which hangs limply at the side.

Thoracic outlet syndrome is compression of the brachial plexus and/or subclavian vessels as they exit the narrow space between the superior shoulder girdle and the first rib. These structures can be affected individually or in combination. Women aged 20 to 50 years are most commonly affected. Etiology may be secondary to congenital abnormalities such as cervical rib or abnormally long transverse process of C7 or an anomalous fibromuscular band in the thoracic outlet. Posttraumatic fibrosis of the scalene muscles is also a possibility.

Peripheral polyneuropathy is "stocking-glove" or distal sensorimotor paresthesia, with diminished or variable deep tendon reflexes. Diabetes mellitus is a frequent cause; early symptoms may respond to a regimen with tighter glucose control. A rapid onset of motor polyneuropathy is seen in Guillain-Barré syndrome, in which an ascending weakness occurs after a viral illness. Other etiologies include alcoholism, vitamin B deficiencies, vitamin B_6 excess, Sjögren's syndrome, AIDS, hypothyroidism, amyloidosis, and renal failure.

MYOFASCIAL PAIN

Myofascial pain is a type of muscle pain that is purportedly caused by the development of "trigger points" within a muscle. A trigger point is an area of local irritation that, when activated, causes referred pain in a characteristic pattern. Trigger points may be felt under the skin in areas where muscles lie close to the surface.

DIFFERENTIAL DIAGNOSIS

Although myofascial pain is a common cause of nonarticular rheumatic pain, it is often misdiagnosed. Trigger points are not visualized on routine imaging studies and cannot be objectively substantiated. Myofascial pain and fibromyalgia may occur together (see Chapter 62).

Treatment includes identifying and eliminating aggravating factors; trigger point injections, in which saline, an anesthetic, or a corticosteroid is injected into the trigger point; dry needling, in which a needle without medication is inserted to deactivate the trigger point; and massage therapy that focuses on releasing the trigger points with specialized techniques. Some evidence suggests that the muscle relaxant tizanidine, a centrally acting alpha$_2$ adrenergic agonist, has shown to be effective in decreasing muscle spasticity, pain, and disability in patients with myofascial pain (Desai et al., 2013). However, muscle relaxants should be used with caution because they have a potential for addiction. Patients need to be aware that this class of drugs is for short-term use because the risk/benefit ratio for prolonged use of muscle relaxants is poorly established. Because muscle relaxants can cause drowsiness and dizziness, patients need to avoid hazardous activities, such as driving or operating machinery, while using these medicines. Patients should also avoid taking them with alcohol or other central nervous system depressants to prevent additive effects. Dry mouth is another side effect of this anticholinergic class of drugs, so frequent mouth rinsing is recommended to prevent dental disease. Topical application of creams such as capsaicin and lidocaine patches may also help to relieve pain.

Some patients achieve relief with NSAIDs or cyclooxygenase-2 inhibitors. Tricyclic antidepressants, such as amitriptyline, and antiepilepsy drugs are sometimes used in cases that do not respond to other treatments. Narcotic analgesics should be avoided if possible because little research supports the use of narcotics in the treatment of soft-tissue injuries.

REGIONAL MUSCULOSKELETAL COMPLAINTS

NECK PAIN

Discomfort and limited ROM arising from the structures in the neck is a common complaint. The pain may originate from any of the musculoskeletal structures, including muscles, ligaments, tendons, cervical vertebrae, nerves, and vasculature. Pain referred to the neck from the temporomandibular joint, pleura, or mediastinum may also be seen. Causes of neck pain are generally

Advanced Assessment 52.4: Spurling's Maneuver

To perform Spurling's maneuver (neck compression), follow this procedure:

1. With the patient's neck in extension, rotate neck to the affected side.
2. Apply downward pressure on the head.
3. Assess for patient complaint of or accentuation of limb pain or paresthesia (a positive finding). Also observe for obvious atrophy in the neck.

structural in nature and most often are the result of trauma, degenerative changes, or muscle spasms. Stress, sedentary occupations, and improper biomechanics are frequently found to be contributing factors; questions regarding these factors should be asked during the history taking. The onset (rapid or insidious), location (arm, shoulder, head, or back), and character (sharp, dull, or aching) of the pain are essential in the differential diagnosis. Of note is pain (in the absence of trauma) that begins gradually and improves with rest, because infection and malignancy in the vertebrae do occur.

Physical examination of the neck begins with the evaluation of ROM, including flexion, extension, rotation, and side bending to determine limitations and the pain-producing movements. Spurling's maneuver should be used to assess nerve root compression (see Advanced Assessment 52.4). This test is widely used in clinical practice; however, a review of studies assessing interrater reliability, sensitivity, and specificity revealed few methodologically sound studies and a need for more research on the usefulness of this test. Palpation of the neck must be done thoroughly, checking for tenderness, muscle spasm, and lymphadenopathy. Lymph nodes in the supraclavicular and axillary regions should be examined carefully; enlarged nodes in the absence of infection may indicate malignancy. The vascular structures and the thyroid should be evaluated. The examination must also include a musculoskeletal and neurovascular assessment of the extremities, including assessments of the muscle strength of biceps, triceps, and handgrips (see Advanced Assessment 52.1). Abnormalities in sensation of any dermatome and altered deep tendon reflexes indicate cervical nerve root compression.

Laboratory studies such as ESR, RF, or ANA test are necessary only if systemic or bone disease is suspected.

DIFFERENTIAL DIAGNOSIS

A common cause of neck pain is cervical *muscle sprain/strain*. However, because it is difficult to differentiate the soft tissues of the neck, these terms also apply to injuries involving the facet joints or ligaments. Hyperextension injuries that occur in motor vehicle collisions (MVCs), often called whiplash, are common neck injuries seen in primary care. Patients presenting with neck pain following an MVC should be carefully evaluated for neurologic dysfunction, dislocations, fractures, and ligamentous tears.

A *spasm* is rigidity or spasticity caused by increased muscle tone. When a muscle is chronically contracted, blood flow is reduced, and ischemia and pain often result. The goal in treating muscle spasm is to induce the muscle to relax, allowing for restoration of internal blood flow, removal of metabolic by-products, and the influx of nutrients.

Degenerative changes affecting the cervical vertebrae are called *spondylosis*. These changes may cause thinning of the intervertebral discs and formation of bony spurs called osteophytes. Spondylosis is often a normal result of aging and is usually asymptomatic. However, in some individuals, osteophytes may impinge on spinal nerve roots and cause radicular signs and symptoms of tingling, burning, and weakness, and bone spurs in the associated muscles. These differential diagnoses are discussed in more detail in Chapter 53.

BACK PAIN

About 85% of the adult population experiences lower back pain at some point in their lives. Common causes of lower back pain include lumbar strain and sprains, nerve impingement, nerve compression, radiculopathy, and fractures. Additional causes include infection, tumors, and systemic inflammatory disorders affecting the axial (spinal) and sacroiliac joints. Approximately 20% of acute lower back pain will develop into chronic lower back pain.

The most common cause of acute lower back pain is lumbar strain and sprains (discussed in more detail in Chapter 53). Strain occurs when the muscles or ligaments of the lower back are stretched, causing microscopic tears. Sprains are caused by the overstretching or tearing of ligaments. Lumbar strain and sprains usually occur from improper use, overuse, or trauma to the muscles and connective tissue of the lower back. Similarly, fractures to the vertebrae occur most often as a result of trauma, although they may occur spontaneously in individuals with decreased bone density (e.g., osteopenia or osteoporosis).

Fractures usually present with an acute onset of pain that radiates around the body and is exacerbated with movement. If no accident or trauma is involved, the patient will usually complain of a time-sequence history of symptoms which may be gradual or sudden and may be localized in the lumbosacral area or radiating. If a vertebral disc syndrome is present, the patient may complain of radiation of pain into the leg, sensory changes, motor weakness, or difficulties with bowel or bladder function. Lesions with mass effects may present similarly, due to localized effects on the spinal cord. For example,

the patient with cauda equine syndrome typically presents with leg weakness, saddle area anesthesia, bowel or bladder incontinence/retention, or impotence. Similarly, symptoms of radiculopathy may include pain, numbness, and a tingling sensation that radiates down the nerve distribution, for example, from the lower back and down the leg in lumbar radiculopathy (sciatica).

Malignancies and localized infections (e.g., spinal abscess) may cause back pain and neurologic symptoms such as weakness or decreased sensation due to swelling and resultant mass effects, which compromise spinal cord or nerve root function. Radiculopathy (dysfunction of one or more nerve roots) is a condition caused by spinal nerve root compression, injury, or inflammation, most commonly due to vertebral disc herniation or spinal stenosis (narrowing of the vertebral canal) from degenerative joint disease. For example, cauda equina syndrome involves compression of multiple lumbar nerve roots and is a medical emergency.

Initial examination should include inspection of the spine, lower extremities, and gait. The clinician should palpate areas of concern and perform an appropriate musculoskeletal, neurologic, and vascular evaluation of the back and lower extremities. The back, spine, and legs should be inspected for asymmetry, atrophy, lesions, trauma, and leg length should be measured from the front (anteriorly), laterally, and posteriorly. The inspection should include standing, sitting with the knees and hips bent at 90 degrees, and lying in a prone position. Forward flexion, lateral flexion, extension, and rotation of the lumbar spine should be evaluated for pain and limitations in ROM and strength, while the clinician is behind the patient stabilizing the hips at the iliac crest. With the patient in a supine position and the examiner's hand stabilizing the patient's pelvis, hip flexion, internal and external rotation of the hip, and knee flexion should be evaluated for ROM, pain, and strength. Chest wall expansion should be assessed by measuring chest circumference before and after maximal inspiration. Vascular examination should include palpation of the dorsalis pedis and posterior tibial pulses in both lower extremities, as well as capillary refill of the toes.

The clinician should perform a neurologic examination of the lower extremities that will detect the small deficits produced by disc disease and the large deficits produced by such problems as compression of the cauda equina due to spinal tumors. The lower extremities should be evaluated and compared for sensation, which may help localize the level of nerve root lesions. Nerve root compression tests including the straight-leg-raise test can be used to evaluate lumbar nerve root impingement or irritation (see Advanced Assessment 52.5), as palpation of the spine cannot confirm the diagnosis of radiculopathy. A positive straight-leg-raise test result is reproduction of pain when the leg is raised 70 degrees or less.

Vertebral disc herniation resulting in radiculopathy of lumbar spinal nerves L4 to L5 and L5 to S1 are particularly common sources of acute back pain, often due to trauma.

Advanced Assessment 52.5:
Straight-Leg Test

To perform this test, follow this procedure:

1. The patient is placed in a supine position.
2. Grasp the heel of the leg to be tested and raise the leg by flexing the hip.
3. Assess for pain or reproduction of symptoms before the end of the normal range of motion (70 degrees).

L4 to L5 and L5 to S1 radiculopathy (sciatica) may be objectively assessed in terms of dermatome sensory deficit, myotome muscle weakness, and deep tendon reflex deficits. The clinician should assess for the inability of the patient to walk on the toes or heels and the inability to dorsiflex the great toe, which may relate to specific lumbar spinal nerve involvement. Lower back pain may be less serious than with other etiologies, with or without pain radiating down one leg.

DIFFERENTIAL DIAGNOSIS

Diagnostic testing varies depending on the history and physical examination findings. Laboratory tests including CBC, urinalysis, ESR, and CRP may be helpful in determining an infectious or inflammatory etiology. Additional laboratory tests such as autoantibody panels may help rule out autoimmune disorders, although positive tests may be nonspecific. Of note, ankylosing spondylitis is characterized by inflammatory back pain in the absence of RF (in contrast to RA) and with most patients demonstrating elevations in acute phase reactants such as CRP and expression of the HLA-B27 genetic haplotype.

In addition to laboratory tests, imaging modalities and procedures may be helpful in making a diagnosis. X-ray is a convenient technique to visualize bony structures if a fracture (traumatic or spontaneous) or misalignment is suspected. CT scan produces a three-dimensional image that is often more helpful than an x-ray in identifying disc rupture, spinal stenosis, or tumors. Ultrasound can show ligament, tendon, and muscle tears, or may be used to identify an intra-abdominal etiology (e.g., gall bladder dysfunction, abdominal aneurysm). Bone scans can be used to measure abnormal metabolic activity seen with tumors, infection, and fractures.

MRI is usually unnecessary, but it may be useful if the clinician suspects soft-tissue injuries, such as nerve impingement, tumor, infection, disc herniation, disc rupture, or trauma to ligaments, tendons, muscles, or blood vessels. MRI is also appropriate for patients who are surgical candidates or who have evidence of systemic disease. Electromyography (EMG) and nerve conduction studies may be used to diagnose a radiculopathy.

Low back pain has a number of potential causes. Common differential diagnoses for back pain include the following:

- Ankylosing spondylitis: back pain and stiffness over several months; relief with exercise; reduced mobility of spine; painful or ankylosed sacroiliac joints; and reduced chest wall expansion. It occurs most often with an insidious onset after age 40 years.
- Cauda equina syndrome: acute urinary or rectal incontinence, with or without paraplegia.
- Dissecting aortic aneurysm: sudden onset of severe low back pain in older adults; pain that is not relieved with rest; pallor, diaphoresis, and confusion may be present; possible asymmetrical pulses and blood pressure in extremities.
- Gallstones: pain follows ingestion of a fatty meal and radiates around trunk to right scapula; belching, bloating, and stomach acid are present, along with right upper quadrant pain.
- Gynecological disorders: vaginal discharge; pain worse around menstruation or ovulation.
- Herniated disc: often preceded by years of recurrent episodes of localized back pain; leg pain overshadows back pain.
- Infection: unremitting or progressive pain at rest; tender spinous process at level of involvement; fever; history of drug use; diabetes; immunosuppression or suspected systemic infection; previous genitourinary or spinal surgery.
- Musculoskeletal strain: often no precipitating event; pain is over lower back and muscles without sciatica; aggravated by sitting, standing, and certain movements; alleviated with rest. Palpation localizes pain and muscle spasms may be seen. Insidious onset; progressive improvement.
- Prostatitis: constant low back pain; urinary hesitancy; change in sexual frequency.
- Pyelonephritis: ill-appearing patient with nausea and vomiting; back and flank pain excruciating with direct percussion.
- Sciatica: pain radiating into the buttocks, thighs, and/or below the knees as the result of L5 or S1 nerve root irritation, compression, or disc prolapse.
- Spinal fracture: pain felt near the site of injury; history of major trauma to the back or (in older adults) a history of strenuous lifting or a minor fall.
- Spinal stenosis: gradual onset in older adults; often mimics intermittent claudication, except pain is usually in buttocks, thigh, or calf, worsens with exertion and back extension (leaning backward or walking downhill), and is relieved with sitting, walking uphill, or leaning forward; weakness and/or bowel and bladder dysfunction may be present.
- Spondylolisthesis: systemic inflammatory condition of the vertebral column and sacroiliac joints; most frequently affects men aged 20 to 30; chronic low back

pain, worse in morning; excessive thoracic kyphosis is present.

- Tumor: unremitting or progressive pain at rest, night pain; tender spinous process at level of involvement; variable neurologic findings; weight loss, fever, or other systemic symptoms; known or suspected malignancy.
- Given the variable etiology of back pain, in the majority of cases, a precise determination of the cause of a patient's pain cannot be made, although the initial history and physical examination usually lead to the diagnosis in cases in which the cause can be identified. The challenge is to identify patients who require more extensive or urgent evaluation. Once emergent causes and systemic disease are ruled out, medical treatment for lower back pain is dictated by the underlying pathology (see Chapter 53).

SHOULDER PAIN

Pain and dysfunction localizing in and around the shoulder girdle are common presenting musculoskeletal complaints. Shoulder pain affects patients of various ages and activity levels. Although shoulder pain can be referred from the neck, chest, or diaphragmatic region, it is most commonly caused by a local process. The shoulder joint includes three large bones (clavicle, scapula, and humerus) and four joints (sternoclavicular, acromioclavicular [AC], glenohumeral, and thoracoscapular). The shoulder is a ball-and-socket joint, like the hip, but the two joints differ significantly in that the hip is a weight-bearing joint and the shoulder is a suspension joint, maximizing mobility. The two chief presenting complaints are usually related to pain and/or instability. Symptoms of decreased motion, power, or function can accompany complaints of pain or instability, but they are rarely the chief complaint.

Common conditions affecting the shoulder include acute injuries (less than 2 weeks' duration; common in younger patients), which include fractures, dislocations, and acute tendon rupture; chronic or repetitive injuries (impingement syndromes, most rotator cuff tears and biceps tendon ruptures); and degenerative, inflammatory, or idiopathic conditions (glenohumeral and AC arthritis, frozen shoulder). Although there have been many technological advances in diagnostic aids, most shoulder disorders can be diagnosed with careful history, clinical examination, and plain radiographs.

In the history, the patient should be asked about the precipitating injury and onset of pain, the location of pain, and the factors that aggravate or alleviate it. The relationship of the pain to the time of day, to active or passive movement, and to body position is significant. The patient's age, occupation, activities, medical history, and social factors will also be important in making a diagnosis. Patients with acute symptoms usually have an injury, such as a fracture, dislocation, or rotator cuff tear.

For patients with chronic shoulder pain, activities related to the onset of symptoms may be useful to the diagnosis.

Instability, another common complaint, occurs most frequently in younger adults and can be classified by the frequency of symptomatic episodes, as well as the direction and degree of instability:

- Frequency: acute injuries may be a first-time dislocation or a recurrent episode.
- Degree: partial (subluxation) with spontaneous reduction or complete (dislocation).
- Location: anterior, posterior, inferior, or multidirectional. Most traumatic dislocations are anterior. Multidirectional instability should be considered in patients who present with recurrent episodes of subluxations or dislocations and no history of significant trauma.

The physical examination of the shoulder should begin with inspection of the shoulder for swelling, color, edema, and symmetry, followed by palpation for tender areas, crepitus, temperature, and deformity. The shoulder should be inspected anteriorly and posteriorly, particularly to observe scapular winging. Both active and passive ROM movements should be tested while comparing the painful shoulder to the unaffected side. When testing ROM of the shoulder, it is important to determine if there is a discrepancy between active and passive motion. Disuse can cause some passive ROM loss; equal losses of active and passive ROM can be secondary to soft-tissue contracture, as in frozen shoulder, or the result of joint incongruity from trauma or arthritis. The most common ROM movements tested include the following:

- The Apley scratch test: this measures abduction and external rotation by having the patient reach behind the head and touch the superior aspect of the opposite scapula. Conversely, internal rotation and adduction of the shoulder are tested by having the patient reach behind the back and touch the inferior aspect of the opposite scapula. External rotation should be measured with the patient's arms at the side and elbows flexed to 90 degrees.
- Internal/external in flexion: with the patient's elbow flexed at the side, thumb pointing up, internally and externally rotate the elbow, taking care to keep the elbow against the body.
- Internal/external in abduction: abduct the patient's shoulder to 90 degrees, keeping the elbow flexed at 90 degrees, and then have the patient lower his or her forearm from the horizontal plane, then raise the forearm, keeping the upper arm parallel to the ground.

Pain with abduction from 45 to 120 degrees (painful arc) indicates supraspinatus tendinitis and subacromial bursitis, which are early rotator cuff injuries. Muscle and bursae involvement produces pain only on active motion, whereas pain with passive ROM may involve tendons, bursae, or restricted joint movement and is generally indicative of more pathology. In an acute anterior dislocation, pain is severe and ROM is limited. The patient will usually hold the arm slightly abducted and externally rotated.

Muscle strength should be assessed and compared with the opposite shoulder. Pain can affect the accuracy of muscle testing. Tears of rotator cuffs and neurologic injury can produce weakness. Functional status should also be assessed, although this may be affected by motivation and ability to adapt to impairment. The level of functional disability will depend on the normal intensity of activities that the patient performs. Resistive muscle testing, reflex testing, and an assessment of the neurosensory and neurovascular status complete the examination.

Because shoulder pain can be referred from other areas, the patient should be evaluated for cardiac, pulmonary, and abdominal causes, as well as neurologic disease or injury and spine. Pain caused by bony malignancy is usually gnawing, constant, and unrelated to movement. Malignant tumor is usually evident by a lytic lesion in the bone on x-ray film.

Plain x-ray films, including the anteroposterior projection and an axillary lateral view, are sufficient to reveal most fractures and dislocations. Additional views may include a transthoracic lateral, which images the glenohumeral joint at a 45-degree posterior oblique, or a 60-degree anterior oblique (Y view). A new view—the apical oblique—is suggested to reveal shoulder instability. This view is simple to obtain and painless for the patient. In addition to the standard x-ray studies, there are other diagnostic tests used in diagnosing shoulder pain. Regular MRI is sufficient for patients with intractable shoulder pain unless they have dislocation. For suspected dislocations, MRI, arthrography, and (if nerve involvement is suspected) EMG are indicated. Although the standard x-ray studies will often be normal, they should be done to rule out structural abnormalities, especially if there is history of trauma or if the problem is persistent. C-spine films and chest films may also be necessary if involvement in those areas is suspected. Laboratory studies should be done in accordance with the patient's history.

DIFFERENTIAL DIAGNOSIS

A summary of common differential diagnoses for shoulder pain is provided in Differential Diagnosis 52.3. A concise differential diagnosis is often obtained by evaluating the patient's chief complaint in the context of its chronicity and the patient's age. Patients younger than 30 years, for example, commonly present with traumatic injuries or instability such as glenohumeral dislocations and AC joint separation. Impingement syndromes and rotator cuff tears are more commonly seen in middle-aged patients. These must be distinguished from frozen shoulder, which produces a global loss of passive and active ROM. Glenohumeral

---

✿ Differential Diagnosis 52.3: Shoulder Pain

Musculoskeletal problems	Adhesive capsulitis (frozen shoulder) Rotator cuff syndrome Impingement Calcific tendinitis Subacromial bursitis Degenerative arthritis: glenohumeral, acromioclavicular
Trauma	Fractures: humerus, clavicle, acromion Acromioclavicular joint sprains Rotator cuff tear Dislocation: glenohumeral Nerve injuries: compression
Neurovascular problems	Reflex sympathetic dystrophy (shoulder–hand syndrome) Thoracic outlet syndrome Cervical root compression Brachial plexus injury
Systemic disease	Inflammatory disease Cancer

---

dislocations are much less common in older patients and must be treated with a high index of suspicion for a concomitant rotator cuff tear (50% of patients older than 40 years will have an acute tear). Older patients (older than 55 years) are more likely to have rotator cuff tears or degenerative arthritis. Fractures and dislocations related to falls also occur in this age-group.

ELBOW PAIN

Usually, elbow complaints in the adult occur because of overuse. The most commonly seen complaint is lateral epicondylitis of the humerus. Although this condition is often called "tennis elbow," it occurs frequently in patients who do not play tennis. It is associated with repeated extension of the wrist and pronation and supination of the forearm, particularly against resistance, which occurs in movements such as opening jars, hammering, and turning doorknobs. The common complaint is pain in the elbow that radiates into the forearm. There is pain and weakness with gripping objects ("coffee cup" sign). Tenderness is present over the lateral epicondyle, and wrist extension against resistance produces the pain. Rest, ice, NSAIDs, and physical therapy are generally effective; corticosteroid injections and wrist splinting may be considered in some cases and have been shown to be effective for short-term relief of lateral epicondylitis. Physical therapy is more efficacious than steroid injection if symptoms persist longer than 6 weeks (Saunders & Longworth, 2012). Surgery is reserved for cases refractory to conservative treatments

Medial epicondylitis is less common; this condition is often referred to as "golfer's elbow." It is a result of overuse or strain of the muscle group arising from the medial epicondyle, which is used in wrist flexion. Tenderness and pain is over the medial epicondyle and is exacerbated by wrist flexion. Diagnosis can be generally made via clinical examination; findings include pain with resisted wrist flexion, tenderness to palpation of the medical epicondyle, and pain with resisted elbow pronation. Treatment is the same as for lateral epicondylitis.

Bursitis of the olecranon is often the cause of pain and swelling in the posterior aspect of the elbow. This may occur with forced extension of the elbow joint. ROM is generally normal, but caution is needed to rule out a septic bursitis. Monitor for fever, redness, heat, and warmth at the site. Synovial fluid aspiration can provide evidence of infection. Radiography is indicated to exclude bone infection. Empiric treatment with antibiotics is not recommended. If cellulitis, constitutional symptoms, or abrasions are present, aspiration and culture are warranted with possible referral to an orthopedic specialist. If none of these symptoms are present, the bursitis is likely caused by inflammation and can be treated with NSAIDS, ice for 15 to 20 minutes several times a day, and rest.

Assessment of position of computer keyboards or other workstation corrections may be helpful. NSAIDs are useful, and splinting with an elbow strap may ease pain by exerting counterpressure on the soft tissue below the lateral epicondyle, or short-term use of a wrist splint may reduce pain from lateral epicondylitis. Physical and/or occupational therapy may also be helpful. These measures are effective in 80% of cases. If the patient is still symptomatic, referral to a specialist is warranted. Surgical procedures are a last resort.

WRIST AND HAND PAIN

Pain in the wrist and hand Allen's test, Phalen's maneuver, the percussion test for Tinel's sign, and/or Finkelstein's test (see Advanced Assessment 52.6) are used to assess the wrist and hand. When assessing and/or treating a patient with an injured hand, the patient should remove all rings as soon as possible. Inflammation secondary to most injuries will precipitate edema, making removal of rings difficult. A tight-fitting ring may cause arterial compression and ischemia if not removed. Usually soap or lubricant jelly will be sufficient to remove the ring. If this does not work, several other techniques may be used (see Therapeutic Procedure 52.1).

ROM of the fingers and wrists should be assessed as follows:

- Have the patient make a fist with the thumb across the knuckles.
- Have the patient extend and widely spread the fingers.
- Have the patient touch each finger with the thumb of the same hand.
- With the palms facing down, passively move the fingers laterally and medially.
- Have the patient flex and extend the hands, with and without resistance.

⁙ **Advanced Assessment 52.6: Tests for Wrist and Hand Problems**

Test	Comments
Allen's test	*Purpose:* Assesses patency of radial and ulnar arteries and the arterial arch. *Procedure:* Compress the radial artery at the wrist. Have patient rapidly open and close his or her hand several times. Then have the patient open the hand. (Hand should be pale or white.) Release pressure from the artery. The hand should flush, indicating patency.
Phalen's test	*Purpose:* Assesses for median nerve compression. *Procedure:* Have the patient maintain forced flexion of the wrist for 1 minute or more, with the dorsal surface of each hand pressed together. If the patient complains of numbness and paresthesias in fingers, the test is considered positive.
Tinel's sign	*Purpose:* Assesses for compression neuropathy. *Procedure:* Percuss the median nerve at the wrist. If the patient complains of tingling in the digits (positive Tinel's sign), compression at the site of percussion is likely.
Finkelstein's test	*Purpose:* Assesses for de Quervain's disease. *Procedure:* Have patient touch thumb into palm and make a fist. Test is positive if moving the wrist into ulnar deviation causes pain.

Therapeutic Procedure 52.1: Removing Rings

	STRING TECHNIQUE
Equipment: 2–0 or 3–0 nylon suture (string technique), rubber tourniquet (tourniquet technique), lubricant (tourniquet technique), mechanical ring cutter (ring cutter technique)	**1.** In a distal direction, wrap 2–0 or 3–0 nylon suture tightly around the finger just distal to the ring. 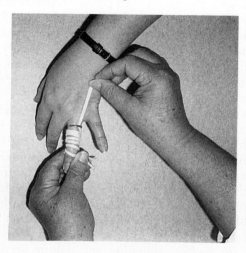 **2.** Slip the proximal end of the string under the ring. **3.** Pull the proximal end of the suture over the ring and firmly retract it distally over the axis of the finger. As each coil of the suture unwinds, it pulls the ring slightly over the coiled suture until it is free 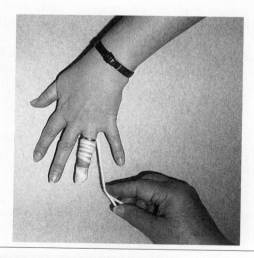

TOURNIQUET TECHNIQUE	**MECHANICAL RING CUTTER TECHNIQUE**
1. Carefully wrap the finger with a rubber tourniquet, starting at the fingertip and working up to the edge of the ring.	**1.** Advise patient that the ring will be cut and obtain his or her consent.
2. Have the patient lie supine on the examination table, with his or her arm pointed straight upward at the ceiling for about 5 minutes. **3.** As soon as the patient lowers his or her arm, remove the tourniquet, apply copious amounts of lubricant, and slide the ring off.	**2.** Follow the manufacturer's directions. Postprocedure: Give ring to patient, or secure as per institution policy and document.

DIFFERENTIAL DIAGNOSES

Wrist injuries are common after falling on an outstretched hand. Patients present after trauma with pain and swelling in the distal forearm or wrist. Numbness may be present if the medial nerve is affected. The mechanism of injury will often provide important clues to the diagnosis. The examination begins with gentle palpation to locate the area of point tenderness and includes a thorough neurovascular assessment. A radiograph of the wrist (including an oblique view) may be necessary to rule out fracture. Common fractures are the Colles fracture of the distal radius and the navicular (scaphoid) fracture of the anatomical snuffbox. It is not unusual to have a navicular fracture missed on radiography, so an orthopedic referral should be provided when the presenting complaint is pain and trauma to the soft-tissue area of the anatomical snuffbox.

A common wrist ligamental injury is an ulnar collateral ligament tear at the base of the thumb. Often seen with ski-pole injury, this condition is related to repetitive gripping, and surgery is necessary to repair a tear in this area. Therefore, when the presenting complaint is pain and trauma to the proximal thumb, an orthopedic referral for stress testing is appropriate even if the x-ray result is negative.

HIP PAIN

Hip pain is discomfort within or around the hip. The largest joint in the body, the hip is subject to stress from ambulation and weight-bearing; it may suffer trauma and chronic mechanical stress. Pain in and around the hip can often be felt in the groin or the buttock, or it can be referred to the thigh or knee. Conversely, pain may be referred to the hip if irritation to the femoral, sciatic, or obturator nerve roots occurs. These may be the result of herniation of lumbar disc, spinal stenosis, retroperitoneal tumor, or femoral hernia.

DIFFERENTIAL DIAGNOSIS

The history should ascertain if pain is focal, as in bursitis, or diffuse, as in synovitis. The presence of stiffness should raise the suspicion of degenerative disease. Inquire about trauma, involvement of other joints, infection, fever, and relation of pain to activity.

Physical examination of the hip must first assess position at rest because fracture of the femoral head results in external rotation and flexion, and an internally rotated shortened leg may be a posterior dislocation. These patients should not have the hip moved until radiographic studies have ruled out fracture or dislocation. Performing palpation of the joint allows recognition of focal tenderness and swelling.

The ROM examination begins with assessment of gait, if possible. Next, the extremity should be put through passive ROM to detect crepitus, limitation of movement, muscle spasm, flexion contracture, or guarding. Flexion and extension need to be performed with the knee straight as well as flexed. Abduction, adduction, and internal and external rotation are assessed. Femoral and pedal pulses (posterior tibial, dorsalis pedis) should be auscultated for strength and bruits. Neurologic testing for sensation and deep tendon reflexes concludes the examination.

Diagnostic testing should include hip x-ray films. Other x-ray studies, such as spine or sacroiliac films or weight-bearing films, may be indicated in special circumstances. MRI, ultrasonography, and joint aspiration are other diagnostic techniques to be considered in special circumstances.

Possible causes are processes in the hip joint, the surrounding muscles, the soft tissues, or the neurovascular system. Diagnosis needs to consider the patient's age because certain problems are more prevalent in different age-groups. In adults, common problems include OA, RA, fractures, referred pain, bursitis, and avascular necrosis. Cancer is a possible differential diagnosis with hip pain. Initially no signs may be present with malignancy; however, tenderness and palpable swelling may develop later over bony prominences. Pain that occurs at night, systemic symptoms, and fractures may eventually occur.

The location of the patient's pain can give valuable clues about the etiology. If the patient's pain is located in the groin or inguinal fold, hip pathology should be considered in the evaluation. If the patient's pain is along the anterior hip, radicular lower back pain or trochanteric bursitis, now referred to as greater trochanteric pain syndrome, may be considered. If the patient's pain is posterior, radicular lower back pain or muscle strain (gluteus, hamstring) is a possible diagnosis. Vascular insufficiency of the aortoiliac area may result in hip and buttock pain as well. Avascular necrosis appears as abrupt hip pain followed by progressive, intermittent episodes. Pain is worsened with motion and activity and often is worse at night. A limp, along with limited abduction and internal rotation, is present. Some AVN can be seen on x-ray, MRI is the gold standard test needed for diagnosis, and an orthopedic referral is indicated. It often occurs as a serious complication of hip trauma, but it may occur unrelated to trauma. It is related to alcoholism, chronic prednisone use, and trauma.

KNEE PAIN

The knee is a complex, modified hinge joint consisting of three bones, three articulations, five major tendons, four major ligaments, and two menisci. The lateral and medial articulations are between the femoral and tibial condyles. The intermediate articulation exists between the patella and the femur. The knee is a relatively weak joint that gains its strength from the strong ligaments that attach the femur to the tibia. There are five intrinsic ligaments that assist in strengthening the articular capsule. The cruciate ligaments connect the femur and tibia within the articular capsule, crossing each other in the form of an X.

As a major weight-bearing joint, the knee is susceptible to many injuries. Torsion is limited in the joint, and any motion that extends beyond the defined range results in a ligamentous injury. Because the knee joint depends on the integrity of the ligaments to provide it with stability, an injury to the knee may be a calamitous event.

The arrangement of three articulations allows a combination of rolling, gliding, and rotation, in addition to flexion and extension. Although it is attached to the lateral tibia, the fibula does not articulate with the knee joint. The anatomy of the knee includes bony structures, ligaments, tendons, bursae, and cartilage. The femoral condyles and the tibial plateaus are capped by the patella and cushioned by the menisci, whereas the ligaments, muscles, tendons, and bursae provide stability.

DIFFERENTIAL DIAGNOSIS

The knee joint is a common site for discomfort due to trauma (24% of all activity-related musculoskeletal injuries in men, the highest of all sites), degenerative disease, and/or rheumatological conditions. Acute pain in the knee may be related to any of the following:

- Fractures
- Meniscal injuries
- Ligamentous injuries
- Musculotendinous strains
- Extensor mechanism injuries
- Contusions

Many knee complaints by adults are the result of overzealous exercise and sports activity. Fractures can involve the distal femur, patella, proximal tibia, and fibula. Inspect for swelling and deformity, palpate for tenderness in the bone itself, and obtain appropriate radiographs. Patellar fractures can result from indirect forces, such as falls, but fractures of the tibia and femur at the knee usually result from major trauma. Patellar dislocations are often reduced at the scene of injury when the knee is extended for transport.

Obtaining a history of the mechanism of injury is key in diagnosing meniscal tears. A history of a twisting injury sustained with the foot planted on the ground and locking (inability to extend the knee completely) with localized pain and tenderness along the joint are indicative of meniscal pathology. Some patients report that manipulating or pushing on the knee enabled them to "unlock it." The patient should be asked if he or she heard or felt a "pop" when the injury occurred.

Patients with ligamentous injuries have acute pain, swelling, and instability. Strains of various musculotendinous structures around the knee also cause acute pain and swelling, but most do not result in instability. Patients with an injury to the extensor mechanism report a fall with a sudden weakness or collapse. Contusions are from direct blows and cause localized pain and tenderness. Contusions are injuries to the leg by a direct blow. Disability may be minor; however, contusions can be quite painful, with significant swelling and tenderness. There may be ecchymosis, and active and passive stress will be painful.

Chronic knee pain is often unrelated to recognized injury or overuse. Conditions that cause chronic knee pain include the following:

- Arthritis
- Tumors
- Sepsis
- Overuse syndromes (including bursitis/tendinitis and anterior knee pain)

Patellofemoral dysfunction encompasses a continuum of disorders, including chondromalacia patellae and patellofemoral arthralgia. It is an overuse syndrome. Pain typically occurs when climbing stairs or when standing up after a period of sitting. Pain is often reproduced by direct pressure on the patella when the patient is supine with knee extended. X-ray films may reveal irregularity of the patella. Management is conservative; NSAIDs and quadriceps-strengthening exercises, such as tensing of quadriceps and straight-leg raising, are indicated.

Tumors are characterized by night pain and often can be palpated or identified on radiograph. Sepsis in the knee joint is rare; it is more commonly located in the prepatellar bursa. Inspection and palpation of the involved area easily determine the location of the infection. Bursitis/tendinitis and anterior knee pain have similar characteristics: both usually are chronic, often secondary to overuse, and often bilateral. The pain typically is worse with rising or walking after sitting, at night, and with prolonged exercise or use.

The physical examination of the knee begins with the patient standing. Both knees should be inspected anteriorly and posteriorly. Inspect the knees for swelling, ecchymosis, erythema, abrasions, puncture wounds, and active ROM. Assess the popliteal space for swelling that may occur with popliteal aneurysm, Baker's cyst, and tumors. It is important to assess movement in both the standing and supine positions and to note any limping, pain, locking, or giving way of the knee. As the patient lies supine, palpate the joint line, muscles, tendons, ligaments, and bones to localize tenderness. An effusion may be demonstrated by eliciting the *bulge sign*: with the patient lying supine, massage the medial knee toward the head, then stroke the lateral aspect of the knee toward the medial aspect. A bulge sign or effusion is indicated if fluctuance occurs over the medial aspect. Palpation for crepitus while the knee is passively flexed and extended helps to determine if meniscal injury is present. Muscle testing of the quadriceps and hamstrings should be performed, as well as a gait should be assessment

A complete physical examination is also important to rule out the presence of systemic disease associated with knee pathology. Many specialized assessment techniques can be used to evaluate the knee. Most are specific and technique driven, requiring practice to master them. The Lachman test should be done on most patients with knee pain; it is 94% specific and is helpful in diagnosing ACL injury. The McMurray and Apley tests are indicated in diagnosing meniscal tears. The anterior drawer test has a low sensitivity and high specificity for confirming ACL pathology, so a positive test strongly suggests a problem, but a negative test does not rule out an ACL tear. The posterior drawer test is used to diagnose posterior cruciate ligament injury. The collateral ligament stress test, also known as the valgus and varus stress tests, evaluates the intact function of the MCL and the LCL, respectively. The Fairbank test, also known as the Apprehension test, can identify dislocation of the patella (see Advanced Assessments 52.7 and 52.8).

Diagnostic testing includes the use of radiographs if mechanical injury or trauma is suspected. Specific weight-bearing views and sunrise or skyline views can be performed. MRI is helpful in diagnosing a torn meniscus or cruciate ligament injury.

ANKLE PAIN

Most ankle pain is the result of ankle injury that results in ligamental damage (a *sprain*). A sprain occurs when the ankle is positioned in an unstable way, causing the ligaments to overstretch. Repeated ankle sprains may result in chronic tendon laxity (see Advanced Assessment 52.9). Ankle pain may be referred pain secondary to disc herniation at the level of L5 to S1. Signs and symptoms include a sensory deficit over the malleolus, weak eversion, and a decreased Achilles reflex.

DIFFERENTIAL DIAGNOSIS

In addition to sprains and fracture, ankle pain has several differential diagnoses. Nerve entrapment may occur secondary to ankle fracture, dislocation, or traction injury. If the tibial nerve is affected, there would be a loss of ankle plantar flexion, toe flexion, and weak ankle inversion.

Posterior impingement syndrome is most commonly seen in ballet dancers. It manifests with pain and swelling of the posterior ankle and worsens with plantar flexion or dorsiflexion of the great toe. Os trigonum is present on lateral x-ray film.

Peroneal tendon subluxation may occur secondary to trauma; it will present with pain and a "snapping" over the posterior distal fibula. Pain will increase with active eversion of the dorsiflexed foot, and there may be palpable/visible movement of tendons.

⁂ Advanced Assessment 52.7: Assessing the Meniscus and the Patella—Special Tests

Test	Comments
McMurray circumduction test—to test for meniscal tear	Flex the knee to the maximum pain-free position. Hold that position while externally rotating the foot, and then gradually extend the knee while maintaining the tibia in external rotation. This maneuver stresses the medial meniscus and often elicits a localized medial compartment click and/or pain in patients with a posterior tear. The same maneuver performed while rotating the foot internally will stress the lateral meniscus. Pain-free flexion beyond 90 degrees is necessary for this test to be useful.
Apprehension sign—to test patellar instability	Have the patient seated with the quadriceps relaxed. Place the knee in extension. Displace the patella laterally and then flex the knee to 30 degrees. With instability, this maneuver displaces the patella to an abnormal position on the lateral femoral condyle. The patient often perceives pain and demonstrates apprehension.
Bulge sign—to assess for effusion	Apply lateral pressure to the area adjacent to the patella. Medial bulge will appear if fluid is in the knee joint.
Inspect/palpate—to assess for effusion	First, inspect the suprapatellar region. A large knee effusion will be visible. Subtle knee effusions can be demonstrated by "milking down" the joint fluid from the suprapatellar pouch. Hold the fluid wave in place with one hand and ballot the patella. Excessive fluid will create a spongy feeling as the patella is pushed down.

✸ Advanced Assessment 52.8: Assessing Knee Ligaments—Special Tests

Test	Comments
Valgus stress test—assess the medial collateral ligament (MCL) stability.	Support thigh to relax the quadriceps muscle. Apply stress initially with the knee extended and then flexed to 25 degrees. With the thigh supported and the knee extended, place one hand on the lateral side of the knee, grasp the medial distal tibia with one hand on the lateral side of the knee, grasp the medial distal tibia with the other hand, and abduct the knee. If the knee opens in a valgus direction more than the opposite knee, the patient has either a complete or partial tear of the MCL.
Varus stress test—assess the lateral collateral ligament (LCL) stability	Assess LCL stability with the knee in extension and 25-degree flexion by reversing the stress pattern used for the MCL. If the knee opens more than the opposite knee in a varus direction, the patient has either a complete or partial tear of the LCL.
Lachman test—anterior cruciate ligament (ACL)	With the patient supine and the knee flexed 15–20 degrees, grasp the calf, wrapping your hand around the leg, with your thumb on the tibial tubercle. With your other hand, stabilize the distal femur, pressing your thumb through the quadriceps tendon while the rest of your hand encircles the thigh above the patella. The knee should be relaxed so that you feel the full weight of it. Simultaneously apply pressure to the tibia posteriorly, attempting to move it forward while pushing backward on the femur, feeling for any anterior excursion of the tibia. The normal response is no forward translation of the tibia. With an ACL tear, there is anterior excursion of the tibia.
Thumb sign—posterior cruciate ligament (PCL)	With the patient supine, flex the knee to 90 degrees with the foot supported. Normally, the anterior tibial plateaus sit 1 cm anterior to the femoral condyles, and you may place your thumbs on top of the medial and lateral tibial plateaus. If the PCL is injured, the proximal tibia falls back and the area available to your thumbs decreases. When the tibial plateaus are flush with the femoral condyles, there is 10 mm or more of posterior laxity, consistent with a complete tear of the PCL.

✸ Advanced Assessment 52.9: Assessing Ankle Ligaments—Special Tests

Test	Comments
Anterior drawer test—to test stability of anterior talofibular ligament; place the ankle in approximately 20 degrees of plantar flexion	Stabilize the tibia, grasp the hindfoot, and pull forward. Asymmetrical or excessive motion will occur with chronic ankle laxity and severe ankle sprains.
Varus stress test—to test the stability of the calcaneofibular ligament	With the tibia stabilized and the ankle in neutral, grasp the calcaneus and invert the hindfoot. Excessive or asymmetrical motion will occur with chronic laxity of the calcaneofibular ligament.

the bone. A tendon rupture can occasionally occur spontaneously in healthy individuals from relatively minor trauma. Achilles tendon rupture is also an uncommon but potential side effect of fluoroquinolones. Physical examination will usually reveal swelling, tenderness, and often bruising over the site of rupture. The tendon's continuity can be tested by performing Thompson's test. To do so, have the patient (1) lie prone, (2) bend the knee so that the leg is vertical, and (3) squeeze the calf. The test is positive if squeezing the calf does not produce plantar flexion of the ankle, indicating a rupture of the tendon. Treatment is either surgical repair or immobilization with a cast with the foot plantar flexed.

Chronic ligamentous laxity may produce few symptoms other than an aching and tenderness over ligaments after prolonged activity. Rest and NSAIDs are the treatment of choice.

FOOT PAIN

Foot pain is a common problem among adults. According to the Framingham population study of older adults, approximately 19% of men and 25% of women have significant foot pain on most days of the week that often limits their ability to function. The authors of this study

Achilles tendon rupture causes pain and inability to walk normally. Closed tendon ruptures usually result from a sudden excessive load applied to the musculotendinous unit, with failure occurring either within the tendon's substance (torn fibers) or at its insertion into recommend that clinicians include a foot examination as part of their routine evaluation of older patients. However, many clinicians may not be adequately prepared to perform such an examination because their training in the diagnosis and care of foot problems is limited.

The foot contains 26 bones, 33 joints, and more than 100 ligaments. Foot pain is usually related to an inflammatory process resulting from trauma (13% of activity-related musculoskeletal injuries in men), a deformity, or a foot–shoe incompatibility. The feet are subjected to numerous forces: for example, when an individual is standing, forces exerted on the foot are equivalent to four times the individual's body weight. Any alteration in ability to use the feet for any reason, such as pain secondary to hammer toe or corns and calluses, will have a significant effect on the health and well-being of the patient.

General treatment measures for foot pain include the use of footwear with roomy toes, supportive arches, and low heels. Heel lifts, cushioned inner soles, and arch supports can provide significant relief when used appropriately. Referral to a podiatrist may be necessary.

DIFFERENTIAL DIAGNOSIS

Differential Diagnosis 52.4 presents common differential diagnoses and their treatment.

Forefoot Problems

Common problems in the forefoot are calluses, corns, plantar warts, bunions, neuromas, and stress fractures. The history in patients with calluses, corns, and warts would reveal discomfort related to pressure, whereas

⏚ Differential Diagnosis 52.4: Foot Pain

Differential Diagnosis	Management
Forefoot	
Hallus valgus or bunion	Avoid pressure on the tender bunion, NSAIDs, protective shields, orthotic devices, appropriate footwear; if no relief, consider surgery.
Enlarged bone on the medial side of the first metatarsal	
Corns and calluses with keratinized skin	Moleskin protection, gentle rubbing with pumice, separating toes with cushions or orthotics; if unrelieved, consider surgery.
Sesamoid disorders localized pain and swelling over first metatarsophalangeal joint	Protect the injured part by limiting weight-bearing, wearing protective padding or strapping, and NSAIDs.
Neuromas	Shoe modification: wide toe box, metatarsal bar, and soft inner soles; NSAIDs; and in severe cases, corticosteroid injections to reduce inflammation.
Stress fractures	Rest and efforts to disperse weight-bearing away from the fracture such as stiff-soled shoe, metatarsal bar, walking cast.
Infection	Treatment as appropriate.
Flat feet	Orthotics.
Bunion	Pad; surgery.
Peripheral neuritis	Investigate cause.
Midfoot	
Pes planus	No treatment if asymptomatic; if symptomatic: flexible arch support, heel-cord stretching, and toe exercises such as picking up objects with toes and spreading toes.
Hindfoot	
Achilles tendinitis	Initial treatment: rest, ice, use of NSAIDs, and immobilization. Heel lifts and heel-cord stretching exercises. Corticosteroids are contraindicated.
Plantar fasciitis Infracalcaneal bursitis	Heel lifts, padded heel cups, and orthotic devices. Acute treatment is rest, ice, NSAIDs, and local corticosteroid injections. Heel-cord stretching exercises and use of a nighttime dorsal splint to maintain ankle dorsiflexion and toe extension may be beneficial; surgical release of the plantar fascia is the measure of last resort.

stress fractures cause pain of acute onset involving the metatarsals. An interdigital neuroma causes tenderness in the third and fourth intermetatarsal spaces with radiation into the toes. Physical examination findings in patients with stress fractures include point tenderness and swelling over the involved bone. The hyperkeratotic lesions of calluses and corns may be indistinguishable from each other, but plantar warts can be distinguished by the punctate bleeding associated with the wart. Interdigital neuromas may sometimes produce a tender nodule in the intermetatarsal space. A *bunion* or *hallus valgus* is the deformity of the first metatarsophalangeal joint associated with the lateral drift of the toe. This presents as a painful swelling on the dorsomedial aspect of the first metatarsal head. Foot–shoe incompatibility may produce physical findings such as the toe deformities of hammer toe and mallet toe.

Midfoot Problems

Midfoot problems are generally the result of pes planus, or flat foot. This is likely to produce pain and stiffness in the midfoot region, often associated with degenerative arthritis or laxity of the posterior tibial tendon. Tenderness to palpation usually occurs along the medial plantar border of the sole with flat foot. Flattening of the medial longitudinal arch of the foot and often a valgus deflection of the heel is indicative of this condition.

Hindfoot Problems

Common hindfoot conditions include plantar fasciitis, infracalcaneal bursitis, and posterior heel problems such as Achilles tendinitis and posterior bursitis. The history of individuals with plantar fasciitis includes subcalcaneal pain that sometimes radiates to the arch of the foot while the person is running or walking. The pain is worse in the morning. Infracalcaneal bursitis produces an aching sensation in the midplantar region of the calcaneus that becomes worse the longer the heel is weight-bearing. The pain associated with Achilles tendinitis is at or proximal to the insertion of the Achilles tendon onto the calcaneus. In this condition, the physical examination reveals swelling and erythema. The pain is increased with dorsiflexion of the ankle, and crepitus may be palpated. Infracalcaneal bursitis produces pain and tenderness to palpation in the midplantar aspect of the calcaneus. Plantar fasciitis findings typically include tenderness along the medial plantar aspect of the calcaneus, with forced dorsiflexion of the digits increasing the pain.

REFERENCES

General

Armstrong AD, Hubbard MC, eds. *Essentials of musculoskeletal care.* 5th ed. Rosemont, IL: American Academy of Orthopedic Surgeons; 2016.

Bally M, Dendukuri N, Rich B, et al. Risk of acute myocardial infarction with NSAIDs in real world use: Bayesian meta-analysis of individual patient data. *BMJ.* 2017:357:j19019.

Dowell D, Haegerich TM, Chou R. CDC guidelines for prescribing opioids for chronic pain - United States, 2016. *MMWR Recomm Rep.* 2016;65(No. RR-1):1–49.

Jensen MP, Patterson DR. Hypnotic approaches for chronic pain management. *Am Psychol.* 2014;69(2):167–177.

Liebson C. *Functional training handbook.* Philadelphia, PA: Wolters Kluwer Health; 2014.

Malanga GA, Nadler SF, eds. *Musculoskeletal physical examination: An evidence-based approach.* 2nd ed. Philadelphia, PA: Elsevier; 2017.

McGee S. *Evidence-based physical diagnosis.* 4th ed. St. Louis, MO: Saunders/Elsevier; 2017.

Onks CA, Wawrzyniak J. The physical therapy prescription. *Med Clin North Am.* 2014;98:869–880.

Raj PP, Erdine S. *Pain-relieving procedures: The illustrated guide.* Chichester: Wiley-Blackwell; 2012.

Simel DL, Drummond R. *The rational clinical examination: Evidence-based clinical diagnosis.* New York, NY: McGraw-Hill; 2009.

Sostres C, Lanas A. Appropriate prescription, adherence and safety of non-steroidal anti-inflammatory drugs. *Med Clin (Barc).* 2016;146:267–272.

Vaccarino AL, Sills TL, Evans KR, Kalali AH. Multiple pain complaints in patients with major depressive disorder. *Psychosom Med.* 2009;71:159–162.

Acute Musculoskeletal Injuries

Allen RJ, Wilson AM. Physical therapy agents. In: Fishman SM et al., eds. *Bonica's management of pain.* 4th ed. Philadelphia, PA: Lippincott Williams & Wilkins; 2012.

Bouma AJ, van Wilgen P, Dijkstra A. The barrier–belief approach in the counseling of physical activity. *Patient Educ Couns.* 2015;98:129–136.

Cameron MH. *Physical agents in rehabilitation: From research to practice.* 4th ed. St. Louis, MO: Elsevier; 2012.

Derry MP, Wiffen PJ, Kalso EA, et al. Topical analgesics for acute and chronic pain in adults—an overview of Cochrane reviews. *Cochrane Database Syst Rev.* 2017;5:CD008609.

Ankle Pain

Beckenkamp PR, Lin CC, Macaskill P, et al. Diagnostic accuracy of the Ottawa ankle and midfoot rules: A systematic review with meta-analysis. *Br J Sports Med.* 2017;51:504–510.

Carr JB. Malleolar fractures and soft tissue injuries of the ankle. In: Browner BD, Jupiter JB, Levine AM, Trafton PG, eds. *Skeletal trauma: Basic science, management and reconstruction.* 3rd ed. Philadelphia, PA: Saunders; 2003:2326.

Doherty C, Delahunt E, Caulfield B, et al. The incidence and prevalence of ankle sprain injury: A systematic review and meta-analysis of prospective epidemiological studies. *Sports Med.* 2014;44:123–140.

Faizullin I, Faizullina E. Effects of balance training on post-sprained ankle joint instability. *Int J Risk Saf Med.* 2015;27 (suppl 1):S99.

Grimm NL, Jacobs JC Jr, Kim J, et al. Ankle injury prevention programs for soccer athletes are protective: A level-I meta-analysis. *J Bone Joint Surg Am.* 2016;98:1436–1443.

Hall EA, Docherty CL, Simon J, et al. Strength-training protocols to improve deficits in participants with chronic ankle instability: A randomized controlled trial. *J Athl Train.* 2015;50:36.

Massey T, Derry S, Moore RA, McQuay HJ. Topical NSAIDs for acute pain in adults. *Cochrane Database Syst Rev.* 2010;(6):CD007402.

Niek van Dijk C. Anterior and posterior ankle impingement. *Foot Ankle Clin.* 2006;11:663.

Schiftan GS, Ross LA, Hahne AJ. The effectiveness of proprioceptive training in preventing ankle sprains in sporting populations: A systematic review and meta-analysis. *J Sci Med Sport.* 2015;18:238.

Seah R, Mani-Babu S. Managing ankle sprains in primary care: What is best practice? A systematic review of the last 10 years of evidence. *Br Med Bull.* 2011;97:105.

Sman AD, Hiller CE, Refshauge KM. Diagnostic accuracy of clinical tests for diagnosis of ankle syndesmosis injury: A systematic review. *Br J Sports Med.* 2013;47:620.

Thomas MJ, Roddy E, Zhang W, et al. The population prevalence of foot and ankle pain in middle and old age: A systematic review. *Pain.* 2011;152:2870.

van Ochten JM, van Middelkoop M, Meuffels D, Bierma-Zeinstra SM. Chronic complaints after ankle sprains: A systematic review on effectiveness of treatments. *J Orthop Sports Phys Ther.* 2014;44:862.

Back Pain

Briggs AM, Bragge P, Smith AJ, et al. Prevalence and associated factors for thoracic spine pain in the adult working population: A literature review. *J Occup Health.* 2009;51:177.

Chou R. In the clinic. Low back pain. *Ann Intern Med.* 2014;160:ITC6.

Croft PR, Papageorgiou AC, Ferry S, et al. Psychologic distress and low back pain. Evidence from a prospective study in the general population. *Spine (Phila Pa 1976).* 1995;20:2731.

Deyo RA, Mirza SK, Martin BI. Back pain prevalence and visit rates: Estimates from U.S. national surveys, 2002. *Spine (Phila Pa 1976).* 2006;31:2724.

Govind J, Bogduck N. Neurolytic blockade for noncancer pain. In: Fishman SM et al., eds. *Bonica's management of pain.* 4th ed. Philadelphia, PA: Lippincott Williams & Wilkins; 2009:1467–1485

Hoy D, Bain C, Williams G, et al. A systematic review of the global prevalence of low back pain. *Arthritis Rheum.* 2012;64:2028.

Humphreys SC, Eck JC, Hodges SD. Neuroimaging in low back pain. *Am Fam Physician.* 2002;65(11):2299–2306.

Katz JN. Lumbar disc disorders and low-back pain: Socioeconomic factors and consequences. *J Bone Joint Surg Am.* 2006;88(suppl 2):21.

Papageorgiou AC, Croft PR, Ferry S, et al. Estimating the prevalence of low back pain in the general population. Evidence from the South Manchester Back Pain Survey. *Spine (Phila Pa 1976).* 1995;20:1889.

Robinson JP, Tait RC. Disability evaluation in painful conditions. In: Fishman SM et al., eds. *Bonica's management of pain.* 4th ed. Philadelphia, PA: Lippincott Williams & Wilkins; 2010:279–288.

Sluys KP, Shults J, Richmond TS. Health-related quality of life and return to work after minor extremity injuries: A longitudinal study comparing upper versus lower extremity injuries. *Injury.* 2016;47:824–831.

Steffens D, Ferreira ML, Latimer J, et al. What triggers an episode of acute low back pain? A case-crossover study. *Arthritis Care Res (Hoboken).* 2015;67:403.

van den Bekerom MP, Sjer A, Somford MP, et al. Non-steroidal anti-inflammatory drugs (NSAIDs) for treating acute ankle sprains in adults: Benefits outweigh adverse events. *Knee Surg Sports Traumatol Arthrosc.* 2015;23:2390.

Elbow, Wrist, and Hand Pain

Behr CT, Altchek DW. The elbow. *Clin Sports Med.* 1997;16:681.

Chen PJ, Liu AL. Concurrent flexor carpi radialis tendon rupture and closed distal radius fracture. *BMJ Case Rep.* 2014;2014.

Descatha A, Carton M, Mediouni Z, et al. Association among work exposure, alcohol intake, smoking and Dupuytren's disease in a large cohort study (GAZEL). *BMJ Open.* 2014;4:e004214.

Jie KE, van Dam LF, Verhagen TF, Hammacher ER. Extension test and ossal point tenderness cannot accurately exclude significant injury in acute elbow trauma. *Ann Emerg Med.* 2014;64:74.

Krogh TP, Fredberg U, Christensen R, et al. Ultrasonographic assessment of tendon thickness, Doppler activity and bony spurs of the elbow in patients with lateral epicondylitis and healthy subjects: A reliability and agreement study. *Ultraschall Med.* 2013;34:468.

Lichtman DM, Lesley NE, Simmons SP. The classification and treatment of Kienbock's disease: The state of the art and a look at the future. *J Hand Surg Eur Vol.* 2010;35:549.

McEvenue G, FitzPatrick F, von Schroeder HP. An educational intervention to improve splinting to improve splinting of common hand injuries. *J Emerg Med.* 2016;50(2):228–234.

Rettig AC. Athletic injuries of the wrist and hand: Part II: Overuse injuries of the wrist and traumatic injuries to the hand. *Am J Sports Med.* 2004;32:262.

Saunders S, Longworth S. *Injection techniques in musculoskeletal medicin.* 3rd ed. London: Churchill Livingstone; 2012.

Swigart CR. Hand and wrist pain. In: Firestein GS, Budd RC, Gabriel SE, McInnes IB, O'Dell R, eds. *Kelley's textbook of rheumatology; vol I.* 9th ed. Philadelphia, PA: Elsevier Saunders;2013:718.

Foot Pain

Aranda Y, Munuera PV. Plantar fasciitis and its relationship with hallux limitus. *J Am Podiatr Med Assoc.* 2014;104:263.

Dunn JE, Link CL, Felson DT, et al. Prevalence of foot and ankle conditions in a multiethnic community sample of older adults. *Am J Epidemiol.* 2004;159:491.

Hillstrom HJ, Song J, Kraszewski AP, et al. Foot type biomechanics part 1: Structure and function of the asymptomatic foot. *Gait Posture.* 2013;37:445.

Jenkins DW, Cooper K, O'Connor R, et al. Prevalence of podiatric conditions seen in Special Olympics athletes: Structural, biomechanical and dermatological findings. *Foot (Edinb).* 2011;21:15.

Macdonald DJ, Holt G, Vass K, et al. The differential diagnosis of foot lumps: 101 cases treated surgically in North Glasgow over 4 years. *Ann R Coll Surg Engl.* 2007;89:272.

Menz HB, Dufour AB, Casey VA, et al. Foot pain and mobility limitations in older adults: The Framingham Foot Study. *J Gerontol A Biol Sci Med Sci.* 2013;68:1281.

Menz HB, Tiedemann A, Kwan MM, et al. Foot pain in community-dwelling older people: An evaluation of the Manchester Foot Pain and Disability Index. *Rheumatology (Oxford).* 2006;45:863.

Mootanah R, Song J, Lenhoff MW, et al. Foot type biomechanics Part 2: Are structure and anthropometrics related to function? *Gait Posture.* 2013;37:452.

Thomas MJ, Roddy E, Zhang W, et al. The population prevalence of foot and ankle pain in middle and old age: A systematic review. *Pain.* 2011;152:2870.

Hip Pain

Agten CA, Sutter R, Buck FM, Pfirrmann CW. Hip imaging in athletes: Sports imaging series. *Radiology.* 2016;280:351.

Christmas C, Crespo CJ, Franckowiak SC, et al. How common is hip pain among older adults? Results from the Third National Health and Nutrition Examination Survey. *J Fam Pract.* 2002;51:345.

Frank JM, Harris JD, Erickson BJ, et al. Prevalence of femoroacetabular impingement imaging findings in asymptomatic volunteers: A systematic review. *Arthroscopy.* 2015;31:1199.

Karrach C, Lynch S. Practical approach to hip pain. *Med Clin North Am.* 2014;98:747–754.

Khanna V, Caragianis A, Diprimio G, et al. Incidence of hip pain in a prospective cohort of asymptomatic volunteers: Is the cam deformity a risk factor for hip pain? *Am J Sports Med.* 2014;42:793.

Kolo FC, Charbonnier C, Pfirrmann CW, et al. Extreme hip motion in professional ballet dancers: Dynamic and morphological evaluation based on magnetic resonance imaging. *Skeletal Radiol.* 2013;42:689.

Martin HD. Clinical examination of the hip. *Oper Tech Orthop.* 2005;15:177.

Martin HD, Palmer IJ. History and physical examination of the hip: The basics. *Curr Rev Musculoskelet Med.* 2013;6:219.

Nunley RM, Prather H, Hunt D, et al. Clinical presentation of symptomatic acetabular dysplasia in skeletally mature patients. *J Bone Joint Surg Am.* 2011;93(suppl 2):17.

Paluska SA. An overview of hip injuries in running. *Sports Med.* 2005;35:991.

Rankin AT, Bleakley CM, Cullen M. Hip joint pathology as a leading cause of groin pain in the sporting population: A 6-year review of 894 cases. *Am J Sports Med.* 2015;43:1698.

Rivière C, Hardijzer A, Lazennec J-Y, et al. Spine-hip add understandings to the pathophysiology of femoro-acetabular impingement: A systematic review. *Orthop Traumatol Surg Res.* 2017;103:549–557.

Williams PT. Effects of running and walking on osteoarthritis and hip replacement risk. *Med Sci Sports Exerc.* 2013;45:1292.

Knee Pain

Alba-Martin P, Gallego-Izquierdo T, Plaza-Mazano G, et al. Effectiveness of therapeutic physical exercise in the treatment of patellofemoral pain syndrome: A systematic review. *J Phys Ther Sci.* 2015;27:2387–2390.

Hochberg MC, Martel-Pelletier J, Monfort J, et al. Combined chondroitin sulfate and glucosamine for painful knee osteoarthritis: A multicenter randomized, double-blind, non-inferiority trial versus celecoxib. *Clin Epidemiol Ann Rheumatol Dis.* 2016;75:37–44.

Jinks C, Jordan K, Croft P. Measuring the population impact of knee pain and disability with the Western Ontario and McMaster Universities Osteoarthritis Index (WOMAC). *Pain.* 2002;100:55.

National Clinical Guideline Center. *Osteoarthritis: Care and management in adults.* London: National Institute for Health and Clinical Excellence; 2014. http://www.ncbi.nlm.nih.gov/pubmed/25340227. Accessed on February 6, 2018.

Nguyen US, Zhang Y, Zhu Y, et al. Increasing prevalence of knee pain and symptomatic knee osteoarthritis: Survey and cohort data. *Ann Intern Med.* 2011;155:725.

Muscle Cramps

Alvarez-Nemegyei J, Canoso JJ. Evidence-based soft tissue rheumatology IV: Anserine bursitis. *J Clin Rheumatol.* 2004;10:205.

Corruble E, Guelfi JD. Pain complaints in depressed inpatients. *Psychopathology.* 2000;33:307.

Eisele S, Garbe E, Zeitz M, et al. Ciprofloxacin-related acute severe myalgia necessitating emergency care treatment: A case report and review of the literature. *Int J Clin Pharmacol Ther.* 2009;47:165.

Jacobson TA. Toward "pain-free" statin prescribing: Clinical algorithm for diagnosis and management of myalgia. *Mayo Clin Proc.* 2008;83:687.

Lyman D. Undiagnosed vitamin D deficiency in the hospitalized patient. *Am Fam Physician.* 2005;71:299.

Shapiro MS, Trebich C, Shilo L, Shenkman L. Myalgias and muscle contractures as the presenting signs of Addison's disease. *Postgrad Med J.* 1988;64:222.

Myofacial Pain

Chan Y, Wang T, Chang C, et al. Short-term effect of massage combined with home exercise on pain, daily activity, and autonomic function in patients with myofascial pain dysfunction syndrome. *J Phys Ther Sci.* 2015;27:217–221.

Desai MJ, Saini V, Saini S. Myofascial pain syndrome: A treatment review. *Pain Ther.* 2013;2(1):21–36.

Meeus M, Nijs J, Meirleir KD. Chronic musculoskeletal pain in patients with the chronic fatigue syndrome: A systematic review. *Eur J Pain.* 2007;11:377.

Yuan QL, Wang P, Liu L, et al. Acupuncture for musculoskeletal pain: A meta-analysis and meta-regression of sham controlled randomized clinical trials. 2016;6:30675.

Neck Pain

Alvarez-Nemegyei J, Canoso JJ. Evidence-based soft tissue rheumatology IV: Anserine bursitis. *J Clin Rheumatol.* 2004;10:205.

Eisele S, Garbe E, Zeitz M, et al. Ciprofloxacin-related acute severe myalgia necessitating emergency care treatment: A case report and review of the literature. *Int J Clin Pharmacol Ther.* 2009;47:165.

Horn ME, Brennan GP, George SZ, Harman JS, Bishop MD. Description of common clinical presentations and associated short-term physical therapy clinical outcomes in patients with neck pain. *Arch Phys Med Rehabil.* 2015;96:1756–1762.

Paresthesias

Campbell WW. *DeJong's the neurologic examination.* 7th ed. Philadelphia, PA: Lippincott Williams & Wilkins; 2013.

Hughes R. Investigation of peripheral neuropathy. *BMJ.* 2010;341:c6100.

Jabre JF, Dillard JW, Salzsieder BT, et al. The use of multiple Tinel's sign in the identification of patients with peripheral neuropathy. *Electromyogr Clin Neurophysiol.* 1995;35:131.

Morrison B, Chaudhry V. Medication, toxic, and vitamin-related neuropathies. *Continuum (Minneap Minn).* 2012;18:139.

Singer MA, Vernino SA, Wolfe GI. Idiopathic neuropathy: New paradigms, new promise. *J Peripher Nerv Syst.* 2012;17 (suppl 2):43.

Shoulder Pain

Iannotti JP, Zlatkin MB, Esterhai JL, et al. Magnetic resonance imaging of the shoulder: Sensitivity, specificity, and predictive value. *J Bone Joint Surg Am.* 1991;73:17.

Lafosse T, Fogerty S, Idoine J, et al. Hyper extension-internal rotation (HERI): A new test for anterior gleno-humeral instability. *Orthop Traumatol Surg Res.* 2016;102:3.

Page MJ, Green S, McBain B, et al. Manual therapy and exercise for rotator cuff disease. *Cochrane Database Syst Rev.* 2016;(6): CD012224.

Reinold MM, Escamilla RF, Wilk KE. Current concepts in the scientific and clinical rationale behind exercises for glenohumeral and scapulothoracic musculature. *J Orthop Sports Phys Ther.* 2009;39:105.

Stevenson JH, Trojian T. Evaluation of shoulder pain. *J Fam Pract.* 2002;51:605.

Teefey SA, Rubin DA, Middleton WD, et al. Detection and quantification of rotator cuff tears. Comparison of ultrasonographic, magnetic resonance imaging, and arthroscopic findings in seventy-one consecutive cases. *J Bone Joint Surg Am.* 2004; 86-A:708.

Wright AA, Wassinger CA, Frank M, et al. Diagnostic accuracy of scapular physical examination tests for shoulder disorders: A systematic review. *Br J Sports Med.* 2013;47:886.

RESOURCES

American Academy of Physical Medicine and Rehabilitation
http://www.aapmr.org
American Academy of Physical Therapy
http://www.aaptnet.org
American Academy of Orthopaedic Surgeons
http://www.aaos.org
American Association of Clinical Endocrinologists (AACE)
http://www.aace.com
American Orthopedic Foot and Ankle Society
http://www.aofas.org
Association of Hip and Knee Surgeons
http://www.aahks.org
Ergonomics. Occupational Safety and Health Administration
https://www.osha.gov/SLTC/ergonomics/
Ergonomics and Musculoskeletal Disorders, Centers for Disease Control and Prevention/National Institute of Occupational Safety and Health
https://www.cdc.gov/niosh/topics/ergonomics/default.html
Fitness Partner
http://www.primusweb.com/fitnesspartner
Muscle Spasms. Cleveland Clinic.
https://my.clevelandclinic.org/health/diseases/15466-muscle-spasms
Musculoskeletal Disorders. Centers for Disease Control and Prevention/National Institute for Occupational Health and Safety.
https://www.cdc.gov/niosh/programs/msd/default.html
National Institute of Arthritis and Musculoskeletal and Skin Diseases
http://www.nih.gov/niams
National Library of Medicine
http://www.nim.nih.gov/melineplus
Orthogate: The Gateway to the Orthopedic Internet
https://www.orthogate.org/patient-education/shoulder/acromio-clavicular-joint-separation
Physical Therapy Association
http://www.apta.org
Physician and Sports Medicine
https://physsportsmed.org
Rehabilitation Foundation
http://www.rfi.org
Symptoms of Peripheral Neuropathy. The Foundation for Peripheral Neuropathy.
https://www.foundationforpn.org/what-is-peripheral-neuropathy/symptoms/
Trigger Points: Diagnosis and Management. *American Family Physician*
https://www.aafp.org/afp/2002/0215/p653.html
Work-Related Musculoskeletal Disorders (WMSDs). Canadian Centre for Occupational Health and Safety
https://www.ccohs.ca/oshanswers/diseases/rmirsi.html

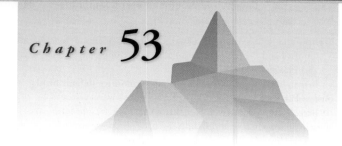

Chapter 53

Spinal Disorders

Patricia Vanhook, PhD, MSN, APRN, FNP-BC, FAAN, FAANP

Lynne M. Dunphy, PhD, APRN, FNP-BC, FAAN, FAANP

Brian Oscar Porter, MD, PhD, MPH, MBA

Conor Luskin, PA-C

CERVICAL MUSCLE SPRAIN/STRAIN

Cervical muscle sprain/strain is a muscle injury in the neck, a common and largely self-limited condition. The soft-tissue muscles of the neck are deeply buried and protected, and it is often difficult to differentiate injuries to the neck by either physical examination or more sophisticated imaging modalities. Thus, this term is also used to describe ligamentous injuries of the facet joints or intervertebral discs. After ruling out neurologic dysfunction and unstable injuries, the treatments for a neck sprain or strain are similar.

"Whiplash" describes an acceleration–deceleration of the neck with rapid flexion–extension and is a common sequela of motor vehicle accidents. Despite no apparent instability, these injuries may cause prolonged disability, probably related to a combination of relatively severe ligamentous/muscle injury with nonorganic overlay.

EPIDEMIOLOGY AND CAUSES

Cervical pain is common in both men and women and is usually described as lasting 2 weeks or longer. Mechanical disorders of the cervical spine are the most common cause of neck pain. Information on the prevalence and incidence of cervical pain is available from multiple sources but varies across a wide range. Consistent reporting of occurrence rates is also hampered by the lack of a reproducible definition of cervical pain across multiple studies. Terms such as *whiplash, acute neck sprain, neck spasm,* and *cervical strain* are frequently used to describe what seems to be a single condition. The prevalence of cervical pain in men and women is

approximately 8% among persons aged 25 to 74 years. The highest prevalence (10%) is among persons aged 45 to 64 years.

It has been estimated that 85% of all neck injuries presenting to primary-care providers result from automobile accidents. The National Safety Council estimates that 20% of all automobile accidents are rear-end impacts that can cause whiplash. Approximately one-third of people will develop neck pain within 24 hours of the injury. The natural history of hyperextension cervical muscle strain and spasm injuries is that 60% get better within the first year, 32% get better within the next year, and 8% have permanent problems.

The relationship between occupational factors and cervical pain is difficult to study because exposure to those factors is usually difficult to quantify. Workers may be exposed to multiple risk factors both on the job and at home. Most of work-related cervical injuries are diagnosed as a sprain or strain, and certain occupations appear to have a predisposition to cervical symptoms. Workers who do repetitive tasks with their upper extremities and prolonged sitting with their head in a flexed position are at risk of developing mechanical neck pain; these include machine operators, carpenters, office workers, dentists, and keyboard operators.

PATHOPHYSIOLOGY

Cervical sprain is a clinical condition describing a nonradiating discomfort or pain in the neck area associated with a concomitant loss of neck motion and stiffness. The major biomechanical function of the cervical spine is to support the skull and provide movement in flexion, extension, and rotation. The supporting structures of the cervical spine are relatively unprotected; thus, injury to the muscles and ligaments that provide these motions can easily occur. Specific abnormalities in cervical strain can almost never be identified, except in traumatic injury to a specific structure.

Normal posture should be effortless and painless. Abnormal forward posture of the head results in chronic strain on the posterior structures of the neck. A variety of daily activities may result in chronic abnormal posture, such as the prolonged use of a computer with a screen below eye level, a faulty sitting position, or the use of bifocal glasses. A variety of factors extraneous to the muscles also can affect muscle tension, including fatigue, pain, anger, emotional stress, anxiety, and depression.

Whiplash injuries are most commonly caused by rear-end motor vehicle collisions (MVCs) when the driver of a stationary car is struck from behind by another vehicle. The driver is usually relaxed and unaware of the impending collision. The sudden acceleration of the struck vehicle pushes the back of the car seat against the driver's torso. This force pushes the driver's torso and shoulders forward while the head remains static but moves posteriorly, causing hyperextension of the neck. This injury is most common in Western societies and metropolitan areas, where there are more automobiles.

CLINICAL PRESENTATION

Subjective

Pain is the most common presenting symptom although the associated complaint of a headache, usually occipital, which may persist for months, is not unusual. The pain is usually located in the middle to lower part of the posterior neck. The area of pain may be limited, or it may cover a large area. The pain may radiate toward the shoulders but usually will not radiate down into the arm. The pain associated with a cervical strain is most often dull and aching and is exacerbated by neck motion and alleviated by rest or immobilization. The pain may follow a significant trauma or may be spontaneous in onset; pain following trauma often persists longer than sprains of spontaneous onset. Nonradicular, nonfocal neck pain is most common and may be noted anywhere from the base of the skull to the cervicothoracic junction. Pain is often worse with motion and may be accompanied by paraspinal spasm and discomfort in the region of the trapezius muscle. Pain may be accompanied by fatigue, sleep disturbance, irritability, and difficulty concentrating. Work tolerance may be impaired.

Cervical pain from an MVC usually does not appear for about 12 to 14 hours after the collision. The driver is often unaware at first of having been injured but later begins to feel stiffness in the neck. The pain at the base of the neck increases and is made worse by head and neck movement. Pain patterns should be evaluated carefully to differentiate muscular pain from radicular symptoms that typically radiate down the upper extremities.

Objective

Physical examination shows decreased neck range of motion (ROM) with poor quality of movement. With typical cervical muscle strain or spasm, Spurling's sign (radicular pain reproduced when the examiner exerts downward pressure on the vertex while tilting the head toward the symptomatic side) is usually negative.

Frequently, there is tenderness to palpation over both the anterior and posterior structures of the cervical spine, specifically the paraspinous muscles, spinous processes, interspinous ligaments, or medial border of the scapula. The intensity of pain is variable, and the loss of cervical motion correlates with intensity of pain. Active motion of the cervical spine against any type of resistance causes an increase in pain. The shoulder examination, as well as the remainder of the physical examination, is typically normal.

DIAGNOSTIC REASONING

Diagnostic Tests

Any evidence of neurologic deficit merits further diagnostic testing, such as radiographs or magnetic resonance imaging (MRI), which is needed to determine the cause. Hyperextension cervical injuries cause only soft-tissue damage, but plain x-ray films of the cervical spine should be obtained in all instances. It is important to include radiographic studies so that unsuspected fractures or dislocations of the cervical spine, facet fractures, odontoid fractures, or spinous process fractures that might otherwise be missed in the neurologically intact patient can be identified or ruled out.

All seven cervical vertebrae must be visualized. Anterior displacement of the pharyngeal air shadow indicates soft-tissue swelling and possible disruption of the intervertebral disc or anterior longitudinal ligament and requires further evaluation. The width of the prevertebral soft tissue at the level of C3 should not exceed 7 mm in normal adults. The normal lordotic curve may be straightened or reversed with muscle spasm, but this limited finding is noted in approximately 10% of normal adults. Preexisting degenerative disease may be noted, most frequently at C5 to C6 or C6 to C7 and is usually age related. In a patient with severe pain, the screening radiographs should be examined for signs of instability.

Differential Diagnosis

The diagnosis of cervical muscle strain is based on the history of localized neck pain and a compatible physical examination demonstrating localized pain, muscle spasm, and a normal neurologic examination. Trauma to the cervical spine may result in major neural damage with paralysis; if the history reveals a significant trauma, a thorough evaluation with x-ray examination should be performed. Because of the significant consequences of potential damage to the spinal cord, referral to an orthopedic surgeon or neurosurgeon should be sought. Potential differential diagnoses include the following:

- Cervical disc herniation presents with associated radicular pain and neurologic findings.
- Cervical spine tumor is accompanied by a history of night pain and weight loss.
- Cervical spine infection is accompanied by fever, sweats, and chills. Consider if the patient has a history of IV drug use.
- Dislocation or subluxation of the spine would be evident on radiographs.
- Inflammatory conditions of the cervical spine (rheumatoid arthritis) would be accompanied by abnormal radiographs.
- Spinal fracture would be evident on radiographs.
- Malingering is accompanied by exaggerated symptomatology and evidence of secondary gain.

MANAGEMENT

Reassurance is a cornerstone of treatment in uncomplicated cases. A decrease in activity allows the injured tissues to heal.

Nonnarcotic analgesics such as NSAIDs are helpful in making the patient more comfortable. NSAIDs can be continued until symptoms have resolved. However, long-term use of NSAIDs can lead to serious gastrointestinal disease, such as ulcers, gastritis, and hemorrhage. Creams, patches, gels, and other topical medications may be helpful for some patients.

Short-term use of muscle relaxants may be helpful if palpable spasms are seen on physical examination, but they have potential for addiction, and several studies have failed to show their efficacy beyond NSAIDs alone. Drowsiness and dizziness are common side effects, and patients should be cautioned not to drive or operate machinery while taking them and to avoid alcohol and other central nervous system (CNS) depressants to prevent additive effects. Opioids should be avoided because of their potential for abuse and lack of research supporting their efficacy in the treatment of soft-tissue injuries.

Neck pain and mobility are improved with physiotherapy. The goal of therapy is to maximize function of the cervical spine. Physical therapy modalities may take the form of cold (ice) initially or heat (warm bath) to help relieve pain and spasm. Activity should be encouraged as determined by the severity of the symptoms. Cervical traction may also be used to diminish pain and spasm if no improvement is seen with heat and medication. Aerobic activity, such as walking, should be started as soon as possible. Once improvement is seen, a course of isometric exercises should begin. Encourage an early return to work and activities.

FOLLOW-UP AND REFERRAL

Usually the course of cervical muscle strain is one of progressive improvement with complete resolution of symptoms over several weeks. Recovery is usually complete without any lasting impairment; however, a small percentage of patients may continue to experience cervical spine pain despite treatment.

Patient Education: Cervical Muscle Sprain/Strain

If neck pain and restricted range of motion are still present after patients have received analgesics and physical therapy and the findings on computed tomography scan or magnetic resonance imaging are normal, referrals for psychiatric support or vocational rehabilitation may be indicated to assist in recovery.

Knowing how a healthy neck works can help patients understand their cervical spine problems and how to care for them. It is important for patients to understand the concepts behind their treatments to receive the greatest benefits. They must also learn appropriate body mechanics to help protect the cervical spine from further damage by preventing its misuse or overuse. Stress from home or work can also lead to muscle tension and other symptoms, so the patient may need professional guidance in relieving or controlling these stressors.

CERVICAL SPONDYLOSIS

Spondylosis (also called *degenerative arthritis*) is a blanket term for a group of chronic degenerative processes that affect the vertebrae and facet joints and cause pain, stiffness, and disability. Spondylosis can occur in the lumbosacral and cervical regions of the spine. *Cervical spondylosis* (also known as *in the cervical vertebrae*) is a common cause of neck pain in older patients.

EPIDEMIOLOGY AND CAUSES

Cervical spondylosis is extremely common. Degenerative changes on radiography are found in 40% of the population at age 50 and in 70% of the population at age 65. It affects both sexes equally, but degenerative changes may start earlier in men. Spondylosis is usually asymptomatic, meaning that a finding on x-ray study does not necessarily account for the patient's pain. Spondylotic changes are cumulative over time, but the onset of symptoms can be accelerated by trauma, poor body mechanics, postural changes, or disc injury.

PATHOPHYSIOLOGY

Changes in the intervertebral discs caused by aging include a loss of water and elasticity, which can make the disc vulnerable to injury and surrounding ligaments less able to support the surrounding structures. As a result of these changes, the disc may collapse and herniate. A herniating disc may impinge on a spinal nerve root and cause radiculopathy, a characteristic pattern of numbness and tingling caused by compression of the cervical nerve roots. Facet hypertrophy and hypertrophy of the uncinate processes can compress the spinal nerves as they exit the foramina, which may also lead to cervical radiculopathy. The pain and numbness typically occur in a dermatomal pattern of the affected nerve root. The most commonly involved nerve roots are C6 and C7, which produce pain and paresthesias into the lower lateral arm, thumb, and middle finger.

In addition, as degeneration progresses, the facet joints may undergo posterior hypertrophy, and the ligamentum flavum may thicken. Both changes may cause a narrowing of the spinal canal. If the secondary bony changes of cervical spondylosis encroach on the spinal cord, a pathological process called *myelopathy* develops. If this process involves both the nerve roots and spinal cord, it is called *myeloradiculopathy*. Regardless of its etiology, radiculopathy causes shoulder and/or arm pain, as well as numbness and/or tingling ("pins and needles"). Fewer than 5% of patients with cervical spondylosis develop myelopathy, and they are usually between ages 40 and 60. Acute myelopathy is most often the result of central soft-disc herniation, which may be visualized on MRI. Herniation may require surgical decompression. If pain is unremitting and cervical nerve-root compression is present, a neurosurgical consultation should be sought immediately.

CLINICAL PRESENTATION

Subjective

Common symptoms are recurring neck stiffness and mild aching discomfort, especially with activity. At rest, the patient may report neck stiffness and trouble turning the neck from side to side. Pain and limited ROM occur with lateral rotation and lateral flexion of the neck toward the affected side. Paresthesias may also occur that follow the dermatome pattern of affected nerve roots.

Objective

In patients with radicular symptoms, testing may reveal characteristic findings of weakness in shoulder abduction (which indicates involvement of the C5 nerve roots), biceps weakness (indicating C6 involvement), and triceps weakness (indicating C7 involvement). Myelopathy signs and symptoms include leg weakness, gait disturbances, balance problems, difficulty performing fine motor tasks, and, in severe cases, loss of bowel and bladder control (see Advanced Assessment 52.3).

DIAGOSTIC REASONING

Diagnostic Tests

Diagnostic tests include radiological assessment of the cervical spine, and if radicular pain is severe or if there is motor or sensory deficit or hyporeflexia, MRI is indicated. Radiographs will determine if subluxation and other osteoarthritic components are present, but an MRI is necessary to identify disc herniation and soft-tissue or spinal cord abnormalities.

Differential Diagnosis

Differential diagnoses include vertebral fractures, cervical stenosis, cervical disc pathology, brachial plexus lesions, and Parsonage-Turner syndrome. If symptoms are bilateral, disc herniation should be considered in the differential diagnosis. Other causes of bilateral parenthesis or weakness that can mimic spine pathology include central neurologic diseases such as multiple sclerosis, Guillain-Barré syndrome, amyotrophic lateral sclerosis, or brain tumor. In patients presenting with radicular or myelopathy signs and symptoms, an MRI is warranted to assess the source of the symptoms and determine severity.

MANAGEMENT

If only radiculopathy is present, a conservative trial of cervical traction may be warranted. Physical therapy to strengthen the neck musculature and teach proper body mechanics may be helpful. Treatment may also include pain relievers, such as NSAIDs. If these conservative measures do not work and radicular symptoms persist, a trial of oral steroids may be tried. Steroid epidural injections are an intermediate treatment for radiculopathy. These injections are done under fluoroscopic guidance by a physiatrist or radiologist. Surgery is indicated in cases of myelopathy, intractable pain, or severe disability. Moist heat may sometimes be helpful.

FOLLOW-UP AND REFERRAL

If conservative measures do not improve symptoms after 6 weeks, consultation with an orthopedic specialist is recommended.

Patient Education: Cervical Spondylosis

Most (75% to 90%) patients with cervical spondylosis improve with conservative treatment. The remaining subset of patients will experience no change in their symptoms or a worsening of symptoms. Patients should be counseled that in the absence of myelopathy, conservative treatment is recommended as a first-line therapy and that surgery is indicated for spinal cord compression and myelopathy. Patients should be instructed to report any worsening of their symptoms or development of myelopathy to their health-care providers.

LOW BACK PAIN

Low back pain (LBP), also referred to as low back sprain or lumbar sprain, is, strictly speaking, an injury to the paravertebral spinal muscles. The term is also used to describe ligamentous injuries to the facet joints or annulus fibrosus. Because of the deep location of the lumbar soft tissues, localizing an injury to a specific structure is difficult if not impossible. Whether muscle or ligamentous structures are involved, the treatment is similar.

LBP occurs in almost 70% of adults at some point in their lives. About 90% of patients with acute LBP will spontaneously recover activity tolerance within 1 month. However, back pain associated with a neurologic deficit, decreased or absent pulses, or bowel and bladder dysfunction is potentially life-threatening and warrants immediate referral. Acute low back pain (ALBP) is pain that persists for less than 6 weeks. Chronic low back pain (CLBP) is defined as pain lasting longer than 3 months; symptoms are typically recurrent and episodic but may be unremitting.

EPIDEMIOLOGY AND CAUSES

LBP is one of the most frequent reasons that patients visit primary-care providers and is the most common reason for loss of work time and disability in adults younger than 45 years. Most symptoms are of limited duration, with 85% of patients demonstrating significant improvement and returning to work within the month. The 4% of patients whose symptoms persist longer than 6 months generate 85% to 90% of the costs to society for treating LBP. Repetitive episodes, however, are common. Back pain is second only to headache as the reason for a complaint of pain. At any given time, 31 million Americans will be experiencing some sort of ALBP. ALBP occurs most frequently in adults in between ages 20 and 50 years. CLBP typically is seen between the third and sixth decades of life, or even older for women.

The overall incidence of LBP is equal in men and women, but women report more LBP after age 60, most likely due to osteoporosis; these women are at risk for vertebral compression fracture. In addition, a woman's likelihood of experiencing LBP is increased after two or more pregnancies. Approximately 2% of patients with ALBP have lumbar radiculopathy, sciatica with or without a disc herniation (see next section on herniated disc).

There are two categories of risk factors that influence LBP: occupational and patient related. Occupations that require hard labor and heavy exertion have been associated with increased risk of LBP. Lifting, pulling and pushing, twisting, slipping, sitting for an extended period, and exposure to prolonged vibration (such as driving or riding in a motor vehicle for long periods of time, as truck drivers do) have been attributed to the development of LBP. In addition, patients who view their occupations as boring, repetitive, or dissatisfying have been associated with a higher rate of LBP indicating a possible psychological component in some patients. LBP is the most frequent cause of lost workdays in the United States.

There is a higher risk of LBP in obese persons and in tall persons. No studies have proven posture as a definite risk factor for LBP, but spine pain from scoliosis is well known and is the basis of this risk factor. Many studies have shown decreased strength of abdominal and spinal muscles in patients with LBP. Physical fitness and conditioning have been found to have a preventive effect on low back injuries. Smoking has been shown to increase one's risk of LBP. Aging increases the risk for CLBP. Psychosocial factors such as depression, anxiety, and alcoholism, among others, have been reported with higher frequency in patients with chronic LBP.

The cause of back pain is not always clear, but it may be related to ligamentous or muscular strain resulting from either a specific traumatic episode or an incompetence of the soft-tissue structure (ALBP). Degeneration of the intervertebral disc, a physiological event of aging, modified by such factors as injury, repetitive trauma, infection, heredity, and tobacco use, may lead to CLBP.

PATHOPHYSIOLOGY

The lumbosacral spine supports the upper body in a balanced, upright position while allowing locomotion. In a static, upright position, maintenance of erect posture is achieved through a balance among the expansile pressure of the intervertebral discs, the stretch placed on the anterior and posterior longitudinal and facet joint ligaments, and the sustained involuntary tone generated by the surrounding lumbosacral and abdominal muscles. The balance of the spine is also related to the reciprocal physiological curves in the cervical, thoracic, and lumbosacral areas of the vertebral column. The balance in curvature results in an individual's posture. Proper alignment is also influenced by structures in the pelvis and lower extremities. Movement of the lumbar spine is associated with a lumbar pelvic rhythm that results in the simultaneous reversal of the lumbar lordosis and rotation of the hips. During flexion and extension of the lumbar spine, tension is produced in the paraspinous, hamstring, and gluteal muscles, the fasciae that surround the muscles, and the ligaments that support the vertebral bodies and discs. In addition to the normal stresses placed on these structures with lowering and raising of the torso, the stresses on these anatomical structures are increased to an even greater degree when an individual is required to lift a heavy object.

The most common cause of ALBP is lumbar strain and sprains. LBP that is associated with back strain may be related to anatomical structures that are tonically contracted in the resting position. Strain occurs when the muscles or ligaments of the lower back are stretched, causing microscopic tears. Sprains are caused by the overstretching or tearing of ligaments. LBP may also occur during motion if the stress is greater than the supporting structures can sustain or if the components of the lumbosacral spine are abnormal. Although the precise pathophysiology of uncomplicated lumbar strain (back strain) is not well characterized, damage may occur in lumbosacral spinal structures if the amount of force generated exceeds the stress capacity of the spine for an individual patient. If the lumbosacral spine is in a mechanically disadvantaged position (e.g., rotated or flexed) the force may not need to be that great to cause a disruption of annular fibers. These fibers may tear when stressed, which in turn causes degeneration of the disc.

Several other less common spinal conditions exist that produce LBP. Spinal stenosis results in nerve impingement with back and lower extremity (calf) pain on extension of the spine owing to the narrowed spinal canal, because this maneuver lengthens and further narrows the canal. Osteoarthritis typically produces erosion with irregular bony deposition known as osteophytes at the articular sites of the vertebrae that may also result in nerve impingement and pain because of degeneration of the joint. Significant scoliosis can predispose a person to osteoarthritis and may result in chronic LBP resulting from a fundamental derangement of vertebral biomechanics, that is, the ability of the axial musculoskeletal system to appropriately distribute mechanical loads placed on the spine. Spondylolisthesis is a slipping (displacement) of one vertebral body either anteriorly or posteriorly relative to another and may be a congenital or acquired condition. Spinal hyperextension often causes increased or repeated stress on the bilateral pars interarticularis, the posterior bony plate connecting the superior and inferior articular facets of an intervertebral joint. A lesion or fracture of the pars interarticularis that causes the facet to separate without actual anterior or posterior slippage of a vertebral body is known as spondylolysis. Either of these conditions may result in nerve impingement with lower back and extremity pain. Although spondylolysis may be asymptomatic, this condition may progress to spondylolisthesis.

CLINICAL PRESENTATION

While lower back pain is a common symptom that may result from many causes, specific characteristics of the pain as well as its accompanying signs and symptoms relate to the underlying etiology.

Subjective

The patient with an acute onset of LBP caused by lumbar strain or sprain will usually present with localized discomfort that occurs shortly after the lumbar tissue has been mechanically stressed. The most commonly reported histories include lifting and/or twisting while carrying a heavy object, prolonged sitting, MVCs, falls, or operation of a vibrating machine, but LBP may be precipitated by something as minor as a sneeze or cough. Patients may have difficulty standing erect and often change position frequently for comfort. There may be associated grimacing and generalized hypersensitivity to light touch. The pain often radiates into the buttocks and posterior thigh. The injury may also result in lower back muscle spasms, with the sudden onset of recurrent pain.

Initial assessment of a patient with activity intolerance resulting from LBP consists of a focused medical history, including a history of the present illness and past medical, family, occupational, and social history. A review of systems, especially description of any injury, is essential and may alert the provider to possible "red flags" warranting immediate attention (see Table 53.1).

Some questions to consider while evaluating the patient's responses include the following:

- Is there a serious systemic disease causing the pain?
- Is there neurologic compromise that might require surgical evaluation?
- Is there social or psychological distress that may amplify or prolong pain?

Focus on History: Low Back Pain

For the patient who complains of low back pain, focus the history by asking questions that will obtain the following information:

1. Mode of onset (abrupt or insidious?)
2. Characteristics:
   - Provoking factors

TABLE 53.1	Red Flags When Assessing a Patient With Low Back Pain		
Suspect Trauma	*Suspect Tumor*	*Suspect Infection*	*Suspect Radiculopathy or Cauda Equina Syndrome*
Severe trauma: • Sports injury • Fall from elevated height • Recent motor vehicle accident Minor trauma (in elderly with osteoporosis): • Coughing • Sneezing • Heavy lifting	• Advanced age (>50 years) • Unexplained fever >38°C (100.4°F) • Night sweats requiring changing of night wear several times • Pain with lying flat • Severe pain at night • Unintended weight loss ≥10% of body weight in 6 months	• Intense pain at night • History of bacterial infection • History of spinal procedure • IV substance abuse • Immune compromised • International travel • Immigrant background • History of malignant pathology	Radiculopathy: • Nerve root compression demonstrated by segmental pain with paraesthesia and loss of strength (Grade 3 or less) Cauda equina: • Sudden loss of bowel or bladder function • Perianal/perineal anesthesia • Improvement of pain with loss of muscle caused by death of nerve root

Source: Casser H, Seddigh S, Raushmann M. Acute lumbar back pain: Investigation, differential diagnosis, and treatment. *Dtsch Arztebl Int.* 2016;113(13): 223–234.

- Aggravating factors
- Relieving factors
3. Effects of activities
   - Posture
   - Coughing, sneezing, straining
   - Exercise, exertion, rest
   - Sleep
4. History
   - Similar or different pains
   - Course (progressive, decreasing, increasing, fluctuating, episodic?)
   - Associated limb and/or neurologic symptoms (pain, paresthesias, numbness, weakness, atrophy, cramps, fasciculations?)
5. Associated symptoms
   - Urinary problems (frequency, urgency, retention, incontinence?)
   - Bowel problems (incontinence or constipation?)
6. Previous back pain history and treatment (medications, types of surgery, nonpharmacologic management, lifestyle and work modifications, litigation or compensation issues?)

The hallmark symptom of CLBP is recurrent LBP that often radiates to one or both buttocks. The pain may be described as "mechanical" in that it is aggravated by activities such as bending, stooping, or twisting. There may be stiffness and a history of intermittent sciatica (i.e., pain radiating down the back of the leg), but discomfort in the lower back remains the predominant symptom. This may be relieved with lying down or a good night's sleep, although if the pain is severe enough it may awaken the patient at night. Psychosocial indicators should be assessed because they can be barriers to recovery in all cases of LBP, both acute and chronic. Consider factors such as fear, financial problems, anger, depression, job dissatisfaction, family problems, or stress that can contribute to prolonged disability.

Objective

There is often diffuse tenderness in the lower back. ROM of the lumbar spine, particularly flexion, is typically reduced and elicits pain. Patients may exhibit a side or forward list from muscle spasm. The degree of lumbar flexion and the ease with which the patient can extend the spine are helpful parameters by which to evaluate progress. Although not characteristic, nonorganic findings, such as widespread sensitivity to light touch, nonanatomical localization of symptoms, inappropriate grimacing, inconsistent actions, and exaggerated pain behaviors, may be seen. In most cases of uncomplicated LBP, the motor and sensory functions of the lumbosacral nerve roots and reflexes of the lower extremities are normal. Negative straight-leg-raise rules out surgically significant disc herniation in 95% of cases (see Advanced Assessment 53.1).

 Advanced Assessment 53.1: Assessing the Lower Back—Special Tests

Test	Comments
Straight-leg raising—places the L5 and S1 nerve roots and the sciatic nerve under tension	With the patient supine and relaxed, elevate the leg until either the leg begins to bend or the patient reports severe pain in buttock or back. Record degree of elevation at which pain occurs. It is considered positive when the pain is elicited below the level of the knee when the leg is raised less than 60 degrees. Next, dorsiflex the ankle to determine whether this motion increased pain (further stretch of the L5 and S1 nerve roots). Plantar flexion of the ankle relieves sciatic tension. Increased back pain with this maneuver is probably nonorganic. The straight-leg-raising test is very sensitive, but not very specific. To increase specificity, raise the leg until pain is felt below the knee, then lower the leg about 5 degrees, which should eliminate the pain. Then, have patient dorsiflex the ipsilateral foot while the leg is raised. This should cause more traction on the sciatic nerve and reproduce the symptoms.
Reverse straight-leg raising—places the L1–L4 nerve roots under tension	With the patient prone, lift the hip into extension while keeping the knee straight. Increased pain suggests compression of the upper lumbar nerve roots.
Prone rectus femoris test—places the L1–L4 nerve roots under tension	With the patient prone, maintain the hip in a neutral position while flexing the knee. Increased pain suggests compression of the upper lumbar nerve roots.

DIAGNOSTIC REASONING

Diagnostic Tests

In cases of CLBP, anteroposterior and lateral radiographs often show age-appropriate changes, such as anterior osteophytes and reduced height of intervertebral discs on the lateral view. ALBP does not warrant radiographs except in the following circumstances:

- Unrelenting night pain or pain at rest
- Fever above 38°C (100.4°F) for greater than 48 hours
- Progressive neuromotor deficit
- Pain with distal numbness or leg weakness
- Loss of bowel or bladder control (retention or incontinence)
- Significant trauma

- History of suspicion of cancer
- Osteoporosis
- Chronic oral steroid use
- Immunosuppressed or immunosuppressive medication
- Drug or alcohol abuse
- Clinical suspicion of ankylosing spondylitis

The following laboratory tests may be considered if there is indication of systemic pathology. These tests would include complete blood count with differential, and erythrocyte sedimentation rate (ESR) if there is suspicion of cancer or infection. Routine imaging is not indicated in diagnosis of patients with nonspecific LBP (Chou et al., 2011).

Differential Diagnosis

LBP is a diagnosis of exclusion. The diagnosis of back strain is based on the history of localized LBP and a compatible physical examination demonstrating localized pain, muscle spasm, and a normal neurologic examination. CLBP is recurrent and has lasted for a longer period of time, and the patient may also demonstrate mildly restricted straight-leg-raising and spinal motion.

Differential diagnoses for ALBP/CLBP include the following (see Differential Diagnosis 53.1):

- Ankylosing spondylitis (family history, morning stiffness, limited mobility of the lumbar spine)
- Drug-seeking behavior (exaggerated symptoms, inconsistent and nonphysiological examination)
- Extraspinal causes (ovarian cyst, nephrolithiasis, pancreatitis, ulcer disease, abdominal aortic aneurysm)
- Fracture of the vertebral body (major trauma or minimal trauma with osteoporosis)
- Herniated nucleus pulposus or ruptured disc (unilateral radicular pain symptoms that extend below the knee and are equal to or greater than the back pain)

- Infection (fever, chills, sweats, elevated ESR)
- Myeloma (night sweats, men older than 50 years)

Differential diagnoses for CLBP that are different than ALBP include the following:

- Depression (abnormal Beck Depression Inventory, sleep disturbances)
- Illness behavior (multiple surgeries, multiple illnesses)
- Inflammatory arthritis (morning stiffness for more than 30 minutes, positive human leukocyte antigen–B27, increased ESR)
- Intervertebral disc infection or vertebral osteomyelitis (history of excruciating pain, recent IV drug use, fever, recent infection/hospitalization, open wound)
- Metastatic tumors, myeloma, lymphoma (pathological fractures, severe night pain, weight loss, fatigue)
- Osteoporosis with compression fractures (female gender, previous fracture)
- Spinal tuberculosis (lower socioeconomic groups, history of AIDS)
- Workplace dissatisfaction (discontent with boss, job)

MANAGEMENT

Reassure the patient that most episodes of ALBP are mild and self-limited; almost 90% resolve within 1 to 6 weeks. Symptom control is considered an adjunct to helping the patient to overcome specific activity intolerance. The management of the patient with LBP, especially if pain is recurrent and/or chronic, requires a *Circle of Caring* by the practitioner. Multiple approaches are required to address the "iceberg" of LBP and the ways that it can interfere with the lives of patients and families. The practitioner should use the most current clinical practice guideline to appropriately manage acute and chronic conditions in conjunction with the patient's preferences for care and management.

⁂ Differential Diagnosis 53.1: Low Back Pain

Diagnosis	Spondylolisthesis	Muscle Strain	Scoliosis	Herniated Nucleus Pulposus	Osteoarthritis	Spinal Stenosis
Age	20	20–40	30	30–50	>50	>60
Pain location	Back	Back (unilateral)	Back	Back (unilateral)	Back (bilateral)	Leg (bilateral)
Pain onset	Insidious	Acute	Insidious	Acute (prior episodes)	Insidious	Insidious
Pain increases	When standing, bending	When standing, bending	When standing, bending	When sitting, bending	When standing	When standing
Pain decreases	When sitting	When sitting	When sitting	When standing	When sitting, bending	When sitting, bending
Straight-leg raising	Negative	Negative	Negative	Positive	Negative	Positive (stress)
X-ray (plain film)	Positive	Negative	Positive	Negative	Positive	Positive

The Iceberg of Low Back Pain

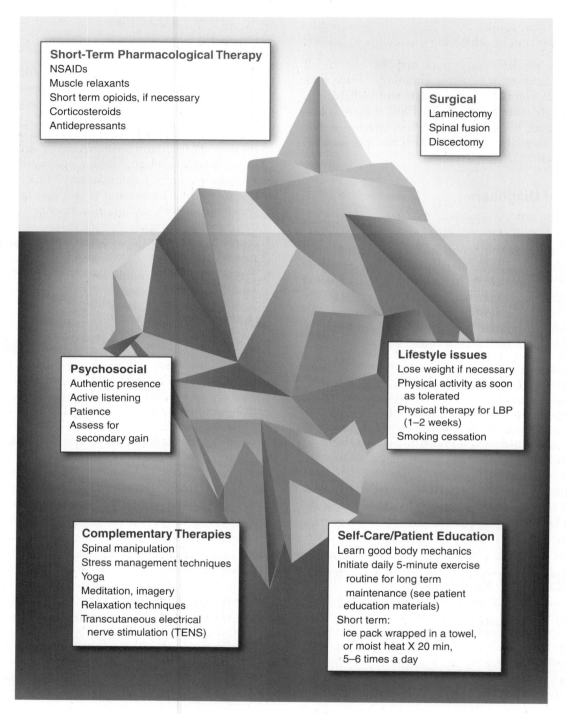

Short-Term Pharmacological Therapy
NSAIDs
Muscle relaxants
Short term opioids, if necessary
Corticosteroids
Antidepressants

Surgical
Laminectomy
Spinal fusion
Discectomy

Psychosocial
Authentic presence
Active listening
Patience
Assess for
    secondary gain

Lifestyle issues
Lose weight if necessary
Physical activity as soon
    as tolerated
Physical therapy for LBP
    (1–2 weeks)
Smoking cessation

Complementary Therapies
Spinal manipulation
Stress management techniques
Yoga
Meditation, imagery
Relaxation techniques
Transcutaneous electrical
    nerve stimulation (TENS)

Self-Care/Patient Education
Learn good body mechanics
Initiate daily 5-minute exercise
    routine for long term
    maintenance (see patient
    education materials)
Short term:
    ice pack wrapped in a towel,
    or moist heat X 20 min,
    5–6 times a day

Nonpharmacologic Management

The initial approach to management of LBP is the utilization of nonpharmacologic approach. There is sufficient evidence to support the following:

- Exercise
- Motor control exercise

- Cognitive behavioral therapy
- Electromyography biofeedback
- Tai chi
- Yoga
- Progressive relaxation
- Superficial heat
- Massage

- Acupuncture
- Spinal manipulation for short-term relief
- Multidisciplinary rehabilitation

Pharmacologic Management

The oral medications used to control the discomfort of LBP primarily include acetaminophen, NSAIDs, and skeletal muscle relaxants. There is fair to good evidence that NSAIDs are effective for reducing pain in patients with LBP. Acetaminophen has not been found to be comparable in efficacy to NSAIDs for treating LBP (Chou et al., 2016; Qaseem et al., 2017). Health-care providers need to be aware that the long-term use of NSAIDs can lead to serious gastrointestinal disease such as ulcers and hemorrhage. NSAIDs also affect renal prostaglandins and may cause fluid retention and edema, so it is also important for patients to monitor for weight gain. The risk of fluid retention and edema may be significant in elderly patients and in those with congestive heart failure. In addition, there is the potential for nephrotoxicity. Patients with gastrointestinal, cardiac, and renal problems should use this drug cautiously. Using the lowest possible effective dose can help to prevent complications. Older adults are more sensitive to the adverse effects of NSAIDs, so it is important to use caution when prescribing NSAIDs for this age group.

There is moderate research evidence showing that skeletal muscle relaxants are more effective than placebo but no evidence that they are better than NSAIDs in relieving symptoms of acute LBP. Multiple trials found skeletal muscle relaxants moderately superior to placebo for short-term relief of LBP (duration less than 1 week) (Qaseem et al., 2017). Patients need to be aware that this class of drugs is for short-term use because the risk/benefit ratio for prolonged use of muscle relaxants is not known. Muscle relaxants cause drowsiness and dizziness, so patients need to avoid hazardous activities when taking them. This class of drug is a CNS depressant, so patients need to avoid taking muscle relaxants with alcohol or other CNS depressants because the combined use will cause additive effects. Dry mouth is another side effect from this antimuscarinic class of drugs, so frequent mouth rinsing is recommended to prevent dental disease.

Research has shown that opioid analgesics do not enhance patients' ability to return to full activity sooner than that of patients taking NSAIDs. In addition, the adverse effects of opioid analgesics were found to be substantial, including the risk for physical dependence.

Activity

It should be stressed that rest has been proven to have little to no effect on the resolution of LBP. Patients should do whatever activities are tolerable. Weight loss, physical activities, and exercise for 30 minutes a day (walking or biking with lumbar flexion and/or extension exercises) are also important. Deconditioning is a real phenomenon that occurs increasingly quickly with increasing age. Lack of activity, leading to deconditioning, becomes a vicious cycle. Reassurance is always appropriate after ruling out more serious causes of back pain. Patients should be encouraged to quit smoking.

FOLLOW-UP AND REFERRAL

The course of patients with back strain is one of gradual improvement, usually over a 1- to 2-week period. The recovery is usually complete, without any lasting impairment. The small percentage of patients who do not make a complete recovery may continue to experience LBP associated with muscle strain. Pain may continue for months or years. These patients are experiencing CLBP, which must be evaluated and treated in a manner that takes into account the special difficulties of individuals with chronic pain. Patients with more severe symptoms can have limited vocational and avocational activities, recreation, and sleep disturbances. Mood, sexuality, and concentration can be adversely affected. Deconditioning can be the result of reduced activities, making both symptoms and any occupational dysfunction worse. Suggest a modified work schedule and more recreational activities that improve general conditioning. Narcotic abuse and dependency can be a problem for patients with chronic pain; refer the patient to a pain management center where a variety of evaluation and treatment modalities are available.

In all patients, preventing recurrence of back pain is another important consideration. The first episode of back pain is usually the briefest and least severe. The vast majority of individuals with an episode of back pain are at risk of developing another episode of back pain that will be more severe and of greater duration. Patients with recurrence are usually resistant to therapies that are beneficial in management of acute back pain, and therefore they may require chronic pain assessment and management strategies (including the use of complementary therapies such as acupuncture or acupressure). Consistent evidence from multiple trials demonstrates that acupuncture is moderately effective for short-term pain relief compared with no treatment or sham transcutaneous electrical nerve stimulation in patients with CLBP. There was no difference in effect between acupuncture and sham acupuncture for long-term pain relief. However, there is moderate evidence supporting acupuncture for long-term pain management compared with patients with chronic back pain receiving no acupuncture (Qaseem et al., 2017).

Referral to a specialist (e.g., neurosurgeon, orthopedic surgeon) is recommended for any patient who has a neurologic deficit or if the patient has a trauma history with x-ray examination revealing instability or fracture that could cause damage to neural elements.

Patient Education: Low Back Pain

Instruct the patient to carefully introduce activities back into his or her day as he or she begins to recover from the worst of the back pain episode. Gradual stretches and regular walking are good activities. There is consistent evidence that application of heat for acute/subacute low back pain is superior to placebo for back functional status and short-term pain relief. Over-the-counter anti-inflammatory medications NSAID may be used if not contraindicated or taking prescription NSAIDs. Provide information on safe back exercises such as modified sit-ups and low back stretches. Encourage patients to make them a regular part of their lifestyle. Emphasize the need to relax. Patients should call if symptoms persist, worsen, or progress; significant pain persists beyond 1 week; or there is no improvement with home management. The American College of Physician Clinical Practice Guideline (Qaseem et al., 2017) reported strong evidence to recommend nonpharmacologic treatment with exercise, multidisciplinary rehabilitation, mindfulness-based stress reduction, tai chi, yoga, motor control exercises, progressive relaxation, electromyography biofeedback, cognitive behavioral therapy, or spinal manipulation for chronic low back pain management.

HERNIATED LUMBAR DISC (HERNIATED NUCLEUS PULPOSUS)

The most common cause of radicular pain to the lower extremities is a herniated lumbar intervertebral disc. Over time, the lumbar discs are subjected to repeated deformations and large loads with physiological motion of the spine. In some individuals, fragmentation of the disc may result, followed by annular rupture, and finally a herniation of the nucleus pulposus into the lumbar canal. The resultant herniated disc syndrome (commonly called "sciatica" or "lumbar radiculopathy") may cause pain and/or numbness and/or weakness in one or both lower extremities. The pain results in part from direct mechanical compression of the nerve root and in part from chemical irritation of the nerve root by substances in the nucleus pulposus.

EPIDEMIOLOGY AND CAUSES

Disc herniation occurs most commonly at the L4 to L5 or L5 to S1 levels with subsequent irritation of the L5 and S1 nerve root. Herniations at more proximal intervertebral levels constitute only 5% of all lumbar disc herniations. Fewer than 2% of patients with LBP have infections, neoplasms, or inflammatory spondyloarthropathies. Spinal stenosis is more likely to be the etiology of radicular pain in patients older than 55 years. Disc disease affects males and females equally.

Risk factors include age-related degenerative changes (it is often difficult to distinguish between normal aging of the spine and pathological changes), cigarette smoking, a narrowed lumbar vertebral canal, obesity, osteoporosis, stress, and muscle tension. Causes include trauma (sudden or over time), frequent lifting without proper utilization of body mechanics, and vibration, such as driving and/or riding in a motor vehicle for prolonged periods of time.

PATHOPHYSIOLOGY

An intervertebral disc is located between each vertebra and is connected to the vertebral body. The discs have a strong outer layer, the *annulus fibrosus*, and the inner *nucleus pulposus*, which is a jellylike material that moves in the center of the annulus and redistributes itself as different stresses are placed on the disc, acting like a shock absorber. Disc anomalies begin when there is injury or degeneration of the annulus fibrosus—the outer portion of the disc. Bulging is an initial indication that the disc is showing signs of wear and tear.

The size of the individual's spinal canal becomes an important consideration when diagnosing a disc problem. A small canal will tolerate less disc material that is bulging or herniated, ruptured, or extruded. A small herniated disc in one patient will not be a problem; in another, the same size disc may cause significant compression of the neural structures. When a disc herniates, the nucleus pulposus pushes through a tear in the annulus fibrosis. The location and amount of disc material in the canal will determine the symptoms. Most discs will rupture more to one side than the other, producing more symptoms in the affected side via compression of a unilateral nerve root. Significant herniations may also bulge bilaterally, producing symptoms on both sides of the body. Thus, the nature of the symptoms is determined by the vertebral level of disc herniation.

In turn, radicular symptoms are the hallmark of disc herniation, and their absence makes this diagnosis highly unlikely. Lesions involving the L5 nerve root produce symptoms extending to the dorsum of the foot with weakened dorsiflexion of the large toe and weakened heel walking. Lesions involving both L5 and S1 nerve roots manifest with symptoms in the lateral and posterior calf, with S1 nerve root lesions extending to the heel, as well as gastrocnemius weakness, impaired toe walking, and a reduced or absent ankle reflex. Less common lesions affecting the L4 and L3 nerve roots include a diminished patellar reflex with symptoms extending to the anterior shin and thigh, with quadriceps weakness and difficulty rising from a squatted position.

CLINICAL PRESENTATION

Subjective

The onset of symptoms may be abrupt but is more likely to be insidious. Unilateral radiculopathy is frequently accompanied by LBP. Some patients report that preexisting back pain disappears when leg pain begins signaling the herniation. The pain is often severe and exaggerated by sitting, walking, standing, coughing, and sneezing. Most often, the pain radiates down from the buttock to the posterior or posterolateral leg to the ankle or foot. These patients typically cannot find a position of comfort. Lying on their side in a fetal position or on their back with a pillow under the knees may afford some relief. Upper or midlumbar radiculopathy (L1–L4 nerve root compression) refers pain to the anterior aspect of the thigh and often does not radiate below the knee.

Compression of the root may also cause paresthesias, loss of deep tendon reflex, and weakness of specific muscle groups. A herniated nucleus pulposus is most commonly seen in patients aged 20 to 50 years.

Objective

Most disc ruptures are posterolateral and press on a lumbar nerve root, which produces radiating pain. There may be paraspinal muscle spasm and lumbar scoliosis, with the trunk tilted away from the affected side. Patients may seem to "list" to one side when standing. When sitting, the patient may have pain and spinal extension (leaning back) when the leg is raised (flip sign). When coupled with reproduced back pain with supine straight-leg raising limited to less than 45 degrees of leg elevation, these signs are highly reliable for herniated disc.

Motor and sensory function of the lumbosacral nerve roots and the deep tendon reflexes should be evaluated. The straight-leg-raise test should be done on both the involved and uninvolved limbs with the patient in the supine position. This test places stress on the L5 and S1 nerve roots. Ipsilateral restriction on straight-leg raising is common with a variety of lumbar spine problems, but a positive crossed straight-leg-raising test (pain in the involved leg or buttock that occurs when lifting the uninvolved leg) is highly specific for nerve root entrapment. To stretch the upper lumbar nerve roots, reverse straight-leg raising test should be performed (see Advanced Assessments 53.1 and 53.2).

DIAGNOSTIC REASONING

Diagnostic Tests

Age-appropriate changes are usually demonstrated on radiograph. MRI might be useful if there is an unclear diagnosis or if the patient is being readied for surgery but otherwise is not indicated.

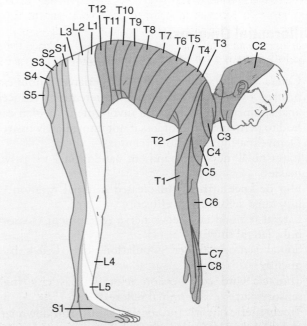

Advanced Assessment 53.2: Classic Findings of Disc Herniation

Nerve Root	Findings
L3–L4 (L4 nerve root)	Weakness in the anterior tibialis, numbness in the shin, thigh pain, and an asymmetrical knee reflex (5% of all herniations)
L4–L5 (L5 nerve root)	Weakness in the great toe extension, numbness top of the foot and first web space, and posterolateral thigh and calf pain
L5–S1 (S1 nerve root)	Weakness in the great toe flexor and gastrocsoleus with inability to sustain tiptoe walking, numbness in the lateral foot, posterior calf pain and ache, and an asymmetrical ankle reflex

Dermatome map. A dermatome map shows the distribution of the spinal nerves. When the body is placed in the quadruped position, the sequence of the dermatomes becomes orderly, starting with C2 (there is no C1 dermatome) at the skull and progressing to S5 at the "tail." (Source: Starkey C, Brown SD. *Orthopedic & athletic injury.* 3rd ed. Philadelphia. PA: F.A. Davis; 2015.)

The majority of patients who present with LBP do not require any imaging studies; however, there are several exceptions that warrant further diagnostic testing and immediate treatment. Patients who have recently experienced a trauma should be considered for radiographic evaluation. Imaging studies are used to evaluate the extent of ligamentous, neural, osseous, and soft-tissue injuries. Patients suspected of having an infection or tumor should be initially screened with plain radiographs followed by MRI.

MRI should also be considered for patients with neurologic symptoms, specifically weakness, loss of deep tendon reflex, or bilateral symptoms.

In cases of neurologic deficit, computed tomography (CT) and/or MRI should be obtained. The superiority of CT at capturing details of osseous structures allows for thorough assessment of fractures. However, CT is not as useful as MRI in visualizing conditions of soft-tissue structure. MRI should be generally ordered first to evaluate the spine. CT is generally used to complement information obtained from other diagnostic imaging studies such as myelography, MRI, and radiographs. The value of CT is its ability to demonstrate the osseous structures of the lumbar spine and their relationship to the neural canal. CT is helpful in the diagnosis of tumors, fractures, partial or complete dislocations, and spondylolisthesis

Differential Diagnosis

The following is a list of differential diagnoses:

- Cauda equina syndrome (CES) (perianal numbness, urinary overflow incontinence or retention, reduced anal sphincter tone, bilateral involvement), which can lead to permanent motor loss if not immediately treated
- Demyelinating conditions (clonus)
- Extraspinal nerve entrapment (abdominal or pelvic masses)
- Hip or knee arthritis (decreased internal rotation of hip, knee deformity or effusion)
- Lateral femoral cutaneous nerve entrapment (sensory only, lateral thigh)
- Spinal stenosis (older population, discussed subsequently)
- Thoracic cord compression (clonus, spasticity, high sensory pattern, abdominal reflexes)
- Trochanteric bursitis (no tension signs, pain down lateral thigh and leg, exquisite tenderness over trochanter)
- Vascular insufficiency (absent posterior tibial pulse, claudication, trophic changes)

MANAGEMENT

Control of symptoms, relief of pain, and improved mobility are all goals of management. Most episodes improve with conservative treatment.

NSAIDs should be given for pain with 1 to 3 days of bedrest. If the pain is severe in the acute phase, which it can be, a short, limited course of muscle relaxants or opioids may be considered. Although not recommended as first-line therapy for ALBP, opioids are sometimes used for short-term relief of severe back pain; however, the potential for abuse and addiction is high with prolonged use. In addition, the use of opiates for long-term pain relief is similarly controversial because this practice may lead to abuse and diversion of prescribed medications, as evidenced by the significant rise in deaths in recent years due to both prescribed and illicit opiate abuse and overdose (see Chapter 78 for chronic pain management).

The patient should be taught to limit sitting, prolonged standing, or walking and to take frequent rest breaks when resuming activity. Most disc herniations resolve without residual problems. Even ruptures with a significant inflammatory component should improve within 3 to 6 weeks. Refer if the problem persists longer than that, if pain increases, or if there is evidence of any "red flags" (see Table 53.1). A short course of oral steroids (5 days) or an epidural injection may reduce leg pain within the first 2 weeks after herniation, although some recent studies have indicated that epidural steroids do not significantly alter pain that has persisted for more than 2 weeks or influence the outcome of the syndrome. Persistent numbness, progression of neurologic deficits, and weakness can occur despite treatment.

Surgical options may need to be considered if symptoms persist for more than 3 months and other underlying causes are ruled out. Intolerable pain, multiple episodes of radiculopathy, severe postural tilt, and persistent dysfunctional pain are all indications for surgery.

FOLLOW-UP AND REFERRAL

Most cases of acute back pain (90%) and/or radiculopathy (60% to 80%) resolve with conservative treatment; the same is true of most cases of chronic back pain and radiculopathy. The patient should return in 7 to 10 days for evaluation of pain and function, and the patient should be monitored every 2 weeks until the patient returns to normal function. A progressive walking program should be initiated after pain is controlled (usually within 7 to 10 days). It is best to start with short walks initially, up to four times per day, lengthening the walks as tolerated. The patient should return to full activity as soon as possible but avoid high-risk activities such as heavy lifting and long car rides.

Progression of any neurologic deficits, such as loss of ankle jerk; bladder and rectal sphincter weakness with retention or incontinence; foot drop with weakness of the anterior tibial, posterior tibial, or peroneal muscles; narcotic addiction in cases of chronic pain; limitation of movement; and restricted activity all warrant referral for further evaluation and treatment.

Patient Education: Herniated Lumbar Disc

Patients should be reassured that most disc herniations resolve without residual problems within 3 to 6 weeks. Cessation of smoking, weight reduction, good posture and body mechanics, and adherence to an exercise regimen are all ways to improve health and prevent recurrence. Modification of the work environment may be necessary.

LUMBAR SPINAL STENOSIS

Lumbar spinal stenosis is narrowing of one or more levels of the lumbar spinal canal and subsequent compression of the nerve roots. In the order of descending likelihood, L4 to L5, L3 to L4, and L1 to L2 are the levels most commonly involved. At L1 to S1, the stenosis is usually not central but foraminal, involving the same root (L5) as central canal stenosis at the L4 to L5 level. Typically, the stenosis must be severe before symptoms occur.

EPIDEMIOLOGY AND CAUSES

Anatomically, as many as 30% of the population may have spinal stenosis after age 60, yet only a portion of this population has symptoms. Obesity is a predisposing factor, as is osteoporosis.

PATHOPHYSIOLOGY

Lumbar spinal stenosis is defined as narrowing of the spinal canal with compression of the nerve roots. It may be congenital or acquired. It most frequently results from enlarging osteophytes at the facet joints, hypertrophy of the ligamentum flavum, and protrusion or bulging of the intervertebral discs. Lumbar spinal stenosis may produce symptoms by directly compressing nerve roots or by compressing nutrient arterioles that supply the nerve roots.

CLINICAL PRESENTATION

Subjective

Onset of symptoms may follow a lifting incident or minor trauma or may gradually emerge. Often there is pseudoclaudication causing radicular complaints (with or without associated back pain) in the calves, buttocks, and upper thighs of one or both legs. Symptoms progress from a proximal to distal direction. Walking or prolonged standing causes pain and weakness in the legs and buttocks. In cases of vascular claudication, the pain stops when the patient stops walking, but pseudoclaudication does not immediately subside when walking stops. The patient may obtain short-term relief by leaning forward (manifested as "stooping"); when grocery shopping, the patient will be leaning on the cart. Relief after sitting is variable, depending on the degree of neural compression. Patients who sleep on their backs, meaning with the spine extended, might awaken after several hours with back and leg pain. Lumbosacral pain is associated with walking and standing. A vague aching in the legs or leg weakness may also be present. Spondylolisthesis (degenerative or spondylolytic), vascular insufficiency, and osteoarthritis of the hips are often associated with spinal stenosis, as well as obesity.

Objective

Muscle weakness of the legs is a subtle phenomenon. This may be best elicited after walking on a treadmill. Proprioception can be impaired; there may be a positive Romberg test. In this test, the patient stands with the feet together and is asked to shut the eyes. The test is positive if the patient sways or loses balance. There may be sensory changes, and these are usually segmental and may involve more than one spinal level. Reflexes are often diminished. Some patients will have a lumbar scoliosis. With bowel or bladder symptoms, sphincter tone may be decreased. However, because many elderly patients have concomitant prostate problems or urinary incontinence, genitourinary evaluation may be necessary to differentiate these processes.

DIAGNOSTIC REASONING

Diagnostic Testing

Patients presenting with signs and symptoms of spinal stenosis should have imaging studies. Radiographs may provide some evidence of spinal stenosis. Anteroposterior and lateral view radiographs (up to L10 in the lateral view) may show significant narrowing of the intervertebral disc or spondylolisthesis. There may be osteopenia or an old burst fracture of the vertebral body. MRI is considered superior to CT scans for visualizing potential causes of stenosis that involve soft tissues, such as a disc bulge or herniation. CT is most useful in delineating osseous causes of stenosis.

Differential Diagnosis

The following is a list of differential diagnoses:

- Abdominal aortic aneurysm (palpable pulsatile mass)
- Arterial insufficiency (distance to claudication constant, recovery after rest, absent or diminished pulses)
- Diabetes mellitus (abnormal glucose metabolism, nonsegmental numbness, skin changes)
- Folic acid or vitamin B_{12} deficiency (confirmed by laboratory tests, anemia)
- Infection (fever, elevated ESR, intervertebral disc narrowing)
- Tumor (patchy neurologic deficit, bone destruction, severe night pain)

MANAGEMENT

Any neurologic deficit, gait disturbance, or bowel and bladder dysfunction should be evaluated further. These changes may not be reversed following surgery for decompression; thus, the goal of the treatment is to prevent progression.

Intermittent use of NSAIDs may be helpful, as well as folic acid or vitamin B_{12} supplementation in some cases depending on results of laboratory tests. However, most management revolves around physical therapy or an exercise program that focuses on flexing the spine. Flexion of the spine increases intraspinal volume. Bicycling is one exercise that is done with the spine in flexion. Improving abdominal muscle tone lifts the pelvis anteriorly and flexes the lumbar spine. Reduction of intra-abdominal fat is critical to achieving the objective. Thus, weight loss may be pivotal. Lumbar flexion exercises increase spinal canal volume. Examples include exercise on all fours, arching the back, or in the fetal position. Exercises that extend the spine should be avoided (swayback).

Lumbar epidural corticosteroid injection may provide some immediate relief for approximately 50% of patients and more sustained relief for approximately 25%. When disabling symptoms persist, decompression laminectomy provides at least short-term relief in some patients but does not always rehabilitate lost function.

FOLLOW-UP AND REFERRAL

The rate of progression is variable from rapid to none. Many patients never develop any neurologic deficits and tolerate the condition well. Pain and limited function, however, can become severe and lead to a secondary depression. Standing erect may become impossible, and the patient may be forced to adopt a stooped posture. Claudication may develop after walking only a few feet. CES develops in some patients, leading to loss of bowel and bladder function.

If nonoperative treatment is ineffective, specialty consultation is warranted. Night pain that disturbs sleep tends to be a sign of advancing disease and also indicates a need to refer and/or consult. Prolonged use of NSAIDs can cause renal failure, hepatotoxicity, and gastrointestinal ulcer disease and can exacerbate existing cardiac disease.

Patient Education: Lumbar Spinal Stenosis

The patient and family should be educated about potentially serious symptoms, such as changes in bowel and bladder function, change in neurologic status, and gait disturbance. The patient should be informed about the side effects of NSAIDs. Weight loss may be helpful, and patients should be provided with dietary instructions and clear guidelines for activity and exercise. Because many of these patients are older adults, they may need a range of services arranged to accomplish these goals.

CAUDA EQUINA SYNDROME

EPIDEMIOLOGY AND CAUSES

CES is rare and occurs in approximately 1 in 65,000 (0.1% to 2%) cases of herniated lumbar disc. A retrospective review of U.S. military service men and women serving from 2001 to 2010, 7 in 100,000 developed CES (Schoenfeld, 2012), Schoenfeld's sample also identified women, age, and rank had implications for higher incidence of CES.

PATHOPHYSIOLOGY

The *cauda equina* is a continuation of the spinal cord below the first lumbar level in the adult. The "horse's tail" consists of an array of nerves that exit the conus of the spinal cord and continue down the lumbar spine, exiting at different lumbar and sacral levels through foramina. These nerves are responsible for specific sensory and motor functions, including perineal sensation and both bladder and anal sphincter functions. The syndrome is divided into two categories cauda equina syndrome-incomplete (CES-I) and cauda equina syndrome with retention (CES-R).

CES-I accounts for 40% of presentations with CES-R the remaining 60%. There is perianal/saddle anesthesia without urinary incontinence or retention with CES-I and fully developed urinary retention or incontinence with CES-R. Pressure or compression on the nerve roots is the ultimate cause of the syndrome. There are multiple etiologies that may cause this syndrome (see Table 53.2); however, the most common is disc herniation at L4–L5 and L5–S1. Whatever the pathology, CES is a medical emergency and requires immediate decompression.

CLINICAL PRESENTATION

Cauda equina compression is characterized by bilateral lower extremity weakness, anesthesia, or paresthesia of the perineum and buttocks (saddle anesthesia). There may or may not be bowel or bladder incontinence or bladder

TABLE 53.2 Cauda Equina Syndrome Etiologies	
Etiology	*Pathology*
Degenerative disease	Disc herniation (L4/5; L5/S1) Lumbar spinal stenosis Spondylolisthesis Cysts Perineural cysts Facet joint cysts
Inflammatory	Acute and chronic ankylosing spondylitis
Traumatic	Spinal fracture Epidural hematoma Postprocedure Post–spinal manipulation
Infectious	Epidural abscess Tuberculosis (Pott's disease)
Malignant	Lymphoma Metastases Primary central nervous system malignancies (schwannoma, neurofibroma, etc.)
Vascular	Aortic dissection Arteriovenous malformation
Other space occupying lesion(s)	Sarcoid

retention. When there is neurologic deficit affecting the bowel or bladder, these changes may not be reversed with surgical decompression,

Subjective

The presenting symptoms may be acute onset or insidious. The patient may complain of pain in both legs that may be more severe in one extremity. He or she may also complain of numbness in the lower extremities, difficulty in voiding, or loss of bowel or bladder control.

Objective

The patient may have a stumbling gait from leg weakness. Quadriceps and/or hip extensor weakness may be observed as the patient has difficulty arising from a chair and uses the arm rests or seat to push self into standing position. The patient is unable to walk on heels and toes due to ankle dorsiflexor and plantar flexor weakness. Bilateral footdrop may be observed. Motor and sensory lumbosacral nerve root examination should be performed as well as an assessment of sphincter tone (via rectal examination) and perianal paresthesia.

DIAGNOSTIC REASONING

Diagnostic Tests

MRI is the diagnostic test of choice. In patients who cannot tolerate or in whom MRI is contraindicated, CT myelogram is warranted, which should be performed by a specialist.

Differential Diagnoses

Differential diagnoses of CES are as follows:

- Guillain-Barré syndrome
- Herniated disc
- Metastatic disease
- Multiple sclerosis
- Pernicious anemia
- Tabes dorsalis
- Spinal cord tumor
- Hysteria and other psychiatric disorders

MANAGEMENT

If cauda equina compression is confirmed, surgical lumbar decompression is necessary to halt neurologic deterioration unless surgery is contraindicated for other medical reasons.

FOLLOW-UP AND REFERRAL

CES patients may have varying levels of postsurgical recovery including ongoing chronic pain and residual neurologic deficits. One in five patients may have physical or psychosocial issues after CES decompression. The need for intensive rehabilitation, learning self-catheterization,

colostomy care, sexual dysfunction, depression, and loss of employment are all issues that the primary-care provider should include as part of the office follow-up evaluation after discharge from surgery. Ongoing support for the patient with linkage to community resources and support groups assists in the long-term recovery process.

Patient Education: Cauda Equina Syndrome

The initial patient education is to explain the syndrome and the sense of urgency for surgical intervention. Post neurosurgical discharge the ongoing patient education should focus to support any knowledge needed for self-care, ongoing health maintenance, community resources, and assuring the social determinants of health are explored with the patient to address needs beyond physical health.

VERTEBRAL FRACTURE

The cervical spine is the most commonly injured part of the spinal column, due to its exposed location above the torso and its inherent flexibility. Within the cervical spine, the most common sites of injury are around the second cervical vertebra (C2, or axis) or in the region of C5, C6, and C7. In contrast, the thoracic spine is rigidly fixed, as the thoracic ribs articulate with the respective transverse processes and sternum. Thus, a great amount of force is necessary to damage the thoracic spine of an otherwise healthy adult. In older adults with osteoporosis or patients with bone disease or metastatic lesions, minor trauma may be sufficient to cause a compression fracture.

The orientation of the facet joints at the TL junction may concentrate forces created from traumatic impact at this level; thus, the second most commonly injured region is the thoracolumbar (TL) junction. At the TL junction, the spinal column changes from a kyphotic to a lordotic curve. Ninety percent of all TL spine injuries occur in the region between T11 and L4. However, these injuries rarely result in complete cord lesions as the spinal canal is relatively wide at this level.

EPIDEMIOLOGY AND CAUSES

Vertebral fractures are most commonly associated with osteoporosis. Osteoporosis is a worldwide public health burden. The International Osteoporosis Foundation estimates that more than 200 million people worldwide are affected by this disease. In the U.S. Agency for Health Care Research and Quality reports 52 million people in the United States have low bone density, and 55% older than 50 years are threatened by osteoporosis. Osteoporosis is caused by hereditary factors, medications such as prolonged use of steroids, smoking, alcoholism, renal disease, other chronic wasting diseases, and lifestyle.

Injuries are the second cause for vertebral fractures. The injuries may be from car or motorcycle accidents, falls from a height, blunt force trauma, gunshot wounds, and sports injuries. Approximately 11,000 spinal cord injuries occur each year in the United States. The average age of spinal cord injury patients is 32, and 80% are men.

Vertebral fractures may also be related to other pathology such as neoplastic disease, infection, tuberculosis (Pott's disease), or other calcium or bone demineralization disease process such as renal failure.

PATHOPHYSIOLOGY

The anatomic theory published by Francis Denis (1983) describes the vertebrae and the attached ligaments that are involved during injury and divides the spinal column into three sections: anterior, middle, and posterior. The anterior contains the anterior half of the vertebra and the anterior longitudinal ligament. The middle is the posterior half of the vertebral body and the posterior longitudinal ligament. The posterior is the pedicles, the facet joints, and supraspinous ligaments.

The Denis Classification classifies injuries into major and minor categories. Major injuries carry a higher risk for instability, whereas minor injuries are deemed simple fractures of the processes of the posterior column. Major injuries are defined by the nature of the involvement of the anatomical structures. Major injury categories are compression, burst, seat-belt–type, and fracture dislocation. Each of these categories is further classified into subcategories to define the structural involvement associated with the fracture (see Table 53.3).

CLINICAL PRESENTATION

Subjective

The patient may present after a fall, motorcycle or car accident with a complaint of midlevel back pain. The pain is associated with movement, and generally the patient can specifically locate the point of pain upon palpation. The pain may be described as aching, stabbing, and/or so severe that the patient cannot continue to do their daily activities. Complaints of lower extremity weakness is significant indication nerve involvement.

Objective

For traumatic injuries, the trunk, chest, and abdomen are examined for ecchymosis and swelling. Lap-belt injuries will have contusions or ecchymosis over the anterior iliac spines. Hematoma and forward shift of the spinous processes are an indication of an unstable flexion distraction or burst fracture. Many vertebral compression fractures may be found incidentally on other radiology examinations. An acute onset of vertebral compression fracture may occur from coughing, sneezing, or lifting. The fractures commonly occur between T8 and L4. Examination may be normal or patient may have kyphosis and midline spine tenderness to palpation. The location of the pain is specific to the level of injury and

TABLE 53.3 Denis Classification of Vertebral Fractures

Major Type	*Subtype*
Compression (wedge) fracture: compression of anterior column	Type A: includes both endplates Type B: involves superior end plate Type C: inferior end plate Type D: anterior cortex buckling with endplates intact
Burst fracture: failure of anterior and middle columns at the level of one or both end plates under axial load	Type A: fracture of both endplates; bone is pushed into canal Type B: fracture of superior endplate Type C: fracture of inferior endplate Type D: burst rotation caused from axial load with rotation Type E: burst lateral flexion; seen as increase on interpediculate distance on anterior-posterior radiograph
Seatbelt-type injury: both posterior and middle columns fail due to hyperflexion and tension forces	One-level injury: chance fracture going through bone or posterior ligamentous tear and disc rupture Level two: middle column is ruptured through the bone or the disc
Fracture-dislocations: injury through all three columns	Flexion-rotation: complete disruption of posterior and middle columns under tension and rotation Flexion-distraction: disruption of both posterior and middle columns under tension with tear of anterior annulus fibrosus, and stripping of anterior longitudinal ligament during subluxation or dislocation Shear: extension injury with disruption of anterior ligament

Source: Denis F. The three column spine and its significance in the classification of acute thoracolumbar spinal injuries. *Spine.* 1983;8:817–831.

correlates well with radiology findings. Perform a full motor and neurologic examination below the level of injury. Any weakness or neurologic deficits are suggestive of spinal cord injury and warrants referral.

DIAGNOSTIC REASONING

Given the patient history, presenting symptoms, and physical examination, diagnostic considerations should include:

- Pott's disease
- Renal failure
- Spinal malignancy
- Osteomyelitis
- Hemangioma of vertebral body

DIAGNOSTIC TESTS

The standard imaging study for vertebral fractures is the anterior–posterior/lateral views of the lumbar and thoracic spine. Changes in vertebral body height, increased interpedicular space, or wedge fractures will be visible on plain films. The films may also identify additional fractures above or below the area identified as suspect for fracture.

CT scan provides further diagnostic value when assessing the fractures for stability or when suspected fracture was not visible on plain films. CT provides optimal views for posterior vertebrae and the neural arch and is comparable to MRI for traumatic injuries; MRI with contrast is indicated for those patients who have lower extremity loss of sensation or muscle weakness. MRI is more specific to identify bleeding, tumor, or infection

Differential Diagnoses

Differential diagnoses include the following:

- Coccyx pain
- Degenerative disc disease
- Vertebral facet arthropathy
- Spondylolysis
- Spondylolisthesis
- Osteoporosis
- Hyperparathyroidism
- Musculoskeletal pain

MANAGEMENT

Vertebral compression fractures are commonly seen and managed by the primary-care provider. The goal for treatment and management should be based on patient preference and knowledge of current evidence-based practice and clinical guidelines.

The primary goals for vertebral compression fractures are pain relief, maintaining function, prevention, and quality of life. With acute vertebral compression fractures with onset of clinical symptoms and diagnosis of 5 days or less, the American Academy of Orthopaedic Surgeons (AAOS) recommends calcitonin for promotion of bone both pain management and to increase function (moderate strength). Calcitonin has also demonstrated faster healing of spinal fractures in osteoporotic patients (Pagonis et al., 2014). A short course of opioids or tramadol may be warranted to assist the patient in mobility and avoid bedrest. Lidocaine patches are used in practice but have not been tested in clinical trials. The standard medication management for back pain is no different with this disorder. Pain relief or pain tolerance assists the patient to tolerate increased mobility and physical therapy with the goal to increase core strength. AAOS guidelines review of the evidence is inconclusive for bedrest, back brace, unsupervised exercise program, electrical stimulation, or opioids or other analgesics for pain management. However, patient preference, other medical conditions, and drug interactions should provide guidance to the provider for pain management for the first week to 10 days. A back brace may provide support but also may further weaken trunk and abdominal muscles. Evidence for surgical intervention is mixed. The AAOS provides a strong recommendation against vertebroplasty and indicates that there is limited evidence to support kyphoplasty. However, when traditional medical treatment has failed to manage patient's pain or pain is substantially altering quality of life then vertebroplasty or kyphoplasty should be considered (Barr et al., 2014).

FOLLOW-UP AND REFERRAL

Any patient with a neurologic deficit on examination should be referred to specialist for further evaluation. Depending on the availability of specialist to the provider, the specialist could include orthopaedic, neurosurgeon, or intervention neuroradiologist.

For conservative management, the patient should be seen within 1 week of the first visit to assess pain level, function, and neurologic integrity. Physical therapy referral should be made as soon as pain is managed. The goal of physical therapy is to strengthen trunk flexion and extensor muscles.

Prevention of other fractures is warranted. Prevention includes weight-bearing exercises and various medications, including bisphosphonates, calcitonin, parathyroid hormone, denosumab, and teriparatide, a daily subcutaneous injection (see Chapter 55 for more information about osteoporosis).

Patient Education: Vertebral Fracture

During recovery, patients should avoid bending, stooping, twisting, or lifting anything over 10 pounds. Additional patient education should include smoking cessation and avoidance of excessive alcohol. Weight-bearing and muscle-strengthening exercises should be encouraged when healing of the fracture is complete. A fall-risk assessment should be performed as part of a fall-prevention strategy.

REFERENCES

Cauda Equina Syndrome

American Society for Radiation Oncology. Evidence-based guideline on palliative radiation therapy for bone metastases, update. 2016.

Cancer Care Ontario. Updated systematic review and clinical practice guideline for the management of malignant extradural spinal cord compression, 2011. Published 2012.

Chau X, Pelzer, G. Timing of surgical intervention in cauda equine syndrome: A systematic clinical review. *World Neurosurg.* 2014;81(3–4):640–650.

Gardner A, Gardner E, Morley T. Cauda equine syndrome: A review of current medico-legal position. *Eur Spine J.* 2011;20:690–697.

Gitelman A, Hishmeh S, Morelli BN, et al. Cauda equina syndrome: A comprehensive review. *Am J Orthopaed.* 2009;37(11):556–562.

National Comprehensive Cancer Network. Clinical practice guidelines in oncology on central nervous system cancers. 2017.

Schoenfeld J. Incidence and epidemiology of cauda equina syndrome: A review of 976 patients from a complete American population. Poster presented at NASS 27th Annual Meeting; Dallas, TX.

Cervical Muscle Sprain/Strain

American College of Radiology, American Society of Neuroradiology, Society for Pediatric Radiology. Practice parameter for the performance of magnetic resonance imaging (MRI) of the head and neck. 2012, amended 2014.

Anderson SE, Boesch C, Zimmermann H, et al. Are there cervical spine findings at MR imaging that are specific to acute symptomatic whiplash injury? A prospective controlled study with four experienced blinded readers. *Radiology*. 2012;262:567.

Bronfort G, Evans R, Anderson AV, et al. Spinal manipulation, medication, or home exercise with advice for acute and subacute neck pain: A randomized trial. *Ann Intern Med*. 2012;156:1.

Cohen SP. Epidemiology, diagnosis, and treatment of neck pain. *Mayo Clin Proc*. 2015;90:284.

Côté P, Hogg-Johnson S, Cassidy JD, et al. Initial patterns of clinical care and recovery from whiplash injuries: A population-based cohort study. *Arch Intern Med*. 2005;165:2257.

Deyo RA. Drug therapy for back pain. Which drugs help which patients? *Spine (Phila Pa 1976)*. 1996;21:2840.

Ferrari R, Lang C. A cross-cultural comparison between Canada and Germany of symptom expectation for whiplash injury. *J Spinal Disord Tech*. 2005;18:92.

Ferrari R, Obelieniene D, Russell A, et al. Laypersons' expectation of the sequelae of whiplash injury: A cross-cultural comparative study between Canada and Lithuania. *Med Sci Monit*. 2002;8:CR728.

Guzman J, Haldeman S, Carroll LJ, et al. Clinical practice implications of the Bone and Joint Decade 2000–2010 Task Force on Neck Pain and Its Associated Disorders: From concepts and findings to recommendations. *Spine (Phila Pa 1976)*. 2008;33:S199.

Japanese Spinal Disease Society. Cervical spondylotic myelopathy clinical practice guidelines. 2015.

Kasch H, Qerama E, Kongsted A, et al. The risk assessment score in acute whiplash injury predicts outcome and reflects biopsychosocial factors. *Spine (Phila Pa 1976)*. 2011;36:S263.

Krakenes J, Kaale BR. Magnetic resonance imaging assessment of craniovertebral ligaments and membranes after whiplash trauma. *Spine (Phila Pa 1976)*. 2006;31:2820.

Motor Accidents Authority of New South Wales. *Guidelines for the management of acute whiplash associated disorders for health professionals*. 3rd ed. 2014.

Muzin S, Isaac Z, Walker J, Abd OE, Baima J. When should a cervical collar be used to treat neck pain? *Curr Rev Musculoskel Med*. 2008;1(2):114–119.

Nordin M, Carragee EJ, Hogg-Johnson S, et al. Assessment of neck pain and its associated disorders: results of the Bone and Joint Decade 2000–2010 Task Force on Neck Pain and Its Associated Disorders. *Spine (Phila Pa 1976)*. 2008;33:S101.

Peloso P, Gross A, Haines T, et al. Medicinal and injection therapies for mechanical neck disorders. *Cochrane Database Syst Rev*. 2007;(5):CD000319.

Walton DM, Macdermid JC, Giorgianni AA, et al. Risk factors for persistent problems following acute whiplash injury: Update of a systematic review and meta-analysis. *J Orthop Sports Phys Ther*. 2013;43:31.

Cervical Spondylosis

American College of Radiology, American Society of Neuroradiology, Society for Pediatric Radiology. Practice parameter for the performance of computed tomography (CT) of the extracranial head and neck. 2016.

Baron EM, Young WF. Cervical spondylotic myelopathy: A brief review of its pathophysiology, clinical course, and diagnosis. *Neurosurgery*. 2007;60:S35.

Carette S, Fehlings MG. Clinical practice. Cervical radiculopathy. *N Engl J Med*. 2005;353:392.

Chiles BW 3rd, Leonard MA, Choudhri HF, Cooper PR. Cervical spondylotic myelopathy: Patterns of neurological deficit and recovery after anterior cervical decompression. *Neurosurgery*. 1999;44:762.

Hehir MK, Figueroa JJ, Zynda-Weiss AM, et al. Unexpected neuroimaging abnormalities in patients with apparent C8 radiculopathy: Broadening the clinical spectrum. *Muscle Nerve*. 2012;45:859.

Iyer S, Kim HJ. Cervical radiculopathy. *Curr Rev Musculoskelet Med*. 2016;9:272.

Japanese Spinal Disease Society. Cervical spondylotic myelopathy clinical practice guidelines. 2015.

Johnson MI, Paley CA, Howe TE, Sluka KA. Transcutaneous electrical nerve stimulation for acute pain. *Cochrane Database Syst Rev*. 2015;(6):CD006142.

Karpova A, Arun R, Davis AM, et al. Predictors of surgical outcome in cervical spondylotic myelopathy. *Spine (Phila Pa 1976)*. 2013;38:392.

Lee MJ, Konodi MA, Cizik AM, et al. Risk factors for medical complication after cervical spine surgery: A multivariate analysis of 582 patients. *Spine (Phila Pa 1976)*. 2013;38:223.

North American Spine Society. Clinical guidelines for diagnosis and treatment of cervical radiculopathy from degenerative disorders. **https://www.spine.org/Documents/ResearchClinicalCare/Guidelines/CervicalRadiculopathy.pdf**. Published 2010.

Rubinstein SM, Pool JJ, van Tulder MW, et al. A systematic review of the diagnostic accuracy of provocative tests of the neck for diagnosing cervical radiculopathy. *Eur Spine J*. 2007;16:307.

Herniated Lumbar Disc

Cloyd JM, Acosta FL Jr, Ames CP. Complications and outcomes of lumbar spine surgery in elderly people: A review of the literature. *J Am Geriatr Soc*. 2008;56:1318.

Hofstee DJ, Gijtenbeek JM, Hoogland PH, et al. Westeinde sciatica trial: Randomized controlled study of bed rest and physiotherapy for acute sciatica. *J Neurosurg*. 2002;96:45.

Jönsson B, Annertz M, Sjöberg C, Strömqvist B. A prospective and consecutive study of surgically treated lumbar spinal stenosis. Part II: Five-year follow-up by an independent observer. *Spine (Phila Pa 1976)*. 1997;22:2938.

Park DK, An HS, Lurie JD, et al. Does multilevel lumbar stenosis lead to poorer outcomes? A subanalysis of the Spine Patient Outcomes Research Trial (SPORT) lumbar stenosis study. *Spine (Phila Pa 1976)*. 2010;35:439.

Pinto RZ, Maher CG, Ferreira ML, et al. Drugs for relief of pain in patients with sciatica: Systematic review and meta-analysis. *BMJ*. 2012;344:e497.

Quaseem A, Wilt TJ, McLean RM, et al. Noninvasive treatments for acute, subacute, and chronic low back pain: A clinical practice guideline from the American College of Physicians. *Ann Intern Med*. 2017;166:514.

Radcliff KE, Rihn J, Hilibrand A, et al. Does the duration of symptoms in patients with spinal stenosis and degenerative spondylolisthesis affect outcomes? Analysis of the Spine Outcomes Research Trial. *Spine (Phila Pa 1976)*. 2011;36:2197.

Rasmussen-Barr E, Held U, Grooten WJ, et al. Non-steroidal anti-inflammatory drugs for sciatica. *Cochrane Database Syst Rev*. 2016;10:CD012382.

Serinken M, Eken C, Gungor F, et al. Comparison of intravenous morphine versus paracetamol in sciatica: A randomized placebo controlled trial. *Acad Emerg Med*. 2016;23:674.

Weinstein JN, Lurie JD, Tosteson TD, et al. Surgical versus nonsurgical treatment for lumbar degenerative spondylolisthesis. *N Engl J Med*. 2007;356:2257.

Weinstein JN, Lurie JD, Tosteson TD, et al. Surgical compared with nonoperative treatment for lumbar degenerative spondylolisthesis. Four-year results in the Spine Patient Outcomes Research Trial (SPORT) randomized and observational cohorts. *J Bone Joint Surg Am*. 2009;91:1295.

Low Back Pain

Armstrong AD, Hubbard MC, eds. *Essentials of musculoskeletal care*. 5th ed. Rosemont, IL: American Academy of Orthopedic Surgeons; 2016.

Casser, H. Seddigh, S., Raushmann, M. Acute lumbar back pain: Investigation, differential diagnosis, and treatment. *Dtsch Arztebl Nit*. 2016;113(13):223–234.

Chou R, Deyo R, Friedly J, et al. *Noninvasive treatments for low back pain* (Comparative Effectiveness Review No. 169). (Prepared by the Pacific Northwest Evidence-based Practice Center under Contract No. 290-2012-00014-I.) AHRQ Publication No. 16-EHC004EF. Rockville, MD: Agency for Healthcare Research and Quality. http://www.effectivehealthcare.ahrq.gov/reports/final.cfm. Published February 2016.

Chou R, Naseem A, Owens DK, et al. Diagnostic imaging for low back pain: Advice for high-value health care from the American College of Physicians. *Ann Intern Med*. 2011;154:181–189.

Dowell D, Haegerich TM, Chou R. CDC Guideline for prescribing opioids for chronic pain—United States, 2016. *MMWR Recomm Rep*. 2016;65(No. RR-1):1–49. doi: http://dx.doi.org/10.15585/mmwr.rr6501e1

Friedman BW, Izarry E, Solorzano C, et al. Diazepam is no better than placebo when added to naproxen for acute low back pain. *Ann Int Med*. 2017;70(2):169–176.

National Institute for Health and Care Excellence. Guideline on low back pain and sciatica in over 16s—Assessment and management. 2016.

Qaseem A, Wilt TJ, McLean RM, Forciea MA. Noninvasive treatments for acute, subacute, and chronic low back pain: A clinical practice guideline from the American College of Physicians. *Ann Intern Med*. 2017;116(7):514–530.

Reese C, Mittag O. Psychological interventions in the rehabilitation of patients with chronic low back pain: Evidence and recommendations from systematic reviews and guidelines. *Int J Rehabil*. 2013;36(1):6–12.

Reed SJ, Pearson S. Institute for Clinical and Economic Review. Choosing Wisely® recommendation analysis: Prioritizing opportunities for reducing inappropriate care: Imaging for nonspecific low back pain. http://icer-review.org/wp-content/uploads/2016/01/FINAL-Imaging-for-Low-Back-Pain-final-analysis-November-28.pdf. Published 2015.

Witenko C, Moorman R, Motycka C, et al. Muscle relaxants for the management of acute low back pain. *P T*. 2014 39(6):427–435.

Lumbar Spinal Stenosis

Ammendolia C, Stuber K, de Bruin LK, et al. Nonoperative treatment of lumbar spinal stenosis with neurogenic claudication: A systematic review. *Spine (Phila Pa 1976)*. 2012;37:E609.

Ammendolia C, Stuber KJ, Rok E, et al. Nonoperative treatment for lumbar spinal stenosis with neurogenic claudication. *Cochrane Database Syst Rev*. 2013;(8):CD010712.

Atlas SJ, Delitto A. Spinal stenosis: Surgical versus nonsurgical treatment. *Clin Orthop Relat Res*. 2006;443:198.

Katz JN, Harris MB. Clinical practice. Lumbar spinal stenosis. *N Engl J Med*. 2008;358:818.

Lee MJ, Dettori JR, Standaert CJ, et al. The natural history of degeneration of the lumbar and cervical spines: A systematic review. *Spine (Phila Pa 1976)*. 2012;37:S18.

Vertebral Fracture

Barr JD, Jensen ME, Hirsch JA, et al. Position statement on percutaneous vertebral augmentation: A consensus statement developed by the Society of Interventional Radiology (SIR), American Association of Neurological Surgeons (AANS), Congress of Neurological Surgeons (CNS), American College of Radiology (ACR), American Society of Neuroradiology (ASNR), American Society of Spine Radiology (ASSR), Canadian Interventional Radiology Association (CIRA) and the Society of NeuroInterventional Surgery (SNIS). *J Vasc Interv Radiol*. 2014;26(2):171–181.

Denis F. The three column spine and its significance in the classification of acute thoracolumbar spinal injuries. *Spine (Phila Pa 1976)*. 1983;8:184–201.

Esses SI, McGuire R, Jenkins J, et al. *The treatment of symptomatic osteoporotic spinal compression fractures: Guidelines and evidence report*. Rosemont, IL: American Academy of Orthopaedic Surgeons; 2010.

Gardner A, Grannum S, Porter K. Thoracic and lumbar spine fractures. *Trauma*. 2005;7:77.

Greenbaum J, Walters N, Levy PD. An evidenced-based approach to radiographic assessment of cervical spine injuries in the emergency department. *J Emerg Med*. 2009;36:64.

McCarthy J, Davis A. Diagnosis and management of vertebral compression fractures. *Am Fam Physician*. 2016;94(1):44–50.

Pagonis TA, Givissis PK, Christodoulou AC. Calcitonin promotes faster healing of spinal fractures in osteoporotic patients. *Int J Orthop*. 2014;1(2).

Savitsky E, Votey S. Emergency department approach to acute thoracolumbar spine injury. *J Emerg Med*. 1997;15:49.

Sherman AL, Razack N. Lumbar compression fracture. Medscape. http://emedicine.medscape.com/article/309615. Published January 20, 2017.

RESOURCES

Choosing Wisely. Back Pain Tests and Treatments
http://www.choosingwisely.org/patient-resources/back-pain-tests-and-treatments

Herniated Disc. National Library of Medicine/PubMed Health
https://www.ncbi.nlm.nih.gov/pubmedhealth/PMHT0024495

Herniated Disk. OrthoInfo/American Academy of Orthopedic Surgeons
https://orthoinfo.aaos.org/en/diseases--conditions/herniated-disk/

Lumbar Spinal Stenosis. OrthoInfo/American Academy of Orthopedic Surgeons
https://orthoinfo.aaos.org/en/diseases--conditions/lumbar-spinal-stenosis/

Lumbar Spine. National Library of Medicine/PubMed Health
https://www.ncbi.nlm.nih.gov/pubmedhealth/PMHT0024393

Neck Sprain. OrthoInfo/ American Academy of Orthopedic Surgeons
https://orthoinfo.aaos.org/en/diseases--conditions/neck-sprain/

Spinal Stenosis. Cleveland Clinic
https://my.clevelandclinic.org/health/diseases/17499-spinal-stenosis

Spine. National Library of Medicine/PubMed Health
https://www.ncbi.nlm.nih.gov/pubmedhealth/PMHT0024395

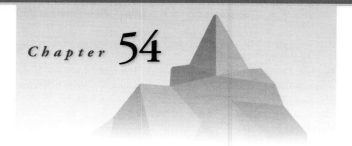

Soft-Tissue Disorders

Patricia Vanhook, PhD, MSN, APRN, FNP-BC, FAAN, FAANP

Lynne M. Dunphy, PhD, APRN, FNP-BC, FAAN, FAANP

Conor Luskin, PA-C

Soft-tissue disorders are extremely common and frequently present in primary care. These disorders are nonsystemic, focal, pathological syndromes involving periarticular tissues that include muscles, tendons, ligaments, fascia, aponeurosis, retinaculum, bursa, and subcutaneous tissue. These disorders are classified as "nonarticular" disorders. Patients who present with a soft-tissue disorder will frequently complain of "hip pain," or "elbow pain," for example; however, this complaint often refers to pain in the general region of these joints, not in the joints themselves. Some may be a consequence of chronic, repetitive, low-grade trauma and overuse; many respond to conservative measures.

A general initial approach to these patients in the primary-care setting is as follows:

- Exclude systemic disease.
- Eliminate aggravating factors.
- Explain the disorder.
- Provide pain relief on a short-term basis.
- Educate about self-care and prognosis.

Underlying structural disorders are not uncommon even in healthy young adults and often contribute to pain syndromes. Body asymmetry is a common cause of many regional pain disorders.

BURSITIS

Bursitis, or inflammation of a bursa, is a common cause of painful musculoskeletal syndromes. Bursae are sacs filled with synovial fluid, located between muscles, tendons, and bony prominences. Bursae cushion bony prominences from overlying muscles (deep bursae) or surface skin (superficial bursae); they may or may not communicate with the adjacent joint space. The bursa provides lubrication for movement of tendons over bones and can be affected by trauma, as in overuse, and by infection,

inflammation, and neoplasms. The total number of bursae varies from person to person, but on average, this figure approaches 160. Some cases of bursitis may result from rheumatic disease and others from a pathological condition of adjoining tissues. It may be acute or chronic.

EPIDEMIOLOGY AND CAUSES

Bursitis is a common complaint, seen most often in patients who are skeletally mature. It is more common in males and tends to be more commonly associated with trauma (including overuse syndrome) in patients younger than 35 years. It is one of the most common reasons for visits to the primary-care setting; the incidence is clearly related to increasing age. The incidence of bursitis of the lower extremities is increased by obesity.

Bursitis commonly develops in the subdeltoid and subacromial bursa of the shoulder, the olecranon bursa of the elbow, the greater trochanteric bursa that is lateral to the hip, the ischial bursa, the prepatellar bursa of the knee, the anserine bursa that lies between the pes anserine tendons, and the retrocalcaneal bursa.

Trauma in the form of repetitive motion injury is probably the most common cause of bursitis, as a result of constant friction between a bursa and musculoskeletal tissues surrounding it. Friction in turn causes irritation, edema, and, over time, inflammation and subsequent degeneration. The end result is an engorged bursal sac with surrounding tissue that has become tender and painful. Movement around the bursa may result in increased pain and pressure. In turn, flexion and extension of the closest joint may be limited by the affected bursa. Aging connective tissues are at a higher risk for microtears with bursitis.

PATHOPHYSIOLOGY

Bursitis is an inflammatory process that may be acute or chronic; the exact etiology is often unknown. Bursitis may be caused by an infectious process, trauma (more common in patients younger than 35 years), repetitive movement disorders, pseudogout, gout, or neoplastic disease. Less often, it may be attributed to rheumatoid disease (especially with nodular or bilateral bursitis) or infection by *Mycobacterium tuberculosis* or Candida fungal infection. Far more commonly, however, septic bursitis is due to bacterial infection.

Up to 80% of septic bursitis cases are due to infection by *Staphylococcus aureus*, with 5% to 20% due to *Streptococcus* and other gram-positive skin flora, which are typically introduced via direct trauma that compromises the protective skin barrier. Immunocompromised conditions such as diabetes mellitus, HIV infection, chronic steroid use, or autoimmune conditions such as rheumatoid arthritis (RA) may all predispose the individual to septic bursitis, and causative trauma to the overlying skin surface may even be microscopic in nature.

Bursitis is essentially a soft-tissue problem rather than a joint problem such as arthritis and often coexists with tendinitis or tenosynovitis. Overuse injury is characterized by repeated cycles of degeneration and regeneration with new collagen deposition. Synovial cells increase in thickness, and the normal bursal lining may be replaced by granulation tissue before eventual fibrosis. In turn, the bursa may become filled with transudative fluid with a high concentration of fibrin. At the conclusion of this inflammatory process, calcium deposition may occur proximal to the affected bursa.

CLINICAL PRESENTATION

Subjective

The presenting symptoms are usually pain and sometimes swelling over the known locations of bursal sacs, which may be accompanied by swelling and warmth over the involved bursa. When the subcutaneous bursal sacs (olecranon and prepatellar) are inflamed by systemic illnesses such as RA, gout, or infection, additional clues to diagnosis may include fever, chills, and arthralgias. The prepatellar and olecranon bursae frequently present with local redness, swelling, and warmth that must be distinguished from septic arthritis. Patients who develop subcutaneous bursitis may have a family history of articular problems. An occupational history may provide a clue to diagnosis. Some examples include "weaver's bottom" (ischial-gluteal bursitis), "miner's elbow" (olecranon bursitis), and "housemaid's knee" (prepatellar bursitis). Bursitis of a deep bursa is manifested by pain over the bursa with activity or direct pressure. The pain may radiate some distance, as in the case of gluteal bursitis, in which the patient may complain of pain in a sciatic distribution. In retrocalcaneal bursitis, there will be pain anterior to the Achilles tendon, just above its insertion into the calcaneus; the pain is aggravated by squeezing the area anterior to the tendon, as well as by dorsiflexion of the ankle.

Objective

Pain may be referred to other musculoskeletal structures contiguous to the bursa; therefore, careful examination is necessary to identify the source of the pain. Clinical signs and symptoms include induration, erythema, and effusion over the olecranon and prepatellar bursae. Gross distention of the bursal sac may be apparent. If there is significant limitation of range of motion (ROM) or pain on flexion, a coincident arthritis must be suspected. Bursitis may also develop from repeated

microtrauma, leading to effusion and thickening of the bursal sac. When irritation and inflammation continue, the bursa is at risk for calcification and development of adhesions around the bursa, thereby limiting tendon movement.

DIAGNOSTIC REASONING

Diagnostic Tests

Laboratory findings will usually be normal. Erythrocyte sedimentation rate and C-reactive protein may be elevated by gout, RA, or infection. In cases of gout, uric acid levels would be elevated. In infectious leukocytosis, the white blood cell (WBC) count may be elevated. Diagnosis of noninfected bursitis should be made based on clinical examination and patient symptomatology.

Differential Diagnosis

When formulating a diagnosis, RA, gout or pseudogout, and septic arthritis must be ruled out. A diagnosis is generally determined from an x-ray film showing the involved joint or bursa, with or without calcified deposits. Further diagnosis is determined from the aspiration of fluid in the affected joint. The fluid is cultured, and a WBC count is done to assess the presence of bacterial infection. An elevated red blood cell count is associated with trauma.

MANAGEMENT

Medical management and treatment of bursitis includes avoidance of activities that can lead to constant irritation of the bursa and application of moist heat or ice to the affected area every 4 hours for 15 to 20 minutes. The use of moist heat versus ice is an individual preference. Immobilization of the affected area to reduce edema and provide support is recommended, along with ROM exercises to prevent loss of mobility and to help maintain motion. It has also been recommended in certain cases that an NSAID along with ultrasound therapy be used. If symptoms recur, an injection of a long-acting corticosteroid (triamcinolone 2 to 10 mg, hydrocortisone 25 to 37.5 mg, methylprednisolone 20 to 40 mg, or dexamethasone 4 to 16 mg, each mixed with an equal volume of lidocaine hydrochloride 1%) into the affected bursa is recommended, followed by application of ice for 10 to 20 minutes. Injections should not be repeated more than every 12 weeks. Injection into a fluid-filled bursa such as in the olecranon and prepatellar bursa is not recommended. Physical therapy in the case of shoulder and hip bursitis can be helpful. Failure of conservative therapy for 6 weeks should warrant orthopedic referral.

Patient Education: Bursitis

Patient education is vital to ensure a rapid recovery. Encouraging a patient to decrease certain activities will speed up recovery. Encourage preliminary stretching and warm-up exercises before activities to maintain flexibility and strength. If medications are a part of the treatment regimen, reinforcement of proper administration and a discussion of their side effects are recommended.

TENDINITIS/TENOSYNOVITIS

Tendinitis is the inflammation of a tendon, which usually occurs at its point of insertion into bone or at the point of muscular origin. The term *tenosynovitis* refers to inflammation involving synovial sheaths surrounding the tendon in addition to the tendons. Common tenosynovitis syndromes, also referred to as overuse syndromes or repetitive motion syndromes, include supraspinatus tendinitis, lateral epicondylitis or "tennis elbow," bicipital tendinitis, de Quervain's tenosynovitis (inflammation of the abductor pollicis longus [APL] and extensor pollicis longus and brevis tendons; discussed separately later in the chapter), "trigger finger" (volar flexor tenosynovitis; discussed separately later in the chapter), patellar tendinitis (patellar tendinosis or "basketball player's knee"), and Achilles tendinitis. Table 54.1 presents common sites for overuse injuries.

EPIDEMIOLOGY AND CAUSES

Overuse injuries are a common cause of tendinitis and occur in both athletes and nonathletes. It is difficult to determine the true incidence because frequently overuse injuries are not brought to the attention of a health-care provider. Despite this, such injuries account for more than 50% of the injuries seen in a primary-care setting and are the most frequently encountered athletic injury. This problem occurs with a slightly increased frequency in men and is most likely related to sports or repetitive activity. It occurs at all ages.

Athletes and manual laborers are especially prone to tendinitis because of repetitive use. Painful areas of tendon are often labelled *tendinitis*, implying an inflammatory nature of the lesion; however, it is unclear whether inflammation is truly present in all forms of the pathology, especially in more chronic situations, which tend to have a more degenerative component. Some sources advocate the use of the term *tendinosis* for this reason. *Tenosynovitis* may result from inflammatory arthropathies such as RA or from gout. Adults who overuse a joint with repeated motion are most likely to develop a *tendinitis*. Some classifications are based on degree of function and whether there is a partial or complete rupture of the tendon.

The potential for repetitive use injury is enhanced by a wide variety of predisposing factors. Underlying anatomical imperfections aggravated by exercise or repeated motions, and obesity have all been identified as risk factors. In addition, poor cardiovascular or musculoskeletal conditioning, underlying cardiovascular disease, arthritis (osteoarthritis [OA] or RA), gout, and stress may all contribute to the development of overuse syndrome. In athletes, overtraining, running on uneven surfaces, poor equipment, inadequate footwear, and leg-length discrepancy may all contribute; in workers, unhealthy work environments both physically and emotionally are thought to contribute. Repeatedly performing arm and hand movements with a very short repetitive cycle of less than 30 seconds during one's daily job is a risk factor. Repeatedly performing the same task over and over in a short period of time in a factory can impose the same level of risk. Vibration, cold environment, and use of some specific hand tools also are considered risk factors (see Risk Factors: Overuse Syndrome.)

TABLE 54.1 Common Anatomical Sites: Overuse Syndrome	
Anatomical Site	*Overuse Syndrome*
Shoulder	Rotator cuff tendinitis Thoracic outlet syndrome
Forearm	Lateral epicondylitis Medial epicondylitis Ulnar nerve entrapments
Hand and wrist	Carpal tunnel syndrome de Quervain's syndrome "Trigger finger"
Leg and foot	Chondromalacia patellae Iliotibial band syndrome Shin splints Achilles tendinitis Plantar fasciitis Stress fracture

Risk Factors: Overuse Syndrome

- Arthritis (OA and RA)
- Congenital defects
- Diabetes mellitus
- Ganglia
- Gout
- Hobbies (knitting, musical instruments, electronic games)
- Hormonal factors (pregnancy, oral contraceptive use, menopause, thyroid disorders, hysterectomy with bilateral oophorectomy)
- Hypertension
- Impaired circulation
- Inflammation of tendons and tendon sheath
- Obesity
- Occupational activities (computer usage, cash registers)
- Paget's disease

- Raynaud's phenomenon
- Renal disease
- Sports (racquet sports, golf, softball, running)
- Underlying anatomical abnormalities

PATHOPHYSIOLOGY

Exact pathophysiological entities involved with tendinitis and tenosynovitis have not been clearly established. It is understood that tenosynovitis involves inflammation of the synovial-lined sheath around one or more tendons, whereas tendinitis involves inflammation of the tendinous tissue itself. Inflammation may be caused by repetitive microtrauma, which leads to repeated cycles of inflammation and tissue regeneration, characterized by fibroblast proliferation, collagen production, and resultant tissue contraction. Because flexor tendons typically run in tight fibro-osseous tunnels, thickening of the surrounding sheath caused by inflammatory changes may in turn limit movement and cause pain as the trapped tendon attempts to glide within the thickened, tight sheath. The parietal and visceral layers of the synovium that surround flexor tendons typically provide nutrition and stability to the tendons, and they also allow for smooth movement of these connective tissues without extensive friction. Tenosynovitis may also be associated with an inflammatory or infectious process.

Tendinitis is usually associated with degenerative changes in the tendon. Calcium deposits may also be noted along the length of the tendon, known as calcific tendinitis; this is especially common in the shoulder joint and Achilles tendon. These tendons tend to stiffen without treatment. Loss of function often follows because they become progressively weaker and may eventually rupture.

CLINICAL PRESENTATION

Subjective

Patients typically complain of pain and swelling over a localized area of tendon, usually in a region where the tendon passes through a tunnel. Pain is usually worse with motion, especially motion that stretches the involved tendon. A squeaking or rubbing and sometimes a triggering or catching sensation will be described by patients who have significant tenosynovitis.

Objective

The diagnosis of tendinitis is clinically driven. Early imaging is usually of minimal benefit, except for in calcific tendinitis where calcium deposits are seen on routine x-rays. A thorough history is essential, including all extracurricular activities. The physical examination should include palpating any tender areas and ruling out any articular involvement of pain. Swelling is usually minimal in tendinitis, but it may be pronounced in cases of infection or with inflammatory causes of tenosynovitis. Examination may reveal localized pain, swelling, and tenderness. The pain will be worsened with certain motions, such as stretching the involved tendon, or with active work or activity that involves use of the tendon, especially against a resisting force. Crepitus and sometimes triggering can be palpated if a significant tenosynovitis has developed. These signs vary depending on the anatomical site of the tendinitis:

- Tendinitis of finger flexors: fingertip numbness from median nerve compression may be present.
- Rotator cuff tendinitis: pain and tenderness are felt over the subacromial space with active motion of the shoulder external rotation and abduction of shoulder. Pain can be triggered by overhead lifting. Lateral arm pain also may be present. An "empty can" test is positive for pain and negative for weakness. In this test, the patient's affected arm is abducted to 90 degrees, in neutral rotation (the thumb is pointed toward the ground). The patient is instructed to turn his or her arm and hand forward as if emptying a can. The examiner places his or her fingers on the outstretched arm near the hand and applies downward pressure.
- Lateral epicondylitis: pain over lateral epicondyle is worse with gripping or shaking hands. The patient may complain of stiffness at night and difficulty extending the arm in the morning.
- Achilles tendinitis: pain is felt with pushing off heel while walking or running.
- Patella tendinitis: pain is felt over the anterior aspect of the knee anteriorly with jumping or running.

If an inflammatory disease is present, associated redness, soft-tissue swelling, and warmth may be present. Inflammatory processes of the tendon sheaths most commonly involve the dorsum of the hands, feet, and ankle and may cause marked soft-tissue swelling. The ROM of contiguous joints may be limited by pain.

DIAGNOSTIC REASONING

Diagnostic Tests

Plain films may be useful to rule out other potential causes of pain in areas in question, but they will not show tendinitis. An exception is calcific tendinitis, for which plain radiography can reveal calcium in the Achilles tendon or in the rotator cuff tendon. Magnetic resonance imaging (MRI) is the diagnostic gold standard for tendinitis but should be reserved for patients who have failed conservative treatment or have weakness of the extremity. Generally, the diagnosis can almost always be made clinically without the need for MRI.

Differential Diagnosis

Differential diagnoses to rule out include fracture, avulsion of the tendon, inflammatory arthritis, RA, and compartment syndrome. It often is not possible to differentiate tendinitis from bursitis, and because the two conditions are treated identically, it is clinically not necessary to do so. The pain in tendinitis is localized to the side of the joint where tendon insertion occurs. Infectious tenosynovitis occurs primarily in the hand. In addition, the tenderness and swelling are located along the synovial lines proximally instead of at the insertion site and the pain is more marked, as are swelling and erythema. Erythrocyte sedimentation rate, C-reactive protein and WBC count will likely to be elevated in the case of infection.

Essentially, definitive diagnosis of tenosynovitis requires careful musculoskeletal examination, confirming the tendon source of the symptoms and excluding pathology from other contiguous musculoskeletal structures, including joints, bursae, and nerves. However, an inflammatory tenosynovitis of the dorsum of the hand or foot may require aspiration of synovial fluid, examination, and culture to confirm the diagnosis.

MANAGEMENT

Treatment depends on the stage of healing of the damaged tissue of the musculoskeletal system. There are three phases of healing: (1) inflammation, (2) proliferation of new collagen and ground substance, and (3) scar remodeling and maturation.

Initial management should include protection, rest, ice, compression, and elevation (PRICE). The injury should be protected and rehabilitated in parallel with the healing process. The injured tissue needs to be stressed to activate collagen remodeling and realignment but also protected from overstress, which will cause reinjury and incite a further inflammatory response. Taping and bracing can both be helpful in providing protection. Ice is useful for treating pain, hemorrhage, and edema. It induces vasoconstriction, which results in a decrease in local blood flow. Ice should be applied for 15 to 20 minutes; direct contact with the skin should be avoided to prevent injury. Treatment may be repeated every 1 to 2 hours in acute cases. In lowering the temperature, ice decreases metabolism and enzymatic function; further, it slows down the inflammatory process. It is useful during the first 48 hours in acute cases.

Compression in concert with cold therapy helps to reduce swelling. Elevation decreases edema by aiding lymphatic and venous return. In acute ankle sprains, for example, elevation has been shown to be the most effective method of reducing swelling. The objective is to treat the initial symptoms with these techniques to prevent prolonged inflammation and avoid new tissue disruption. In addition, measures of relative rest are used to protect the tissue from further injury.

In the second stage of healing, the objective is to gradually introduce stress and apply modalities to increase collagen production, size, cross-linking, and alignment. The rate of collagen fiber formation is directly related to the functional state of the affected area. The collagen fibers reorient themselves in line with the tensile force applied to the tissue. In the third stage, the objective is to make the collagen as elastic as possible and decrease formation of scar tissue. Progressive stress is placed on tissue to promote an increase in collagen fibril size and to increase cross-linking in tissues. Flexibility training is needed to decrease cross-linking in the joint capsule. Home exercises or formal physical therapy can assist healing in stages 2 and 3.

Immobilization may be counterproductive, and absolute rest should be limited to 1 to 2 days at most until the inflammation response has settled or in severe, chronic cases of tendinitis, after active rest has failed. *Active rest* means that the injured area can be used, but it should be protected from significant stress, which may cause further damage. The frequency and intensity of an activity may be decreased or altered, for example, but all activity should not be completely eliminated. Physical therapy is a cornerstone of treatment and can aid in the development of an individualized plan for the patient. Ice plays an important role once exercise and activity are resumed. It should be applied at the end of every exercise session to help prevent recurrence of inflammation and swelling.

Heat is effective after 48 hours in the acute phase and in the chronic phase. After the acute phase of the healing process, heat is useful in improving blood flow, relieving muscle spasm, and decreasing tissue stiffness, allowing greater ease of deformation. The most beneficial form of deep heat is ultrasound because the high-frequency waves render the tissues less stiff and more susceptible to remodeling by applied tensile forces. Ultrasound also increases local circulation.

NSAIDs can also help with tendinitis on two fronts. First, they decrease inflammation in the affected area, second; they help with palliative relief for the patient. NSAIDs are probably best prescribed at maximum dose for 10 to 14 days. If no benefit is noted in the first 3 days, it is unlikely further benefit will be gained. Although widely prescribed, they have not been shown to effectively shorten recovery time; they may be useful in their analgesic effect in supporting a patient's compliance with physical therapy.

Corticosteroids are occasionally indicated in cases of chronic overuse syndromes. They should never be injected directly into a tendon, because this can lead to rupture. In addition, activity needs to be decreased for 5 to 10 days after injection. Tendon sheath injections, by contrast, are quite effective in treating tenosynovitis of the ankle or wrist. Steroid injections can also be given intra-articulately when there is significant reactive synovitis with effusion but should be reserved for providers who have been taught the proper injection technique for the given joint.

FOLLOW-UP AND REFERRAL

Soft-tissue injuries cause considerable pain, discomfort, and potential dysfunction. A comprehensive team approach, structured in a *Circle of Caring* model, is necessary for these patients to avoid significant sequelae. As noted in the section on management, interventions need to be geared toward the stage of healing to be effective. The balance between rest and healing and the danger of erring in either direction can be great without thoughtful consideration by a team of providers, as well as maximum hearing of the patient's voice. Athletes may be overanxious and overdo; unhappy employees might have more of a psychogenic component to their pathology.

Referral to physical therapy is essential, as is referral to an orthopedic specialist if there is any question as to nature of pathology. Treatment must be individualized, and the patient must be a chief architect in the plan of care. Patients requiring corticosteroid injections should be referred. Occupational therapists can assist with fitting of splints if necessary. Treatment should be conservative for approximately 4 to 6 weeks. If the patient still has pain or dysfunction despite conservative treatment, orthopaedic referral should be considered.

Patient Education: Tendinitis and Tenosynovitis

It is important that patients understand the nature of their injury and be involved in the plan of care. In the case of athletes, careful evaluation of training schedules and circumstances surrounding the injury is essential so that appropriate preventive measures can be put in place to support healing and avoid future injury. In the case of a work-related repetitive motion injury, evaluation of the workplace may be necessary.

In cases in which the patient's job is the source of repetitive strain injury, restrictions on work activity may be necessary. A careful and thorough occupational history can help make determinations about the contributing factors in the patient's job environment. A comprehensive ergonomic worksite evaluation may be conducted by a physical or occupational therapist in identifying specific problems. Ultimately, however, patients with severe forms of repetitive strain injury may need to change occupations.

HAND AND WRIST DISORDERS

CARPAL TUNNEL SYNDROME

Carpal tunnel syndrome (CTS) is the most common cause of peripheral nerve compression, affecting approximately 3% to 6% of adults. Pain and/or numbness affects some part of the median nerve distribution. Symptoms tend to affect the dominant hand, but more than half the patients experience bilateral symptoms. Women are three times more likely than men are to be diagnosed with CTS.

EPIDEMIOLOGY AND CAUSES

CTS is most common in persons aged 40 to 60 years and affects females significantly more frequently than males, most commonly middle-aged and pregnant women. Roughly 80% of patients are older than 40 years. Any condition that reduces the size or space of the carpal tunnel can cause compression of the medial nerve. Any movement that causes the wrist to repeatedly flex or extend out of the neutral position or that places pressure on the median nerve may contribute to the development of CTS. Direct compression may result from neoplasms, a misaligned fracture, or trauma to the carpal tunnel. The greatest risk is found in occupations that require repeated flexion or extension of the wrist, use of hand tools that require forceful gripping, or use of hand tools that vibrate. CTS has been reported to occur spontaneously, most often during conditions that affect hormone balance (e.g., pregnancy, menopause, myxedematous hypothyroidism, diabetes mellitus) or in patients with other underlying musculoskeletal disorders (e.g., gout, RA, acute injury, acromegaly). Although the mechanism is unclear, it is thought that the generalized fluid increase or deposition of matrix substances (e.g., myxedema, amyloidosis) in the body tissues causes impingement on the median nerve within the carpal tunnel. This is also likely to underlie the association of CTS with fluid overload in end-stage renal disease and chronic dialysis.

Past history of wrist trauma or Colles fracture, degenerative (and inflammatory) joint disease, ganglionic cysts, obesity, fibromyalgia, and scleroderma are other risk factors for this disorder. There is no universal agreement that CTS is work related. Although no genetic mutations have been identified other than a rare chromosome 17 deletion that leads to an autosomal dominant neuropathic disorder prone to pressure-related nerve palsies, CTS is well known to occur in families and likely has a strong genetic component.

PATHOPHYSIOLOGY

The anatomy of the wrist extends from the distal radius and ulna to the carpometacarpal joint. The eight small carpal bones of the wrist, arranged in two rows, account for numerous articulations and enable the wrist to perform a wide ROM. The wrist is the second most mobile joint in the body, allowing for the exceptional mobility of the hand. Radial ligaments and the triangular fibrocartilage complex maintain the stability of the carpal bones. The carpal tunnel is formed by the arrangement of the wrist bones and the inelastic flexor retinaculum ligament. Through this tunnel run the finger flexor tendons and the median nerve. Any source of inflammation or pressure within this canal can result in symptoms of CTS.

Patients with CTS are prone to developing increases in pressure within the carpal tunnel during wrist flexion and extension. In turn, this may lead to edema within the nerve tissue. These mechanisms may also result in venous congestion and stasis, compression of the median nerve, and resultant ischemia, leading to the pain and paresthesias associated with CTS.

CLINICAL PRESENTATION

Subjective

Typically, the patient will present with an aching sensation that radiates into the thenar area. A hallmark symptom is nighttime awakening with pain and numbness. Paresthesias and numbness in the median distribution (medial thumb second one-third and medial portion of the fourth digit) typically accompany the pain. In later disease, patients often report that they frequently drop objects and that they cannot open jars or twist off lids. Repetitive motions of the hand or stationary tasks with the wrist held flexed or extended for a period of time (such as when driving) worsen pain and numbness. Patients report that they must rub or shake the hand to "get the circulation" going. Persistent numbness and thenar atrophy can occur when the compression is severe and/or long-standing.

Objective

Examination of the patient with suspected CTS should include inspection of the wrist and hand for swelling, redness, nodules, deformity, and muscle atrophy. The thenar eminence (at the base of the thumb) is the best location to assess for atrophy. If the thenar eminence is atrophied or flattened, chronic CTS should be suspected. Palpation of the hand and wrist should be done to check for swelling, bogginess, or tenderness. Each distal interphalangeal (DIP), proximal interphalangeal (PIP), and metacarpophalangeal (MCP) joint should be palpated, as well as the wrist bones. Capillary refill time should be determined, and the radial and ulnar arteries should be assessed for patency. Allen's test, Phalen's maneuver, and Tinel's sign (see Advanced Assessment 52.6) should be performed to determine individual patency of both the radial and ulnar arteries. In addition, the carpal compression test should be done. In this test, the examiner places the thumbs over the flexor retinaculum and applies even pressure over the area of the median nerve for 30 to 60 seconds. A positive test is indicated by the occurrence of paresthesia in the hand or first three digits. Finally, the patient should draw the pattern of numbness and tingling in his or her hand or indicate it on a preprinted picture of the hand and wrist.

The performance of sensory testing to aid in the diagnosis is of little clinical value. Many patients who do not have CTS have diminished ability to differentiate sharp and dull sensations on the fingers and therefore yield a high false-positive rate for this testing. Also remember that occupation and handedness may affect the muscular symmetry of the hands and wrists in the absence of a musculoskeletal condition.

DIAGNOSTIC REASONING

Diagnostic Tests

Radiographs should be done if the patient has limited wrist movement; however, the most useful diagnostic test is a median nerve conduction velocity study. By measuring the velocity of sensory conduction, nerve entrapment may be conclusively validated. It is important to remember that this is an invasive test and that it is considerably more expensive than other diagnostic methods. In addition, a patient may have an abnormal nerve conduction velocity study but have no clinical symptoms; conversely, 5% to 10% of patients with CTS have normal test results.

Differential Diagnosis

The following is a list of differential diagnoses:

* Arthritis of the carpometacarpal joint of the thumb (painful motion)
* Cervical radiculopathy affecting the C6 nerve root (neck pain, numbness in the thumb and index finger only)
* Diabetes mellitus with paresthesias (determine on history)
* Median nerve compression at the elbow (tenderness at the proximal forearm)
* Wrist arthritis (limited motion, evident on radiograph)

MANAGEMENT

Conservative treatment is recommended for patients who present with acute symptoms. It has been reported that 50% to 75% of conservatively treated patients will attain symptom relief. The goal of treatment is to prevent the flexion and extension movements of the wrist. This is best accomplished through use of a splint that allows free movement of the fingers and the thumb while maintaining the wrist in the neutral position. Recommendations for wearing of the splint vary from constantly (day and night) to nighttime only. Some providers recommend using the splints day and night for 3 weeks, then nightly only for 3 more weeks. Splinting can be a cost-effective method for symptom control. Maximum results from splinting are attained if it is instituted within the first 3 months of symptom onset.

Oral NSAIDs are another conservative measure that can be used in conjunction with splinting. These drugs are often prescribed for patients who experience pain as part of the syndrome, but they may have some general usefulness in controlling edema in the carpal tunnel.

Corticosteroid injections, although used by some providers, are discouraged for treatment of CTS. Although the injections provide temporary relief, there is a concern that the median nerve could sustain damage and scarring or that infection may occur.

The use of vitamin B$_6$ (pyridoxine) in CTS has been reported in the literature over the past several years. Although there are no conclusive studies on the utility of this medication in treating or preventing CTS, use of this vitamin is becoming more prevalent. Care should be taken with dosing because larger doses may result in neuropathies. It is also important to determine whether the patient is on any other medications that may be affected by pyridoxine; for example, serum concentrations of phenytoin and phenobarbital may be decreased with pyridoxine.

Management of concurrent disease (e.g., hypothyroidism, diabetes mellitus) is an important aspect of the conservative treatment of CTS. Treatment that diminishes fluid retention, when used with other conservative methods, will produce better results in relieving the symptoms of CTS.

CTS that occurs during pregnancy usually resolves after pregnancy. Treatment consists of splinting and other nonoperative measures such as corticosteroid injections. CTS that is work related may respond to ergonomic modifications.

FOLLOW-UP AND REFERRAL

The presence of thenar atrophy or unremitting symptoms with conservative treatment warrant referral for surgical evaluation. Carpal tunnel release is one of the most commonly performed hand surgeries; it is usually done with local anesthesia on an outpatient basis. The surgery may be performed by a hand specialist, plastic surgeon, or neurosurgeon.

Patient Education: Carpal Tunnel Syndrome

Workers who are exposed to occupational risks for CTS should be educated on the causes and prevention of CTS. The work environment should be assessed for ergonomic risks to workers; often an ergonomic specialist is needed to perform these assessments. *Ergonomics* means fitting the job to the worker, as opposed to the worker accommodating to the workspace. Special attention should be paid to jobs with a known ability to produce extreme or repeated flexion of the wrist. Ergonomic evaluations and recommendations include the following:

- Evaluating the workstations of computer keyboard workers in regard to the height of the keyboard, chair, and monitor.
- Teaching lifting techniques and reviewing them annually.
- Rotating jobs for workers who perform repetitive tasks.
- Resting frequently or wearing specially designed hand wear; for example, workers who use vibrating tools should wear anti-vibration gloves or should be given frequent, short rest breaks.

Outside of workplace risks, patients should be educated to consider the stress on the wrist during everyday activities such as gardening and cleaning. Knitting, sewing, and playing musical instruments may put tension on the wrist. Patients should be advised to avoid carrying heavy briefcases, packages, or purses with the hands. Bags with shoulder straps, backpacks, or bags with wheels should be recommended to patients with risk factors for CTS.

DE QUERVAIN'S TENOSYNOVITIS

EPIDEMIOLOGY AND CAUSES

De Quervain's tenosynovitis is condition in which the APL and the extensor pollicis brevis (EPB) tendons exert excessive friction on their synovial sheath, causing inflammation. It is characterized by pain at the base of the thumb or at the radial styloid process on abduction and extension of the thumb and commonly occurs in patients who perform pinch-grip activities such as using hand tools with extreme pressure, carrying trays with a pinch grip, assembly work, and sewing/cutting activities. It is more common in middle-aged women and is often precipitated by repetitive use of the thumb.

PATHOPHYSIOLOGY

Within the wrist, there are six dorsal tunnels that transport the extensor tendons. The first tunnel transports the APL and EPB tendons, which form the radial border of the anatomical snuffbox. The APL and EPB tendons are responsible for thumb flexion and extension and for establishing a grip. De Quervain's tenosynovitis occurs when the synovial lining of the tunnel becomes inflamed. The opening of the canal narrows, causing stenosis. This results in pain when the tendons move.

CLINICAL PRESENTATION

Subjective

De Quervain's tenosynovitis presents with pain at the radial side of the wrist, usually with lifting. This pain is aggravated by attempts to move the thumb or make a fist. Patients may complain of pain while turning a key or a doorknob or while attempting to open a jar. Often the condition occurs as the result of lifting infants with the second metacarpals (web between the thumb and the index finger) under the baby's axillae. Chronic pain, loss of strength, and loss of thumb motion can occur. If there is a possible relationship to the patient's occupation/hobby, ask about the specifics of these activities.

Objective

The history and physical examination should proceed as described for CTS. Assessment for crepitation should be performed over the radial styloid. On palpation, the tendon sheath may feel thickened.

DIAGNOSTIC REASONING

Diagnostic Tests

Allen's test, Phalen's maneuver, and Tinel's sign should be negative. The confirmation test for de Quervain's tenosynovitis is Finkelstein's test (see Advanced Assessment 52.6). There is usually no need for additional diagnostic testing. Wrist x-ray studies are indicated only if there is a history of trauma. Calcification associated with tendinitis occasionally can be seen on radiographs.

Differential Diagnosis

The differential diagnoses include CTS, carpometacarpal joint arthrosis of the thumb, scaphoid fractures, and arthritis of the thumb and/or wrist.

MANAGEMENT

Noninvasive treatment includes rest, splinting, and NSAIDs. A 2-week course of NSAIDs is usually helpful (see discussion about NSAIDs in Chapter 52). Splints that are used are either a radial gutter splint or a customized long opponens splint. The splint should immobilize both the wrist and the thumb. Splinting is used for 3 to 6 weeks. Invasive treatments include corticosteroid injections into the tendon sheath performed by an orthopaedist or experienced provider.

FOLLOW-UP AND REFERRAL

Patients with unremitting symptoms after 6 to 8 weeks of conservative treatment should be referred for orthopaedic consultation and possible surgery.

Patient Education: De Quervain's Tenosynovitis

Patients should be educated regarding the cause of de Quervain's tenosynovitis. Modifications to hand tools or the work environment may need to be made. For example, hand tools may be retrofitted with a larger grip surface, so that pressure is more evenly distributed over the palmar surface of the hand. Avoidance of the precipitating factor is often enough to permanently resolve early symptoms.

GANGLION CYST

A *ganglion* is a cyst that develops on or in a tendon sheath. It is filled with a thick, gel-like material that leaks from the joint into the weakened tendon sheath and forms a cyst sac. A ganglionic cyst is usually caused by frequent strains and contusions, resulting in joint inflammation. The most common sites are on the dorsum of the wrist over the radiocarpal joint or on the volar surface of the wrist near the flexor carpi radialis tendon. The ganglion can be asymptomatic, or it may be associated with dull aching and weakness. It can be distinguished from a tumor by its soft consistency and transillumination. Treatment includes aspiration or surgical removal, although a conservative approach is appropriate because spontaneous disappearance may occur.

TRIGGER FINGER

"Trigger finger" or "locked finger" is a common name for *stenosing tenosynovitis of the flexor tendons*. This problem can be painful and functionally limiting. Any digit can be affected, although it most commonly affects the ring or middle finger. Inflammation at the MCP joint pulley causes a size discrepancy between the tendon and the pulley. Because the tendon no longer slides freely through the pulley, there is a snapping or locking phenomenon. The digit remains flexed or extended until the tendon pops through the pulley, causing severe pain. Tenderness with palpation of the flexor tendon over the MCP joint is noted. There is a higher prevalence of trigger finger in patients with CTS and de Quervain stenosing tenosynovitis.

Trigger finger may be idiopathic (more common in middle-aged women) or associated with RA or diabetes. Patients typically report pain and catching when they flex the finger and may describe the finger as going "out of joint." They may awaken with the finger locked in the palm, although the finger gradually unlocks during the day. Physical examination reveals tenderness in the palm at the level of the distal palmar crease, usually overlying the MCP joint. A nodule may also be palpable. The nodule moves, and the finger may lock when the patient flexes and extends the affected finger. This movement is almost always painful. Full flexion of the finger may not be possible.

The most effective therapy for this problem is local anaesthetic and corticosteroid injection into the tendon sheath, plus a modification of activities for about a month. A small number of patients require surgical release of the tendon. Splinting and NSAIDs have not proven effective.

TENDON INJURIES OF THE HAND

Several finger deformities are caused by traumatic tendon ruptures of avulsions. The appearance of each type of deformity depends on the affected tendon:

- Jersey finger is caused by avulsion or rupture of the flexor digitorum profundus tendon and is characterized by inability to actively flex the DIP joint (Fig. 54.1).
- Mallet finger is caused by rupture or avulsion of the extensor digitorum tendon and is characterized by inability to actively extend the DIP. The joint typically rests at 30 degrees of flexion (Fig. 54.2).
- Boutonniere deformity is caused by rupture of the central portion of the extensor tendon at its insertion into the middle phalanx. The finger is held partially flexed at the PIP joint and extended or hyperextended at the DIP joint. Flexion contracture of the PIP joint and extension contracture of the DIP joint are possible (Fig. 54.3). This injury is most commonly seen in patients with advanced RA (see Chapter 62).

Partial tendon injuries are treated with splinting and exercises to restore function to the tendons. However, complete tears and avulsions require surgical repair. The PIP joint should be splinted in extension for 6 weeks in a young patient and for 3 weeks in an elderly patient. The DIP joint is left free. Active and passive ROM should be initiated at the DIP joint. If the injury is already 1 to 2 weeks old, this may not be possible.

DUPUYTREN'S CONTRACTURE

Sometimes referred to as "Viking disease" or palmar fibromatosis, this condition affects the palmar tissue between the skin and the distal palm and fingers, most often in the fourth and fifth fingers but also in the thumb–index

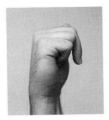

Figure 54.1 Jersey finger.

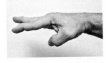

Figure 54.2 Mallet finger.

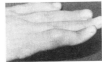

Figure 54.3 Boutonniere deformity.

finger web space. Visible, palpable fibrous bands, reminiscent of tendons, can extend from the palm to the PIP joint of Dupuytren-affected fingers. It is a progressive condition that results in flexor contracture while not affecting the flexor tendons. As the contractures increase, patients have trouble grasping objects, pulling on gloves, and putting hands in pockets. Sensation in the affected fingers usually is normal. It occurs most frequently in persons aged 40 to 60 years and is a familial disorder, most commonly affecting males of northern European ancestry. It is dysfunctional and disfiguring but does not cause pain. Injections or surgery are the only therapeutic options. Patients should be referred to an orthopedic specialist for treatment

SHOULDER DISORDERS

ADHESIVE CAPSULITIS

Often referred to as a "frozen shoulder," adhesive capsulitis is defined as idiopathic loss of both active and passive ROM, with no clear predisposition based on gender, arm dominance, or occupation. Patients aged 40 to 60 years are more likely to be affected; diabetes mellitus (especially type 1) is the most common risk factor. Patients with diabetes tend to be refractory to treatment, and 40% to 50% will have bilateral involvement. Other underlying conditions related to frozen shoulder include hypothyroidism, Dupuytren disease, cervical disc herniation, Parkinson's disease, stroke, and tumors. In a short period of time, immobility will result in a tight, painful shoulder joint that has limited active ROM (a "freezing" phase of pain) and then typically progresses to a "thawing" phase of decreasing discomfort associated with a steady improvement in function. This process may take anywhere from 6 months to 2 years. Although adhesive capsulitis may result from any condition that produces pain and immobility, in older patients and individuals without predisposing factors, the possibility of underlying organic or neoplastic disease should be considered.

Physical examination typically reveals a loss in both active and passive ROM. Pain and tenderness are common with motion and at the deltoid insertion. Diffuse tenderness about the shoulder may also be present. AP and axillary radiographs of the shoulder are indicated to ensure that smooth, concentric joint surfaces with an intact cartilage space are present and to rule out other pathology such as osteophytes, loose bodies, calcium deposits, or tumors. Other studies, such as arthrography, CT, or MRI, are rarely indicated if radiographs are normal.

Adhesive capsulitis is differentiated from chronic posterior shoulder dislocation, tumor, and OA on radiograph. Posttraumatic shoulder stiffness is, obviously, related to a history of trauma. Rotator cuff tear is differentiated because of the presence of normal passive ROM.

Treatment consists of the application of moist heat and use of analgesics (NSAIDs and nonnarcotic analgesics. Physical therapy is recommended to restore function, along with gentle stretching exercises that can be performed at home. The patient should be advised that recovery time is often lengthy, and there is potential for chronic stiffness and residual pain. If improvement is not seen within 6 to 12 weeks, the patient should be referred to an orthopedic specialist.

ROTATOR CUFF SYNDROME

Rotator cuff syndrome may include impingement problems, calcific tendinitis, and subacromial bursitis (shoulder bursitis). The term *impingement syndrome* refers to pathological changes that result when the subacromial bursa and/or rotator cuff becomes inflamed because of compression under the acromion or "roof" of the shoulder joint (rotator cuff tendinitis). It is the leading cause of shoulder pain, ranging from bursitis to rotator cuff tendinitis and, eventually, degenerative tears of the rotator cuff. In addition, the biceps tendon may be impinged (in bicipital tendinitis).

The rotator cuff covers the anterior, superior, and posterior aspects of the humoral head and is formed by the coming together of four muscles. These muscles assist in the elevation of the arm. Inflammation of the subacromial bursa and underlying rotator cuff tendons is a common cause of shoulder pain in middle-aged patients. Rotator cuff pathology presents a continuum from edema and hemorrhage to chronic inflammation and fibrosis to microscopic tendon fiber failure progressing to full-thickness rotator cuff tears. The etiology is multifactorial. A loss of microvascular blood supply to the tendon and repeated mechanical insults as the tendon passes under the coracoacromial arch combine to cause damage over time.

The history is usually one of gradual onset of anterior and lateral shoulder pain exacerbated by overhead activity. Typical presenting pain is lateral arm pain radiating from the shoulder to elbow; if pain radiates past the elbow, cervical spine pathology should be considered. Night pain and difficulty sleeping on the affected side are also common. Atrophy of the muscles about the top and back of the shoulder may be apparent if the patient has had problems over a period of several months, although this may also indicate a chronic rotator cuff tear or neuropathic disorder.

On physical examination, palpation over the greater tuberosity and subacromial bursa commonly elicits tenderness and crepitus with shoulder motion. Pain will be elicited by having the patient slowly lower the abducted arm against downward resistance. Neer and Hawkins signs are generally positive. Impingement testing involves locally anesthetizing the shoulder. If the patient is then stronger and without pain after subacromial injection, pain inhibition from inflammation and fibrosis is likely rather than full-blown tear. AP and axillary radiographs are usually negative; narrowing of the space between the head of the humerus and the undersurface of the acromion suggests a long-standing rotator cuff tear.

Frozen shoulder is ruled out if active and passive ROM loss is not present; a rotator cuff tear will not improve with subacromial injection of local anesthetic; glenohumeral arthritis is evident on radiograph and there is pain on motion; acromioclavicular (AC) arthritis presents with tenderness over the AC joint.

Treatment includes resting from the offending activity and NSAIDs. The patient should begin a stretching program with emphasis on posterior capsule stretching. If home therapy of three to four times a day over a period of 6 weeks does not result in improvement, a subacromial corticosteroid injection can be administered, followed by continued stretching. Steroid injections should not be repeated if the previous injection does not produce significant and sustained (more than 3 months) relief. Significant rotator cuff weakness or failure to improve after 6 weeks of rehabilitation (with or without subacromial steroid injection) is an indication for further evaluation and operative consideration.

CALCIFIC TENDINITIS

Calcific tendinitis is a degenerative process accompanied by a local deposit of calcium that develops in the rotator cuff. The calcified material often creates inflammatory changes in the subdeltoid bursa and is frequently asymptomatic until an acute event or overuse exacerbates the condition. The symptom of calcific tendinitis is severe, localized pain that occurs with any movement of the shoulder usually acute onset with extreme pain, patients often go to the ER. With the arm in a dependent position, the pain is absent or minimal. The shoulder is acutely tender and can be warm to the touch or swollen. X-ray films usually demonstrate the deposit. A transaxillary view is necessary if the deposit is anterior or posterior to the joint in the subscapularis muscle.

Minor or mild cases of calcific tendinitis rarely need invasive treatment. Anti-inflammatory medications, ultrasound, physical therapy, and rest are usually effective in ameliorating the pain. Some deposits appear soft, fluffy, or irregular on x-ray examination. Aspiration by a radiologist to remove some of the material while concurrently injecting an anesthetic with corticosteroid preparation can provide immediate relief. In more severe cases or those that fail to respond to conservative treatment, corticosteroid infections can be considered.

ROTATOR CUFF TEAR

Rotator cuff tear may occur secondary to trauma or from degenerative, calcific changes, chronic mechanical impingement, and altered blood supply to the tendons over time. The rotator cuff muscles insert into the tuberosities of the humerus and tightly hold the ball-and-socket joint of the shoulder together. Rotator cuff injuries are considered to be more serious than other soft-tissue injuries of the shoulder. Most full-thickness rotator cuff tears occur spontaneously in patients older than 50 years, presumably because of age-related changes in vascularity and tissue degeneration. The supraspinatus tendon is most often affected. Older people with rotator cuff tear may have only mild, disabling symptoms, or may even be asymptomatic. This injury can occur in individuals younger than 40 years, usually because of aggressive physical injury and repeated trauma from contact sports (e.g., football).

The patient will usually report a lateral deltoid pain, and weakness may be present. There may be a history of reaching overhead and feeling "something give" in the shoulder and then noting that the ipsilateral arm drops to the side. Thereafter it is difficult and very painful to abduct the arm. The pain is often worse at night, and the patient may report difficulty sleeping. To reach behind to scratch his or her back causes extreme pain.

The "empty can" test also isolates the mechanism of the rotator cuff (see description above). The examiner places his or her fingers on the outstretched arm near the hand and applies pressure to assess if the patient can maintain position against resistance. If the patient reports pain but no weakness is evident, tendinitis is probable. Most tears are relatively small, however, and the patient is often able to maintain some control. It is clinically very difficult to differentiate tendinitis from a tear. The back of the shoulder may appear sunken, indicating atrophy of the supraspinatus and infraspinatus muscles following a long-standing cuff tear. If patient has pain and weakness, a tear is more likely.

A suspected rotator cuff tear can be confirmed by performing the "drop arm" test. The examiner abducts the patient's shoulder to 90 degrees and instructs the patient to lower his or her arm slowly. If the arm drops to the side rapidly, the test is considered positive. However, this finding is indicative of late disease or a severe tear.

Soft-tissue injuries do not show up on plain x-rays; therefore, findings are usually reported as within normal limits even though the films may demonstrate calcification from previous or chronic injuries. There may be spurring of the acromion process or calcium deposits in the soft tissue, as well as bony deformities from previous dislocations. Lytic lesions indicating metastatic disease can also show up on radiography. More aggressive diagnostic testing such as MRI, ultrasonography, or arthrography may be indicated in patients with a history of acute trauma or if there is no response to conservative treatment.

Nonoperative treatment includes icing the shoulder (most commonly in cases of acute injury), NSAIDs, physical therapy with stretching and strengthening exercises, and avoiding overhead activities. Ice should be applied to the entire shoulder for 15 to 20 minutes twice daily. Corticosteroid injections should be used judiciously. Over time, steroid injections further weaken the tendon and can accelerate propagation of the rotator cuff tear. Patients should never receive more than three subacromial injections. Patients with significant failure and failed rehabilitation should be considered candidates for surgery. The exception to this rule is the patient younger than 60 years who has an acute traumatic cuff tear, in whom recovery is best accomplished within 6 weeks of the injury.

SHOULDER SPRAINS

AC sprains often occur in young men and are typically associated with a fall while the arm is adducted, causing trauma to the AC joint, although the injury may occur because of indirect trauma. The patient will present with pain, especially on adduction or abduction past 90 degrees, point tenderness over the ACJ, swelling, and possible deformity.

Acromioclavicular joint (ACJ) sprain are classified as follows into six grades:

1. AC ligament strain.
2. Slight disruption of ACJ; coracoclavicular (CC) ligament strain.
3. Dislocation of AC joint with AC ligament disruption and torn CC ligaments; deltoid and trapezius may be detached.
4. All of 3, but the CC ligaments are completely torn, clavicle is displaced posteriorly, and deltoid and trapezius are detached.
5. All of 4, with CC distance 100% to 300% greater than normal side; deltoid and trapezius are detached from distal half clavicle.
6. All of 4, with clavicle in subcoracoid position.

HIP DISORDERS

Hip pain is a common symptom with a number of possible causes. In a survey of 6,596 adults ages 60 years and older, 14.3% reported significant hip pain on most days over the past 6 weeks.

GREATER TROCHANTERIC PAIN SYNDROME

Greater trochanteric pain syndrome (GTPS) is a combination of both gluteal (buttock) tendon injuries (tendinopathy) and bursitis (inflammation of the bursa) surrounding the hip joint. In most instances, GTPS is due to a gluteus medius or minimus tendinopathy, with variable involvement of the regional bursae. It may also be associated with lumbar spondylosis, degenerative arthritis of the hip, and lower limb–length discrepancy. This category also includes external coxa saltans, known as "snapping hip." Two or more of these disorders often co-occur in patients. Historically, the term "trochanteric bursitis" was used to describe any pain around the lateral hip. However, advanced imaging and histopathological studies have shown that involvement of the trochanteric bursae in patients with lateral hip pain is variable, and when present, exists as a secondary or associated finding. Bursitis is inflammation of tissue that reduces friction around a tendon, but practically, this problem involves the tendon insertion, such as the gluteus medius tendon. Thus, trochanteric bursitis is a misnomer when it used to describe all causes of lateral hip pain. In fact, primary trochanteric bursitis is rare and is typically of microbial etiology.

GTPS is characterized by chronic, intermittent, aching pain over the lateral aspect of the hip, and some patients report numbness in the upper thigh. Pain will increase with movement, especially external rotation and abduction, and can be triggered by prolonged standing or lying on the affected side. Other signs and symptoms include pain on forced hip abduction, distinct tenderness around the greater trochanter, and pain extending down the lateral aspect of the thigh.

GTPS is treated with NSAID therapy (e.g., naproxen [Naprosyn] 375 to 500 mg by mouth two times daily for 1 to 2 weeks). Persistent cases may require corticosteroid injections.

OSTEOARTHRITIS

OA usually causes stiffness or pain with use that is felt in the morning and improves during the day. Pain referred to the groin, thigh, knee, and lateral side of the leg may occur. Often pain or stiffness affects other joints as well. For more information, see the section on OA in Chapter 55.

RHEUMATOID DISEASE

With rheumatoid disease, the hip pain is bilateral, and characteristics include morning stiffness and limited ROM that does not resolve with activity. The hip is generally not the first joint affected. During an acute phase, there is tenderness and fullness or thickening seen in the joint.

PROXIMAL HIP FRACTURE

Hip fractures are one of the most common of all adult fractures, accounting for at least half of all hospital days related to fracture care in the United States. The two primary types of hip fractures are *femoral neck* (intracapsular) and *intertrochanteric*, both of which occur most frequently in older adults who have sustained a fall at home or similar low-energy trauma. The incidence of hip fractures doubles for each decade of life after age 50 years, with women affected twice as often as men are.

Risks for hip fractures include physical activity, previous fracture, visual impairment, institutionalization, and osteoporosis. Pain in the hip area after trauma, such as a fall or motor vehicle collision, especially in patients older than 50 years, should give rise to the suggestion of fractures. Neither a lack of trauma nor a long-standing history of hip pain rules out a fracture. In some cases, a fracture may occur as a pathological fracture secondary to an underlying neoplasm or chronic corticosteroid usage. The patient should be admitted to the hospital.

Obtain a history of how the injury occurred and whether the fall was witnessed by anyone other than the patient. A loss of consciousness for any period would necessitate a cardiac and neurologic referral, as well as referral for orthopedic care. Determine the patient's mental status, and try to obtain a realistic assessment of the preinjury functional status.

Physical examination typically reveals an externally rotated and shortened injured leg. Any motion to this extremity will produce severe pain centered around the affected groin. Examine the pelvic bony prominences for tenderness because pubis ramus fractures may also be present or may be confused with the hip injury. It is important to check for lower extremity pulses and neurologic function. The entire limb should be assessed for points of tenderness or deformity that may indicate the presence of other fractures at sites such as the femur, tibia, or ankle. An anteroposterior view of the pelvis and "shoot-through" lateral views of the affected hip can provide definitive radiographic evidence to confirm the diagnosis. In most cases, surgical repair of the fracture is the treatment of choice.

MERALGIA PARESTHETICA

Caused by compression of the lateral femoral cutaneous nerve, meralgia paresthetica is commonly seen in overweight middle-aged men. Symptoms include pain or paresthesias over the anterior superior iliac spine and the anterior lateral thigh, with decreased touch and pinprick sensation. Treatment includes analgesics and avoiding tight clothing around the waist.

AVASCULAR NECROSIS

Avascular necrosis appears as abrupt hip pain followed by progressive, intermittent episodes. Pain is worsened with motion and activity and often is worse at night. A limp, along with limited abduction and internal rotation, is present. MRI is needed for diagnosis, and an orthopedic referral is indicated. It often occurs as a serious complication of hip trauma, but it may occur unrelated to trauma.

MALIGNANCY

Initially no signs may be present with malignancy; however, tenderness and palpable swelling may develop later over bony prominences. Night pain, systemic symptoms, and fractures may be seen.

ANKLE DISORDERS

Approximately 50% of sports-related injuries are related to overuse. Of injuries seen in running clinics, the majority are due to overuse with about half involving the lower leg. Many such injuries involve a tendinopathy. The clinical presentation and management of tendinopathies involving ankle tendons other than the Achilles is typical of the care for tendinitis as presented for other anatomical areas discussed. Achilles tendinopathy, as well as acute ankle injuries, is discussed separately. Fifteen percent of overuse injuries affect the ankle, most commonly the Achilles, posterior tibialis, peroneus longus, and peroneus brevis tendons. Tendinopathy can develop in both the athletic and sedentary patients but is uncommon in children. Extrinsic factors that can predispose to ankle tendinopathy include improper training, poor biomechanics (e.g., running technique), and improper footwear. Intrinsic factors can include foot malalignment, leg length discrepancy, joint laxity, and obesity.

ANKLE SPRAINS

Ankle ligaments provide mechanical stability, proprioceptive information, and directed motion for the joint. Recurrent ankle sprains can lead to functional instability and loss of normal ankle kinematics and proprioception, which can result in recurrent injury, chronic instability, early degenerative bony changes, and chronic pain. Acute ankle sprains can result in lost days of work and inability to participate in sports.

EPIDEMIOLOGY AND CAUSES

Over 3 million ankle sprains occur each year in the United States, which translates to an incidence of 2.5 ankle sprains per 1,000 individuals. Men and women are affected equally except in two age ranges: men aged 19 to 24 have significantly higher ankle sprain rates than women of the same age, and women older than 30 years have significantly higher rates than similarly aged men. One-half of all ankle sprains occur during athletic activity.

PATHOPHYSIOLOGY

Most ankle pain is the result of ankle injury that results in ligamental damage (a *sprain*). A sprain occurs when the ankle is positioned in an unstable way, causing the ligaments to overstretch. A *first-degree sprain* involves stretching of ligamentous fibers; a *second-degree sprain* involves a tear of part of the ligament, with pain and swelling; and a *third-degree sprain* results in complete ligamentous separation (see Table 54.2). Inversion injury is most common, causing damage to the lateral ligaments of the ankle. By contrast, the medial ligaments are tight and allow for much less motion than the lateral ligaments.

CLINICAL PRESENTATION

Subjective

During the history, the patient should be asked open-ended question about how the injury occurred and what happened after the injury. If the patient was able to walk and continue activity, a serious ligamental injury or fracture is less likely. If the ankle became swollen and discolored within minutes after injury, a severe soft-tissue injury or even a fracture can be suspected.

Objective

The physical examination should include inspection and palpation. Swelling in the area of the internal and external malleoli should be assessed by comparing the landmarks with those of the opposite foot. The location of a deformity helps to localize the injury, and the degree of discoloration is associated with the extent of the injury. The ankle and foot should be palpated to localize the tenderness. It is also helpful to compare the passive ROM in one leg with the opposite extremity. It is important to note crepitus because it is often a sign of fracture. The anterior drawer test should be performed to test the stability of the anterior talofibular ligament,

TABLE 54.2   Ankle Sprains

Classification	First Degree	Second Degree	Third Degree
Type of pain	Stretching, minor tearing of ligament fibers	Partial tearing of ligament fibers	Complete tear of ligament
Clinical manifestations			
Pain	Minimal	Mild to moderate	Severe
Swelling	Mild	Moderate	Significant; occurs rapidly, usually within the first 30 minutes
Ecchymosis	Mild	Moderate	Severe; occurs rapidly, usually within the first 30 minutes
ROM	Full, nonpainful	Slightly limited, painful	Limited; loss of function
Point tenderness	Mild	Point tenderness	Severe
Joint stability	Stable	Mild joint laxity	Abnormal
Weight-bearing	Able to bear weight	Painful or inability to bear weight	Inability to bear weight
Management	RICE Active ROM Partial weight-bearing activity Return to sports in 2–3 weeks with ankle support	RICE Active ROM Non–weight-bearing activity as tolerated Gradual return to sports with Aircast or taping	Refer to orthopedic specialist; surgery may be required Cast for 4–6 weeks No weight-bearing; rehabilitation Return to sports in 4–8 weeks with support
Complications	Recurrent sprains within 1 month if not fully rehabilitated	Recurrent sprains Joint instability Traumatic arthritis	Persistent instability Traumatic arthritis

Abbreviations: RICE, rest, ice, compression, elevation; ROM, range of motion.

and the varus stress test should be performed to test the stability of the calcaneofibular ligament (see Advanced Assessment 52.8).

DIAGNOSTIC REASONING

Diagnostic Testing

The Ottawa Rule lists criteria that should be met for radiographic examination of the ankle or foot (see Advanced Assessment 54.1). These guidelines are commonly used to determine the utility of radiography in diagnosing a fracture in the assessment of ankle and foot injuries. However, these guidelines should not be used for pregnant women, children younger than 6 years, and those who have head injuries or who otherwise cannot follow the directions.

Differential Diagnosis

Acute trauma to the ankle is common and raises suspicion for a lateral ankle sprain or fracture, rather than

 Advanced Assessment 54.1: Ottawa Ankle and Foot Rules

If a patient meets any of the following criteria, a radiograph should be performed:

- An ankle radiograph is indicated when ankle pain is present and there is tenderness over the posterior 6 cm or tip of the posterior or lateral malleolus.
- A foot radiograph is indicated when midfoot pain is present and there is tenderness over the navicular or the base of the fifth metatarsal.
- A radiograph of the painful area is indicated when ankle or midfoot pain is present and the patient is unable to take four steps both immediately and in the emergency department.

Source: Stiell IG, Greenberg GH, McKnight RD, Nair RC, McDowell I, Worthington JR. A study to develop clinical decision rules for the use of radiography in acute ankle injuries. *Ann Emerg Med.* 1992;21(4):384–390.

tendinopathy. Most acute fractures are apparent on diagnostic imaging (typically a plain radiograph), while most ankle sprains that cause patients to seek medical attention occur from trauma and cause immediate symptoms or pain and instability, rather than worsening over weeks as is typical with peroneal tendinopathy. Symptoms from a chronic ankle injury, especially an ankle sprain, can mimic peroneal tendinopathy. Patients with a chronic ankle sprain typically complain of turning or "rolling" their ankle frequently and manifest laxity with performance of the anterior drawer or talar tilt examination maneuvers, features absent with peroneal tendinopathy.

MANAGEMENT

Initial management should include PRICE. Ice application or immersion in an ice water should occur immediately after injury and then every few hours for the next 48 hours. An elastic bandage or splint may be applied to stabilize the ankle against inversion and eversion stresses. Activity should be limited until the pain and swelling subside. NSAIDs can be used for pain relief.

FOLLOW-UP AND REFERRAL

Acute pain typically decreases quite rapidly in the first 2 weeks after the injury, although true healing of the underlying injury may take as long as 3 years. As many as 5% to 33% of patients report that pain is still present 1 year postinjury. For patients with persistent symptoms, balance and resistance training have been shown to improve ankle strength and stability, but whether such training reduces pain is unclear. As many as 30% of all patients develop some type of chronic ankle instability often leading to reinjury. There is currently no clear evidence for which patients will progress to chronic ankle instability upon initial injury. Chronic ankle instability unresponsive to appropriate physical therapy, including proprioceptive and strength training, should be referred. In patients with symptoms that persist for more than 6 to 8 weeks, obtaining an MRI can help to rule out conditions such as talar dome fractures or syndesmosis injury.

Patient Education: Ankle Sprains

Patients and families should be taught that for prevention of ankle reinjury, supports such as semirigid orthoses, lace-ups, and high-top shoes, and/or taping may be effective during high risk activities. Stretching, strengthening, and proprioceptive ankle training using a wobble board under the guidance of a physical therapist are often effective in preventing reinjury.

REFERENCES

General

McNab JW. *A practical guide to joint and soft tissue injections.* 3rd ed. Philadelphia, PA: Wolters Kluwer; 2015.

Wilder RP, Sethi S. Overuse injuries: tendinopathies, stress fractures, compartment syndrome, and shin splints. *Clin Sports Med.* 2004;23:55.

Ankle

Cooper M, Mait A, Nie JP, et al. Deltoid ligament injury patterns in external rotation ankle injuries: A cadaveric study. *Foot Ankle Surg.* 2017:23(Suppl. 1):26.

Dizon JM, Reyes JJ. A systematic review on the effectiveness of external ankle supports in the prevention of inversion ankle sprains among elite and recreational players. *J Sci Med Sport.* 2010;13:309.

Doherty C, Delahunt E, Caulfield B, et al. The incidence and prevalence of ankle sprain injury: A systematic review and meta-analysis of prospective epidemiological studies. *Sports Med.* 2014;44:123.

Fulton J, Wright K, Kelly M, et al. Injury risk is altered by previous injury: A systematic review of the literature and presentation of causative neuromuscular factors. *Int J Sports Phys Ther.* 2014;9:583.

Gribble PA, Bleakley CM, Caulfield BM, et al. 2016 consensus statement of the International Ankle Consortium: Prevalence, impact and long-term consequences of lateral ankle sprains. *Br J Sports Med.* 2016;50:1493.

Gribble PA, Bleakley CM, Caulfield BM, et al. Evidence review for the 2016 International Ankle Consortium consensus statement on the prevalence, impact and long-term consequences of lateral ankle sprains. *Br J Sports Med.* 2016;50:1496.

Hansrani V, Khanbhai M, Bhandari S, Pillai A, McCollum C. The role of compression in the management of soft tissue ankle injuries: A systematic review. *Eur J Orthopaed Surg Traumatol.* 2015;25(6):987–995.

Kuwada GT. Surgical correlation of preoperative MRI findings of trauma to tendons and ligaments of the foot and ankle. *J Am Podiatr Med Assoc.* 2008;98:370.

Park HJ, Cha SD, Kim HS, et al. Reliability of MRI findings of peroneal tendinopathy in patients with lateral chronic ankle instability. *Clin Orthop Surg.* 2010;2:237.

Sman AD, Hiller CE, Refshauge KM. Diagnostic accuracy of clinical tests for diagnosis of ankle syndesmosis injury: A systematic review. *Br J Sports Med.* 2013;47:620.

Tendford AS, Yin A, Hunt KJ. Foot and ankle injuries in runners. *Phys Med Rehabil Clin N Am.* 2016;27(1):127–137.

van Dijk CN, Lim LS, Bossuyt PM, Marti RK. Physical examination is sufficient for the diagnosis of sprained ankles. *J Bone Joint Surg Br.* 1996;78:958.

Bursitis

Khodaee M. Common superficial bursitis. *Am Fam Physician.* 2017;95(4):224–231.

Hand and Wrist

Adams JE, Hubbard MC. Hand and wrist. In: Armstrong AD, Hubbard MC, eds. *Essentials of musculoskeletal care.* 5th ed., 422–548.

Alba-Martin P, Gallego-Izquierdo T, Plaza-Mazano G, et al. Effectiveness of therapeutic physical exercise in the treatment of patellofemoral pain syndrome: a systematic review. *J Phys Ther Sci.* 2015;27:2387–2390.

American Academy of Orthopaedic Surgeons. Management of carpal tunnel syndrome evidenced based clinical practice guideline. **http://www.aaos.org/ctsguideline.** Published February 29, 2016.

Fowler JR, Baratz ME. Percutaneous trigger finger release. *J Hand Surg Am.* 2013;38:2005.

Griffin LY, et al. Overuse syndromes. In: Armstrong AD, Hubbard MC eds. *Essentials of musculoskeletal care.* 5th ed. 166–172.

Guigale JM, Fowler JR. Trigger finger: Adult and pediatric treatment strategies. *Orthop Clin North Am.* 2015;46:561–569.

Huang HK, Wang JP, Wang ST, et al. Outcomes and complications after percutaneous release for trigger digits in diabetic and non-diabetic patients. *J Hand Surg Eur Vol.* 2015;40:735.

Kise NJ, Risberg MA, Stensrud S, et al. Exercise therapy versus arthroscopic partial meniscectomy for degenerative meniscal tear in middle aged patients: randomized controlled trial with two-year follow-up. *Br J Sports Med.* 50(23):1473–1480.

Melton JK, Memarzadeh A, Dunbar WH, Cross MJ. Semimembraneous tenosynovitis: Diagnosis and management of a commonly missed cause of posteromedial knee pain. *Knee.* 2017; 24:305–309.

McMurty JT, Isaacs J. Extensor tendons injuries. *Clin Sports Med.* 2015;34:167–180.

Rizzo M, Stern PJ, Benhaim P, Hurst LC. Contemporary management of Dupuytren contracture. *Instr Course Lect.* 2014;63:131–142.

Wang J, Zhao JG, Liang CC. Percutaneous release, open surgery, or corticosteroid injection, which is the best treatment method for trigger digits? *Clin Orthop Relat Res.* 2013;471:1879.

Werner BC, Boatright JD, Chhabra AB, Dacus AR. Trigger digit release: Rates of surgery and complications as indicated by a United States Medicare database. *J Hand Surg Eur Vol.* 2016;41:970.

Hip

Anderson BC. *Office orthopedics for primary care: Diagnosis and treatment.* 2nd ed. Philadelphia, PA: WB Saunders; 1999.

Fearon AM, Scarvell JM, Neeman T, et al. Greater trochanteric pain syndrome: Defining the clinical syndrome. *Br J Sports Med.* 2013;47:649.

Fearon AM, Cook JL, Scarvell JM, et al. Greater trochanteric pain syndrome negatively affects work, physical activity and quality of life: A case control study. *J Arthroplasty.* 2014;29:383.

Ho GW, Howard TM. Greater trochanteric pain syndrome: More than bursitis and iliotibial tract friction. *Curr Sports Med Rep.* 2012;11:232.

Reich MS, Shannon C, Tsai E, Salata MJ. Hip arthroscopy for extra-articular hip disease. *Curr Rev Musculoskelet Med.* 2013;6:250.

Rivière C, Hardijzer A, Lazennec J.-Y, et al. Spine-hip add understandings to the pathophysiology of femoro-acetabular impingement: A systematic review. *Orthop Traumatol Surg Res.* 2017;103:549–557.

Woodley SJ, Mercer SR, Nicholson HD. Morphology of the bursae associated with the greater trochanter of the femur. *J Bone Joint Surg Am.* 2008;90:284.

Shoulder

de Castro Veado MA, Prata EF, Gomes GC. Rotator cuff injury in patients over the age of 65 years: Evaluation of function, integrity, and strength. *Revista Bras Ortoped.* 2015;50(3):318–323.

Page MJ, Green S, McBain B, et al. Manual therapy and exercise for rotator cuff disease. *Cochrane Database Syst Rev.* 2016;(6):CD012224.

RESOURCES

American Academy of Orthopaedic Surgeons
  www.aaos.org
American Academy of Physical Medicine and Rehabilitation
  www.aapmr.org
American Academy of Physical Therapy
  www.aaptnet.org
American Association of Clinical Endocrinologists (AACE)
  www.aace.com
American Orthopedic Foot and Ankle Society
  www.aofas.org
Association of Hip and Knee Surgeons
  www.aahks.org
American Physical Therapy Association
  www.apta.org
National Institute of Arthritis and Musculoskeletal and Skin Diseases
  www. niams.nih.gov/

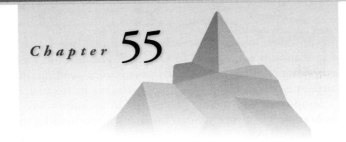

Chapter 55

Osteoarthritis and Osteoporosis

Patricia Vanhook, PhD, MSN, APRN, FNP-BC, FAAN, FAANP

Lynne M. Dunphy, PhD, APRN, FNP-BC, FAAN, FAANP

Lori Martin-Plank, PhD, APRN, FNP-BC, GNP-BC, FAANP

Conor Luskin, PA-C

OSTEOARTHRITIS

Osteoarthritis (OA), also known as *degenerative joint disease* (DJD) or "wear and tear" arthritis, is the most common articular disease in adults older than age 45. It is the most widespread form of arthritis and is a significant cause of functional impairment, chronic pain, and disability in the older population.

OA is a gradual and progressive joint disease typically found in middle-aged to elderly patients. OA is a joint condition in which loss of articular cartilage and degeneration occur, which leads to pain and often deformity. Although symptoms of OA occur earlier in women, the prevalence among men and women is equal. In addition to age, risk factors include genetics, female sex, joint injury, past trauma, advancing age, obesity, and mechanical stress (Glyn-Jones et al., 2015).

Often, OA is classified as "primary" or idiopathic, resulting from one or more of the following:

- Advancing age
- Obesity
- Occupational overloading of joints
- Familial type II collagen gene polymorphisms

In contrast, secondary OA develops at varying intervals after trauma, infection, osteonecrosis, congenital malalignment, or in the setting of inflammatory arthritis or metabolic disease. In reality, primary and secondary OA may coexist.

OA encompasses a group of subtypes with different etiological factors but a common response pattern in joint tissues, which is primarily noninflammatory and involves a combination of biomechanical stresses and biochemical changes in articular cartilage and synovial membrane. There is erosion and fibrillation of cartilage, with joint space narrowing and osteophyte formation. Principal sites for OA are the distal interphalangeal (DIP) joints, the proximal interphalangeal (PIP) joints, and the carpometacarpal (CMC) joint of the thumb in the hand; the first metatarsophalangeal or great toe joint; and the hips, knees, and cervical and lumbar spine. Although hand joints associated with the pincer grasp and lower-extremity weight-bearing joints are affected, the ankle, wrist, shoulder, and elbow are usually not, unless the cause of the arthritis is traumatic or occupational.

Although both osteoarthritis and rheumatoid arthritis (RA) affect the phalanges, they occur in different locations. RA usually presents as bilateral pain, swelling, and stiffness of the metacarpophalangeal and PIP joints with characteristic deformities and spares the DIP joints. Generally, other systemic complaints will occur, and joints other than just those in the hand will be affected as well. (See Chapter 62 for a full discussion of RA.) Osteoarthritis affects the distal interphalangeal joints (Heberden's nodes) and PIP joints (Bouchard's nodes) and presents with swelling, stiffness, pain, and deformity.

EPIDEMIOLOGY AND CAUSES

OA affects approximately 60 million Americans. Radiographic evidence of OA is present in about 33% to almost 90% of people older than age 65. Gender differences are not apparent before age 45. After age 50, however, women are more likely to have OA, with women representing 74% of cases, according to the Arthritis Foundation. The actual numbers are probably grossly underreported because many older adults are asymptomatic or do not report symptoms, which they mistakenly believe to be an inevitable consequence of aging, or for which they believe there is no treatment.

Age is a risk factor, with a sharp increase in the middle to late years of life. The Framingham Osteoarthritis Study and the English twin study have identified a genetic component in hand arthritis in women.

Genetic research on families with a preponderance of arthritis has demonstrated mutations of the *col2A1* gene, the precursor to type II collagen. Other genetic influences also have been identified, but the current approach to the study of genetics and OA is fraught with inconsistencies in defining the disease. Patients who have parents who developed OA at middle age or earlier or parents with polyarticular disease are considered at high risk for developing the disease themselves.

Obesity is a risk factor for arthritis in weight-bearing joints such as the knee. Exercise, including recreational jogging, has not been shown to increase the risk of OA. Muscle weakness around the joints, abnormal gait pattern or weight-bearing, local joint injury, and repetitive occupational joint use are contributing factors. Cruciate ligament damage or meniscal tears, particularly when accompanied by partial or total meniscectomy, increase the risk of knee OA. Low levels of vitamin C and/or vitamin D have also been implicated as a risk factor for OA. Estrogen replacement therapy is associated with a reduced risk of knee and hip OA; it was also shown to have a moderately protective but not statistically significant effect against worsening of radiographic knee OA in a group of white American women enrolled in the Framingham study. Although all of these factors have been cited as having a role in OA, the definitive cause of the disease is not known. In general, biomechanical, biochemical, inflammatory, and immunological factors are all implicated in the pathogenesis of OA.

PATHOPHYSIOLOGY

The exact pathophysiology of OA is still under study, with many promising developments on the horizon. Normal cartilage derives its viscoelastic and compressive characteristics from cellular and matrix components. Chondrocytes synthesize type II collagen and glycosaminoglycans to maintain the integrity of the extracellular matrix. These chondrocytes are also responsible for balancing cartilage degradation and repair. In contrast to the autoreactive inflammatory pathology associated with rheumatoid arthritis, systemic lupus erythematosus, and other inflammatory arthritides, in OA articular cartilage is thought to be initially damaged due to repetitive microtrauma or a single inciting macro-traumatic event. Bone and joint malalignment, ligamentous laxity, weakness in muscle groups that provide counterforce against the involved joint (e.g., quadriceps for the knee joint), and any type of underlying structural defect may magnify the damage imparted by this repetitive physical trauma. Proprioception is also impaired in affected knee joints. This diminishes muscular reflexes that normally provide compensatory mechanical mechanisms to counter destructive load-bearing forces on arthritic joints. In addition, underlying genetic defects in cartilage formation (e.g., type II collagen defects, ochronotic cartilage with abnormal pigment deposition) may lead to tissue damage from normal wear and tear in the absence of inciting physical trauma.

Mechanical loading of the joint has been shown to increase macromolecule formation by the chondrocyte within the extracellular matrix as a function of both load intensity and frequency of load-bearing, affecting not only the concentration of matrix proteoglycans but also the integrity of the collagen meshwork. The act of mechanical forces triggering biochemical reactions has been termed *mechanotransduction* and is only now beginning to be characterized within the chondrocyte. Although much of this pathogenesis is poorly understood and stems from preclinical animal studies, we know that cartilage matrix degradation predominates in OA, with greater fluid loss from joint cartilage in response to mechanical loading. In turn, attempts at repair by chondrocytes are ineffectual.

In addition, the disease process of OA includes sclerosis of underlying subchondral bone and abnormalities in the juxta-articular bone marrow. Abnormal bone deposition within the degenerating joint, which impinges on the joint space, is known as osteophyte formation. These osteophytes may give the impression of external bulging within the joint space, which may sometimes be mistaken for the inflammatory joint pathology of rheumatoid arthritis. However, if spinal osteophytes impinge on nerve roots, they may produce radicular symptoms, similar to those seen in intervertebral disc herniation.

Crystal deposition into the synovial fluid of osteoarthritic joints, particularly calcium pyrophosphate dihydrate and basic calcium phosphate crystals, also correlates with worsening degrees of radiographic joint pathology and cartilaginous fissuring. Although evidence for the pathophysiological nature of these crystals is primarily circumstantial, these crystals appear to initiate an inflammatory synovitis, MMP secretion, and synovial proliferation with subsequent cartilaginous destruction. Moreover, patients with an inherited predisposition to calcium pyrophosphate dihydrate deposition also develop severely degenerative OA.

CLINICAL PRESENTATION

Subjective

Patients typically present with slowly developing, localized pain in the affected joint or joints that interferes with their usual activities. The onset is subtle, and the pain may be ignored initially. Patients with OA in the weight-bearing joints may have early morning stiffness or stiffness after inactivity, which subsides after 30 minutes, also referred to as the "gel phenomenon." Pain and stiffness are also present in hand OA, often accompanied by bony deformities such as Heberden's nodes, which affect the DIP joints, and Bouchard's nodes, which affect the PIP joints. Internal derangement in weight-bearing joints may cause them to "lock" or "buckle," increasing the risk for falls; patients often report that their knee "gave way" or "wouldn't bend." In the later stages of OA, pain may be also present at rest. OA may present as monoarticular or polyarticular.

The history should include information on the onset, location, and duration of pain; any self-care measures the patient has taken to alleviate pain and the effectiveness of these measures; and associated symptoms such as joint stiffness, swelling, or deformity. Does the pain interfere with sleep or awaken the patient at night? Inquire if there is a family history of OA. An occupational history should be explored for evidence of overuse; any trauma or surgery to the joint should be noted. A history of activity/

exercise patterns, any changes in activities of daily living (ADLs) or instrumental ADLs, and weight changes, especially a gain in weight should be noted. Socioeconomic factors and vocational issues should be explored. It is also important to obtain a past or present history of any systemic illness or chronic disease state, along with a list of current medications, including over-the-counter (OTC) preparations, herbal remedies, and nutraceuticals. OA of the wrists, ankles, and shoulder is usually related to trauma or other secondary causes.

Objective

Typical clinical findings of OA include minimal or no swelling of affected joints, tenderness on direct palpation, crepitus, and reduced passive and active ROM. Crepitus is a common, although late, finding and a sensitive criterion for OA. There may be effusions in the large joints.

Physical exam findings include the following:

- Hands: enlargement of the DIP and/or PIP joints. The CMC joint of the thumb may also be enlarged and in general there may be pain on motion.
- Feet: swelling (bunion) of the big toe and DIP joints.
- Knees and hips: possible pain and crepitus on passive range of motion (ROM). There may be tenderness to palpation along the joint line, and some muscle atrophy may be present. Hard swelling, if present, is usually a result of bone spurs, whereas soft swelling is related to effusion. There may be significantly decreased ROM, both active and passive. The hip of any patient who complains of knee pain should be examined as well; pain referred to the knee may be the only symptom of hip OA. Hip OA usually causes pain in the inguinal fold and patient has pain with internal/external rotation of the hip.
- Spine: degenerative changes are common. There may be limited motion and stiffness of the neck and/or lower back. Bony spurs at the facet joints may produce pain and compression of spinal root nerves.
- Shoulder: atrophy of the shoulder muscles may be noted during physical exam. Palpation may elicit tenderness over the front and back of the shoulder. Crepitus is commonly present with rotation or flexion; ROM is usually decreased.

The physical exam should include a functional status evaluation in the older adult. Gait abnormalities such as a limp are significant. Evaluation for spinal and hip alignment and leg-length discrepancy is helpful initially to detect contributing factors. Affected joints should be examined for tenderness, bony deformities, swelling, redness, warmth, and ROM. Tenderness along the joint line, crepitus, and limited ROM are typical but nonspecific findings. Knee joint effusion may also be seen, as well as Baker's cysts in the posterior popliteal area. Muscle strength, especially that of the quadriceps muscles, and joint stability should be assessed. The presence of fever or

weight loss, especially when accompanied by fatigue and poor appetite, is suggestive of a systemic problem rather than OA; these symptoms need further investigation.

The most common symptom of OA is joint pain. OA pain tends to worsen with activity, more often following a period of rest. OA can also cause morning stiffness and generally lasts less than 30 minutes, unlike rheumatoid arthritis, which can cause stiffness for 45 minutes or longer (Glyn-Jones et al., 2015). Frequently, the patient may report joint locking or joint instability. These symptoms result in loss of function, with patients limiting their ADLs due to the pain and stiffness. Early in the disease process, the joints may appear normal. However, the patient's gait may be antalgic if weight-bearing joints are involved.

The joints most commonly affected are the hands, knees, hips, and spine, but any joint can be involved. OA is often asymmetrical, whereas RA is normally symmetrical and bilateral, especially in the hands. Pain on ROM and limitation of ROM are common to all forms of OA. Box 55.1 explains the unique physical exam findings for common joints.

DIAGNOSTIC REASONING

Diagnostic Tests

Clinicians can make the diagnosis of OA based on the history and physical exam because OA is primarily a clinical diagnosis. Plain radiographs can be helpful in confirming the diagnosis and in ruling out other conditions (Griffin et al., 2016). No laboratory tests are required to make the diagnosis.

Radiographic testing may be useful in the following situations:

- To establish diagnosis at the hip
- To assess disease severity at other joints
- To screen for other types of bone and joint pathology if pain is severe enough and disrupts sleep
- To determine baseline status to assess change over time

Early changes often do not appear, but as the disease progresses, x-ray findings include:

- Asymmetrical joint space narrowing
- Bony cysts and osteophytes
- Subchondral sclerosis

Radiographic findings are poorly correlated to symptomatology. Further x-ray studies may be ordered to document progression of the disease if symptoms increase markedly, ability to perform ADLs changes dramatically, or the patient is being evaluated for surgical intervention. Magnetic resonance imaging (MRI) and computed tomography (CT) scans may be ordered for patients with suspected spinal stenosis.

Laboratory testing is helpful in ruling out other conditions such as RA, gout, lupus, sepsis, or polymyalgia

Box 55.1   Physical Findings of Common Joints for Osteoarthritis

Hand

Pain on range of motion
Hypertrophic changes at distal interphalangeal and proximal interphalangeal joints
(Heberden nodes and Bouchard nodes)
Tenderness over carpometacarpal joint of thumb

Shoulder

Pain on range of motion
Limitation of range of motion, especially external rotation
Crepitus on range of motion

Knee

Pain on range of motion
Joint effusion
Crepitus on range of motion
Presence of popliteal cyst (Baker cyst)
Lateral instability
Valgus or varus deformity

Spine

Pain on range of motion
Limitation of range of motion
Lower extremity sensory loss, reflex loss, motor weakness caused by nerve root impingement
Pseudoclaudication caused by spinal stenosis

Hip

Pain on range of motion
Pain in buttock
Limitation of range of motion, especially internal rotation

Foot

Pain on ambulation, especially at first metatarsophalangeal joint
Limited range of motion of first metatarsophalangeal joint, hallux rigidus
Hallux valgus deformity (bunion)

---

rheumatica but has little place in establishing a diagnosis of OA. Complete blood count (CBC), C-reactive protein, and erythrocyte sedimentation rate (ESR) are usually normal; the ESR in older patients is more likely to be elevated. Rheumatoid factor, antinuclear antibody (ANA), serum uric acid, or 24-hour urinary uric acid levels may be ordered to rule out RA, lupus, or gout, depending on the clinical presentation, but again may yield significant false-positive results. Synovial fluid analyses may be useful in ruling out inflammatory and/or infectious arthritis (see Differential Diagnosis 55.1).

The American College of Rheumatology (ACR; Zandany et al., 2013) published *Five Things Physicians and Patients Should Question* as a part of the American Board of Internal Medicine (ABIM) Choosing Wisely program to inform clinicians and the public about evidence-based practice. The five recommendations include:

1. Don't test ANA sub-serologies without a positive ANA and clinical suspicion of immune-mediated disease.
2. Don't test for Lyme disease as a cause of musculoskeletal symptoms without an exposure history and appropriate exam findings.
3. Don't perform MRI of the peripheral joints to routinely monitor inflammatory arthritis.
4. Don't prescribe biologics for rheumatoid arthritis before a trial of methotrexate (or other conventional nonbiologic disease-modifying antirheumatic drug).
5. Don't routinely repeat dual-energy X-ray absorptiometry (DXA) scans more often than once every 2 years.

Differential Diagnosis 55.1: Osteoarthritis

- Rheumatoid arthritis
- Crystalline arthropathies (i.e., gout and pseudogout)
- Inflammatory arthritis
- Seronegative spondyloarthropathies (e.g., psoriatic arthritis and reactive arthritis)
- Septic arthritis or postinfectious arthropathy
- Fibromyalgia
- Tendinitis
- Ankylosing spondylitis
- Avascular necrosis
- Patellofemoral arthritis
- Bursitis
- Lupus erythematosus
- Lyme disease
- Neuropathy
- Neuromuscular disease
- Parkinson's disease
- Osteopenia or osteoporosis
- Paget's disease
- Bone malignancy

The ACR has identified classification criteria for the diagnosis of OA of the hand, knee, and hip that uses a stepwise progression for diagnosis based on patient history, physical exam, laboratory studies if available, and radiology studies if indicated and/or completed (see Table 55.1).

TABLE 55.1	American College of Rheumatology Osteoarthritis Diagnosis Criteria for Hand, Knee, and Hip		
	Hand	*Knee*	*Hip*
History	Pain, aching, stiffness in the hand and three of the following	Pain in the knee and three of the following	Pain in the hip and the following
Physical Exam	1. Hard tissue enlargement of two or more of the following joints: • Second and third interphalangeal • The second and third proximal interphalangeal joints • The first carpometacarpal joint of both hands 2. Hard tissue enlargement of distal interphalangeal joints 3. Less than three swollen metacarpophalangeal joints 4. Deformity in at least one of the joints above	1. Age over 50 years 2. <30 minutes morning stiffness 3. Crepitus on active motion 4. Bony tenderness 5. Bony enlargement 6. No palpable warmth or synovium 7. Joint effusion may be present (balloon sign) picture*	1. Internal rotation <15° AND/OR 2. Hip flexion ≤115° if ESR not available OR 3. Internal hip rotation ≥15° AND pain associated with internal rotation AND morning stiffness of the hip ≤60 minutes 4. AND age ≥50 years
Laboratory Findings	NA	If using laboratory findings: pain in the knee and five of the following: 1. Age over 50 years 2. <30 minutes morning stiffness 3. Crepitus on active motion 4. Bony tenderness 5. Bony enlargement 6. No palpable warmth or synovium 7. Erythrocyte sedimentation rate <40 mm/hr 8. Rheumatoid factor: <1:40 9. Synovial fluid signs of osteoarthritis	ESR ≤45 mm/hr
Radiology Findings	NA	If using radiology findings: 1. Pain in knee and one of the following: • Age over 50 • <30 minutes of morning stiffness • Crepitus on active motion • Osteophytes	If using radiology findings: 1. Pain in the hip and two of the following: • ESR <20 mm/hr • Radiographic femoral and/or acetabular osteophytes • Radiographic joint space narrowing (superior, axial, and/or medial)

Sources: Altman R, Alarcón G, Appelrouth D, et al. The American College of Rheumatology criteria for the classification and reporting of osteoarthritis of the hand. *Arthritis Rheum.* 1990;33(11):1601–1610; Altman R, Alarcón G, Appelrouth D, et al. The American College of Rheumatology criteria for the classification and reporting of osteoarthritis of the hip. *Arthritis Rheum.* 1991;34:505; Altman R, Asch E, Bloch D, et al. Development of criteria for the classification and reporting of osteoarthritis. Classification of osteoarthritis of the knee. Diagnostic and Therapeutic Criteria Committee of the American Rheumatism Association. *Arthritis Rheum.* 1986;29(8): 1039–1049.

MANAGEMENT

The principles of management of OA are to control pain and other symptoms, to maximize functional independence and mobility, to minimize disability, and to preserve quality of life. The Osteoarthritis Research Society International's guidelines for conservative management of osteoarthritis with and without comorbidities are presented in Table 55.2.

Management choices can be categorized as nonpharmacological, pharmacological, complementary and alternative, and surgical. In general, treatment should begin with the safest and least invasive therapies before proceeding to more invasive therapies. All patients with OA should receive treatment from the first two categories. Surgical management for end-stage/severe OA of hip and knee has been shown to be cost effective and improve quality of life (Kamaruzaman, Kinghorn, & Oppong, 2017).

TABLE 55.2 Osteoarthritis Research Society International Conservative Management of Osteoarthritis

Core Treatments for All OA Patients*			
Land-based exercise Strength training Weight management		Water-based exercise Self-management Education	
KNEE ONLY OA WITHOUT COMORBIDITIES	**KNEE ONLY OA WITH COMORBIDITIES**	**MULTIPLE JOINT OA WITHOUT COMORBIDITIES**	**MULTIPLE JOINT OA WITH COMORBIDITIES**
Biomechanical interventions	Biomechanical interventions	Oral COX-2 inhibitors (selective NSAIDs)	Balneotherapy
Intra-articular corticosteroids	Walking cane	Intra-articular corticosteroids	Biomechanical interventions
Topical NSAIDs	Intra-articular corticosteroids	Oral nonselective NSAIDs	Intra-articular corticosteroids
Capsaicin	Topical NSAIDs	Duloxetine	Oral COX-2 inhibitors (selective NSAIDs)
Duloxetine		Biomechanical interventions	Duloxetine
Acetaminophen			Acetaminophen

Abbreviations: COX-2, cyclooxygenase-2; OA, osteoarthritis.
*Refer to orthopedic for consideration of surgery if conservative management is ineffective.
Source: Osteoarthritis Research Society International (OARSI). OARSI guidelines. https://www.oarsi.org/education/oarsi-guidelines.

Nonpharmacological Management

Self-Care Strategies

Initial management of OA includes educating the patient about the nature of the disease, delineating the role of the patient in self-management, and providing sources of information and support for the patient. The Arthritis Foundation is an excellent resource and offers information sheets, local support groups, and an arthritis self-help course that includes exercise, joint protection, and relaxation techniques, along with information on medications that are typically used to manage symptoms. Weight loss is often an important component of the plan of care (see Table 55.2).

Involvement of the patient's spouse or significant other in the education and support of the individual with arthritis, specifically in helping him or her to develop coping skills, has proven superior to working with the patient alone. In a recent study of patients with OA, an informal network of social support appeared to be effective in mitigating the depression and functional limitations imposed by the disease and significantly enhancing quality of life. Trials of regular monthly phone calls by trained lay personnel to patients, discussing issues such as pain, medication, and treatment adherence, access to medical services, and functional concerns, were also effective. Patients experienced improvement in pain status and function with specific counseling; medical costs were negligible (see Evidence-Based Nursing Practice 55.1).

Physical Therapy

Nonpharmacological management strategies include physical therapy for muscle strengthening, particularly quadriceps strengthening for patients with knee OA.

The physical therapist also evaluates mobility and the need for assistive devices such as canes or walkers to reduce load-bearing on the arthritic joint. The physical therapist may recommend environmental modifications to maximize functional independence and safety. Other orthotic devices, such as shoe lifts, splints, or bracing, may be prescribed to improve biomechanics. Heat, ice, or ultrasound may be applied locally to decrease pain. Whenever feasible, a supervised exercise program incorporating aerobic and resistive components should be instituted. Several significant studies of arthritis patients utilizing comparison groups attest to the safety and efficacy of fitness training programs versus ROM and health education alone. Participants in the fitness program experienced better task performance and reported less physical disability, less pain, and improved psychological functioning. Aquatic exercise programs are also excellent, particularly those that are tailored to the needs of arthritic patients.

Transcutaneous electrical nerve stimulation is sometimes used for arthritic pain, but studies to date have not established its effectiveness. Use of pulsed electric and electromagnetic fields (PEMF), more commonly used for the treatment of nonunion fractures, has shown some promise in preliminary studies of patients with knee OA, but further studies are needed before PEMF can be recommended as adjunctive treatment for OA.

Occupational Therapy

Short-term occupational therapy to maximize ADL abilities and evaluate the need for adaptive devices is often overlooked, but it can be invaluable to the patient with arthritis. Devices such as a raised toilet seat, toilet side

Evidence-Based Nursing Practice 55.1

Davis GC, White TL. A goal attainment pain management program for older adults with arthritis. *Pain Manag Nurs.* 2008;9(4):171–179.

The purpose of this study was to test the effectiveness of the Goal Attainment Pain Management Program (GAPMAP) for promoting the self-efficacy of older adults in managing chronic musculoskeletal pain associated with rheumatic disease. Seventeen older adults living in independent-living residential settings were included in the study, with an average age of 79.29 years. The GAPMAP intervention took place over a 3-month period and initially involved small group meetings to discuss pain management strategies and potential barriers to pain management. Participants then met with the nurse researchers individually to set personalized pain management goals. Attainment of these goals was assessed at the end of the 3 months. Participants received follow-up phone calls at weeks 1, 4, and 8 to assess progress and allow for discussion.

A significant finding of this study was that 13 of the 17 participants either met or exceeded their expected goals, examples of which include "pain reduction, pacing activities, walking, weight loss, performing selected exercises, and community participation" (p. 176). Additionally, participants were more likely to use "exercise" and "a heated pool, tub, or shower" as pain management strategies after the intervention. "Exercise and distraction" were found to be more helpful for participants after intervention, and there was a significant improvement in both the "experience of living with persistent pain" and "expected outcomes of pain management" (p. 177). The results of this study, although preliminary, highlight goal setting as a tool that nurses can use to help older adults take greater control over their own pain management. Supporting older adults to maintain their autonomy and participate in their own care through programs such as GAPMAP is an important part of nursing practice. More research with a larger sample size would be important for assessing the generalizability of these findings when applied to other aspects of the care of older adults.

---

rails, elastic shoelaces, reachers, and various kitchen accessories can enhance functional capacity and independence.

Complementary Therapy

Acupuncture and nutritional therapy (including vitamin supplementation) are alternative therapies used for the management of OA and other musculoskeletal problems (see Complementary Therapies 55.1). Although some studies suggest that acupuncture may be beneficial as an adjunctive treatment for OA, results are inconclusive. The American Academy of Orthopedic Surgeons (AAOS) does not recommend for or against acupuncture in OA of the knee due to conflicting evidence. Methylsulfonylmethane and *S*-adenosyl methionine are other dietary supplements some patients find beneficial, although at present no evidence exists to support this. Therapeutic magnets also appear helpful to some patients anecdotally.

Pharmacological Management

The ACR has issued guidelines for pharmacological treatment of OA of the hand, hip, and knee. For *hand* osteoarthritis, the ACR conditionally recommends using one or more of the following:

- Topical capsaicin
- Topical NSAIDs
- Oral NSAIDs
- Tramadol

The ACR conditionally recommends against using intra-articular therapies or opioid analgesics for hand OA. For patients 75 years and older, the ACR conditionally recommends the use of topical, rather than oral, NSAIDs.

 Complementary Therapies 55.1: Osteoarthritis and Musculoskeletal Problems

Acupuncture

Acupuncture has been used for treatment of chronic low back pain and osteoarthritis (OA) in Asia for hundreds of years. It is now being used more frequently in other regions as a complementary modality for OA and chronic low back pain. Numerous studies have shown acupuncture to be an effective treatment in many pain syndromes; however, the quality of some of the research is questionable. Studies in which patients were treated with standard medical therapy and acupuncture have demonstrated significant improvement in functional status and pain relief. There studies using acupuncture as an adjuvant to standard therapy have shown positive results as have studies using acupuncture compared to no treatment. Although additional controlled studies on efficacy are needed, acupuncture can be used and is safe and well tolerated.

Massage may be especially helpful. Acupressure may also be considered as adjunctive therapy for patients with chronic cervical spine pain.

Source: Liu L, Skinner M, McDonough S, Mabire L, Baxter GD. Acupuncture for low back pain: An overview of systematic reviews. *Evid Based Complement Alternat Med.* 2015;2015:328196.

For *knee* osteoarthritis, the ACR conditionally recommends using one of the following:

- Acetaminophen
- Oral NSAIDs
- Topical NSAIDs
- Tramadol
- Intra-articular corticosteroid injections

For *hip* osteoarthritis conservative therapy, the AAOS conditionally recommends using one or more of the following for initial management:

- Obesity management (moderate evidence)
- Nonnarcotic management (strong evidence): oral NSAIDs improve short-term pain function
- Physical therapy (strong evidence)
- Intra-articular corticosteroid injections (strong evidence)
- Mental health disorder (moderate evidence): management of depression, anxiety, and psychosis impact pain relief, function, and ADL

Acetaminophen

The goal of pharmacological management is pain control, with acetaminophen (Tylenol) as the first-line agent. Two tablets of Tylenol—regular strength (325 mg) or extra strength (500 mg)—may be taken every 4 to 6 hours as needed, or two tablets of Tylenol Arthritis Extended Relief Caplets (650 mg) may be taken every 8 hours as needed, not to exceed 3,000 mg in 24 hours. The maximum daily dose of acetaminophen in patients receiving warfarin therapy should not exceed 2,500 mg by mouth. Patients should be cautioned about using alcohol with acetaminophen. Hepatotoxicity is a serious potential adverse effect.

Nonsteroidal Anti-Inflammatory Drugs

NSAIDs actually comprise several categories of pharmacological agents, all sharing comparable anti-inflammatory properties. Although each class acts in an individual manner, all inhibit the production of prostaglandins, which are inflammatory mediators. Cyclooxygenase (COX), or prostaglandin endoperoxide synthase, is the first enzyme in the prostaglandin synthesis pathway. This enzyme transforms arachidonic acid into other prostaglandin breakdown products. Two forms of COX are present: COX-1 is normally present in blood vessels, stomach, and kidney and promotes the normal functioning of those systems; COX-2 is generated in inflammatory settings by cytokines and inflammatory mediators. NSAIDs can be selective and nonselective COX inhibitors. All possess antipyretic, analgesic, and anti-inflammatory properties. Inhibition of COX-1 is largely responsible for the adverse effects associated with NSAID therapy, including gastrointestinal (GI) bleeding, ulcerogenic activity, fluid retention, and blockade of platelet aggregation. Patients on NSAIDs are four to five times more likely to have GI bleeding than individuals who are not taking the drugs. The risk of bleeding is increased during the first month of treatment and with increased dosages of the NSAID; older age and polypharmacy are also risk factors. It was hoped that the use of the COX-2 inhibitors would be equally effective for pain while curbing GI side effects or platelets; however, subsequent data regarding the increased risk of vascular events such as myocardial infarction (MI) or transient ischemic attack (TIA)/stroke

have resulted in withdrawal of several of these agents from the market. NSAIDs also interact with several other classes of medication. In addition, NSAIDs are known to cause fluid retention, as well as having the potential to cause nephrotoxicity.

When initiating NSAID therapy, it is best to begin with the lowest dose possible and increase as needed. It is important to question the patient about use of OTC medications because many patients with OA take ibuprofen (e.g., Advil, Nuprin, Motrin IB) in a nonprescription strength for headache, fever, or other minor discomforts and do not associate the OTC form with prescribed medication. If the patient is intolerant of one medication in a specific class, another one in the same class may prove to be satisfactory. Individualization of therapy is the key to successful management.

Because of emerging data indicating that the COX-2 inhibitor celecoxib may be associated with increased risk of serious cardiovascular events (MI, TIA), especially when used for long periods of time or in high-risk settings (such as after surgery), the U.S. Food and Drug Administration (FDA) has issued a recommendation that prescribers consider this emerging information when weighing risks versus benefits for individual patients. According to the FDA, patients who are at high risk of GI bleed have a history of intolerance to nonselective NSAIDs, or are not doing well on nonselective NSAIDs may be appropriate candidates for COX-2 inhibitor therapy; also, individual patient risk for cardiovascular events and other risks commonly associated with NSAIDs should be considered. There is considerable variability among patients in both effectiveness and tolerance of NSAIDs. If one particular drug proves ineffective or unacceptable, benefit may be obtained by changing to a drug of a different class. The doses of these drugs should be individualized. The addition of a proton pump inhibitor, histamine-2 blocker (H_2 blocker), or the prostaglandin analog misoprostol to NSAID therapy helps protect against gastroduodenal ulceration. In addition, meloxicam (Mobic) is a preferential inhibitor of COX-2, but it is not a true COX-2 inhibitor according to FDA criteria. It appears to be well tolerated with few drug–drug interactions. The American Academy of Family Practice Physicians has issued the following recommendations regarding NSAID use:

- Initiate therapy with acetaminophen, and if NSAIDs are needed, use the lowest dose for the shortest duration possible.
- Avoid NSAIDs in patients with preexisting renal disease, congestive heart failure, or cirrhosis.
- Avoid NSAIDs and aspirin in patients taking anticoagulants.
- Creatinine should be monitored for patients on angiotensin-converting enzyme inhibitors or angiotensin receptor blockers who are prescribed NSAIDs on a regular basis.

Recommendations from other medical experts emphasize that conservative treatments such as physical therapy and exercise should be first-line management. If NSAIDs must be used, those with the highest COX-1 selectivity should be tried initially (ibuprofen, aspirin, naproxen).

Additional Pain Relievers

Tramadol hydrochloride (Ultram) is an opioid pain reliever that is indicated for moderate to moderately severe pain. It is available as a combination drug with acetaminophen that works synergistically; it can also be taken with NSAIDs. It is contraindicated in patients who use alcohol and who are taking hypnotics and other narcotic medications and should be used with caution in patients with the potential to abuse it. Caution also should be used in patients who also are taking selective serotonin reuptake inhibitors due to the risk of serotonin syndrome. There is no evidence that this medication is more effective than NSAIDs. Any prescription for opioids should be considered only if expected pain and function are anticipated to outweigh the risks to the patient, and should be combined with non-pharmacologic therapy (CDC Guidelines for Prescribing Opioids for Chronic Pain, 2018).

There is no clear evidence that muscle relaxants or benzodiazepines are helpful adjuncts, although some clinicians continue to prescribe them because actual spasms of the paraspinous muscles are elicited on physical exam in the case of vertebral OA.

Other medications such as gabapentin (Neurontin), selective serotonin reuptake inhibitors, and tricyclic antidepressants have also proven effective in the management of patients with OA who have chronic pain.

Glucosamine with or without chondroitin, a dietary supplement not regulated by the FDA, has been found in systematic review to have medium-term effects for pain and function but no long-term effect (Newberry et al., 2017).

Topical agents such as capsaicin (Zostrix) cream, applied three to four times daily to painful areas, either alone or in concert with oral pharmacotherapy, may be helpful. The patient should be cautioned to avoid rubbing the cream in the eyes and to wash hands carefully after using capsaicin to avoid irritation. Some redness and burning at the site of application is normal initially, but it should disappear after 3 to 5 days. If irritation persists, the medication should be discontinued. Other topical agents, such as BENGAY, Icy Hot, and similar preparations, are menthol based and have a temporary, local effect. Topical preparations also give the patient a sense of control over his or her own treatment (see Drugs Commonly Prescribed 55.1).

Drugs Commonly Prescribed 55.1: Pharmacological Treatment of Osteoarthritis

DRUG/USAGE	INDICATION	ADVERSE REACTIONS AND PRESCRIBING CONSIDERATIONS
Acetaminophen (Tylenol)	Treatment of mild to moderate pain; fever; does not have anti-inflammatory properties	Monitor alcohol intake and limit to <3 drinks/day; hepatotoxicity may occur with chronic use or in doses >3 g/day. Low cost, easy availability, overall safety profile.
Capsaicin cream	Topical for pain	Naturally occurring substance that seems to interfere with transmission of painful stimuli.
NSAIDs	Acute and chronic pain	Renal and/or platelet dysfunction; GI bleeding. Risk factors for GI bleed: older age, comorbidity, history of peptic ulcer, history of GI bleed, glucocorticoids, anticoagulation, combination NSAID therapy, and increased dose.
Tramadol HCl (Ultram; available in immediate and extended release); also available with acetaminophen (Ultracet)	Relief of moderate to moderately severe pain Opioid analgesic	Low abuse potential; nonscheduled; do not use with SSRIs, TCAs, MAO inhibitors to avoid serotonin syndrome. Do not use extended-release form with hepatic or renal disease. CNS depression, caution in elderly, use lowest dose initially.
Codeine (Tylenol with codeine)	Analgesic, opioid. Treatment of mild to moderate pain is last choice.	Weak opioid; side-effect profile not good for older adults; also increased risk of hip fracture. Use with caution in head injury; constipation.
Hyaluronic acid (viscosupplement injection)—used as joint injection for pain relief for OA of knee only	Either three injections over 15 days or weekly injections for 5 weeks	Expensive; mild adverse effects include injection site inflammatory/allergic reaction, transient worsening of symptoms; systemic include occasional muscle cramps (not common); always risk of infection with intra-articular injection.

Continued

Drugs Commonly Prescribed 55.1: Pharmacological Treatment of Osteoarthritis—cont'd

DRUG/USAGE	INDICATION	ADVERSE REACTIONS AND PRESCRIBING CONSIDERATIONS
Corticosteroids—hydrocortisone (Cortisol)	Symptom relief for weeks to months; intra-articular injection—dose depends on anatomical site and medication	Duration of relief may be short (1–2 weeks) in lower extremities, shoulder, or elbow; may be effective in hand for several months; always risk of infection with intra-articular injection; local reaction at injection site. Can increase blood glucose in diabetics.
Prednisolone tebutate (Hydeltra)		
Methylprednisolone acetate (Depo-medrol)	No more than two injections should be given in any weight-bearing joint.	
Triamcinolone acetonide (Kenalog)		
Triamcinolone hexacetonide (Aristospan)		
Betamethasone (Celestone)		

Abbreviations: CNS, central nervous system; GI, gastrointestinal; MAO, monoamine oxidase; OA, osteoarthritis; SSRI, selective serotonin reuptake inhibitor; TCA, tricyclic antidepressant.

Corticosteroid Intra-articular Injections

Intra-articular steroids have been used for some time in the treatment of OA of the knee. Several controlled studies document their efficacy for up to 4 weeks, although some patients report a response for up to 6 months after injection. Agents include triamcinolone hexacetonide, triamcinolone acetonide, and methylprednisolone (Solu-Medrol). A 1% lidocaine solution is usually mixed with the steroid before injection. Patients are instructed to rest the joint for a day and to limit physical activity for 48 to 72 hours after the injection. The hip may also be injected, but this procedure should be done under ultrasound or fluoroscopic guidance. Joint injection is also used in these and other joints for bursitis or tendinitis.

The use of intra-articular injections of corticosteroids should be judicious: No more than three to four injections should be done per year, and they should be used only in episodes of acute flare-up. If steroid injections are administered excessively, they can accelerate joint deterioration and increase the risk of avascular necrosis. Research about the effectiveness of corticosteroid injections is inconclusive. For this reason, the AAOS is unable to recommend for or against the use of intra-articular corticosteroids for patients with symptomatic osteoarthritis of the knee; providers must use their best judgment and the patient's preferences when making the decision for joint injections.

Viscosupplementation

Viscosupplementation with intra-articular hyaluronic acid is also used for treatment of knee OA. Hyaluronic acid is a naturally occurring component of synovial fluid; its purpose is to lubricate the joint for low-impact activities and potentially prevent mechanical joint damage during high-impact activities. In patients with OA, the viscosity and elasticity of synovial fluid are decreased; there may be a lower concentration and limited distribution of hyaluronic acid. Consequently, all of the rheological features of synovial fluid, such as shock absorption, lubrication, and protection, may be decreased, further increasing the risk of damage to synovial tissue and the articular cartilage surface. Hyaluronan (Hyalgan), hylan G-F 20 (Synvisc), and hyaluronic acid (Orthovisc, a highly purified, high molecular weight form of hyaluronic acid) are intended to restore all of the protective functions found in normal synovial fluid. They are indicated for pain relief of knee OA that has failed to respond to conservative measures. Intra-articular injections of hyaluronic acid are marketed as medical devices, not medications, and may be used in conjunction with NSAIDs. Hyaluronic acid is injected once a week for 3 to 5 weeks depending on the preparation, and it may provide benefit for 6 months or longer. Adverse effects of hyaluronic acid injections include transient, localized pain, burning, and swelling at the injection site. Several studies have demonstrated the efficacy of viscosupplementation as equal to or better than continuous NSAID therapy, with significant improvement in pain at night or at rest as well as improvement of pain on motion, including walking pain. Duration of benefit was 8 to 12 months. Intra-articular injection has not been shown to be 100% effective; some studies suggested that the benefit was confined to patients with mild degenerative arthritis. Other conflicting information about viscosupplementation indicates the need for more studies and more rigorous methodology. The AAOS does not recommend for or against viscosupplementation due to inconclusive results. Viscosupplementation is costly and is often not used unless the patient has insurance that will cover this cost.

Surgical Intervention

If nonsurgical strategies fail to provide sufficient pain relief and maintenance of function, referral to an orthopedic surgeon for surgical evaluation is indicated. Arthroscopic procedures can include joint lavage, partial medial or lateral meniscectomy or chondroplasty as indicated, lateral patellar retinacular release, fracture drilling of full-thickness defects, or chondral grafts. The AAOS does not currently recommend joint lavage or debridement; partial meniscectomy is advised only when there is strong evidence of a torn meniscus in addition to the OA. Large or open surgical procedures could include osteotomy and partial or total joint arthroplasty. For maximum success, ongoing communication among patients, medical and surgical providers, and physical therapists is essential in identifying appropriate candidates for surgery, treating comorbidities, and establishing rehabilitation goals. Outcomes following total hip and knee replacement demonstrated a higher level of postoperative function and better quality of life in candidates who had surgery earlier rather than waiting until the pain was intolerable and functional abilities had declined. It is also known that psychosocial factors such as motivation and emotional and social functioning (measured at baseline) are strong predictors of postoperative recovery. Annual radiographs to evaluate the position and fixation of the prosthetic components may also be recommended.

Surgery should be reserved for patients whose symptoms have not responded to other treatments. Indication for surgery is continued pain and disability despite conservative treatment. Arthroplasty consists of the surgical removal of joint surface and the insertion of a metal and plastic prosthesis. The prosthesis is held in place by cement or by bone ingrowth into a porous coating on the prosthesis. The most effective surgical intervention is total joint replacement, with excellent patient outcomes following total joint replacement of the hip, knee, and shoulder. Most current joint prostheses function well for 15 to 20 years. After joint replacement, patients require partial weight-bearing, which progresses to full weight-bearing in 1 to 3 months; ROM and strengthening exercises are started within a few days after joint-replacement surgery and continued until the patient has good ROM and strength.

Long-Term Pain Management

For patients who are not candidates for surgery and who have intractable pain, long-term pain management is necessary. Goals of long-term pain management are to maximize quality of life and minimize pain and functional loss. Consultation with a pain management specialist for collaborative management may be beneficial; the use of alternative treatments, including massage therapy, acupuncture, or acupressure, can further enhance pain management and promote a feeling of relaxation and well-being. Pharmacological management should be individualized; it should take into consideration comorbidities, other medications, age, and functional abilities.

New technologies continue to be developed for this disabling disorder. Newer medications, complementary therapies, different prosthetic joint components, osteochondral replacement procedures, and gene therapy for rare hereditary forms of OA are some promising new directions.

FOLLOW-UP AND REFERRAL

Patients with OA may be referred to a rheumatologist or orthopedic surgeon for collaborative management. If conservative measures fail, the patient's quality of life can be markedly diminished. Frequent or constant disabling pain, especially pain at rest, and functionally limiting symptoms are the most important criteria for orthopedic referral. Patients may also be referred to physical therapy or occupational therapy for functional evaluation, education in joint preservation, and recommendations for environmental modifications to maximize function. Other options include referral to a pain management specialist, a professional massage therapist, or a licensed acupuncturist. Referral to the Arthritis Foundation for patient education and support is also valuable. The patient should be seen for follow-up at 3- to 6-month intervals and should be instructed to contact his or her primary health-care provider if pain increases or functional status declines. ROM and functional status should be assessed at each visit. There are a number of scales, such as the Arthritis Impact Measurement Scale 2, that allow the clinician to monitor the patient's perception of his or her progress with greater accuracy. A shorter version of this scale is also available. A variety of other scales measure function and disability, such as the Pain Disability Index and the Stanford Health Assessment Questionnaire. It is important to monitor all patients on aspirin or NSAID therapy for GI blood loss and cardiac, renal, and mental status. Practitioners should order periodic CBC, renal function tests, and tests for occult blood in stool.

Patient Education: Osteoarthritis

Education of the patient and support persons is essential to successful management of OA. The Arthritis Foundation is an excellent resource for patient education, as well as a variety of services that are provided at the local and national level. In addition, courses such as the Arthritis Self-Help Course (ASHC) and People with Arthritis Can Exercise are available. Research has shown that patients who complete the ASHC show a decrease in pain and physician visits, even with increased physical disability. The improvements, sustained over a 4-year period, are attributed to these patients' feelings of enhanced self-efficacy.

Exercise programs should be individualized, with protection of the weight-bearing joints. Swimming or water exercise (which minimizes impact on joints) is especially recommended. Rest after exercise is also important.

The patient with OA needs to be aware of potential adverse effects of medications and drug interactions. Key areas for education include acceptance of the chronic nature of OA and lifestyle management to maximize function and minimize pain and the preservation of joint function. Vocational rehabilitation may also be necessary.

OSTEOPOROSIS

Osteoporosis is a generalized skeletal disorder characterized by normal bone mineralization but low bone mass (bone mineral density [BMD]) and disruption of the bony architecture, both of which result in an increased risk of fractures. Its chief clinical manifestations are vertebral and hip fractures, although fractures can occur at any skeletal site. This is contrasted with *osteopenia,* which is a less severe form of decreased bone mineral density, and *osteomalacia,* which denotes a decrease in actual bone mineralization. Fractures associated with osteoporosis may place significant physical and psychosocial stress on individual patients and caregivers. Osteoporosis is now recognized as a significant public health concern with potentially devastating consequences in both human and economic terms. Increasing attention to women's health issues, the application of epidemiological research in prioritizing public health problems, and the need to minimize health-care expenditures have all contributed to recent efforts aimed at the prevention, identification, and effective treatment of this condition to avoid fractures.

EPIDEMIOLOGY AND CAUSES

Osteoporosis is characterized by microarchitectural deterioration of bone tissue, which leads to low BMD and fragility and a consequent susceptibility to fractures. Epidemiological studies in Europe, Japan, and the United States reveal that an estimated 75 million people are affected by osteoporosis. Roughly 4 out of 10 white women older than age 50 in the United States will experience a hip, spine, or wrist fracture during the remainder of their lives. Looking ahead, the lifetime risk of fractures will increase for all ethnic groups as people live longer. Approximately 10 million individuals older than age 50

in the United States have osteoporosis of the hip. An additional 33.6 million individuals older than age 50 have low bone mass, or osteopenia, of the hip and thus are at risk of developing osteoporosis and its potential complications later in life. Common consequences of osteoporosis are vertebral fractures and fracture of the hip and distal radius. In addition, a diagnosis of osteoporosis can lead to depression, loss of independence, body deformities, and a fear of initial or subsequent osteoporotic fractures.

As a result of both the aging of the population and the rise in the age-specific incidence of osteoporosis, the number of osteoporotic fractures has been increasing annually. Approximately 1.5 million osteoporotic fractures of the vertebral body, proximal femur, or distal radius occur each year in the United States. In 2005, osteoporotic fractures accounted for an estimated annual cost in excess of $19 billion per year. Proximal femur fractures, associated with the greatest health-care costs, are accompanied by a 50% risk of dying within 1 year of the fracture and impair the ability to perform ADLs in up to 75% of patients who survive.

Women are more likely to have osteoporosis, but men also may be affected. Women have a two to four times greater lifetime risk of sustaining an osteoporotic fracture than men do because of the loss of BMD following the cessation of ovarian estrogen production at menopause. Bone loss after menopause is caused predominantly by estrogen deficiency and is most rapid (up to 7% per year) in the first decade after menopause. Postmenopausal osteoporosis is more prevalent in white and Asian women than in women of other races, with the majority of white women developing osteoporosis by the end of the first postmenopausal decade. By age 65, one-third of women will have had a vertebral fracture, and by the ninth decade of life, one in three will have had a hip fracture. The incidence, prevalence, and pathogenesis of bone loss in men are incompletely understood, and more research is called for in this area. Fractures of any type from osteoporosis are associated with a significantly higher likelihood of both physical and functional limitations. Patients who have already sustained a fracture from osteoporosis have a more than a fivefold increase in the risk of sustaining another osteoporotic fracture.

The cause of osteoporosis is multifactorial. Although genetic factors are important determinants of bone density, other lifestyle, disease-related, and medication-related factors also contribute to an individual's risk for having osteoporosis.

Risk Factors: Osteoporosis

Lifestyle

- Low body weight
- Cigarette smoking
- Excessive alcohol intake

- Low dietary calcium intake
- Vitamin D deficiency

Disease-related risk factors

- Thyrotoxicosis
- Hyperparathyroidism
- Cushing's disease
- Hypogonadism
- Rheumatoid arthritis
- Inflammatory bowel disease
- Chronic renal insufficiency
- Malabsorptive diseases
- Secondary estrogen deficiency resulting from anorexia or overexercise

Medication-related risk factors

- Glucocorticoids
- Excessive thyroxine
- Long-term use of phenytoin

Other risk factors

- Advanced age
- Family history of osteoporosis
- Postmenopausal
- Genetic predisposition

Although genetic factors may account for up to 70% to 75% of the variance in peak bone mass, many lifestyle factors play a significant role, and most are amenable to interventions aimed at primary and secondary prevention and treatment of osteoporosis. Regular exercise has been shown to preserve BMD, whereas a sedentary lifestyle probably contributes to osteopenia. Weight-bearing exercise, such as walking, is considered one of the best forms of activity for prevention of osteoporosis and is associated with higher bone density. There is increasing evidence that muscle strength training may prevent further loss of BMD in postmenopausal women. Furthermore, the improved mobility, agility, and muscle strength that occur in people who engage in regular exercise may help to prevent falls and associated fractures.

The primary dietary risk factor for osteoporosis is lack of adequate calcium intake throughout the life cycle. The majority of cross-sectional studies support the supposition that long-term inadequate dietary calcium has a deleterious effect on skeletal mass. The importance of adequate calcium, phosphorus, and vitamin D intake for children, adolescents, and young adults should not be underestimated, because studies have indicated that women begin losing bone mass (albeit at a rate of less than 1% a year) in their early 30s. There is increasing evidence that vitamin D deficiency is more prevalent than previously thought, particularly among individuals at increased risk, such as the elderly; those living in northern latitudes; and in individuals with poor nutrition, malabsorption, or chronic liver or renal disease. Modest vitamin D deficiency can lead to a compensatory, secondary hyperparathyroidism and is an important risk factor for osteoporosis and fractures.

Cigarette smoking is an established risk factor for loss of bone density. The proposed mechanism of action is a reduction in circulating estrogen levels, as well as smoking's toxic effects on osteoblasts.

Among the medications associated with the development of osteoporosis, long-term use of glucocorticoids (steroids) has been shown to cause bone loss both rapidly and dramatically. Patients who take 7.5 mg or more of prednisone per day for more than 1 month have been identified as being at higher risk. Long-term excessive thyroid hormone may also potentiate bone loss, reinforcing the need to routinely monitor thyroid-stimulating hormone (TSH) levels in patients who require thyroid hormone replacement. Cyclosporine, cytotoxic drugs, anticonvulsants, excessive alcohol intake, heparin, and lithium are medications that have potentially detrimental effects on the skeleton. Long-term use of proton pump inhibitors for gastroesophageal reflux disease has been implicated in contributing to osteoporosis by inducing hypochlorhydria that interferes with calcium absorption.

In men, testosterone deficiency from primary or secondary hypogonadism is a common cause of osteoporosis, although few large-scale studies have been done in this area. One small cross-sectional study found that men who had undergone orchiectomy for prostate cancer had significantly higher rates of severe osteoporosis, some of which developed before castration. Research identifying the causes of and treatment for osteoporosis in men is both increasing and necessary, because preliminary data have shown a higher mortality rate in men with hip fractures compared with women. Measurement parameters for osteoporosis and osteopenia in men are different than women and controversy exists regarding the most accurate measurement factors. There is general agreement that osteoporosis in men occurs a decade or so after that in women.

PATHOPHYSIOLOGY

Normal bone contains an abundance of intracellular mineral salts (calcium phosphate and calcium carbonate) referred to as *hydroxyapatites*. As hydroxyapatites are deposited in collagenous fibers within immature bone cells (osteoblasts), the tissue becomes hardened, or ossified. Essentially, two types of bone are formed—cancellous or dense. Cancellous bone tissue is spongy, containing many open spaces filled with marrow. It consists of an irregular latticework of thin plates of bone called *trabeculae* and provides some skeletal support. Overlying spongy bone is dense bone that is much more compact, providing substantial skeletal support.

Bone tissue is continuously remodeled throughout life. In this process, osteoclasts release proteolytic enzymes that break down osseous tissue, and new bone tissue is formed in its place by osteoblasts. At menopause, the remodeling process becomes less homeostatic, and osteoclastic activity begins to predominate, while the rate of bone turnover increases. Bony spicules are reduced in number and size, and horizontal spicules acting as struts do not fully extend to contralateral supporting structures from their sites of origin, thus drastically reducing structural support. This leads to a decrease in cortical thickness and both the number and size of trabeculae in cancellous bone, leading to a decrease in bone density.

Osteoporosis is likely to be a multifactorial process related to increased bone resorption, decreased bone formation, and an overall decrease in peak bone mass at baseline (largely determined by genetic predisposition). Each of these physiological processes may predominate to a different extent in different osteoporotic individuals. New bone formation also appears to be impaired in estrogen-deficient states because estrogen has been shown to mediate transforming growth factor–β secretion by osteoblasts. Interestingly, androgen (e.g., testosterone) deficiency similarly results in increased bone turnover and can predispose an individual to osteoporosis as well.

Because serum hormone levels often do not differ between osteoporotic individuals and age-matched controls, changes in bone resorption and formation appear to be mediated largely by local factors, including mechanical loads on the bones themselves, as well as changes in the concentrations of local growth factors and their receptor proteins. Excesses in both exogenous (therapeutic) and endogenous (stress- or disease-related) glucocorticoids are well-known causes of osteoporosis, but unlike the role of sex hormones, glucocorticoids appear to be most involved in the regulation of new bone formation by osteoblasts. This growth effect is mediated largely by the inhibition of local growth factors including insulin-like growth factor and its cognate receptor binding proteins, as well as prostaglandins.

Research on the effects of prostaglandins and NSAIDs on osteoporosis is not definitive. It appears that excess prostaglandin (PG) production (especially that of PGE_2) may increase bone resorption, whereas significant inhibition of prostaglandins may lead to reduced bone formation in response to mechanical weight-bearing. Interleukin (IL)-6 produced by osteoblasts and other marrow-derived cells has been shown to increase osteoclastogenesis via a PG-dependent mechanism, leading to increased bone resorption in osteoporotic individuals. In contrast, IL-4 and IL-13 appear to inhibit bone resorption by decreasing PG synthesis, whereas IL-7 may contribute to bone loss. Finally, excess production of parathyroid hormone (PTH; as seen in primary hyperparathyroidism) and PTH-related protein (produced by bone and cartilage cells and the mammary gland in lactating women) both lead to increased bone resorption via their effects on downstream growth factors, possibly including fibroblast growth factor. Importantly, however, this complex set of interactions by secreted growth factors on bone resorption and formation has yet to be fully

characterized, and the importance of various cytokines and growth factors can only be suggested by the current literature.

CLINICAL PRESENTATION

Subjective

There are usually no clinical symptoms with the onset of osteoporosis until a fracture occurs. The only "early" symptom that may be noticed is the gradual development of upper or midthoracic back pain associated with activity or long periods of sitting or standing, which is relieved with rest in the recumbent position. To emphasize the importance of taking a comprehensive history, a strong predictor for future osteoporosis-related fractures is a history of previous fractures, notably those occurring from minimal trauma.

Objective

Acute vertebral compression fractures generally occur in the thoracic or high lumbar region, with the patient experiencing a more sudden, severe onset of pain (see Chapter 53). With acute compression fractures, point tenderness in the specific area of the fracture can be elicited during the physical exam. As bone density decreases, microfractures of the anterior vertebral bodies in the thoracic spine are likely to accumulate over time, leading to the characteristic dorsal kyphosis (or "dowager's hump"). The resultant exaggerated kyphosis produces a loss of height, which is generally not a "complaint," per se, but may be only casually mentioned by a patient during the course of a health-care visit. This may be the only verbal cue the practitioner receives to help identify that patient as being at risk for having osteoporosis. As kyphosis worsens over time, impairment of rib mobility, a decrease in lung volumes, and an increase in respiratory complaints may occur.

DIAGNOSTIC REASONING

Diagnostic Tests

For the practitioner, assessing a patient's risk for osteoporosis and signs of the disease based on the physical exam and history can provide support for the decision to proceed with further diagnostic testing. Risk assessment tools are currently available and may be used by clinicians as a quantitative means to support the need for additional diagnostic testing. The Simple Calculated Osteoporosis Risk Estimation (SCORE) instrument, for example, is estimated to have 90% sensitivity and approximately 40% specificity for identifying individuals with low BMD at the hip. The Fracture Risk Assessment tool (FRAX®) was developed to evaluate fracture risk of patients. It is based on individual patient models that integrate the risks associated with clinical risk factors as well as BMD at the femoral neck. It is a useful tool to aid clinical decision-making about the use of pharmacological therapies in patients with low bone mass.

The U.S. Prevention Task Force (USPTF) recommends osteoporosis screening in women 65 years and older and in younger women whose fracture risk is equal to or greater than that of a 65-year-old white woman who has no additional risk factors (Grade B).

The goal of screening for osteoporosis is to identify persons at increased risk of sustaining a low-trauma fracture and who would benefit from intervention to minimize that risk.

Standard radiographs are considered insensitive for detecting bone loss, with films typically indicating bone loss only when it exceeds 30% or more. No biochemical marker currently exists that is used to detect bone loss; however, preliminary evidence from clinical trials suggests that such markers may be used in the future to evaluate early response to therapy.

The physiological process of bone turnover may be assessed with a variety of serum or urinary markers, allowing the monitoring of bone loss and reformation, although these markers do not provide bone mass density, which is considered the definitive test for diagnosis. However, these markers are useful in monitoring treatment and can serve as useful adjuncts in the original diagnosis of osteoporosis. In general, serum markers provide information about bone formation, whereas urinary markers supply evidence of bone resorption.

Bone alkaline phosphatase (BAP) is the most commonly available serum indicator of osteoblastic activity. These levels should be obtained before the initiation of therapy and then at 3- to 6-month intervals to monitor response. BAP levels that drop significantly may indicate lack of compliance with treatment. Urinary N-telopeptide is the most specific and newest urinary bone resorption marker available. This assay, which measures the urinary excretion of cross-linked N-telopeptide of type I collagen, is useful in identifying individuals with osteoporosis who have high rates of bone resorption and who might be good candidates for antiresorption therapy.

BMD measurement by densitometry is currently considered the gold standard diagnostic test for definitively diagnosing either osteopenia or osteoporosis. *Osteopenia* is the diagnostic term used when BMD is found to be less than normal but not severe enough to be considered osteoporotic. BMD densitometry is non-invasive and can be completed in 5 to 15 minutes. A number of BMD measurement technologies are available, including dual-energy x-ray absorptiometry (DXA)—the "gold standard" for documenting osteoporosis of the proximal femur and lumbar spine; single-energy x-ray absorptiometry and peripheral DXA for the radius and calcaneus (heel); ultrasonography for the heel, fingers, and tibia; and quantitative CT (QCT), including peripheral QCT for the spine, hip, and radius.

These technologies use a variety of anatomical sites from which to measure BMD and emit very low radiation

doses (less than or equal to a standard chest x-ray study). Although all methods are considered accurate, the DXA method is most widely accepted because prospective epidemiological studies have found it to be most precise for reproducibility in both the short and long term, making it an excellent method for monitoring responses to interventions over time. DXA densitometry measures BMD at the central skeletal sites of the lumbar spine and hip (including both the femoral neck and greater trochanter).

BMD measurement reports are interpreted by using the calculated Z-scores and T-scores. Both use a normally distributed bell curve in determining how any one individual compares to a reference population, with Z-scores representing age- and sex-matched distributions and T-scores representing mean peak bone mass of a young adult distribution. The T-score is the most clinically relevant value on the BMD report and is used to confirm the presence of osteoporosis and to determine fracture risk. For every standard deviation below the young-adult matched mean, there is a significant increase in fracture risk. The World Health Organization's diagnostic criteria for osteoporosis are presented in Table 55.3.

Medicare-approved indications for BMD testing include (1) estrogen-deficient women at risk for osteoporosis, (2) patients with vertebral abnormalities, (3) patients receiving or needing to be on long-term glucocorticoids, (4) patients with primary parathyroidism, and (5) patients being monitored for response or efficacy of an approved osteoporosis drug therapy.

Secondary causes of osteoporosis should be considered in all patients with low BMD. The American Association of Clinical Endocrinologists recommends CBC, serum chemistry panel (calcium, phosphate, liver enzymes, total alkaline phosphatase, creatinine, electrolytes), and urinalysis, including pH to exclude secondary causes of osteoporosis. Additional laboratory analysis may be warranted if there are abnormalities in these test results or if there is additional evidence to suspect specific secondary causes for bone loss. These analyses include sensitive

TABLE 55.3 World Health Organization Diagnostic Criteria for Osteoporosis	
Diagnosis	*Diagnostic Findings*
Normal	BMD within 1 SD of young adult reference mean
Osteopenia	BMD >1 SD below young adult reference mean (21)
Osteoporosis	BMD >2.5 SD below young adult reference mean (22.5)
Osteoporosis (severe)	BMD >2.5 SD below young adult reference mean (22.5) AND presence of osteoporotic fractures

Abbreviation: BMD, bone mineral density.

TSH, 24-hour urinary calcium excretion, ESR, parathyroid hormone concentration, 25-hydroxyvitamin D concentration, dexamethasone suppression and other tests for hyperadrenocorticism, acid–base studies, serum or urine protein electrophoresis, and bone marrow examination or bone biopsy.

Differential Diagnosis

If a fracture has occurred, it is important to distinguish the underlying cause. Was it related to trauma, or was there an underlying pathological condition such as osteoporosis or neoplasm? Similarly, skeletal changes could result from a variety of underlying conditions, including a neoplasm, such as multiple myeloma or other neoplasias; osteomalacia; osteogenesis imperfecta tarda (type I); skeletal hyperparathyroidism (primary and secondary); and hyperthyroidism.

Screening for fracture risk involves appropriate history, physical examination, standard biochemical and hematologic studies, and measurement of BMD. The clinical history should include inquiring about possible secondary causes of bone loss, such as use of medications with potential adverse effects on bone health and family history of osteoporosis. Approaches to BMD screening vary from country to country, in part due to cost and questions regarding the efficacy of a broad population screening policy.

MANAGEMENT

The goals for prevention or treatment of osteoporosis are to prevent fractures, stabilize or improve bone mass, maximize physical functioning, relieve symptoms of fractures and resulting skeletal deformity, and maximize psychosocial functioning and coping.

The ability to meet these goals is dependent on both the patient and the practitioner's dedication to work as a team, first in determining what therapeutic regimen will be most beneficial and acceptable to the patient. Following this is the long-term commitment to continuing treatment, evaluating the therapeutic response, and assessing for the need to redirect the management plan based on the response. An algorithm outlining prevention, detection, and management strategies for osteoporosis is presented in Figure 55.1.

In addition to the physical and functional limitations that can be quantified, practitioners must also address the human and emotional aspects of being diagnosed with osteoporosis. Although not often the direct cause of death, and often identified as a "silent disease" until the patient sustains a fracture, for many individuals a fracture can lead to a downward spiral in physical and mental health and well-being. There may be an abrupt descent into disease and disability. From an individual's perspective, osteoporosis can have a devastating effect on patients and their families and can dramatically affect functional status, leaving the patient feeling vulnerable, isolated, and uncertain of the future.

Lifestyle Management

For both the prevention and treatment of osteoporosis, smoking cessation, moderation of alcohol use, weight-bearing exercise, and adequate calcium and vitamin D intake are advised. In addition, avoidance of falls by eliminating hazards in the home and gait training or other exercises that improve strength and agility through physical therapy are important considerations. Nursing research has found that women with osteoporosis seek interventions that promote the ability to better care for themselves, reduce stress and isolation, and prevent further disability (Oh et al., 2014). Weight training and walking are effective interventions for prevention and/or treatment. An active lifestyle, including safe and appropriate exercise, should be actively encouraged by the provider. Protective pads worn around the outer thigh, which cover the trochanteric region of the hip, can prevent hip fractures in elderly residents in nursing homes. Patients with pain from osteoporotic fractures may find therapies such as massage, music, or acupuncture helpful.

Pharmacological Management

Calcium and Vitamin D

Optimal calcium intake varies according to age, sex, and other conditions (see Table 55.4).

Adequate intake of calcium and vitamin D is necessary for both the prevention and treatment of osteoporosis when consumed during childhood, adolescence, and early adulthood. An optimal diet for treatment (or prevention) of osteoporosis includes an adequate intake of calories (to avoid malnutrition), calcium, and vitamin D. Postmenopausal women who are getting adequate calcium from dietary intake alone (approximately 1,200 mg daily) do not need to take calcium supplements. Women with inadequate dietary intake should take supplemental elemental calcium (generally 500–1,000 mg/day), in divided doses at mealtime, so that their total calcium intake (diet plus supplements) approximates 1,200 mg/day. There is considerable controversy about the calcium supplements and the risk of cardiovascular disease; additionally, the evidence that ingestion of calcium supplementation is truly preventative of fractures is weak. The trend is to lessen emphasis on ingestion of calcium supplementation. Women should also ingest a total of 800 international units of vitamin D daily. Higher doses are required if they have malabsorption or rapid metabolism of vitamin D due to concomitant anticonvulsant drug therapy. Most postmenopausal women with osteoporosis require vitamin D supplementation because it is difficult to achieve goals with diet alone.

Supplemental calcium and vitamin D has shown to decrease falls and fractures in institutionalized elder adults.

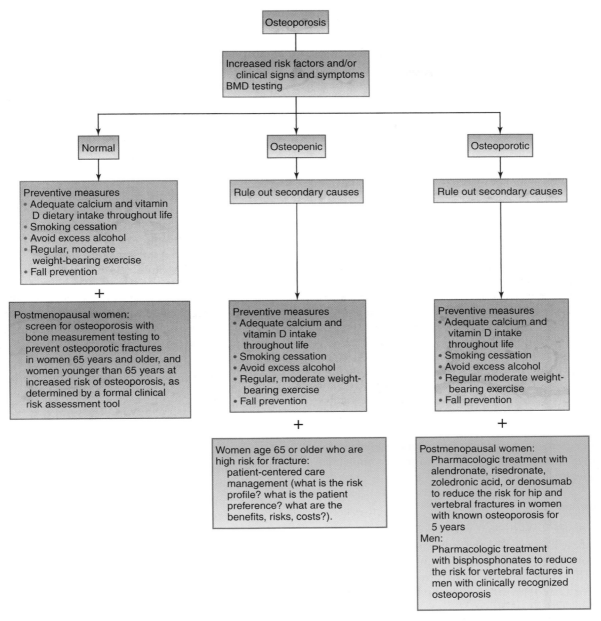

Figure 55.1 Prevention, detection, and management of osteoporosis.

TABLE 55.4	Recommended Daily Calcium Intake
Women	**Amount**
50 years and younger	1,000 mg daily
51 years and older	1,200 mg daily
Men	**Amount**
70 years and younger	1,000 mg daily
71 years and older	1,200 mg daily

Source: Committee to Review Dietary Reference Intakes for Vitamin D and Calcium, Food and Nutrition Board, Institute of Medicine. *Dietary reference intakes for calcium and vitamin D.* Washington, DC: National Academy Press; 2010.

Systematic review of 26 studies found that vertebral fractures were reduced by supplementation of calcium and vitamin D but not fractures at other sites. Yet four trials with minimal bias that included nearly 45,000 participants demonstrated no effect for supplementation at any site. The U.S. USPTF concluded evidence is insufficient to support the recommendation of calcium (at more than 1,000 mg/day) and vitamin D supplementation (at more than 400 IU/day).

In general, the best source of calcium is from dietary sources. The National Institutes of Health Office of Dietary Supplements provides a detailed list of food sources. If the need for OTC supplementation, calcium is available in many forms, and patients may be confused about which type or brand is best. The majority of commercially available supplements contain similar amounts of elemental calcium per calcium weight in milligrams, and patient choice should depend on affordability, number of tablets per day necessary, and whether it is convenient for the patient to take them with food. Calcium carbonate is less expensive and more easily absorbed with meals. Individuals with hypochlorhydria may absorb calcium citrate more efficiently, and it can be taken with or without food. Inadequate levels of vitamin D interfere with the body's absorption of calcium. The National Osteoporosis Foundation recommendations is as follows:

- Adults younger than age 50: 400 to 800 IU of vitamin D daily
- Adults older than age 50: 800 to 1,000 IU of vitamin D daily

Estrogen Therapy

Estrogen was the mainstay of treatment for osteoporosis for many years, until data from the Women's Health Initiative (WHI) suggested that estrogen-progestin therapy reduced fracture risk at a cost of increases in the incidence of breast cancer, coronary heart disease (CHD), stroke, and venous thromboembolism, or in the case of unopposed estrogen, an increase in stroke and thromboembolism risk (but not CHD or breast cancer). As a result, the 2017 American College of Physicians (ACP) treatment of low bone density or osteoporosis to prevent fractures in men and women recommends against using menopausal estrogen or estrogen plus progesterone and raloxifene for treatment of osteoporosis in women (strong recommendation; moderate quality of evidence).

Bisphosphonates

Pharmacologic treatment with bisphoshonates are now the first line treatment for women with osteoporosis according to the 2017 America College of Physicians (ACP) statement on the Treatment of Low Bone Density or Osteoporosis to Prevent Fractures in Men and Women. Specifically, this guideline recommends that clinicians use pharmacologic treatment with alendronate, risedronate, zoledronic acid, or denosumab to reduce the risk for hip and vertebral fractures in women who have known osteoporosis. Further, it recommends pharmacologic therapy for five years with no bone density monitoring during this period. Likewise, clinicians should offer pharmacologic treatment with biophosphates to reduce the risk for vertebral fracture in those who have clinically recognized osteoporosis (see Table 55.5).

Alendronate sodium (Fosamax), a third-generation bisphosphonate, has been approved by the FDA for the prevention and treatment of osteoporosis. It binds to bone hydroxyapatite and specifically inhibits the activity of osteoclasts, thus reducing bone turnover. Treatment with alendronate sodium has been shown to increase BMD of the vertebrae, femoral neck, and femoral trochanter by 5% to 10% and to reduce hip, vertebral, and wrist fractures by approximately 50% over a 3-year study period.

Like other bisphosphonates, alendronate sodium has the potential to irritate upper GI mucosa and is contraindicated in patients who have abnormalities of the esophagus that delay esophageal emptying or in patients who are unable to take the medication exactly as directed. Because of the specific manner in which alendronate sodium needs to be taken, some individuals initially perceive it as an inconvenience they would rather avoid; with careful patient teaching and the willingness to try this medication, however, many patients find no difficulty incorporating it into their daily routine. Risedronate (Actonel) is another drug in this category, also available in weekly dosing, as is ibandronate (Boniva), which is available in monthly dosing. Only bisphosphonates have been demonstrated in large clinical trials to reduce the risk of fractures in patients being treated with glucocorticoid therapy.

TABLE 55.5	ACP Recommendations for Treatment of Low Bone Density or Osteoporosis to Prevent Fractures in Men and Women
Recommendation 1	Pharmacological treatment with alendronate, risedronate, zoledronic acid, or denosumab to reduce the risk for hip and vertebral fractures in women with osteoporosis
Recommendation 2	Clinicians treat osteoporotic women with pharmacologic therapy for five years
Recommendation 3	Clinicians offer pharmacologic treatment with biophosphates to reduce the risk for vertebral fracture in men who have clinically recognized osteoporosis
Recommendation 4	Recommends against bone density monitoring during the five-year pharmacologic treatment period for osteoporosis in women
Recommendation 5	Recommends against using estrogen plus progesterone therapy or raloxifene for the treatment of osteoporosis in women
Recommendation 6	Clinicians should make the decision to treat osteopenic women 65 years of age or older who are at a high risk for fracture based on patient preferences, fracture risk profile, and benefits, harms, and costs of medications

Adapted from The American College of Physician treatment of low bone density or osteoporosis to prevent fractures in men and women: A clinical practice guideline update from the American College of Physicians. *Ann Intern Med.* 2017; 166:166:818-839; doi:10.73226/M15-1361

Risedronate (Actonel) prevents bone loss and reduces vertebral fracture risk by about 70%. Similar effects have been noted in alendronate (Fosamax) and etidronate disodium (Didronel). Zoledronic acid (Reclast, Zometa) is an IV third generation bisphosphonate. A once-yearly dosage of zoledronic acid (Reclast) 5 mg IV has been noted to reduce the incidence of bone fracture in the hip, spine, and other sites in postmenopausal women with osteoporosis. Adequate calcium and vitamin D must be maintained before, during, and after treatment. Zoledronic acid is approved for prevention and treatment of postmenopausal osteoporosis and glucocorticoid osteoporosis, as well as treatment of osteoporosis in men and treatment of Paget's disease.

American College of Physicians (ACP) treatment of low bone density or osteoporosis to prevent fractures in men and women advises providers to consider biophosphates for men with clinical osteoporosis. The discussion with the patient should include the risks and benefits of therapy. There is a moderate-quality of evidence that vertebral fractures in osteoprotic men were reduced by zoledronic acid (see Drugs Commonly Prescribed 55.2).

Androgen Supplementation

Few studies have examined pharmacological therapy effectiveness in osteoporotic men. Preliminary data from one study showed an increase in BMD in men with idiopathic primary osteoporosis when treated with

---

Drugs Commonly Prescribed 55.2: Osteoporosis

DRUG	INDICATION	ADVERSE REACTIONS AND PRESCRIBING CONSIDERATIONS
Bisphosphonates: therapy for five years		
Risedronate (Actonel) Available in daily, weekly, twice-monthly, and once-monthly dosage forms	Prevention and treatment of post-menopausal osteoporosis; increase bone mass in men with osteoporosis	• Swallow whole; take in the morning with a full glass of water before other food or drink; remain in upright position for at least 30 minutes. • Caution with other GI irritants such as aspirin. • May cause abdominal pain, atrial fibrillation, and esophageal ulceration. • Hypocalcemia is an absolute contraindication for all bisphosphonates.
Alendronate (Fosamax) Also available with vitamin D; daily or once-weekly dosage	Prevention and treatment of post-menopausal osteoporosis and osteoporosis in men	• Take on an empty stomach at least 30 minutes before a meal; drink full glass of water and remain upright for at least 30 minutes. • Can increase toxic effects of aspirin; can decrease absorption of calcium supplements and vitamin D. • See adverse effects above.
Ibandronate (Boniva) Available in oral daily or monthly preparations and IV preparation for every 3-month dosing	Prevention and treatment of post-menopausal osteoporosis, osteoporosis in women with breast cancer on specific therapy, and treatment of hypercalcemia in malignancy	• Swallow oral whole; take in the morning with full glass of water; remain upright and do not eat or drink for an additional 60 minutes; take on same day each month. • See adverse effects above. • The IV form may cause bone pain, arthralgia, and atrial fibrillation.
Zoledronic acid (Reclast)	Prevention and treatment of osteoporosis in post-menopausal women; increase bone mass in men with osteoporosis	• Yearly injection. • Obtain baseline renal function parameters within 10 days before initial dose. • Avoid in renal disease. • Adequate hydration is important • Concomitant administration of calcium and vitamin D before, during, and after drug administration. • Osteonecrosis of the jaw has been seen; also, arthralgia, atrial fibrillation, and bone pain can occur. • Consider an IV zoledronic acid holiday after 3 annual doses in moderate-risk patients or after 6 annual doses in higher-risk patients.

Continued

Drugs Commonly Prescribed 55.2: Osteoporosis—cont'd

DRUG	INDICATION	ADVERSE REACTIONS AND PRESCRIBING CONSIDERATIONS
Parathyroid Hormone		
Teriparatide (Forteo)	Treatment of osteoporosis in post-menopausal women at high risk for fracture (prior fracture and *T*-score less than −3)	• Daily subcutaneous injection for up to 24 months • Stimulates bone formation more than bone resorption • Contraindicated in hyperparathyroidism. Adverse reactions include dizziness, orthostatic hypotension, arthralgia, injection site reaction, secondary malignancy • Limit treatment to 2 years
Monoclonal Antibody		
Denosumab (Prolia)	Treatment of osteoporosis in post-menopausal women at high risk for fracture, prior fracture, or failure on other therapy	• Subcutaneous injection every 6 months • Contraindicated in hypocalcemia • Increases risk of serious infection • A drug holiday not recommended

intramuscular testosterone over 6 months. Although no adverse cardiovascular events were found in the treatment group, studies of longer duration are indicated in this area to better estimate the risks versus benefits of testosterone supplementation in men.

Fluoride

Oral sodium fluoride has been used extensively in Europe for the treatment of osteoporosis and has been found to significantly increase vertebral bone density by increasing the number of osteoblasts. Large, prospective studies have not shown a concurrent reduction in fractures, however; and until future research shows otherwise, it is believed the quality of bone produced by fluoride is more brittle than that formed by antiresorptive agents. Therefore, in the United States, sodium fluoride is currently not approved for the prevention or treatment of osteoporosis by the FDA.

FOLLOW-UP AND REFERRAL

Perhaps the most important part of managing the treatment of osteoporosis is improving adherence to treatment by individualizing the plan of care according to what is most effective in terms of increasing BMD and preventing fractures and what is most acceptable to the patient. There are currently no well-accepted guidelines for monitoring treatment of osteoporosis. Repeat BMD testing to monitor treatment response in osteoporotic patients should be limited to at least 2-year intervals. For patients with osteopenia or a normal

baseline BMD, repeat measurement every 2 to 3 years is indicated to monitor for either stabilization or progression of the disease. Referral to an endocrinologist is warranted any time secondary causes of osteoporosis cannot be excluded or if the response to treatment is less than expected for the type of therapy instituted.

Patient Education: Osteoporosis

A number of informative patient education materials are available from a variety of sources, including pharmaceutical companies. Extensive, individualized education should be given to individuals when BMD results are available. This is particularly true for patients who are found to be osteoporotic and who have an array of interventions available to them.

Reviewing potential hazards that may lead to falls and reinforcing the importance of maintaining agility are equally important in the ongoing care and management of patients who are at increased risk for fractures. Referral to a physical therapist and/or a home-care nursing evaluation is often of value in this area. Referral to local support groups, national osteoporosis education groups, and mental health counseling may also be of benefit for patients who seek further assistance in either learning about their condition or coping with their situation. Active exercise, such as weight training and/or walking, should be encouraged and supported.

For additional resources please visit
https://davisedge.fadavis.com/

REFERENCES

Osteoarthritis

Altman R, Alarcón G, Appelrouth D, et al. The American College of Rheumatology criteria for the classification and reporting of osteoarthritis of the hand. *Arthritis Rheum*. 1990;33(11):1601–1610.

Altman R, Alarcón G, Appelrouth D, et al. The American College of Rheumatology criteria for the classification and reporting of osteoarthritis of the hip. *Arthritis Rheum*. 1991;34:505.

Altman R, Asch E, Bloch D, et al. Development of criteria for the classification and reporting of osteoarthritis. Classification of osteoarthritis of the knee. Diagnostic and Therapeutic Criteria Committee of the American Rheumatism Association. *Arthritis Rheum*. 1986;29(8):1039–1049.

American Academy of Orthopaedic Surgeons. Management of osteoarthritis of the hip: Evidence-based clinical practice guidelines. **https://www.aaos.org/uploadedFiles/PreProduction/Quality/Guidelines_and_Reviews/OA%20Hip%20CPG_3.13.17.pdf**

Barbour KE, Lui LY, Nevitt MC, et al. Hip osteoarthritis and the risk of all-cause and disease-specific mortality in older women: A population-based cohort study. *Arthritis Rheumatol*. 2015;67:1798–1805.

Bruyère O, Cooper C, Arden N, et al. Can we identify patients with high risk of osteoarthritis progression who will respond to treatment? A focus on epidemiology and phenotype of osteoarthritis. *Drugs Aging*. 2015;32:179–187.

Centers for Disease Control and Prevention. Guidelines for prescribing opioids for chronic pain. Retrieved **https://www.cdc.gov/drugoverdose/pdf/Guidelines_Factsheet-a.pdf**.

Chapple CM, Nicholson H, Baxter GD, Abbott JH. Patient characteristics that predict progression of knee osteoarthritis: A systematic review of prognostic studies. *Arthritis Care Res (Hoboken)*. 2011;63:1115–125.

Chen L, Michalsen A. Management of chronic pain using complementary and integrative medicine. *BMJ*. 2017;357:j1284. doi:10.1136/bmj.j1284.

Collins JE, Katz JN, Dervan EE, Losina E. Trajectories and risk profiles of pain in persons with radiographic, symptomatic knee osteoarthritis: Data from the osteoarthritis initiative. *Osteoarthritis Cartilage*. 2014;22:622–630.

Davis GC, White TL. A goal attainment pain management program for older adults with arthritis. *Pain Manag Nurs*. 2008;9(4):171–179.

de Rooij M, van der Leeden M, Heymans MW, et al. Prognosis of pain and physical functioning in patients with knee osteoarthritis: A systematic review and meta-analysis. *Arthritis Care Res* (Hoboken). 2016;68:481–492.

Dowell D, Haegerich TM, Chou R. CDC Guideline for Prescribing Opioids for Chronic Pain — United States, 2016. MMWR Recomm Rep 2016;65(No. RR-1):1–49. DOI: **http://dx.doi.org/10.15585/mmwr.rr6501e1**.

French SD, Bennell KL, Nicolson PJ, et al. What do people with knee or hip osteoarthritis need to know? An international consensus list of essential statements for osteoarthritis. *Arthritis Care Res (Hoboken)*. 2015;67:809–816.

Gandek B. Measurement properties of the Western Ontario and McMaster Universities Osteoarthritis Index: A systematic review. *Arthritis Care Res (Hoboken)*. 2015;67:216.

Glyn-Jones S, Palmer R, Agricola R. Osteoarthritis. *Lancet*. 2015;386:376–387.

Haugen IK, Ramachandran VS, Misra D, et al. Hand osteoarthritis in relation to mortality and incidence of cardiovascular disease: Data from the Framingham heart study. *Ann Rheum Dis*. 2015;74:74–81.

Hawker GA, Croxford R, Bierman AS, et al. All-cause mortality and serious cardiovascular events in people with hip and knee osteoarthritis: A population based cohort study. *PLoS One*. 2014;9:e91286. **https://doi.org/10.1371/journal.pone.0091286**

Henrotin Y, Raman R, Richette P, et al. Consensus statement on viscosupplementation with hyaluronic acid for the management of osteoarthritis. *Semin Arthritis Rheum*. 2015;45(2):140–149.

Hochberg MC, Martel-Pelletier J, et al. Combined chondroitin sulfate and glucosamine for painful knee osteoarthritis: A multicenter randomized, double-blind, non-inferiority trial versus celecoxib. *Clin Epidemiol Ann Rheumatol Dis*. 2016;75:37–44. doi:10.1136/annrheumdis-2014-206792.

Holla JF, van der Leeden M, Heymans MW, et al. Three trajectories of activity limitations in early symptomatic knee osteoarthritis: A 5-year follow-up study. *Ann Rheum Dis*. 2014;73:1369–75. doi: 10.1136/annrheumdis-2012–202984.

Hunter DJ, Nevitt M, Losina E, Kraus V. Biomarkers for osteoarthritis: Current position and steps towards further validation. *Best Pract Res Clin Rheumatol*. 2014;28:61–71. doi: 10.1016/j.berh.2014.01.007.

Kamaruzaman J, Kinghorn P, Oppong R. Cost-effectiveness of surgical interventions for the management of osteoarthritis: A systematic review of the literature. *BMC Musculoskelet Disord*. 2017;18:183. doi: 10.1186/s12891-017-1540-2

Kluzek S, Sanchez-Santos MT, Leyland KM, et al. Painful knee but not hand osteoarthritis is an independent predictor of mortality over 23 years follow-up of a population-based cohort of middle-aged women. *Ann Rheum Dis*. 2016;75:1749–56. doi: 10.1136/annrheumdis-2015-208056.

Kroon FP, van der Burg LR, Buchbinder R, et al. Self-management education programmes for osteoarthritis. *Cochrane Database Syst Rev*. 2014;(1):CD008963.

Kwok WY, Plevier JW, Rosendaal FR, et al. Risk factors for progression in hand osteoarthritis: A systematic review. *Arthritis Care Res (Hoboken)*. 2013;65:552–62. doi: 10.1002/acr.21851

Leyland KM, Hart DJ, Javaid MK, et al. The natural history of radiographic knee osteoarthritis: A fourteen-year population-based cohort study. *Arthritis Rheum*. 2012;64:2243–51. doi: 10.1002/art.34415.

Messier SP, Mihalko SL, Legault C, et al. Effects of intensive diet and exercise on knee joint loads, inflammation, and clinical outcomes among overweight and obese adults with knee osteoarthritis: The IDEA randomized clinical trial. *JAMA*. 2013;310:1263–73. doi: 10.1001/jama.2013.277669.

McAlidon TE, Bannaru RR, Sullivan MC, et al. ORASI guidelines for non-surgical management of knee osteoarthritis. *Osteoarthritis Cartilage*. 2014;22:363–388.

McCaffrey R. The effect of music on acute confusion in older adults after hip or knee surgery. *Appl Nurs Res*. 2006;22:107–112.

Newberry SJ, FitzGerald J, SooHoo NF, et al. Treatment of osteoarthritis of the knee: An update review. Comparative effectiveness review no. 190. (Prepared by the RAND Southern California Evidence-based Practice Center under Contract No. 290-2015-00010-I.) AHRQ Publication No.17-EHC011-EF. Rockville, MD: Agency for Healthcare Research and Quality. **https://effectivehealthcare.ahrq.gov/sites/default/files/pdf/osteoarthritis-knee-update_research-2017.pdf**. Published May 2017.

Neogi T. The epidemiology and impact of pain in osteoarthritis. *Osteoarthritis Cartilage.* 2013;21:1145–1153 doi: 10.1016/j.joca.2013.03.018

Perry LA, Mosler C, Atkins A, Minehart M. Cardiovascular risks associated with NSAIDs and COX-2 inhibitors. *US Pharmacist.* 2014;39(3):35–38.

Scarpignato C, Lanas A, Blandiza C, et al. Safe prescribing of non-steroidal anti-inflammatory drugs in patients with osteoarthritis-an expert consensus addressing benefits as well as gastrointestinal and cardiovascular risks. *BMC Med.* 2015;13:55. doi: 10.1186/s12916015-0285-8.

Tanamas S, Hanna FS, Cicuttini FM, et al. Does knee malalignment increase the risk of development and progression of knee osteoarthritis? A systematic review. *Arthritis Rheum.* 2009;61:459–467.

Wesseling J, Bastick AN, ten Wolde S, et al. Identifying trajectories of pain severity in early symptomatic knee osteoarthritis: A 5-year followup of the Cohort Hip and Cohort Knee (CHECK) Study. *J Rheumatol.* 2015;42:1470–1477. doi: 10.3899/jrheum.141036

Zandany J, et al. Choosing wisely: The American College of Rheumatology's top 5 list of things physicians and patients should question. *Arthritis Care Res.* 2013;65(3):329–339. doi: 10.1002/acr.21930.

Osteoporosis

Adler RA, El-Hajj Fuleihan G, Bauer DC, et al. Managing osteoporosis in patients on long-term bisphosphonate treatment: Report of a Task Force of the American Society for Bone and Mineral Research. *J Bone Miner Res.* 2016;31(1):16–35.

The American College of Physician treatment of low bone density or osteoporosis to prevent fractures in men and women: A clinical practice guideline update from the American College of Physicians. *Ann Intern Med.* 2017;166:166:818–839; doi:10.73226/M15–1361

Barr RJ, Stewart A, Torgerson DJ, Reid DM. Population screening for osteoporosis risk: A randomised control trial of medication use and fracture risk. *Osteoporos Int.* 2010;21:561–568. doi: 10.1007/s00198-009-1007.

Basedow M, Esterman A. Assessing appropriateness of osteoarthritis care using quality indicators: A systematic review. *J Eval Clin Pract.* 2015;21:782. doi.org/10.1111/jep.12402

Berry SD, Samelson EJ, Pencina MJ, et al. Repeat bone mineral density screening and prediction of hip and major osteoporotic fracture. *JAMA.* 2013;310:1256–1262 doi:10.1001/jama.2013.277817

Bolland MJ, Leung W, Tai V, et al. Calcium intake and risk of fracture: systematic review. *BMJ.* 2015;351:h4580.

Buckley L, Guyatt G, Fink H, McAlindon T. 2017 American College of Rheumatology guideline for the prevention and treatment of glucocorticoid-induced osteoporosis. *Arthritis Care Res (Hoboken).* 2017;69(8):1095–1110.

Camacho PM, Petak SM, Binkley N, et al. American Association of Clinical Endocrinologists and American College of Endocrinology Clinical Practice Guidelines for the diagnosis and treatment of postmenopausal osteoporosis—2016. *Endocrinol Pract.* 2016;22(suppl 4):1–42.

Committee on Practice Bulletins-Gynecology, The American College of Obstetricians and Gynecologists. ACOG practice bulletin n. 129. Osteoporosis. *Obstet Gynecol.* 2012;120(3):718–734.

Cosman F, Crittenden DB, Adachi JD, et al. Romosozumab treatment in postmenopausal women with osteoporosis. *N Engl J Med.* 2016;375:1532–1543. DOI: 10.1056/NEJMoa1607948

Cosman F, de Beur SJ, LeBoff MS, et al. Clinician's guide to prevention and treatment of osteoporosis. *Osteoporosis Int.* 2014;25(10):2359–2381.

Eisman JA, Bogoch ER, Dell R, et al.; ASBMR Task Force on Secondary Fracture Prevention. Making the first fracture the last fracture: ASBMR Task Force report on secondary fracture prevention. *J Bone Miner Res.* 2012;27(10):2039–2046.

Fernandes L, Hagen KB, Bijlsma JW, et al. EULAR recommendations for the non-pharmacological core management of hip and knee osteoarthritis. *Ann Rheum Dis.* 2013;72:1125–35. doi: 10.1136/annrheumdis-2012-202745

Genant HK, Engelke K, Bolognese MA, et al. Effects of romosozumab compared with teriparatide on bone density and mass at the spine and hip in postmenopausal women with low bone mass. *J Bone Miner Res.* 2017;32:181–187. doi: 10.1002/jbmr.2932

Golden NH, Abrams SA; Committee on Nutrition. Optimizing bone health in children and adolescents. *Pediatrics.* 2014;134(4):e1229–1243.

Gourlay ML, Fine JP, Preisser JS, et al. Bone-density testing interval and transition to osteoporosis in older women. *N Engl J Med.* 2012;366:225–233. doi: 10.1056/NEJMoa1107142.

Hochberg MC, Altman RD, April KT, et al. American College of Rheumatology 2012 recommendations for the use of nonpharmacologic and pharmacologic therapies in osteoarthritis of the hand, hip, and knee. *Arthritis Care Res (Hoboken).* 2012; 64:465–474.

Ito K, Elkin EB, Girotra M, Morris MJ. Cost-effectiveness of fracture prevention in men who receive androgen deprivation therapy for localized prostate cancer. *Ann Intern Med.* 2010; 152:621–629. DOI: 10.7326/0003-4819-152-10-201005180-00002.

Langdahl BL, Libanati C, Crittenden DB, et al. Romosozumab (sclerostin monoclonal antibody) versus teriparatide in postmenopausal women with osteoporosis transitioning from oral bisphosphonate therapy: a randomised, open-label, phase 3 trial. *Lancet.* 2017;390:1585–1594. doi: 10.1016/S0140-6736(17)31613-6.

Leslie WD, Morin SN, Lix LM. Manitoba Bone Density Program. Rate of bone density change does not enhance fracture prediction in routine clinical practice. *J Clin Endocrinol Metab.* 2012;97:1211–1218.

Mirza F, Canalis E. Secondary osteoporosis: Pathophysiology and management. *Eur J Endocrinol.* 2015;173(3):R131–R151. doi:10.1530/EJE-15-0118.

Oh EG, Yoo JY, Lee JE, et al. Effects of a three-month therapeutic lifestyle modification program to improve bone health in postmenopausal Korean women in a rural community: A randomized controlled trial. *Res Nurs Health.* 2014;37(4):292–301.

Qaseem A, Forciea MA, McLean RM, Denberg TD; Clinical Guidelines Committee of the American College of Physicians. Treatment of low bone density or osteoporosis to prevent fractures in men and women: A clinical practice guideline update from the American College of Physicians. *Ann Intern Med.* 2017;166(11):818–839.

Rabar S, Lau R, O'Flynn N, et al. Risk assessment of fragility fractures: Summary of NICE guidance. *BMJ.* 2012;345:e3698.

Saag KG, Petersen J, Brandi ML, et al. Romosozumab or alendronate for fracture prevention in women with osteoporosis. *N Engl J Med.* 2017;377:1417–1427. doi: 10.1056/NEJMoa1708322.

Shifren JL, Gass ML; NAMS Recommendations for Clinical Care of Midlife Women Working Group. The North American Menopause Society recommendations for clinical care of midlife women. *Menopause.* 2014;21(10):1038–1062.

Tai V, Leung W, Grey A, Reid IR, Bolland MJ. Calcium intake and bone mineral density: Systematic review and meta-analysis. *BMJ.* 2015;351:h4183. doi: https://doi.org/10.1136/bmj.h4183

US Preventive Services Task Force. Screening for Osteoporosis to Prevent FracturesUS Preventive Services Task Force Recommendation Statement. JAMA. 2018;319(24):2521–2531. doi:10.1001/jama.2018.7498

Watts NB, Adler RA, Bilezikian JP, et al.; Endocrine Society. Osteoporosis in men: An Endocrine Society clinical practice guideline. *J Clin Endocrinol Metab.* 2012;97(6):1802–1822.

RESOURCES

Arthritis Foundation
  www.arthritis.org
Calcium Fact Sheet for Health Professionals. National Institutes of Health Office of Dietary Supplements
  https://ods.od.nih.gov/factsheets/Calcium-HealthProfessional

National Osteoporosis Foundation
  www.nof.org
National Women's Health Resource Center (NWHRC)
  www.healthywomen.org
Osteoporosis. American College of Obstetricians and Gynecologists
  https://www.acog.org/Patients/FAQs/Osteoporosis
Osteoporosis. National Institute of Arthritis and Musculoskeletal Diseases
  https://www.bones.nih.gov/health-info/bone/osteoporosis
Osteoporosis. OrthoInfo/American Academy of Orthopedic Surgeons
  https://orthoinfo.aaos.org/en/diseases—conditions/osteoporosis
Osteoporosis and Arthritis: Two Common But Different Conditions. National Institute of Arthritis and Musculoskeletal Diseases
  https://www.bones.nih.gov/health-info/bone/osteoporosis/conditions-behaviors/osteoporosis-arthritis#b
Osteoporosis Society of Canada
  www.osteoporosis.ca

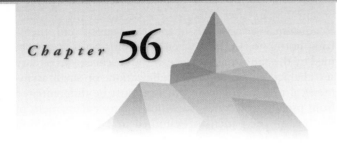

Chapter **56**

Common Endocrine and Metabolic Complaints

Debera J. Thomas, DNS, RN, FNP/ANP

Brian Oscar Porter, MD, PhD, MPH, MBA

HYPOCALCEMIA

Hypocalcemia is defined as a calcium level of less than 8.5 mg/dL. In response to hypocalcemia, secretion of parathyroid hormone (PTH) increases, which leads to mobilization of calcium stores from the bone and an increase in the absorption of calcium in the intestines. Neuromuscular signs and symptoms may occur in the presence of hypocalcemia because calcium is an important mediator in neuromuscular transmission and other intracellular biochemical activities.

Acute neuromuscular irritability occurs when the serum calcium drops abruptly by 2 to 3 mg/dL. Neuromuscular signs and symptoms include the following:

- *Carpopedal spasm (Trousseau's sign)* is a violent, painful contraction of the hands or feet. It is one of the neuromuscular signs indicating hypocalcemia and is a significant sign of tetany. It is often preceded by muscle cramps in the legs and feet. Carpal spasm consists of a flexed elbow and wrist, adducted thumb over the palm, flexed metacarpophalangeal joints, adduction of hyperextended fingers, and extended interphalangeal joints. The response is elicited by inflation of a blood pressure cuff to 20 mm Hg above the level of the systolic blood pressure. Inflation is maintained for 3 minutes to elicit the response, which is secondary to ulnar and median nerve ischemia.
- *Chvostek's sign* is the second neuromuscular sign associated with hypocalcemia. It is an abnormal unilateral spasm of the facial muscle when the facial nerve is tapped below the zygomatic arch anterior to the earlobe. In severe hypocalcemia, spontaneous spasms may also occur in the lower extremities and feet.

Other symptoms of hypocalcemia include various neuropsychiatric disorders, including irritability, emotional instability, problems with memory, and psychosis. Complaints of paresthesias, fatigue, muscle cramps, or muscle weakness may be elicited on history. Gastrointestinal manifestations include dysphagia, nausea, vomiting, biliary colic, and abdominal pain or cramping. Patients may also complain of chronic constipation or diarrhea. Cardiovascular symptoms include hypotension, bradycardia, congestive heart failure (CHF), and dysrhythmias. Prolonged QT intervals may be seen on the electrocardiogram.

Chronic hypocalcemia may cause the skin to be coarse, dry, and scaly. Alopecia may present with thinning of the eyebrows and eyelashes. Nails are often rigid, brittle, and thin, with transverse grooves. Subcapsular cataracts, optic neuritis, intracranial calcification, papilledema, and parkinsonian-type movements may also be present in chronic hypocalcemia.

DIFFERENTIAL DIAGNOSIS

Patients exhibiting the above signs and symptoms should be immediately assessed for hypocalcemia. Normal serum calcium values in adults range from 9 to 11 mg/dL. Immediate medical treatment is indicated in patients with marked hypocalcemia (less than 6.5 mg/dL).

PTH deficiency disease or inadvertent damage to the parathyroid glands during neck surgery may cause acute severe hypocalcemia. Acute transient hypocalcemia may occur in burns, severe sepsis, pregnancy, extensive blood transfusions with citrated blood, acute pancreatitis, and acute renal failure.

Aggressive treatment of hypercalcemia with plicamycin (Mithracin), bisphosphonates, and calcitonin (Cibacalcin, Calcimar) may result in acute hypocalcemia. Other drugs that may produce hypocalcemia include radiographic contrast dyes that contain the calcium-chelating agent EDTA and antiviral medication foscarnet (Foscavir).

Chronic hypocalcemia is usually caused by the absence of PTH, ineffective PTH, vitamin D deficiency, chronic renal failure, hypomagnesemia, or hypoalbuminemia. Other potential causes of chronic hypocalcemia include alkalosis, malabsorption syndromes, chronic pancreatitis, laxative abuse, chronic liver failure, phosphate excess, and osteomalacia.

A focused history, clinical examination, and subsequent laboratory tests may determine the cause of hypocalcemia. In the absence of a clearly identifiable etiology such as a medication, chronic liver or renal disease, or an acute disease process, additional laboratory studies are needed. Further laboratory evaluation should begin with serum magnesium, serum phosphorus, and albumin levels. Depending on these findings, the clinician should initiate treatment if indicated. A serum PTH level will assist in the diagnosis of parathyroid disease. A direct measure of serum vitamin D levels is the 25-hydroxycholecalciferol (25-[OH]D$_3$) assay.

Patients exhibiting either Trousseau's or Chvostek's sign accompanied by respiratory distress (e.g., stridor, loud crowing noises, and cyanosis) require immediate referral for emergency care because the neuromuscular irritation produced by hypocalcemia may progress rapidly to laryngospasms, seizures, and dysrhythmias. If the serum calcium levels have gradually declined, symptoms are usually subtle.

GYNECOMASTIA

Gynecomastia is the enlargement of glandular breast tissue in men, resulting in increased breast size. True gynecomastia involves enlargement of the stromal and ductal tissues; it may present unilaterally and progress to bilateral symmetrical or asymmetrical enlargement. Gynecomastia results from an imbalance of androgen and estrogen or an increase in prolactin. Growth hormones, estrogen, and corticosteroids stimulate ductal growth in the breasts. Progesterone and prolactin stimulate alveolar lobular growth of the breasts.

Gynecomastia is estimated to affect 12% to 40% of the male population in the United States and is present in approximately 60% of men older than 50 years, due to a decrease in testosterone levels. Transient gynecomastia occurs in male neonates (60% to 90%) and at puberty (50% to 60%).

DIFFERENTIAL DIAGNOSIS

Asymptomatic gynecomastia may be an incidental finding on routine examination. It may also present as an acute unilateral (or bilateral) painful tender mass beneath the areola or as a progressive painless enlargement of breast tissue. The enlargement may be obvious by observation alone; however, less severe cases are noted only during palpation. Pain in the nipple or breast and tenderness often accompany gynecomastia. Gynecomastia lasting longer than 1 year is usually asymptomatic. Nipple discharge is rare (present in fewer than 5% of cases).

Gynecomastia associated with puberty has an age at onset of 12 to 14 years. The duration is approximately 6 months, followed by spontaneous regression. Gynecomastia that presents before or after puberty and cannot be

associated with physiological aging, a drug side effect, or chronic disease requires further investigation by an endocrinologist. Associated symptoms may assist in identifying the cause. Attention to any impact on body image, especially in adolescents, is important A referral to an endocrinologist is required for all cases in which gynecomastia appears before puberty, if gynecomastia does not resolve within 2 years after puberty, if it occurs in the presence of abnormal serum levels of free testosterone and luteinizing hormone (LH), or when gynecomastia is accompanied by the abnormal presence or the absence of secondary sex characteristics, undermasculinization, or small asymmetrical testes. True gynecomastia must be differentiated from pseudo-gynecomastia, which is fatty enlargement of the breast. The patient is examined in a supine position while the examiner grasps breast tissue between the thumb and forefinger and gently moves the two digits toward the nipple. A firm or rubbery, mobile, disclike mound of tissue at least 2 to 4 cm in diameter arising concentrically from beneath the nipple and areolar region confirms gynecomastia. The glandular enlargement of gynecomastia is usually resistive and ropy in texture. Severe cases present with more extensive enlargement.

Lack of a disc of tissue suggests the enlargement is the result of adipose tissue deposition (pseudogynecomastia). Mammography will distinguish between the two if the clinical examination is inconclusive. When gynecomastia is accompanied by other breast abnormalities, especially if they are unilateral, a mammogram is indicated to rule out a neoplasm. In addition, a disc that is greater than 4 cm in diameter should be evaluated via mammography.

When true gynecomastia has been established, the patient is evaluated for physiological (developmental) or pathological causes. Although physiological causes of gynecomastia are most common cause, pathological causes should always be ruled out with a thorough history and physical examination. The most common causes of gynecomastia are puberty (25%), idiopathic (25%), drug related (15%), cirrhosis or malnutrition (10%), and testicular failure (10%). Other causes include renal failure, thyroid disease, neoplasms (including testicular cancer), hyperprolactinemia, Klinefelter's syndrome, and gonadotropin deficiency. Decreased libido and impotence may accompany gynecomastia and may indicate the presence of chronic pulmonary, renal, or liver disease; testicular failure; or endocrine pathology. Idiopathic and pubertal gynecomastia should resolve spontaneously within 1 to 2 years and require no medication. The patient should be followed every 3 to 6 months, and the size of the disc should be measured until it has resolved.

Medications implicated in gynecomastia include highly active antiretroviral therapy for HIV infection, calcium channel blockers, tricyclic antidepressants, and selective serotonin reuptake inhibitors. Less common medication causes include amiodarone, human growth hormone, amphetamines, and diazepam.

Malignant breast tumors (which represent about 3% of all cases of gynecomastia) in men are typically unilateral, firm, and immobile; they grow rapidly and are often painful. Nipple retraction and discharge, skin dimpling, and axillary lymphadenopathy may also accompany breast neoplasms. Mammography and fine-needle biopsy are essential for confirming the diagnosis.

Of note, surgery for breast reduction in adult males with gynecomastia recently increased by 5% in just 1 year, which has been suggested to be due to the decreasing stigma for men seeking cosmetic surgery (Delgado, 2016).

HIRSUTISM

Hirsutism is an increase in terminal hair growth on the face, chest, back, lower abdomen, pubic area, axilla, and inner thighs. It is present in approximately 5% of women. Almost 25% of these women have terminal hair growth on the face, especially on the upper lip. Hirsutism is caused by increased secretion of androgens by the ovary or adrenal glands or an increased sensitivity to androgens. It is often accompanied by menstrual irregularities.

There are two major types of hair: vellus and terminal. Vellus hair is found over most of the body and is fine, soft, and unpigmented. During puberty, vellus hair often changes to terminal hair in the presence of increased androgens. Terminal hairs are characteristically dark, coarse, pigmented, and thicker compared with vellus hair. Terminal hairs are found on the scalp, eyebrows, and the axillary and pubic areas after puberty. They are found in lesser abundance on the extremities.

DIFFERENTIAL DIAGNOSIS

Androgen-dependent terminal hair growth may be caused by pathology in the adrenal glands or ovaries or by exogenous androgen administration. The age, associated symptoms, and rapidity of onset are critical factors in differentiating potential causes. The characteristic increase in terminal hair growth occurs in areas most sensitive to androgen: the upper lip, chin, chest, upper arms, upper abdomen, lower abdomen, thighs, and upper and lower back.

Although most (90%) cases of hirsutism are idiopathic or result from polycystic ovary syndrome (PCOS), more serious underlying disease entities must be ruled out. A targeted history with emphasis on when hirsutism was first recognized and how rapidly it has progressed, a detailed menstrual history, and a review of associated symptoms may provide some insight into the cause of hirsutism. When the cause of hirsutism is determined to be of adrenal or ovarian origin, the patient is referred to an endocrinologist for treatment.

The physical examination should focus on signs of adrenal disease and virilization that may further clarify possible causes. For example, accompanying signs of virilization, hoarseness of the voice, clitorimegaly, receding temporal hairline, acne, loss of body fat, and breast atrophy may be due to an ovarian or adrenal tumor. Markedly increased levels of plasma androgens often accompany this virilization.

Laboratory evaluation of hirsutism is indicated in women with menstrual irregularities, a history of sudden onset or rapid progression of hirsutism, associated symptoms of ovarian or adrenal pathology, and moderate to severe presentations. Evaluation of free testosterone levels, androstenedione, total testosterone, 17-hydroxyprogesterone, urine 17-hydroxycorticosteroids, thyroid-stimulating hormone, prolactin levels, LH, follicle-stimulating hormone (FSH), and dehydroepiandrosterone sulfate (DHEA-S) will provide insights into possible causes or the need for further evaluation. Slightly elevated levels of serum androgens (free testosterone) are found in 40% of women with idiopathic hirsutism, whereas LH/FSH levels are increased in 75% of cases of PCOS. Testosterone levels greater than 200 ng/dL (in women) and/or DHEA-S levels greater than 700 ng/dL indicate the need for an ovarian and adrenal work-up because these levels are rarely seen in idiopathic hirsutism or PCOS.

Idiopathic hirsutism in women is the result of excessive androgenic activity and begins during puberty. There is a gradual development over 2 to 3 years followed by a period of stability. There is a familial tendency toward hirsutism. Women of eastern European or Mediterranean descent are likely to have increased terminal hair growth. Idiopathic hirsutism usually occurs in women aged 15 to 25 years without symptoms of virilization. It is usually mild and not accompanied by menstrual irregularities. Weight reduction may assist patients, since if the woman is obese, androgen production may be reduced with weight loss. Obese women have increased androgen levels due to insulin-stimulated androgen production in ovarian theca cells. Hirsutism can also present in pregnancy owing to the production of androgens by the placenta and corpus luteum. Postmenopausal women experience an increase in androgen production, with 75% experiencing noticeable growth of facial hair.

Mild cases of hirsutism can be managed by cosmetic therapy, including physical hair removal, chemical depilatories, and bleaching. Electrolysis and laser therapy are more permanent solutions but are costly. Estrogen-dominant oral contraceptives are effective and will increase levels of sex hormone–binding globulin, which in turn, reduces free (unbound and biologically active) testosterone levels. Progesterone-dominant contraceptives will increase clearance of testosterone. Medroxyprogesterone is also effective.

Of note, hormonal therapy will stop further hair growth but will not reverse the present hair growth, which must be treated cosmetically. It may take 6 to 24 months to detect results of hormonal treatment, which may need to be lifelong. Eflornithine 13.9% (Vaniqa) cream is Food and Drug Administration–approved to reduce unwanted facial hair in women and has shown evidence of reducing hair growth on the upper lip, especially when combined with laser therapy.

INCREASED NECK SIZE

Along with an extensive muscular, vascular, and neurologic network, the neck contains approximately 75 lymph nodes, the trachea, larynx, pharynx, the submandibular and salivary glands, cervical vertebrae, and the parathyroid and thyroid glands. Pathology in one of these structures or in an area that is drained by one of the many cervical lymph node chains may increase neck size.

A patient with increased neck size may present with complaints that shirt collars have become too tight. The patient should be evaluated immediately for difficulty swallowing or problems with breathing, as a rapid diagnostic work-up with specialty referral is indicated in the presence of either symptom. Some patients may also complain of neck pain.

DIFFERENTIAL DIAGNOSIS

Increased neck size may be caused by a mass in any structure in the neck, including glands, lymph nodes, the larynx, or pharynx. Cysts may also develop in the neck and increase its size. Blockage of the salivary glands produces neck enlargement. The most common cause of increased neck size is an enlarged thyroid gland. Other potential causes include trauma, masses, neoplasms, cysts, and lymph node enlargement. In addition, a patient with an increase in neck size may exhibit sleep apnea (see Chapter 29 for a full discussion).

A thorough history can assist in diagnosing the cause of increased neck size. For example, patients reporting a recent fall, automobile accident, or injury may have sustained cervical trauma, while a recent infection may cause lymph node enlargement. The patient should be questioned about a history of thyroid problems or recent surgeries, allergies, sinus problems, and any complaints of headaches. Symptoms of dysphagia, dyspnea, chest tenderness, cough, and hoarseness should be addressed. Complaints of neck pain should be investigated, including if the pain is aggravated by range-of-motion movements, breathing, swallowing, or chewing.

The physical examination should assess whether the swelling (enlargement) of the neck is focal or diffuse. One or more focal masses may be enlarged lymph nodes related to Hodgkin's disease, sarcoidosis, a thyroglossal cyst, thyroid adenoma, or carcinoma. If the swelling is diffuse, venous distention of CHF, Graves' disease (autoimmune hyperthyroidism), subacute thyroiditis, superior vena cava syndrome, or subcutaneous emphysema (which is usually accompanied by subcutaneous crepitus) may be suspected. If the swelling is focal, it should be noted if the lesion is midline or lateral. Midline masses may indicate thyroglossal cysts or adenoma of the thyroid; lateral masses are more likely related to Virchow's node (a single lymph node in the left supraclavicular fossa that takes its supply from lymph vessels in the abdomen and when enlarged may signify serious abdominal pathology), Hodgkin's lymphoma, bronchial cysts, a pharyngeal pouch, or a stone of Wharton's duct (submandibular salivary duct).

Intermediate swelling suggests venous congestion of CHF, a bronchial cyst, a stone of Wharton's duct, or an aneurysm.

A technique for detecting thyromegaly as the cause of neck swelling is to have the patient sit upright for examination. During examination, the neck is exposed down to the sternal notch while the examiner stands directly in front of the patient with the thyroid gland at the examiner's eye level. The patient should take several sips of water while the examiner observes for an enlarged thyroid gland. After visual examination, the thyroid is palpated anteriorly and posteriorly.

Thyroid nodules can be palpated in about 5% of Americans. Women are more likely to have palpable thyroid nodules, and the frequency of nodules increases with age. Fewer than 10% of singular nodules are malignant. Thyroid-stimulating hormone and free thyroxine (T_4) levels should be obtained on the patient with enlargement or any abnormalities of the thyroid.

A single enlarged lymph node is unlikely to result in a significant increase in neck size. Sudden complaints of a lymph node enlargement suggest an infectious process. Patients who present with enlargement of a node over several months or multiple nodal involvement are more likely to have neoplastic disease. A hard, immobile mass is also suggestive of a neoplastic process. A referral is indicated for biopsy of the nodes. Laryngeal cancer also produces cervical lymphadenopathy and an increase in neck size, which may be accompanied by pain, dyspnea, dysphagia, hemoptysis, stridor, or hoarseness.

POLYDIPSIA, POLYPHAGIA, AND POLYURIA

Polydipsia is excessive thirst; it is associated with several endocrine diseases and certain drugs. Polydipsia may accompany increased urine output (polyuria), which can be related to excessive loss of water and salt.

Polyphagia refers to excessive eating before satiety. This symptom can present as a persistent or intermittent condition, resulting from endocrine and psychological disorders. Certain drugs are also known to cause polyphagia. Elevated thyroxine (T_4) levels increase metabolism and thus the body's need for calories, often causing polyphagia.

Polyuria is a condition associated with increased urine production; it is defined as excretion of more than 3,000 mL (3 L) of urine per day. Any condition that increases hyperosmolar states will increase urination as a consequence of osmotic diuresis. The patient with polyuria is at risk for developing a fluid volume deficit that could result in hypovolemia.

DIFFERENTIAL DIAGNOSIS

Differential diagnoses for the patient with symptoms of polydipsia, polyphagia, and polyuria (also known as "The 3 P's") include diabetes mellitus (DM), diabetes insipidus, diuretic abuse, head trauma, and psychiatric disorders. See Figure 56.1 for other cause of these symptoms.

Diagnostic Reasoning Algorithm: Polydipsia, Polyphagia, and Polyuria

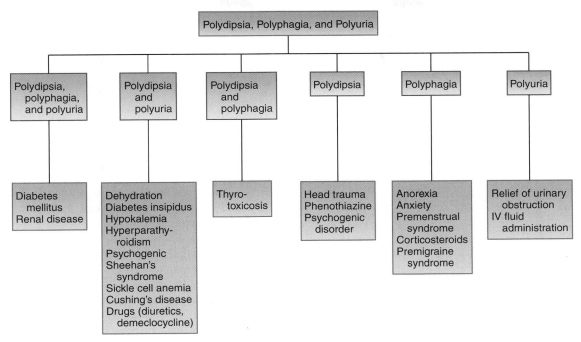

Figure 56.1 Diagnostic algorithm: polydipsia, polyphagia, and polyuria.

The patient should be questioned about any history of head trauma, weight changes, thyroid disease, hypertension, and family history of diabetes. The patient should also be questioned about any history of psychiatric illnesses or changes in mental status, such as decreases in alertness or memory, as well as symptoms of fatigue. A detailed 48-hour history of intake and output should be obtained, including the type of fluid intake over 48 hours, as well as the characteristics of urine output. Urine output is often difficult for patients to estimate and objective measurement may be needed. A weight history should also be obtained.

The patient should be assessed for signs of dehydration and malnutrition. Weight and vital signs are assessed. Initial laboratory testing includes urinalysis, urine specific gravity, serum electrolytes, blood urea nitrogen, serum creatinine, complete blood count, fasting serum glucose level, and glycosylated hemoglobin A1c (HbA1c) percentage.

Polydipsia, polyphagia, and polyuria are the classic symptoms of DM. Blood glucose levels should be evaluated in patients who experience these three symptoms. A HbA1c equal to or greater than 6.5%, a fasting (following 8 hours of no caloric intake) blood glucose level equal to or greater than 126 mg/dL, a 2-hour postprandial plasma glucose level equal to or greater than 200 mg/dL following a 75-g oral glucose tolerance test, a random blood glucose level greater than 200 mg/dL in persons with classic symptoms of hyperglycemia (polyuria, polydipsia, polyphagia, weight loss), or hyperglycemic crisis confirms the diagnosis of DM. Additional symptoms indicating DM include weakness, fatigue, increased susceptibility to infections, and nocturia.

REFERENCES

Gynecomastia

Ansstas G, Ansstas M. Gynecomastia. http://emedicine.medscape.com/article/120858-overview. Published 2013.

Delgado M. American Society of Plastic Surgeons Report 2015 statistics. https://www.gynecomastia.org/doctors/migueldelgado/blog/american-society-plastic-surgeons-report-2015-statistics. Published 2016, March 11. Accessed August 29, 2017.

Hirsutism

Griffing GT. Hirsutism. http://emedicine.medscape.com/article/121038-overview. Updated March 24, 2017. Accessed September 7, 2017.

Hypocalcemia

John DR, Suthar P. Radiological features of long-standing hypoparathyroidism. *Pol J Radiol.* 2016;81:42–45.

Polydipsia, Polyphagia, and Polyuria

American Diabetes Association. Classification and diagnosis of diabetes. *Diabetes Care.* 2017;40(Suppl 1): S11–S24. https://doi.org/10.2337/dc17-S005. Accessed September 7, 2017.

RESOURCES

American Association of Clinical Endocrinologists
www.aace.com

National Institute of Diabetes and Digestive and Kidney Diseases: Endocrine Diseases
https://www.niddk.nih.gov/health-information/endocrine-diseases/hashimotos-disease

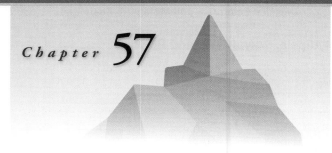

Chapter 57

Glandular Disorders

Debera J. Thomas, DNS, RN, FNP/ANP

Brian Oscar Porter, MD, PhD, MPH, MBA

HYPERTHYROIDISM

Hyperthyroidism, a common clinical condition, includes a heterogeneous group of conditions characterized by the excessive secretion and synthesis of one or both of the thyroid hormones thyroxine (T_4) and triiodothyronine (T_3). Although many clinicians use the terms interchangeably, *thyrotoxicosis* is a more general term that encompasses hyperthyroidism, as well as exogenous thyroid hormone intake and subacute thyroiditis, in which acute inflammation of the thyroid gland results in the rapid excretion (rather than overproduction) of stored thyroid hormones.

The clinical manifestations of hyperthyroidism result from the effects of excessive thyroid hormone on bodily tissues, resulting in alterations in growth, metabolism, and development. These manifestations are sometimes mistaken for signs of psychiatric illnesses. The long-term effects of inadequately treated overt hyperthyroidism are heart disease, osteoporosis (in postmenopausal women), mental illness, and infertility.

EPIDEMIOLOGY AND CAUSES

Hyperthyroidism occurs in 1.2% of the U.S. population. It may occur at any age but peaks in persons aged 20 to 40 years. Only 10% to 15% of hyperthyroidism is diagnosed in older adults. The prevalence of hyperthyroidism is 2% in women older than 70 years of age and 4% in women aged 40 to 60 years, with an overall prevalence of 1% to 3%. Hyperthyroidism is much more common in women than men (8:1).

Hyperthyroidism often occurs spontaneously from overproduction of thyroid hormones, but it can also result from the excessive intake of thyroid hormones. Graves' disease is by far the most common cause of spontaneous hyperthyroidism in the United States. An autoimmune disorder characterized by autoreactive, agonistic antibodies to the thyroid-stimulating hormone (TSH) receptor,

Graves' disease accounts for 80% to 90% of hyperthyroid cases, peaking in young adults aged 20 to 40 years. It is also the most common form of hyperthyroidism that occurs during pregnancy.

Subacute thyroiditis is the most common cause of thyrotoxicosis, accounting for 15% to 20% of cases. Characterized by glandular inflammation and follicular cell destruction, it is thought to be of viral etiology, frequently occurring following an acute viral infection. More common in middle-aged adults between 40 and 50 years of age, subacute thyroiditis is more likely to develop in women than in men. Silent thyroiditis is a form of subacute thyroiditis in which the thyroid gland is moderately enlarged and nontender. It usually occurs in adults between 30 and 40 years of age and is also more common in women.

Toxic multinodular goiter (Plummer disease) is as common as subacute thyroiditis, accounting for 15% to 20% of thyrotoxicosis cases. This type of goiter is more common in older adults and is a complication of chronic, inactive nodular goiter. This condition is more common in other parts of the world where dietary iodine deficiency is prevalent. A single, toxic thyroid adenoma is the next most common cause of thyrotoxicosis, accounting for 3% to 5% of all cases.

The inappropriate use of thyroid replacement therapy or treatment errors may also produce symptoms of hyperthyroidism. Thyrotoxicosis factitia is a form of thyrotoxicosis in which a patient takes excessive amounts of either thyroxine (T_4) or triiodothyronine (T_3). This condition should be considered in a patient with access to hormone supplements or with psychiatric problems. An excess of dietary iodine may also precipitate symptoms of hyperthyroidism.

A tumor of the pituitary gland causing hypersecretion of TSH (thyrotropin) is a rare cause of hyperthyroidism. Other uncommon causes include metastatic follicular thyroid carcinoma, ingestion of iodine-containing drugs (e.g., certain expectorants, amiodarone, seaweed-containing health food supplements) or iodinated radiocontrast media, choriocarcinoma, or hydatidiform molar pregnancy producing high amounts of human chorionic gonadotropin that can weakly activate the receptor for TSH, struma ovarii (ectopic thyroid tissue) that is associated with dermoid tumors and ovarian teratomas, and testicular embryonal carcinoma (see Table 57.1).

PATHOPHYSIOLOGY

All types of hyperthyroidism are a result of overproduction, overexposure (exogenous sources), and/or secretion of thyroid hormones, and the clinical manifestations of hyperthyroidism are a direct result of the effect of excessive thyroid hormones on essentially all organ systems and bodily tissues. Although thyroid hormones are required to regulate normal growth and development, excessive

TABLE 57.1	**Hyperthyroidism: Common and Rare Causes**	
	Disorder/Problem	*Etiology/Comments*
Common Causes	Graves' disease	Autoimmune disease
	Toxic nodular goiter	Unknown development of nodules that progress from nontoxic to toxic over time
	Subacute thyroiditis	Thought to be caused by viral infection
	Thyrotoxicosis factitia	Excessive ingestion of exogenous thyroid hormones
	Jod-Basedow phenomenon	Large intake of dietary iodine or iodinated radiocontrast dye exposure in a person with thyroid disease
Rare Causes	Pituitary adenoma	Rare tumor of the pituitary gland
	Struma ovarii	Rare secretion of thyroid hormones by thyroid tissue located in ovarian dermoid tumors
	Metastatic thyroid cancer	Very rare cause
	High-dose amiodarone	Excessive dosage of iodine-containing amiodarone
	Pregnancy and trophoblastic tumors	Very high serum levels of human chorionic gonadotropin

release of T_4 and T_3 from the thyroid into the circulation upregulates metabolism, leading to an increase in total body heat production, heart rate and contractility, and vasodilation. This explains the clinical manifestations of thyrotoxicosis, which include palpitations, diaphoresis, heat intolerance, and anxiety.

T_3 is normally 20 to 100 times more biologically active than T_4, which is converted to T_3 in peripheral tissues. Interestingly, the degree of symptomatology does not consistently correlate with the extent of thyroid hormone overproduction. In general, younger patients tend to have symptoms more reflective of sympathetic activation (e.g., tremors, anxiety, and hyperactivity), whereas older patients manifest more cardiovascular symptoms, including atrial fibrillation and dyspnea, as well as weight loss.

Graves' disease is an autoimmune disorder that results from aberrantly produced thyroid-stimulating immunoglobulins activating TSH receptors in the thyroid gland, overriding the gland's normal regulatory mechanisms, and thereby leading to thyroid hyperplasia (goiter) and increased synthesis of T3. Thyroid hormone levels are typically highest with this form of thyrotoxicosis, and excessive thyroid hormone levels result in thyroid growth (hypertrophy), hypermetabolism, and sympathetic overactivity.

Graves' disease has a higher prevalence in people with human leukocyte antigen (HLA)–DRw3 and HLA-B89. It also strongly correlates with other autoimmune conditions including vitiligo, type 1 diabetes mellitus (DM), pernicious anemia, myasthenia gravis, and adrenal insufficiency. A diffusely enlarged goiter involving both thyroid lobes, hyperthyroid ophthalmopathy (e.g., periorbital edema, conjunctival edema and injection known as chemosis, proptosis, lid lag, and even diplopia), and excessive uptake of radioactive iodine on diagnostic testing are all common characteristics. Circulating antithyroperoxidase (anti-TPO) is another common finding.

In contrast, subacute thyroiditis produces symptoms of thyrotoxicosis via the release of preformed thyroid hormones, in response to an inflammatory response after an acute viral infection. Thus, unlike other common causes of thyrotoxicosis including toxic multinodular goiter and an isolated toxic adenoma that involve increased production and hypersecretion of thyroid hormones, subacute thyroiditis demonstrates a very low uptake of radioactive iodine on diagnostic testing. Subacute painful or granulomatous thyroiditis is associated with HLA-Bw35.

Toxic multinodular goiter typically arises in geographic areas where dietary iodine is deficient. As scattered portions of the thyroid gland increase in activity in an attempt to compensate for insufficient iodine, hormonal excess develops slowly over time. In fact, this condition may be asymptomatic at the time of diagnosis, especially in older individuals in whom the classic symptoms of hyperthyroidism may be blunted—a condition termed *apathetic hyperthyroidism*.

Nuclear scintigraphy demonstrates scattered areas of both increased and decreased iodine uptake, which reflect the increased thyroidal activity that manifests in the setting of adequate dietary iodine. In contrast, a single hyperfunctioning monoclonal follicular adenoma will show only a single focus of increased uptake on a radioactive thyroid scan. Such nodules tend to be functional only once they reach at least 2.5 cm in size. As pituitary TSH production is suppressed by the adenoma, the remaining glandular tissue becomes hypofunctional and actually demonstrates decreased uptake on nuclear scintigraphy.

Autoregulation of the thyroid normally prevents thyrotoxicosis in the face of dietary iodine excess. However, in the setting of a particularly concentrated iodine load (such as with iodinated radiocontrast media), patients with one or more autonomous thyroid nodules may lose this adaptive capability and be thrown into thyrotoxicosis (Jod-Basedow effect or Jod-Basedow syndrome).

CLINICAL PRESENTATION

The clinical presentation of hyperthyroidism depends on the duration and the amount of excessive thyroid hormone secretion. Symptoms vary, depending on the cause and organ systems affected. Patients may be asymptomatic in the presence of mild elevations of thyroid hormones; they are more likely to remain asymptomatic at increasing levels if the increased secretion has been gradual.

Subjective

Because thyroid hormones affect most organ systems, a complete history and review of systems is indicated. Most patients with hyperthyroidism will complain of some combination of anxiety, nervousness, diaphoresis, fatigue, heat intolerance, palpitations, weight loss, and insomnia. In situations in which the thyroid tissue has become enlarged, the patient may complain of fullness or pressure in the neck. Additional symptoms include

weakness, exercise intolerance, tremors, lower extremity edema, weight loss in the presence of an increased appetite, menstrual irregularities, frequent bowel movements or diarrhea, and exertional dyspnea.

Eye complaints include blurred vision, proptosis (downward displacement of the eyeball), photophobia, and double vision. Patients may also report that they are unable to concentrate, extremely irritable, and emotionally labile. Older patients may present with vague symptoms such as unexplained weight loss, apathy, worsening of angina, depression, change in bowel habits, and weakness. A summary of potential signs and symptoms of hyperthyroidism is presented in Table 57.2.

Patients should be questioned about current and prior endocrine diseases (in the patient and family), as well as a personal or family history of thyroid nodules, goiter, use of iodide-containing drugs, and thyroid neoplasms. Radiation to the head and neck increases the risk of thyroid cancer, which can rarely be associated with hyperthyroidism. A weight history should be obtained, including recent and

TABLE 57.2	**Hyperthyroidism: Clinical Presentation**	
Bodily System	**Subjective**	**Objective**
General	Fatigue Weight loss Increased appetite	Muscle atrophy Tremors
Integumentary	Diaphoresis Heat intolerance	Warm, flushed, moist skin Onycholysis Hyperpigmentation Fine and silky hair Thinning hair Dermopathy of legs Pretibial myxedema Urticaria Pruritus Vitiligo
Gastrointestinal	Diarrhea Increased bowel movements Increased appetite	Increased liver function
Eye	Blurred vision Increased tearing Double vision Decreased visual acuity Photophobia Feelings of increased orbital pressure	Increased exophthalmos Lid lag and edema Corneal ulceration
Neurological	Tremors of hands	Hyperactive reflexes Tremor
Cardiopulmonary	Palpitations Exertional dyspnea Breathlessness	Sinus tachycardia Elevated blood pressure Symptoms of congestive heart failure Dysrhythmias (atrial fibrillation)
Genitourinary	Menstrual irregularities (decreased menstrual flow)	Gynecomastia
Head and neck	Pressure in neck Increased neck size	Enlarged thyroid gland

TABLE 57.2 Hyperthyroidism: Clinical Presentation—cont'd

Bodily System	Subjective	Objective
Psychosocial	Anxiety Nervousness Insomnia Irritability Emotional lability Restlessness	Increased pulse rate Increased respiratory rate Increased blood pressure
Musculoskeletal	Weakness	Proximal muscle weakness Loss of muscle tone Osteoporosis (in postmenopausal women)
Laboratory findings		Normochromic normocytic anemia Hypercalcemia Potassium wasting Increased alkaline phosphatase

long-term weight patterns. If the patient is currently taking thyroid hormone replacement medication, how the medication is being taken should be assessed. Patients should also be questioned about any recent viral infections or the possibility of pregnancy, as well as use of other medications.

Objective

Signs of thyrotoxicosis are associated with the various forms of hyperthyroidism and range from overt manifestations in young adults with an acute onset to a subtler presentation in older adults. Often, an older adult will present with symptoms typically diagnosed as failure to thrive.

The neck should be examined for visual enlargement of the thyroid and palpated for lymphadenopathy. The thyroid must be palpated thoroughly, noting any nodules or enlargement, both anteriorly and posteriorly. On physical examination, the thyroid may be enlarged, nodules may be palpable, and a bruit may be heard over the thyroid gland with the bell of a stethoscope. Whereas the goiter of Graves' disease is typically firm, the thyroid in toxic multinodular goiter may be softer, but with several palpable nodules. The neck should be moderately extended during examination, and water should be provided to the patient to aid swallowing. The thyroid gland moves with swallowing; however, a very large goiter or a large thyroid mass may prevent movement.

In subacute thyroiditis, the patient will present with a firm, painful, thyroid gland enlargement, fatigue, and possibly a low-grade fever. An enlarged painful thyroid gland is also consistent with degeneration or hemorrhage into a thyroid nodule, as well as either granulomatous or suppurative thyroiditis. In contrast, in silent thyroiditis or subacute lymphocytic thyroiditis, the gland is swollen but not usually tender.

Cardiovascular manifestations include tachycardia (resting heart rate greater than 90 beats per minute), irregular pulse, systolic murmurs, and widening of the pulse pressure. Although rare, an infiltrative dermopathy may be present in the lower extremities, which includes myxedema (i.e., deposition of glycosaminoglycan material in the dermis of the lower extremities causing nonpitting pretibial edema), erythema due to an inflammatory cell infiltrate, and skin thickening along the ankles and pretibial areas.

Visual acuity should be tested and lid lag assessed by instructing the patient to slowly gaze up and down. As the patient gazes downward, the upper lid will lag behind the eye movement. Lid lag can also be detected by the eyeball lagging behind the lower lid as the patient gazes upward. Hyperthyroid ophthalmopathy occurs in 40% of patients with Graves' disease and is rare in patients with subacute thyroiditis. The conjunctiva may be inflamed, and visual acuity may be affected. Exophthalmos, excessive lacrimation, lid retraction, and lid lag may be present.

The examiner should assess the skin and extremities for edema, general appearance, and signs of thinning hair. The skin may be moist and velvety to the touch, with increased pigmentation, spider angiomata, and vitiligo. Onycholysis (splitting and spooning of the nails) may also be present. Deep tendon reflexes may show a rapid relaxation of the reflexes, and the most predominant hyperactive reflex is usually the Achilles tendon reflex. The patient may have decreased strength in the extremities and fine tremors, especially of the hands when the arms are fully outstretched. Lymphadenopathy and splenomegaly may also be present.

Patients with long-standing hyperthyroidism may also have clubbing of the digits and signs of new bone growth in the hands, termed *thyroid acropachy*. Older adults with hyperthyroidism often appear apathetic. Physical examination may reveal atrial fibrillation (present in one-third of all older adults with hyperthyroidism), fine skin, brittle nails, and symptoms of congestive heart failure. The thyroid gland is often not enlarged in older adults.

Thyroid storm or crisis is a severe and sometimes fatal form of hyperthyroidism that requires immediate emergency medical care. Assessment, contributing factors, and treatments for thyroid storm are shown in Table 57.3.

TABLE 57.3	Thyroid Storm/Crisis
Contributing Factors	Acute infection Trauma Stress trigger in patient with hyperthyroidism Uncontrolled diabetes mellitus Severe drug reaction Withdrawal of antithyroid medication or radioactive iodine therapy
Symptoms: Initial	Fever (usually first symptom), often >100.4°F (38°C) Nausea, vomiting Abdominal pain
Symptoms: Progressive	Severe agitation, occasional psychosis Elevated temperature Diaphoresis Tachycardia, heart failure Dysrhythmia (atrial fibrillation of flutter) Confusion Cardiovascular collapse Malignant exophthalmos
Laboratory Findings	Elevated free thyroid hormone (T_4) levels, but no more increased than typical hyperthyroidism (thyroid storm is predominantly a clinical diagnosis, rather than biochemical or laboratory-based)
Management	Hospitalization and aggressive reversal of thyrotoxins 1. To block thyroid hormone synthesis, propylthiouracil (PTU) is given daily in two to four divided doses; methimazole is typically not used during thyroid storm because it does not prevent peripheral conversion of T_4 to T_3. 2. To alleviate the beta-adrenergic symptoms, beta blockers are given (propranolol [Inderal] IV). 3. To block conversion of T_4 to T_3, hydrocortisone is given IV. 4. If radioactive iodine is prescribed but not given for a few days, concentrated potassium iodide oral solution or Telepaque may be given. 5. Supportive measures: decrease fever, treat underlying infection, administer IV fluids and glucose as needed.

DIAGNOSTIC REASONING

Diagnostic Tests

Initial Testing

National organizations differ in their recommendations for routine screening of asymptomatic patients. In 2015, the U.S. Preventive Services Task Force (USPSTF)

reviewed the 2004 recommendations for thyroid screening and reaffirmed that there is insufficient evidence for or against routine screening for thyroid disease in adults without symptoms, and the USPSTF has not updated this recommendation. If the patient is symptomatic or in a high-risk category, such as having a family history of thyroid disease or a previous history of thyroid disease or autoimmune disorders, screening is appropriate.

Levels of thyroid hormone often do not correlate reliably with the clinical presentation of hyperthyroidism. The initial screening tests for suspected hyperthyroidism are the sensitive serum TSH assay to detect suppressed levels in the setting of elevated thyroid hormones, as well as measurement of T_4 and T_3 levels. Laboratory protocols that include free thyroxine (FT_4) immunoassay and T_3 if the TSH is low can prevent additional blood draws and expense. If the protocol is not in place, FT_4 and T_3 levels should be tested next. The sensitive TSH assay has a functional sensitivity of 0.02 mcg/dL or less, although units for this test are typically expressed as mIU/L, milli-units/L, or mcIU/mL.

In most cases of hyperthyroidism, a TSH level of less than 0.35 mIU/L usually accompanies an elevated FT_4 measurement (>12.5 mcg/dL). Measurement of FT_4 is generally preferred to total T_4 because it measures the level of T_4 unbound to carrier proteins that is, therefore, biologically active. A significant number of medications may alter laboratory results due to alterations in protein binding. These include anabolic steroids, androgens, estrogens, heparin, iodine-containing compounds, phenytoin (Dilantin), rifampin (Rimactane, Rifadin), and salicylates. In addition, in the setting of a low TSH level, T_3 levels should be obtained because approximately 5% of hyperthyroid patients have normal T_4 levels but elevated T_3 levels. Normal levels for T_3 range from 100 to 200 ng/dL.

Subsequent Testing

In Graves' disease, antithyroglobulin and antimicrosomal antibodies are elevated. A TSH receptor antibody test is usually elevated in Graves' disease and is part of subsequent testing. The diagnosis of thyrotoxicosis is considered in cases of hyperthyroidism when TSH levels are depressed and measurements of T_4 are normal. Subacute thyroiditis may also have laboratory abnormalities of elevated erythrocyte sedimentation rate and C-reactive protein. Mild anemia is also common.

Nuclear scintigraphy with radiolabeled iodine (^{123}I) or technetium (^{99}Tc) helps in assessing the functional status of the thyroid gland. A 24-hour radioactive iodine uptake (RAIU) test can differentiate Graves' disease from subacute thyroiditis and toxic nodular goiters, thereby refining treatment recommendations. It identifies areas of increased and decreased thyroid function, often termed *hot* and *cold* spots, within the gland. Patients with toxic nodular goiter and Graves' disease have a high

RAIU, whereas in subacute thyroiditis, iodine uptake is low. Importantly, however, toxic adenoma and toxic multinodular goiter both present with areas of decreased isotope uptake as well, because the hyperfunctioning nodules lead to suppression of TSH via negative hormonal feedback. A thyroid scan is critical to determining functionality of any dominant thyroid nodule in a patient presenting with thyrotoxicosis because cold nodules are highly suspicious for concomitant malignancy and must be evaluated further.

An ultrasound of the thyroid will assist in differentiating a cyst from a nodule. A pure thyroid cyst is less likely to be malignant than a nodule. A fine-needle biopsy is the preferred initial diagnostic technique for evaluation of thyroid masses, particularly solid masses, to rule out malignancy. Magnetic resonance imaging (MRI) is the preferred test to assess for ophthalmopathy resulting from Graves' disease. It is especially beneficial in ruling out an orbital tumor.

Differential Diagnosis

Thyrotoxicosis, due to high levels of TSH, is seen in rare pituitary tumors. Excessive exogenous thyroid administration will produce the same symptoms seen in thyrotoxicosis. Thyroid cancer must be considered when the thyroid gland is hard and enlarged or when nodules are palpated.

T_4 levels may be elevated in acute illnesses such as hepatitis, in the presence of elevated estrogen levels, acute psychiatric problems, hyperemesis, familial thyroid hormone binding abnormalities, and autoimmunity. Dopamine (Intropin, Dopastat) and high dosages of glucocorticoids may decrease TSH levels. Drugs that may increase T_4 levels include amiodarone (Cordarone), amphetamines, clofibrate (Atromid-S), high-dose glucocorticoids, heparin administered during dialysis, heroin, levothyroxine (Synthroid), methadone (Dolophine), and perphenazine (Trilafon).

MANAGEMENT

Treatment of hyperthyroidism differs depending on the cause and patient characteristics. A euthyroid state is the goal of treatment, while minimizing the adverse effects of treatment and decreasing the incidence of iatrogenic hypothyroidism.

Emergency treatment is necessary if the patient presents in thyroid storm (see Table 57.3). The patient should be hospitalized for oral and IV hydration, if needed, and immediately begin thyroid-blocking medications, beta-adrenergic blockers, and corticosteroids if signs of ophthalmopathy are present. Iodine blocks the release of stored thyroid hormones, and glucocorticosteroids block the conversion of T_4 to T_3. Patients intolerant of beta blockers (e.g., asthmatics, patients with chronic obstructive pulmonary disease [COPD]) may be treated with calcium channel blockers as an alternate therapy. Supportive measures include treating any underlying infection, managing fever with antipyretics, hydration, and cooling blankets, and correcting any fluid and electrolyte imbalances. In critically ill patients, plasmapheresis or hemodialysis may reduce the circulating levels of T_3 and T_4.

Multinodular and uninodular goiters should be referred to an endocrinologist for evaluation of possible malignancy. Nonmalignant thyroid nodular disease with laboratory evaluations indicating hyperthyroidism is most often treated with radioactive iodine.

Treatment of Graves' Disease

The three treatment options for Graves' disease are antithyroid drugs, radioactive iodine, or surgery. None of these treatments alters the underlying autoimmune process of Graves' disease. The most successful treatment in achieving a permanent euthyroid state is surgery; however, it is rarely the preferred method of treatment unless the thyroid gland is extremely enlarged and is pressing on other structures in the neck. Many patients treated with radioactive iodine will experience a relapse and require a second treatment. Radioactive iodine also may worsen ophthalmopathy if present. Currently the majority of endocrinologists use an ablative dose of radioactive iodine. This allows the resolution of hyperthyroidism, although patients then become hypothyroid and require thyroid replacement therapy for life.

Pharmacological Therapy

Patients experiencing tachycardia, palpitations, or tremors benefit from the introduction of a beta blocker during the initiation of therapy. Beta blockers provide effective, short-term relief of hyperadrenergic symptoms. Use of a beta blocker is contraindicated in patients with COPD, bronchospasm, or uncompensated heart failure. They are used cautiously in patients who take insulin because it may block symptoms of hypoglycemia. Beta-adrenergic blockers often require higher and more frequent dosing because of the frequent resistance to usual doses. Once ablative treatment is completed, beta blockers will be tapered and discontinued. As stated previously, calcium channel blockers are an option in patients for whom beta blockers are contraindicated; however, this class of drug should also be avoided in patients with uncompensated heart failure, given their propensity to decrease cardiac contractility.

Antithyroid medications work by inhibiting thyroid hormone synthesis at multiple steps. They are used as a primary treatment to reduce the level of thyroid hormone on the initiation of radioactive iodine therapy, as well as before and after thyroid surgery. These drugs take time to achieve their peak effect, however, and hormone levels may not be significantly decreased for 2 to 8 weeks. These medications are not used as the primary or sole treatment in the majority of patients.

Two antithyroid drugs are used—propylthiouracil (PTU) and methimazole (MMI). These drugs are the treatment of choice for pregnant women—especially PTU, because it is less likely to cross the placenta than MMI. As a pregnancy progresses, the dose of PTU often decreases and can frequently be discontinued before delivery. It is important to remember that all antithyroid drugs do cross the placental barrier to some extent, and overtreatment can have adverse effects on a fetus. Therefore, a clinical endocrinologist should be part of the pregnant woman's care.

PTU has an added therapeutic effect of inhibiting T_3 activity and preventing peripheral conversion of T_4 into T_3—the more biologically active of the two main thyroid hormones. Thus, it is useful in cases of thyrotoxicosis to rapidly reduce hyperthyroid symptoms. These drugs are also often used in persons awaiting surgical intervention and in patients of childbearing age. Antithyroid drug treatment may also be the preferred treatment in patients without significant thyroid gland enlargement.

PTU is usually started at doses of 50 to 150 mg by mouth (PO) two or three times per day (150 to 300 mg per day). MMI (Tapazole) is given at an initial dose of 10 to 40 mg orally or rectally daily. The dosage is titrated every 3 to 4 weeks based on thyroxine levels and TSH levels. TSH and T_4 levels are evaluated every visit, and a targeted history and physical examination is performed to monitor therapeutic response (see Drugs Commonly Prescribed 57.1).

These drugs are not indicated for long-term use because more than one-half of patients on these drugs alone experience resumption of symptoms. Once the patient has achieved a euthyroid state, the frequency of follow-up visits is extended to every 4 to 6 weeks for a period of 3 to 4 months. If the TSH and free T_4 remain stable during this time, the follow-up is extended to every 3 to 4 months. In patients taking antithyroid medication, a serum FT_4 level should be evaluated with TSH levels because the TSH level may remain suppressed due to chronic hyperthyroidism long after T_4 levels are decreased.

Common adverse reactions to antithyroid medications include rash, urticaria, and arthralgias, which may occur in 1% to 5% of patients. Rare but serious adverse reactions include agranulocytosis, aplastic anemia, and hepatitis, which may occur in up to 0.5% of patients taking antithyroid medications. Except for agranulocytosis, which is more common with MMI, these reactions are more likely to occur with PTU. Thus, patients taking these drugs should be instructed to report immediately any signs of infection, especially fever, sore throat, malaise, or mouth sores. The antithyroid medication must be discontinued immediately if any of these symptoms occur. The patient is often changed to a regimen of radioactive iodine to produce a euthyroid state. Agranulocytosis may take up to 10 to 14 days to resolve fully after the medication is stopped and may require concomitant administration of granulocyte colony-stimulating factor (filgrastim).

Before initiation of antithyroid therapy, a baseline complete blood count (CBC) and liver function tests including hepatic aminotransferases (aspartate aminotransferase, alanine aminotransferase) should be obtained. During therapy, the white blood cell count is checked every 2 weeks during the first month and then every 4 to 6 months thereafter. Liver enzymes should be evaluated every 3 to 6 months.

Antithyroid drugs are used for 6 to 24 months after achievement of a euthyroid state. The dosage is then gradually decreased until the drug is withdrawn. The patient is followed every 1 to 2 months initially after cessation of therapy for a possible relapse. Many patients will experience a permanent remission after a 1- to 2-year course of antithyroid medications.

Radioactive Iodine

Radioactive iodine–131 (^{131}I; Iodotope) is the treatment of choice for hyperthyroidism in the United States, especially in middle-aged or older adults. Typically, a 24-hour radioiodine uptake dose of 75 to 200 mcCi (microcuries) per gram of estimated thyroid tissue is administered orally, which concentrates in overactive thyroid cells, where it emits radiation, causing inflammation and the ultimate destruction of the pathological cells. It is less invasive than thyroidectomy, is a targeted therapy that is

---

⬤ Drugs Commonly Prescribed 57.1: Hyperthyroidism

DRUG	INDICATIONS	ADVERSE REACTIONS AND PRESCRIBING CONSIDERATIONS
Propylthiouracil (PTU)	Hyperthyroidism	Common: pruritus, drowsiness, allergic dermatitis, nausea, vomiting, arthralgia Rare: agranulocytosis Note: onset of drug action is 1 week, peaking in 4–10 weeks with a duration of 1–4 weeks
Methimazole (MMI) (Tapazole)	Hyperthyroidism	Common: pruritus, drowsiness, allergic dermatitis, nausea, parotitis, arthralgia Rare: agranulocytosis Note: onset of drug action is 1 week, peaking in 4–10 weeks with a duration of 36–72 hours

focused solely on the thyroid, and does not require hospitalization.

Although response to this therapy is slower than with antithyroid drugs or surgical excision, radioablation is indicated in patients who have a poor response to antithyroid medication, as well as in cases of toxic multinodular goiter. Radioiodine is contraindicated in pregnancy and breastfeeding. The recurrence rate for hyperthyroidism is relatively low with this treatment. For patients with Graves' disease, there is a 5% recurrence 1 year after treatment, which remains steady for 5 years. This is in contrast to patients with uninodular or multinodular toxic goiter, who have a 6% to 7% recurrence rate initially and a 30% recurrence rate after 5 years.

Women receiving radioactive iodine therapy should not become pregnant until at least 4 months after therapy. T_4 levels need to be checked monthly for 3 months after the administration of radioactive iodine in patients receiving radioactive thyroid ablation therapy. Euthyroid patients should be assessed every 3 to 6 months for hypothyroidism by monitoring the FT_4 and sensitive TSH levels. Hypothyroidism may occur at any time, but it is most likely to present during the first year. Some patients will fail treatment and require a second dose. First-time failure rates may be as high as 45%, but about 70% of patients receiving radioactive iodine therapy eventually develop hypothyroidism.

Hyperthyroid ophthalmopathy is often exacerbated with radioactive iodine treatment; however, research has found that the incidence of ophthalmopathy is reduced when prednisone (0.4 mg/kg) is given concurrently with radioactive iodine treatments. If ophthalmopathy occurs, the patient requires referral to an ophthalmologist. Treatment often includes diuretics and ophthalmic prednisone. Methylcellulose eye drops (Tear Naturale) are useful to protect against excessive ocular dryness.

A nonradioactive alternative to thyroid radioablation for severe Graves' disease or subacute thyroiditis involves administering a large quantity of concentrated iodine as a saturated solution of potassium iodide (SSKI, 35–50 mg iodide per drop, 1–2 drops in water orally twice daily; Lugol solution, 8-mg iodide per drop, 3–5 drops in water orally 3 times daily) or iopanoic acid (Telepaque, 1–3 g orally or 0.5 g orally twice daily). These concentrated iodine therapies effectively block the conversion of T_4 to T_3 and inhibit the release of thyroid hormones. SSKI and Lugol solution should not be used when autonomous thyroid nodules are present, however, such as in toxic multinodular goiter or toxic adenoma, because they may worsen thyrotoxicosis. In addition, these therapies are generally used only in severe cases of thyrotoxicosis because their use precludes definitive therapy with radioactive iodine for several months as the thyroid processes the iodine load. In addition, concentrated iodine is less expensive and more readily available than radioactive iodine formulations and, thus, are more common in resource-limited settings.

Surgery

Surgery (subtotal or total thyroidectomy) is required for patients with compressive symptoms of the neck due to thyroid enlargement, such as hoarseness (from compression of the recurrent laryngeal nerve) or respiratory stridor, which indicates displacement of the trachea. Surgery may also be considered for cosmetic reasons in patients who have failed other treatment options and patients with refractory amiodarone-induced hyperthyroidism. Surgery is often recommended in patients with a large multinodular goiter or if thyroid cancer is suspected. It is also indicated in individuals who cannot tolerate antithyroid medications; however, an antithyroid medication may be administered during the presurgery stage to prevent excessive release of stored thyroid hormones during the procedure. In addition, propranolol is typically used to decrease the resting heart rate to below 80 beats per minute, and SSKI may be administered (1–2 drops orally twice daily) for 2 weeks before surgical resection.

Before the development of these preoperative pharmacotherapies, thyroidectomy was one of the most common causes of thyroid storm. Today, important complications of surgery include permanent hypothyroidism, which requires lifelong thyroid hormone replacement, and laryngeal paralysis via damage to the recurrent laryngeal nerve. Hypoparathyroidism may also result if one or more of the parathyroid glands is inadvertently resected during surgery.

Treatment of Subacute Thyroiditis

Subacute thyroiditis is a self-limited condition treated with beta-adrenergic blocking medications and NSAIDs. If patients have moderate to severe symptoms or do not respond to beta blockers and NSAIDs, they are candidates for treatment with corticosteroids. Subacute thyroiditis often follows a viral illness. After the thyroiditis, some patients may experience a transient hypothyroid state. These patients will need thyroid hormone until they return to a euthyroid state. For the patient with pain, NSAIDs may help. Short-term use of oral prednisone may be indicated for severe inflammation and pain; doses of 40 mg daily for 1 to 2 weeks with a gradual taper over 2 to 4 weeks are usually effective.

Treatment of Subclinical Hyperthyroidism

Subclinical hyperthyroidism is characterized by subnormal TSH levels in the face of normal concentrations of T_4 and T_3. Emerging research indicates that subclinical hyperthyroidism is associated with a higher mortality rate in persons older than 65 years of age. The Third National Health and Nutrition Examination Survey found that 0.7% of participants had subclinical hyperthyroidism (persons with known thyroid disease were excluded from the study). There is an increased risk of atrial fibrillation, particularly in postmenopausal women, as well as decreased bone density. Consultation with an endocrinologist is indicated for these patients. If treatment is not initiated, the patient should be monitored every 6 months for overt hyperthyroidism and assessed for the cardiac and bone effects of excess thyroid hormone.

Patients experiencing symptoms of infiltrative ophthalmopathy will need to be followed by an ophthalmologist. Glucocorticoids, diuretics, and methylcellulose eyedrops may provide symptomatic relief. Radiation or surgical decompression may be initiated by the ophthalmologist in severe cases.

FOLLOW-UP AND REFERRAL

Given the importance of both acute and long-term follow-up in the ongoing management of hyperthyroidism and its complications, appropriate referrals and follow-up schedules are discussed above in the section on Management. In general, the complex nature of thyrotoxicosis requires collaboration and referral to an endocrinologist for effective management and close follow-up.

Importantly, up to half of all patients with Graves' disease who enter remission after starting antithyroid pharmacotherapy without definitive thyroid ablation will have a second attack of thyrotoxicosis within 1 year. In addition, all patients with Graves' disease should be referred to an ophthalmologist for full evaluation, because up to half of these patients have some form of ophthalmopathy, which may present subclinically. However, Graves' disease ophthalmopathy may also present before the patient develops symptoms of full-blown thyrotoxicosis.

Specific time frames for follow-up are dependent on the choice of treatment and patient response, as described in the section on Management. TSH, FT_4, and T_3 levels should be monitored at each follow-up visit, as well as measurements of blood pressure, pulse, weight, and character of the thyroid gland. General guidelines for long-term follow-up include the following:

1. Monitor thyroid function tests at least twice a year.
2. Initial treatment should be evaluated at 1 month and at 6 months or more frequently if the patient is symptomatic.
3. Therapy with antithyroid medications should continue for 3 to 24 months.
4. After radioiodine ablative therapy, thyroid function tests should be performed at 4 to 6 weeks, 12 weeks, 6 months, and annually thereafter, if stable.

Patient Education: Hyperthyroidism

After diagnosis, the patient with hyperthyroidism should be given information about various treatment options, including the risks and benefits of each treatment and the consequences of no treatment. The importance of strict adherence to provider guidelines for follow-up must be stressed to each patient. If the treatment regimen has produced a state of hypothyroidism, the patient should be informed that thyroid hormone replacement therapy must continue for life.

Patients need to know that it may take 4 to 6 weeks after starting medication to notice an improvement in symptoms because of the amount of stored hormone in the thyroid gland. Patients who are unaware of this phenomenon may not comply with the treatment regimen. Patients need written instructions to monitor for the signs and symptoms of thyroid storm, as well as signs of hypothyroidism once treatment is initiated. The patient should be informed of the potential adverse reactions of all medications, particularly antithyroid preparations, and to discontinue the medication and to notify their primary-care practitioner if fever, sore throat, or malaise develops. Patients taking antithyroid medications should wear a medical identification bracelet.

Persons receiving radioactive iodine therapy should avoid contact with infants, children, and pregnant women for 7 days after ingestion. Women who receive this treatment postpartum must not breastfeed for at least 3 to 6 months, because radioactive iodine is excreted in breast milk and can ablate the infant's thyroid.

The need for adequate rest and exercise after ablative therapy should be stressed. Patients will need adequate sleep, as well as relaxation time, and should be taught methods to promote relaxation, such as biofeedback, music, or guided imagery. Patients should be encouraged to express their concerns regarding psychosocial implications of their disease, and the physiological basis for their symptoms should be reinforced.

Patients who complain of heat intolerance may benefit from wearing or sleeping on natural fabrics during the summer months and should remain adequately hydrated. Patients who have experienced significant weight loss may benefit from a high-carbohydrate, high-calorie diet. A patient with Graves' disease may benefit from dividing food intake into six smaller meals daily. If diarrhea is a problem, discourage foods that increase peristalsis such as highly seasoned foods and bulky or fiber-rich foods. Stimulants such as caffeine should be avoided.

The patient should check his or her weight daily and immediately report any weight loss of more than 4 pounds in 1 day. A consistent weight loss of 1 to 2 pounds daily should also be reported. Once treatment is initiated and the patient is euthyroid, caloric needs decrease but the patient may still have an increased appetite. A sensible diet low in fat and sugar with adequate protein may avoid significant unwanted weight gain during this period. The patient should be instructed to check his or her weight frequently and adjust dietary intake to maintain an ideal weight.

A supplemental multivitamin, particularly with vitamin B complex, is needed to prevent nutrient deficiencies in times of severe hyperthyroidism because of a high level of vitamin consumption during hyperthyroid states. For example, patients suspected of having long-standing hyperthyroidism may benefit from vitamin D and calcium supplementation because osteoporosis is a complication of elevated thyroid hormones.

Some patients may experience depression as the level of thyroid hormones change. This should be discussed with patients who should be instructed to report any worsening of symptoms of depression or anxiety to ensure prompt evaluation. If reassurance of such patients does not relieve anxiety, temporary symptomatic treatment with low-dose anxiolytics may be indicated.

Patients with exophthalmos should wear dark protective lenses when outdoors during the day. The use of artificial tears may relieve feelings of dryness and provide some corneal protection. Glasses or other eye protection should be worn during any activity that may introduce dust or dirt into the eyes. A sleeping mask should be worn at night if the patient cannot close the eyes adequately.

HYPOTHYROIDISM

Hypothyroidism is a common, treatable disorder in which there is a slow progression of thyroid hypofunction, followed by signs and symptoms indicating thyroid failure. It is a disease of various causes that lead to inadequate amounts of thyroid hormone being produced and/or secreted, resulting in a slowing of many bodily functions and metabolic processes. Because hypothyroidism has an insidious onset and progresses slowly, the clinical manifestations may go unrecognized.

EPIDEMIOLOGY AND CAUSES

The incidence of hypothyroidism varies with age, gender, and geographic and environmental factors. The incidence from numerous surveys ranges from 3 to 14 cases per 1,000 women, with significantly fewer cases reported in men. In fact, the incidence in women is 2 to 8 times greater than it is in men. It is estimated that as much as 4.6% of the U.S. population has an elevated TSH with a higher incidence in European Americans (5.1%) than in either Hispanics (4.1%) or African Americans (1.7%).

Thyroid hormone deficiency present at birth is known as *congenital hypothyroidism*. Affecting 1 in 4,000 newborns, the causes of congenital hypothyroidism include developmental abnormalities of the thyroid gland, enzymatic defects, iodine deficiency, maternal antibodies to thyroid hormones, and excessive intake of goitrogens by the mother. In such instances, the mother may also suffer from thyroid deficiency. Thyroid hormone deficiency beginning in early infancy and childhood is characterized by growth retardation, mental deficiency, and delayed dentition. Adolescents with primary hypothyroidism may present with an enlarged sella turcica and, rarely, precocious puberty, in addition to growth retardation. Growth retardation is treatable with hormone replacement therapy at this stage, but mental retardation persists.

The most common worldwide cause of thyroid disorders is iodine deficiency, with a worldwide prevalence of 2% to 5%. In the United States, where iodine ingestion is usually adequate due to the ready availability of iodized salt, autoimmune processes are the primary cause of thyroid disease. Hashimoto's thyroiditis, a type of primary hypothyroidism, is the most common form of autoimmune thyroid disease. This type of hypothyroidism occurs at least four times more often in women than in men, with the average age at onset from 30 to 60 years.

Subclinical hypothyroidism is the presence of normal free thyroxine immunoassay (FT_4) with an elevated TSH. As many as 15% of patients older than 65 years of age have this profile, as do many other adults. However, few of these patients report symptoms or their symptoms are nonspecific.

Iatrogenic hypothyroidism, which occurs after treatment with radioactive iodine (for hyperthyroidism) or surgery (for hyperthyroidism, thyroid nodules, or thyroid carcinoma), is the next most common cause of hypothyroidism, accounting for 30% to 40% of cases. Hypothyroidism also becomes increasingly common with age; in individuals older than 50 years of age, up to 10% may have elevated TSH levels.

More than 95% of patients with hypothyroidism have primary or thyroidal hypothyroidism, involving dysfunction or atrophy of the thyroid gland. When the thyroid dysfunction is caused by failure of the pituitary gland, the hypothalamus, or both, it is known as central hypothyroidism. More specifically, failure of the pituitary gland to secrete adequate amounts of TSH is known as secondary hypothyroidism, whereas tertiary hypothyroidism results from inadequate secretion of thyrotropin-releasing hormone (TRH) by the hypothalamus or failure of TRH to activate its cognate receptors within the pituitary gland (peripheral resistance). Table 57.4 summarizes the causes of hypothyroidism.

Risk factors for thyroid failure include a family history of thyroid disease, personal history of thyroid disease, presence of antithyroid antibodies, radiation treatment to the head, neck, or chest, other autoimmune diseases, advanced age, and the use of lithium, amiodarone (Cordarone), or iodine.

Although production of T_4 decreases with age, serum T_4 and TSH levels remain stable, whereas T_3 levels may decrease in persons older than 80 years of age. In many cases, hypothyroidism in the older adult is characterized by symptoms that may be subtle and similar to the normal signs of aging, thus making it easy to overlook. Common symptoms include hoarseness, deafness, confusion, frank psychosis, dementia, ataxia, depression, constipation, intolerance of cold temperatures, dry skin, and hair loss.

PATHOPHYSIOLOGY

Normal thyroid function is required for every metabolic process in the human body. Growth and development, protein synthesis, and cell metabolism are all dependent on an adequate supply of thyroid hormone to the

TABLE 57.4 Causes of Hypothyroidism

Cause	Etiology
Loss of functional thyroid tissue	Idiopathic hypothyroidism: atrophy (probably autoimmune), TSH receptor–blocking antibodies Chronic autoimmune thyroiditis (Hashimoto's disease) Amiodarone External radiation Status—post-radioiodine (^{131}I) treatment Status—post-thyroidectomy Infiltrating disorders: malignancy, granulomatous disease Thyroid dysgenesis
Biosynthetic defects in thyroid hormone production	Inherited defects in hormone synthesis Iodine deficiency Antithyroid agents: thioamides, lithium, iodide
Central hypothyroidism	TSH deficiency caused by pituitary disease: postpartum infarction (Sheehan syndrome), tumors (e.g., craniopharyngioma, pituitary adenoma), granulomatous disease (sarcoidosis), and irradiation TSH deficiency caused by hypothalamic disease: tumors, irradiation, and transiently occurring nonthyroidal illness Generalized resistance to thyroid hormones in both the pituitary and peripheral tissues
Transient hypothyroidism	Postpartum thyroiditis Subacute thyroiditis (usually viral) Withdrawal of thyroid hormone therapy in a euthyroid patient

Abbreviation: TSH, thyroid-stimulating hormone.

peripheral tissues. The thyroid plays an essential role in fetal development, oxygen consumption, heat production, sympathetic nervous system function, and cardiovascular, hematopoietic, pulmonary, and renal system function. Because of the multiple physiological effects of the thyroid gland, a deficiency of the T_4 hormone can lead to a complex array of clinical findings.

Localized thyroid disease is the most common cause of hypothyroidism in the United States, namely Hashimoto's autoimmune thyroiditis. Worldwide, iodine deficiency is the most common etiology, because this element is a critical component of all thyroid hormones and incorporation of iodide molecules is a critical step in thyroid hormone synthesis. Under normal circumstances, the thyroid secretes 100 to 125 mcg of T_4 per day but only minute amounts of T_3. T_4 is converted to T_3 in peripheral tissues, and T_3 is 20 to 100 times more biologically active than T_4.

When the production of T_4 is inadequate, the thyroid gland enlarges in response to increasing levels of pituitary TSH. This stimulates hypertrophy and hyperplasia of the thyroid gland, resulting in a *goiter*. In addition, deiodinase activity within the thyroid is increased, allowing for greater conversion of T_4 to T_3. Thus, the thyroid attempts to compensate by secreting increased amounts of T_3. However, in areas where the soil and water are deficient in iodine and iodized salt is not commonly available, inadequate substrate exists for these compensatory mechanisms, and endemic goiter results. Thus, simple (nontoxic) goiter is the most common type of thyroid enlargement.

Hashimoto's thyroiditis is the most common etiology of hypothyroidism in the United States. The pathogenesis of this autoimmune form of hypothyroidism is not fully understood but develops in individuals with genetic susceptibility coupled with environmental factors. Recent research has revealed that CD4+ Th17 T cells that secrete interleukin (IL)-17 may play a role in the induction of autoimmune disorders. Hashimoto's thyroiditis results when the body pathologically recognizes thyroid antigens as foreign, leading to a chronic immune response involving lymphocytic infiltration, vacuolization, and fibrosis of the thyroid parenchyma, which eventually leads to atrophy of the thyroid follicles.

Autoantibodies may be undetectable early on in the disease process. However, over the course of the disease, up to 95% of these patients develop serum antibodies to thyroid tissue, including antimicrosomal (anti-TPO) antibodies in 95% of patients and antithyroglobulin antibodies in 60% of patients. Over time, however, these autoantibodies usually become undetectable, and it is unclear whether these autoantibodies are truly pathogenic or simply reflect the underlying autoimmune process.

Inflammatory hypofunctioning thyroiditis may also result from other etiologies. Destructive thyroid inflammation may occur due to immune cross reactivity after viral infections, producing transient forms of hypothyroidism including the painful de Quervain thyroiditis, as well as subacute thyroiditis. In addition to having a painful and tender thyroid gland, these patients are often significantly fatigued.

Lymphocytic thyroiditis and transient hypothyroidism also occur in up to 10% of new mothers between 2 and 10 months postpartum. This figure may rise as high as 25% in those with other autoimmune conditions such as type 1 DM. This condition is usually transient, lasting less than 4 months, and responds well to short courses of thyroid hormone replacement. However, postpartum thyroiditis predisposes women to long-term hypothyroidism in the future.

Several iatrogenic causes of hypothyroidism have been recognized. Amiodarone (Cordarone), an iodine-containing antiarrhythmic, can have direct inhibitory effects on the thyroid gland. Interferon-α, thalidomide, and the antiretroviral agent stavudine have also been associated with primary hypothyroidism. Both dopamine and lithium are associated with central (secondary or tertiary) hypothyroidism due to their effects on the hypothalamic-pituitary axis and the secretion of TRH from the hypothalamus or TSH from the pituitary gland. As a noniatrogenic cause, central hypothyroidism may also result from direct impingement by tumors on the pituitary gland (e.g., a pituitary adenoma that fails to produce TSH) or the hypothalamus. Brain irradiation has also been associated with subsequent defects along the hypothalamic-pituitary hormonal axis.

By far, however, the most common reason for iatrogenic hypothyroidism is the therapeutic result of previously treated hyperthyroidism (see previous section on hyperthyroidism in this chapter). Radioactive iodine treatment (^{131}I, Iodotope), concentrated iodine therapy (SSKI, Lugol solution), therapeutic surgical resection, or treatment for head and neck cancer involving external beam irradiation to the neck or surgical excision of a cancerous mass may all result in permanent hypothyroidism. Thus, these patients require close follow-up to detect clinical or biochemical evidence of hypothyroidism.

Low levels of thyroid hormones affect virtually every bodily system, resulting in an overall decrease in basal metabolic rate. An insufficient amount of thyroid hormone causes abnormalities in lipid metabolism, with an increase in total cholesterol, low-density lipoproteins (LDLs), and triglycerides. These increases are associated with the development of atherosclerosis and cardiac disease in the hypothyroid patient. The gastrointestinal (GI) tract may be slowed in both gastric emptying and intestinal transit time, and gastric parietal cell dysfunction may result in achlorhydria and impaired digestion. Deficiencies in vitamin B_{12}, iron, and folate may also occur. Endocrine abnormalities of hypothyroidism include menstrual irregularities, infertility, delayed onset of puberty, and insulin resistance. Adequate amounts of thyroid hormone are also necessary for optimal erythropoiesis, and anemia is common in patients with hypothyroidism.

A characteristic pathophysiological change of hypothyroidism is the accumulation of hydrophilic proteoglycans within the interstitial space, which causes an increase in interstitial fluid. Pleural, cardiac, and peritoneal effusions are a common result of this process, as is the characteristic mucinous edema seen in long-standing hypothyroidism, known as myxedema. In a general sense, myxedema denotes infiltration of various bodily tissues with glycosaminoglycan substances, which may have widespread effects. In the heart, this infiltration decreases both chronotropy and inotropy, leading to cardiac hypertrophy as the body attempts to compensate for the decreased cardiac output.

CLINICAL PRESENTATION

Subjective

The clinical presentation of the patient with hypothyroidism varies with the age at onset, duration of illness, and severity of disease. Regardless of the type or cause of hypothyroidism, the symptoms are similar. Because this can be an insidious disease, the early symptoms are often subtle and nonspecific, increasing the risk of a missed diagnosis. The severity of symptoms may be related to the duration of hypothyroidism. A rapid onset of hypothyroidism is associated with more recognizable symptoms than is a gradual onset. The symptoms are directly related to the inadequate amount of thyroid hormone in the peripheral tissues.

Classic early symptoms include fatigue, dry skin, slight weight gain, cold intolerance, constipation, and heavy menses. Myalgia, muscle cramps, headaches, and weakness may also be present. Later symptoms include very dry skin, coarse hair, loss of lateral eyebrows, alopecia, hoarseness, continued weight gain, slight impairment in mental ability, depression, decreased libido, and hypersomnia. Many of the symptoms are common complaints, which are not specific by themselves but together make up the manifestations of clinical hypothyroidism. Subclinical disease may be even more subtle or asymptomatic.

A complete review of systems is needed because symptoms are often subtle and may involve every bodily system. The presence of pain and swelling or enlargement in the neck, a history of radiation to the neck, and previous endocrine problems in the past medical history or family history should be elicited. It is also important to obtain a complete medication history, and, for women, a complete menstrual history is essential, including the most recent date, characteristics, and duration of the last menstrual period. Some findings are more specific for Hashimoto's thyroiditis including painless thyroid enlargement, neck pain, sore throat, a feeling of fullness in the throat, low-grade fever, and exhaustion.

Patients with hypothyroidism often experience decreased motility of the GI system, and constipation may be present. Researchers have found a link between patients with autoimmune thyroid disease and atrophic gastritis who also present with pernicious anemia.

Objective

The physical examination should begin with an observation of the overall appearance of the patient, noting slow movements and dull facies. The blood pressure, resting pulse, respiratory rate, and weight should be compared with previous examinations.

The hair may become coarse and thin, and thinning of the eyebrows may occur. Patients with hypothyroidism frequently have a thickened tongue, evidenced by indentations from the teeth around the tongue edges. The character of the thyroid is variable and may be enlarged and tender with a visible goiter or, alternatively, nonpalpable. The consistency, size, and nodularity (focal or diffuse) of the thyroid should be noted, as well as any scars present on the neck that could signify past thyroid surgery.

The heart may be hypertrophic, which may be identified by noting a laterally displaced point of maximal impulse. The patient is usually bradycardic and may have a pericardial effusion. Similarly, the lung examination may reveal a pleural effusion. The abdominal examination usually reveals diminished or hypoactive bowel sounds. On neurological examination, the patient may be hypotonic and hyporeflexic with a prolonged relaxation phase and/or ataxic.

The patient with hypothyroidism may have facial puffiness, periorbital edema, dry and thick skin, dry and coarse hair, brittle nails, slow speech, bradykinesia, hoarseness, an enlarged tongue, bradycardia, mild diastolic hypertension, psychological disorders, and pitting edema of the lower extremities. Myxedematous changes occur in the later stages of hypothyroidism, with thickened, scaly, and "doughy" skin, an enlarged tongue, muscle weakness, joint complaints, a hearing impairment, and ascites. Table 57.5 summarizes the clinical presentation of hypothyroidism.

DIAGNOSTIC REASONING

Diagnostic Tests

Initial Testing

Although one in five women will develop an alteration in thyroid function in her lifetime, recently published clinical guidelines do not recommend routine screening of asymptomatic women before age 50 years. Many clinicians, however, still use age 40 years as their criterion to begin screening. Although there are no universally accepted screening recommendations for hypothyroidism, the American Thyroid Association recommends baseline screening at age 35 years, with close attention to high-risk patients (e.g., pregnant women, women older than 60 years of age, persons with other autoimmune diseases). The American Association of Clinical Endocrinologists recommends assessing TSH in women of childbearing age before pregnancy and in the first trimester. Women experiencing unexplained infertility should be screened for thyroid dysfunction, and postpartum women with vague complaints may benefit from screening. In addition, congenital hypothyroidism is routinely screened for in neonates, as mandated in most states because failing to treat hypothyroidism promptly in this group may have serious sequelae (e.g., intellectual and developmental disabilities).

In 2015, the USPSTF reviewed the 2004 recommendations for thyroid screening and reaffirmed that there is insufficient evidence for or against routine screening for thyroid disease in adults without symptoms. In turn, the USPSTF does not recommend routine screening in adults without specific risk factors. However, all patients with an abnormal thyroid examination or prior history of

TABLE 57.5 Clinical Presentation: Hypothyroidism		
Bodily System	**Subjective**	**Objective**
General	Fatigue Lethargy Mild weight gain Cold intolerance Mild depression Decreased libido Hypersomnia Muscle weakness and cramping	Slowing of mental processes Dull facial expression Periorbital puffiness Hypothermia Yellow skin (carotenemia) Facial pallor/swelling (myxedema)
Integumentary	Decreased sweating Hair loss Ankle swelling	Dry, cool, rough skin Alopecia Dry, coarse, thick hair Nonpitting edema
Gastrointestinal	Constipation Nausea	Hypoactive bowel sounds Large tongue Ascites
Neurological	Memory deficits Personality changes	Hyporeflexia Bradykinesia Delayed relaxation of reflexes Slowing of mental processes
Cardiopulmonary	Inability to exercise	Bradycardia Cardiac enlargement Pleural effusion
Genitourinary	Menorrhagia, irregular menses	Decrease in fertility
Head and neck	Enlargement of the neck	Enlarged tongue (late stage) Hoarseness

any medically or surgically treated thyroid disease should be screened with a yearly serum TSH measurement while stable. In addition, patients with other autoimmune diseases such as DM type 1 or pernicious anemia, unexplained depression or other psychiatric diagnoses, cognitive dysfunction, prior external beam irradiation to the head and neck, previous radioablation of the thyroid, hypercholesterolemia, chronic amiodarone or lithium use, or a first-degree relative with autoimmune thyroid disease or other autoimmune disorders should be screened with TSH measurements.

The diagnosis of hypothyroidism is made by measuring serum TSH. TSH and FT_4 should also be used to monitor treatment. When autoimmune thyroiditis is the suspected underlying cause of hypothyroidism, confirmation should be sought by performing antithyroid antibody titers—either for antimicrosomal (anti-TPO) antibodies or antithyroglobulin antibodies. The antimicrosomal antibody test is more sensitive and specific. If the TSH is low, inappropriately normal, or insufficiently elevated in the presence of low T_4 values, central hypothyroidism caused by hypothalamic or pituitary disease should be excluded before starting thyroid replacement therapy.

The sensitive thyrotropin assay is the most specific test for diagnosing primary hypothyroidism. A rise in the TSH will precede any other abnormality of thyroid function as the first evidence of primary hypothyroidism. Hypothyroidism caused by primary thyroid failure can be confirmed by a concomitant finding of a decrease in serum FT_4. Patients in an early stage of hypothyroidism may present with an increase in serum TSH level together with a normal or low-normal serum FT_4 level

By radioimmunoassay, primary hypothyroidism is associated with low FT_4 with an elevated TSH level. Values will differ depending on the laboratory method used. The normal range of ultrasensitive TSH is 0.4 to 4.0 milliunits/L. The elderly have a slightly higher normal range. TSH levels from 4.5 to 10 milliunits/L have varied treatment recommendations. Absent cardiovascular disease, there are no outcome data to suggest that treatment for levels between 2.5 and 4.5 milliunits/L is beneficial. An elevated TSH (up to 15 to 20 milliunits/L) may be temporarily observed in euthyroid patients with a systemic illness. In this situation, the TSH and T_4 should be repeated in 2 to 3 weeks for confirmation.

Patients with secondary or tertiary (central) hypothyroidism show a low, normal, or mildly elevated TSH level with low FT_4 and T_3 by radioimmunoassay. In subclinical hypothyroidism, these laboratory values show a mildly increased TSH level with a normal FT_4 concentration. Measurement of FT_4 is always preferred over total T_4, because of alterations in the protein-binding of thyroid hormone levels that can result in large fluctuations in total serum T_4 levels. The free thyroxine index (FTI), although not the test of choice, may be used if laboratories that do not have the capacity to measure FT_4. FTI

uses a T_3 resin uptake test to calculate the percentage of hormone-binding sites available and multiplies this by the total T_4 level to give an estimation of the free T_4 level.

A high (1:400) antimicrosomal (anti-TPO) antibody titer is diagnostic for Hashimoto's thyroiditis. The degree of antibody elevation correlates directly with clinical hypothyroidism, although it is unclear whether the antibodies themselves are pathogenic because clinical disease may also be apparent with low or absent titers. When hypothyroidism is present for a long period of time, antibody titers typically fall. The antithyroglobulin antibody is also increased, but it is not as specific for Hashimoto's thyroiditis. If no antibodies are identified at the time of diagnosis, the condition is called *idiopathic hypothyroidism,* which is also considered a form of autoimmune thyroiditis. Antimicrosomal antibody titers and thyroid hormone (TSH and FT_4) levels should also be evaluated in patients with repeat miscarriages.

Medications such as metoclopramide (Reglan) increase TSH levels. Dopamine (Intropin), glucocorticoids, NSAIDs, and somatostatin decrease TSH levels. Other medications, such as phenytoin (Dilantin), amiodarone (Cordarone), and lithium carbonate, can also affect thyroid function tests. Smoking (nicotine) also impacts thyroid hormone levels. These medication and chemical exposures act via a number of mechanisms to affect thyroid function. A drug may bind with albumin and displace thyroid hormone off carrier proteins, or it may prevent albumin from binding with T_3 or T_4, in each case resulting in more active hormone in circulation. Some drugs may cause an upregulation in metabolic processing proteins (i.e., different cytochrome P oxidase isomers), which normally inactivate thyroid hormones; thus, their upregulation can lead to more rapid processing of thyroid hormones and, in turn, affect TSH levels.

Subsequent Testing

Once a diagnosis of hypothyroidism is confirmed, additional testing may be necessary to determine the effect of the disease on other bodily systems. Because the T_3 level is nonspecific and insensitive, it is not routinely used as an initial diagnostic tool. In the early stages of hypothyroidism, T_3 levels may be normal because of TSH-induced hyperstimulation. T_3 levels may not fall until late in the disease. Because the T_3 level correlates well with clinical status, the patient will not be as severely hypothyroid in clinical presentation until the T_3 falls to significantly low levels. In addition, the T_3 level may be below normal or elevated in patients with chronic disease.

Because anemia is a frequent complication of hypothyroidism, a CBC should be done. In addition, a blood chemistry profile should be done to assess for alterations in serum electrolytes, blood urea nitrogen, creatinine, serum osmolarity, and glucose, because glomerular filtration rate (renal function) can be decreased. A urinalysis should also be performed, with specific attention to the presence of protein (indicating possible renal impairment). Changes in blood chemistry may be an indication of deteriorating thyroid function leading to myxedema.

Patients with mild to moderate hypothyroidism have a tendency to develop hypertension (especially diastolic hypertension); therefore, blood pressure should be monitored. Interestingly, patients with long-standing or severe hypothyroidism tend to be normotensive or hypotensive. Depression of the uptake of LDL cholesterol by the liver in hypothyroid patients due to decreased LDL receptor expression (among other mechanisms) causes a decreased rate of cholesterol catabolism that leads to hypercholesterolemia. These patients tend to have elevated triglycerides and elevated LDL cholesterol. The combination of hypertension and hyperlipidemia increases the risk of atherosclerotic heart disease in hypothyroid patients. Thus, an annual lipid profile and an electrocardiogram (ECG) should be done. As the cardiac system continues to deteriorate, the ECG may show nonspecific ST and T-wave changes or low-voltage QRS complexes.

Unless there is reason to suspect a thyroid nodule or to confirm multinodular goiter, radioactive iodine scans and uptake are not usually necessary in hypothyroidism. As part of a complete examination of the patient with hypothyroidism, patients should have an annual chest x-ray examination to rule out cardiopulmonary complications, including cardiomegaly, congestive heart failure, and pleural effusion.

Ultrasound studies of the thyroid may be useful if a nodular thyroid is detected or if infiltrative disease is suspected (e.g., amyloidosis, sarcoidosis, or tuberculosis). Fine-needle aspiration (FNA) is indicated for suspicious nodules, which may be found in patients with hypothyroidism, hyperthyroidism, or euthyroidism. In fact, 5% to 6% of isolated nodules are malignant, especially larger ones, and ultrasound may reveal suspicious findings for cancer such as irregular margins or microcalcifications.

Differential Diagnosis

Marked variations in TSH may occur in the setting of an acute illness or psychiatric disorder when the body's metabolic demands are altered. TSH levels normally peak in the evening and are at their lowest in the afternoon. Nonthyroidal illness is often associated with decreased TSH, T_3, and FT_4 levels without clinical hypothyroidism, with a reduction in the conversion of T_3 from T_4. In addition, usually the TSH level is normal or mildly increased during recovery from nonthyroidal illness.

In euthyroid hypothyroxinemia, the patient is euthyroid with a decreased T_4 level due to a decreased concentration of thyroid-binding globulin caused by nephrotic syndrome, exogenous testosterone exposure, or high-dose corticosteroids. Also, drugs that inhibit T_4 binding, such as phenytoin, phenobarbital, and salicylates, may decrease the total T_4 level.

MANAGEMENT

The goal of thyroid hormone replacement in primary hypothyroidism is to normalize, not suppress, the TSH, given the risks of overtreatment. Suppressed TSH, particularly in postmenopausal women or individuals with levothyroxine over-replacement, causes decreased bone mineral density after several years, leading to osteoporosis. Hypothyroidism is typically treated medically (see Drugs Commonly Prescribed 57.2). However, surgery may be indicated for particularly large, nonfunctional goiters that impair tracheoesophageal functioning. The replacement goal in central hypothyroidism is to normalize the FT_4 because the TSH is not a reliable indicator of euthyroidism. The usual medication is levothyroxine (Levothroid, Levoxyl, Synthroid), a synthetic preparation of T_4, which has generally replaced desiccated bovine thyroid preparations, given their greater purity and consistency of dosing. Levothyroxine preparations are manufactured in numerous dosages, allowing for specific, precise titration to meet individual patient requirements.

Drugs Commonly Prescribed 57.2: Hypothyroidism: Lifelong Pharmaceutical Treatment

DRUG	INDICATIONS	ADVERSE REACTIONS AND PRESCRIBING CONSIDERATIONS
Synthetic L-thyroxine* T_4 (Levothroid, Levoxyl, Synthroid)	Patients with increased TSH level, usually three times the upper limit of the assay Overt hypothyroidism Goal: administer enough thyroid supplement orally to result in normal free T_4 and TSH levels	Monitor antihyperglycemics, oral anticoagulants, and potential sympathomimetics. Wait 4–5 hours after cholestyramine ingestion. Not to be prescribed for obesity. Use with caution in patients with cardiovascular disease, diabetes mellitus, adrenal insufficiency. Increased sensitivity in myxedema and severe hypothyroidism. Start with the lowest dose and increase by 0.025 mg/day every 3–6 weeks as needed, to no more than a maximum of 0.3 mg per day. Older adults require slightly lower initial doses.

*Synthetic T_3 supplements (Cytomel) are not recommended as a drug of choice.

According to the medical guidelines developed by the American Association of Clinical Endocrinologists, the usual dose is 1.6 mcg/kg per day for full replacement. Otherwise healthy patients younger than 60 years may receive 50 to 100 mcg daily as a full replacement dose. Patients who are older or have coronary artery disease should begin with one-half of the expected replacement dose or 25 to 50 mcg/day orally, increasing the dose gradually by 25 mcg/day once every 4 to 6 weeks. The TSH level should be measured every 4 to 8 weeks after initiating therapy and before each dosage increase. The common dosage is 75 to 150 mcg/day. Dosing is best done in the morning to avoid nighttime insomnia. Many other medications and mineral supplements interfere with GI absorption of thyroid hormone replacements, including iron, calcium carbonate, aluminum hydroxide, sucralfate, and tube feedings. Thus, these medications require separation of dosing in time, whereas patients receiving continuous tube feedings require IV thyroxine dosing.

Replacement with T_3 preparations (liothyronine [Cytomel, Triostat]) is usually not indicated; however, anecdotal reports exist that indicated combination T_3/T_4 therapy may be helpful in patients who do not respond adequately to T_4 replacement alone. Although T_3 is better absorbed via the GI tract than T_4, the appropriate ratio of triiodothyronine preparations versus thyroxine in combination therapy has not been well established, and such treatment decisions require expert input from an endocrinologist.

Another treatment of historical importance that is still used today in some settings owing to its relative lower cost is desiccated bovine thyroid (Armour Thyroid). Obtained from pooled thyroid extracts from cows, these preparations contain multiple foreign antigens, and the specific levels of active hormone are difficult to control. Some manufacturers standardize preparations based on bioassays, whereas others use iodine content as a surrogate measure of activity. T_3 and T_4 are both present, usually in a 1:4 ratio. Although some older patients who have been treated for many years with desiccated thyroid are wary of changing medications after decades of replacement therapy at stable doses, few clinicians in the United States will start new patients on these preparations. They should not be used for patients with underlying cardiac disease, given the varied concentrations of highly active T_3, which poses a greater risk of over-replacement and iatrogenic thyrotoxicosis.

Regardless of choice of replacement therapy, all patients should be monitored for signs of thyrotoxicity, especially angina pectoris and arrhythmias, because optimizing thyroid replacement dosing can be difficult and time consuming. If significant adverse symptoms occur during levothyroxine replacement, the dose should be decreased and the patient should be referred to an endocrinologist for evaluation before reattempting replacement therapy at the original higher dose.

Concurrent severe illness or major surgery may alter dosing requirements in either direction in the hypothyroid patient. Pregnancy is also well known to increase replacement therapy requirements. Some clinicians suggest increasing replacement dosing by 30% upon confirmation of pregnancy, with subsequent adjustments guided by TSH levels because untreated hypothyroidism in pregnancy is associated with preeclampsia, postpartum cardiac dysfunction, anemia, miscarriage, and low birth weight. The levothyroxine dose should be returned to the pre-pregnancy dose after delivery, and a serum TSH level should be obtained at 6 to 8 weeks postpartum.

Untreated hypothyroidism may progress steadily for 10 to 15 years before resulting in *myxedema coma*—a life-threatening state of multiorgan failure, characterized by progressive respiratory depression, decreased cardiac output, and fluid and electrolyte abnormalities (including hyponatremia)—or even death. Box 57.1 presents the assessment and management of patients with myxedema coma.

Treatment of Subclinical Hypothyroidism

Treatment for subclinical hypothyroidism has varied recommendations. The American Thyroid Association and the American Association of Clinical Endocrinologists recommend treating subclinical disease when there is presence of antithyroid antibodies, when evidence of atherosclerotic cardiovascular disease exists, when heart failure exists, or if the patient is symptomatic at the respective TSH level.

Some patients with subclinical hypothyroidism feel better when treated with levothyroxine. Medication therapy has potentially dangerous adverse effects but may improve subtle abnormalities, prevent goitrous growth, and prevent the development of frank hypothyroidism. Therapy is advisable especially if thyroid autoantibodies are positive, because overt hypothyroidism frequently develops in these patients.

In young patients or patients with goiter and subclinical hypothyroidism, levothyroxine therapy should be considered. If the decision is made not to treat these patients, they should be evaluated at 6- to 12-month intervals for evidence of more severe clinical disease or biological loss of thyroid function as reflected in worsening laboratory indices. A lower dose (0.5–1.0 mcg/kg) of levothyroxine may be given for the treatment of subclinical hypothyroidism. If the diagnosis of hypothyroidism is uncertain in a patient who is already on levothyroxine, the dose can be reduced by one-half, and FT_4 and TSH levels can be reassessed in 6 to 8 weeks. If the TSH level is increasing, the patient should resume the previous higher dose. If the TSH is normal, the patient should discontinue the levothyroxine, and the TSH level should be rechecked in 6 to 8 weeks for any increase.

Box 57.1 Assessment and Management of Myxedema Coma

Untreated hypothyroidism may progress steadily for 10 to 15 years before resulting in myxedema coma (a life-threatening condition characterized by progressive respiratory depression, decreased cardiac output, and fluid and electrolyte abnormalities) or death. Myxedema coma is severe hypothyroidism, most commonly seen in older adult women, presenting with altered mental status (profound lethargy or coma), hypothermia, bradycardia, hypoventilation, hypoglycemia, and adrenal insufficiency. It is usually triggered by a precipitating factor such as noncompliance with levothyroxine therapy, ingestion of narcotics or analgesics, sepsis, cerebrovascular accident (stroke), myocardial infarction, trauma, or severe stress. The mortality rate can be greater than 50% despite emergency medical intervention.

Assessment

The patient is usually pale with periorbital edema, dry skin, decreased temperature, macroglossia, distant heart sounds, bradycardia, and delayed deep tendon reflexes. The patient may have hyponatremia, seizures, and hypotension, with secondary respiratory acidosis, hypoxia, and retention of CO_2. A clinical diagnosis is required, in addition to laboratory confirmation, as T_4 is usually low while TSH is high.

Management

Provide ventilatory support if indicated, treat hypothermia, and administer levothyroxine (Synthroid, Levothroid) IV 300 to 500 mcg over 15 minutes and then IV 100 mcg every 24 hours to bring thyroxine concentrations back to normal levels quickly. Glucocorticoids should also be administered until coexistent adrenal insufficiency can be ruled out. Hydrocortisone hemisuccinate 100 mg IV bolus is initially given, followed by 50 mg IV every 12 hours or 25 mg IV every 6 hours until the plasma cortisol level is confirmed as within normal limits. Administer IV hydration to correct hypotension, adding dextrose if hypoglycemia is present. Avoid overhydration because clearance of free water is impaired in these patients. Rule out and treat precipitating factors (e.g., if septic or otherwise infected of bacterial origin, treat with antibiotics). Patients with myxedema coma need emergency medical intervention and should be treated by an endocrinologist in an intensive care setting.

FOLLOW-UP AND REFERRAL

After therapy has been initiated with levothyroxine, the primary-care practitioner should monitor the impact of therapy in 4 to 8 weeks by evaluating the TSH level to determine whether adjustment of the levothyroxine dose is necessary. The target TSH level is 0.3 to 2.4 mIU/L. Increasing the levothyroxine dose more often than at 6-week intervals may lead to thyroid hormone over-replacement. Once a stable dose of levothyroxine has been established, the TSH level in primary hypothyroidism or the FT_4 level in central hypothyroidism can be checked biannually or annually.

The patient should be examined annually for manifestations of thyrotoxicity (e.g., tachycardia, nervousness, or tremor) before increasing thyroid hormone replacement dosages. Laboratory values (FT_4 and TSH levels) within normal limits and a satisfactory clinical examination suggest that treatment is adequate. For maintenance treatment, the medication should be titrated to the lowest dose required to maintain euthyroidism, with a normal TSH level and a normal or slightly elevated T_4 concentration. Undetectable TSH levels suggest overtreatment, and the dose of thyroid hormone replacement should be decreased in these patients. TSH levels greater than 10 mIU/L indicate undertreatment, in which case the dose of hormone replacement medication should be increased.

Referral to an endocrinologist is necessary if the patient has cardiac disease, symptoms of myxedema, or central (secondary or tertiary) hypothyroidism. After starting hormone replacement therapy, if signs or symptoms of myxedema, chest pain, or thyrotoxicosis develop, an endocrinologist should be consulted. These patients are at a high risk for serious complications related to hypothyroidism or its treatment. Hypothyroid patients with severe illness or those who present with unusual or confusing laboratory findings should be referred to an endocrinologist. Referral to an endocrinologist is also indicated in patients younger than 18 years of age, in those with evidence of pituitary disease, in pregnant and postpartum patients, and in patients taking lithium or amiodarone (Cordarone).

For asymptomatic patients with subclinical hypothyroidism who (after consultation) are not being treated with medication, a TSH should be performed yearly, along with a focused history and physical examination to monitor for disease progression that may require the initiation of therapy.

Patient Education: Hypothyroidism

During follow-up visits, emphasis should be placed on compliance with lifelong thyroid therapy (if indicated), reviewing the symptoms of hypothyroidism and hyperthyroidism, and stressing the importance of adherence to the follow-up schedule. Instructions should be simple and repeated frequently with written information in the patient's primary language. An older adult or patient with decreased mental status or depression with hypothyroidism may need additional emotional support, reinforcement, and follow-up teaching. Support in the home setting may be necessary until the symptoms of slowed mental processes and depression abate. Initially, a family member may be needed to remind the patient to take his or her daily dose of medication (see The Patient's Voice 57.1).

Patients should be encouraged to wear an extra layer of clothing if they have cold intolerance and should be warned not to use a heating pad, since patients with diminished mental status, deceased sensitivity, and slowed responses may be at risk for thermal burns. If psychomotor symptoms are present, the patient should be cautioned against operating dangerous machinery or driving a motor vehicle until the symptoms have resolved.

Patients who are at high risk for hypothyroidism (e.g., those who have had previous thyroid surgery, radioactive iodine treatment, a history of thyroiditis, and postpartum women) should be taught the common symptoms of hypothyroidism (e.g., lethargy, fatigue, cold intolerance, constipation, weight gain, dry skin). The patient and family should be instructed that hypothyroidism is a chronic, sometimes progressive disease requiring monitoring every 6 to 12 months to monitor response to therapy. Patients and their families should be reassured that as the treatment progresses, the symptoms will resolve. Because heredity is implicated in hypothyroidism, patients with children should be instructed to advise their child's primary-care practitioner of their diagnosis.

Practitioners are encouraged to write prescriptions for thyroid hormone replacement therapy that do not allow for substitution and use the same medication brand for the patient throughout treatment to maintain consistency of dosing. The same brand of thyroid preparation is recommended because the bioavailability, stability, and content of active thyroid hormone may vary with different formulations. Patients should be given the rationale for their choice treatment, potential adverse effect profile, and dosage of their medication. Emphasis should be on the realization that medication use is lifelong. The patient should understand that as the body ages or as there are changes in body weight (including loss in body mass from bulky surgical amputations), pregnant or non-pregnant state, or other significant changes in metabolic demand, the dosage of thyroid replacement medication may need to be adjusted.

The patient should be taught the signs of iatrogenic hyperthyroidism (thyrotoxicity) due to thyroid replacement overdosage (e.g., nervousness, palpitations, insomnia, tremor). It is important to explain that it will take 1 to 2 weeks for the medication to be effective. During this time, patients may experience an increase in urination and a decrease in periorbital puffiness.

The absorption of levothyroxine from the GI tract may be slowed by concurrent use of certain drugs, such as ferrous sulfate, sucralfate (Carafate), or antacids. The dose of thyroid hormone should be taken 2 hours before or 4 hours after ingestion of these medications. Because levothyroxine supplements may increase blood glucose levels, patients with diabetes mellitus should carefully monitor their blood sugar levels, as doses of insulin or oral hypoglycemic agents may need to be adjusted. Thyroid hormones may also affect the levels of phenytoin (Dilantin), lithium, tricyclic antidepressants, estrogen, digitalis, anticoagulants, and indomethacin (Indocin). The appropriate blood tests and screenings should be performed, and patients should be instructed on key adverse reactions of thyroid hormone replacement to report, should they occur.

Because of increased sensitivity to certain medications in hypothyroid patients, patients should be cautioned against the use of analgesics and sedatives. Even in small dosages, these medications can cause severe somnolence and respiratory depression. Infrequently, a patient treated for hypothyroidism with normal TSH levels may continue to feel fatigued but should be discouraged from increasing the dose of thyroid hormone without consultation with a clinician, which some patients may be tempted to do. Persistent fatigue warrants further investigation as to the underlying cause and should be discussed during a clinic visit. In cases where patient compliance may be a problem, weekly dosing can be established with the guidance of an endocrinologist because the half-life of T_4 is approximately 1 week.

Patients should be taught to follow a healthy diet, with an emphasis on low-fat, high-fiber foods. Some patients may need to follow a diet that promotes weight loss once medication has been started. Because many patients with hypothyroidism experience constipation, they should increase their intake of raw fruits and vegetables and bran or high-fiber cereals and breads, and add unprocessed bran (two tablespoons daily) to cereal or liquids. A bulk-forming laxative containing psyllium may also be taken on a daily basis. Increasing water intake to six to eight glasses a day is often beneficial in reducing constipation, as is increasing physical activity. A low-fat diet is recommended because there is a high incidence of atherosclerotic heart disease in patients with hypothyroidism.

Once therapy with levothyroxine is initiated, the patient should be able to resume all previous activities. Initially, rest periods with a gradual increase in exercise and activity, as tolerated, may be indicated. The patient must be instructed that if he or she develops any signs or symptoms of cardiac or respiratory difficulty, it is essential to seek immediate medical attention.

 The Patient's Voice 57.1

I pretty much had a normal life. I was working in an administrative job, was in a bad relationship, and was perimenopausal. I would get home from work, and it was a struggle to make dinner and clean up. I was exhausted all the time. I had trouble getting out of bed in the morning even after going to bed at 7:00 p.m.! On the weekends I would sleep for 14 hours a night and still wake up tired. At meetings, where I had once been quick with suggestions, I couldn't seem to think and put two sentences together. I had trouble finding the right words. I thought I was getting early Alzheimer's.

I was 50 years old, and I felt like 100! I was constipated, cold all the time, and in a mental fog every day. I saw my primary-care practitioner. She told me I was probably depressed because of my life situation and being perimenopausal and prescribed an antidepressant. After taking that for more than a month, I was not feeling any better and saw a different provider. That provider did a bunch of tests, and a TSH level was one of them. The results were through the roof. My thyroid was almost entirely shut down. If someone had just done the test earlier, I could have been spared a few years of total exhaustion.

THYROID CANCER

Thyroid cancer is classified as differentiated (papillary and follicular) or undifferentiated (medullary and anaplastic) forms. Approximately 60% of thyroid cancers are papillary, 20% are follicular, and the remaining 20% of cases are medullary or anaplastic.

EPIDEMIOLOGY AND CAUSES

Thyroid cancer is the most common endocrine-related cancer. The incidence of thyroid cancer in the United States is low, with an approximate lifetime risk of 1.2%. The National Cancer Institute estimates there were 56,870 new cases of thyroid cancer diagnosed in 2017. The incidence increases with age and is more common in adults aged 20 to 54 years, but thyroid cancer can occur at any age and is three times more common in women than in men.

Most thyroid cancers are small and slow growing. Nodules are often found on routine physical examinations, by the patient, or via imaging done for other purposes. Thyroid nodules found in persons younger than 20 years of age or in adults older than 60 years of age are more likely to be cancerous. Anaplastic tumors are the fastest growing of all thyroid neoplasms; they are more common in older adults and are associated with a high mortality rate. Overall, thyroid cancer accounts for 0.3% of all cancer deaths per year.

The major risk factor for developing thyroid cancer is exposure to ionizing radiation. Several historical incidents resulting in high-dose radiation exposure have been linked to an increased incidence of papillary thyroid malignancies in children, including the atomic bombings of the Japanese cities of Hiroshima and Nagasaki during World War II, military testing of the atomic bomb near the Marshall Islands, and the nuclear power plant meltdown in the Russian city of Chernobyl.

Moreover, until the 1950s, radiation treatments were given to children as treatment for an enlarged thymus, enlarged tonsils, and acne. It is estimated that 1 to 2 million individuals were exposed to this risk factor. Studies have estimated that one-third of patients who received radiation therapy to the head and neck will develop a thyroid nodule, and one-third of those patients will later develop a thyroid malignancy. Thus, it may be advisable for patients who received head and neck irradiation as children to have an thyroid ultrasound for screening purposes.

Importantly, low-dose radiation exposure associated with routine radiographic imaging studies has not been shown to be tumorigenic. Interestingly, ^{131}I radioablation therapy for thyrotoxicosis and high-dose external beam radiotherapy have not been associated with papillary thyroid carcinoma, presumably because of the greater amount of cellular apoptosis associated with these doses of radiation.

There is also an increased incidence of follicular and anaplastic thyroid carcinoma in areas where iodine deficiency and goiter are more prevalent. Thyroid cancer is also more common in persons with autoimmune disease. Medullary carcinoma is an inherited form of familial thyroid cancer, with 90% of those inheriting the autosomal dominant gene ultimately developing cancer. Metastatic cancer of the thyroid is less common, but renal cancer, breast cancer, lung cancer, and malignant melanoma can all metastasize to the thyroid gland.

PATHOPHYSIOLOGY

Thyroid carcinomas are relatively rare in the United States, but benign thyroid disease is significantly more common. An estimated 10% of the general adult population develops thyroid nodules; although the vast majority of these nodules represent benign disease, it is estimated that 5% to 6% of isolated nodules are malignant. Thus, distinguishing nonmalignant from malignant cases requires careful clinical evaluation. Thyroid cancers range from those that are well differentiated and slow growing to those that are poorly differentiated and aggressive. As with other malignancies, poorly differentiated thyroid cancers have an unfavorable prognosis.

Cancers of the thyroid gland are typically classified into primary or secondary (metastatic) tumors. Primary tumors include papillary (80% of cases), follicular (10% of cases), anaplastic (2% of cases), and medullary (5% to 10% of cases) tumors, as well as sarcomas and rare cases of primary non-Hodgkin's thyroid lymphomas (2% to 5% of cases), which should be considered in persons with a rapidly growing goiter. Hürthle cell carcinoma is another rare type of thyroid malignancy (2% to 3% of thyroid cancers) that is often considered a variant of follicular carcinoma. Consisting almost exclusively of Hürthle cells (also called oxyphilic or oncocytic cells) that contain abundant granular acidophilic cytoplasm, these malignancies are highly aggressive, metastasize in more than half of cases, and are difficult to follow because they do not respond to TSH or take up radioiodine.

Papillary, follicular, and anaplastic tumors arise from endodermally derived thyroxine and thyroglobulin-producing follicular epithelium, whereas medullary tumors arise from neuroendocrine-derived parafollicular or C cells. Thyroid lymphomas arise from intrathyroid lymph tissue and are strongly associated with chronic lymphocytic thyroiditis (Hashimoto's autoimmune thyroiditis), whereas sarcomas are derived from the vascular and connective tissue interwoven throughout the thyroid gland.

As with all types of malignancies, thyroid cancer is believed to develop from a series of mutational events producing an immortalized cell that is genetically different from its source. This explains the strong association of thyroid cancer with radiation exposure, which increases the incidence of DNA mutations and leads to transformation of normal thyroid cells into malignant clones. Similarly, germline mutations in the *RET* proto-oncogene have been associated with the inherited cancer syndromes of multiple endocrine neoplasia (MEN) 2A, MEN 2B, familial adenomatous polyposis, and familial medullary thyroid carcinoma (FMTC) syndrome—all of which are associated with medullary thyroid carcinoma.

CLINICAL PRESENTATION

Subjective

The major symptom of thyroid cancer is a lump or nodule in the neck, which is usually painless. Patients may also complain of a tight or full feeling in the neck, difficulty breathing or swallowing, hoarseness, hemoptysis, and swollen lymph nodes. In particular, the new onset of hoarseness with hemoptysis is strongly suggestive of a malignant growth. Progressive dysphagia and shortness of breath may indicate invasiveness. Neck pain is usually a late symptom with thyroid cancer.

Objective

Differentiated thyroid carcinomas most commonly present as a thyroid mass or nodule. However, almost 10% of the adult U.S. population has a palpable thyroid nodule, making clinical examination of the thyroid an ineffective method of screening. Although malignant neoplasms of the thyroid are more likely to be fixed, nontender, firm, and irregular in shape, only a biopsy can rule in malignancy. The physical examination should also include evaluation of the tongue, oropharynx, and cervical spine for swelling, nodules, or tenderness, which may suggest extension of disease or alternative pathology.

DIAGNOSTIC REASONING

Although there are typical presentations of benign versus malignant nodules of the thyroid, many malignant lesions have an atypical presentation. Thus, a biopsy is the only reliable method of differentiating benign from malignant lesions, and patients should be referred for evaluation and probable biopsy upon palpation of a nodule. Fewer than 5% of nodules are malignant, and multiple nodules of the same consistency are more likely to be benign.

Diagnostic Tests

Initial Testing

High-resolution ultrasonography is beneficial in identifying thyroid nodules but is not reliable in differentiating benign from malignant lesions. Ultrasound is indicated when there is suspicion of multinodular disease or when the thyroid is difficult to evaluate clinically. Radioactive iodine uptake testing is a means of determining functionality of a thyroid nodule; positive uptake portends a more favorable prognosis in thyroid cancer, owing to the ability to treat such tumors with high-dose radioactive iodine therapy.

Subsequent Testing

FNA biopsy is usually successful in differentiating benign from cancerous lesions of the thyroid gland and has 83% sensitivity and 92% specificity. Thus, the FNA will not capture all cases, and repeat biopsy may be necessary. The sensitivity of FNA is increased if it is ultrasound-guided. Nondiagnostic FNA biopsies may require surgical lobectomy to confirm that the nodule is not, in fact, malignant. Psammoma bodies are found in 50% of papillary carcinomas; they are circular, laminated bodies found in the stroma of the tumor.

Thyroid function tests typically show levels within the normal range in the setting of thyroid cancer, unless the patient also has thyroiditis. Elevated serum calcitonin is a strong tumor marker of medullary thyroid carcinoma, but these cancers are somewhat rare overall, so this test is not usually used in the initial work-up. For the inherited cancer syndromes MEN 2A, MEN 2B, and FMTC, polymerase chain reaction assays are used to detect germline mutations in the *RET* oncogene.

Computed tomography (CT) and MRI are used when the tumor is large or recurrent or when there is suspected extrathyroidal extension of the tumor, but these imaging modalities are not helpful for evaluating a simple, isolated nodule. However, they can be used to assess for distant metastases and regional lymph node involvement. Spread to the lymph nodes is more common with papillary than follicular carcinomas, and if distant metastasis occurs, the lung and bone are the most common sites. Interestingly, lymph node metastases are not an important prognostic factor, but distant metastasis is associated with a nearly 70-fold increase in death.

Differential Diagnosis

Differential diagnoses of thyroid cancer include lymphocytic thyroiditis, multinodular goiter, a benign thyroid nodule, cystic nodules, and regional lymphadenopathy. Mass-related effects may be similar to those associated with laryngeal carcinoma or other forms of head and neck cancer (e.g., dysphagia or hoarseness due to recurrent laryngeal nerve involvement with vocal cord paralysis, hemoptysis due to local invasion through the trachea).

If medullary thyroid carcinoma is diagnosed, it is critical to take a thorough family history to assess whether this presentation occurs as a component of several inherited cancer syndromes, including MEN 2A or Sipple syndrome (which may present with concurrent pheochromocytoma and hyperparathyroidism), MEN 2B (which may present with concurrent pheochromocytoma, a tall and slender Marfanoid body habitus, and ganglioneuromas), or FMTC syndrome.

MANAGEMENT

Initial Management

Any swelling suggestive of malignancy should be referred for evaluation of the mass. Early referral of patients with thyroid nodules to an endocrinologist for evaluation and treatment reduces costs, decreases patient hospital time, and increases the precision of the diagnosis. The prognosis is good for thyroid cancer that is found early, is less than 2 cm in diameter, is of a favorable histological type, and has not invaded locally or metastasized.

A surgeon and an oncologist (possibly a radiation or medical oncologist) will be necessary for determining the diagnosis and treatment plan, as thyroidectomy is the treatment of choice. The decision is based on the type of tumor, the size, and whether the tumor is compressing other structures. A surgeon with expertise in thyroid surgery should perform the procedure because of the potential to damage the laryngeal nerves and parathyroid glands. For small, noninvasive tumors, some surgeons prefer to perform a lobectomy as a more conservative approach. However, if there is local invasion by the tumor, there is a greater possibility of recurrence. Thus, radical neck surgery may be indicated for tumors with extensive local invasion.

Subsequent Management

After a total thyroidectomy, patients are often treated with radioactive iodine therapy to ablate any remnant thyroid tissue. Thyroid replacement therapy is initiated to suppress TSH to a goal of 0.1 mIU/L, and patients are monitored closely for response to therapy. Patients are subsequently followed every 6 to 12 months by an endocrinologist. A thorough neck examination, chest x-ray, and physical examination are performed to assess for evidence of thyrotoxicosis. Thyroglobulin levels may also be measured for well-differentiated carcinomas. The endocrinologist may perform a follow-up ^{131}I scan 6 to 12 months after a total thyroidectomy and may initiate further radioactive iodine ablation therapy if indicated. A follow-up ^{131}I scan is not useful in medullary cancer because medullary carcinoma does not take up the radioactive isotope.

Some forms of thyroid malignancy have unique treatments. In addition to thyroidectomy and postoperative radiation therapy, thyroid lymphomas may also require chemotherapy directed by a medical oncologist. Sarcomas are particularly aggressive and, after thyroidectomy, are poorly responsive to chemotherapy and carry a poor prognosis.

Long-term prognosis of thyroid malignancy depends on the tumor cell type, the size of the primary growth, gender (men are twice as likely to die from thyroid cancer as women), age at diagnosis (death is more common in patients diagnosed younger than 20 years of age or older than 40 years of age), and the extent of metastasis at the time of excision. Fortunately, papillary thyroid cancer is rarely fatal.

FOLLOW-UP AND REFERRAL

Follow-up is directed by the knowledge that no single diagnostic tool is sufficient to evaluate for recurrent disease. The follow-up of patients who have been treated for thyroid cancer includes periodic clinical examinations, serum thyroglobulin measurements, chest x-rays, and ultrasound examination to assess for recurrence. The patient is followed closely during the first 3 to 4 years after surgery because recurrence is more likely within this time period. The patient with a total thyroidectomy will also require thyroid hormone replacement for life, as described in the section on Management. Patients with medullary carcinoma MEN2 should be offered *RET* (rearranged during transcription) proto-oncogene testing. Provided the mutation is identified, all first-degree relatives should be offered *RET* mutational testing as well.

Patient Education: Thyroid Cancer

Patients with a family history of thyroid cancer should be advised to perform a "neck check" monthly. Patients with a history of goiter or irradiation should also perform this screening technique. The check is performed at home with a glass of water and a handheld mirror. The patient should be instructed to hold the mirror to visualize the area between the Adam's apple and clavicle. Then the head should be tilted backward, enough to adequately visualize the area without producing coughing or choking. As a sip of water is swallowed, the patient should observe the area for any bulging. The maneuver should be repeated several times. Any signs of bulging should be reported immediately. An instruction card on how to perform the *Neck Check* can be obtained through ThyCa: Thyroid Cancer Survivors' Association, Inc.

CUSHING'S SYNDROME

Cushing's syndrome includes myriad symptoms and physical features produced by persistent inappropriate hypercortisolemia. The condition was named after Harvey Cushing, a physician who found pituitary adenomas in six of eight patients with symptoms of adrenocortical hyperfunctioning in 1932.

EPIDEMIOLOGY AND CAUSES

Cushing's syndrome can be caused by cortisol hypersecretion by the adrenal cortex due to cortical hypertrophy or to a tumor of the adrenal gland. However, the prolonged administration of large doses of exogenous glucocorticoid hormones will also cause this cluster of signs and symptoms and simulate dysfunctional adrenal overactivity. The term *Cushing's disease* refers specifically to excess secretion of adrenocorticotropic hormone (ACTH) caused by a pituitary adenoma, which results in overproduction of cortisol by the adrenal gland.

Cushing's syndrome may be classified mechanistically as ACTH-dependent or ACTH-independent hypercortisolemic states. The former mechanism results in adrenocortical hyperplasia and is most frequently (70% of cases) due to an ACTH-secreting pituitary adenoma in Cushing's disease, which occurs more commonly in women. These tumors are usually small (microadenomas) and may not be recognizable on pituitary imaging, with some patients demonstrating only hyperplasia of pituitary corticotrophs. Fewer than 10% of affected patients have a tumor greater than 10 mm in diameter. The tumors are not encapsulated and present in the anterior pituitary gland. Spontaneous cases of Cushing's syndrome are rare, occurring in 2.6 persons per 1,000,000 patient years. Malignant pituitary tumors are particularly rare.

Nonpituitary tumors account for ectopic ACTH secretion in 10% to 15% of ACTH-dependent cases of Cushing's syndrome. In contrast, excessive administration of exogenous ACTH (as a therapeutic) and ectopic secretion of corticotropin-releasing hormone (CRH) by nonhypothalamic tumors each account for less than 1% of ACTH-hypersecretion cases.

The majority of ACTH-independent cases of Cushing's syndrome are due to iatrogenic administration of glucocorticoid hormones for therapeutic purposes. However, tumors of the adrenal cortex account for up to 20% of ACTH-independent cases, and both micronodular and macronodular dysplasia of the adrenal gland have been observed, although these etiologies are both quite rare, accounting for fewer than 1% of cases of Cushing's syndrome.

PATHOPHYSIOLOGY

A basic knowledge of the hypothalamic-pituitary-adrenal neurohormonal axis is required to properly understand the pathophysiology of Cushing's syndrome. Ultimately regulated by the central nervous system, CRH is first produced by the hypothalamus and released into the hypophyseal portal circulation, where it stimulates the production of proopiomelanocortin (POMC) by corticotrophs in the anterior pituitary gland, from which ACTH (also called corticotropin) is derived as a cleavage product. ACTH then acts directly on the adrenal cortex to stimulate the production of cortisol and other adrenal hormones that act at peripheral tissue sites as intranuclear transcription factors for steroid-responsive genes. Cortisol is then metabolized by the liver and kidneys, and its breakdown products are secreted in the urine as 17-hydroxycorticosteroids, 17-ketogenic steroids, and 17-ketosteroids.

A key regulatory mechanism of this neuroendocrine axis is the negative feedback exerted by each downstream product on its preceding hormone—namely, the inhibitory effects of ACTH on CRH secretion, as well as serum cortisol on the secretion of ACTH and CRH at the level of the pituitary and hypothalamus, respectively. The pituitary is also likely subject to other forms of positive feedback from additional secretagogues. For example, pituitary corticotrophs have been shown to express receptors for growth hormone–releasing peptide (GHRP) and increase ACTH production in response to GHRP secretion.

The secretion of ACTH (and, subsequently, serum cortisol) is normally pulsatile in nature in terms of frequency and remains constant. However, the extent of ACTH release with each pulse varies according to the body's circadian rhythms (sleep–wake cycles), which accounts for the variation in serum cortisol levels observed through serial measurements at different times of the day. Physical and emotional stressors that increase the body's metabolic demands also increase ACTH and cortisol secretion. In the normal diurnal sleep–wake cycle, levels are highest in the early morning on awakening and are lowest late in the evening and during the very early morning hours after midnight.

In patients with Cushing's disease, pituitary adenomas secrete excessive amounts of ACTH. The hypersecretion is random, episodic, and does not follow the usual circadian rhythm of ACTH secretion in terms of amplitude and duration. ACTH stimulates the secretion of glucocorticoids, mineralocorticoids, and androgenic steroids from the adrenal cortex. As cortical hyperplasia increases, the adrenal glands secrete increasing amounts of cortisol in response to each incremental pulse of ACTH. Moreover, in the presence of an adenoma, the usual negative feedback mechanism of excessive glucocorticoid secretion does not suppress ACTH production to the same extent as in unaffected persons, possibly owing to a defect in the glucocorticoid receptor in adenomatous corticotrophs. In turn, these patients present with hypercortisolemia and elevated levels of ACTH—particularly those with macroadenomas.

Importantly, however, in contrast to the ACTH-producing cells of relatively rarer ectopic nonpituitary adenomas that remain virtually unresponsive to negative feedback mechanisms, pituitary adenomatous corticotrophs appear to still retain a threshold level, albeit a higher one than in normal corticotrophs, for cortisol-mediated negative feedback. This allows a high-dose dexamethasone suppression test to differentiate between pituitary and nonpituitary sources of ACTH hypersecretion. With ectopic nonpituitary ACTH secretion, both hypothalamic CRH secretion and pituitary ACTH secretion from normal corticotrophs are suppressed. A number of tumor types have been implicated with ectopic ACTH hypersecretion, most commonly small oat-cell carcinoma of the lung and carcinoid tumors of the thymus or pancreas, all of which arise from neuroendocrine cell precursors. Interestingly, most of these tumors secrete a greater proportion of POMC precursors than ACTH itself.

In patients with Cushing's syndrome, cortisol measurements taken at various times during a 24-hour period will demonstrate prolonged elevations of cortisol levels, even though some readings may be within the normal range. The normally tight regulatory relationship between ACTH and cortisol secretion is lost, with late evening cortisol levels being particularly high. This excessive production of cortisol over the entire 24-hour sleep–wake cycle results in the clinical signs and symptoms of Cushing's syndrome.

The most frequent cause of Cushing's syndrome, however, is prolonged administration of exogenous glucocorticoid hormones—an iatrogenic etiology that is ACTH-independent. Thus, any medical problem requiring the prolonged use of corticosteroids predisposes the patient to develop this syndrome. Examples include autoimmune disorders, reactive airway disease, and COPD—all of which may involve long-term systemic corticosteroid use as maintenance therapy or for recurrent exacerbations. Rarely, megestrol acetate (Megace), which has intrinsic glucocorticoid activity, may also lead to Cushing's syndrome. Exogenous corticosteroid administration leads to suppression of CRH and ACTH excretion, as well as corticosteroid production by native adrenal tissue. This results in bilateral adrenocortical atrophy and low salivary and urinary levels of 17-hydroxycorticosteroid and cortisol, unless cortisol itself is the steroid being administered.

Primary adrenocortical disease including cortical tumors and both micronodular and macronodular hyperplasia is much less common. Adrenal tumors may be benign adenomas or malignant carcinomas. Both types of tumors demonstrate altered expression of genes involved in apoptosis and telomeric function, which appears to underlie clonal immortalization. However, a number of significant differences exist between benign and malignant tumors. Adrenal adenomas produce cortisol from cholesterol backbones very efficiently, secreting relatively low levels of the cortisol precursors dehydroepiandrosterone (DHEA-S) and 17-ketosteroids. Benign adenomatous cells have also been shown to respond to beta-adrenergic agonists and multiple cytokines, including IL-1, gastric inhibitory peptide, vasopressin, and serotonin.

In contrast, adrenal carcinomas are far less efficient at producing cortisol and secrete cortisol precursors at disproportionately higher concentrations. Adrenal carcinomas are still capable of leading to Cushing's syndrome, however, owing to their size and secretory cell mass. They are also more likely than adrenal adenomas to produce elevated levels of the aldosterone precursor corticosterone and its hydroxy and deoxy variants. Adrenal carcinomas also produce high levels of vascular endothelial growth factor–A, insulin-like growth factor (IGF)–1, IGF-2, IGF-2 receptor, cell cyclins, cyclin-dependent kinase, and the chemokines IL-8 and epithelial neutrophil-activating protein–78. In contrast, levels of the antiangiogenic factor thrombospondin-1 are reduced.

With primary adrenocortical tumors, hypercortisolemia allows for negative feedback of both CRH and ACTH secretion. Thus, pituitary corticotrophs atrophy, as do the normal adrenal cells of the zona fasciculata and zona reticularis. In contrast, macronodular adrenal hyperplasia results in glands weighing 25 to 500 g or more, with multiple benign nodules greater than 5 mm in diameter and a hypertrophic (rather than atrophic) internodular cortex.

CLINICAL PRESENTATION

Subjective

The clinical presentation of Cushing's disease is usually gradual, developing over months or years. Signs and symptoms of Cushing's disease are those of hypercortisolism and androgen excess. The presentation of patients with Cushing's syndrome is similar. Common complaints include weight gain, back pain, headaches, skin changes, and muscle weakness. Women may complain of menstrual irregularities and hirsutism, and men often report decreased libido and impotence. Patients may also complain of emotional lability, increased appetite, increased irritability, anxiety, poor concentration and memory, and sleep disturbances.

Objective

Patients with Cushing's syndrome usually present with generalized or central obesity. In fact, obesity is the most common and often the first clinical manifestation of this disorder. Excessive accumulation of fat in the face leads to the typical "moon face" appearance. Facial plethora often accompanies the moon facies. The "buffalo hump" appearance is caused by excessive accumulation of fat in the supraclavicular and dorsocervical area.

Most patients will have readily recognizable skin changes. There is atrophy of the epidermis and connective tissue, producing a thinning of the skin and easy bruising. Fungal infections of the skin, nails, and oral mucosa are common. Skin wounds heal slowly in the presence of excessive cortisol. Additional skin changes include hirsutism, acne, and striae (stretch marks). Striae are typically red to purple and usually are present on the abdomen but may be present on the hips, buttocks, thighs, breast, and axillae. Hyperpigmentation, commonly found in some types of Cushing's syndrome, is rare in patients with Cushing's disease.

Most patients have muscle weakness, which is more prominent proximally and in the lower extremities. The extremities are usually thin, with muscle wasting.

Osteoporosis is common in patients with prolonged elevated cortisol levels, and pathological fractures may be evident on radiographic examination.

Other manifestations include glaucoma, leukocytosis, granulocytosis, lymphopenia, and psychiatric symptoms. Less common clinical findings include renal calculi and edema. Hypokalemic alkalosis is rare in Cushing's disease but is often seen in Cushing's syndrome. Hypertension is often present secondary to sodium and water retention. Glucose intolerance and hyperglycemia result because cortisol interferes with the transfer of insulin across the cell membrane.

DIAGNOSTIC REASONING

Diagnostic Tests

Initial Testing

Cushing's syndrome and disease are diagnosed via a combination of laboratory testing and radiographic examinations. The Endocrine Society has released diagnostic guidelines recommending that one of four tests be used in the initial testing for Cushing's syndrome: urine free cortisol (at least two measurements), late-night salivary cortisol (two measurements), 1-mg overnight dexamethasone suppression test (DST), or a longer low-dose DST (2 mg/day for 48 hours). Additional laboratory tests should include a CBC, blood glucose level, and comprehensive metabolic panel. Hypercortisolemia impairs glucose tolerance and often produces hypokalemia and leukocytosis.

Initial tests to assess cortisol levels include serum cortisol levels and urinary cortisol. The overnight DST assists in the confirmation of hypercortisolemia. In this test, the patient ingests 1-mg of dexamethasone (Decadron) orally at 11:00 p.m., and the plasma cortisol level is measured at 8 a.m. the next morning. A normal finding is a value below 1.8 mcg/dL, whereas an elevated morning cortisol level would indicate that the patient's endogenous cortisol secretion is insensitive to the negative feedback imparted by the exogenous dexamethasone dose. False-positive results may occur, however, in patients who are obese, depressed, or under extreme stress, given the elevated cortisol levels seen in these conditions. Medications that can also produce high cortisol levels include estrogens, antiseizure medications, and rifampin. Phenytoin (Dilantin), phenobarbital (Luminal), and primidone (Mysoline) accelerate the metabolism of dexamethasone and can also produce a false-positive dexamethasone test.

A nighttime (11:00 p.m.) salivary cortisol level is normally below 4.2 nmol/L, and obtaining two samples within this range excludes the diagnosis of Cushing's syndrome. In contrast, levels twice this high are suggestive of Cushing's syndrome. Although this is a relatively easy test to perform (samples are stable at room temperature), it requires special sample collection tubes and a nighttime collection schedule. The test has a sensitivity of 93% to 100%.

A urinary free cortisol 24-hour collection test requires the patient to collect urine for 24 hours, which is often not a practical expectation, unless the collection is done in an inpatient setting. The majority of patients with Cushing's syndrome will have an elevated level; if it is four-fold the upper limit of normal, this result is considered diagnostic for Cushing's syndrome. However, mild Cushing's syndrome may still have normal levels; thus, normal urinary free cortisol levels (<50 mcg/24 h) do not rule out Cushing's syndrome entirely. If the test result is positive for Cushing's syndrome, the patient should be referred to an endocrinologist, who will conduct further testing to determine the cause and subtype of Cushing's syndrome. If symptoms of Cushing's syndrome are present but tests do not confirm the diagnosis of hypercortisolism, a low-dose DST should be performed.

Subsequent Testing

The low-dose DST involves administration of dexamethasone 0.5 mg PO every 6 hours for 48 hours. Urine is collected on day 2 of the test. Urinary free cortisol above 20 mcg/dL or a 17-hydroxycorticosteroid level above 4.5 mcg/dL confirms the diagnosis of hypercortisolism. Many medications, including corticosteroids, phenothiazines, phenytoin, diuretics, quinidine, penicillin G, oral contraceptives, lithium, acetylsalicylic acid, and monoamine oxidase inhibitors, may affect the accuracy of test results.

Baseline plasma ACTH levels should be assessed once hypercortisolism is confirmed. Levels are highest between 7:00 and 10:00 a.m. (8 to 80 pg/mL) and lowest just before bedtime (less than 10 pg/mL). Generally, levels below 20 pg/mL indicate a possible adrenal tumor, and levels exceeding 20 pg/mL are indicative of a pituitary or ectopic secreting ACTH tumor.

After completion of hormonal studies, radiological assessments are performed to localize the possible source of excess cortisol production. Most microadenomas of the pituitary gland are detected by imaging. An abdominal CT scan of the adrenal glands is done to detect adrenal tumors. In Cushing's disease, the adrenal glands are enlarged. A CT scan of the chest and abdomen is also beneficial in detecting possible sites of ectopic secretion. Because the lung is the most likely source of ectopic secretion, special attention to the chest is indicated. If the source is determined to be the pituitary gland, an MRI assessment is indicated.

Patients should also be assessed for other sequelae of Cushing's syndrome such as hypokalemia, anemia, metabolic alkalosis, hyperglycemia, and hypercholesterolemia. Except for initial testing, the diagnosis of Cushing's syndrome and the differentiation as to cause are best accomplished either by an endocrinologist or in collaboration with an endocrinologist.

Differential Diagnosis

Pregnancy, obesity, and excessive physical activity may produce elevated serum cortisol levels. Other conditions that may produce elevated cortisol levels are alcoholism, severe depression, obesity, hypertension, DM, glucocorticoid therapy, estrogen replacement therapy, and oral contraceptives. There are also various familial (genetic) predispositions to hypercortisolemia. Type 1 MEN 1 syndrome presents with pituitary corticotroph adenomas in 2% of cases, whereas Carney's syndrome is a rare autosomal dominant complex consisting of bilateral micronodular dysplasia, pigmented lentigines, and blue nevi on the head and trunk, as well as multiple endocrine and nonendocrine neoplasms.

MANAGEMENT

The goals of treatment are to normalize the cortisol level and treat the underlying cause of hypercortisolemia. The initial clinical management of patients with Cushing's syndrome should be handled by an endocrinologist. Despite successful treatment, some patients may relapse, so the patient must be evaluated for recurrence of hypercortisolemia.

Initial Management

Transsphenoidal pituitary microsurgery is the treatment of choice for pituitary adenoma causing Cushing's disease. If surgery is unsuccessful, irradiation of the pituitary may be considered. Complications from surgery include transient diabetes insipidus, visual disturbances, cerebrospinal rhinorrhea, and meningitis. After microsurgery, 75% of patients will experience dramatic decreases in cortisol and will require exogenous glucocorticoid therapy for 6 to 36 months after surgery. For patients who fail to respond or who have a recurrence, treatment may include stereotactic pituitary radiosurgery (gamma knife) or laparoscopic bilateral adrenalectomy. Conventional pituitary irradiation therapy has a 23% cure rate. Failure rates with both types of treatment increase over time.

Diagnostic errors (e.g., depression with a lack of pituitary adenoma) increase failure rates of patients treated with surgery. After transsphenoidal pituitary microsurgery, 25% of patients have persistent signs and symptoms. This is more likely to occur if the tumor was not completely removed and in patients with corticotrophic hyperplasia. These patients require a second pituitary operation, radiotherapy, or bilateral total adrenalectomy.

In younger patients who are not surgical candidates, mitotane (Lysodren) or alternatively ketoconazole (Nizoral) 200 mg every 6 hours can be used alone or in combination to reduce cortisol overproduction, as inhibitors of steroidogenesis. Older adults who are not surgical candidates may tolerate the use of ketoconazole; however, liver enzymes may be elevated with this treatment and need to be monitored.

Subsequent Management

After resection of a pituitary adenoma, corticotropins are suppressed, and temporary cortisone replacement therapy is indicated as directed by an endocrinologist for 9 to 12 months, but may be as long as 36 months. The drugs of choice for adrenal replacement therapy are hydrocortisone (Cortef), prednisone (Deltasone), and fludrocortisone (Florinef). Dexamethasone (Decadron) is an alternative. The lowest dose effective in maintaining hormone levels is recommended. Complications of untreated or inadequately treated Cushing's disease are increased susceptibility to infections, nephrolithiasis, hypertension, and osteoporosis. Inadequate treatment may also lead to psychosis or uncontrolled DM. Medications for corticosteroid replacement are listed in Drugs Commonly Prescribed 57.3.

FOLLOW-UP AND REFERRAL

The follow-up for each patient depends on the selected therapy and is critical, since excessive corticosteroid treatment should be avoided as much as possible. The disorder is usually chronic and characterized by periods of cyclic exacerbation and rare remissions. Complications include osteoporosis, increased susceptibility to infection, hirsutism, and metastases of malignant tumors, depending on causality. Thus, the patient should be followed monthly for the first year and checked for signs of adrenal hypofunction, and then every 6 to 12 months.

An endocrinology referral is critical to establish and proper diagnosis and treatment plan, although ongoing management requires the close coordination with the primary-care practitioner. Referrals are suggested for surgical intervention for the following conditions associated with Cushing's syndrome:

1. *Primary hypersecretion of ACTH.* Transsphenoidal microsurgery is recommended and is often followed by radiation and sometimes by medication (adrenocortical inhibitors).
2. *Adrenocortical tumors.* Surgery is recommended, but prognosis is poor. Replacement therapy is used but usually for only 3 to 12 months. The patient may need treatment with adrenocortical inhibitors if not treated with surgery, which should be managed by an endocrinologist.
3. *Ectopic ACTH production.* Surgery is recommended for removal of neoplastic tissue to manage symptoms, although surgical cure is unlikely. Sometimes a bilateral adrenalectomy is performed. Follow-up for these patients would depend on causality and recommended treatment.

Drugs Commonly Prescribed 57.3: Corticosteroid Replacement Therapy

DRUG	INDICATION	ADVERSE REACTIONS AND PRESCRIBING CONSIDERATIONS
Prednisone (Deltasone, Meticorten) oral	Adrenalectomy Pituitary resection	Glucocorticoid activity: moderate Mineralocorticoid activity: weak Use the lowest effective dose to prevent side effects such as diabetes mellitus, psychosis, osteoporosis, and infections.
Prednisolone (Delta-Cortef, Prelone)	Adrenalectomy Pituitary resection	Glucocorticoid activity: moderate Mineralocorticoid activity: weak Use the lowest effective dose to prevent side effects such as diabetes mellitus, psychosis, osteoporosis, and infections.
Methylprednisolone oral (Medrol), IM or IV (Depo-Medrol)	Adrenalectomy Pituitary resection	Glucocorticoid activity: moderate Mineralocorticoid activity: none Use the lowest effective dose to prevent side effects such as diabetes mellitus, psychosis, osteoporosis, and infections.
Hydrocortisone (Cortef, Hydrocortone) oral, IM, IV, topical, and ophthalmic	Adrenalectomy Pituitary resection	Glucocorticoid activity: high Mineralocorticoid activity: yes Use the lowest effective dose to prevent side effects such as diabetes mellitus, psychosis, osteoporosis, and infections.
Cortisone acetate (Cortone) oral and IM	Adrenalectomy Pituitary resection	Glucocorticoid activity: high Mineralocorticoid activity: yes Use the lowest effective dose to prevent side effects such as diabetes mellitus, psychosis, osteoporosis, and infections.
Dexamethasone (long-acting) oral, IM, and IV (Decadron)	Adrenalectomy Pituitary resection	Glucocorticoid activity: very high Mineralocorticoid activity: weak Use the lowest effective dose to prevent side effects such as diabetes mellitus, psychosis, osteoporosis, and infections.
Fludrocortisone (Florinef) oral	Adrenalectomy Pituitary resection	Glucocorticoid activity: none Mineralocorticoid activity: high Use the lowest effective dose to prevent side effects such as sodium and water retention, edema, hypertension, and hypokalemia.

There is the potential for failure of any surgical intervention. Thus, the patient must be instructed to report any return of symptoms if he or she has been asymptomatic for a period after the operation.

Patient Education: Cushing's Syndrome

The patient will need education to cope with lifelong symptomatology (e.g., information on the importance of early interventions for infections), strategies to manage overwhelming stress and emotional lability, use of potassium supplements, and maintenance of a high-protein diet.

Although patients with Cushing's syndrome will be managed initially by an endocrinologist, the primary-care practitioner often manages other aspects of the patient's health. The patient should understand that it is important to work collaboratively with the primary-care practitioner in managing symptoms successfully.

Patients need a thorough understanding of their medications and the warning signs of undertreatment or overtreatment with cortisone. Cortisone preparations should be taken with food. Patients need to be told that they should consult with the primary-care practitioner when initiating additional medications, both by prescription or over the counter. Patients on high doses of corticosteroids should wear a medical identification bracelet. Because these patients are prone to infections, they should be instructed on how to avoid common infections, both bacterial and fungal. Patients cannot rely on fever to indicate the seriousness of infection, given the anti-inflammatory effects of corticosteroids; therefore, they need to report any initial signs of infection promptly to the primary-care practitioner.

Nutritional counseling may be indicated, including information on avoidance of excessive sodium and on a well-balanced, low-fat diet. Many patients are obese, and the importance of weight loss must be addressed.

Patients should monitor their glucose levels at least weekly. During periods of stress or medication adjustment, glucose levels will need to be tested more frequently. Patients should assess their glucose levels daily during periods of medication adjustment. If levels are stable and within normal levels, patients may continue testing glucose levels until at least 1 week after the final dose adjustment. Patients should resume daily glucose testing in times of stress or if any signs of infection are present. If the morning glucose level at any time is above normal, more frequent testing is indicated. The patient should be given a log to record the glucose test results and instructed to bring the log to each primary-care visit.

Patients with Cushing's syndrome will need to have their blood pressure monitored weekly. As with glucose monitoring, the frequency will depend on their symptoms and coexisting cardiovascular disease. More frequent monitoring will be needed during times of stress. The patient should obtain a sphygmomanometer for home use and keep a log of his or her blood pressures so that the primary-care practitioner can see the pattern.

The patient should be instructed about fall prevention. Because of the potential for osteoporosis with chronic corticosteroid treatment, the patient should avoid activities that are likely to cause falls. Simple environmental changes can be made in the home to increase safety, such as removing small rugs, placing rails around the bathtub, and using a shower chair.

Patients should also report any symptoms of GI upset (nausea, bloating, vomiting) and monitor themselves for signs of GI bleeding (vomiting blood, tarry stools, increasing fatigue).

Instructions on skin care are essential. Older adults with a history of long-term corticosteroid use are more prone to pressure ulcers. Thin, easily traumatized skin must be protected. These individuals should avoid applying tape and adhesive bandages directly to their skin. They should wear protective clothing for outdoor activities such as gardening.

ADRENAL INSUFFICIENCY

Low levels of cortisol secretion by the adrenal glands can result from inadequate stimulation of the adrenals by ACTH from the anterior pituitary or because the adrenals are unable to produce adrenocortical hormones. *Addison's disease*, also known as primary adrenal insufficiency, is relatively rare and results from a failure of the adrenal glands to produce hormones because of a problem in the gland rather than a problem with the pituitary or ACTH production. Other types of adrenal insufficiency, or hypocortisolism, occur from secondary sources, such as a failure of the pituitary gland to produce adequate levels of the adrenal-stimulating hormone ACTH or the abrupt withdrawal of exogenously administered glucocorticoids, which previously suppressed endogenous adrenal hormone production.

EPIDEMIOLOGY AND CAUSES

Addison's disease is primarily caused by autoimmune destruction of the adrenal cortex in 80% of cases in the United States. Although it can occur at any age, Addison's disease most often occurs in persons 30 to 60 years of age. The prevalence of Addison's disease is 40 to 60 cases per 1,000,000 persons in the United States. Risk factors for Addison's disease include having a first- or second-degree relative with the disease.

Other causes of (secondary) adrenal insufficiency are chronic corticosteroid use followed by a physiologically stressful event, such as severe infection, trauma, or a surgical procedure, in which adrenal hormone levels are inadequate due to the iatrogenic suppression of endogenous hormone production. Tuberculosis infection is the most common infectious cause of adrenal insufficiency worldwide, whereas HIV is the most common infectious cause in the United States, resulting from the direct effects of infection on the adrenal glands themselves. Other causes include bilateral adrenal hemorrhage and infarction, tumors of the adrenal gland causing decreased function, anti-steroidogenic drugs (e.g., ketoconazole [Nizoral], etomidate [Amidate]), sarcoidosis, hemochromatosis, amyloidosis, and congenital causes.

PATHOPHYSIOLOGY

Idiopathic Addison's disease is an autoimmune disorder that can occur at any age. Adrenal-specific autoantibodies are present in 50% to 70% of cases and are more likely to be present in younger patients and those with other autoimmune diseases. These autoantibodies are specific for cells of the adrenal cortex and for the enzyme(s) responsible for the production of cortisol and aldosterone. A combination of autoantibodies and cell-mediated immune responses is responsible for this disease. Frequently, idiopathic Addison's disease appears with other autoimmune diseases, which are collectively termed *autoimmune polyendocrine syndrome* (APS). Type 1 APS is an inherited autosomal recessive disease and, along with Addison's disease, includes hypoparathyroidism and mucocutaneous candidiasis. Type 2 APS is the more common type, with a constellation of disorders that includes Addison's disease, DM, celiac disease, immune thyroid disease, and hypogonadism.

Secondary hypocortisolism is usually a result of low ACTH levels and subsequent adrenal atrophy. The resulting hypocortisolism causes clinical manifestations similar to Addison's disease. However, in this type of hypocortisolism, there is no hyperpigmentation as typically seen in Addison's disease, and the renin-angiotensin system functions normally, resulting in normal aldosterone and potassium levels.

CLINICAL PRESENTATION

Clinical manifestations of Addison's disease include fatigue, weakness, anorexia, weight loss, nausea, abdominal pain, diarrhea, hypoglycemia, and hypotension (particularly orthostatic hypotension), which are primarily the result of hypocortisolism and hypoaldosteronism. Patients with Addison's disease typically exhibit hyperpigmentation due to elevated levels of ACTH, which is derived from the precursor protein POMC that also gives rise to melanocyte-stimulating hormone. In severe cases, when a patient has Addison's disease that is well managed but the patient subsequently experiences a physiological stressor of some kind (e.g., infection, surgery), the requirement for cortisol increases and the patient may experience an Addisonian crisis, manifesting as severe hypotension and vascular collapse. The decreased adrenal androgen secretion associated with Addison's disease results in the loss of secondary sex characteristics (loss of pubic and axillary hair) in women, but because the adrenals are not a major source of androgens in men, male patients do not experience any loss of secondary sex characteristics.

DIAGNOSTIC REASONING

Diagnostic Tests

When Addison's disease or other forms of hypocortisolism are suspected, a plasma cortisol level should be obtained. A morning (8:00 a.m.) cortisol level of less than 3 mcg/dL is consistent with Addison's disease, especially if accompanied by a plasma ACTH level greater than 200 pg/mL. Diagnosis is confirmed by a cosyntropin stimulation test, in which a synthetic form of ACTH is given intramuscularly (IM) and a serum cortisol level is obtained 45 minutes later. In Addison's disease, the exogenous ACTH dose does not result in a corresponding increase in cortisol secretion, demonstrating primary failure of the adrenal glands to respond to ACTH. Small, noncalcified adrenal glands on CT scan are indicative of autoimmune Addison's disease.

Differential Diagnosis

Patients with Addison's disease generally have an elevated ACTH level, which is associated with hyperpigmentation of the skin. In contrast, if a patient has hypocortisolism that is a result of hypopituitarism resulting in a low ACTH level, he or she will have normal pigmentation. In any patient with unexplained hypotension, Addison's disease and other forms of hypocortisolism should be considered. Other nonspecific clinical manifestations that may be associated with Addison's disease but are also common in other conditions are nausea, unintentional weight loss, weakness, and anorexia. Hypocortisolism should be considered when other causes for the constitutional symptoms have been ruled out.

MANAGEMENT

Initial therapy for adrenal insufficiency consists of hydrocortisone 15 to 30 mg in two divided doses, with two-thirds of the dose given in the morning and one-third given in the early evening. Prednisone can be used if the patient does not respond well to hydrocortisone. The dose of prednisone is 2 to 4 mg in the morning and 1 to 2 mg in the evening. The dose is adjusted based on the clinical response.

Stress hormone supplementation is necessary for patients who experience significant physiological stressors, such as serious infection, trauma, or surgery. In cases of severe stress, hydrocortisone is given IV or IM every 6 hours at a maximum dose of 50 mg. Oral medication at lower doses can be prescribed if the stress is less severe and then reduced to normal when the stress subsides.

In addition to hydrocortisone (glucocorticoid), mineralocorticoids must be replaced, although not all patients require daily therapy. Fludrocortisone (Florinef) acetate is the drug of choice and has a potent sodium-retaining effect. The usual dosage is 0.05 to 0.2 mg PO daily, which should be determined in conjunction with an endocrinologist. Symptoms of fatigue, postural hypotension, hyponatremia, or hyperkalemia may indicate the need for a higher dosage. Of note, in contrast to glucocorticoid requirements, increased mineralocorticoid supplementation is not required during times of increased physiological stress.

Some patients require androgen therapy along with the medications mentioned above. Dehydroepiandrosterone (DHEA) 25 to 50 mg PO daily has been shown to improve sense of well-being, increase muscle mass, and reverse bone loss. When prescribed DHEA, older women should be monitored for masculinizing effects.

FOLLOW-UP AND REFERRAL

Patients with adrenal insufficiency require chronic glucocorticoid and mineralocorticoid supplementation and are prone to Addisonian crises, due to the inability to mount an appropriate stress hormone response with endogenous cortisol. Determination of an appropriate replacement dose and regimen requires periodic assessment for signs of both underdosing (weakness, dizziness, and headaches on waking) and overdosing (Cushingoid features).

Once chronic maintenance dosing is established in conjunction with an endocrinologist, the primary-care provider will be able to meet most of the patient's ongoing health-care needs but should also evaluate for iatrogenic complications of chronic corticosteroid use, including cataract formation (requiring annual ophthalmological examinations) and the development of osteopenia/osteoporosis (requiring periodic dual-energy x-ray absorptiometry scanning). Expert consultation with an endocrinologist should be sought if dose adjustments or a change in class of hormone replacement is indicated.

Patient Education: Adrenal Insufficiency

Any patient with Addison's disease or adrenal insufficiency needs to be well informed about this condition and the potential implications for Addisonian crisis if the patient should develop a serious infection or experience other physiological stressors. Given the significant risk from systemic illness, patients should be instructed to see their health-care provider practitioner during times of illness. In these instances, additional corticosteroid (stress hormone) supplementation may be required—for example, a doubling or tripling of the dose of hormone replacement therapy in the setting of an illness, surgery, or dental procedure. This may require parenteral (IM) dosing if oral supplementation is not possible (e.g., due to significant nausea, vomiting, or diarrhea). Thus, if possible, patients should be trained to self-administer IM injections and may be given a reserve prescription for parenteral hydrocortisone or similar agent to be used in these situations.

REFERENCES

Adrenal Insufficiency

Bancos I, Hahner S, Tomlinson J, Arlt W. Diagnosis and management of adrenal insufficiency. *Lancet Diabetes Endocrinol.* 2015;3(3):216–226.

Falorni A, Minarelli V, Morelli S. Therapy of adrenal insufficiency: An update. *Endocrine.* 2013;43(3):514–528.

Griffing GT. Addison disease. http://emedicine.medscape.com/article/116467-overview. Updated March 23, 2017. Accessed October 8, 2017.

Cushing's Syndrome

Afshari A, Ardeshirpour Y, Lodish MB, et al. Facial plethora: A modern technology for quantifying an ancient clinical sign and its use in Cushing syndrome. *J Clin Endocrinol Metab.* 2015;100(10):3928–3933.

Lacroiz, A, Feelders, RA, Stratakis CA, Nieman LK. Cushing's syndrome. *Lancet.* 2015;386(9996):913–927.

Nieman LK, Biller B, Findling JW, et al. Treatment of Cushing's syndrome: an Endocrine Society Clinical Practice Guideline. *J Clin Endocrinol Metab.* 2015;199(8):2807–2831.

Pivonello R, DeLeo M, Cozzolino A, Colao A. The treatment of Cushing's Disease. *Endocr Rev.* 2015;36(4):385–486.

Hyperthyroidism

Endocrine Society. Endocrine facts and figures. http://endocrine-facts.org/health-conditions/thyroid/4-hyperthyroidism/#top. Published 2015. Accessed September 23, 2017.

Ross DS. Subclinical hyperthyroidism in nonpregnant adults. UpToDate. https://www.uptodate.com/contents/subclinical-hyperthyroidism-in-nonpregnant-adults. Accessed September 24, 2017.

Ross DS, Burch HB, Cooper DS, et al. 2016 American Thyroid Association guidelines for diagnosis and management of hyperthyroidism and other causes of thyrotoxicosis. *Thyroid.* 2016;26(10):1343–1421. http://online.liebertpub.com/doi/pdf/10.1089/thy.2016.0229. Accessed September 24, 2017.

Hypothyroidism

Garber JR, Cobin RH, Gharib H, et al. ATA/AACE guidelines: Clinical practice guidelines for hypothyroidism in adults: Co-sponsored by the American Association of Clinical Endocrinologists and the American Thyroid Association. *Endocr Pract.* 2012;18(6):e1–e45.

Grossman A, Weiss A, Koren-Morag N, et al. Subclinical thyroid disease and mortality in the elderly: A retrospective cohort study. *Am J Med.* 2016;129(4):423–430.

Ritchie M, Yeap BB. Thyroid hormone: Influences on mood and cognition in adults. *Maturitas.* 2016;81(2):266–275. https://ac.els-cdn.com/S0378512215006064/1-s2.0-S0378512215006064-main.pdf?_tid=0cece936-a166-11e7-98ed-00000aab0f6b&acdnat=1506284713_4e7fb3816091c9ec9f7c319d55890033. Accessed September 24, 2017.

U.S. Preventive Services Task Force. Thyroid dysfunction: Screening. https://www.uspreventiveservicestaskforce.org/Page/Document/UpdateSummaryFinal/thyroid-dysfunction-screening?ds=1&s=thyroid%20screening. Published 2015. Accessed September 23, 2017.

RESOURCES

American Cancer Society
http://www.cancer.org/search/index?QueryText=Endocrine+diseases

Adrenal Disorders

National Adrenal Diseases Foundation (NADF)
http://www.nadf.us/

Thyroid Disorders

American Thyroid Association
www.thyroid.org

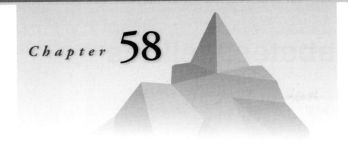

Chapter **58**

Diabetes Mellitus

Angela K. Golden, DNP, APRN, FNP-C, FAANP

Debera J. Thomas, DNS, RN, FNP/ANP

Brian Oscar Porter, MD, PhD, MPH, MBA

Diabetes mellitus (DM) is a syndrome of disordered carbohydrate, fat, and protein metabolism resulting in hyperglycemia that is caused by deficits in insulin secretion, insulin action, or a combination of both. The majority of patients with DM have type 1 DM or type 2 DM, each of which has a distinct epidemiology and etiology. *Impaired fasting glucose* is a prediabetic state where a person's fasting glucose is consistently elevated above the normal range, but below the level of 100 and 125 mg/dL for a formal diagnosis of diabetes mellitus. *Impaired glucose tolerance (IGT)* describes a prediabetic state of hyperglycemia where a 2-hour post-glucose load glycemic level is 140 to 199 mg/dL. DM is the most common endocrine disorder, affecting 30.3 million people in the United States. Up to 7.2 million people may not be aware that they have DM. The National Diabetes Statistics report for 2017 estimated that 9.4% of the adult population in the United States has DM. Tight control of blood glucose levels reduces the morbidity and mortality rates associated with DM. The complications of inadequately treated DM include cardiovascular and peripheral vascular disease (PVD), decreased immune system functioning, renal failure, retinopathy, and nephropathy. Indeed, DM is now the leading cause of both end-stage renal disease and acquired blindness in the United States.

DIABETES MELLITUS TYPE 1

Diabetes mellitus type 1 is a metabolic disorder characterized by severe insulin deficiency resulting from beta cell destruction, which produces hyperglycemia due to the altered metabolism of lipids, carbohydrates, and proteins. This chronic hyperglycemia results in damage to various bodily organs, especially the eyes, kidneys, nerves, heart, and both small and large blood vessels. Loss of vision, renal failure, loss of a lower extremity, and chronic foot ulcers due to peripheral neuropathy are common sequelae of long-term hyperglycemia. Such complications result in significant social, economic, and psychological demands on patients and their families.

EPIDEMIOLOGY AND CAUSES

Type 1 DM occurs in approximately 1.25 million Americans, and it is estimated that 5 million Americans will have type 1 DM by 2050. Type 1 DM was previously known as insulin-dependent DM or juvenile-onset diabetes. Although 60% of patients are younger than 18 years of age on first presentation, cases may occur at any age with a fairly abrupt onset. It is uncommon in children younger than 1 year and in adults older than 30 years of age. In nonpediatric patients, type 1 DM is sometimes known as latent autoimmune diabetes of adults (LADA). Although there is no gender predisposition, marked variations in gender predominance have been observed across ethnocultural groups, correlating with differential expression of human leukocyte antigen (HLA) haplotypes. In turn, type 1 DM is 1.5 to 2 times more common in Caucasians of European descent than in non-Caucasians.

Type 1 DM has two forms—*immune-mediated DM* (type 1A) and *idiopathic DM* (type 1B). Immune-mediated DM accounts for 90% of cases and is generally referred to as type 1 DM. It is caused by autoimmune destruction of insulin-producing pancreatic beta islet cells. The triggering factor in the development of type 1 DM is thought to be an infection or toxic insult in persons with a genetic predisposition. The most commonly identified infectious agents are congenital rubella (associated with the development of type 1 DM and other autoimmune syndromes up to 5 to 20 years later), Coxsackie B4 virus, cytomegalovirus, adenovirus, and mumps virus. Although it is unclear whether direct viral infection of pancreatic beta cells plays a role, infections with these agents are believed to cause a cross-reactive autoimmune response against pancreatic beta cell antigens. In turn, sensitized immune cells may release destructive cytotoxins and antibodies that contribute to the development of type 1 DM. Of note, immunization with viral or bacterial antigens does not increase the risk of developing autoimmune DM.

High birth weight greater than 4,000 g and higher than expected weight gain in the first year of life are associated with an increased risk of type 1 DM, but viral antigens and certain dietary influences appear to have the strongest impact. Although food epitopes may not mimic beta cell antigens directly, proteins from other animal species may trigger autoimmune reactions leading to type 1 DM. Epidemiological research from at least 10 countries implicated protein components of cow's milk (e.g., bovine serum albumin, beta-casein) as the most likely dietary triggers, but cross-sectional and prospective

909

The Iceberg of Diabetes Mellitus

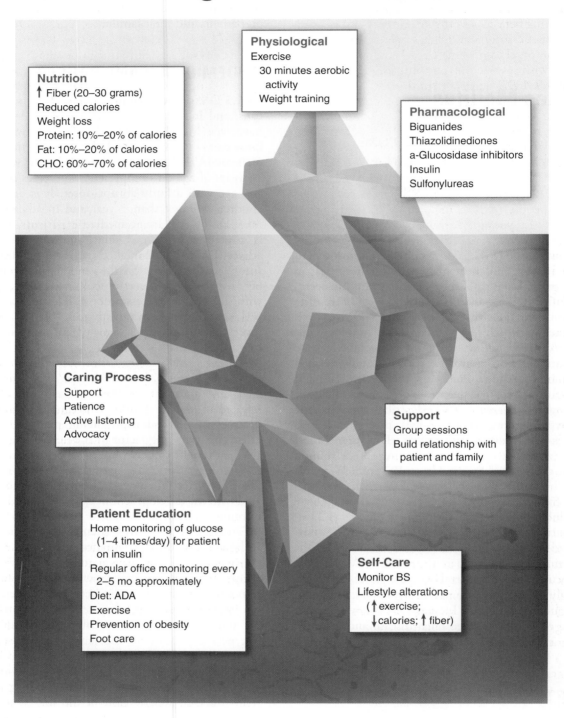

Physiological
Exercise
   30 minutes aerobic
     activity
   Weight training

Nutrition
↑ Fiber (20–30 grams)
Reduced calories
Weight loss
Protein: 10%–20% of calories
Fat: 10%–20% of calories
CHO: 60%–70% of calories

Pharmacological
Biguanides
Thiazolidinediones
a-Glucosidase inhibitors
Insulin
Sulfonylureas

Caring Process
Support
Patience
Active listening
Advocacy

Support
Group sessions
Build relationship with
   patient and family

Patient Education
Home monitoring of glucose
   (1–4 times/day) for patient
   on insulin
Regular office monitoring every
   2–5 mo approximately
Diet: ADA
Exercise
Prevention of obesity
Foot care

Self-Care
Monitor BS
Lifestyle alterations
  (↑ exercise;
   ↓ calories; ↑ fiber)

studies did not confirm these associations (with some work suggesting a protective effect of vitamin D). The early introduction of gluten and rice-containing cereals into an infant's diet before 3 months or after 7 months of age has also been implicated in increasing type 1 DM risk.

Patients with immune-mediated DM are rarely obese and are prone to other autoimmune diseases such as Graves' disease, Hashimoto's thyroiditis, Addison's disease, vitiligo, and pernicious anemia. In contrast, idiopathic type 1B DM, which accounts for less than 10% of type 1 DM cases, shows no evidence of autoimmunity and has no known cause. It is a rare form of DM that is inherited and more common in people of Asian, African, or Hispanic origin.

PATHOPHYSIOLOGY

Type 1 DM is characterized by a reduction or absence of functioning beta cells in the pancreatic islets of Langerhans. Genetic susceptibility has been mapped to the HLA region on chromosome 6p, with an increased risk associated with specific polymorphisms in several *HLA-DQ* and *HLA-DR* genes, preproinsulin (the primary protein product of the insulin gene), and PTPN22 (a tyrosine phosphatase involved in T-cell receptor signaling). Inheritance of type 1 DM appears to be polygenic, as expression of a particular HLA allele is insufficient by itself to lead to autoimmune beta cell destruction. However, there are rare forms of monogenic diabetes that account for 1% to 5% percent of all cases in young people (e.g., neonatal DM, maturity-onset diabetes of the young). Although other genes within the major histocompatability complex (MHC) loci and some non-MHC genes (e.g., cytotoxic T lymphocyte–associated antigen 4) influence type 1 DM risk, class II HLA genes have the greatest effect. In fact, certain non-MHC genes confer an increased risk only in the presence of particular HLA haplotypes, showing the importance of polygenic interactions.

Much of our understanding of the pathogenesis of autoimmune DM stems from studies in diabetogenic rodent models. Animal studies demonstrate that a triggering mechanism, such as a viral infection or other environmental factor, can stimulate an inflammatory response and autoimmune infiltration of pancreatic beta cells—a process termed *insulitis*. Islet cell antigens are presented by macrophages and other antigen-presenting cells within the context of class II MHC proteins to autoreactive T cells that mediate subsequent beta cell destruction. Alterations in just one or two amino acid positions within certain class II MHC proteins can markedly increase or decrease their capacity to present autoantigens to autoreactive T cells, presumably by altering binding affinity. Molecular mimicry is often cited as the mechanism by which seemingly innocuous environmental (e.g., food-based epitopes) or infectious (e.g., viral) antigens that share homology with islet cell antigens initiate a destructive autoimmune process.

Type 1 DM is clearly associated with an increased incidence of other autoimmune disorders, including thyroid, adrenal, and gonadal insufficiency. The coexistence of these conditions has been termed *polyglandular autoimmune disease type 2*. Other rare autoimmune syndromes involving insulitis include autoimmune polyendocrine syndrome type 1, which results from a mutation in the *AIRE* gene that normally allows for expression of autoantigens in the thymus (including insulin) to mediate T-cell self-tolerance and IPEX syndrome, which involves mutations in *foxp3*—a master control gene for regulatory T cells—that lead to DM and potentially fatal fulminant enteritis in affected infants.

Both Th1 and Th2 cells are capable of inducing beta cell destruction, underscoring the importance of both cell-mediated and humoral immune processes in the pathogenesis of type 1 DM. The presence of functional autoreactive B lymphocytes and islet cell–specific autoantibodies has been shown to both increase the incidence and shorten the time to progression of type 1 DM. Islet cell–specific antibodies may be identified in 70% to 80% of individuals with prediabetes and in those newly diagnosed with type 1 DM. Antibodies specific for insulin are usually detected first, followed by antibodies against the islet cell enzyme glutamic acid decarboxylase (GAD; which shares homology with the proteins of certain viruses implicated in the development of type 1 DM, such as Coxsackie B4 virus), and later antibodies specific for insulinoma-associated protein 2 (IA-2; a tyrosine phosphatase). Development of two of these three types of autoantibodies is strongly predictive of progression to type 1A DM in genetically predisposed individuals. However, it is unclear if these autoantibodies are pathogenic or simply formed as a consequence of immunological upregulation, as they are not essential for the pathogenesis of type 1 DM.

Genetic predisposition alone does not fully account for disease pathogenesis, however. Identical (monozygotic) twin studies reveal only a 30% lifetime risk of developing type 1 DM in twin siblings of probands, compared to a 5% risk in nonidentical siblings. Twin studies also demonstrate that autoantibodies against beta islet cells may be present for years in the sibling of a proband before autoimmune diabetes develops. Thus, destruction of a significant amount of beta cell mass may take months to years before resulting in a lack of insulin. The inflammatory cytokine milieu plays an important role in diabetic pathogenesis, and some patients with type 1 DM may have a reversible component to their disease if the autoinflammatory process can be stopped early enough and an adequate number of beta cells salvaged (e.g., insulin-like growth factor–1 has a role in preserving beta cell function).

Progressive beta cell destruction remains the hallmark of type 1 DM, with hyperglycemia typically developing once 80% to 90% of a patient's beta cells have been destroyed. This hyperglycemia leads to both microvascular and macrovascular complications, which underlie long-term diabetic damage. Vascular endothelial dysfunction and inflammation result in fibrosis and intimal thickening in blood vessels, leading to progressive narrowing of the vascular lumen. The resultant decreased blood flow through the microvasculature leads to tissue ischemia throughout the body and functional impairment of multiple end organs. Several clinical trials have demonstrated that careful glycemic control reduces the development and delays the progression of microvascular manifestations of DM, including nephropathy and retinopathy.

CLINICAL PRESENTATION

Subjective

Although the symptom manifestations of type 1 DM vary, the majority of patients seek medical attention due to symptoms related to hyperglycemia, with the initial diagnosis in children often being made when patients present in frank diabetic ketoacidosis (DKA). The classic symptoms of type 1 DM are polyuria (increased urination), polydipsia (increased fluid intake due to excessive thirst), nocturnal enuresis, polyphagia with paradoxical weight loss (due to reduced glucose metabolism, despite increased consumption), visual changes (especially blurred vision), and eventual fatigue, weakness, and anorexia. Polyuria results from osmotic diuresis secondary to sustained hyperglycemia; this loss of glucose, free water, and electrolytes in the urine induces a hyperosmolar state, which causes excessive thirst and compensatory polydipsia. Blurred vision results from the lens and retina being exposed to hyperosmolar fluids. A decreased plasma volume resulting from significant fluid losses may cause dizziness and fatigue, while weakness results from the catabolism of muscle proteins and potassium loss.

Because hyperglycemia worsens humoral immunity and leukocyte function, patients with DM may present with repeated or complicated infections, decreased wound healing, or infections that are uncommon in the general public, such as serious staphylococcal and *Klebsiella pneumoniae* infections, malignant (necrotizing) otitis externa due to *Pseudomonas aeruginosa*, or rhinocerebral mucormycosis, which occurs almost exclusively in patients with DM. Pathogens are able to multiply rapidly because the increased glucose in bodily fluids acts as an energy source. If a patient complains of nausea, abdominal pain, or genitourinary discomfort, urinary tract infection must be ruled out because individuals with DM are more likely to experience serious complications of pyelonephritis, such as renal papillary necrosis, emphysematous (necrotizing) pyelonephritis, or progression to gram-negative bacterial sepsis. Female patients may also present with complaints of vaginal pruritus or burning caused by vulvovaginitis.

Objective

Signs of dehydration such as poor skin turgor and dry mucous membranes may be present. Weight loss despite a normal or increased appetite may be noted, as water, glycogen, and triglyceride stores are depleted and glucose cannot be metabolized for its nutritional value due to insulinemia. A reduction in muscle mass may be seen, as muscle proteins are broken down to generate amino acids used by the liver for gluconeogenesis, resulting in the formation of ketone bodies. Thus, ketoacidosis is usually present and may be mild to severe.

Signs of severe ketosis known as diabetic ketoacidosis (DKA) include extreme fatigue, abnormal cramping, and alterations in breathing pattern. In addition, a telltale sign of ketosis is halitosis, which smells like a combination of nail polish (acetone) and rotting fruit. In contrast, hyperosmolar hyperglycemic state (HHS) is a serious form of nonketotic acidosis resulting from prolonged hyperglycemia that is less common than DKA but has a higher mortality rate. HHS is seen most frequently in adults who have a restriction in fluid intake for some reason, such as a concurrent illness, impaired physical function, or reduced cognition.

The physical examination should include a funduscopic examination, as patients with long-standing DM frequently develop diabetic retinopathy, as a result of retinal ischemia. Five stages of retinopathy are evident on physical examination: (1) dilation of retinal venules and retinal capillary microaneurysms; (2) increased vascular permeability; (3) retinal ischemia due to vascular occlusion; (4) angiogenesis (proliferation of new retinal surface blood vessels); and (5) retinal hemorrhage with fibrovascular proliferation and contraction, which may lead to retinal detachment. Such findings are discernible on funduscopic examination and require expert evaluation by an ophthalmological specialist.

Patients with poorly controlled DM can present with various skin complications, such as chronic pyogenic infections or necrobiosis lipoidica diabeticorum, which consists of well-demarcated plaques with a shiny yellow surface that occur on the anterior surfaces of the legs or dorsal aspect of the ankles. The physical examination must include a comprehensive foot evaluation because patients can present with paresthesias related to dysfunction of peripheral sensory nerves, which can decrease sensitivity to extremity trauma. The typical stocking-glove distribution of anesthesia classically leads to unrecognized foot ulcers or burns on the hands from cooking or smoking. Thus, diabetic foot ulcers result from a combination of factors, including decreased circulation, infection, decreased immune responses, and peripheral neuropathy. Moreover, neurological complications may also impact the cranial nerves, for example, third (oculomotor), fourth (trochlear), or sixth (abducens) cranial nerve palsies resulting in deviations in gaze of the affected eye.

DIAGNOSTIC REASONING

Diagnostic Tests

The American Diabetes Association (ADA) does not recommend screening for type 1 DM in apparently healthy individuals who have no risk factors for this disorder. However, if suspected, point-of-care testing can be accomplished by utilizing a portable blood glucose monitor to determine capillary blood glucose level as a random plasma glucose measurement taken without regard to the timing of a patient's last meal. If elevated, the patient's urine should be tested for ketones and additional plasma glucose testing should be initiated.

Initial Testing

Current guidelines for the diagnosis of DM include any one of the following:

- Glycosylated hemoglobin (A1C) of 6.5% or higher
- Symptoms of diabetes (e.g., polyuria, polydipsia, weight loss) plus a random plasma glucose level of 200 mg/dL or higher
- Fasting plasma glucose level of 126 mg/dL or higher (following 8 hours of no caloric intake)
- Two-hour plasma glucose level of 200 mg/dL or higher during an oral glucose tolerance test (OGTT) with a 75-g glucose load

The first three criteria listed above should be confirmed by repeat testing (preferably with the same test) without delay, except in the setting of unequivocal hyperglycemia with acute metabolic decompensation.

Patients with borderline glucose intolerance at risk for developing type 1 DM or those with suspected LADA can be tested for antibodies against GAD, insulin, tyrosine phosphatases (e.g., IA-2), or zinc transporters (e.g., ZnT8), as these autoantibodies help differentiate LADA from type 2 DM. If two or more of these antibody classes are positive in the setting of diagnostic hyperglycemia, then the diagnosis of type 1 DM is confirmed. However, such antibodies are not a diagnostic requirement for type 1 DM.

Another test to assess beta cell function and insulin production in a patient with type 1 DM is the C-peptide level. Proinsulin is cleaved into insulin and C-peptide, the latter being biologically inactive. Therefore, C-peptide levels are found in amounts equal to endogenous insulin. However, exogenous insulin preparations do not include C-peptide. Thus, a patient with residual pancreatic beta cell function will have decreased but nonetheless detectable levels of C-peptide, whereas if no insulin is being produced, the levels of C-peptide will be negligible (normal fasting level = 0.51–2.72 ng/mL or 0.17–0.90 mmol/L).

The International Expert Committee on Diabetes recommends that an A1C of 6.5% or greater can be used to diagnose DM with a repeat level obtained for confirmation. Confirmatory testing is not needed, however, if a patient has the clinical symptoms of DM or the random plasma glucose level is greater than 200 mg/dL. Of note, this test cannot be used for diagnosis in the setting of pregnancy, hemoglobinopathy, or other situations with abnormal rates of erythrocyte turnover.

Subsequent Testing

A1C determination gives valuable insight into the mean plasma glucose concentration over the preceding 2 to 3 months and is helpful in documenting the degree of glycemic control at the time of diagnosis and as part of continuing care. The risk of developing complications of type 1 DM, such as retinopathy, nephropathy, and neuropathy, are significantly reduced when A1C levels are maintained below 7%, which is recommended as a treatment goal by the ADA. The A1C level roughly correlates to mean plasma glucose concentration: 6% = glucose of 135 mg/dL; 7% = 170 mg/dL; 8% = 205 mg/dL; 9% = 240 mg/dL; 10% = 275 mg/dL; 11% = 310 mg/dL; 12% = 345 mg/dL. A1C testing should be done at least twice a year in patients with good glycemic control and quarterly in patients whose therapy has changed or in patients who have not yet achieved their glycemic goals.

Additional laboratory tests that are appropriate to the evaluation of the patient's general medical condition and cardiovascular risk status should be performed. These include a fasting lipid profile (total cholesterol, high-density lipoprotein [HDL], low-density lipoprotein [LDL], and triglyceride levels), urinalysis, microalbuminuria, thyroid function tests (thyroid-stimulating hormone, free T_4), liver enzymes (aspartate aminotransferase, alanine aminotransferase [ALT], gamma glutamyltransferase), and blood urea nitrogen and serum creatinine if proteinuria is present. Urine cultures may be obtained if indicated by symptom complaints or urinalysis results. A 12-lead electrocardiogram (ECG) should be done in adults at the time of diagnosis, and screening for other autoimmune diseases (e.g., vitamin B_{12} deficiency, celiac disease, hypothyroidism, hyperthyroidism) should be considered as well.

Differential Diagnosis

With the classic symptoms of DM confirmed by blood plasma glucose testing, a diagnosis of DM can be made; however, other potential causes of hyperglycemia should be considered. Hyperglycemia and glucosuria are present in patients with Cushing's disease, pheochromocytoma, and acromegaly. Extreme stress or trauma, such as that seen in extensive burns, may produce transient hyperglycemia. Renal tubular disease may produce glycosuria without concurrent hyperglycemia. Several pharmacological agents can cause hyperglycemia, including glucocorticoids, furosemide (Lasix), thiazide diuretics, sympathomimetic agents, estrogen-containing products, beta blockers, and nicotinic acid.

Non-immune secondary causes of hyperglycemia may mimic either type 1 or type 2 DM, depending on whether the mechanism is destruction of beta islet cells with subsequent insulin deficiency or peripheral insulin resistance in which the body produces insulin that is utilized inefficiently by the peripheral tissues. Non-immune mechanisms of beta cell destruction that produce a type 1 DM-like state include hemochromatosis, cystic fibrosis, and pancreatitis.

MANAGEMENT

Type 1 DM is a chronic illness that requires ongoing health-care and patient education to prevent acute and chronic complications. The complexity and lifelong management regimens necessitate that the patient and clinician work as a team to develop and implement the treatment plan. The ADA recommends a team approach to care, including the primary-care practitioner, an endocrinologist for periodic evaluation, a certified diabetes educator, a dietitian, the patient, and the patient's family. Essential to successful implementation of the treatment plan is the plan's fit with the patient's lifestyle to the extent possible. This is where a diabetes educator is of the most assistance. Children with type 1 DM will also need school personnel involved in the treatment team.

A comprehensive treatment program requires exogenous insulin, frequent self-monitoring of blood glucose (SMBG), medical nutrition therapy, regular exercise, continuing education in the prevention and treatment of diabetic complications (e.g., cardiovascular disease [CVD]), and the periodic reassessment of treatment goals. As with any chronic illness, a diagnosis of DM requires incorporation of the diagnosis and subsequent management strategy into the patient's lifestyle. Often, it may take a traumatic event or "turning point" in a patient's management to break the complacency of a treatment plan to one that focuses on lifestyle changes. The principles of assessment and management of type 1 DM are summarized in Table 58.1.

Of note, while type 1A DM is essentially insulin-dependent, the need for insulin replacement therapy in patients with type 1B DM is variable. Clinical trials are currently evaluating prevention strategies to delay the onset of clinical disease in type 1B DM, and the ADA is hopeful that effective preventive therapies will eventually be found.

Initial Management

Insulin Therapy

The initial goal of treatment for type 1 DM is to normalize the elevated blood glucose level. This is best accomplished by intensive insulin regimens to achieve the following goals: plasma glucose levels of 80 to 130 mg/dL before meals, peak postprandial (1–2 hours after the beginning of a meal) glucose levels of less than 180 mg/dL, and an A1C below 7% for adults with type 1 DM. The patient with new-onset type 1 DM often presents in crisis and requires hospitalization. These patients should be managed by or in close collaboration with an endocrinologist and a comprehensive health-care team. When patients present in acute hyperglycemia, it is essential not only to treat the hyperglycemia but also to determine its underlying cause (e.g., medication nonadherence, dietary indiscretions, or underlying infection, which is the most common cause of DKA, the inpatient treatment of which is detailed in Table 58.2).

The Diabetes Control and Complications Trial conclusively demonstrated that in patients with type 1 DM, the risk of development or progression of retinopathy, nephropathy, and neuropathy is reduced by 50% to 75% with intensive insulin regimens compared with conventional treatment regimens. Individual treatment goals should, however, take into account the patient's capacity to understand and carry out the treatment, the risk for severe hypoglycemia, and any other factors that increase risk or decrease benefit. Tight glycemic control increases the chance of hypoglycemic episodes and may not be

---

TABLE 58.1   Outpatient Assessment and Management of the Patient With Type 1 Diabetes Mellitus

Assessment	*Laboratory Monitoring*	*General Health Maintenance*
Every visit: • Symptoms of hypoglycemia and hyperglycemia • Results of SMBG • Any self-adjustments based on SMBG or symptoms • Problems with adherence • Symptoms of complications • Any other medical illnesses • Medications (prescription and over the counter) • Height and weight • Blood pressure • Cardiovascular assessment • Thyroid examination • Ophthalmic examination (with an annual dilated retinal eye examination) • Peripheral vascular assessment • Feet and skin assessment • Neurological assessment • Oral examination	A1C every 3 months during the first year of initiation of insulin therapy and during periods of insulin dosage adjustment. In patients who have met treatment goals, measure A1C twice a year, if stable. Initially upon diagnosis and annually, if stable: • Lipid profile • Urinalysis • Serum creatinine Microalbuminuria screening annually: • Method 1: spot UACR (can be performed in clinic; first morning void is preferred because of diurnal variation in albumin excretion; >30 mcg albumin/mg creatinine indicates microalbuminuria) • Method 2: 24-hour urine collection	Immunizations and prophylaxis: • Pneumococcal vaccine • Influenza vaccine annually • Cardioprotective aspirin in patients >40 years Patient education: • Preconception or contraceptive counseling (initial and quarterly, when applicable) • Smoking cessation, if applicable

TABLE 58.2   Diabetic Ketoacidosis (DKA)

Overview	Clinical Presentation	Management
DKA is an acute life-threatening decompensation of glucose metabolism seen in DM (most commonly in type 1) that requires immediate medical attention. The cardinal features of DKA include the following: • Hyperglycemia—blood glucose level >359 mg/dL • Ketonemia—plasma ketone level >5 mmol/L • Acidosis—plasma bicarbonate level <9 mEq/L Causes: • Lack of insulin • Stress (physical or emotional), even with continued insulin therapy Pathophysiology: • As insulin levels decrease, concentrations of glucagon rise, which increases glucose levels. • Epinephrine inhibits glucose transport in peripheral tissues, thereby stimulating the production of glucose from non-carbohydrate substrates in the liver. • Free fatty acids from adipose stores are oxidized in the liver for energy, causing release of ketones and resultant acidosis.	Initial signs of DKA: • Anorexia • Increased thirst • Nausea/vomiting • Abdominal cramping • Increased urine formation • Fatigue Later signs: • Kussmaul respiration • Signs of dehydration (usual fluid deficit of 3–5 L) • Oliguria • Altered consciousness Left untreated: • Coma • Vascular collapse • Renal shutdown • Blood glucose increases from 300–800 mg/dL Diagnostic tests: • Serum glucose • Sodium potassium • Phosphate • Bicarbonate • Beta-hydroxybutyrate • Osmolarity • pH • Calculated anion gap	Goals: • Correct hyperglycemia • Correct dehydration • Normalize electrolytes (replenish deficiencies) • Correct acidosis First line of treatment is insulin: • Continuous-dose insulin infusion: 0.1–0.2 units/kg/hr Correct dehydration and electrolyte imbalance: • Rapid IV infusion of normal saline (0.9% NaCl) or Ringer's lactate: 1–2 L • Potassium replacement 3–4 hours after initiation of insulin and fluid therapy • Phosphorus replacement • Bicarbonate therapy if pH is 7.0 or below After recovery, causes of DKA should be explored. Patients should be taught about increased insulin needs during periods of illness and stress.

appropriate for many elderly patients, patients with coronary artery disease (CAD) who may be prone to hypoglycemia, or those with diabetic neuropathy who may lack the early neurological (adrenergic) warning signs of hypoglycemia.

The initiation of insulin therapy in newly diagnosed type 1 DM patients should be managed by or in close collaboration with an endocrinologist. The majority of insulin used today is made chemically identical to human insulin by recombinant DNA technology or by chemical modification of pork insulin; however, beef and pork insulin preparations are still available. Insulin is available in rapid, short, intermediate, and long-acting forms. The optimal dosage is highly individualized and can depend on the site and depth of injections, skin temperature (related to subcutaneous and superficial blood circulation in the skin), and exercise. Human insulin is preferred for patients newly beginning insulin therapy, pregnant women, and persons with allergies.

In the United States, insulin is available in concentrations of 100 or 500 U/mL, but highly concentrated preparations are used only in rare cases of insulin resistance, when a patient requires large doses. The 2017 ADA Standards of Medical Care in Diabetes state that the majority of patients with type 1 DM should be treated with multiple daily injections of prandial insulin and daily basal insulin or with a continuous subcutaneous insulin infusion pump. Both strategies require diligent and frequent blood glucose monitoring by the patient and should be selected on the basis of what is most appropriate for the patient's current or future lifestyle choices, given the severe consequences of therapeutic nonadherence. Commercially mixed neutral protamine Hagedorn (NPH) and regular insulin preparations are also available to reduce the number of injections needed, or the patient can custom mix his or her own insulin preparation. Both insulin dosage and timing should be individualized for the patient according to his or her health needs and lifestyle choices (see Drugs Commonly Prescribed 58.1).

Some patients may experience early morning hyperglycemia due to complete absorption of the evening insulin dose before the early morning hours (the dawn phenomenon), particularly if an intermediate-acting form of insulin is used, such as NPH, which has a peak effect at 6 to 10 hours after subcutaneous injection and a duration of action of 10 to 16 hours. In addition,

Drugs Commonly Prescribed 58.1: Diabetes Mellitus Type 1 Insulin Regimens

SINGLE-DOSE THERAPY

Single Injection

- Intermediate or long-acting insulin with or without regular insulin in the morning *or* Intermediate or long-acting insulin at bedtime
- Recommend at a minimum SMBG in the morning and at bedtime

CONVENTIONAL SPLIT-DOSE THERAPY

Two Injections

- Mixture of NPH and regular insulin in the morning and evening
- Recommend at a minimum SMBG before each dosing and at bedtime

INTENSIVE INSULIN THERAPY

Three Injections

- NPH and regular insulin in the morning; regular insulin at dinner; NPH insulin at bedtime
- Monitor for increased risk of hypoglycemic episodes

Four Injections

- Regular or lispro insulin before meals and long-acting insulin to maintain basal insulin levels
- Monitor for increased risk of hypoglycemic episodes

TYPES OF INSULIN	SPECIES	ONSET, PEAK, AND DURATION*	ROUTE
Insulin Glulisine			
Apidra	Recombinant DNA (usually used in combination with longer-acting insulins)	<5 min, 1–2 hr, 2–3 hr	SC
Insulin Aspart			
Novolog	Recombinant DNA (usually used in combination with longer-acting insulins)	<10 min, 1–3 hr, 3–5 hr	SC
Insulin Lispro			
Humalog	Recombinant DNA (usually used in combination with longer-acting insulins)	<15 min, 1–2 hr, 3–4 hr	SC
Regular Insulin			
Humulin R	Human	30–60 min, 2–6 hr, 6–8 hr	SC, IM, IV
Iletin II Regular	Pork	30–60 min, 2–6 hr, 6–8 hr	SC, IM, IV
Novolin R	Human	30–60 min, 2–6 hr, 6–8 hr	SC, IM, IV
Purified Pork Regular	Pork	30–60 min, 2–6 hr, 6–8 hr	SC, IM, IV
Velosulin	Human	30–60 min, 2–4 hr, 6–8 hr	SC, IM, IV
Insulin Isophane Suspension (NPH)			
Humulin N	Human	1–1.5 hr, 4–12 hr, 18–24 hr	SC
Iletin II NPH	Pork	1–1.5 hr, 4–12 hr, 18–24 hr	SC
Novolin N	Human	1–1.5 hr, 4–12 hr, 18–24 hr	SC
Purified Pork NPH	Pork	1–1.5 hr, 4–12 hr, 18–24 hr	SC
Insulin Isophane Suspension (NPH)/Regular Insulin			
Humulin 70/30	Human	30–60 min, 2–12 hr, 24 hr	SC
Humulin 50/50	Human	30–60 min, 3–5 hr, 24 hr	SC
Novolin 70/30	Human	30–60 min, 2–12 hr, 24 hr	SC
Insulin Glargine			
Lantus	Insulin analog	Slowly absorbed with gradual onset, peakless, lasting up to 24 hr	SC
Insulin Detemir			
Levemir	Insulin analog	Slowly absorbed with gradual onset, relative constant concentration with peak at 6–10 hr, lasting up to 24 hr	SC

Abbreviations: IM, intramuscular; IV, intravenous; NPH, neutral protamine Hagedorn; SC, subcutaneous; SMBG, self-monitoring of blood glucose.
*General guidance, affected by multiple factors.

humans have an increased insulin requirement in the morning because of early morning secretion of growth hormone and cortisol. Thus, increasing the nighttime insulin dose to address early morning hyperglycemia may lead to late evening hypoglycemia, in the absence of an adequate insulin effect in the early morning hours. Therefore, if NPH is being used, the evening dose should be given later. Alternatively, it may be more efficient to prevent early morning hyperglycemia by switching the regimen from NPH to a longer-acting form of insulin, such as glargine (Lantus) or detemir (Levemir).

Self-Monitoring of Blood Glucose Levels

Self-monitoring of blood glucose (SMBG) is the testing of capillary blood to determine blood glucose level. Typically, plasma venous glucose measurements are within 15% of the results of whole blood capillary test results. SMBG is recommended for patients with type 1 DM to evaluate the effectiveness of the insulin regimen, medical nutrition therapy, and exercise. Used properly, it is the most practical mechanism to maintain glucose levels as close to normal as possible and to prevent the most common complication of DM therapy—hypoglycemia.

The frequency and timing of blood glucose monitoring are dependent on the needs and goals of the individual patient. Optimal SMBG for patients with type 1 DM is three to four times a day—before each meal and before bedtime, but with intensive control, blood glucose checks could be up to 10 times a day, as postprandial assessment is added. Common barriers to frequent SMBG in patients with type 1 DM include cost (e.g., test strips, multiple glucometers), inconvenience, and the discomfort produced by the finger pricks. The benefit versus cost ratio must be thoroughly explored with each patient, as a treatment plan is developed, and individualized goals are established. Table 58.3 presents the goals of glucose management for patients without symptoms of hypoglycemia.

Continuous Glucose Monitoring

Continuous glucose monitoring (CGM) utilizes a device that measures interstitial glucose concentration and can be utilized with intensive insulin therapy. This measurement correlates with SMBG. Such devices have been studied in adults older than 25 years of age and found to reduce the amount of time type 1 DM patients experience hyperglycemic and hypoglycemic episodes. The measurement of CGM must be calibrated with SMBG, however, and SMBG should be used to make acute treatment decisions. Patients who have limited awareness of hypoglycemic episodes or experience them frequently may also benefit from CGM.

There are many different types of blood glucose meters, and one should be selected that best fits the needs and resources of the patient. Many glucometers have the ability to download records into personal computers, which allows clinicians to readily review the data. This can provide helpful information regarding trends in SMBG. The patient should, nevertheless, be instructed to keep a log of results along with insulin doses so that adjustments can be made to the treatment plan. There are more than 1,100 smartphone apps available to help manage DM. The proper function of the glucometer, as well as the patient's SMBG testing technique, should be assessed for accuracy at each visit while the patient's ideal dose is being adjusted and then annually once the patient's regimen is stabilized.

Management of Hypoglycemia

Hypoglycemia is a common occurrence in patients with type 1 DM and occurs for a variety of reasons: excessive exogenous insulin, missed meals or inadequate food intake, excessive exercise, alcohol ingestion, drug interactions, or decreases in liver or kidney function. Signs and symptoms include diaphoresis, tachycardia, hunger, shakiness, altered mentation (ranging from an inability to concentrate to frank coma), slurred speech, and seizures. The signs and symptoms exhibited by the patient are highly individual and can vary from mild to severe. In 2017, the International Hypoglycemia Study Group of the ADA Standards of Medical Care in Diabetes classified a plasma glucose level of less than 54 mg/dL as serious, clinically significant hypoglycemia. A blood glucose level of 70 mg/dL is considered a threshold level that requires intervention.

The goal of treatment is to normalize the plasma glucose level promptly. If the patient is conscious and able to swallow, this is best accomplished by the prompt ingestion of glucose or carbohydrate-containing food with a high glycemic index for rapid absorption. Pure glucose is the treatment of choice according to the ADA, but any carbohydrate that can increase the blood glucose level can be given. Food with significant fat content may delay the glycemic response. Examples of appropriate foods include one-half cup of any fruit juice (with no additional sugar added), 6 ounces of regular soda (not diet or sugarless), 1 cup of milk, or glucose tablets. Candy (other than chocolate) can be used in dire situations but is not recommended when other sources of sugar are available. Blood glucose should be checked 15 minutes after treatment, and additional carbohydrates should be given if the blood glucose remains less than 70 mg/dL. For severe

TABLE 58.3 Goals of Glucose Management*	
Time	*Goal*
Before meals	80–120 mg/dL
Postprandial	<180 mg/dL
Bedtime	100–140 mg/dL

*Goals are for glucose management without symptoms of hypoglycemia.

hypoglycemia in a patient who is unconscious or unable to swallow, 1 mg of glucagon can be given subcutaneously to mobilize hepatic glucose stores. An alternative treatment in the inpatient setting is to administer 50 mL of a 50% dextrose solution intravenously.

Nocturnal hypoglycemia can occur if the predinner, intermediate-acting insulin dose is too high or if the patient skips dinner or eats an inadequate amount of food. The patient may not awaken with symptoms but on arising may note an increased fasting glucose level. This is due to a compensatory mechanism in the liver, which responds by mobilizing glucose from hepatic glycogen stores in response to sustained hypoglycemia. After the hypoglycemia has been resolved, the possible causes should be reviewed with the patient and preventive measures discussed. The Somogyi effect, for example, is a unique combination in which a diabetic patient develops hypoglycemia during the night with rebound hyperglycemia in the morning. Although several studies have failed to confirm the validity of this pathological process, many clinicians still feel the Somogyi effect exists and is most commonly observed in children with type 1 DM.

Diet

Once the patient has been educated in insulin therapy, SMBG, and the treatment of hypoglycemia, subsequent management includes education in meal planning and dietary practices. Meal planning or medical nutritional therapy is one of the most challenging aspects of diabetes management because achievement of treatment goals may require substantial lifestyle changes related to food intake. The goals of nutritional therapy are to maintain normal blood glucose levels, prevent hypoglycemia, maintain normal serum lipid levels, attain or maintain a reasonable body weight, and promote healthy eating practices. The meal plan should be based on the patient's food choices, exercise habits, medical history, current and goal weight, and lifestyle, cultural, ethnic, and financial factors.

Most patients will benefit from a referral to a certified diabetic educator for a group program or individual counseling; thus, referral to a dietitian for an initial consultation should be ordered for all diabetic patients at a minimum.

The first step of a nutritional consultation is the initial assessment of the patient's nutritional status, including a detailed diet history. Recommendations for dietary changes should not be made until the patient's current eating patterns are determined. Individuals on insulin should eat at consistent times that are synchronized with their insulin administration. Most patients with type 1 DM are lean, so weight loss is generally not a major factor in meal planning. The following formulas can be used to determine the total number of kilocalories needed to maintain current weight:

- For men: 66 + 13.7 (weight in kg) + 5 (height in cm) − 6.8 (age)

- For women: 65 + 9.6 (weight in kg) + 1.7 (height in cm) − 4.7 (age)

Multiply the result by 1.2 for a fairly active person and by up to 1.5 for an ill person, given increased caloric requirements.

A nutritionally balanced meal plan is important for the patient with type 1 DM, which should take into account the higher prevalence of atherosclerosis typically seen in patients with DM. The ADA acknowledges that no single dietary plan is appropriate for all patients and that each patient needs an individualized eating plan. The current recommendation is for each patient to receive medical nutrition therapy provided by a registered dietician knowledgeable in diabetes management. The goals of the eating plan are to maintain a healthy body weight, support glycemic control, facilitate blood pressure and lipid goals, and delay or prevent the complications of DM. Examples of nutrient dense, high-quality eating plans for DM are the Mediterranean Diet, Dietary Approaches to Stop Hypertension, and plant-based diets.

Nutritive sweeteners (such as fructose, dextrose, and maltose) and sugar alcohols (such as sorbitol, mannitol, and xylitol) have not demonstrated a significant advantage over sucrose in improving overall diabetes control, and sugar alcohols in excessive amounts may have a laxative effect. The caloric and carbohydrate content of all these sweeteners should be taken into account in the meal plan. Non-nutritive sweeteners such as saccharin, aspartame, acesulfame potassium, sucralose, and the Latin American herb stevia are noncaloric and do not affect the blood glucose level. The majority of patients with type 1 DM can safely use them. It is unclear, however, whether nonnutritive sweeteners and the products that contain them (e.g., sugarless diet sodas) provide any advantage over nutritive sweeteners, in terms of weight management.

Although soluble fiber can inhibit the absorption of glucose from the small intestine, the amount of fiber contained in most foods will not have a significant effect on blood glucose levels. Fiber recommendations for individuals with DM, therefore, are the same as for the general population (20 to 35 g/day).

Vitamin and mineral supplementation is not generally recommended for persons whose dietary intake is adequate. For example, chromium replacements have no known benefit except for the patient who may be chromium deficient as a result of long-term parenteral nutrition. In addition, magnesium and sodium replacement should be given only if medically warranted.

The same recommendations for the general population concerning alcohol ingestion are appropriate for the patient with type 1 DM. Alcohol consumption in some patients can increase hypoglycemia with insulin or insulin secretagogues; diabetic patients should be made aware of this and instructed to drink alcohol cautiously. Additionally, calories from alcohol should be included as part of the total caloric intake. Heavily sweetened alcoholic drinks should be avoided, and alcohol intake should be considered as part of the meal plan.

Exercise

According to ADA standards, all patients should undergo a careful evaluation of their medical history and assessment for cardiovascular risk factors (hypertension, hyperlipidemia, family history, etc.) before being provided assistance in developing a regular exercise program. If the patient is determined to be at high risk for cardiovascular disease, they should be referred for a more thorough evaluation before starting an activity program. However, in the absence of other risk factors, the patient with type 1 DM can perform all levels of exercise and physical activity, as long as glycemic control is established and there is no evidence of complications that would preclude exercise.

Because the metabolic adjustments that maintain blood glucose levels during exercise in a nondiabetic individual are impaired in patients with type 1 DM, exercise can exacerbate hyperglycemia if the diabetic patient has too little insulin available. Conversely, if there is too much insulin present, hypoglycemia may occur. Thus, the diabetic patient must use the following general guidelines regarding exercise to regulate the glycemic response:

- Check blood glucose before, every 30 to 60 minutes during, and after exercise.
- Avoid exercise if fasting glucose is more than 250 mg/dL and ketosis is present or if the glucose level is more than 300 mg/dL, regardless of whether ketosis is present.
- Consume additional carbohydrate if the glucose level is less than 100 mg/dL and as needed to avoid hypoglycemia.
- Identify when changes in insulin dose or food intake are necessary.

Any exercise program should be individualized to take into account the patient's activity interests, lifestyle, physical condition, and motivation. The program should include at least 150 minutes per week of moderate-intensity aerobic activity. Muscle-strengthening exercises can also be added.

Urine Ketone Testing

Urine ketone testing is recommended for patients with type 1 DM when the patient experiences documented hyperglycemia or stressful events that can lead to hyperglycemia. For instance, during an acute illness, particularly if the patient is nauseated and vomiting, urine ketones can be monitored, especially if the patient is ketosis prone and has had documented ketotic episodes in the past. Because pregnancy places stress on the diabetic patient, it may also be recommended that pregnant patients perform periodic ketone assessments. Ketonuria can reflect dehydration and the need for increased fluid intake, as well as increased insulin requirements.

FOLLOW-UP AND REFERRAL

Continuity of care is essential in the management of type 1 DM, and patients typically benefit from a long-term relationship with their primary-care practitioner. Long-term surveillance for potential complications of DM demands almost as much daily attention by the patient and office time of the primary-care practitioner as do the daily insulin regimens needed to manage the disease effectively.

The frequency of follow-up visits depends on the degree to which blood glucose levels are controlled, changes in insulin therapy, and the presence and severity of complications or other medical conditions. If the patient uses SMBG effectively, telephone consultations instead of clinic visits may be possible. Once glycemic levels are effectively regulated (e.g., A1C consistently below 7%) and insulin regimens are stabilized, diabetic patients may be seen at least quarterly. These visits should include a discussion of SMBG results, adjustments to therapy made by the patient, symptoms of DM and its complications, problems with adherence to the treatment plan, changes in lifestyle behaviors, any modifications to the patient's medications, and the frequency, causes, and severity of hyperglycemia or hypoglycemia.

The National Institutes of Health has created a multicenter program called the Type 1 Diabetes Trial-Net, which is an international research network that accepts referral of relatives of patients with type 1 DM for screening with islet cell antibody measurements. It offers treatment with various agents that are being investigated as potentially preventing the development of the disease.

The potential for the development of long-term complications of DM affecting almost every major organ system necessitates regular follow-up of all diabetic patients. For example, diabetic retinopathy remains the leading cause of new-onset blindness among adults 20 to 74 years of age, and at 20 years postdiagnosis of type 1 DM, nearly all patients have some degree of retinopathy. In addition, growth impairment, an increased susceptibility to infection, and autonomic neuropathy may occur, resulting in gastrointestinal, genitourinary, and cardiovascular symptoms, including sexual dysfunction. Indeed, persons with DM have an increased incidence of atherosclerotic heart disease, PVD, and cerebrovascular disease. The development of the life-threatening sequelae of hyperglycemia, DKA (more common in type 1 DM), and HHS (more common in type 2 DM) may first be detected by the primary-care practitioner at unscheduled sick visits; however, these conditions call for immediate referral to the emergency department (see Tables 58.2 and 58.4 for more information on these serious complications).

If any of these complications are detected or suspected, referral to a specialist to guide management may

TABLE 58.4 Hyperosmolar Hyperglycemic Syndrome (HHS)

Overview	Clinical Presentation	Management
HHS is characterized by: • Severe hyperglycemia—blood sugar >600 mg/dL • No ketosis • Hyperosmolality • Dehydration • High mortality rate Occurs in: • Older diabetics who develop infection or other illness • Undiagnosed diabetics • Patients with diabetes mellitus diagnosed after a prolonged period of hyperglycemia Precipitating factors: • Peritoneal dialysis • Hemodialysis • Tube feeding with high-protein formulas • Mannitol infusion • Phenytoin (Dilantin) • Corticosteroids • Immunosuppressive agents • Diuretics • Surgery • Myocardial infarction • Sepsis • Renal insufficiency • Congestive heart failure	Insidious onset with subtle initial symptoms; history may indicate decreased fluid intake. Patients may present with: • Polyuria • Polydipsia • Weakness • No ketoacidosis • Lethargy and confusion develop when serum osmolality >310 mOsm/kg • Coma Laboratory tests: • Severe hyperglycemia—blood glucose >600 mg/dL • Initial serum sodium decreased • Serum sodium increases as dehydration progresses • Serum osmolality >400 mOsm/kg	Goals: • Correct dehydration • Normalize electrolytes (replenish deficiencies) Correct dehydration and electrolyte imbalance: • Rapid infusion of hypotonic saline (0.45% NaCl) • In cases of hypovolemia, use normal saline (0.9% NaCl) • Fluid needs may be 4–6 L in 8–10 hours • Correct serum sodium with the following equation: corrected sodium = measured sodium + (0.8 × every 50 mg/dL increment of plasma glucose above 100 mg/dL) • Once blood glucose is <250 mg/dL, fluid replacement should be with 5% dextrose in 0.45% saline solution or normal saline • End point of fluid therapy is to return urine output to ≥50 mL/hr • Less potassium replacement is typically needed than in diabetic ketoacidosis

be indicated. Key follow-up and management principles with respect to the diabetic patient are as follows:

• *Retinopathy:* The ADA recommends that adults with type 1 DM should be seen by an ophthalmologist or optometrist and have a dilated comprehensive eye examination within the first 5 years of diagnosis. If there is no retinopathy at the first evaluation, an eye examination should be done every 2 years. If retinopathy is detected, a full eye examination should be done by an ophthalmologist or optometrist at least annually.

• *Hyperlipidemia:* Adults with type 1 DM should be tested annually for lipid disorders with a complete fasting lipid profile, given the increased risk in these individuals for CAD.

• *Nephropathy:* The ADA recommends assessing urinary albumin to monitor for developing nephropathy at least once a year in patients with type 1 DM. Screening with a spot urinary albumin-to-creatinine ratio (UACR) and an estimated glomerular filtration (eGFR) rate should be done after a disease duration of 5 years or sooner if the patient has hypertension. Persistent albuminuria (greater than 30 mg/g of creatinine) is the earliest stage of diabetic nephropathy, and overt nephropathy with

albuminuria equal to or greater than 300 mg/g creatinine will develop over a period of 10 to 15 years in approximately 80% of patients with microalbuminuria, many of whom will also present with hypertension.

Transient elevations of albumin excretion occur with acute febrile illnesses, marked hypertension, short-term hyperglycemia, exercise, urinary tract infections, and heart failure. Angiotensin-converting enzyme inhibitors (ACEIs) have been found to postpone the progression of microalbuminuria and, ultimately, nephropathy. Thus, they are suggested as part of the initial therapy for diabetic patients with nephropathy. Their use is contraindicated in women who are pregnant, however, and they should be used with caution in women of childbearing age. ACEI may also exacerbate hyperkalemia in patients with advanced renal insufficiency or hyporeninemic hypoaldosteronism. Older adults with advanced renal disease and patients with renal artery stenosis may experience a decline in renal function with ACEI. If a patient does not tolerate the use of ACEI, angiotensin receptor blockers (ARBs) can be used. Some studies suggest these agents can be used together in diabetic patients with nephropathy because they act by different, albeit related, mechanisms.

- *Hypertension:* In a patient with type 1 DM, hypertension is often a manifestation of nephropathy. Control of hypertension has been demonstrated to reduce the rate of progression of nephropathy and to reduce the complications of CVD. ADA guidelines recommend that the goal for blood pressure control in nonpregnant adults is to maintain the systolic blood pressure at less than 140 mm Hg and the diastolic blood pressure at less than 90 mm Hg. Even lower systolic and diastolic blood pressure should be target in patients that are at high risk of cardiovascular disease. The goal for patients with isolated systolic hypertension is also less than 140 mm Hg. Patients at high risk for CVD may target a lower goal of 130/80 mm Hg, if this can be achieved without significant side effects. Studies have shown that the closer patients with DM approach the target blood pressure, the less likely they are to develop cardiac sequelae. Initial treatment for diabetic patients with hypertension should include lifestyle management and, if medication is required, an ACEI or ARB should be started, unless contraindicated. Patients with signs of congestive heart failure and an abnormal ejection fraction should be immediately referred for a cardiology consult.
- *Macrovascular disease:* Diabetic patients are at risk for developing macrovascular complications including stroke, PVD, CAD, and other forms of CVD. Evidence of uncontrolled angina, carotid bruits, and ECG abnormalities may require advanced intervention. Daily intake of aspirin has been shown to reduce cardiovascular events in patients with DM. Patients with disabling claudication or nonhealing ulcers require a vascular consultation for their PVD. All diabetic patients should be screened for these diseases, because symptoms may not be present until late in the course of the disease process.
- *Neuropathy:* One-half of the patients with hyperglycemia extending over 15 years will develop some degree of neuropathy. Foot ulcers and related problems resulting from the decreased peripheral sensation in diabetic patients with significant neuropathy are a major cause of morbidity in DM, with potentially life-threatening consequences if such infections spread systemically. Peripheral neuropathy may result in pain, loss of sensation, and muscle weakness. The feet and ankles are affected most often, but many patients also complain of pain in the knees and upper extremities. Severe pain from neuropathy can lead to sleep and mood disturbances. A thorough initial foot examination followed by annual follow-up foot examinations are indicated in asymptomatic patients. A 10-g Semmes-Weinstein monofilament should be used to assess sensation at least annually. Abnormal findings indicate the need for a thorough vascular, neurological, musculoskeletal, and soft tissue evaluation.

Many patients take several medications to control the pain or discomfort of neuropathy. Non-opioid analgesics, calcium channel blockers, narcotic analgesics, tricyclic antidepressants, antiarrhythmics, and local anesthetics are frequently prescribed. Pregabalin (Lyrica) and duloxetine (Cymbalta) have received U.S. Food and Drug Administration (FDA) approval for the treatment of neuropathic pain in DM. The opioid tapentadol (Nucynta, Palexia, Tapal) has also received FDA approval, but the evidence is weaker related to its effectiveness in diabetic neuropathy. Tricyclic antidepressants are commonly prescribed for painful neuropathies, as are gabapentin (Neurontin), venlafaxine (Effexor), carbamazepine (Tegretol), tramadol (Ultram), and topical capsaicin. Patients with chronic pain syndromes may benefit from a referral to a chronic pain clinic.

Patients with neuropathy require professional nail and callus care because most ulcers begin at the site of a callus. Supportive athletic shoes are recommended for all patients for walking. Extra-depth shoes and custom-molded shoe inserts are indicated for patients who are at high risk for foot ulcers. Patients at high risk include those with neuropathy, structural deformities of the feet, skin, or nails, and those with a history of previous ulcers. Charcot foot disorders occur in 9% of patients with neuropathy, which may be confused with those of cellulitis. This highly morbid condition leads to bony destruction, joint subluxation, and bony remodeling of the foot. Patients with abnormal findings on radiological examination should be referred to an orthopedist for further evaluation.

- *Pregnancy:* Of the 10% of all pregnancies that are complicated by DM, 0.2% to 0.5% are in women with type 1 DM. There is an increased risk for pregnancy-related complications in these patients, including preeclampsia, preterm delivery, intrauterine fetal demise, and cardiac and renal malformations. These women should undergo preconception counseling and then frequent follow-up to stress the importance of extremely tight glucose control.
- *Diabetes distress:* This distinct psychological disorder related to DM is very common. The constant demands of medication dosing, monitoring of blood glucose, food tracking, and increased attention to physician activity have an adverse psychological impact on up to 45% of patients. Annual screening for this disorder should be done with a validated measurement tool, such as the Diabetes Distress Scale for Adults With Type 1 Diabetes. If the patient screens positive for this condition, he or she should be referred to a mental health professional. In some cases, the demands of glycemic control on the patient's lifestyle can lead to depression, and patients should be evaluated for depression by the primary-care practitioner following the initial diagnosis of DM and then annually.
- *Other:* Autonomic involvement can affect gastrointestinal, cardiovascular, and genitourinary function. Sexual dysfunction, particularly erectile dysfunction, occurs frequently in older patients.

Patient Education: Diabetes Mellitus Type 1

A key focus in the education of patients with type 1 DM is insulin self-injection and the appropriate use of insulin syringes and autoinjectors. Insulin administration involves the use of subcutaneous syringes marked in insulin units. Regulations governing the purchase of syringes vary greatly from state to state. Although syringe manufacturers recommend that syringes be used only once, it appears safe and practical for the patient to reuse the syringe if needed, but it should be discarded if the needle integrity is compromised. Syringes should be recapped by the patient using a one-handed technique, and they should be discarded according to state requirements. Patients with visual or dexterity difficulties may benefit from prefilling syringes. Prefilled insulin syringes may be stored in a vertical position in the refrigerator for up to 30 days with the needle pointing upward.

Alternatives to syringes include jet injectors and penlike autoinjector devices. Jet injectors are useful for patients who have needle phobias, but they are expensive. Penlike devices hold insulin cartridges and are useful if the patient is visually or neurologically impaired, and they help to increase the accuracy of insulin administration. Unlike older insulins, newer varieties of insulin do not require constant refrigeration, which makes them more convenient for patients. Another alternative insulin delivery device is the implanted insulin pump, which is a small device that is worn externally. Continuous subcutaneous insulin is delivered from the pump via tubing attached to the pump reservoir. Use of the insulin pump requires oversight by skilled professionals, the careful selection of patients, frequent blood glucose monitoring, and comprehensive patient education.

Insulin should be injected at room temperature, but insulin storage bottles not in use should be refrigerated. Insulin should be injected into the subcutaneous tissue of the upper arm, anterior or lateral aspects of the thigh, the buttocks, or the abdomen. Rotation of the site within one area is recommended rather than rotating to a different site with each injection.

Education in foot care should also be reviewed at each visit. Patients at high risk for foot ulcer development should be encouraged to follow through with periodic professional foot care and daily foot hygiene. Patients at low risk should be encouraged to continue good hygiene, wear properly fitting footwear, avoid trauma to the feet, stop smoking if applicable, and immediately report any blisters, macerated skin, or hemorrhage into a callus, as well as limit weight-bearing on the affected extremity.

Patients should understand that any illness maximizes stress, and this is especially true for individuals with DM. When acutely ill, all patients must continue to take their insulin and increase blood glucose monitoring to every 2 hours. Supplemental dosages of regular insulin may be needed to control blood glucose levels. If the patient's blood sugar is higher than 240 mg/dL, the urine should be checked for ketones every 4 hours. A caloric intake of 50 g of carbohydrates every 4 hours should be maintained. A variety of clear fluids, including some with glucose, should be encouraged, as well as gelatin, ice pops, regular soda, soup, and toast, if tolerated. Patients should be encouraged to maintain an oral fluid intake of 6 to 9 oz/hr to avoid dehydration. If the illness is accompanied by vomiting or diarrhea for more than 2 hours, a fever of 101°F (38.3°C) or higher, or blood glucose of 240 mg/dL or higher and ketones continue to appear in the urine despite additional insulin, the patient should be instructed to seek medical attention immediately, given the risk of developing DKA.

DIABETES MELLITUS TYPE 2

Type 2 DM is characterized by the abnormal secretion of insulin, resistance to the action of insulin in the target tissues, and/or an inadequate response at the level of the insulin receptor. Type 2 DM reduces life expectancy because of complications that are affected by the duration of DM, the degree of blood glucose control, and other cardiovascular risk factors such as smoking and hypertension.

EPIDEMIOLOGY AND CAUSES

According to the Centers for Disease Control and Prevention (CDC), the prevalence of type 2 DM in the United States is 9.4%. Approximately 95% of all Americans diagnosed with DM have this form of diabetes. Approximately 28 million American adults have type 2 DM, but nearly 24% of individuals are unaware that they have the disorder. The disease is often asymptomatic in its early stages; as a result, individuals can remain undiagnosed for many years. However, chronic hyperglycemia is associated with long-term damage and dysfunction of various organs, including the kidneys, liver, eyes, nerves, heart, and blood vessels. In turn, type 2 DM is the seventh leading cause of death in the United States, as it contributes to many other diseases of major organ systems, such as cardiovascular, cerebrovascular, and kidney disorders. The comorbidities associated with type 2 DM are extensive and are reflected in the per capita health-care costs of people with DM in the United States, which are five times higher than those without DM.

Type 2 DM has a stronger genetic association than type 1 DM. First-degree relatives of patients with type 2 DM have a 5- to 10-fold higher lifetime risk of developing DM than age-matched control subjects with no family history. Moreover, nearly 40% of patients have at least one affected parent with the disease, and monozygotic twin studies have demonstrated between 60% and 90% concordance.

Risk Factors: Diabetes Mellitus Type 2

Family history (first-degree relative)
Body mass index >25 kg/m² (lower for Asian Americans)
Age >45 years
Impaired fasting glucose or A1C >5.7%
History of gestational diabetes
Hypertension (>140/90 mm Hg or on antihypertensive therapy)
Hyperlipidemia (high-density lipoprotein <35 mg/dL, triglycerides >250 mg/dL)
Women with polycystic ovarian syndrome
Race/Ethnicity

- African American
- Latino
- Native American
- Asian American
- Pacific Islander

The overall prevalence of type 2 DM is increasing in the U.S. general population, as well as among certain ethnic minority groups. A disproportionate number of African Americans, Latinos, Native Americans, Asian Americans, and Pacific Islanders have type 2 DM compared with the general population. Native Americans and Alaskan Natives have the highest prevalence of diagnosed type 2 DM. Along with genetic differences, additional factors that may underlie this disparity in disease prevalence include socioeconomic factors, differential health-care practices, unequal access to health-care resources, and ethnocultural influences in diet and activity level.

Unlike type 1 DM, the incidence of type 2 DM increases with age, reaching 25% in individuals aged 65 years and older. However, it is important to note that this form of DM may be diagnosed at any age. Rates of newly diagnosed cases of type 2 DM among children are on the rise, reflecting the marked increase in childhood obesity over the past several decades. Indeed, the CDC estimates that the prevalence of type 2 DM in children and adolescence will quadruple over the next 40 years.

Several pharmacological agents are associated with iatrogenic hyperglycemia and the eventual development of overt DM. These include glucocorticoids, hormonal therapies such as oral contraceptives, the immunosuppressants tacrolimus and cyclosporine, nicotinic acid (niacin), antiretroviral protease inhibitors used for HIV (which also cause central fat redistribution known as lipodystrophy syndrome), several atypical antipsychotic agents including clozapine and olanzapine, and certain antihypertensives including beta blockers, calcium channel blockers, clonidine, and thiazide diuretics. In contrast, both ACEIs and ARBs appear to improve insulin sensitivity and reduce the development of type 2 DM in hypertensive nondiabetic patients.

PATHOPHYSIOLOGY

Type 2 DM is associated with two physiological abnormalities: insulin resistance and impaired insulin secretion by the beta islet cells of the pancreas. Initially, as insulin resistance increases, insulin levels begin to rise but the glucose level remains normal, resulting in a state of hyperinsulinemia. Insulin resistance worsens in conjunction with hyperinsulinemia, eventually resulting in the development of fasting hyperglycemia, as hepatic gluconeogenesis increases due to glucagon being produced in response to the hyperinsulinemia. Hyperglycemia is ultimately toxic to pancreatic beta cells and, over time, results in relative hypoinsulinemia, which ultimately necessitates exogenous insulin in cases of advanced type 2 DM.

Unlike the pathophysiology in type 1 DM, there is no autoimmune destruction of pancreatic beta cells in type 2 DM. Rather, there is a decline in beta cell function, with impaired insulin secretion in response to a glycemic load, which results in elevated plasma glucose levels. This first manifests as postprandial elevated glucose levels, and because insulin also supports the transport of amino acids and fatty acids, alterations in lipids and proteins may be seen. Thus, multiple processes are affected.

The sequence of impaired insulin secretion preceding worsening insulin resistance has been observed in prospective studies, although other studies have indicated these two pathophysiological mechanisms are independent risk factors for the development of type 2 DM and occur in concert, rather than sequentially. Although insufficient to cause DM alone, insulin resistance appears to be the strongest predictor of type 2 DM development, an observation that is reinforced by the importance of insulin resistance as a component of metabolic syndrome (see Chapter 35).

Insulin resistance is primarily thought to be caused by toxicity due to elevated levels of free fatty acids and pro-inflammatory cytokines that are associated with acquired traits, such as aging and obesity, in which these substances are produced by adipose tissue. Obesity is characterized by low-grade systemic inflammation, which has been linked to beta cell dysfunction. For example, adipocyte-derived tumor necrosis factor–α has been positively correlated with increasing insulin resistance, as has the adipocyte-derived hormone resistin. In contrast, the adipocyte-derived hormone adiponectin appears to be negatively correlated with insulin resistance.

Obesity is a major modifiable risk factor for type 2 DM, affecting up to 90% of individuals with the disease. Physical exercise with a corresponding weight loss of just 5% to 10% of total body weight can prevent or delay the development of type 2 DM in individuals with obesity, generating marked improvement in insulin resistance. Patients who are not obese but who have a disproportionate percentage of body weight distributed in the visceral area rather than at the hips are also at greater risk of developing type 2 DM.

The interaction of genetic and environmental factors may be responsible for producing epigenetic changes that underlie the heterogeneity of type 2 DM. More than 40 single nucleotide polymorphisms have been identified that increase the risk of developing type 2 DM. Genetic variants have been identified that affect incretin hormones (which normally decrease glucose levels), beta cell function, and key protein regulators. The intestinal microbiome may also play a role in the risk of developing type 2 DM, as the gut flora impacts nutrient absorption. Studies demonstrate the ability to improve insulin sensitivity by altering the gut biome.

Elevated plasma glucose levels may be tolerated for many years by the patient with DM who, in turn, may not seek treatment until significant complications result. Eventually, insulin secretion will become insufficient to compensate for insulin resistance. Moreover, hyperinsulinemia and hyperglycemia increase lipid synthesis, raising serum levels of fatty acids, triglycerides (greater than 150 mg/dL), and LDL cholesterol, while lowering HDL cholesterol. This increase in lipids is also toxic to beta cells and is referred to as lipotoxicity.

Overall, the pathogenesis of type 2 DM has been labeled the "ominous octet," consisting of eight distinct factors: 1) beta cell failure; 2) insulin resistance in muscle cells; 3) insulin resistance in liver cells; 4) adipocyte resistance to the antilipolytic effect of insulin, which results in increased plasma free fatty acids; 5) decreased incretin; 6) increased glucagon secretion and enhanced hepatic sensitivity to glucagon; 7) enhanced renal glucose reabsorption; and 8) resistance of the central nervous system to the anorectic effect of insulin, which results in appetite dysregulation and weight gain.

The gastrointestinal tissues contribute to this pathophysiology through the actions of the incretins glucagon-like peptide-1 (GLP1) and gastric inhibitory polypeptide (GIP). These two hormones play a significant role in glucose absorption. In type 2 DM, GLP1 is deficient, while there is resistance to the GIP effect on the stimulation of insulin secretion. GLP1 normally inhibits glucagon secretion postprandially. Pancreatic alpha cells stimulate glucagon secretion and are normally responsive to beta cell function. In type 2 DM, this communication becomes dysfunctional, and alpha cells begin to hypersecrete glucagon.

The kidneys are designed to filter glucose through the sodium-glucose transport 2 (SGLT2) transporter system. A small amount of glucose is also filtered through the SGLT1 transporter located in the descending proximal tubule of the renal nephron. The kidneys reabsorb even more glucose in hyperglycemic states. Eventually, this hyperglycemia leads to renal microvascular damage and eventually diabetic kidney disease.

CLINICAL PRESENTATION

Because the onset of type 2 DM may occur years before a diagnosis is made, individuals who are asymptomatic tend to be diagnosed during a routine physical examination or during treatment for another condition.

Subjective

Because the onset of type 2 DM is usually insidious, only a minority of patients are initially symptomatic. A patient may, however, present with pruritus, fatigue, neuropathic complaints such as numbness and tingling, or blurred vision. The symptoms of type 1 and type 2 DM are essentially the same due to hyperglycemia (see the previous section on type 1 DM for a complete discussion), although the severe ketoacidosis that may occur in type 1 DM is rare in patients with type 2 DM. Thus, some patients present with increased urination, nocturia, thirst, or polydipsia. In many cases, type 2 DM initially presents as an infection, such as vaginitis (candidiasis) in women, balanitis (especially in elderly men), or a skin infection. Cardiovascular symptoms such as angina may also prompt a heretofore undiagnosed patient with type 2 DM to seek health care.

Objective

There may be no dramatic change in objective findings with type 2 DM, although the typical patient is often obese, with a history of dyslipidemia, hypertension, and CAD. Abnormal healing and an increased occurrence of infection, especially yeast infection, may also be present.

In severe cases, patients may present with HHS, in which profound dehydration results from prolonged hyperglycemia (see Table 58.4). Formerly known as hyperosmolar hyperglycemic nonketotic coma, HHS is associated with a high mortality rate and is typically seen in older diabetic adults who have developed an infection, such as pneumonia, or other illness. Patients with undiagnosed DM may develop this condition due to prolonged hyperglycemia in the absence of treatment. Other risk factors for developing HHS in the diabetic patients include peritoneal dialysis, hemodialysis, tube feedings with high-protein formulas, and the use of mannitol, phenytoin, corticosteroids, immunosuppressive agents, and diuretics. Symptoms of HHS are dramatic, including severe hyperglycemia (greater than 600 mg/dL), plasma or serum hyperosmolality (more than 340 mOsm), and profound dehydration. Although classically thought of as a nonketotic condition, ketosis may or may not be present in HHS, and neurological symptoms range from a clouded sensorium to frank coma. HHS requires immediate referral for acute care management.

DIAGNOSTIC REASONING

Diagnostic Tests

Because early detection and prompt treatment may reduce the complications of type 2 DM, screening for DM as part of routine medical care is appropriate under certain circumstances. Screening for prediabetes and DM should be considered in all individuals who are overweight or obese, regardless of age, and for all adults aged 45 years and older. Testing should be repeated at a minimum of 3-year intervals, with several laboratory approaches capable of diagnosing type 2 DM, as described in the following section.

Initial Testing

Immediate testing for hyperglycemia in the clinical setting can be accomplished by using a portable monitor to assess capillary blood glucose level. This test is referred to as a random capillary blood glucose measurement and may be taken without regard to timing of the patient's last meal. It is important to note that certain drugs can produce hyperglycemia, including glucocorticoids, furosemide (Lasix), thiazide diuretics, phenytoin (Dilantin), estrogen-containing products, beta blockers, and nicotinic acid. A result of 200 mg/dL or greater should be followed-up by screening for elevated blood glucose using a whole blood sample. If the random plasma glucose level is elevated, additional blood glucose testing should be done.

There are four laboratory-based criteria to confirm DM:

1. Glycosylated hemoglobin (A1C) level greater than or equal to 6.5%*
2. Random plasma glucose level of 200 mg/dL in the presence of classic symptoms of hyperglycemia or a hyperglycemic crisis*
3. Fasting plasma glucose level of 126 mg/dL or higher on two occasions; *fasting* is defined as no caloric intake for at least 8 hours
4. Two-hour postload plasma glucose level of 200 mg/dL or higher during an OGTT, following consumption of a glucose load containing the equivalent of 75 g of anhydrous glucose dissolved in water (OGTT is also used to screen for diabetes during pregnancy)

*In the absence of unequivocal hyperglycemia, results should be confirmed by repeat testing on a new blood sample without delay, preferably using the same type of test.

Subsequent Testing

An A1C determination gives valuable insight into the mean glycemic level over the preceding 2 to 3 months and is helpful in documenting the degree of glycemic control at the time of diagnosis and as part of continuing care. An A1C value of less than 7% indicates strong control; however, a value of less than 6.5% has been shown to significantly decrease the occurrence of complications, provided this can be achieved without hypoglycemia or other adverse effect.

Additional laboratory tests that are appropriate to the evaluation of the patient's general medical condition should be performed at the time of diagnosis and at least annually thereafter. These include a fasting lipid profile, serum creatinine, eGFR, liver function tests, and spot urinary UACR. A C-peptide measurement (reflecting endogenous insulin production) may be ordered if the diagnosis between type 1 and 2 DM is unclear. In type 2 DM, the C-peptide level is normal or elevated, while it is decreased in type 1 DM, given the lack of insulin production.

Specific evaluations that should be performed to assess for end-organ damage at diagnosis and annually thereafter. These include, but are not limited to, body mass index assessment, blood pressure measurement including orthostatic blood pressure (especially in older adults), funduscopic eye examination, thyroid palpation, full skin examination to evaluate for acanthosis nigricans, and a comprehensive foot examination to assess for diabetic ulcers.

Differential Diagnosis

Differential diagnoses for type 2 DM include prediabetes (glucose intolerance), gestational diabetes (new-onset DM developing at any stage of pregnancy), Cushing's syndrome, pheochromocytoma, and drug-induced hyperglycemia. In addition, a patient who fails to respond to metformin or other antihyperglycemic agents should be evaluated for the possibility of type 1 DM. Although type 1 DM occurs infrequently in older adults, it should be considered in patients with other autoimmune disorders, patients without a family history of type 2 DM, or patients of normal weight.

Increasing evidence points to linkages among CAD, hyperlipidemia, obesity, and type 2 DM; thus, such comorbidities must be ruled out in all diabetic patients. A prediabetic state of glucose intolerance has also been associated with hypertension, obesity, and hyperlipidemia as a collection of comorbidities known as metabolic syndrome, which is a strong predictor of eventual development of DM and CVD (see Chapter 35 for further information on metabolic syndrome).

MANAGEMENT

Type 2 DM is a chronic, complex illness that requires ongoing health care and education to prevent acute and chronic complications. Interventions should include treatments directed at both risk reduction and glycemic control. Lifestyle management is an important part of treatment and comprises nutrition therapy, activity prescriptions for exercise, decreased prolonged sitting, and, in older adults, training in balance and flexibility. Lifestyle management should also focus on mental health, sleep, and smoking cessation.

Preventing or delaying complications is accomplished by active screening and frequent clinical assessments, as well as the use of medications. Obesity management has become a high-level target in the treatment of patients with type 2 DM, including the possible use of medications and surgery for the treatment of obesity. The pharmacologic approach to antihyperglycemic treatment changes rapidly as new medications and drug classes are approved and older medications are combined with newer agents.

Although the primary-care practitioner's focus is often on glycemic control and risk reduction, the patient's focus is typically on the need to fit these treatment interventions into an acceptable lifestyle for the patient and ensure that they are minimally disruptive. Research has identified that dietary modifications, the need for frequent blood glucose monitoring, and subsequent follow-up with health-care providers place a financial and psychological burden on patients and their families.

Lifestyle Management

Lifestyle management encompasses nutritional education including the treatment of obesity, physical activity, adequate sleep and sleep hygiene practices, the evaluation of psychosocial status and stress reduction, and smoking cessation if applicable.

The 2017 ADA Standards of Care recommend that every patient receive diabetes self-management education (DSME) and diabetes self-management support (DSMS) at the time of diagnosis. Patients should be evaluated for the need for specialty referrals annually and with the onset of any new complication or transition in care. Comprehensive diabetes treatment programs are designed to be patient centered and to provide patients with the information they need to be empowered to self-treat and to become the leader in their own DM management. Studies of patients who complete DSME demonstrate lower A1C values, lower weight, and improved quality of life. Unfortunately, in contrast to newly diagnosed (mostly pediatric) patients with type 1 DM, not many patients with type 2 DM receive formal DSME and DSMS.

Nutritional Therapy

Meal planning or nutritional therapy is one of the most fundamental and challenging components of DM management. The goal of nutritional therapy is to achieve and maintain body weight goals, blood glucose and lipid levels, and blood pressure goals, and to delay or prevent the complications of DM. Most patients with type 2 DM are obese or overweight; therefore, weight loss is generally a significant factor in meal planning. Although hypocaloric diets and weight loss usually improve blood glucose control, traditional dietary strategies have not proven to be particularly effective in achieving long-term weight loss.

As research continues to explore why weight loss and weight maintenance are so difficult, the emphasis of dietary counseling should be on the consumption of nutrient-dense foods in appropriate portion sizes to control serum glucose levels and promote healthy eating practices. The meal plan should be based on the patient's food preferences, activity level, medical history, and both current and target weights, as well as lifestyle, cultural, ethnic, and financial factors. Ideally, a registered dietician or certified diabetes educator should be consulted to assist patients. It is important for the clinician to be nonjudgmental and to help patients enjoy their healthy food choices.

If weight loss is indicated, a moderate caloric restriction of 500 to 750 calories less than the patient's average daily intake, as calculated from a detailed food history (which can be tracked with a food diary), can be instituted. A hypocaloric diet, independent of weight loss, is associated with increased insulin sensitivity and the improvement of blood glucose levels. Moderate weight loss, irrespective of the patient's starting weight, has significant benefits, especially in decreasing morbidity and mortality rates. In fact, weight loss is a primary intervention because it improves the serum lipid profile, reduces blood pressure, decreases insulin resistance, and ameliorates glucose intolerance.

Individuals on most oral glucose-lowering agents and/or insulin therapy should eat at consistent times that are synchronized with their medication administration. A nutritionally balanced meal plan is important for the patient with type 2 DM and should take into account the higher prevalence of atherosclerosis in patients with DM. Specific diets for patients with diabetes are no longer recommended by the ADA; instead, the ADA recommends that macronutrient distribution within the diet is individualized for each patient, with total calorie and metabolic needs used as guides (see Table 58.5 for nutritional information on different classes of macronutrients).

Physical Activity

Physical activity is an integral component of the management of type 2 DM. Activity-based interventions include increasing general movement through activities of daily living and decreasing sedentary behavior. Exercise is a specific type of physical activity, and the recommendation is 150 minutes per week of moderate to intensive physical effort. The exercise should occur at least 3 days per week, with no more than 2 consecutive days without exercise. In addition, decreasing sedentary behavior is critical, and not sitting for more than 30 minutes at a time is recommended. Older adults should have flexibility and balance training two to three times per week. Also, studies have demonstrated that older adults have improved A1C control if resistance training is added 2 days per week to their exercise routine.

Before beginning an exercise program, patients should be screened for the presence of macrovascular and/or microvascular complications that may be worsened by exercise. These include CAD, PVD, retinopathy, nephropathy, and peripheral or autonomic neuropathy. The patient with type 2 DM can perform all levels of exercise, as long as glycemic control is adequate and there is no evidence of DM complications. If there are complications, consultation with the appropriate specialists should be completed before starting an exercise program. If the patient is taking particular oral antidiabetic agents (e.g., sulfonylureas) or is on insulin therapy,

TABLE 58.5	Macronutrient Information	
Macronutrient	*Recommend*	*Avoid*
Carbohydrates	Whole grains Vegetables (fresh preferred) Fruits (fresh preferred) Legumes Emphasis on high fiber content	Refined (simple) sugars Refined flour Sugar-sweetened beverages Minimize foods with added sugar
Protein	Daily intake: 1–1.5 g/kg Daily intake with chronic kidney disease: 0.8 g/kg	Do not use protein foods to treat or prevent nocturnal hypo-glycemia
Fats	Monounsaturated fats Foods rich in long chain omega-3 fatty acids Daily intake: 25%–30% of total calories	Trans fatty acids

exercise can lead to hypoglycemia. Thus, patients initiating an exercise regimen should be aware of the signs and symptoms of hypoglycemia and be prepared to treat such an event. Any exercise prescription should be individualized to take into account the patient's level of interest in physical activity, lifestyle practices, physical condition, financial situation, and motivation.

Psychosocial Issues

Appropriately addressing psychosocial issues is included in ADA treatment guidelines. The ADA suggests screening patients for depression, diabetes distress, anxiety, eating disorders, and impaired cognitive function at least annually. For patients to provide their own self-care, they need to have emotional well-being. DM is a risk factor for depression and anxiety. Thus, screening and appropriate referrals to mental health providers are important for the overall care and support of diabetic patients and their families.

Monitoring Blood Glucose Levels

The optimal monitoring of blood glucose levels in patients with type 2 DM has not been clearly established. SMBG is useful for guiding the effectiveness and safety of treatment with anti-hyperglycemic medications or insulin, especially in patients who have not consistently achieved blood glucose treatment goals. These patients should be instructed to keep a log of their results for periodic review by the primary-care practitioner.

CGM may play a role in patients who have difficulty achieving glycemic control or who are using an intensive insulin regimen. Patients who are unaware of their hypoglycemic episodes may also benefit from CGM, given the life-threatening risk of hypoglycemia and the need for immediate intervention. Both types of blood glucose monitoring can assist patients and their health-care providers in understanding the patient's individual response to treatment. Continuous monitoring requires more intensive education than SMBG, however.

Pharmacological Therapy

Pharmacological therapy for type 2 DM is required when lifestyle management does not result in adequate blood glucose control. Drug therapy should always be considered an adjunctive therapy to lifestyle management, as the latter is typically initiated first. However, for particular patients with significant disease, the American Association of Clinical Endocrinologists (AACE) and American College of Endocrinology agree with the ADA Standards of Care that pharmacotherapy can be initiated at the time of diagnosis simultaneously with lifestyle management.

Selecting a medication for glycemic control involves analyzing the risks and benefits of the agent according to patient age, comorbidities, and hypoglycemia risk. Basic recommendations from professional organizations differ with regard to initiating pharmacologic therapy. The AACE recommends that patients with recent-onset type 2 DM or mild hyperglycemia (A1C <7.5%) start with lifestyle treatment and monotherapy. The ADA and AACE recommend metformin if there are no contraindications, such as renal disease or abnormal creatinine clearance, acute myocardial infarction, or septicemia. The AACE recommends adding a second agent to lifestyle treatment and metformin if the A1C is more than 7.5% at the time of diagnosis or after 3 months of monotherapy without achievement of the patient's blood glucose goals. In contrast, the ADA does not recommend dual-agent pharmacotherapy until the A1C is 9.0% or greater. This differs from AACE guidelines, which recommend starting insulin if the patient's A1C is 9.0% or higher at the time of presentation and if the patient is symptomatic. The ADA, on the other hand, recommends starting insulin when the A1C is 10% or greater with symptoms.

Current therapy for type 2 DM includes drugs that alter insulin action, stimulate insulin secretion, affect the absorption of glucose, mimic the effects of incretin, act as an insulin secretagogue, or suppress postprandial glucagon release. Insulin itself is also a treatment for type 2 DM. Both AACE and ADA guidelines list (in no selected order) sulfonylureas, thiazolidinediones, dipeptidyl peptidase-4 inhibitors (DPP4-Is), SGLT2 inhibitors, GLP1 receptor agonists, and insulin.

Metformin (Glucophage) is a biguanide that works by suppressing excessive hepatic glucose production and by increasing glucose utilization in peripheral tissues. Metformin reduces fasting and postprandial hyperglycemia and reduces hepatic gluconeogenesis. It may also improve glucose levels by reducing intestinal glucose absorption. Metformin does not stimulate endogenous insulin secretion, but it can provide cardiovascular protection and contribute to weight loss.

Metformin can be used as a monotherapy unless the patient has contraindications or intolerance. Although metformin is the first-line medication recommended by the ADA and the AACE for DM type 2, it should be used only in patients with adequate renal function and should not be used in patients with an eGFR below 45 mL/min/1.73 m². Metformin also has a boxed warning in its FDA-approved prescribing information for lactic acidosis, although this side effect is very rare. Patients at risk for developing lactic acidosis include those with liver impairment, alcohol abuse, and cardiopulmonary insufficiency. Metformin should be discontinued 24 to 48 hours before diagnostic and surgical procedures due to the risk of decreased kidney function, and its administration should not be resumed for at least 6 hours after these procedures or until the patient is adequately hydrated.

Initial dosing is 500 mg once a day with breakfast or dinner for 1 week, then twice daily with breakfast and dinner. The dosage should be titrated up to a maximum dose of 2,000 mg. Several weeks of therapy may be needed to achieve maximum effects of the given dose. Common adverse reactions include diarrhea, nausea, anorexia, and abdominal discomfort, which usually resolve with a gradual increase of dosage. Metformin has been shown to cause decreased vitamin B_{12} absorption, and patients on long-term metformin therapy should undergo periodic testing for B_{12} deficiency, especially if the patient complains of peripheral neuropathy. At the maximum dose, the monthly cost of metformin in the United States is approximately $4 on many generic formularies. Metformin is currently found in 20 combination formulations with other medications (see Drugs Commonly Prescribed 58.2).

Sulfonylureas work by stimulating pancreatic insulin secretion; thus, pancreatic beta cells must still be producing insulin in order for sulfonylureas to be effective, as they do not reduce insulin resistance. The advantages of second-generation sulfonylureas over older first-generation agents include their improved safety profile, shorter half-life, and relatively higher effects on A1C, with an approximate 1.5% decrease. However, these agents carry a higher risk of hypoglycemia and weight gain than other medications. In addition, patients with severe insulin resistance may respond better to treatment with metformin or thiazolidinediones than with sulfonylureas.

Therapy with sulfonylureas should be initiated at the lowest possible dose and usually begins with a once-daily dose before breakfast. The dosage can be increased every 2 weeks until the desired response is achieved, the maximum dosage is reached, or side effects preclude further increases. Common adverse reactions are mild gastrointestinal upset, weight gain, and skin rashes. Serious effects include hypoglycemia and severe anemias. Sulfonylureas

are metabolized in the liver, and their use should be avoided in persons with significant hepatic dysfunction. Sulfonylureas are not recommended for use during third trimester of pregnancy or for women who are planning a pregnancy.

Numerous drugs can interfere with the metabolism of sulfonylureas and can alter their effects. Nonsteroidal anti-inflammatory agents, azole antifungal drugs, salicylates, sulfonamides, warfarin (Coumadin), monoamine oxidase inhibitors, quinolones, and beta-blockers can all potentiate the effects of sulfonylureas and lead to hypoglycemia. In contrast, thiazide diuretics, corticosteroids, phenothiazines, oral contraceptives, nicotinic acid, sympathomimetics, calcium channel blocking drugs, and isoniazid (INH) can reduce the effects of sulfonylureas and result in loss of glycemic control.

Acarbose (Precose) and miglitol (Glyset) are alpha-glucosidase inhibitors that slow the breakdown of complex carbohydrates into monosaccharides. This effect occurs on the brush border of the small intestine, thus reducing postprandial blood glucose levels. The recommended initial dosage of acarbose is 50 mg/day, which should be slowly titrated up to the maintenance dosage of 50 to 100 mg three times daily with meals. Miglitol also delays absorption of carbohydrates, thereby lowering the postprandial glucose level. Therapy is initiated with the lowest effective dosage of 25 mg three times daily, eventually increasing to the maintenance dose of 50 mg three times daily. Both drugs have similar common adverse effects—flatulence and diarrhea—which are thought to be caused by the osmotic effect of undigested carbohydrates in the distal bowel. Contraindications to alpha-glucosidase inhibitors include any chronic intestinal disease that could be worsened by increased bowel gas formation.

The thiazolidinediones, pioglitazone (Actos) and rosiglitazone (Avandia), work by sensitizing peripheral tissues to insulin by activating the nuclear glitazone receptor (also known as peroxisome proliferator-activated receptor-γ), which lowers serum glucose levels without increasing pancreatic insulin secretion. The thiazolidinediones can decrease A1C from 0.5% to 1.4%, with a low risk of hypoglycemia. They can be used either alone or in combination with other antihyperglycemic medications, including insulin. Thiazolidinediones should be used cautiously in patients at risk for fractures. Common side effects include significant weight gain, upper respiratory tract infection, edema, fluid retention, anemia, and hypoglycemia. These medications carry a boxed warning for congestive heart failure in their prescribing information. In addition, due to possible liver damage, hepatic enzyme levels should be monitored before their initiation and during treatment.

There are two categories of incretin mimetics: DPP4-Is and GLP1 analogues. DPP4-Is prolong and enhance the activity of incretins, which suppresses glucagon secretion and modestly reduces A1C by 0.5% to 0.8%. Although medications from this class can be used as monotherapy,

Drugs Commonly Prescribed 58.2: Noninsulin Agents for Diabetes Mellitus Type 2

DRUG CLASS AND EXAMPLES	INDICATION	ADVERSE REACTIONS AND PRESCRIBING CONSIDERATIONS
Biguanides		
• Metformin (Glucophage)	Monotherapy; may be used as an adjunct to diet in type 2 DM or with a sulfonylurea or insulin therapy	Monitor for hypoglycemia, especially in older adults. Adverse reactions include gastrointestinal disturbances and metallic taste. Contraindicated in renal disease; renal function should be assessed before starting.
First-Generation Sulfonylureas (*no longer recommended, given newer agents*)		
• Chlorpropamide (Diabinese) • Tolbutamide (Orinase)	For use as an adjunct to diet and exercise in type 2 DM (largely replaced by second-generation sulfonylureas)	Adverse reactions include hypoglycemia with high doses or in fasting patients, weight gain, headache, gastrointestinal upset, skin rashes, severe anemia, and hypersensitivity. Increased risk of cardiovascular mortality. Contraindicated for patients with impaired liver or kidney function, given the increased risk of hypoglycemia; not for use in type 1 DM or DKA. Worse safety profile than second-generation sulfonylureas, so no longer recommended.
Second-Generation Sulfonylureas		
• Glimepiride (Amaryl; sometimes considered as third-generation) • Glipizide (Glucotrol) • Glyburide (Diaßeta, Micronase)	For use as an adjunct to diet and exercise in type 2 DM	Same as for first-generation sulfonylureas, but with relatively improved safety profile than older agents. Increased potency by weight compared to first-generation drugs.
Alpha-Glucosidase Inhibitors		
• Acarbose (Precose) • Miglitol (Glyset)	For use as an adjunct to diet and exercise in type 2 DM; used as monotherapy or added to insulin, metformin, or a sulfonylurea	Adverse reactions include flatulence, diarrhea, and abdominal pain (advise patient to take with first bite of main meal, starting with a low dose and gradually increasing). Contraindicated in DKA and in patients with inflammatory bowel disease, colonic ulceration, intestinal obstruction, and chronic intestinal diseases impacting digestion. Do not use if serum creatinine is greater than 2 mg/dL. Use glucose (tablets, gel), not fructose (such as in fruit juices), to treat hypoglycemia, as the metabolism of complex carbohydrates will be inhibited.
Thiazolidinediones		
• Pioglitazone (Actos) • Rosiglitazone (Avandia)	For use as an adjunct to diet and exercise in type 2 DM; used as monotherapy to reduce insulin resistance or added to metformin; not for use with type 1 DM or DKA	Adverse reactions include exacerbation of congestive heart failure, swelling of legs, fluid retention, weight gain, upper respiratory tract infection, and hypersensitivity. Increased risk of bladder tumors reported. Do not give to patients with liver disease or if ALT is greater than 2.5 × upper limit of normal; monitor transaminases at baseline, every 2 months for first 12 months, and then periodically; discontinue if levels increase or jaundice occurs. Contraindicated in New York Heart Association Class III or IV heart failure. May cause resumption of ovulation in an anovulatory patient (and thus may result in unintended pregnancy).

Continued

Drugs Commonly Prescribed 58.2: Noninsulin Agents for Diabetes Mellitus Type 2—cont'd

DRUG CLASS AND EXAMPLES	INDICATION	ADVERSE REACTIONS AND PRESCRIBING CONSIDERATIONS
Dipeptidyl Peptidase-4 Inhibitors		
• Alogliptin (Nesina) • Linagliptin (Tradjenta) • Saxagliptin (Onglyza) • Sitagliptin (Januvia)	Can be used as monotherapy as incretin mimetic, but usually used as an add-on drug for type 2 DM; available in combination with metformin, thiazolidinediones, and sodium-glucose transport-2 inhibitors	Adverse reactions include Stevens-Johnson Syndrome, nasopharyngitis, diarrhea, abdominal pain, pancreatitis, joint pain, and renal failure. May cause hypoglycemia when used with sulfonylureas.
Glucagon-like Peptide-1 Analogues		
• Albiglutide (Tanzeum) • Dulaglutide (Trulicity) • Exenatide (Byetta/Bydureon) • Liraglutide (Victoza) • Lixisenatide (Adlyxin)	Can be used as monotherapy as incretin mimetic, but usually used as an add-on drug for type 2 DM; available in combination with insulin	Adverse reactions include severe pancreatitis, nausea, dyspepsia, injection site reactions, and arthralgia. Do not use with gastroparesis, and use with caution in patients with renal impairment. Contraindicated for patients with a family history of multiple endocrine neoplasia syndrome type 2 or medullary thyroid carcinoma, given an increased risk of thyroid C-cell tumors.
Sodium-Glucose Transport-2 Inhibitors		
• Canagliflozin (Invokana) • Dapagliflozin (Farxiga) • Empagliflozin (Jardiance)	Can be used as monotherapy, but usually used as an add-on drug for type 2 DM	Adverse reactions include acute renal failure, ketoacidosis, hypotension, urinary and/or genital fungal infections, and nausea. Contraindicated in patients with congestive heart failure, nephrotoxicity, or volume depletion.
Meglitinides		
• Mitiglinide (Glufast) • Nateglinide (Starlix) • Repaglinide (Prandin)	For use as an adjunct to diet and exercise in type 2 DM; used as monotherapy as an insulin secretagogue or can be added to a thiazolidinedione; not for use with type 1 DM or DKA	Adverse reactions include weight gain, gastrointestinal complaints, hypoglycemia, cardiovascular events, and hypersensitivity. Contraindicated in patients taking gemfibrozil.

Abbreviations: DKA, diabetic ketoacidosis; DM, diabetes mellitus.

they are more likely to be used as add-on therapy to metformin. Common adverse effects include nasopharyngitis, abdominal pain, and hypoglycemia when used with sulfonylureas. Severe adverse effects include pancreatitis, Stevens-Johnson syndrome, and renal failure. In 2015, the FDA issued a warning for this medication class because it can cause severe joint pain. DPP4-Is are given once daily and are available in combination with metformin, thiazolidinediones, and SGLT2-Is.

GLP1 analogues enhance insulin secretion in a glucose-dependent manner in response to food intake. GLP1 analogues also improve insulin sensitivity, increase beta cell mass, and decrease glucagon secretion. GLP1 analogues affect satiety and hunger by decreasing the hedonic value (appeal) of food, prolonging the time food remains in the stomach, and decreasing the patient's motivation to eat. GLP1 analogues are injected with daily or weekly

dosing and must be slowly increased over time from initial dosing. The 2016 LEADER trial demonstrated a reduced risk of mortality from cardiovascular causes with these medications, while the 2017 CSALE trial demonstrated a delayed onset of DM for patients with prediabetes taking these medications. Common side effects include gastrointestinal distress (e.g., nausea, vomiting, and diarrhea), headache, fatigue, and pancreatitis. There is also a boxed warning in their prescribing information for an increased risk of thyroid C-cell tumors with these medications due to studies in rodents; they are contraindicated in patients with medullary thyroid carcinoma and multiple endocrine neoplasia type 2. A modest reduction in A1C of 0.5% to 0.8% can be expected with their use.

SGLT2-Is block the activity of SGLT proteins in the renal proximal tubule, thereby reducing glucose reuptake and increasing the secretion of glucose in the urine. The medication is given once daily. Patients often lose weight due to the loss of sugar through the kidney. The 2015 EMPA-REG OUTCOME study demonstrated a reduced rate of cardiovascular events and a slowed progression of kidney disease with this class of medication. Common adverse effects include mycotic urinary and genital infections. Severe adverse reactions include renal failure, ketoacidosis, and pancreatitis. SGLT2-Is are contraindicated in patients with congestive heart failure, nephrotoxicity, and volume depletion.

Meglitinides are insulin secretagogues that act similarly to sulfonylureas but with a greater effect in reducing A1C and with a lower risk of hypoglycemia than sulfonylureas. Side effects include weight gain and gastrointestinal complaints, and they are not intended for patients with type 1 DM or DKA. Dosing is multiple times a day before meals. Certain drugs such as gemfibrozil (which are contraindicated with meglitinides) and azole antifungals can markedly increase the level of these drugs and increase their risk of hypoglycemia.

There are several other medications that are infrequently used for type 2 DM. Bromocriptine is a dopamine agonist and increases insulin sensitivity at the dopamine receptors. Common side effects are nausea and orthostatic hypotension. Colesevelam is a bile acid sequestrant that binds bile acid in the intestinal tract, increasing hepatic glucose production and incretin levels. Hypoglycemia is rare with this agent, although LDL levels often decrease; other side effects include constipation and decreased absorption of other medications.

Individual treatment goals should take into account the patient's capacity to understand and carry out the management plan, the risk of severe hypoglycemia, and any other factors that increase risk or decrease benefit of selected treatments. When lifestyle management plus antidiabetic agents fail to control blood glucose levels, or if the patient's A1C at diagnosis is high, the addition of insulin is recommended. Relatively large doses of insulin may be required for type 2 DM patients, given their degree of insulin resistance, in comparison to patients with type 1 DM. The 2018 Standards of Diabetes Care published by the ADA recommends starting at 0.1 to 0.2 U/kg/day of basal insulin (approximately 10 U) and increase the dosage by 10% to 15% or 2 to 4 units once or twice a week, as guided by fasting blood glucose levels. The normal target fasting blood glucose level is less than 140 mg/dL. Metformin and thiazolidinediones can be used with insulin therapy, as they facilitate lower doses of insulin in maintaining glycemic control; however, sulfonylureas should be discontinued, given the significant risk of hypoglycemia when combined with exogenous insulin. A description of the properties of long-acting basal insulin formations can be found in the earlier section on type 1 DM (see Drugs Commonly Prescribed 58.1).

Because several types of oral antidiabetic agents can be used as monotherapy, in combination with one another, or with insulin therapy, treatment decisions in type 2 DM can be complex. The following is a synopsis of treatment recommendations in type 2 DM. Each patient's treatment plan will require individualization that is dependent on the starting A1C value at the time of pharmacotherapy initiation and specific lifestyle issues or comorbidities:

- Immediately upon diagnosis of type 2 DM, begin lifestyle therapy with medically assisted obesity treatment.
- If glycemic goals are still not met 3 months later, begin single-agent or dual therapy with oral antidiabetic agents, depending on whether A1C is less than or greater than 7.5%.
- If glycemic goals are not met in 3 months, initiate triple therapy.
- If after 3 additional months (or at the time of diagnosis) A1C is 9.0% or higher and the patient is symptomatic, add insulin therapy.

The ADA Standards of Care differ slightly from these guidelines. Dual therapy is not started at diagnosis unless A1C greater than or equal to 9.0%, and insulin therapy is not initiated until A1C greater than or equal to 10% and the patient is symptomatic.

Monitoring for Hypoglycemia

Hypoglycemia (defined as a plasma glucose less than 54 mg/dL, although the glucose alert value is defined as <70 mg/dL) may occur in patients with type 2 DM for a variety of reasons: excessive exogenous insulin, excessive dosing of oral antidiabetic agents, missed meals or inadequate food intake, excessive exercise, alcohol ingestion, drug interactions, and a decrease in liver or kidney function. When using two oral antidiabetic agents, the potential for hypoglycemic episodes is greater, and the patient and family members should be aware of this. Signs and symptoms include diaphoresis, tachycardia, hunger, shakiness, altered mentation (ranging from an inability to concentrate to coma), slurred speech, and seizure. The signs and symptoms exhibited by the patient are highly individualized and can vary from mild to severe. If the patient becomes acutely ill for any reason, blood glucose levels will need closer monitoring, given the body's increased metabolic demands. Parenteral insulin may be necessary in this situation, if oral agents cannot be tolerated due to nausea, vomiting, or impaired oral intake.

FOLLOW-UP AND REFERRAL

Because type 2 DM is a chronic disease, continuing care is essential, and the goal of treatment is to prevent or slow the development of diabetic complications. The frequency of patient visits depends on the degree to which blood glucose levels are controlled, changes in antihyperglycemic therapy, and the presence and degree of complications or other medical conditions. If the patient is performing SMBG, telephone consultations may be possible instead of clinic visits. Once glycemic levels are adequately regulated, the patient should be seen at least quarterly. These visits should include a discussion of the results of SMBG, symptoms of hypoglycemia and other illnesses, patient adjustments to therapy and changes in lifestyle due to disease management, problems with adherence to the treatment plan and medications, as well as the frequency, causes, and severity of hyperglycemia or hypoglycemia if the patient is on insulin therapy and/or antidiabetic agents.

On initial diagnosis, the patient should be referred to a dietitian and a certified diabetes educator. Effective dietary modification as directed by a qualified nutritionist may also be a key factor in preventing the development of DM type 2 in a prediabetic patient. A1C determination should be performed at least twice a year in patients with adequate glycemic control and quarterly in patients whose therapy has changed or who are not meeting glycemic goals. Patients should also undergo annual examinations of the feet and eyes (including funduscopy), the latter of which requires referral to a qualified ophthalmologist or optometrist.

If any of the following complications are detected or suspected, referral to a specialist to guide management may be indicated. Key follow-up and management principles with respect to the diabetic patient are as follows:

- *Retinopathy:* Type 2 DM is the leading cause of acquired blindness in adults aged 20 to 74 years, and up to 25% of newly diagnosed patients may present with retinopathy at the time of diagnosis. Comprehensive visual eye examinations and dilated retinal examinations should be performed at the time of diagnosis by an ophthalmologist or optometrist who is knowledgeable and experienced in the management of diabetic retinopathy. If the examination is normal, follow-up examinations can be conducted every 2 years, but if there is any concern for abnormalities, then the examinations should be done annually. Optimizing blood pressure and lipid levels can reduce the risk or slow the progression of retinopathy.

- *Hyperlipidemia:* Adults with type 2 DM should be tested at diagnosis for lipid disorders and every 5 years thereafter if the initial lipid panel is normal. The AACE recommends an annual fasting lipid profile, including serum cholesterol, triglyceride, HDL, and calculated LDL cholesterol measurements. Some patients can achieve recommended lipid goals with lifestyle management (i.e., modifications to diet and physical activity), but the majority will need pharmacologic therapy. The purpose of treatment is to reduce cardiovascular events. ADA guidelines suggest that the emphasis in clinical management be based on risk profiles using the American College of Cardiology (ACC) Atherosclerotic Cardiovascular Disease (ASCVD) risk calculator. Aggressive therapy is indicated because it has been shown to lower the risk of CAD. The LDL level should be less than 100 mg/dL in a patient with no overt CVD and less than 70 mg/dL with overt CVD. In patients with extreme risk of CVD, the LDL level should be less than 55 mg/dL. The use of statins (HMG CoA-reductase inhibitors) as antihyperlipidemic therapy is indicated in these patients, with nutritional treatment (dietary modification) initiated as first-line therapy. Moderate- to high-intensity dosing is based on patient age and cardiovascular risk level.

- *Diabetic kidney disease:* A routine spot UACR (normal <30 mcg albumin/mg creatinine) and eGFR should be performed annually on all diabetic patients. Screening for the patient with type 2 DM should begin at the time of diagnosis because it is not known how long the patient has had DM before his or her formal diagnosis. The ADA recommends screening at the time of diagnosis, followed by annual screening. Albuminuria is found more often in patients with DM and hypertension. Thus, in addition to maintaining normal serum glucose levels, controlling BP is the most effective method to slow or reduce the risk of diabetic kidney disease. ACEIs or ARBs are the recommended treatment for patients with DM and hypertension, abnormally high UACR, or a lower than normal eGFR.

- *Hypertension:* In a patient with type 2 DM, hypertension is often part of a syndrome that includes glucose intolerance, insulin resistance, obesity, dyslipidemia, and CAD. It is present in one-third of patients diagnosed with type 2 DM, and control of hypertension has been shown to reduce the rate of progression of nephropathy and to reduce the complications of CVD. Systolic blood pressure should be less than 140 mm Hg and diastolic blood pressure below 90 mm Hg. A lower blood pressure goal of 130/80 mm Hg may be appropriate for patients at high risk for cardiovascular events but only if this can be achieved without significant risk or burden to the patient. Treatment can be with ACEIs, ARBs, thiazide-like diuretics, or dihydropyridine calcium channel blockers.

- *Macrovascular disease:* Evidence of uncontrolled angina, carotid bruits, or ECG abnormalities may require advanced intervention and calls for referral to a cardiologist. Daily aspirin is recommended for cardiac prophylaxis in patients with a 10-year risk of CVD greater than 10% at a dose of 81 to 165 mg/day. Given the increased risk of bleeding due to its antiplatelet effects, aspirin is not recommended in low-risk patients with a 10-year CVD risk of less than 5%. Diabetic patients are at risk for developing macrovascular complications including stroke, PVD, and CAD. All diabetic patients should be screened for these diseases, because symptoms may not be present until late in the course of the disease process. Patients with disabling claudication or nonhealing ulcers require a vascular consultation for their PVD. Type 2 DM is the leading cause of nontraumatic lower extremity amputation due to PVD and peripheral neuropathy. Problems involving the feet may require care by a podiatrist, orthopedic surgeon, vascular surgeon, or rehabilitation specialist.

- *Neuropathy:* All patients should be screened for neuropathic symptoms at the time of diagnosis and then at least annually. Peripheral neuropathy may result in pain, loss of sensation, and muscle weakness. Its incidence increases over time in patients with type 2 DM, and it is more prevalent in patients with low serum insulin concentrations and poor glycemic control. Autonomic involvement can affect gastrointestinal, cardiovascular, and genitourinary function. Patients with significant urinary symptoms or impotence should be referred to a urologist.

- *Pregnancy:* To reduce the risk of fetal malformation and maternal and fetal complications, every pregnancy in a woman with type 2 DM should be planned in advance. Insulin is the first-line medication for the treatment of diabetes in pregnancy. No long-term pregnancy studies of oral diabetic agents have been conducted. A pregnant patient with type 2 DM requires tight blood glucose control and should be monitored closely by a multidisciplinary team, including the obstetrician or certified nurse midwife. Maintaining A1C at less than 6.0% during pregnancy is recommended to prevent adverse fetal outcomes, although this goal increases the risk of hypoglycemia.

Patient Education: Diabetes Mellitus Type 2

Successful diabetes management involves a team effort to achieve mutually agreed upon treatment goals. To achieve these goals, it is crucial that the patient, family, or significant others be educated in all aspects of the treatment plan. The following list is a synopsis of the salient topics for patient education in type 2 DM:

- *Introduction:* Definition and causes of type 2 DM; function of the pancreas in insulin production
- *Regulation of blood glucose:* Role of food, physical activity, and insulin in glucose utilization; signs and symptoms, causes, treatment, and prevention of hyperglycemia and hypoglycemia; guidance on when to contact the primary-care practitioner
- *Blood glucose monitoring and urine testing:* How to perform SMBG and how often to test; recording and reporting blood glucose results; urine ketone testing
- *Medication and insulin administration:* Actions and adverse reactions of antidiabetic agents; actions and types of insulin, including effects on blood glucose; storage of medication supplies; drawing, mixing, and injecting insulin and GLP1 analogues; injection site selection and rotation; needle disposal
- *Meal planning:* Types of macronutrients (carbohydrates, proteins, fats); dietary practices, including timing of meals, portion control, use of sweeteners, dining out, consumption of alcohol, and dietary modification during acute illness

- *Physical activity:* Benefits of exercise; types of activity best suited to the patient; effects on blood glucose; planning and measuring exercise effort, including snack intake
- *Prevention of long-term complications:* Importance of blood glucose control; periodic eye examinations and regular foot care; prevention of infection; early detection of the signs and symptoms of complications

HYPOGLYCEMIA

Hypoglycemia is a clinical syndrome of subnormal plasma glucose concentration that may affect infants through the elderly, although the primary etiology of the disorder differs markedly among various age groups. Adult hypoglycemia is characterized by blood glucose levels of less than 55 mg/dL, whereas neonatal hypoglycemia is defined as a level below 30 mg/dL in the first 24 hours of life. There is no universal agreement about hypoglycemia thresholds, however, with some research supporting a level of less than 50 mg/dL for men, 45 mg/dL for women, and 40 mg/dL for infants and children. Regardless, clinical hypoglycemia occurs when the blood glucose level is low enough to cause signs or symptoms.

EPIDEMIOLOGY AND CAUSES

Classic hypoglycemia denotes a low plasma glucose level in the setting of insulin-dependent DM. Inconsistent subcutaneous absorption of insulin, decreased food intake, missed meals, increased insulin secretion during exercise, physical and emotional stress, and antidiabetic medications such as sulfonylureas can all produce hypoglycemia in patients with DM. However, hypoglycemia occurs more commonly with insulin-treated type 1 DM.

Hypoglycemia with DM is the most commonly occurring endocrine emergency; however, it is not common in patients without DM. Hypoglycemia as a separate disease entity is most common in the elderly and is more prevalent in women overall. About 1% of the nondiabetic population is affected. Although endocrine disorders are the most frequent cause of hypoglycemia, bariatric surgery, insulinomas, non–islet cell neoplasms, liver disease, pregnancy, certain medications, and alcohol consumption are also causes. Hypoglycemia in neonates is a unique phenomenon, largely related to the immature developmental stage of the neonatal endocrine system.

There are three types of hypoglycemia—fasting, reactive, and induced—the causes of which are summarized in Table 58.6. Fasting hypoglycemia is a low blood sugar level more than 5 hours after eating; it can be subacute or chronic, but blood glucose does not return to normal levels without glucose ingestion or administration. The possible causes of fasting hypoglycemia include pancreatic beta cell tumors, extrapancreatic tumors, hypopituitarism,

TABLE 58.6 Causes of Hypoglycemia

Type of Hypoglycemia	Causes
Fasting hypoglycemia	Renal failure (decreases urinary excretion of insulin) Hepatic disease Insulinomas Pancreatic tumors Autoimmune disease Hypopituitarism Extrapancreatic tumors Ethanol intake Septicemia
Reactive hypoglycemia	Postgastrectomy Gastric bypass surgery Hereditary fructose intolerance Congenital enzyme deficiency Pancreatic beta cell dysfunction Meals high in carbohydrates Exercise Pregnancy
Drug-induced hypoglycemia	Exogenous insulin Sulfonylureas Propranolol Salicylates Quinine Pentamidine Disopyramide

myxedema, glycogen storage diseases, medications, ethanol-induced hypoglycemia, severe malnutrition, septicemia, pregnancy, and renal failure, which results in decreased insulin clearance from the body. In adrenocortical insufficiency, there is a decreased production of cortisol that is required for gluconeogenesis, thus leading to hypoglycemia. Liver diseases including hepatitis, cirrhosis, hepatomas, and hepatic congestion interfere with the uptake and release of glycogen from the liver and can ultimately lead to hypoglycemia.

The list of drugs that can cause fasting hypoglycemia is lengthy: insulin, sulfonylureas, fluoroquinolones, propranolol (Inderal), salicylates, quinidine, pentamidine (Pentam 300, NebuPent), warfarin (Coumadin), sulfonamides, tricyclic antidepressants, disopyramide (Norpace), didanosine, ritodrine, chlorpromazine, INH, selective serotonin reuptake inhibitors, clofibrate, thiazide diuretics, lithium, and ACEIs. Poisoning with organophosphate and carbamate-based pesticides also results in hypoglycemia. The illegal sexual-enhancement drug methylenedioxymethamphetamine (MDMA; ecstasy) has also been associated with severe hypoglycemia.

Reactive or postprandial hypoglycemia is less common than fasting hypoglycemia and is most often acute in nature. Reactive hypoglycemia usually produces symptoms 2 to 4 hours after a carbohydrate-rich meal, and symptoms in these patients rarely occur in a fasting state. Within 5 to 6 hours after a meal, the blood glucose level will return to normal. Reactive hypoglycemia may also be caused by gastrointestinal surgery or any other alimentary tract disorder that affects carbohydrate absorption, congenital deficiency of any of the enzymes necessary for carbohydrate metabolism, and late insulin release caused by beta cell dysfunction. Postprandial hypoglycemia is an early manifestation of type 2 DM and has also been seen with extreme exertion in untrained, physically unfit persons, as well as in patients with sepsis or heart failure. Idiopathic or functional postprandial hypoglycemia also exists that cannot be ascribed to any discrete cause.

Induced hypoglycemia is the most common form of hypoglycemia. Medications and alcohol are the most frequent causes of induced hypoglycemia, which may be factitious or self-induced by the excessive intake of sulfonylureas or insulin. The timing of these types of hypoglycemic events is unrelated to food intake. If this type of hypoglycemia is suspected in patients with known access to these drugs (e.g., health-care workers, caregivers of diabetic patients), serum and urine sulfonylurea levels should be obtained. A very low or nonexistent serum C-peptide level confirms that insulin is being injected exogenously, rather than being produced endogenously.

Lifestyle patterns may contribute to hypoglycemia in nondiabetic patients as well. The excessive consumption of simple sugars, an excessively refined and processed diet, excessive exercise, stress, irregular eating patterns, or missing meals can all cause abnormal fluctuations in blood sugar levels. Nutrient deficiencies, food allergies, and poor digestion also contribute to hypoglycemia, and cigarette smoking and high caffeine intake can produce instability in blood glucose levels.

PATHOPHYSIOLOGY

To understand the clinical and biochemical phenomenon of hypoglycemia, it is important to grasp the mechanics behind the body's careful maintenance of euglycemic plasma glucose levels between 80 and 90 mg/dL. After a carbohydrate-containing meal in which glucose is absorbed from the gut into the bloodstream, plasma glucose levels transiently increase to 120 to 140 mg/dL. Glucose subsequently enters pancreatic beta cells via the glucose transporter 1 (GLUT1) and GLUT2 cell membrane transporters, where the enzyme glucokinase phosphorylates it to glucose-6-phosphate. This acts as a glucose sensor and triggers the passive entry of calcium into beta cells, causing insulin secretion. Insulin lowers plasma glucose levels by decreasing hepatic glycolysis (glycogen breakdown) and gluconeogenesis (de novo glucose synthesis), driving glucose uptake by skeletal muscle and adipose tissue via the translocation of intracellular GLUT molecules to the cell membrane surface, and decreasing both proteolysis and lipolysis, which reduces the number of gluconeogenic precursors. In turn, plasma glucose concentration typically returns to a normal level within several hours after a carbohydrate-containing meal.

Hypoglycemia is sensed by central nervous system receptors in the hypothalamus as well as peripheral receptors that act via afferent nerves to trigger an appropriate hormonal response to maintain glucose homeostasis. The body counters glucose levels below 80 mg/dL by decreasing pancreatic insulin production and eventually secreting several counterregulatory hormones at levels below 70 mg/dL. These include glucagon from pancreatic alpha cells that acts directly on the liver and epinephrine from the adrenal medulla that acts similarly to glucagon via hepatic beta-adrenergic receptors, mediates the autonomic (i.e., sympathetic, adrenergic) symptoms of hypoglycemia (e.g., diaphoresis, tachycardia, anxiety), and inhibits insulin secretion via alpha-2-adrenergic receptors. If the hypoglycemia becomes severe (less than 60 mg/dL) or persists for several hours, additional counterregulatory hormones are mobilized, including cortisol from the adrenal cortex and growth hormone from the pituitary gland.

Counterregulatory hormones increase hepatic glucose production via a number of mechanisms, including glycogen breakdown (glycogenolysis) into individual glucose monomers and, once intrahepatic glycogen stores are depleted, de novo glucose synthesis (gluconeogenesis) from amino acids, pyruvate, glycerol, and free fatty acid precursors. The body also metabolically shifts away from glucose utilization toward alternate sources of fuel to maintain euglycemia, such as proteins and ketone bodies converted from fats. Increased lipolysis is reflected in increased plasma free fatty acids, and increased protein breakdown is reflected in higher concentrations of the amino acids alanine and glutamine.

The brain uses glucose almost exclusively as its fuel source; however, it is not capable of synthesizing or storing it. Thus, the brain is particularly sensitive to dramatic changes in blood glucose concentration. Hypoglycemia, in which plasma glucose falls below 60 mg/dL, prevents the brain from receiving an adequate supply of blood glucose, thereby impairing function. In adults, cognitive dysfunction can be detected in otherwise normal individuals at plasma glucose levels between 50 and 55 mg/dL; older men are particularly prone to this type of neurological impairment. At levels between 45 and 50 mg/dL, lethargy and obtundation follow, with coma occurring at levels below 30 mg/dL, followed by convulsions below 20 mg/dL and eventually death. Severe hypoglycemia has also been associated with cardiovascular dysfunction. Even in infants and children, otherwise asymptomatic hypoglycemia has been associated with neurocognitive impairment.

The histological structure of the pancreas is specifically designed to prevent these events, however. Within the pancreas, each islet of Langerhans consists of several hundred cells, including a core of insulin-producing beta cells surrounded by glucagon-secreting alpha cells and an outer layer of somatostatin-producing delta cells and PP cells, which make pancreatic polypeptide. As arterial blood enters the islet core, the beta cells are the first to encounter plasma glucose concentrations. Thus, the function of alpha cells is determined largely by the normal activity of beta cells. For example, insulin directly inhibits glucagon secretion by pancreatic alpha cells.

In adults, reactive hypoglycemia occurs when these counterregulatory responses fail after the person consumes a carbohydrate load, causing blood glucose to fall 2 to 5 hours after eating. Patients with decreased glucagon and epinephrine responses to low blood glucose levels have up to a 25-fold greater risk of experiencing hypoglycemia, particularly during sleep, as sleep itself decreases counterregulatory hormonal responses.

Unfortunately, an initial hypoglycemic episode appears to contribute to a vicious cycle of hypoglycemia, as recurrent hypoglycemia has been associated with autonomic failure and a delay in onset of the early warning signs associated with subsequent hypoglycemic episodes. This may relate to an increased production of cortisol, which decreases glucagon and epinephrine responses, as well as an upregulation of glucose transport in the brain, which renders the central nervous system less sensitive to producing neuroglycopenic symptoms.

CLINICAL PRESENTATION

The clinical presentation of hypoglycemia, especially subjective symptoms, varies depending on the physical status of the person. For example, older adults with neuropathy may lack awareness of hypoglycemic symptoms unless they are severe. In addition, with accidental exposures to hypoglycemic agents, symptoms are often neither recognized nor associated with hypoglycemia.

Subjective

Symptoms of hypoglycemia may be present when blood glucose levels fall below 60 mg/dL, and brain function is often impaired when glycemic levels fall below 50 mg/dL. Moreover, some patients exhibit symptoms with abnormal fluctuations of glucose and insulin. Symptoms vary from very mild to severe and are classified as adrenergic or neuroglycopenic. Adrenergic symptoms include sweating, tremulousness, dizziness, confusion, anxiety, and palpitations. Neuroglycopenic symptoms include headaches, fatigue, weakness, drowsiness, syncope, diplopia, blurred vision, and personality changes. Seizures and coma are severe presentations. The medical history should focus on eating habits, mealtimes, exercise habits, alcohol intake, any history of liver or renal disease, and any family history of endocrine disorders, including DM and hypoglycemia. Hypoglycemic symptoms are often relieved with the ingestion of carbohydrates. The neurological manifestations of hemiparesis, convulsions, confusion, and coma are more common in patients with DM.

Objective

Objective findings that accompany hypoglycemia include tachycardia with or without premature ventricular contractions, diaphoresis, hypothermia or hyperthermia, coma, seizures, tremors, positive Babinski's sign, aphasia, and hemiparesis. A physical examination with special attention to objective signs of endocrinological disease is indicated initially. Assessment for an enlarged liver and neurological signs of chronic alcohol abuse should also be performed to evaluate for this key cause of hypoglycemia. In patients unable to provide an adequate medical history, the skin should be examined for needle marks, which may reflect possible insulin injections.

DIAGNOSTIC REASONING

Diagnostic Tests

Blood glucose levels are used to diagnose hypoglycemia, which is suspected if a random level is between 45 and 60 mg/dL or if an overnight fasting glucose level is less than 60 mg/dL. Hypoglycemia is considered present if the blood glucose level is 45 mg/dL or less. Evaluation of the etiology, when not attributed to the treatment of DM, requires subsequent laboratory evaluations.

Initial Testing

Initial testing for suspected hypoglycemia includes measurement of the blood glucose level. Chronic hypoglycemia may be evident by measuring a low glycohemoglobin (A1C) level; however, the most informative time to obtain a blood glucose level is when the patient is experiencing acute symptoms. If hypoglycemia and symptoms occur concurrently and if both are relieved with eating, the diagnosis of postprandial hypoglycemia is confirmed. Of note, finger-stick monitors are not highly accurate at extremes of high or low glucose concentrations. Thus, they are helpful in detecting high and low blood glucose levels in general, but the specific numerical result may not accurately reflect the true blood glucose concentration. It is also important to recognize that whole blood glucose levels are 10% to 15% lower than serum glucose levels, because red blood cells consume glucose.

More than one-third of normal patients have hypoglycemia with or without symptoms during a short-term 4-hour fasting test. Thus, as an alternative, a 5-hour OGTT may be done using a 100-g glucose load, by taking hourly glucose and insulin measurements. Hypoglycemia is typically diagnosed if the patient experiences a decrease in blood glucose concentration of greater than 100 mg/dL per hour or a blood glucose level of less than 50 mg/dL at any point during the test. However, overinterpretation of this test may lead to an overdiagnosis of hypoglycemia. In turn, some experts caution the use of the OGTT as a diagnostic test for hypoglycemia, requiring that low blood glucose levels be accompanied by clinical signs and symptoms of hypoglycemia, which must ameliorate upon subsequent glucose ingestion in order to diagnose hypoglycemia. These three criteria are known as Whipple's triad.

In turn, for a definitive diagnosis of hypoglycemia, the patient should have (1) documented occurrences of low blood glucose levels, (2) symptoms that occur when the blood glucose level is low, (3) evidence that symptoms are relieved by sugar or other carbohydrate-containing foods, and (4) identification of the particular type of hypoglycemia. The most reliable method of diagnosing hypoglycemia is a supervised 72-hour fasting plasma glucose test. During this test, the patient is allowed calorie- and caffeine-free fluids, while she or he fasts at least overnight and up to 72 hours to detect symptoms develop in the presence of hypoglycemia. Before and after the fast, baseline measurements of serum glucose, insulin, proinsulin, and C-peptide concentration are obtained. Urine is tested for ketones throughout the test, and capillary glucose measurements are taken every 6 hours. The test is terminated when symptoms of hypoglycemia appear, and a blood glucose level is measured immediately. A positive test result for men is considered to be a blood glucose level of less than 55 mg/dL and in women, of less than 45 mg/dL. If after 72 hours of fasting and light exercise, hypoglycemia (less than 60 mg/dL) is not demonstrated, the test is negative. This test is performed in a hospital setting under close observation, as either glucagon or glucose must be administered after the symptomatic blood draw to reverse hypoglycemic manifestations.

Subsequent Testing

The following laboratory tests assist in the diagnostic reasoning during a hypoglycemic episode: plasma insulin level, insulin antibodies, plasma and urine sulfonylurea levels, and C-peptide concentration. Other tests include a blood urea nitrogen, serum creatinine, blood alcohol level, and liver function tests. Fasting insulin levels range from 8.0 to 16.0 mcU/mL or 3.0 to 0.6 ng/mL. An abnormally elevated insulin level in the absence of blood glucose variation is suggestive of an insulinoma, exogenous insulin administration, insulin resistance syndrome, or reactive hypoglycemia in developing DM. Elevated insulin levels in response to glucose fluctuations suggests functional or reactive hypoglycemia. To rule out endocrinological pathology if suspected, cortisol and adrenocorticotropic hormone levels are obtained. The first morning void can be tested for ketones, as a lack of ketone bodies implies a defect in the fatty acid oxidation pathway.

C-peptide analysis is done via radioimmunoassay and provides an index of beta cell function; normal values range from 0.9 to 4.2 ng/mL. A low C-peptide level with an elevated insulin level confirms exogenous insulin administration. In contrast, C-peptide levels are elevated with insulinomas. To differentiate the effects of an insulinoma from factitious hypoglycemia, the ratio of insulin to C-peptide is determined. If the insulin to C-peptide ratio is equal to or less than 1.0, the hypoglycemia is a result of endogenous insulin secretion; if it is greater than 1.0, then exogenous insulin administration is confirmed.

Differential Diagnosis

Differential diagnoses that share many of the same signs and symptoms of hypoglycemia include generalized anxiety disorder, panic attacks, hyperventilation, pheochromocytoma, drug or alcohol intoxication, transient ischemic attack, cerebrovascular accident, and psychosis. Causes of reactive hypoglycemia include meals high in refined carbohydrates, since certain nutrients such as fructose and galactose can cause a burst of insulin secretion. Certain drugs (e.g., sulfonylureas, salicylates) can cause excess glucose utilization or deficient glucose production, resulting in hypoglycemia. Oral diabetic medications are especially prone to causing reactive hypoglycemia when used in combination therapy, especially with concurrent insulin treatment. Insulinomas (i.e., adenomas of the islets of Langerhans), although rare, should be considered in an otherwise healthy adult who is found to have fasting hypoglycemia.

MANAGEMENT

The goal of the management of hypoglycemia is to normalize blood glucose levels and treat the underlying cause of hypoglycemia. As acute severe hypoglycemia may be life-threatening, treatment to increase low glycemic levels must occur immediately and should be administered locally wherever the hypoglycemia is first detected, in the field by emergency medical services first responders, in an emergency department, or in an urgent care setting. Following stabilization, the patient with identifiable pathology is typically referred to an endocrinologist for further evaluation and treatment. In cases of functional and idiopathic hypoglycemia, the management plan may be developed by the primary-care practitioner in consultation with an endocrinologist.

Initial Management

The treatment of acute hypoglycemia for alert patients who can ingest by mouth is 6 to 12 ounces of orange juice or other fruit juice without additional sugar. One cup (8 oz) of milk can be substituted if juice is unavailable. Glucose tablets or gel, if available, can also be used as rapidly absorbed glucose sources. In acute care settings, glucose is provided emergently as standardized IV bolus preparations of dextrose diluted to various concentrations in water (e.g., D25% or D50%), as opposed to standardized hypotonic saline solutions with lower amounts of dextrose that are used primarily for maintenance glucose requirements (e.g., D5% 0.45% NaCl). The blood glucose level should be monitored closely after IV bolus administration of dextrose and then periodically while the patient is on a dextrose-containing continuous IV drip. Glucagon hydrochloride (0.03 to 0.1 mg/kg per dose; 1 to 2 mg in adults; 1 mg in children older than 5 years or weighing more than 20 kg; 0.5 mg in children younger than 5 years or weighing less than 20 kg) may be given IM, SC, or IV if the patient is unresponsive. Doses may be repeated as needed every few hours in adults and even more frequently in children (up to every 20 to 30 minutes initially).

Hypoglycemia is a medical emergency because of the seriousness of potential sequelae (e.g., seizures, coma, cardiovascular dysfunction, death). Thus, even if euglycemia is readily restored, patients must be evaluated for potential hospital admission for inpatient care and close observation if there is any concern for the recurrence of hypoglycemia. Patients requiring hospital admission include those with hypoglycemia without an obvious cause or with severe or persistent neurological deficits.

Subsequent Management

The long-term management of hypoglycemia includes treatment of its underlying causes and dietary modifications as needed. If hypoglycemia is a result of pancreatic or extrapancreatic tumors, surgical excision is recommended. Although the treatment of choice for insulinoma is surgical resection, there is only an 85% success rate with an experienced surgeon. If the tumor is small, it may not be found on an exploratory laparotomy. When surgery is unsuccessful, an endocrinologist may initiate diazoxide (Hyperstat, Proglycem; 3–8 mg/kg per day orally in divided doses three times daily or 200 mg every 4 hours in adults) therapy to reduce insulin secretion. If hypoglycemia is caused by rapid gastric emptying following a gastrectomy, an anticholinergic drug may provide relief by delaying gastric emptying and decreasing intestinal motility.

In patients with inoperable pancreatic tumors or in whom resection has been unsuccessful, small frequent feedings that are high in carbohydrates (every 2–3 hours) may be effective in preventing acute hypoglycemic episodes. In patients with renal failure, frequent small high-carbohydrate meals may prevent hypoglycemic episodes. Similarly, in patients with pseudohypoglycemia or idiopathic hypoglycemia, in which a cause cannot be identified, treatment consists primarily of dietary modifications. A high-protein, low-carbohydrate diet divided into six small meals per day often relieves symptoms. Caffeine, refined sugars, and alcohol should be restricted. If food allergies are suspected, allergy testing may be indicated to identify offending foods to avoid. If a medication is suspected as a causative factor, alternative agents must be considered.

SMBG is the cornerstone of long-term self-management of hypoglycemia. Patients may need to monitor blood glucose levels frequently during the initiation of lifestyle changes or dietary modifications to evaluate success. Monitoring glucose levels during exercise, eating at regularly scheduled intervals, and understanding the importance of SMBG to self-diagnosis and early detection may prevent severe hypoglycemic reactions.

FOLLOW-UP AND REFERRAL

Patients with a history of hypoglycemic events require frequent follow-up and evaluation, as determined on an individual basis. More frequent SMBG may be indicated, especially from 12 to 24 hours after a hypoglycemic event. At each visit, the patient's record of cumulative hypoglycemic events should be reviewed for patterns or clues as to triggering factors, such as postprandial associations. Patients who continue to experience hypoglycemic episodes despite intervention should be referred to an endocrinologist.

Patient Education: Hypoglycemia

The importance of dietary modifications must be stressed. Nondiabetic patients with reactive, functional, or fasting hypoglycemia should eat five or six small meals daily to steady the release of glucose into the blood. These meals should be balanced with carbohydrates, protein, and some fat. Patients who experience symptoms after a meal that is high in refined sugar but not after a nonsugary meal should restrict refined sugars in the diet. Patients who cannot eat small meals throughout the day should be encouraged to carry raw seeds and nuts mixed with dried fruits for periodic snacking.

Patients with DM who experience hypoglycemia should be instructed to maintain their glycemic goals, report all episodes of hypoglycemia, and monitor blood glucose levels at bedtime and before, during, and after exercise to assist in glycemic management. Alcohol, cigarette smoking, and caffeine should be avoided in these patients.

REFERENCES

Type 1 Diabetes Mellitus

Aathira R, Jain V. Advances in management of type 1 diabetes mellitus. *World J Diabetes.* 2014;15(5):689–696.

American Diabetes Association. Standards of medical care in diabetes—2017. *Diabetes Care.* 2017;40(Suppl 1).

Dhatariya KK, Vallanki, P. Treatment of diabetic ketoacidosis (DKA)/ hyperglycemic hyperosmolar state (HHS): Novel advances in management of hyperglycemic crisis (UK versus USA). *Curr Diab Rep.* 2017;17(5):33.

Funnell MM, Piatt GA. Incorporating diabetes self-management education into your practice: When, what and how. *J Nurse Pract.* 2017;13(7):466–474.

Havas S, Donner T. Tight control of type 1 diabetes: Recommendations for patients. *Am Fam Physician.* 2006;74:971–978, 983–984.

Type 2 Diabetes Mellitus

Carmichael KA. What is a logical approach for choosing among new agents for patients with type 2 diabetes? *Consultant.* 2013;53(2):100–102.

DeFronzo RA. From the triumvirate to the ominous octet: A new paradigm for the treatment of type 2 diabetes mellitus. *Diabetes.* 2009;58:773–795.

Ely EK, Gruss SM, Luman ET, et al. A national effort to prevent type 2 diabetes: Participant-level evaluation of CDC's National Diabetes Prevention Program. *Diabetes Care.* 2017;40(10):1331–1341.

Garber A, Abrahamson MJ, Barzilay JI, et al. Consensus statement by the American Association of Clinical Endocrinology and American College of Endocrinology on the comprehensive type 2 diabetes management algorithm. *Endocr Pract.* 2017;23(2):207–238.

Hinen D. Glucagon-like peptide 1 receptor agonists for type 2 diabetes. *Diabetes Spectr.* 2017;30(3):202–210.

Kahn C, Cooper ME, Del Prato S. Pathophysiology and treatment of type 2 diabetes: Perspectives on the past, present, and future. *Lancet.* 2014;383(9922):1068–1083.

Le Roux CW. 3 years of liraglutide versus placebo for type 2 diabetes risk reduction and weight management in individuals with prediabetes: A randomized, double-blind trial. *Lancet.* 2017;389(10077):1399–1409.

Marso SP, Daniels GH, Brown-Frandesen K, et al. Liraglutide and cardiovascular outcomes in type 2 diabetes. *N Engl J Med.* 2016;375:311–322.

Smith D. The dyslipidemia of type 2 diabetes: Treatment strategies. *Consultant.* 2013;53(3):137–144.

Sola D, Rossi L, Schianca GP, et al. Sulfonylureas and their use in clinical practice. *Arch Med Sci.* 2015;11(4):840–848.

U.S. Food & Drug Administration. FDA drug safety communication: FDA warns that DPP-4 inhibitors for type 2 diabetes may cause severe point pain. https://www.fda.gov/Drugs/DrugSafety/ucm459579.htm. Published 2016. Accessed October 20, 2017.

RESOURCES

ACC AHA ASCVD Risk Calculator
http://tools.acc.org/ASCVD-Risk-Estimator-Plus/#!/calculate/estimate/

American Association of Diabetes Educators
www.diabeteseducator.org

American Diabetes Association
www.diabetes.org

American Dietetic Association
www.eatright.org

Centers for Disease Control and Prevention—Diabetes
https://www.cdc.gov/diabetes/pdfs/data/statistics/national-diabetes-statistics-report.pdf

Indian Health Services Diabetes Program
www.ihs.gov/MedicalPrograms/Diabetes

Juvenile Diabetes Foundation International
http://www.jdrf.org/about/fact-sheets/type-1-diabetes-facts/

National Diabetes Information Clearinghouse
http://diabetes.niddk.nih.gov

National Eye Institute—National Eye Health Education Program
www.nei.nih.gov

National Institute of Diabetes and Digestive and Kidney Diseases
www.niddk.nih.gov

Scales and Measures (Diabetes Distress Scales)
http://behavioraldiabetes.org/scales-and-measures/#1448434304201-ce67e63c-8e90

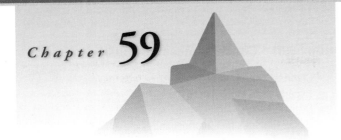

Chapter **59**

Metabolic Disorders

Debera J. Thomas, DNS, RN, FNP/ANP

Brian Oscar Porter, MD, PhD, MPH, MBA

OBESITY

Obesity, defined as an excess amount of adipose tissue (body fat), is a chronic disease that is multifactorial and neurobehavioral in nature. The World Health Organization classifies obesity as one of the world's most neglected public health problems. It is associated with multiple comorbidities, including an increased risk of cancer, cardiovascular disease, disability, diabetes mellitus, gallbladder disease, high blood pressure, osteoarthritis, sleep apnea, and cerebrovascular accident (stroke). The increase in body fat promotes adipose tissue dysfunction that results in significant adverse metabolic, biomechanical, and psychosocial health consequences.

EPIDEMIOLOGY AND CAUSES

The American Medical Association classified obesity as a disease in 2013. The U.S. Centers for Disease Control and Prevention (CDC) bases its classifications of overweight and obesity on body mass index (BMI). Although not an entirely accurate reflection of increased bodily fat, the BMI provides a "ballpark" figure from which to estimate obesity. See Table 59.1, Calculating Body Mass Index and Classifying Obesity.

Published clinical guidelines on the identification, evaluation, and treatment of overweight and obesity cite the complex etiology of overeating that makes this chronic illness poorly understood and often intractable to medical management. The two major types of obesity are central (apple-shaped) and lower body (pear-shaped) obesity. Patients with central obesity have excessive body fat in the abdomen and flank areas and are at a greater risk for type 2 diabetes mellitus, coronary artery disease (CAD), stroke, and early death, compared with those with lower body obesity who have excessive adipose tissue in the buttocks and thighs.

Overweight and obesity are epidemic in the United States today and rates are increasing across the globe.

TABLE 59.1 Calculating Body Mass Index and Classifying Obesity	
Calculating Body Mass Index	
The most recent formula for calculating body mass index (BMI) was developed by a panel convened by the National Heart, Lung, and Blood Institute and the National Institute of Diabetes and Digestive and Kidney Diseases of the National Institutes of Health. The equation for BMI is weight (kg) divided by height (m) squared (kg/m^2).	
Classifying Obesity Classification	BMI
Overweight	25–29.9 kg/m^2
Obesity Class 1 Class 2 Class 3 (severe, extreme)	30–34.9 kg/m^2 35–39.9 kg/m^2 >40 kg/m^2

Obesity has tripled worldwide since 1975. In the United States, obesity affects 36.5% of adults, with more than one-third being overweight with a BMI between 25 and 29.9 kg/m^2. Thus, overall 70.2% of American adults are overweight or obese. Moreover, the World Health Organization reports that 41 million children younger than 5 years of age were overweight or obese in 2016. More women than men are obese across all age-groups, and African American women are more likely to be obese than European American women. However, the incidence of obesity is higher in those of lower socioeconomic status, regardless of race.

The health-care costs of obesity in the United States are estimated to be between $147 billion and $210 billion annually. Job absenteeism as a result of obesity and its related comorbidities costs about $4.3 billion each year. Moreover, Americans spend more than $64 billion a year on diets, weight-loss supplements, and low-calorie food products in an attempt to treat obesity. In fact, obesity kills more people than does being underweight. In addition, the psychological costs of obesity, which are difficult to quantify in impact, include stigmatization, discrimination, and social isolation.

The main causes of obesity are considered extragenetic (nongenetic in etiology) and epigenetic (heritable changes or alterations in gene expression and/or function without modification of the DNA-based genetic code). In addition, more than 100 genetic variants have been identified that are associated with obesity risk; however, these genetic variants account for only a small percentage of obesity risk. Indeed, secondary causes of obesity due to medical conditions are rare and include various endocrine and neurological diseases.

Extragenetic causes of obesity include cultural and environmental factors (e.g., geographic location, family structure, socioeconomic status), suboptimal nutrition and physical inactivity, disrupted sleep cycles, medication side effects, stress, neurologic dysfunction (e.g., central nervous system trauma, hypothalamic inflammation, leptin resistance), viral infections, and alterations in the gut microbiome. In fact, a diet that is energy dense and combined with a sedentary lifestyle is the main causes of obesity in the United States, and an environment that supports a sedentary lifestyle and facilitates access to fatty foods, processed foods, and refined sugars has contributed to the high incidence of obesity today.

Epigenetic causes of obesity include developmental events that occur pre-pregnancy, during gestation, and post-pregnancy. For example, having a parent (either a father or mother) who is overweight or obese prior to pregnancy increases the risk of overweight or obese offspring, as well as the risk of other related diseases, such as type 2 diabetes mellitus, cardiovascular disease, and certain types of cancer. During gestation, unhealthy maternal nutrition, particularly in pregnant women who are overweight or obese, may increase nutrient transfer through the placenta into the fetal circulation, causing alternations in fetal gene expression that may increase the child's predisposition to being overweight or obese. As a postpregnancy example, early exposure to antibiotics in childhood has also been shown to be a risk factor in the development of overweight and obesity later in life, although the mechanism is unclear.

PATHOPHYSIOLOGY

Obesity affects almost every bodily system and is associated with an increased risk of multiple comorbid diseases (see Box 59.1). The health risks associated with obesity are directly correlated with its severity and include metabolic and structural impacts on the body, as well as psychosocial disability that results from the social stigma attached to obesity. Mortality risk increases as complications of obesity develop and approaches 50% when a patient's weight is 30% to 40% above his or her ideal body weight. Obesity is associated with an increased risk of colon, rectal, and prostate cancer in males, and uterine, gallbladder, biliary tract, breast, and ovarian cancer are more prevalent in obese females. Patients who are obese also have increased surgical and obstetrical risks. A reduction in body weight of 5% to 20% significantly decreases these comorbid risk factors in obese individuals.

Obesity is a complex, multifactorial disease that involves interactions among lifestyle, behavioral, genetic, and environmental factors. An increase in weight, and ultimately obesity, result when one's intake of calories persistently exceeds energy expenditures. The control of appetite and the mechanisms that govern food intake are complex and incompletely understood. The hypothalamus controls certain aspects of appetite and appears to have a role in an individual's food preferences. Other important central nervous system sites include the solitary tract of the hindbrain, the arcuate and

---

Box 59.1   Consequences of Obesity

- Coronary heart disease/congestive heart failure
- Hypertension
- Dyslipidemia/hyperlipidemia
- Type 2 diabetes mellitus/insulin resistance
- Metabolic syndrome
- Sleep apnea
- Restrictive lung disease
- Asthma
- Varicose veins and venous insufficiency
- Gout/hyperuricemia
- Osteoarthritis
- Reflux esophagitis
- Gallbladder disease
- Thromboembolic disease
- Cancers: Endometrial, breast, prostate, colon

---

paraventricular nuclei, and the amygdala. Mediated by several neurotransmitters including norepinephrine, dynorphin, hypocretin, serotonin, neuropeptide Y, and ghrelin, both the central and peripheral nervous systems produce and integrate a complex array of neural inputs that regulate appetite, energy metabolism, and body fat mass.

The body is known to have neuroendocrine homeostatic feedback control mechanisms involving both the peripheral and central nervous systems, which seek to maintain adequate nutrient intake and an ideal body weight. Examples include glycemic levels (hypoglycemia is a trigger to eat), serum leptin concentrations, glucocorticoids that act as appetite stimulants, sympathomimetic hormones that act as appetite suppressants, and the peptide ghrelin—a ligand for the growth hormone secretagogue receptor that increases appetite (ghrelin levels increase in anticipation of a meal and in response to diet-induced weight loss).

Differences in fat-free body mass also correlate strongly with differences in energy expenditure among different individuals. In particular, weight gain is associated with increased metabolic demands and energy expenditure that retard further weight gain, whereas weight loss is associated with reductions in energy expenditure that counter further weight loss. Thus, a formerly obese individual who loses weight will experience a relative decrease in energy expenditure compared with a nonobese individual and will thus require 15% fewer calories to maintain his or her reduced weight. In turn, failing to reduce one's caloric intake appropriately may result in progressive weight gain.

Adipocytes, the cellular basis of obesity, secrete hormones and cytokines known as adipokines, which form the basis of neuroendocrine regulatory mechanisms that contribute to obesity if dysregulated. These include leptin (which inhibits hunger), adiponectin (which is insulin-sensitizing, anti-inflammatory, and anti-atherogenic), resistin (which causes insulin resistance and is a feedback regulator for adipogenesis), apelin (which regulates blood sugar), visfatin (which mimics insulin and comes from visceral fat), vaspin (which is insulin-sensitizing and anti-inflammatory), and retinol-binding protein 4 (which promotes insulin resistance and fat deposition). Adipokines also include regulators of lipoprotein metabolism (e.g., lipoprotein lipase, lipotransin, apolipoprotein E, cholesterol ester transfer protein) and inflammatory cytokines (e.g., prostaglandins, tumor necrosis factor-α [TNF-α], interleukins, plasminogen activator inhibitor 1, monocyte chemoattractant protein 1).

Expressed by adipose, intestinal, and placental cells, the leptin gene has been the subject of much controversy in human obesity. Serum leptin concentrations strongly correlate with body fat content, and leptin-deficient mice demonstrate insulin resistance, hyperinsulinemia, and hyperphagia. Leptin has been shown to reduce levels of neuropeptide Y, a potent stimulus for food intake produced in the brain's arcuate nucleus. Human obesity due to leptin deficiency has been identified in two consanguineous families, as has obesity due to leptin receptor deficiency. However, leptin overexpression has not been shown to reduce appetite or weight, and most obese patients express normal levels of this protein, albeit with decreased sensitivity to leptin. Thus, decreased leptin levels appear to signal that fat stores are insufficient for growth and reproduction; however, the hormone itself is not a negative regulator of appetite or weight gain.

There is a well-documented genetic predisposition for the development of obesity. Twin studies have revealed strong correlations in obesity prevalence between siblings raised together by the same set of parents, as well as apart in separate households. In contrast, the BMIs of adoptees correlate more closely with those of their biological parents rather than their adoptive parents. Moreover, obesity is a presenting feature of at least 24 genetic syndromes, displaying an entire range of heritability patterns. These syndromes are relatively rare, but the most common are Prader-Willi syndrome, a neurodegenerative disorder resulting from genetic abnormalities in the long arm of chromosome 15q11 to 13, and the autosomal recessive Bardet-Biedl syndrome involving concurrent hypogenitalism, mental retardation, and renal abnormalities.

On a molecular level, the bulk of our understanding of the pathophysiology and genetics of obesity stems from preclinical animal models—particularly that of the obese mouse, for which a number of genetically altered strains are available. Through genetically engineered knockout mice that lack one or more target genes, as well as transgenic models that overexpress either a functional or nonfunctional version of a target gene, researchers have identified several single gene defects that result in obesity. Some of these genetic findings have been further generalized to humans.

There is recent evidence that alterations in the gut microbiome are linked to obesity. Research is ongoing, but evidence obtained thus far shows a parallel between the obesity pandemic and the increase in antibiotic use and the development of microbial resistance. Antibiotic use, diet, and bariatric surgery alter the gut microbiome, which in turn alters energy metabolism and body habitus. The gut microbiome is likely a factor in the complex interplay of genetics, environment, and gut permeability in the development of obesity and other chronic diseases.

CLINICAL PRESENTATION

Subjective

Patients often present to their health-care provider with some or all of the following symptoms as a result of obesity: fatigue, decreased energy, weakness, joint pain, shortness of breath, increased daytime sleepiness, and depression. Most will seek help for another medical condition or present with one or more of the aforementioned complaints. A comprehensive history includes probing for a weight history and attempts at weight loss, as patients often report several attempts with repeated dieting. Family history of obesity and cultural food preferences must be addressed in the assessment, and the amount of control the patient maintains in food purchasing and preparation should also be considered. The patient should be questioned about any periods of rapid weight gain and environmental or psychosocial changes in lifestyle or behavior during these periods. An exercise history should also be obtained, with special emphasis on the relationship of any weight gain or weight-loss periods to exercise. Specific questions to assess current or past eating disorders are essential.

Objective

A complete physical examination, with a focus not only on body weight, but also on signs of possible secondary causes (e.g., Cushing's syndrome, thyroid disease) and complications (e.g., diabetes mellitus, peripheral vascular disease) of obesity should be done. The diagnosis of obesity is based on a BMI of 30 kg/m^2 or greater (see Table 59.1). However, in extremely muscular individuals, BMI is not an accurate gauge of obesity; in such cases, a body-fat analysis will yield more accurate information about body composition. In children, obesity is diagnosed as a BMI in the 95th percentile or higher on age- and gender-specific pediatric growth charts.

Historically, ideal body weight has been calculated by comparing actual body weight to population tables from the Metropolitan Life Insurance Company. Weights for the original and updated tables were calculated based on data from middle-class Americans seeking insurance; as Americans grew heavier, the weights in the table increased. Measurements of weight and height are used to calculate the BMI for the precise classification of obesity. BMI is calculated by taking the body weight in kilograms divided by the height in meters squared.

BMI remains the measurement most frequently used in research and clinical practice to assess overweight and obesity because it is easily calculated without laboratory equipment. In clinical studies, BMI correlates with measurements of body fat percentage taken with underwater displacement weighing, but is not as reliable in older adults.

Two methods can be used to assess for central obesity, which is the type of obesity most associated with significant complications. The first is to measure waist circumference, with values greater than 40 inches in men and more than 35 inches in women indicating central obesity. The second method is to calculate a waist-to-hip ratio using the following formula:

$$\text{Waist-to-hip ratio} = \frac{\text{Waist measurement at smallest part}}{\text{Hip measurement at largest circumference}}$$

A ratio of greater than 1.0 in males and more than 0.8 for females indicates central truncal obesity.

DIAGNOSTIC REASONING

A complete history and physical examination with anthropometric measurement are essential elements of the initial assessment. A past medical history and complete medication profile are also necessary, especially regarding the intake of corticosteroids or appetite stimulants, as well as past use of appetite suppressants, laxative, diuretics, or herbal supplements as evidence of past weight-loss attempts.

Diagnostic Tests

Initial assessment of the obese patient should include the following laboratory tests: thyroid-stimulating hormone (TSH), fasting glucose and glycosylated hemoglobin A1c, fasting lipid profile, liver function tests with an alkaline phosphatase and total bilirubin, serum electrolytes, creatinine, blood urea nitrogen, uric acid, vitamin D level, and general laboratory tests, including a complete blood count, urinalysis, and urinary microalbumin. An electrocardiogram should also be obtained to assess cardiac health.

Also included in initial testing may be an evaluation of bodily composition (body fat percentage) using calipers or bioelectrical impedance. Both are inexpensive assessment methods; however, calipers are not as accurate in patients with a high BMI, while the impedance-based measurement is hydration-dependent. Dual-energy x-ray absorptiometry (DXA) is accurate but relatively expensive, and DXA machines may not accommodate very obese patients.

Differential Diagnosis

The diagnosis of obesity is usually straightforward, although underlying causes may not always be evident. Thus, the differential diagnosis of obesity is geared toward determining the underlying etiology. Secondary causes of obesity, such as Cushing's syndrome, hypothalamic injury, and hypothyroidism, must be ruled out before initiating a treatment plan with the patient. For example, edematous states and water balance must be considered, as acute or chronic fluid retention should be distinguished from increased adiposity. Although the vast majority of obesity cases are due to non-nutritive dietary choices and sedentary lifestyle behaviors, certain medical conditions such as hypothyroidism can be ruled out with simple laboratory tests (e.g., TSH). However, in general, an extensive laboratory work-up is not necessary. Rare syndromes may also be associated with severe or morbid obesity, such as Pickwickian syndrome that consists of hypersomnia, congestive heart failure, and hypertension in an obese patient.

Patients should also be evaluated for other risk factors associated with obesity—especially those implicated in CAD, such as hyperlipidemia and insulin resistance associated with type 2 diabetes mellitus. *Metabolic syndrome* is a constellation of risk factors including hypertension, hyperlipidemia, insulin resistance, and overweight/obesity that significantly increases an individual's risk of cardiovascular disease and diabetes mellitus (see Chapter 35 for more information on metabolic syndrome). The American Diabetes Association has published a statement with multiple professional societies addressing metabolic syndrome, and the Endocrine Society has a practice guideline stressing the importance of recognizing these at-risk patients.

MANAGEMENT

Whether weight gain is related to exogenous or endogenous factors is an important determination in developing a comprehensive treatment plan, as many secondary causes of obesity may be treatable. For example, if obesity is caused by hypothyroidism, treating the thyroid issues may solve the weight gain problem. Ultimately, the clinical management of obesity requires the balancing of energy intake versus expenditure. Current clinical evidence suggests that successful treatment must include a combination of diet, exercise, and behavioral interventions, as multidisciplinary approaches to weight loss have a higher success rate. Continued close contact with a health-care provider is more important for long-term success than any particular diet program. Given the chronic nature of obesity, the patient must learn long-term weight management skills. Cognitive therapy in conjunction with education is effective in increasing self-esteem, improving depression, and decreasing patients' dissatisfaction with their bodies.

The management plan should focus on reducing comorbidity and visceral obesity, not solely on improving cosmetic outcomes. Dietary instructions are essentially the same for the obese individual as they are for a healthy nonobese person. The National Heart, Lung, and Blood Institute of the National Institutes of Health (NIH) recommends following a heart-healthy eating plan with an emphasis on portion control that includes abundant fruits and vegetables, whole grains, low-fat protein sources, and small amounts of foods containing high levels of monounsaturated and polyunsaturated fats, such as nuts and seeds. A management plan that is realistic, that can fit into the patient's lifestyle, and that includes gradual changes in diet and activity is more likely to be successful than extremely or fad dieting.

Cultural and socioeconomic factors affect not only the prevalence of obesity but also attitudes as to acceptable weight and its implications. For example, some cultures view being overweight as a sign of good health and prosperity. In many Western cultures, obesity is seen more as a cosmetic problem than a major health problem. Thus, patient counseling should stress the health benefits of weight loss, such as reductions in blood pressure, serum triglycerides, and blood glucose levels (especially in patients with type 2 diabetes mellitus who may experience decreased A1c levels), as well as an increase in the level of cardioprotective high-density lipoprotein cholesterol. In addition, assisting the patient to identify reasons for overeating may benefit the patient in managing his or her dietary behaviors. Being tired, anxious, socially isolated, and angry are all major triggers for overeating, as denoted by the HALT acronym, which stands for Hungry, Angry, Lonely, and Tired.

Management should be directed toward an initial goal of decreasing the patient's weight by 10% over 6 months. Subsequent goals are set after achieving this initial weight-loss goal. Treatment guidelines include measuring BMI at each patient encounter. If a patient has a BMI of 25 kg/m^2 or more or a waist circumference greater than 35 inches in females or greater than 40 inches males, care should be taken to assess for comorbidities and cardiovascular risk factors. All patients, regardless of their BMI, should be counseled about healthy lifestyle behaviors, including healthy dietary and exercise habits. Weight loss goals and treatment plans should be made in consultation with the patient, in order to devise a program that is practical and feasible for the patient. If on repeated visits, the patient has failed to lose weight, the provider should explore barriers to behavioral change and alternative approaches with the patient.

Dietary Management

Before dietary modifications are initiated, a 3- to 7-day diet history should be evaluated. The patient should keep a diary, recording all oral intake, including water and drinks. It is often beneficial to have the patient record daily activities along with food intake. Clues as to lifestyle patterns and behavioral eating patterns can be assessed more adequately with both sets of data. The overall goal of weight loss depends on a calorie deficit in which caloric expenditure exceeds caloric intake. A daily caloric deficit of 500 to 750 calories has been shown to be effective in achieving weight loss regardless of the manipulation of macronutrients (fats, carbohydrates, and protein). Thus, the goal is to create a caloric deficit following a healthy eating plan. Besides calorie restriction, dietary recommendations must consider minimum recommended daily nutrient requirements, the patient's food preferences, and the patient's lifestyle.

Physical Activity

Physical activity is a significant part of a weight loss and maintenance program. It is especially beneficial in the long-term management of weight loss, lowering blood pressure, increasing muscle mass, increasing insulin sensitivity, improving the lipid profile, and improving glucose metabolism. Unless specific contraindications exist, physical activity should be prescribed for all patients. The NIH recommendation for physical activity for everyone is 150 minutes of moderate-intensity aerobic physical activity per week. Moderately intense physical exertion is equal to a brisk walk of 3 to 4 miles per hour. Patients are more likely to continue low-intensity physical activity than high-intensity physical activity. A 20-minute walk is usually acceptable to most patients as a starting point. Including resistance exercises in the physical activity prescription will also help maintain lean body mass.

Younger patients with obesity may begin an aerobic exercise program if physical examination results are within normal levels. Older, sedentary patients should begin with walking programs. Exercise tolerance testing may be indicated for older adults and adults at risk for CAD before beginning a physical activity program.

Behavior Modification

Behavior modification is essential for initial weight loss and weight maintenance. Unless the patient can identify eating patterns and lifestyle patterns that have contributed to weight gain and change those within his or her control, long-term weight management will not be achieved. Restrictive eating behavior control includes cognitive strategies for portion control and healthy food selections. The need to identify impulsive and binge eating is also important. Behavioral management is enhanced by avoiding high-risk environments or altering the environment to reduce triggers to overeating.

Stress has a significant impact on eating behavior. During times of stress, the patient may find it impossible to implement behavior modification techniques. Relaxation techniques can assist in managing stress. Relaxation techniques must be practiced frequently in times of low stress so they can be effectively used in times of excessive stress.

Pharmacological Management

Pharmacological therapy for obesity has been available for decades, although the medications currently approved by the U.S. Food and Drug Administration (FDA) for use in overweight and obesity all have notable side-effect profiles. Medications approved by the FDA for weight loss include orlistat (Xenical, Alli [lower dose available without a prescription]), lorcaserin (Belviq), phentermine plus extended-release (ER) topiramate (Qsymia), naltrexone-bupropion (Contrave), and liraglutide (Saxenda).

Orlistat functions by blocking the absorption of fat in the gastrointestinal (GI) tract. Orlistat 60 mg is available as an over-the-counter formulation (Alli) and is taken with each fat-containing meal to inhibit gastric and pancreatic lipases, thereby reducing fat absorption. It is also available by prescription (Xenical) at a dose of 120 mg. Demonstrated results are a weight loss of 2 to 4 kg maintained for 2 years. Adverse effects of orlistat at either dose include diarrhea, gas, and abdominal cramping. Some studies suggest it may also inhibit the absorption of fat-soluble vitamins.

Lorcaserin (Belviq) is a selective serotonin 5-HT2C agonist and acts on the hypothalamus to reduce appetite. Lorcaserin should be used with a reduced-calorie diet and increased physical activity for chronic weight management at a dose of 10 mg orally twice a day. It should be discontinued if a 5% weight loss is not achieved by week 12 because it is unlikely to have any future effect on weight loss. Side effects include constipation, dry mouth, fatigue, nausea, headache, and cough.

Phentermine-topiramate (Qsymia) suppresses appetite and increases feelings of satiety. Phentermine-topiramate has four dose formulations to allow for titration of the medication when starting and stopping the drug. The usual dose for weight loss is 7.5 mg/46 mg or 15 mg/92 mg. It is taken each morning to suppress the appetite (phentermine component) and increase satiety, decrease food appeal, and increase metabolic rate (topiramate component). In studies, patients lost approximately 8% of their starting body weight using this combination medication. Side effects include dry mouth, paresthesia, constipation, insomnia, changes in taste sensation, and seizures if abruptly discontinued.

Naltrexone-bupropion (Contrave) works by targeting the hypothalamic melanocortin system and the mesolimbic reward system to affect weight loss, but the exact mechanism of action is not fully characterized. Naltrexone-bupropion is supplied in tablets that contain 8 mg of naltrexone and 90 mg of bupropion. One tablet should be taken during week 1 and then increased by one tablet per day in subsequent weeks to reach a maintenance dose of

2 tablets twice a day at week 4. Side effects include constipation, dry mouth, headache, diarrhea, hypertension, insomnia, liver damage, tachycardia and nausea and vomiting.

Liraglutide (Saxenda) is an injectable glucagon-like peptide 1 (GLP-1) analog that causes weight loss by slowing gastric emptying and suppressing food intake; it is also approved to treat diabetes mellitus (Victoza). The starting injection dose of liraglutide (Saxenda) is 0.6 mg daily for the first week. The dose is increased by 0.6 mg daily per week until the full dose of 3.0 mg is achieved by week 5. Side effects include nauseas, diarrhea, constipation, abdominal pain, headache, and tachycardia. Liraglutide may also cause medullary thyroid carcinoma in rodents and has been associated with postmarketing cases of pancreatitis.

Surgical Intervention

Surgical intervention for obesity should be reserved for those patients who have a BMI over 40 kg/m² or over 35 kg/m² with comorbid conditions. Surgery is usually not considered until the obese patient has failed more conventional weight-loss methods. The rate of bariatric surgery is increasing in the United States today. The most common surgical procedure is the roux-en-Y gastric bypass (RYGB), which may be done laparoscopically. Gastric banding is another option, but the weight-loss results are less dramatic than with RYGB. However, short-term complications of gastric banding are fewer than with RYGB. A third surgical option that is gaining in popularity is a sleeve gastrectomy. In this procedure, about 75% of the stomach is removed but the rest of the GI tract is left intact. Weight loss is less than with RYGB but greater than with gastric banding, with a lower complication rate than RYGB.

Some studies have shown that weight-loss surgery can produce up to a 50% loss of initial body weight. Complications may occur in up to 40% of patients after surgery and include peritonitis, abdominal wall hernia, dumping syndrome, infection, acute cholecystitis, hypoglycemia, pyloric outlet obstruction, chronic diarrhea, nausea, and vomiting. Patients should be counseled regarding these potential complications of surgical interventions. They should also be informed of the possibility of regaining much of the lost weight if lifestyle changes are not also undertaken and sustained.

Additional Clinical Considerations

The increasing number of obese and morbidly obese patients brings a challenge to primary-care practitioners. Caring for patients who are obese certainly includes treating the obesity, but many of these patients have diseases and illnesses that will bring them to the provider's office. The National Institute of Diabetes and Digestive and Kidney Diseases Weight-Control Information Network offers suggestions for health-care providers in the care of these individuals separate from the need to treat the underlying obesity. Health-care providers and clinic staff need to receive education related to respect for patients, the need for size-appropriate equipment in the clinic, and providing the same level of care for obese patients as nonobese patients. Box 59.2 provides details to guide providers in creating an accessible and comfortable clinic environment for obese patients, including medical equipment that can accurately assess patients who are obese and ways to reduce patient fears about their weight.

FOLLOW-UP AND REFERRAL

Most patients on weight-loss programs require close follow-up. The severity of the problem and the nature of the interventions should govern how frequently the primary-care practitioner sees the patient, but clearly, patients are more successful in maintaining weight loss with frequent follow-up visits. Many patients will benefit from frequent clinician visits that provide medical guidance, goal-setting, and emotional support throughout the weight-loss process. In addition, the importance of clinical follow-up once weight-loss goals have been achieved should be emphasized, because recurrent weight gain following periods of significant weight loss is common. The patient should be seen for a weigh-in, blood pressure measurement, and discussion of progress at least monthly, but once a week is often most beneficial until the patient has developed habituated lifestyle changes.

Specialty referrals are driven by the identification of underlying causes of overweight and obesity, such as endocrinological causes that may be reversible or genetic etiologies that may require further counseling for the patient and his or her family (if heritable). In addition, patients may benefit from a referral to a dietitian who specializes in weight loss. A surgical referral may be indicated for morbidly obese patients if nonsurgical interventions have proven unsuccessful. In addition, referrals to comprehensive weight-loss programs at specialized weight-loss centers have become increasingly popular, although such programs are often not covered by health insurance plans or other third-party payors and, thus, may prove costly for the patient. Referrals to weight-loss support groups may be beneficial regardless of the type of weight-loss interventions selected.

In addition, given the critical role that maladaptive psychosocial coping mechanisms play in driving the behavior of many obese patients, referrals to mental health professionals specializing in weight-loss assessment and counseling are typically indicated. For example, weight-loss surgery will typically not be attempted unless a thorough psychological evaluation of the patient and his or her social support network has been completed and the patient's psychological status is deemed capable of supporting the postsurgical practices needed to maintain weight loss.

Box 59.2 Provider's Guide to Caring for Obese Patients

Create an accessible and comfortable clinic environment:

- Provide sturdy, armless chairs and high, firm sofas in waiting rooms.
- Provide sturdy, wide examination tables that are bolted to the floor to prevent tipping.
- Provide a sturdy stool or step with handles to help patients get on the examination table.
- Provide extra-large examination gowns.
- Install a split lavatory seat and provide a specimen collector with a handle.

Use medical equipment that can accurately assess patients who are obese:

- Use large adult blood pressure cuffs or thigh cuffs on patients with an upper-arm circumference greater than 34 cm.
- Have extra-long phlebotomy needles, tourniquets, and large vaginal speculae on hand.
- Have a weight scale with adequate capacity (greater than 350 pounds) for obese patients.

Reduce patient fears about weight assessment:

- Weigh patients only when medically appropriate.
- Weigh patients in a private area.
- Record weight without comments.
- Ask patients if they wish to discuss their weight or health.
- Avoid using the term *obesity*. Your patients may be more comfortable with phrases such as "difficulties with weight" or "being overweight." You may wish to ask your patients what terms they prefer when discussing their weight.

Patient Education: Obesity

Patient education includes instruction on how to maintain a balance between caloric intake and energy expenditure. Physical activity, a healthy diet, and lifestyle changes should be emphasized. Many patients are unaware of techniques to reduce fat in their diet by cooking methods alone, for example, the use of nonstick cookware that obviates the need to use fat or grease in the pan. Other suggestions are to bake, broil, and braise foods rather than to fry them with oil or solid animal and dairy fats such as lard, shortening, margarine, or butter. In addition, many obese persons skip breakfast and eat more in the late afternoon and evening, which is not helpful.

Obese patients must be guided to set realistic weight-loss goals and educated about the importance of combining therapeutic approaches (e.g., dietary changes plus increased physical activity, even if pharmaceutical or surgical approaches are utilized). Sustaining weight loss requires behavioral changes, and patients should plan out their weight-loss strategy in writing. The plan should include dietary modifications, a physical activity routine, and behavioral strategies. A calendar should be developed outlining the schedule. If lapses in the plan are experienced, the patient should explore the reasons for the lapse. The primary-care practitioner should review the plan and schedule outline at each visit.

Adequate social support is a key element to successful weight loss. Patients who feel "sabotaged" or undermined by family members who do not support the same type of effective weight loss behaviors as the patient (especially home-based dietary practices) will need to explore methods for support outside of the family. Patients typically benefit from weight-loss support groups, and the primary-care practitioner can use online resources to find a support group in the patient's geographic area. Finding a walking partner and initiating a walking program immediately after work before returning home are strategies that can be suggested.

GOUT

Gout is a metabolic disease that produces an inflammatory arthritis. Gout was characterized as far back as the time of Hippocrates and has been referred to as "the disease of kings" because of its prevalence in the wealthy, who were able to afford the traditionally expensive, purine-rich foods that typically trigger this disorder. Once a disabling chronic disease, current medical diagnostics and treatment modalities have decreased its disabling effects.

EPIDEMIOLOGY AND CAUSES

Persons from the United States, the Pacific Islands, and countries with abundant lifestyles have an increased incidence of gout. In the United States, gout affects 8.3 million adults. Gout rarely occurs in children, premenopausal women, or men younger than 30 years of age. Seventy percent of people with gout are men, with a peak incidence between 40 and 50 years of age. The increased incidence of gout in older adults has been associated with an increased use of diuretics. Twenty percent of patients who present with gout have a family history of the disease. Gout is more prevalent in African American men, possibly because of the increased prevalence of hypertension in this group.

Hyperuricemia (i.e., uric acid levels exceeding 7 mg/dL in men and 6 mg/dL in women) occurs in 5% to 10% of the U.S. population. Most of these adults, however, are asymptomatic. One in five persons with hyperuricemia will develop urate deposits in a joint, soft tissues, or cartilage. Patients with gout may experience an acute attack with rapid fluctuations of serum urate levels. Surgery, dehydration, binge alcohol consumption, emotional stress, infections, diuretics, and uricosuric drugs can all cause rapid fluctuations in serum urate levels.

Predisposing risk factors for the development of gout are listed in Risk Factors: Gout. Causes of primary gout include idiopathic inborn errors of purine metabolism, decreased renal clearance of uric acid, and specific enzymatic defects such as those resulting in Lesch-Nyhan syndrome and glycogen storage disease. Secondary causes of gout include other disease processes and medications, such as thiazide diuretics, that result in an overproduction or underexcretion of uric acid.

PATHOPHYSIOLOGY

Overproduction and/or underexcretion of uric acid with tissue deposition of monosodium urate crystals is the metabolic disorder underlying gout. Most individuals (90%) with gout have inappropriate underexcretion of uric acid. At the time of puberty, serum uric acid levels are known to increase in males; however, most (90%–95%) men remain asymptomatic throughout life. In addition, estrogen is believed to be protective from hyperuricemia in women.

Gout is a direct result of hyperuricemia (high serum uric acid) and the increased saturation of urate in the plasma and other bodily fluids. Supersaturation of bodily fluids results in a precipitation of monosodium urate crystals out of bodily fluids and into the joints, soft tissues, and cartilage. This leads to the symptoms and clinical findings of gout, as the deposition and crystallization of urate in the joints trigger an inflammatory response. Thus, the arthritis produced by gout is characterized by recurrent, painful attacks of monoarticular joint inflammation caused by the phagocytosis of urate crystals, which deposit in joints, soft tissues, and cartilage.

Risk Factors: Gout

Primary Risk Factors

- Decreased renal clearance of uric acid
- Enzyme defects (Lesch-Nyhan syndrome, glycogen storage diseases)

Secondary Risk Factors

- Excessive (daily) intake of purine-rich foods
- Obesity
- Starvation
- Dehydration
- Alcohol abuse
- Medications: thiazide diuretics, ethambutol, nicotinic acid, pyrazinamide, low-dose salicylates, cyclosporine

- Paget's disease
- Chronic hemolytic anemia
- Psoriasis
- Cytotoxic drugs
- Sarcoma and other carcinomas
- Chronic renal disease
- Hypothyroidism
- Lead poisoning
- Hyperparathyroidism
- Diabetes insipidus
- Diabetic ketoacidosis

Several mechanisms may trigger an acute attack of gout, the most common being trauma or surgery. Gout attacks may also be paradoxically triggered by prophylactic or uricosuric agents, which are known to lower serum uric acid levels. Acute attacks are also more likely to occur at lower serum uric acid levels in persons with alcoholism due to decreased urinary excretion. There is also an increased incidence of hypothyroidism in persons with

crystal aspirates in synovial fluid. Of note, although gout is frequently cited as a risk factor for the development of CAD, subsequent studies did not confirm these initial findings from the Framingham Heart Study that raised concerns.

Gouty arthritis may extend to several joints and is classified into four stages based on timing and clinical presentation (see Table 59.2): asymptomatic, acute phase, intercritical, and chronic tophaceous. For unclear reasons, gouty arthritis has a predilection for the first metatarsophalangeal joint (the great toe)—a condition known as podagra. This may result from the relative coolness of this peripheral joint that allows for greater crystal deposition, the constant microtrauma to which this joint is subjected, and the differential impact that weight-bearing alternating with recumbency has on the resorption of joint fluid and intra-articular urate.

In general, urate crystallization is more likely to occur at lower temperatures. Noninflamed synovial fluid in the knee is significantly cooler (90–91°F [32.2–32.78°C]) than core body temperature. Thus, although a serum uric acid concentration of 7 mg/dL appears to be the threshold level above which gout is more likely to

TABLE 59.2 Stages of Gout			
Stage	*Subjective Findings*	*Objective Findings*	*Diagnostic Findings*
I. Asymptomatic	None	None	Microtophaceous deposits of urate in joints and bursae
II. Acute phase (inflammatory phase)	Extremely painful monoarticular or polyarticular attack Pruritus and desquamation of the skin surrounding affected joints as the inflammation subsides	Affected joints are red, warm, and swollen Early acute attack subsides within a few days, but may last up to 2 weeks, as inflammation gradually subsides 10% of patients experience only one acute attack during their lifetime	Elevated WBC count Elevated temperature Elevated serum uric acid or normouricemia
III. Intercritical (interval between acute attacks)	None; patient is asymptomatic	Duration of intervals between attacks decreases as the disease progresses. If a second acute attack occurs, it usually presents within the first year after the initial attack	Microtophaceous deposits of urate in joints and bursae Serum urate levels should be below 6 mg/dL if adequately treated
IV. Chronic tophaceous (results from recurrent attacks with multiple sites of urate deposits [tophi] in articular and periarticular tissue)	May restrict movement of affected joints Chronic pain, stiffness, decreased joint function, joint derangement, and secondary joint degeneration affecting the upper and lower extremities	More than 50% of patients progress to this stage within 20 years of the initial attack if not properly managed Occasionally, tophus ulceration and erosion with chalk-textured drainage observed Uric acid kidney stones in 5%–10% of patients	Tophi

develop, crystallization may be more likely to occur at lower urate concentrations intra-articularly. In addition, hyperuricemia alone is insufficient to lead to crystallization. As part of the inflammatory process, urate-specific immunoglobulin (Ig) molecules coat monosodium urate crystals in gouty synovial fluid, likely serving as a promoter of nucleation for urate crystal formation.

As gout progresses, crystals are deposited into multiple bodily tissues. In severe cases with repeated attacks, monosodium urate monohydrate crystals form into a nodular deposit known as a *tophus,* surrounded by granulomatous inflammation consisting of monocytes and giant cells. In addition to the skin and joints, *tophaceous* swellings may be found in a number of bodily tissues, including the heart valves, kidneys, and larynx, capable of leading to significant pathology. Microtophi, consisting of collections of urate crystals surrounded only by a thin fibrocytic ring, may also be present in gouty synovial fluid. Some research has suggested that these microtophi release their urate crystals into the joint fluid after the initiation of synovial inflammation in the early stages of a gout attack.

Urate crystals induce intra-articular inflammation via a number of mechanisms. Synovial lining cells, monocytes, and endothelial cells have all been shown to phagocytose urate crystals in vitro and subsequently increase their production of inflammatory mediators via transcriptional upregulation and mRNA stabilization, including interleukin (IL)-1, IL-6, IL-8, and TNF-α. Blockade of IL-8 and TNF activity has been further shown to counter urate-induced inflammation.

Neutrophilic migration into affected joints and their subsequent phagocytosis of urate crystals appears to play a central role in the pathogenesis of gouty arthritis. Neutrophils undergo an oxidative burst during this process, releasing lysosomal enzymes, superoxide anions, leukotriene B4, and IL-1, among other inflammatory mediators. Indeed, the complexities of neutrophilic chemotaxis and function within gouty joints have been a central focus of gout research. Studies have indicated tyrosine kinases, phospholipases, adhesion molecules such as E-selectin, and several chemotactic factors play key roles in neutrophilic recruitment and activation by urate crystals. This explains the efficacy of colchicine in treating acute attacks, because it inhibits neutrophil tyrosine kinase activity in response to both gout and pseudogout crystals, as well as downregulates the activity of adhesion molecules on both neutrophils and endothelial cells.

A number of proteins interact with urate crystals to increase their pro-inflammatory properties. For example, immunoglobulins bound to urate crystals lead to a greater release of lysosomal and superoxide enzymes by neutrophils. The complement and kinin systems have also been implicated in urate crystal pathology, but they are not requisite for acute gouty inflammation. Although acute attacks of gout typically resolve spontaneously within several weeks, if left untreated or if inadequately treated, gout leads to chronic arthritis and bony erosions within 5 to 10 years, resulting in joint deformities and ultimately restricting function.

The self-limited nature of an acute gout attack involves several mechanisms. Neutrophil mediators have been shown to cleave Ig molecules from urate crystals to reduce their inflammatory nature. The inflammatory properties of tophaceous urate crystals are also reduced after protease treatment in vitro. Lipoproteins (specifically apolipoprotein B) reduce the inflammatory potential of urate crystals after binding, indicating that they may be involved in the self-limited resolution of acute attacks. In addition to the deactivation and death of inflammatory cells and the inactivation of secreted pro-inflammatory mediators, leukocytes, monocytes, and macrophages have been shown in vitro to alter their cytokine transcriptional activity over time. In turn, they secrete several anti-inflammatory cytokines upon resolution of an acute gout attack, including IL-1 receptor antagonist, transforming growth factor–β, and peroxisome-proliferator-activated receptor–γ.

CLINICAL PRESENTATION

Subjective

A thorough evaluation of the onset, characteristics, and potentiating causes of gouty joint pain is completed on initial evaluation. The patient will present during an acute attack with pain, tenderness, erythema, and swelling of the affected joints. The usual presentation is monoarticular, and the joint most frequently affected is the first metatarsophalangeal joint of the great (big) toe; however, the midfoot, knees, fingers, wrists, and elbows may also be affected. The typical presentation is excruciating pain that awakens the patient at night. Patients often describe the pain as throbbing, crushing, and pulsating. The pain is not relieved by rest or positional changes and prevents weight-bearing on the affected limb. Often the patient cannot tolerate anything coming in contact with the affected joint—even bed clothing touching the limb can be extremely painful.

The patient's past medical history, including any joint or musculoskeletal trauma, should be reviewed, along with any family history of gout. The patient may also report an episode of recent trauma to the affected joint, a recent drinking binge, or an eating binge of gout-triggering foods before the acute attack. Patients may report a recent operation or severe illness, especially one producing a shift in fluid balance. Because gout is more prevalent in patients with hypertension, obesity, and hyperlipidemia, history-taking should focus on these contributing factors. In addition, a drug history, specific for recent increased intake of aspirin or cyclosporine, should also be obtained.

Objective

Even though, typically, a patient with gout initially presents with monoarticular joint complaints, a complete bilateral examination of all joints should be performed.

Bilateral joints should be assessed for symmetry in appearance and range of motion. Asymmetrical presentation of joint inflammation, redness, tenderness, and limitations in range of motion are typical of gout. On physical examination, the affected area is warm or hot to the touch. The patient will complain of pain on palpation, and range of motion will be limited. Skin overlying the affected area is often red and taut. Several days after an acute attack, desquamation over affected joints may be evident.

The joint most frequently affected in the initial attack of gout is the first metatarsophalangeal joint, known as podagra. The manifestation of podagra is experienced by approximately 90% of patients with gout. Subsequent attacks may progress to include several joints (polyarticular disease). Other joints that are frequently affected include the instep of the ankle, the heels, knees, wrists, fingers, and elbows. Peripheral joints are more likely to be involved because central joints are warmer and less conducive to crystal formations. In polyarticular episodes or if a large joint is involved, the patient may have an elevated temperature, tachycardia, anorexia, malaise, headache, and/or chills.

Patients who have progressed to the chronic tophaceous stage of gout will have palpable tophi. *Tophi* are nodular deposits of monosodium urate monohydrate crystals that initiate the inflammatory process. Most tophi are firm and movable, whereas the overlying skin is thin and red. Tophi are most likely to develop on the pinnae of the ears, olecranon tips, and the distal interphalangeal joints of the hands and feet. Extensive tissue deposits of urate may also occur on the helix and antihelix of the ear, the eyelids, the sclera, and cornea.

DIAGNOSTIC REASONING

Diagnostic Tests

The clinical presentation and medical history findings are often sufficient to diagnose gout. Serum uric acid levels and radiographic imaging may provide supportive evidence; however, a definitive diagnosis is only made with identification of sodium urate crystals in the aspirated fluid from affected joints.

Initial Testing

Initial testing for gout includes a serum uric acid level. Most patients will have an elevated serum urate level in the absence of elevated blood urea nitrogen because serum urate is above 7.5 mg/dL in up to 95% of persons with gout. However, some studies have suggested that serum urate levels may be normal in up to 15% of patients at the time of an acute gout attack. Thus, elevated serum urate levels are not diagnostic of gout in the absence of characteristic joint signs and symptoms, and the clinician should look for other supportive laboratory findings. The erythrocyte sedimentation rate and white blood cell (WBC) count may also be elevated during an acute attack. The WBC count is typically greater than 10,000 cells/mcL, but values up to 100,000 cells/mcL may occasionally be observed.

The classic radiographic findings of gout are tophi, normal mineralization of bone, joint space preservation without narrowing, an asymmetrical polyarticular distribution, an overhanging edge cortex, and punched-out erosions of bone. However, radiographs of affected joints may show no changes in early stages of disease. The only radiographic evidence of gout in its early stages may be asymmetrical soft-tissue swelling. With recurrent attacks and progressive disease, however, radiolucent urate tophi and punched-out appearing areas become apparent in bone. Tophi appear as cloudlike increases in density, which may show signs of calcification. Urate crystals may also be seen in subcutaneous tissue, cartilage, joints, and other tissues. In the very late stages of gout, demineralization and loss of articular structures may be apparent on radiographic examination. Most changes are asymmetrical and occur predominantly in the feet, ankles, and knees. Patients with severe disease often have involvement of the hands and elbows as well.

Subsequent Testing

The definitive test to confirm the diagnosis of acute gout is microscopic observation of urate crystals in aspirated joint fluid. The synovial fluid will be turbid during an acute attack, and needle-shaped uric acid crystals are identified as strongly negatively birefringent when examined by compensated polariscopic examination of wet smears of aspirated joint fluid. This means that when examined with a polarizing filter and red compensator filter, uric acid crystals appear yellow when aligned in parallel to the slow axis of the red compensator and blue when aligned perpendicularly to the direction of polarization. Of note, patients who present with gout and comorbid symptoms of abdominal pain, peripheral neuropathy, and proteinuria should be assessed for lead exposure, as hyperuricemia has been associated with acute exposure to high lead levels.

Differential Diagnosis

Differential diagnoses for gout include other arthritides and infectious musculoskeletal and skin conditions, including septic arthritis, rheumatoid arthritis, psoriatic arthritis, bursitis, fracture, cellulitis, acute joint trauma, pseudogout (i.e., joint inflammation due to calcium pyrophosphate crystal deposition), and reactive arthritis (a postinfectious forms of arthritis previously known as Reiter's syndrome).

Septic arthritis should be considered when a patient presents with joint pain, swelling, and erythema. Septic arthritis occasionally coexists with gout and should also be strongly considered when a patient does not respond to initial management for gout. Septic arthritis more commonly occurs in larger joints. Gram stains and cultures of synovial fluids are positive for bacteria in septic arthritis, and patients often present with fever and chills.

Radiographic examination often reveals joint-space narrowing and erosions within 1 to 2 weeks of the onset of septic arthritis.

A rheumatoid factor titer may help rule out rheumatoid arthritis, as either rheumatoid factor or antibodies against citrullinated cyclic peptides are more likely to be positive in rheumatoid arthritis than gout. Clinically, rheumatoid arthritis may resemble gout, but it typically has a symmetrical joint presentation, including clinical signs, symptoms, and radiographic findings. Joint-space narrowing is also typical of rheumatoid joint disease but not in gout. Psoriatic arthritis may resemble gout in its early stages; however, the initial joints affected are frequently in the hands, feet, sacroiliac and spinal joints. Fusiform soft-tissue swelling is typical of psoriatic arthritis, and early joint-space narrowing is also common as a differentiating trait from gout.

Pseudogout is an inflammatory joint pathology that presents with many similar characteristics to gout. However, polarized microscopic examination of joint fluid aspirate reveals rhomboid-shaped calcium pyrophosphate dihydrate crystals that are weakly positively birefringent, rather than the strongly negatively birefringent needle-shaped uric acid crystals associated with gout. Thus, the calcium pyrophosphate crystals of pseudogout appear blue when aligned in parallel to the slow axis of the red compensator and yellow when aligned perpendicularly to the axis of polarization. Pseudogout usually presents at a later age, and the symptoms are characteristically less acute and less severe than gout. Pseudogout is polyarticular in approximately 75% of patients and typically affects the knees and larger joints. Pseudogout is associated with hyperthyroidism and hypothyroidism, hypomagnesemia, amyloidosis, hypercalcemia, hypophosphatemia, and hemosiderosis.

The development of an inflamed joint in a young man or woman following a GI (e.g., *Campylobacter, Salmonella, Shigella*) or genitourinary (e.g., *Chlamydia trachomatis*) infection would raise suspicion for reactive arthritis. In its typical presentation, this form of autoimmune joint inflammation is accompanied by conjunctivitis and noninfectious urethritis, comprising the classic triad of reactive arthritis.

MANAGEMENT

The goals of clinical management are to terminate an acute attack, prevent future attacks, normalize hyperuricemia, and prevent potential complications of urate deposits. Management of gout includes pharmacological treatment of acute attacks and long-term medical and pharmacological treatment of hyperuricemia. Acute management of gout includes generalized rest, elevation and immobilization of affected joints, and pharmacological treatment. Prevention of disability due to gout is a reality today because of advances in pharmacological treatment; however, the patient must

become an active participant in the long-term treatment plan (Table 59.3).

Initial Management

Pharmacological treatment for an acute attack includes NSAIDs, colchicine (if the onset of symptoms is less than 36 hours), and corticosteroids.

Nonsteroidal Anti-inflammatory Drugs

The initial medication of choice for acute gout attacks is an NSAID. Traditionally, indomethacin (Indocin) has been the most commonly prescribed NSAID for an acute attack of gout, but other NSAIDs are just as effective. Indomethacin 25 to 50 mg every 8 hours is given until symptoms subside, usually for 5 to 10 days. An effective alternative to indomethacin is naproxen (Naprosyn). The first dose of naproxen is 750 mg, followed by 250 mg every 8 hours for 5 to 10 days. NSAIDs are discontinued after the pain has dissipated.

Contraindications to the use of NSAIDs include active peptic ulcer disease, impaired renal function, and allergic reactions to NSAIDs. Potential adverse reactions of NSAIDs include GI bleeding, nausea, rash, hypertension (especially in the elderly), hepatic impairment, fluid retention, and acute tubular necrosis with subsequent acute renal insufficiency (particularly at high doses or with chronic use).

TABLE 59.3	Management of Gout
Acute attack	NSAIDs (avoid aspirin, given unpredictable effects on serum uric acid levels) Colchicine Corticosteroids Rest
If no further attacks develop	Avoid excessive alcohol consumption Dietary modification to avoid purine-rich foods (total elimination is not necessary)
If an additional acute attack develops	NSAIDs Colchicine Corticosteroids Rest Avoid alcohol and binge eating Low-purine diet
If two or more additional attacks develop	Uric acid secretion <1,000 mg/ 24 hr: probenecid Uric acid secretion >1,000 mg/ 24 hr: allopurinol Dietary modification to avoid purine-rich foods Lifestyle modification Colchicine

Colchicine

Colchicine is an effective medication to terminate an acute attack of gout if administered within 36 hours of the initial onset of symptoms. If administered within this time frame, it is effective in 90% of all patients. Colchicine can be administered orally or IV. The IV route is rarely used due to its low therapeutic index (i.e., benefit vs. toxicity ratio). In acute attacks, 1 to 1.2 mg of oral colchicine should be administered at the first sign of an attack, followed by 0.5 to 0.6 mg every hour or 1 to 1.2 mg every 2 hours until the pain is relieved. The cumulative dose of colchicine should not exceed 4 to 6 mg during one course of treatment for an acute attack.

Adverse reactions include nausea, vomiting, diarrhea, abdominal pain, and cramping; these side effects are more pronounced at higher doses. Colchicine usually provides relief within 18 hours; however, many patients will experience diarrhea or nausea within 24 hours of the first dose. Colchicine is contraindicated in patients with a hypersensitivity to colchicine, blood dyscrasias, and severe cardiovascular, renal, or GI disease. Patients with renal or hepatic disease require a decreased total dose. In addition, colchicine must be used with caution in older adults.

Corticosteroids

Corticosteroids can provide dramatic systematic relief and can be administered orally, intramuscularly, or intra-articularly. In most cases, corticosteroids are reserved for refractory cases or cases where the use of colchicine and NSAIDs is contraindicated. Corticosteroids are contraindicated in septic conditions; therefore, they should not be administered before analysis of the synovial aspirate to assess for bacteria or other signs of infection. For polyarticular gout, prednisone 40 to 60 mg orally taken daily usually produces a good response. The dose should be tapered quickly over 5 to 7 days. Patients with mono-articular disease who cannot tolerate oral corticosteroids or NSAIDs may benefit from intra-articular steroid injection, which is typically given as triamcinolone 10 to 40 mg, depending on the size of the affected joint.

Subsequent Management

The long-term management of gout includes pharmacological agents, dietary modifications, activity evaluation, and education regarding the prevention of gout. Patients with extensive or large tophi may benefit from surgical excision of these lesions.

Pharmacological Management

Pharmacological prophylaxis should be initiated after the second or third attack. In patients with hyperuricemia and a history of only one acute attack, lifestyle modifications may prevent further attacks. Alternatives to thiazide diuretics, which can precipitate gout, should be considered. Pharmacological prophylaxis should be considered in patients with polyarticular gout and patients with consistent hyperuricemia greater than 8 mg/dL. Colchicine and NSAIDs may be continued in lower doses for up to 12 months after an acute attack.

Colchicine is often used to prevent further acute attacks triggered by changes in uric acid levels; however, colchicine does not correct the underlying causes of an acute attack. In addition, adverse effects of long-term colchicine use include bone marrow suppression, peripheral neuritis, and GI symptoms, especially diarrhea. The dosage of colchicine for long-term preventive management ranges from 0.5 to 1.2 mg daily. Colchicine is also often used to prevent acute attacks of gout that may be precipitated by the initiation of urate-lowering medications (e.g., probenecid, allopurinol), due to the rapid decrease in serum urate levels that can precipitate intra-articular uric acid crystallization. Before scheduled surgery, colchicine 0.5 to 0.6 mg orally three times daily for 3 days before and 3 days after surgery can be used to prevent acute attacks of gout precipitated by surgical trauma.

Three classes of agents are currently available to lower uric acid levels. Probenecid (Benemid) is a uricosuric agent that blocks tubular reabsorption of filtered urate; allopurinol (Zyloprim) and febuxostat (Uloric) are xanthine oxidase inhibitors that lower plasma urate and urinary uric acid levels; and the intravenous agent pegloticase (Krystexxa) is a uricase that is used to treat high serum uric acid levels that are refractory to other treatments. These should not be started during or within 1 month after an acute attack. Before initiation, a 24-hour urinary uric acid excretion test should be performed to differentiate between patients who are hypersecretors versus hyposecretors, because pharmacological management of the two conditions differs. Uric acid excretion greater than 1,000 mg in 24 hours is abnormal, and levels between 800 and 1,000 mg in 24 hours are considered to be borderline.

Probenecid is indicated in patients whose urinary uric acid excretion is below 700 to 800 mg in 24 hours. It is the drug of choice in persons younger than 60 years of age without a history of blood dyscrasias, renal failure, or kidney stones. An initial daily dosage of 500 mg (250 mg twice daily) is recommended, increasing gradually to 1 to 2 g after 1 week. Dosage is increased based on uric acid levels, to a maximum dose of 2 g daily. Major adverse reactions of this drug include skin rash, uric acid stones, and GI upset. It may also precipitate an exacerbation of gout if it produces rapid shifts in uric acid levels. Probenecid inhibits the excretion of penicillin, indomethacin (Indocin), and acetazolamide (Diamox).

Allopurinol (Zyloprim) is used to decrease uric acid production in patients who are unable to take probenecid. It is indicated in patients whose 24-hour uric acid secretion is greater than 1,000 mg. The initial dose is 100 to 200 mg daily, with the average daily dose ranging from 200 to 300 mg. Dosages of 400 to 600 mg daily are indicated only in severe gout. The maximum daily dose is 800 mg. The goal of therapy is to decrease the serum uric acid levels below 6 mg/dL. Dosage should be adjusted based on serum uric acid levels every 2 to 6 months. Adverse reactions include GI upset, headache, rash, bone marrow suppression, fever, liver or kidney failure, vasculitis, lymphadenopathy, hepatitis, alopecia, and dermatitis. It is contraindicated in persons with idiopathic hemochromatosis and renal and hepatic disease, and the safety of its use in pregnant or lactating women has not been established. Serious hypersensitivity reactions to allopurinol may occur but are rare. However, patients should be cautioned to discontinue use and immediately report any rash or fever that occurs after starting the drug. Twenty percent of patients on both allopurinol and ampicillin develop a rash.

Febuxostat (Uloric) is also used to lower serum uric acid levels by blocking uric acid production through the inhibition of the xanthine oxidase enzyme. The dosage is 40 to 80 mg daily to achieve a serum uric acid level of 6 mg/dL or lower. Serious adverse reactions may occur including hypersensitivity, rhabdomyolysis, interstitial nephritis, stroke, and myocardial infarction.

Pegloticase (Krystexxa) is a recombinant uricase enzyme that catalyzes the oxidation of uric acid to allantoin, thereby lowering serum uric acid levels. The optimal dose is 8 mg IV given every 2 weeks. If serum uric acid levels increase above 6 mg/dL while on treatment, discontinuation of the treatment should be considered. Given the risk of severe hypersensitivity, including anaphylaxis, pegloticase should be administered following premedication with corticosteroids and antihistamines. Its use is contraindicated in glucose-6-phoshate dehydrogenase deficiency, given the increased risk of hemolysis and methemoglobinemia.

Dietary Modifications

Dietary modifications include avoiding purine-rich foods, maintaining adequate fluid intake, and moderating alcohol intake. Complete dietary restriction of purine-containing foods has not proven effective; therefore, a moderation of purine in the diet, but not complete restriction, is recommended. Foods high in purine content are listed in Box 59.3. Fluid intake should be sufficient to maintain an output of 2,000 mL/day. Patients should force fluids to exceed 3,000 mL/day, especially if they are prescribed a uricosuric agent to facilitate urinary excretion.

Box 59.3   Foods High in Purines

- All meats and seafoods (especially organ meats such as liver, kidneys, and sweetbreads [thymus, pancreas])
- Meat extracts and gravies
- Yeast and yeast extracts (brewer's and baker's)
- Beer and alcoholic beverages
- Beans, peas, lentils, oatmeal, spinach, asparagus, cauliflower, and mushrooms
- Mussels and scallops
- Anchovies, herring, and sardines
- Trout, haddock, mackerel, and tuna

Lifestyle Modifications

Physical activity must be restricted during an acute gout attack, and bedrest should be maintained for 24 hours following an acute attack. The joint should be immobilized; if a lower extremity is involved, no weight-bearing should be allowed during the acute attack. During intercritical periods, physical therapy may be indicated to maintain or improve function. Hot compresses may promote comfort after an acute attack but should not be instituted until the acute pain subsides, usually 24 to 72 hours after the initiation of therapy. The patient should apply heat for 20 minutes two to three times daily through the use of moist heating pads, warm showers and baths, or moist towels heated in a microwave. Relief may also be obtained using ice packs during an acute attack. Patients should be instructed to apply packs for only 10 to 20 minutes sessions at a time to avoid thermal damage to the skin; ice packs should be discontinued if pain is not relieved. Long-term management includes dietary moderation of purine-containing foods (limited to no more than one to two servings of purine-rich foods per day), moderating alcohol intake, maintaining weight, and sufficient physical activity to maintain joint mobility during quiescent periods between gout flares.

FOLLOW-UP AND REFERRAL

The patient should be evaluated 1 to 2 weeks after an acute attack. If antihyperuricemia therapy is initiated, the patient needs to be followed every 4 to 6 weeks to adjust medications and review the goals of treatment. For long-term management, annual follow-up is recommended. Special attention is given to previously affected joints, as to their range of motion and stability. Joints should be symmetrically evaluated for tophi. Annual serum uric acid levels are indicated in all patients, and evaluation of renal function is indicated for patients on prophylactic antihyperuricemic therapy.

An evaluation of the patient's diet (including specific questions about alcohol intake) and physical activity should be conducted during the annual exam. Reinforcement of previous education is essential to increase adherence to medication and physical activity regimens during intercritical periods. Patients who are overweight will need continued reinforcement to lose weight and reduce stress on weight-bearing joints. Patients younger than 35 years of age, premenopausal women, patients with frequent acute attacks despite prophylactic treatment, and patients with renal insufficiency should be referred to a rheumatologist for an initial evaluation. Some patients may benefit from a physical therapist's exercise prescription or evaluation by a podiatrist for joint disease primarily affecting the feet. In addition, patients with extensive or large tophi may require surgical referral for possible excision of cosmetically troublesome lesions or especially tophi that interfere with joint function.

Patient Education: Gout

Patients need instructions on the avoidance of triggers for acute gout attacks. Excessive exercise, trauma, dehydration, and alcohol or eating binges may precipitate an acute attack. Patients need explicit information on the potential adverse reactions of their medication regimens (as well as the propensity for some medications, such as thiazide diuretics, to trigger acute attacks) and measures to allay potentially preventable adverse effects.

Fluid intake should exceed 2,000 mL daily to prevent the formation of uric acid kidney stones and to avoid dehydration, which may precipitate an acute attack. Dietary modifications must be reviewed with patients in detail, and written information should be provided on foods to avoid. Because both wine and alcoholic spirits in excessive amounts impair the kidney's ability to excrete uric acid, they should be consumed only in moderation (patients must be made aware that binge drinking may provoke an acute attack). If the patient is obese, weight loss should be encouraged because loss of excess body fat may normalize serum uric acid levels without pharmacological intervention. However, caution against extreme or rapid weight loss should be given because secondary hyperuricemia may result. A very low calorie diet may also precipitate an acute attack.

Importantly, weight loss will also decrease stress on weight-bearing joints, thus reducing pathological joint damage due to gout. Good posture and protection of weight-bearing joints are essential. Because the feet are most frequently affected, the patient should wear supportive and properly fitting shoes. At the first signs of an acute attack, the patient should limit all activity, limit weight-bearing if appropriate, and contact the primary-care practitioner for guidance on acute intervention. Patients may need to take colchicine before having elective surgery if they are not already taking it regularly. These patients should also be instructed to avoid aspirin, given that it may increase or decrease uric acid levels in the blood.

 For additional resources please visit
https://davisedge.fadavis.com/

REFERENCES

Gout

Khanna PP, FitzGerald J. Evolution of management of gout: A comparison of recent guidelines. *Curr Opin Rheumatol.* 2015;27(2):139–146.

Stewart S, Dalbeth N, Rome K. The impact of gout on the foot: A review. *Gout Hyperuricemia.* 2016;3(1):1–8. https://www.researchgate.net/profile/Sarah_Stewart13/publication/298352850_The_impact_of_gout_on_the_foot_a_review/links/56e8736b08aec65cb45ec6fd.pdf. Accessed November 4, 2017.

Obesity

Centers for Disease Control and Prevention. Defining adult overweight and obesity. https://www.cdc.gov/obesity/adult/defining.html. Updated June 16, 2016. Accessed October 30, 2017.

Centers for Disease Control and Prevention. Adult obesity facts. https://www.cdc.gov/obesity/data/adult.html. Updated August 2017. Accessed October 31, 2017.

Centers for Disease Control and Prevention. Disability and obesity. https://www.cdc.gov/ncbddd/disabilityandhealth/obesity.html. Updated August 1, 2017. Accessed November 1, 2017.

Centers for Disease Control and Prevention. Adult obesity causes & consequences. https://www.cdc.gov/obesity/adult/causes.html. Updated August 29, 2017. Accessed October 30, 2017.

Garvey WT, Mechanick JI, Brett EM, et al. American Association of Clinical Endocrinologists and American College of Endocrinology comprehensive clinical practice guidelines for medical care of patients with obesity. *Endocr Pract.* 2016;22(suppl 3):1–203.

Gerard P. Gut microbiota and obesity. *Cell Mol Life Sci.* 2016;73:147–162.

Kalish VB. Obesity in older adults. *Prim Care.* 2016;43(1):137–144.

Ladenheim EE. Liraglutide and obesity: A review of the data so far. *Drug Des Devel Ther.* 2015;9:1867–1875.

Marchesi JR, Adams DH, Fava F, et al. The gut microbiota and host health: A new clinical frontier. *Gut.* 2016;65(2):330–339.

National Heart, Lung, and Blood Institute, National Institutes of Health. Physical activity. https://www.nhlbi.nih.gov/health/health-topics/topics/heart-healthy-lifestyle-changes/physical-activity. Updated June 22, 2016. Accessed November 4, 2017.

National Institute of Diabetes and Digestive and Kidney Diseases, National Institutes of Health. Overweight & obesity statistics. https://www.niddk.nih.gov/health-information/health-statistics/overweight-obesity. Updated August 2017. Accessed October 31, 2017.

Rodriguez JE. Past, present, and future of pharmacologic therapy in obesity. *Prim Care.* 2016;43(1):61–67.

Schwartz J. Nutritional therapy. *Prim Care.* 2016;43(1):97–107.

Smith KB, Smith MS. Obesity statistics. *Prim Care.* 2016;43(1):121–135.

Spieker EA, Pyzocha N. Economic impact of obesity. *Prim Care.* 2016;43(1):83–95.

Van Dijk SJ, Tellam RL, Morrison JL, et al. Recent developments on the role of epigenetics in obesity and metabolic disease. *Clin Epigenetics.* 2016;7(66):1–13. https://clinicalepigeneticsjournal.biomedcentral.com/articles/10.1186/s13148-015-0101-5. Accessed November 2, 2017.

Waleh MQ. Impacts of physical activity on the obese. *Prim Care.* 2016;43(1):97–107.

World Health Organization. *Obesity and overweight.* http://www.who.int/mediacentre/factsheets/fs311/en/. Updated October 2017. Accessed November 1, 2017.

RESOURCES

Gout

Arthritis Foundation
www.arthritis.org

National Institute of Arthritis and Musculoskeletal Disorders
www.niams.nih.gov

Obesity

American Society of Bariatric Physicians
www.asbp.org

Overeaters Anonymous
www.oa.org

Obesity Society
www.obesity.org

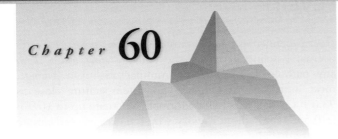

Chapter **60**

Common Hematological and Immunological Complaints

Jacinta D. Elder, MD, MSc

Jill E. Winland-Brown, EdD, APRN, FNP-BC

Brian Oscar Porter, MD, PhD, MPH, MBA

BRUISING

A *bruise* (ecchymosis) is an integumentary manifestation of extravasated blood. Discoloration of the skin is attributed to a local interstitial pool of erythrocytes, which causes a light to dark blue skin color associated with red pigment. The bruise sets off a local inflammatory event that includes macrophage invasion and histamine release, which may be associated with edema. Macrophages engulf red blood cells (RBCs) to clear the area of extravasated blood.

Macrophages that contain the RBCs excrete hemosiderin and hematoidin. Hemosiderin is brown, and hematoidin is yellow. The release of these molecules from macrophages accounts for the characteristic color changes of bruises during their resolution. In general, the initial redness of a bruise transitions into a blue or purple hue in 1 to 2 days and may even darken to a black color several days later. Following this, a color change to green occurs approximately one week after the initial onset of the bruise, and then a yellowish-brown appearance, which gradually fades over time. Hematomas (larger bruises resulting from collections of blood that pool under the skin) require lengthier periods of time to resolve than smaller bruises.

Bruising may result from blunt trauma or occur spontaneously in the absence of trauma. Thrombocytopenia (platelet counts below 50,000 cells/mL) predisposes an individual to bruise formation with minor trauma, given the integral role of platelets in the formation of blood clots. Spontaneous bruising may be seen with platelet counts below 30,000 cells/mL, particularly on the arms and legs. Spontaneous bruising may also be associated with the chronic use of corticosteroid or anticoagulant therapies. Corticosteroids weaken the vascular walls, making them prone to release erythrocytes. Anticoagulants, when their levels exceed the therapeutic range, can permit microvascular ruptures to spill blood into interstitial spaces.

One of the most common forms of anticoagulant therapy consists of warfarin (Coumadin) in oral dosages that are intended to keep the international normalized ratio (INR) between 2.0 and 3.0 for most disease-related prophylaxis, such as the prevention of valvular thrombus in atrial fibrillation. Although dosing guidelines must be individualized for each patient, initial dosing of warfarin is typically 2 to 5 mg per day for 3 days, followed by measurement of prothrombin time (PT) and INR. This initial loading dose starts the process of anticoagulation. Dosages thereafter range from 2 to 7.5 mg daily, although dosages can be higher than 10 mg if the INR dictates. Excessive dosing of warfarin or other anticoagulants may lead to easy bruising as one of the most obvious clinical signs of overdose. If the INR is above the therapeutic target, the clinician should consider withholding one or more days of anticoagulant therapy and possibly starting reversal therapy with vitamin K if active bleeding is present. PT and INR should be reevaluated within 3 to 5 days of the dosage adjustment, and treatment should be restarted at a lower dose after a hiatus of therapy.

DIFFERENTIAL DIAGNOSIS

Unexplained or suspicious bruising may be the primary-care practitioner's first clue to an underlying medical condition or to physically dangerous circumstances in a patient's life. A thorough history and physical examination by the clinician should focus on the cause of the bruising and distinguish between extrinsic versus intrinsic causes. The differential diagnoses of the causes of bruising include chronic use of corticosteroid and anticoagulant therapies, thrombocytopenia, hemolytic anemia, domestic violence, self-inflicted injury or other blunt trauma, and hypersensitivity vasculitis.

955

FATIGUE

Fatigue presents as a complaint of tiredness that cannot be explained on the basis of exercise or other activity. It may be either acute or chronic, associated with a disease or independent of other pathophysiology.

Acute fatigue is most often associated with viral or bacterial infections and may serve as a harbinger of impending symptoms such as fever. Determining the etiology of chronic fatigue that may last for months is far more complex. A patient seeking relief from chronic fatigue may see their clinician during many times before the cause can be identified. The patient usually cannot explain the cause of chronic fatigue without the clinician asking appropriate assessment questions.

The clinical history of fatigue offers insights into the nature of the cause. Patient reports of fatigue that increases over the course of a day and abates after rest suggests an underlying medical condition that may account for the fatigue. For example, fatigue may reflect hematological abnormalities associated with other disease conditions, such as chronic anemia that results in decreased oxygen-carrying capacity, which makes the patient less tolerant of physical exertion and may contribute to persistent fatigue.

Functional fatigue is more typically characterized by fatigue on awakening that may improve after exercise. The close associations of depression and anxiety with fatigue make for a difficult task in distinguishing functional causes of fatigue from the fatigue itself. Depression has been cited as one of the most common comorbidities underlying complaints of fatigue in the primary-care setting. Mental health disorders, in general, are more likely to be found in patients reporting significant fatigue to primary-care practitioners, whereas underlying serious somatic disorders may be found in only a small percentage of these patients. Nonetheless, the strong association between fatigue and haematological abnormalities, in particular, should raise suspicion for easily ruled out physical conditions, such as anemia, as contributing factors.

DIFFERENTIAL DIAGNOSIS

Fatigue by itself presents a complicated differential, as it seldom presents without additional comorbidities. Acute fatigue is perhaps the simplest type to diagnose and treat. For example, acute fatigue typically appears in a clinical history that is positive for viral or bacterial exposure, combined with examination findings of fever and other systemic abnormalities. Chronic fatigue has many causes, including chronic anxiety or stress reactions, lack of restorative sleep due to poor sleep hygiene or sleep apnea, depression, infectious mononucleosis, hepatitis, tuberculosis, anemia, heart disease, lung disease, electrolyte disturbances, rheumatoid diseases, and cancer. Thus, a detailed history and physical examination are key to distinguishing these underlying conditions. For instance, in the case of

anemia, a detailed history may reveal fatigue that worsens with exertion, and physical examination may demonstrate findings of conjunctival pallor and pale nailbeds, gingivae, or tongue, along with sinus tachycardia.

FEVER

Fever is defined as a temperature elevation above a patient's normal baseline in which the etiology may result from any pathology and is often multifactorial. On average, most individuals maintain a body temperature close to 98.6°F (37°C), which may normally fluctuate up to ±0.9°F (± 0.5°C) throughout the day. Physical exertion can elevate body temperature temporarily, followed by a return to baseline after the activity ends. A persistent elevation in temperature clearly reflects an underlying pathology, however.

Fever may be either acute or chronic. If acute, body temperature tends to be greater than 101.3°F (38.5°C). Acute fever is associated with upper respiratory infections that are either bacterial or viral in etiology, drug reactions, gastroenteritis, or urinary tract infections. Physiologically, fever is associated with the release of inflammatory immune mediators (e.g., interleukin-6, tumor necrosis factor–α) that act as pyrogens, presumably to create an environment within the body that is not conducive to microbial growth and replication. The ability of the body to elevate the temperature in the event of infection diminishes with advancing age, due to a weakening of the immune system as one gets older. Therefore, acute fever in an elderly adult might not be as elevated compared with that in a younger patient. Quite often, the older patient may not even mount a febrile response; therefore, other symptoms may be more commonly indicative of an infection, such as malaise, decreased appetite, decreased mentation, delirium, or confusion.

Chronic fevers tend to be low-grade temperature elevations. Temperatures rise to 100.4°F (38°C), for example, in cases of infectious hepatitis, infectious mononucleosis (especially in the third and fourth weeks after the onset of symptoms), cancer, sinusitis, dental abscess, prostatitis, and tuberculosis (TB).

The origin of a fever may not be apparent from the patient's history, physical examination, or laboratory testing. If the cause is not evident after a thorough work-up, a persistent fever should be classified as a *fever of unknown origin* (FUO). Specifically, FUO is defined as a fever of greater than 101.3°F (38.5°C) that occurs on at least three occasions over a 3-week period in an ambulatory patient. A hospitalized patient is diagnosed with FUO if the unexplained fever persists for 1 week.

DIFFERENTIAL DIAGNOSIS

The differential diagnosis of fever is extremely broad, with FUO alone having several hundred potential causes. Thus, the primary-care practitioner should approach diagnostic decision-making for fever with several large etiological categories in mind, such as infection, malignancy, noninfectious inflammatory diseases (e.g., rheumatologic disorders), drug or environmental exposures, thromboembolic disease, and even factitious causes.

The magnitude of fever elevation may guide the clinician in differentiating its cause. Fevers can vary widely, however, based on the patient's age, history of pathogenic exposure, and many other factors. Fevers in excess of 104°F (40°C) tend to be associated with pancreatitis, pyelonephritis, and intracranial pathology (e.g., bacterial meningitis). Fevers between 101.3°F (38.5°C) and 104°F (40°C) are associated with urinary tract infections and some acute viral syndromes. Fevers less than 101.3°F (38.5°C) are characteristic of infectious hepatitis, some acute viral infections, and TB.

Differentiations in fever elevation guide the decision-making process of which laboratory evaluations to recommend. Correlated with history and physical examination findings, fever elevation determines the type of sampling of blood or other bodily fluids to be ordered. In addition, in the absence of definitive test results, knowledge of the categories of fever elevation may help guide the clinician toward a more specific differential diagnosis. For example, a middle-aged woman with a 3-day fever of 102.2°F (39°C) who presents with a nonproductive cough, chills, inspiratory chest discomfort, and clear lungs that are dull to percussion at the bases raises the suspicion for a pulmonary consolidative process that should prompt the clinician to order a chest x-ray and complete blood count. However, the clinician may decide not to order blood cultures for this patient because there are focal symptoms to explain the fever and the fever is not high enough to suggest systemic infection, for which blood cultures would be indicated.

Mediations and environmental toxins may also cause fever. When this etiology is suspected, the history should focus on exposure to drugs (prescribed medications or illicit drugs) and industrial chemicals, including pesticides and herbicides used in animal husbandry and agriculture. Fevers of environmental origin tend to follow an indolent course, often showing peaks and troughs. Physical signs may also be absent, thus adding to the indolence of the presentation.

LYMPHADENOPATHY

The term *lymphadenopathy* is used in clinical practice to designate any abnormality of lymph nodes and, in particular, enlarged lymph nodes. *Lymphadenitis* is a term that suggests that inflammation is the cause of the lymph node enlargement. Lymph node enlargement may be regionally or systemically associated with inflammation. If the inflammation is regional, the lymph nodes that are proximal to a site of infection will show enlargement. If the disease process is systemic, lymph nodes in three or more sites that are dispersed across the body may become enlarged. An example of regional lymph node enlargement is cervical lymphadenopathy associated with pharyngitis. An example of systemic lymphadenopathy is HIV infection, in which there may be lymphadenopathy in three or more extrainguinal lymphatic chains.

Lymphadenopathy follows the course of the underlying disease. Thus, lymph nodes may be acutely or chronically enlarged depending on actual disease pathology, the natural history of the disease, as well as the duration of the disease. Acute infection often leaves the regional nodes tender to touch. Chronically enlarged nodes may be nontender.

DIFFERENTIAL DIAGNOSIS

The differential diagnosis for lymphadenopathy depends on the location of involvement, patient characteristics, and associated findings. Neck masses, for example, involve a differential that is based on node location in the neck, the age of the patient, and associated morbidities such as tobacco use. The clinician should distinguish between slow growth in nodes and rapid or acute onset of lymphadenopathy. Acute onset is characteristic of inflammation or acute infection, whereas slow-growing nodes in the neck suggest neoplasm, such as lymphoma. However, there are exceptions. For example, a young patient with no history of tobacco or ethanol use may present with slow-growing cervical lymphadenopathy, but the possibility of neoplasm is minimal in a patient of this age and with this history. Nonetheless, an adult older than age 70 years with even a remote history of tobacco use is likely to be diagnosed with lymphoma if there is slow-growing neck lymphadenopathy. Thus, the patient's age is an important consideration in the differential diagnosis of neck lymphadenopathy.

HIV-associated lymphadenopathy presents challenges to the differential diagnosis. The average HIV-infected patient is younger than 50 years of age, has a history of alcohol and/or tobacco use, and may also be antibody-positive to other sexually transmitted diseases. Lymphadenopathy can affect the neck, axillae, inguinal region, breasts, and thorax. Reactive lymphadenopathy is characteristic of early and middle stages of the disease attributable to HIV infection itself. Later disease findings contributing to lymphadenopathy may include lymphoma or infection with cytomegalovirus, human papillomavirus, toxoplasmosis, or *Mycobacterium avium* complex. Persistent slow-growth enlargement, therefore, is reason to consider lymph node aspiration and cytological evaluation in this setting.

REFERENCES

Bruising

Neutze D, Roque J. Clinical evaluation of bleeding and bruising in primary care. *Am Fam Physician*. 2016;93(4):279–286.

Fatigue

Stadje R, Dornieden K, Baum E, et al. The differential diagnosis of tiredness: A systematic review. *BMC Fam Pract*. 2016;17:147.

Fever

Hersch E, Oh R. Prolonged febrile illness and fever of unknown origin in adults. *Am Fam Physician*. 2014;90(2):91–96.

Lymphadenopathy

Mohseni S, Shojaiefard A, Khorgami Z, et al. Peripheral lymphadenopathy: Approach and diagnostic tools. *Iran J Med Sci*. 2014;39(2):158–170.

RESOURCES

American Society of Hematology
    http://www.hematology.org/patients/
Rare Disease Report Resource Guide for Physicians
    http://www.raredr.com/resource-guide/2016/hematological

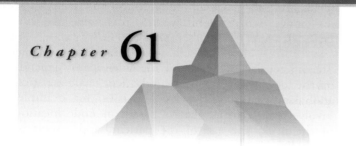

Chapter **61**

Hematological Disorders

Jacinta D. Elder, MD, MSc

Jill E. Winland-Brown, EdD, APRN, FNP-BC

Brian Oscar Porter, MD, PhD, MPH, MBA

ANEMIA

Evaluation of anemia is extremely common in clinical practice and is one of the most common laboratory abnormalities encountered in the primary-care setting. *Anemia* can mean any of several problems that involve suboptimal red blood cell (RBC) number or function. The diagnosis suggests low hemoglobin, low hematocrit (Hct), and/or a low number of RBCs. All of these problems involve a reduced amount of oxygen circulating in the body, because RBCs carry oxygen to tissues and cells. The World Health Organization (WHO) identifies anemia as a hemoglobin of less than 13.0 g/dL (less than 42% Hct) in men and less than 12.0 g/dL (less than 36% Hct) in women. Slightly higher normal ranges of hemoglobin and Hct values are considered standard in developed versus underdeveloped regions of the world.

The evaluation of anemia may be uncomplicated, unless the patient has comorbidities that can impact the evaluation of anemia, including the interpretation of laboratory results. Past medical history, family history, concurrent medical problems, and predisposing risk factors for anemia are important to consider in the evaluation of all forms of anemia and other hematologic disorders. It is important to determine whether the anemia is due to decreased RBC production, maturation defects of RBC precursors, destruction (hemolysis) of RBCs in the peripheral blood, or acute blood loss.

MICROCYTIC ANEMIAS

Microcytic anemia is a category of anemia based on the small size (*micro-*) of RBCs (*-cytic*). It has been linked to nutritional deficiencies, particularly a deficiency in dietary intake or gastrointestinal (GI) uptake of iron. The small size of RBCs is identified via the mean corpuscular volume (MCV). Microcytosis, therefore, refers to an MCV value of less than 80 fL.

EPIDEMIOLOGY AND CAUSES

Microcytic anemia related to iron deficiency is one of the most common anemias throughout the world. The incidence is high among women of childbearing age, with up to one-third of pregnant women developing anemia in the third trimester. Worldwide, the ratio of incidence between women and men is 4:1, but in the United States, 20% of adult women are affected by the condition compared with 3% of adult men. These statistics have remained constant for the past decade. The main causes of microcytic anemia include (1) inadequate oral intake or GI uptake of dietary iron, (2) anemia of chronic disease (ACD), (3) thalassemia, and (4) sideroblastic anemias.

The incidence of iron-deficiency anemia has been estimated to be 1:2.0 to 2.5 among pregnant women and 1:6 in persons older than age 75 years. Iron-deficiency anemia is often the easiest type of anemia to correct, unless it is caused by a GI malignancy. Iron deficiency is, therefore, straightforward to identify and remains the most common cause of microcytic anemia. Most adults in the United States ingest and absorb an adequate amount of iron in their diets. It is estimated that the average dietary intake of iron in the United States is 10 to 15 mg per day, of which not more than 10% is absorbed in the stomach, duodenum, and jejunum. The average healthy adult, therefore, absorbs approximately 1 to 2 mg of iron per day. In addition, the same adult loses an amount of iron equal to that ingested and absorbed, thereby maintaining homeostasis.

ACD, unlike iron-deficiency anemia, presents a more complex diagnostic picture because of the many and varied causes of inflammatory disorders in chronic disease, which include rheumatoid arthritis, malignancies, and serious infections. Given its complex diagnostic picture, ACD must always be considered in the differential for microcytic anemia, the precise incidence and prevalence of ACD are unknown.

The thalassemias are a group of inherited diseases of alpha- or beta-globin chains. Microcytic anemia is caused by hemolysis that results from the suboptimal synthesis of alpha- or beta-globin chains, known as alpha- or beta-thalassemias. Beta-thalassemia is associated with descendants of individuals who originated in areas around the Mediterranean Sea. Alpha-thalassemia is far more widespread, occurring in individuals with ancestry from the Asian continent, including China and Southeast Asia. A high prevalence of alpha-thalassemia has also been noted among persons living along the western coast of Africa.

Sideroblastic anemia results from a disorder of heme synthesis, resulting in abnormal hemoglobin and disordered RBC function. It may be caused by chronic alcoholism or lead poisoning or may be a stage in the evolution of a generalized bone marrow disorder that may progress to acute leukemia.

PATHOPHYSIOLOGY

Normal Hemoglobin Formation

The predominant normal adult hemoglobin (hemoglobin A; hemoglobin A_1; $\alpha_2\beta_2$) comprises one pair of alpha-globin chains and one pair of beta-globin chains, accounting for 90% to 95% of total adult hemoglobin. Each of these globin chains is linked to an individual heme group, which consists of a protoporphyrin IX molecule bound to a ferrous (Fe^{2+}) reduced iron ion. It is this heme unit that reversibly binds oxygen, allowing for transport of oxygen by the hemoglobin tetramer to the bodily tissues.

Several other forms of hemoglobin are formed during human development. At least three distinct forms of hemoglobin consisting of different combinations of zeta (ζ), epsilon (ε), gamma (γ), and alpha (α) chains present themselves throughout embryonic development in the following order: hemoglobin Gower I ($\zeta_2\varepsilon_2$), hemoglobin Portland ($\zeta_2\gamma_2$), and hemoglobin Gower II ($\alpha_2\varepsilon_2$). In contrast, the predominant normal hemoglobin form in infancy is hemoglobin F or fetal hemoglobin (approximately 80%), which has two gamma-globin chains substituted for the beta-chains ($\alpha_2\gamma_2$). Hemoglobin F has a stronger affinity for oxygen than hemoglobin A does, allowing for oxygen transport across the placenta from the mother to the developing fetus. As a newborn ages, this form of hemoglobin slowly clears from the circulation, accounting for less than 1% of hemoglobin by 6 months of age, with a corresponding increase in hemoglobin A. Finally, an additional form of adult hemoglobin known as hemoglobin A_2 also exists, which is present in far smaller amounts than hemoglobin A (about 2% to 5% of total adult hemoglobin). With a slightly higher oxygen affinity than hemoglobin A, hemoglobin A_2 has two delta (δ)-globin chains substituted for the beta-globin chains ($\alpha_2\delta_2$).

Iron-Deficiency Anemia

Because the reduced ferrous (Fe^{2+}) ion is a critical component of the heme moiety in hemoglobin, sufficient iron stores are critical for adequate erythropoiesis in the bone marrow. In low-iron states, the production of hemoglobin is severely reduced, resulting in marked microcytosis. Iron deficiency remains the most common cause of microcytic anemia in the United States. Because most adults receive enough iron in their diets to prevent microcytosis (other than strict vegan vegetarians, who consume no animal-based products of any kind), the clinician's attention should turn to malabsorption or occult loss of blood as the primary causes of iron-deficiency anemia.

The majority of iron uptake occurs in the duodenum and upper jejunum. Thus, malabsorption of iron is linked to underlying GI problems such as celiac sprue, surgical resections involving the stomach, duodenum, or jejunum, inflammatory bowel disease such as Crohn's disease, rapid GI motility, gastroenteritis, and selected drugs such as the histamine receptor 2 (H_2) antagonist cimetidine (Tagamet). Decreased levels of iron can also occur as the result of molecular bonds between plasma iron stores and certain drugs. These bonds develop during the distribution phase of pharmacokinetics, sequestering iron ions and decreasing the plasma pool available for integration into heme molecules. For example, sulfonamide drugs such as sulfamethoxazole-trimethoprim (co-trimoxazole, Bactrim, Septra) can cause decreased plasma levels of iron.

Iron deficiency resulting from acute or chronic (occult) blood loss with inadequate iron intake to compensate is perhaps the most prevalent cause of microcytic anemia. A net loss of blood depletes iron stores and impairs the bone marrow's ability to synthesize new RBCs, due to progressively decreased heme synthesis. Thus, RBCs are decreased not only in number but also in size, producing a characteristic microcytic anemia. Common sites of bleeding (which may be either painless or painful) include the GI tract (e.g., upper GI tract lesions such as peptic ulcers or gastritis; lower GI tract lesions such as colon cancer, ulcerative colitis, Crohn's disease, diverticulosis, and ruptured hemorrhoids) and the genitourinary tract (e.g., heavy endometrial bleeding known as menorrhagia, hematuria from bladder cancer). In fact, microcytic anemia may be the first laboratory finding that initiates a line of investigation identifying underlying malignancy. For example, heme-positive stools or melena are strong indications for colonoscopic cancer screening in men and women older than 50 years or in younger individuals with a strong family history.

Anemia of Chronic Disease

ACD may cause microcytic or normocytic anemia. ACD as a cause of microcytic anemia results from mechanisms that involve inflammation, infection, and/or underlying malignancy. Inflammation may lead to occult and progressive blood loss, because microvascular eruptions may result from histamine-release and immune complexes that physically invade the involved region. When these eruptions occur in the GI tract, occult blood escapes through the intestines. Thus, of particular concern is the relationship of occult blood in the stool to GI malignancy. Alternatively, chronic use of NSAIDs such as ibuprofen (Motrin, Advil) and aspirin for chronic pain conditions (e.g., routine management of rheumatoid arthritis and osteoarthritis) must also be considered as a cause of occult blood loss. Blood loss results from erosion of the protective mucosal lining of the stomach due to decreased production of prostaglandin formed by the enzymes cyclooxygenase-1 and cyclooxygenase-2—the molecular targets inhibited by NSAIDs.

Thalassemias

The pathology of thalassemia is related either to depletion or mutation in the genes that code for the subunits of the protein component of adult hemoglobin—the alpha- and beta-globin chains. Alpha-thalassemia is caused by gene depletion that leads to a reduction of alpha-globin chain synthesis. Because two copies of the alpha-globin chain gene are inherited from each parent on chromosome 16, mutations or deletions may exist in one or more of these four genes, producing distinct clinical manifestations. Mutations or deletions in all four genes results in alpha (O)–thalassemia or alpha-thalassemia major. No hemoglobin A, A_2, or F can form in this disorder, which

is incompatible with extrauterine life. Rather, there is an excess of Bart's hemoglobin, which consists of gamma chain tetramers (γ_4). Bart's hemoglobin has an oxygen affinity at least 10-fold greater than that of hemoglobin A and, thus, cannot effectively release oxygen to fetal tissues. This causes severe anemia with resultant congestive heart failure, widespread capillary leak, and anasarca known as hydrops fetalis (i.e., widespread edema of all fetal tissues), typically resulting in fetal demise by the third trimester of pregnancy.

Mutations in three of the four alpha genes results in hemoglobin H disease, characterized by the widespread formation of hemoglobin H, which consists of a tetramer of four beta-globin chains (β_4). This results in moderate to severe lifelong hemolytic anemia, which typically requires repeated blood transfusions. Mutations in only two of the four alpha genes is called alpha-thalassemia minor or alpha-thalassemia-1 trait. This results in a mild anemia with only minor clinical manifestations. Mutation in only one of the four alpha-globin genes is a silent carrier state called alpha-thalassemia minima or alpha-thalassemia-2 trait and can be diagnosed only through DNA analysis because it has no clinical manifestations.

In contrast, only one gene for the beta-globin chain is inherited from each parent. Mutation or deletion of one of these genes results in beta-thalassemia minor or beta-thalassemia trait, characterized by a mild anemia that is typically asymptomatic. Deletions or severe mutations in both beta-globin genes result in beta-thalassemia major (Cooley's anemia), characterized by a severe transfusion-dependent, lifelong anemia with skeletal abnormalities due to bone marrow expansion in the body's attempt to increase hematopoiesis. An intermediate form of the disorder known as beta-thalassemia intermedia also exists in which a patient inherits two mutated, albeit expressed, beta-globin genes, each with a different type of mutation (a compound heterozygote) that results in varied levels of expression or functionality. Clinical manifestations may be worsened by acute illness or infection that impairs erythropoiesis and exacerbates the anemia.

Sideroblastic Anemias

Sideroblastosis and its resulting microcytic anemia are caused by a host of molecular defects that affect the biosynthesis of the heme moiety of hemoglobin. Heme is normally formed first by the creation of 5-aminolevulinic acid (ALA) from glycine and succinyl-coenzyme A by the erythroid isoform of the mitochondrial enzyme ALA synthase, which requires vitamin B_6 (pyridoxine) as a cofactor. Although the underlying genetic defects in many forms of hereditary sideroblastic anemia have not been characterized, known mutations occur most commonly in the genes for the erythroid form of ALA synthase (located on the X chromosome), the mitochondrial transporter ABC7, pyridoxal 5-phosphate (resulting in a reversible form of the disease responsive to pyridoxine therapy), ferrochelatase, the copper-dependent enzyme cytochrome oxidase, and pseudouridine synthase–1.

In most forms of sideroblastic anemia, elemental iron is typically delivered appropriately to erythrocyte precursors. However, underlying enzymatic mutations prevent or reduce the ability of heme to incorporate into protoporphyrin IX. A reduced number of RBCs form from ring sideroblast precursors (a diagnostic hallmark) found in the bone marrow, because peripheral reticulocytosis is markedly diminished. Despite an increase in the RBC growth factor erythropoietin, anemia results from the destruction of abnormal erythroid precursors in the bone marrow via apoptosis and intramedullary hemolysis.

Sideroblastic mutations result in excessive iron deposition in the mitochondria of affected erythrocytes (erythropoietic hemochromatosis) which, nonetheless, are hypochromic and microcytic because this form of mitochondrial ferritin cannot be utilized for cytoplasmic maturation in the developing erythrocyte. Intestinal iron absorption is actually increased in sideroblastic anemia, owing to ineffective erythropoiesis, as is also observed in the thalassemias. Thus, iron overload occurs not only in erythroid cells but throughout the body, similar to genetic (familial) hemochromatosis, with predictable end-organ damage due to iron deposition (e.g., cirrhosis [liver], cardiomyopathy [heart], and endocrine defects [pancreas and adrenal glands]).

Acquired forms of sideroblastic anemia also exist. The most common causes include chronic alcoholism, which results in a multifactorial pathogenesis including many of the hypoproliferative mechanisms previously cited, iatrogenic associations with the antituberculous drug isoniazid and the antibiotic chloramphenicol, zinc toxicity, in which zinc ions preferentially bind to protoporphyrin in place of iron, and copper deficiency, which leads to decreased intestinal absorption of iron and diminished reduction of iron ions from the ferric (3+) state to the bioavailable ferrous (2+) form as a result of reduced cytochrome oxidase activity. Lead poisoning is also often cited as an acquired cause of sideroblastic anemia because lead inhibits ALA synthase. However, with lead toxicity, true ring sideroblasts are typically not seen in the bone marrow, owing to the inhibitory effect of lead on the enzyme ferrochelatase, thereby preventing the integration of ferrous ions into heme. Idiopathic acquired sideroblastic anemia may also occur when a single erythroid progenitor cell develops a mutation affecting the heme synthesis pathway but is also conferred a survival advantage. As clonal proliferation of this precursor cell ensues, the bone marrow is largely replaced by cells of this single sideroblastic lineage that is prone to apoptosis, which results in a myelodysplastic anemia.

CLINICAL PRESENTATION

Subjective

Overall, patients with microcytic anemia present with subjective findings of tachycardia, fatigue, shortness of breath, dyspnea on exertion, palpitations, listlessness, poor concentration, anorexia, and dizziness or lightheadedness. Because similar subjective findings as these are also associated with many additional diagnoses other than microcytic anemia, the history of patient complaints is unlikely to be conclusive.

Objective

As the patient's hemoglobin drops below 10 g/dL (approximately 30% Hct), many patients present with a facial mask of fatigue, sallow-colored skin, pale mucous membranes, tachycardia, and tachypnea at rest. It is possible also to note a prolonged blanching response in the nailbeds (more than 3 seconds), although many patients never present with this sign. Severe iron-deficiency anemia can also cause progressive skin and mucosal changes, such as brittle nails, cheilosis (reddened appearance of the lips, with fissures formed at the angles of the mouth), and a smooth appearance to the tongue. In addition, pica is considered an objective finding associated with severe iron deficiency. *Pica* is identified as an eating disorder of craving for food substitutes, such as clay, dirt, ice chips, or cotton.

DIAGNOSTIC REASONING

Diagnostic Tests

Knowing when to screen for anemia is key. Screening is recommended in pregnant female patients and in children at one year of age when metabolic demands are extremely high and the individual appears otherwise healthy. Men and postmenopausal women should not be routinely screened for anemia unless the clinical picture suggests it is the possible cause of symptomatology, such as fatigue, generalized weakness, shortness of breath with exertion, pallor, dizziness, fainting, headaches, chest pain, or evidence of GI bleeding (either occult or gross bleeding).

Initial diagnostic testing is focused on obtaining a complete blood count (CBC), including RBC count and RBC indices (MCV, mean corpuscular hemoglobin [MCH], and mean corpuscular hemoglobin concentration [MCHC]). A low RBC count, hemoglobin level, and/or Hct identify anemia (see Table 61.1). As a rule of thumb, Hct is three times the value of the hemoglobin. For example, a hemoglobin value of 13.0 g/dL suggests an estimated Hct of 39%.

TABLE 61.1   Classification of Anemias

Anemia	Examples of Causes	Mean Corpuscular Volume (fL)	Mean Corpuscular Hemoglobin (pg/cell)	Mean Corpuscular Hemoglobin Concentration (%)
Microcytic, hypochromic	Iron deficiency, lead poisoning, thalassemia, rheumatoid arthritis	50–80	12–25	25–30
Microcytic, normochromic	Renal disease, infection, liver disease, malignancies	<80	20–25	27
Normocytic, normochromic	Sepsis, hemorrhage, hemolysis, drug-induced aplastic anemia, radiation, hereditary spherocytosis	82–92	25–30	32–36
Macrocytic, normochromic	Vitamin B_{12} and folic acid deficiency, some drugs, pernicious anemia	95–150	30–50	32–36

INDICATIONS FOR HEMOGLOBIN ELECTROPHORESIS

- Suspected thalassemia, especially in individuals with positive family history for the disorder
- Differentiation among the types of thalassemias
- Evaluation of a positive sickle cell anemia screening (Sickledex) test to differentiate sickle cell trait (20%–40% Hgb S) from sickle cell disease (>70% Hgb S)
- Diagnosis of hemoglobin C disease or combined hemoglobin C/sickle cell anemia (hemoglobin SC disease)
- Identification of the numerous types of abnormal hemoglobin, most of which do not produce clinical disease

Hemoglobin Electrophoresis	Percentage of Hemoglobin	Comments
Hgb A_1 (adults) Infants	>95 10–30	Low: alpha- and beta-thalassemia major and minor
Hgb A_2 (adults) Cord blood Birth–6 months >6 months	2–5 0–1.8 0–3.5 1.5–3.5	Elevated: beta-thalassemia major and minor up to 9%
Hgb F (adults) Neonates 1 month 2 months 3 months 6 months–1 year	<10 70–80 70 50 25 3	Elevated: beta-thalassemia minor up to 9% Elevated: thalassemia major and minor (after 6 months)
Hgb C	Absent	Usually asymptomatic, but can cause red blood cells to sickle due to osmotic fragility; occurs in 2%–3% of black individuals
Hgb D	Absent	Rarely occurs alone but worsens disease when in combination with sickle cell anemia or thalassemia
Hgb E	Absent	Rarely occurs alone but worsens disease when in combination with sickle cell anemia or thalassemia
Hgb H	Absent	Unstable tetramer of beta-hemoglobin chains; 30% of hemoglobin in severe alpha-thalassemia with three of four mutated alpha genes (hemoglobin H disease)
Hgb M	Absent	Any of several mutated forms of hemoglobin that cannot be reduced to an oxygen-carrying state, resulting in congenital methemoglobinemia
Hgb S	Absent	Elevated in sickle cell anemia: <40% in sickle cell trait; 85%–95% in sickle cell disease. Most common beta-hemoglobin chain variant: if both beta-chain genes are affected, then sickle cell anemia (0.25% of African Americans); if only one gene affected, then sickle cell trait (8%–10% of African Americans)

Abbreviation: Hgb, hemoglobin.

Iron-Deficiency Anemia

The diagnostic tests for iron-deficiency anemia are relatively simple to perform and are readily available to the primary-care practitioner. Serum ferritin is a reliable test of low iron stores, provided the patient does not have advanced liver disease. A serum ferritin value of less than 30 mg/L is considered pathological. As the ferritin level falls, the total iron-binding capacity (TIBC) rises above the normal range. If the drop in ferritin and rise in TIBC continue without intervention, the serum iron level will eventually fall (to less than 30 mg/L), as will the transferrin saturation (to less than 15%). In addition, secondary testing should focus on the RBC morphology indices from the CBC. Findings such as anisocytosis (variable RBC size), poikilocytosis (variable RBC shape), and hypochromasia (pale-colored RBCs) may be seen when severely iron-deficient samples are microscopically evaluated.

Anemia of Chronic Disease

Diagnostic tests for ACD focus on distinguishing ACD from iron-deficiency anemia. Unlike iron-deficiency anemia, ACD presents with a low serum iron level, along with a low TIBC. The serum transferrin level is either normal or increased in patients with ACD. Finally, the clinician should expect the transferrin saturation to be low, as it is in iron-deficiency anemia.

Thalassemias

The diagnosis of both alpha- and beta-thalassemias require a CBC and hemoglobin electrophoresis to identify the type and amount of each hemoglobin chain. The CBC is essential to determine the diagnosis of microcytic anemia, as the hemoglobin and MCV are low for each type of thalassemia. In alpha-thalassemia trait, the hemoglobin electrophoresis reveals no increase in hemoglobin A_2 or hemoglobin F. In addition, no hemoglobin H is present. Plasma iron parameters are normal. The level of anemia in alpha-thalassemia is modest, as evidenced by an Hct between 27% and 40%.

Beta-thalassemia minor patients have modest anemia. Unlike those with alpha-thalassemia trait, hemoglobin electrophoresis in these patients reveals elevated hemoglobin A_2 and, in some cases, elevated hemoglobin F. Neither type of hemoglobin will typically be elevated to greater than 9%, however.

Patients with beta-thalassemia major present very differently from patients with other forms of thalassemia, as the degree of anemia is severe. If left untreated, Hct levels fall to less than 10%. Electrophoresis reveals little to no hemoglobin A, with variable amounts of hemoglobin A_2 present. The clinician should expect hemoglobin F to be the primary hemoglobin detectable in these patients. As with all of the thalassemias, findings in patients with beta-thalassemia will include abnormal RBC morphology, such as poikilocytosis and anisocytosis.

Sideroblastic Anemia

A diagnosis of sideroblastic anemia is confirmed by a Prussian blue stain of a bone marrow aspirate. The Prussian blue stain reveals tinged sideroblasts, which have iron deposits located in the mitochondria that surround the RBC nucleus. In addition, erythroid hyperplasia is present in the aspirate from patients with sideroblastic anemia. A high level of serum iron and a high transferrin saturation should accompany these findings. Without a stain of the bone marrow aspirate, the laboratory profile could mimic iron-deficiency anemia, with a moderately low Hct of 20% to 30% and a low MCV.

Differential Diagnosis

The differential diagnosis as to the type of microcytic anemia depends on blood work results. Microcytic anemia is typically distinguished as to its four predominant etiologies, as discussed above: iron-deficiency anemia, ACD, thalassemias, and sideroblastic anemia. The ultimate goal of the diagnostic evaluation is to identify the underlying cause of the microcytic anemia, such as GI malignancy, iron malabsorption, blood loss, menorrhagia, and so forth. For example, iron-deficiency anemia in a man or woman over 50 years of age should be ruled out as GI malignancy with a screening colonoscopy as soon as possible.

MANAGEMENT

The management of microcytic anemia focuses on treating and eradicating the cause of the anemia. If amelioration of the cause is not possible, symptomatic care is indicated. The severity of the anemia will direct the intervention. For example, the decision to transfuse a patient with RBCs is a major clinical step that may be indicated if the Hct is 27% or less. This decision requires a thoughtful analysis of the overall clinical setting and hemodynamic status of the patient, which may not be severely compromised, even at low hemoglobin levels. For instance, transfusing patients with volume-sensitive comorbidities, such as congestive heart failure, calls for great caution, given the risks of fluid overload and high output cardiac failure. In addition, the risk of iron overload following repeated RBC transfusions must be carefully considered. Therefore, more conservative treatments are initiated in nonemergent settings.

Iron-Deficiency Anemia

Iron-deficiency anemia is first treated with an increase in dietary iron and thereafter with supplemental iron. Foods rich in iron should be recommended, such as animal proteins, legumes, and dark green leafy vegetables, such as spinach. Diet alone may be sufficient in treating iron deficiency if the patient is either young or middle-aged or the cause of the anemia is short-lived. However, as the patient ages (particularly beyond the age 65 of years) and if the cause of the anemia is chronic, iron deficiency must be treated with either supplemental oral or parenteral iron.

Supplemental oral iron is best given as ferrous sulfate 325 mg three times daily; 10 to 20 mg will be absorbed from the total daily regimen if the serum iron level is moderately low. In more severe cases, however, the level of absorption will increase. The clinician should recheck the RBC indices and iron values in 2 to 4 weeks after starting the regimen to ascertain the effectiveness of the oral regimen. The patient's adherence to the regimen could be complicated by the requirement that iron supplements be taken on an empty stomach to achieve maximal absorption. Some individuals have GI intolerance to oral iron or some may develop constipation on oral iron. Both of these can lead to difficulty for the patient in adhering to the regimen.

Therefore, if no measured improvement in anemia (Hct elevated by one-half of baseline), MCV, and iron stores appears after 1 month of therapy, the clinician should confirm adequate adherence to the iron regimen along with the underlying cause of the iron deficiency. The patient should continue to take supplemental iron for 3 to 6 months after normal levels in the blood and serum indices have been restored. Within 1 to 2 weeks there should be an increase in hemoglobin (reticulocytes begin to increase within 3 to 4 days). Thereafter, the clinician should recheck laboratory values as indicated by the clinical assessment.

It is uncommon that the patient will not respond to oral iron, unless the patient is on hemodialysis or there is severe recurrent blood loss, such as with GI or uterine hemorrhage or if a malabsorption syndrome present. However, if the patient does not respond to supplemental iron, and none of the confounding factors mentioned play a role, the clinician should doubt the initial diagnosis of iron-deficiency anemia. In particular, ACD should be suspected as the cause, or the clinician should reconsider whether the rate of GI or uterine blood loss might exceed stem-cell deployment from the bone marrow.

Given the risk of anaphylaxis, supplemental parenteral iron is indicated only when there is documented failure of therapy with oral iron supplements. The clinician should calculate the daily dose by subtracting the patient's measured MCV from the normal lower range value (which varies by age and gender). This value is considered the total number of milligrams of iron to add according to the MCV. In addition, the clinician must add 1,000 mg to the delivered dose to cover the storage of iron in the body. Overall, the daily dosage of supplemental parenteral iron is approximately 1,300 to 2,000 mg (1.3–2.0 g) of iron. The preferred parenteral route of administration is IV. Because anaphylaxis is possible with IV iron, the initial dose should be delivered over 4 to 6 hours to minimize adverse effects; some practitioners advocate giving 50 mg over the first hour as a trial.

Anemia of Chronic Disease

Treatment of ACD is focused on treating the underlying cause (i.e., the precipitating illness). Because these patients are less likely to respond to oral iron supplementation, parenteral iron is recommended. Red blood cell transfusions may become necessary for symptomatic treatment if Hct falls to 27% to 30%. In most cases of ACD, however, Hct will stay above 30%. ACD due to chronic renal failure, human immunodeficiency virus (HIV) infection and cancer chemotherapy (not anemia related to the cancer itself) might require treatment with drugs that stimulate erythropoiesis given subcutaneously, such as erythropoietin alfa or darbepoetin alfa. The dosage varies according to patient tolerance and hematological requirements. The U.S. Food and Drug Administration recommends the lowest possible dose necessary to eliminate the need for transfusions, so as to prevent dangerously high increases in hemoglobin.

To protect against a potentially dangerous rise in hemoglobin, it is recommended that the hemoglobin be checked twice weekly for 2 to 6 weeks after an increase in dose in these erythropoietic agents. Administration should be held for hemoglobin that exceeds 12 g/dL or rises more than 1 g/dL in any 2-week period. Erythropoietin alfa (Epogen, Procrit) is given three times weekly and then adjusted in dose according to therapeutic response. Darbepoetin alfa (Aranesp) may initially be given weekly and then adjusted to dosing every 2 weeks. These medications can be administered IV in the hospital or clinical setting. In addition, patients can learn to self-inject these medications subcutaneously, just as diabetic patients learn to self-inject insulin.

Thalassemia

Thalassemia often requires no treatment other than vigilance by the clinician concerning hematological markers. If a clinician diagnoses microcytosis with mild anemia, the patient should not be subjected to further checks for iron deficiency if there is a distinct thalassemic etiology. Thus, clinical vigilance may be all that is required for microcytosis with mild anemia.

Patients with severe anemia, however, such as that associated with beta-thalassemia major and hemoglobin H disease, require regular transfusion with packed RBCs. In addition, these patients require folate supplementation and possibly oral iron chelation therapy to prevent hemosiderosis and hemochromatosis resulting from multiple transfusions. Hemosiderosis of chronic standing may also require referral for a splenectomy.

Sideroblastic Anemia

There are few options for the treatment of sideroblastosis. Depending on the severity of anemia, RBC transfusions may be required. Large doses (200 mg/day) of vitamin B_6 (pyridoxine, e.g., Beesix) have benefited some patients. Erythropoietin alfa (Epogen) has proven to be of little aid in supporting these patients.

FOLLOW-UP AND REFERRAL

Mild iron-deficiency anemia necessitates follow-up every 4 to 6 months. There should be no need to retest iron stores after the first follow-up visit following the initial diagnosis, unless indicated by patient complaints or physical examination findings. Thus, typical follow-up testing may consist only of serial CBCs. A referral to an appropriate specialist may be necessary if a thorough work-up identifies serious pathology that accounts for the iron-deficiency anemia, such as GI malignancy or other type of occult blood loss. These patients may require upper and/or lower endoscopy or other type of work-up to exclude serious pathology. Anyone 50 years or older with heme-positive stools or evidence of iron-deficiency anemia should be referred for a colonoscopy unless the risks of colonoscopy outweigh the potential benefits of catching a GI cancer early—such as in elderly patients with an increased risk of intestinal perforation that could prove fatal.

In general, the plan of referral for microcytic anemia should isolate the cause of the anemia, initiate treatment in the primary-care setting, and involve specialty care referral only as needed. The primary-care practitioner, therefore, has the responsibility to perform all screening tests and to seek to determine the underlying cause. In turn, referral to a specialist for iron-deficiency anemia is almost never required unless it is complicated by concurrent diagnoses, including other causes of microcytic anemia. For example, iron-deficiency anemia secondary to menorrhagia would necessitate appropriate gynecological referral if procedural interventions, such as uterine ablation or hysterectomy, are indicated.

ACD follow-up can be more complicated than follow-up of iron-deficiency anemia. If the patient requires erythropoietin injections, he or she should be maintained on a 30-day follow-up schedule once the hemoglobin level is acceptable and has stabilized, to continue for approximately 6 months after initiating therapy. In most cases, only a CBC will be required to determine the effectiveness of therapy. It is exceptional for patients with ACD to require transfusions. The clinician should refer patients with ACD to gastroenterologists, hepatologists, oncologists, rheumatologists, hematologists, or other specialists depending on the suspected underlying pathology based on initial evaluation by the primary-care practitioner. For example, if the clinician were to detect occult blood in the stool of a patient with microcytic anemia and the history did not reveal a likely cause, referral to a gastroenterologist would be warranted.

Patients diagnosed with one of the thalassemias may or may not require referral to a hematologist. Although patients with more aggressive thalassemias (such as beta-thalassemia major or hemoglobin H disease) must be referred promptly to a hematologist, who will be entrusted with managing the plan of care, patients with alpha- or beta-thalassemia minor may be managed by the primary-care practitioner following initial diagnosis. In these patients, it may only be necessary to monitor serial CBCs every 3 to 4 months. More frequent observation and intervention is required, however, for the other types of thalassemias, which require transfusion therapy, and the plan of care established by the hematologist will dictate the follow-up schedule.

Because sideroblastosis is diagnosed by examination of a bone marrow aspirate, early referral to a hematologist is required for suspected sideroblastic anemia. The hematologist may also perform tests to determine lead exposure and resultant damage from lead toxicity, a common etiology of sideroblastic anemia. Follow-up evaluation will become the responsibility of the primary-care practitioner, however, and CBCs in these patients should be monitored every 2 to 3 months.

Patient Education: Microcytic Anemias

Education should focus on self-care and primary-care management of the underlying cause of microcytic anemia. Self-care encompasses topics such as adherence to the medication regimen, dietary changes, level of activity, self-monitoring for signs and symptoms of anemia, and adjustment to the requirements of new health-related practices. For example, patients with iron-deficiency anemia must be educated to perform the following self-care behaviors: (1) take ferrous sulfate (supplemental iron) on an empty stomach or at most with a small snack; (2) eat foods that are rich in iron, vitamin C, and B-complex vitamins, which are all necessary for proper RBC development; (3) remain as active as possible, and if fatigued, rest before resuming activity; (4) self-monitor for fatigue, shortness of breath, pale-colored stools (before initiating supplemental iron), and palpitations or tachycardia, which may all be associated with decreased oxygen-carrying capacity due to anemia; and (5) share information about iron deficiency so that friends and/or family can assist in lifestyle adjustments that new health-related behaviors will require.

Additional patient education focuses on primary-care management. Patients need to understand the importance of timely clinical laboratory evaluations, return follow-up visits, recognizing signs and symptoms of recurrent anemia that should be reported to the clinician, and proper techniques for administering or receiving drugs that must be delivered via a parenteral route, such as erythropoietin or IV iron supplements. The need to remain vigilant for the signs of potential iron overload in patients with severe anemia who are receiving chronic blood transfusions is key, including monitoring for the signs of liver dysfunction, such as nausea, loss of appetite, weight loss, yellowing of the skin, and swelling of the lower legs.

NORMOCYTIC ANEMIA

Normocytic anemia is defined as an anemia associated with normally sized RBCs (MCV = 81–99 fL), although normal ranges vary with age. Many forms of normocytic anemia have normally shaped RBCs as well, although some conditions are recognized by typical abnormal morphological findings on a peripheral blood smear. Most commonly, this type of anemia results from chronic disease states that lead to a hypoproliferative anemia. However, acute blood loss, hemolysis, and volume overload are other important etiologies of normocytic anemia.

EPIDEMIOLOGY AND CAUSES

Normocytic anemias cover a broad range of diseases and conditions, each with its own epidemiology and prevalence rate. Nonetheless, it is possible to estimate the incidence of normocytic ACD by recognizing that at least half of all patients with an underlying chronic disease will develop normocytic anemia over the course of their illness, while some will develop a microcytic ACD as discussed previously.

PATHOPHYSIOLOGY

One of the ways in which normocytic ACD develops is through the reduction of the erythrocyte life cycle. The presumed mechanism for this is through increased phagocytosis by macrophages, which results in increased clearance of erythrocytes from the circulation. It is not known how or why this happens because there appears to be no intrinsic defects in the erythrocyte that have yet to be found. ACD can also be considered to be a hypoproliferative anemia because of bone marrow suppression (myelosuppression) resulting from the effects of inflammatory cytokines on the bone marrow. Animal studies have shown that certain inflammatory cytokines such as tumor necrosis factor–α, interferon (IFN)-β, and IFN-γ may underlie these mechanisms of hypoproliferation in normocytic ACD.

The combination of reduced cell life and impaired stem cell production (hypoproliferation) associated with chronic illness typically results in a normocytic, normochromic anemia. Any condition that creates inflammation can therefore cause ACD. These include but are

not limited to chronic infection, chronic inflammatory disorders, autoimmune activation, malignancy (with or without bone marrow invasion), cardiac disease, diabetes mellitus, endocrine disorders (e.g., hypothyroidism, hypoadrenalism, hypopituitarism, hypogonadism), acute renal insufficiency (due to the accumulation of uremic metabolites that decrease RBC life span), and chronic renal insufficiency (due to impaired erythropoietin synthesis by the kidneys). Severe trauma, surgery, or major acute disease states such as sepsis and myocardial infarction may also result in normocytic anemia, possibly due to the significant tissue damage and inflammatory response associated with these events.

Most importantly, iron metabolism plays a critical role in the pathogenesis of ACD. The human body does not have a defined pathway to excrete excess iron. Thus, it is essential to life that the absorption of dietary iron be regulated efficiently. Decreased dietary ingestion or decreased absorption could lead to iron deficiency and excess ingestion or absorption to iron overload. This regulation is mediated by the iron-regulatory hormone hepcidin, which binds to the iron export protein, ferroportin, and induces its internalization and degradation, thus limiting the amount of iron released into the blood.

The major factors that are implicated in hepcidin regulation include tissue iron stores, transferrin saturation, hypoxia, inflammation, and erythropoiesis. Upregulated by the pro-inflammatory cytokines interleukin (IL)-6, IL-1, and the bacterial superantigen lipopolysaccharide (LPS), hepcidin has been shown in animal models to directly inhibit iron absorption by the gut, resulting in decreased plasma iron levels. It is known that the erythropoietic demand reduces hepcidin levels to increase iron availability for the production of RBCs; however, the molecular details of this mechanism are still being elucidated. Moreover, patients with ACD are less capable of adequate erythropoietin upregulation in response to their anemic state, compared with patients with non–iron-sequestering anemias (e.g., iron-deficiency anemia). Although absolute erythropoietin levels may be increased in ACD compared with nonanemic normal values, the bone marrow demonstrates a decreased erythropoietic response to this growth factor

Aplastic anemia also results in a hypoproliferative normocytic anemia. This may be a primary condition affecting only the erythroid lineage or it may encompass more than one cell line (e.g., white blood cells [WBCs] or platelets), which would indicate a proliferative defect in an earlier common progenitor cell that gives rise to more than one bone marrow lineage. Aplastic anemia may also be secondarily associated with certain types of viral infections in high-risk individuals, such as parvovirus B19 infection in patients with sickle cell disease or hereditary spherocytosis. A failure of erythropoietin production by the kidneys, as is also observed in chronic renal insufficiency, will similarly result in reduced RBC production and decreased reticulocytosis.

Normocytic anemia may also be caused by a relative increase in plasma volume, such as that which occurs in pregnancy or iatrogenic parenteral overhydration. This results in a dilutional drop in plasma hemoglobin, which may be physiological, as in pregnancy, or which may be reversible via pharmacological diuresis, as in the case of fluid overload.

Increased blood loss, such as from acute bleeding or hemolysis, is another major cause of normocytic anemia. As bleeding progresses and the marrow undergoes reticulocytosis, MCV may be transiently increased due to the relatively larger size of reticulocytes. However, once plasma and bone marrow iron stores are exhausted, hemoglobin production decreases, and this anemia transitions to a normocytic state and then eventually into a microcytic anemia characteristic of iron-deficiency anemia.

If hemolysis occurs intravascularly, fragmented RBCs termed *schistocytes* are seen on peripheral blood smear. This type of anemia is most commonly associated with hemolytic uremic syndrome (HUS), thrombotic thrombocytopenic purpura (TTP), disseminated intravascular coagulation (DIC), or heart valve abnormalities that cause mechanical RBC shearing. Hemolysis may also occur extravascularly with clearance of RBCs by the reticuloendothelial system. This is characterized by rounded RBCs termed *spherocytes* on peripheral blood smear and occurs most commonly due to splenic removal of RBCs, as seen in hypersplenism or autoimmune hemolytic anemia (AIHA).

Immune-mediated hemolysis typically occurs when RBC-specific antibodies coat erythrocytes, rendering them prone to splenic removal or direct hemolysis by antibody-mediated complement fixation. RBC-specific antibodies may form as a consequence of antibody upregulation from viral infections such as mononucleosis, malignancies (especially chronic lymphocytic leukemia), or autoimmune disorders such as systemic lupus erythematosus. When these antibodies are primarily of the immunoglobulin (Ig)G class, they are known as warm agglutinins because they result in RBC aggregation (agglutination) at warmer temperatures, due to the binding of two RBCs at a time (one to each of the IgG molecule's two antigen-binding sites). In contrast, IgM RBC-specific antibodies, such as those associated with *Mycoplasma* infection, are called cold agglutinins because they are capable of causing RBC aggregation at relatively lower temperatures by virtue of a greater number of antigen-binding and complement fixation sites that results from their tendency to cluster in pentamers (i.e., aggregates of 5 IgM molecules with a total of 10 antigen-specific binding sites).

Extravascular hemolysis may also result from a whole host of intrinsic RBC membrane defects, such as mutations in the membrane protein spectrin that cause hereditary spherocytosis. In addition, mutations in certain cytoplasmic enzymes render RBCs more prone to hemolysis. A prime example are disorders of glucose-6-phosphate dehydrogenase (G-6-PD), an enzyme critical to the production of glutathione, a powerful reducing agent and the RBC's main protective mechanism against highly oxidizing compounds such as naphthalene (the active chemical agent found in mothballs) or certain drugs such as trimethoprim-sulfamethoxazole (Bactrim), primaquine, and dapsone.

CLINICAL PRESENTATION

Subjective

The patient presentation will depend on the severity of the anemia. Because normocytic anemia rarely presents with a moderate to severe anemia of less than 30% Hct, many patients with the diagnosis do not report subjective findings. On closer questioning, however, they might note malaise or fatigue.

Objective

The objective findings of normocytic anemia are the same as for microcytic anemia.

DIAGNOSTIC REASONING

Diagnostic Tests

Initial testing begins with a CBC. The clinician should expect the finding of anemia not to be accompanied by an alteration in RBC indices (MCV, MCH, MCHC) to establish a diagnosis of normocytic normochromic anemia, such as that associated with acute blood loss, sepsis, underlying malignancy, mechanical shearing of RBCs from prosthetic heart valves, aplastic anemia, or normocytic ACD.

Subsequent testing includes an absolute reticulocyte count (normal range for adults is 0.5%–2.5% of the total RBC count). Reticulocytes are the less mature stage of RBCs. They acquire their name from their fine cytoplasmic network of ribosomal RNA used for hemoglobin synthesis, which is called a *reticulum;* this network appears when stained with certain dyes such as new methylene blue. The reticulum is lost as the RBC matures but is prominent in these less mature cells of the RBC lineage, which are larger than their mature RBC counterparts. Thus, the reticulocyte count is always higher than normal in any proliferative condition (i.e., proliferative normocytic anemia). While overall MCV may be elevated due to this abundance of immature reticulocytes in some forms of anemia, MCV may paradoxically be normal in a true microcytic anemia with a significant reticulocytosis, because the average (mean) RBC size may appear normal in the face of both small and large cells. Thus, the clinician must keep in mind that size descriptions such as normocytic and microcytic are typically referring to the RBC itself, whereas MCV is an average size assessment of the overall erythroid cell lineage.

Proliferative microcytic anemia may be difficult to diagnose solely from laboratory testing. If the patient has a recent history of trauma, the diagnosis of proliferative microcytic anemia secondary to hemorrhage should be considered. However, when hemorrhage is not part of the clinical picture, attention should turn to evaluating the patient for hemolysis as a potential etiology. Testing for hemolysis requires a peripheral smear, as RBC morphology is useful in determining the cause of the hemolysis. Possible morphological changes in RBC appearance include spherocytes, sickle cells, and schistocytes. Spherocytes are erythrocytes shaped like rounded spheres or globes, which are abnormal shapes for an erythrocyte. Sickle cells assume the shape of a quarter moon or the curved metal blade instrument known as a sickle, from which these erythrocytes take their name. Schistocytes, on the other hand, are classically called "fragmented" and appear as many varied shapes.

Further genetic testing may be required if these abnormal RBC morphologies are detected on a peripheral smear. The presence of sickle cells on the smear implies a sickle cell anemia diagnosis or one of its variants, such as sickle beta-thalassemia, or sickle C disease. The presence of spherocytes necessitates obtaining a Coombs' test to detect anti-RBC antibodies, because a positive Coombs' test suggests hemolysis due to an AIHA, whereas a negative test may suggest hereditary spherocytosis. Schistocytes require the clinician to order a prothrombin time (PT) and partial thromboplastin time (PTT), because elevated PT/PTT values may reflect DIC if there is also thrombocytopenia, given that platelet consumption from widespread thrombi and microthrombi is characteristic of this disorder. This results in bleeding and/or oozing, which may be refractory to treatment and ultimately prove fatal. Normal PT/PTT values in the presence of schistocytes suggests any one of several diagnoses, including severe hypertension, HUS/TTP, heart valve abnormalities (such as mitral valve stenosis), vasculitis, or hemolysis with concurrent elevated liver enzymes and low platelets (HELLP) syndrome. HELLP syndrome is typically associated with pregnancy, especially later-term pregnancies; delivery of the baby is the primary intervention.

Although the peripheral smear typically reveals morphological changes in RBCs in the patient with hemolysis, RBC shape may be normal in some forms of hemolysis, such as with deficiency in the enzyme glucose-6-phosphodiesterase (G-6-PD). A low level of G-6-PD in the absence of morphological changes in the peripheral blood smear of a patient with normocytic anemia strongly implicates the lack of this enzyme as the cause for the hemolysis. However,

G-6-PD levels measured during an acute attack of hemolytic anemia may appear paradoxically elevated in patients with G-6-PD deficiency because of the relatively higher concentration of G-6-PD found in reticulocytes, which are upregulated during acute hemolysis as the bone marrow attempts to compensate for the loss in hemolyzed RBCs. Thus, serum levels are often normal during acute hemolytic attacks, and the diagnosis of G-6-PD deficiency must be confirmed by redrawing G-6-PD levels several weeks after the acute anemia has resolved.

Should the G-6-PD level be within normal limits in a patient who reports voiding dark red urine in the morning, then it is necessary to consider conducting the Ham acidified serum lysis test, as dark red urine raises suspicion of paroxysmal nocturnal hemoglobinuria (PNH). The traditional Ham acidified serum lysis test may provide a definitive diagnosis, although state-of-the-art diagnostic testing typically involves flow cytometric analysis, which directly evaluates RBCs for reduced or absent levels of the cell surface molecules CD55 and CD59 that result from the genetic defects underlying PNH.

In patients diagnosed with a hypoproliferative normocytic anemia with a normal MCV and low reticulocyte count, attention should turn to the WBC count and platelet count. If both are low, the clinician should suspect pancytopenia affecting all the major bone marrow lineages. If the WBC and thrombocyte counts are high, however, then either ACD or renal disease is the likely cause of the normocytic anemia. Subsequent tests, therefore, involve renal function studies (e.g., blood urea nitrogen [BUN] and creatinine) and a careful review of the patient's medical history. Assessing endogenous erythropoietin levels is an important part of this work-up as well.

Differential Diagnosis

The differential for normocytic anemia includes mixed anemias of other classifications. Differentiation should be made between three major causative mechanisms: *deficiency* of various factors needed for normal RBC development (e.g., iron, vitamin B_{12}, folic acid, pyridoxine [vitamin B_6]); *central* RBC production abnormalities— caused by impaired bone marrow function (e.g., anemia of chronic disease, anemia of the elderly, malignant blood disorders); and *peripheral* disorders of RBC loss (e.g., bleeding, hemolysis). Mixed anemias may appear normocytic because the MCV is within normal range, even though iron-deficient RBCs may be small and vitamin B_{12} or folate-deficient RBCs are megaloblastic. Moreover, because ACD is part of the differential for microcytic anemia as well as normocytic anemia, the clinician must distinguish between the RBC indices of these two forms of ACD, in addition to focusing on the underlying chronic pathology.

MANAGEMENT

The management of normocytic anemia focuses on the cause of the disorder. In the initial phase of management, treatment should be symptomatic, alleviating the common downstream effects of anemia. Subsequent management consists of correcting, stabilizing, or preventing the underlying cause of the normocytic anemia (e.g., ACD, AIHA, heart valve abnormalities, vasculitis, severe hypertension, HELLP syndrome, and DIC).

Apart from appropriately treating the underlying disease pathology, management of ACD may sometimes be only watchful waiting; however, if the patient's Hct drops below 30%, the clinician may consider using recombinant erythropoietin (rhEPO) or darbepoetin. Dosing with rhEPO or darbepoetin for ACD is highly individualized and is dependent on the underlying causative disease pathology. In general, treatment should be targeted to increase hemoglobin to 10 to 12 g/dL, but not by more than 1 g/dL in a 2-week period.

Starting doses range from 50 to 150 U/kg subcutaneously (SC) three times per week (or 50–200 microgram every 2 weeks for darbepoetin), depending on the underlying pathology, and should only be initiated after carefully reviewing dosing guidelines in the specific product labeling. For the first 3 weeks of therapy, the clinician should check the Hct twice weekly until the dosage level is stabilized. Two to 6 weeks may pass before the Hct undergoes an appreciable elevation. These agents should ideally be used with oral iron supplementation if the patient is able to tolerate. If there is no response after 6 weeks, the physician should confirm compliance with iron therapy. If noncompliance with iron is noted, the patient should restart iron supplementation if possible. If there is no response after 6 weeks, the patient may receive a trial of IV iron supplementation.

Endogenous erythropoietin levels do not aid in determining the starting dose of exogenous erythropoietin alfa therapy. Moreover, the clinician may increase the dosage and frequency of administration until the Hct rises to an appropriate level. As the dosage level rises, however, it is possible that polycythemia (i.e., Hct greater than 60%–65%) may develop as a side effect of exogenous erythropoietin usage. Thus, if hemoglobin rises to 12 or 13 g/dL or the patient becomes frankly polycythemic, the drug should be discontinued. Within a week of discontinuing therapy, the Hct should start to decline. Otherwise, in rare cases, it may be necessary to phlebotomize the patient, removing enough volume to cause a drop in the Hct.

After the clinician achieves and maintains a normal Hct, the dosage level may be reduced and/or the frequency of administration changed. Thus, the management of dosing of exogenous RBC growth factors such as erythropoietin alfa (Epogen, Procrit) or darbepoetin-alfa (Aranesp) requires expert consultation with a hematologist or other appropriate specialist, given the significant risks of overdosage associated with polycythemia, including thrombosis, stroke, and myocardial infarction. As a result, RBC growth factors are rarely used to treat anemia outside of chronic kidney disease.

First-line treatment of AIHA consists of oral or intravenous corticosteroid therapy, such as prednisone 1 to 2 mg/kg per day in divided doses. Thus, an adult who weighs 70 kg would receive between 70 and 140 mg of prednisone in two or three divided doses each day. After an initial response is documented, the prednisone dose is decreased to 20 to 30 mg/day within several weeks, followed by a slow taper over several months to prevent recurrence of the condition. As for other patients on chronic corticosteroid therapy, supplementation with calcium, vitamin D, and folic acid may be initiated, along with bisphosphonate therapy, as prophylaxis against osteoporosis. If transfusion is required for severe anemia, the clinician should be aware that the risk of transfusion reaction is very high owing to crossmatching difficulties for these patients, given their Coombs' test positivity. The clinician should expect that the transfused cells will survive no better than the patient's own erythrocytes if the underlying AIHA is left untreated.

Surgical consultation is required for possible splenectomy should prednisone become ineffective or too toxic from chronic administration. In emergency situations, short-term hemolytic control in 1 to 3 weeks may be achieved with IV immune globulin (500 mg/kg per day for 1 to 4 days). In addition, off-label use of rituximab (Rituxan), an anti-CD20 B-cell–depleting monoclonal antibody therapy, has been used as second-line therapy for AIHA.

Heart valve abnormalities require an individualized plan of care developed with referral to an interventional cardiologist, which may include surgical correction of the abnormality. Many patients with heart valve abnormalities will have already started taking warfarin sodium (Coumadin) to prevent embolism formation. They should not stop taking anticoagulant therapy unless their platelet counts fall along with the Hct or active bleeding is present. Anticoagulation should also be stopped in the face of a rapidly falling hemoglobin, even in the setting of a normal platelet count.

Treatment of vasculitis consists of high-dose prednisone, and it may be necessary to raise the prednisone dose to 60 mg daily. The clinician should slowly taper the corticosteroid dose as the lesions of vasculitis heal, fever declines, and other symptoms abate. Additional immunosuppressive therapy may also be required to augment the prednisone. Cyclophosphamide (Cytoxan) in a dose range of 1 to 2 mg/kg per day may be added to the prednisone regimen. These drugs should be taken either along with or following a meal to avoid GI upset. If the dosage of cyclophosphamide exceeds 100 mg, the clinician can anticipate that only 75% of the dose will be absorbed via the GI tract. Therefore, for doses that exceed 100 mg, the dose should be split. Weekly or biweekly monitoring of the patient's

CBC, liver and renal function tests, and uric acid level are necessary, given the potential toxicities of these agents.

Severe hypertension (greater than 180 mm Hg systolic and 110 mm Hg diastolic) can be treated with one antihypertensive agent or a combination of agents. Hemolysis that is secondary to severe hypertension may present in a patient that is known to the clinician, in which case drug therapy should be adjusted according to the history of treatment for the individual patient. (See the section on management of hypertension in Chapter 35.)

HELLP syndrome typically occurs during the third trimester of pregnancy. Because of its late onset in pregnancy, delivery of the infant is the treatment of choice. Most hematological indices return to baseline within 2 to 3 days after delivery; however, thrombocytopenia may persist for a week or more.

DIC requires treatment with heparin and platelet transfusions (replacement therapy). Platelet transfusion thresholds run as low as 20,000/mcL to minimize the risk of spontaneous bleeding, 50,000/mcL in the setting of active bleeding, or higher in the anticipation of invasive procedures. Platelet transfusions, however, are often futile because of severe consumptive coagulopathy that quickly extracts platelets from the circulation.

Although the role of heparin is controversial, especially before or after surgery, heparin is mandated if thrombus is diagnosed in DIC. In addition, fresh frozen plasma is an important therapy in DIC. It is often used empirically, rather than waiting for tests that specifically confirm deficits in certain clotting factors. Before symptoms are present, anticoagulation in the form of low molecular weight heparin (LMWH) such as enoxaparin (Lovenox) is an accepted therapy for patients at risk of postoperative deep vein thrombosis, provided renal function is normal (since LMWH is renally cleared). There are also recombinant versions of certain human clotting factors such as factor VIII that are available for use in significant bleeding disorders.

Because patients who require heparin therapy for DIC require around-the-clock nursing care, they should be admitted to a hospital, where they can receive 500 to 750 U/hr of heparin, according to established weight-based dosing nomograms. Platelet transfusions should be used to maintain the thrombocyte count. In addition, cryoprecipitate should be given to raise the fibrinogen level to 150 mg/dL or more.

Prevention of hemolysis caused by low levels of G-6-PD by avoiding hemolytic triggers is preferred to treating hemolysis once an attack has initiated; however, the primary-care clinician must understand both prevention and treatment strategies for hemolysis resulting from G-6-PD deficiency. Avoidance of oxidant drugs, such as dapsone (Avlosulfon), quinidine (Quinaglute Dura-tabs), and sulfonamide drugs (e.g., sulfamethoxazole/trimethoprim), as well as environmental triggers such as naphthalene (moth balls), is critical to prevent hemolysis in patients who are G-6-PD-deficient. Treatment for acute hemolytic attacks consists of discontinuing all oxidant drugs, increasing oral and/or IV fluids, and administering RBC transfusions as indicated by the Hct level. Screening for G-6-PD among patients who may require one or more oxidant drugs has become standard in the management of patients with HIV/AIDS (sulfamethoxazole/trimethoprim prophylaxis or treatment for *Pneumocystis jiroveci* pneumonia) and patients such as elderly women who are susceptible to urinary tract infections (UTIs) and may require frequent antibiotic treatment.

FOLLOW-UP AND REFERRAL

If normocytic anemia is not accompanied by an abnormal reticulocyte count or abnormal erythrocyte morphology, then follow-up every 6 months is sufficient for most patients, and no referral is required for these patients. Follow-up should consist of a history and physical examination, along with a CBC and reticulocyte count. The patient's records should be constructed so that these values are readily retrievable to allow for long-term monitoring.

If the peripheral smear is positive for spherocytes, sickle cells, or schistocytes, the primary-care practitioner should refer the patient to a hematologist for further diagnostic evaluation and management. The hematologist will create a plan of care, which the primary-care practitioner can co-manage. Routine follow-up with the hematologist should occur every 3 to 6 months, depending on the severity and chronicity of the underlying pathologic mechanism of the anemia, such as hemolysis.

If the reticulocyte count is low and the clinician discovers a low WBC and platelet count as well, the patient is diagnosed with pancytopenia, and referral to a hematologist is indicated. If the evaluation of a bone marrow aspirate suggests the need for treatment, the hematologist will determine the plan of care. Normal or high WBC and platelet counts rule out pancytopenia, which suggests the need for referrals to specialists who can diagnose and treat the underlying cause of the normocytic anemia. These referrals may include gastroenterologists, hepatologists, rheumatologists, infectious disease specialists, nephrologists, or cardiologists.

Patient Education: Normocytic Anemia

Education for patients should follow the pattern outlined in the section on microcytic anemia, addressing self-care regimens and primary-care management. Self-care of normocytic anemia is similar to that for other anemias. The patient should be instructed to remain as active as possible, and, if he or she becomes fatigued, to rest. In addition, the patient must remain vigilant for the signs and symptoms of a declining Hct—malaise, fatigue, shortness of breath, tachycardia, and palpitations. If a deficiency in G-6-PD is diagnosed, the patient should be made aware of this and of all the potential oxidant drugs and chemical exposures that could trigger hemolysis and should be avoided.

Patient education concerning primary-care management should address topics including their underlying cause of normocytic anemia. Because of the chronicity of several of these causes, patients must be instructed at every visit to adhere to their treatment regimens and follow-up plan, including pertinent laboratory testing. For example, sickle cell disease patients require frequent follow-up, infectious disease prophylaxis, and assistance from their families during sickle crises. Establishing a plan for the management of sickle cell crises is an important preparatory step in anticipation of an event and is discussed in greater detail later in this chapter in the section on sickle cell anemia.

MACROCYTIC ANEMIA

Macrocytic anemia (or megaloblastic anemia) is defined as anemia with an MCV equal to or greater than 100 fL. These anemic states are typically normochromic and may be normoblastic or megaloblastic with large erythroid precursors. Macrocytic anemias result most commonly from defects in DNA metabolism or changes in RBC membrane structure.

EPIDEMIOLOGY AND CAUSES

The prevalence of macrocytic anemia is greatest among people of northern European and Caucasian descent. Incidence increases past 60 years of age, but it has been observed in all age-groups. Overall, both sexes are equally affected by macrocytic anemia, although certain forms show a gender predisposition, particularly as related to autoimmune phenomena that are more common in women.

Macrocytic anemia has four general categories of causes: (1) vitamin B_{12} deficiency, (2) folate deficiency, (3) antimetabolite drugs such as methotrexate, and (4) miscellaneous etiologies. The most common cause of megaloblastic anemia is a hereditary autoimmune disorder called pernicious anemia, which results in vitamin B_{12} deficiency, a critical component to the RBC maturation pathway and effective erythropoiesis. In contrast to other forms of macrocytic anemia, pernicious anemia affects women more than men at a rate of 5:1, with peak onset occurring in midlife, often after the age of 40 years.

PATHOPHYSIOLOGY

Vitamin B_{12} Deficiency

Pernicious anemia is a macrocytic anemia caused by a hereditary autoimmune disorder in which destructive antibodies are directed against intrinsic factor, a 45 kDa protein produced by gastric parietal cells that binds to dietary vitamin B_{12} (cobalamin) during the digestion and absorption of nutrients, which is critical to DNA synthesis and RBC maturation. Under normal conditions, dietary vitamin B_{12} is cleaved from carrier proteins in the acidic environment of the stomach by the protease pepsin. It is then rapidly bound by cobalamin-binding factors known as R-proteins, which are found in gastric secretions and the saliva. As these complexes are not absorbable, they pass out of the stomach and into the duodenum. However, the alkaline environment produced by pancreatic proteases in the duodenum allows for the release of vitamin B_{12} from R-factor and its subsequent rapid, high-affinity binding to intrinsic factor. This newly formed vitamin B_{12}–intrinsic factor complex then binds to specific receptors for this complex (e.g., cubilin) in the ileum, where absorption into ileal enterocytes is mediated primarily by transcobalamin II (complexes bound to transcobalamin I and transcobalamin III are metabolically inert).

Vitamin B_{12} is essential to the maturation of erythrocytes via the conversion of homocysteine into methionine and the demethylation of tetrahydrofolate. Demethylated tetrahydrofolate is a key component in the conversion of deoxyuridate to thymidylate and in purine synthesis involved in DNA metabolism. Anti-intrinsic factor antibodies are present in up to three-fourths of all patients with pernicious anemia and act either by blocking the binding of vitamin B_{12} to intrinsic factor or by blocking the binding of the cobalamin-intrinsic factor complex to ileal enterocyte receptors. In addition, autoantibodies produced against gastric parietal cells and pathogenic $CD4^+$ T cells act in concert to destroy gastric parietal cells, producing a morphological change in the stomach lining known as atrophic gastritis.

A subsequent decrease in gastric acid production compounds vitamin B_{12} deficiency, as cobalamin cannot be freed from its carrier proteins in the less acidic stomach environment, thereby preventing its subsequent binding to intrinsic factor in the duodenum. Prolonged use of medications that counter gastric acid production such as histamine-2 blockers (e.g., ranitidine, famotidine, cimetidine) and proton pump inhibitors (e.g., esomeprazole, omeprazole, pantoprazole) have a similar effect. The widely used diabetic drug metformin (Glucophage) also decreases vitamin B_{12} absorption in up to one-third of patients taking this medication.

Thus, insufficient levels of vitamin B_{12} cause erythrocytes to expand in size compared with normal RBCs, thereby producing a characteristic megaloblastic anemia. In turn, pernicious anemia is characterized by a macrocytic anemia, a low serum level of vitamin B_{12}, atrophic gastritis, achlorhydria secondary to gastric atrophy, and a greater probability of other autoimmune diseases, such as hypothyroidism and vitiligo.

Normally, the complex of vitamin B_{12} and intrinsic factor is absorbed through the terminal ileum and then travels to the liver where it is stored. Studies have estimated that the liver may store up to 5,000 mcg/day of vitamin B_{12}. Because the body requires no more than

10 mcg/day, liver stores of vitamin B_{12} typically last for several years before anemia ensues. Therefore, megaloblastic anemia is insidious in onset. In patients with HIV disease and liver dysfunction, both the depletion of liver stores of vitamin B_{12} and the destruction of storage sites within the liver have been identified as underlying causes of megaloblastic anemia.

Dietary deficiency of vitamin B_{12} in the typical American diet is rare because of its rich supply of animal proteins. However, because meats and dairy products are the only dietary source of vitamin B_{12}, vegetarians and particularly vegans (who completely avoid all meat and dairy products) may consume inadequate amounts of vitamin B_{12}. Other reasons for poor absorption include a number of mechanical causes, such as those associated with surgical GI resections (e.g., partial or total gastrectomy, resections of the terminal jejunum or proximal ileum) and Crohn's disease, which can destroy sections of the small intestine where absorption of vitamin B_{12} would otherwise occur.

Folic Acid Deficiency

Folic acid is a critical nutrient that acts in concert with vitamin B_{12} to further nuclear maturation in erythrocytes. Folate deficiency leads to decreased levels of tetrahydrofolate, an important building block of DNA. As with vitamin B_{12} deficiency, abnormal erythroid precursors deficient in folate are prone to intramedullary hemolysis within the bone marrow, leading to a characteristic anemia clinically indistinguishable from that of vitamin B_{12} deficiency. Animal models have also demonstrated that RBC precursors in folate deficiency are more prone to apoptosis (programmed cell death), although human studies are less definitive. However, in contrast to vitamin B_{12} deficiency, folic acid deficiency does not produce neurological sequelae.

Macrocytic anemia due to folate deficiency presents with a low serum folate level and a normal level of vitamin B_{12}. It is almost always related to inadequate dietary intake, although folic acid is found in citrus fruits, dark green leafy vegetables, and animal proteins. Adequate dietary intake is 50 to 100 mcg/day, except in pregnant women who need 800 mcg/day to prevent neural tube defects during fetal development. Even in developed countries such as the United States, pregnant patients may not consume adequate amounts of folate in their diets, with folic acid deficiency increasing in incidence in multigravid patients and with multigestational pregnancies.

Less common causes of folic acid deficiency are impaired metabolism and storage of folate. The liver typically stores enough folic acid as N^5-methyltetrahydrofolic acid (approximately 5,000 mcg) to serve the body's needs for several months, given the body's use of 50 to 100 mcg/day, as long as hemolysis and increased erythrocyte production are not issues, as in sickle cell anemia. There are many causes of impaired folate metabolism and hepatic storage, including chronic alcohol use resulting in decreased enterohepatic cycling and drugs such as phenytoin (Dilantin), sulfamethoxazole/trimethoprim (Bactrim), methotrexate, and oral contraceptives, which contribute to folic acid deficiency via a variety of mechanisms.

Impaired absorption of folic acid is another cause of folic acid deficiency. Tropical sprue, surgical removal of even part of the GI tract, inflammatory bowel diseases such as Crohn's disease and ulcerative colitis, and some intestinal parasitic infections are the primary causes of impaired folic acid absorption. Unlike vitamin B_{12}, however, folic acid can be absorbed along the entire GI tract.

Antimetabolite Drugs

Any chemical that serves as a potential inhibitor of DNA or RNA synthesis is a potential cause of macrocytic anemia. Drugs such as hydroxyurea (an inhibitor of ribonucleotide reductase), the antiviral zidovudine, and the chemotherapies methotrexate, azathioprine, and 6-mercaptopurine can all cause macrocytosis, with methotrexate being best known for leading to anemia. Methotrexate interrupts purine metabolism in the liver by competitively preventing molecular binding of folic acid with dihydrofolate reductase, an enzyme required for the storage of folic acid. Thus, less folic acid can be stored, thereby leading to a reduction in serum folate levels.

Miscellaneous Etiologies

Various unrelated causes of macrocytic anemia include thiamine or pyridoxine-responsive anemias and Lesch-Nyhan syndrome. Macrocytic anemia may also be caused by chronic alcoholism (i.e., ingestion of at least 80 g of alcohol per day), possibly via changes in RBC membranes caused by the alcohol breakdown product acetaldehyde. In addition, liver disease may lead to macrocytic anemia, possibly via increased lipid deposition in RBC membranes and myelodysplasia, which causes a normoblastic (albeit macrocytic) anemia.

CLINICAL PRESENTATION

Subjective

Patients with macrocytic anemia may present with stomatitis, glossitis, nausea, anorexia, diarrhea, peripheral neuropathies, and malaise if they have pernicious anemia. Macrocytic anemia due to other causes will present similarly. Patients may also have complaints consistent with peripheral neuropathy (e.g., numbness of tingling of the hands and feet, decreased reflexes, positive Babinski sign [upward plantar flexion]), which does not occur in folate deficiency, but is part of the symptom constellation associated with chronic vitamin B$_{12}$ deficiency.

Objective

The clinician may note any of the following findings on physical examination: pale or icteric mucosa, a dry and cracked oropharynx, a thickened and smooth-surfaced tongue, tachycardia, a systolic ejection murmur, tachypnea, and diffuse abdominal tenderness without organomegaly. Long-standing vitamin B$_{12}$ deficiency may also result in a variety of neurological signs and pathological manifestations, including peripheral neuropathy in a glove and stocking distribution on the distal extremities, increased or decreased deep tendon reflexes, impaired position sense, diminished vibratory sensation in the lower extremities, a positive Romberg sign, a variable Babinski sign, and pronounced irritability or other mental status changes, including frank dementia in severe cases. Of the megaloblastic anemias, neurological signs related to myelin defects in the dorsal and lateral spinal columns present only in vitamin B$_{12}$ deficiency and not with isolated folic acid deficiency.

DIAGNOSTIC REASONING

Diagnostic Tests

Initial testing involves confirmation of a megaloblastic macrocytic anemia on a peripheral blood smear. Expected findings include anemia and an elevated MCV (greater than 100 fL). MCHC is typically within normal limits, as the anemia is usually normocytic. It is important to note that the pathological processes that underlie macrocytic anemia may occur simultaneously with causes of microcytic or normocytic anemia, such as iron deficiency and thalassemia (microcytic) or ACD (normocytic). In these mixed anemias, MCV may actually be within a normal range, and the RBC indices are difficult to predict, typically requiring referral to a hematologist.

Reticulocytes may be either low or normal in number, depending on the cause of the anemia. If the cause of macrocytosis is a deficiency in vitamin B$_{12}$, then the serum level should be less than 0.1 mcg/mL and hypersegmented neutrophils will be present on the peripheral smear. Macro-ovalocytes will also be evident. In the case of folic acid deficiency, the serum folate level will typically be less than 3 ng/mL, although levels may vary in patients with chronic deficiency. Homocysteine and methylmalonic acid levels can distinguish between these two etiologies, with both values being elevated in vitamin B$_{12}$ deficiency, whereas only homocysteine levels are elevated in folic acid deficiency. Common to both etiologies is a high serum iron level and findings consistent with mild hemolysis, including low

haptoglobin, elevated lactate dehydrogenase (LDH), and mildly increased unconjugated bilirubinemia.

The Schilling test is rarely performed today but was classically used to diagnose GI malabsorption as a common etiology of vitamin B$_{12}$ deficiency. The Schilling test uses orally administered radiolabeled vitamin B$_{12}$ to measure the ability of the small intestine to absorb vitamin B$_{12}$, which is subsequently secreted in the urine. It involves a two-stage 24-hour urine collection that needs to be done before any radioactive diagnostic scans are performed, as the material used in these scans may confound measurements of the radiolabeled vitamin B$_{12}$.

When diagnosing iatrogenic etiologies of macrocytic anemia, it is important to recognize that blood levels of specific drugs such as the antimetabolite methotrexate may vary according to individual laboratory standards. Additional tests may be indicated to assess for changes in liver function that may also be impaired by drugs, as reflected in elevations of hepatic transaminases (alanine aminotransferase [ALT] and aspartate aminotransferase [AST]), bilirubin, and LDH. Urobilinogen may also be identified in the urinalysis.

Differential Diagnosis

The differential diagnoses for macrocytic anemia include all of the causes identified in this section: vitamin B$_{12}$ deficiency, folate deficiency, antimetabolite drugs, and miscellaneous causes. In addition, the differential diagnosis includes anemia of chronic liver disease and myelodysplasia.

A thorough patient history often leads the clinician to the cause of the anemia even when diagnostic laboratory results might be equivocal. For example, if the patient is pregnant, then the clinician should suspect folate deficiency over vitamin B$_{12}$ deficiency. In addition, megaloblastic anemia due to vitamin B$_{12}$ or folate deficiency is also often characterized by thrombocytopenia and neutropenia due to defects in megakaryocyte and myeloid precursors. This same pancytopenia is also commonly seen in the various types of myelodysplasia.

MANAGEMENT

A general management approach to the patient with macrocytic anemia should address the cause of the anemia, as well as the downstream effects of the anemia itself. Thus, the goal is to correct or ameliorate the underlying cause while addressing clinically significant sequelae of the anemia. For example, it might be appropriate to deliver supplemental vitamin B$_{12}$ or folate while providing RBC transfusions as needed. Transfusion is rarely indicated for macrocytic anemia, other than in severe cases. These patients are often elderly and unable to handle large-volume transfusions, given the risk of fluid overload.

If the cause of vitamin B_{12} deficiency anemia is not pernicious anemia and malabsorption, then the clinician may follow these guidelines for oral supplementation: prescribe up to 1,000 mcg/day of oral cobalamin until normal serum levels of vitamin B_{12} are achieved (usually in 6 to 12 weeks after the initiation of therapy). High doses such as these may even be effective in some cases of pernicious anemia, despite the lack of intrinsic factor, given the presence of an additional, albeit less efficient, GI absorption pathway that functions independently of intrinsic factor and does not require absorption through the terminal ileum. Daily oral therapy, however, requires a high degree of patient commitment and compliance.

In most cases of pernicious anemia, especially if neurological symptoms are present, more aggressive therapy is warranted. In these cases, the preferred route of administration is parenteral with 1,000 mcg of vitamin B_{12} intramuscularly daily for the first 7 days, then weekly for 1 month, followed by once monthly administration for life. Lower parenteral doses of 100 mcg have been advocated, although toxicity related to vitamin B_{12} overtreatment is not typically observed, as excess vitamin B_{12} is excreted in the urine. After depleted stores are replaced, patients may transition to oral, sublingual, or nasal preparations of vitamin B_{12} for ease of administration; however, serum levels of vitamin B_{12} and methylmalonic acid should still be followed periodically to ensure compliance with these medication regimens.

For folic acid deficiency, the clinician should prescribe 1 mg/day of supplemental folic acid. The effects of therapy should be reassessed after 2 to 3 months. It is critical to understand that treatment of folic acid deficiency will reverse many of the hematological defects shared with vitamin B_{12} deficiency; however, the neurological manifestations of cobalamin deficiency will progress and may be devastating if treated inappropriately with folic acid supplementation alone. Thus, it is important to rule out vitamin B_{12} deficiency before starting a folate replacement regimen, and if empiric therapy must be started before testing is available, patients should be treated with both folic acid and vitamin B_{12} supplements until each deficiency is ruled out. Patients suspected of having either condition who do not respond with a significant reticulocytosis after 1 week of therapy should be evaluated further for a mixed anemic process, which may have been originally masked by megaloblastic manifestations. Note that occasionally even one nutritious and well-balanced meal can normalize folate levels in a person with true deficiency.

If the cause of the macrocytic anemia is an antimetabolite drug or other iatrogenic drug toxicity, the patient should discontinue all suspected drugs. Laboratory tests for elevated drug levels should be ordered; liver transaminases (AST, ALT) should also be monitored for evidence of liver dysfunction, as well as coagulation times (PT/INR and PTT) as an indication of hepatic synthetic function. For patients with macrocytic anemia from miscellaneous causes, the individual etiologies and underlying disorders must be addressed.

It is also important to evaluate serum potassium levels in profoundly anemic patients once they start treatment, as increased erythropoiesis will markedly increase potassium utilization. As a result, as the anemia corrects, these patients may become significantly hypokalemic, requiring oral potassium repletion.

FOLLOW-UP AND REFERRAL

Follow-up of the patient with vitamin B_{12} deficiency involves assessing the severity of the anemia. Serial CBCs and monitoring of vitamin B_{12} levels are required on a monthly basis after starting oral cobalamin therapy. If parenteral therapy is initiated, more frequent testing is required (e.g., every 2 weeks). Additional testing includes liver function tests; if these reveal elevated transaminase levels before cobalamin replacement is started, then their course should be evaluated every 2 to 4 weeks. If liver enzyme levels rise after the start of therapy, more frequent testing might be required, as well as additional diagnostic testing for evolving hepatotoxicity.

Referral for vitamin B_{12} deficiency is often not required unless the diagnosis is pernicious anemia or the patient suffers from a particularly difficult to diagnose mixed anemic process. A hematologist and gastroenterologist should be consulted in the event of pernicious anemia, as these patients are at greater risk for gastric cancer, carcinoid tumors, and colorectal carcinoma. Thus, stool should be monitored periodically for occult blood as a trigger for colonoscopy. In addition, the hyperhomocysteinemia that accompanies vitamin B_{12} or folic acid deficiency is a risk factor for atherosclerosis and venous thromboembolism and should be addressed as an independent risk factor.

Follow-up of the patient with folic acid deficiency consists of a CBC and serum folate level drawn 2 to 3 months after starting therapy. The problem should be corrected by this point if the patient has adhered to the daily regimen of folic acid replacement. No referrals are indicated unless the anemia does not resolve.

Patient Education

Patients need to learn how to enrich their diets with folic acid and vitamin B_{12}. Increasing dark green leafy vegetables in one or two meals daily can support supplements and other therapies. In addition, patients should be educated about the basic signs and symptoms of macrocytic anemia so that they can self-monitor the effectiveness of therapy and possible recurrence of the anemia.

SICKLE CELL ANEMIA

Sickle cell anemia is an autosomal recessive disorder. The disease is caused by a point mutation in the DNA sequence of the gene for the beta-hemoglobin chain (termed the *hemoglobin S gene*), resulting in a marked hemoglobinopathy in which intracellular hemoglobin molecules form abnormal polymers that cause gross sickling of RBCs under hypoxic conditions. It is therefore diagnosed by the detection of sickled (scythe-shaped) cells on peripheral blood smear, a positive family history, recurrent painful episodes of vaso-occlusive pain, and a pattern demonstrating mutated hemoglobin S on a hemoglobin gel electrophoresis profile.

EPIDEMIOLOGY AND CAUSES

Sickle cell anemia and sickle cell trait are inherited conditions that occur most commonly in people of West African descent. The disease has also been identified in persons of European or Middle Eastern ancestry, although these cases are extremely rare. The disease is not prevalent among persons of Asian or Pacific Island descent.

Initial symptoms appear within the first year of life for those born with sickle cell anemia. Given the perinatal manifestations and associated comorbidities, prenatal screening is now available for at-risk couples, consisting of DNA analysis from fetal cells. The procedure should be offered to these couples as part of their prenatal counseling. If both the father and mother have sickle cell trait and each carries one copy of the mutated hemoglobin S gene, their offspring have a one in four chance of developing true homozygous sickle cell anemia. In more than 40 states, newborns undergo universal neonatal screening for hemoglobinopathies, including hemoglobin protein electrophoresis screening for sickle cell disease, the thalassemias, and other variant hemoglobinopathies.

Autosomal recessive genes for hemoglobin S are distributed equally between both sexes. Individuals who are homozygous for the hemoglobin S gene will develop sickle cell anemia and experience recurrent sickle cell crises throughout their lives. In addition, overall life expectancy is typically reduced to between 40 and 50 years of age. Those who are heterozygous for the hemoglobin S gene are said to carry the sickle cell trait, which is asymptomatic because hemoglobin A accounts for more than half of their hemoglobin. Approximately 8% to 10% of persons of West African descent in the United States carry the sickle cell trait, whereas 1 in 400 African Americans suffers from actual sickle cell anemia. Sickle cell disease also affects individuals of other ethnicities, but at much lower rates, with approximately 100,000 Americans in total affected by the disease, the vast majority of which being of African descent.

PATHOPHYSIOLOGY

The cause of sickle cell anemia is a point mutation in the genetic sequence of the beta-chain hemoglobin gene, which results in the replacement of glutamic acid by valine at the N-terminal amino acid position 6 of this protein chain. The substitution of valine leads to the production of hemoglobin S, which is poorly soluble and prone to rigid polymerization when in its deoxygenated state. This typically occurs under conditions of physiological stress, such as physical overexertion, muscle tissue ischemia causing lactic acidosis, dehydration, infection, or exposure to cold environmental temperatures. However, the majority of acute sickling events have no identifiable cause.

Polymerized deoxyhemoglobin S takes on a rope-like form, aligning itself with other polymerized strands and transforming erythrocytes into a rigid, sickled, crescent-like shape. In turn, these sickled erythrocytes regularly become lodged in the microvasculature of various organs and bodily tissues, causing small but highly symptomatic infarcts throughout the body. Sickled cells adhere rigidly to the inner membranes lining small blood vessels, inducing intimal hyperplasia that contributes to the obstruction of free blood flow in the smaller capillaries, as well as RBC hemolysis due to adherence to the inner vessel wall. In turn, RBCs in patients with sickle cell disease have an average life span of 17 days, versus the normal length of 100 days.

Sickled cells become lodged in the microvasculature as small thrombi. Once the thrombi are situated against the vascular membrane, they attract plasma proteins, leukocytes, and platelets, creating an occlusion to blood flow. This inflammatory process escalates, as ischemia to the surrounding tissue unfolds. Ischemic injury and infarcts cause pain as perimeter tissue is increasingly starved for oxygen and other nutrients. The rate of sickling increases as tissues become more hypoxic and acidotic. Erythrocytes, with or without hemoglobin S, that are lodged in and around the microthrombi lose intracellular water, which results either in hemolysis occurring before RBC sickling or in escalated sickle cell formation and plasma hyperviscosity. As hypoxia and acidosis increase, more erythrocytes begin to sickle, and nearly all sickled cells in the area of the thrombus will eventually hemolyze.

The body attempts to compensate for this resultant anemia (which is typically normocytic, unless also associated with iron deficiency or a form of thalassemia) with expansion and upregulation of the bone marrow, which has several pathological implications. Chronically elevated WBC counts result in the production of inflammatory cytokines, which further complicates vaso-occlusive crises. The additional blood cell production and vascular flow may also lead to cardiomegaly and eventually high-output congestive heart failure. This results in greater metabolic and caloric requirements as the affected individual ages, leading to stunted growth and lower than average adult weight if the condition is poorly controlled and nutritional requirements are not met with dietary supplements.

Anemia is also worsened by impaired production of the RBC growth factor erythropoietin (which is normally produced in the kidney), due to progressive renal disease from microinfarction of the vasa recta capillaries in the renal medulla. Hemolysis results in hyperbilirubinemia, which predisposes to the development of pigmented cholelithiasis (gallstones). In turn, cholecystectomy is the most common surgical procedure in patients with sickle cell anemia.

The formation of microthrombi occurs in many parts of the body but is especially prone to occur in the chest, vertebrae, and long bones of the legs. In pediatric patients, swelling, tenderness, and inflammation of the hands and feet (especially the fingers and toes, termed *dactylitis*), known as hand–foot syndrome, is a common manifestation before age 2 years. Leg ulcers are also common, typically affecting the skin over the lateral and medial malleoli and subject to infection by *Staphylococcus aureus, Pseudomonas, Streptococcus* species, or *Bacteroides*.

Bone manifestations also occur. As ischemia progresses due to vaso-occlusion, the affected bone eventually infarcts and becomes susceptible to osteomyelitis by *Salmonella* species and, less commonly, *S. aureus*. Severely debilitating noninfectious aseptic necrosis of the hip or shoulder joints may also occur due to vaso-occlusion of the arterial supply to the femoral or humeral heads, resulting in eventual loss of the entire joint.

Organs including the heart, liver, penis, and kidney also tend to be affected by vaso-occlusive crises, particularly during childhood and adolescent years. Priapism (painful and sustained penile erection often lasting several hours) is an emergent condition requiring inpatient treatment with hydration, transfusion, and in some cases surgical intervention to release engorged blood, as ischemia of the penis can lead to tissue necrosis. Retinopathy and its associated complications caused by microvascular ischemia increase in prevalence with age as well, including proliferative retinopathy, retinal hemorrhage and detachment, as well as retinal artery occlusion. Such changes may begin in childhood, and in turn, many patients with sickle cell anemia become blind before the age of 40 years.

Splenic sequestration results when large numbers of sickled erythrocytes become lodged in an engorged, functional spleen during early childhood, resulting in severe anemia and potentially fatal hypovolemic shock, with a mortality rate of 10% to 15%. Because this condition tends to be recurrent, splenectomy is often performed after the first episode. Later in adult life, vaso-occlusive episodes in the spleen lead to autoinfarction, with replacement of the splenic parenchyma by fibrotic tissue, resulting in functional asplenia. Although this precludes the occurrence of splenic sequestration syndrome, splenic autoinfarction results in increased susceptibility to infection by encapsulated organisms, such as *Streptococcus pneumoniae* and *Haemophilus influenzae*.

In addition to splenic sequestration, severe anemia may also result from aplastic crises, in which patients experience extreme suppression of bone marrow erythropoiesis. This is often a postinfectious phenomenon that may follow infection with Epstein-Barr virus, *S. pneumoniae, Salmonella,* and especially parvovirus B19, seen classically in pediatric patients, which directly infects erythroid progenitors. The bone marrow is also susceptible to infarction, which may further exacerbate the chronic anemia.

Sickle cell disease patients are at risk for other life-threatening conditions, as well. In *acute chest syndrome*, bilateral pulmonary infiltrates occur with fever and significant pleuritic chest pain, resulting in a "splinting" pattern of respirations that consists of shallow breaths of suboptimal volume, which leads to progressive atelectasis and hypoxia. This condition may be triggered by vaso-occlusion, pulmonic infection, in situ thrombus formation with pulmonary infarction, or pulmonary emboli associated with bone marrow infarction (including fat emboli). Respiratory failure can occur if the condition is not treated aggressively with IV hydration, RBC transfusion, pain management to relieve respiratory splinting, supplemental oxygen, and antibiotics for documented infection (e.g., community-acquired pneumonia or less commonly bacteremia).

Another serious complication of sickle cell disease is the tendency for cerebrovascular accidents (e.g., strokes, transient ischemic attacks). In fact, a significant percentage of these patients will experience strokes before reaching adulthood, some repeatedly—with the first episode most commonly occurring between 2 and 8 years of age. Myocardial infarction may also occur in the presence or absence of documented coronary artery disease, believed to be due either to vaso-occlusion of the coronary vasculature or to severe hypoxemia resulting from the reduced oxygen-carrying capacity of the blood.

CLINICAL PRESENTATION

Subjective

Subjective findings are associated with the severity of the anemia and with pain. Pain is evident only when there is a crisis, but the subjective findings of anemia may be apparent without concurrent crisis. Thus, apart from sickle cell crises, the subjective findings of sickle cell anemia are similar to those of other types of chronic anemia.

The cardinal subjective symptom of a sickle cell crisis is pain. Pain appears suddenly in the back, chest, abdomen, or extremities, which patients typically characterize as excruciating. It may last for several hours or several days and is unrelieved by rest or change in body position. Massaging the site is of little value in relieving pain.

Other subjective findings may include nausea, anorexia, light-headedness, significant anxiety or panic, heart palpitations, and shortness of breath. Personality traits characteristic of patients who have lived with a chronic debilitating disease may also be present, including depression, anxiety, negative thinking, catastrophizing, delayed psychological maturation, learned helplessness, and addiction disorders involving alcohol or opioid use as a means of self-medicating.

Objective

The patient may present with a low-grade fever (less than 101.3°F [38.5°C]) during and preceding a sickle cell crisis. Additional symptoms may include point tenderness and guarding at the sites of pain, pinpoint pupils, an inability to follow commands, photophobia, tachycardia and a systolic murmur, tachypnea, diminished respiratory excursion, hepatomegaly, a nonpalpable spleen (due to infarction and fibrosis), and pretibial leg ulcers affecting the skin and underlying tissue.

Outside of a sickle cell crisis, the clinician may note characteristic physical findings resulting from chronic bone marrow expansion including a lengthened tower-shaped skull, frontal bossing of the forehead, and fish-mouth deformities of the vertebrae. During the objective examination, the clinician may note chronic effects of hemolysis, such as jaundice or a sallow color to the skin. The patient may appear older than his or her stated years.

DIAGNOSTIC REASONING

Diagnostic Tests

Initial testing involves a CBC and a peripheral blood smear. It should be clear, however, that adults with sickle cell disease do not present de novo. They are typically diagnosed soon after birth and learn to cope with sickle cell crises even as they face delayed physical and psychological maturation. Postnatal infant screening in the United States, therefore, typically includes a hemoglobin electrophoresis to detect sickle cell disease and the various thalassemias, as well as a CBC and peripheral blood smear, although the specific panel of postnatal screening tests differ by state.

Sickled cells will constitute 5% to 10% of the peripheral blood smear in most patients. The elevated reticulocyte count (>10% of the total erythrocyte count) is characteristically accompanied by the presence of Howell-Jolly bodies, which are small remnants of nuclear material from hemolyzed erythrocytes that reflect hyposplenia from autoinfarction, as well as target cells, which are erythrocytes with a deeply stained core surrounded by a lighter-stained margin that resemble a target with a bull's eye. The clinician should also expect the WBC count to be elevated to 12,000 cells/mcL or greater, especially during and soon after a sickle cell crisis.

Further testing may include an indirect bilirubin level, which will be elevated after a sickle cell crisis due to hemolysis. Conversely, haptoglobin, a glycoprotein that binds free hemoglobin released from hemolyzed erythrocytes, will be significantly decreased, as it cannot be replaced quickly enough after a severe hemolytic episode.

Differential Diagnosis

The differential diagnosis for sickle cell anemia includes anemia resulting from other causes, sickle thalassemia (a combination of the hemoglobin S and one of the various thalassemia mutations), hemoglobin C disease (a glutamic acid to lysine mutation in the sixth position residue of the beta-hemoglobin chain), nonspecific abdominal pain, UTI, poisoning, and diabetes mellitus. Each of these mimics some or all of the subjective and objective findings elicited from the history and physical examination in sickle cell anemia patients.

Sickle cell anemia is differentiated from sickle thalassemia by the MCV. The MCV will be low if there is any combination of sickle cell anemia and beta-thalassemia (a microcytic anemia) or normal if only sickle cell anemia is present. Sickle beta-thalassemia is typically a milder but nonetheless significantly morbid condition compared with homozygous sickle cell disease. If there is no production of protein from the other beta hemoglobin gene (known as *sickle beta thal⁰*), these patients will be the most symptomatic, as all of their hemoglobin will be of the S form. Alternatively, reduced but detectable protein production from the other beta-chain gene (*sickle beta thal⁺*) results in a milder condition, as some functional hemoglobin A remains present.

A combination of sickle cell anemia with alpha-thalassemia may cause a slower rate of sickling due to a reduced MCHC in the erythrocytes due to the concurrent alpha-thalassemia. Therefore, the sickle cell crises in these patients are typically less damaging and possibly less painful than those in patients without this sickle thalassemia combination.

Hemoglobin C disorders are differentiated by a milder course of anemia than sickle cell anemia. Indeed, some patients with hemoglobin C disorders may pass their lives without any crises caused by the disorder. The underlying pathology is differentiated from sickle cell anemia by the substitution of lysine instead of valine at amino acid position 6 of the beta-hemoglobin chain. Morphological differentiation between these disorders comes with a peripheral blood smear, which reveals rectangular crystals of hemoglobin C in erythrocytes. With heterozygous sickle cell/hemoglobin C disease (sickle C disease or SC disease), adult patients may still be prone to splenic sequestration crises, as their spleens typically do not autoinfarct and fibrose. There are also rarer forms of doubly heterozygous hemoglobinopathies in which hemoglobin S is combined with hemoglobins A, G, or O.

Nonspecific abdominal pain that mimics sickle cell anemia will have none of the characteristic laboratory markers of sickle cell anemia, other than possibly an elevated WBC count or a low Hct. Sickle cell anemia in crisis usually also manifests with extra-abdominal pain. UTI is linked to sickle cell anemia, as these patients experience UTIs more frequently than other individuals. A UTI can present with excruciating abdominal pain and referred pain to the back and chest. The WBC count is typically elevated, and there could be a low-grade fever with either frank or microscopic blood present in the urine. Thus, the distinguishing differences between isolated cases of UTI and those associated with sickle cell anemia include the history and laboratory markers of sickle cell anemia.

Poisoning with certain agents may present with hypoxemia and acidosis that are similar to what is observed in a sickle cell crisis. For example, ingestion of strong alkalines, such as those contained in household cleaning compounds, causes nausea, vomiting, acute abdominal pain, and dyspnea. The history and CBC should aid in the rapid and almost certain differentiation of poisoning from sickle cell anemia. Diabetes mellitus is also in the differential for sickle cell anemia because of the similarities in blood chemistries in these conditions, including renal and hepatic function tests and an acidic blood pH, as well as urinalysis results and physical examination findings. Again, as is the case with the other differential diagnoses, the history, CBC, and peripheral blood smear should readily differentiate these etiologies, even in an emergent situation.

MANAGEMENT

Initial Management

Folic acid supplementation of 1 mg/day by mouth is indicated, along with a diet that is rich in the B complex vitamins and vitamin C. Significant rehydration is needed as a part of management and is a key to reversing sickle cell crises. It aids in keeping the blood pH normal, thereby preventing acidosis and the sequela of RBC sickling. Hydroxyurea, a chemotherapeutic agent, is a common treatment to increase hemoglobin F levels, an infant hemoglobin form with a higher affinity for oxygen than hemoglobin A or S, which results in less hypoxemia and less sickling of RBCs. In turn, this reduces the frequency of painful sickle cell crises.

Although packed RBC transfusions may be indicated in sickle cell anemia treatment to decrease the fraction of hemoglobin S prone to polymerization, especially in children, transfusions are less commonly used in adults and must always be weighed against the risks of infection (especially with hepatitis C), transfusion reactions, and iron overload. Anemia with a hemoglobin of less than

7 g/dL has been associated with a greater risk of stroke, severe vaso-occlusive episodes, acute chest, and death in children. Chronic transfusions, however, lead to iron overload and iatrogenic hemochromatosis, which can destroy solid organs such as the liver and adrenal glands. Exchange transfusion may be used when the clinical manifestations of sickle cell anemia (e.g., acute chest, priapism) are severe and refractory to initial treatment, in order to decrease hemoglobin S to less than 50% of total hemoglobin.

If osteomyelitis is confirmed with magnetic resonance imaging (MRI), which is the diagnostic imaging test of choice, then antibiotic therapy is required. *Salmonella* predominates in osteomyelitis of sickle cell patients over *S. aureus,* which is seen more commonly in non–sickle cell patients. Dactylitis (painful swelling of the feet and hands during the first several years of life in children with sickle cell anemia) requires urgent treatment, as do aseptic necrosis of the hip and priapism.

Subsequent Management

Management of sickle cell crises often requires hospitalization. General goals include symptomatic control of pain with opioid-type drugs, IV rehydration, oxygen supplementation to re-establish normal or near-normal oxygen tension and to prevent or control acidosis, and vigilance against possible damage to vital organs such as the heart, liver, lungs, and kidneys. Parents or other family members should also be taught how to assess for splenic size so that they can recognize the early signs of splenic sequestration syndrome in affected individuals.

Given the increased risk of infection by encapsulated organisms (e.g., *Streptococcus pneumoniae, Haemophilus influenzae*) in sickle cell anemia patients, prophylactic penicillin should be used in children 2 months to 5 years of age and lifelong in children and adults who have had a splenectomy secondary to splenic sequestration crises. In addition, patients should receive all age-appropriate immunizations according to current vaccine guidelines, including both protein-conjugate (13-valent Prevnar, in infants 2 months and older, children, and adults) and polysaccharide (23-valent Pneumovax in children 2 years and older and adults) antipneumococcal vaccines, Haemophilus influenzae type b (Hib) vaccine, influenza (trivalent inactivated) vaccine, and meningococcal vaccine.

Given the chronicity of sickle cell anemia and the propensity for recurrent sickle cell crises, there is a phenomenon of learned helplessness, narcotic addiction, and drug-seeking behavior that may develop in sickle cell disease patients who are afflicted with chronic pain. These are critical conditions that must be considered when developing a treatment plan for the management of sickle cell anemia, because they can significantly affect the patient's capacity for effective self-care.

Currently, the only cure for sickle cell disease and the other hemoglobinopathies previously discussed is transplantation of hematopoietic stem cells from a human leukocyte antigen–identical related donor, which is the major factor limiting its use, given the paucity of matched donors. However, the ethical challenge of balancing transplant-related morbidity and mortality, which includes strokes and seizures in the early years, has led to changes in transplant protocols in the United States, with the avoidance of total body irradiation in preparing the patient's bone marrow to receive transplanted stem cells as well as the use of less toxic conditioning regimens (such as cyclophosphamide, busulfan, and T-cell depletion using antithymocyte globulin or Campath). A combination of methotrexate and cyclosporine or cyclosporine and prednisone is used for prophylaxis against graft-versus-host disease. The success rate with these techniques is now at least 93%, with a graft rejection rate of 5% to 7%.

FOLLOW-UP AND REFERRAL

Follow-up visits with sickle cell anemia patients should occur every 3 months during periods of stability when patients have not been in crisis for a period of 6 months or more; however, the frequency and duration of crises may increase the required frequency of follow-up examinations with appropriate laboratory evaluations. Routine clinical markers to be assessed at follow-up include a CBC, fasting blood sugar, serum electrolyte panel, renal and liver function studies, and urinalysis. Annual or biannual 12-lead electrocardiograms are also necessary to screen for cardiac pathology.

Every patient with sickle cell anemia should be evaluated at least twice per year by a hematologist. In addition, retinal examinations should be performed by an ophthalmologist on an annual basis. Retinal photographs may be required once retinopathies have been diagnosed. Other referrals become evident as organ function decreases, which may include cardiologists, gastroenterologists, nephrologists, orthopedic surgeons (for aseptic joint necrosis), and general surgeons (for splenectomy).

Patient Education: Sickle Cell Anemia

Education for patients with sickle cell disease should focus on the patient's maturation and personality development, within the context of living with this chronic disease. Secondary gains (in the form of extra attention) that the patient received due to the illness early in life may result in the patient regressing to childish behaviors and coping mechanisms during sickle cell crises. In turn, these patients often present with poor coping skills. Patients who exhibit such regressive behavior should understand that friends, acquaintances, and particularly prospective life partners and spouses may be offended by these behaviors. The patient and his or her family, therefore, should be educated in ways that provide anticipatory guidance to others who witness such events.

Self-care behaviors that may prevent sickle cell crises should be reinforced regularly. These include adequate hydration, folic acid supplementation, avoidance of situations that tax the patient's physical and emotional stamina, and adequate sleep and rest as part of everyday activities. Additional self-care actions include participation in peer support groups, pregnancy prevention unless the patient is prepared for the possibility of additional sickle cell crises during pregnancy and lactation, prenatal counseling and testing of the fetus for DNA evidence of sickle cell disease, and avoidance of alcohol and adrenergic dietary elements, such as caffeine, that can cause diuresis and dehydrate the body.

Self-care also involves the patient's own spiritual practices. Spiritual beliefs and practices provide a unique contribution to the course of disease adaptation. In light of the early death of sickle cell anemia patients compared with the general population, spiritual practices may enhance personal acceptance of the disease. In addition, spiritual practices can marshal inner resources to resolve feelings of hopelessness and helplessness during sickle cell crises.

Because sickle cell disease is a lifelong condition, problems unique to children and adolescents with chronic disease are abundant. There is an important transition period in which the specialty care of these patients typically transitions from a pediatric to an internal medicine setting. Thus, these patients are often shocked to find that they are treated differently in an adult medicine setting, with more stringent requirements for adhering to a chronic treatment plan—especially regarding patient compliance and its relationship to the emergent treatment of chronic pain exacerbations. Peer support groups can be particularly helpful for these patients.

POLYCYTHEMIA

Polycythemia involves an increase in erythrocyte number or concentration, which results in an increase in blood viscosity. The disorder may be either relative or absolute. An Hct greater than 51% in women and 54% in men is characteristic of the condition. The term *polycythemia* is somewhat misleading, as it literally means too many blood cells (*poly* = "many"; *cythemia* = "blood cells"), rather than too many erythrocytes, in particular. Nevertheless, the name is only associated with an increase in erythrocytes.

EPIDEMIOLOGY AND CAUSES

The incidence of polycythemia increases with age. It is more prevalent in men older than 70 years of age compared with women of similar age by a ratio of 2:1. Overall, the incidence is 1.9:100,000 persons. These statistics have remained stable for the past 60 years, according to multiple retrospective analyses. The incidence and prevalence of polycythemia increase among persons who reside at high altitudes, given the body's compensation for the relatively lower environmental oxygen tension through the upregulation of erythropoiesis.

Causes of relative polycythemia include decreased fluid intake, increased fluid loss from the body, and extravasation (redistribution) of vascular fluid into the tissues. Absolute polycythemia, on the other hand, may be caused by either primary or secondary mechanisms. Primary polycythemia involves the proliferation of stem cells independent of erythropoietin and is termed *polycythemia vera*. In contrast, causes of secondary absolute polycythemia include Cushing's syndrome, erythropoietin-secreting tumors, and chronic hypoxia, such as that associated with carboxyhemoglobinemia and residence at high altitudes.

PATHOPHYSIOLOGY

Relative Polycythemia

Relative polycythemia is a condition in which there is a decrease in plasma volume while the total number of circulating erythrocytes remains constant. The underlying pathology is almost always dehydration, which may be either acute or chronic. Acute dehydration is associated with vomiting, burns, crush-type injuries, and fevers, whereas chronic dehydration is an outcome of long-term use of diuretics, such as furosemide. Another chronic cause of dehydration is decreased oral fluid intake, a condition frequently encountered in older adults. Cigarette smoking, though also an important cause of absolute polycythemia, is known to decrease plasma volume. Interestingly, this reduction reverses on cessation of smoking (with a reduction in Hct of 4 or more percentage points in just a matter of days). Terms such as *pseudo-* or *spurious polycythemia, stress erythrocytosis,* and *Gaisböck's disease* have all been used to label chronic states in which plasma volume is reduced while Hct and hemoglobin are elevated.

Absolute Polycythemia

Absolute polycythemia is a condition in which the actual numbers of circulating erythrocytes are increased with a corresponding increase in measured RBC mass. (One exception is *inapparent polycythemia* in which the increase in RBC numbers is counterbalanced by an increase in plasma volume, thereby masking polycythemia on standard blood tests.)

Absolute polycythemia may be divided into primary and secondary categories. Many diagnosticians consider primary disease to be polycythemia vera, which is a chronic myeloproliferative disorder caused by an abnormally dividing pluripotential stem cell that leads to a clonal erythrocytosis that is erythropoietin independent, as well as a variable leukocytosis (increased myelocytes)

and thrombocytosis. Aberrant cell signaling pathways involving tyrosine kinases, tyrosine phosphatases, insulin-like growth factor–1 (IGF-1), and transcriptional dysregulation have all been suggested as causative factors, although 96% of polycythemia vera cases have mutations in Janus Kinase 2 (JAK2). The erythropoietin–erythropoietin receptor pathway does not appear to be affected, however, because erythropoietin levels are typically low in these patients.

Physiologically, erythropoietin has many functions: (1) stimulating mitogenicity (cell division) of progenitor cells, (2) protecting progenitor cells from apoptosis, and (3) inducing specific proteins involved in the differentiation and terminal maturation of erythrocytes, such as ankyrin and spectrin (structural membrane proteins) and the oxygen-binding hemoglobin chains. In turn, primary polycythemia may result from congenital or acquired mutations in erythroid progenitor cells that affect the erythropoietin–erythropoietin receptor pathway. For example, primary familial and congenital polycythemia (also called benign erythrocytosis) is an autosomal dominant disorder thought to result from mutations in the erythropoietin receptor that lead to increased responsiveness of erythrocytes to this growth factor. However, the specific molecular defect remains undefined in many patients.

There are several causes of secondary absolute polycythemia—chronic hypoxia, carboxyhemoglobinemia, Cushing's syndrome, chronic corticosteroid use, erythropoietin-secreting tumors, and cardiopulmonary diseases (the most common cause of secondary polycythemia), which decrease oxygen saturation or diminish renal blood flow. Acquired forms include polycythemia due to chronic hypoxia, such as that associated with prolonged high-altitude living, where the partial pressure of ambient oxygen is decreased. In addition, carboxyhemoglobinemia is a condition associated with tobacco use, in which carbon monoxide–containing cigarette smoke increases levels of carboxyhemoglobin (hemoglobin bound stably to carbon monoxide). This prevents the binding of oxygen to hemoglobin and results in a leftward shift of the hemoglobin-oxygen dissociation curve. This shift reflects a decrease in oxygen delivery to the tissues that is, in turn, compensated by polycythemia.

Cushing's syndrome (abnormal corticosteroid production arising from the pituitary gland [ACTH overproduction], adrenal glands, or a hormonally active tumor [cortisol overproduction]) and chronic exogenous steroid use (either of corticosteroids or anabolic steroids) are both erythrogenic and, if left unchecked, may lead to polycythemia. In addition, the act of blood doping, in which RBC infusions are administered before sporting events by athletes to increase their oxygen-carrying capacity, is an important iatrogenic source of polycythemia. Finally, erythropoietin-secreting tumors tend to be located in the kidneys (e.g., renal cell carcinoma), liver (e.g., hepatocellular carcinoma, hepatoma), uterus (e.g., leiomyomata or fibroids), or central nervous system (CNS) vasculature (e.g., hemangioblastoma).

Although these forms are rare, secondary polycythemia may also be congenital, caused by inborn mutations that alter the oxygen affinity of hemoglobin, leading to decreased oxygen delivery to peripheral tissues with resultant hypoxemia. These include mutations in the alpha- and beta-globin genes that cause a marked increase in oxygen affinity with compensatory polycythemia, congenital methemoglobinemia in which the iron moiety in hemoglobin is trapped in the oxidized ferric state and therefore unable to bind oxygen (mutations in cytochrome b5 reductase prevent reduction of ferric ions back to the oxygen-binding ferrous form), and mutations that lower levels of 2,3-bisphosphoglycerate, a key molecule involved in oxygen delivery to peripheral tissues.

Several other erythroid growth factors have also been shown to exist. Stem cell factor, granulocyte-macrophage colony-stimulating factor, and IL-3 are responsible for the growth of early pluripotent stem cells that give rise to the erythroid lineage. In addition, IGF-1 also stimulates erythropoiesis in early progenitors and appears particularly important in patients with end-stage renal disease who no longer produce adequate amounts of erythropoietin due to parenchymal kidney damage. Type 1 receptors for angiotensin II have also been identified on erythroid progenitor cells, and both angiotensin-converting enzyme (ACE) inhibitors and angiotensin II receptor blockers (ARBs) have been shown to counteract erythrocytosis in renal transplant patients.

Thus, secondary polycythemia may result from any number of mutations that affect these different growth factors, although these molecular lesions tend to be rare and many have only been identified in familial cohorts. Along this same line, iatrogenic polycythemia secondary to excessive use of exogenous RBC growth factors such as erythropoietin-alpha and darbepoetin-alfa should always be considered in patients on medications of this class (either via prescribed or surreptitious use, such as in the case of sports-related doping).

CLINICAL PRESENTATION

Subjective

Because cardiopulmonary disease is the most common cause of polycythemia, the clinician should elicit any history of pulmonary symptoms such as chronic cough, cyanosis, hypersomnolence, shortness of breath, or dyspnea on exertion. Many subjective complaints do not arise until the Hct is greater than 60%. Common complaints include headache, blurred vision, weakness, fatigue, irritability, dizziness, and, on occasion, tinnitus. Epistaxis, however, may be the main presenting complaint, as epistaxis can occur due to mucosal engorgement of the nares and irregularities in clotting. After a warm bath or shower, patients may complain of generalized pruritus, which is caused by the release of histamine from basophils that redistribute from the vascular compartment to the tissues or pool along dilated vascular walls.

Eliciting a detailed smoking history is crucial, as well as an occupational history of persistent exposure to air pollutants. In particular, the constellation of symptoms that reflect chronic carbon monoxide exposure should be assessed in patients with high-risk occupations, such as taxi and bus drivers, toll-booth operators, and underground tunnel or parking garage attendants.

Objective

The clinician should assess for erythromelalgia (burning pain in the hands and feet that is pathognomonic for polycythemia vera), as well as a tendency toward venous and arterial thrombosis or hemorrhage due to thrombocytosis and hyperviscosity. GI manifestations are also common, including peptic ulcer disease and gastroduodenal erosions. These are believed to be from hyperviscosity and increased histamine release. On ocular examination, the clinician may note new vessel growth on the retinae as well as vascular engorgement. Splenomegaly is almost always present. Tenderness may be elicited on palpation of both upper abdominal quadrants. The left quadrant may be tender because of gastric ulceration and the right quadrant because of duodenal ulcers or, infrequently, due to hepatomegaly.

The skin (especially on the face) and mucous membranes have a dark, flushed (plethoric) appearance. The skin appears purplish or cyanotic as a result of inadequate tissue oxygenation, and a ruddy cyanosis may be apparent on the fingers and toes. In addition, Cushingoid features (e.g., round and reddened "moon" facies with acne, high blood pressure, abdominal obesity with thin and weak extremities, a prominent fat pad on the back between the shoulders, reddish stretch marks, osteoporotic bones, hirsutism and irregular menses in women) may be present if Cushing's syndrome or chronic corticosteroid use is the cause of secondary absolute polycythemia.

DIAGNOSTIC REASONING

Diagnostic Tests

Polycythemia tends to be suspected when Hct is greater than 48% or hemoglobin is greater than 16.5 g/dL in women or Hct is greater than 52% or hemoglobin is greater than 18.5 g/dL in men. These levels should always be age-adjusted. Thus, initial testing includes a CBC, which begins the process of differentiating absolute from relative polycythemia.

If the patient has polycythemia vera or one of the other absolute polycythemias, the Hct is typically greater than 55% for women and 60% for men. In fact, if the Hct is not greater than these percentages, Cushing's disease and overuse of steroids should be ruled out, as both cause milder degrees of polycythemia.

By definition, there is an elevated RBC count in absolute polycythemia, but RBC morphology is classically normal on the peripheral blood smear. In the absence of concurrent infection, the WBC count in absolute polycythemia typically ranges between 10,000 and 20,000 cells/mcL. The differential is usually unremarkable except for occasional basophilia. The clinician should expect the platelet count to be elevated and to vary—at times exceeding 1 million cells/mcL.

Secondary tests aid in the differentiation of primary versus secondary causes of absolute polycythemia. The diagnosis of polycythemia vera is based on detecting splenomegaly in combination with an elevated Hct and platelet count. However, a definitive diagnosis of polycythemia vera may call for bone marrow biopsy if other biochemical studies are inconclusive. Erythropoietin levels are usually low in polycythemia vera, and a normal or elevated erythropoietin level necessitates a search for other causes. Secondary testing is directed by the suspected underlying pathology. Pulse oximetry should be measured after minimal exertion as an important part of the diagnostic work-up. In addition, an arterial blood gas drawn to measure the partial pressure of oxygen in arterial blood (PaO_2) and co-oximetry to assess for the effects of carbon monoxide exposure (carboxyhemoglobin) or oxygen-poor methemoglobin may be indicated. Carboxyhemoglobin levels greater than 5% suggest CO poisoning.

If the patient has relative polycythemia, the CBC will reveal an elevated RBC mass, but the Hct will often not be as high as 55% to 60%. Plasma volume may also be measured to help distinguish relative versus absolute polycythemia, but values are not always predictable. In addition, the WBC and platelet counts are lower for relative polycythemia compared with absolute polycythemia.

Differential Diagnosis

The differential diagnoses for polycythemia vera include chronic myeloid leukemia, myelofibrosis, and essential thrombocytosis. Chronic myeloid leukemia has a highly elevated WBC count (30,000 cells/mcL). Myelofibrosis presents with a normal or decreased Hct and an abnormal RBC morphology. Essential thrombocytosis would have a normal Hct with a markedly elevated platelet count. Spurious polycythemia, in which there is a contracted plasma volume rather than a true increase in RBC mass, may be due to diuretic therapy, dehydration, or decreased fluid intake.

MANAGEMENT

In general, the principles of polycythemia management concern the difference between relative and absolute causes. This section, therefore, presents management of polycythemia according to the underlying pathology.

Initial Management

Relative Polycythemia

Relative polycythemia is associated with dehydration; therefore, the key objective is to rehydrate the patient. Rehydration in the primary-care setting generally consists of oral hydration and medication adjustment if the cause of dehydration is related to a pharmaceutical agent, such as a diuretic. Thus, the clinician must decide whether the patient is able to adhere to instructions regarding oral fluid intake and changes in his or her drug regimen. Should IV rehydration be required, other factors must also be considered, such as the patient's age, associated comorbidities (e.g., cardiopulmonary disease such as congestive heart failure), ability to adhere to self-care instructions, and availability of outpatient nursing care to provide adequate monitoring. Because of the complexity of care required for IV rehydration, an acute care or in-hospital setting with adequate nursing management is often the preferred context for IV fluid therapy. Central to the decision to initiate oral versus IV hydration is the capacity of family or other caregivers to assist in the patient's rehydration.

Absolute Polycythemia

Absolute polycythemia management begins with progressive phlebotomies if the Hct is greater than 55% to 60%. Phlebotomy is required to prevent thrombus formation, which can lead to a fatal embolic event, cerebrovascular accident, or myocardial infarction in a polycythemic patient. The goal of phlebotomy is to decrease the Hct to 45% or lower. This goal can be achieved by the weekly removal of 500 mL of whole blood. For example, if the starting Hct is 65% and 3% to 4% Hct is lost with each 500 mL of blood, the goal of a 45% Hct can be reached after five to six phlebotomies. Maintenance of an Hct at or below 45% will require subsequent phlebotomies, and iron deficiency would be expected to develop after repeated phlebotomy.

Patients will report an abatement of symptoms as the Hct falls. Should iron deficiency occur, iron supplementation should not be started because supplements can stymie therapeutic gains achieved by phlebotomy. Despite potential iron deficiency, the fatigue associated with polycythemia should improve once an Hct of 45% or less has been reached.

Initial management of all forms of absolute polycythemia follows the path of phlebotomy outlined above. However, additional guidelines for initial management are specific to the underlying cause, for example, Cushing's disease, corticosteroid use, erythropoietin-secreting tumor, hypoxia, carboxyhemoglobinemia. Surgical resection of the glandular source may be indicated for Cushing's syndrome depending on the source of the excess corticosteroids, for example, the pituitary gland, the adrenal glands, or another tumor site. Tapering of corticosteroids, if possible, is the management of corticosteroid-induced polycythemia. Tumor excision or reduction is the management for erythropoietin-secreting tumors. Oxygen supplementation may be the initial management for chronic hypoxia (if Pao_2 is less than 60 mm Hg), and cessation of smoking is the management for carboxyhemoglobinemia due to tobacco use.

Given the significant risk of clot formation with polycythemia, hydroxyurea (Hydrea) is particularly useful in patients at risk for thrombosis, and low-dose aspirin should be started in all patients (especially those with thrombocytosis) unless contraindicated by another condition. IFN-α is useful in patients refractory to other treatments or in those with significant refractory pruritus, although it may cause troublesome side effects such as flu-like symptoms and depression. Antihistamines may be helpful in treating the pruritus associated with polycythemia vera, although some patients experience significant sedation with these medications (especially older first-generation antihistamines with greater CNS penetration).

Anagrelide (Agrylin) is an antiplatelet agent that reduces platelet count and can be useful in patients with thrombocytosis, although it should be used in caution in patients with coronary artery disease. Allopurinol should be used in patients with significantly elevated uric acid levels due to high RBC turnover, provided any acute gout attack has already been treated with colchicine, as allopurinol may precipitate uric acid deposition in the joints.

Subsequent Management

Subsequent management follows the steps taken in initial management. Patients with polycythemia vera will require repeated phlebotomies. Nonalkylating agents may be employed to suppress stem cell formation, such as hydroxyurea (Hydrea) 60 to 80 mg/kg three times per week. Alkylating agents such as busulfan (Myleran) may also be used (1–3 mg/day as maintenance, with higher doses for induction), but these medications carry a risk of long-term leukemia development. Also, the risks of myelosuppression, such as systemic infection, must be considered with all of these agents, particularly if used at higher doses.

Secondary maintenance of patients with absolute polycythemia may also include antiplatelet aggregation therapy with aspirin, although this treatment is controversial because the risk of thrombosis is decreased with phlebotomy alone. If aspirin is used, a dose in the range of 81 to 325 mg/day should be sufficient, although there is no consensus among hematologists and oncologists regarding the effectiveness of long-term aspirin or the most appropriate dose in this population.

FOLLOW-UP AND REFERRAL

Relative Polycythemia

After dehydration has been treated, usually no long-term follow-up or referral is required in these patients, provided the underlying cause of the dehydration has been addressed. However, follow-up of patients who receive diuretics should be based on the need to monitor electrolytes and the therapeutic aims of diuretic therapy (e.g., follow-up of cardiac function). In turn, evaluating for normal potassium and sodium levels is an important goal of follow-up visits typically scheduled at 3-month intervals for patients maintained on chronic diuretic therapy.

Absolute Polycythemia

Because weekly phlebotomies are required to achieve and maintain an Hct of 45% or less, weekly CBC assessments and a brief office visits are needed in these patients. An initial referral to a hematologist is also required to confirm the diagnosis and establish the plan of care. If secondary management strategies such as myelosuppression are required, the primary-care practitioner should rely on the hematologist for recommendations and co-management. Specialty referral is also important because polycythemia vera carries a significant risk of transforming over time into myelofibrosis with myeloid metaplasia or acute myeloid leukemia.

Referrals to surgeons are required for tumor excision or pituitary resection, if indicated. A positive finding on computed tomography of the abdomen or MRI of the brain should involve an immediate surgical consultation. A pulmonary referral may be necessary if the clinician does not detect lower carboxyhemoglobin levels as expected after a patient stops smoking.

Patient Education: Polycythemia

Patients should learn that absolute polycythemia reduces life span. On average, patients live for less than 15 years after this diagnosis because of the risks of thrombosis. Despite this prognosis, however, patients should be reassured that active participation in their care may extend the quality of their lives and increase longevity.

Increased quality of life is associated with improvement in the subjective presentation of the disease. Points to address in patient education include adherence to fluid intake requirements, drug regimens, exercise recommendations, laboratory evaluations, and adherence to follow-up visit schedules with the primary-care practitioner and all specialty referrals.

Fluid intake requirements may fluctuate according to the stage and duration of treatment. As the disease progresses and phlebotomies occur repeatedly, the daily fluid intake should average 2 L for a 70-kg adult. Earlier in the treatment before blood volume is reduced, the necessary fluid intake is likely to be less at 1 to 1.5 L/day. Drug regimen adherence may require learning how to self-medicate with a parenteral agent such as IFN-α. Therefore, teaching the patient and/or caregiver how to deliver the drug is essential to the educational plan.

Instruction regarding exercise is dependent on the patient's level of tolerance for physical activity. The objective, however, should remain clear that increasing the patient's level of activity can reduce thrombosis formation. Simplest among exercise plans for persons older than 60 years of age is regular walking. The clinician should recommend that the patient walk with a partner in a safe place, such as an indoor shopping mall. An alternative is walking from side to side in a pool of waist-high water. This form of aquatic exercise can be helpful for patients with joint and bone-related problems who otherwise experience increased pain when walking out of water.

Adherence to laboratory evaluations may diminish over time as the patient copes with this chronic and indolent fatal disease. Drawing the patient's family and network of social supports into the circle of education may enhance the patient's adherence to follow-up regimens. Call-back schedules for laboratory evaluations that fit with the patient's daily activities and provide rhythm to the patient's life are more likely to generate improved adherence.

Finally, visits to the clinician and specialists are times when patient education should be reinforced. Importantly, addressing and treating depression—an anticipated outcome of absolute polycythemia—can enhance adherence to all other elements of patient education. Therefore, teaching the patient and loved ones to recognize and report depression is a critical component of the educational plan.

LEUKEMIA

Leukemia is a neoplastic disease of malignant hematopoietic stem cells that differentiate and proliferate according to specific lineage trajectories that distinguish the types of leukemia as either acute or chronic. Further classification of leukemia specifies the stage of development and type of WBC (immunophenotype) that is involved in the malignant transformation (see Table 61.2). The involved leukocytes proliferate and occupy space previously filled by nonmalignant cell lines. Thus, one significant outcome of the malignancy is the suppression of nonmalignant blood cells.

EPIDEMIOLOGY AND CAUSES

The incidence of leukemias varies according to childhood and adult age groups. Overall, there is a slight predominance of male to female cases. Acute lymphoblastic (lymphocytic) leukemia (ALL) is the predominant form in children between 2 and 15 years of age, with a higher prevalence among children younger than 5 years of age. Other types of leukemia more commonly strike adults. Acute myelogenous (myelocytic/myeloid) leukemia (AML) may be seen in adults of all ages, but its incidence increases after 40 years of age. Chronic lymphocytic leukemia (CLL) is more prevalent among adults older than 60 years of age; however, it may appear in persons of any age. CLL is the most common leukemia in Western (developed) countries, with a median age of onset of

TABLE 61.2 **Types of Leukemia and General Treatment Considerations**			
	Age at Onset	*Combination Chemotherapy**	*Treatment—Other**
ACUTE LEUKEMIA			
Acute myelogenous leukemia (AML)	All adults but more prominent at >40 years	Daunorubicin (Cerubidine) OR Idarubicin (Idamycin) OR Mitoxantrone PLUS Cytarabine (Ara-C)	Autologous or allogeneic Bone marrow transplantation (BMT) for high-risk patients in first remission
Acute lymphoblastic leukemia (ALL)	2–15 years, rarely in adults	*Induction:* 4-drug regimen Daunorubicin (Cerubidine) Vincristine (Oncovin) Prednisone (Deltasone) Asparaginase (DVP L-asp) *Consolidation:* Daunorubicin (Cerubidine) Cytarabine (Ara-C) *Maintenance:* 4-drug regimen	Central nervous system intrathecal methotrexate and cranial irradiation Allogeneic BMT in high-risk patients in first remission

TABLE 61.2 Types of Leukemia and General Treatment Considerations—cont'd

	Age at Onset	Combination Chemotherapy*	Treatment—Other*
CHRONIC LEUKEMIA			
Chronic myelogenous leukemia (CML)	All patients, but more prominent at >60 years Median age 42 years	Imatinib (Gleevec) PLUS Hydroxyurea (Hydrea)	Allogeneic BMT in chronic phase (greater success in younger patients)
Chronic lymphocytic leukemia (CLL)	>60 years	Cladribine OR Fludarabine (Fludara) OR Chlorambucil (Leukeran) PLUS Cyclophosphamide May be used in combination with rituximab (Rituxan) or alemtuzumab (Campath)	Allogeneic BMT

*For all leukemias, the need for epoetin (Epogen, Procrit), darbepoetin (Aranesp), and/or pegfilgrastim (Neulasta) must be assessed.

70 years. Chronic myelogenous (myelocytic/myeloid) leukemia (CML) strikes middle-aged persons, with a median age of onset of 42 years.

The etiology of leukemia is complex and not fully understood. Researchers have linked leukemia to environmental toxins such as chemical solvents, petroleum products, and insecticides, as well as heredity factors, although familial leukemias are rare. It is unclear whether the incidence of leukemia is higher among adult identical twins compared with other adults; however, CLL in particular appears to have a familial predisposition.

The complications of mutagenic pharmacotherapies used to treat lymphoma, rheumatoid arthritis, or to maintain immunosuppression post-transplantation have provided insight into disease etiology. For example, alkylating agents such as melphalan (Alkeran) and cisplatin (Platinol) have been associated with a 5% to 10% increased incidence of leukemia among patients who have been receiving them for an extended period of time. Likewise, prolonged exposure to high doses of ionizing radiation is also associated with the later development of leukemia. In cases of prolonged toxin and radiation exposure, a latency period of up to 20 years may pass before a leukemia diagnosis develops. Shorter latency periods are seen following exposure to chemotherapeutic agents that inhibit the DNA-splicing enzyme topoisomerase II, such as etoposide, doxorubicin, and mitoxantrone.

PATHOPHYSIOLOGY

There are two staging and classification systems for leukemia. The French-American-British (FAB) classification system, which was first described in 1976, is based on morphology and cytochemical features of the leukemia cells. It is still in use today despite the emergence of cytogenetics and immunophenotyping as important markers in the diagnosis and prognosis of leukemia. A newer, more commonly used classification system was generated by the WHO, which incorporates morphological features, cytochemistry, immunophenotyping, cytogenetics and clinical features.

The 2016 revision to the WHO classification of tumors of the hematopoietic and lymphoid tissues reflects numerous advances in the identification of biomarkers associated with some myeloid neoplasms, lymphoid neoplasms, and AML. These have been derived in large part from gene expression analysis and next-generation sequencing. This update enables the implementation of improved diagnostic criteria, as well as genetic factors of prognostic significance to guide therapy, for the disease entities present in the previous WHO classification.

For example, AML now has several subcategories, one of which is AML with recurrent genetic abnormalities. Within this subcategory alone, there are now eleven types of AML:

- AML with t(8;21)(q22;q22.1); RUNX1-RUNX1T1
- AML with inv(16)(p13.1q22) or t(16;16)(p13.1;q22); CBFB-MYH11
- Acute promyelocytic leukemia (APL) with PML-RARA
- AML with t(9;11)(p21.3;q23.3); KMT2A-MLLT3
- AML with t(6;9)(p23;q34.1); DEK-NUP214
- AML with inv(3)(q21.3q26.2) or t(3;3)(q21.3;q26.2); GATA2, MECOM
- AML (megakaryoblastic) with t(1;22)(p13.3;q13.3); RBM15-MKL1
- Provisional entity: AML with BCR-ABL1

- AML with mutated NPM1
- AML with biallelic mutations of CEBPA
- Provisional entity: AML with mutated RUNX1

Thus, the full complexity of the revised WHO classification system is beyond the scope of this text. However, an overview of the FAB classification system of myeloid and lymphocytic leukemias in both acute and chronic forms is illustrative of the genetic mutations and prognostic factors that underlie the wide variety of leukemias and help to explain their underlying pathophysiology.

Acute Nonlymphocytic Leukemia

By far, the largest number of adults with acute leukemia (as high as 80%) suffer from acute nonlymphocytic leukemia (ANLL), which mainly presents after 40 years of age and increases in incidence with each year thereafter. It originates in the malignant transformation of a single stem cell or a few select cells. At least 85% of all cases have been associated with defined clonal karyotypic abnormalities in all cells of the progenitor line.

ANLL is a category that includes the leukemias also known as AML and acute granulocytic leukemia (AGL), although some classification systems have eliminated the ANLL and AGL nomenclature altogether, in favor of a more comprehensive classification system that categorizes all acute leukemias of non-lymphocytic origin as forms of AML. In the FAB system, ANLL is divided into eight distinct morphologic classes (M0 to M7), with classes M3 to M5 further subdivided into two subclasses each. Each of these subtypes is characterized by one or more cytogenetic abnormalities that can be used to predict prognosis and guide treatment, as they can determine responsiveness to specific chemotherapies. Some of these same genetic abnormalities are incorporated into the revised 2016 WHO classification system. For example, acute promyelocytic leukemia (AML class M3) is associated with a translocation between chromosomes 15 and 17 that juxtaposes the promyelocytic leukemia (PML) and retinoic acid receptor-alpha (RARA) genes, repressing the latter and preventing retinoic acid–induced differentiation of promyelocytes. Nonetheless, this mutation portends a favorable prognosis, as promyelocytic M3 cells are particularly sensitive to therapy with all-trans retinoic acid.

Genetic abnormalities that carry a particularly poor prognosis in ANLL include mutations resulting in monosomy (an entire chromosomal deletion) of chromosomes 5 or 7 or trisomy of chromosome 8. The former monosomies are particularly associated with AML resulting from previous chemotherapy with alkalinizing agents or exposure to ionizing radiation. In contrast, AML associated with past exposure to topoisomerase II inhibiting agents is often associated with mutations in chromosome 11.

Acute myeloblastic leukemia (AML class M2) and acute myelomonocytic leukemia (AML class M4) have both been associated with a balanced translocation between chromosomes 8 and 21, which juxtaposes the transcription factor genes *AML1* and *ETO*, leading to dysregulated transcription of genes directly involved in myeloid cell division (e.g., granulocyte-monocyte colony stimulating factor [GM-CSF], IL-3, and the antiapoptotic gene *BCL-2*). AML class M4 has also been associated with inversions or translocations in chromosome 16, creating a fusion of the genes *CBFB* and *MYH11*, which leads to repressed transcription of genes involved in myelocytic differentiation. Acute monoblastic leukemia (AML class M5) is associated with rearrangements of chromosome 11, whereas mutations in chromosome 3 appear to confer thrombocytosis in the setting of AML.

Acute Lymphoblastic Leukemia

ALL can appear among persons of all ages but is clearly a disease predominantly of early childhood, as noted earlier. B-cell lymphoblasts or, in far fewer cases, T-cell lymphoblasts increase in number after a single hematopoietic stem cell undergoes transformation (immortalization). Interestingly, the cytogenetics of ALL in children differs from that in adults. For instance, the Philadelphia chromosome (a balanced translocation between chromosomes 9 and 22 that juxtaposes and activates the *BCR* and *ABL* oncogenes) is seen in only 5% of childhood cases, while this is the most common abnormality in adult ALL and is found in up to 40% of cases. In contrast, hyperdiploidy (in which greater than 50 chromosomes are found in malignant clones) is seen in up to 30% of childhood cases but in no more than 5% of affected adults.

In contrast to CML (see next section), the presence of the Philadelphia chromosome is a poor prognostic indicator in ALL, contributing to dysregulated activation of the RAS intracellular signaling pathway that leads to uncontrolled cell division. These patients often have additional karyotypic abnormalities such as monosomy of chromosome 7. Studies have shown that ALL patients with the Philadelphia chromosome may be divided into two subsets that are distinguished by differing translocation breakpoints along the BCR gene—one in which this karyotypic abnormality appears restricted to a B lineage lymphoblastic cell clone and another in which the Philadelphia chromosome is further identified in myelogenous cell lines as well, indicating these patients may have a indolent form of CML that underwent a B lineage lymphoblastic crisis at the time of diagnosis.

As with AML, different forms of ALL have been distinguished on the basis of morphology, with certain cytogenetic profiles correlating with each presentation. For instance, ALL of L3-type B-cell origin often shares a translocation of chromosomes 8 and 14 that is also seen in B-cell-derived Burkitt's lymphoma, suggesting that these cancers are varied manifestations of the same underlying malignant transformation event. Pre–B-cell ALL has been associated with translocations between chromosomes

1 and 19, which lead to a fusion protein between the highly active transcription factors *E2A* and *PBX1*, with subsequent immortalization of this early B-cell progenitor that portends a particularly poor prognosis. Infantile ALL has been associated in up to 80% of cases with translocations involving the mixed lineage leukemia (MLL) gene at chromosome 11q23, which is thought to regulate a number of downstream genes involved in lymphocyte differentiation, thereby resulting in extremely poor outcomes. A poor prognosis is also seen in ALL associated with translocations between chromosomes 4 and 11, a mutation that is commonly seen in AML class M5.

A translocation between chromosomes 12 and 21 that produces a fusion protein between the transcription factors *TEL* and *AML1* is the most common mutation seen in childhood ALL. Fortunately, this translocation confers a favorable prognosis in ALL, as does the presence of hyperdiploidy (with 50–60 chromosomes) with occasional structural abnormalities such as partial chromosomal duplications and translocations. Multiple copies of chromosome 21 and the X chromosome are the most common findings in hyperdiploidy, but several other duplications have been noted as well (e.g., chromosomes 4, 6, 10, and 14). The high prevalence of these karyotypic abnormalities in childhood ALL underlies the generally favorable outcomes associated with this form of leukemia in children.

T-cell ALL is a less common entity that typically strikes young men. Related to T-cell lymphomas, these patients may present with particularly high WBC counts, invasion of malignant cells into the CNS via the cerebrospinal fluid, and the presence of a mediastinal tumor. Well over half of these cancers are characterized by mutations in genes coding for the various protein components of the T-cell receptor—alpha, beta, gamma, or delta subunits. The T-cell receptor is a heterodimeric protein composed of either alpha–beta or gamma–delta subunit pairs expressed on the surface of the T cell, which allow for the recognition of specific antigens. Mutations commonly occur in chromosome 14, which encodes the alpha and delta receptor subunits, or chromosome 7, which encodes the genes for the beta and gamma chains. Translocations at these sites typically juxtapose these genes with various transcription factors that lead to dysregulated expression of the receptor subunit and proliferation of the T-cell clone. Mutations in these same chromosomes that do not involve these receptor subunits, as well as in others such as chromosomes 6 and 11, have also been identified in T-cell ALL. Interestingly, prognosis does not appear tied to these particular cytogenetics, and outcomes are generally favorable in both adults and children with T-cell ALL.

Chronic Myelogenous Leukemia

CML (chronic myelocytic leukemia, chronic myeloid leukemia) is most commonly associated with the development of the Philadelphia chromosome in a hematopoietic stem cell that commits to the myeloid lineage. Although differentiation is typically unaffected, the leukemic stem cell is self-renewing and produces a tremendous number of daughter cells, with the same leukemic clone dominating up to 90% of the bone marrow at the time of diagnosis. In this mutation, breaks occur in the DNA resulting in an equivalent exchange of genetic material between chromosomes 9 and 22. Oncogene activation occurs, as the reciprocal translocation [t(9;22)(q34;q11)] juxtaposes the *BCR* and *c-ABL* genes, creating a BCR–ABL fusion protein that confers a proliferative advantage to the leukemic clone, even in the absence of cellular growth factors.

The functions of the native BCR and ABL proteins are not fully elucidated, and neither gene alone is capable of malignant transformation; however, the fusion protein is oncogenic, giving rise to malignant clones through upregulated tyrosine kinase (phosphorylation) activity within a number of intracellular signaling pathways contributing to cell division (e.g., RAS, c-Myc, and JAK/STAT molecular pathways). This explains the effectiveness of treatment with the tyrosine kinase inhibitor imatinib (Gleevec). Depending on the site of the chromosomal breaks, various types of the BCR-ABL fusion protein may be formed. In turn, cells transformed by these different species of fusion protein appear to respond differentially to specific therapies.

Although IL-3 and G-CSF mRNA transcripts are both upregulated in leukemic cell clones, the precise role of cytokines in the dysregulated growth of these cells remains unclear. As with other forms of leukemia, leukemic cell clones appear to arise from a self-renewing pool of mutated leukemic stem cells, which are typically less mature than the differentiated granulocytic leukemic clones themselves. In fact, the Philadelphia chromosome has been identified in a number of cell lineages in CML, including granulocyte, macrophage, erythrocyte, megakaryocyte (platelet), and B-lymphocyte precursor cells, indicating that the mutation first occurs in an early, noncommitted, multilineage hematopoietic stem cell.

The creation of the Philadelphia chromosome may predate the onset of disease symptoms by many years—a pattern suggesting that the disease progresses through a latent or asymptomatic phase before becoming active. For example, the karyotypic abnormality may first arise in the third decade of life, with symptom onset as much as 10 to 20 years later. In fact, normal bone marrow function is characteristic of the disease trajectory in the early years after development of the Philadelphia chromosome. The pool of leukemic stem cells may not be expanded in number; however, leukemic daughter cells undergo clonal expansion and eventually crowd out normal bone marrow components. In addition, cell surface adhesion factors (e.g., beta-1 integrin) are down-regulated, eliminating adhesion-dependent growth inhibition in which normal cells are triggered to stop proliferating after coming into contact with one another.

As with any chronic leukemia, a dreaded complication of CML is degeneration into a leukemic blast crisis, in which leukemic progenitor cells develop self-renewing properties as they undergo further mutations resulting in clonal proliferation of either myeloid or lymphoid (almost exclusively B lineage) blasts, given the widespread presence of the Philadelphia chromosome in multiple lineages. Most commonly, the additional mutations described include trisomies of chromosomes 8 or 19, duplication of the Philadelphia chromosome itself, or mutations in the *p53* tumor suppressor gene on chromosome 17.

These blast cells may express many of the same proteins as hematopoietic stem cells, such as the transcription factor beta-catenin. Both leukemic stem cells and their progeny appear more resistant to apoptosis than wild-type (nonmutated) cells, but the significance of this to the pathogenesis of CML is not fully known. However, resistance to apoptosis appears to be important, as the lifespan of leukemic cell clones is not significantly greater than that of wild-type granulocytes and does not appear to account for their increase in number.

Finally, CML may also occur in the absence of the Philadelphia chromosome mutation, which is known as atypical CML. Up to 15% of CML patients may suffer from this condition, although some hematologist-oncologist specialists have chosen to classify these patients as having a distinct myeloproliferative disease, rather than true CML. For reasons that are poorly understood, these patients have a worse prognosis with a poorer response to therapy and shorter survival times.

Chronic Lymphocytic Leukemia

CLL is a chronic lymphoproliferative disorder typically associated with increased numbers of small B lymphocytes and is clinically indistinguishable from small lymphocytic B-cell lymphoma. After a malignant alteration occurs in a B-cell precursor, thus forming a malignant cell line, the clonal abnormality is passed on to slowly replicating progeny that are functionally incompetent.

The genetics of the malignant alteration in CLL are not as well established as they are for CML. Malignant B-cell clones are known to be frozen in a state of differentiation somewhere between the pre-B- and mature B-cell phase, with rates of proliferation and cell death varying widely among different individuals. These cells express very low levels of surface immunoglobulin, with various B lineage–specific cell surface proteins (e.g., CD19, CD20, CD21), as well as CD5, which is primarily considered a T-cell marker. Variant forms exist that do not adhere to these criteria, although some hematologist-oncologists feel that a proliferation of non–CD5-expressing B cells represents a leukemic phase of non-Hodgkin's lymphoma, rather than true CLL.

The relative percentages of both T cells and natural killer cells are reduced in CLL, although absolute numbers of T lymphocytes may be increased, given the tremendous expansion of lymphocytes. Moreover, some CLL patients demonstrate unusual forms of T cells with low levels of surface CD4 and CD8 proteins. Such nonclassical T cells are also found in other autoimmune diseases. In addition, although hypogammaglobulinemia is common in patients with CLL, immunoglobulin receptors on leukemic cells may demonstrate autoimmune specificity, which may explain the increased frequency of AIHA, idiopathic thrombocytopenic purpura, and pure red cell aplasia in persons with CLL. Given their lack of protective antibodies, infection by Gram negative or encapsulated organisms is the most frequent cause of morbidity and mortality in persons with CLL.

Cytogenetic analysis of CLL cell clones has revealed chromosomal abnormalities in up to 70% of cases. The most frequent karyotypic abnormalities include trisomy of chromosome 12, partial deletions in chromosome 13 that affect the tumor suppressor retinoblastoma (*Rb*) gene, and partial deletions in chromosomes 11 and 17 that are associated with a particularly poor prognosis and shorter survival. The *p53* tumor suppressor gene located on chromosome 17 is often affected, either by deletion or expression of a mutated nonfunctional protein, with both conditions leading to unregulated cellular proliferation. In contrast, the overexpression of survival factors has also been identified in B lineage CLL, including the anti-apoptotic molecules BCL-2 and inducible nitric oxide synthetase.

CLINICAL PRESENTATION

Subjective

Patients with acute leukemia commonly complain of bone and joint pain, as well as fevers, chills, palpitations, shortness of breath, and signs of infection. Patients may also have gingival bleeding associated with gingival hyperplasia. Complaints of skin eruptions, easy bruising, or prolonged bleeding from simple wounds form a significant part of the subjective history.

Patients with chronic leukemia complain of fatigue, night sweats, and low-grade fevers. Although there is no clear differentiation in subjective findings between CML and CLL, CML may present with the symptoms of leukostasis associated with very high WBC counts (greater than 500,000 cells/mcL). The syndrome of leukostasis is characterized by blurred vision, respiratory distress, and occasionally priapism (prolonged and painful erections that last for several hours). Nausea and vomiting may be associated with organomegaly in both types of chronic leukemia. Bone and joint pain are typically limited to the myeloproliferative stages of CML.

Objective

The clinician will often note a high fever in patients with acute leukemia. Tachycardia and tachypnea are related findings. Patients appear pale due to anemia and manifest skin eruptions related to impaired platelet function, such as petechiae and purpura. Confusion due to hypoxemia and fever may be revealed using standardized evaluation tools such as the Folstein Mini-Mental State Exam.

In chronic leukemia patients, heart and lung sounds are typically within normal limits except during states of infection, in which case the lungs may reveal adventitious sounds. Splenomegaly may be evident and variably associated with hepatomegaly and/or lymph node enlargement. Temperature may not be elevated in chronic leukemia, as it often is in acute leukemia, unless the disease has progressed or there is a concurrent infection. In addition, the patient's skin color varies between pale and normal in chronic leukemia, and few, if any, skin eruptions are evident.

DIAGNOSTIC REASONING

Diagnostic Tests

Initial testing for suspected acute leukemia includes a CBC with peripheral blood smear and platelet count. The WBC count may be significantly elevated (more than 300,000 cells/mcL). Granulocytes (polysegmented and banded forms) are typically diminished in number, as are platelets (often less than 50,000/mcL). An Hct of less than 30% is a common finding, especially if the WBC count is markedly elevated. The peripheral smear reveals a blastocystosis of greater than 25% in almost all cases.

Initial tests for suspected chronic leukemia are the same as for acute leukemia: CBC, peripheral blood smear, and platelet count. The WBC count should be elevated in CML and CLL, but typically more so in CML (elevations >100,000 cells/mcL are common). Lymphocytosis, however, differentiates CLL from CML. Lymphocytes occupy as much as 90% of the peripheral smear in CLL. The peripheral smear of CML is characterized by a left-shifted myeloid series, with mature forms of myeloid cells predominant in the smear. Platelets may be elevated and are rarely diminished.

Once leukemia is suspected in the primary-care setting, referral to a hematologist should be initiated in order to conduct further specialized testing, such as a bone marrow aspirate and morphological, immunophenotypic, and cytogenetic studies to determine the specific type of leukemia and guide treatment based on prognostic factors in the updated 2016 WHO classification system. Results should parallel the peripheral blood smear, thus confirming the initial diagnosis with greater accuracy in quantitative and qualitative indices.

For example, in acute leukemia, the bone marrow aspirate reveals hypercellular components, which are dominated by blasts. At least 30% of bone marrow cells must be blasts to diagnose acute leukemia. Auer bodies are rod-shaped structures, present in the cytoplasm of myeloblasts, myelocytes, and monoblasts in leukemic patients. They predominate among myeloblasts in the bone marrow aspirates of patients with AML. Serum chemistry profiles are critical for secondary testing in acute leukemia patients because of rapid cell turnover in the WBC population, which liberates intracellular uric acid and leads to significant increases in serum uric acid concentration.

In CML, bone marrow evaluation typically reveals the presence of the Philadelphia chromosome, along with a left-shifted myelopoiesis. Blasts occupy less than 5% of the aspirated sample. Subsequent testing of CML also includes measuring leukocyte alkaline phosphatase, which is usually low, thus reflecting the abnormal function of neutrophils. Additional testing includes measuring the vitamin B_{12} level and serum chemistries. The vitamin B_{12} level is typically elevated, as is the uric acid level.

In CLL, bone marrow biopsy results confirm the initial peripheral blood smear as well, as small, mature lymphocytes dominate the field. Monoclonal surface immunoglobulin on the malignant lymphocytes aids in distinguishing these small cells from their normal counterparts. Another secondary test, immunoelectrophoresis, further supports the diagnosis of CLL in about half of patients, as the profile from the electrophoresis demonstrates hypogammaglobulinemia.

Molecular methods of cytogenetic analysis (e.g., fluorescent in situ hybridization, Southern blot, reverse transcriptase–polymerase chain reaction) to identify the Philadelphia chromosome and other karyotypic abnormalities are critical for predicting prognosis and determining the most effective treatment plan for each type of leukemia. These analyses have revolutionized leukemia treatment by facilitating the use of individualized, directed therapy and form the basis of the revised 2016 WHO classification system for these blood cancers.

Differential Diagnosis

Acute Leukemia

The left-shifted (immature) bone marrow aspirate of acute leukemia must be distinguished from the left-shifted aspirates that are associated with recent exposure to toxic chemicals and radiation. The clinician should expect that the full recovery period after certain toxic exposures will be at least 6 weeks and may extend to 12 weeks. If exposure to toxins and not monoclonal malignant transformation was the cause of the cellular left-shift, then subsequent testing should reveal maturing cell lines. It is also important to rule out false-positive left-shifted aspirates by repeating the procedure several days later, although some patients may not want to be subjected to this invasive procedure again so rapidly, unless the results will influence imminent treatment decisions.

Acute leukemias must be distinguished from their chronic counterparts and from similar myeloproliferative disorders, such as polycythemia. ALL may also resemble other lymphoproliferative diseases, such as lymphoma and mononucleosis. Therefore, a skilled pathologist is required to differentiate these lymphoproliferative conditions, given their differences in prognosis and treatment plans.

Chronic Leukemia

The Philadelphia chromosome of CML distinguishes this disease from myeloproliferative responses to infection, systemic inflammation, and other malignancies. Clinical wisdom will also help the practitioner to distinguish the leukocytosis of CML from other reactive states. CML will likely present with more than 50,000 cells/mcL, but reactive states will not mount as great an immune response. In addition, CML differs from other myeloproliferative diseases, as the erythrocyte count, RBC indices, and Hct are generally normal in CML.

Microscopic evaluation of a bone marrow aspirate differentiates CLL from other lymphocytic disorders, such as viral infections. In addition, unlike CLL, viral infections will present with flu-like symptoms, which include fever, chills, myalgias, and arthralgias. Thus, CLL is perhaps the easiest among the leukemias to distinguish.

MANAGEMENT

The probability of successful treatment and subsequent cure for acute leukemia decreases with advancing age. In addition, a cure for acute leukemia is less probable if the patient is diagnosed late in the disease trajectory, after several physiological systems have become involved. In general, treatment begins with combination chemotherapy to induce remission (i.e., induction phase), followed by a stage of chemotherapy called the consolidation phase, and finally a prolonged maintenance phase. Unlike the acute leukemias, chronic leukemias usually follow an indolent course, which means that myelosuppressive chemotherapy may not be initiated until symptoms necessitate intervention. Symptoms, therefore, are managed as they appear.

Acute Leukemia

AML patients typically receive combination chemotherapy (see Table 61.2). The oncologist will set the dose ranges for at least two drugs—daunorubicin (Cerubidine) or idarubicin (Idamycin) or mitoxantrone plus cytarabine (Ara-C). The primary-care practitioner should monitor hepatic function throughout the course of combination therapy, which may run in 3- to 6-day cycles every 3 to 4 weeks for a total of 3 to 6 months, depending on successful remission and patient tolerance. Combination therapy produces bone marrow aplasia, which abates after 2 weeks following the conclusion of therapy. Aplastic patients, therefore, require supportive antibiotic prophylaxis, vigorous stoma care due to severe denuding of mucosal surfaces, and possible RBC transfusions. The primary-care practitioner's role is to co-manage the adverse effects of chemotherapy and to monitor serum chemistries, including liver function tests.

Adult patients with ALL may enter remission with initial management (albeit not as quickly or as easily as children with ALL) without the aplastic disorders associated with the initial treatment of AML. Combination four-drug chemotherapy is the mainstay for initial management of ALL, including vincristine (Oncovin), daunorubicin (Cerubidine), prednisone (Deltasone), and asparaginase (DVP L-asp). Other combinations are under investigation. Co-management with the oncologist is the same as for patients with AML, except that vigorous stoma care and associated weight reduction may not figure as prominently in ALL management. Glucose intolerance may develop due to prednisone therapy, particularly in patients suffering from diabetes mellitus at baseline. Thus, the primary-care practitioner is responsible for making adjustments to antidiabetic agents during chemotherapy.

After remission has been achieved for the patient with acute leukemia, a consolidation course of treatment is begun. Consolidation cycles differ for the acute leukemias (see Table 61.2). AML patients receive one complete chemotherapy consolidation cycle. Alternatively, they may receive a bone marrow transplantation to consolidate the gains of earlier therapy. Transplantation may be autologous (an individual's own marrow saved before treatment), allogeneic (marrow donated by another individual), or syngeneic (marrow donated by an identical twin). Therapeutic Procedure 61.1 presents information that should be provided to the patient who will be undergoing bone marrow transplantation.

Patients with ALL, on the other hand, face different challenges during the consolidation phase of management. They must receive CNS prophylaxis against malignant lymphocytes that may have crossed the blood–brain barrier to hide in meningeal crypts, which typically consists of intrathecal methotrexate and cranial irradiation.

Chronic Leukemia

Patients with CML are initially managed with watchful vigilance. Should treatment be required for symptoms related to hyperleukocytosis, such as blurred vision and respiratory distress, leukophoresis may be initiated. In addition, depending on the severity of symptoms, hydroxyurea (Hydrea) may be started at 2 to 4 g/day PO, followed by maintenance therapy of 0.5 to 2 g/day. The

Therapeutic Procedure 61.1: Bone Marrow Transplantation

The following information should be provided to patients undergoing bone marrow transplantation (BMT).

What Is It?

BMT consists of the intravenous administration of 500 to 700 mL of bone marrow. The patient is "conditioned" to receive the bone marrow through a regimen of immunosuppressive therapy (chemotherapy or radiation). This conditioning eradicates malignant cells, provides immunosuppression, and creates a space for the bone marrow to engraft the transplanted marrow stem cells. The marrow is usually infused 48 to 72 hours after the patient's last dose of chemotherapy or radiation.

The bone marrow is "harvested" from a donor. It may be an autologous transplant (aspirated from the pelvic bones of the patient during a remission), an allogeneic transplant (from a compatible donor such as a parent or sibling with a similar tissue type), or a syngeneic transplant (from an identical twin). Peripheral stem cell transplants are currently the state of the art in bone marrow reconstitution, in which rare, peripherally circulating stem cells are collected from the donor through an apheresis procedure, rather than harvesting whole bone marrow directly from the pelvic bones. This has greatly reduced the pain, discomfort, and complications associated with bone marrow (i.e., hematopoietic stem cell) donation.

What Will Happen Before the Procedure?

- The clinician should provide complete information about the specific procedure (e.g., pretreatment, medication and activity restrictions), answer any questions, and provide emotional support.
- The patient should prepare for an extended hospital stay.

- The patient should prepare for side effects that are anticipated with immunosuppressant and cytoablative therapies (e.g., nausea, vomiting, cataracts, sterility, hair loss).
- What Will Happen During the Procedure
- The nursing staff will do the following:
  1. Observe vital signs and monitor for complications (e.g., allergic reactions, fluid overload, pulmonary embolism)
  2. Provide support and reassurance

What Will Happen After the Procedure?

- The nursing staff will monitor the following:
  1. Routine vital signs
  2. Signs and symptoms of infection (e.g., fever, chills)
  3. Potential complications from chemotherapy given to prevent graft-versus-host disease
  4. Signs and symptoms of graft-versus-host disease (e.g., rash, jaundice, joint pain, diarrhea, failure to engraft [pancytopenia])
- Mouth and skin care will be provided every 2 hours to help prevent ulcers and infection
- Intramuscular injections will be avoided because they may lead to increased bleeding into the muscles, due to thrombocytopenia

What to Do After Discharge?

- Avoid infection by staying away from crowds and people with known infections
- Avoid sharp objects (for example, shave with an electric razor rather than an exposed razor blade)
- Avoid eating fresh fruits and vegetables if neutropenic (given the risk of infection)

leukopenic goal of 5,000 to 10,000 WBCs/mcL requires frequent monitoring to track the decreasing WBC count.

Symptom management and clinical vigilance are the initial therapies for patients with CLL. Conditions that typically require intervention include thrombocytopenia (less than 50,000 platelets/mcL), anemia (less than 27% Hct), lymphadenopathy that impedes activities of daily living, and fatigue that reduces nutritional intake and immobilizes the patient. Of note, most oncologists tolerate lower platelet thresholds before transfusing platelets to as low as 10,000/mcL, provided there is no active bleeding. If combination chemotherapy is utilized, the monitoring of platelet and erythrocyte counts is required given the risk of myelosuppression secondary to chemotherapy. Exogenous erythropoietin (Epogen, Procrit, Aranesp) may assist in countering chemotherapy-induced anemia. In addition, the use of pegfilgrastim (Neulasta) and other granulocyte colony-stimulating factors may counter neutropenia and decrease the associated risk of serious infection.

FOLLOW-UP AND REFERRAL

All patients with suspected leukemia require immediate referral to an oncologist. For patients with acute leukemia, co-management of adverse effects from combination chemotherapy will require monthly follow-up with the primary-care practitioner during the course of chemotherapy. The oncologist will direct treatment recommendations and chemotherapy adjustments, as well as supervise laboratory analyses. The primary-care practitioner will provide oversight of these same monitoring laboratory results, along with recommendations for symptom management.

For the patient with chronic leukemia, if clinical vigilance is all that is required per recommendation of the oncologist, the primary-care practitioner should order laboratory evaluations including a CBC, platelet count, and peripheral blood smear every 6 weeks. Depending on symptom onset and severity, physical examinations may be done as infrequently as every 2 to 3 months, if the patient is otherwise stable. Once chemotherapy intervention begins, however, the oncologist will make treatment recommendations and alterations to the management plan, as needed.

Patient Education: Leukemia

The patient may not be prepared for diseased-based education soon after receiving a clinical diagnosis of leukemia; therefore, it is important to involve not only the patient but also his or her significant others in any education provided. Particular attention should be focused on treatment recommendations and their proposed impact on daily life and the patient's state of well-being. Treatment recommendations that include myelo-suppressive therapies will require self-care activities for which the patient may not have the capacity. Thus, education should begin with an assessment of the patient's ability to monitor for infection, adverse effects of treatments, integrity of the skin and mucous membranes, and fluid/nutritional status. Any deficits in the patient's ability to follow through with these self-assessments should raise concern for an increased risk of complications from treatment. Thus, resources that can aid the patient in performing these self-assessments should be arranged well before treatment is initiated.

In addition to self-assessment, patient education must also address the anticipated burden on caregivers. Older patients and family members may not be able to adapt to the demands of treatment schedules, aplastic crises, and treatment complications. In turn, the clinician should plan teaching sessions with both the patient and caregivers present. The information should be repeated in subsequent sessions, and the patient and caregivers should be asked to recall and repeat instructions provided in earlier sessions to confirm proper understanding. In addition, the clinician should monitor both the patient and caregivers for signs of emotional strain and possible depression.

Patients need to be reassured that for all forms of leukemia, clinical vigilance is a form of treatment just as surely as is chemotherapy. Thus, if clinical vigilance is indicated, the patient and caregivers should learn the reasons to withhold pharmacological interventions while maintaining a watchful eye. Finally, patient education may require referral to support groups with other patients who have learned to live with cancer. Thus, referrals can include connections to other patients with leukemia within a primary-care practice as well as support groups convened by local chapters of the American Cancer Society. The goal of support group referral is to advance the patient's connection with others who can share treatment-related information and advance coping strategies. Caregivers may require a separate support group where they can discuss issues that are unique to their role.

REFERENCES

General

Young N, Gerson S, High K, eds. *Clinical hematology: Text with CD-ROM*. Mosby; 2006.

Anemia

Gunder LM. What you can learn from RBC analysis. *Clin Advisor*. 2008;11(12):19–23.

Muncie H, Campbell J. Alpha and beta thalassemia. *Am Fam Physician*. 2009;80(4):339–344, 371.

Short M, Domagalski J. Iron deficiency anemia: Evaluation and management. *Am Fam Physician*. 2013;87(2):98–104.

Stabler S. Vitamin B12 deficiency. *N Engl J Med*. 2013;368: 149–160.

Leukemia

Arber DA, Orazi A, Hasserjian R, et al. The 2016 revision to the World Health classification of myeloid neoplasms and acute leukemia. *Blood*. 2016;127(20):2391–2405.

Davis A, Viera A, Mead M. Leukemia: An overview for primary care. *Am Fam Physician*. 2014;89(9):731–738.

Polycythemia

Tefferi A, Barbui T. Essential thrombocythemia and polycythemia vera: Focus on clinical practice. *Mayo Clin Proc*. 2015;90(9): 1283–1293.

Tefferi A, Barbui T. Polycythemia vera and essential thrombocythemia: 2015 update on diagnosis, risk-stratification and management. *Am J Hematol*. 2015;90:163–173.

Sickle Cell Anemia

Piel F, Steinberg M, Rees D. Sickle cell disease. *N Engl J Med*. 2017;376:1561–1573.

RESOURCES

Leukemia

American Cancer Society
https://www.cancer.org/cancer/leukemia.html

Sickle Cell Anemia

Sickle Cell Disease Association of America
http://www.sicklecelldisease.org

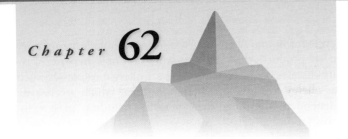

Chapter 62

Immunological Disorders

Brian Oscar Porter, MD, PhD, MPH, MBA
Jill E. Winland-Brown, EdD, APRN, FNP-BC

ALLERGIC REACTIONS

Allergy is defined as an immune-mediated reaction to a foreign environmental allergen. It is characterized by an inflammatory response to allergen exposure to the body. Typical sites for allergen exposure are the skin and respiratory tree, where local reactions may occur. Allergen exposure may also lead to a systemic response, however, in which multiple organs and the circulatory system may become involved. Allergenic shock or anaphylaxis is an extreme example of this systemic response.

Atopy is a term used to characterize an immunoglobulin (Ig)E-mediated immune response that is exaggerated or out of character for exposure to what appear to be innocuous environmental allergens. Whereas allergic skin reactions are classically characterized by raised, erythematous wheal and flare reactions termed urticarial plaques, another common allergic skin condition, atopic dermatitis, has several different manifestations whose pathophysiology extends beyond IgE-mediated allergic processes (see Chapter 16).

EPIDEMIOLOGY AND CAUSES

In contrast to autoimmune reactions, which tend to have a female predominance, allergic reactions are equally distributed between the sexes, affecting men as often as women, without regard to race or ethnicity. The incidence of allergies is greater in children than in adults, perhaps because of the immaturity of immune responses in children and the tendency toward humorally mediated T helper cell–2 (Th2)-type responses.

Seasonal allergies vary according to hemispheric geography, which means that pollen, mold, and fungal spores affect individuals according to seasonal patterns of exposure in the Northern and Southern hemispheres. In North America, pollen counts rise and fall in a May to September pattern, whereas molds follow a March through December pattern in outdoor environments; therefore, there are only 2 to 3 months of the year, in the late winter, when pollens and molds tend not affect the population. During cold weather, however, individuals remain indoors for longer periods of time, which can increase the risk of more frequent exposure to dust mites and other indoor allergens, including indoor mold species that tend to propagate in cool, dark interior environments, such as damp basements or bathrooms.

Causes of allergies include a wide array of environmental allergens and the corresponding intrinsic immune complexes formed by the body as it mounts a vigorous response to allergenic exposure. Environmental allergens include natural *inhalants* such as pollen, mold, and fungal spores, *ingestants* such as food and drug allergens, *injectants* such as animal or insect venoms, and *contactants* including dust mites and their feces, animal hair and dander, as well as chemical components in hair- and skin-care products. Regardless of the source, the allergen invades the body, either locally or systemically, eliciting a complex immune-regulated response that results in either local or systemic effects.

PATHOPHYSIOLOGY

All allergens are foreign substances to the body. Cellular and humoral immune responses occur after initial exposure to a foreign substance. Immune responses result from a complex, coordinated set of events requiring several cell types, cell surface signaling proteins, and secreted regulatory cytokines. Key cell types involved in the allergic response include histamine-containing mast cells and basophils, as well as highly granular eosinophils. Also important are antibody-secreting plasma cells that are specialized, differentiated B-lineage cells designed to produce monoclonal antibodies of a single antigenic specificity. Additionally, CD4+ T helper cells are also antigen-specific and produce an array of regulatory cytokines after their T-cell receptors encounter specific allergens. Helper T cells of the Th2 class produce cytokines (e.g., interleukin [IL]-4, IL-5, IL-13) that upregulate humoral antibody-mediated immune responses, whereas Th1 helper T cells predominantly produce a separate set of cytokines (e.g., interferon [IFN]-γ IL-12) that upregulate cell-mediated antibody-independent cytotoxic responses.

According to the Gell-Coombs classification system, there are four basic types of immune responses to allergens (termed *hypersensitivity responses*, as a group), categorized by whether they are dependent on circulating antibodies (types 1–3) or only on cellular immune components (type 4). Type 1 immune responses are considered classic allergic hypersensitivity reactions. However, type 3 immune responses often underlie what are termed *drug and food allergies*, whereas type 4 immune reactions mediate contact dermatitis, a pathological response to certain skin irritants, such as the allergens in poison ivy and poison oak.

Type 1: Immunoglobulin E-mediated Immediate Hypersensitivity Response

In the first step of initial exposure to an allergen, the immune system must recognize that the allergen is foreign. Immunoglobulin E (IgE) is a class of antibody present in relatively low concentration in the circulation. As with all immunoglobulins, IgE molecules are antigen specific in their variable arms, allowing for binding of more than one IgE molecule to a single circulating antigenic molecule. However, the constant portion of the IgE molecule (Fc) allows for its binding to the surface of cells specifically expressing high-affinity receptors for the IgE molecule (FcεRI). IgE molecules are bound to tissue-derived mast cells located primarily in the skin, respiratory system, and gastrointestinal (GI) tract, where external environmental allergens are most likely to contact or invade the body. In addition, allergen-specific IgE molecules are bound to circulating basophils.

Antibody cross-linking is the process by which two or more cell surface-bound IgE molecules bind a common antigen, thereby triggering intracellular signaling and degranulation of the immune cell, with the release of cytokine mediators. Such responses do not typically occur on initial exposure to an allergen. On first exposure, specific IgE molecules are formed via class-switching of monoclonal antibodies produced by pre-existing antigen-specific B cells from the IgG or IgM classes to IgE, based on the constant Fc portion of cell surface antibody molecules. Once secreted by the B cell, these IgE molecules then bind to mast cells and basophils. Upon re-exposure (when the same allergen binds to cell-bound antigen-specific IgE), a cascade of cellular events occurs, resulting in intracellular calcium shifts that facilitate cyclic nucleotide signaling molecules to trigger degranulation of the immune cell.

Degranulation results in the excretion of preformed inflammatory mediators from the immune cell, including histamine, heparin, tryptase, other proteolytic enzymes, thromboxane, arachidonic acid, prostaglandins, superoxides, and several eosinophilic and neutrophilic chemotactic factors. In addition, the synthesis of newly formed inflammatory mediators, including leukotrienes and certain cytokines, is also triggered.

These inflammatory mediators cause venules, capillaries, and arterioles to dilate and become hyperpermeable. The mucous membranes are triggered to increase mucus excretion and the walls of hollow visceral structures to spasm as a result of smooth muscle contraction. Dehydration may result from the relative shift of fluid that follows intravascular proteins out of the vasculature and into the extravascular space, thus potentially lowering blood pressure. Hypotension may also be aggravated by environmental factors, such as relative heat and humidity.

IgE activation and cellular excretion of inflammatory mediators may take place within seconds to minutes after antigenic exposure. Whereas the effects of initially released inflammatory mediators may last for 30 minutes or less, repeated allergenic exposure can prolong the inflammatory

cycle for hours. A prolonged and intractable inflammatory cycle produces the clinical picture of atopic hypersensitivity diseases characterized by type 1 allergic responses, such as allergic rhinitis and allergic asthma, which are heavily dependent on inflammatory cells, including mast cells, eosinophils, and Th2 cells.

A second category of type 1 allergic reaction is *anaphylaxis*. Unlike atopic diseases, which are typically characterized by localized effects in the skin or respiratory tract, anaphylaxis produces systemic effects. All of the inflammatory processes of hypersensitivity become exaggerated, leading to life-threatening hypotension, bronchospasm, laryngospasm, angioedema, smooth muscle and visceral organ contractions, and raised inflammatory skin eruptions (generalized urticaria or hives). Anaphylaxis may follow exposure in susceptible individuals to well-known allergens, such as insect venom (bee or wasp stings) or certain drugs such as penicillin. However, these responses are not limited to individuals with a history of atopic disease and may occur unexpectedly in any individual. Therefore, a history of atopy does not predict anaphylaxis. If left untreated, anaphylaxis is typically fatal. Therapeutic Procedure 62.1 describes a seven-step treatment algorithm for anaphylaxis.

 Therapeutic Procedure 62.1: Seven-step Treatment for Anaphylaxis

- Step 1: Administer aqueous epinephrine 1:1,000 dilution 0.3–0.5 mg (0.3–0.5 mL) intramuscularly into the upper lateral thigh, in a supine position with the head below heart level, if possible.
- Step 2: Repeat epinephrine every 5–15 minutes as required by the clinical presentation. If hypotensive, position the patient supine with feet elevated.
- Step 3: Support bronchodilation if patient is without laryngospasm by administering albuterol 3 mL (2.5 mg) inhalation via nebulizer.
- Step 4: If patient is in laryngospasm or pulmonary arrest, perform emergency endotracheal intubation and provide respiratory support.
- Step 5: Start IV fluids using normal saline or Ringer's lactate solution to maintain systolic blood pressure greater than 90 mm Hg. The rate of flow should be determined by the blood pressure reading but typically may be bolused.
- Step 6: If the patient is conscious and without laryngospasm, administer diphenhydramine (Benadryl) 25–50 mg to relieve cutaneous symptoms. H_2-blockers may also be added (particularly if GI symptoms are present) but have not been shown to be as effective as H_1-blockers.
- Step 7: Transfer the patient to an acute-care emergency center for continued support and observation. Add corticosteroids (IV or PO) to prevent late-phase anaphylactic reactions, which may be as severe as early-phase reactions.

See text regarding teaching about injectable epinephrine (EpiPen).

Type 2: Antibody-mediated Cellular Cytotoxicity Response

Type 2 antibody-mediated cellular cytotoxicity responses introduce an immune mechanism different from type 1 immediate hypersensitivity responses. Type 2 responses involve the activation of antigen-specific IgM and IgG molecules. These humoral immune molecules bind to foreign antigens and activate serum immune complement. This leads to destruction of any cell to which an allergen-antibody complex is bound; thus, a type 2 immune response is cytotoxic. Examples of such type 2 responses include neonatal Rh (Rhesus blood group factor)-incompatibility hemolytic disease and immune-mediated hemolytic anemia. In addition, if when these antibodies bind to foreign antigens such as microbial cell surface proteins, the invading microbes become prone to phagocytosis and destruction by host immune cells—a process known as opsonization.

Type 3: Antibody–Allergen Immune Complex Response

The third category of immune responses also requires IgM and IgG activation, as is characteristic of a type 2 immune response. However, type 3 responses denote a free-standing immune complex that is formed between these immunoglobulins and the allergen. These complexes become deposited into the various tissues of the body, activating serum complement that in turn triggers multiple inflammatory mediators. These reactions tend to be systemic, as immune complexes affect multiple organs and tissue types throughout the body. The reaction is not immediate, and in fact, may occur up to 2 to 3 weeks after antigenic exposure. Hypersensitivity-type pneumonitis secondary to an inhaled allergen and serum sickness are two examples of type 3 immune responses. Delayed drug reactions are also classic examples of type 3 responses, with the most common offenders being the antiepileptic drugs phenytoin, phenobarbital, and carbamazepine, as well as various antibiotics.

Type 4: Delayed-type Cellular Hypersensitivity Response

The fourth category of immune responses is defined as a cell-mediated delayed-type immune response that is unlike the three previous categories, which are all mediated by humoral factors (antibody-dependent). The other three categories directly involve few, if any, T lymphocytes. However, type 4 reactions are T cell–dependent and usually begin in the skin, where large numbers of T cells are found. Antigen contacting the skin is endocytosed (taken up) by antigen-presenting cells, which process and relocate small antigenic peptides to the cell surface, coupled to antigen-presenting proteins known as major histocompatibility complex (MHC) molecules.

Antigen-specific T-cell receptors recognize and bind to these antigenic peptide–MHC complexes, which leads to a series of inflammatory reactions including cellular lysis of the antigen-presenting cell and cytokine production. Because of this delay in cellular lysis, which may occur up to 2 to 3 days after antigenic exposure, skin eruptions do not appear immediately. Contact dermatitis (e.g., poison ivy, chemical irritations, nickel metallic allergies) is the classic example of a type 4 immune response, typically referred to as delayed-type hypersensitivity. In addition, the positive wheal-and-flare response to *Mycobacterium tuberculosis* (TB) purified protein derivative (PPD) used in TB screening is also a type 4 immune response, which is why the tuberculin skin test (TST) is read 48 to 72 hours after it is administered.

CLINICAL PRESENTATION

Subjective

Patients with classic atopic disease report fatigue and/ or malaise, irritability, itchy and watery eyes, sneezing, rhinorrhea, nasal congestion, coughing without sputum production (unless a secondary bacterial infection accompanies the allergy), pruritus, and, in more severe cases, wheezing. Two elements are common to subjective complaints associated with allergies. First, an exposure to an allergen precedes the onset of symptoms. Thus, allergic rhinitis can be distinguished from perennial rhinitis because environmental seasonal allergen exposure precedes the former. Second, patients typically attempt to control their symptoms with self-care. For example, their subjective picture usually includes self-medication and may be somewhat controlled with over-the-counter (OTC) agents. A history of subjective allergic symptoms, therefore, requires accompanying inquiry concerning the use of OTC antihistamines and decongestants.

Objective

The sinuses may be tender to percussion if nasal congestion has predisposed a patient to sinusitis (due to impeded mucous drainage); otherwise, the sinuses are typically nontender in uncomplicated allergic rhinitis. The conjunctivae and mucous membranes in general will be injected. Nasal turbinates are erythematous. Cervical nodes may feel small and hard ("shotty"), with few greater than 1 cm in size. Postauricular nodes and thoracic nodes are less commonly involved. Tympanic membranes may appear dull to light but will be otherwise unremarkable.

Tachycardia typically accompanies OTC decongestant use, but fever does not contribute to the tachycardia, as it is almost always absent. Drowsiness is also typical with OTC antihistamine use (especially with first generation H_1-blocking agents with greater central nervous system [CNS] penetration). Lungs will be clear after several deep breaths and coughs, unless allergic asthma results in wheezing. Except in patients with anaphylaxis or allergenic invasion of the GI tract, the abdominal examination will be unremarkable. In these exceptional cases, profound abdominal tenderness may inhibit deep palpation.

Skin eruptions will depend on the type of allergic reaction and may include urticaria (type 1 response), fissures, circumscribed papules, bullae, and petechiae. The clinician should expect no singular picture of skin eruptions that corresponds with the allergenic source; however, there are associations in skin presentation and history that may lend themselves to diagnostic conclusions. For example, a history of exposure to poison ivy and multiple circumscribed papules in the anatomic place of exposure provides an association that is diagnostic of delayed-type hypersensitivity to a specific exposure. Poison ivy, poison oak, and poison sumac all produce contact dermatitis caused by the oily irritant substance urushiol, which is contained in the leaves of these plants, leading to a delayed, cell-mediated (type 4) immune response.

If the patient's sensorium is affected, an objective mental status examination may reveal diminished problem-solving ability, impairment in recent recall, and unfocused attention. These signs are particularly evident in older adults and others who practice polypharmacy with combination OTC agents. Thus, it may be difficult to distinguish between the sedative effects of anti-allergy medications (in particular, antihistaminic agents) versus the impact of a chronic atopic condition that is affecting the patient's sleep–wake cycle, such as severe allergic rhinitis or night-time asthma.

DIAGNOSTIC REASONING

Diagnostic Tests

Initial evaluation begins with the clinical history. The clinician should ask the patient to describe any changes in diet, skin-care products, or activities involving environmental exposures that preceded the onset of allergic symptoms. Suspicions raised by the history will often be confirmed or at least supported by subsequent diagnostic testing. Thus, particularly with regard to the evaluation of environmental exposures, a detailed history informed by the clinical presentation should largely drive diagnostic allergy testing.

Type 1 Response

Some clinicians recommend initial testing with skin tests by allergists to diagnose the response to specific allergens. Skin tests involve first pricking the epidermis with a small amount of a liquid extract of each allergen of interest. Later, to test suspicious allergens that initially result as negative on prick testing, small amounts of these extracts can be injected into the intradermal layers of the skin, which is believed to be a more sensitive form of skin testing than prick testing. (Patch testing, in which small amounts of emulsions of potential allergens are applied

directly to the skin and left in place for 24–48 hours, is generally performed to diagnose contact dermatitis and other manifestations of type 4 hypersensitivity reactions.) Skin pricking testing is the first stage of allergen testing because of the very slight but potentially fatal risk that the applied allergen could cause a serious systemic allergic response (anaphylaxis). Thus, for every negative prick test, an intradermal injection may be placed as a more sensitive, albeit potentially higher risk, method of allergen testing.

The selection of antigens to be tested follows a pattern of reasoning based on the question: What are the most likely culprits? The exact composition of skin-test panels is determined by regional and patient-specific determinants. An allergist will expose the patient to small amounts of regional and suspected environmental allergens in skin test panels by prick or injection. If the test is positive, a wheal should appear in 15 to 20 minutes. The reliability and sensitivity of skin testing make it the preferred test for initial diagnosis. Skin tests are done with both positive (histamine) and negative (inert substances, such as saline) controls, and results must be judged against these controls as some individuals are sensitive to any kind of scratching or pricking of the skin, just by the nature of the insult to the skin, and not due to hypersensitivity to the antigen.

The rate of false-positive responses in allergen skin testing is high. Testing should not be done indiscriminately or overinterpreted. In fact, many environmental and food allergens may test positive in up to half of the general population who otherwise demonstrate no other manifestations of hypersensitivity to these antigens. In turn, skin tests are far more useful in ruling out (i.e., excluding, rather than confirming) specific antigenic hypersensitivities, when reactions are negative.

Alternatives to allergen skin testing include in vitro serum-based testing methods, such as the radioallergosorbent test (RAST), the enzyme-linked immunosorbent assay (ELISA), and the fluorescent antibody staining technique (FAST). These serum tests reduce the risk of hypersensitivity-type reactions from allergens as seen in skin testing because they only measure antigen-specific IgE levels in the blood, rather than assess for functional hypersensitivity responses. Thus, skin tests are typically more sensitive than serum RAST tests in detecting true hypersensitivity responses because more atopic individuals will be positive on skin tests than will have elevated antigen-specific IgE serum levels. RAST tests are usually considered more specific than allergen skin testing, as nonatopic individuals are unlikely to have high allergen-specific IgE levels, which must be balanced with their relatively decreased level of diagnostic sensitivity.

Consideration of sensitivity and specificity of allergy testing is particularly important for food challenge testing, which often uses skin prick testing as an initial screen to rule out specific food allergies, given its high sensitivity. Some clinicians also complement skin testing with

RAST testing because although some food allergies may be type 3 immune complex responses, others are type 1 anaphylactic food allergy reactions that are IgE-mediated and clinically severe. Definitive testing for such reactions may take place via blinded food challenges in an office setting by an allergy specialist (with ready access to endotracheal intubation supplies and injectable epinephrine) in the presence of physicians or other persons qualified to treat anaphylactic reactions. Set amounts of food are given to persons suspected of food allergy (typically children) in progressively increasing amounts, and individuals are subsequently monitored for several hours for any reaction. This is a highly specific test and is thus very effective in ruling out food allergies. Obviously, however, this testing method carries a risk of anaphylaxis. Thus, RAST testing may be done instead of an observed food challenge to avoid needlessly subjecting individuals with high food-specific IgE levels to intentional exposure with that food trigger.

The most common form of asthma is an allergen-driven atopic disease characterized by type 1 immune responses to environmental allergens, although it is distinct from systemic anaphylaxis. Atopic airway hyperreactivity may also be triggered by environmental irritants, such as tobacco smoke, which is not a true allergen. Thus, these individuals do not express tobacco-specific IgE levels, although smoke and other environmental pollutants may trigger an asthma attack. Reactive airway disease (bronchial hyper-responsiveness), therefore, may be either allergic or nonallergic in origin. As asthma is largely an atopic, allergen-driven disease, sputum from an asthmatic patient may reveal eosinophils after staining with methylene blue dye, because sputum from atopic individuals typically demonstrates higher levels of eosinophils than in the nonatopic population.

Type 2 Response

Rh testing of blood during pregnancy is the initial test to determine prospective Rh incompatibility. In infants with suspected immune-mediated hemolytic anemia, an elevated indirect bilirubin level indicates hemolysis. Red blood cell (RBC) hemolysis is further associated with decreased serum haptoglobin levels. Autoimmune haemolytic anemia is also associated with a positive Coombs' test, which detects RBC-specific antibodies in the blood.

Type 3 Response

Initial tests are employed to detect complement activation, as an underlying step in immune-complex reactions. A complement-based ELISA will give specific evidence of complement activation and consumption of complement proteins. For example, the ELISA might show lower levels of C_3 and/or C_4, which are two complement factors that may be diminished if an allergic inflammatory reaction has activated the complement system. Similarly, the CH50 test, which is a measure of overall complement protein levels, will also be low

in this setting. Skin manifestations in type 3 immune responses may be biopsied and stained for immune complex deposition, which is a hallmark of such reactions.

Type 4 Response

Skin testing is the initial test of preference for cell-mediated hypersensitivity, e.g., tuberculin skin testing. Allergens are either injected intradermally or applied topically onto patches of skin. Results are then read 48 to 72 hours after application to assess for a delayed-type hypersensitivity reaction. Positive responses consist of induration (for injected allergens) and erythema and papules (for topically applied allergy skin patch testing).

Antigen-specific serum IgE levels may aid in distinguishing allergic from nonallergic immune responses. For example, classic type 1 hypersensitivity reactions are IgE-mediated, whereas cell-mediated type 4 responses are not. Although both type 2 and type 3 responses are antibody-mediated, the IgE immunoglobulin class is not typically involved in those reactions. An elevated peripheral eosinophil count may also provide secondary confirmation of recent IgE-mediated atopic disease.

Differential Diagnosis

Clinical history is the mainstay of differentiating allergic disease. Allergies are triggered by exposure to environmental antigens. The history, therefore, must support allergenic exposure proximal to the onset of symptoms and may often reveal partial or temporary relief of symptoms from OTC allergy remedies, as well as possible familial allergic patterns. Additional differentiation of classical allergic disease from other types of immune responses comes from skin test results, antigen-specific IgE levels, and other diagnostic tests aimed at identifying antibody-mediated immune responses.

Alternatively, irritants that enter the body but do not initiate classical immune-mediated hypersensitivity responses include nonallergic sources, such as air pollutants and tobacco smoke. In addition, some research has suggested that susceptible asthmatic patients may experience worsening of symptoms associated with barometric changes in the atmosphere, although it is unclear whether this weather-related phenomenon may actually be due to increases in airborne pollen levels associated with atmospheric pressure changes.

MANAGEMENT

Allergy management requires both symptomatic relief and prevention of exposure to specific allergens. Following the initial diagnosis and treatment of acute symptoms, priority should be given to identifying and avoiding triggering allergens, whether with respect to respiratory symptoms (asthma, allergic rhinitis), cutaneous manifestations (urticaria), ocular allergies, or systemic allergic reactions (anaphylaxis). (Atopic dermatitis, another core atopic disorder, is covered in detail in Chapter 16.) For both allergic rhinitis and asthma patients, long-term immunomodulatory therapy with allergy vaccines (i.e., allergen immunotherapy) offers both effective prophylaxis and attenuation of future atopic symptoms.

Initial Management

The patient must become vigilant in avoiding further allergenic exposure. After clinical history, skin testing, and antigen-specific IgE levels have identified likely triggering allergens, avoidance behaviors should be initiated. For example, individuals diagnosed with hypersensitivity to penicillin must avoid not only penicillin but also cephalosporins, given the likelihood of cross reactivity. However, although penicillin remains one of the most common triggers of antibiotic hypersensitivity, penicillin allergy is typically overdiagnosed based on limited self-reported history. Thus, a detailed patient history should focus on whether an anaphylactic reaction to penicillin truly occurred, as research involving confirmatory skin testing and antibiotic challenge has consistently demonstrated that most patients who report penicillin allergies do not have true penicillin hypersensitivity reactions or contraindicating anaphylaxis. Moreover, when use of a specific antibiotic class is deemed essential in an allergic patient, desensitization to penicillin or other antibiotics can be performed in a controlled clinical environment with the capacity to treat anaphylaxis and other forms of hypersensitivity (e.g., intensive care or step-down unit).

Along the same lines, bee venom reactions can be avoided in venom-allergic patients by not disturbing beehives or wasp nests. Dust mite–allergic patients may use specially designed mattress and pillow covers that seal in dust mites and their allergenic fecal matter, avoid dust-collecting ceiling fans, remove carpets from bedrooms to limit dust mite exposure during sleeping hours, and regularly wash plush toys and any other potential dust reservoirs in hot water. Patients with pollen allergies should keep windows closed in favor of using air conditioning in both the home and car, as well as bathe soon after outdoor exposure to pollen, which can adhere to clothes and hair. Air-conditioning filters should be changed regularly, although high-efficiency particulate air (HEPA) filters and chemical agents purported to reduce the concentration of aeroallergens have not been shown to be consistently effective.

Subsequent Management

Subsequent management consists of ongoing symptom control and immunotherapy. Symptom control can be achieved either through prescribed or OTC agents for common respiratory, ocular, and cutaneous manifestations. There are many classes of drugs that have demonstrated efficacy for symptom management in allergic disease, for example, sympathomimetics (used as decongestants), antihistamines (both oral and topical), corticosteroids (topical, inhaled, or systemic), cromolyn, and theophylline. Newer generation antihistamines have been designed to have less anticholinergic effects and CNS penetration and, therefore, cause less tachycardia and sedation than first-generation agents.

Of note, in addition to future allergen avoidance, the most severe form of allergic disease, anaphylaxis, requires emergent treatment (e.g., epinephrine, IV fluids) for immediate life-threatening manifestations caused by preformed inflammatory mediators, as well as prophylactic treatment (e.g., corticosteroids) for delayed, late phase manifestations caused by de novo (newly formed) immune mediators, as described in Therapeutic Procedure 62.1. Because late phase anaphylactic reactions may occur up to 24 hours following allergen exposure and can prove fatal, prophylactic corticosteroids should be given, although they are ineffective in treating acute symptoms, given their slow onset of action.

Symptom Control

Many OTC oral and topical agents are sympathomimetic (alpha-receptor agonist) in activity. Common examples of oral drugs in this class include pseudoephedrine (Sudafed) and chlorpheniramine (Chlor-Trimeton), and intranasal oxymetazoline (Afrin) spray is also widely used on an as needed basis. In addition, epinephrine (Primatene Mist) was previously available OTC as an inhalational therapy in the same class of sympathomimetic drugs. However, sale of the chlorofluorocarbon (CFC)–containing formulation of inhaled epinephrine was prohibited by the U.S. Food and Drug Administration (FDA) in 2012, as the FDA ultimately phased out all CFC-containing inhalant formulations from the U.S. market, given environmental concerns over the impact of CFC on ozone levels.

Sympathomimetic agents may display both alpha-adrenergic and beta-adrenergic properties. They vasoconstrict engorged mucosa (an alpha-adrenergic property) and dilate the bronchioles by relaxing smooth muscle (a beta-adrenergic property). Therefore, they support antihistamines in drying secretions while opening the airways of the nasopharynx and bronchial tree. In addition, however, they also typically increase heart rate and may lead to palpitations (a beta-adrenergic effect). Because of their low molecular weight and solubility, sympathomimetics may cross the blood–brain barrier, resulting in irritability, anxiety, and addiction potential, particularly when combined with other psychoactive substances such as ethanol. In addition, topical intranasal agents such as oxymetazoline are well known to induce tachyphylaxis (i.e., a decreased response to the drug following frequent use over a relatively short period of time), resulting in rebound nasal congestion upon withdrawal after chronic use (rhinitis medicamentosum).

The abuse potential of OTC sympathomimetics remains high for many reasons. They are available for purchase and consumption without professional supervision, are relatively inexpensive, provide rapid symptomatic relief, and are heavily marketed. In addition, sympathomimetic formulations may be readily manipulated to form highly addictive illicit drug substances, such as methamphetamine (which in recent years has resulted in increasing restrictions on the OTC availability of some of these drugs, such as pseudoephedrine). In addition, regular use of short- and long-acting beta-adrenergic inhalants, such as albuterol (Proventil) and salmeterol (Serevent, Advair) may increase disease-related morbidity in asthmatic patients, including both exacerbations and asthma-related deaths.

Another class of agents widely used for allergic reactions and chronic atopic disease are the antihistamines. With both first and second-generation agents now available OTC, antihistamines are widely used in allergic disease for their ability to block H_1-histamine receptors, thereby reducing the effects of histamine released early in the inflammatory cascade. The blockade of H_1-receptor sites also contributes to the therapeutic effect of drying secretions. Adverse effects include over-dryness and sedation. The risk of sedation, particularly in older adults and children, may require dose reduction or a limited drug trial. Newer generation antihistamines such as desloratadine (Clarinex), fexofenadine (Allegra), and cetirizine (Zyrtec) are typically less sedating than first-generation agents (diphenhydramine [Benadryl], hydroxyzine [Atarax]). At prescribed doses, second-generation agents dry secretions without causing excessive drowsiness in most patients and can be dosed once daily. They are also not associated with untoward cardiac events (e.g., QTc prolongation, fatal arrhythmias), which had been observed with other long-acting second-generation antihistamines now withdrawn from the market (astemizole [Hismanal], terfenadine [Seldane]), particularly when used in combination with macrolide antibiotics or azole antifungals. Anticholinergic agents such as intranasal ipratropium (Atrovent) are also effective at drying secretions.

H_2-receptor antagonists such as cimetidine (Tagamet) and Ranitidine (Zantac) may also be useful in managing mild allergic reactions, although they are primarily used to decrease the production of stomach acid for GI symptoms. In some cases when allergy patients have failed to improve after receiving epinephrine and diphenhydramine, they have responded to cimetidine. However, H_2 blockers are known to cross the blood–brain barrier and may have mood-altering and significant anticholinergic effects, particularly in elderly patients.

Corticosteroids form a third group of drugs used in symptom control. Given their long onset of action (several hours), they have little role in the acute treatment of symptoms. However, they may prevent the recurrence of symptoms in patients with mild allergic reactions, such as urticaria. They also constitute part of the long-term treatment regimen of life-threatening allergic reactions, such as the manifestations of systemic anaphylaxis, including severe laryngeal edema, bronchospasm, and hypotension. For most hypersensitivity reactions, a dosage of 1 to 2 mg/kg per day of prednisone for 4 or 5 days is usually sufficient to prevent recurrent or late-onset symptoms. Short-term pulse dosing such as this does not require tapering. However, the clinician should consider tapering the regimen if the patient has received corticosteroid therapy in the recent past or if there are plans to continue therapy for more than several weeks. When given as short-term therapy, prednisone and other corticosteroids have benign adverse effect profiles. However, prolonged use of systemic corticosteroids has several implications, including the development of Cushingoid syndrome, adrenal insufficiency, and hyperglycemia.

Inhaled corticosteroids such as fluticasone propionate (Flovent) are used as standard prophylactic controller medications in allergic asthma (see Chapter 31). Intranasal corticosteroids such as mometasone furoate (Nasonex) are extremely effective for long-term control of both nasopharyngeal and ocular allergic rhinitis symptoms (see Chapter 24). Because corticosteroids are immunosuppressive anti-inflammatory agents, they effectively down-regulate the allergic immune responses characteristic of atopic disease.

Immunotherapy

Allergen immunotherapy (allergy vaccine) offers the patient long-term control of atopic disease. Given the small, albeit well documented, risk of anaphylaxis or other hypersensitivity reactions associated with allergen immunotherapy, its use is usually limited in scope to patients with intractable allergic rhinitis or asthma whose disease fails to be controlled with symptom management or for whom consistent allergen avoidance is not possible. Immunotherapy regimens should be prescribed and administered by a qualified specialist with expert knowledge in allergic diseases, as the first step is the proper identification of key allergens, which are the patient's most troublesome environmental triggers. Depending on the number of allergens identified, these extracts are combined into one or more allergy vaccine admixtures, taking into account both cross-reactivity of individual allergens and the reduced stability of certain allergen extracts (e.g., plant pollens, animal dander) in combination with others, given the presence of proteolytic enzymes in many fungal and insect (e.g., dust mite, wasp or bee venom) extracts.

Injections of commercially prepared extracts of these allergens are given subcutaneously in 0.5 mL allotments of diluent that progress from minimal dilutional strength to higher concentrations. The weekly injections continue, increasing in concentration until symptoms are controlled and/or the maximum concentration of allergen extract is achieved, at which time the frequency of injections may be decreased to once monthly. Immunotherapy may require more than 12 months of treatments before maximal effects are observed. There are also "rush immunotherapy" protocols that are being evaluated, which are shorter-course regimens that escalate a patient to maximal allergen extract concentrations more quickly than traditional regimens.

Current guidelines recommend continuing allergen immunotherapy for 3 to 5 years, after which many individuals experience lasting suppression of allergic hypersensitivity, allowing for the tapering and eventual cessation of extract injections. However, many patients experience recurrence of allergic symptoms when they attempt to stop or even taper the frequency of maintenance immunotherapy. Thus, although not generally recommended, some patients may continue immunotherapy for life.

Injection allergen immunotherapy has been used for over a century. However, a newer development is sublingual formulations, in which liquid extract is administered in drops under the tongue. The concept behind these regimens is the same as traditional subcutaneous and intradermal injection immunotherapy, although the convenience of this dosing route is self-evident, particularly given the potential for self-administration in nonclinical settings. Although sublingual immunotherapy has gained acceptance in Europe, its use is not as widespread in the United States, and evaluations of its safety and efficacy are ongoing.

Other forms of biologic immunotherapy exist for allergic diseases. For extremely refractory cases of atopy, such as severe allergic asthma with atopic dermatitis, the anti-IgE monoclonal antibody omalizumab (Xolair) may be effective. Xolair is FDA-approved for moderate to severe persistent asthma in persons 12 years and older. This therapy acts by binding circulating IgE and preventing its interaction with cell-surface molecules on blood cells that mediate allergic hypersensitivity responses, including mast cells, basophils, and eosinophils, thereby preventing initiation of the allergic cascade.

Nursing Situation: Immunotherapy

A 55-year-old woman has severe and persistent allergic rhinitis refractory to both OTC and prescription controller medications. Her primary triggering allergens are dust mites, ragweed pollen, egg, and *Aspergillus*. Food-based allergen immunotherapy is not considered an acceptable therapeutic strategy, given the relatively higher risk of anaphylaxis to food antigens. Thus, she completely avoids egg in her diet. To avoid dust mite exposure, she has removed all carpeting from her bedroom and replaced her curtains with window blinds. However, she cannot relocate from her home in the midwestern United States, where ragweed pollen levels are elevated between July and October. Her husband cleans the bathroom tiles and kitchen cabinets where *Aspergillus* might grow.

For the past 3 months, she has seen her primary-care practitioner on six occasions. Her medication regimen includes a prescribed inhaled intranasal corticosteroid and both long- and short-acting antihistamines. Despite treatment, her symptoms keep her awake at night, and recently she has started to wheeze, requiring use of an albuterol metered-dose inhaler. Her primary-care practitioner referred her to an allergist, who identified her specific allergens and recommended allergen immunotherapy on the basis of the severity and recurrence of her symptoms, as well as her refractoriness to other medications. Because of the risk of anaphylaxis associated with allergen immunotherapy, the risk–benefit ratio of this approach is discussed extensively with the patient before she initiates an immunotherapy regimen. The patient undergoes allergen skin testing; the results confirm allergic sensitivity to ragweed, dust mites, egg, and *Aspergillus*. The patient initiates weekly injections of an individual prepared allergy admixture at the lowest dilution. She continues this therapy and notes that after 3 months, she is able to control her symptoms with the inhaled intranasal corticosteroid and no longer needs the albuterol inhaler. The allergist recommends continuation of the immunotherapy for at least 1 year, after which the patient's condition and treatment regimen will be reassessed.

FOLLOW-UP AND REFERRAL

Follow-up of the patient with an allergic reaction is directly dependent on the severity and chronicity of the atopy and may consist of both regular visits and increased consultations during seasonal allergy periods, depending on symptoms. Follow-up tests include a complete blood count (CBC) to evaluate for leukocytosis and eosinophilia, as well as fasting blood sugar tests to assess for hyperglycemia if the patient requires systemic corticosteroids.

An allergist should be consulted if the symptoms cannot be controlled. The allergist is responsible for ordering and evaluating skin tests and for prescribing, administering, and evaluating the effectiveness of immunotherapy.

Patient Education: Allergic Reactions

Depending on the patient's clinical manifestations, she or he must know what foods or other environmental allergens to avoid. The patient and clinician should decide together how to identify and control exposure to triggering allergens that may have been unknown by the patient before the diagnosis. For example, few patients know the places that dust mites hide or understand how to eradicate *Aspergillus* with simple household chemicals.

Patients with significant respiratory symptoms may need to learn how to use nasal inhalants for significant rhinitis symptoms or metered-dose inhalers (MDIs) for bronchial/pulmonary symptoms. Initial use under the clinician's supervision can provide both the patient and clinician with reassurance that the drug will be delivered correctly. For patients with asthma, the use of spacers for MDIs should be taught and encouraged as a means of maximizing medication delivery (see Chapter 31). The patient should learn which drugs may be taken together without significant risk of interaction and which should be administered alone or with food to facilitate absorption. The narrow therapeutic index of some drugs, such as theophylline, requires vigilance on the part of the patient to report the early symptoms of drug toxicity.

Patients with a history of anaphylaxis must have epinephrine available at all times for emergencies should they encounter offending allergens. The immediate use of epinephrine after any exposure to a known anaphylactic triggering agent is crucial. The clinician should prescribe self-administered intramuscular epinephrine (EpiPen autoinjector) and have the patient demonstrate an understanding of its use before leaving the office. The patient should be instructed that whenever a dose is self-administered, emergency department care should be sought in case the reaction worsens or recurs, requiring more advanced therapy such as IV epinephrine or crystalloid infusion. Given the life-threatening nature of anaphylaxis, susceptible individuals with a history of systemic hypersensitivity reactions to environmental triggers must always have access to a readily available source of epinephrine.

Many patients will take OTC agents to help with allergy symptoms and should be taught to read and interpret drug labels correctly to check for ingredients that might cause tachycardia, drowsiness, or other adverse effects. Given safety concerns with several adrenergic agents when used in combination with other drugs, patients should be cautioned to be alert for any OTC formulations containing ephedrine, phenylephrine, phenylpropanolamine, or pseudoephedrine.

RHEUMATOID ARTHRITIS

Rheumatoid arthritis (RA) is a chronic, progressive, systemic inflammatory disease that primarily affects the synovial joints, although it may affect many organ systems. Joints are destroyed over a long course of disease remissions and exacerbations. Structural deformities, which create emotional as well as physical trauma for the patient, are common as the disease progresses. *Healthy People 2020* has three objectives related to this chronic debilitating condition: (1) increasing the proportion of adults with chronic joint symptoms who have seen a health-care provider for their symptoms, (2) increasing the proportion of adults with physician-diagnosed arthritis who have had effective evidence-based arthritis education as an integral part of the management of their condition, and (3) reducing the proportion of adults with physician-diagnosed arthritis who find it "very difficult" to perform specific joint-related activities.

EPIDEMIOLOGY AND CAUSES

RA is one of the most common connective tissue diseases in the United States and one of the most destructive to the joints. Women with the disease outnumber men at a ratio of 2.5 to 3.1:1, with a worldwide incidence of approximately 3 in 10,000 persons. Prevalence increases with age, with a peak of cases occurring between ages 40 and 60 years after an onset of disease between 20 and 40 years of age. RA has been observed across all racial and ethnic groups, but familial patterns have been observed, with first-degree relatives of affected patients having approximately a twofold to threefold higher risk of developing disease. Characterizing the genetic predispositions for disease remains an area of active research, and an association between RA and the human leukocyte antigen (HLA) system, a series of linked genes on the sixth chromosome, has been observed. Although genetic risk factors have been identified, the cause of the disease is unknown. Most therapies target the inflammatory pathways that mediate disease manifestations. Other potential etiological factors that have been implicated include infection, autoimmunity, environmental triggers, and hormonal influences.

PATHOPHYSIOLOGY

Rheumatoid arthritis causes joint destruction through many immunopathogenic mechanisms. Proteolytic enzymes (proteases) digest the tissue components of affected joints. This is speculated to occur due to local antigens that evoke the inflammatory cascade in the joint space; however, the source of these antigens is not fully characterized. These antigens may be autoimmune targets (e.g., type II collagen found only in articular cartilage and the vitreous of the eye, glycoprotein-39 found in cartilage, citrulline-containing peptides [CCPs] including citrullinated fibrin, and glucose-6-phosphate isomerase), which activate self-reactive T cells that initiate the inflammatory cascade.

T cells comprise nearly half the immune cells in an inflamed rheumatoid joint and are characterized by an activated T helper phenotype based on the cell surface expression of HLA-DR (MHC class II) antigens, CD27, CD4, as well as the costimulatory molecules CD28 and CD40. However, it has been difficult to characterize the antigenic specificity of the initial set of T cells that trigger this immune response, because the inflammatory cascade is characterized by widespread recruitment of so-called "bystander T cells" that do not express autoantigen specificity but, nonetheless, proliferate and contribute to the destruction of the affected joint through cytokine expression. Interestingly, some evidence indicates that it may not be the antigens themselves that trigger self-reactive T cells, but rather genetic mutations that alter specific amino acids within MHC class II antigen-presenting molecules (such as HLA-DRβ1) found on antigen-presenting cells. Other work has implicated superantigen interactions, in which several different T-cell clones are activated independent of their association with MHC class II molecules.

Cells of the synovial (joint) lining including joint endothelium, T cells, and fibroblast-like cells proliferate, producing cytokines (e.g., IL-1, IL-6, IL-8, IL-15, IL-18, IFN-γ), neuropeptides such as substance P, and chemotactic factors that induce expression of cell adhesion molecules (e.g., intercellular adhesion molecule [ICAM]–1, vascular cell adhesion molecule [VCAM]–1, P-selectin, E-selectin). This leads to increased recruitment of an array of immune cells into the affected joint, including mast cells that produce histamine, tryptase, leukotrienes, cytokines, and chymase; multinucleated cells and macrophages, which are the main source of potentially toxic nitric oxide and destructive matrix metalloproteinases (MMP) (e.g., collagenase [MMP-1], stromelysin [MMP-3], macrophage elastase [MMP-12]); and self-reactive plasma cells capable of producing autoantibodies (e.g., rheumatoid factor). Synovial fibroblasts further produce MMP-13, which has great specificity for type II collagen and is primarily responsible for soft tissue invasion in the affected joint.

Particularly noteworthy in the pathogenesis of RA is the production of rheumatoid factor—polyclonal antibody species typically of the IgM class that have specificity for the constant Fc region of IgG. Rheumatoid factor forms large immune complexes capable of activating complement proteins that themselves are cytolytic and chemotactic. The production of these antibodies is enhanced by cytokines secreted by regulatory CD4+ T helper cells. The plasma cell genes that encode rheumatoid factor (RF) undergo somatic mutations that increase their affinity for IgG, a process known as affinity maturation. Although RF is not pathognomonic of RA (as it may also be present in scleroderma, systemic lupus erythematosus [SLE], and even some viral infections) and may be absent in up to 25% of RA cases, the presence of these antibodies in the peripheral circulation correlates with invasive disease of greater severity.

Another type of autoantibody found in the blood of RA patients, anti-CCP antibodies (primarily specific for the connective tissue protein filaggrin) are considered more specific for RA than RF and are now widely used in the diagnosis of early RA. However, they do not appear to play as significant a role in joint destruction and the immunopathogenesis of RA as rheumatoid factor, because citrullinated peptides (which are the target of anti-CCP antibodies) are not typically found in the synovia of affected joints.

Tumor necrosis factor–alpha (TNF-α) is one of the main cytokines that trigger the proliferative rheumatoid synovium, which explains the efficacy of anti–TNF-α immunotherapies in treating RA. However, in addition to TNF-α, a wide array of cytokines has been implicated in the pathophysiology of the rheumatoid joint, including granulocyte-macrophage colony-stimulating factor, IL-2, IL-13, IL-17, and transforming growth factor–beta. Moreover, cells of the synovial lining undergo transformation into a rapidly proliferating state (although incapable of true metastasis) in which several types of transcription factors (NF-κB, Fos, Jun, Raf, Myc)

and intracellular kinases (e.g., mitogen-activated protein kinase) are upregulated.

As these various inflammatory pathways manifest over time, joints are progressively destroyed by an invasive rheumatoid pannus. The rheumatoid pannus consists of granulated vascular tissue extending from the vascular bed into the joint space. Acting similarly to a destructive malignancy, the pannus is characterized by increased angiogenesis (new blood vessel formation), which is mediated by the upregulation of several angiogenic cytokines and growth factors, including hypoxia-inducible factor–1, vascular endothelial growth factor, heparin-binding growth factors, macrophage angiogenic factor, epithelial neutrophil activating peptide-78, TNF-α, prostaglandin E$_1$ (PGE$_1$), PGE$_2$, and IL-8. Despite this increased vascularity, circulation is often inadequate for the exaggerated level of cellular proliferation in the rheumatoid synovium. In addition, the increased intra-articular pressure within the affected joint resulting from cellular proliferation, fibrin and clotting factor deposition, and fluid accumulation may compress articular vessels, resulting in progressive joint ischemia.

Mutations and overexpression of certain cell cycle regulatory proteins such as the *p53* tumor suppressor gene have been identified in cells of the rheumatoid synovium, which may render them less susceptible to apoptosis (programmed cell death). Proteolytic enzymes (e.g., MMP, glycosidases) released by cells in the pannus destroy the connective tissue matrix, including glycosaminoglycans, fibronectin, proteoglycans such as chondroitin sulfate, collagen, and eventually subchondral bony structures. In addition, certain components of the rheumatoid pannus, such as regulatory T cells and bone marrow stromal cells, induce differentiation and proliferation of bone osteoclasts, which leads to further joint destruction. However, the pannus remains responsive to antiproliferative immunosuppressant treatments.

Within the synovial fluid, an inflammatory response also ensues but with a notably different distribution of immune cells. Polymorphonuclear neutrophils are the most prominent cellular infiltrate, numbering upwards of one billion in severely inflamed joints. These cells secrete a host of proteolytic enzymes into the joint fluid (e.g., myeloperoxidase, collagenase and other MMPs, elastase, and lysozyme), as well as inflammatory cytokines (e.g., prostaglandins, IL-1β), and chemotactic factors (e.g., leukotriene B4, platelet activating factor). Because accumulation of joint fluid distends the joint capsule and contributes greatly to articular pains, aspiration of this exudative fluid may provide immediate relief.

The immunopathology of RA is widespread and extends beyond the joint synovium. Constitutional signs and symptoms including fever, anorexia, weight loss, and fatigue may be prominent during acute flares, reflecting the systemic nature of the disease, which may involve layers of the heart muscle, cardiac valves, pulmonary visceral pleura, spleen, larynx, dura mater, and sclera (extra-articular manifestations). Other organ manifestations of RA may include pericardial effusions, cardiac dysfunction (including myocardial infarction), and rarely pericarditis. Lung manifestations may include pleural effusion, pleuritis, interstitial fibrosis, and bronchiolitis obliterans with organizing pneumonia. Hematological findings are not uncommon and may include anemia of chronic disease or thrombocytosis. RA associated with both splenomegaly and neutropenia is termed *Felty's syndrome*. Ocular manifestations include keratoconjunctivitis associated with dry eye syndrome (sicca), as well as episcleritis, uveitis, and nodular scleritis, which can lead to blindness.

Rheumatoid nodules are another common extra-articular manifestation of RA. These nodules typically appear on the elbows but may be found on any extensor surface of the body that is subject to repeated mechanical stress, pressure, or irritation. Found in up to 25% of RA patients, these initially microscopic nodules are subcutaneous and may form into larger granulomas, characterized by a central section of fibrinoid necrosis that is surrounded by a palisade of radially arranged, elongated connective tissue cells enveloped by chronic granulation tissue.

CLINICAL PRESENTATION

Subjective

In the early stages of the disease, the RA patient may complain of malaise, diffuse arthritis, weight loss, anorexia, and low-grade fever. In addition, the patient may complain of neuropathic pain in the extremities, ocular pain, and chest pain on deep inspiration.

The patient typically awakens with joint pain and stiffness but reports that it improves as the day progresses. Not only does pain subside, but the swelling associated with joints in the early morning also abates with moderate activity, thereby leading to decreased joint stiffness. As the disease progresses over time, recurrent pain and swelling in both small and large peripheral joints may result in diminished activity and worsening pain and immobility.

Objective

Key physical findings of RA are peripheral symmetric polyarthritis and morning stiffness, which typically last longer than 1 hour. The clinician may note that certain joints are affected more than others, such as the proximal interphalangeal (PIP) and metacarpophalangeal (MCP) joints in the hands and wrists, as well as the knees. The toes and ankles also tend to be affected. The clinician should expect the affected joints to be tender (painful to pressure), edematous, and partially immobile. Radiographic x-ray changes in early disease may be nondescript or absent even though synovial changes have already begun. However, advanced magnetic resonance imaging (MRI) has shown promise as an imaging modality capable of detecting early joint manifestations with increased sensitivity compared with x-ray studies.

As the disease progresses, affected joints will appear more deformed and rigid, with diminished range of motion. Characteristic findings of advanced disease include Boutonnière deformity of affected fingers, in which the PIP joint is in a nonreducible state of flexion with hyperextension of the distal interphalangeal (DIP) joint, as well as the associated swan neck deformity, in which the PIP joint is hyperextended and the DIP joint is in a constant state of flexion. The most severe form of structural joint damage in the hands is known as arthritis mutilans, which is characterized by extensive bone resorption, complete loss of the joint space, shortening and malpositioning of the fingers, and almost complete loss of function. In contrast to small joint involvement, monoarticular arthritis of a large joint is a far less common presentation in RA and is more suspicious for reactive arthritis, which does not typically manifest with morning stiffness.

Physical examination may also reveal additional significant findings associated with extra-articular organ manifestations of the disease. A cardiac rub associated with pericarditis may be detected. A pulmonary friction rub or diminished respiratory excursion may suggest inflammation of the visceral pleura, as well as involvement of the bony structures of the ribs and sternum. Dry crackles may reflect an interstitial pulmonary process in advanced chronic disease. A finding of injected sclera suggests scleritis. Loss of sensation, especially in the lower extremities, indicates peripheral neuropathy, and ecchymotic lesions may appear on the arms and legs. Rheumatoid nodules are commonly observed over the olecranon process or other extensor surfaces of the limbs and may be tender.

DIAGNOSTIC REASONING

Diagnostic Tests

The preferred initial test for diagnosis of RA is measurement of peripherally circulating RF, an IgM class autoantibody that binds to the Fc portion of IgG molecules. The test result provides both qualitative and quantitative information that is useful in correlating with physical markers of RA. For example, a positive RF titer of greater than 1:150 indicates a poorer prognosis and is often accompanied by findings of severe disease, such as rheumatoid nodules. It is necessary to interpret both the presence of RF (qualitative) with the dilutional titer (quantitative) because RF may be present in other diseases and its incidence increases with age. It is estimated that only 75% of RA patients are positive for RF.

Because RF alone is not diagnostic of RA, a more specific test is for circulating anti-CCP antibodies in the peripheral blood. This autoantibody species is more specific for RA than RF and may be detected earlier in the disease process. However, anti-CCP titers correlate less well with severity of disease or prognosis, compared with RF.

Initial testing should also include an erythrocyte sedimentation rate (ESR), which will be elevated if the disease is active. C-reactive protein (CRP) is an acute-phase reactant, which, like ESR, is reflective of a heightened inflammatory state. Thus, CRP may be evaluated in addition to or in place of ESR as a nonspecific indicator of inflammation. Other tests include a CBC to rule out anemia as a potential cause of fatigue and to evaluate for an associated leukocytosis or, alternatively, neutropenia. A platelet count (showing normal or high values) will become more elevated as joints become more inflamed. In addition, joint fluid analysis may aid in distinguishing RA from other causes of joint inflammation, such as infection. Aspirates from rheumatoid joints will show between 2,000 and 50,000 white blood cells (WBCs) per mcL, with a pronounced neutrophil component (see Table 52.2).

Subsequent laboratory tests may be used as markers of disease progression. For example, ESR and CRP act as markers of inflammation, which may be helpful in tracking the course of disease and response to therapy. Quantitative antinuclear antibodies (ANAs) may also help in differentiating RA from SLE, because lower titers suggest rheumatoid disease. If the diagnosis is in doubt, a comprehensive autoantibody panel may be done to help distinguish RA from other autoimmune connective tissue disorders, such as Sjögren's syndrome, although interpretation of such panels typically requires expert rheumatologic knowledge.

Radiographic x-ray changes in the joints may not be evident in the initial phases of the disease. However, after the disease has run its course for 6 months or more, radiographs will reveal bone erosions in the joints of the hands and feet. Plain films may show bony erosions in up to 30% of patients within 1 year of diagnosis and in up to 90% of cases after the first 2 years. MRI has gained wider acceptance in recent years as a more sensitive (albeit more expensive) detection method for joint changes in early disease. Research is ongoing into the cost-benefit assessment of early disease detection with MRI as a trigger for earlier medical intervention that could potentially lead to decreased disease progression and subsequent complications over time, thereby off setting the initial expense.

Differential Diagnosis

In general, an array of connective tissue diseases must be considered in the differential diagnosis of RA. These include osteoarthritis, gout, chronic Lyme disease, SLE, infection by human parvovirus B19, polymyalgia rheumatica, Sjögren's syndrome, sarcoidosis, and various neoplasms. Osteoarthritis almost never affects the wrists and the metacarpophalangeal joints. Osteoarthritis is classically known for affecting the DIP joints with Heberden's nodes (hard, bony swellings) in the fingers. In contrast,

the distal joints are less commonly affected in RA, and there are typically no Heberden's nodes in the hands. Within the thumb, the carpophalangeal joint is typically affected in osteoarthritis, whereas the interphalangeal joint is more often affected in RA.

A diagnosis of gout is confirmed by the finding of urate crystals in synovial aspirate. For crystalline arthritides, gout crystals are negatively birefringent, whereas pseudogout has positively birefringent calcium pyrophosphate crystals. Chronic Lyme disease usually involves only a single joint. A characteristic expanding bull's-eye rash known as erythema migrans is typical, and positive serological markers against the causative agent (*Borrelia burgdorferi*) distinguish Lyme disease from RA.

Infection with human parvovirus B19 may also manifest with joint pain. Serological evidence of antiparvovirus B19 IgM antibody and a characteristic rash with an erythematous "slapped cheek" appearance distinguish this infection from RA. When considering acute viral polyarthritis, other causative infections include hepatitis C and rubella (rubeola virus), which may be distinguished from RA via specific immunoassays and organism-specific antibody titers.

SLE arthritic changes are almost never deforming and erosive changes are absent on radiographs. Patients with polymyalgia rheumatica are usually negative for RF or have low titers. In addition, this disease usually affects persons older than 50 years of age. Whereas qualitative RF positivity increases with age and may be nonspecifically present in older adults, patients with polymyalgia rheumatica may report myalgias but not distinctive arthralgias or arthritis.

A more challenging disease to distinguish from RA is psoriatic arthritis, because joint manifestations may not occur concurrently with cutaneous psoriatic findings in these patients. However, if psoriatic lesions are not present at the time of evaluation, a family history of psoriasis and joint manifestations in one or more relatives usually supports this diagnosis. Another form of seronegative (RF-negative) spondyloarthritis, ankylosing spondylitis, may also present with peripheral arthritis; however, the predominant feature of this condition is axial (spinal) stiffness due to arthritis and dysfunctional bony changes in the vertebral joints, which is not typically seen in RA. Finally, some neoplasms can mimic rheumatoid disease, but again, RF is typically negative or quantitatively low in this setting.

MANAGEMENT

The management of RA progresses from conservative interventions to aggressive symptom management. Although the disease is debilitating over time, clinicians also recognize the potential adverse effects of immunosuppressive and anti-inflammatory therapies, including increased infection risk and hepatotoxicity. Thus, systemic therapy is typically initiated in response to symptom manifestations, thereby sparing the liver and GI tract from prolonged use of potentially toxic agents.

The overall goals of management are to reduce pain and inflammation and to preserve joint function. It is possible to achieve these goals in early management without pharmacological agents. This section on management, therefore, includes nonpharmacological interventions as therapy for RA, particularly early in the disease process.

Initial Management

Joint swelling and immobility on rising, which abate or diminish throughout the day, characterize early rheumatoid disease. Early disease symptoms can be managed by one or a combination of the following: physical and occupational therapies, heat and cold applications, exercise, rest, assistive devices, splints, meditation, chiropractic adjustments, and weight loss.

Physical and occupational therapists are educated to identify strategies that promote function and prevent immobility. Their special skills in motivating patients to remain active should not be underestimated in early disease management. Often patients attend therapy sessions and derive accompanying educational and emotional benefits from associating with other patients diagnosed with RA.

Heat and cold applications provide analgesia and relaxation to muscles and connective tissue. It is usually necessary to try both heat and cold therapy with individual patients because some patients respond better to one rather than the other. Application in anticipation of exercise may enhance joint mobility during exercise. Particularly helpful to some patients is to remain seated in warm water for 10 to 30 minutes.

Exercise reduces pain and inflammation only if the affected joints are not stressed during an inflammatory period. Outside of an inflammatory event, the joints may undergo judicious stress through an increase in resistance exercises to promote strength and endurance. Thus, isometric exercises (in which the joint angle and muscle length are held constant) should be prescribed for inflamed joints, and isotonic exercises (in which muscle length is shortened with contractions against a constant load) should be done at other times. Patients may also benefit from low-resistance aerobic exercise at the shallow end of a swimming pool.

Rest reduces pain and inflammation by controlling joint movement. However, one must distinguish between systemic rest and resting of the joints. Systemic rest signifies a prescribed period of relaxation that may involve sleep. Patients with mild inflammation may benefit from systemic rest in the prone position for 1 to 2 hours per day; the rest period may extend to 2-hour periods three or four times daily during waking hours, as necessitated by severe inflammation. Like systemic rest, resting of the joints should be done in a prone position to avoid

hip contractures; however, the duration of rest is much shorter than with systemic rest, usually lasting only 20 to 40 minutes. In either case, the patient should prepare a method for awakening to avoid excessive systemic rest, as excessive rest may signal depression or other underlying disease.

Assistive devices include those that the patient requires to complete activities of daily living. Canes or crutches can relieve stress on affected weight-bearing joints during periods of acute inflammation. Once the inflammation subsides, the patient may walk without such devices. When the clinician or physical therapist recommends using a cane or crutches, it is important to the patient's self-esteem and inner hope to explain that these may be needed only temporarily. Other assistive devices for the home include bars for gripping the inside of a shower or bathtub or beside the toilet, a raised toilet seat, retrieval–extension devices for picking up items from the floor or at a distance, and an electronic chair lift to help the patient manage stairs.

Splints reduce pain, promote function, and stabilize involved joints. The hands and wrists are the preferred regions for splints, which are usually applied at night. Splints of the hips and knees are usually not preferred over lying prone. The position of optimal function should be considered when applying the splint. Moreover, the material of the splint should be lightweight, non-abrasive, and durable enough to withstand frequent applications. Because self-application is preferred, the splint should be structured so that the patient can apply it without assistance.

Meditation may be helpful in relieving depression and anxiety associated with chronic disease and disability. In addition, it promotes self-care practices and self-efficacy. Meditation may follow traditional spiritual paths, whereby patients learn from teachers in traditional religious communities. Alternatively, meditation may involve guiding the attention using restful music, images, spiritual charms, and breath work. Patients with RA should meditate in a prone position to prevent postmeditation joint stiffness and pain.

The role of chiropractic adjustment remains controversial among traditional Western medicine practitioners; however, its benefits to the patient with RA must be considered. Chiropractors can relieve pressure to unaffected joints that compensates for decreased weight-bearing or activity in the affected joints. Although adjustments may require repeated manipulations and therapeutic benefits may be short-lived, other benefits include an increased sense of well-being and improved quality of life.

Weight loss reduces pressure on weight-bearing joints in the lower extremities and enhances activity. Alternatively, overeating may be a sign of depression. Thus, weight gain must be addressed in an overall plan of encouraging weight reduction (if applicable) to achieve ideal body weight.

Subsequent Management

Drug therapies include analgesics, NSAIDs, corticosteroids, nonbiologic and biologic disease-modifying antirheumatic drugs (DMARDs), and older therapies as described in the following sections.

Analgesics

Analgesics such as acetaminophen (Tylenol) or capsaicin cream, gel, lotion, or roll-on may be effective, even though they have no anti-inflammatory effects. Although aspirin has been the mainstay of therapy for RA, acetaminophen may be helpful for mild pain. Of note, opioid analgesics have also been used for more significant pain although these agents are addictive and are not disease modifying in RA. Given the public health risks associated with the overuse of prescription opioids, reliance on narcotic analgesics as primary RA therapy is strongly discouraged and presents a significant danger for the patient.

NSAIDs

Subsequent management begins with a consideration of cyclooxygenase inhibitors, which include aspirin and other NSAIDs. Drugs of this class may not need to be used daily during the early stages of disease. Rather, the patient can take them only for pain that is unrelieved by nonpharmacologic means. Patients may be individually more responsive to one type of NSAID than another, and trial courses are sometimes required to determine the most effective agent although simultaneous use of multiple NSAIDs is discouraged. Different NSAIDs may also differ in their side effect profiles (e.g., sulindac 150 mg by mouth [PO] twice daily, conferring fewer GI side effects than other NSAIDs). However, the adverse effects of NSAIDs as a class are well documented, including renal toxicity, GI side effects, platelet inhibition, and idiosyncratic hypersensitivity reactions. Thus, they should not be used indiscriminately.

Extra-strength (1,000 mg) aspirin can be used up to three to four times per day if baseline liver function studies, platelet count, renal function studies, and hemoglobin level are within normal limits. Caution must be exercised when prescribing 4 g of aspirin per day to persons older than 65 years of age, however, as their hepatic and renal function may be impaired by age. Dose reductions are warranted if adverse effects ensue or laboratory markers dictate. Aspirin should always be taken with 8 ounces of water or milk to avoid pill erosion or ulceration of the gastric mucosa. Enteric-coated aspirin is preferred to prevent gastric erosion. Concurrent anticoagulant therapy is a relative contraindication to aspirin and other NSAID use. Patients on anticoagulant therapy should avoid these medications or, if benefits of these medications are thought to outweigh their risks, lower doses may be used.

If adverse effects of aspirin occur or if the therapeutic efficacy diminishes, other NSAIDs may be used. With chronic use, individual drugs of the same NSAID class can lose their effectiveness in a specific patient. However, many different NSAIDs are available, and clinicians may recommend a different NSAID in these cases.

The primary adverse effect of the NSAIDs is GI discomfort. Their inhibition of gastric prostaglandin E (a natural stomach protectant) predisposes the gastric mucosa to erosion. Most of the NSAIDs can be taken with an H_2-blocker such as ranitidine (Zantac) to reduce dyspepsia; however, H_2-blockers do not reduce hemorrhage or mucosal erosions. Proton pump inhibitors such as omeprazole (Prilosec) OTC or esomeprazole magnesium (Nexium) suppress gastric acid secretion and may be preferred to H_2-blockers for GI prophylaxis with NSAID use.

Minimal elevations in serum transaminase levels are to be expected at daily doses of 2,400 mg ibuprofen (Motrin, Advil) for adults younger than 65 years of age; the maximum dose may be as high as 3,200 mg/day if no adverse effects are apparent, but prolonged use of such doses may confer significant renal, hepatic, or GI toxicity, as well as iatrogenic hypertension. Should transaminase levels exceed two times the upper limit of normal, a dose reduction is indicated, along with laboratory evaluation for infectious causes of elevated liver enzymes, such as screening for hepatitis B and C.

Toxicity from prolonged NSAID use may result in renal impairment and present with acute renal failure requiring emergent care, as patients are prone to overuse NSAIDs, given their OTC availability and highly marketed nature. Thus, renal toxicity is as important a consideration as gastritis and ulcer formation. A rise in serum creatinine or blood urea nitrogen after starting NSAID therapy is an indication for further testing and initiating a possible dose reduction or cessation. Should renal failure develop, it is usually reversible after withdrawing the agent, given the proper supportive care.

Corticosteroids

Corticosteroids (up to 7.5 mg prednisone daily by mouth or injected intra-articularly, such as triamcinolone) may be helpful in RA. However, side effects of prolonged corticosteroid use include adrenal insufficiency, hyperglycemia, osteoporosis, increased infection risk, and skin discoloration, which explains why maximal daily therapy is not recommended for more than 6 months. In addition, calcium, vitamin D, and bisphosphonates are indicated with prolonged corticosteroid use to mitigate bone demineralization. (The adverse effect profile of corticosteroids is thoroughly covered in the atopic dermatitis section of Chapter 16.)

Disease-modifying Antirheumatic Drugs

DMARDs include immunosuppressants and immunomodulators of various types, many of which have been used for decades. However, the newest class of DMARDs are biologic immunotherapeutic agents, including anticytokine immunotherapies (TNF-α inhibitors, IL-1 inhibitors, IL-6 inhibitors) and anti–B cell and anti–T-cell agents (see Drugs Commonly Prescribed 62.1). Active disease should be treated early with DMARDs within

Drugs Commonly Prescribed 62.1: Disease-modifying Antirheumatic Drugs (DMARDs)

DRUG	ADVERSE REACTIONS AND PRESCRIBING CONSIDERATIONS
Aminoquinoline	
Hydroxychloroquine (Plaquenil)	May cause irreversible retinopathy, alopecia, and blood dyscrasias.
Immunosuppressant	
Cyclosporine (Neoral)	Indicated only in patients who have not responded to methotrexate. Should not be used in pregnancy unless benefits of using the drug outweigh potential risks to the fetus. Monitor renal and hepatic function. Reduce dose if hypertension occurs.
Pyrimidine Synthesis Inhibitors	
Leflunomide (Arava)	Monitor liver function. May cause GI upset, leukopenia, thrombocytopenia.
Salicylate Sulfonamides	
Sulfasalazine (Azulfidine)	Monitor liver function. May cause nausea, dyspepsia, abdominal pain, vomiting, leukopenia, thrombocytopenia, and urine or skin discoloration.
Folic Acid Antagonist	
Methotrexate (Rheumatrex)	Monitor liver function. May cause blood dyscrasias, GI upset, hepatotoxicity, opportunistic infections, fatal skin reactions.
Tumor Necrosis Factor (TNF)-α Blockers	
Caution with all TNF-α blockers for reactivation of TB and hepatitis B, predisposition to serious infection, development of lupus-like syndrome, development of selective cytopenias and pancytopenias, worsening of demyelinating syndromes, worsening of heart failure, increased malignancy rates, and cautious use in patients at risk for hepatic injury or with elevated liver function enzymes.	
Adalimumab (Humira)	May be used with or without methotrexate in moderate to severe RA.
Etanercept (Enbrel)	May be used with or without methotrexate in moderate to severe RA.
Infliximab (Remicade)	Should be used in combination with methotrexate for moderate to severe RA.
Certolizumab (Cimzia)	May be used with or without methotrexate in moderate to severe RA.
Golimumab (Simponi)	Should be used in combination with methotrexate for moderate to severe RA.
Interleukin-1 Receptor Antagonist	
Anakinra (Kineret)	May cause predisposition to infections, headache, nausea, vomiting, diarrhea, stomach pain, neutropenia.
Interleukin-6 Receptor Antagonists	
Tocilizumab (Actemra)	May be used with or without methotrexate in patients with an inadequate response to one or more DMARDs, including TNF-α blockers. May predispose to infections, hyperlipidemia, GI perforation in at-risk patients.
Sarilumab (Kevzara)	May be used with or without methotrexate in patients with an inadequate response to one or more DMARDs, including TNF-α blockers. May predispose to infections, hyperlipidemia, GI perforation in at-risk patients.
Anti–B Cell Agents	
Rituximab (Rituxan)	Indicated for use with methotrexate in patients who do not respond to TNF-α blockers. Stop hypertension medications during treatment. May cause angioedema; abdominal pain or black, tarry stools; blood dyscrasias.
Anti–T Cell Agents	
Abatacept (Orencia)	May be used as monotherapy or with other DMARDs, other than TNF-α blockers. May predispose to infections, headache, or respiratory adverse events in COPD patients.

Continued

Drugs Commonly Prescribed 62.1: Disease-Modifying Antirheumatic Drugs (DMARDs)—cont'd	
DRUG	**ADVERSE REACTIONS AND PRESCRIBING CONSIDERATIONS**
Tyrosine Kinase Inhibitor	
Tofacitinib (Xeljanz)	May be used as monotherapy or with other DMARDs, other than TNF-α blockers or potent immunosuppressants such as azathioprine or cyclosporine. May predispose to infections, hepatic enzyme elevations, neutropenia, anemia, GI perforation in at-risk patients.

3 months of disease onset and even more aggressively in severe disease. Because anti–TNF-α therapy inhibits cell-mediated immunity, a potential side effect of this therapy is reactivation of latent (dormant) TB infection. TB screening should be instituted in all patients before starting biologic immunosuppressive agents.

Combination therapy with DMARDs is more effective than monotherapy, and several different combinations have been tested. There is strong evidence for the greater efficacy of the combination of three DMARDs—methotrexate, sulfasalazine, and hydroxychloroquine—versus methotrexate monotherapy or dual therapy with only sulfasalazine and hydroxychloroquine. There is also a strong evidence for adding a TNF-α blocking agent to methotrexate therapy in patients with moderately or highly active disease after 3 months of methotrexate monotherapy.

Although the anti–TNF-α agents are considered first-line biologic DMARDs, other biologic agents have been approved for use in RA patients with an inadequate therapeutic response or intolerance to anti–TNF-α agents (e.g., abatacept, rituximab, tocilizumab, sarilumab), as well as the small molecule tyrosine kinase inhibitor tofacitinib. It is not recommended, however, that immunosuppressive biologic agents with different mechanisms of action be used in combination, given the risk of serious infection. Thus, therapies should be crafted based on the patient's tolerance of side effects and the presence of comorbid conditions.

Older Therapies

Other DMARDs are possible options in the event of treatment failure with aspirin and other NSAIDs, but these are used less often now, given their low therapeutic index (higher toxicity risk) and the development of the newer biologic agents discussed previously. These include azathioprine (Imuran), gold sodium thiomalate (Myochrysine), antimalarials, penicillamine (Depen), sulfasalazine (Azulfidine), and minocycline hydrochloride (Minocin). Hydroxychloroquine (Plaquenil) is an antimalarial usually used in milder disease, compared with sulfasalazine, which is used more often in moderate disease. Most of the COX-2 inhibitors, which were a mainstay of therapy in the past, are no longer marketed because of their cardiovascular risks. Celecoxib (Celebrex) is one of the last remaining.

Methotrexate is an older agent that is also used in many common chemotherapeutic regimens for the treatment

of cancer. In contrast to many other older DMARDs, methotrexate remains highly effective in RA, including low-dose regimens early in the disease process. It may be administered in adults younger than age 65 years at an initial weekly dose of 7.5 mg PO. The dosage may be doubled during the second week if tolerance and therapeutic aims necessitate, although its full therapeutic effect may take 4 to 6 weeks to manifest. Maximum dosage for RA is typically 25 mg per week.

The potential toxic effects of methotrexate include interstitial pneumonitis, hepatic cirrhosis, and teratogenicity. It is therefore not used in women who may become pregnant or in patients with chronic liver disease or elevated hepatic function enzymes. Combined use of methotrexate with NSAIDs, sulfonamides (e.g., sulfamethoxazole/trimethoprim [SMX/TMP]), or sulfonylureas such as glipizide (Glucotrol) increases the chance of hepatotoxicity, so concurrent use of these drugs is discouraged. Increased risk of hepatotoxicity is also seen with diabetes, obesity, and renal disease. The decisions to initiate methotrexate therapy must be weighed against its potential risks and the availability and appropriateness of alternative therapeutic options.

FOLLOW-UP AND REFERRAL

The follow-up of patients with RA requires routine clinical laboratory evaluation and episodic adjustments in interventions. Routine clinical laboratory evaluation is performed every 90 days and includes CBC, platelet count, serum liver and renal function studies, and fasting blood sugar. Most of the adverse effects of drugs used in the management of RA can be monitored with this routine panel. If methotrexate is used, a serum albumin level should be added to the routine panel of tests to monitor hepatic synthetic function.

The CRP blood test is a nonspecific method for evaluating the severity and course of the inflammatory process. CRP is normally less than 0.8 mg/dL and is typically elevated in RA before treatment. Failure to decrease the CRP level after initiating treatment may thus indicate a lack of efficacy of the therapeutic agent or the presence of an underlying infection or tissue necrosis; therefore, CRP should be monitored to determine the effectiveness of therapy. ESR may follow this same pattern during treatment and may serve as a less technically involved, and therefore less expensive and more widely available, alternative test of inflammation compared with CRP. However, many clinicians question the utility of the ESR, as an elevated value is highly nonspecific and the assay itself is highly subjective.

Following scheduled laboratory evaluations, each visit to the clinician should address the interim clinical history since the last visit. Attention should focus on the efficacy of relief measures and the onset, duration, and frequency of pain and swelling of the joints. Standardized and validated disease assessment tools may be completed by the clinician at each visit to assess how well treatment interventions have achieved the targeted goals of low disease activity and complete disease remission, commonly known as "treating to target."

The primary-care practitioner should refer the patient to a rheumatologist if initial management (including aspirin or NSAID therapy) fails. The rheumatologist is responsible for initiating therapies such as methotrexate and other DMARDs, including newer biologic agents. Co-management may mean that the rheumatologist will evaluate the patient twice each year once stable or more frequently, as signs and symptoms necessitate. In particular, specialist input is typically required to effectively "treat to target."

Patient Education: Rheumatoid Arthritis

Patient education focuses on the goals of therapy, which are reduction of pain, control of inflammation, and preservation of function. Many of the key patient education topics were covered under the earlier section on Initial Management. In addition, education should address the therapeutic and adverse effects of all drugs used. Because RA is a chronic disease, education should also encompass the emotional, social, and spiritual sequelae of living with recurrent bouts of pain and disability.

The goals of therapy are best realized by promoting self-care. Education concerning self-care should include caregivers who must share common therapeutic goals for the patient before they can support the patient's self-care practices. To help keep the patient from sinking into a cycle of seeking secondary gains from the "sick" role, the caregiver should support normal social role behaviors by encouraging self-care. The caregiver, therefore, becomes integral to achieving the therapeutic goals of therapy, which should be reviewed at each visit. This is an ideal context to employ the *Circle of Caring* model involving all medical modalities, nursing modalities, complementary therapies, and the patient's family.

CHRONIC FATIGUE SYNDROME AND FIBROMYALGIA SYNDROME

Myalgic encephalomyelitis/chronic fatigue syndrome (ME/CFS) remains poorly understood, despite abundant attention in the scientific and lay press. Although a recent Institute of Medicine report recommended this condition be renamed systemic exertion intolerance disease, the lack of agreement as to its cause, laboratory markers, and clinical course may explain why the syndrome is not discussed in some medical texts. There appears to be significant overlap between CFS and fibromyalgia syndrome (FMS), another controversial chronic pain syndrome. Most patients with CFS meet criteria for FMS, and at least 70% of patients with FMS meet criteria for CFS. Moreover, both disorders have been widely recognized in persons with comorbid psychiatric illness, because nearly two-thirds of CFS patients and one-third of FMS patients meet criteria for depression, or anxiety disorders. Many authors have criticized the historical and physical diagnostic criteria for both conditions as having a strong potential for overlap with somatization disorders.

EPIDEMIOLOGY AND CAUSES

Without a generally accepted working definition of CFS, it is difficult to systematically ascertain its epidemiology. Chronic fatigue is an initial complaint in up to 25% of patients in ambulatory care settings, and it is estimated that approximately 10% of these individuals meet diagnostic criteria for CFS. One source sites that 2.5 million Americans suffer from ME/CFS (National Academies of Sciences Engineering Medicine, 2015). Numerous books in the popular press have advanced the belief that women are affected two times more often than men. The same references tend to agree that younger women are affected more often. CFS has been hypothesized to be autoimmune and infectious in etiology; however, the causes for the syndrome have yet to be determined. Importantly, it is a diagnosis of exclusion, with the incidence ranging from 4 to 8.6 cases per 100,000 adults.

More epidemiological data for FMS exist in the medical literature. An estimated 11 million people in the United States have FMS, and 80% to 90% are women. The prevalence of FMS has been estimated at 0.5% for men and 3.4% for women, with some studies claiming an increased prevalence in women compared with men of up to 10:1. Prevalence is higher in older patients, at more than 7% for women aged 60 to 79 years.

These numbers are reflected in the clinical impact of FMS, as up to 20% of all patient visits to rheumatology practices are for FMS. It is now considered the most common cause of generalized musculoskeletal pain in women aged 20 to 55 years. FMS may occur with greater frequency in patients with disorders characterized by systemic inflammation, including RA, SLE, and hepatitis C infection. However, an underlying inflammatory etiology to FMS is unclear, because relatives of patients with fibromyalgia are seven times more likely than relatives of patients with RA to have FMS. In addition, several studies have shown that up to 50% of patients with FMS have a history of sexual and/or physical abuse, suggesting the importance of psychological factors in the development of FMS.

PATHOPHYSIOLOGY

Despite extensive investigation, the pathophysiology of CFS and FMS are unclear. It has been hypothesized that both syndromes may be disorders of muscle energy metabolism, inflammatory or immunopathological diseases of muscle, generalized disorders of pain perception, neuronally mediated hypotension, neuroendocrine disturbances, dysregulated serotonin secretion, sleep disturbances, or a sequela of sexual abuse or domestic violence. Although depression and anxiety disorders demonstrate great overlap with both CFS and FMS, it is controversial as to whether these conditions occur concurrently, whether CFS and FMS lead to psychiatric sequelae, or whether these chronic conditions are somatic manifestations of underlying mood disorders. Patients commonly experience accusations of malingering (intentionally fabricating symptoms for secondary gain).

Extensive work has explored a potential infectious etiology for CFS, focusing on Epstein-Barr virus (EBV), retroviruses, and human herpesvirus–6 (HHV-6) as causative agents. However, there has been difficulty in reproducing positive results across different laboratories. Moreover, no consistent serological profile has been identified that distinguishes patients with CFS from control groups across multiple studies.

Several studies, however, have demonstrated qualitative and quantitative differences in immune function between patients with CFS and controls, including reduced numbers of natural killer cells with depressed function, reduced levels of immunoglobulin and immune complexes, and increased numbers of cell surface adhesion molecules, among others. However, the differences are of questionable clinical significance and have been inconsistent and even conflicting among different studies.

Studies that have examined neuroendocrine differences between affected patients and controls have produced similarly inconclusive results. Although some evidence points to diminished secretion of adrenocorticotropic hormone and reduced serum cortisol levels, these findings are not specific for CFS and have also been observed in FMS, as well as in healthy subjects with altered sleep patterns related to overnight work shifts.

Studies attempting to clarify the etiology of FMS have also not been definitive. For many years, FMS was considered a disorder of muscle metabolism, possibly related to chronic hypoxia of muscular tissue. However, studies of lactate levels, muscle force studies, and postexertional pain have demonstrated a marked similarity between patients with FMS and sedentary controls. Thus, the most current theories suggest that patients with FMS have disproportionate perceptions of pain, exacerbated by muscle inactivity and deconditioning. In fact, lower pain perception thresholds have been documented in first-degree relatives of patients with FMS.

Although no studies have been conclusive, altered pain perception is more likely to be a central rather than peripheral nociceptor (pain receptor) phenomenon. This is supported by observations in FMS patients of altered patterns of sleep and mood, decreased blood flow to pain centers in the brain, and alterations in serotonin secretions and the pituitary-hypothalamic-adrenal neuroendocrine axis. In addition, autonomic dysregulation of heart rate and systemic blood pressure has also been implicated on the basis of tilt-table testing for orthostatic hypotension; again, these findings have not been consistently reproduced. An inflammatory component to the myalgias of FMS has never been shown, which likely explains the lack of efficacy of NSAID and corticosteroid therapies in this condition.

CLINICAL PRESENTATION

Subjective

The symptomatic presentation of CFS and FMS may overlap considerably. Patients may report postexercise malaise, fatigue, polyarthralgia, headaches, impaired memory and concentration, depressed mood, cognitive disturbances, sore throat, restless and disordered sleep, and myalgias. Often the patient will also report having consulted one or more specialists concerning these vague symptoms.

Objective

The onset of CFS is sudden and may be preceded by a mononucleosis-like illness or by significant GI findings. This same type of preceding event may also herald the onset of FMS. The patient will appear tired, and the skin may be pale. Cervical lymph nodes, if enlarged, will be shotty and nontender. Otherwise, the examination may be unremarkable. Despite complaints of impaired memory and concentration, the results of objective mental status assessments may vary with reference to recent recall and problem-solving abilities.

For a diagnosis of FMS to be made, the patient must have widespread muscular pain that has been present for at least 3 months. The pain should be present in at least 11 of 18 tender points on digital palpation with an applied pressure of 4 kg/cm (enough force to whiten the examiner's nailbed). The 18 tender points are bilateral sites at nine key locations (see Table 62.1). Pain at these sites should be significantly greater than at control sites, which are not expected to be tender, such as the patient's thumbnail or mid-forearm.

DIAGNOSTIC REASONING

Diagnostic Tests

CFS tends to affect active, highly functional adults. The physical examination for CFS is typically normal. Advanced imaging tests such as computed tomography (CT) and MRI are not indicated in the absence of significant physical findings. In addition, virus-specific serologies against EBV or Lyme disease are also not recommended without a strong suspicion from history or

TABLE 62.1	Diagnostic Criteria for Fibromyalgia*
History Criteria	Pain is considered widespread when ALL of the following are present: Pain in the left side of the body Pain in the right side of the body Pain above the waist Pain below the waist Axial skeletal pain (cervical spine, anterior chest, thoracic spine, or lower back)
Pain Criteria	Pain exists in at least 11 of 18 tender points on digital palpation (at a force of at least 4 kg/cm): • Occiput: bilateral, at the suboccipital muscle insertions • Low cervical: bilateral, at the anterior aspects of the inter-transverse spaces at C5–C7 • Trapezius: bilateral, at the midpoint of the upper border • Supraspinatus: bilateral, at the origins above the scapular spine near the medial border • Second rib: bilateral, at the second costochondral junctions, just lateral to the junctions on upper surfaces • Lateral epicondyle: bilateral, 2 cm distal to the epicondyles • Gluteal: bilateral, in upper quadrants of the buttocks in anterior fold of muscle • Greater trochanter: bilateral, posterior to the trochanteric prominence • Knee: bilateral, at the medial fat pad proximal to the joint line For a tender point to be "positive," the client must state that the palpation was painful. A statement of "tender" is not considered "painful."

*Client must have a history of widespread pain (present for at least 3 months) in specific anatomic areas and must exhibit this pain during an examination of tender points.
Source: Running AF, Berndt AE: *Management guidelines for nurse practitioners working in family practice.* Philadelphia, PA: FA Davis; 2003:586.

physical examination findings, because any positive result is likely to be falsely positive in the setting of low suspicion.

Laboratory testing for FMS should include the same screening tests as for CFS, as well as muscle enzymes (creatine kinase, aldolase). Antinuclear antibody testing is typically not helpful unless an autoimmune disorder such as SLE is strongly suspected because it may generate a false-positive result that incorrectly labels these patients as having lupus.

Differential Diagnosis

There is a wide differential diagnosis for both CFS and FMS. Many diagnoses can be ruled out with basic laboratory studies mentioned in the preceding text. The differential includes rheumatic diseases, such as SLE, RA, and polymyalgia rheumatica; endocrinological diseases, such as thyroid and parathyroid disease; metabolic myopathies; neuropathies; infectious diseases, such as Lyme disease; mood disorders and psychiatric illnesses, including depression, persistent depressive disorder, personality disorders, and psychosis; malingering; and other conditions such as irritable bowel syndrome, cancer, and parkinsonism.

Myofascial pain syndrome involves a more limited number of tender muscular trigger points than FMS, as well as involuntary constrictions of muscular fascia (fibrous connective tissue that surrounds muscles). This condition has been considered either a separate clinical entity or a regional variant of FMS. Sjögren's syndrome should also be considered in the differential diagnosis, as many CFS patients also present with anhydrosis.

ME/CFS may severely affect a person's ability to conduct activities of daily living. Patients have profound fatigue, cognitive dysfunction, sleep abnormalities, overall pain, and any type of exertion exacerbates these symptoms. Sjögren's syndrome should also be considered as a differential diagnosis as many patients with ME/CFS also present with anhydrosis.

MANAGEMENT

The management of CFS and FMS remains controversial. A supportive approach to the patient–clinician relationship is critical for effective treatment, as this reinforces that CFS or FMS is a genuine diagnosis and, thus, avoids the debate between psychological and "organic" etiologies. Ultimately, the goal of therapy is to enable the patient to have the best quality of life possible within the limitations of chronic disability related to pain.

The two therapies that have been shown to be beneficial in terms of symptom relief and increased function (albeit not curative) are cognitive behavior therapy, which changes beliefs and behaviors that are barriers to recovery, and graded exercise. Increased bedrest should not be encouraged.

The following pharmacotherapies have been tried with little consistent success: galantamine (Reminyl), a drug used to treat Alzheimer's disease; intravenous immune globulin (IVIG); acyclovir (Zovirax); and selective serotonin reuptake inhibitors (SSRIs), such as citalopram (Celexa), fluoxetine (Prozac), and paroxetine (Paxil). Corticosteroids have shown some benefit in uncontrolled studies but increase the risk of adrenal suppression; controlled, blinded studies have not confirmed these benefits.

The long-term prognosis of CFS is better than the short-term prognosis. However, certain factors have been cited as predicting a poor prognosis: (1) having more than eight medically unexplained physical symptoms, other than the ones cited as CFS diagnostic criteria, (2) lifetime history of dysthymia, (3) chronic fatigue lasting more than 1.5 years, (4) less than 16 years of formal education, and (5) age greater than 38 years at the onset of disease.

For FMS, acetaminophen (Tylenol; 650 mg 4 times daily) and tramadol (Ultram; 75 mg 4 times daily) as combination therapy may be helpful analgesics, but there is little to no evidence that NSAID or corticosteroid therapy is beneficial. Tramadol is a synthetic opioid that carries some abuse potential, but it is generally considered less than for oxycodone, hydrocodone, or morphine. Amitriptyline (Elavil) 75 mg daily in divided doses remains one of the medications most frequently prescribed for FMS. Although it helps some patients, studies have shown that after 3 months, it has no greater effect than placebo. Additionally, this and other tricyclics have anticholinergic side effects.

A similar transient therapeutic effect has also been seen with cyclobenzaprine (Flexeril), which appears effective for the first 3 months, initially taken at 5 mg three times daily and then increasing to 10 mg three times daily. The adage of "start low and go slow" applies to this medication as well. Desipramine (Norpramin) is an alternative tricyclic agent with fewer side effects and may work in patients who respond to amitriptyline but cannot tolerate it. Of all the SSRIs, fluoxetine has been most promising when taken in doses from 20 to 80 mg daily. Dual norepinephrine and serotonin reuptake inhibitors, such as duloxetine (Cymbalta) 40 to 60 mg daily, have shown some benefit as well. Although management guidelines are not well established, tramadol should probably be added only after psychotropic medications are tried first. In addition, low-dose clonazepam (Klonopin; 0.5 mg at bedtime) may be helpful, and research is also being done on the usefulness of antiseizure medications. Pregabalin (Lyrica), approved for FMS in 2007, may be started at 75 mg twice daily and increased to a maintenance dose of 150 to 225 mg twice daily. Pregabalin may cause dizziness or somnolence, however, and has the potential to cause severe allergic reactions.

An ongoing low-impact aerobic (cardiovascular) exercise program (walking, swimming, biking, water aerobics) with cognitive-behavioral therapy, hypnotherapy, or electromyogram biofeedback therapy may be a useful adjunct in certain patients, because these therapies have been shown in limited trials to increase quality of life (although not affecting symptom severity). Chiropractic and massage therapies are only weakly supported. Trials with ultraviolet light (especially blue-spectrum light) exposure have shown mixed results. Vitamin supplementation also has received mixed results in small clinical trials.

FOLLOW-UP AND REFERRAL

Follow-up for CFS and FMS should occur according to the symptoms reported. Because many of these patients have been treated for affective psychiatric disorders in the past, they may already know what psychological manifestations should trigger professional assistance.

Typically, patients are referred to rheumatologists initially to assist in confirming the diagnosis by ruling out autoimmune syndromes. Referral to regional specialists who study and treat CFS and FMS may be required. Psychiatric referral could be necessary if mood disorders are apparent or mental status test results warrant.

Patient Education: Chronic Fatigue Syndrome and Fibromyalgia Syndrome

For both CFS and FMS, management relies on helping the patient cope with a chronic condition by learning methods to deal with the long-term symptoms. While validating its impact on the patient's life, clinicians should stress that the patient does not have a fatal disease. Although symptomatic, it may be relatively benign in terms of the risk of complications, and the patient can live a normal and productive life. Living with the uncertainty of the diagnosis and the chronicity of the problem are continuing challenges for both the patient and clinician. This is illustrated in The Patient's Voice 62.1.

Patients may be encouraged to use whatever alternative means they believe might assist them with pain relief such as chiropractic, therapeutic touch, guided imagery, and hypnosis. At present, there are no definitive answers or standard treatments for these conditions. Pain is as the patient perceives it, and any treatment may relieve the pain if the patient believes it to be helpful. Patients should understand that physical and emotional stress can worsen their symptoms. Patient education has been shown in unblinded studies to improve FMS symptoms and quality of life and is a critical component of treatment. The *Circle of Caring* model is tested in cases in which a patient is frustrated and experiences daily pain. It is especially trying when a patient outwardly appears to be fine but is mentally suffering internally. Conditions such as these may require multiple resources and for all those involved with the patient to focus on finding what works best for each individual patient. Evidence-Based Nursing Practice 62.1 describes the responses of parents and families to the presence of CFS as a chronic illness.

SJÖGREN'S SYNDROME

Sjögren's syndrome (SS) is a chronic inflammatory autoimmune disorder caused by exocrine dysfunction. It presents as dryness in all areas of the body where there are exocrine glands associated with mucous membranes, most notably the salivary and lacrimal glands. However, SS has the potential to affect a wide array of organ systems including the skin, lung, kidney, and heart. In addition, the hematopoietic system may be affected with a propensity for lymphoma.

EPIDEMIOLOGY AND CAUSES

SS has a worldwide distribution with an annual incidence of 4 in 100,000 people; 70% of these cases may be primary, whereas the others are associated with comorbid

The Patient's Voice 62.1: Chronic Fatigue Syndrome

I have been chronically tired for years. It started out that I would drive the kids to school in my nightgown, then I'd go back to bed. I had given up my job the year before. Thank goodness we could afford it. My husband thought that I was depressed, so I went to doctor after doctor and tried all sorts of antidepressant medications with no relief. One doctor suggested that I needed to see a psychiatrist because the antidepressants were not working, and he said I was obviously depressed. I knew "deep down" that I wasn't depressed, but I also knew that something wasn't right. I knew I had to do something when I overheard one of my kids on the phone telling his friend not to come over because his mom was just "having another lazy day in her PJs."

That same week, I heard an ad on the radio inviting participants for a study on chronic fatigue syndrome. I had heard about the syndrome vaguely and thought it was just a "catch-all term" for tiredness. I didn't really think it was a medical condition. I called the phone number given for the study and after answering just a few questions over the phone, I felt 200 percent better! There actually is a medical name for the condition that I know I have. Now, I know I'm not crazy or just lazy. I can't wait to participate in the study. Even if it doesn't help me, I'll feel better knowing that what I have is "real."

Evidence-Based Nursing Practice 62.1

Donalek JG. When a parent is chronically ill: Chronic fatigue syndrome. *Nurs Res.* 2009;58(5):332–339.

Because chronic illness may reshape not only the life of the ill parent but also that of the entire family, this study was undertaken to describe the responses of parents and the ensuing family system responses to the presence of chronic fatigue syndrome as a chronic parental illness. This qualitative study involved eight ill parents and multiple members of their families. After interviews were conducted, thematic analyses at the individual, intrafamily, and across-family levels were used to explore the phenomena. The parents described the onset of illness, an ongoing struggle to receive an appropriate diagnosis and care, and the significance of the illness in transforming present and future roles of family members. Multiple members of their family together with the ill parent described how they struggled with the reality of the illness, the shifting roles and responsibilities of the parents and their children, the reduced family income, and the frequent social isolation that could be exacerbated by the controversial nature of the illness. Families described and demonstrated their struggles to maintain a normal family life and make plans in the face of ongoing uncertainty. Recommendations are made for future directions in family nursing research exploring the responses of families in which a parent is chronically ill.

conditions and are considered secondary. Accurate estimates of disease prevalence are complicated by a lack of agreement as to the defining diagnostic criteria of the disease. However, it is generally agreed that SS affects women nine times more often than men. The typical age range for disease onset is 40 to 60 years. The cause of the syndrome has not been fully characterized, although it is generally considered autoimmune in nature. Because SS typically accompanies underlying rheumatic diseases (e.g., RA, SLE, systemic sclerosis), investigations evaluating the etiological links among these conditions are ongoing.

PATHOPHYSIOLOGY

As an autoimmune disorder, lymphocytic infiltration in all affected organs is the pathophysiologic hallmark of SS. Pooling of lymphocytes and plasma cells in the lacrimal glands causes the characteristic dry eye conjunctivitis of the syndrome called keratoconjunctivitis sicca, while parotid enlargement and diminished salivary excretions result from a similar infiltrate within the salivary glands along with hyperplasia of the ductal epithelium, which produces characteristic dry mouth (xerostomia).

At least three-quarters of these infiltrating cells are T lymphocytes, primarily of the CD4+ T-helper subset, with classical TCRαβ receptors and expressing a memory cell phenotype including LFA-1 surface adhesion molecules. About 10% of the infiltrating cells are B lymphocytes and plasma cells that produce significant amounts of oligoclonal immunoglobulin. The adjacent glandular epithelium expresses high levels of class II MHC (HLA-DR) and costimulatory molecules such as B7, suggesting antigenic T-cell stimulation is central to the pathogenesis of SS. It is unclear whether these stimulatory antigens are autoantigens and/or specific viral antigens.

Evidence for a genetic predisposition to SS is supported by studies that recognize a familial propensity for specific HLA-DR3, HLA-DR5, and HLA-DRB3 alleles in affected patients and their relatives. Primary SS has also been linked to genetic polymorphisms in regulatory DNA sequences of the IL-10 gene, a cytokine that influences cell-mediated immunity. However, IFN-γ and IL-2 appear to be the primary immunomodulatory cytokines in SS. Produced by ductal epithelium, IFN-γ upregulates the expression of HLA-DR molecules on epithelial antigen presenting cells and potentiates T lymphocyte cellular cytotoxicity. Cytolytic destruction of exocrine gland tissue does not appear to explain the full pathology of SS, however, because decreased saliva and tear production does not correlate well with the degree of histological damage on glandular biopsies.

The importance of autoantibodies in the pathophysiology of SS has long been emphasized. Autoantibodies specific for acetylcholine receptors in salivary glands have been suggested to impair the secretion of saliva in histologically normal glands. Far more common, however, are autoantibodies to specific nucleoproteins associated with RNA, including anti-Ro (SSA) antibodies seen in up to 90% of SS cases and anti-La (SSB) antibodies seen in up to half of cases. Although the pathogenetic role of these antibodies is unclear, the same antibodies can be found in a variety of other autoimmune disorders, including neonatal lupus in which they mediate complete heart block after crossing the placenta from mother to child. Anti-α-fodrin antibodies may be even more sensitive and specific for SS than anti-Ro or anti-La antibodies, but their pathological significance is not fully established.

Infection by various viruses, including EBV, retroviruses such as human T-cell lymphotropic virus (HTLV-1), hepatitis C virus, and coxsackievirus, has been suggested as an underlying cause of primary SS. In vitro studies and preclinical animal models have demonstrated that infection with these viruses is capable of leading to lymphocytic infiltrates of the salivary and lacrimal glands, recreating many of the same symptoms as SS. Although viral particles are typically not present in high numbers, viral infection has been suggested to break tolerance to autoantigens and lead to SS via autoimmune activation. The relationship between SS and viral infection is not entirely clear, however, because much of the etiological evidence is indirect and does not predominate for any single virus.

Disorders of estrogen have also been indirectly implicated because primary SS is seen predominantly in women. Postmenopausal women taking estrogen therapy have a higher incidence of ocular dryness compared with controls. This evidence remains circumstantial, however.

CLINICAL PRESENTATION

Subjective

A patient may complain of dryness of the eyes and the feeling that a particulate is in them. Keratoconjunctivitis sicca is dryness of the cornea caused by a deficiency of tear secretion in which the corneal surface appears dull and rough and the eye feels gritty and irritated. The patient may also complain of dryness of the mouth caused by cessation of normal salivary secretions. In addition, the patient may complain of loss of taste and smell, recurrent dental caries, dysphagia, vaginismus, and rectal bleeding. Associated complaints can include RA symptoms of joint swelling, pain, and malaise, as well as low-grade fever. Fatigue is another important aspect of the presentation, due to disrupted sleep patterns from mucosal dryness or accompanying systemic symptoms such as arthralgias and myalgias.

Objective

The patient may appear chronically ill, particularly if RA precedes SS. The patient's breath may smell fetid because of dental caries and mucosal dryness, and the mucosal beds of the nose and throat will be pale and may reveal small fissures. The tongue can be beefy red because of dryness. Similar findings are associated with the vagina and anus.

Many other systemic, albeit rare, manifestations of SS may be present: a macular, papular, vesicular, or purpuric skin rash; arthralgias and myalgias; cardiopulmonary manifestations such as pericarditis or pulmonary hypertension from lymphocytic interstitial pneumonitis; pulmonary emboli due to circulating antiphospholipid/anticardiolipin antibodies; interstitial nephritis leading to renal tubular acidosis or glomerulonephritis (similar to that of SLE); gastroesophageal reflux disease (GERD); hypothyroidism due to autoimmune thyroiditis; neurological sequelae including peripheral (mononeuritis multiplex or symmetric neuropathies) and autonomic neuropathies, CNS manifestations mimicking multiple sclerosis, transverse myelitis, optic neuritis, or ischemic strokes that may be due to vasculitis, thrombosis, or demyelination.

DIAGNOSTIC REASONING

Diagnostic Tests

SS is diagnosed via clinical and laboratory findings, rather than identification of a single causative agent. Clinical diagnosis of SS includes six defining criteria:

1. Inadequate tear production (evaluated using the Schirmer test with filter paper to blot tears on the lateral third of the lower eyelid [less than 5 mm of wetting in 5 minutes is abnormal] or using artificial replacement tears more than 3 times daily)
2. Signs of corneal epithelial damage from dry eye using Rose-Bengal or fluorescein staining and slit-lamp examination
3. Decreased saliva production
4. Lymphocytic infiltration of labial salivary gland tissue on histopathology following labial gland biopsy—the closest test to a gold standard for diagnosis (greater than 50 immune cells surrounding an intact glandular lobule)
5. Impaired salivary gland function by objective testing via radionuclide technetium scanning (quantitative salivary gland scintigraphy demonstrating poor uptake), parotid sialography with parotid gland cannulation and injection of oil-based contrast material, or spontaneous saliva production of less than or equal to 1.5 mL/15 min
6. Autoantibodies including anti-Ro and/or anti-La

Initial laboratory tests include a CBC, RF, ANA, and γ-globulin profile. The CBC may reveal anemia of chronic disease that is typically mild, leukopenia, and/or eosinophilia. The eosinophilia is caused by autoimmune factors and not by external antigens. RF is positive in three-fourths of samples. ANA is typically elevated, as are γ-globulin levels.

Electrophoresis studies are required to determine whether SS is present alone or in combination with other rheumatoid disease. SS alone typically manifests more specific autoantibodies—anti-Ro and anti-La—whereas SS and rheumatoid disease together may reveal antibodies against exocrine ducts and RA-associated nuclear antigens.

Differential Diagnosis

Because patients with SS have a higher prevalence of hypothyroidism, this should be screened via a thorough history and thyroid-stimulating hormone (TSH)/free T_4 level. Further laboratory work-up includes a basic metabolic panel with hepatic function tests (liver transaminases), RF (to assess for RA), and ANA (to assess for SLE). HIV and hepatitis C testing may also be indicated. Sarcoidosis could be evaluated with a chest x-ray examination to evaluate for hilar lymphadenopathy or interstitial lung disease. An MRI or ultrasound and biopsy should be done if there is unilateral salivary gland enlargement to rule out malignancy or specific glandular pathology, such as acute bacterial sialadenitis. Bilateral salivary gland swelling may be due to acute viral infection (e.g., mumps, coxsackievirus, echovirus, or EBV) or chronic infection with HIV or hepatitis C; granulomatous diseases such as sarcoidosis, amyloidosis, or TB; malnutrition; alcoholism; and eating disorders such as bulimia or anorexia with purging features.

Additional differential diagnoses for SS include other autoimmune disorders that may exist concurrently, such as SLE, scleroderma, or RA. In fact, RF may be positive in up to 75% of cases. It is also critical to distinguish SS from patients with FMS or depression who may have significant anticholinergic toxicities from psychiatric medications, which can lead to dry eyes and especially dry mouth. Dry eyes may also result from impaired blinking due to muscular or neurological disorders, vitamin A deficiency leading to mucin deficiency (xerophthalmia), conjunctivitis, infiltration of the lacrimal glands (from sarcoidosis, lymphoma, or amyloidosis), or blepharitis from Meibomian gland dysfunction. Dry mouth can also result from sialadenitis from obstructing salivary gland stones, chronic viral infections (e.g., hepatitis C, HIV), and iatrogenic anticholinergic drug effects. In fact, the following conditions are exclusion criteria for SS: previous head/neck irradiation or preexisting lymphoma, comorbid infection with hepatitis C or HIV with AIDS, sarcoidosis, graft versus host disease, or recent use of anticholinergic medications. Symptoms of mucosal dryness are also common in liver disease and depression, which should also be considered as part of the differential.

MANAGEMENT

The management of this syndrome consists primarily of symptom-directed supportive care, although research into immunomodulatory therapies is ongoing.

To address the primary manifestations of dry eyes and dry mouth, saline eye drops can relieve lacrimal dryness, while hard candies and gum may be used to stimulate salivation but should be sugar-free to avoid worsening dental caries. Dried fruits that contain malic acid may also be helpful in stimulating salivation. In extreme cases of salivary dryness, the patient should be encouraged to apply an artificial salivary gel or use a mouth spray. Fluids can also keep the mouth well lubricated as long as they do not contain caffeine (a diuretic) or ethanol (as used in mouthwash), which can be drying. Special toothpastes and toothbrushes designed for a dry mouth are also available. Quarterly dental evaluations, along with vigorous flossing and regular brushing, may prevent dental caries. Dry lips may be treated with petroleum jelly (Vaseline), dry skin with moisturizing lotions, and vaginal dryness with intravaginal lubricant gel.

Artificial tears and salivary gels containing hypromellose (0.3%) or methylcellulose (0.3%) and may be used every 2 to 4 hours if needed. Several of these can be irritating to certain individuals. Pilocarpine (Salagen) 5 mg PO three to four times daily and cevimeline (Evoxac) 30 to 60 mg PO three times daily are specific cholinergic (muscarinic) agonists (parasympathomimetics) for stimulating aqueous secretions. These drugs are contraindicated in persons with narrow-angle glaucoma or iritis, owing to their mydriatic effects. Cevimeline should not be used if a patient has asthma, because it can worsen respiratory secretions.

Acetylcysteine can be used as a mucolytic if thick mucus fibers coat the eye, but it may be unacceptable to some patients because of its characteristic "rotten egg smell" due to its sulphur content. Spreading agents such as polyethylene glycol and dextran-70 0.1% drops are also available for dry eyes. Topical cyclosporine 0.05% 1 gtt every 12 hours is FDA-approved to increase tear production, presumably by decreasing T-cell infiltration within the conjunctivae. If these treatments prove ineffective, the patient may undergo punctal occlusion, in which collagen plugs are placed by an ophthalmologist into the lacrimal puncta on the inferior eyelid so that tears (artificial or natural) cannot drain into the nasolacrimal duct.

The following are rarer systemic manifestations of SS, along with specific treatments:

- Macular, papular, vesicular, or purpuric skin rashes may require biopsy and treatment as a form of vasculitis.
- Arthralgias and myalgias may respond to NSAIDs or hydroxychloroquine.
- Inflammatory cardiopulmonary manifestations such as pericarditis or pulmonary hypertension from lymphocytic interstitial pneumonitis may require treatment with corticosteroids (prednisone) or other immunosuppressants (azathioprine, chlorambucil, cyclophosphamide).

- Interstitial nephritis leading to renal tubular acidosis or glomerulonephritis (similar to that of SLE) may require corticosteroid or immunosuppressant therapy (cyclophosphamide, mycophenolate).
- Rare neurological sequelae such as peripheral mononeuritis multiplex or symmetrical neuropathies and autonomic dysfunction (confirmed by tilt-table tests) may require mineralocorticoid therapy.
- Neuropathies and CNS manifestations mimicking multiple sclerosis, transverse myelitis, optic neuritis, or ischemic strokes may be due to vasculitis, thrombosis, or demyelination and require treatment with immunosuppressants.

Most recently, treatment guidelines from the Sjögren's Syndrome Foundation have put forth the anti-CD20 monoclonal antibody therapy rituximab (Rituxan) for patients with systemic symptoms severe enough to require biologic therapy. However, this therapy is not yet FDA-approved for Sjögren's syndrome. Multiple biologic therapies are currently in development for this significant area of unmet medical need.

FOLLOW-UP AND REFERRAL

Follow-up of SS consists of ongoing evaluation to assess the effectiveness of symptom management and the need for alterations in treatment. If SS presents as an isolated condition, follow-up evaluations may occur as infrequently as twice per year. However, more frequent evaluations are necessitated by the presence of concurrent disease. Referrals may not be necessary except when this syndrome accompanies other diseases. The clinician may consult with a rheumatologist initially to differentiate the disease from other rheumatic conditions and to confirm the diagnosis.

During follow-up examinations, it is important to monitor for dental caries or oral candidiasis, which can lead to severe mouth pain and requires antifungal therapy. It is also important to screen for infectious conjunctivitis and complications from nasal dryness and laryngotracheal reflux, which can stimulate vagal responses and mimic allergic or recurrent sinusitis symptoms, including repeated throat clearing and postnasal drip–like symptoms. This type of reflux may be treated with proton pump inhibitors (similar to GERD), with referral to an ear, nose, and throat specialist if needed.

Patient Education: Sjögren's Syndrome

The patient should learn that mucosal dryness can be controlled with conservative interventions. Regular application of artificial lubricants locally can prevent the soreness and untoward effects of dry mucosae. The patient should be encouraged to wear sunglasses to protect the eyes from strong light, wind, and dust, as well as to avoid low-humidity environments that exacerbate dryness. If the patient has sore lesions in the mouth, tobacco, alcohol, and both spicy and salty foods should be avoided. OTC medications that decrease pharyngeal secretions, such as antihistamines, antidepressants, anticholinergics, and atropine derivatives, should be avoided. Patients should be warned that they are at greater risk for complications from surgeries requiring general anesthesia and intubation, given their increased risk for thick, inspissated mucus and atelectasis.

SYSTEMIC LUPUS ERYTHEMATOSUS

SLE is an inflammatory autoimmune disease that affects many organ systems. Spontaneous remissions and exacerbations characterize the clinical picture. SLE can be mild or aggressive and even life-threatening in presentation.

EPIDEMIOLOGY AND CAUSES

The prevalence of SLE is 40 to 50 cases per 100,000 people and is associated with age, gender, race, and genetics. Nearly 85% of patients with SLE are women, most often in their third or fourth decade of life. However, 15% of cases present after the age of 55 years. Juvenile cases are not uncommon, however, with 20% of diagnosed patients being younger than 16 years. In children, the female to male ratio is 3:1 and in adults, it is 10 to 15:1. Epidemiological studies have identified sex hormones as potential causative factors for SLE, because onset of the disease in women typically occurs before menopause. Estrogen has been shown to stimulate T cells, B cells, and macrophages, as well as to increase the expression of cytokines, endothelial cell adhesion molecules, and antigen-presenting MHC molecules. SLE flares have also been associated with hyperprolactinemia.

In contrast, androgenic hormones such as testosterone tend to be immunosuppressive, which may also contribute to the gender specificity of SLE. Although men with lupus typically experience less photosensitivity than women, they are often considered to have more severe disease manifestations, with a greater incidence of serositis and a higher 1-year mortality rate, although they tend to present at an older age of onset.

Persons of African descent are four times more likely to develop the disease compared with Caucasians. SLE also disproportionately affects patients of Asian ancestry, and some studies show higher rates of disease in Hispanic patients compared with the general population. Several lines of evidence have demonstrated a genetic component to SLE, such as a high concordance rate between monozygotic twins, a propensity for specific HLA-DR class II MHC genes in affected individuals, and positive gene linkage studies in affected siblings. Poor prognostic factors include concurrent hypertension, male gender, developing active disease at a young age, low socioeconomic status, and being African American.

Trends related to ethnic background (i.e., higher disease rates in people of color) have been observed with many chronic diseases and are multifactorial in nature. They must not be attributed solely to "genetic differences between the races" because worse outcomes are also associated with the presence of prothrombotic antiphospholipid antibodies (e.g., lupus anticoagulant, anticardiolipin) and highly active inflammatory disease, both of which may be addressed through individualized treatment plans to decrease the risk of morbidity.

Although not causative of SLE, several triggering factors for acute exacerbations have been identified. These include exposure to ultraviolet (UVB and UVA) rays, which is believed to cause increased cytokine and cell adhesion molecule expression; certain infections (e.g., EBV, *Mycobacteria,* trypanosomes) that may stimulate cross-reacting autoantibodies; emotional stress, which, although controversial, has been tied to mild disease flares; pregnancy and postpartum hormonal fluctuations; and surgery, which may increase the formation of autoantibody-containing immune complexes via the release of intracellular antigens into the circulation from tissue trauma. Exposure to cigarette smoke or silica dust also increases the risk of developing SLE, which implicates inflammatory lung pathology.

PATHOPHYSIOLOGY

The pathophysiology of SLE is best understood by a review of the diagnostic criteria. The diagnosis of SLE is made after 4 or more of the following 11 criteria are met in the absence of medications or other disorders known to induce these effects, as defined by the American College of Rheumatology:

- Arthritis—nonerosive and usually involving two or more joints
- Photosensitivity—often triggering skin rashes, exposure to the sun's UVB rays may be a triggering event for SLE exacerbations
- Oral (or nasal) ulcers—typically painless
- Malar rash—bilateral butterfly formation across the cheeks and nasal bridge
- Discoid rash—raised red patches, sometimes with denuded central areas
- Serositis (inflammation) of the pleura or pericardia
- Renal disease (any one of three indicators): more than 0.5 g/day proteinuria, 3+ or more proteinuria (as detected by dipstick), or cellular casts
- Hematological disorders (any one of four indicators): hemolytic anemia, leukopenia (less than 4,000 WBCs/mcL), lymphopenia (less than 1,500 lymphocytes/mcL), thrombocytopenia (less than 100,000 platelets/mcL)

- Neurological disease (e.g., seizures, psychoses) not otherwise explained by iatrogenic or metabolic causes
- Positive ANA antibodies
- Immunological abnormalities (any one of four indicators): positive antiphospholipid antibodies such as anticardiolipin or lupus anticoagulant, antibody to double-stranded native DNA (anti-dsDNA), anti-Sm (Smith) antibody, false-positive serological test for syphilis (VDRL, RPR)

SLE is, at its core, a condition of disordered immunity in which mechanisms that normally prevent immune cell activation by autoantigens are eliminated. Many factors have been identified that contribute to this autoimmune activation, for example, an inhibition of suppressor T cells that normally downregulate immune responses, an increase in CD4+ T helper cells, increased cytokine production (e.g., IFN-α, IL-4, IL-6, IL-10), polyclonal B cell activation, and dysregulated intracellular signaling (particularly pathways involving cytosolic calcium). These changes contribute to a significant production of autoantibodies that are considered a hallmark of the disease. Mouse models of SLE have demonstrated dysregulated apoptosis in which nuclear antigens (e.g., DNA, ribonucleoprotein, histones) are exposed on the cell surface, which are capable of recognition by autoreactive lymphocytes. In turn, autoantibodies often appear in the serum years before the actual onset of SLE symptoms.

Autoantibodies are also formed against cell surface antigens, including antibodies specific for RBCs and WBCs, platelets, and neuronal and renal cells. These antibodies mediate cellular destruction via complement activation, antibody-dependent cellular cytotoxicity, and opsonization. Although not seen universally, autoantibody-derived immune complexes are believed to underlie the pathology of most of clinical manifestations of SLE. Histochemical staining has identified immune complex deposition along the basement membrane in nephritic kidneys, at the dermal–epidermal junction in skin lesions, within the choroid plexus, as well as the pleural cavity and pericardium—all major sites of SLE pathology. The biochemical nature of both the autoantigen and autoantibody (e.g., size, charge, binding affinity, rate of phagocytic clearance, ability to be neutralized by complement proteins) determines where these complexes form and the extent of tissue damage after their deposition.

One of the organ systems most severely affected by immune complex deposition is the renal system. In addition to the deposition of circulating immune complexes along the glomerular basement membrane, autoreactive IgG$_1$ and IgG$_3$ anti-DNA antibodies also bind directly to autoantigens in the basement membranes, serving as a nidus for complement activation. These chemotactic complement proteins then attract leukocytes and mononuclear cells that phagocytose the immune complexes, releasing cytokines and clotting factors that lead to fibrinoid necrosis, ongoing inflammation, renal scarring, and kidney dysfunction. Diffuse proliferative glomerulonephritis is the most common histological form of lupus nephritis, which results from this inflammation. In contrast, lupus membranous nephropathy is not associated with inflammation. Rather, in this setting, immune complex activation is separated physically from circulating immune cells by the glomerular basement membrane, resulting in epithelial injury and proteinuria without active inflammation.

A subset of individuals with SLE is also prone to developing antiphospholipid antibodies, including antibodies against the β_2-glycoprotein I complex and cardiolipin, as well as the lupus anticoagulant. These individuals have more severe disease, related primarily to an increased thrombogenic state, which predisposes to both venous and arterial thromboembolism, resulting in a greater incidence of deep venous thrombosis, pulmonary embolism, cerebrovascular accidents (strokes and transient ischemic attacks), and recurrent first-trimester miscarriages due to placental infarcts. Normally, β_2-glycoprotein has an anticoagulant effect, which is abrogated by these antiphospholipid antibodies.

One of the most characteristic physical findings of SLE is a bilateral malar rash, often called a "butterfly rash" for its characteristic location across the nose and cheekbones. This and other SLE skin rashes are exacerbated by sun exposure, largely due to ultraviolet damage to DNA in skin keratinocytes and alterations in membrane phospholipid metabolism. Thus, anti-DNA, anti-RNA, anti-Ro, anti-La, and antiphospholipid autoantibodies form that mediate keratinocyte destruction and local skin inflammation. IL-1 production from cutaneous keratinocytes and antigen-presenting Langerhans cells potentiates this inflammatory response.

CLINICAL PRESENTATION

Subjective

The patient may complain of malaise, fever, anorexia, and unplanned weight loss. The patient may also complain of blurred vision and conjunctival swelling. Sleeplessness and depression are also common complaints. Joints may be reported to be swollen and painful by history, but this may not be evident on examination. Shortness of breath and painful inspiration may be present if lung pathology exists. Vague abdominal pain and/or abdominal cramping may also be part of the history.

Objective

Integumentary findings may include the following:

- A characteristic "butterfly" rash, as well as other photosensitive rashes, are common.
- Alopecia and scalp exanthema are typical findings.
- Splinter hemorrhages, periungual erythema, and fingertip lesions may be observed on the fingers and toes.

- Lymphadenopathy in several regions of the body indicates systemic disease.
- Discoid lupus presents with scarring and highly inflammatory (even ulcerating) skin lesions, but often does not present with the familiar autoantibodies of SLE, such as ANA, anti-dsDNA, and anti-Smith antibodies.
- Raynaud's phenomenon, a vascular condition, may be seen in up to 40% of patients as whitish-blue skin color changes in response to cold temperatures, which then change to red upon rewarming, often predating other symptoms.

Musculoskeletal findings may include the following:

- Musculoskeletal joint pains (asymmetrical, nondeforming, migratory arthritis—often in the hands and fingers) occur in 90% of cases and are often the presenting complaint.
- Swollen joints may not follow a particular pattern, as in other rheumatic diseases; joint inflammation is typically nonerosive on radiographs.

Neurological findings may include the following:

- Cognitive thought processes may be impaired. Therefore, the clinician should carefully listen to the patient's explanations in response to questioning to establish lapses in logic; however, these deficits often are not evident in mental functioning assessments commonly used in primary-care settings, such as the Folstein Mini-Mental State Exam.
- Evidence of peripheral paresthesias and diminished deep tendon reflexes may be present.

Cardiac findings may include the following:

- A systolic murmur may be present.
- Distended jugular veins suggest right-sided cardiac failure, which may be seen with pulmonary hypertension or interstitial lung disease.

GI findings may include the following:

- Painless oral and nasal ulcers may be seen.
- Right upper abdominal quadrant tenderness may accompany the finding of hepatomegaly; hepatitis is a common finding.
- Right lower quadrant tenderness suggests right colon enlargement, which may be caused by intestinal vasculitis.

DIAGNOSTIC REASONING

Diagnostic Tests

Initial testing should include a CBC with platelet count, basic metabolic panel (serum electrolytes and kidney function tests), serum albumin (which will be reduced in nephropathy), ANA, urinalysis, and screening tests for anti-dsDNA antibodies (highly specific, with 75% to 95% sensitivity), antiphospholipid antibodies, and anti-Sm antibodies (highly specific, but with only 25% sensitivity). Other common autoantibodies include those against single-stranded DNA and nucleoprotein, including antiribonucleoprotein as seen in scleroderma and both anti-Ro (SSA) and anti-La (SSB) as seen in SS.

The CBC may reveal either anemia or leukopenia or both. If the patient is leukopenic, the differential count may reveal lymphocytopenia. One-third of patients with SLE will be thrombocytopenic. ANA results are likely to be elevated in more than 90% of cases; however, this finding is not specific for SLE. Numerous other inflammatory diseases are also associated with an elevated ANA. Changes in serum levels of autoantibodies (increasing anti-dsDNA levels) or complement (decreasing CH50, C3, and C4 levels) correlate with active SLE disease. Elevated ESR and CRP levels are nonspecific markers of active inflammation. Proteinuria is a possible finding on urinalysis in nephrotic or nephritic patients, with hematuria in the latter.

All test results should be interpreted in conjunction with clinical presentation (history and physical examination) to evaluate for worsening of the disease state and should not be overinterpreted or underinterpreted in isolation. These initial laboratory tests, along with characteristic clinical manifestations, should be sufficient to confirm a diagnosis of SLE. Of note, as reflected in the SLE diagnostic criteria, RPR tests for syphilis may be falsely positive due to anticardiolipin antibodies or other SLE-related phenomena.

Pertinent imaging tests should be guided by clinical presentation, such as a chest radiography for pulmonary symptoms, renal ultrasound in the face of renal failure, and plain films for arthritic joints. If indicated in the setting of pulmonary findings, pulmonary function tests often have a restrictive pattern, given inflammation and scarring in the lungs. More invasive procedures such as renal biopsy are indicated when histology is needed to determine prognosis and guide therapy. Electrocardiography and echocardiography are indicated to evaluate for pericarditis and other cardiac pathology, and specific tests such as ventilation–perfusion scans or high-resolution spiral CT scans of the lungs are used to evaluate for pulmonary emboli in prothrombotic patients. As with other thrombotic phenomena, a negative D-dimer test may effectively rule out thrombosis; however, the nonspecific nature of this test in inflammatory conditions typically decreases its diagnostic utility in SLE.

As with SS, keratoconjunctivitis sicca may be present, as can pathognomonic (albeit rare) cotton wool retinal exudates from retinal vasculitis. Scleritis and anterior uveitis may also occur but are both uncommon. Mild to moderate cytopenias may affect all three major cell lines (i.e., leukopenia, anemia, thrombocytopenia), with thrombocytopenia leading to easy bruising and purpura. Rarely, severe autoimmune hemolytic anemia can also result.

In contrast, thrombophilia may also occur, increasing the risk of thrombosis, including deep vein thrombosis and arterial blood clots, especially if antiphospholipid antibodies or lupus anticoagulant are present (the latter being paradoxically named, as it increases the risk of thrombosis). This prothrombotic state is the cause of recurrent miscarriages (abortions) early in pregnancy, usually in the first trimester. Thus, such an obstetric history should always make the clinician think of antiphospholipid syndrome and SLE as potential underlying diagnoses.

Differential Diagnosis

The differential diagnosis for SLE includes vasculitis, RA, scleroderma, SS, juvenile idiopathic arthritis (particularly the systemic form), chronic active hepatitis, drug reactions, drug-induced lupus, and polyarteritis. The diagnostic criteria described in the section on Pathophysiology should aid in distinguishing SLE from these other diseases. Hypothyroidism also needs to be ruled out as a cause of fatigue via a TSH and free T_4 level. Drug-induced lupus has a milder presentation and is associated predominantly with procainamide, hydralazine, and minocycline, as well as the anti-TNF biologic immunomodulators.

MANAGEMENT

The principal goal of therapy in SLE is symptom control, as current treatment is not curative. Many patients require little or no intervention. Mild joint pain may be managed with nonpharmacological interventions, as described in the section on RA. Emotional support and referral to SLE support groups are both helpful in establishing control over some symptoms. Dietary modifications should consider the specific clinical presentation. For example, active inflammatory states may require higher-calorie diets if weight loss is a concern; in contrast, corticosteroid-induced surges in appetite may call for lower-calorie diets. Corticosteroid- or NSAID-induced hypertension and hyperlipidemia (or that accompanying lupus nephritis) may call for low-salt and low-fat/low-cholesterol diets, respectively. Likewise, a lack of sun exposure because of photosensitivity may require vitamin D and calcium supplements to prevent bone loss, especially given chronic corticosteroid use. If conservative management fails, however, the patient may require antimalarials, corticosteroids, immunosuppressants, or immunomodulatory biologic agents.

Constitutional symptoms are often the most troubling for patients. Fatigue is the most common symptom and tends to be the most debilitating. It can happen even in the absence of signs of active inflammation. Fatigue may be multifactorial, but if due predominantly to SLE, it tends to respond to treatment with hydroxychloroquine, corticosteroids, or dehydroepiandrosterone. In addition to weight loss associated with hyperinflammatory states, weight gain may also occur due to generalized edema (anasarca) resulting from hypoalbuminemia in nephrotic syndrome or fluid retention and increased appetite associated with glucocorticoid use. If fever is present, it is important to deduce whether it is due to the SLE itself, infection (more likely if fever is episodic and occurs while the patient is on active corticosteroids or immunosuppressive therapies), or a drug reaction that may also present with a morbilliform rash and be prolonged, without an antipyretic response to NSAIDs or acetaminophen.

NSAIDs are effective for mild musculoskeletal symptoms and mild serositis (inflammation of serosal layers, such as the pleura or pericardia). Cyclooxygenase-1 (COX-1) inhibitors are used most frequently, as several COX-2 inhibitors have been withdrawn from the market due to serious cardiovascular health risks. In turn, the remaining COX-2 inhibitors (e.g., celecoxib) should be used with caution.

Cutaneous manifestations of lupus, including discoid lupus, respond well to antimalarials such as hydroxychloroquine (Plaquenil), which are also second-line agents for joint pains and myalgias. Antimalarials are also effective in treating serosal inflammation (pleuritis and pericarditis) and constitutional symptoms including fatigue and fever. Given their association with the long-term reduction of multiple SLE-related complications, their use is recommended in nearly all SLE patients. However, these agents are not without side effects and require appropriate monitoring, including for potential ocular toxicity.

When multiple organ systems are involved or manifestations within a given organ system are moderate to severe, glucocorticoids may be given alone or in combination with another immunosuppressant. Prednisone and other glucocorticoids are effective at treating and preventing relapses if started as soon as a marked rise in anti-dsDNA antibodies is observed in the setting of clinical disease manifestations. Many SLE patients can be maintained on low doses of corticosteroids. However, although these medications are often considered a mainstay of SLE treatment, the clinician must be aware of the important side effects of systemic (both IV and PO) corticosteroids, which include avascular necrosis (i.e., a reduction in blood supply to a major joint such as the knee or hip that results in joint necrosis), osteopenia and osteoporosis with bone fractures or vertebral collapse, growth inhibition in children, glaucoma and cataracts, hyperglycemia and diabetes mellitus, hypertension, weight gain, early atherosclerosis that can lead to long-term coronary artery disease and cardiac damage, as well as cognitive dysfunction and behavioral changes, which may be associated with both short-term and chronic use of corticosteroids. Thus, although corticosteroid therapy is associated with a delayed onset of organ damage after diagnosis, the side effects and health risks of corticosteroids are well documented and may cause significant morbidity in SLE patients. Many lupus specialists strive to decrease corticosteroid use whenever possible by use of steroid-sparing agents.

One of the newest drugs approved by the FDA for SLE treatment is the biologic immunomodulatory agent belimumab (Benlysta), a monoclonal antibody therapy that binds the soluble B cell growth factor B-lymphocyte stimulator (BLyS), thereby preventing signaling through its cognate B cell surface receptor. As BLyS is known to support autoreactive B cells in SLE, belimumab effectively inhibits the production of autoantibodies capable of mediating organ damage and inflammation. Although not a curative therapy for SLE and not indicated to treat acute flares, belimumab has been shown to decrease disease activity, reduce symptom flare rates, and improve symptoms in autoantibody-positive lupus patients, as well as lead to reductions in corticosteroid controller therapy.

Persistent evidence of SLE-related organ damage or symptomatic flares in the face of NSAID or antimalarial therapy may signal the need for more aggressive immunosuppressive therapy, such as higher-dose glucocorticoid pulse therapy or the addition of other immunosuppressants such as mycophenolate mofetil (CellCept), azathioprine (Imuran), methotrexate, and cyclophosphamide (Cytoxan). For example, pulmonary manifestations related to lung inflammation may include pleuritis with a pleural friction rub, lung effusions, pneumonitis, interstitial lung disease, alveolar hemorrhage, or eventually pulmonary hypertension.

Of note, GI manifestations often relate to SLE treatments, rather than to the disease itself, such as gastritis and peptic ulcers resulting from chronic NSAID and corticosteroid use. However, SLE-related vasculitis can lead to inflammation of the pancreas, large intestine, and serosal layers of the peritoneum, as well as to esophagitis and GERD. In addition, both hepatomegaly and splenomegaly may be detected, along with lymphadenopathy.

The cardiovascular system may manifest with pericarditis or a verrucous form of nonbacterial endocarditis known as Libman-Sacks endocarditis. This is associated with antiphospholipid antibodies and can produce emboli due to valvular insufficiency and turbulent blood flow. There is also a well-documented phenomenon of transmission of anti-Ro and anti-La anti-single-stranded DNA antibodies from a mother with SLE to her developing fetus, which can result in potentially fatal third-degree heart block in newborns. This is known as neonatal lupus, which is not a manifestation of primary lupus in the fetus, however, and is different from pediatric manifestations of SLE.

CNS and psychiatric manifestations of SLE are quite varied and may require aggressive immunosuppressive treatment. These may include cognitive defects, delirium, depression, mania, anxiety, psychosis (which may also result iatrogenically from corticosteroid use), headache, aseptic meningitis, and various neuropathies. Ischemic CNS damage from a thromboembolic cerebrovascular accident may underlie these symptoms as well.

Kidney involvement may be clinically apparent in up to one-half of all SLE patients and is the primary reason for lupus-related hospitalization. Renal biopsy may reveal several histological subtypes of lupus nephritis. Type I is normal. Type II is pure mesangial and carries with it a good prognosis. Type III is segmental and focal proliferative lupus nephritis and usually responds to corticosteroids. Type IV is diffuse proliferative lupus nephritis, which is typically considered to carry the worst prognosis, presenting with hypertension and leading to end-stage renal disease (ESRD) or death in up to 50% of cases. Type IV patients typically require an induction of remission and maintenance treatment regimen with high-dose corticosteroids and immunosuppressants such as azathioprine (Imuran), mycophenolate mofetil (CellCept), or cyclophosphamide (Cytoxan). Type V is membranous nephritis with a variable presentation that worsens as complement levels decrease due to immune complex formation and organ deposition. One-third of Type V patients need no treatment other than that for other SLE symptoms, one-third require low to moderate dose corticosteroids, and one-third need high-dose corticosteroids. Type VI is advanced sclerosing lupus nephritis, which nearly always leads to ESRD, given the irreversibility of renal fibrosis.

Although SLE-related organ damage often signals the need for aggressive immunosuppressive therapy, the severity of organ damage does not always correlate with the severity of inflammation. For instance, kidney dysfunction may relate to irreversible scarring from past kidney inflammation that has since resolved and, in turn, may not be effectively treated with immunosuppressants. This is an important distinction for the clinician to make because worsening or ongoing inflammation may be treated with corticosteroids or immunosuppressants, whereas treating noninflammatory organ damage with this same regimen just increases the risks of side effects and iatrogenic complications due to immunosuppression, without improving the underlying organ damage.

Disease progression in the face of potent immunosuppressants, such as cyclophosphamide, portends a particularly poor prognosis. Several immunomodulatory treatments are being explored, including immune system ablation with high-dose chemotherapy, with or without stem cell transplantation. In addition, although not FDA-approved to treat lupus, the anti-B cell (anti-CD20) monoclonal antibody immunotherapy rituximab (Rituxan) is often used in refractory SLE patients, given its familiar side-effect profile and relatively long record of clinical use in other indications.

Five-year survival in SLE has greatly improved in recent decades, given the therapeutic advances discussed in this section, and is currently greater than 90%. However, the course of SLE tends to be relapsing and remitting, characterized by recurrent flares with intermittent periods of quiescence, sometimes resulting in prolonged periods of remission lasting several years. CNS and renal involvement, especially diffuse proliferative nephritis or advanced sclerosing nephritis, portend the worst prognosis. Indeed, most SLE inpatients are admitted to inpatient care for renal complications, whereas patients with isolated cutaneous and joint/muscle manifestations have the best prognosis. Short-term risk of death is also often due to infection related to immunosuppression by multiple classes of SLE medications, in addition to organ involvement associated with active inflammation in the heart, kidney, or CNS.

FOLLOW-UP AND REFERRAL

Follow-up of SLE patients is critical to track the course of the disease, which is highly variable. SLE patients who require only nonpharmacological management should still be seen at least twice per year to assess for disease progression. Patients requiring medication are typically seen at least every 3 months after stabilization on an optimal controller regimen. Before consultation with a rheumatologist, patients should receive laboratory evaluation in the primary-care setting including CBC, urinalysis, CRP, and ANA to follow the course of the disease.

In addition, SLE patients have a greater risk of lymphoma. A greater risk of breast cancer, abnormal Pap smears, and squamous cell skin cancer has also been suggested. Thus, appropriate cancer screening in the primary-care setting is critical.

Referral to a rheumatologist is indicated if antimalarials, corticosteroids, immunosuppressants, or biologic immunomodulators are to be prescribed.

Patient Education: Systemic Lupus Erythematosus

Newly diagnosed patients should receive referrals to information hotlines for SLE and an array of patient advocacy groups, given the potential life-changing impact of this disease. These organizations provide patients with access to materials that support symptom control and facilitate social supports. In addition, patients should learn their individualized trajectory of disease progression and prognosis, depending on their clinical manifestations.

Patients should learn that rest is essential during disease exacerbations (lupus flares). The need for increased oral fluids and appropriate dosing of NSAIDs during such flares are also essential parts of the educational plan. Patients should understand the need for professional intervention when their temperature escalates beyond 101.5°F (38.5°C), because fevers can signal the onset of an opportunistic infection or a lupus flare, for which the primary-care practitioner should be consulted immediately.

Immunizations have not been shown to induce SLE flares and should not be avoided, except for live attenuated vaccines in immunocompromised hosts. If possible, sulfonamide antibiotics (e.g., trimethoprim/sulfamethoxazole [Bactrim]) and tetracyclines should be avoided, because they may lead to adverse effects in SLE patients, including exacerbation of photosensitivity. Women should be encouraged to avoid pregnancy until the disease is in remission for at least 6 months because there are high miscarriage rates due to thromboembolic complications. In addition, birth control pills may exacerbate disease manifestations, although low-dose estrogen pills appear to be better tolerated. Corticosteroids, NSAIDs, and hydroxychloroquine are usually used to treat pregnant women, whereas other immunosuppressants such as methotrexate and cyclophosphamide are contraindicated in pregnancy due to potential teratogenic effects.

REFERENCES

Allergic Reactions

Bernstein IL, et al. Allergy diagnostic testing: An updated practice parameter. *Ann Allergy Asthma Immunol.* 2008;100(3 suppl 3): S1–S148.

Lieberman P, et al. Anaphylaxis—a practice parameter update 2015. *Ann Allergy Asthma Immunol.* 2015;115:341–384.

Schrijvers R, et al. Pathogenesis and diagnosis of delayed-type drug hypersensitivity reactions, from bedside to bench and back. *Clin Transl Allergy.* 2015;5:31.

Chronic Fatigue Syndrome and Fibromyalgia Syndrome

Donalek JG. When a parent is chronically ill. *Nurs Res.* 2009; 58(5):332–339.

Ganiats TG. Redefining the chronic fatigue syndrome. *Ann Intern Med.* 2015;162:653–654.

Institute of Medicine. *Beyond myalgic encephalomyelitis/chronic fatigue syndrome: Redefining an illness.* Washington, DC: The National Academies; 2015.

Jain R, Jain, S. Fibromyalgia: Management strategies for the primary care practitioner. *Adv Prim Care Med Clin Update.* 2008;15–18.

Kodner, C. Common questions about the diagnosis and management of fibromyalgia. *Am Fam Physician.* 2015;91(7):472–478.

Marter A, Agruss JC. Solving the riddle of fibromyalgia: An evidence-based practice protocol for the advanced practice nurse. *J Nurse Pract.* 2008;4(6):424–437.

Menzies V, Jallo N. Guided imagery as a treatment option for fatigue: A literature review. *J Holist Nurs.* 2011;29(4):279–286.

National Academies of Sciences Engineering Medicine. Beyond myalgic encephalomyelitis/chronic fatigue syndrome: Redefining an illness. http://www.nationalacademies.org/hmd/Reports/2015/ME-CFS.aspx. Published February, 10, 2015.

Okifuji A, Gao J, Bokat C et al. Management of fibromyalgia syndrome in 2016. *Pain Manag.* 2016;6(4):383–400.

Rheumatoid Arthritis

Furfaro, N. Rituximab for rheumatoid arthritis—Practical guidance for optimizing treatment. *Adv Nurse Pract.* 2008;16(1):61–64.

Singh JA, et al. 2012 update of the 2008 American College of Rheumatology recommendations for the use of disease-modifying antirheumatic drugs and biologic agents in the treatment of rheumatoid arthritis. *Arthritis Care Res.* 2012;64(5):625–639.

Smolen J, et al. EULAR recommendations for the management of rheumatoid arthritis with synthetic and biological disease-modifying antirheumatic drugs: 2016 update. *Ann Rheum Dis.* 2017;76(6):960–977.

Wasserman A. Diagnosis and management of rheumatoid arthritis. *Am Fam Physician.* 2011;84(11):1245–1252.

Sjögren's Syndrome

Kruszka P, et al. Diagnosis and management of Sjögren syndrome. *Am Fam Physician.* 2009;79(6):465–470, 472.

Sjögren's Syndrome Foundation. Clinical practice guidelines: Systemic manifestations in Sjögren's patients. https://www.sjogrens.org/home/research-programs/clinical-practice-guidelines. Published 2017. Accessed November 13, 2017.

Stefanski AL, Tomiak C, Pleyer U, Dietrich T, Burmester GR, Dörner T. The diagnosis and treatment of Sjögren's syndrome. *Dtsch Arztebl Int.* 2017;114:354–361.

Systemic Lupus Erythematosus

Hui-Yuen J, et al. Belimumab in systemic lupus erythematosus: A perspective review. *Ther Adv Musculoskel Dis.* 2015;7(4):115–121.

Lam N, et al. Systemic lupus erythematosus: Primary care approach to diagnosis and management. *Am Fam Physician.* 2016;94(4): 284–294.

Tunnicliffe D, et al. Diagnosis, monitoring, and treatment of systemic lupus erythematosus: A systematic review of clinical practice guidelines. *Arthritis Care Res.* 2015:67(10):1440–1452.

RESOURCES

Allergic Reactions

National Institute of Allergy and Infectious Diseases, National Institutes of Health
http://www.niaid.nih.gov

Chronic Fatigue Syndrome and Fibromyalgia Syndrome

American Fibromyalgia Syndrome Association, Inc.
http://www.afsafund.org
Chronic Fatigue and Immune Dysfunction Syndrome Association of America
http://www.cfids.org
National Fibromyalgia Association
http://www.fmaware.org

Sjögren's Syndrome

American College of Rheumatology
http://www.rheumatology.org

Systemic Lupus Erythematosus

American Autoimmune Related Disease Association
http://www.aarda.org
Arthritis Foundation
http://www.arthritis.org
Lupus Foundation of America
http://www.lupus.org
Lupus Research Alliance
http://www.lupusresearch.org

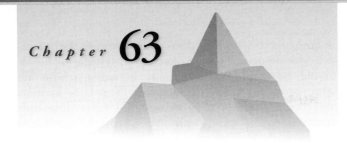

Infectious Disorders

Virginia Sheikh, MD, MHS

Jill E. Winland-Brown, EdD, APRN, FNP-BC

Brian Oscar Porter, MD, PhD, MPH, MBA

INFECTIOUS MONONUCLEOSIS

Infectious mononucleosis, formerly called "glandular fever," is a viral syndrome characterized by prolonged malaise and fatigue, fever, sore throat, and tender cervical lymphadenopathy. The majority (90%) of infectious mononucleosis cases are caused by infection with Epstein-Barr virus (EBV). Cytomegalovirus (CMV) is a less common viral cause.

EPIDEMIOLOGY AND CAUSES

Both EBV and CMV infections are widespread; up to 95% of adults are seropositive for EBV exposure and 59% of individuals aged 6 or older are seropositive for CMV exposure. Both EBV and CMV are members of the Herpesviridae family of viruses and cause lifelong, usually asymptomatic infection. Humans are the major reservoir for latent EBV infection, which typically spreads through intimate contact with asymptomatic viral shedders. Humans, along with monkeys, are the major reservoir for CMV infection, which can be transmitted to others by direct contact with urine or saliva (especially from babies and young children), through sexual contact, and via breast milk.

Symptomatic cases of infectious mononucleosis are most common in teenagers and young adults, for whom the most important mode of transmission is kissing. Preadolescent children, especially those who live in crowded living conditions, are commonly infected with EBV and CMV through saliva, although they are typically asymptomatic. The incidence of infectious mononucleosis is equal among genders, economic classes, and educational levels, although the incidence of clinical infection is up to 30 times higher in whites than blacks. There is no seasonal variation in rates of infectious mononucleosis infection.

PATHOPHYSIOLOGY

EBV is most commonly spread through saliva. Once inside the oral cavity, the virus initially infects and replicates in oropharyngeal epithelial cells. Infectious virions then infect B cells, which migrate and disseminate infection widely throughout the lymphoreticular system, which includes the lymph nodes, spleen, and liver. At the time of infectious mononucleosis symptom onset, high levels of EBV can be detected in the blood. The immune response to EBV viremia includes an atypical peripheral lymphocytosis, which is characterized by a large number of activated CD8+ T cells and natural killer cells. These cells are key to preventing the acute lysis of virally infected cells (i.e., the lytic phase of infection) and establishing nonlytic, subclinical lifelong infection. CMV is transmitted through close contact with body fluids (saliva, urine, and stool), blood or tissue exposure, sexual exposure, or perinatal exposure.

Although the majority of individuals with chronic EBV and/or CMV infection remain asymptomatic throughout their lifetimes, both viruses have the potential to cause serious disease. For example, many cases of Hodgkin's and non-Hodgkin's lymphoma are associated with EBV. Babies born to women who experienced infectious mononucleosis caused by CMV during pregnancy are at risk of congenital CMV infection, which can cause serious complications, including preterm birth, seizures, and central nervous system impairment. CMV reactivation causes significant disease in severely immunosuppressed patients, such as those with HIV/AIDS and bone marrow transplant recipients.

CLINICAL PRESENTATION

Subjective

Patients with infectious mononucleosis typically present with complaints of fever, sore throat, adenopathy, and fatigue. Gastrointestinal (GI) manifestations including nausea, vomiting, and anorexia may also be present, as may hepatosplenomegaly, headache, and, occasionally, a morbilliform viral exanthem (rash). Patients may also report neuropathies, headache, photophobia, dysphagia, sore throat, diffuse chest pain, dyspnea, cough, nausea, myalgia, and arthralgia. They usually cannot identify a known contact with EBV infection before the onset of symptoms.

Objective

Children and teenagers with mononucleosis may present with fevers as high as 39°C (greater than 102.5°F). Almost all patients with infectious mononucleosis will have tender, cervical lymphadenopathy, although this finding is not specific. Posterior cervical, axillary, and inguinal adenopathy are more specific findings. Nuchal stiffness associated with painful lymph nodes may be present, although not as rigid as in meningitis. The pharynx is typically infected. The tonsils may be enlarged, and tonsillar exudate may be present. Splenomegaly is present in up to 60% of patients. The liver may also be enlarged and tender to deep palpation, but jaundice is uncommon. Patients with infectious mononucleosis as a result of CMV infection are less likely to develop lymphadenopathy, tonsillitis, or splenomegaly.

Patients with infectious mononucleosis may present with a fine, maculopapular rash (viral exanthem). More commonly, patients with infectious mononucleosis who have been treated with antibiotics (usually amoxicillin or ampicillin) develop a pruritic, morbilliform rash that can be mistaken for antibiotic allergy.

DIAGNOSTIC REASONING

The symptoms of mononucleosis are seen in many diseases; therefore, laboratory findings play an important role in the differential diagnosis. Although limited diagnostic testing may establish the diagnosis in straightforward cases, additional testing may be required for certain presenting symptoms (e.g., pharyngitis) and in more complex situations.

Diagnostic Tests

Often the diagnosis of infectious mononucleosis can be made with clinical symptoms and with results from a complete blood count (CBC), serum chemistries, and a heterophile antibody test (Monospot). The CBC usually shows at least 50% lymphocytes, including 10% "atypical" lymphocytes. Mild thrombocytopenia and neutropenia are frequent transient findings. Liver enzyme levels, particularly serum transaminase levels, are mildly or moderately elevated in about 90% of patients.

The Monospot test detects heterophile antibodies, which are circulating immunoglobulin (Ig)M antibodies that target red blood cell antigens. Heterophile antibodies are present in 80% to 90% of patients with acute infectious mononucleosis, although they are not specific and may take several weeks to become positive. The Monospot test is less sensitive in younger patients (75% sensitivity in children aged 24–28 months and 25% in children aged 10–24 months); therefore, EBV-specific serologies should be checked in children. In fact, further testing of EBV-specific serum IgM antibodies may prove useful in adult patients as well if the diagnosis based on initial testing is questionable. Anti-EBNA and anti-VCA are two specific anti-EBV serology tests that are widely available, although they are also less sensitive in younger patients (60% sensitivity in infants but up to 100% sensitivity in young adults). False-positive results for EBV have been noted in HIV-infected individuals but are considered rare.

For patients with infectious mononucleosis with negative Monospot test results, serological testing for CMV should be considered, especially in patients who are immunocompromised or pregnant. The U.S. Centers for Disease Control and Prevention (CDC) recommends measurement of IgG (commonly via an enzyme-linked immunosorbent assay or ELISA) in paired samples taken 1 to 3 months apart following initial presentation. Evidence of seroconversion (i.e., first sample IgG negative and second sample IgG positive) establishes the diagnosis of acute CMV infection.

Differential Diagnosis

Although infectious mononucleosis due to EBV or CMV occurs relatively commonly, the differential diagnosis for the common presenting symptoms of fever, pharyngitis, and lymphadenopathy is broad. Other important considerations include streptococcal infection, peritonsillar abscess, and acute HIV. Acute leukemia, which is uncommon, may also present with these symptoms. Certain medications such as isoniazid, phenytoin, or carbamazepine may induce a mononucleosis-like illness. Acute toxoplasmosis, caused by infection with the parasite *Toxoplasma gondii*, can also cause fever and cervical adenopathy in immunocompetent individuals.

Throat culture and/or rapid antigen detection testing should be performed routinely in these cases to rule out group A streptococcal disease. Peritonsillar abscess should be suspected in patients who present with severe unilateral sore throat, drooling, muffled voice, or trismus (lockjaw). For cases in which acute HIV is a possibility, a fourth-generation combined antigen/antibody immunoassay assay should be ordered to detect recent HIV infection (refer to the section on Human Immunodeficiency Virus for more information on acute HIV infection and HIV testing). Acute infection with *T. gondii*, which is uncommon, can typically be excluded with serologic testing, as the absence of anti-*Toxoplasma* IgM and IgG antibodies essentially excludes the diagnosis.

Table 63.1 presents a comparison of the signs and symptoms of EBV-related syndromes. Glandular variant infectious mononucleosis, in which lymphadenopathy is out of proportion to the pharyngitis, differs from systemic variant mononucleosis that presents with fever and fatigue and typically has mild or absent lymphadenopathy and pharyngitis.

MANAGEMENT

The mainstay of management of infectious mononucleosis is supportive care. No effective antiviral medications are available for the treatment of infectious mononucleosis caused by EBV infection. Infectious mononucleosis caused by CMV is typically self-limited, and therefore, antiviral therapy is not typically indicated. NSAIDs or

TABLE 63.1 Infectious Mononucleosis Symptoms

	EBV-Related Infectious Mononucleosis	CMV-Related Infectious Mononucleosis	Oral Hairy Leukoplakia	Duncan's Disease (X-linked Lymphoproliferative Disorder)
Malaise	+	+	+/−	+
Lymphadenopathy	+	+/−	+	+
Fever	+	+	+/−	+/−
Splenomegaly	+ (50% of cases)	+/−	+/−	+
Pharyngeal exudate	+	−	−	−

+ present; − absent.

acetaminophen (in the absence of significant liver injury) can help minimize fever and discomfort. Adequate hydration and nutrition should be emphasized. Supportive measures such as gargling with warm salt water and throat lozenges may alleviate throat pain. Although strict bed rest is not required, adequate rest to support recovery is recommended.

FOLLOW-UP AND REFERRAL

Because patients with infectious mononucleosis are at risk of serious sequelae including splenic rupture, airway compromise, bone marrow suppression, and neurologic complications, patients should be followed regularly until symptom resolution. Repeat laboratory testing may also be necessary if significant abnormalities were present at the time of initial diagnosis, such as elevations in liver-associated enzymes. The primary-care practitioner should provide the patient with a full clinical picture of the disease, including its prolonged course of recovery, so that the patient may play an active role in self-assessment during the follow-up period.

Although severe complications are unlikely, prompt referral may be necessary. Splenic rupture is a rare (2 in 1,000) but potentially fatal complication of infectious mononucleosis. Patients with splenic rupture may experience abdominal pain and or progressive anemia. Patients with these symptoms should be referred for surgical consultation on an urgent or emergent basis depending on the acuity of the symptoms. Patients with infectious mononucleosis who complain of difficulty breathing should be evaluated for airway obstruction, caused by cervical lymphadenopathy or mucosal swelling. Emergent consultation with an otolaryngologist and corticosteroid therapy are warranted in these cases.

Other uncommon but serious sequelae may develop and require ongoing monitoring and/or referral to a specialist. Rare hematologic complications may include hemolytic or aplastic anemia, thrombocytopenia, thrombotic thrombocytopenic purpura, hemolytic uremic syndrome, or disseminated intravascular coagulation. Cardiovascular complications include myocarditis. Renal and genitourinary complications include glomerulonephritis or genital ulceration, and GI complications include pancreatitis. Neurological complications of infectious mononucleosis include Guillain-Barré syndrome, facial nerve palsy, meningoencephalitis, aseptic meningitis, transverse myelitis, or optic neuritis. Any patient with encephalitis will require an immediate neurological consultation.

Patient Education: Infectious Mononucleosis

Young, school-age patients must be warned of the dangers of contact sports and rough-housing for at least 4 weeks after the onset of symptoms because splenic rupture occurs predominantly within 3 weeks of symptom onset and may occur in the absence of frank splenomegaly (50% of splenic rupture cases). In addition, up to one-half of all splenic rupture cases may occur without any preceding trauma, and rupture does not correlate with symptom severity or abnormal laboratory results. A good rule of thumb is that the patient's energy level must be at baseline before the resumption of strenuous or risky physical activity, and this must not occur before 4 weeks. However, strict bedrest is not required during this entire period and will be driven largely by the patient's energy level.

Patients must learn that their recurrent fevers will typically disappear long before they feel recovered; fevers will typically subside after 10 to 14 days, although energy level will not rebound to baseline until 1 to 3 months postinfection. Therefore, teenagers and young adults who typically manage busy schedules and active lives will need to accept that they require rest for a prolonged recovery period that will last weeks, rather than days.

Other elements to consider in patient education include providing information about prescribed drugs, such as the appropriate dosage and adverse effects. The primary-care practitioner should also caution patients to avoid alcohol and cigarette use because they aggravate coughing and nausea. Alcohol should be avoided for a minimum of 3 months after liver function tests return to normal. In addition, patient education should include age-appropriate counseling regarding sexual practices and the risk of sexually transmitted infections other than EBV-associated infectious mononucleosis that may impact future fertility (e.g., pelvic inflammatory disease) or even be life-threatening (e.g., HIV).

LYME DISEASE

Lyme disease is a multisystem inflammatory disease caused by *Borrelia burgdorferi,* a tick-borne spirochete (bacteria). Most of the early signs and symptoms are nonspecific including fever, chills, headache, fatigue, myalgia, arthralgia, and lymphadenopathy. Some patients, however, experience the erythema migrans ("bulls-eye") rash, which is classically associated with Lyme disease. Later manifestations of Lyme disease include meningitis, arthritis, facial palsy, arrhythmias, nerve pain, and short-term memory loss.

EPIDEMIOLOGY AND CAUSES

B. burgdorferi is transmitted to humans primarily through the bite of the *Ixodes scapularis* (black-legged or deer) tick, which is common throughout wooded areas in the eastern part of the United States. The tick survives on bloodmeals from mammals, birds, reptiles, and amphibians at each stage of its life, and it is through these bloodmeals that the tick is infected with *B. burgdorferi.*

Most human infections occur in the late spring, summer, and early fall and are a result of tick nymph bites. The tick eggs hatch in springtime and develop into larvae over the following summer. The tick larvae acquire spirochetes upon taking their first blood meal from infected mice, birds, or other small mammals. The larvae eventually detach from their hosts to molt and emerge the following spring as infected nymphs. Nymph ticks are very small (less than 2 mm), and, therefore, humans are less likely see or remove nymphs after a bite. Nymphs detach and molt into adults in the early fall.

Adults survive throughout fall and winter, feeding exclusively on large mammals, primarily on white tailed deer, before laying eggs in the spring. Although infected adult ticks are also able to transmit the infection, adult ticks are larger and, therefore, more likely to be recognized and removed by humans. Thus, the tick life cycle and the ability to identify bites from larger adult ticks help to explain the seasonal preference for Lyme disease being spread by nymphs in the summer months, rather than in the winter.

Although Lyme disease is named for a town in Connecticut (Old Lyme), where it was isolated among residents in the 1970s, it is prevalent in much of the northeastern and mid-Atlantic United States. In 2015, 95% of Lyme disease cases were reported in the following 14 states: Connecticut, Delaware, Maine, Maryland, Massachusetts, Minnesota, New Hampshire, New Jersey, New York, Pennsylvania, Rhode Island, Vermont, Virginia, and Wisconsin. Up to one-half the ticks found in these states may be infected with the spirochete. In Europe and Asia, other species of *Borrelia* cause disease with somewhat different clinical manifestations.

According to the CDC, the incidence of Lyme disease rose steadily over 10 years to a peak in 2009 and has remained relatively constant through 2015. The diagnosis of Lyme disease, which can be challenging and is described subsequently, causes some difficulty in collecting reliable incidence data. Lyme disease affects individuals with exposure to *B. burgdorferi* via a tick bite, without regard to race, gender, or other demographic traits.

PATHOPHYSIOLOGY

After the bite of an infected tick, the likelihood of *B. burgdorferi* infection depends on the duration of tick exposure. The infected tick must feed for at least 24 to 48 hours before it transmits the spirochete to the host. After infection, spirochetes are believed to bind fibronectin and epithelial cell–derived proteoglycans (e.g., heparin, dermatan sulfate) in the extracellular matrix via glycosaminoglycan receptors. This initiates a mild local inflammatory response that causes cutaneous erythema at sites of spirochetal invasion and centrifugal (outward) spread from the original tick bite, resulting in the rash termed erythema migrans. Subsequent spirochetemia and tissue-specific binding may cause neurological sequelae, vasculopathy, and cardiac conduction defects in certain individuals. Arthritis is thought to be due to joint inflammation from localized exposure to spirochetal antigens, such as outer surface protein A (OspA) or the heat shock protein groEL.

B. burgdorferi has been shown to exert immunomodulatory influences on host cells, including both decreased MHC class II antigen-presenting molecules on Langerhans cells isolated from late-phase cutaneous skin lesions and upregulation of the class II MHC molecules HLA-DR1, HLA-DR2, and HLA-DR4 on synovial endothelial cells in arthritic joints. The role of cytokines in this disease has not been fully elucidated, but several studies have demonstrated increased levels of macrophage-derived tumor necrosis factor–alpha, interleukin (IL)-1, and IL-6 in the blood, synovial fluid, and cerebrospinal fluid (CSF) of affected persons.

In addition, an autoimmune pathology has also been implicated in late disease manifestations. Most notably, the predominant T-cell receptor found on activated T lymphocytes after infection is specific for an epitope of OspA presented within certain class II MHC molecules that are upregulated in affected patients. Moreover, this OspA epitope has been shown to be cross-reactive with the leukocyte adhesion molecule human lymphocyte function associated antigen–1 (LFA-1), which is highly expressed on T lymphocytes. Studies of transgenic mice tolerant to OspA suggest that this protein does not fully explain these autoimmune phenomena.

Some evidence suggests the importance of a *Borrelia*-specific superantigen. In addition, IgM antibodies against the spirochete protein flagellin are cross-reactive with human axonal proteins and myelin; these have been suggested to mediate the neurological sequelae of Lyme disease. Several other types of autoantibodies have been identified in the CSF of Lyme disease patients. However, it is not known whether these antibodies play a role in the actual pathogenesis of the disease or are simply a benign secondary consequence of infection.

CLINICAL PRESENTATION

Subjective

Early in the course of the disease, the patient typically complains of a flu-like illness, including fever, chills, and myalgia. The patient may report a rash that grew in size. Most patients with Lyme disease do not recall a tick bite.

Later in the course of the disease, malaise, fatigue, headache, neck pain and stiffness, and generalized pain may constitute presenting symptoms. Left untreated, the disease may progress to include arthritis of one or more joints. Late in the disease trajectory, the patient may complain of memory loss, cognitive disturbances, mood changes, and peripheral neuropathy in addition to arthritis.

Objective

In early-localized disease, occurring 3 to 30 days after exposure, 70% to 80% of Lyme disease presentations include an erythema migrans rash. Erythema migrans is typically located on parts of the body where the tick selectively feeds, such as the axilla, groin, and waistline. The bull's-eye–appearing rash grows in size as it spreads from the site of the bite. This classic rash is occasionally pruritic and/or burning, may develop central clearing, and is typically greater than 5 cm in size. The presence of this rash is essentially diagnostic of Lyme disease and should prompt treatment in the appropriate clinical and epidemiologic setting, without the need for serological confirmation.

It should be noted that another tick-borne disease (southern tick-associated rash illness or STARI) associated with *Amblyomma americanum* (lone star tick) bites can also present with a similar rash. Although the cause of STARI is not known, patients with STARI appear to respond to the same treatment for Lyme disease (doxycycline). The patient may have a low-grade fever, and the physical examination may reveal lymphadenopathy.

In early disseminated disease, which occurs days to 10 months after infection and often in the absence of erythema migrans, infected patients may present with systemic manifestations including carditis (less than 10% of cases) and neurological manifestations (10% of cases) such as lymphocytic meningitis, cranial nerve (CN) palsies (especially of CN VII), and radiculoneuritis. This neurological triad is known as Bannwarth syndrome and is more common in European cases of Lyme disease than in the United States.

Objective findings later in the disease include regional or organ-specific physical abnormalities. In late disease, which may be months to years after exposure, symptoms are characterized by intermittent arthritis (50% of cases, which respond to oral antibiotic therapy) and arthralgias (20%), with 10% having monoarthritis of the knee. Very late in the disease trajectory, musculoskeletal findings predominate. In particular, joints become edematous and are associated with pain to touch. Gait disturbance may occur in association with encephalopathy.

Patients may have neurological manifestations known as tertiary neuroborreliosis, including encephalopathy, neurocognitive impairment, and peripheral neuropathy. Objective findings may include nuchal rigidity, sensorimotor disturbances, and paresthesias. Mental status examination may be positive for impaired problem resolution. Cardiac findings include dysrhythmias and a prolonged P-R interval. A rare finding is third-degree heart block. Skin eruptions resembling the erythema migrans of early infection may recur later, as well.

DIAGNOSTIC REASONING

Diagnostic Tests

As discussed earlier, the presence of an erythema migrans rash in a Lyme-endemic area should prompt a clinical diagnosis of Lyme disease, regardless of laboratory testing results. Because erythema migrans typically occurs in the first 1 to 2 weeks following *B. burgdorferi* infection before many patients develop antibodies, serologic testing is only 40% sensitive in this setting. Although STARI presents similarly, Lyme remains more common than STARI in Lyme-endemic areas; therefore, patients in these areas with erythema migrans lesions should be presumed to have Lyme disease.

For patients who present with extra-cutaneous symptoms concerning for Lyme disease such as arthritis, carditis, or facial palsy, laboratory testing is necessary to make a Lyme disease diagnosis. Currently, the CDC recommends a two-step process for testing blood for antibodies to *B. burgdorferi*. The first step is an enzyme immunoassay (EIA) and the second step, performed only if the EIA is positive, is a confirmatory Western blot assay. Often, laboratories will offer "reflex" tests that automatically proceed with Western blot testing of positive EIA samples.

Serologic testing performed within the first few weeks of symptoms (and presumably *B. burgdorferi* infection) should assay IgM antibodies, whereas serologic testing performed later in infection should assess IgG antibodies, which develop approximately 1 month after initial exposure. IgM levels can remain elevated for more than a year, so they cannot be used to make a diagnosis of active disease. Repeated serologic testing 4 to 6 weeks after exposure (during the convalescent period) may be appropriate if early serologic testing is negative.

A Western blot is considered positive if two of three of the following IgM bands are positive (OspC/24, 39, 4) or if five of the following IgG bands are positive (18, 23, 28, 30, 39, 41, 45, 58, 66, and 96). False-positive Western blot results are relatively common in uninfected individuals; therefore, the CDC does not recommend performing Western blot testing unless the screening ELISA result is positive. In addition, Lyme disease serologic testing should only be performed with findings that clearly suggest this disease, rather than with only nonspecific chronic complaints. Testing results should be measured against CDC testing standards because results may vary significantly between individual laboratories. When used appropriately, Lyme disease serologic testing is highly sensitive and specific for the diagnosis of Lyme disease.

For a number of reasons, the following tests for Lyme detection are not widely accepted and are considered experimental, rather than confirmatory or diagnostic: variable surface antigen ELISA, polymerase chain reaction (PCR), urinary antigen testing, T-cell proliferative responses, and immune complex disruption. Thus, providers should not use these tests to confirm a diagnosis of Lyme disease.

For patients who present with symptoms suggestive of infection of the CNS (e.g., neuroborreliosis), lumbar puncture should be performed. Analysis of the CSF typical reveals modest pleocytosis (up to several hundred white blood cells [WBCs]) and moderately elevated protein. CSF glucose is typically normal. CSF should be sent for antibodies against *B. burgdorferi,* and positive results are highly specific for the diagnosis of Lyme meningitis. Negative results do not, however, rule out the diagnosis. Testing for other etiologic causes of the patient's symptoms, such as herpes simplex virus, West Nile virus, and syphilis, should also be performed on the CSF fluid.

Because Lyme arthritis is a late manifestation of *B. burgdorferi,* IgG antibodies to *Borrelia* are almost always strongly positive. Therefore, the two-step serologic testing of the blood may be adequate to establish the diagnosis of Lyme arthritis in the appropriate clinical setting. Arthrocentesis may be appropriate to rule out other causes of arthritis. Synovial fluid analysis typically reveals characteristics consistent with any inflammatory arthritis; WBCs are typically elevated with a neutrophilic predominance. *B. burgdorferi* rarely grows in culture. PCR testing of *B. burgdorferi* has not been validated.

Differential Diagnosis

For patients who present with a viral-like illness and skin lesions within one month of tick bite, human granulocytic anaplasmosis (HGA), babesiosis, and STARI should be considered as alternative or comorbid diagnoses. Both HGA and babesiosis are transmitted by Ixodes ticks. HGA is caused by *Anaplasma phagocytophilum* and may present with high fever and severe constitutional complaints, elevated liver enzymes, and leukopenia and/or thrombocytopenia. Babesiosis is caused by infection of the parasite *Babesia microti* and can present with fatigue, high fever, headache, and myalgia. As mentioned earlier, the cause of STARI is not known, but patients may experience erythema migrans–like rashes.

Differential diagnoses for Lyme disease also includes viral syndromes, Rocky Mountain spotted fever, and relapsing fever. It is important not to confuse fibromyalgia syndrome (FMS) or chronic fatigue syndrome (CFS or myalgic encephalomyelitis), which are not inflammatory disorders and have never been shown to be clearly infectious in etiology. Although FMS may develop after the onset of Lyme disease, it is important not to simply accept a diagnosis of chronic Lyme disease made previously by another clinician, because there is little evidence that this condition actually exists, as opposed to the late manifestations of the disease, which are considered genuine aspects of the disease process.

MANAGEMENT

The goal of management for the infected patient is to minimize the manifestations of the disease at the time of diagnosis, although protective measures to prevent primary infection are a key component of any comprehensive management program to benefit others. Patients living in Lyme-endemic areas should be advised to avoid tick bites by use of both protective clothing and tick repellents. After outdoor activities, patients should check for ticks daily and remove attached ticks promptly.

For children 8 years of age and older and nonpregnant adult patients with attached ticks, the Infectious Disease Society of America (IDSA) suggests that clinicians offer a single dose of doxycycline (200 mg) when *all* the following circumstances are met: (a) the attached tick can be identified as an *Ixodes scapularis* nymph or adult tick that has been attached for 36 hours or longer based on the degree of engorgement and exposure, (b) prophylaxis can be started within 72 hours of the time the tick was removed, (c) ecologic information indicates the local rate of infection is 20% or greater, and (d) doxycycline is not contraindicated.

Approximately 90% of early-localized Lyme disease responds to antibiotic therapy. The duration of treatment depends on the extent of involvement. Regimens for early localized disease should last for 10 to 14 days, whereas 30 days of therapy are required for cardiac, neurological, and arthritic manifestations. IDSA recommends doxycycline (Vibramycin) 100 mg twice daily for the initial management of erythema migrans. Doxycycline, or any tetracycline, is not recommended for children younger than 8 years of age or in pregnant women, given the risk of tooth discoloration. The dosage is 2 mg/kg for children older than 8 years. Doxycycline is also effective against ehrlichiosis. Alternative agents include amoxicillin (Amoxil), cefuroxime (Ceftin), and erythromycin (E-Mycin). Cefuroxime is typically more expensive than doxycycline or amoxicillin. The amoxicillin dose is 500 mg three times daily (50 mg/kg per day divided every 8 hours, with this same maximum dose in children). The cefuroxime dose is 500 mg twice daily in adults and up to 30 mg/kg per day divided twice daily, with the same maximum dose in children.

Up to 15% of patients may display worsening of symptoms with rigors, fever, or hypotension in the first 24 hours of antibiotic therapy due to acute inflammatory cytokines. This is referred to as the Jarisch-Herxheimer reaction and is well documented in tick- and louse-borne relapsing fever conditions. Macrolides such as erythromycin are not as effective as doxycycline, amoxicillin, or cefuroxime and should be used only for patients intolerant to these other first-line antibiotic choices. A first-generation cephalosporin such as cephalexin (Keflex) should not be used because these are not active against *Borrelia.*

Early disseminated disease with mostly musculoskeletal manifestations should be treated with the same oral agents for 2 to 3 weeks, as long as meningitis or third-degree heart block is not noted. If neurological sequelae (other than isolated facial nerve palsy) or third-degree heart block is noted, IV antibiotic therapy should be started with ceftriaxone (2 g daily) or cefotaxime (2 g three times daily) for 2 to 4 weeks. First- and second-degree heart block and isolated facial nerve palsy can be treated with 3 weeks of oral antibiotics.

A lumbar puncture should be done to analyze the CSF for anti-*Borrelia* antibodies or inflammatory cells (WBCs), because neurological manifestations may be subclinical. If subclinical meningitis is suspected with elevated WBCs in the CSF, IV antibiotic therapy is required. Third-degree heart block should be treated with IV ceftriaxone or cefotaxime; prednisone 40 to 60 mg/day in divided doses may be added if patients do not respond within 4 days, but this approach has not been validated in randomized trials. Late Lyme disease is treated with amoxicillin or doxycycline for at least 4 weeks if arthritis is the primary manifestation. If patients fail one or two courses of oral antibiotic therapy or if late disease presents with neurological sequelae (or if a lumbar puncture shows subclinical meningitis with WBC or autoantibodies), IV antibiotic therapy of ceftriaxone or cefotaxime for 4 weeks should be used.

All IV antibiotic therapy may be completed on an outpatient basis if the patient has reliable IV access (e.g., a peripherally inserted central catheter or a central venous catheter, as opposed to a peripheral IV line) and a stable social situation. In addition, at least the first IV dose should be given in a monitored setting to evaluate for drug hypersensitivity. Weekly CBCs should be done to monitor for leukopenia, which may be seen with ceftriaxone and cefotaxime. Ceftriaxone may cause biliary sludging, which can be monitored with weekly hepatic panels to evaluate for hyperbilirubinemia. If this occurs, the patient should be switched to cefotaxime. GI effects, including *Clostridium difficile* colitis, may also occur. Doxycycline causes photosensitivity, and amoxicillin and cefuroxime can cause drug rashes.

Combination antibiotic therapy, an oral course of antibiotics following IV courses, pulse therapy with weekly IV treatments, and extended regimens lasting beyond 2 to 4 weeks have never been validated for Lyme disease through randomized trials and should be avoided. These are only likely to increase drug toxicity. There is also no evidence that pharmacological treatment of asymptomatic seropositivity, found on routine "screening" for instance, provides any benefit. These patients should be thoroughly evaluated, however, to determine whether an asymptomatic phase is actually latent infection that will eventually manifest as late disease, because such individuals typically do not progress through early disease manifestations.

Symptoms may persist after appropriate antibiotic treatment. Some Lyme disease symptoms such as headache, fatigue, and malaise commonly take months or years to resolve following treatment. In other cases, persistent symptoms may be attributable to another, untreated, tick-borne pathogen, such as *Ehrlichia* species. Continued infection with *B. burgdorferi* after appropriate Lyme treatment should only be suspected if Lyme-specific symptoms worsen after treatment or if new Lyme-specific signs or symptoms develop.

FOLLOW-UP AND REFERRAL

Follow-up for symptomatic presentations, before an actual diagnosis is made, may require weekly sessions. Thus, antibiotic therapy may be started after initial laboratory testing, if Lyme disease is highly suspected, and later stopped if the diagnosis is not confirmed on follow-up.

The rash of erythema migrans begins to resolve after the fifth dose of oral antibiotics, whereas fibromyalgic and CFS-like symptoms (e.g., headache, weakness, fatigue, arthralgias) may persist for years after infection. Actual FMS is also recognized as a postinfectious complication of Lyme disease.

Referral to a specialist may not be required if the diagnosis is straightforward. However, if the diagnosis is unclear, rather than overtreating with antibiotic therapy, a referral to an infectious disease specialist is indicated for further evaluation and recommendations. Neurological, cardiac, and other serious manifestations may necessitate appropriate specialist referrals, should these manifestations persist, despite primary-care management.

Patient Education: Lyme Disease

People should be encouraged to avoid foliage (where ticks may reside), especially at the ankle level, along wooded paths and to walk in the center of the path to avoid low-lying brush. Hikers should wear clothing that can prevent ticks from attaching to the skin. When planning an activity in the woods, the patient should wear long pants and boots, and pants should be tucked inside the boot lip. Shirt collars should be closed. Tick repellent should be applied to any exposed skin and the scalp. After removing clothing, the patient should inspect the axillae, groin, and waistband areas, in particular, for evidence of attached ticks or bites.

If infection has already occurred, the patient needs to understand the course of the disease and that recurrence of symptoms after initial treatment might occur. Patients who are seropositive are not necessarily immune from reinfection. Reinfection is possible with *Borrelia* of a different strain if the patient remains exposed to high-risk environments.

HUMAN IMMUNODEFICIENCY VIRUS INFECTION

More than one million people in the United States are living with human immunodeficiency virus (HIV) infection, and about 15% of them are unaware of their infection. Although patients may experience a flu-like illness with acute HIV infection, many patients are asymptomatic for years, despite having high levels of HIV in the blood and other bodily fluids such as semen. HIV infects key immune cells called CD4+ T cells, leading to death of most of these infected cells. Over a period of months or decades, HIV kills more CD4+ T cells than the body can produce, and the patient's CD4+ T-cell count begins to decline. When the CD4+ T-cell count drops below 200 cells/mcL, the patient becomes particularly susceptible to opportunistic infections and is considered to have acquired immunodeficiency syndrome (AIDS). Table 63.2 presents the CDC HIV classification system for adults and adolescents.

This section of the chapter covers screening, preexposure prophylaxis (PrEP), and postexposure prophylaxis (PEP). In addition, the section discusses the diagnosis and management of HIV infection in the acute setting and before the progression to AIDS. Refer to the section on acquired immunodeficiency syndrome for the diagnosis and management of AIDS and opportunistic infections.

TABLE 63.2   Centers for Disease Control and Prevention HIV Classification System for Adults and Adolescents

This system emphasizes the importance of CD4+ T-lymphocyte testing in clinical management of HIV-infected persons. The system is based on three ranges of CD4+ T-cell counts and three clinical categories, giving a matrix of nine exclusive categories.

Criteria for HIV Infection

Persons aged 13 years or older with repeatedly (two or more) reactive screening tests (ELISA and HIV-specific antibodies identified by a supplemental test such as the Western blot). Other specific methods of diagnosis of HIV-1 include virus isolation, antigen detection, and detection of HIV genetic material by PCR or bDNA assay.

AIDS-defining Conditions

The term *AIDS-defining illness* refers to any of a list of infections, diseases, or conditions that, when occurring in an HIV-infected person, leads to a diagnosis of AIDS, the most advanced stage of HIV infection. AIDS is also diagnosed if an HIV-infected person has a CD4+ T-cell count below 200 cells/mcL, regardless of whether that person has an AIDS-defining condition. Twenty-six conditions were identified and classified as AIDS-defining conditions in 1993 by the CDC.

Clinical Category	CD4+ T cell Count*	Clinical Manifestations
A1	≥500 cells/mcL	Category A consists of one or more of the conditions listed below in a person with documented HIV infection. Conditions listed in Categories B and C must not have occurred. • Asymptomatic HIV infection • Persistent generalized lymphadenopathy (noted in two or more extra-inguinal sites, at least 1 cm in diameter for ≥3 months) • Acute (primary) HIV infection with accompanying illness or history of acute HIV infection
A2	200–499 cells/mcL	See A1
A3	<200 cells/mcL	See A1
B1	≥500 cells/mcL	Symptomatic HIV infection (but not A or C conditions) Examples include but not limited to: • Bacillary angiomatosis • Candidiasis, vulvovaginal: Persistent >1 month, poorly responsive to treatment • Candidiasis, oropharyngeal • Cervical dysplasia, severe, or carcinoma *in situ* • Constitutional symptoms such as fever or diarrhea >1 month (The above must be attributed to HIV infection or have a clinical course or management complicated by HIV.)
B2	200–499 cells/mcL	See B1
B3	<200 cells/mcL	See B1

TABLE 63.2 **Centers for Disease Control and Prevention HIV Classification System for Adults and Adolescents—cont'd**

Clinical Category	CD4+ T cell Count*	Clinical Manifestations
C1	≥500 cells/mcL	Category C includes the clinical conditions listed below; for classification purposes, once a Category C condition has occurred, the person will remain classified as category C: • Bacterial pneumonia, recurrent (≥2 episodes in 1 year) • Candidiasis: esophageal, tracheal, bronchi, lungs • Cervical cancer, invasive • Coccidioidomycosis, disseminated or extrapulmonary • Cryptococcosis, extrapulmonary • Cryptosporidiosis, chronic intestinal (>1 month) • Cytomegalovirus disease in other than liver, spleen, nodes (e.g., CMV retinitis) • Encephalopathy, HIV-related • Herpes simplex with mucocutaneous ulcer >1 month, bronchitis, pneumonia, esophagitis • Histoplasmosis, disseminated or extrapulmonary • Isosporiasis, chronic intestinal >1 month • Kaposi's sarcoma • Lymphoma: Burkitt's, immunoblastic, primary CNS • *Mycobacterium avium* complex or *M kansasii,* disseminated or extrapulmonary • *M tuberculosis,* pulmonary or extrapulmonary • *Mycobacterium,* other species, disseminated or extrapulmonary • *Pneumocystis jiroveci* pneumonia (PCP) • Progressive multifocal leukoencephalopathy (PML) • *Salmonella* bacteremia, recurrent • *Toxoplasma gondii* (brain) • Wasting syndrome due to HIV (involuntary weight loss >10% of baseline body weight) with either chronic diarrhea (≥2 loose stools per day for ≥1 month) or chronic weakness and fever ≥1 month
C2	200–499 cells/mcL	See C1
C3	<200 cells/mcL	See C1

*There is diurnal variation in CD4+ counts, averaging slightly higher in the afternoon, in HIV-positive persons. Blood for sequential CD4+ counts should be drawn at the same time each day.
Source: Selik R, Mokotoff ED, Branson B, et al. Revised surveillance case definition for HIV infection—United States, 2014. *MMWR Recomm Rep.* 2014;63(RR03);1-10.

EPIDEMIOLOGY AND CAUSES

In 2016, an estimated 36.7 million people were living with HIV worldwide but only 19.5 million of them were receiving antiretroviral therapy (ART). The same year, 1.8 million people were newly infected, and 1.0 million people died from AIDS. HIV has affected all regions of the world. According to the World Health Organization, almost two-thirds of new HIV infections occur in Africa. More than 3 million children are living with HIV.

Although HIV was primarily associated with gay men in the early 1980s, today's HIV epidemic in the United States affects people of any sexual orientation, gender, race, and ethnicity. Men who have sex with men still account for the majority (70%) of new infections, but nearly a quarter (23%) of new infections occurs in individuals who are heterosexual. Although more than quarter (27%) of newly infected individuals are white, African Americans (45%) and Hispanic/Latinos (24%) are disproportionately affected, relative to the demographic distribution of the U.S. population at large. Young people aged 13 to 24 years are particularly affected by HIV infection. Although the number of new HIV diagnoses has declined among women in recent years, women made up 19% of new HIV diagnoses in the United States in 2015.

There are two strains of HIV: HIV-1 and HIV-2. HIV-1 is the predominant strain of HIV worldwide and in the United States. HIV-1 has been genetically divided into groups or subtypes M, N, and O. Group M has been further subdivided into subclasses known as clades, designated A through J. In the United States, nearly all HIV infections are caused by HIV-1 clade B. HIV-2, found most commonly in West Africa, results in slower disease progression and appears less readily transmissible. HIV-2 infection should be considered in patients who were born in Africa, have traveled in Africa, or have had sexual contact or shared needles with someone from Africa. Coinfection with both strains of HIV may occur. As is discussed under Diagnostic Tests, the CDC now recommends screening for HIV using an antigen/antibody combination immunoassay, most of which detect both HIV-1 and HIV-2.

HIV cannot be transmitted by casual contact (e.g., handshakes, closed or open-mouth kissing, hugs). HIV is acquired through sexual intercourse, exposure to infected blood or tissue, perinatal transmission, or breastfeeding. HIV is considered a sexually transmitted infection because both HIV and infected CD4+ T cells may be present in semen and vaginal secretions. During vaginal or anal sex, friction can cause minute tears to these highly vascular mucous membranes. These tears can allow systemic exposure to HIV-infected bodily fluids during penetrative intercourse, particularly on ejaculation. The use of latex condoms can help prevent the exchange of secretions.

Anyone who has had unprotected sex (without a condom or other adequate form of barrier protection) is considered potentially at risk for HIV infection. The risk of HIV transmission from a single episode of unprotected receptive vaginal intercourse with a known HIV-positive sexual partner is estimated to be between 0.08% and 0.2%, and the infection risk associated with a similar episode of receptive anal intercourse is 0.1% to 0.3%. The risk of HIV transmission from oral sex (mouth to genital or mouth to anal contact) is difficult to determine because most people who practice oral sex also practice other forms of sex during the same encounter. Oral to vaginal (cunnilingus), oral to anal (anilingus), and receptive oral to penile (fellatio) sex carry little risk of HIV transmission. The highest risk of HIV transmission from oral sex is to a person performing fellatio on an HIV-infected man who ejaculates. Factors that increase the risk of HIV transmission from oral sex include oral or genital ulcers or cuts, bleeding gums, and concurrent STIs.

HIV can also be transmitted through the sharing of needles with an HIV-infected person; therefore, people who inject illicit drugs (i.e., IV drug abusers) are a high-risk group for HIV infection, as well hepatitis B and C infection. The use of a new, sterile needle and syringe for every injection can substantially reduce the risk of acquiring and transmitting these viruses. These sterile supplies are often available through pharmacies without a prescription or through syringe services programs, also called needle exchange programs.

Before blood banks began universal testing for HIV, people who had blood transfusions were at high risk for HIV infection (e.g., individuals with hemophilia), given the presence of contaminated blood products in the blood banking system. Routine testing of all blood products for HIV-1 and HIV-2 has now virtually eliminated this route of transmission in the United States and other developed nations with universal blood testing standards. However, given the potential of an HIV-positive individual to donate blood during the asymptomatic and undetectable window period before seroconversion with the presence of HIV-specific antibodies has occurred, transmission rates as low as 1 in 1,000,000 to 1 in 2,000,000 transfusion procedures are typically cited during informed consent procedures for transfused blood products.

HIV can be maternally transmitted from mother to newborn. Current guidelines that employ elective cesarean delivery to avoid birth canal exposure, prenatal STI screening and treatment, as well as updated prenatal and perinatal antiretroviral (ARV) regimens for both mother and child, have decreased this rate to less than 1% in some centers. HIV is present in the breast milk of infected mothers and can be a mode of HIV transmission, so breastfeeding by an HIV-infected woman is not recommended in the United States and other countries where women have ready access to formula and clean water.

PATHOPHYSIOLOGY

HIV infection begins with the transfer of the virus from one host to another. In the case of sexual transmission, infectious virus is exposed to mucocutaneous tissue, such as in the genital tract or anus. Dendritic cells called Langerhans cells found within the mucosal epithelium are believed to be the earliest targets of HIV infection. After these cells are infected with HIV, they bind to CD4+ T cells and subsequently migrate to draining lymph nodes via regional lymphatic channels. Within these lymph nodes, HIV further infects follicular dendritic cells capable of presenting virus to circulating CD4+ T cells. HIV, both as free virus and in CD4+ T cells, then enters the blood stream and disseminates vis lymphatic tissues throughout the body. These events are responsible for the fever, malaise, and lymphadenopathy associated with acute HIV infection.

Initial HIV infection of a human CD4+ T cell requires several steps. First, the gp120 molecule of HIV attaches to the CD4 receptor. This interaction causes a conformational change in gp120 that allows for additional interaction with co-receptors CXCR4 or CCR5. X4-tropic viruses bind to CXCR4 co-receptors, and R5 viruses bind to CCR5 co-receptors. Engagement of one of these two co-receptors promotes membrane fusion and internalization of the HIV virion and its components. Humans cells that lack the CCR5 receptor cannot be infected by R5-tropic viruses, and the drug maraviroc (Selzentry), which blocks the human CCR5 receptor, is an effective antiviral drug in patients infected with R5-tropic virus. Maraviroc is not effective, however, in the treatment of patients infected with X-4 tropic virus or dual-tropic viruses.

Once HIV infects the CD4+ T cell, HIV begins its replication activities by converting its genetic material (RNA) into complementary DNA strands, using the RNA-dependent DNA polymerase enzyme reverse transcriptase (RT)—the hallmark of retroviruses. Because mammalian cells do not express RT, this enzyme was the first retrovirus-specific therapeutic target for HIV medications in the form of nucleoside (and nucleotide) RT inhibitors (NRTIs), as well as the nonnucleoside RT inhibitors (NNRTIs). These agents either serve as competitive chain terminators of elongating viral DNA strands (NRTIs) or interfere with the DNA template-primer activity of RT (NNRTIs). Importantly, RT lacks the histone repair enzymes characteristic of mammalian DNA polymerases. This results in a high rate of uncorrected mutations during each cycle of viral DNA replication. In turn, this leads to the rapid development of resistance by HIV to most ARV agents, particularly if used suboptimally as monotherapy or, alternatively, as combination therapy with a high degree of patient nonadherence.

Viral DNA then becomes double-stranded and is incorporated into the host cell genome by viral integrase. This new DNA acts as a blueprint for replication, directing the infected host cell to make new viral particles of HIV. Integrase inhibitor ARVs, such as raltegravir (Isentress) and dolutegravir (Tivicay), inhibit the genomic integration step in the viral replication process.

In addition to genomic replication, a large portion of viral DNA is transcribed and subsequently translated into a large polyprotein, which must then be activated by the HIV protease enzyme. This enzyme acts like "chemical scissors" and catalyzes the cleavage of polyproteins into mature structural proteins and enzymes. This process results in formation of a large number of infectious viral particles, which bud from the host cell and seek out new cells to infect. The HIV protease enzyme is the target of one of the most potent classes of ARV agents—the protease inhibitors (PIs).

CLINICAL PRESENTATION

Subjective

Most patients with HIV infection are minimally symptomatic or asymptomatic for years after initial infection, so routine HIV screening should be part of regular health maintenance for all healthy adults. Providers should discuss risk behaviors with their patients and test patients at high risk of HIV annually. The following Focus on History provides a template for the discussion of HIV risk factors. Patients who present with STIs should be tested for HIV. See the section "Management" for specific risk factors that should prompt annual testing.

Focus on History: Evaluating Risk of HIV Infection

Sexual History and Sexually Transmitted Diseases

- Describe your sexual relationships.
- Describe your sexual orientation.
- Describe your sexual practices. Have you ever had anal sex?
- Have you ever had a sexually transmitted disease (STD)?
- Have you ever had a vaginal discharge or other problem (for women)? Penile discharge or other problem (for men)?
- Have any of your sexual partners been tested for STDs?
- Do you practice safer sex, such as using condoms or other forms of barrier protection?
- What form of birth control do you use, if any?
- Have any of your sexual partners been told that they were HIV positive or had AIDS?

- Would you expect any of your sexual partners to have been exposed to an STD or HIV? Why or why not?

Substance Abuse

- Have you ever injected drugs (legal or illegal [street])?
- Have you ever shared needles, such as for injections, piercings, or tattoos?
- Have you ever used (in any form) illegal or street drugs?
- Do you drink alcohol? If so, how much?

Transfusion History

- Did you receive any blood or blood products between 1977 and 1985?
- Are you or any of your sexual partners a hemophiliac?
- Have you ever received any donor sperm during artificial insemination?

Infection History

- Have you or any of your sexual partners ever had any form of hepatitis?
- Have you or anyone close to you been diagnosed with tuberculosis (TB)? If so, what is (or was) the treatment?
- Have you ever had a positive test for TB?
- Have you ever taken medications for TB?

Occupational History

- Do you work in the health-care field? In a long-term residential facility? In a jail or prison?
- Are you exposed to blood or other body fluids while on the job?
- Have you ever had a needle-stick injury?

After acute HIV infection, approximately 8% of patients experience flu-like symptoms such as fever, sore throat, myalgia, headache, cervical lymphadenopathy, and night sweats. Although the differential diagnosis for this constellation of symptoms is very broad, providers should keep this diagnosis in mind, because early HIV treatment leads to better health outcomes for patients. The symptoms associated with acute HIV infection may be the only symptoms the patient has before developing AIDS years later, so recognition of the infection during this phase may prevent subsequent morbidity and mortality and prevent transmission of HIV to the patient's sexual partners.

In the years that follow initial HIV infection, as the disease slowly progresses, HIV-infected patients may become more vulnerable to outbreaks of common infections. For example, they may experience herpes zoster (i.e., shingles or reactivation of varicella zoster virus) or unusually aggressive or frequent outbreaks of herpes labialis. Patients may also present with oral candidiasis (thrush). Although these infections also occur in individuals without HIV infection (e.g., in patients prescribed corticosteroids) and are not considered AIDS-defining illnesses, providers should consider testing for HIV in this setting.

Objective

Many patients with HIV infection will have no objective signs of infection. However, the following physical or laboratory signs should prompt consideration of HIV testing.

- Persistent generalized lymphadenopathy: This is a relatively common feature in early HIV infection, when the patient is often asymptomatic. During the assessment, the clinician must be alert for enlarged lymph nodes involving two noncontiguous sites, other than inguinal nodes. The clinician should measure and record the size of nodes if palpable, although significant nonpalpable lymphadenopathy may also be evident on imaging exams.
- Localized *Candida* infections: Thrush is a common finding in HIV infection. The presence of thrush indicates advanced immunosuppression, with a high probability of a serious or opportunistic infection (OI) within 3 years. The clinician should carefully assess the oral cavity, using a high-quality flashlight and look for the presence of white plaques (thrush), dark purplish lesions (possibly Kaposi's sarcoma), or a whitish hair-like growth on the tongue (oral hairy leukoplakia caused by EBV, seen in advanced states of immunosuppression). If white plaque is found, the clinician should attempt to lightly scrape off a portion with a tongue blade. If thrush is present, the plaque will bleed as it is scraped off. *Candida* esophagitis is a late complication of HIV infection; the usual presentation is thrush with odynophagia. *Candida* vaginitis in women with HIV infection is more likely to be recurrent or refractory to therapy than in other women.
- Sexually transmitted infectious: STIs increase the likelihood of HIV transmission or acquisition. The clinician should do a thorough examination of the rectal and genital area, inspecting for perianal and genital herpes simplex lesions, as well as penile or vaginal discharge reflective of gonorrhea or other STI.
- Weight loss: The clinician should document the patient's height and weight at the time of the examination and record the patient's description of weight loss (i.e., amount lost over what period of time) because this is a common presenting sign in patients with undiagnosed HIV infection and may herald progressive immunosuppression.
- Cytopenias: Anemia, leukopenia, and/or thrombocytopenia often complicate HIV infection. The clinician should check the CBC with leukocyte differential, in addition to specific T lymphocyte subset (CD4+ and CD8+) counts to assess the level of HIV-associated immunosuppression.

DIAGNOSTIC REASONING

HIV testing should be part of routine care for individuals aged 15 to 65 years. Patients with risk factors for HIV infection should be tested annually.

Diagnostic Tests

In 2013, the CDC updated its guidelines for the diagnosis of HIV to recommend the use of an U.S. Food and Drug Administration (FDA)-approved HIV-1/2 antigen/antibody combination immunoassay (sometimes referred to as a fourth-generation HIV immunoassay) for the initial screening of HIV. Unlike previous serologic tests used to screen for HIV that relied solely on an individual's antibody response to HIV infection, the HIV-1/2 antigen/antibody combination immunoassay detects an HIV antigen (p24) in addition to IgM and IgG antibodies to HIV-1 and HIV-2. Detection of the p24 antigen, which is present in the blood earlier than HIV antibodies, allows for earlier detection of HIV and shortening of the "window period" between HIV infection and a positive HIV test result. For specimens that are positive by the HIV-1/2 antigen/antibody combination immunoassay, HIV infection is then confirmed with an additional immunoassay to distinguish between HIV-1 and HIV-2 antibodies or, if the distinguishing assay is inconclusive, nucleic acid amplification testing (NAT, often referred to as HIV viral load testing).

Several rapid HIV serologic tests are available for use in high-throughput clinical settings (such as emergency departments or labor and delivery units) or at home. Numerous portable, rapid HIV tests are commercially available. Two home HIV tests are currently available in the United States. The Home Access HIV-1 Test System tests blood from a finger prick, and the OraQuick in-Home HIV Test uses oral fluid from a mouth swab.

Before 2014, routine screening for HIV was performed using a two-tiered algorithm, which used an enzyme-linked immunosorbent assay (ELISA) followed by a confirmatory Western blot if the initial ELISA was positive. Both of these tests rely on presence of host's antibodies. This approach was sensitive and specific overall, but failed to identify many cases of acute HIV infection and misdiagnosed HIV-2-infected patients as having HIV-1.

Using the new algorithm, nucleic acid testing (NAT) to determine HIV viral load is not needed to establish the diagnosis of HIV, except in certain circumstances. First, as described above, NAT testing of HIV-1 is used when the HIV-1/HIV-2 antibody distinguishing assay is inconclusive. Second, NAT testing is used for screening of blood donors. Third, the diagnosis of neonatal HIV infection in infants born to HIV-infected mothers is made using NAT because maternal antibodies are present in infants' blood for the first 6 to 12 months of life. Lastly, NAT testing may be considered when acute HIV is suspected, although HIV-1 RNA is present in the blood only 1 or 2 days before the rise in p24 antigen, which is detected in the HIV-1/2 antigen/antibody immunoassay. Of note, detectable RNA at low levels may represent false-positive results in some cases.

All states, the District of Columbia, and United States territories require that laboratories report positive HIV test results to the public health authority serving the patient's geographic area. However, primary-care practitioners should become familiar with the specific reporting requirements of their states and local health departments because they may differ.

Differential Diagnosis

The signs and symptoms of acute HIV infection are very similar to those seen in other common diseases such as infectious mononucleosis (due to EBV or CMV and described earlier in this chapter), toxoplasmosis, rubella, viral hepatitis, and drug reactions. The symptoms and signs seen in chronic HIV, before AIDS, are commonly seen in other immunosuppressed patients, such as those on chemotherapy, radiation therapy, or long-term corticosteroids. Certain cancers can also cause a decrease in the CD4+ T-cell count. Cytopenias including lymphopenia may be due to a primary or infiltrative bone marrow disorder and may require bone marrow biopsy if an HIV test is negative.

There is also a well-documented condition known as idiopathic CD4 lymphocytopenia (ICL) that was first noted around the same time HIV infection was characterized. In ICL, patients present with the same laboratory profile as HIV-infected patients (low CD4+ T-cell counts), but with no direct evidence of HIV infection, that is, no virus is detectable in the blood of ICL patients even using the most sensitive assays. In turn, this condition is not attributed to HIV nor to any other infectious agent as yet identified, although patients may suffer from the same opportunistic infections and AIDS-defining illnesses as seen with advanced HIV infection.

MANAGEMENT

This section addresses screening for HIV in at-risk patients, pre-exposure prophylaxis (PrEP), postexposure prophylaxis (PEP), and the management of HIV in infected patients who have not yet developed AIDS.

Screening

Approximately 166,000 people in the United States are living with HIV but are unaware of their status. Most of these individuals are likely asymptomatic. The CDC recommends HIV screening of all adults, adolescents, and pregnant women in health-care settings for HIV after the patient is notified that testing will be performed unless the patient declines (opt-out screening). Although many states previously required written consent prior to HIV testing, most states have eliminated this requirement because it was a barrier to early diagnosis. Primary-care practitioners should inform themselves of state laws regarding HIV testing.

People with any of the following risk factors should be tested annually: men who have sex with men, sex (anal or vaginal) with an HIV-positive partner, more than one sexual partner since their last HIV test, injected drugs or shared needles or works (e.g., water or cotton), exchanged sex for drugs or money, diagnosed with viral hepatitis or tuberculosis, sex with someone who falls into one or more of the previous categories. Testing is the first step toward

earlier HIV treatment. Results from the recent START study demonstrated that earlier treatment of HIV offered patients clear health benefits.

Pre-exposure Prophylaxis

Recent clinical trials have demonstrated that certain populations at very high risk of HIV can reduce their likelihood of acquiring the infection by taking certain antiviral drugs daily (PrEP) in combination with condoms and other preventative safer sex measures. In 2014, the U.S. Public Health Service released the first comprehensive guidelines for PrEP and recommended consideration of PrEP for all HIV-negative individuals who are at substantial risk of acquiring HIV infection. Risk groups include HIV-uninfected individuals for whom one of the following is true:

- Man or woman in an ongoing relationship with an HIV-infected partner
- Gay or bisexual man who has anal sex without a condom and is not in a mutually monogamous relationship with a HIV-uninfected man or has been diagnosed with an STI in the past 6 months
- Gay or bisexual man who has been diagnosed with an STI in the past 6 months
- Heterosexual man or woman who does not regularly use condoms during sex with partners of unknown HIV status or who are at substantial risk of HIV infection
- Individual who has injected illicit drugs in the past 6 months and shared injection equipment or has been in drug treatment for injection drug use in the past 6 months

Candidates for PrEP must be willing to adhere to PrEP daily and follow-up with a provider every 3 months for repeat HIV testing and other follow-up assessments.

Before the initiation of PrEP, the following laboratory tests should be performed: HIV testing, hepatitis B virus (HBV) serology, hepatitis C virus (HCV) serology, and serum chemistry for estimation of renal function. The only drug combination currently approved by the FDA for PrEP is emtricitabine 200 mg/tenofovir 300 mg (Truvada). Because tenofovir treatment is associated with renal toxicity, individuals with creatinine clearance lower than 60 mL/min should not be offered PrEP with emtricitabine/tenofovir. Because these individuals are at high risk of HBV infection, all individuals who are susceptible (nonimmune) should be vaccinated. For individuals who are HBV-infected, emtricitabine and tenofovir are both active against HBV. Individuals with HBV who stop emtricitabine/tenofovir are at risk for a HBV flare, which is characterized by elevations in hepatic enzymes. Therefore, liver function tests should be monitored in these patients.

Postexposure Prophylaxis

PEP should be considered after an HIV-uninfected individual has a recent (less than 72 hours) exposure that carries a substantial risk of HIV infection. Substantial risks include percutaneous contact or exposure of mucosal surfaces (e.g., vagina, eye, or nonintact skin) with blood, semen, vaginal secretions, rectal secretions, breast milk, or any body fluid contaminated with blood from a source known to be HIV infected.

PEP should be provided only for infrequent exposures. Individuals who engage in high-risk behaviors may be offered PEP, but PEP should be followed by PrEP, as described in the preceding section. Nonoccupational HIV exposures might include sexual assault or a nonoccupational needle-stick. The most common cause of occupational exposure to HIV is a needle-stick injury in a health-care setting. Although the risk of acquiring HIV through a single occupational or nonoccupational exposure is low (e.g., approximately 0.3% for an occupational needle stick from an HIV-positive patient, 0.08% for receptive penile-vaginal intercourse), exposed individuals may experience significant anxiety. The Patient's Voice 63.1 presents one health-care worker's perspective when faced with such a situation.

PEP should be initiated within 72 hours of exposure and is unlikely to be effective when started later. The following laboratory tests should be performed upon presentation: HIV antibody/antigen testing, HBV serology (HBsAg, HBsAb, and HBcAb), HCV serology, serum creatinine, alanine transaminase (ALT), and aspartate aminotransferase (AST). For those who have been sexually exposed, testing for syphilis, gonorrhoea, chlamydia, and pregnancy should be performed. If the individual who is the source of the exposure is available, the following tests should be performed on the source: HIV antibody/antigen testing (for those with unknown HIV status) or HIV viral load and HIV genotypic testing (for those with known HIV infection), HBV serology (HBsAg, HBsAb, and HBcAb), and HCV serology.

In 2016, the CDC published updated guidance for nonoccupational PEP and recommended that all PEP

regimens should include a 28-day course of a three-drug ARV regimen. For adults and adolescents aged 13 years and older with creatinine clearance 60 mL/min or greater, the CDC recommends emtricitabine 200 mg/tenofovir 300 mg (Truvada) once daily and either raltegravir 400 mg twice daily or dolutegravir 50 mg once daily for adults and adolescents aged 13 years and older with creatinine clearance 60 mL/min or greater. The recommended alternative regimen is a four-drug combination of emtricitabine 200 mg/tenofovir 300 mg once daily, darunavir 800 mg once daily, and ritonavir 100 mg once daily.

For adults and adolescents aged 13 years and older with creatinine clearance £59 mL/min, the CDC recommends zidovudine and lamivudine (both adjusted as indicated for impaired renal function) and either raltegravir 400 mg twice daily or dolutegravir 50 mg once daily. Again, the recommended alternative regimen is a four-drug combination of emtricitabine 200 mg/tenofovir 300 mg once daily, darunavir 800 mg once daily, and ritonavir 100 mg once daily.

The most recent updates to the recommendations for occupational PEP were published in 2013. All recommended regimens contain three or more ARV drugs. The preferred PEP regimen is raltegravir 400 mg twice daily with emtricitabine 200 mg/tenofovir 300 mg once daily. Most clinicians, however, would likely consider dolutegravir 50 mg once daily with emtricitabine 200 mg/tenofovir 300 mg once daily. Of note, preliminary data from an observational surveillance study of birth outcomes among pregnant women receiving HIV treatment in Botswana suggest that dolutegravir exposure at the time of conception, but not later in pregnancy, may be associated with an increased risk of neural tube defects in infants born to these women. Before prescribing dolutegravir or another integrase strand transfer inhibitor (INSTI) to an individual of childbearing potential, please refer to the Department of Health and Human Services Guidelines at AIDSinfo for updated information on this topic. Immediate expert consultation may be appropriate before the initiation of PEP. The CDC guidance provides recommended regimens for children younger than 13 years of age. However, a pediatric HIV expert may be better equipped to manage the dosing, administration challenges, side effects, and counseling in this population. Expert consultation is also indicated when the exposed individual is pregnant. When the source individual is HIV infected with a viral strain with known resistance mutations, consultation with an HIV expert is advised. Abacavir sulfate should not be included in any PEP regimen because the rapid initiation of PEP does not allow sufficient time to perform HLA-B*5701 testing. Patients with the HLA-B*5701 allele are at high risk of abacavir hypersensitivity syndrome, which can lead to death.

Health-care providers prescribing PEP should educate their patients regarding the potential risks of each of the components of their PEP regimens and provide counseling on ways to prevent transmission of HIV. Because many exposed individuals feel considerable stress at the time of exposure, providers should consider scheduling an early

---

 The Patient's Voice 63.1: HIV Infection

I am furious! I've been a nurse for 20 years and have always been proud of my skills and techniques. I have been stuck by needles, but only a few times during my career . . . usually when a patient suddenly moved and not through negligence on my part. I thought nothing of it until last month when I went to my doctor because I was feeling so tired and run down. He asked if I had been tested for HIV, and I said no. Just to appease him, I had the test done, and it was positive.

The only thing I can relate it to is a needle stick that occurred when I was working in home health several years ago. I didn't even think anything of it at the time, and I didn't even fill out an incident report. I don't have any recourse now since I can't prove I was infected "on the job." Now, I hear about the needleless syringes and all the safe guards in place. If I had them back then, I probably wouldn't be in the situation I am now. I am so angry! What do I do now?

follow-up visit (3–7 days) and be prepared to reiterate some of the initial counseling discussion. Providers should also assess patients' needs for mental health and other services

Four to six weeks after the HIV exposure, HIV antigen/antibody testing should be repeated, along with other tests such as serum creatinine, ALT, and AST, as appropriate based on the PEP regimen. Exposed individuals whose HIV testing is negative should undergo repeat testing again 3 months and 6 months after exposure. For exposed individuals with positive HIV testing, HIV treatment should be continued. The management of acute and early HIV infection is discussed next.

Treatment for Acute HIV and Early HIV Infection (Prior to AIDS)

All patients with HIV should be treated with ART, regardless of CD4+ T-cell count. Although there is no cure at this time for HIV infection, numerous effective combinations of ART are available, and early HIV treatment provides patients with health benefits. With early detection and early initiation of treatment, HIV infection can be managed as a chronic but controllable infectious disease.

The key goals of ART are to durably suppress HIV viral load and improve the patient's immune system, thereby preventing AIDS-related events such as opportunistic infections (OIs) and death. Principles of management for early HIV infection include (1) initial disclosure of HIV status, (2) initiation of drug therapy to suppress the virus, and (3) monitoring of viral activity to determine any need to modify or revise drug therapy.

Initial Disclosure

Disclosure of HIV test results is a critical event in the clinician–patient relationship. Disclosure counseling sets the tone and foundation for the patient's acceptance, knowledge base, and attitudes about his or her HIV infection (see The Iceberg of Living with HIV). Disclosure of HIV test results is typically a stressful period for the patient, who may experience significant denial toward a positive test result. Some guidelines and concepts for disclosure counseling are summarized here:

- Disclosure counseling should be done face-to-face. In planning the disclosure of the patient's HIV status, the clinician should assess the degree to which the patient or parent/guardian is prepared to receive the results. The clinician should also assess the patient's social, demographic, cultural, and psychological characteristics, which may relate to coping with a positive HIV test. During the disclosure session, the provider should discuss the natural history of HIV infection, the potential effects of HIV infection on physical and mental health, the role of health maintenance practices, the availability of treatment, and the need to practice HIV transmission prevention behaviors.
- The disclosure counseling process is an opportunity to provide immediate interventions and involve the

patient in ongoing medical, mental health, social, and family support networks. Immediate interventions may include the following: assessing the patient for the risk of inflicting violence to themselves or others; ensuring that the patient will receive a thorough medical evaluation for staging and initial care; informing the patient of ongoing availability of services; scheduling the next appointment; addressing prevention of further HIV transmission; assessing the availability of an immediate support person and other care providers; providing local and national resources for information on HIV infection; and making appropriate referrals for any ongoing services that cannot be provided on site.

- The provider must reassure the newly diagnosed patient that medical advances have led to the availability of numerous ARV drugs, which have led to prolonged survival and improved quality of life for HIV-infected patients. In fact, some recent studies have suggested that with early and attentive medical care, optimized medication adherence, and healthy lifestyle habits, HIV-infected patients may enjoy nearly the same life expectancies as noninfected individuals in the United States. Many newly diagnosed patients and their family members think that HIV is a "death sentence," so learning the facts about the effectiveness of modern HIV treatments can provide patients with great relief.
- Clinicians should assist patients in understanding the advantages and disadvantages of disclosing their HIV status to others by providing counseling, factual information regarding legal aspects of disclosure, opportunities for patient education and dialogue, and referrals as needed.
- The patient should be strongly advised and encouraged to disclose their HIV status to significant others, particularly sexual and needle-sharing partners. Some local and state health departments will do partner notification without disclosing the name of the HIV-positive person, providing partners with the knowledge that they have been exposed to a sexually transmitted disease and that HIV testing is advised. Some patients prefer to have a provider present at the time of disclosure to significant others.
- The prevention of HIV transmission must be discussed at the time of the initial diagnosis of HIV infection. The patient's blood and semen become infectious to others shortly after the patient is initially infected, so risky sexual behaviors need to be addressed immediately. The patient should also be advised against donating blood, plasma, tissue, body organs, sperm, or eggs.
- The patient must also understand that the virus mutates or changes within each person; therefore, the HIV-infected person remains at risk of acquiring a slightly different HIV strain from another HIV-infected individual—a phenomenon known as superinfection. The existence in the patient of a second viral strain with a different mutation profile can complicate the selection of an appropriate ARV regimen, increase the likelihood of infectious complications, and hasten the progression of disease. Patients from West Africa are also at risk of coinfection with strains of both HIV-1 and HIV-2.

The Iceberg of Living with HIV

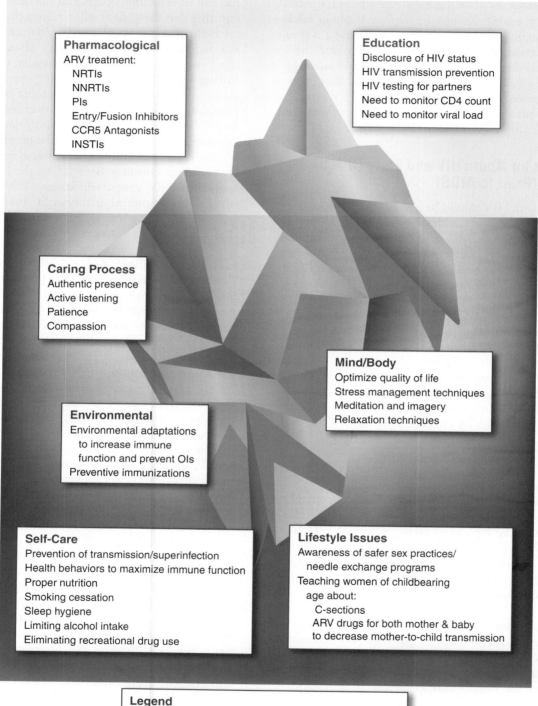

Pharmacological
ARV treatment:
  NRTIs
  NNRTIs
  PIs
  Entry/Fusion Inhibitors
  CCR5 Antagonists
  INSTIs

Education
Disclosure of HIV status
HIV transmission prevention
HIV testing for partners
Need to monitor CD4 count
Need to monitor viral load

Caring Process
Authentic presence
Active listening
Patience
Compassion

Mind/Body
Optimize quality of life
Stress management techniques
Meditation and imagery
Relaxation techniques

Environmental
Environmental adaptations
  to increase immune
  function and prevent OIs
Preventive immunizations

Self-Care
Prevention of transmission/superinfection
Health behaviors to maximize immune function
Proper nutrition
Smoking cessation
Sleep hygiene
Limiting alcohol intake
Eliminating recreational drug use

Lifestyle Issues
Awareness of safer sex practices/
  needle exchange programs
Teaching women of childbearing
  age about:
    C-sections
    ARV drugs for both mother & baby
    to decrease mother-to-child transmission

Legend
ARV = antiretroviral
INSTIs = integrase strand transfer inhibitors
NRTIs = nucleoside reverse transcriptase inhibitors
NNRTIs = non-nucleoside reverse transcriptase inhibitors
PIs = protease inhibitors
OIs = opportunistic infections

Initial Laboratory Testing (Patients Newly Diagnosed With HIV)

Some key diagnostic tests for patients newly diagnosed with HIV are listed in Table 63.3 (see also Fig. 63.1). HIV drug-resistance testing is recommended for all patients before initiating ART to help guide the choice of ARV regimen. The most common form of resistance testing is known as HIV genotyping, in which specific viral mutations are detected via DNA sequence analysis compared with a "wild-type" (nonmutated) HIV reference sequence. HIV phenotyping assays are also available in which drug resistance is measured by growing viral isolates from a patient in the presence of individual ARV

TABLE 63.3 Diagnostic Tests for a Newly Diagnosed HIV Patient	
Test	**Interpreting the Results**
CD4+ T-cell count	>500 cells/mcL: at low risk for opportunistic infections. 500–200 cells/mcL: low to moderate risk for opportunistic infections <200 cells/mcL: AIDS, high risk for opportunistic infections; prophylaxis for *Pneumocystis jiroveci pneumonia* (PCP) and *Mycobacterium avium* complex (MAC) may be needed while awaiting increase in T-cell count in response to effective ART [To calculate absolute CD4+ count: number of WBC × % lymphocytes × % CD4+ = absolute CD4+ T cell count]
HIV viral load	The baseline viral load will be a bench mark for evaluating the patient's response to ART. A decrease in the HIV viral load indicates a therapeutic response to ART; an increase in viral load indicates disease progression.
Genotyping resistance testing	Viral resistance testing will guide the choice of ARV regimen. Although drug resistance mutations accumulate over time and are more common in patients who have been on ARV drugs in the past, drug-resistant HIV strains can be transmitted from one individual to another. Viral amplification for resistance testing may not always be possible for patients who have HIV RNA levels <500 to 1,000 copies/mL
Tropism testing (if considering treatment with CCR5 antagonist)	Maraviroc is not a preferred ARV drug for patients starting ART for the first time, so this test is likely not needed unless genotypic resistance testing reveals an extensive resistance profile. Patients who are infected with X4 or dual-tropic viruses should not be treated with a CCR5 antagonist. Tropism can change over time in the same individual.
Hepatitis A, B, and C serologies	Patients who are nonimmune to viral hepatitis should be vaccinated with hepatitis A and B vaccines. Patients with HBV and HCV need additional liver health monitoring. HBV coinfection is an important factor to consider in selection an ART regimen and, subsequently, in withdrawing or changing ART. Several ARV drugs (e.g., emtricitabine, lamivudine, tenofovir disoproxil fumarate, and tenofovir alafenamide) have activity against HBV.
Complete blood count with differential	Anemia is common; may be related to HIV disease, underlying infection, or medication (particularly zidovudine [AZT]). Bone marrow biopsy may be done to check for fungi, *M. avium* or tuberculosis, CMV, parvovirus, or malignancy. Thrombocytopenia is often seen. In early infection, idiopathic thrombocytopenia purpura may be seen; in later infection, thrombocytopenia may be because of bone marrow suppression. Thrombocytopenia may also be seen with Kaposi's sarcoma. Leukopenia is common; WBC counts less than 2,000 cells/mcL are common and, in isolation, are not cause for alarm. If using medications that cause neutropenia, may need to prescribe colony-stimulating factors such as filgrastim (Neupogen).
Basic serum chemistry	Renal function may be impaired because of HIV nephropathy, volume depletion from diarrhea, or wasting.
Liver associated chemistries	Liver associated enzymes (AST, ALT, alkaline phosphatase) may be elevated as a result of HBV or HCV coinfection, medications, alcohol abuse, or non-alcoholic fatty liver disease (NAFLD), which is common in HIV-infected patients. Elevations in bilirubin may indicate disseminated MAC infection. Bilirubin may also become elevated after starting certain ARV drugs (atazanavir). Elevated lactate dehydrogenase (LDH) may be nonspecific or related to PCP, lymphoma, hemolysis, muscle wasting, or may be caused by HIV or AZT. Low albumin levels may indicate malnutrition.

Continued

TABLE 63.3 Diagnostic Tests for a Newly Diagnosed HIV Patient—cont'd	
Test	*Interpreting the Results*
Fasting lipid profile	Patients infected with HIV are at high risk of metabolic diseases, obesity, and cardiovascular disease. Elevated triglycerides may be a response to cytokine activation.
Hemoglobin A1c	Patients infected with HIV are at high risk of metabolic diseases, such as type II diabetes mellitus.
Interferon-gamma release assay or purified protein derivative tuberculin skin test (TST)	A positive interferon-gamma assay result or TST induration of 5 mm or more is considered a positive reaction (no reaction may be due to anergy); evaluate for signs/symptoms of active TB with physical examination and chest x-ray.
HLA-B*5701 testing (if considering treatment with abacavir)	Abacavir and abacavir-containing regimens should not be prescribed in patients who are positive for HLA-B*5701 or in whom testing has not been performed, given the increased risk of abacavir hypersensitivity.
Urinalysis	Patients infected with HIV are at risk of renal disease both from HIV and from some ARV drugs (e.g., tenofovir).
STI screening, including rapid plasma reagin screening	Patients with HIV are at risk for other sexually transmitted infections.
Pregnancy test	For women of childbearing potential.

agents and comparing these growth rates to those of a wild-type HIV strain. Given the higher cost of HIV phenotyping tests, these tests are done much less frequently than HIV genotyping tests.

Monitoring HIV viral load is an essential part of HIV management after the initiation of ART. Box 63.1 describes some of the features of viral load testing and some of the differences between the various laboratory tests that are available for viral load testing.

Initiation of Drug Therapy

All patients with HIV infection should be offered ART. Fundamental concepts that underlie the foundation of ART include the following:

- Complete eradication of HIV infection cannot be achieved with current HIV drug therapy.
- Suppression of HIV RNA strongly predicts a reduced likelihood of disease progression and death. Ideally, HIV patients on ART should achieve suppression of HIV RNA to levels below the limit of detection within the first several months of ART initiation.
- Viral replication, especially while on ART, leads to viral resistance mutations. Viral resistance mutations confer resistance to one or more ARV drugs, reducing the effectiveness of ART.
- Complete immune reconstitution, particularly for those who have advanced HIV disease, may not be possible. Regeneration and increases in CD4+ T-cell counts are typically seen in patients receiving ART; however, the loss of CD4+ T lymphocyte may not be entirely reversible. Especially in patients with severe

immunosuppression (CD4+ T cells <50 cells/mcL), CD4+ T-cell counts may not rise above the key threshold of 200 cells/mcL until several years after ART initiation.

ARVs for Initial HIV-1 Infection

In the United States, approximately 30 agents in seven mechanistic drug classes are approved for the treatment of HIV. These classes NRTIs, NNRTIs, PIs, fusion inhibitors, INSTIs, chemokine (C-C motif) receptor 5 (CCR5) antagonists, and CD4-directed post-attachment HIV-1 inhibitors. An additional class of medications, pharmacokinetic (PK) enhancers, functions to "boost" the level of other ARVs to therapeutic concentrations by inhibiting metabolism of the other ARVs.

Guidelines for the Use of Antiretroviral Agents in HIV-1 Infected Adults and Adolescent Living With HIV is a "living document" that is updated regularly, based on new safety and efficacy information on ARVs. These guidelines are produced by the Panel on Clinical Practices for Treatment of HIV Infection, convened by the U.S. Department of Health and Human Services, and may be obtained online at http://AIDSinfo. nih.gov, a public access Web site. Providers prescribing HIV treatment should refer to this document for the most up-to-date information on ART. The Panel currently recommends patients be placed on two NRTIs in combination with a third active ARV drug from one of three drug classes: INSTIs, NNRTIs, or a protease inhibitor (PI) with a pharmacokinetic (PK) enhancer (cobicistat or ritonavir).

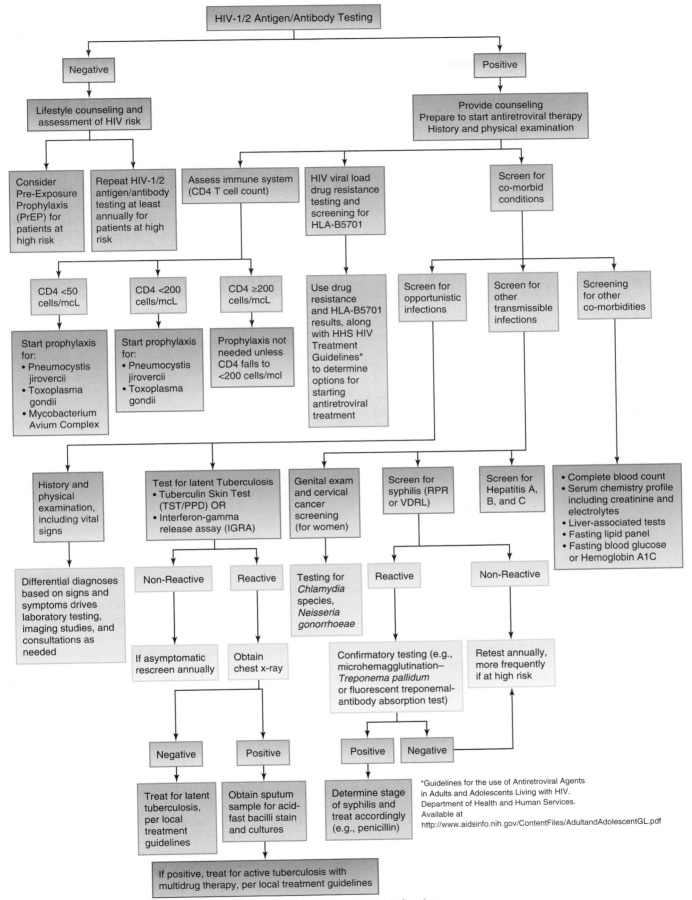

Figure 63.1 Treatment flowchart for management of early HIV infection

Treatment Standards/Guidelines Initiation of ARV Therapy

Source: U.S. Department of Health and Human Services. *Guidelines for the Use of Antiretroviral Agents in HIV-1 Infected Adults* and *Adolescents Living With HIV*. https://aidsinfo.nih.gov/guidelines/html/1/adult-and-adolescent-arv/0. Published 2017.

ART is recommended for all HIV-infected individuals, regardless of CD4+ T-cell count, to reduce the morbidly and mortality associated with HIV infection and to prevent HIV transmission. INSTI-based regimens are recommended as initial therapy for most people with HIV, although in certain clinical situations a PI- or an NNRTI-based regimen may be preferred.

PREFERRED REGIMENS

INSTI-Based Regimens

- Bictegravir/tenofovir alafenamide/emtricitabine
- Dolutegravir/abacavir/lamivudine—**only** for patients who are HLA-B*5701 negative
- Dolutegravir plus either tenofovir disoproxil fumarate/emtricitabine or tenofovir alafenamide/emtricitabine
- Elvitegravir/cobicistat/tenofovir alafenamide/emtricitabine
- Elvitegravir/cobicistat/tenofovir disoproxil fumarate/emtricitabine
- Raltegravir plus either tenofovir disoproxil fumarate/emtricitabine or tenofovir alafenamide/emtricitabine

PI-Based Regimens

- Darunavir/ritonavir plus either tenofovir disoproxil fumarate/emtricitabine or tenofovir alafenamide/emtricitabine

NRTIs were the first effective class of ARV drugs developed for HIV infection and are active against both HIV-1 and HIV-2. The nucleoside analogs work by incorporating themselves into elongating DNA strands of HIV during the viral replication cycle. Given their unique chemical structure, NRTIs cause a termination of the growing DNA strand immediately after incorporation. Because the resulting DNA strand is incomplete, it cannot contribute to the formation of a new viral particle. Drugs in this class and their common brand names and abbreviations include zidovudine (Retrovir; ZDV; AZT), lamivudine (Epivir; 3TC), didanosine (Videx; ddI), ddI-EC (Videx EC), zalcitabine (Hivid; ddC), stavudine (Zerit; d4T), Combivir (combination drug containing AZT and 3TC), abacavir (Ziagen; ABC), Epzicom (combination drug containing ABC and 3TC), Trizivir (combination drug containing ABC, 3TC, and AZT), emtricitabine (Emtriva; FTC), tenofovir disoproxil fumarate (Viread; TDF), tenofovir alafenamide (Vemlidy; TAF), Truvada (combination drug containing FTC and TDF), and Descovy (combination drug containing FTC and TAF).

NNRTIs are called nonnucleoside inhibitors because although they work at the same stage as nucleoside analogs, they have a different mechanism of action. NNRTIs

stop HIV-1 production by binding directly to the reverse transcriptase enzyme and preventing the transcription of viral DNA from RNA (i.e., the unique action of the HIV reverse transcriptase enzyme). The NNRTIs are generally effective in crossing the blood–brain barrier and may be useful in managing HIV-associated dementia. The drugs in this category include nevirapine (Viramune), delavirdine (Rescriptor), efavirenz (Sustiva), etravirine (Intelence), and rilpivirine (Edurant). Agents in this category are specific for the reverse transcriptase enzyme of HIV-1 and are ineffective against HIV-2 infection.

PIs work at the end of the viral replication cycle by restricting the action of the HIV protease enzyme, which processes viral parent proteins into smaller functional component proteins. Thus, PIs prevent the successful assembly and release of new HIV virions from infected CD4+ T cells. The development of this class of drugs gave rise to ART, as combination regimens containing three agents from two distinct ARV classes were shown to be effective in reducing HIV viral load to below the limit of detection of currently available viral load tests. The drugs in this category include saquinavir (Invirase; SQV), indinavir (Crixivan; IDV), ritonavir (Norvir; RTV), nelfinavir (Viracept; NFV), fosamprenavir (Lexiva; LXV; prodrug of amprenavir [Agenerase]), atazanavir (Reyataz; ATV), tipranavir (Aptivus; TPV), and Kaletra (lopinavir/ritonavir; LPV/r). PI drugs are typically given in conjunction with a PK enhancer (often called a "booster"), such as low-dose ritonavir or cobicistat. PK enhancers inhibit the metabolism of the therapeutic drug (the PI in this case), allowing for higher blood levels of the drug. PIs are active against both HIV-1 and HIV-2.

Fusion inhibitors work by stopping the virus from attaching to target cells. Enfuvirtide (Fuzeon; T-20) was the first FDA-approved drug in this category and, in contrast to other ARVs, is administered in adults via subcutaneous injection twice daily.

CCR5 antagonists prevent the binding of R5-tropic HIV strains to the cellular co-receptor CCR5. Maraviroc (Selzentry) was the first drug to be FDA-approved in this category. Of note, before initiating CCR5 antagonist therapy, a patient must undergo a test of viral tropism. Patients who are infected with X4 or dual tropic-viruses that bind to the cellular co-receptor CXCR4 should not be treated with a CCR5 antagonist. Given the cost of commercial tropism tests such as the Trofile Assay, this therapeutic option may be impractical in resource-limited settings.

INSTIs, also known as integrase inhibitors, directly inhibit the DNA strand transfer function of the HIV integrase enzyme, which allows incorporation of newly transcribed HIV DNA into the host cell genome. Inhibition of this critical step in the HIV replication cycle prevents the production of new HIV virions. INSTIs include raltegravir (Isentress), elvitegravir (Vitekta), dolutegravir (Tivicay), and bictegravir (available only in combination with tenofovir alafenamide and emtricitabine in Biktarvy). Of note, preliminary data from an observational surveillance study of birth outcomes among pregnant women receiving ARV drugs in Botswana suggest that dolutegravir exposure

---

Box 63.1 Viral Load Tests

- Viral load monitoring can establish the prognosis of a patient with HIV infection. Rising viral load indicates disease progression; falling viral load indicates a favorable prognostic trend.
- Plasma viral load may range from a few hundred virions (also called viral copies or viral equivalents) to more than a million per mL—a 10,000-fold range. Such large ranges are easiest to express in logarithmic (log) form.
- To express a number in logarithmic form, a base value is raised to a power. The latter exponent is the logarithm. The base 10 is commonly used in medicine without being explicitly specified; often, only the power (the exponent or log) of 10 is shown. For example, a viral load of 10,000 copies/mL is 10^4 copies/mL or

4 logs, while a viral load 10 times higher than that (100,000 copies/mL or 10^5 copies/mL) is 5 logs.
- Changes in viral load are commonly expressed in either numerical or logarithmic terms. For example, a twofold change is equal to approximately a 0.3 log change.
- In viral load measurements, the sum of laboratory variation (due to intrinsic variability in the test itself) and biological variation (due to variation in viral load concentration in the body) is generally assumed to be 0.3–0.5 log (twofold to three-fold). Therefore, only changes in viral load greater than this are considered to be clinically meaningful.

Type	Manufacturer	Name	HIV Detection Range
Polymerase chain reaction (PCR)	Roche Diagnostics	Amplicor HIV-1 Monitor Test 1.5	400–750,000 copies/mL
PCR	Roche Diagnostics	Amplicor HIV-1 Monitor Test 1.5 Ultra Sensitive	50–75,000 copies/mL
Branched DNA PCR	Chiron/Bayer	VERSANT HIV-1 RNA 3.0 Assay (bDNA)	<50–500,000 copies/mL
Nucleic acid sequence–based amplification	Organon Teknika	NucliSens HIV-1 QT	80–10,000 copies/mL

---

at the time of conception, but not later in pregnancy, may be associated with an increased risk of neural tube defects. Before prescribing an INSTI to an individual of childbearing potential, please refer to the *Guidelines for the Use of Antiretroviral Agents in HIV-1 Infected Adults and Adolescents Living With HIV* for updated information on this topic.

The most recent category of ARV drugs is the CD4-directed post-attachment HIV-1 inhibitor class. The only FDA-approved drug in this class is ibalizumab (Trogarzo), which is a monoclonal IgG4 antibody that binds to domain 2 of the human CD4 molecule, thereby interfering with the post-attachment steps that are required for HIV entry. Ibalizumab, in combination with other ARV drugs, is approved for the treatment of heavily treatment-experienced adults with multidrug resistant HIV-1 infection who are failing their current antiretroviral regimen.

In addition to the ARV agents described earlier, numerous combination products are now available for convenient dosing. Many of the regimens recommended by the Panel are available in a single pill as a once-daily oral regimen or as a two-pill once-daily regimen (e.g., Atripla containing efavirenz, emtricitabine, and tenofovir disoproxil fumarate; Stribild (Quad pill) containing elvitegravir, cobicistat, emtricitabine, and tenofovir disoproxil fumarate).

ARVs for Initial HIV-2 Infection

In contrast to HIV-1, far less is known about effective treatments against HIV-2. Given the slower progression

and decreased virulence of HIV-2 compared with HIV-1, treatment guidelines regarding when to initiate therapy for HIV-2 infection are less established. Treatment decisions regarding HIV-2 infection should be referred to an infectious disease specialist.

Management of Medication Side Effects and Drug–Drug Interactions

This section describes important side effects of several ARV drugs included in the preferred regimens for patients initiating ART. ARV drugs have the potential to cause more side effects than are described here, and clinicians should refer to the *Guidelines for the Use of Antiretroviral Agents in HIV-1 Infected Adults and Adolescents Living With HIV* and to the prescribing information in product labeling (package inserts) for both common and uncommon side effects to particular ARV drugs. In addition, the Guidelines include extensive tables describing the potential drug–drug interactions that may occur with ARVs. Providers should consider referral to HIV experts for HIV patients taking numerous other medications to avoid these interactions.

Abacavir has been associated with a serious hypersensitivity syndrome characterized by influenza-like symptoms, including fever, malaise, rash, myalgias, headache, nausea, vomiting, and diarrhea. This syndrome is not mediated by drug-specific IgE antibodies and is not considered an immediate hypersensitivity reaction, although it typically manifests within days of starting abacavir, requiring the medication to be stopped immediately. In addition, abacavir hypersensitivity syndrome may present with severe and life-threatening symptoms such as hypotension, particularly on drug re-exposure. Thus, abacavir should never be restarted in these patients. Genetic testing has revealed that the B*5701 allele of the human leukocyte antigen (HLA) gene complex has a strong association with this syndrome. Testing for this allele is indicated before starting abacavir, and presence of the allele is a contraindication for this drug.

Tenofovir disoproxil fumarate (TDF) has been associated with renal impairment and decreases in bone mineral density (BMD). TDF is a commonly prescribed ARV, as it is a component of some of the most widely used combination ARV products, such as Truvada and Atripla. Tenofovir alafenamide fumarate (TAF) is a prodrug of TDF that was approved by the FDA in 2015. Several combination products are now available with TAF, rather than TDF. Although TAF appears to be less likely to cause renal impairment and decreases in BMD, the FDA still recommends monitoring for both these adverse reactions. Patients on TDF or TAF should be monitored routinely with tests of creatinine clearance (calculated), serum phosphorus, and urine protein. For HIV-infected patients who have a history of pathologic bone fracture or who are at risk for osteopenia, BMD monitoring should be considered. Although the effect of supplementation with calcium and vitamin D has not been studied in this setting, supplementation may nonetheless be beneficial.

Designing a Compatible Medication Regimen

The patient's ability to adhere to a potent combination drug regimen (or drug "cocktail") must be discussed in detail before initiating therapy. Once a patient is started on drug therapy, there is a risk of developing drug resistance if viral suppression is not maintained through careful medication adherence. Viral mutations causing drug resistance can rapidly occur within 2 weeks to as little as 2 days of a patient stopping ARV medications or failing to take the full set of prescribed doses. ARVs have varying requirements regarding dosing, dietary restrictions, numbers of pills to be taken each day, and drug interactions. The clinician must prescribe an ART regimen that is compatible with the patient's day-to-day activities, including lifestyle choices, eating habits, social habits, and any limitations related to the patient's work and home environments.

Evidence-Based Nursing Practice 63.1 discusses an alternative methodology for the prediction of adherence to anti-HIV treatment. Effective treatment is fundamental to controlling the progression of HIV infection to AIDS, and helping a patient to live with HIV requires a multidisciplinary approach.

Assessment of Treatment Effectiveness

The goal of HIV therapy is to render the patient's HIV viral load so low that it cannot be measured by the test

 Evidence-Based Nursing Practice 63.1

Thompson IR, Bidgood P, Petróczi A, Denholm-Price JC, Fielder MD; EuResist Network Study Group. An alternative methodology for the prediction of adherence to anti-HIV treatment. *AIDS Res Ther.* 2009;6:9. http://www.aidsrestherapy.com/content/6/1/9.

Successful treatment of HIV-positive patients is fundamental to preventing the progression to AIDS. Treatment failure may be related to the development of drug resistance and/or insufficient drug levels in the blood. Severe side effects, coupled with the intense nature of many ARV drug regimens, can lead to treatment fatigue and consequently to periodic or permanent medication nonadherence. Although nonadherence is a recognized problem in HIV treatment, it is poorly detected in both clinical practice and health outcomes research and is often based on unreliable information such as self-reports, or in a clinical research setting, indirectly through Medication Events Monitoring System pill bottles or prescription refill rates. To meet the need for objective information on adherence, this study proposes a method using viral load and HIV genome sequence data to identify nonadherence among patients.

With nonadherence operationally defined as a sharp increase in viral load in the absence of drug resistance mutations, it was hypothesized that periods of nonadherence can be identified retrospectively based on the observed relationship between changes in viral load and HIV mutations. It was suggested that validation of the hypothesized approach would serve as a first step on the road to clinical practice. The information inferred from clinical data on adherence would be a crucial feature of treatment prediction tools to aid practitioners in daily clinical practice. In addition, distinguishing characteristics of biological markers routinely used to assess the progression of HIV disease may be identified in adherent and nonadherent groups. This latter approach would directly help clinicians to differentiate between nonresponding (albeit adherent) versus nonadherent patients.

being used (i.e., below the level of detection). Several commercial assays measure HIV viral load, varying in cost and sensitivity (i.e., with lower detection limits). At present, the standard commonly adopted in the United States is a lower detection limit of 20, 40, or 50 copies/mL, although less expensive assays with decreased sensitivity (detection limits of 400–500 copies/mL) are commonly used in developing countries, given resource limitations. Highly sensitive detection assays capable of measuring HIV viral load down to a single copy per milliliter have been developed for research purposes.

A baseline viral load is determined by taking two separate viral load tests approximately 2 to 3 weeks apart. If the results of the two tests are similar, a stable baseline is established and used to monitor the effects of drug therapy. The viral load should be repeated 4 to 6 weeks after the initiation of drug therapy or after any alteration in an ARV regimen is made. The initiation of ARV therapy should correspond with a decrease in viral load, typically by a factor of 10 after 2 to 4 weeks. Effective ART will often suppress viral load fully after 8 to 12 weeks of therapy.

Thus, if viral load is about the same or higher than the baseline level after initiating treatment, changes in the drug regimen or counseling regarding adherence are likely needed. It should be noted that reestablishment of complete suppression of the virus to below the detection limit of established viral load assays (e.g., HIV RNA less than 20, 40, or 50 copies/mL, depending on the assay) should remain the primary goal of ARV therapy. Once adequate viral suppression has been achieved, a viral load test should be repeated every 3 to 6 months to confirm chronic viral suppression.

CD4+ T-cell count is typically followed with similar frequency to assess for adequate immune reconstitution after initiating ART, although cellular immune reconstitution typically lags behind decreases in viral load, with an expected increase in CD4+ T cells of 100 to 150 cells/mL annually in adequately treated patients. Immunological nonresponders who fail to undergo adequate cellular immune reconstitution on ART, despite viral load suppression, remain at increased risk for opportunistic infection and may require alterations in their ARV regimen, as directed by an HIV specialist.

FOLLOW-UP AND REFERRAL

Follow-up for a patient infected with HIV will be required for the rest of the patient's life. In general, a primary-care practitioner should refer the patient to an HIV specialist. Often HIV specialists are trained in infectious diseases; however, many primary-care providers, nurse practitioners, and physician assistants are experienced and well trained in the care of the HIV-infected patient. Stable patients with suppressed viral loads and adequate CD4+ T-cell counts may be seen every 3 to 4 months for ongoing monitoring, provided medication adherence and social stability are apparent. However, the clinician caring for HIV-infected patients must always be vigilant for the need for rapid evaluation if patients develop intercurrent complaints that could signal breakthrough viral replication or other forms of disease progression.

For patients with CD4+ T-cell counts below 200 cells/mcL (see the following section, "Acquired Immunodeficiency Syndrome"), prophylactic medications against common opportunistic diseases, including pneumocystis pneumonia (PCP) and mycobacterial infections, may be necessary. In addition, concurrent chronic viral infections, such as hepatitis B or hepatitis C, require specialty referral to an appropriate clinical specialist (such as a hepatologist) because these infections are typically more aggressive with a worse prognosis in the HIV-infected patient.

Recent studies have demonstrated that, in the era of effective ART, HIV-infected patients are at high risk of morbidly and mortality from non-AIDS conditions, such as cardiovascular disease, diabetes mellitus, or liver disease. The prevention and treatment of many of these chronic diseases that are also seen in the general population are now a large focus of HIV management. Tobacco, alcohol, and drug use should be discouraged, and a healthy diet and exercise should be encouraged.

Health maintenance of the HIV-infected patient also requires close attention to preventive immunizations, which may include pneumococcal vaccine (23-valent polysaccharide vaccine; Pneumovax) that may be re-administered after 5 years, annual influenza vaccination, tetanus toxoid boosters every 10 years, human papillomavirus (HPV) vaccine, and vaccination for both hepatitis A (two vaccinations spaced 6 months apart) and hepatitis B (three vaccinations spaced 1 and 6 months apart). Importantly, attenuated live virus vaccines including measles, mumps, rubella (MMR), oral polio virus (OPV), bacillus Calmette-Guérin anti-TB vaccine (BCG), intranasal influenza vaccine, and those for varicella (chickenpox) and yellow fever are contraindicated in HIV-infected patients with advanced disease and significant immunosuppression. However, the MMR and varicella vaccines may be given early in the course of the disease to non-immunosuppressed HIV-infected individuals.

Patient Education: Human Immunodeficiency Virus Infection

HIV infection is a chronic lifelong disease. Education may facilitate self-care activities that can decrease the risk of superinfection with other HIV strains, hepatitis viruses, and opportunistic pathogens. The HIV-infected patient requires extensive personalized education for his or her specific medical conditions and therapeutic ART regimen, including specific drug contraindications and interaction warnings. It is also critical to provide adequate support to facilitate adherence to what may be a demanding ART regimen.

Likewise, the patient will need continual reinforcement and education on the need to attain and maintain effective HIV transmission prevention behaviors, such as safer sex practices (e.g., barrier protection, a single exclusive sexual partner) to decrease the potential of transmitting HIV to others or acquiring new HIV strains. A wide variety of patient education materials are available from pharmaceutical companies, AIDS support organizations, and government and health-care agencies (see Resources at the end of this chapter). Educational programs for clinicians are also available through the Association of Nurses in AIDS Care (ANAC) at 1-800-260-6780.

ACQUIRED IMMUNODEFICIENCY SYNDROME

A person with HIV is classified as having progressed from HIV infection to AIDs if the CD4+ T-cell count falls below 200 cells/mcL or he or she develops an opportunistic infection or other AIDS-defining illness.

EPIDEMIOLOGY AND CAUSES

Despite the availability of sensitive and specific HIV testing and numerous effective ART options, more than 18,000 people were diagnosed with AIDS in the United States in 2015 and more than 6,000 people died as a result of HIV disease. Worldwide, one million people died due to AIDS, including more than 120,000 children.

PATHOPHYSIOLOGY

HIV is well recognized for its lengthy latency period after acute infection, in which infected persons remain relatively asymptomatic in the absence of ART, despite persistent low-level viremia and progressive $CD4^+$ T-cell destruction (approximately 40–80 $CD4^+$ T cells/mcL per year in untreated patients). Over a period of months or years, however, the replication activities of the virus supersede the capacity for $CD4^+$ T-cell regeneration, except in rare cases. As the $CD4^+$ T-cell count declines, patients become increasingly susceptible to opportunistic infections and malignancies.

The natural history of HIV infection can vary significantly from one patient to another. Thus, it is impossible to predict precisely when HIV will progress to AIDS in a person infected with HIV without treatment. Studies conducted in the 1980s to the mid-1990s, before the availability of effective ART, indicated the usual survival time after the diagnosis of AIDS was just 3 years. It is clear, however, that effective ART has dramatically improved the survival and quality of life for many HIV-infected persons, including those with AIDS.

CLINICAL PRESENTATION

Subjective

Patients with AIDS may present with a variety of viral, bacterial, fungal, and/or protozoal opportunistic infections. Common viral infections include CMV, herpes simplex virus, varicella zoster virus, and progressive multifocal leukoencephalopathy (PML, which is caused by infection with the John Cunningham or JC virus). Common bacterial infections include *Mycobacterium avium* complex (MAC, which is caused by *M. avium* and *Mycobacterium intracellulare*) and tuberculosis. Common fungal infections include candidiasis, PCP, histoplasmosis *(Histoplasma capsulatum)*, and cryptococcosis *(Cryptococcus neoformans)*. Common protozoal infections include cryptosporidiosis, which causes chronic diarrhea, and cerebral toxoplasmosis (*T. gondii* infection of the CNS), which can be life-threatening. Other potential problems include malignancies such as Hodgkin's and non-Hodgkin's lymphoma and AIDS wasting syndrome.

In assessing the patient with AIDS, it is important to realize these patients may have more than one, and sometimes several, active opportunistic infections. Therefore, a careful history, thorough review of systems, physical examination, and frequent follow-up assessments are extremely important. Advanced Assessment 63.1 provides a framework for the evaluation of an HIV-infected patient with advanced disease.

The patient may complain of visual problems, such as a loss of central or peripheral vision, blurring of vision, loss of visual acuity, eye pain, photophobia, or the development of "floaters." Such complaints should raise

Advanced Assessment 63.1: HIV-positive Individual

HISTORY	
Present Illness	When were you diagnosed with HIV? Why did you take the HIV test? Why did you come to the doctor today? How are you feeling physically? How are you feeling emotionally?
Past Medical History	Have you been to a health-care provider for HIV care? Do you know what your viral load is? What your $CD4^+$ T-cell count is? When were these tests last done? Have you had any opportunistic infections, such as PCP or thrush? Were you ever hospitalized for these infections? What is your past medical history? Surgical history? Are you using any nontraditional (alternative or complementary) therapies? If so, please explain. Have you ever had heart problems or a history of high cholesterol?
Social Support History	What is your living situation (e.g., home life, support system [friends, relatives], financial situation, emotional situation, occupational situation, sexual relationships)? What do you know about HIV infection? Are you sexually active? Do you know how to prevent the spread of HIV from one person to another? If so, do you use those methods?

✤ Advanced Assessment 63.1: HIV-positive Individual—cont'd

Medication History	What HIV drugs have you taken in the past? How long were you on them? How long have you been off them? Have you been taking any medications for prophylaxis? Do you take them all of the time or just some of the time? What other medications are you taking (prescription, over-the-counter drugs, herbal remedies)?
Nutritional History	Tell me about your usual diet. Do you eat raw eggs or raw fish? How do you cook your meat? Do you take any appetite enhancers? Do you take any nutritional supplements?
Travel History	Do you travel often? If so, where? Have you traveled or lived in other states or out of the country? If so, when, where, and for how long?

PHYSICAL EXAMINATION

General Overview and Mental Status	Level of consciousness Confusion Difficulty in remembering Change in mental status or mood Fatigue Change in activities of daily living
Neurological System	Headaches and associated signs and symptoms Neurological examination; cranial nerve examination
Respiratory System	Shortness of breath or dyspnea and associated signs and symptoms Cough and associated signs and symptoms Hiccups Lung sounds Respiratory rate, rhythm, characteristics; use of accessory muscles
Cardiovascular System	Heart sounds Pulse rate, rhythm, characteristics
Hematological and Lymphatic System	Swollen, enlarged, or tender glands Fever
Gastrointestinal System and Nutrition	Sores or white spots in the mouth or lips; dental assessment Problems eating or swallowing Nausea/vomiting Change in weight or appetite Change in bowel habits (diarrhea, constipation) Nutritional intake Anorectal symptoms, lesions, masses, or warts
Dermatologic	Active rash, evidence of previous rashes (herpes zoster) Kaposi's sarcoma
Genitourinary	Abnormal Pap smear Condyloma acuminata Signs or symptoms of other sexually transmitted infections (e.g., discharge, dysuria, pruritus, rash)

suspicion for CMV retinitis or fungal endophthalmitis (ocular histoplasmosis).

Neurological symptoms or alterations in mental status, including headaches, confusion, mood swings, personality changes, dizziness, neck stiffness, fever, lethargy, malaise, nausea, vomiting, photophobia (intolerance of light due to resulting eye pain), neurological deficits,

hemiparesis, ataxia, cranial nerve palsies, or seizures may be the result of herpes encephalopathy, PML, cryptococcal meningitis, or cerebral toxoplasmosis.

GI problems such as diarrhea and abdominal pain may be present concurrently with unintentional weight loss, fever, chills, or night sweats, as a result of CMV enterocolitis, viral gastroenteritis, pancreatitis, AIDS wasting syndrome, MAC, *Salmonella* or other enteric bacterial infection, cryptosporidiosis, giardiasis, isosporiasis, or histoplasmosis. Dermatological problems may develop, such as stinging or burning papules or bumpy rashes in a linear or clustered pattern, which may be indicative of herpes simplex or HPV infection, particularly if located in the anogenital region. Other painless lesions, such as the purplish plaques of Kaposi's sarcoma, may go unnoticed in areas poorly visible to the patient (e.g., the back).

The patient may also complain of pulmonary symptoms, such as shortness of breath or a persistent cough. These symptoms may be accompanied by fever, chills, night sweats, weight loss, purulent or blood-tinged sputum, or chest pain, which may be indicative of PCP, bacterial pneumonia, or active TB. The clinician should determine the onset of pulmonary symptoms, because PCP and TB are usually insidious in presentation, with worsening of symptoms over days to weeks, whereas pulmonary toxoplasmosis progresses more rapidly. In addition, nonspecific complaints of fatigue, weakness, and fever with anemia and leukopenia could signify disseminated MAC with bone marrow involvement.

Objective

A complete physical examination is indicated for the patient with AIDS because an array of opportunistic infections and malignancies may affect literally any organ system. Some of the most common physical presentations of AIDS are described in this section by organ system.

With CMV retinitis, retinal changes are seen on ophthalmoscopic examination. With toxoplasmosis encephalitis (the most common presentation of *Toxoplasma* infection), the clinician should check for altered level of consciousness, impaired cognition, and any stroke-like symptoms. Of note, the physical examination findings of cryptococcal meningitis are typically not as striking as the fulminant meningitic symptoms of bacterial meningitis.

Oropharyngeal examination may reveal erythematous mucosal ulcers, which should raise suspicion for herpes simplex or CMV, or if patchy white lesions are present, candidiasis or EBV-associated oral hairy leukoplakia, which is typically limited to the tongue, gingivae, and/ or buccal mucosa.

A wide variety of skin lesions may present with AIDS. Herpes simplex lesions are initially papulovesicular (fluid-filled), painful, and pruritic; these clustered lesions become progressively erythematous and ulcerated, eventually crusting over before healing. The lesions of shingles are exquisitely painful papules and vesicles, which present with a burning sensation and are distributed over a well-demarcated region of the skin known as a dermatome, corresponding to the cutaneous area innervated by a single spinal nerve. Genital warts associated with HPV infection (condyloma acuminata) appear as raised, flesh-colored papules, with or without stalks, in isolation or in clusters. Cutaneous Kaposi's sarcoma presents with

one or more raised, dark-colored lesions that may occur anywhere on the body, whereas cutaneous cryptococcosis usually presents as a single ulcerated nodule at the site of infection. Papular pruritic eruption (PPE) of HIV is a highly pruritic rash that presents as widespread papular to nodular skin lesions; as a diagnosis of exclusion, the etiology of PPE is unclear but has been suggested to be due to a dysregulated immune response to arthropod bites because it often improves after initiating ART. Eosinophilic folliculitis is an overlapping diagnosis with PPE in which biopsy confirms perifollicular eosinophilic infiltration that has been suggested to be of autoimmune etiology.

Findings on pulmonary examination may be nonspecific in the setting of a wide variety of infectious processes, such as PCP, TB, or community-acquired pneumonia. Therefore, physical examination findings should be considered within the context of a careful medical history detailing clinical presentation and timing of symptom onset, along with appropriate diagnostic imaging and laboratory studies. Advanced Assessment 63.1 presents additional history and physical examination information to be gathered from the HIV-positive patient.

DIAGNOSTIC REASONING

Diagnostic Tests

Table 63.4 includes some of the diagnostic tests a provider should consider in evaluating an HIV-infected patient with AIDS, including CD4+ T-cell count and HIV viral load, as well as additional laboratory tests to perform and how to interpret them, as guided by the patient's presenting signs and symptoms.

For patients with suspected TB or PCP, the clinician should order a purified protein derivative, chest x-ray, and sputum examination for smear and culture or a molecular test for TB screening if available. Tests for acid-fast bacilli (AFB) are done for TB, and a silver stain or direct fluorescent antibody (DFA) test will detect fungal forms in PCP. PCR tests are becoming increasingly available and can be helpful. In addition to sputa, bronchoalveolar lavage fluid (from bronchoscopy) may be examined, as well as specific blood cultures.

For patients with neurological symptoms, a referring physician should order a computed tomography scan or magnetic resonance imaging of the brain to check for the presence of ring-enhancing lesions, which could be associated with *T. gondii* or CNS lymphoma, or nonenhancing areas of white matter (demyelination), which could indicate PML. A lumbar puncture may be indicated.

If diarrhea is present, with or without other GI symptoms, the clinician should send stool cultures for infectious organisms, including examination for protozoal forms, ova, and parasites. Viral infections such as CMV colitis may require colonoscopic biopsy of the GI mucosa for a definitive diagnosis.

TABLE 63.4   Diagnostic Tests for the HIV-Infected Patient With AIDS

Test	Interpreting the Results
CD4+ T-cell count	<200 cells/mcL or <14%: Prophylaxis for PCP <100 cells/mcL or <14%: Prophylaxis for toxoplasmosis (often the same as PCP prophylaxis) <50 cells/mcL or <14%: Prophylaxis for *Mycobacterium avium* complex (MAC) CD4+ T-cell counts may also help narrow or broaden the differential diagnosis of a presenting complaint because some opportunistic infections (OIs) are rare at higher CD4+ T-cell counts.
HIV viral load	An increase in viral load while on ART indicates poor adherence, poor absorption, and/or emergence of drug resistance mutations.
Genotypic resistance testing	If a change in regimen is required, viral resistance testing will guide the choice of components in the next ART regimen. Viral amplification for resistance testing may not always be possible for patients who have HIV RNA levels <500 to 1,000 copies/mL.
Tropism testing (if considering treatment with CCR5 antagonist)	Patients who are infected with X4 or dual-tropic viruses should not be treated with a CCR5 antagonist. Tropism can change over time in the same individual; therefore, this test may need to be repeated if significant time has elapsed since the last test.
HLA-B*5701 testing (if considering treatment with abacavir)	Abacavir and abacavir-containing regimens should not be prescribed in patients who are positive for HLA-B*5701 or in whom testing has not been performed, given the increased risk of abacavir hypersensitivity.
Hepatitis A, B, and C serologies	HBV coinfection is an important factor to consider in selecting an ART regimen and, subsequently, in withdrawing or changing ARV components. Several ARV drugs (e.g., emtricitabine, lamivudine, tenofovir disoproxil fumarate, and tenofovir alafenamide) have activity against HBV, and HBV-infected patients are at risk for an HBV flare after withdrawal of these ARV drugs.
Complete blood count with differential	Anemia is common; may be related to HIV disease, underlying infection, or medication (particularly zidovudine [AZT]). Bone marrow biopsy may be done to check for fungi, *M. avium* or tuberculosis, CMV, parvovirus, or malignancy. Thrombocytopenia is often seen. In early infection, idiopathic thrombocytopenia purpura may be seen; in later infection, thrombocytopenia may be because of bone marrow suppression. Thrombocytopenia may also be seen with Kaposi's sarcoma. Leukopenia is common; WBC counts less than 2,000 cells/mcL are common and, in isolation, are not cause for alarm. If using medications that cause neutropenia, may need to prescribe colony-stimulating factors such as filgrastim (Neupogen).
Basic serum chemistry	Renal function may be impaired because of HIV nephropathy, ARV drugs, dehydration, or volume depletion from diarrhea, or wasting. Electrolytes may need repletion due to diarrhea or malnutrition. Low phosphorus may indicate Fanconi Syndrome, due to tenofovir-containing regimens.
Liver-associated chemistries	Liver associated enzymes (AST, ALT, alkaline phosphatase) may be elevated as a result of HBV or HCV coinfection, medications, alcohol abuse, or nonalcoholic fatty liver disease (NAFLD), which is common in HIV-infected patients. Elevations in bilirubin may indicate disseminated MAC infection. Bilirubin may also become elevated after starting certain ARV drugs (atazanavir). Elevated lactate dehydrogenase (LDH) may be nonspecific or related to PCP, lymphoma, hemolysis, muscle wasting, or may be caused by HIV or AZT. Low albumin levels may indicate malnutrition.
Interferon-gamma release assay or purified protein derivative, tuberculin skin test (TST)	A positive interferon-gamma assay result or TST induration of 5 mm or more is considered a positive reaction (no reaction may be due to anergy); evaluate for signs/symptoms of active TB with physical examination and chest x-ray.
Urinalysis	Patients infected with HIV are at risk of renal disease both from HIV and from some ARV drugs (e.g., tenofovir).

Differential Diagnosis

The differential diagnoses for AIDS-associated illnesses are extensive, particularly with regard to pulmonary, neurological, and GI manifestations, and are geared toward identifying underlying disease processes and infections. In the pulmonary differential, the clinician should consider TB, PCP, MAC, histoplasmosis, or other bacterial, viral, fungal, or protozoal infections of the pulmonary system, as well as internal Kaposi's sarcoma affecting the lungs. Regarding the neurological system, the clinician should consider CNS lymphoma or other malignancy, in addition to the cerebral infections discussed earlier of toxoplasmosis and PML. In the GI system, CMV must be considered, as well as protozoal infections (e.g., cryptosporidiosis, isosporiasis, giardiasis) and malabsorption syndromes. Pancytopenia should raise suspicion of disseminated MAC infection in the bone marrow.

MANAGEMENT

The overall focus of HIV management is to help the patient maintain HIV viral suppression, thereby improving the immune system and preventing AIDS-defining illness and improving quality of life. Providing support for ART adherence is essential to that goal.

However, opportunistic infections still affect a substantial number of HIV patients, even in resource-abundant settings, given factors such as therapeutic nonadherence, barriers to health-care accessibility, and comorbid medical conditions that interfere with effective HIV treatment. Thus, correctly identifying the causative organism of a presenting opportunistic infection is crucial to initiating appropriate treatment in a timely fashion. Because CD4+ T-cell count serves as the major clinical indicator of immunocompetence in HIV-infected individuals, when CD4+ T-cell count falls below 200 cells/mcL, the HIV-positive patient becomes increasingly prone to opportunistic infections. PCP prophylaxis is required for CD4+ T-cell counts of less than 200 cells/mcL, *T. gondii* prophylaxis for counts less than 100 cells/mcL, and MAC prophylaxis for counts less than 50 cells/mcL.

Candidiasis

The diagnosis of oral candidiasis can generally be made clinically without laboratory testing. Oral candidiasis can be treated with fluconazole 100 mg/day for 1 to 2 weeks. Esophagitis can be treated similarly, except with a 3-week duration.

Chronic Diarrhea

Patients with AIDS are at risk of many opportunistic infections associated with diarrhea. Work-up should include stool for ova and parasites (cryptosporidiosis, isosporiasis, giardiasis, strongyloides), stool culture, and testing for *Clostridium difficile*. For diarrhea that persists and for which a diagnosis is not made, CMV colitis (discussed subsequently) should be considered. Colonoscopy with biopsy may be necessary.

Cytomegalovirus

CMV viremia is common in HIV-infected patients and should not be treated in the absence of end-organ disease, which may include colitis, pneumonitis, or sight-threatening retinitis. The diagnosis of CMV end-organ disease generally requires a tissue biopsy or, in the case of eye disease, ophthalmologic consultation. Ganciclovir (Cytovene) may be given at 5 mg/kg IV every 12 hours for 14 days or foscarnet (Foscavir) 90 mg/kg IV every 12 hours for 14 days. The dose of either drug should be reduced in patients with renal failure. Valganciclovir is an oral formulation of the drug ganciclovir and is now used frequently when a patient's disease is managed in the outpatient setting. Valganciclovir is used at 900 mg by mouth (PO) every 12 hours for induction therapy and 900 mg PO once daily for maintenance therapy. In addition, cidofovir (Vistide) 5 mg/kg IV may be given with probenecid (Benemid) for 1 week, then reduced to every 2 weeks. Cidofovir should not be used in patients with renal insufficiency. Also, a combination of foscarnet/ganciclovir, or intravitreal injections or implants of ganciclovir (which treat only the affected area) may be tried. For maintenance, ganciclovir 5 mg/kg IV daily or foscarnet 90 to 120 mg/kg IV daily may be given.

Cryptococcosis

For acute treatment of *Cryptococcus neoformans* infection, amphotericin B deoxycholate (Fungizone) 0.7 to 1.0 mg/kg IV daily for 14 days with or without 5-flucytosine 100 mg/kg PO divided four times daily and then fluconazole 400 mg daily or itraconazole 200 mg PO two times daily for 8 weeks is used. In milder cases, fluconazole 400 to 800 mg daily for 8 to 12 weeks may be used, although inadequate treatment may lead to antifungal resistance. CNS infection (cryptococcal meningitis) should be treated with an initial period of IV induction therapy. Serum cryptococcal antigen titers should be followed, as well as CSF titers if applicable, to evaluate response to therapy. Secondary antifungal prophylaxis with fluconazole 200 mg PO daily is typically continued for life or until the CD4+ T-cell count is greater than or equal to 200 cells/mcL for at least 6 months.

Cryptosporidiosis

There is no effective treatment for *Cryptosporidium* infection other than immune reconstitution with continued ART. In severe cases, nitazoxanide 500 to 1,000 mg PO two times daily given with food for 14 days may help to clear the infection.

Herpes Simplex

For treatment of acute herpes simplex virus manifestations, the clinician should prescribe acyclovir 200 to 400 mg PO three times daily for 7 to 10 days, famciclovir 250 mg PO three times daily, or valaciclovir (Valtrex) 1 g PO two times daily for 7 to 10 days. For suppressive treatment, acyclovir 400 mg PO two times daily for 3 to 7 days per week should be given. Foscarnet 40 mg/kg IV every 8 hours for 10 days can be used for acyclovir-resistant herpes.

Herpes Zoster

Herpes zoster (varicella zoster virus, shingles) should be treated with acyclovir (Zovirax) 800 mg PO five times daily for 7 to 10 days or famciclovir (Famvir) 500 mg PO three times daily for 7 days plus topical silver sulfadiazine for skin lesions. In severe cases, the patient may require IV acyclovir (10 mg/kg per dose) every 8 hours. Valaciclovir (Valtrex), a prodrug of acyclovir, may also be used at 1 g PO every 8 hours for 7 days; although more expensive than acyclovir, its simplified dosing regimen may result in greater adherence.

Histoplasmosis

Primary prophylaxis with itraconazole 200 mg PO daily is indicated for patients with CD4+ T cell counts less than 150 cells/mcL who live in endemic areas. Disseminated *Histoplasma capsulatum* infection is treated with a 2-week induction period of liposomal amphotericin B 3 mg/kg IV daily (5 mg/kg for meningitis), followed by itraconazole 200 mg PO three times daily for 3 days and then two times daily for at least 1 year. Secondary prophylaxis with itraconazole 200 mg PO daily, initiated after resolution of initial histoplasmosis infection, is often continued for life.

Kaposi's Sarcoma (Human Herpesvirus-8)

Although Kaposi's sarcoma has been associated with underlying HHV-8 infection, herpes-specific antiviral therapies are not utilized in current treatment regimens. Rather, cutaneous Kaposi's sarcoma typically improves on ART, as HIV viral load is suppressed and immune status improves. However, disseminated disease may require more aggressive treatment, particularly if any internal organs are affected. Local treatment consists of cryotherapy, excision, intralesional vinblastine, or radiation. Systemic chemotherapy for more severe disease may include vinblastine, vincristine, doxorubicin, liposomal doxorubicin, liposomal daunorubicin, bleomycin, or paclitaxel. For more severe cases requiring chemotherapy, treatment is typically guided by a qualified oncology specialist.

Mycobacterium avium Complex

For acute treatment, at least two drugs should be used for initial therapy with clarithromycin 500 mg PO twice daily or plus ethambutol 15 mg/kg PO per day OR azithromycin 500 to 600 mg PO daily plus ethambutol 15 mg/kg PO per day. The duration of treatment is at least 12 months and should not be discontinued unless signs and symptoms of MAC have resolved and CD4+ T-cell count is greater than 100 cells/mcL in response to ART.

Mycobacterium tuberculosis

Most public health departments manage or co-manage the treatment of active TB infection. Several ARV drugs are contraindicated or require dosage adjustments when coadministered with TB medications capable of affecting the cytochrome p450 enzymatic pathway, such as rifampin and rifapentine. Thus, it is critical to review current guidelines for each HIV drug the patient is prescribed using a frequently updated resource such as AIDSinfo (www.aidsinfo.nih.gov), the official Web site sponsored by the National Institutes of Health, which posts national treatment and prevention guidelines for HIV infection.

To reduce the risk of secondary reactivation TB, patients with latent TB infection (LTBI) diagnosed by a positive tuberculin skin test greater than or equal to 5 mm or a positive interferon-gamma release assay in the absence of active pulmonary disease (i.e., negative radiological imaging, absence of clinical signs and symptoms) should take isonicotinoylhydrazine (INH; Isoniazid, Laniazid) 300 mg daily with pyridoxine 500 mg PO daily for 9 months. LTBI treatment with rifapentine is contraindicated for patients on PIs and most NNRTIs.

For active TB infection, patients should be started on INH 300 mg daily plus rifampin 600 mg plus pyrazinamide 15 to 30 mg/kg daily plus either ethambutol (Myambutol) 15 mg/kg daily or streptomycin 15 mg/kg intramuscularly daily (maximum 1 g). ARV regimens should be modified to avoid potentially dangerous drug interactions between certain agents, such as rifampin and PIs/NNRTIs. Rifabutin may be used as an alternative to rifampin, given its improved drug interaction profile. Patients on pyrazinamide should undergo regular serum uric acid monitoring, whereas ethambutol use requires periodic visual acuity and red-green color perception testing, given risks of ocular toxicity. Pyrazinamide and ethambutol may be discontinued after 2 months to minimize toxicity, if supported by TB susceptibility testing. Thus, it is critical to send sputum AFB cultures as soon as possible. Combination treatment for active TB infection should be continued for at least 6 months after conversion to negative sputum cultures.

Oral Hairy Leukoplakia (Epstein-Barr Virus Infection)

These common oral lesions found mainly on the tongue typically improve after the initiation of effective ART.

Pneumocystis jiroveci Pneumonia

There are several options for prophylaxis of PCP at CD4+ T-cell counts of less than 200 cells/mcL. The first is trimethoprim-sulfamethoxazole (TMP/SMX, Bactrim, Septra), one double-strength (DS) tablet daily or three times per week. Prophylaxis may be better tolerated when begun with small doses leading to incremental increases, such as TMP/SMX suspension 1 mL PO daily for 3 days, then 2 mL PO daily for 3 days, then 5 mL PO daily for 3 days, then 10 mL PO daily for 3 days, then 20 mL PO daily for 3 days, and then 1 DS TMP/SMX tablet daily.

Between 10% and 40% of all patients on this oral course will develop an allergic reaction with fever and a pruritic morbilliform rash and will have to stop treatment. However, this reaction is typically not IgE mediated, nor is it considered an immediate hypersensitivity reaction. It may be mediated by an allergic reaction to the sulfa moiety, particularly in individuals of the slow acetylation phenotype who metabolize sulfonamides at slower rates. Given the effectiveness of TMP/SMX for PCP prophylaxis, rechallenge with TMP/SMX may be attempted at a later date.

Dapsone (Avlosulfon) 100 mg PO daily, inhaled nebulized pentamidine (NebuPent) 300 mg every month, or atovaquone (Mepron) 1,500 mg PO daily can also be used for PCP prophylaxis, although these regimens are not as effective as TMP/SMX prophylaxis. PCP prophylaxis may be stopped if CD4+ T-cell counts increase above 200 cells/mcL for more than 3 months.

For the treatment of mild to moderate PCP, the clinician may prescribe TMP/SMX at 15 mg TMP/kg total daily dose, divided three times daily PO or IV. A typical adult dose is 2 DS tablets of TMP/SMX PO every 8 hours. Other treatments include pentamidine 4 mg/kg daily IV; dapsone 100 mg daily (check glucose-6-phosphate dehydrogenase level before dosing, given the risk of anemia) plus TMP 15 mg/kg total daily dose, divided three times daily; clindamycin 600 mg PO or IV three times daily plus primaquine 30 mg daily; atovaquone (Mepron) 750 mg PO two times daily with meals plus pyrimethamine (Fansidar) 50 to 75 mg PO daily; or trimetrexate (Neutrexin) plus dapsone plus leucovorin (folinic acid; Wellcovorin), with continuation of therapy for 3 weeks before switching to maintenance therapy.

Patients with acute PCP who develop respiratory distress will require hospitalization. If patients develop hypoxia as documented on a room air arterial blood gas with a Pao$_2$ of less than 70 mm Hg or an arterial-alveolar O$_2$ gradient greater than 35 mm Hg, patients should also be started on corticosteroids (prednisone 40 mg PO 2 times daily for 5 days, then 40 mg PO daily for 5 days, then 20 mg PO daily for 11 days—all doses given 30 minutes before TMP/SMX dosing) to reduce pulmonary inflammation associated with PCP.

Progressive Multifocal Leukoencephalopathy

There is no treatment for this progressively deteriorating disease caused by JC virus infection of the CNS. Some patients improve on ARV therapy for the underlying HIV infection, which adequately suppresses HIV viral load. In advanced or progressively deteriorating cases, however, the clinician and referring physician should consider discussing hospice care with the patient, family, or significant others, because the prognosis is nearly uniformly fatal.

Toxoplasmosis

Prophylaxis against *T. gondii* at CD4+ T cell counts of less than 100 cells/mcL, TMP/SMX is 1 DS tablet PO daily or three times per week or dapsone 50 mg PO daily plus pyrimethamine 50 mg PO every week with folinic acid (Wellcovorin) 25 mg PO per week. Prophylaxis may be stopped if CD4+ T cell counts increase above 200 cells/mcL for more than 3 months.

For acute treatment, pyrimethamine 75 to 100 mg PO daily plus folinic acid 10 to 20 mg PO daily plus either sulfadiazine 1 to 1.5 g PO four times daily or clindamycin 600 to 900 mg PO four times daily for 6 to 8 weeks is used. Maintenance suppressive therapy is pyrimethamine 25 to 50 mg PO daily plus either sulfadiazine 1 g PO twice daily or clindamycin 300 to 450 mg PO four times daily.

FOLLOW-UP AND REFERRAL

Clinical status, medication adherence, and the availability of social supports all determine how often the patient will need follow-up appointments. Follow-up visits should be more frequent at the time of initiation of ART or any new medications to assess for response to therapy, as well as drug tolerance. A CD4+ T-cell count should be obtained every 3 to 6 months. HIV viral load should be determined when initiating or switching ARV regimens, and a follow-up viral load must be done in 2 to 8 weeks to determine effectiveness of the medication regimen; viral load should fall by at least a factor of 10 after 2 weeks of ART. Resistance testing should be considered if a therapeutic response is not noted with ART or HIV viral rebound occurs despite adequate medication adherence. In stable patients, HIV viral load may be checked every 3 to 4 months. The goal of ART should be complete viral suppression to below the limit of detection on standardized commercial HIV viral load assays.

Specialty referrals are unique to each patient and are guided by HIV-related complications, such as opportunistic infections and malignancies, which develop in the immunosuppressed individual. For example, in addition to periodic visits to an infectious disease or HIV specialist, a referral should be made to an ophthalmologist whenever the patient complains of visual problems, whereas unresolved diarrhea or GI problems may require referral to a gastroenterologist. Similarly, an oncology referral may be necessary for patients with Kaposi's sarcoma or if there is a suspicion of malignancy.

Patient Education: Acquired Immunodeficiency Syndrome

Patient education is an ongoing process and does not end with counseling after the initial diagnosis. Patient-centered education should include an ongoing review of health maintenance and HIV transmission prevention behaviors because sexual abstinence should not be assumed for any patient, regardless of HIV status. Patient education is particularly important regarding the early detection of visual problems. Other healthful behaviors, such as smoking cessation and limiting alcohol intake, should be discussed within the larger context of HIV infection, given the increased morbidity and mortality risk imparted by these behaviors.

The clinician should also work with the patient to convey the risks of drug interactions, given the complicated nature of ARV metabolism and both prophylactic and treatment regimens for opportunistic infections. Because blood levels of ARV medications may be increased or decreased by several other common medications, the patient must understand the need to discuss any other medications being taken simultaneously. In addition, a thorough understanding of self-care practices to avoid opportunistic infections is critical.

Because AIDS has taken on a "female face" over the past decade, as an increasing number of women have become affected, the need for women to use effective contraception and infection prevention methods has taken on a new urgency in recent years. Women with HIV should have regular age-based cervical cancer screening. If abnormalities are present, they tend to be more severe and progress more rapidly in HIV-infected women.

All patients should be encouraged to complete advance directives early in the course of HIV infection. If the clinician broaches this topic at a later stage of the disease (i.e., after a patient has developed AIDS), the patient may mistakenly assume that the clinician has additional information regarding his or her prognosis of which the patient is unaware. Thus, lines of communication need to be kept open between the clinician, the patient, significant others, and family members, depending of the extent of diagnosis disclosure by the patient.

REFERENCES

HIV and AIDS

American College of Obstetricians and Gynecologists' Committee on Practice Bulletins–Gynecology. Practice bulletin no. 167: Gynecologic care for women and adolescents with human immunodeficiency virus. *Obstet Gynecol.*

Centers for Disease Control and Prevention. Update to interim guidance for preexposure prophylaxis (PrEP) for the prevention of HIV Infection: PrEP for injecting drug users. MMWR Morb Mortal Wkly Rep. 2013;62:463–465.

Centers for Disease Control and Prevention. Laboratory testing for the diagnosis of HIV infection: Updated recommendations. https://stacks.cdc.gov/view/cdc/23447. Published June 27, 2014. Accessed October 6, 2017.

Centers for Disease Control and Prevention. HIV surveillance report, 2015;27. http://www.cdc.gov/hiv/library/reports/hiv-surveillance.html. Published November 2016. Accessed October 6, 2017.

Centers for Disease Control and Prevention. Updated guidelines for antiretroviral postexposure prophylaxis after sexual, injection drug use, or other nonoccupational exposure to HIV—United States, 2016. *MMWR Morb Mortal Wkly Rep.* 2016;65:458.

Insight Start Study Group, Lundgren JD, Babiker AG, et al. Initiation of antiretroviral therapy in early asymptomatic HIV infection. *N Engl J Med.* 2015;373:795–807.

Lifson AR, Grund B, Gardner EM, et al. Improved quality of life with immediate versus deferred initiation of antiretroviral therapy in early asymptomatic HIV infection. *AIDS.* 2017;31:953–963.

Kuhar DT, Henderson DK, Struble KA, et al. Updated U.S. Public Health Service guidelines for the management of occupational exposures to human immunodeficiency virus and recommendations for postexposure prophylaxis. *Infect Control Hosp Epidemiol.* 2013;34(9):875–892.

Masur H, Brooks JT, Benson CA, et al. Prevention and treatment of opportunistic infections in HIV-infected adults and adolescents: Updated Guidelines from the Centers for Disease Control and Prevention, National Institutes of Health, and HIV Medicine Association of the Infectious Diseases Society of America. *Clin Infect Dis.* 2014;58:1308–1311.

Panel on Opportunistic Infections in HIV-Infected Adults and Adolescents. Guidelines for the prevention and treatment of opportunistic infections in HIV-infected adults and adolescents: Recommendations from the Centers for Disease Control and Prevention, the National Institutes of Health, and the HIV Medicine Association of the Infectious Diseases Society of America. http://aidsinfo.nih.gov/contentfiles/lvguidelines/adult_oi.pdf. Accessed October 6, 2017.

Swan AM. Acute HIV infection in primary care. *Adv Nurse Pract.* 2009;17(9):49–54.

Thompson IR, Bidgood P, Petróczi A, Denholm-Price JC, Fielder MD; EuResist Network Study Group. An alternative methodology for the prediction of adherence to anti-HIV treatment. *AIDS Res Ther.* 2009;6:9. http://www.aidsrestherapy.com/content/6/1/9.

Infectious Mononucleosis

Balfour HH Jr, Dunmire SK, Hogquist KA. Infectious mononucleosis. *Clin Transl Immunol.* 2015;4:e33.

Bartlett A, Williams R, Hilton M. Splenic rupture in infectious mononucleosis: A systematic review of published case reports. *Injury.* 2016;47:531–538.

De Paor M, O'Brien K, Fahey T, Smith SM. Antiviral agents for infectious mononucleosis (glandular fever). *Cochrane Database Syst Rev.* 2016;12:CD011487.

Ebell MH, Call M, Shinholser J, Gardner J. Does this patient have infectious mononucleosis?: The rational clinical examination systematic review. *JAMA.* 2016;315:1502–1509.

Griffiths P, Lumley S. Cytomegalovirus. *Curr Opin Infect Dis.* 2014;27:554–559.

Lennon P, Crotty M, Fenton JE. Infectious mononucleosis. *BMJ.* 2015;350:h1825.

Rezk E, Nofal YH, Hamzeh A, Aboujaib MF, AlKheder MA, Al Hammad MF. Steroids for symptom control in infectious mononucleosis. *Cochrane Database Syst Rev.* 2015;(11):CD004402.

Rinderknecht AS, Pomerantz WJ. Spontaneous splenic rupture in infectious mononucleosis: Case report and review of the literature. *Pediatr Emerg Care.* 2012;28:1377–1379.

Staras SA, Dollard SC, Radford KW, Flanders WD, Pass RF, Cannon MJ. Seroprevalence of cytomegalovirus infection in the United States, 1988–1994. *Clin Infect Dis.* 2006;43:1143–1151.

Vouloumanou EK, Rafailidis PI, Falagas ME. Current diagnosis and management of infectious mononucleosis. *Curr Opin Hematol.* 2012;19:14–20.

Yager JE, Magaret AS, Kuntz SR, et al. Valganciclovir for the suppression of Epstein-Barr virus replication. *J Infect Dis.* 2017; 216:198–202.

Lyme Disease

Berende A, ter Hofstede HJ, Vos FJ, et al. Randomized trial of longer-term therapy for symptoms attributed to Lyme disease. *N Engl J Med.* 2016;374:1209–1220.

Butler T. The Jarisch-Herxheimer Reaction after antibiotic treatment of spirochetal infections: A review of recent cases and our understanding of pathogenesis. *Am J Trop Med Hyg.* 2017;96:46–52.

Cadavid D, Auwaerter PG, Rumbaugh J, Gelderblom H. Antibiotics for the neurological complications of Lyme disease. *Cochrane Database Syst Rev.* 2016;12:CD006978.

Chaaya G, Jaller-Char JJ, Ali SK. Beyond the bull's eye: Recognizing Lyme disease. *J Fam Pract.* 2016;65:373–379.

Cutler SJ, Rudenko N, Golovchenko M, et al. Diagnosing *Borreliosis. Vector Borne Zoonotic Dis.* 2017;17:2–11.

Eisen L, Dolan MC. Evidence for personal protective measures to reduce human contact with blacklegged ticks and for environmentally based control methods to suppress host-seeking blacklegged ticks and reduce infection with Lyme disease spirochetes in tick vectors and rodent reservoirs. *J Med Entomol.* 2016. [Epub ahead of print.]

Lantos PM. Chronic Lyme disease. *Infect Dis Clin North Am.* 2015;29:325–340.

Lantos PM, Shapiro ED, Auwaerter PG, et al. Unorthodox alternative therapies marketed to treat Lyme disease. *Clin Infect Dis.* 2015;60:1776–1782.

Puius YA, Kalish RA. Lyme arthritis: Pathogenesis, clinical presentation, and management. *Infect Dis Clin North Am.* 2008; 22:289–300, vi–vii.

Sanchez E, Vannier E, Wormser GP, Hu LT. Diagnosis, treatment, and prevention of lyme disease, human granulocytic anaplasmosis, and babesiosis: A review. *JAMA.* 2016;315:1767–1777.

Shen AK, Mead PS, Beard CB. The Lyme disease vaccine—a public health perspective. *Clin Infect Dis.* 2011;52(suppl 3):s247–s252.

Theel ES. The past, present, and (possible) future of serologic testing for Lyme disease. *J Clin Microbiol.* 2016;54:1191–1196.

Tilly K, Rosa PA, Stewart PE. Biology of infection with *Borrelia burgdorferi. Infect Dis Clin North Am.* 2008;22:217–234, v.

Waddell LA, Greig J, Mascarenhas M, Harding S, Lindsay R, Ogden N. The accuracy of diagnostic tests for Lyme disease in humans, a systematic review and meta-analysis of north american research. *PLoS One.* 2016;11:e0168613.

Wormser GP, Dattwyler RJ, Shapiro ED, et al. The clinical assessment, treatment, and prevention of lyme disease, human granulocytic anaplasmosis, and babesiosis: Clinical practice guidelines by the Infectious Diseases Society of America. *Clin Infect Dis.* 2006;43:1089–1134.

RESOURCES

HIV/AIDS

AIDSinfo: U.S. Department of Health and Human Services
www.AIDSinfo.nih.gov

AIDS Resource List
https://npin.cdc.gov/

Center for AIDS
www.centerforaids.org

Centers for Disease Control and Prevention (CDC), National Prevention Information Network
www.cdcnpin.org

HIV Consumer Council
www.hivcouncil.org

H.O.P.E. Foundation
www.hopedc.org

National Pediatric AIDS Network
www.npan.org

Lyme Disease

American Lyme Disease Foundation
http://www.aldf.com/

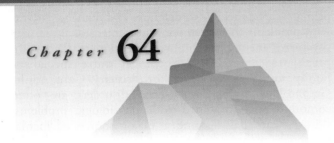

Chapter **64**

Common Psychosocial Complaints

Beth M. King, PhD, APRN, PMHCNS-BC, PMHNP-BC

Timothy Wilson, DNP, APRN, FNP, PMHNP

Lynne M. Dunphy, PhD, APRN, FNP-BC, FAAN,

FAANP

OVERVIEW

In the past decade, there has been a substantial increase in the number of people living with serious mental illness and substance use disorders who receive care from primary-care providers and emergency department services. This increase is often related to the long wait times for initial evaluation by mental health providers and the nationwide shortage of such providers, particularly in rural communities. The chronic debilitating nature of serious mental health disorders places a heavy emotional and financial burden on the individual, his or her family, community, and society. A mental health disorder affects the patient's functional capacity, family relationships and economic stability, and can often lead to the development of comorbid chronic diseases and premature mortality, as well as real-life suffering on a day-to-day level for the individual and family.

Thomas Insel, former Director of the National Institute of Mental Health, provides this description of the numbers associated with mental disorders; "The number of adults with any diagnosable mental disorder within the past year is estimated to be nearly 1 in 5, or roughly 43 million Americans. Although most of these conditions are not disabling, nearly 10 million American adults (1 in 25) have serious functional impairment due to a mental illness, such as a psychotic or serious mood or anxiety disorder. Fully 20 percent—1 in 5—of children ages 13–18 currently have and/or previously had a seriously debilitating mental disorder. By comparison, 8.3 percent of children under age 18 have asthma and 0.2 percent have diabetes" (Insel, 2015).

According to the Centers for Disease Control and Prevention, 42,773 individuals committed suicide in the United States in 2014, which is approximately the same number of deaths from breast cancer in the United States, more than deaths from prostate cancer, six times the number of deaths from HIV, and three times the number of deaths from homicide. Furthermore, the suicide rate in the United States increased by 24% from 1999 through 2014. Some theorize that the economic recession of the late 2000s and the increase in incidence of substance use are some of the factors leading to more frequent incidents of suicide (Asar, 2016). The increase in suicide rate is higher among females (45% increase) than males (16% increase), narrowing the suicide rate gap between the two genders. However, as of 2014, the suicide rate in men is still three times higher than that in women (Curtain, Warner, & Hedegaard, 2016).

Walker, McGee, and Druss (2015) provided a systematic review of publications related to mortality associated with mental illness estimated that the median reduction in life expectancy among those with mental illness was 10.1 years (range 1.4–32 years). Most of this early mortality is attributed to "natural causes," such as acute and chronic comorbid conditions including heart, pulmonary, and infectious diseases. On the basis of the prevalence of mental illness globally, the authors concluded that 8 million deaths occur each year that could have been averted if people with mental illness died at the same rate as the general population. For the United States, this translates to approximately 350,000 deaths that could be averted each year.

The economic impact of treating these disorders has increased over the past decade. In the United States, spending on mental health services is expected to be approximately $234 billion by 2020, accounting for 6.5% of all health-care expenditures (Substance Abuse and Mental Health Services Administration, 2014) These disorders comprise one of the five most costly medical conditions, extracting a severe cost burden on the nation and on the families and systems that provide support and care for people with serious mental illnesses.

Psychological and physical health influence each other greatly and are best approached effectively in an integrated manner. The signs and symptoms of mental disorders exist on a continuum and affect patients, families, and society, each in a unique way. What determines the burden of illness is the severity of symptoms, their duration, and the level of functional impairment. The *Diagnostic and Statistical Manual of Mental Disorders* (fifth edition; *DSM-5*) notes the relevance and significance of cultural factors and their influence on the expression and management of psychosocial illness. The Cultural Formulation Interview in the *DSM-5* (2013, p. 749–759) provides a mechanism for assessing the impact of culture on an individual's clinical presentation and course. For individuals and families for whom English is not their first language, it is crucial that a bicultural, appropriately trained interpreter be provided for all interviews, ideally one with specialized expertise and training in interpreting mental health issues.

All primary-care clinicians should be familiar with the *DSM-5* (see Advanced Assessment 64.1 for an overview of the *DSM-5* diagnostic classification system). For purposes of this textbook, the primary behavioral health

diagnoses are discussed; various clinical subtypes can be referenced directly from the *DSM-5*. The chapters in this psychosocial section have been organized based on the 2016 *International Classification of Diseases*, Tenth Revision, Clinical Modification (*ICD-10-CM*) Classifications of Mental and Behavioral Disorders.

Advanced practice registered nurses (APRNs) are ideal primary-care providers to diagnose and manage patients with problems that often are multidimensional, be they psychiatric mental health nurse practitioners (PMHNP), psychiatric mental health clinical nurse specialists, family nurse practitioners, or Primary Care Adult-Gerontology NPS. Psychosocial disorders are often comorbid and combined with physiologic problems. Primary care has become a major source of mental health treatment in recent years. The underdiagnosis and undertreatment of mental health disorders is a common

---

⁘ Advanced Assessment 64.1: The *Diagnostic and Statistical Manual of Mental Disorders,* Fifth Edition *(DSM-5)*

The *DSM-5* is a descriptive manual of mental disorders authored by the American Psychiatric Association. The *DSM-5* addresses the scientific and practice advances and was 15 years in the making. It provides the diagnostic criteria for each mental disorder. These descriptions enable clinicians to diagnose, communicate about, and treat people with various mental disorders. It has been demonstrated that the use of such criteria enhances agreement among clinicians.

Precise *DSM-5* criteria have been defined for each diagnosis with the addition of and reorganization of some previously identified conditions. This manual is divided into three sections: Section I contains user information, Section II contains the diagnostic criteria, and Section III addresses cultural aspects and conditions that need further research, including emerging measurement tools.

Effective October 2016, the *International Classification of Diseases*, 10th Edition, Clinical Modifications (*ICD-10-CM*), Classification of Mental and Behavioral Disorders was published, which is correlated to the *DSM-5*. Providers of mental health will need to be knowledgeable about both sets of codes. Both the *DSM* and *ICD* codes are used for diagnosis, and they are actually the same codes: the *DSM* is simply a guide to picking the right ICD code. *DSM-5* guides the provider to the applicable *ICD-10-CM* codes that are used for billing.

Nonaxial System

The first category combines the clinical disorder(s) and/or the personality and/or the developmental disorder with the known medical conditions; category two identifies the applicable environmental and psychosocial stressors; and category three provides a global assessment of functioning. In previous editions, a companion resource for primary care was developed. There are no plans to provide such a companion because one of the goals of the *DSM-5* revision was to reorganize the text to incorporate

clinical decision-making for the disciplines of psychiatry and primary care, where many individuals seek and receive mental health care. Accurate identification and treatment has the potential to improve morbidity and mortality from mental health disorders.

Using *DSM-5* Symptom Criteria

Specific symptom criteria are listed and defined for all *DSM-5* disorders and problems. In most cases, these criteria include symptom type, number, intensity, and duration. To meet the symptom criteria for a particular disorder, the patient must have experienced the minimal number of specified symptoms for a defined period of time, and the symptoms experienced should be sufficient to cause distress or impair psychosocial functioning. Persons who have fewer symptoms of less duration or less intensity may have an atypical form of the disorder, or their condition may be described as subclinical. The term *subclinical* does *not* imply that treatment is unnecessary. Atypical symptoms and subclinical symptoms can cause significant distress.

Using *DSM-5* Distress Criteria

Symptomatic patients typically report subjective distress. However, a patient's distress may also be observed by others or assessed by the practitioner. There are no absolute measures of symptom-induced distress: Symptoms that are highly distressing to one person may be only mildly distressing to another. The experience of distress should not be confused with the manner in which a person expresses his or her distress. It is possible for a highly distressed person who is suffering a great deal to have trouble expressing his or her distress, whereas others may be able to describe their distress in painful detail. Whether or not a distressed person is expressive should not overly influence the assessment. Often, simple verbal statements of symptom-related discomfort and suffering are sufficient.

phenomenon in primary care. It is important that the primary care APRN have a high index of suspicion regarding mental health problems. Patients may present to primary care with a constellation of signs and symptoms that have medical and psychological underpinnings. It is important both to consider previously identified psychosocial issues and to evaluate for undiagnosed mental health disorders. Patients benefit from continuity of care and from the nursing emphasis on patient-centered care.

Models of integrated and collaborative care are effective and lead to better outcomes for patients with mental health problems. Patient-centered medical homes have assumed prominence in our health-care delivery system, providing continuity of care over time as well as access to an entire health-care team. The collaborative method is based on Wagner's Chronic Care Model and emphasizes behavioral change, use of information systems such as electronic health records, and a team approach, utilizing high-level expertise for illness management and strong community linkages. Patients score higher on scales for quality of life and social role function, as well as for management of specific illnesses in practices using chronic care collaborative models compared with other care approaches. The collaborative model is one with which APRNs are familiar and in which they can use to best advantage a combination of their clinical and relationship skills.

This chapter presents some of the most common psychosocial concerns that the APRN is most likely to encounter in practice. It gives a general overview of each complaint and a discussion of the potential differential diagnoses that should be considered. These specific diagnoses are presented in detail in subsequent chapters within this section.

STRESS AND ANXIETY

Anxiety affects approximately 40 million adults; thus, it is the most common psychiatric disorder in the United States. Data from the National Comorbidity Survey indicate a 24.9% lifetime and an 18.2% 1-year prevalence rate for any anxiety disorder. Anxiety most commonly presents in individuals aged 20 to 45 years and is more frequently seen in women. For most people, anxiety is an unpleasant state of physical and psychological arousal that interferes with effective psychosocial functioning. Occasional, mild anxiety is a normal fact of life and can be positive; however, severe or chronic anxiety can become debilitating. Although anxiety disorders were once thought to be of minor clinical significance, it is now clear that they are serious illnesses, responsible for substantial morbidity and, possibly, mortality.

Anxiety symptoms are typically manifested in several dimensions: affective, cognitive, behavioral, and somatic. Affectively, anxiety is an experience of dread, foreboding, or panic, often accompanied by autonomic hyperactivity—primarily sympathetic—manifested as bodily symptoms. The patient may attempt to counter

the affective component of anxiety by cognitive thoughts that seek to make sense of or minimize the discomfort. Additional affective symptoms of anxiety are apprehension, fear, irritability, intolerance, frustration, and overreaction or hypersensitivity to personal feelings of shame. Behaviors such as avoidance, distractibility, and restlessness reflect the anxiety or may evolve in response to it. Behavioral symptoms of anxiety may include apathy, compulsions, rigidity, overreactions, preoccupation, and repetitive actions such as hair pulling or nail biting. Somatic symptoms of anxiety range in intensity from a loss of appetite, dry mouth, and fatigue, to diarrhea, sweating, chest pain, hyperventilation, vomiting, and paresthesias. Highly anxious persons may experience the full range of anxiety symptoms or may have only one or two symptoms. The classification of anxiety disorders is largely based on clinical presentation and is discussed in depth in Chapter 68.

DIFFERENTIAL DIAGNOSIS

Anxiety disorder encompasses a variety of disorders (see Differential Diagnosis 64.1):

- *Specific phobia disorders,* such as agoraphobia, social phobias, and assorted specific phobias

---

 Differential Diagnosis 64.1: Anxiety Disorders

- Realistic worries.
- Adjustment disorders (usually transient).
- Panic disorder: the specific worry is focused on the symptoms of panic.
- Social anxiety disorder (social phobia): the worry is about social situations.
- Obsessive-compulsive disorder: the worry becomes focused on a specific object or activity.
- Separation disorder: the worry is about being away from parents and caregivers.
- Somatic symptoms disorder: the worry is focused on physiologic symptoms.
- Body dysmorphic disorder: the worry is focused on a perceived defect in physical appearance.
- Post-traumatic stress and acute stress disorder: the worry is focused on reminders of a traumatic event.
- Anxiety disorder due to another medical condition (for example, hyperthyroidism)
- Psychotic anxiety disorders: the worries are not reality tested (delusions).
- Substance-induced anxiety disorder: the anxiety is caused by substance intoxication (stimulants, caffeine) or substance withdrawal (alcohol, alprazolam, fluoxetine).

Source: Adapted from American Psychiatric Association. Anxiety disorders. *Diagnostic and statistical manual of mental disorders: DSM-5.* 5th ed. Washington, DC: American Psychiatric Association; 2013:189–234.

- *Other anxiety disorders*, such as panic disorder, generalized anxiety disorder, and other mixed anxiety disorders (see Chapter 68)
- A variety of *obsessive-compulsive disorders*, both specified and unspecified (see Chapter 69)
- Stress-related and adjustment disorders, such as post-traumatic stress and adjustment disorders such as grief reaction (see Chapter 68)
- *Dissociative and conversion disorders*
- *Somatoform disorders*, such as body dysmorphic disorder (see Chapter 69) and hypochondriasis
- *Nonpsychotic mental disorders*, such as depersonalization-derealization syndrome

The extreme variability of anxiety presentations in primary care makes it one of the most commonly seen complaints. In addition, like the mood disorders, anxiety disorders can also be viewed on a continuum. The primary-care provider must differentiate between patients with a relatively mild and transient anxiety state, often externally situated, and patients with a pervasive and more debilitating anxiety disorder. Screening questions may include the following: *Are you a constant worrier, unnecessarily anxious all the time about a lot of different things? How long have you felt like this? Does this interfere with your day-to-day functioning?* A diagnosis of generalized anxiety disorder is reserved for those patients who experience extensive, pervasive, and disabling anxiety that lasts for more than six months. These criteria are necessary to avoid overdiagnosis of the "worried well."

The age of the patient is important in considering the differential diagnoses. Young and middle-aged patients are more likely to have a true anxiety disorder, whereas older patients may be more likely to have an underlying physiological component, such as a vascular dementia, that must be ruled out. Undiagnosed arrhythmias and metabolic conditions, as well as drug reactions, may all manifest as anxiety. Many medical conditions involving stimulation of the sympathetic nervous system may produce anxiety symptoms, complicating the diagnosis. Anxiety caused by a medical disorder may be intermittent, such as anxiety associated with transient cardiac arrhythmias or abrupt changes in blood glucose levels. In all cases, potential physical explanations for anxiety symptoms should be evaluated first. Patients with constant anxiety may warrant an ECG, a drug screen, and a thyroid profile, especially if there is accompanying weight loss.

A variety of psychiatric disorders, such as mood disorders, certain psychoses, dementias, and substance-induced disorders may present with anxiety as a prominent part of their constellation of symptomatology. For example, anywhere from 42% to 100% of depressed patients (average 67%) have anxiety symptoms, and 33% of depressed patients have panic attacks. In addition, 17% to 65% (average 40%) of anxious patients and 33% of patients with panic disorder have depressive symptoms. The complexity of these disorders can pose considerable diagnostic and treatment challenges for the primary-care clinician. Referral for psychiatric evaluation may be needed to establish a correct diagnosis and offer treatment guidance.

DEPRESSED MOOD

A common psychosocial condition seen in primary-care settings is depression or sadness. Depression is common for many reasons. People use the term "depression" to describe a wide variety of negative emotional experiences, ranging from sadness to disinterest in pleasurable activities to self-hate. The hallmarks of major depression are sadness and apathy, although symptoms presented in primary care may be *fatigue, loss of appetite, and change in sleep*. In most cases, the sadness and apathy associated with major depression can be distinguished from ordinary changes in mood. A number of screening tools can be utilized (Table 64.1).

No description of depression, whether as a symptom or disorder, is complete without addressing the psychological pain and suffering of depression. The pain of depression can become so severe that some depressed persons

TABLE 64.1 Screening Tools			
Mental Health Criterion	**Resource**	**Screening Tool**	**Links**
General Overview of Tools	Substance Abuse and Mental Health Services Administration (SAMHSA)	Mental Health Screening Tools: Links & Descriptions	https://www.integration.samhsa.gov/clinical-practice/screening-tools
	American Psychiatric Association	Assessment measures for baseline and to monitor treatment progress. Includes Adult and Child/Adolescent tools	https://www.psychiatry.org/psychiatrists/practice/dsm/educational-resources/assessment-measures#Disorder
	Medicare Preventative Services	Screening ICD-10 codes, overview of coverage for depression, alcohol misuse, other medical screenings	https://www.cms.gov/Medicare/Prevention/PrevntionGenInfo/medicare-preventive-services/MPS-QuickReferenceChart-1.html

Mental Health Criterion	**Resource**	**Screening Tool**	**Links**
	Health Measures Northwestern University/ NIH Grant	PROMIS Tools	http://www.healthmeasures.net/ explore-measurement-systems/ promis
	World Health Organization	World Health Organization Disability Assessment Schedule (WHODAS 2.0)	http://www.who.int/classifications/ icf/whodasii/en/
Anxiety	Pfizer	Generalized anxiety disorder 7-item scale (GAD-7)	http://www.phqscreeners.com/ sites/g/files/g10016261/f/201412/ GAD-7_English.pdf
	Adult attention-deficit/hyperactivity disorder (ADHD) Toolkit Assessment Tools	Hamilton Anxiety Rating Scale	http://naceonline.com/ AdultADHDtoolkit/assessment-tools/hama.pdf
Depressed Mood	Pfizer	Screener Overview: Patient Health Questionnaire (PHQ)-several versions	http://www.phqscreeners.com/ select-screener/41
		PHQ-9: Common screening tool for depression	http://www.phqscreeners.com/ sites/g/files/g10016261/f/201412/ PHQ-9_English.pdf
	Substance Abuse and Mental Health Services Administration (SAMHSA)	Mood Disorder Questionnaire (MDQ)	https://www.integration.samhsa. gov/images/res/MDQ.pdf
Bipolar	American Psychiatric Association	Young Mania Rating Scale	http://dcf.psychiatry.ufl.edu/ files/2011/05/Young-Mania-Rating-Scale-Measure-with-background.pdf
Suicide	SAMHSA	SAFE-T	https://www.integration.samhsa. gov/images/res/SAFE_T.pdf
		Columbia Suicide Severity Rating Scale (C-SSRS)	https://www.integration.samhsa. gov/clinical-practice/Columbia_ Suicide_Severity_Rating_Scale.pdf
Substance Use Disorder	SAMHSA	SBIRT: Screening, Brief Intervention, and Referral for Treatment	https://www.integration.samhsa. gov/clinical-practice/sbirt
		AUDIT: Alcohol Use Disorders Identification Test	https://www.integration.samhsa.gov/ AUDIT_screener_for_alcohol.pdf
		AUDIT-C	https://www.integration.samhsa. gov/images/res/tool_auditc.pdf
		CAGE-AID	https://www.integration.samhsa. gov/images/res/CAGEAID.pdf
	National Institute on Alcohol Abuse and Alcoholism	Alcohol Screening and Brief Intervention for Youth Guide: A Practitioners Guide	https://pubs.niaaa.nih.gov/ OrderForm/EncForm/Youth_ Guide_Order_Form
	National Institute on Alcohol Abuse and Alcoholism	TWEAK	https://pubs.niaaa.nih.gov/ publications/AssessingAlcohol/ InstrumentPDFs/74_TWEAK.pdf

are willing to go to any length to obtain even a moment of relief. Depression-related thoughts of death or suicide are not uncommon and should be assessed by asking the question, "Are you thinking of harming yourself or committing suicide?" However, the pain of depression can be difficult to articulate: The depressed person may only be able to make vague references to "hurting" or "feeling bad." The US. Preventative Services Task Force (USPSTF; 2016) recommends "screening for depression in the general adult population, including pregnant and postpartum women." Chapter 67 discusses screening tools for depression.

Individual variations in the clinical presentation of depression can be great, sometimes making the condition difficult to recognize. The more common patient presentation of depression in primary-care settings is the person who has moderate to severe feelings of sadness or apathy that he or she may, or may not, attribute to depression. Common presentations also include complaints of unexplained fatigue, insomnia, irritability, anger, anxiety, and hyperactivity. Many deeply depressed persons are unaware of the level of impairment resulting from their illness. Slowed thinking and emotional numbness—two severe symptoms of depression—can contribute to minimal self-awareness of depression. Gender can affect presentation, but gender should not influence assessment.

Cultural variations in the presentation of depression are also individualized, based on the person's perception of depression. Patients may focus less on personal experiences and more on physical aches and pains. Ethnic and cultural norms concerning privacy, embarrassment, and disclosure will have an impact on the patient's presentation and willingness to discuss symptoms.

Depression belongs to a broad category called *mood (affective) disorders*, which encompass bipolar disorder, major depressive disorder, atypical depression, and persistent mood (affective) disorders such as dysthymic disorder. See Chapter 67 for an in-depth discussion of the mood-disorders.

DIFFERENTIAL DIAGNOSES

A pertinent screening question for an individual presenting with depression is *"Do you ever get so depressed that you can't function?"* The clinician needs to be aware that depression can be heterogeneous in presentation; it may, for example, contain a seasonal component, such as seasonal affective disorder; it may be a "reactive depression," triggered by external stressors and more responsive to context (see "Grief" later in this chapter); and in some cases, depressive preoccupations can become delusional convictions (see Differential Diagnosis 64.2).

The clinician should rule out organic causes—is there a headache or focal neurological symptoms? Are there endocrine changes? Several endocrine conditions, such as hyperthyroidism, menopause, myxedema, and Cushing's disease, may present with depression. Additional questions include: Is there a loss of appetite, weight, or libido? Is there sleeplessness or hypersomnia? To rule out organic causes, laboratory studies, such as a drug screen, chemistry panel, thyroid panel, Venereal Disease Research Laboratory Test for syphilis, and complete blood count, may be considered. If Cushing's syndrome is suspected, serum cortisol and cortisol suppression test should be ordered; if menopause is suspected, a serum follicle-stimulating hormone and estradiol level should be ordered. Screening tests to evaluate nonorganic depression include the PRIME-MED and Patient Health Questionnaire-9 (see Chapter 67). A referral to a psychiatrist and/or PMHNP should be

Differential Diagnosis 64.2: Types of Depression

- Uncomplicated bereavement (see "Grief" in this chapter).
- Depressive disorder due to another medical condition: consider in older patients.
- Substance-induced mood disorder: most common in younger patients.
- Brief psychotic disorder: occurs without a clear episode of depression; may resolve quickly and be a response to stress.
- Bipolar disorders: recurrent or previous symptoms of hypomania or hypermania, such as racing thoughts, impulsivity, spending sprees, not needing sleep.
- Persistent depressive disorder (dysthymia): depressive symptoms are milder than those of major depressive disorder but may persist for years.
- Schizophrenia, schizoaffective disorder, or delusional disorder—delusions and hallucinations occur during periods with no mood symptoms.

Source: Adapted from American Psychiatric Association. Depressive disorders. *Diagnostic and statistical manual of mental disorders: DSM-5.* 5th ed. Washington, DC: American Psychiatric Association; 2013:155–188.

considered if the depression is severe, or if there is suicidal ideation (see Chapter 67 for Acute Suicide Risk).

GRIEF

Grief, mourning, and *bereavement* are terms that define a universal human response to loss. Loss may be defined broadly. Typically, we think of loss of a spouse, a child, a sibling, a parent, as most associated with this concept; however, *grief* may be triggered by the loss of a variety of things of value to an individual: loss of a pet, a home, social status, occupation and/or job, imprisonment, or loss of a homeland. Many things may trigger grief.

Grieving is both an emotional and a physiological response. In acute grief, as in cases of other stressful events, there may be a disruption of biological rhythms. It is well documented that grief is accompanied by impaired immune function, specifically decreased lymphocyte proliferation and impaired functioning of natural killer cells, although it is not known how clinically significant these changes are. Manifestations of grief reflect cultural context, the individual's personality, previous life experiences, the significance of the loss, past psychological history, the relationship with the deceased, existing family and social networks, other life events, resources, educational level, and general state of health.

The stages of grieving, identified in the classic work of Elisabeth Kübler-Ross (1965), are as follows:

- Denial
- Anger

- Bargaining
- Depression
- Acceptance

Grief is identified when the onset of a patient's symptoms is associated with the death of a loved one, either recent or past. Grief, however, may not be limited to the physical death of a loved one. Grief can also result from the loss of a significant relationship or the loss of an important aspect of one's identity.

Each person grieves in a manner that is, for him or her, meaningful and effective. With normal grief, there is consistent progress toward acceptance.

Grief consists of three distinct phases: avoidance, confrontation, and accommodation.

- Acknowledging the loss
- Reacting to the separation—feeling the pain, expressing reactions
- Recollecting and reexperiencing the deceased and the relationship—realistically reviewing and remembering the deceased
- Relinquishing attachment to the deceased while still acknowledging a loving connection to the deceased
- Readjusting to move adaptively into the new reality without forgetting the old
- Reinvesting; redirecting one's energy to new goals, pursuits, hopes, causes, beliefs, activities

Grief can be understood as a journey along a well-marked psychological path: each person travels in his or her own way and at his or her own speed. The way a person grieves, and, consequently, the amount of time a person needs to move from agony to acceptance is heavily influenced by personal, social, cultural, religious, and spiritual norms.

Lifestyle is also a factor to be considered. Individuals who live in social isolation may find it more difficult to grieve a loss without close significant others who can offer comfort and assistance. Grieving for a loss alone can drain psychosocial resources that are needed for day-to-day functioning. An equally difficult modern problem is the overvaluation of immediacy. Living with technology has increased our cultural expectations for speed. Human experiences that require time may appear suspect in this context. Busy employers, families, and friends may support grieving, if (in their perceptions) it does not take too long—the implication being that personal grief should not take too much time, or demand too many valuable social resources. After a year has passed, family and friends may begin to ask why the grieving person is not "over" his or her loss yet.

Grief can present in many ways. It can range from absent or delayed grief to excessively intense and prolonged emotions, or to complicated grief associated with suicidal ideation or frank psychosis. The risk factors for a more complicated grief reaction include (1) sudden and/or violent death, (2) social isolation, (3) individuals who believe that they are in some way responsible for the death (real or imagined), (4) individuals with a history of traumatic losses, and (5) individuals who had an intensely ambivalent or dependent relationship with the deceased. In some instances, reduced or absent grief may be an appropriate reaction.

DIFFERENTIAL DIAGNOSIS

Cultural, ethnic, religious, and social beliefs, community and family traditions, and personal characteristics all determine how and when a person, a couple, or a family will mourn a loss. For some people, grieving is a well-defined, highly satisfying ritual. For others, particularly those who have never suffered a major loss before, grief can be confusing and disturbing. In terms of psychosocial health and well-being, the process of mourning should allow the person to experience pain but achieve acceptance.

Grief and depression share many of the same characteristics, and it can sometimes be difficult to evaluate exactly when the scope of normal grieving has slipped into a pathological realm. It is important to distinguish the grieving process from a major depressive episode. The *DSM-5* points out several features that help to define each process. In addition, an individual with a history of depression is at risk for depression during times of major loss. The mood disturbance in depression is typically pervasive and unrelenting, whereas fluctuations of mood in grief are common.

Early detection of grief and preventive interventions can alleviate suffering and lead to earlier and more effective treatment. This includes preparing (if possible) the person and family for the normal stages of grieving—normalizing grief. In the case of terminal illness, early and ongoing bereavement assessment and a collaborative process are essential components of a preventive approach to bereavement care. Interventions include bereavement education and counseling that assist in facilitating communication with the dying person. There is strong evidence that involvement and caregiving benefits survivors.

Primary-care clinicians can assist bereaved individuals by doing the following:

- Validating pain and distress related to loss
- Providing appropriate pharmacological therapy
- Making bereaved patients aware of the many supportive therapies available and having ready a list of referrals

Utilizing the *Circle of Caring* model, community services that focus on grief, especially traumatic grief (miscarriage, death of a child at birth, death from violence or war), church resources, family support, and other support services to deal with special issues, for example, single parenting, may all be beneficial. Appropriate medical therapy should be given as indicated, depending on symptomatology and history. For example, a brief course of a short-acting sedative may be appropriate during acute grief to induce sleep or to get through the funeral and burial, especially when supportive interventions have not succeeded. The use of drugs such as tranquilizers or alcohol, which numb emotions, should be discouraged. Antidepressant therapy may be considered for patients with particularly prolonged or complex grief reactions, even when it may be difficult to differentiate depression from a normal grief response. Clinical data suggest that selective serotonin reuptake inhibitors (referred to as SSRIs) may be beneficial and assist the patient to mobilize the energy necessary to progress through the stages of mourning and grief.

Specific counseling sessions for the bereaved may be extremely valuable and may assist in the prevention of pathological mourning or depressive reactions. These sessions, with trained counsellors/therapists, can assist the grieving person in recognizing and expressing angry or ambivalent feelings toward a deceased person. Group counseling, as well as self-help groups, can be important adjunctive therapies.

The goals for treating complicated grief reactions include facilitating mourning and helping the patient to find new activities and relationships to substitute for the loss. Studies have found that effective treatment of depressive syndromes, even as early as 6 to 8 weeks after the death of a loved one, reduces suffering and facilitates the work of grief. The notion that medications or psychotherapy impede the process of grief is unsubstantiated and may, at times, serve to prolong suffering and disability. Obviously, elements of psychosis clearly indicate a need for more aggressive treatment: Some patients may even become suicidal and should be referred for psychiatric care for further assessment and treatment.

SUBSTANCE USE DISORDER

The primary-care provider has an obligation to inquire about, provide information about, and make appropriate referrals for substance-related or behavioral addictions. All agents in the substance use disorder (SUD) category can cause tolerance, habituation, and physical dependence. The legal substances that fall into this category include tobacco, alcohol, and in some states cannabis; illicit substances include cannabis in some jurisdictions, cocaine, opioids without medical prescription or necessity, hallucinogens, certain inhalants, and stimulants such as methamphetamine. Sedatives, hypnotics, and anxiolytics may be prescribed for a variety of reasons on a short-term basis, but these substances also can lead to dependence and subsequent abuse, causing the user to seek the substance through illegal channels. The use of substances to enhance cognitive function as well as athletic performance, some of which are legal, all have the potential to veer for overuse. Caffeine is unique in that it is not classified as an SUD agent, but symptom criteria for intoxication and withdrawal are provided. Additionally, the *DSM-5* includes the behavioral addiction of gambling. There has been lobbying for inclusion of

diagnoses for additional behavioral addictions such as "Internet shopping," but evidence is lacking for many of these diagnoses

The science of addictions has grown over the past 20 years, and evidence suggests a common neurophysiological basis to all addictive behaviors. These disorders are considered chronic and relapsing because despite significant negative consequences, the behaviors continue. It is now recognized that dopamine is vital in this process, and thus pharmacological agents have been introduced to target certain areas of the brain. Targeted treatments, often referred to as medically assisted treatments (MATs) for tobacco, alcohol, and opioids are now available. There has been resistance to MATs by some members of the recovery community, especially those dedicated to the abstinence model from all substances and recovery through interpersonal support, spiritual growth, and the shared self-help community. However, as has been well documented, areas in the United States are in the grip of a multifactorial epidemic of opioid addiction, with multiple deaths documented from overdoses. The reality of this epidemic, combined with increasing biological knowledge and superior pharmacological products, have led to an increasing acceptance by the recovery community that a combined approach of MAT with behavioral and psychological support recovery may be a superior approach for many.

DIFFERENTIAL DIAGNOSIS

For some individuals, substance use is recreational and does not cause impairment or distress. Substance use disorders are recognized when a person's use of a substance affects a person's relationships or work or school obligations. The hallmarks of a substance use disorder are tolerance (the person needs more and more of the substance for same effect), withdrawal (stopping brings on painful physical and/or psychological symptoms), and compulsive use. The person no longer just enjoys the substance; they *need it* (see Differential Diagnosis 64.3). Screening questions that may uncover a substance abuse problem include the following: *Has anyone ever suggested that you have an alcohol or drug problem?* or *Have you ever gotten into trouble because of alcohol or drugs?*

Chapter 65 discusses substance use disorder in greater depth and includes a section dedicated to opioid use. The use of MATs are emphasized as a primary arm of potential management plans.

INTIMATE PARTNER VIOLENCE

Intimate partner violence (IPV) is defined as a pattern of assaultive and coercive behaviors that may include inflicted physical injury, psychological abuse, sexual

Differential Diagnosis 64.3: Substance Use Disorders

- Recreational use: Substance use—even heavy substance use—that does not cause clinically significant impairment or distress.
- Substance dependence: tolerance, withdrawal, and/or a pattern of compulsive use are present.
- Substance intoxication: a set of symptoms and behaviors that occurs shortly after taking the substance. Each substance tends to have a pattern of intoxication but for this diagnosis to be applied, there must be evidence of clinically significant distress or behavioral impairment to distinguish it from recreational use.
- Substance withdrawal: signs and symptoms that occur when an individual attempts to stop using a substance. A screening question might be: *Do you ever get troubling symptoms when you try to stop drinking or using a drug?*
- Substance-induced mental disorders: substance abuse can amplify many psychiatric disorders and needs to be considered in many instances of altered mental status and function.

Source: Adapted from American Psychiatric Association. Substance-related and addictive disorders. *Diagnostic and statistical manual of mental disorders: DSM-5* 5th edition. Washington, DC: American Psychiatric Association; 2013:481–590.

assault, progressive social isolation, stalking, deprivation, intimidation, and threats perpetrated by someone who is, was, or wishes to be involved in an intimate relationship with an adult or adolescent, and aimed at establishing control by one partner over the other. IPV is not associated with any ethnic group, religion, socioeconomic level, level of education, employment, or sexual orientation. However, typically the victim is a child, a woman, or an elderly person, and the typical perpetrator is a man (in the case of partner abuse), a parent or other trusted adult (in the case of child abuse), or an adult child or other caregiver (in the case of elder abuse). Although alcohol/substance abuse and a history of childhood abuse are important correlates of IPV, they do not cause or explain IPV.

Estimates of the prevalence of IPV in the United States are that 1 to 4 million women per year are physically, sexually, or emotionally abused by their partners; however only a small percentage of IPV is ever reported, so numbers are often unreliable.

More than one type of violence may occur in any given family; for example, in one study, 45% to 70% of battered women reported that their batterer also abused their children. In 2013, the World Health Organization (WHO), the U.S. Preventive Services Task Force (USPSTF), and Cochrane Reviews released identification and treatment recommendations for IPV. All guidelines encourage clinicians to be alert to physical and behavioral signs of abuse such as trauma or somatic symptoms.

DIFFERENTIAL DIAGNOSIS

It is difficult to know when to include violence in the differential diagnosis. Recognition of IPV continues to be difficult because the victim and the abuser often conspire to conceal it. The partner, if present, may be suspicious. Symptoms or behaviors that may signal abuse include exacerbation or poor control of chronic illness, sleep disturbances, chronic pain, or frequent unexplained appointment changes. Behavioral red flags are (1) a patient who is reluctant to speak in front of her partner or gives evasive answers and (2) an overly protective or controlling partner. Any patient presenting with multiple complaints or whose symptoms are not consistent with her history should be assessed for violence at least once and reassessed if she fails to respond to therapy appropriately (see Box 64.1). Exposure to IPV is frequently linked with mental health issues such as depression, anxiety, suicide attempts, and/or substance abuse. Problems or injuries during pregnancy should raise the level of suspicion, as should delays in seeking medical care.

Box 64.1 Advanced Practice Nursing Interventions for Intimate Partner Violence

Prevention:

- Teach conflict resolution skills.
- Create a safety plan to remove the individual(s) from the violent situation.
- Inquire about the abuse. Questions to ask include the following:
  1. Has the physical violence increased in frequency/severity over the past year?
  2. Have you ever been choked?
  3. Has a weapon or threat with a weapon been used?
  4. Have you been threatened with death, or do you believe the individual could kill you?
  5. Is there a gun in the house?
  6. Have you ever been forced to have sex when you did not wish to?
  7. For women, have you ever been abused while you were pregnant?
  8. Is alcohol or substance abuse a factor? How often is the alcohol or substance used?
  9. Have your daily activities been controlled?
  10. Is the individual violent and constantly jealous of you?
- Provide community resources.
- Provide counseling and other therapy as indicated (e.g., crisis intervention, post-traumatic stress disorder therapy, physical rehabilitation).
- Document findings and interventions.

Source: Adapted from Jezierski M. Abuse of women by male partners: Basic knowledge for emergency nurses. *J Emerg Nurs.* 1994;20(5):361–368.

The first goal of assessment is to determine whether an individual is a target of violence. The second goal is to evaluate the level of danger. The patient must be seen alone. The partner, children, and family members should be asked to leave the room. If an interpreter is needed, a professional interpreter of the same sex as the patient should be used rather than a family member. If the partner refuses to leave, the clinician should avoid confrontation and instead strategize a way to get the patient alone later. Requesting a urinalysis or chest x-ray exam is often an effective approach.

Routine screening for IPV is recommended by the USPSTF for all women of childbearing age at initial visits and periodically (Feltner et al., 2018). The USPSTF found insufficient evidence to routinely screen the elderly or other vulnerable populations, Of utmost importance is that safety and confidentiality are established before asking questions about abuse. The clinician should always preface IPV questioning with an appropriate and nonthreatening explanation such as, "I ask all my patients these questions because these problems affect many people's health." Avoid using stigmatizing words such as *domestic violence* or *abuse*. In some instances, a patient may disclose a past experience with violence that may provide useful information in providing appropriate care.

The clinician must communicate concern and caring and tell each woman that all women are assessed for abuse. The seriousness of the issue cannot be underscored enough. Although it may be necessary to obtain specific information, the clinician should try to limit data gathering to essentials. Some sources suggest "funneling," beginning with innocuous questions and progressing to more directed approach. Use of a validated instrument should be considered; the USPSTF (2013) reports that that following instruments are those with the highest levels of sensitivity and specificity for identifying IPV: Hurt, Insult, Threaten, Scream (HITS); Ongoing Abuse Screen/Ongoing Violence Assessment Tool (OAS/OVAT); Slapped, Threatened, and Throw (STaT); Humiliation, Afraid, Rape, Kick (HARK); Modified Childhood Trauma Questionnaire–Short Form (CTQ-SF); and Woman Abuse Screen Tool (WAST). Many patients will disclose emotional abuse long before they are comfortable disclosing physical abuse, even if both are occurring. A key component of the abuse experience is intrusion; many patients who are in an abusive relationship may perceive questioning as intrusive. Again, sensitivity is crucial.

Any evidence of IPV requires full compliance with local reporting and referral laws. Local and state agencies for victims have established protocols and systems for providing services that include emergency housing, health care, foster care, and displacement counseling. Despite the significant incidence of IPV, there is still a shortage of referral services for violent offenders. Violent individuals who are motivated to stop their violence may benefit from community support groups. Local crisis services and police hotlines should be contacted to protect victims of domestic violence. Victims of IPV should have the phone number and address for local emergency services, legal advocacy programs, and support groups, or at least be informed regarding how to obtain this information.

Clinicians should consider referral for mental health evaluation for associated psychiatric problems. Those living with abuse may have associated major depression, panic disorder, post-traumatic stress disorder, suicidal thoughts, and co-occurring substance abuse. A patient who may refuse referrals for domestic violence services may accept a referral to obtain help with abuse-related depression and anxiety.

Clinicians may also want to consider participating in preventive services by working with local and state coalitions against domestic violence, child abuse, and elder abuse. In addition, the work environment should have clear policies and procedures defining abuse-reporting procedures. This is important in every office, because primary-care clinicians are often the "first stop" for victims of abuse.

REFERENCES

General

American Psychiatric Association. *Diagnostic and statistical manual of mental disorders.* 5th ed. Arlington, VA: American Psychiatric Association; 2013.

Asar S. Suicide rates on the rise in the U.S. *USA Today.* https://www.usatoday.com/story/news/2016/04/22/suicide-rate-rise-us/83284568/. Published April 22, 2016.

Sadock BJ, Sadock VA. *Kaplan and Sadock's synopsis of psychiatry.* 11th ed. Philadelphia, PA: Wolters Kluwer; 2015.

Substance Abuse and Mental Health Services Administration. Projections of national expenditures for treatment of mental and substance use disorders, 2010–2020. https://store.samhsa.gov/shin/content//SMA14-4883/SMA14-4883.pdf. Published 2014.

Tavernise S. US suicide rate surges to a 30-year high. *New York Times.* April 22, 2016. https://www.nytimes.com/2016/04/22/health/us-suicide-rate-surges-to-a-30-year-high.html.

Woltmann E, Grogan-Kaylor A, Perron B, Georges H, Kilbourne AM, Bauer MS. Comparative effectiveness of collaborative chronic care models for mental health conditions across primary, specialty, and behavioral health care settings: Systematic review and meta-Analysis. *Am J Psychiatry.* 2012;169:790–804.

Depressed Mood

Substance Abuse and Mental Health Services Administration. Patient health questionnaire (PHQ-9). http://www.integration.samhsa.gov/images/res/PHQ%20-%20Questions.pdf. Accessed December 8, 2014.

Grief

Bolton JM, Au W, Walld R, et al. Parental bereavement after the death of an offspring in a motor vehicle collision: A population-based study. *Am J Epidemiol.* 2014;179:177–185.

Bonanno GA, Papa A, Lalande K, et al. Grief processing and deliberate grief avoidance: A prospective comparison of bereaved spouses and parents in the United States and the People's Republic of China. *J Consult Clin Psychol.* 2005;73:86–98.

Collier R. Prolonged grief proposed as mental disorder. *CMAJ.* 2011;183:E439–E440.

Currier JM, Neimeyer RA, Berman JS. The effectiveness of psycho-therapeutic interventions for bereaved persons: a comprehensive quantitative review. *Psychol Bull.* 2008;134:648–661.

Curtain SC, Warner M, Hedegaard H. Increase in suicide in United States, 1999–2014 (NCHS Data Brief No. 241). https://www.cdc.gov/nchs/products/databriefs/db241.htm. Published 2016.

Jones MP, Bartrop RW, Forcier L, Penny R. The long-term impact of bereavement upon spouse health: A 10-year follow-up. *Acta Neuropsychiatr.* 2010;22:212–217.

Kersting A, Brähler E, Glaesmer H, Wagner B. Prevalence of complicated grief in a representative population-based sample. *J Affect Disord.* 2011;131:339–341.

Kübler-Ross E. *On death and dying.* (1965). New York, NY: Basic Books.

Lee M-A, Carr D. Does the context of spousal loss affect the physical functioning of older widowed persons? A longitudinal analysis. *Res Aging.* 2007;29:457–487.

Li J, Precht DH, Mortensen PB, Olsen J. Mortality in parents after death of a child in Denmark: A nationwide follow-up study. *Lancet.* 2003;361:363–367.

Lobb EA, Kristjanson LJ, Aoun SM, et al. Predictors of complicated grief: A systematic review of empirical studies. *Death Stud.* 2010;34:673–698.

Maciejewski PK, Zhang B, Block SD, Prigerson HG. An empirical examination of the stage theory of grief. *JAMA.* 2007;297:716.

Mancini AD, Griffin P, Bonanno GA. Recent trends in the treatment of prolonged grief. *Curr Opin Psychiatry.* 2012;25:46–51.

Nagraj S, Barclay S. Bereavement care in primary care: a systematic literature review and narrative synthesis. *Br J Gen Pract.* 2011;61:e42–e48.

Näppä U, Lundgren AB, Axelsson B. The effect of bereavement groups on grief, anxiety, and depression—a controlled, prospective intervention study. *BMC Palliat Care.* 2016;15:58e1–e8.

Newson RS, Boelen PA, Hek K, et al. The prevalence and characteristics of complicated grief in older adults. *J Affect Disord.* 2011;132:231–238.

Onrust SA, Cuijpers P. Mood and anxiety disorders in widowhood: a systematic review. *Aging Ment Health.* 2006;10:327–334.

Schut H, Stroebe MS. Interventions to enhance adaptation to bereavement. *J Palliat Med.* 2005;8(suppl 1):S140.

Shah SM, Carey IM, Harris T, et al. The effect of unexpected bereavement on mortality in older couples. *Am J Public Health.* 2013;103:1140–1145.

Simon NM. Is complicated grief a post-loss stress disorder? *Depress Anxiety.* 2012;29:541–544.

Simon NM. Treating complicated grief. *JAMA.* 2013;310:416–423.

Simon NM, Wall MM, Keshaviah A, Dryman MT, LeBlanc NJ, Shear MK. et al. Informing the symptom profile of complicated grief. *Depress Anxiety.* 2011;28:118–126.

Tol WA, Barbui C, van Ommeren M. Management of acute stress, PTSD, and bereavement: WHO recommendations. *JAMA.* 2013;310:477–478.

van Denderen M, de Keijser J, Kleen M, Boelen PA. Psychopathology among homicidally bereaved individuals: A systematic review. *Trauma Violence Abuse.* 2015;16:70–80.

Warner J, Metcalfe C, King M. Evaluating the use of benzodiazepines following recent bereavement. *Br J Psychiatry.* 2001;178:36–41.

Wittouck C, Van Autreve S, De Jaegere E, et al. The prevention and treatment of complicated grief: a meta-analysis. *Clin Psychol Rev.* 2011;31:69–78.

World Health Organization. WHO guidelines for the management of conditions specifically related to stress. http://www.who.int/mental_health/resources/emergencies/en/. Published 2013.

Interpersonal Violence

Breiding MJ, Smith SG, Basile KC, et al. Prevalence and characteristics of sexual violence, stalking, and intimate partner violence victimization—national intimate partner and sexual violence survey, United States, 2011. *MMWR Surveill Summ.* 2014;63:1.

Buller AM, Devries KM, Howard LM, Bacchus LJ. Associations between intimate partner violence and health among men who have sex with men: A systematic review and meta-analysis. *PLoS Med.* 2014; 11:e1001609.

Devries KM, Mak JY, Bacchus LJ, et al. Intimate partner violence and incident depressive symptoms and suicide attempts: A systematic review of longitudinal studies. *PLoS Med.* 2013;10:e1001439.

Feltner C, Wallace I, Berkman N, et al. Screening for Intimate Partner Violence, Elder Abuse, and Abuse of Vulnerable AdultsEvidence Report and Systematic Review for the US Preventive Services Task Force. *JAMA.* 2018;320(16):1688–1701. doi:10.1001/jama.2018.13212

Gracia E, López-Quílez A, Marco M, et al. The spatial epidemiology of intimate partner violence: Do neighborhoods matter? *Am J Epidemiol.* 2015;182:58.

Insel T. Mental health awareness month: By the numbers. https://www.nimh.nih.gov/about/directors/thomas-insel/blog/2015/mental-health-awareness-month-by-the-numbers.shtml. Published 2015.

Khalifeh H, Oram S, Trevillion K, et al. Recent intimate partner violence among people with chronic mental illness: findings from a national cross-sectional survey. *Br J Psychiatry.* 2015;207:207.

Kimerling R, Iverson KM, Dichter ME, et al. Prevalence of intimate partner violence among women veterans who utilize veterans health administration primary care. *J Gen Intern Med.* 2016;31:888.

Lehrer JA, Buka S, Gortmaker S, Shrier LA. Depressive symptomatology as a predictor of exposure to intimate partner violence among US female adolescents and young adults. *Arch Pediatr Adolesc Med.* 2006;160:270.

Ludermir AB, Lewis G, Valongueiro SA, et al. Violence against women by their intimate partner during pregnancy and postnatal depression: a prospective cohort study. *Lancet.* 2010;376:903.

McFarlane J, Malecha A, Watson K, et al. Intimate partner sexual assault against women: Frequency, health consequences, and treatment outcomes. *Obstet Gynecol.* 2005;105:99.

Moyer VA; U.S. Preventive Services Task Force. Screening for intimate partner violence and abuse of elderly and vulnerable adults: U.S. Preventive Services Task Force recommendation statement. *Ann Intern Med.* 2013;158(6):478–486.

O'Doherty L, Hegarty K, Ramsay J, Davidson L, Feder G, Taft A. Screening women for intimate partner violence in healthcare settings [review]. *Cochrane Database System Rev.* 2015;7:CD007007. doi:10.1002/14651858.CD007007.pub3

Reddy KS. Global Burden of Disease Study 2015 provides GPS for global health 2030. *Lancet.* 2016;388(10053):1447–1449.

Rees S, Silove D, Chey T, et al. Lifetime prevalence of gender-based violence in women and the relationship with mental disorders and psychosocial function. *JAMA.* 2011;306:513.

Roberts AL, Gilman SE, Fitzmaurice G, et al. Witness of intimate partner violence in childhood and perpetration of intimate partner violence in adulthood. *Epidemiology.* 2010;21:809.

Roberts AL, McLaughlin KA, Conron KJ, Koenen KC. Adulthood stressors, history of childhood adversity, and risk of perpetration of intimate partner violence. *Am J Prev Med.* 2011;40:128.

Sprague S, Madden K, Simunovic N, et al. Barriers to screening for intimate partner violence. *Women Health.* 2012;52:587.

Sugg N. Intimate partner violence: prevalence, health consequences, and intervention. *Med Clin North Am.* 2015;99:629–649.

Screening for intimate partner violence and abuse of vulnerable adults: U.S. Preventive Services Task Force recommendation. *Ann Intern Med.* 2013;158:1–28.

Sumner SA, Mercy JA, Dahlberg LL, et al. Violence in the United States: Status, challenges, and opportunities. *JAMA.* 2015;314:478–488.

Swailes AL, Lehman EB, McCall-Hosenfeld. Intimate partner violence discussions in the healthcare setting: A cross-sectional study. *Prev Med Rep.* 2017;8:215–220.

U.S. Preventative Task Force. Final recommendation statement: Depression in adults: Screening. https://www.uspreventiveservicestaskforce. org/Page/Document/RecommendationStatementFinal/depression-in-adults-screening1. Published 2016.

U.S. Preventive Services Task Force. Draft Update Summary: Intimate Partner Violence, Elder Abuse, and Abuse of Vulnerable Adults: Screening. https://www.uspreventiveservicestaskforce.org/Page/Document/UpdateSummaryDraft/intimate-partner-violence-and-abuse-of-elderly-and-vulnerable-adults-screening. Published May 2016.

Walker ER, McGee RE, Druss BG. Mortality in mental disorders and global disease burden implications. *JAMA Psychiatry.* 2015;72(4):334–341.

Wallace ME, Hoyert D, Williams C, Mendola P. Pregnancy-associated homicide and suicide in 37 US states with enhanced pregnancy surveillance. *Am J Obstet Gynecol.* 2016;215:364.e1–10.

World Health Organization. Responding to intimate partner violence and sexual violence against women: WHO clinical and policy guidelines. http://apps.who.int/iris/bitstream/10665/85240/1/9789241548595_eng.pdf. Published 2013.

World Health Organization. Responding to intimate partner violence and sexual violence against women (WHO Clinical and Policy Guidelines). http://www.who.int/reproductivehealth/publications/violence/9789241548595/en. Published 2013. Accessed August 29, 2013.

World Health Organization. Chapter 4: Violence by intimate partners. In *World Report on Violence and Health*. Geneva, Switzerland: World Health Organization. Retrieved from http://www.who.int/violence_injury_prevention/violence/global_campaign/en/chap4.pdf. Published 2002.

Substance Use Disorder

See Chapter 65 for references.

RESOURCES

General

Mental Health Statistics. National Institute of Mental Health. https://www.nimh.nih.gov/health/statistics/index.shtml

NIH Psychiatric Genomics Symposium. National Institutes of Health. https://videocast.nih.gov/Summary.asp?File=23388&bhcp=1

Anxiety

Advice for Parents of Children With Anxiety Disorders. Brain & Behaviour Research Foundation. https://www.bbrfoundation.org/blog/advice-parents-children-anxiety-disorders

Anxiety Disorders. National Alliance on Mental Illness. https://www.nami.org/Learn-More/Mental-Health-Conditions/Anxiety-Disorders/Overview

https://www.nimh.nih.gov/health/topics/anxiety-disorders/index.shtml

Generalized Anxiety Disorder: When Worry Gets Out of Control. National Institute of Mental Health https://www.nimh.nih.gov/health/publications/generalized-anxiety-disorder-gad/index.shtml

Panic Disorder: When Fear Overwhelms. National Institute of Mental Health. https://www.nimh.nih.gov/health/publications/panic-disorder-when-fear-overwhelms/index.shtml

Social Anxiety Disorder: More Than Just Shyness. National Institute of Mental Health https://www.nimh.nih.gov/health/publications/social-anxiety-disorder-more-than-just-shyness/index.shtml

Child Abuse

Child Development Positive Parenting Tips. (2017). Centers for Disease Control and Prevention. https://www.cdc.gov/ncbddd/childdevelopment/positiveparenting/index.html

Child Maltreatment. U.S. Department of Health & Human Services. https://www.acf.hhs.gov/cb/resource/child-maltreatment-2016

Child Welfare Information Gateway. U.S. Department of Health & Human Services. https://www.childwelfare.gov/

Children Benefit When Parents Have Safe, Stable, Nurturing Relationships. Centers for Disease Control and Prevention/National Center for Injury Prevention and Control. https://www.cdc.gov/violenceprevention/pdf/SSNRs-for-Parents.pdf

Preventing Child Abuse and Neglect: A Technical Package for Policy, Norm, and Programmatic Activities. Centers for Disease Control and Prevention/National Center for Injury Prevention and Control. https://www.cdc.gov/violenceprevention/pdf/CAN-Prevention-Technical-Package.pdf

Depression

Adult Depression in Primary Care. U.S. Department of Health and Human Services/Agency for Healthcare Research and Quality. https://www.guideline.gov/summaries/summary/50406?

Depression. National Institute of Mental Health (NIMH). https://www.nimh.nih.gov/health/topics/depression/index.shtml#part_145398

Depression Basics. National Institute of Mental Health (NIMH). https://www.nimh.nih.gov/health/publications/depression/index.shtml

Depression in Adults: Screening (2016). U.S. Preventative Services Task Force. https://www.uspreventiveservicestaskforce.org/Page/Document/UpdateSummaryFinal/depression-in-adults-screening1

Depression in Children and Adolescents: Screening (2016). U.S. Preventative Services Task Force. https://www.uspreventiveservicestaskforce.org/Page/Document/UpdateSummaryFinal/depression-in-children-and-adolescents-screening1

Depression in Women. National Institute of Mental Health (NIMH). https://www.nimh.nih.gov/health/publications/depression-in-women/index.shtml

Depression: What You Need to Know. National Institute of Mental Health (NIMH). https://www.nimh.nih.gov/health/publications/depression-what-you-need-to-know/index.shtml

Final Recommendation: Depression in Adults: Screening. U.S. Department of Health and Human Services/Agency for Healthcare Research and Quality
> https://www.guideline.gov/summaries/summary/49978?

Men and Depression. National Institute of Mental Health (NIMH)
> https://www.nimh.nih.gov/health/publications/men-and-depression/index.shtml

Non-pharmacological Versus Pharmacological Treatment of Adults With MDD. U.S. Department of Health and Human Services/Agency for Healthcare Research and Quality.
> https://www.guideline.gov/summaries/summary/50075?

Older Adults & Depression. National Institute of Mental Health (NIMH)
> https://www.nimh.nih.gov/health/publications/older-adults-and-depression/index.shtml

Suicide Risk in Adolescents, Adults, and Older Adults: Screening (May, 2014). U.S. Preventative Services Task Force.
> https://www.uspreventiveservicestaskforce.org/Page/Document/UpdateSummaryFinal/suicide-risk-in-adolescents-adults-and-older-adults-screening

Teen Depression. National Institute of Mental Health (NIMH)
> https://www.nimh.nih.gov/health/publications/teen-depression/index.shtml

VA/DoD Clinical Practice Guideline for the Management of Major Depressive Disorder (2016). Department of Veterans Affairs and Department of Defense
> https://www.healthquality.va.gov/guidelines/MH/mdd/MDDCPGClinicianSummaryFINAL1.pdf

VA/DoD/Pocket Card (April, 2016). Department of Veterans Affairs and Department of Defense.
> https://www.healthquality.va.gov/guidelines/MH/mdd/MDDCPGPocketcardFINAL1.pdf

Domestic Assault-Intimate Partner Violence (IPV)

Dating Matters: Strategies to Promote Healthy Teen Relationships. Centers for Disease Control and Prevention/Division of Violence Prevention
> https://www.cdc.gov/violenceprevention/pdf/DatingMatters_flyer-a.pdf

Domestic Violence. American Academy of Family Physicians
> https://familydoctor.org/domestic-violence-protecting-yourself-and-your-children/

Domestic Violence Against Men. Mayo Clinic
> https://www.mayoclinic.org/healthy-lifestyle/adult-health/in-depth/domestic-violence-against-men/art-20045149?p=1

Domestic Violence: Threat for Women. Mayo Clinic
> https://www.mayoclinic.org/healthy-lifestyle/adult-health/in-depth/domestic-violence/art-20048397?p=1

Evaluating What Works for Victims and Offenders: The Domestic Violence Homicide Prevention Demonstration Initiative. National Institute of Justice.
> https://www.nij.gov/topics/crime/intimate-partner-violence/Pages/evaluation-of-domestic-violence-homicide-prevention-demonstration-initiative.aspx

Family Context Is an Important Element in the Development of Teen Dating Violence and Should Be Considered in Prevention and Intervention (2017). National Institute of Justice.
> https://www.nij.gov/topics/crime/intimate-partner-violence/teen-dating-violence/Pages/family-context-in-development-of-teen-dating-violence.aspx

Intimate Partner Violence. SAMHSA-HRSA for Integrated Health Solutions
> https://www.integration.samhsa.gov/clinical-practice/intimate-partner-violence

Intimate Partner Violence and Sexual Violence Victimization Assessment Instruments for Use in Healthcare Setting. Centers for Disease Control and Prevention/Division of Violence Prevention
> https://www.cdc.gov/violenceprevention/pdf/ipv/ipvandsvscreening.pdf

Intimate Partner Violence Screening & Counselling: Research Symposium (2013). U.S. Department of Health and Human Services/Office of Women's Health.
> https://sis.nlm.nih.gov/outreach/2013ipv/IPV%20screening%20bibliography.pdf

Intimate Partner Violence, Sexual Violence and Stalking (2010-2012). Centers for Disease Control and Prevention/Division of Violence Prevention.
> https://www.cdc.gov/violenceprevention/pdf/NISVS-infographic-2016.pdf

IPV Web site. IPV Health Partners.
> http://ipvhealthpartners.org/

NSVRC Home Page. National Sexual Violence Resource Center (NSVRC).
> https://www.nsvrc.org/

Preventing Intimate Partner Violence Across the Lifespan (2017). Centers for Disease Control and Prevention/Division of Violence Prevention.
> https://www.cdc.gov/violenceprevention/pdf/ipv-technicalpackages.pdf

Protecting Students From Sexual Assault. National Institute of Justice
> https://www.justice.gov/ovw/protecting-students-sexual-assault

Risks in Adolescence That Lead to Intimate Partner Violence in Young Adulthood (2017). National Institute of Justice.
> https://www.nij.gov/topics/crime/intimate-partner-violence/Pages/risks-in-adolescence-that-lead-to-intimate-partner-violence-in-young-adulthood.aspx

Talking Points: NISVS State Report. Centers for Disease Control and Prevention

Division of Violence Prevention.
> https://www.nsvrc.org/sites/default/files/nsvrc_publications_talking-points-nisvs_state_report_0.pdf

National Intimate Partner and Sexual Violence Survey. 2010-2010 State Survey (April, 2017). Centers for Disease Control and Prevention/Division of Violence Prevention
> https://www.cdc.gov/violenceprevention/pdf/NISVS-StateReportBook.pdf

Elder Abuse

Elder Abuse. National Institute on Aging (NIH).
> https://www.nia.nih.gov/health/elder-abuse#caregiver

Elder Abuse & Neglect. HelpGuide.org
> https://www.helpguide.org/articles/abuse/elder-abuse-and-neglect.htm

Elder Abuse: Risk and Protective Factors. Centers for Disease Control & Prevention (CDC).
> https://www.cdc.gov/violenceprevention/elderabuse/riskprotectivefactors.html

NCEA: What We Do. National Center on Elder Abuse (NCEA).
> https://ncea.acl.gov/whatwedo/practice/prevention-strategies.html

Grief

Aging With Dignity. Five Wishes.
> https://agingwithdignity.org/

American Hospice Foundation
   https://americanhospice.org/
Coping With Loss of Your Loved One. American Psychological Association.
   http://www.apa.org/helpcenter/grief.aspx
Elizabeth Kübler-Ross Foundation
   http://www.ekrfoundation.org/
Five Stages of Grief
   https://grief.com/the-five-stages-of-grief/
National Hospice & Palliative Care Organization.
   https://www.nhpco.org/
Supporting Someone Who Is Grieving. National Hospice & Palliative Care Organization.
   http://www.caringinfo.org/files/public/brochures/Supporting_Someone_Who_is_Grieving.pdf

The Grieving Process. American Cancer Society.
   https://www.cancer.org/treatment/end-of-life-care/grief-and-loss/grieving-process.html
There Is No Right or Wrong Way to Grieve After Loss. National Hospice & Palliative Care Organization.
   http://www.caringinfo.org/files/public/brochures/There_is_no_Wrong_or_Right_Way_to_Grieve_After_a_Loss.pdf
What Is Grief? Mayo Clinic.
   https://www.mayoclinic.org/patient-visitor-guide/support-groups/what-is-grief

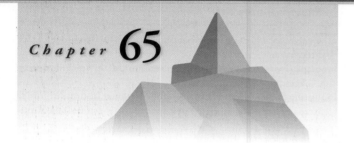

Chapter **65**

Substance Use Disorders

Cesar Benarroche, MD

Lynne M. Dunphy, PhD, APRN, FNP-BC, FAAN, FAANP

Dianne M. Loomis, DNP, APRN, FNP-BC

Kim S. Griswold, MD, MPH, AS, RN

Patricia A. Pastore, MS, APRN, FNP-BC

The fifth edition of the *Diagnostic and Statistical Manual of Mental Disorders (DSM-5)* replaced the term *addiction* with the term *substance use disorder (SUD)*. The core features of SUDs include a triad of behavioral, physiological, and cognitive symptoms. A basic understanding of several terms is essential. Soon after consuming an agent, *intoxication* occurs. This process is considered reversible; as the effect of the substance wears off, a return to baseline generally occurs. Intoxication can occur in individuals without an SUD as well as in individuals with an SUD. Several symptoms of intoxication include impaired judgment, psychomotor and interpersonal behavioral changes, and alertness. Substance *withdrawal* is characterized by functional impairment related to the cessation or reduction of a substance, which is demonstrated in physiological, cognitive, and behavioral symptoms.

Use is defined as sporadic or intermittent utilization of alcohol or drugs with no adverse consequences. *Abuse* is defined as utilization of drugs or alcohol that causes the user some type of adverse consequence. *Dependence* involves physiological and/or psychological components. *Physical dependence* refers to the physiological effects of withdrawal from rapid dose reduction, abrupt cessation of the drug, or administration of an antagonist. *Psychological* or *behavioral dependence* emphasizes pathological use patterns and substance-seeking activities; it is a subjective need for the substance. *SUD* is a chronic illness characterized by impaired control, social impairment, and use despite significant consequences, tolerance, and withdrawal.

The risk of SUD is directly related to the properties of the drug of choice, such as availability, cost, how quickly the brain perceives the substance, and its ability to produce gratification or pleasure, as well as various environmental factors. A person may initially consume a drug for any number of reasons. However, people continue using a drug based on the actual or perceived rewards of substance use. Denial and rationalization of substance use, substance effects, or consequences of substance use make it possible for an individual to continue to use a substance as though he or she is immune to unexpected or dangerous consequences. The current opioid epidemic with skyrocketing death rates bears witness to this sad fact. Substance-related disorders that may be seen in a primary-care setting and that are included in this chapter are nicotine, alcohol, cannabis, hallucinogen, inhalant, opioid, sedative and hypnotic, and stimulant disorders. In many instances patients may have multiple addictions. Caffeine is discussed in the intoxication and withdrawal section.

EPIDEMIOLOGY AND CAUSES

The highest prevalence rates for substance use occur in persons aged 18 to 24 years. In 2016, 24.6% of adults in the United States reported tobacco use, a slight decline from 2012 statistics. Tobacco use is the leading preventable cause of death and disability. The total direct and indirect costs incurred by the United States are nearly $200 billion annually. Nicotine and tobacco contribute to deaths from cancer, heart and lung disease, and infant mortality attributable to maternal smoking. More than 31% (129.47 million) of persons aged 12 and older reported current alcohol use (one or more drink in the past month). Alcohol remains the primary substance of abuse and dependence; 15.1 million persons are dependent on or abuse alcohol alone, a slight increase from the 2012 survey; 2.8 million persons are dependent on or abuse alcohol plus illicit drugs. Illicit drugs are defined as including prescription drugs used for off-prescription purposes—for example, opioids who were prescribed but are used by someone else or are used by a person for other than what prescribed. For persons aged 12 years and older, 28.6 million persons had utilized an illicit substance in the previous month (SAMHSA, 2016). Current illicit drug use among persons aged 12 years and older increased from 8.1% in 2008 to 10.6% in 2016 (SAMHSA, 2016). Substance use is estimated at 7.5% (20.1 million) persons aged 12 or older. The total annual cost to society of substance use problems is estimated at almost $740 billion in health-care costs, loss of productivity, and crime-related costs annually (National Institute on Drug Abuse [NIDA], 2017).

The survey further identified that male sex, ethnicity, and education level seem to correlate with current alcohol use. Caucasians (56.3%) followed by individuals belonging to more than two races (47.3%) reported the highest alcohol use. The rates of alcohol use for other groups, in declining order, were as follows: Hispanics 42.5%, African Americans 41.7%, Asians 35.5%, and American Indians or Native Alaskans 34.4%. With increasing levels of education in adults age 18 or older, alcohol use increased; in addition, among adults with less than 12 years of education only 32.7% currently used alcohol versus 67.0% of college graduates. College students were more likely to use alcohol, binge drink, and drink heavily than their peers who were not full-time students and those not in college; these rates have remained stable for some time (see Table 65.1).

Binge alcohol use peaks in 18- to 25-year-olds with rates of 38.4%. More men aged 18 to 25 years 56% (62.9% of males) reported alcohol use than women (55%). Increased volume of alcohol consumption correlates with increased use of illicit substances and tobacco use, as well as traffic-related fatalities. In 2016, 10,497 people died in alcohol-impaired driving crashes, accounting for 28% of all traffic-related

TABLE 65.1   Prevalence of Drinking, Binge Drinking, and Heavy Drinking in the Past Month Among College and Students

Adults Aged 18–22	Drinking	Binge Drinking	Heavy Drinking
College students	50%	37.9%	12.5%
Non college students	48.2%	32.6%	8.5%

Source: Substance Abuse and Mental Health Services Administration, 2015.

deaths in the United States (National Highway Traffic Safety Administration, 2016). Self-reported drinking and driving has declined since it peaked in 2006 with 161 million compared with 111 million in 2014 (CDC, 2018). Underage drinking (aged 12–20) is of particular concern, with current drinking rates estimated to be 9.3 million persons. These values have slowly declined over the past 10 years.

Several recent studies have raised the alarm about rises in alcohol use disorders (AUDs), especially in woman, older adults, and minorities. Grant et al. (2017) documented that drinking in older adults and women and minorities of all ages is on the rise. One large-scale epidemiologic study from the National Institute of Alcohol Abuse and Alcoholism comparing survey data from 2001–2002 and 2012–2013 documented alarming increases in alcohol use (11.2%), high-risk drinking (29.9%), and alcohol dependence or abuse (49.4%). Women specifically had increases in use (15.8%), high-risk drinking (57.9%), and dependence or abuse (83.7%), as well as older adults (over 65), with use increasing 22.4%, high-risk drinking increasing 65.2%, and alcohol dependence and abuse increasing 106.7%, respectively, double that of the general population. Every racial and ethnic group in this study had increases in the prevalence of use, high-risk drinking, and alcohol dependence and abuse. Taken altogether, these statistics document that millions more Americans are using and abusing alcohol, constituting a true public health crisis. The incidence of drinking among women especially has also increased worldwide (Slade et al., 2016). In 2010 it was documented that alcohol-related problems cost the United States more than $250 billion per year. It is clear these dollar costs will also increase with increased use and abuse (Schuckit, 2017).

Despite the increases in both use of many of these substances and associated mortality, alcohol and drug use disorders continue to be undertreated. According to the 2012–2013 National Epidemiologic Survey on Alcohol and Related Conditions III, only 19.8% of respondents with lifetime AUD were ever treated for their disorder. Many individuals who are untreated identify stigma as a major barrier.

Marijuana is now legal in some states, and the trend appears to be toward more widespread legalization. Marijuana's current use increased from 5.8% to 8.9% from

2007 to 2016. It is estimated that 4.3 million persons aged 12 years or older were classified having a marijuana use disorder meaning dependent on or an abuser of marijuana. Additionally, 2.1 million persons aged 12 years and older were classified as dependent on or an abuser of prescription drugs such as pain relievers; and 867,000 million persons were classified as dependent on or an abuser of cocaine (Substance Abuse and Mental Health Services Administration, 2016).

Age is a factor in substance use disorders. In youth aged 12 to 17 years, concurrent use of illicit substances was greater in those who used tobacco or alcohol. The rate for substance use disorder is highest for adults aged 18 to 25 years at nearly 15.1%, compared with youth aged 12 to 17 years at 4.3% and adults older than age 26 years at 6.6%. In addition, rates of nonmedical use (off-label) of prescription drugs increased from 4.1% to 4.6% in young adults aged 18 to 25 years. In adults aged 26 to 59 years, there has been a gradual increase in illicit use, with marijuana and nonmedical (off-label) use of prescription drugs being the most prevalent. Some of this increase is suspected to be related to the aging baby boomers, who are known to have had increased exposure. Research in those over age 65 for marijuana and illicit drugs is not as well documented. If it mirrors increases in alcohol use and abuse, it would be frightening, and all primary-care providers should maintain a high index of suspicion for drug use and abuse in all ages and both sexes. Male sex, ethnicity, education, employment status, and criminal justice population correlate overall with illicit substance use. In summary, national statistics indicate that the most commonly used legal substances are caffeine, alcohol, and nicotine; the most commonly used illegal substances are marijuana, prescription pain relievers used for off-label reasons, and cocaine.

Comorbidities (also known as "dual diagnosis") are common in persons with substance abuse. The most common comorbidities are substance abuse with more than one substance and mood disorders including bipolar disorder, anxiety disorders, antisocial personality, and schizophrenia. People who abuse substances are about 20 times more likely to die from suicide than are those in the general population. About 15% of people with alcohol abuse or dependency commit suicide. The frequency of suicide among individuals in this group is second only to that among patients with major depression; many individuals with alcohol abuse or dependency may have underlying depression, further increasing their suicide risk.

Different population-based causes for substance use have been described. As with all psychiatric disorders, the initial causative theories evolved from psychodynamic models; subsequent models include behavioral, genetic, and neurochemical explanations. According to one NIDA survey, family transmission is a core risk factor for substance abuse. Both social learning and genetic models have been developed to explain the increased risk and incidence of substance abuse in the children of substance-abusing parents. Compared with earlier generations, however, Americans today are more likely to seek the immediate gratification and immediate solutions offered by drugs.

PATHOPHYSIOLOGY

Controversy continues to surround the disease concept of addiction despite compelling scientific evidence, and acceptance by the public, largely due to the recovery movement in the treatment community (Alcoholics Anonymous [AA], Narcotics Anonymous [NA]), that addiction is a disease. Nonetheless, some legal experts and criminologists view the use and abuse of drugs as intentional acts related to a lack of self-restraint and willpower (Wilbanks, 1989). Philosopher Herbert Fingarette (1988), for example, maintains that the "disease" model, fundamentally reductionistic, is a myth, and limits treatment options, individual autonomy, and self-efficacy. Peele (1985) provides a useful distinction for thinking about various disease models. The *susceptibility* variant emphasizes that genetic factors play an important role in the development of substance dependence, influencing the individual's vulnerability. In contrast, the *exposure* construct holds that chemicals and their actions on the brain are the primary causes of addiction. These are not in conflict; they simply represent different emphasis.

The disease model espoused by AA stresses the importance of spirituality in the etiology of, and recovery from, alcoholism, for example. In contrast, the medical community tends to point to the significance of biological factors: genetic *susceptibility* and brain abnormalities from substance *exposure*.

There is increasing understanding that genetics *and* the environment interact in an individual. There is strong evidence of familial transmission based on a confluence of both genetic and psychosocial pathways. The inherited characteristic is not a disease but a predisposition, or *susceptibility*. There is not one specific gene that "causes" addiction; rather addiction is a complex disorder influenced by many factors. Indeed, it may be discovered some day that some genetic factors may ultimately prove protective against certain addictions. Recognition of genetic risk factors does not require that alcoholism and drug dependencies be defined as disease states. A wide range of human traits are influenced by genetics, including physical endurance. An often repeated saying sums this up with the adage that genetics "loads" the gun; lifestyle pulls the trigger.

One characteristic that all commonly abused drugs share is their ability to stimulate reward centers in the brain. Anatomical pathways, neurotransmitter dysregulation, and imbalance and neuroadaptation are important neurophysiological components of addiction. These dopaminergic pathways in the brain are believed to be essential for the feelings of pleasure, reward, motivation, and incentive salience (whereby exposure to a stimulus is transformed from a pure sensory experience to one that brings it to the forefront of consciousness and causes it to be sought out). Recent brain imaging studies of addicted individuals confirm underlying disruption to these brain regions that are important in motivation, reward, and pleasure. In addition, this area is essential for learning and memory, executive decision-making, and behavior control. This documents the effects of drugs on brain structure and function, or the *exposure* model of addiction.

All addictive substances/behaviors involve increases in dopamine levels in the mesolimbic dopamine system, the reward system of the brain. The ventral tegmental area, located at the origin of the mesolimbic dopamine system, consists of gamma-aminobutyric acid (GABA) interneurons, and dopamine and glutamate neurons. When a "drug"—a substance or a behavior—binds GABA receptors on GABA interneurons, they decrease the release of GABA onto dopamine neurons. This lowers the inhibitory effect of GABA interneurons on dopamine neurons, leading to increased dopamine transmission, a process called "disinhibition." Drugs and behaviors bind a pocket between the alpha and gamma subunits on GABAA receptors, and the alpha-1 subunit isoform and are believed to be responsible for addictive behavior. GABAA receptors with the alpha-1 subunit are abundant in GABA interneurons in the ventral tegmental area of mice.

Addictive drugs can cause long-lasting changes to the reward system. Synaptic plasticity, or changes in synaptic strength determined by prior synaptic activity, is thought to underlie learning and memory processes. Early in this process, alpha-amino-3-hydroxy-5-methyl-4-isoxazole propionic acid (AMPA) receptors move from the interior to the surface of dopamine neurons, which leads to greater susceptibility to be stimulated by the excitatory neurotransmitter glutamate. Because of the AMPA receptor migration, future use of addictive drugs can lead to even greater dopamine transmission. The majority of genetic risk factors for substance use disorder is believed to be non–substance specific and thus shared among different substances. In two twin studies, genetic influences were shared across multiple substances including sedatives, cannabis, and stimulants and not specific to substance. Twin studies also suggest that the majority of environmental risk factors for substance use disorders shared between twin pairs, such as family environment, is not specific to substance. Tolerance and dependence are believed to be related to the alteration of the neurochemical pathways, as well as overall cellular changes of the brain. This process of neuroadaptation can be persistent and permanent. These changes affect how the brain functions and have been the focus of research to describe the compulsive and harmful effects of addiction.

Deleterious effects are seen in all individuals exposed to substance use. In infants exposed in utero, prematurity and developmental issues are seen; adolescents demonstrate poor school performance and high dropout rates, as well as an increased risk of violence, infectious diseases, and in the case of opioid usage, death. Further, adults demonstrate poor concentration, coping, and interpersonal skills, which adversely affect employment, family dynamics, and parenting. Current knowledge helps to identify the differences in the brains of those with addiction and those without addiction. This ongoing research and understandings of neurobiology has helped to provide targeted treatments, often referred to as medically assistive therapy (MAT), for specific disorders. There is increased understanding that addiction is a chronic, in most cases, progressive, and frequently relapsing disease, warranting management more similar to treatment of physical diseases such as hypertension and diabetes and require systematic and longitudinal care.

CLINICAL PRESENTATION

Patients who ask questions about their personal substance use may have used substances for a relatively short period of time; more often, however, patient questions are motivated by having recently suffered negative consequences from long-standing substance use. Routine substance use and abuse screening have become a standard of practice in primary care. The most consistent identifier for substance abuse may be the numerous health consequences of abusing drugs and alcohol. Personal characteristics are not reliable indicators. Persons of all ages, races, religions, and every socioeconomic status are susceptible to substance abuse, and substance dependence typically follows substance abuse.

The clinical presentation of a person with substance intoxication, abuse, or withdrawal will vary depending on the substance abused. Box 65.1 presents a summary of the clinical presentation of an individual with cannabis, cocaine, stimulant, nicotine, caffeine, or alcohol intoxication and withdrawal.

DIAGNOSTIC REASONING

Symptoms

The *DSM-5* divides the substance-related disorders into two groups: *substance use disorders* (those pathological behaviors associated with substance-seeking activities) and *substance-induced disorders* (intoxication, withdrawal, and mental disorders caused by a medication or a substance). Substance use disorders are marked by continual use of a substance despite significant related problems. Patients develop a tolerance for the substance and require progressively greater amounts to elicit the effects desired. In addition, patients experience physical and psychological signs and symptoms of withdrawal if the agent is not used. They are classified as mild (two to three symptoms),

Box 65.1   Clinical Presentation: Selected Substance Intoxication and Withdrawal

Cannabis-Related Disorders

- *Cannabis Intoxication:* Intoxication typically includes euphoria, alterations in mood and judgment, and changes in sensory perception, cognition, and coordination. Driving and machine-operating skills may be impaired.
- *Cannabis Withdrawal:* Transient symptoms occur on withdrawal, usually within 1 week of stopping after prolonged use, and include irritability, cravings, anxiety, sleep problems, and decreased appetite.

Stimulant-Related Disorders

- *Stimulant Intoxication:* Symptoms include euphoria; increased wakefulness; decreased appetite; and increased breathing, heart rate, blood pressure, and body temperature.
- *Stimulant Withdrawal:* Symptoms occur within hours or days of last use and include severe depression, anxiety, fatigue, psychosis, and intense craving for the drug. Experienced heavy users may plan their drug use to include substances that can prevent or minimize withdrawal.

Tobacco-Related Disorders

- *Tobacco Intoxication:* No characteristics for intoxication.
- *Tobacco Withdrawal:* Cessation of daily tobacco use produces symptoms within 24 hours. Withdrawal symptoms include intense cravings, depressed mood, sleep problems, impaired concentration, anxiety, increased appetite, and irritability.

Hallucinogen-Related Disorders

- *Phencyclidine or Other Hallucinogen Intoxication:* Several behavioral symptoms occur shortly after use of phencyclidine, including hallucinations, delusions, paranoia, and a sense of being outside one's body. For other hallucinogens, symptoms include rapid mood swings and inability to think rationally, communicate with others, or recognize reality. Physical symptoms include increased heart rate, body temperature, and blood pressure; dizziness, loss of appetite, tremors, pupil enlargement.

- *Phencyclidine or Other Hallucinogen Withdrawal:* There are no established withdrawal symptoms.

Inhalant-Related Disorders

- *Inhalant Intoxication:* Intoxication can include confusion, nausea, slurred speech, lack of coordination, euphoria, dizziness and lightheaded, drowsiness, lack of inhibition, delusions or hallucinations, and headache.
- *Inhalant Withdrawal:* Generally mild; not recognized as a specific disorder.

Opioid-Related Disorders

- *Opioid Intoxication:* Intoxication typically includes a sudden change in behavior, which can include euphoria, drowsiness, confusion, nausea, and slowed breathing. Constipation is a commonly recognized side effect of opioid use.
- *Opioid Withdrawal:* Withdrawal symptoms include muscle and bone pain, sleep disturbances, nausea and diarrhea, and intense cravings.

Sedative, Hypnotic, or Anxiolytic Disorders

- *Sedative, Hypnotic, or Anxiolytic Intoxication:* Symptoms include slurred speech, confusion, trouble concentrating, dry mouth, decreased blood pressure and breathing rate, dizziness and lightheadedness, headache, and slowed movements and thinking.
- *Sedative, Hypnotic, or Anxiolytic Withdrawal:* Symptoms may include seizures; shakiness; trouble sleeping; agitation; increased heart rate, blood pressure, and body temperature accompanied by sweating; hyperreflexia, and intense cravings.

Caffeine-Related Disorders

- *Caffeine Intoxication:* Symptoms include increased alertness and muscle movements, increased urination, sleeplessness, increased heart rate, and sweating.
- *Caffeine Withdrawal:* Suddenly stopping or reducing daily caffeine use may cause withdrawal symptoms within 12-24 hours, which may include fatigue, headache, and insomnia.

Sources: Substance Abuse and Mental Health Services Administration (SAMHSA). Join the Voices for Recovery. Commonly misused substances. https://recoverymonth.gov/sites/default/files/toolkit/recovery_month_2018_full_toolkit.pdf; National Institute on Drug Abuse (NIDA). DrugFacts. 2016-2018. https://www.drugabuse.gov/publications/finder/t/160/DrugFacts; National Institute on Drug Abuse for Teens. Is caffeine really addictive? 2016. https://teens.drugabuse.gov/blog/post/caffeine-really-addictive

moderate (four to five symptoms), or severe (six or more symptoms). See the *DSM-5* for the complete diagnostic criteria.

The existence and prevalence of significant comorbidities may make the "primary" disorder difficult to identify. However, it is always necessary to concurrently treat the substance use and dependence issues, regardless of the comorbidity. Evidence shows that unless the comorbid condition is also addressed and treated, recurrence of the substance use is likely.

Differential Diagnosis

Opioid Use Disorders

Opioid use disorders (OUD) include (1) opioid abuse, (2) opioid dependence, and (3) opioid use. OUD is also categorized as *mild, moderate,* or *severe.* In 1997, the United States became one of only two developed countries in the world that made it legal for pharmaceutical companies to advertise drugs directly to consumers, including children. Evidence shows that the opioid epidemic of the last 12 years is a particularly American phenomenon (Shipton et al., 2018). Since then prescription drug addiction and prescription drug overdoses have skyrocketed. Drug overdose is now the leading cause of accidental death in the United States. Since 2000, deaths from opioid overdoses have nearly quadrupled overall. This problem is not only affecting the young. Opioid overdose deaths have seen an eightfold increase in those aged 55 to 64; ages 65 to 74 have seen a sevenfold increase. Four out of five people who become addicted to heroin start out with a legal prescription from a licensed prescriber—a result of injury, chronic pain like arthritis, postoperative care, or a medical procedure. Substance-abuse disorders affect 20.8 million people in the United States—as many as those with diabetes and 1.5 times as many as those with cancer. Yet only 1 in 10 people receives treatment. Opioids—prescription and illicit—are the main driver of drug overdose deaths. Opioids were involved in 42,249 deaths in 2016, and opioid overdose deaths were five times higher in 2016 than 1999. In 2016, the five states with the highest rates of death due to drug overdose were West Virginia (52.0 per 100,000), Ohio (39.1 per 100,000), New Hampshire (39.0 per 100,000), Pennsylvania (37.9 per 100,000), and (Kentucky (33.5 per 100,000) (CDC, 2017).

Opioid abuse can include both prescription and/or illicit drugs such as heroin, and combinations thereof. Indeed, this current epidemic is blamed on overprescription of opioids, as well as oversupply and production. Drug manufacturers chose to provide a cheaper form of certain opioid pills that could be crushed and then injected. The most frequent drugs of abuse include hydrocodone, fentanyl, oxycodone, oxymorphone, morphine, and methadone.

Opioids can both relieve pain and cause euphoria. The pain relief effect of opioids is achieved by the drug attaching to the opioid receptor and thus blocking the subjective feeling of pain. Particular populations at risk for prescription opioid abuse include women, adolescents and young adults, and older adults. In the 1990s, attention to adequate pain management had become recognized as the standard of care. It is the clinician's responsibility to adequately evaluate, assess, and prescribe appropriate therapy for pain. This can be a daunting task in primary care. Several strategies may be helpful. Current guidelines are available from the CDC in dealing with chronic nonmalignant pain. It is critically important for all providers to be aware of these prescribing guidelines. Overprescribing leads to addiction, which often leads to escalating use, overdose, and unexpected death.

Heroin (also known as smack, H, ska, junk) abuse results in significant costs related to medical care, criminal justice, and lost productivity; it is estimated to cost the United States billions of dollars annually. Heroin can be injected, snorted, or smoked. The opioid crisis continues to grow worse, in part because new types of drugs are finding their way onto the streets. Fentanyl, heroin's synthetic cousin, is among the worst offenders. According to the CDC, fentanyl is up to 100 times more potent than morphine and many times more than heroin. Drugs users generally do not know when their heroin is laced with fentanyl or fentanyl analogues, so when they inject their usual quantity of heroin, they can inadvertently take a deadly dose of another substance. In addition, although dealers may try to include these substances to improve potency, their measuring equipment usually is not fine-tuned enough to ensure they stay below the levels that could cause users to overdose. The fentanyl and like substances sold on the street are almost always made in a clandestine lab; it is less pure than the pharmaceutical version, and thus its effect on the body can be more unpredictable. Heroin and fentanyl may look identical; with drugs purchased on the street, users often do not know what they are taking. In a PBS Newshour segment from 2016 on the opioid crisis in the New England states, Tim Pifer, the director of the New Hampshire State Police Forensic Laboratory, is quoted stating "You're injecting yourself with a loaded gun."

On July 11, 2018, the CDC issued an official CDC Health Update regarding a dramatic rise in the supply of illicitly manufactured fentanyl and fentanyl analogs, as well as an equally dramatic rise in deaths involving synthetic opioids other than methadone. The rate of synthetic opioid overdose deaths in the U.S. rose from 3.1 to 6.2 deaths per 100,000 between 2015 and 2016, marking the first year that synthetic opioids became the most common type of opioid involved in all opioid overdose deaths (CDC, 2018). The National Center for Health Statistics indicated that more than 55% of opioid overdose deaths (27,000 overdose deaths) involved synthetic opioids, exceeding the number of *all* opioid deaths in 2013 (NCHS, 2017).

Medical issues related to heroin use involve HIV/AIDS, hepatitis B and C, and tuberculosis, to name a few; social issues involve justice issues, interference with education and employment, and significant family distress. Neonatal issues such as low birth weight and abstinence (withdrawal) symptoms can be addressed during pregnancy, with the mother receiving prenatal care in addition to comprehensive drug treatment and methadone maintenance.

Traditional rehabilitation measures have proven spectacularly unsuccessful in dealing with moderate to severe OUD, with people going to "rehab" as many as 30 times and continuing to relapse. "Rehabilitation mills" have proliferated, especially in places like Florida, reimbursement may be available, or families may self-pay any price to save their family member. There has been increasing recognition in the rehab community about the benefits of pharmacological treatment, known as medication-assisted therapy (MAT), that uses buprenorphine/naloxone or methadone in a supervised treatment program administered either in an outpatient or inpatient setting. There is insufficient evidence to recommend for or against most psychosocial interventions in the case of OUD (Department of Veteran Affairs, 2015).

Nicotine Dependence

Nicotine is the addictive substance in tobacco and is present in cigarettes, cigars, chewing tobacco, pipes, and snuff. This topic is covered in detail in Chapter 33, "Smoking Addiction."

A new "delivery model" for nicotine was introduced to the mass market in the United States in 2007 in the form of e-cigarettes. E-cigarettes do not produce tobacco smoke but rather an aerosol, which actually consists of fine particles and often is mistaken for water vapor. The term "vaping" is the act of inhaling and exhaling this aerosol, or vapor, produced by an e-cigarette or similar device. E-cigarettes, which resemble smoked cigarettes, and "vape" pens, which resemble large fountain pens, have become increasingly popular. Vaping devices include not just e-cigarettes but also vape pens and advanced personal vaporizers (also known as "MODS").

Generally, a vaping device consists of a mouthpiece, a battery, a cartridge for containing the e-liquid or e-juice, and a heating component for the device that is powered by a battery. When the device is used, the battery heats up the heating component, which turns the contents of the e-liquid into an aerosol that is inhaled into the lungs and then exhaled. The e-liquid in vaporizer products usually contains a propylene glycol or vegetable glycerin-based liquid with nicotine, flavoring, and other chemicals and metals, but not tobacco. Some people use these devices to vape THC, the chemical responsible for most of marijuana's mind-altering effects, or even synthetic drugs such as flakka, instead of nicotine. The health risks and benefits of using these relatively new devices are still being evaluated. However, there is a growing body of evidence indicating that the chemicals in these products may be dangerous. Health advocates are recommending caution in using them and calling for additional research into their potential risks versus benefits.

According to NIDA (2017), nearly one in three students in 12th grade reported use of some kind of vaping device in the past year, raising concerns about the impact on their health. What is in the device ranges from nicotine, to marijuana, to "just flavoring." The use of hookahs and regular cigarettes continues to decline. The survey indicated that 51.8% of the students said it was "just flavoring" that they "vaped," 32.8% said "nicotine," and 11.1% said marijuana. As first-time nicotine users, there is a risk that these young people may begin to smoke regular cigarettes.

In 2017, 79.8% of eighth graders reported that they disapproved of regularly vaping nicotine, declining in 12th graders to 71.8%. Only 14.1% of 12th graders see great risk in marijuana smoking according to this survey,

down from 17.1% the year before and down from a staggering 40.6% rate of disapproval in 1991. Twenty-three percent of 10th graders reported that it was "easy" to get tranquillizers, up from 20.5% the year before.

Alcohol-Related Disorders

Problem drinking that becomes severe is given the medical diagnosis of alcohol use disorder (AUD). AUD is a chronic relapsing progressive brain disease characterized by compulsive alcohol use, loss of control over alcohol intake, and a negative emotional state when not using. Alcohol use disorder includes (1) alcohol abuse and (2) alcohol dependence. It is also classified as mild, moderate, and severe. It is characterized by a problematic pattern of alcohol use, leading to clinically significant impairment or distress, as manifested by multiple psychosocial, behavioral, or physiological features. An estimated 16 million people in the United States have AUD. Approximately 6.2% or 15.1 million adults in the United States aged 18 and older had AUD in 2015. This includes 9.8 million men and 5.3 million women. Adolescents can be diagnosed with AUD as well, and in 2015, an estimated 623,000 adolescents ages 12 to 17 had AUD.

Alcohol consumption is extremely variable, as is its effect on the health and well-being of an individual. Currently, approximately 85,000 deaths a year are attributable to alcohol use, and its economic cost is projected to be $250 billion a year. According to the National Institute on Alcohol Abuse and Alcoholism (NIAAA), the younger the age at drinking onset, the greater the chance that at some point in life, an individual will develop an alcohol disorder. The person who begins drinking before age 15 is four times more likely to develop an alcohol disorder as an adult. Researchers have found that the risk of adult alcohol disorders *decreases* by 14% for each additional year of age drinking onset is delayed. Individuals who start drinking at age 21 to 22 years have significantly lower risks for developing adult alcohol dependence. Alcohol disorders are family disorders. It is estimated that one in five adults in the United States has lived with an alcoholic while growing up. Children who grow up with alcoholism are at risk for being abused and becoming problem drinkers in adulthood. Concurrent depression, anxiety, or personality disorder; evidence of a family history of alcohol disorder; or evidence of early age at drinking onset are critical risk factors for alcohol disorder. Although there is little debate that alcohol is an addictive drug, there is a great deal of debate regarding the nature of alcoholism. The core of the debate has to do with significant evidence of alcoholism as a genetic disorder, a biological disease, and as a maladaptive behavior. Alcoholism cannot be fully explained by any one of these models. What is not clear is how these different factors interact. What is clear, however, is that significant exposure to high blood alcohol levels increases the risk of uncontrolled, compulsive, or problem drinking.

The unique biochemical effects of alcohol are related to the drug's ability to produce both short- and long-term changes in neuron membranes and the enhancement and inhibition of critical ion channels. As a central nervous system (CNS) depressant, alcohol can be compared to drugs such as barbiturates and benzodiazepines. It is readily absorbed from the stomach and small intestine into the bloodstream and is metabolized by the liver.

Alcohol intoxication is greatest when blood alcohol levels are increasing. In other words, alcohol intoxication is a manifestation of the rate at which alcohol is consumed.

- A blood alcohol level of 0.05 causes disruptions in thinking, judgment, and inhibition.
- A blood alcohol level of 0.1 produces obvious intoxication.
- A blood alcohol level of 0.2 results in depression of motor functioning and emotional/behavioral dysfunction.
- A blood alcohol level of 0.3 produces stupor and confusion. Blood alcohol levels of 0.4 and higher produce coma.

There is currently dispute in the literature regarding "safe" alcohol intake. According to the Dietary Guidelines for Americans 2015-2020, U.S. Department of Health and Human Services and U.S. Department of Agriculture, Appendix 9, "If alcohol is consumed, it should be in moderation—up to one drink per day for women and up to two drinks per day for men—and only by adults of legal drinking age." The Dietary Guidelines does not recommend that individuals who do not drink alcohol start drinking for any reason.

A 2018 large-scale, worldwide epidemiologic study reports there is no "safe" level of alcohol. The global research team calculated that alcohol was the seventh leading risk factor for both premature death and disability. Alcohol use was responsible for over 2% of all deaths in women and just under 7% of deaths in men. Alcohol-related death and disability were particularly pronounced among younger people. This study suggests that the safest level of alcohol intake is *none*, despite the identification of certain health-protective factors also identified in the study. The trend is essentially toward lower levels of "safe" use, more similar to the "Dietary Guidelines for Americans 2015-2020."

Several terms are used in the literature to describe alcohol disorders, and it is important to understand the various definitions. The NIAAA defines *low-risk drinking* for men as less than drinks per day and no more than 14 drinks per week, and for all women and men aged 65 and older no more than 3 drinks per day and no more than 7 drinks per week. *At-risk drinking* is consuming volumes greater than these guidelines. *Harmful drinking,* on the other hand, occurs when alcohol is causing physical, psychological, or social harm exhibited by zero to two dependence criteria and zero to one abuse criteria, according to this agency. The *DSM-5* also categorizes

disorders as alcohol-use disorder, alcohol intoxication, and alcohol withdrawal.

Other terms are frequently seen in the literature. The term *problem drinker* refers to persons who do not meet the diagnostic criteria for abuse or dependence but who experience problems related to alcohol, and the World Health Organization uses the term *harmful use,* which can be defined as drinking that is causing either physical or psychological harm. In addition, the term *hazardous drinking* is characterized by the risk of harmful consequences (physical, mental, or social) related to alcohol use. Binge drinking (i.e., consuming 5 or more alcoholic beverages within 2 hours for men and more than 4 alcoholic beverages for women) often results in acute impairment and causes a large portion of alcohol-related deaths.

Alcohol affects circulation and cardiac functioning and dilates skin blood vessels, thereby producing flushing and a decrease in body temperature. Reduction in risk of coronary artery disease has been proposed as a benefit of light to moderate consumption. The rationale for this proposal is based on the finding that in low doses, alcohol can increase high-density lipoprotein and decrease low-density lipoprotein. This benefit is canceled out, however, by common unhealthy behaviors such as poor diet, smoking, or excessive use.

Alcohol-use disorder typically has a slow, progressive course; persons generally present for care after 10 to 20 years of use. At-risk drinking may progress to an alcohol use disorder with its attendant morbidity and mortality. Components of the history can include driving under the influence (DUI), work issues, and relationship issues, and, as noted earlier, family history is important. Alcohol disorders have several deleterious health consequences that affect multiple organ systems. Some of these multiple health effects related to alcohol are listed as follows:

- Cardiovascular system: hypertension, arrhythmias, dyslipidemia, cardiomyopathy, and stroke
- Gastrointestinal system: dyspepsia progressing progress to gastritis, peptic ulcers, abnormalities of the liver enzymes, alcoholic hepatitis, fatty liver, pancreatitis, esophageal varices, and cirrhosis
- Neuropsychiatric changes: peripheral neuropathy, memory impairment, suicidality, cortical atrophy, and dementia
- Neoplastic: increased risk of cancer, particularly oral, pharyngeal, laryngeal, esophageal, and possibly breast and colon cancer
- Safety issues: increased number of motor vehicles accidents, falls, burns, episodes of violence, and risky sexual behaviors

It is important to understand that an individual's sex plays a part in alcohol disorders. Recommendations about the daily use of alcohol for women are less than for men because of women's smaller body mass and less efficient ability to metabolize alcohol. Among heavy drinkers (men and women), women develop problems with alcohol at an accelerated rate and are at greater risk for cirrhosis. Increased rates of miscarriage among heavy drinkers are also seen.

To meet the diagnosis of AUD, individuals must meet certain criteria outlined in the *DSM-5*. In *DSM-5*, anyone meeting any two of the 11 criteria during the same 12-month period receives a diagnosis of AUD. The severity of AUD—mild, moderate, or severe—is based on the number of criteria met. See the *DSM-5* for complete diagnostic criteria.

Knowledge of alcohol withdrawal symptoms and appropriate therapy is essential. Abrupt cessation of alcohol in dependent persons can range from mild (characterized by symptoms such as irritability, tremulousness, and insomnia) to severe symptoms (characterized by withdrawal seizures, delirium tremens [disorientation, diaphoresis, visual hallucinations, tachycardia, hypertension, and agitation]); if left untreated, death is a potential complication in severe withdrawal.

Treatment may occur in both the outpatient and the inpatient settings. Pharmacological therapy of withdrawal includes intermediate- or long-acting benzodiazepines such as lorazepam, oxazepam, diazepam, or chlordiazepoxide. Carbamazepine has also been shown to be effective in mild to moderate symptoms of withdrawal and has the added advantage to decrease craving. In addition, adjunctive medications include antipsychotic medications such as haloperidol, which is used in patients with significant hallucinations and agitation. Cardiovascular stabilization with beta blockers needs to be considered in patients with coronary heart disease. When beta blockers are used with oxazepam, stabilization of vital signs and decreased craving have been demonstrated. In addition, clonidine has been found helpful in controlling hypertension and tachycardia. Phenytoin may be appropriate for patients with an underlying seizure disorder, but it is not effective for withdrawal seizures.

It has been estimated that one in five patients presenting to primary care has a current problem or past problem with alcohol abuse. Primary care provides an excellent opportunity to address alcohol-related issues, provides education and information, and offers therapeutic modalities. Screening and behavioral interventions for alcohol disorders are recommended by the U.S. Preventive Services Task Force for all adults. The NIAAA recommends screening as part of routine evaluations and in response to medical conditions that are affected by alcohol, as well as before prescribing medications that may interact with alcohol.

Several screening tools are available such as CAGE, AUDIT, and others. NIAA specifically recommends annually administering the Single Item Alcohol Screening Questionnaire. Patients are asked a single screening question: "How many times in the past year have you had X or more drinks in a day?" where X is five for men and four for women, and a response of >1 is considered positive. This question not only provides information to the clinician but also informs the patient of safe amounts of alcohol consumption. For patients without a documented AUD, who screen positive for unhealthy alcohol use, an initial brief alcohol intervention outlining the risks of drinking and advice to abstain or drink within nationally established guidelines and gender-specific limits for daily and weekly consumption.

The clinician may use a more specific tool or refer the patient to a specialist to properly identify the severity of the disorder. Proper identification of at-risk drinking and alcohol abuse is important so that proper treatment can be initiated. Unhealthy alcohol use was defined as the presence of an AUD, as determined by a standardized diagnostic interview, or risky consumption, as determined using a validated 30-day calendar method. Psychosocial interventions for patients who test positive for AUD include behavioral couple therapy, cognitive behavioral therapy, community reinforcement approach, motivational enhancement therapy, and/or 12-step facilitation. Pharmacological therapy (referred to throughout this chapter as MAT) has been found to be helpful for dependent and chronic dependent drinking, those identified as having moderate-severe AUD.

Cannabis Disorders

The psychoactive effects of marijuana are produced by cannabinoids, of which tetrahydrocannabinol (THC) is the active ingredient. Specific receptors for cannabis have been identified in the brain, particularly in the basal ganglia, hippocampus, and cerebellum. Tolerance and psychological dependence on cannabis have been reported, and abrupt discontinuation of high daily doses can produce withdrawal symptoms that include irritability, insomnia, and mild nausea. The euphoric effects of marijuana can last for hours. These effects include distortions of time, sound, color, and taste; changes in the ability to concentrate; and dreamlike states. Studies of the mental status changes produced by smoking marijuana indicate that the drug affects behavior by increasing brain cell–receptor sensitivity to dopamine. THC can create a mellow mood state by increasing GABA activity. THC impairs short-term memory by decreasing brain acetylcholine activity. High doses of marijuana are associated with red eye; mild increases in heart rate; orthostatic hypotension; increased appetite; dry mouth; and disruptions in recall, memory storage, and sensory-input coding. Memory impairment appears to be the most significant long-term effect of marijuana use.

Marijuana is most commonly smoked either through cigarettes (joints, nails, and reefer) or pipes (bongs or bowls); a potent marijuana resin (hashish) is also smoked. Likewise marijuana can be "vaped." Ingestion is not as common but may be seen in foods and teas. Marijuana is commonly smoked, and it is very well absorbed from the pulmonary system to the circulatory system to the brain. Behavioral effects tend to develop immediately. Absorbed

THC is distributed throughout the body but concentrates in body fat. THC crosses the blood–brain barrier with ease and efficiency. THC also crosses the placenta and affects the fetus. Ingested THC is slowly metabolized and eliminated by the liver over a period of 1 to 4 days. Chronic marijuana smokers can test positive for THC metabolites for weeks, despite brief drug-free periods.

Smoked marijuana has been shown to improve appetite in persons with HIV and AIDS and to reduce nausea and vomiting in chemotherapy patients. In recent years, the potency of THC in marijuana has increased from a low of 0.5% in the 1970s to levels from 6% to 10% in 2000. No longer a symbol of social rebellion, marijuana today may be equated by smokers with tobacco, alcohol, and caffeine. As with long-term users of nicotine, alcohol, and caffeine, long-term marijuana smokers who wish to stop usually find it extremely difficult to do so. Heavy daily users of marijuana experience significant withdrawal symptoms and cravings.

Significant health risks are associated with inhalation of marijuana. Fifty to seventy percent more carcinogens are present in cannabis than in tobacco, and thus patients may present to primary care with common respiratory complaints of cough, asthma, and respiratory infections. In addition, there is an increased incidence of head and neck cancers (twofold to threefold increase), as well as lung cancer. Circulatory changes seen include variability of blood pressure, arrhythmias, and cerebellar infarction. Immune system dysfunction and fertility issues of erratic ovulation and reduced sperm count have also been reported. Overall the most significant changes are in mood and cognition. Exacerbation of panic attacks, anxiety, and depression has also been reported. Other behavior changes may include a lack of desire to participate in activities; persistent cognitive and memory impairment, especially if abuse began in adolescence; and psychotic symptoms. In genetically predisposed adolescents, exposure to cannabis has been associated with onset of psychosis and worsening outcomes of schizophrenia. Medical marijuana use for various conditions such as glaucoma, AIDS wasting, neuropathic pain, spasticity, and nausea from chemotherapy has been proposed, but the Food and Drug Administration (FDA) and Drug Enforcement Administration do not support its use at this time, although marijuana use for medical purposes is legal in some states. Limitations currently are related to a lack of valid studies with consistent THC dosage. In addition, the physical risks related to inhalation may further limit its use.

The most important aspect about marijuana use is education of parents and children about the threat marijuana poses to the young brain, not considered fully developed to age 25. Additionally, for those older than age 25, ongoing education and awareness about the risks of marijuana usage should be stressed. Actual declines in IQ scores have been documented related to marijuana use, especially as adolescents and young adults. Additionally,

states that have legalized are still working to develop sensitive and reliable testing for blood and/or breathe levels to assess driving safety and efficacy after smoking marijuana. It is unclear if it will be seriously implicated to rises in motor vehicle accidents and fatalities.

No specific pharmacotherapies are available for cannabis use disorder; there is strong evidence for recommending cognitive behavioral therapy, motivational enhancement therapy, or combining the two approaches, depending on patient preference.

Hallucinogen-Related Disorders

The phencyclidines are synthetic agents that produce a range of feelings from dissociation to stupor and death. The dissociative agents can be smoked, consumed orally, or snorted. These agents include PCP, or angel dust. In addition, several other substances produce similar effects: ketamine (vitamin K, Special K, and Valium K) and *Salvia divinorum*. Persons taking these substances may present with various injuries from falls and accidents. Memory loss and deficits in cognition can last for months with chronic use.

The "other" hallucinogen use disorders involve the following substances: LSD, or lysergic acid diethylamide (acid, blotter, cubes, microdot yellow sunshine, blue heaven); mescaline (buttons, cactus, mesc, peyote); MDMA or ecstasy; and psilocybin (magic mushrooms, purple passion, shrooms, little smoke). These agents can produce hallucinations, nausea, and altered perceptions. These substances are usually taken orally but can be smoked, snorted, or taken by injection. Duration of effect can vary from hours to days depending on the substance. Flashbacks can occur with LSD. Ecstasy possesses stimulant properties and long-term neurotoxic effects in addition to the hallucinogenic properties. Withdrawal symptom criteria have not been established for any of the hallucinogenic agents.

Inhalant-Related Disorders

The exposure to volatile hydrocarbons from solvents (paint thinners, gasoline, glues); gases (butane, propane, aerosol propellants, nitrous oxide); nitrites (isoamyl, isobutyl, cyclohexyl) with street names such as laughing gas, poppers, snappers, and whippets comprise these disorders. These substances can produce neurocognitive problems, as well as pulmonary and cardiac issues. Inhalants have been associated with sudden death related to cardiac arrhythmias but also through respiratory depression and aspiration.

Sedative-Hypnotic or Anxiolytic-Related Disorders

The substances used in this disorder include barbiturates, carbamates such as muscle relaxers, and benzodiazepine and benzodiazepine-like agents. There is only one distinction between the various benzodiazepines. Xanax (alprazolam) and Ativan (lorazepam) are short-acting.

Klonopin (clonazepam) and Valium (diazepam) are longer-acting. These substances are CNS depressants that can be utilized for legitimate medical conditions, but the behaviors of early refills and obtaining prescriptions from multiple providers help to define this disorder. These agents can cause various neurological deficits in memory, coordination, autonomic depression, and cognition, and they produce many of the same effects as alcohol. There is a synergistic effect of use of these products when combined with alcohol and other drugs, that cam prove very dangerous and in some instances, fatal. These substances in their own right can be fiercely addictive as a drug of choice and dose-dependent as well as length of use might warrant in-patient detoxification.

Stimulant-Related Disorders

Cocaine- and amphetamine-related substances are included in this disorder. These substances are typically smoked, snorted, or injected. Diversion of stimulant attention-deficit/hyperactivity disorder medications also contributes to this disorder.

Cocaine Disorders. Cocaine acts as a CNS stimulant by blocking the reuptake of dopamine, thereby increasing dopamine activity in several areas of the brain. Cocaine may also have dopamine-agonist effects. The dopamine effects of cocaine account for most of the immediate and long-term effects of the drug. Biochemical studies of cocaine have shown that cocaine has extremely self-reinforcing, self-rewarding properties, and thus is highly addictive. The euphoria of cocaine intoxication, combined with the dysphoria of cocaine crashing and craving, can lead to compulsive consumption.

Cocaine is available in several forms: the hydrochloride salt that is inhaled or injected; the alkaloid solid, rock crystal (crack) made by combining the salt with baking soda or ammonia that is usually smoked; and freebase that is manufactured by heating the salt form and combining it with ether and then inhaling (freebasing). Intravenous administration and smoking have the most rapid pharmacological and euphoric onset of action (within 10–30 minutes), as well as discontinuation effect, whereas the onset for intranasal usage is 30 to 60 minutes. Compulsive and abusive use is associated with IV and smoking routes of administration.

One of the most important studies of cocaine's effects on the brain and emotional states successfully used functional magnetic resonance imaging (fMRI) to study the rush, high, low, and craving experiences of cocaine-dependent adults. Maximum cocaine blood levels were reached in an average of 7 minutes after infusion, dysphoria and paranoia developed about 11 minutes after infusion, and cravings for more cocaine occurred about 12 minutes after infusion. One of the most impressive indicators of the speed and scope of cocaine's effects on the brain was that subjects reported maximal feelings of euphoria as cocaine was being infused, before maximal

cocaine blood levels had been reached. Cocaine intoxication is characterized by elation, significant increases in self-esteem, and the perception of improved task performance. Intoxication can also produce agitation, irritability, impaired judgment, impulsive sexual behavior, aggression, hyperactivity, and mania. Chronic cocaine use has been associated with the onset of symptoms of thought, personality, and mood disorders and with paranoid psychosis.

Tolerance to cocaine occurs as users are unable to achieve the euphoric effects of the first episode of use and subsequently escalate the dosage. In addition to its stimulant effect, cocaine also has anesthetic and convulsant effects; and sensitization develops even without a change in dosage. It is believed that this has contributed to deaths by cardiac arrest or seizure followed by respiratory arrest that may occur with the first use episode and precipitately with any use thereafter. Cardiovascular conditions such as hypertension, angina, myocardial infarction, and cerebrovascular accident may also be seen. In addition, pulmonary edema and respiratory depression may occur. Potential complications of pregnancy include abruptio placentae, uterine rupture, and hypertension. Higher rates of sudden infant death syndrome have been reported in infants exposed to cocaine prenatally.

Cocaine withdrawal is typically characterized by irritability, depression, and anxiety and generally decreases after the first few weeks of abstinence. Currently, there are no FDA-approved pharmacological agents to assist withdrawal. In early abstinence, insomnia may be problematic, as evidenced by memory and attention deficits that may place the individual at higher risk of relapse. Some infants manifest symptoms such as tremulousness and irritability during the neonatal period.

Over the past few decades, smoked cocaine (crack), an extremely rapid-acting form of the drug, became cheap and easy to obtain. Cocaine has consistently been linked with severe social problems and antisocial behavior, such as gang violence and prostitution. Harmful behaviors such as driving while impaired, sexually transmitted disease exposure, and violence are also reported.

Amphetamine-Type Disorders. Substances include amphetamines, dextroamphetamine, methamphetamine, and methylphenidate. After having been a relatively popular and cheap drug of abuse, amphetamines quickly came to be associated with violent, bizarre behavior at a time when mellow "highs" were more socially acceptable. Decades later, amphetamines, particularly methamphetamine ("crank"), have once again become popular among older adolescents and young adults.

Methamphetamine is a synthetic agent also known as speed, meth, chalk, ice, and crystal. Users describe being high as being "amped" (amplified) or "tweaked." Methamphetamine is a potent, easy-to-make, inexpensive stimulant, which can be snorted or injected. "Crystal-meth" is methamphetamine in a freebase form; "ice" is a high-grade form of "crystal-meth" that is sold in rocks, like crack cocaine. Because of its purity and potency, "ice" is expensive; one hit can deliver an extreme amphetamine high that can last for hours. A methamphetamine rush is intense. Intoxication includes elation, increased self-esteem, increased physical endurance, insensitivity to fatigue, and feelings of being invulnerable. Methamphetamine half-life is 11 hours or more, which far exceeds that of cocaine. This long half-life contributes to the longer neurological changes. But like cocaine, amphetamine increases dopamine activity, is self-reinforcing, and is a highly efficient addictive agent. Several side effects of methamphetamine use are hyperthermia, dehydration, a significant anxiety, insomnia, mood disturbances, and violent behavior, as well as psychosis. These symptoms can persist even after the behavior of abuse has stopped. Additional physical signs and symptoms include dermatological changes such as sores and dental issues, including tooth decay and tooth loss.

Chronic users experience acute episodes of euphoria and dysphoria that can mimic bipolar disorder. Other medical issues that can occur with stimulant use include nasal septum perforation, respiratory and cardiovascular issues such as chest pain, myocardial infarction, arrhythmias, and stroke. Stimulant use produces several adverse pregnancy outcomes.

Caffeine-Related Disorders

Caffeine is present in many products; it is naturally present in coffee, tea, and chocolate. The cola nut extract is commonly used in cola-type beverages. Caffeine added to food is subject to the Federal Food, Drug, and Cosmetic Act. According to 21 CFR 182.1180, caffeine up to a level of 0.02 percent (200 ppm) is generally recognized as safe (GRAS) for use in cola-type beverages (consistent with cGMPs). FDA regulations require beverage companies to list caffeine in the ingredients list on product labels, but there is no FDA requirement to list the precise amount of caffeine present in a product. Soda manufactures voluntarily label the amount of caffeine in accordance with American Beverage Association guidelines. More recently, energy drink manufacturers have begun to use the same guidelines and at times with cautionary statements: *some products contain advisories against use by children, pregnant women, or individuals sensitive to caffeine.* There is concern however products with added caffeine (both liquids and solids) are proliferating in the food supply. Additionally, the patterns of use of caffeine-containing products are changing and not well understood and caffeinated products are readily available and attractive to children and adolescents. It is known that estimates of exposure to caffeine from all sources are approaching health reference values.

The average daily U.S. consumption over the past 10 years has remained stable at 300 mg per person per day. At low doses, caffeine causes symptoms such as insomnia and restlessness. At high doses (greater than 1,000 mg/day),

caffeine may induce arrhythmias, and psychomotor agitation can occur. Death from caffeine can occur with ingestion of 5 to 10 g. Well-known products that contain caffeine are coffee, tea, soft drinks, over-the-counter medications, energy drinks, some snack foods, some ice creams and yogurts, and chocolate. There is great variability in the amount of caffeine present in products as well as the individual's response to a particular dosage. The primary source of caffeine for adults and youths comes from beverages. The caffeine content of coffee can range from 95 to 330 mg depending on the size of the beverage. Even decaffeinated coffee contains small amounts of caffeine ranging from 3 to 12 mg/serving. The caffeine content of tea ranges from 15 to 74 mg/serving. Caffeinated soft drinks include colas, Mountain Dew, and some root beers. The caffeine content of these beverages can range from 22 to 69 mg per 12-ounce serving. Energy drinks can contain anywhere between 33 and 400 mg of caffeine per serving. Over-the-counter medications that contain caffeine include analgesic and weight loss products, as well as agents used to inhibit sleep; caffeine contained in these products can range from 30 to 130 mg/serving. Currently, youth are exposed to caffeine products at younger ages. The American College of Sports Medicine (ACSM) released an official statement with the following recommendations:

- stop marketing to high-risk groups, especially children and teens at sports events
- do not consume energy drinks before, during, or after intense exercise—some deaths have occurred under these circumstances
- educate consumers about the difference between soda, coffee, and energy drinks. This should be included in school nutrition, health and wellness classes.

They also recommend that health-care providers inquire about use of these products, especially in children, teens, and young adults (ACSM, 2018). There is also a call for more research and potential revisiting of regulations. Currently, the impact of long-term, higher caffeine exposure at younger ages poses many unanswered questions.

Gambling Disorder

Gambling disorder is characterized by frequent, compulsive, uncontrolled, or addictive gambling occurring habitually, intermittently, or in isolated episodes. To meet the *DSM-5* criteria for a gambling disorder, four of nine symptom criteria need to be present for 12 months and the disorder must be causing significant distress. See the *DSM-5* for complete diagnostic criteria. What is different about the inclusion of this disorder in the *DSM-5* is that gambling is a *behavior,* not a substance. Engaging in the behavior, however, may cause the same stimulation of the brain's pleasure centers that substances do, and there is the element of compulsivity. This has led to discussion of "internet shopping" also a behavior. This is an ongoing debate.

MANAGEMENT

Primary-care practitioners are often the first health-care professionals to observe the health and psychosocial impact of substance abuse; sometimes the primary-care practitioner is the only health-care professional the patient is willing to talk to. Clinicians can take advantage of this by striving to help patients recognize their substance abuse and take the first steps toward improvement. Several options are available from brief advice, printed information, brief intervention (Center for Substance Abuse Treatment, 1999), professional intervention, peer intervention, and referral to treatment and/or self-help groups. Brief intervention has been most helpful for someone "at-risk"; in a patient testing positive for SUD or the dependent drinker, the role of brief intervention is less clear.

It should always be a goal to promote early engagement and retention of patients with substance use conditions who can benefit from addiction-focused treatment. Many patients may initially decline voluntary referral, or at least express ambivalence, but provider encouragement and support may improve patient willingness to pursue further involvement if they see it as consistent with their other priorities. There is considerable evidence from psychotherapy research that general factors such as therapist skill, the strength of the therapeutic alliance, and the structure provided by regular clinical contact can have as powerful an effect on engagement as the specific content or conceptual approach of specialized interventions. Therefore, attention to these general therapeutic factors is at least as important as the specific treatment approach selected, and is exemplified by the *Circle of Caring* model espoused in this text.

Although some patients with substance-related problems recover without formal treatment, especially as they age, most require a variety of interventions. Some patients are not ready to give up substances or continue to be in denial. With these patients, the following strategies are recommended:

- Use motivational interviewing (MI) (see Chapter 81) and emphasize the common elements of effective interventions including improving self-efficacy for change, promoting a therapeutic relationship, strengthening coping skills, changing reinforcement contingencies for recovery, and enhancing social support for recovery.
- Reiterate to the patient that the most consistent predictors of successful outcome are retention in formal treatment and/or active involvement with community support for recovery.
- Discuss strategies demonstrated to be efficacious to promote active involvement in available mutual help programs (e.g., Alcoholics Anonymous [AA], Narcotics Anonymous [NA]).
- Coordinate addiction-focused psychosocial interventions with evidence-based intervention(s) for other biopsychosocial problems to address identified concurrent problems consistent with patient priorities.
- Provide intervention in the least restrictive setting necessary to promote access to care, safety, and effectiveness.
- If a patient drops out of treatment, the treatment team should make efforts to contact the patient and reengage him or her in treatment. If the patient remains unwilling to engage in any addiction-focused care, maintain MI style of interactions. Emphasize that options remain available in the future and determine whether treatment for medical and psychiatric problems can be effectively and safely provided while looking for windows of opportunity to engage the patient in addiction treatment. Even when patients refuse referral or are unable to participate in specialized addiction treatment, many are accepting of general medical or mental health care. The chronic illness approach is consistent with management approaches for many other disorders treated in medical and psychiatric settings.

Treatment of the severely mentally ill who are also drug dependent continues to pose problems; specialized addiction agencies have trouble treating such patients. Generally, integrated treatment of both the psychiatric disorder and the addiction is more effective than either parallel or sequential treatment. Integrated models of care are limited but increasingly recognized in local and state mental health agencies. Among patients in early recovery from SUDs or following relapse, prioritize other needs through shared decision-making (e.g., related to other mental health conditions, housing, supportive recovery environment, employment, or related recovery-relevant factors) among identified biopsychosocial problems and arranging services to address them.

Patients with poor physical health or severe legal and interpersonal problems will need improvement in these areas to feel able to change their substance abuse behaviors. Substance-related mental disorders should be treated as well. Patients often already have a great deal of information about their substance abuse and the benefits of stopping. The most useful patient education will address the process of stopping. Some people are able to stop on their first try, but the more typical pattern is repeated efforts to stop until the individual is substance free. Specific management of each case will depend on the substance being abused. General indications for the need for inpatient treatment of substance abuse are presented in Box 65.2.

MAT is available for nicotine, alcohol, and opioid disorders. Nicotine agents are listed in Chapter 33 (see Drugs Commonly Prescribed 33.1). Pharmacological options for maintenance of alcohol abstinence in dependent drinkers include disulfiram (Antabuse), oral and extended-release injectable naltrexone (Revia), and acamprosate (Campral). For most, naltrexone is the primary drug choice unless co-occurring opioid use is present. Treatment options for opioid disorders may include

Box 65.2 Indications for Inpatient Withdrawal From Substances Including Alcohol

Several factors need to be considered when identifying the best treatment placement for patients with substance use disorders. Of particular concern is withdrawal from alcohol and from the sedative, hypnotic, and anxiolytic agents. Withdrawal from these agents can cause cardiovascular collapse, delirium, and death. Withdrawal from opiates does not impart the same risk. Cardiac monitoring may be indicated in cocaine intoxication. Assessing medical stability requires evaluation of several factors. These factors include the following:

Current Situation

- Severe illness—unable to tolerate oral medications
- Suicidal and homicidal ideation—either in ideation or intent
- Lengthy and heavy substance abuse
- Prior unsuccessful attempts at ambulatory medically supervised withdrawal
- Social conditions such as homelessness with decreased chance to complete ambulatory medically supervised withdrawal
- Active psychosis or severe cognitive impairment
- Medical conditions—cardiovascular disease, pregnancy, liver disease
- Withdrawal symptoms for the substance *or* taking the same (or closely related) substance to relieve symptoms of withdrawal
- Alcohol withdrawal symptoms as defined by *DSM-5*. Objective measurement of alcohol withdrawal symptoms is recommended. The Clinical Institute Withdrawal Assessment of Alcohol (CIWA-Ar) is commonly utilized. Scores greater than 20 are considered severe; 10–19 moderate withdrawal; and scores less than 10 are interpreted as mild. Consider inpatient management for scores greater than or equal to 10.
- Risk of withdrawal from other substances in addition to alcohol (e.g., sedative hypnotics)

Past History

- History of withdrawal
- History of withdrawal seizures or delirium tremens

Source: Department of Veteran Affairs. *VA/DoD clinical practice guideline for the management of substance use disorders*, version 3. https://www.healthquality.va.gov/guidelines/MH/sud/VADoDSUDCPGRevised22216.pdf. Published 2015; revised 2017.

detoxification (managed opiate withdrawal), behavioral strategies, and pharmacological intervention. Long-term maintenance of abstinence can be achieved by methadone maintenance or buprenorphine (Subutex, Buprenex) alone or with naltrexone. It is imperative for all disorders that behavioral therapies are ongoing.

The first goal of treatment should be the restoration of the physical, psychological, and social well-being of the person and family. Significant damage has often been done to the patient's support system. The family may have additional co-dependent and enabling issues to address and also may need treatment. Sometimes

relationships that have remained intact during the substance abuse phase ultimately falter and disintegrate when one partner becomes engaged in treatment. For many years, the first treatment goal in substance abuse was abstinence. Research for many years had shown that moderation in use is rarely effective for those with a substance abuse problem. However, as more biological and neurophysiologic data are available, and the lack of success in opioid-use disorder (OUD) of this model, increasingly even stalwarts long rooted in this line of thinking have begun to integrate MAT, with the broader goals as stated earlier. Approaches include specific procedures or techniques such as MAT, as well as individual therapy, family therapy, group therapy, relapse prevention, pharmacotherapy, and treatment programs. Treatment programs tend to be multidisciplinary and often include a specific set of procedures. However, there is no standardization of terminology for categorizing treatment programs and procedures, and their effects are difficult to measure. Broadly, some programs focus on controlling acute withdrawal (detoxification), and others aim at long-term behavioral change. Interventions should be provided in the least restrictive setting necessary to promote access to care, safety, and effectiveness. Some programs are residential, with treatment for one to three months. Some use MAT, while others are based on or incorporate individual psychotherapy, AA or other 12-step principles, or therapeutic community principles. Increasingly, multimodal approaches are used, and there must be shared decision-making between the patient and provider about the recommended approach that might work best for this person. Publicly funded treatment programs for drug dependence are categorized as methadone maintenance (mostly outpatient), outpatient drug-free programs, therapeutic communities, or short-term inpatient programs. Substantial reduction in illicit drug use, antisocial behaviors, and psychiatric distress among patients dependent on cocaine or heroin are much more likely following treatment lasting at least 3 months, and programs that include MAT in the case especially of alcohol and opioid abuse, where successful drug treatment is available. Such a time-in-treatment effect is seen across very different modalities, from residential therapeutic communities to ambulatory methadone maintenance programs. Increasingly, the recovery community has embraced integrated and individualized approaches.

FOLLOW-UP AND REFERRAL

In addition to primary care, patients being treated for substance abuse will need access to several information and support resources, which should include education services, treatment programs, and support groups. It is unlikely that any single program or support group will be sufficient, so patients are encouraged to make repeated contact with several different types of programs and groups. Follow-up includes monitoring self-reported use, laboratory markers, and consequences. Follow-up for patients in active treatment includes monitoring adherence, response to treatment, and adverse effects. Education about AUD and/or OUD consequences and treatments should be ongoing. Encouragement to abstain from nonprescribed opioids and other addictive substances is critical in the context of a caring relationship. Encouragement to attend community supports for recovery (e.g., mutual help groups) and to make lifestyle changes that support recovery is also important. None of these options should be either/or. There must be shared decision-making with the patient and family and a variety of approaches tried, monitored, and evaluated. SUD is a chronic, potentially relapsing and progressive disease. There is no end to treatment.

Referral to a specialist should be made immediately when the patient's behavior represents a danger to self or others. Substance abuse, particularly alcohol abuse, is a factor in motor vehicle accidents, family violence, and suicide. It can also be very helpful for patients to have at least one appointment with a specialist to develop a comprehensive assessment of the patient's substance use and abuse. For the patient, this assessment is a critical source of information that can reduce his or her ambivalence toward making needed changes in substance-related behaviors. Seeing a specialist can also be motivational, in that one of the most common reasons for failing to try to make required changes in behavior is the patient's unspoken fears of failure.

Patient Education: Substance Use Disorder

Individuals who have developed psychological and physical needs for a substance often have also formed strong attachments to their substance use lifestyle and substance-based relationships. It may be impossible to effectively address a person's substance abuse without taking into account his or her substance-based relationships and attachments. A person can become strongly attached to the people, places, and community that make up his or her substance abuse lifestyle. From friendships among coworkers that develop at designated smoking areas to football parties and alternative lifestyles, for many people, the thought of giving up their attachments may be more painful than the thought of giving up their actual substances of abuse. The fear of losing these valued attachments is frequently used to rationalize continued substance abuse.

Personal losses may increase or decrease the motivation to significantly change substance use behaviors. Individuals who have not suffered substance abuse–related losses may nevertheless have to deal with significant interpersonal conflicts related to their substance-abuse behaviors. Years of substance abuse can result in the loss of all non–substance-based relationships, significant loss of self-esteem, financial losses, and loss of physical and mental health. These personal losses can have a devastating psychological impact on the individual. The patient may feel that he or she is in a no-win situation: Feelings of hopelessness may manifest as ambivalence about making needed changes in substance use behaviors or bravado about continued substance abuse.

The clinician should educate patients regarding the effects of drugs, especially during pregnancy, and provide information on substance abuse and treatment to patients and their families. Practitioners should provide information regarding danger of exposure to HIV, hepatitis, and other infections and to obtain appropriate testing if there is suspicion of exposure. Care providers should teach family members about the dynamics that may continue to enable substance abuse; often they are unaware of these. The clinician can give family members specific feedback in this area about behaviors that he or she has observed; it is also important to discuss the strategy of using an intervention with the family and how to set up one if indicated.

Codependence is a term that has come to mean the behavioral patterns of family members who have been significantly affected by another family member's substance use or addiction. Related concepts of enabling and denial may characterize family members of patients who abuse substances. Twelve-step programs should be encouraged—for example, NA or AA for the individual with the substance-abuse problem and Al Anon for family members. As noted earlier, family members and significant others need treatment also. The *Circle of Caring* model may be utilized in caring for those with addictions.

Nursing Situation: Substance Abuse and the *Circle of Caring*

The following vignette, abstracted from Smith-Battle L, Drake MA, Diekemper M, The responsive use of self in community health nursing practice. *Adv Nurs Sci* 1997;20(2):85, addresses a person with substance abuse. It is a story that highlights the skills of involvement, coordination, and advocacy that helped to reintegrate this mother into the community and the child into the family. The mother's eventual reintegration was contingent on the APRN's responsiveness and perseverance in a situation with an uncertain outcome, which demonstrates practice within a *Circle of Caring*.

In this situation, an unreceptive new mother tested positive at the birth of her baby for cocaine abuse. The infant was severely injured at 2 months of age in a car accident when, unrestrained, he hit his head against the dashboard. The infant was removed from the mother's care and placed with an aunt. The following account is from a nurse involved with the family:

[In the year after the accident], I saw the baby at the aunt's house and we got him involved with developmental programs . . . I hooked them up with all that . . . Meanwhile, I was visiting mom. [Describes how the mother was in and out of treatment programs.]

I got a phone call from her one morning. She told me that a drug dealer had beat her up and put a gun to her head over a 5-dollar debt. "I'm going to die. I'm either going to get killed or I'm going to die of using cocaine." So I worked with the social worker and we got her into a long-term, 3-month treatment [program] away from the entire environment. And when she came back, I will never forget, I cried when I called her. She had make-up on. She had gained weight . . . I didn't even recognize her . . .

A year later, when she came back, she started visiting with her son at the aunt's house, and gradually the whole team, the social worker, myself, the aunt, and all other interventionists, we had huge meetings and we basically started reintegrating the child into the home. And now she has him full-time. And she's been clean . . . She keeps up with all [her son's appointments] and she goes to Narcotics Anonymous three times a week. She wants to become a treatment counselor and . . . she finished her GED. She's just a total success story . . .

. . . She told me once, "Everyone that ever cared about me has left me or treated me like crap." . . . [it] was the first time in her life where [although] she was down-right obnoxious and hateful [to me], I never bit back or quit coming. I mean, I accepted her behavior because I knew it was the drug use and it wasn't her.

REFERENCES

GBD 2016 Alcohol Collaborators. Alcohol use and burden for 195 countries and territories, 1990–2016: a systematic analysis for the Global Burden of Disease Study 2016. *Lancet*. Sep;392(10152):1015–1035

Allen JP, Litten RZ, Fertig JB, et al. A review of research on the Alcohol Use Disorders Identification Test (AUDIT). Alcoholism. *Clin Exp Res*. 1997;21:613–619.

American Society of Addiction Medicine (ASAM). *The ASAM criteria: treatment for addictive, substance-related, and co-occurring conditions*. Chevy Chase, MD: ASAM, 2013.

Anton RF, et al. Combined pharmacotherapies and behavioral interventions for alcohol dependence: The COMBINE study: A randomized controlled trial. *JAMA*. 2006;295(17):2003–2017.

Argoff CE, Kahan M, Sellers EM. Preventing and managing aberrant drug-related behavior in primary care: Systematic review of outcomes evidence. *J Opioid Manag*. 2014;10:119–134.

Bayard M, et al. Alcohol withdrawal syndrome. *Am Fam Physician*. 2004;69(6):1443–1450.

Beckham N. Motivational interviewing with hazardous drinkers. *J Am Acad Nurse Pract*. 2006;19(2):103–110.

Bendtsen P, Anderson P, Wojnar M, et al. Professional's attitudes do not influence screening and brief interventions rates for hazardous and harmful drinkers: Results from ODHIN study. *Alcohol Alcohol*. 2015;50:430–437.

Blow FC, et al. Brief screening for alcohol problems in elderly populations using the Short Michigan Alcoholism Screening Test—Geriatric Version (SMAST-G). *Alcoholism Clin Exp Res*. 1998;22(suppl):131A.

Bradford T, et al. Methamphetamine abuse. *Am Fam Physician*. 2007;76:1169–1176.

Bradley KA, Bush KR, McDonnell MB, Malone T, Fihn SD. Screening for problem drinking: Comparison of CAGE and AUDIT. Ambulatory Care Quality Improvement Project (ACQUIP). Alcohol Use Disorders Identification Test. *J Gen Intern Med*. 1998;13:379–388.

Cacciola JS, Alterman AI, Dephilippis D, et al. Development and initial evaluation of the Brief Addiction Monitor (BAM). *J Subst Abuse Treat*. 2013;44:256–263.

Califf R, Woodcock J, Ostroff S. A proactive response to prescription opioid abuse. *N Engl J Med*. 2016;374:1480–1485.

Centers for Disease Control and Prevention. Reported law enforcement encounters testing positive for fentanyl increase across US. Atlanta, GA: US Department of Health and Human Services, CDC 2016. http://www.cdc.gov/drugoverdose/data/fentanyl-le-reports.html Accessed February 25, 2018.

Center for Behavioral Health Statistics and Quality. 2015 National survey on drug use and health: Methodological summary and definitions. http://www.samhsa.gov/data. Published 2016. Accessed February 24, 2018.

Centers for Disease Control and Prevention. *Wide-ranging online data for epidemiologic research (WONDER)*. Atlanta, GA: National Center for Health Statistics; 2016.

Centers for Disease Control and Prevention. Annual self-reported alcohol-impaired driving episodes among U.S. adults, 1993–2014. https://www.cdc.gov/motorvehiclesafety/impaired_driving/impaired-drv_factsheet.html. Published 2017.

Centers for Disease Control and Prevention (2017). Drug overdose death data. https://www.cdc.gov/drugoverdose/data/statedeaths.html. Published 2017.

Centers for Disease Control and Prevention. Vital statistics rapid release: Provisional drug overdose death counts. https://www.cdc.gov/nchs/nvss/vsrr/drug-overdose-data.htm6.

Centers for Disease Control and Prevention. NCHS vital statistics rapid release: Provisional drug overdose death counts. https://www.cdc.gov/nchs/nvss/vsrr/drug-overdose-data.htm. Accessed July 9, 2018.

Center for Substance Abuse Treatment. Chapter 2—Brief interventions in substance abuse treatment. *Brief interventions and brief therapies for substance abuse. Rockville*, MD: *Substance Abuse and Mental Health Services Administration (Treatment Improvement Protocol (TIP) Series, No. 34)*. https://www.ncbi.nlm.nih.gov/books/NBK64942/. Published 1999.

CDC. Behavioral Risk Factor Surveillance System (BRFSS), 1993–2014. https://www.cdc.gov/brfss. Accessed Sept. 6, 2018

Chou R, Turner JA, Devine EB, et al. The effectiveness and risks of long-term opioid therapy for chronic pain: A systematic review for a National Institutes of Health Pathways to Prevention Workshop. *Ann Intern Med*. 2015;162:276–286.

Cicero TJ, Ellis MS, Surratt HL, Kurtz SP. The changing face of heroin use in the United States: A retrospective analysis of the past 50 years. *JAMA Psychiatry*. 2014;71:821–826.

Crowley R, Kirschner N, Dunn AS, Bornstein SS. Health and public policy to facilitate effective prevention and treatment of substance use disorders involving illicit and prescription drugs: An American College of Physicians Position Paper. *Ann Intern Med*. 2017;166:733–736.

Dasgupta A. False-positive DOA testing results due to prescription medications. *MLO*. 24–26, 2009. https://www.mlo-online.com/false-positive-doa-testing-results-due-to-prescription-medications.php. Accessed July 19, 2018.

Degenhardt L, Bruno R, Lintzeris N, et al. Agreement between definitions of pharmaceutical opioid use disorders and dependence in people taking opioids for chronic non-cancer pain (POINT): A cohort study. *Lancet Psychiatry*. 2015;2:314–322.

Denis CM, Cacciola JS, Alterman AI. Addiction Severity Index (ASI) summary scores: Comparison of the recent status scores of the ASI-6 and the composite scores of the ASI-5. *J Subst Abuse Treat.* 2013;45:444–450.

Department of Veteran Affairs. VA/DoD clinical practice guideline for the management of substance use disorders, version 3. https://www.healthquality.va.gov/guidelines/MH/sud/VADoDSUDCPGRevised22216.pdf. Published 2015. Revised 2017.

Dowell D, Haegerich TM, Chou R. CDC guideline for prescribing opioids for chronic pain — United States, 2016. *MMWR Recomm Rep.* 2016;65(No. RR-1):1–49. DOI: http://dx.doi.org/10.15585/mmwr.rr6501e1.

Drewnowski A, Rehm CD. Sources of caffeine in diets of US children and adults: Trends by beverage type and purchase location. *Nutrients.* 2016;8(3):154.

Drug Enforcement Administration. Counterfeit prescription pills containing fentanyls: A global threat. DEA intelligence brief. Washington, DC: U.S. Department of Justice, Drug Enforcement Administration. https://www.dea.gov/docs/Counterfeit%20Prescription%20Pills.pdf. Published 2016. Accessed September 5, 2018.

Drug Enforcement Administration. National heroin threat assessment summary—updated. DEA intelligence report. Washington, DC: U.S. Department of Justice, Drug Enforcement Administration. https://www.dea.gov/divisions/hq/2016/hq062716_attach.pdf. Published 2016.

Dube SR, Felitti VJ, Dong M, et al. Childhood abuse, neglect, and household dysfunction and the risk of illicit drug use: the adverse childhood experiences study. *Pediatrics.* 2003;111:564–569.

Els C, Jackson TD, Kunyk D, et al. Adverse events associated with medium- and long-term use of opioids for chronic non-cancer pain: An overview of Cochrane Reviews. *Cochrane Database Syst Rev.* 2017;10:CD012509.

Ewing, JA. Detecting alcoholism. The CAGE questionnaire. *JAMA.* 1984;252:1905–1907.

Fareed A, Vayalapalli S, Casarella J, Drexler K. Treatment outcome for flexible dosing buprenorphine maintenance treatment. *Am J Drug Alcohol Abuse.* 2012;38:155–160.

Fiellin DA, et al. Screening for alcohol problems in primary care: A systemic review. *Arch Gen Psychiatry.* 2000;160:1977–1989.

Fingarette H. *Heavy drinking: The myth of alcoholism as a disease.* Berkeley, CA: University of California Press; 1988.

Frenk SM, Porter KS, Paulozzi LJ. Prescription opioid analgesic use among adults: United States, 1999–2012 (NCHS data brief, no. 189). Hyattsville, MD: National Center for Health Statistics; 2015.

Gassman RA. Practitioner-level predictors of alcohol problems detection and management activities. *J Subst Use.* 2007;12(3):191–202.

Gawin FH. Cocaine addiction: Psychology and neurophysiology. *Science.* 1991;251:1580–1586.

Gibson A, Degenhardt L, Mattick RP, et al. Exposure to opioid maintenance treatment reduces long-term mortality. *Addiction.* 2008;103:462–468.

Goodman JD, McKay JR, DePhillipis D. Progress monitoring in mental health and addiction: A means of improving care. *Prof Psychol Res Pract.* 2013;44:231–246.

Gould RL, Coulson MC, Patel N, Highton-Williamson E, Howard RJ. Interventions for reducing benzodiazepine use in older people: Meta-analysis of randomised controlled trials. *Br J Psychiatry.* 2014;204(2):98–107.

Grant BF, Chou SP, Saha TD, et al. Prevalence of 12-month alcohol use, high-risk drinking, and *DSM-IV* alcohol use disorder in the United States, 2001–2002 to 2012–2013. Results from the National Epidemiologic Survey on Alcohol and Related Conditions. *JAMA Psychiatry.* 2017;74(9):911–923.

Grant BF, Goldstein RB, Saha TD, et al. Epidemiology of *DSM-5* alcohol use disorder: Results from the National Epidemiologic Survey on Alcohol and Related Conditions III. *JAMA Psychiatry.* 2015;72(8):757–766.

Greenwald MK, Comer SD, Fiellin DA. Buprenorphine maintenance and mu-opioid receptor availability in the treatment of opioid use disorder: Implications for clinical use and policy. *Drug Alcohol Depend.* 2014;144:1–11.

Griswold KS, et al. Adolescent substance use and abuse: Recognition and management. *Am Fam Physician.* 2008;77(3):331–336.

Han BH, Moore AA. Prevention and screening of unhealthy substance use by older adults. *Clin Geriatr Med.* 2018;34(1):117–129.

Harwood, GA. Alcohol abuse screening in primary care. *Nurse Pract.* 2005;30(2):56–61.

Hedegaard H, Warner M, Miniño AM. *Drug overdose deaths in the United States, 1999–2016* (NCHS data brief, no. 294). Hyattsville, MD: National Center for Health Statistics; 2017. Accessed September 5, 2018.

Hedlund JL, Vieweg BW. The Michigan Alcoholism Screening Test (MAST): A comprehensive review. *J Operat Psychiatry.* 1964;15:55–64.

Higgins JP, Babu K, Deuster PA, Shearer J. Energy drinks: A contemporary issues paper. *Curr Sports Med Rep.* 2018;17:65–72.

Institute of Medicine. *Improving the quality of health care for mental and substance use conditions* (Quality Chasm series). Washington, DC: The National Academies Press; 2006.

Johnson BA, et al. Topiramate for treating alcohol dependence: A randomized controlled trial. *JAMA.* 2007;298(14):1641–1651.

Jones CM. Heroin use and heroin use risk behaviors among nonmedical users of prescription opioid pain relievers—United States, 2002–2004 and 2008–2010. *Drug Alcohol Depend.* 2013;132:95–100.

Jones CM, Logan J, Gladden RM, Bohm MK. Vital signs: Demographic and substance use trends among heroin users—United States, 2002–2013. *MMWR Morb Mortal Wkly Rep.* 2015;64(26):719–725.

Jones CM, Paulozzi LJ, Mack KA. Sources of prescription opioid pain relievers by frequency of past-year nonmedical use United States, 2008–2011. *JAMA Intern Med.* 2014;174:802–803.

Kalivas PW. The glutamate homeostasis hypothesis of addiction. *Nat Rev Neurosci.* 2009;10:561–572.

Kaner E, Bland M, Cassidy P, et al. Effectiveness of screening and brief alcohol intervention in primary care (SIPS trial): Pragmatic cluster randomised controlled trial. *BMJ.* 2013;346:e8501. https://doi.org/10.1136/bmj.e8501

Kendler KS, Jacobson KC, Prescott CA, Neale MC. Specificity of genetic and environmental risk factors for use and abuse/dependence of cannabis, cocaine, hallucinogens, sedatives, stimulants, and opiates in male twins. *Am J Psychiatry.* 2003;160:687–695.

Kendler KS, Ohlsson H, Maes HH, Sundquist K, Lichtenstein P, Sundquist J. A population-based Swedish Twin and Sibling Study of cannabis, stimulant and sedative abuse in men. *Drug Alcohol Depend.* 2015;149:49–54.

Keyes KM, Hatzenbuehler ML, McLaughlin KA, et al. Stigma and treatment for alcohol disorders in the United States. *Am J Epidemiol.* 2010;172(12):1364–1372.

Knight JR, et al. Validity of brief alcohol screening test among adolescents: A comparison of the AUDIT, POSIT, CAGE, and CRAFFT. *Alcohol Clin Exp Res*. 2003;27:67–73.

Kral LA. Opioid tapering: Safely discontinuing opioid analgesics. Pain treatment topics. **http://paincommunity.org/blog/wp-content/uploads/Safely_Tapering_Opioids.pdf**. Published 2006.

Larson MJ, Mohr MS, Brolin M, et al. High incidence of unhealthy alcohol use in older adult. *Subst Abuse*. 2011;32:50–58.

Mann K, et al. The efficacy of acamprosate in the maintenance of abstinence in alcohol-dependent individuals: Results of a meta-analysis. *Alcohol Clin Exp Res*. 2004;28(1):51–63.

Mattick RP, Breen C, Kimber J, Davoli M. Buprenorphine maintenance versus placebo or methadone maintenance for opioid dependence. *Cochrane Database Syst Rev*. 2014;(2):CD002207.

McCusker RR, et al. Caffeine content of energy drinks, carbonated sodas, and other beverages. *J Anal Toxicol*. 2006;30:112–114.

McGuinness P. Update on marijuana. *J Psychosoc Nurs Ment Health Serv*. 2009;47(10):19–22.

McNeely J, Cleland CM, Strauss SM, et al. Validation of self-administered Single-Item Screening Questions (SISQs) for unhealthy alcohol and drug use in primary care patients. *J Gen Intern Med*. 2015;30:1757–1764.

Meltzer EC, Rybin D, Meshesha LZ, et al. Aberrant drug-related behaviors: Unsystematic documentation does not identify prescription drug use disorder. *Pain Med*. 2012;13:1436.

Mertens JR, Chi FW, Weisner CM, et al. Physician versus non-physician delivery of alcohol screening, brief intervention and referral to treatment in adult primary care: The ADVISE cluster randomized controlled implementation trial. *Addict Sci Clin Pract*. 2015;10:26.

Moyer VA; Preventive Services Task Force. Screening and behavioral counseling interventions in primary care to reduce alcohol misuse: U.S. Preventive Services Task Force recommendation statement. *Ann Intern Med*. 2013;159:210–218.

National Highway Traffic Safety Administration. Traffic safety facts 2016 data: Alcohol-impaired driving. Washington, DC: U.S. Department of Transportation; 2017. **https://crashstats.nhtsa.dot.gov/Api/Public/ViewPublication/812450**. Accessed September 6, 2018.

National Institute on Alcohol Abuse and Alcoholism. Helping patients who drink too much: A clinician's guide. **https://www.niaaa.nih.gov/guide**. Published 2005.

National Institute on Alcohol Abuse and Alcoholism. Drinking levels defined **https://www.niaaa.nih.gov/alcohol-health/overview-alcohol-consumption/moderate-binge-drinking**. Accessed September 6, 2018.

Nunes EV, Selzer J, Levounis P, Davies CA. *Substance dependence and co-occurring psychiatric disorders*. Kingston, NJ: Civic Research Institute; 2010.

O'Regan A, Cullen W, Hickey L, Meagher D, Hannigan A. Is problem alcohol use being detected and treated in Irish general practice? *BMC Fam Pract*. 2018;19:30.

Peele S. The meaning of addiction: Compulsive experience and its interpretation. Lexington, MA: D.C. Health; 1985.

Poston JM, Hanson WE. Meta-analysis of psychological assessment as a therapeutic intervention. *Psychol Assess*. 2010;22:203–212.

PBS. PBC Newshour segment. **https://www.pbs.org/newshour/health/fentanyl-deadlier-heroin-single-photo**. Accessed September 6, 2018.

Reinert DF, Allen JP. The Alcohol Use Disorders Identification Test (AUDIT): A review of recent research. *Alcohol Clin Exp Res*. 2002;26:272–279.

Rigotti NA, Clair C, Munafò MR, Stead LF. Interventions for smoking cessation in hospitalised patients. *Cochrane Database Syst Rev*. 2012;(5):CD001837.

Rigotti NA, Regan S, Levy DE, et al. Sustained care intervention and postdischarge smoking cessation among hospitalized adults: A randomized clinical trial. *JAMA*. 2014;312:719–728.

Rösner S, Hackl-Herrwerth A, Leucht S, Vecchi S, Srisurapanont M, Soyka M. Opioid antagonists for alcohol dependence. *Cochrane Database Syst Rev*. 2010;(12):CD001867.

Rudd RA, Seth P, David F, Scholl L. Increases in drug and opioid-involved overdose deaths—United States, 2010–2015. *MMWR Morb Mortal Wkly Rep*. 2016;65:1445.

Schuckit MA. Remarkable increases in alcohol use disorders. *JAMA Psychiatry*. 2017;74(9):869–870.

Shipton, EA, Shipton, EE, Shipton, AJ. A review of the opioid epidemic: what do we do about it? *Pain Ther*. 2018;7(1):23–36.

Slade T, Chapman C, Swift W, Keyes K, Tonks Z, Teesson M. Birth cohort trends in global epidemiology of alcohol use and alcohol-related harms in men and women: Systematic review and metaregression. *BMJ Open*. 2016;6:e011837.

Smith P, et al. Primary care validation of a single-question alcohol screening test. *J Gen Intern Med*. 2009;24(7):783–788.

Soeffing JM, Martin LD, Fingerhood MI, et al. Buprenorphine maintenance treatment in a primary care setting: Outcomes at 1 year. *J Subst Abuse Treat*. 2009;37:426–430.

Srisurapanont M, Jarusuraisin N. Naltrexone for the treatment of alcoholism: A meta-analysis of randomized controlled trials. *Int J Neuropsychopharmacol*. 2005;8(2):267–280.

Strang J, McCambridge J, Best D, et al. Loss of tolerance and overdose mortality after inpatient opiate detoxification: Follow up study. *BMJ*. 2003;326:959–960.

Substance Abuse and Mental Health Service Administration. Risk and protective factors. **http://www.samhsa.gov/capt/practicing-effective-prevention/prevention-behavioral-health/risk-protective-factors**. Published 2015.

Substance Abuse and Mental Health Services Administration. Table 6.84B. Tobacco product and alcohol use in past month among persons aged 18 to 22, by college enrollment status: Percentages, 2014 and 2015. 2015 National Survey on Drug Use and Health (NSDUH). **https://www.samhsa.gov/data/sites/default/files/NSDUH-DetTabs-2015/NSDUH-DetTabs-2015/NSDUH-DetTabs-2015.htm#tab6-84b**.

Substance Abuse and Mental Health Services Administration. Table 5.6A. Substance use disorder in past year among persons aged 18 or older, by demographic characteristics: Numbers in thousands, 2014 and 2015. 2015 National Survey on Drug Use and Health (NSDUH). **https://www.samhsa.gov/data/sites/default/files/NSDUH-DetTabs-2015/NSDUH-DetTabs-2015/NSDUH-DetTabs-2015.htm#tab5-6a**.

Substance Abuse and Mental Health Services Administration. Table 6.84B. Tobacco product and alcohol use in past month among persons aged 18 to 22, by college enrollment status: Percentages, 2014 and 2015. 2015 National Survey on Drug Use and Health (NSDUH). **https://www.samhsa.gov/data/sites/default/files/NSDUH-DetTabs-2015/NSDUH-DetTabs-2015/NSDUH-DetTabs-2015.htm#tab6-84b**.

Substance Abuse and Mental Health Services Administration. Table 2.50A. Alcohol use in lifetime, past year, and past month among persons aged 12 to 20, by demographic characteristics: Numbers in thousands, 2015 and 2016. 2016 National Survey on Drug Use and Health. https://www.samhsa.gov/data/sites/default/files/NSDUH-DetTabs-2016/NSDUH-DetTabs-2016.pdf. Published September 7, 2017.

Substance Abuse and Mental Health Services Administration. Table 5.2. A substance use disorder for specific substances in past year among persons aged 12 or older, by age group: Numbers in thousands, 2015 and 2016. 2016 National Survey on Drug Use and Health (NSDUH). https://www.samhsa.gov/data/sites/default/files/NSDUH-DetTabs-2016/NSDUH-DetTabs-2016.pdf. Published September 7, 2017.

Substance Abuse and Mental Health Services Administration. Figure 11: Past month binge and heavy alcohol use among people aged 12 or older, by age group: Percentages, 2016. 2016 National Survey on Drug use and Health (NSDH). https://www.samhsa.gov/data/sites/default/files/NSDUH-FFR1-2016/NSDUH-FFR1-2016.htm#alcohol2.

Substance Abuse and Mental Health Services Administration. Table 2.33D: Alcohol use in lifetime among persons aged 12 or older, by age group and demographic characteristics: Standard errors of percentages, 2015 and 2016. 2016 National Survey on Drug use and Health (NSDH). https://www.samhsa.gov/data/sites/default/files/NSDUH-DetTabs-2016/NSDUH-DetTabs-2016.pdf.

Substance Abuse and Mental Health Services Administration. 2016 National Survey on Drug use and Health (NSDH), marijuana use. https://www.samhsa.gov/data/sites/default/files/NSDUH-FFR1-2016/NSDUH-FFR1-2016.htm#illicit2.

Substance Abuse and Mental Health Services Administration. Federal guidelines for opioid treatment programs (HHS Publication No. [SMA] PEP15-FEDGUIDEOTP). https://store.samhsa.gov/shin/content/PEP15-FEDGUIDEOTP/PEP15-FEDGUIDEOTP.pdf. Published 2015.

Substance Abuse and Mental Health Services Administration. Medication-assisted treatment (MAT). https://www.samhsa.gov/medication-assisted-treatment. Published 2018.

Thombs DL. *Introduction to addictive behaviors*. 3rd ed. New York: Guilford Press; 2006.

Tsuang MT, Lyons MJ, Meyer JM, et al. Co-occurrence of abuse of different drugs in men: The role of drug-specific and shared vulnerabilities. *Arch Gen Psychiatry*. 1998;55:967–972.

U.S. Department of Health and Human Services, National Institutes of Health, National Institute on Drug Abuse. Misuse of prescription drugs. http://www.nida.nih.gov/ResearchReports/Prescription/prescription7.html. Published 2018.

U.S. Food and Drug Administration. Caffeine intake by the US population. www.fda.gov/downloads/AboutFDA/CentersOffices/OfficeofFoods/CFSAN/CFSANFOIAElectronicReadingRoom/UCM333191.pdf. Published 2010.

U.S. Preventive Services Task Force. Alcohol misuse: screening and behavioral counseling interventions in primary care. http://www.uspreventiveservicestaskforce.org/uspstf/uspsdrin.htm. Published May 2013.

van Beurden I, Anderson P, Akkermans RP, et al. Involvement of general practitioners in managing alcohol problems: a randomized controlled trial of a tailored improvement programme. *Addiction*. 2012;107:1601–1611.

Weiss RD, Potter JS, Griffin ML, et al. Long-term outcomes from the national drug abuse treatment clinical trials network prescription opioid addiction treatment study. *Drug Alcohol Depend*. 2015;150:112–119.

Wilbanks WL. Drug addiction should be treated as a lack of self-discipline. In: Leone B, ed. *Chemical dependency: Opposing viewpoints*. San Diego, CA: Greenhaven; 1989.

Willenbring ML, et al. Helping patients who drink too much: An evidence-based guide for primary care clinicians. *Am Fam Physician*. 2009;80(1):44–50.

Willenbring ML, Olson DH. A randomized trial of integrated outpatient treatment for medically ill alcoholic men. *Arch Intern Med*. 1999;159(16):1946–1952.

Williams EC, Achtmeyer CE, Thomas RM, et al. Factors underlying quality problems with alcohol screening prompted by a clinical reminder in primary care: A multi-site qualitative study. *J Gen Intern Med*. 2015;30:1125–1132.

Williams EC, Rubinsky AD, Chavez LJ, et al. An early evaluation of implementation of brief intervention for unhealthy alcohol use in the US Veterans Health Administration. *Addiction*. 2014;109:1472–1481.

Zammit S, et al. Maternal tobacco, cannabis and alcohol use during pregnancy and risk of adolescent psychotic symptoms in offspring. *Br J Psychiatry*. 2009;195(4):294–300.

RESOURCES

General

Alcoholics Anonymous
http://www.aa.org/

Narcotics Anonymous
http://www.na.org/

Rethinking Drinking. National Institute on Alcohol Abuse and Alcoholism (NIAAA)
http://rethinkingdrinking.niaaa.nih.gov

Substance Abuse Treatment: Addressing the Specific Needs of Women: A Treatment Improvement Protocol. Substance Abuse and Mental Health Services Administration (SAMHSA)
https://store.samhsa.gov/shin/content//SMA15-4426/SMA15-4426.pdf

Substance Use Disorders. Substance Abuse and Mental Health Services Administration (SAMHSA)
https://www.samhsa.gov/disorders/substance-use

Treatment for Alcohol Problems: Finding and Getting Help. National Institute on Alcohol Abuse and Alcoholism (NIAAA)
http://pubs.niaaa.nih.gov/publications/Treatment/treatment.htm

Alcohol

Alcohol: A Women's Health Issue. National Institute on Alcohol Abuse and Alcoholism
https://pubs.niaaa.nih.gov/publications/brochurewomen/women.htm

Alcohol: Facts on Alcohol and the Impact Abusing Alcohol Can Have on People. Substance Abuse and Mental Health Services Administration
https://www.samhsa.gov/atod/alcohol

Older Adults and Alcohol: You Can Get Help. National Institute on Alcohol Abuse and Alcoholism
https://pubs.niaaa.nih.gov/publications/olderAdults/olderAdults.pdf

Understanding Alcohol Use Disorders and Their Treatment: When Does Drinking Become a Problem? When Should Someone Seek Help? American Psychological Association
http://www.apa.org/helpcenter/alcohol-disorders.aspx

Anxiolytic Drugs

Benzodiazepines: Licit Uses, Illicit Uses, Illicit Distribution, and Control Status. Drug Enforcement Administration
https://www.deadiversion.usdoj.gov/drug_chem_info/benzo.pdf

Benzodiazepines: Profile, History, Methods of Use, Short-Term Effects, Long-Term Effects, Tolerance and Withdrawal. Center for Substance Abuse Research University of Maryland
http://www.cesar.umd.edu/cesar/drugs/benzos.asp

Cannabis

CDC Guideline for Prescribing Opioids for Chronic Pain: Promoting Patient Care and Safety. The US Opioid Overdose Epidemic, Prescription Opioids Have Benefits and Risks. Centers for Disease Control and Prevention
https://www.cdc.gov/drugoverdose/pdf/Guidelines_At-A-Glance-508.pdf

Cocaine: How Does Cocaine Produce Its Effect? National Institute on Drug Abuse
https://www.drugabuse.gov/publications/research-reports/cocaine/how-does-cocaine-produce-its-effects

Drug Facts: What Is Cocaine? How Do People Use Cocaine? What Are the Health Effects of Cocaine Use? Can a Person Overdose on Cocaine? How Can a Cocaine Overdose Be Treated? How Does Cocaine Use Lead to Addiction? National Institute on Drug Abuse
https://www.drugabuse.gov/publications/drugfacts/cocaine

Drugs, Brains, and Behavior: The Science of Addiction. National Institute on Drug Abuse
https://www.drugabuse.gov/publications/drugs-brains-behavior-science-addiction/preface

Marijuana (Cannabis): Get Facts on Marijuana, Surveillance, Laws and Policies, and Preventing Youth Marijuana Use. Substance Abuse Mental Health Service Administration
https://store.samhsa.gov/shin/content//SMA05-4010/SMA05-4010.pdf

Motivational Enhancement Therapy and Cognitive Behavioral Therapy for Adolescent Cannabis Users. Substance Abuse Mental Health Service Administration
https://store.samhsa.gov/shin/content//SMA05-4010/SMA05-4010.pdf

The Brian's Response to Cocaine: Cocaine Can Change the Way the Brain Works, Cocaine Can Tightens Blood Vessels. National Institute of Drug Abuse
https://teens.drugabuse.gov/sites/default/files/cocaine.pdf

Hallucinogenic Drugs

Hallucinogens and Dissociative Drugs: Common Hallucinogens and Dissociative Drugs. Classic Hallucinogens. National Institute on Drug Abuse
https://www.drugabuse.gov/publications/research-reports/hallucinogens-dissociative-drugs/what-are-dissociative-drugs

Hallucinogens: What Are Hallucinogens? National Institute on Drug Abuse
https://www.drugabuse.gov/publications/drugfacts/hallucinogens

Hypnotics

Drug Facts: Club Drugs (GHB, Ketamine, and Rohypnol) How Are Club Drugs Abused? How Do Club Drugs Affect the Brain? What Other Adverse Effects Do Club Drugs Have on Health? How Widespread Is Club Drug Abuse? National Institute on Drug Abuse
https://www.drugabuse.gov/sites/default/files/drugfacts_clubdrugs_12_2014.pdf

MDMA (Ecstasy/Molly): What Is MDMA? How Do People Use MDMA? How Does MDMA Affect the Brain? What Are Other Health Effects of MDMA? National Institute on Drug Abuse
https://www.drugabuse.gov/publications/drugfacts/mdma-ecstasymolly

Substance Abuse (Depressants or Sedative-Hypnotic Drugs): What Is It? Symptoms, Diagnosis, Prevention, Treatment, When to Call A Professional, Prognosis. Harvard Health Publishing
https://www.health.harvard.edu/diseases-and-conditions/substance-abuse-depressants-or-sedative-hypnotic-drugs

Nicotine

Nicotine Addiction: Brain Mechanisms, Nicotine and Neurotransmitter Release, Monoamine Oxidase, Neuroadaptation, Clinical Aspects of Nicotine Addiction, Psychoactive Effects of Nicotine. Genetics of Nicotine Addiction. U.S. National Library of Medicine
https://www.ncbi.nlm.nih.gov/pmc/articles/PMC2928221/

Nicotine Dependence: An Overview, Symptoms and Causes, Diagnosis and Treatment; A Short Film; and Risk Factors, Complications, and Prevention. Mayo Clinic
https://www.mayoclinic.org/diseases-conditions/nicotine-dependence/symptoms-causes/syc-20351584

Tobacco/Nicotine: Is Nicotine Addictive? National Institute on Drug Abuse
https://www.drugabuse.gov/publications/research-reports/tobacco/nicotine-addictive

Opioid Addiction

Effective Treatments for Opioid Addiction. National Institute on Drug Abuse
https://www.drugabuse.gov/publications/effective-treatments-opioid-addiction/effective-treatments-opioid-addiction

Opioid Addiction. American Academy of Family Physicians
https://familydoctor.org/condition/opioid-addiction/

Perception Opioids: About the Problem, Risk Factors, Addiction and Overdose. Centers for Disease Control and Prevention
https://www.cdc.gov/drugoverdose/opioids/prescribed.html

Preventing an Opioid Overdose: Know the Signs. Save a Life. Centers for Disease Control and Prevention
https://www.cdc.gov/drugoverdose/pdf/patients/Preventing-an-Opioid-Overdose-Tip-Card-a.pdf

Principles of Substance Abuse Prevention for Early Childhood. A Research-Based Guide. National Institute on Drug Abuse
https://www.drugabuse.gov/publications/principles-substance-abuse-prevention-early-childhood/index

Promoting Safer and More Effective Pain Management: Understanding Prescription Opioids, Opioids and Chronic Pain. Centers for Disease Control and Prevention
https://www.cdc.gov/drugoverdose/pdf/Guidelines_Factsheet-Patients-a.pdf

Stimulants

Get the Facts on Stimulants: Cocaine and Methamphetamine. Substance Abuse and Mental Health Service Administration
https://www.samhsa.gov/atod/stimulants

Stimulant ADHD Medications: Methylphenidate and Amphetamines. The National Institute on Drug Abuse
https://www.drugabuse.gov/publications/drugfacts/stimulant-adhd-medications-methylphenidate-amphetamines

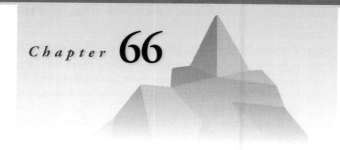

Chapter 66

Schizophrenia Spectrum Disorders

Martin T. Strassnig, MD

Michael E. Thase, MD

Lynne M. Dunphy, PhD, APRN, FNP-BC, FAAN, FAANP

Psychotic disorders are disturbances of thought content and/or process and signal a departure from reality, often accompanied by a combination of hallucinations and delusions, disorganized thinking (speech), disorganized or abnormal motor behavior (including catatonia), and negative symptoms. A person with psychosis may exhibit difficulties with communication, insight, behavior, and relationships. Psychosis may be the direct result of medication effects, such as illicit drugs or prescribed steroids. It may also be confused with delirium, which most often signals a medical rather than psychiatric causes. Psychotic disorders may coexist with other psychiatric and medical disorders. Schizoaffective disorder exhibits symptoms of both schizophrenia and mood disorders. Psychotic disorders can be classified into several categories, as outlined in Table 66.1.

Schizophrenia is among the most disabling and expensive mental illnesses, surpassed only by substance use disorders and depression. The World Health Organization ranks it as one of the top 15 illnesses contributing to the global burden of disease. The cost is staggering. For example, an analysis of insurance claims in the United States found that annual health-related expenses of someone with chronic schizophrenia averaged more than $15,000 (Nicholl, 2010). The cost of schizophrenia-related treatment from 2004–2009 in the U.S. increased from 9.4 billion to 11.5 million (Feldman, 2014).

People with schizophrenia often experience symptoms such as hearing internally generated voices not heard by others or believing that other people are reading their minds, controlling their thoughts, or plotting to harm them. These symptoms may leave them fearful and withdrawn, reluctant to engage in treatment, and/or nonadherent to treatment. Because of its sometimes-disruptive symptoms, a diagnosis of schizophrenia can have serious implications for patients and families. Schizophrenia is a serious disorder of the mind and brain, but it is also

TABLE 66.1 Psychotic Disorders

Psychotic Disorder	Description
Schizophrenia	Onset: Acute or insidious. Symptoms present for at least 6 months with at least two or more positive or negative symptoms present for at least 1 month. Social, employment, or self-care impairment.
Bipolar I disorder, manic, severe, with psychosis	Onset: Variable. Signs and symptoms must be present for 1 week or if hospitalization is required. Psychotic signs and symptoms present only during mood disorder. Social and employment impairment during episode.
Bipolar I disorder, mixed episode, with psychosis	Onset: Variable. Signs and symptoms must be present for 1 week or if hospitalization is required. Meets criteria for depression and mania. Positive signs and symptoms only with mood symptoms. Social and employment impairment during episode.
Major depression, severe, with psychotic features	Onset: Variable. Lasts 2+ weeks. Positive signs and symptoms occur only during mood episode. Impairment during episode (includes postpartum).
Schizoaffective disorder	Presence of psychosis independent and concurrent with major mood symptoms.
Brief psychotic disorder	Onset: Acute. Full expression within 2 weeks and complete remission 1–3 months, lasts at least 1 day but less than 1 month. May have an acute stressor.
Schizophreniform	Usually acute onset of symptoms. Criteria of schizophrenia are met, but for fewer than 6 months.
Delusional disorder	Criteria for schizophrenia are not met. Onset subtle, nonbizarre delusions, symptoms last more than 1 month.

Sources: American Psychiatric Association. *Diagnostic and statistical manual of mental disorders.* 5th ed. Arlington, VA; American Psychiatric Association; 2013. Mojtabai R, Fochtmann LJ, Bromet EJ. Other psychotic disorders. In: Sadock BJ, et al, eds. *Kaplan and Sadock's comprehensive textbook of psychiatry.* Philadelphia, PA: Lippincott Williams & Wilkins; 2017.

highly treatable. Although there is no cure (as of 2018) for schizophrenia, the treatment success rate with anti-psychotic medications and psychosocial therapies can be high.

EPIDEMIOLOGY AND CAUSES

The number of people who will be diagnosed as having schizophrenia in a year is about one in 4,000. So in a given year, about 1.5 million people worldwide and about 100,000 people in the United States are diag-nosed with schizophrenia. The prevalence (how many cases there are at any given time) averages approximately 1.1% of the population over age 18; in other words, at any one time, as many as 51 million people worldwide and 2.2 million people in the United States have schizo-phrenia. The risk of developing the illness over one's life-time averages 0.7%, with minor variations related to race and ethnicity, immigration status, and socioeconomic and geographical factors. Men are 1.4 times more likely to develop schizophrenia than women. Age of onset is typically during adolescence or early 20s; childhood and late-life onset (over 45 years) are rare. Age at onset occurs earlier in men, commonly in late adolescence and early 20s; women tend to present in their late 20s to mid-30s. However, in both males and females, subtle symptoms may occur long before a definitive diagnosis is made, and males tend to have a worse prognosis and more difficult course. The prevalence of schizophrenia in adolescents is low, and although rare, it can occur in childhood before age 13. Early onset tends to point to a poor prognosis; however, early intervention and early use of new medications lead to better medical outcomes for the individual. Recent research increasingly shows that the disease process of schizophrenia gradually and significantly damages the individual's brain, and that ear-lier treatments (medications and other therapies) seem to result in less damage over time. The earlier someone with schizophrenia is diagnosed and stabilized on treatment, the better the long-term prognosis for their illness. There is a higher incidence of co-occuring disorders in those with schizophrenia such as depressive disorders, anxiety disorders, specifically social anxiety, post-traumatic stress, and obsessive-compulsive disorders, as well as alcohol and substance use. Additionally, there are higher rates of metabolic and neurological problems. The rate of suicide is higher in those with schizophrenia; teens with schizo-phrenia have approximately a 50% risk of attempted sui-cide; about 10% of all completed suicides are by people with schizophrenia, and about 5% of all people with schizophrenia commit suicide (Arsenault-Lapierre et al., 2004; Hor & Taylor, 2010).

The disease course is variable, with some patients exhib-iting only mild symptoms, while others follow a chronic course resulting in functional impairment, including an inability to maintain independent housing and gainful employment, and social deficits. Poor engagement in health maintenance initiatives such as cancer screenings, exercise, nutrition, tobacco cessation, and identification of other comorbid chronic medical diseases play a role in poor outcomes. Overall, one-third recover, one-third wax and wane, and one-third have a chronic course and slow deterioration.

Identified but poorly understood risk factors include immigration, living in an urban area, obstetrical compli-cations, late-winter/early-spring births (perhaps related to exposure to influenza virus during neural develop-ment), and advanced paternal age (thought to be related to increased risk of de novo mutations). Leading theories of why people get schizophrenia is that it is a result of a genetic predisposition combined with an environmen-tal exposures and/or stresses during pregnancy or child-hood that contribute to, or trigger, the disorder. Already researchers have identified several of the key genes that, when damaged, seem to create a predisposition, or increased risk, for schizophrenia

PATHOPHYSIOLOGY

Although the pathogenesis of the disorder is unknown, schizophrenia is likely a syndrome comprising multiple diseases that present with similar signs and symptoms. It may run in families. As already noted, living in an urban environment, male gender, and a history of migration are associated with a slightly higher risk for developing the illness. Genetic factors and gene–environment inter-actions together contribute more than 80% of the risk for developing schizophrenia. However, no single gene is responsible for a greater likelihood of developing schizo-phrenia. Environmental factors associated with a higher likelihood of developing schizophrenia include cannabis use, prenatal infection or malnutrition, obstetric compli-cations, and a history of late-winter/early-spring birth. Prenatal maternal stress, including physiologic stress such as in times of famine, as well as psychological stressors, such as prenatal death of the father, and antenatal infec-tion or exposure, have been implicated (Koenig et al., 2005). It is safe to say that various genetic and environ-mental factors combine to cause schizophrenia, but the mechanisms are poorly understood. Several neurotrans-mitter systems are involved in the pathology of schizo-phrenia including dopamine, glutamate, GABA, and acetylcholine. These represent the current best targets for pharmacological intervention in the disorder.

CLINICAL PRESENTATION

The onset of schizophrenia may be abrupt or insidi-ous. The illness begins for many individuals in adoles-cence and shows a slow and gradual development of clinical symptoms, with the first frank episode usually presenting in between 15 and 25 years of age in men and 25 and 35 years of age in women and a second peak for women in their 40s. Depressive symptoms are common, occur in approximately half of cases, and should not habitually be diagnosed as schizoaffective disorder (discussed subsequently). Schizophrenia presents with four symptom clusters that are used to describe the disorder, and each has implications for therapeutic treatment. Positive symptoms, negative symptoms, cognitive impairments, and affective disturbances comprise these clusters.

Positive symptoms refer to the "active" qualities of these symptoms that are abnormal and are synonymous with psychosis. Positive symptoms include delusions, hallucinations, disorganized thinking (speech), and grossly disorganized or abnormal behavior (catatonia). Delusions are the hallmark of positive symptoms, occurring in more than half of patients. Delusions are fixed beliefs that are not amenable to change despite conflicting evidence. They can include persecutory, referential, somatic, religious, or grandiose themes. Hallucinations are sensory impressions without basis of reality. They can be vivid and clear to the individual experiencing them and may occur in any sensory modality such as auditory, visual, somatic, olfactory, or gustatory, with auditory followed by visual hallucinations most common. Auditory hallucinations are distinct from the individual's own thoughts and are the most common type of hallucination They must occur in the context of a clear sensorium. Disorganization is seen in behavior and/or thinking. Disorganized thinking is typically inferred from speech and must substantially impair effective communications. Commonly observed forms of abnormal speech are as follows:

- Tangentiality—getting off topic without answering questions appropriately
- Circumstantiality—will answer question in markedly roundabout manner
- Derailment—switching topics without a logic sequence
- Neologisms—creation of new, idiosyncratic words
- Word salad—words are placed together without any sensible meaning

Grossly disorganized or abnormal motor behavior (including catatonia) may occur with schizophrenia with problems noted in goal-directed activities and activities of daily living.

Negative symptoms represent diminished or a lack of normal characteristics—diminished emotional expression and avolition. *Diminished emotional expression* encompasses reductions in expression of the face, eye contact, intonation of speech, and movements of the hands, head, and face that contribute to emotion of speech. *Avolition* represents decline in motivated self-initiated purposeful activities. This encompasses loss of affective responsiveness, verbal expression, and communication, personal and social motivation, and enjoyment. Primary negative symptoms can be resistant to treatment and closely related to functional outcome. Secondary negative symptoms may be routed in other manifestations such as depression of the illness or treatment including sedating antipsychotics.

Cognitive impairments in schizophrenia often are seen early in life and correlate with everyday functional outcomes such as the ability to keep a job or live independently. Cognitive impairments include difficulties with memory, attention, psychomotor speed, and executive function. Cognitive impairments, along with negative symptoms, are the most common contributors to disability in schizophrenia.

Affective disturbances, which are difficulties with mood and affect, are seen with schizophrenia. Depression and anxiety can be detected before, during or after a psychotic episode, and providers must be alert for risk of suicide, particularly at the initiation of treatment, immediately after an acute psychotic crisis, and throughout outpatient encounters (see Box 66.1).

DIAGNOSTIC REASONING

Symptoms

The Diagnostic and Statistical Manual of Mental Disorders, fifth edition (*DSM-5*) provides detailed symptom criteria for schizophrenia. Two or more of positive or negative symptoms must be present, with one of the positive symptoms being delusions, hallucinations, or disorganized speech. Dysfunction in one or more areas such as interpersonal relations, work or education, or self-care also must be present. Associated features include inappropriate affect, anhedonia, dysphoric mood, abnormal psychomotor activity, cognitive dysfunction, confusion, lack of insight, and depersonalization. Abnormal neurological findings may show a broad range of dysfunction including slow reaction time, poor coordination, abnormalities in eye tracking, and impaired sensory gating.

Schizoaffective disorder appears to be one-third as common as schizophrenia with an estimated prevalence of 0.3% and requires an uninterrupted period of illness during which the criteria for schizophrenia and a major mood disorder are met. There must also be a period of 2 weeks or longer during which there are psychotic symptoms in complete absence of mood symptoms. The incidence is higher in females than in males. Age of onset is typically early adulthood, although it may occur in adolescence to adulthood. Social dysfunction and exclusion of autism spectrum disorder or other communication disorders of childhood onset required for schizophrenia do not have to be met. Occupational function and social functioning are often impaired but need not be defining criteria for diagnosis. This contrasts with schizophrenia. There may be restricted social contact, anosognosia (poor insight), and difficulties with self-care; however, *negative symptoms* may be less severe

Box 66.1 Symptom Clusters of Schizophrenia

Positive Symptoms—exaggeration of normal processes

- Hallucinations: Perception of a sensory process in the absence of an external source; can be auditory (most common), visual, somatic, olfactory, or gustatory, alone or in combination.
- Delusions: Fixed false belief. Classified as bizarre delusion—clearly implausible; or nonbizarre delusions—although not true, is understandable with possibility of being true. Categorized as grandiose, paranoid, nihilistic, and erotomanic.
- Disorganization: Affective or cognitive chaos; manifested in speech and behavior as loose or illogical thoughts lacking connectivity.
- Movement disorders: Grossly disorganized or abnormal motor behavior including catatonia.

Negative Symptoms—absence or diminution of normal processes

- Flat or blunted affect
- Alogia: Poverty of speech
- Asociality/anhedonia: Lack of pleasure in acts that are normally pleasurable; failure to engage with peers socially
- Apathy: Lack of self-motivation, poor grooming and hygiene, anergy

Cognitive Impairments

- Poor executive functioning, concrete thoughts, diminished processing speed
- Difficulty focusing, maintaining attention
- Verbal and visual learning and memory deficits
- Verbal comprehension
- Social cognition

Affective Disturbances

- Blunted or flat affect, loss of affective reactivity, odd affect
- Poor self-esteem
- Depression and anxiety
- Increased risk of suicide

Source: Adapted from American Psychiatric Association. *Diagnostic and statistical manual of mental disorders.* 5th ed. Arlington, VA; American Psychiatric Association; 2013.

and less persistent. Alcohol and substance abuse can be associated with schizoaffective disorder. Individuals may go on to a diagnosis of schizophrenia, major depressive disorder, or bipolar disorder. As with schizophrenia, schizoaffective disorder carries a 10% lifetime risk of suicide, and assessment regarding suicide lethality must be always addressed. Please refer to the *DSM-5* for complete diagnostic criteria.

Table 66.1 briefly identifies other psychotic disorders for consideration.

Differential Diagnosis

Initial presentation may occur in the primary-care setting. The role of the primary-care provider is to identify and refer any suspected or new cases of schizophrenia for urgent psychiatric evaluation. In some settings, especially in rural settings, this may be difficult owing to a paucity of mental health services and psychiatric providers. The primary-care provider is responsible to evaluate the patient's current risk to self and others. Any person presenting with psychosis for the initial or "first break" should be fully evaluated for underlying medical conditions. Consideration of substance abuse should be one of the primary differentials, and toxicology testing should be performed. Alcohol, opioids, cocaine, amphetamines, MDMA-receptor antagonists (ecstasy), and hallucinogens are some of the most common offenders. In addition, it is not only consumption of these agents, but also withdrawal from them, that may precipitate symptoms. Commonly prescribed medications such as anticholinergic agents, phenytoin, steroids, H_2 blockers (cimetidine), and anxiolytics may produce similar symptoms. Other differentials to consider include delirium, in which the onset of symptoms can occur rapidly and are accompanied by confusion, and in which visual hallucinations are more common, versus schizophrenia, in which the sensorium remains clear, symptoms occur over a longer time period and auditory hallucinations occur more frequently. For individuals with acute, later onset psychotic conditions, medical illnesses such as hepatic encephalopathy, hyponatremia, hypoglycemia, hypoxia, intracranial bleed, infection, meningitis/encephalitis, and so forth should also be considered. A complete history and physical exam with attention to neurological and mental status exam are essential. Laboratory evaluation should include complete blood count (CBC) with differential, electrolytes, renal function, liver profile, thyroid function, drug and alcohol toxicology, and pregnancy. Attention should be paid to potential infectious diseases processes with screening for syphilis, HIV, and hepatitis C. It may be determined that further testing for heavy metals, electroencephalogram, or brain imaging with magnetic resonance imaging or computed tomography is warranted.

MANAGEMENT

Depending on the individual long-term course, schizophrenia can be a chronic illness that influences many aspects of everyday life for patients and their families. Treatment goals should include reducing or eliminating symptoms, maximizing quality of life, improving function, and promoting and maintaining recovery within the context of an early intervention model of care. Treatment involves a multidisciplinary approach: assertive outreach approaches, family involvement and interventions, psychological interventions and psychologically informed care, vocational and educational interventions, and antipsychotic medication and monitoring (Scottish Intercollegiate Guidelines Network, 2013).

Pharmacotherapy with antipsychotic medications is the mainstay of treatment for schizophrenia (McDonagh et al., 2017; Scottish Intercollegiate Guidelines Network, 2013). Early therapeutic intervention is important and improves long-term outcomes. Pharmacological intervention is quite effective in addressing the *positive symptoms* of schizophrenia but less successful for negative and cognitive symptoms. The negative and cognitive symptoms are best addressed in a more multifaceted approach including cognitive behavior therapy and cognitive remediation therapy in combination with psychiatric rehabilitation approaches. Strategies to prevent relapse and encourage medication adherence are essential. The Expert Consensus Guideline Series (Velligan et al., 2014) determined that adherence problems in patients with serious mental illness primarily stem from poor insight and lack of illness awareness or distress associated with specific side effects or a general fear of potential side effects.

Social support plays a crucial role in minimizing the social disability associated with schizophrenia. The *Circle of Caring* (see Chapter 1) is essential in helping the patient navigate the complex system of primary care and mental health services, as well as providing education for patients and significant others to access available community resources. Understanding the lived experience of the patient, family, and community of those living with schizophrenia, as well as their definition of wellness and recovery, helps to foster insight and adherence to the treatment plan. Of critical importance is the establishment of the therapeutic alliance, providing a supportive environment, maintaining continuity of provider when possible, and developing a trusting relationship where the patient is the active participant in his or her care. Recovery includes wellness and provision of primary care. Management of comorbid conditions is central to that effort.

Targets of Treatment

The goals of therapy include management of symptoms; evaluation of community issues such as housing, employment, homelessness, justice issues, and victimization; and assessment of co-occurring illnesses such as post-traumatic stress disorder, substance abuse, and depression (McDonagh et al., 2017; Scottish Intercollegiate Guidelines Network, 2013). In addition, it is essential to provide education to significant others to enhance the therapeutic alliance and compliance with the treatment plan (Scottish Intercollegiate Guidelines Network, 2013).

Pharmacological Management

Antipsychotic medications are the primary treatment for psychotic symptoms (McDonagh, 2017; Scottish Intercollegiate Guidelines Network, 2013). These medications help to alleviate the positive symptoms and decrease hospital days and relapse rates. In addition, a greater response to medication is often seen when it is started early in the course of the disease. Initiation of early and effective doses of antipsychotic medication is important because it may influence the effect on the patient and family, as well as decrease the risk of injury to self or others (see Drugs Commonly Prescribed 66.1 and 66.2).

Drugs Commonly Prescribed 66.1: Typical Antipsychotics

DRUG	INDICATION	ADVERSE REACTIONS AND PRESCRIBING CONSIDERATIONS
High Potency		
Perphenazine* (Trilafon)	Psychosis Severe behavioral disturbances due to cognitive impairment Nausea/vomiting	• Risk for neuroleptic malignant syndrome • Monitor for movement disorder (AIMS), CBC, LFTs, annual eye exam, renal function, serum prolactin, photosensitivity • Administration 2×/day
Fluphenazine (Prolixin)*+	Psychosis	• Monitor for movement disorder, CBC, LFTs, annual eye exam, serum prolactin, skin exanthemas • Administration 2×/day
Trifluoperazine (Stelazine)*	Psychosis Anxiety disorder	• Monitor for movement disorder, CBC, LFTs, annual eye exam, serum prolactin • Administration 2×/day
Haloperidol (Haldol)*+	Acute psychosis Schizophrenia ADHD Tourette's disorder	• EPS, hyperprolactinemia • QT prolongation risk: mild if oral, moderate if IV administration • Sedation, weight gain, rare photosensitivity • Monitor for movement disorder, CBC, LFTs, serum prolactin, and urinalysis
Thiothixene (Navane)*	Schizophrenia	• Monitor for movement disorder, CBC, LFTs, annual eye exam, serum prolactin, TFTs, and urinalysis • Photosensitivity

Drugs Commonly Prescribed 66.1: Typical Antipsychotics—cont'd

DRUG	INDICATION	ADVERSE REACTIONS AND PRESCRIBING CONSIDERATIONS
Medium Potency		
Loxapine (Loxitane)*	Bipolar Schizophrenia	• Photosensitivity, seizures • CBC, ophthalmological exam, TFTs, and urinalysis
Low Potency		
Chlorpromazine (Thorazine)*	Acute intermittent porphyria Acute psychosis Nausea/vomiting Tetanus Schizophrenia Hiccups	• Photosensitivity, sulfite sensitivity • AIMS assessment, CBC, ophthalmological exam, and prolactin

Abbreviations: ADHD, attention-deficit/hyperactivity disorder; AIMS, Abnormal Involuntary Movement Scale; CBC, complete blood count; EPS, extrapyramidal symptoms; LFT, liver function test; TFTs, thyroid function tests.
*Black-box warning: dementia.
+Also available as long-acting depot injection to be given biweekly (Prolixin) or monthly (Haloperidol).

Drugs Commonly Prescribed 66.2: Atypical Antipsychotics

DRUG	INDICATION	ADVERSE REACTIONS AND PRESCRIBING CONSIDERATIONS
Clozapine (Clozaril)*	Schizophrenia Schizoaffective disorder	• Agranulocytosis, lowered seizure threshold† • Rare myocarditis • Anticholinergic effects, no EPS, postural hypotension, prolong QT interval, sedation • Metabolic effects: monitor weight gain,++ increased lipids,++ FPG,++ waist circumference, CBC with differential, LFTs, and AIMS
Olanzapine (Zyprexa)*	Bipolar depression Bipolar disorder Depression Mania Schizophrenia	• Anticholinergic effects, dizziness/hypotension • Sedation • Metabolic effect: weight gain++ • Monitor AIMS assessment, body weight, waist circumference, glucose, lipids, LFTs, neurological function
Quetiapine (Seroquel)*	Bipolar depression Bipolar disorder Depression Mania Schizophrenia	• Anticholinergic effects, postural hypotension, somnolence • Metabolic effects: weight gain,++ FPG+ • Monitor AIMS assessment, body weight, waist circumference, glucose, LFTs, neurological function, lipid profile
Risperidone (Risperdal)*	Autism Bipolar disorder Mania Schizophrenia	• Anxiety, agitation, hypotension, sedation • EPS+++ • Metabolic effects: weight gain,+ increased lipids,+ FPG,+ hyperprolactinemia++ • Monitor: AIMS assessment, body weight, waist circumference, glucose, LFTs, neurological function, lipid profile
Aripiprazole (Abilify)*	Autism Bipolar disorder Depression Mania Schizophrenia	• Rarely significant side effects of EPS, weight gain, or prolactin elevation • Monitor: AIMS assessment, body weight, glucose, LFTs, neurological function, lipid profile

Continued

Drugs Commonly Prescribed 66.2: Atypical Antipsychotics—cont'd

DRUG	INDICATION	ADVERSE REACTIONS AND PRESCRIBING CONSIDERATIONS
Ziprasidone (Geodon)*	Bipolar disorder Mania Schizophrenia	• May prolong QT interval • Rarely significant side effects of EPS, weight gain, or prolactin elevation • Monitor: ECG, AIMS assessment, body weight, glucose, LFTs, neurological function, lipid profile
Paliperidone (Invega)*	Schizoaffective disorder Schizophrenia	• May prolong QT interval, EPS, tachycardia • Metabolic effects: weight gain,+ prolactinemia • Monitor AIMS, ECG, body weight, glucose, lipid profile, LFTs, neurological function
Iloperidone (Fanapt)*	Schizophrenia	• Anticholinergic+, dizziness, tachycardia, orthostatic hypotension,+ sedation, EPS+ • Prolong QT interval+++ • Metabolic effects: weight gain,++ prolactinemia+ • Monitor AIMS and ECG

Abbreviations: AIMS, Abnormal Involuntary Movement Scale; CBC, complete blood count; ECG, electrocardiogram; EPS, extrapyramidal symptoms; FPG, fasting plasma glucose; LFT, liver function test.

*Black-box warning: dementia.

†Doses greater than 600 mg.

+Mild, ++moderate, +++high risk.

Because medication-naive patients are more sensitive to the psychotropic effects of medications (they respond to lower doses and may show heightened sensitivity to side effects), initiation at the lower end of standard dose is recommended. Response rates are variable; slow titration of antipsychotic medication is recommended to help reduce the risk of intolerable side effects that may affect long-term adherence, although more rapid dose escalation is sometimes required. Patients who experience a first episode are typically more responsive to treatment than those who have experienced multiple episodes of illness; remission is achieved within 3 to 4 months for 70% of patients, and 83% have a stable remission by 1 year. Unfortunately, some individuals will not seek treatment because of paranoid symptoms or impaired thinking process.

The antipsychotic medications can be divided into two categories: (1) first-generation conventional, or "typical," and (2) the second- or newer generation of "atypical" antipsychotic medications, based on their pharmacology and side-effect profile. The typical, or conventional, antipsychotics have been in wide use since the 1960s. These medications are very effective; however, they are more likely than atypical antipsychotics to cause motor system side effects, nonadherence to a potential consequence (see Table 66.2). All antipsychotic medications primarily exert their beneficial effects by reducing the positive symptoms. The "atypicals" are equally as effective as the older antipsychotics in the treatment of positive symptoms and less likely to cause motor side effects. As a group, however, atypical antipsychotics have

commonly been associated with weight gain and metabolic disturbances such as elevated blood glucose or lipids, type 2 diabetes mellitus, and cardiovascular disease. There are not, however, any medications that can reverse the pathophysiology of schizophrenia in a curative way.

The Clinical Antipsychotic Trials of Intervention Effectiveness project (CATIE) sponsored by the National Institute of Mental Health completed 10 years ago looked at the various antipsychotic medications, comparing a number of the newer drugs with the conventional antipsychotic perphenazine. The newer, "atypical" drugs were not superior to perphenazine, a "typical" antipsychotic, although olanzapine had the highest rate of "persistence" (i.e., was switched less often because of side effects or lack of efficacy). Given the magnitude of the problem of nonadherence with antipsychotic medications, depot medications are particularly important for patients with compliance issues. These are injectable formulations that are given intramuscularly in either biweekly or monthly intervals, ensuring delivery. Adjunctive medications help with controlling side effects and assisting with comorbid illnesses such as anxiety and depression.

Extrapyramidal symptoms (EPS) are potentially troubling side effects of antipsychotics and include Parkinson-like symptoms, akathisia (an inability to sit still), and dystonia (akin to muscle cramps). In some cases, tardive dyskinesia develops (a late-onset and persistent movement disorder attributed to antipsychotic use). It is thought that these symptoms are related to blockade of the dopamine receptors and thus the decreased functional availability of dopamine, and in the case of tardive

TABLE 66.2   Comparison of the First-Generation Antipsychotics and Risk of Side Effects

High Potency	Low Potency	Shared Side Effects
High risk of extrapyramidal effects Moderate risk of sedation Low risk of orthostatic hypotension and tachycardia Low risk of anticholinergic and anti-adrenergic effects Higher risk of neuroleptic malignant syndrome	Lower risk of extrapyramidal effects High risk of sedation High risk of orthostatic hypotension and tachycardia High risk of anticholinergic and antiadrenergic effects Lower risk of neuroleptic malignant syndrome	Moderate risk of weight gain Low risk of metabolic effects High risk of sexual dysfunction Seizures (rare) Allergic and dermatological effects

dyskinesia, dopamine hypersensitivity in central nervous system motor tracts. These symptoms are summarized in Table 66.3. Anticholinergic medications are used to manage the symptoms experienced by many patients treated with antipsychotic medications. Prophylactic treatment with anticholinergics may be used to diminish EPS other than tardive dyskinesia. Patient education is essential in discussing EPS to identify and treat these symptoms and to ensure adherence to the pharmacological regimen. In addition, if anxiety and/or aggressive behaviors are present, treatment with benzodiazepines may be used.

Another set of troubling side effects includes weight gain and metabolic derangements, mostly associated with the use of "atypical" antipsychotics, most commonly olanzapine, clozapine, quetiapine, and risperidone. The majority of chronic patients with schizophrenia are now obese and many have glucose dysregulation, lipid abnormalities, and high blood pressure. Along with unhealthy lifestyles and high rates of smoking, a major consequence of antipsychotic-induced weight gain is that cardiovascular disease–related mortality is much higher in schizophrenia than in the general population, shortening lives by 20 years on average.

Frequent monitoring of body weight, body mass index (BMI), and metabolic parameters is recommended for all people receiving antipsychotics, including people with schizophrenia. Monitoring for diabetes and dyslipidemia is especially important in patients with a positive family history of those conditions and in those receiving a second-generation antipsychotic. Recommendations include sequential measurement of BMI, waist circumference, blood pressure, fasting glucose, and fasting lipid profile at baseline, 1 month, 3 months, and annually. Assess individual and family medical history at baseline and annually.

In addition, the clinician can help encourage the patient to remain compliant with the antipsychotic medication regimen, as well as all nonpharmacological therapies, to prevent relapse. Persons experiencing a first episode should remain on the antipsychotic medication for at least 18 months. Olanzapine (Zyprexa) has been shown to be slightly more effective than haloperidol, although the difference is modest and does not take into account later emerging problems that may result from olanzapine's less favorable metabolic profile. Discontinuation rates for haloperidol are slightly higher due to side effects (Scottish Intercollegiate Guidelines Network, 2013). Although not completely risk free for development of tardive dyskinesia, the second-generation antipsychotics have a significantly lower risk than haloperidol. It is important to note that each medication carries its own side-effect profile and metabolic risks. Adverse effects of medications should be discussed as choice of medication is agreed on.

Among all the antipsychotic medications, clozapine has the lowest risk of causing EPS, although its use is limited by the risk of causing low neutrophils and in the worst case, agranulocytosis. For the latter reason, frequent and ongoing CBC monitoring is mandatory. Nevertheless, when first- and second-line therapies fail, clozapine is helpful in managing previously treatment-resistant symptoms and suicidal behaviors. Myocarditis is a potential adverse reaction to clozapine (Clozaril). Patients presenting with fatigue, tachypnea, chest pain, fever, and dyspnea need emergent evaluation with an electrocardiogram, white blood cell count, and serum troponin levels. If myocarditis is diagnosed, clozapine must be stopped. Treatment of coexisting depression with antidepressants may improve overall functioning.

Currently the manufacturer recommends evaluation of cataracts at baseline and every 6 months for patients taking quetiapine (Seroquel). Ongoing education that builds on previous medical encounters is essential to assist the patient and family with methods to reduce the increased risk of cardiac- and pulmonary-related events. An increased risk of mortality from cancer has been demonstrated in patients with schizophrenia, especially for women with breast cancer and for men with lung cancer.

Nonpharmacological Management

For patients with persistent positive symptoms, CBT has been found to be helpful in the reduction of both symptoms and relapse rates. Patients who have experienced a

TABLE 66.3 Extrapyramidal Symptoms, Description, and Treatment

Movement Disorder/Timing	Description	Treatment
Akathisia Occurs a few days to a few weeks after initiation of medication	Restlessness Subjective: Unable to sit still, unable to remain calm Objective: Pacing, foot-tapping, shifting weight from foot to foot	Discontinue medication Benzodiazepines: lorazepam, diazepam, alprazolam Beta blockers such as propranolol
Dystonia May occur after a single dose of medication to several days later	Involuntary muscle contractions affecting the head and neck (hoarseness, laryngeal spasms, oculogyric crisis, torticollis) May involve the torso and extremities (opisthotonus)	Anticholinergics Antiparkinsonian medication
Pseudoparkinsonism May occur after a single dose, but typically seen a few weeks later as the dosage is increased	Slow pill-rolling tremor of hands, cogwheel rigidity, shuffling gait, mask-like face, loss of arm swing, and bradyphrenia After prolonged use "rabbit syndrome": tremor of lips characterized by constant chewing motion	Anticholinergics
Tardive Dyskinesia Late-appearing manifestation, months to years	Involuntary rapid movements of the face (lip smacking, grimacing, facial distortions), torso, and extremities 6% irreversible	Prevention and screening tools for movement disorders every 3–6 months Anticholinergic agents Antiparkinsonian agents Removal of agent

high incidence of relapse may benefit from an assertive community treatment (ACT) team approach (Scottish Intercollegiate Guidelines Network, 2013). ACT is an evidence-based program that provides culturally sensitive services for individuals with severe and persistent mental illnesses who have not benefited from traditional outpatient mental health programming and who also have a significant history of hospitalizations for mental health reasons. ACT is a comprehensive, multidisciplinary, team-based approach to treatment, with a strong emphasis on recovery principles individualized to meet the patient's needs. Services include case management, medication management, vocational counseling and placement, family counseling and psychoeducation, mental health and substance abuse counseling, and wellness management education. Services are provided in the community in the consumers' natural settings. Services are provided 24 hours a day, 7 days a week, for as long as needed. ACT participation is either voluntary or court mandated. The team approach includes a psychiatrist, psychiatric nurse, counselors, case manager, and peer support. The original ACT model included a nurse practitioner who provided medical care, but this is no longer an integral part of the ACT model. A hallmark of ACT is to develop a positive, trusting relationship with each client to improve his or her

compliance with mental health treatment and focus on mental health and recovery.

FOLLOW-UP AND REFERRAL

Treatment of schizophrenia requires integrated care. Families play the key role in supporting patients to accept treatment, preferably beginning early in the disease course. Patients who present a danger to themselves or others and those who neglect their personal care needs need to be hospitalized.

The course of illness of schizophrenia is variable and often chronic, with symptoms, cognitive deficits, and medical health issues combining to create high levels of disability. Patients with schizophrenia have an average life span that is reduced by 20 years compared with population norms, which is due to suicide, and medical comorbidities that lead to diabetes and cardiovascular disease. Typically, 15% of patients have a good outcome, 30% have an intermediate outcome, and 55% have a poor outcome. Early aggressive treatment, based on the biopsychosocial model, checking for suicidality, developing a healthy lifestyle, and integrated medical care are important to improve prognosis and reduce medical morbidity and mortality. Poor prognosis is indicated by a gradual onset of symptoms, earlier onset, lack of mood symptoms, disorganized thoughts and behavior, and comorbid substance use. Depression is common.

Patient Education: Schizophrenia

Because schizophrenia is best viewed as a chronic and potentially lifelong illness, looking at a variety of strategies to optimize functional status is important. Stigmatization, which represents a chronic negative interaction with the environment that most persons living with schizophrenia deal with on a regular basis, must be recognized. Stigmatization reduces schizophrenia to a stereotyped set of negative attitudes, fears, and incorrect beliefs that affects how the disease is understood. Harmful effects of stigma may increase the schizophrenia liability and have negative effects on the clinical course of the disease. Labels and social disapproval may result in patient anxiety and contribute to negative discrimination. This negativity can influence health-care access, damage self-esteem and self-efficacy, and increase depressive symptoms. Increased likelihood of the misuse of alcohol and drugs may be related to the prejudice and discrimination related to schizophrenia.

The *Circle of Caring* model, encompassing the concepts of authentic presence, advocacy, knowing, commitment, and patience, is the essence of humanistic, quality, medical care for all populations but is critically important for those living with schizophrenia and other serious mental illnesses. This model must be fostered in staff training and incorporated into the culture of your health-care setting to reduce the negative effects of stigma.

There is some evidence that practicing active coping strategies and sharing stories with peers may reduce stigma and facilitate attendance at primary care. Peers have the unique lived experience of being mental health consumers themselves who are in recovery. With peer support training, they are able to share experiences and coping strategies that support recovery for those living with mental illness. Services run by trained peers also include assistance with housing and benefits advisement, employment and career counseling, justice issues, advocacy, and independent living skills. Peer-delivered services have been shown to diminish feelings of isolation, to improve coping skills, and often to decrease the need for hospitalization.

Social skill training improves social adjustment and coping skills. Supportive individual and group psychotherapy along with medications can reduce relapses and enhance occupational and vocational functioning. Employment may de-stigmatize a person coping with both psychiatric disability and a criminal record, and paid employment may aid in community integration. Family education helps to improve communication between the patient and mental health services and subsequently helps to reduce relapse rates and improve family functioning. Social centers aim to address isolation experienced by most patients. Social centers, sometimes called "club houses," provide a voluntary semistructured program wherein patients can meet in a safe environment to share conversation and participate in activities with others having similar concerns. Community resources such as the National Alliance of Mentally Ill are invaluable sources of support for patients and families.

REFERENCES

American Diabetes Association, American Psychiatric Association, American Association of Clinical Endocrinologists, North American Association for the Study of Obesity. Consensus development conference on antipsychotic drugs and obesity and diabetes. *Diabetes Care.* 2004;27:596–601.

American Psychiatric Association. *Practice guideline for the treatment of patients with schizophrenia.* 2nd ed. Complete summary. http://psychiatryonline.org/content.aspx?bookID=28&sectionID=1665359. Published 2006.

Arango C, et al. A comparison of schizophrenia outpatients treated with antipsychotics with and without metabolic syndrome: Findings from the CLAMORS study. *Schizophr Res.* 2008;104(1-3):1–12.

Arsenault-Lapierre G, Kim C, Turecki G. Psychiatric diagnoses in 3275 suicides: A meta-analysis. *BMC Psychiatry.* 2004;4:37.

Barbui C, Girlanda F, Ay E, Cipriani A, Becker T, Koesters M. Implementation of treatment guidelines for specialist mental health care. *Cochrane Database Syst Rev.* 2014;1:CD009780.

Bartels SJ, Pratt SI. Psychosocial rehabilitation and quality of life for older adults with serious mental illness: Recent findings and future research directions. *Curr Opin Psychiatry.* 2009;22(4):381–385.

Bora E, Murray RM. Meta-analysis of cognitive deficits in ultra-high risk to psychosis and first-episode psychosis: do the cognitive deficits progress over, or after, the onset of psychosis? *Schizophr Bull.* 2014;40:744.

Brown AS, Derkits EJ. Prenatal infection and schizophrenia: A review of epidemiologic and translational studies. *Am J Psychiatry.* 2010;167:261.

Buchanan RW, Kreyenbuhl J, Kelly DL, et al. The 2009 schizophrenia PORT psychopharmacological treatment recommendations and summary statements. *Schizophr Bull.* 2010;36:71.

Cantor-Graae E, Selten, JP. Schizophrenia and migration: A meta-analysis and review. *Am J Psychiatry.* 2005;162:12–24.

Chien WT, Yip AL. Current approaches to treatments for schizophrenia spectrum disorders, part I: An overview and medical treatments. *Neuropsychiatr Dis Treat.* 2013;9:1311–1132.

Clemmensen L, et al. A systematic review of the long-term effects of early onset schizophrenia. *BMC Psychiatry.* 2012;12:150.

Courey TC. Detection, prevention, and management of extrapyramidal symptoms. *J Nurse Pract.* 2007;3(7):464–469.

Debbané M, Eliez S, Badoud D, et al. Developing psychosis and its risk states through the lens of schizotypy. *Schizophr Bull.* 2015;41(suppl 2):S396.

Drapalski AL, Lucksted A, Perrin PB, et al. A model of internalized stigma and its effects on people with mental illness. *Psychiatr Serv.* 2013;64:264.

Fantini G, Tibaldi G, Rucci P, et al. Quality of care indicators for schizophrenia: Determinants of observed variations among Italian Departments of Mental Health. Results from the ETAS DSM study. *Epidemiol Psychiatr Sci.* 2016:1–15.

Fearon P, et al. Incidence of schizophrenia and other psychoses in ethnic minority groups: Results from the MRC AESOP Study. *Psychol Med.* 2006;36:1–10.

Feldman R, Bailey RA, Muller J, et al. Cost of schizophrenia in the Medicare program. *Popul Health Manag.* 2014;17:190.

Gough SA, Robert P. Diabetes and its prevention: Pragmatic solutions for people with schizophrenia. *Br J Psychiatry Suppl.* 2004;47: S106-S111.

Griswold KS, et al. Primary care after psychiatric crisis: A qualitative analysis. *Ann Fam Med.* 2008;6(1):38–43.

Haddock G, Eisner E, Boone C, Davies G, Coogan C, Barrowclough C. An investigation of the implementation of NICE-recommended CBT interventions for people with schizophrenia. *J Ment Health.* 2014;23(4):162–165.

Harrison RNS, Gaughran F, Murray RM, et al. Development of multivariable models to predict change in Body Mass Index within a clinical trial population of psychotic individuals. *Sci Rep.* 2017;7(1):14738.

Hor K, Taylor M. Suicide and schizophrenia: A systematic review of rates and risk factors. *J Psychopharmacol.* 2010;24:81.

Kamble P, et al. Use of antipsychotics among elderly nursing home residents with dementia in the US: An analysis of National Survey Data. *Drugs Aging.* 2009;26(6):483–492.

Kane JM, Robinson DG, Schooler NR, et al. Comprehensive versus usual community care for first-episode psychosis: 2-Year outcomes from the NIMH RAISE early treatment program. *Am J Psychiatry.* 2016;173:362.

Kessler RC, et al. The individual-level and societal-level effects of mental disorders on earnings in the United States: Results from the National Comorbidity Survey Replication. *Am J Psychiatry.* 2008;165:703–711.

Kirkbride JB, et al. Heterogeneity in incidence rates of schizophrenia and other psychotic syndromes: Findings from the 3-center AeSOP study. *Arch Gen Psychiatry.* 2006;63:250–258.

Kirkpatrick B, Fenton WS, Carpenter WT Jr, Marder SR. The NIMH-MATRICS consensus statement on negative symptoms. *Schizophr Bull.* 2006;32:214.

Koenig JI, Elmer GI, Shepard PD, et al. Prenatal exposure to a repeated variable stress paradigm elicits behavioral and neuroendocrinological changes in the adult offspring: Potential relevance to schizophrenia. *Behav Brain Res.* 2005;156:251.

Kristensen K, Cadenhead KS. Cannabis abuse and risk for psychosis in a prodromal sample. *Psychiatry Res.* 2007;151:151.

Kuepper R, van Os J, Lieb R, et al. Continued cannabis use and risk of incidence and persistence of psychotic symptoms: 10 year follow-up cohort study. *BMJ.* 2011;342:d738.

Lieberman JA, et al. Effectiveness of antipsychotic drugs in patients with chronic schizophrenia. *N Engl J Med.* 2005;353(12):1209–1223.

Lumby, B. Guide schizophrenia patients to better physical health. *Nurs Pract.* 2007;32(7):30–37.

Lynskey, MT, Strang, J. The global burden of drug use and mental disorders. *Lancet.* 2013;382(9904):1540–1542.

McDonagh MS, Dana T, Selph S, et al. Treatments for schizophrenia in adults: A systematic review (Comparative Effectiveness Review No. 198; prepared by the Pacific Northwest Evidence-based Practice Center under Contract No. 290-2015-00009-I). AHRQ Publication No. 17(18)-EHC031-EF. Rockville, MD: Agency for Healthcare Research and Quality; 2017. http://www.effectivehealthcare.ahrq.gov/reports/final.cfm.

McGurk, SR, Twamley, EW, Sitzer, DI, McHugo, GJ, Mueser, KT. A meta-analysis of cognitive remediation in schizophrenia. *Am J Psychiatry.* 2007;164(12):1791–1802.

McGrath J, Welham J, Scott J, et al. Association between cannabis use and psychosis-related outcomes using sibling pair analysis in a cohort of young adults. *Arch Gen Psychiatry.* 2010;67:440.

McIntyre, RS. Understanding needs, interactions, treatment, and expectations among individuals affected by bipolar disorder or schizophrenia: The UNITE global survey. *J Clin Psychiatry.* 2009;70(suppl 3):5–11.

Miller AL. Implementing treatment guidelines. *Clin Schizophr Relat Psychoses.* 2011;5:15–16.

Morden NE, et al. Health care for patients with serious mental illness: Family medicine's role. *J Am Board Fam Med.* 2009;22(2):187–195.

Moore TA. Schizophrenia treatment guidelines in the United States. *Clin Schizophr Relat Psychoses.* 2011;5:40–49.

Morriss R, Vinjamuri I, Faizal MA, Bolton CA, McCarthy JP. Training to recognise the early signs of recurrence in schizophrenia. *Cochrane Database Syst Rev.* 2013;(2):CD005147.

National Association of State Mental Health Program Directors (NASMHPD) Medical Directors Council. *Morbidity and mortality in people with serious mental illness.* Alexandria, VA: NASMHPD; 2006.

National Institute for Health and Clinical Excellence. *Psychosis and schizophrenia in adults: prevention and treatment.* https://www.nice.org.uk/guidance/cg178. Published March 2014.

National Institute for Health and Clinical Excellence (NICE). *Psychosis and schizophrenia in adults. Treatment and management* (NICE Clinical Guideline 178). London: NICE; 2014.

Newcomer, JW. Comparing the safety and efficacy of atypical antipsychotics in psychiatric patients with comorbid medical illnesses. *J Clin Psychiatry.* 2009;70(suppl 3):30–36.

Nicholl D, Akhras KS, Diels J, Schadrack J. Burden of schizophrenia in recently diagnosed patients: Healthcare utilisation and cost perspective. *Curr Med Res Opin.* 2010;26:943.

Perkins DV, et al. Gainful employment reduces stigma toward people recovering from schizophrenia. *Community Ment Health J.* 2009;45(3):158–162.

Pillinger T, Beck K, Gobjila C, et al. Impaired glucose homeostasis in first-episode schizophrenia: A systematic review and meta-analysis. *JAMA Psychiatry.* 2017;74:261.

Rosen C, Grossman LS, Harrow M, et al. Diagnostic and prognostic significance of Schneiderian first-rank symptoms: A 20-year longitudinal study of schizophrenia and bipolar disorder. *Compr Psychiatry.* 2011;52:126.

Sadock BJ, et al. *Kaplan and Sadock's comprehensive textbook of psychiatry.* 10th ed. Philadelphia, PA: Lippincott Williams & Wilkins; 2017.

Sartorius N. Lessons from a 10-year global programme against stigma and discrimination because of illness. *Psychol Health Med.* 2006;11:383–388.

Schooler N, et al. Risperidone and haloperidol in first-episode psychosis: A long-term randomized trial. *Am J Psychiatry.* 2005;162(5):947–953.

Scottish Intercollegiate Guidelines Network (SIGN). *Management of schizophrenia: A national clinical guideline. Management of schizophrenia* (SIGN publication no. 131). Edinburgh, Scotland, SIGN; 2013. http://www.sign.ac.uk/sign-131-management-of-schizophrenia.html.

Selten JP, Cantor-Graae E. Social defeat: Risk factor for schizophrenia? *Br J Psychiatry.* 2005;187:101–102.

Semisa D, Casacchia M, Di Munzio W, et al. Gruppo SIEP-DIRECT'S. Promoting recovery of schizophrenic patients: discrepancy between routine practice and evidence. The SIEP-DIRECT'S Project [in Italian]. *Epidemiol Psychiatr Soc.* 2008;17:331–348.

Somaiya M, Grover S, Avasthi A, Chakrabarti S. Changes in cost of treating schizophrenia: comparison of two studies done a decade apart. *Psychiatry Res.* 2014;215:547.

Strauss GP, Horan WP, Kirkpatrick B, et al. Deconstructing negative symptoms of schizophrenia: Avolition-apathy and diminished expression clusters predict clinical presentation and functional outcome. *J Psychiatr Res.* 2013;47:783.

Tandon, R, Nasrallah, HA, Keshavan MS. Schizophrenia, "just the facts" 5. Treatment and prevention. Past, present, and future. *Schizophr Res.* 2010;122(1-3):1–23.

Velligan DI, Weiden, PJ, Sajatovic, M. The Expert Consensus Guideline Series: Adherence problems in patients with serious and persistent mental illness. *J Clin Psychiatry.* 2009;70(suppl 4):1–46.

Warner, R. Recovery from schizophrenia and the recovery model. *Curr Opin Psychiatry.* 2009;22(4):374–380.

Ward PB, Firth J, Rosenbaum S, Samaras K, Stubbs B, Curtis J. Lifestyle interventions to reduce premature mortality in schizophrenia. *Lancet Psychiatry.* 2017;4(7):e14.

Werbeloff N, Levine SZ, Rabinowitz J. Elaboration on the association between immigration and schizophrenia: A population-based national study disaggregating annual trends, country of origin and sex over 15 years. *Soc Psychiatry Psychiatr Epidemiol.* 2012;47:303.

Willhite RK, et al. Gender differences in symptoms, functioning and social support in patients at ultra-high risk for developing a psychotic disorder. *Schizophr Res.* 2008;104(1-3):237–245.

World Health Organization. Schizophrenia, schizotypal and delusional disorders. *International statistical classification of disease and related health problems.* 10th revision. http://apps.who.int/classifications/icd10/browse/2015/en#/F20-F29. Published 2015.

Zhao S, Sampson S, Xia J, Jayaram MB. Psychoeducation (brief) for people with serious mental illness. *Cochrane Database Syst Rev.* 2015;(4):CD010823.

Zhuo C, Tao R, Jiang R, Lin X, Shao M. Cancer mortality in patients with schizophrenia: Systematic review and meta-analysis. *Br J Psychiatry.* 2017;211(1):7–13.

RESOURCES

Advice for Parents of Children With Behavioral and Psychiatric Disorders. Brain and Behavior Research Foundation
https://www.bbrfoundation.org/blog/advice-parents-children-behavioral-and-psychiatric-disorders

Coordinated Specialty Care Fact Sheet and Checklist. National Institute of Mental Health
https://www.nimh.nih.gov/health/publications/raise-fact-sheet-coordinated-specialty-care/index.shtml

Delusional Disorder. Harvard Health Publishing
https://www.health.harvard.edu/diseases-and-conditions/delusional-disorder

Delusional Disorder Health Library. Cleveland Clinic
https://my.clevelandclinic.org/health/diseases/9599-delusional-disorder

Delusional Infestation: Overview and Recommendations. DynaMed Plus
http://www.dynamed.com/topics/dmp~AN~T114682/Delusional-infestation#Overview-and-Recommendations

Discussion Groups for Persons and Families With Schizophrenia. National Alliance on Mental Illness
https://www.nami.org/Learn-More/Mental-Health-Conditions/Schizophrenia/Discuss

Expert Q & A: Schizophrenia. Psychiatry.org
https://www.psychiatry.org/patients-families/schizophrenia/expert-q-and-a

Fact Sheet: Early Warning Signs of Psychosis. National Institute of Mental Health
https://www.nimh.nih.gov/health/publications/raise-fact-sheet-early-warning-signs-of-psychosis/raise-early-warning-signs-of-psychosis-fact-sheet_152933.pdf

Fact Sheet: First Episode Psychosis. National Institute of Mental Health
https://www.nimh.nih.gov/health/publications/raise-fact-sheet-first-episode-psychosis/index.shtml

Patient Story: Schizophrenia. Psychiatry.Org.
https://www.psychiatry.org/patients-families/schizophrenia/patient-story

Practice Parameter for the Assessment and Treatment of Children and Adolescents With Schizophrenia. American Academy of Child & Adolescent Psychiatry. AHRQ National Guidelines Clearing House.
https://www.guideline.gov/summaries/summary/48381?

Schizophrenia. Medline Plus Patient Information
https://medlineplus.gov/schizophrenia.html

Schizophrenia. National Alliance on Mental Illness.
https://www.nami.org/Learn-More/Mental-Health-Conditions/Schizophrenia

Schizophrenia. National Institute of Mental Health
https://www.nimh.nih.gov/health/topics/schizophrenia/index.shtml

Schizophrenia Brochure. National Institute of Mental Health
https://www.nimh.nih.gov/health/publications/schizophrenia-basics/index.shtml

Schizophrenia: Overview and Recommendations. DynaMed Plus
http://www.dynamed.com/topics/dmp~AN~T115234#Overview-and-Recommendations

Schizophrenia: Overview Treatment. DynaMed Plus
http://www.dynamed.com/topics/dmp~AN~T115234#Treatment

Schizotypal Personality Disorder. Mayo Clinic.
https://www.mayoclinic.org/diseases-conditions/schizotypal-personality-disorder/symptoms-causes/syc-20353919

Schizotypal Personality Disorder. Medline Plus Health Information
https://medlineplus.gov/ency/article/001525.htm

Schizotypal Personality Disorder. Targeting the D1 Dopamine Receptor to Improve Working Memory in Schizotypal Personality Disorder. Brain and Behavior Research Foundation.
https://www.bbrfoundation.org/content/targeting-d1-dopamine-receptor-improve-working-memory-schizotypal-personality-disorder

Schizophrenia Statistics. National Institute of Mental Health
https://www.nimh.nih.gov/health/statistics/prevalence/schizophrenia.shtml

What is Schizophrenia? A brief video. National Alliance on Mental Illness.
https://www.nami.org/Learn-More/Mental-Health-Conditions/Schizophrenia

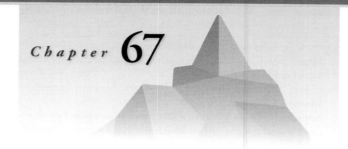

Chapter 67

Mood Disorders

Rehan Aziz, MD, FAPA

Lynne M. Dunphy, PhD, APRN, FNP-BC, FAAN, FAANP

Susan Bulfin, DNP, APRN, FNP-BC

OVERVIEW

The following sections include major depressive, dysthymic, and bipolar disorders. Major depressive disorder is the primary diagnosis in this category. In the *Diagnostic and Statistical Manual of Mental Disorders* (DSM-5), a more chronic form, persistent depressive disorder or dysthymia, is included, as well as information on peripartum mood disorders. Additionally, in this chapter, acute suicide risk is discussed in detail. Many patients see their primary care clinicians in the month before they attempt suicide.

MAJOR DEPRESSIVE DISORDER

Depression is a common condition seen in primary-care settings. People use the term *depression* to describe a wide variety of negative emotional states, ranging from sadness to loss of interest or pleasure in activities to irritability to self-hate. The hallmarks of major depression, however, are sadness and anhedonia (loss of pleasure). In most cases, the sadness and anhedonia associated with major depression can be distinguished from ordinary changes in mood.

Depression causes great psychological pain, prompting many depressed persons to consider any solution that they think may bring relief. Patients may have difficulty describing their pain and may make vague references to "hurting" or "feeling bad." Thoughts of death or suicide are not uncommon. A study of women with postpartum depression revealed the various descriptors with which individuals may characterize signs and symptoms associated with depression (see Evidence-Based Nursing Practice 67.1).

Individual variations in the clinical presentation of depression can be great, sometimes making the condition difficult to recognize. In primary-care settings, patients often present with ambiguous symptoms of unexplained fatigue, changes in appetite, and changes in sleep patterns; only when questioned will they admit to feelings of "sadness." Others will complain of moderate to significant feelings of apathy. Additional presentations include complaints of irritability, anger, anxiety, or hyperactivity. Many deeply depressed persons are unaware of the level of functional impairment resulting from their illness. Slowed thinking and emotional numbness—two significant symptoms of depression—can contribute to a lack of awareness of depression. Gender and culture can impact presentation, but gender should not influence assessment.

Major depressive disorder (MDD) is characterized by substantial negative changes in mood, thinking, and behavior. A person who is severely depressed will have intense feelings of sadness, irritability, or apathy. These feelings may persist and are unrelieved by situational changes, for example, whether at home, at school, at work, or in recreational situations, the mood of the depressed person will vary little. In some cases, the mood of the depressed person may vary slightly but without improving significantly.

Negative changes in thinking associated with depression are common. Depressed thinking can be described as global, distorted, and circular. Rather than dealing with today, the depressed person may instead focus on past events or think about a bleak future. The balance between positive and negative thoughts about self, life, and the future becomes distorted. Negative views can seem more valid than positive views. Global negative thinking can take on a ruminative or circular pattern, so that the depressed person's negative thinking seems to always depart from and arrive at the same painful conclusions.

Major depression interferes with decision-making and concentration. The smallest decision, such as whether to make a phone call, becomes difficult. The depressed person may become alarmed by his or her inability to make choices or to concentrate. Although others may recognize negative changes in the depressed person's thinking, it can develop without warning to the patient. The negative thinking may include thoughts of death and suicide. Some clinicians attempt to make a clear distinction between passive thoughts of death and active thoughts of suicide, but both patterns are alarming.

Changes in behavior may occur. The individual may begin behaving uncharacteristically. For this reason, significant others may become aware of the depression before the patient does. Depression-related behavioral changes range from changes in grooming and in interpersonal interactions to substance abuse, irritability, aggression, and social withdrawal.

Cultural variations in the presentation of depression are also individualized. Based on how traditional or nontraditional the individual's attitudes and behaviors are, patients may focus less on personal experiences and more on physical aches and pains. Ethnic and cultural norms concerning privacy, embarrassment, and disclosure will also have an impact on the patient's presentation.

The Iceberg of Depression

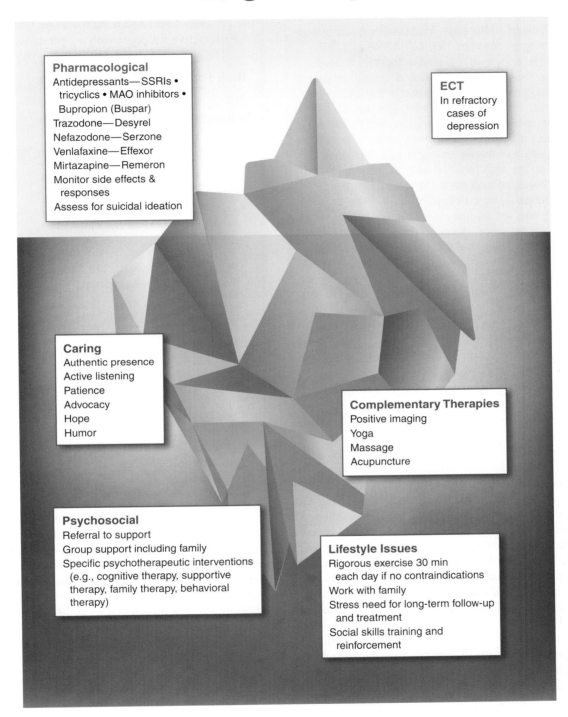

Pharmacological
Antidepressants—SSRIs •
  tricyclics • MAO inhibitors •
  Bupropion (Buspar)
Trazodone—Desyrel
Nefazodone—Serzone
Venlafaxine—Effexor
Mirtazapine—Remeron
Monitor side effects &
  responses
Assess for suicidal ideation

ECT
In refractory
cases of
depression

Caring
Authentic presence
Active listening
Patience
Advocacy
Hope
Humor

Complementary Therapies
Positive imaging
Yoga
Massage
Acupuncture

Psychosocial
Referral to support
Group support including family
Specific psychotherapeutic interventions
  (e.g., cognitive therapy, supportive
  therapy, family therapy, behavioral
  therapy)

Lifestyle Issues
Rigorous exercise 30 min
  each day if no contraindications
Work with family
Stress need for long-term follow-up
  and treatment
Social skills training and
  reinforcement

EPIDEMIOLOGY AND CAUSES

It is estimated that up to 20% of the U.S. population will experience a significant episode of depression at some time during their lives. These rates are consistent across developed European nations. In developing countries such as China, Brazil, and Mexico, prevalence rates are approximately 9%. The lifetime prevalence of an MDD is 16.5% with a 6.7% 12-month prevalence rate. However, the lifetime prevalence of MDD in those 65 years and older is significantly less compared with younger age-groups. In certain segments of the older adult population, usually those who are sicker and/or in pain, the prevalence of depression can be higher. Some studies

Evidence-Based Nursing Practice 67.1 Depression

Beck CT. Teetering on the edge: A substantive theory of post-partum depression. *Nurs Res.* 1993;42(1):42–48.

This classic study used a qualitative approach to develop a theory regarding women's perceptions of postpartum depression. Drawing a sample of 12 from a postpartum support group, the researcher conducted in-depth interviews with the women about their experiences of postpartum depression. What emerged was a rich description of the nature of postpartum depression and how these women managed their depression. "Teetering on the edge" was the hallmark metaphor that the researcher extracted to describe the process that the participants confronted during their depression. They felt "between" sane and insane, and the researcher identified several stages: "Encountering the terror" described the unpredictable nature of feelings that overwhelmed them, anxiety and panic attacks, obsessions, and loss of concentration. In the next stage, called "the dying of self," the women experienced isolation, withdrawal, and feelings of dissociation and depersonalization. Most had suicidal ideation. In the next stage, "struggling to survive," they began to grapple with their feelings. They searched out support groups, used prayer and faith to manage the depression, and began, hesitantly, and with some steps forward and some steps backward, to recover.

document prevalence as high as 40% in nursing home patients and as high as 30% in community-dwelling elders with chronic medical conditions. Older adults have many risk factors for depression because of the frequent losses experienced within this age-group.

There is a higher incidence of depression in women (21%) than in men (13%). Researchers have studied this phenomenon for decades. There does not appear to be a single, universal explanation for women's greater susceptibility to depression. In the United States in 2010, the estimated annual economic consequences of MDD, including direct medical costs and workplace costs, exceeded $200 billion.

Depression may also occur during the peripartum period. Peripartum depression (PPD) usually occurs within 1 to 3 weeks after childbirth, but PPD can occur during pregnancy or up to 4 weeks after delivery. About 3% to 6% of women will develop PPD. Half of all episodes begin before delivery. Risk factors for PPD include a history of depression before, during, or after pregnancy; a current history of depression; unplanned pregnancy; preterm birth; giving birth to a child with a medical condition or birth defect; lack of social, economic, and personal support; and concurrent stressful life events.

Once a person experiences one depressive episode, they are at higher risk for a recurrence, with as many as 50% experiencing another episode; after two occurrences, there is an 80% chance of another recurrence. In the absence of systematic screening, usual care by primary-care providers fails to detect between 30% and 50% of depressed patients. This makes it imperative that primary-care practitioners inquire sensitively about depression and use evidence-based screening tools (see Chapter 64).

Risk factors for depression are presented below.

Risk Factors: Major Depression

Age

- Adolescent or older adult

Gender

- Female

Family History

- Strong family history of depression, suicide or suicide attempts, alcohol abuse, or other substance abuse

History

- History of migraine headaches, back pain, recent myocardial infarction, or peptic ulcer disease

Current Medical Condition

- Current chronic disease (especially multiple diseases)
- Insomnia

Lifestyle

- Stress
- Poverty
- Less than high school education
- Recent traumatic event
- Parent or caregiver of a child or children with behavioral disorders, especially hyperactivity
- Retired

Depression is also an independent risk factor for increased morbidity and mortality from cardiac disease. In patients with coexisting atrial fibrillation and congestive heart failure, even with optimal treatment, a higher rate of depressive symptoms correlates with increased cardiovascular mortality. The World Health Organization (WHO) estimates that by 2020, depression will rank second only to cardiovascular illness in terms of disease burden and as a worldwide cause of disability. Similarly, patients with comorbid diabetes mellitus and depression face increased mortality in comparison to those patients without concomitant disease.

PATHOPHYSIOLOGY

A correlation between the hypersecretion of cortisol and depression is one of the oldest observations in biological psychiatry. Neurovegetative signs and symptoms of depression may correlate with various neuroendocrine abnormalities.

Approximately 5% to 10% of all patients with depression have a coexisting thyroid disorder. Recent research has focused on the theory that a subset of depressed patients may have an unrecognized autoimmune disorder that affects the thyroid gland. Some depressed patients benefit from liothyronine. A thyroid stimulating hormone (TSH) level should be obtained on all depressed patients. The pathophysiology of peripartum depression has included etiological theories of decreased maternal estrogen as well as abnormalities in maternal neurotransmitters.

Alterations in sleep, appetite, and sexual behavior, as well as biological changes in endocrine, immunological, and chronobiological measures in depressed patients, all suggest dysregulation of the hypothalamus. The stooped posture of depressed patients, motor slowness, and minor cognitive impairments are similar to the signs of disorder of the basal ganglia, such as Parkinson's disease and other subcortical dementias.

Genetic factors are strongly implicated in the development of depressive disorders, although it is impossible to rule out psychosocial factors, as well as other non-genetic factors. Adoption studies have provided data supporting a genetic basis for the inheritance of mood disorders. For major depression, the concordance rate in monozygotic twins is about 50%, arguing strongly for a genetic disposition. A recent study indicated that a functional polymorphism in the serotonin transporter gene (5-HTT) may interact with stressful life events to markedly increase the risk for depression and suicide, especially when the stressors are encountered early in life.

Stressful life events commonly precede first episodes of mood disorders. Some speculate that the stress accompanying the first episode results in long-lasting changes in neurocircuitry. Thus, the person is at high risk for subsequent mood episodes, unrelated to an external stressor. The external psychosocial factor most often associated with the onset of a major depressive episode is the loss of a spouse or a parent, especially if it occurs before age 11. Another risk factor is unemployment; persons out of work are three times more likely to report symptoms of an episode of major depression than those who are employed. However, what may seem to be a relatively mild stressor from an outside perspective may be devastating to the person because of whatever personal meaning they assign to the event.

CLINICAL PRESENTATION

A comprehensive MDD assessment extends beyond the presence or absence of sadness or anhedonia. Though, these symptoms may be reported by the patient, observed and reported by significant others, or observed by the practitioner. Two quick questions, recommended by the U.S. Preventive Services Task Force, that provide a preliminary screen for depression are:

- Have you felt down or hopeless over the past few weeks?
- Have you had little interest in doing things over the past few weeks?

A positive response to one or both questions in this screen indicates possible MDD, but the test has a high false-positive rate. Thus, confirmatory testing should be performed using a validated screening instrument and a clinical interview.

The clinical diagnosis of depression can be assisted by the Patient Health Questionnaire-9 (PHQ-9) questionnaire. Its sensitivity (85%) and specificity (84%) make it an excellent tool to utilize in primary care. Consisting of a checklist of nine symptoms, the PHQ-9 provides an effective supplementation to the two-question screen. The patient is asked to indicate the frequency with which depressive symptoms have occurred over the preceding 2 weeks. It can be filled out quickly either in the waiting room or exam room before a primary-care visit. The PHQ-9 may also be used to track the progress of treatment at each follow up visit. A similar measure of symptom severity, the self-rated Quick Inventory of Depressive Symptomatology (QIDS-SR), can be used for the same purpose and has the additional benefit of including symptom severity and thus may provide a sensitive measure of change with treatment.

Other scales frequently employed include the Geriatric Depression Scale (GDS), a widely used and validated screening tool for use in older adults. The Edinburgh Postnatal Depression (EPSD) scale is one of the most commonly used screening tools for PPD. Common presenting symptoms are in Box 67.1.

Some patients with major depression may, as a result of the disorder, find it difficult to list their symptoms. In this case, self-screening assessment tools such as the Zung Self-Rating Depression Scale or Beck Depression Inventory, checklists, direct observations, or yes-or-no questions may be substituted. When yes-or-no assessment questions are used, all yes responses should be explored. Extremely depressed patients may not tolerate assessment in any form that requires effort on their part. They can become irritable and impatient with the practitioner for asking questions that, to them, seem "unnecessary." This situation can sometimes be improved by indicating that the purpose of asking questions is to better understand the patient's situation.

Box 67.1 Components of Depression in Elderly Persons

- Vegetative—poor appetite, disrupted sleep, early morning awakening
- Somatic—pain throughout body or out of proportion with underlying pathology
- Psychological—obsessive feelings of guilt and worry, ruminations throughout the night; suicidal ideation; memory problems
- Psychomotor—anxiety; psychomotor agitation
- Diurnal variation in symptoms—cannot "get moving" in morning, or specific time of day when depression is worst

Programs aimed at enhancing public awareness of depression have been impactful. As such, more patients are likely to seek professional health care for MDD as a result of having self-assessed their symptoms via surveys published in popular magazines, on-line or in local newspapers. Practitioners can help determine symptom intensity, duration, and impact on functioning. It is also valuable to ask patients to identify which symptoms they consider treatment priorities.

DIAGNOSTIC REASONING

Symptoms

The *DSM-5* symptom criteria for a major depressive episode require that five (or more) symptoms have been present during the same 2-week period and represent a change from previous functioning. The symptoms must be present nearly every day. At least one of the symptoms is either (1) depressed mood or (2) anhedonia, meaning loss of interest or pleasure. See the *DSM-5* for complete diagnostic criteria of major depressive disorder.

In patients with comorbid anxiety and depression, the symptom profile may be balanced or either symptom can predominate; in addition, some patients with so-called mixed anxiety and depression may demonstrate symptoms of both disorders but may not meet the full diagnostic criteria for either. Any patient who has symptoms of either depression or anxiety should be evaluated for current symptoms of both disorders. Consensus recommendations from a panel of experts who represent psychiatry, primary care, pharmacy, and managed care state that every patient suspected of having unipolar depression be evaluated for bipolar disorder using a quick screening tool before being treated with antidepressants, in order to prevent a switch into mania (see the Young Mania Assessment Tool). It is also necessary to rule out other medical conditions and substance use. Then the patient's depressive symptoms must be assessed for severity, duration, and recurrence, to differentiate among the depressive disorders. One consideration is persistent depressive disorder or dysthymia, which is distinguished by a protracted time course.

Differential Diagnosis

All patients must be carefully evaluated for underlying medical conditions. Many medical and neurological disorders and pharmacological substances can produce symptoms of depression. Careful medical history and physical examination should be done on all patients, including a neurological exam and routine blood work and urinalysis. The history needs to include the patient's personal as well as family history of depression and suicide. Tests for thyroid and adrenal function should be included because disorders of both of these endocrine systems can mimic depression. Cardiac drugs, antihypertensive agents,

sedatives, hypnotics, antipsychotics, antiepileptics, antiparkinsonian drugs, analgesics, antibacterials, steroids, and antineoplastics have all been associated with depressive symptomatology. A careful medication review, including over-the-counter (OTC) drugs and herbal agents, as well as evaluation of alcohol and substance use, is imperative. The most common neurological disorders that may manifest depressive symptoms are Parkinson's disease (50%–75% of patients have depressive symptoms that do not correlate with physical disability), dementing illnesses (including Alzheimer type), epilepsy, cerebrovascular disease, and tumors. The interictal changes associated with temporal lobe epilepsy can mimic a depressive disorder, especially if the epileptic focus is on the right side. There is increasing evidence of linkages between depression and cardiovascular disease, not limited to sequelae but actually preceding the event. In brain tumors, depression is more common in cases of anterior lobe tumor as opposed to posterior lobe lesions, and in both cases it responds to antidepressants. The "pseudodementia" of MDD can be differentiated from dementia with regard to onset (sudden in the case of pseudodementia) and its co-occurrence with low mood. Patients with depression will sometimes not answer questions, whereas those with dementia may confabulate. Depressed patients may be encouraged into remembering during an interview; those with primary dementia cannot. It is important to differentiate postpartum "blues" from PPD as presenting symptoms are similar. Symptoms of postpartum blues are less severe and transient in nature, although their presence increases the risk of PPD. The main distinguishing features of PPD are the longer duration of symptoms and the severity of symptoms with features of hopelessness and worthlessness.

In terms of mental disorders, depression can be a feature of many disorders listed in the *DSM-5*. Depression has a high comorbidity with the anxiety disorders, as well as alcohol-use disorders, eating disorders, schizophrenia, schizophreniform disorder, and somatic symptom disorders. Bereaved patients also need careful assessment.

MANAGEMENT

Remission of symptoms should be the standard for successful treatment of depression. Remission is defined as a virtual absence of depressive symptoms or a PHQ-9 score of less than 5. Alternatively, response is defined as a substantial reduction in symptoms. On the PHQ-9, it is at least a 50% decrease in the score. In clinical trials, only 25% to 35% of patients experience complete remission of depressive symptoms with an initial course of antidepressant therapy across 4 to 6 weeks. Remission is important though because incomplete relief of symptoms may increase the risk of relapse and further impairment. The mainstays of treatment are the use of antidepressants and/or psychotherapy. For mild to moderate depression, either medication or psychotherapy is recommended; if the depression is more severe, evidence-based guidelines support the simultaneous use of both (Institute for Clinical Systems Improvement, 2016; Michigan Quality Improvement Consortium, 2016). If a patient expresses suicidal intent or plan or has a history of suicidal attempt, consultation with a psychiatric mental health nurse practitioner (PMHNP) or psychiatrist may become important. In addition, treatment of a mood disorder such as major depression requires a *Circle of Caring* (see Chapter 1). For patients from differing ethnic groups or cultures, discussion of acceptable treatments should form the basis of therapeutic management (Michigan Quality Improvement Consortium, 2016; Trangle et al., 2016).

Pharmacological Management

With pharmacological therapy, about 7 out of 10 patients with severe major depression ultimately will obtain symptom relief, although it may take several trials to find the right medication. Agents that are effective in the front-line treatment of MDD are the selective serotonin reuptake inhibitors (SSRIs), serotonin-norepinephrine reuptake inhibitors (SNRIs), tricyclic antidepressants (TCAs), bupropion, which is a norepinephrine dopamine reuptake inhibitor, among others (Michigan Quality Improvement Consortium, 2016).

Antidepressant medications can be prescribed based on their half-life, neurotransmitter or receptor activity, side-effect profile, and/or clinical efficacy. The half-life for newer antidepressant medications ranges from hours to several days. Neurotransmitter or receptor activity accounts for differences in medication effects, including sedation, activation, and anxiolytic (antianxiety) activity. In general, antidepressant medications with significant norepinephrine effects (e.g., bupropion) tend to be activating.

Important common side-effect risks with serotonin-specific antidepressants include decreased sexual desire, decreased sexual response, headache, stomach upset, sedation, fatigue, or nervousness. For some patients, dramatic decreases in adverse effects can be obtained by adjusting the time of day the medication is taken. Patients who are bothered by adverse effects when they take an antidepressant in the morning may experience milder side effects if they take the same medication with dinner or at bedtime. Extremely low starting doses may be necessary when it is clear that a patient seems able to benefit from an antidepressant but cannot tolerate medication side effects during the early stages of treatment. Absolute medication dose limitations have been defined for patients with seizure disorders, renal disease, and liver disease. Some antidepressants, such as bupropion, are contraindicated for persons with bulimia, and some drugs, such as paroxetine, fluoxetine, and fluvoxamine, have significant liver CYP P450 interaction effects. In elders, antidepressants should be started at lower doses and titrated slowly. For some pregnant women, antidepressants are a safer option than untreated depression. For breastfeeding mothers, sertraline and paroxetine have demonstrated undetectable serum levels in infants with no short-term effects, further research is needed on the long-term effects. TCAs are not less effective than newer antidepressant medications, but they can produce more side effects and have greater lethality in overdose.

Regarding efficacy, a meta-analysis by Cipriani et al. (2009), comparing efficacy and acceptability of second-generation antidepressants, indicated that sertraline and escitalopram should be considered for initial therapy for adults with moderate to severe depression. When an agent does not seem to be effective after a full trial of 4 to 6 weeks, switching, either between or within classes, is recommended. Switching between SSRIs and SNRIs can be done by prescribing the new drug at equivalent dosage. Switching from SSRI to TCA or SNRI can be accomplished through cross-tapering, where the SSRI is gradually reduced over a 1- to 2-week period as the new drug is introduced and gradually increased to therapeutic levels. Cross-tapering is also recommended for mirtazapine. Because paroxetine possesses the most distressing discontinuation symptoms, one approach may be to switch to fluoxetine and then slowly taper. Discontinuation symptoms are generally not a problem for bupropion because it does not possess strong serotonergic properties. It is recommended to taper bupropion over a 1-week period while initiating the new drug at full dosage. Paroxetine, fluvoxamine, and fluoxetine are metabolized by the liver and could potentially increase the blood level of bupropion and the risk of seizures, especially at high doses of bupropion. Refer to specific prescribing considerations and patient information regarding monoamine oxidase inhibitors. The most important aspect is to warn patients about abrupt cessation and formulate a plan to discontinue by tapering over a 2- to 3-week period.

Providers are advised to identify all supplements or medications the patient is currently taking before starting an antidepressant medication, particularly if the patient has not taken a psychotropic medication previously. This list should include all compounds—prescribed and self-administered. Many people take OTC products—vitamins, minerals, herbal remedies—that they may not consider "medications." The high number of such products available makes this information vital. Patient use of megadose vitamin and mineral supplements, weight-loss or weight-gain products, and nutritional supplements should also be noted. At present, the standard of practice regarding the use of prescribed and herbal compounds is that the two treatments should not be used simultaneously. For example, there is no compelling evidence for the efficacy of St. John's wort in either mild or moderate depression; neither is the herb recommended in cases of more serious major depressive disorder. St. John's wort, however, when taken with an antidepressant can precipitate serotonin syndrome. It also induces the hepatic metabolism of many drugs. For information on specific drugs for major depression, see Drugs Commonly Prescribed 67.1.

Lastly, each patient should be given information to ensure that he or she understands the potential benefits of taking medication, the specific medication being prescribed, possible adverse effects and how to handle them, and what to do in an emergency. When possible, this information should be made available in writing. Effective patient education makes it possible for patients to participate in their care and decreases the risks of having a patient agree to take medications without being fully informed of the medication's risks and benefits

Nonpharmacological Management

Both interpersonal and cognitive behavior therapy have been shown to be effective for the treatment of depression, and there is evidence that the combination of psychotherapy and pharmacotherapy may be more effective than either alone. Patients with major depression need

Drugs Commonly Prescribed 67.1: Major Depressive Disorder

DRUG	INDICATION	ADVERSE REACTIONS AND PRESCRIBING CONSIDERATIONS
Selective Serotonin Reuptake Inhibitors (SSRIs)		
All SSRIs		Common to most SSRIs: • Response rates: 60%–70% • Remission rates: 20%–35% • Safest class of antidepressants in overdose • Avoid sudden discontinuation due to possible withdrawal syndrome • Do not prescribe with MAOIs due to risk of serotonin syndrome • Agitation, dizziness, headache, drowsiness (dose in evening), insomnia (dose in morning), nausea/vomiting (self-limiting 1–3 weeks), and xerostomia • SIADH, risk is highest in the elderly • Serotonin syndrome (caution with "triptans") • SSRI-induced mania in BD patients • If anxiety/panic disorder develops or patient has a history of these disorders, start low and adjust dose slowly • Increased risk of suicidal behavior in children, adolescents, and young adults • Absent or slight weight gain except for paroxetine • Sexual dysfunction in 30%–40%, resolving after medication is discontinued • Wait 2 weeks after discontinuing an SSRI to start an MAOI (wait 5 weeks after fluoxetine is discontinued) • Wait 2 weeks after discontinuing an MAOI to start an SSRI
citalopram (Celexa)*	Depression SAD† Panic disorder† PTSD†/OCD† Hot flashes*,† PMDD†	• Tolerability similar to sertraline • Minimal CYP P450 effects • Causes dose-dependent QT interval prolongation, which can cause torsades de pointes, ventricular tachycardia, and sudden death • Monitor weight
escitalopram (Lexapro)*	Depression Generalized anxiety disorder Depression in children aged 12–17 years	• Minimal CYP 450 effects • Insomnia increases 50% with each 20-mg dose • Monitor weight
fluoxetine (Prozac)*	Bulimia Depression OCD Panic disorder PMDD Depression and OCD in children	• Less severe discontinuation syndrome due to long half-life • Nausea (20%), headache, GI complaints (10%), anxiety, nervousness, insomnia, drowsiness, fatigue, dizziness, tremor • Strong inhibition of CYP 2D6 can lead to drug–drug interactions • Monitoring parameters: weight and growth rate • Must wait 5 weeks after discontinuing before initiating MAOI
fluvoxamine (Luvox)*	OCD Social anxiety disorder	• More side effects than other SSRIs • Inhibition of CYP 1A2 and 3A4 results in high potential for drug–drug interactions • Monitor growth rate and weight

Drugs Commonly Prescribed 67.1: Major Depressive Disorder—cont'd

DRUG	INDICATION	ADVERSE REACTIONS AND PRESCRIBING CONSIDERATIONS
paroxetine (Paxil)*	Depression GAD Hot flashes Menopause OCD Panic PTSD PMDD SAD	• Most severe discontinuation syndrome • Causes the most weight gain of the SSRIs • Nausea/vomiting (25%), xerostomia, sedation, insomnia, tremor • Strong inhibition of CYP 2D6 can lead to drug–drug interactions • Exposure to paroxetine in the first trimester has been associated with an increased risk of cardiac birth defects
sertraline (Zoloft)*	Depression OCD Panic PTSD PMDD SAD	• Nausea, vomiting, diarrhea, drowsiness, headache • Monitor weight • Considered the safest for pregnancy and nursing
fluoxetine/ olanzapine (Symbyax)	Bipolar depression Treatment-resistant depression (treatment failure with two separate antidepressants)	• Remission rate: 25.5% • Side effects—see individual medications
Serotonin-Norepinephrine Reuptake Inhibitors (SNRIs)		
All SNRIs		Common to most SNRIs: • Response rates: 60%–70% • Remission rates: up to 50% • Safety in overdose is intermediate, between SSRIs and TCAs • Avoid sudden discontinuation • Do not prescribe with MAOIs • Agitation, weakness, dizziness, headache, drowsiness, insomnia, nausea/vomiting (self-limiting 1–3 weeks), and xerostomia. • Increased risk of suicidal behavior in children, adolescents, and young adults • SIADH, risk is highest in elders • Serotonin syndrome (caution with "triptans") • SNRI-induced mania in BD • If anxiety/panic disorder develops or if the patient has a history of these disorders, start low and adjust dose slowly • Contraindicated in uncontrolled closed-angle glaucoma • Sexual dysfunction, resolving in days after medication discontinuation • Monitor blood pressure for diastolic hypertension • Wait 2 weeks after discontinuing an SNRI to start an MAOI • Wait 2 weeks after discontinuing an MAOI to start SNRI.
desvenlafaxine (Pristiq)*	Depression	• Dose adjustment required with renal impairment
duloxetine (Cymbalta)*	Depression Diabetic neuropathy Fibromyalgia GAD Musculoskeletal pain Osteoarthritis	• Do not use with hepatic impairment or seizure disorder • May cause rare hepatotoxicity, monitor LFTs periodically • May cause orthostatic hypotension • May cause hypertension
venlafaxine (Effexor)*	Depression GAD Panic disorder SAD	• Monitor blood pressure due to risk of hypertension • Insomnia, nervousness

Continued

Drugs Commonly Prescribed 67.1 Major Depressive Disorder—cont'd

DRUG	INDICATION	ADVERSE REACTIONS AND PRESCRIBING CONSIDERATIONS
Tetracyclic Antidepressants		
All Tetracyclic Antidepressants		Common to Most Tetracyclic Antidepressants: • Increased risk of suicidal behavior in children, adolescents, and young adults
mirtazapine (Remeron)*	Depression	• Response and remission rates: 53%–63% • Somnolence (high incidence) and weight gain • Precautions include dizziness, increased cholesterol levels, and orthostatic hypotension • Can cause rare agranulocytosis • Monitor glucose, lipids
maprotiline (Ludiomil)*	Depression	• Seizure precaution; caution with CVD • Risk of extrapyramidal symptoms, including tardive dyskinesia • Monitor ECG
Serotonin Modulators		
Serotonin Modulators		Common to Most Serotonin Modulators: • Increased risk of suicidal behavior in children, adolescents, and young adults
nefazodone (Serzone)*	Depression	• Risk of hepatic failure; as a result, it is rarely prescribed • Response rate—35%–67% • Remission—35%–52% • Considered the safest for pregnancy and nursing • Modest antidepressant; used mainly for hypnotic and anxiolytic effects. • Allow washout period when discontinuing fluoxetine and starting nefazodone (at least 1 week) • Monitor liver transaminases
trazodone (Desyrel)*	Depression	• Rarely used as an antidepressant; often prescribed at low doses for insomnia in depressed patients • Do not give after myocardial infarction • Potentiates alcohol, other CNS depressants; sedative effect
Norepinephrine-Dopamine Reuptake Inhibitor (NDRIs)		
bupropion (Wellbutrin, Zyban)*	Depression Smoking cessation SAD ADHD	• Response rate: 52%–70% • May cause weight loss • Fewer sexual side effects • Avoid use in patients with seizure disorders, history of eating disorders, or history of alcohol dependence/withdrawal due to increased risk of seizures • Increased risk of suicidal behavior in children, adolescents, and young adults
Tricyclic Antidepressants (TCAs)		
All TCAs	In addition to major indications may be used in conjunction with mood stabilizers and antipsychotics to treat concomitant depression	Common to most TCAs: • Response rates: 43%–70% • Remission rates: 25%–60% • High lethality with overdose • Analgesic, anticholinergic, and antimuscarinic actions; high side-effect burden • Avoid in patients with narrow angle glaucoma or prostatic hypertrophy • Risk of cardiotoxicity, QTc prolongation • Wait 2 weeks to start after discontinuation of fluoxetine, MAOIs • Do not use with history of seizures, glaucoma, urinary retention • Increased risk of suicidal behavior in children, adolescents, and young adults • Drug levels helpful to monitor for some agents • Monitor ECG and blood pressure • Treat constipation with fiber and exercise
amitriptyline (Elavil)*	Depression	• Monitor BP, HR, ECG, serum concentrations

Drugs Commonly Prescribed 67.1 Major Depressive Disorder—cont'd

DRUG	INDICATION	ADVERSE REACTIONS AND PRESCRIBING CONSIDERATIONS
amoxapine (Asendin)*	Depression	• Moderate sedation. Monitor orthostatic blood pressure, may cause tardive dyskinesia and neuromuscular symptoms • Monitor ECG
clomipramine (Anafranil)*	OCD	• Strong anticholinergic effect sedation, orthostatic hypotension • Monitor BP, ECG and liver transaminases if hepatic disease
desipramine (Norpramin)*	Depression	• Less sedating • Monitor ECG and serum concentrations
doxepin (Sinequan)*	Anxiety Atopic dermatitis Depression Eczema Insomnia Lichen simplex	• Strong sedation and orthostatic hypotension • Monitor ECG
imipramine (Tofranil)*	Depression Enuresis	• Moderate sedation and hypotension • Monitor ECG and serum concentrations
nortriptyline (Pamelor)*	Depression	• Monitor ECG and serum concentrations
protriptyline (Vivactil)*	Depression	• Strong anticholinergic effects • Activating • Monitor ECG
trimipramine (Surmontil)*	Depression	• Strong sedation effect, monitor orthostatic blood pressure • Monitor ECG
Monoamine Oxidase Inhibitors (MAOIs)		
All MAOIs		Common to most MAOIs: • Increased risk of suicidal behavior in children, adolescents, and young adults
isocarboxazid (Marplan)*	Depression	• 60%–70% remission rates; may be better in atypical depression • Requires dietary (tyramine) restrictions: Aged, smoked or fermented meat; aged cheeses; tap/unpasteurized beers; sauerkraut; soy/tofu • Avoid dextromethorphan, other serotoninergic compounds • Potential for hypertensive crisis • Potential for serotonin syndrome • Because of the potential for serious adverse effects, drug interactions, and necessity of dietary restrictions, MAOIs (e.g., phenelzine, tranylcypromine) generally are not used as initial therapy for major depressive disorders • Monitor liver transaminases and for orthostatic hypotension
tranylcypromine (Parnate)	Depression	Monitor liver transaminases and blood pressure
phenelzine (Nardil)*	Depression	Monitor liver transaminases and blood pressure

*Black-box warning: children, suicide ideation.
†Not Food and Drug Administration approved for this indication.
Abbreviations: CNS, central nervous system; Cr, creatinine; ECG, elctrocardiogram; GAD, generalized anxiety disorder; GI, gastrointestinal; LFTs, liver function tests; MAOI, monoamine oxidase inhibitor; OCD, obsessive compulsive disorder; PMDD, premenstrual dysphoric disorder; PTSD, post-traumatic stress disorder; SAD, social anxiety disorder; SIADH, syndrome of inappropriate antidiuretic hormone secretion; SNRI, selective norepinephrine reuptake inhibitor; SSRI, selective serotonin reuptake inhibitor; TCA, tricyclic antidepressant; TFTs, liver function tests; TSH, thyroid stimulating hormone.

hope and reassurance. Both are particularly important with patients who may have lived with untreated depression. Informing a person that his or her disorder is major depression and that the disorder can be treated sets the stage for patients to define goals for improvement and begin to combat the demoralization that can develop after months of untreated depression. False reassurances and unrealistic expectations must be avoided, however.

The support needs of patients with major depression can be significant. It is unlikely that, in a primary-care setting, practitioners will be able to meet all of a patient's needs. For this reason, new sources of support should be identified. Friends, relatives, and spouse or partners are important potential sources of information, comfort, and assistance. Professional-led support groups and peer self-help groups are also highly effective.

Support is an important resource for all depressed patients, but patients who are anxious or irritable may require a great deal of practitioner patience. Anxious, irritable patients can be indecisive, critical, and demanding and can appear uncooperative or uninterested. Every effort must be made to avoid getting into a power struggle or challenging upset patients. In the long run, reassuring acceptance is easier and more effective.

Establishing a routine and focusing on increasing activities and behaviors may be a constructive approach. Massage, relaxation therapies, exercise, good nutrition, and a variety of forms of self-care should also be initiated and supported.

For some patients, the only important outcome of treatment for major depression is symptom relief. Normalized sleep, appetite, mood, energy, and concentration should, however, be viewed as minimal patient outcomes. If the patient's risk for future episodes of depression is to be significantly lowered, additional outcomes need to be addressed. Improved patient depression awareness is important. Patients treated for major depression should, as a stated outcome of treatment, increase their understanding of their illness and improve their abilities to cope with depression. The most important outcome is that the patient will immediately seek help should symptoms of major depression return. Depressive episodes that persist for months despite an adequate course of therapy, relapse despite ongoing treatment or are characterized by extremely high symptom levels, including inability to function or thoughts of suicide, require referral and specialized care, sometimes in an inpatient setting.

FOLLOW-UP AND REFERRAL

Follow-up during treatment of depression and/or anxiety is absolutely necessary to ensure adherence to therapy. The patient must be monitored to ensure that the prescription was filled and that the medication was taken. Treatment outcome should be assessed regularly using formal diagnostic assessment tools. Target symptoms are used to evaluate the effectiveness of medication during early stages of treatment and until full symptom remission is obtained. In moderate to severe depression, follow-up is determined by the severity of the initial PHQ-9.

A reasonable criterion for extending the initial treatment is to assess whether the patient is experiencing a 50% or greater reduction in baseline symptom severity at 6 weeks of therapeutic dose. If the patient's symptoms are reduced by 50% or more, but the patient is not yet at remission, and if medication has been well tolerated,

continue to prescribe. Raising the dose is recommended. In the acute phase of treatment and recovery, the patient should be seen or contacted every 1 to 2 weeks within the first month of therapy and at least once in the succeeding 4 to 8 weeks. For persons who can be treated effectively with antidepressant medication, satisfactory symptom relief often is achieved within 4 to 6 weeks. Many patients begin to feel better in 2 to 3 weeks. When the patient reports target symptom relief or the assessment indicates symptom remission has been achieved, the practitioner and patient develop a treatment and discontinuation plan. The duration of medication treatment for uncomplicated major depression is at a minimum 6 to 12 months at the treatment dose (Michigan Quality Improvement Consortium, 2016). A longer treatment period is recommended for patients with complicated or multiple disorders or patients who have a history of one or more years of untreated depression. In these instances, treatment duration should extend from 15 months to indefinite. Short half-life antidepressants are discontinued gradually over a period of 2 to 3 weeks. Persons who experience significant discontinuation symptoms may report flu-like symptoms that last a few days. Consultation with a specialist should be considered if discontinuation symptoms appear to be significant or persistent.

Patient Education: Major Depressive Disorder

It is important for the provider to teach the patient and significant other(s) to report signs of increased agitation, irritability, and suicidality. Emergency phone numbers (such as crisis services) and tertiary care sites need to be given to the patient and significant others should such symptoms emerge. It has been known for some time that some patients may experience an increase in suicidal thoughts or urges during the first few weeks of treatment. Danger signs and symptoms include the following:

- Hallucinations or delusions
- Severe adverse effects from antidepressant medications (e.g., severe urinary retention, fluctuation in blood pressure, seizures, cardiac complications)
- Suicidal thoughts
- Extreme self-care deficits (e.g., not able to care for basic needs)

The person and their family should understand that depression generates feelings of helplessness, powerlessness, and pessimism; major decisions should be delayed. The practitioner should reassure the patient that current feelings will change. All side effects of drugs should be clearly understood, and the provider should stress the importance of taking medication daily as ordered for maximum effect. The clinician should advise the patient and family that drugs to offset adverse effects are available, or that medication can be changed. Patients should be encouraged to maintain a schedule of activities and to maintain their regularly scheduled visits with their primary-care clinician.

BIPOLAR AND RELATED DISORDERS

Bipolar disorder (BD) is characterized by cyclic episodes of mania and depression. Mania is characterized by excessive excitement, elation, delusions of grandeur, distractibility, restlessness, agitation, flight of ideas, frenzied movement, decreased sleep, and poor judgment.

BD is commonly seen in the primary-care setting and is frequently mistaken for other conditions, often MDD. The spectrum of bipolar disorder includes bipolar I (BD I), in which the essential feature is mania; bipolar II (BD II), characterized by recurrent moods of hypomania (a persistent period of excitement or hyperactivity with a moderate change in behavior) and depression; cyclothymic disorder, characterized by alternating cycles of hypomania and depressive episodes, but of lesser severity than those of manic or major depressive disorders; substance/medication-induced bipolar disorder; and bipolar and related disorders due to another medical condition. The three major categories—BD I, BD II, and cyclothymic disorder—are discussed here.

Clinicians must be able to distinguish between depressive episodes occurring in the context of unipolar depression and bipolar mood disorders because patients with BD require mood-stabilizing pharmacological therapy, and their symptoms may worsen with antidepressant monotherapy. Emerging data from a variety of sources have confirmed a typical delay between symptom onset and diagnosis of 5 to 10 years, with patients seeing an average of four health-care providers before the correct diagnosis is given. MDD is a common misdiagnosis, the treatment for which (e.g., antidepressant monotherapy) may induce mania in BD patients. Over a 5-year period, 85% of patients with BD will have a relapse after one affective episode. During interepisode periods, half of the patients may experience subsyndromal symptoms, such as cognitive impairment and impulsivity; the length of interepisode intervals tends to decrease progressively across multiple recurrences. Inappropriate pharmacological treatment for BD is associated with increases in morbidity and mortality and with suicide.

EPIDEMIOLOGY AND CAUSES

The pathogenesis of bipolar disorder is unknown, but biological, psychological, and social factors are thought to contribute. Depression and BD differ significantly in their genetics, prognosis, and treatment. BD is the sixth leading cause of disability worldwide in patients aged 15 to 55. The financial burden of this disorder eclipses that of diabetes, and the impact on occupational function due to BD is more extensive than in major depressive disorder. Two-thirds of patients with BD are substantially adversely affected by their illness; but the negative impact of BD goes beyond its morbidity rate. Twenty-five percent to 50% of patients with BD have a lifetime risk of suicide attempt; up to 15% of patients will complete suicide. Attempts can occur during the manic, hypomanic, depressed, or mixed phases of BD but are most likely to occur in depressed or mixed states.

BD I has a lifetime prevalence of 1% to 3%; when the entire spectrum of bipolar disorder is included, the prevalence may approach 7% to 10%. Men and women are equally affected, although BD II is more common in women. The mean age of onset of BD I is 18 years of age, and for BD II it is 20 years of age. It can occur in early childhood, adolescence, or as late as the sixth or seventh decades of life. New onset of mania after age 40 is rare and should prompt consideration of a medical condition, such as neurological disease, thyroid dysfunction, or substance abuse or withdrawal.

Genetic components play a significant role in transmitting BD. In monozygotic twins, concordance rates approach 70%, indicating that BD is highly heritable, though its expression is also influenced by environmental factors. If one parent has BD, then their offspring will have a 20% risk of developing it. It is unknown how culture affects the expression of bipolar disorder.

PATHOPHYSIOLOGY

Depression and mania are affective states that are sometimes viewed as existing on a continuum of mood disorders. As such, many current biological theories of depression also apply to mania. Several genetic variants have been associated with bipolar disorder in genome-wide association studies. Greater understanding of the complex gene–environment interactions for these disorders is likely to emerge in the future and holds promise for attaining a clearer understanding of affective illnesses.

CLINICAL PRESENTATION

BD may be viewed as a disorder of "elevated mood" or "energy" that manifests as euphoria, irritability, or dysphoria. Approximately 25% of all patients experience episodes of pure mania, 40% demonstrate mixed (dysphoric) mania, and 10% to 25% are "rapid cyclers," manifesting quick shifts from mania to depression.

An initial manic episode may be related to an adverse life event or stressor; however, subsequent episodes may occur without an identifiable trigger. Seasonal changes may result in fall or winter depression and spring or summer mania. Light exposure can trigger manic episodes. Many women with BD report mood changes related to the menstrual cycle. Manic episodes usually last 3 to 6 months if untreated, and the symptoms typically escalate rapidly over a period of days. Psychotic symptoms may be present in the acute manic phase or in the depressive phase. Psychotic depression should raise an index of suspicion that the patient may have an underlying bipolar disorder. Older adult patients may manifest irritability rather than elated mood. Untreated depressive episodes can last 6 to 12 months, and some treatment-resistant patients with depression actually have BD. Almost 90% of all persons with BD experience depression, and most BD patients present for treatment during a depressive episode. In *all* patients presenting with depression, clinicians should inquire specifically about symptoms of past manic or hypomanic episodes, past treatment and responses, and family history. Patients may be asymptomatic during interepisode periods.

Over a 5-year period, 85% of patients with BD will have a relapse after one affective episode. Although some patients experience limited functional recovery despite successful syndrome treatment, early intervention is associated with improved outcomes. Most commonly patients will present for treatment for a depressive episode rather than for the euphoria associated with a manic or hypomanic episode. Often patients, for a variety of reasons, will leave out these episodes when reviewing their medical history and clinicians may fail to query or recognize previous hypomanic or manic symptoms. Some patients even identify periods of normal mood as depressed when compared with mania.

DIAGNOSTIC REASONING

A complete physical exam is needed, as well as neurological assessment, to exclude other etiologies of mood symptoms or psychosis. The patient's mental status should be assessed, including general appearance, attitude, behaviors, mood, affect, speech, thought processes and content, concentration, and memory. Focus the physical and neurological exam (e.g., cranial nerves, reflexes, muscle tone, gait) on identifying or excluding a medical cause of the patient's symptoms. Comorbidity, and the possibility of precipitating factors such as thyroid disorder, head injuries, or substance abuse should also be considered.

Diagnostic testing includes a complete blood count (CBC) with differential, platelet count, comprehensive blood chemistry panel, free thyroxine (T_4), thyroid-stimulating hormone (TSH), rapid plasma reagin (RPR), HIV antibody test, urinalysis, urine toxicology screen, and pregnancy test. In the setting of HIV/AIDS, hepatitis C, and other infectious causes, new-onset mood or bipolar-like symptoms require further studies to exclude identifiable causes of mood changes. Consider conducting a Mini-Mental State Exam to assess cognition. Refer to neurology or infectious disease to assist with diagnosis if indicated.

Box 67.2 DIGFAST Mnemonic for Bipolar Disorder

The following mnemonic, DIGFAST, is useful for identifying BD:

- **D**istractibility
- **I**nsomnia (decreased need for sleep)
- **G**randiosity (inflated self-esteem)
- **F**light of ideas (racing thoughts, negative for rumination)
- **A**ctivities (increased, goal directed)
- **S**peech (pressured, increased talkativeness)
- **T**houghtlessness (pleasure-seeking activities that show poor judgment such as spending sprees, sexual indiscretions, reckless driving, arguments if irritable)

Brain magnetic resonance imaging or computed tomography scans may be helpful if clinical findings suggest an underlying central nervous system (CNS) disorder.

Symptoms

Three major categories of bipolar disorder are recognized:

- Bipolar Disorder I: Patients with BD I have had at least one episode of mania. A major depressive episode is not required for diagnosis.
- Bipolar Disorder II: BD II is characterized by a history of both depression and hypomania.
- Cyclothymic Disorder: Cyclothymia involves 2 years of symptoms of hypomania and depression that do not meet the full criteria for either mood episode.

A mnemonic for bipolar disorder is presented in Box 67.2. Complete diagnostic criteria can be found in the *DSM-5*.

Differential Diagnosis

Bipolar I Disorder

The differential diagnoses to consider are the following: MDD, other bipolar disorder, schizophrenia, anxiety disorders, attention-deficit/hyperactivity disorder, personality disorders, and substance use. It is essential to obtain a full psychiatric history and also, if the patient consents, to interview family and friends to corroborate information and help establish the diagnosis of BD. Patients with mania often lack insight into their symptoms and do not report them. They feel euphoric during a manic episode and value their productivity during an episode of hypomania. Family members and friends may be able to report historical clues, personal factors, and suicidal ideation that may be associated with increased suicide risk and point to a diagnosis of BD. To help differentiate between bipolar and unipolar depression, as part of the history, ask about the onset, frequency, and duration of symptoms, as well as about distractibility, seasonality, and other characteristics of a depressed patient's high and low moods (see Box 67.3).

> ## Box 67.3 Distinguishing Between Bipolar and Unipolar Depressive Episodes
>
> - Ask all depressed patients about history of mania and hypomania.
> - Ask about family history of bipolar disorder—"loaded" family history is a clue to bipolarity in "unipolar" patients.
> - Involve family member and/or significant other in screening process.
> - Administer a screening instrument for bipolar disorder, such as the Mood Disorder Questionnaire.
> - Early age at onset (<25 years) is another clue for bipolarity.
> - Psychotic features are another clinical clue for bipolarity in the seemingly unipolar patient, as is seasonal pattern.
> - Adverse and/or inadequate antidepressant response such as treatment-emergent hypomania or agitation, erratic or uneven antidepressant responses, multiple antidepressant failures, or "treatment-resistant depression."

Sources: Hirschfeld RM, Vornik LA. Recognition and diagnosis of bipolar disorder. *J Clin Psychiatry.* 2004;65(suppl 15):5–9; Lohano K, Loganathan M, Roberts RJ, Gao Y. When to suspect bipolar disorder. *J Fam Pract.* 2010;59(12):682–688.

Bipolar II Disorder

The differential diagnosis of Bipolar II disorder is the same as BD I. However, because of some patients' reluctance to view hypomania as a pathological state, it can be difficult to distinguish from other forms of recurrent depression. It is essential to inquire about suicide, because most suicide attempts are associated with depressive episodes or mixed episodes.

Cyclothymic Disorder

Differentiating the milder, subsyndromal form of bipolar disorder can be challenging, especially in determining the length of previous episodes. In addition, borderline personality disorder and substance-induced mood disorders need to be considered.

General Considerations for All Bipolar Disorders

Among those patients who have not experienced psychotic symptoms or classic recurrent episodes of MDD, two diagnoses that are sometimes confused with bipolar disorders are substance abuse and cluster B personality disorders, and there may be comorbidities with these entities. However, in substance abuse, euphoria/dysphoria is temporally related to drug intoxication and withdrawal state. In cluster B personality disorders, "mood swings" last from minutes to hours to days, not weeks to months, and are typically closely associated to interpersonal disruptions or alliances.

Clinicians should inquire about chronic or recurrent nonspecific physical symptoms (e.g., fatigue, headache, or gastrointestinal distress) and about depressive or manic feelings and behaviors. Medical disorders that may coexist or appear similar to BD should be considered, including thyroid dysfunction, vasculitis, chronic infection, malignancies, and metabolic disorders. Clinical and laboratory findings may help to exclude these causes. Family history, particularly of first-degree relatives should be reviewed. Recent medications, including hormonal contraceptives, and treatment during prior episodes should be noted, especially any temporal association between drugs and symptoms; many drugs can induce or exacerbate manic or depressive symptoms. Levodopa and corticosteroids are the most common causes of drug-induced mania; these agents can also cause depressive symptoms.

Patients with BD often self-medicate with drugs and alcohol to relieve anxiety, insomnia, agitation, and excessive fatigue. Drugs, alcohol, and some medications may also contribute to these symptoms. More than one-half of those patients who meet the criteria for bipolar disorder have an alcohol or substance use disorder or other mental health disorder, increasing the risk for suicide attempt. Clinicians should assess the severity, frequency, and longitudinal course of depressive and manic episodes and determine whether the symptoms meet the specific diagnostic criteria for bipolar or another psychiatric disorder. Patients should be asked about deterioration in the baseline level of functioning at work or school or in personal relationships.

Patients with BD appear especially sensitive to sleep deprivation, which may occur in conjunction with stressors such as bereavement, childbirth, vacation, longer work hours, and shift changes. They may experience periods of decreased need for sleep while manic. Disrupted sleep can also precipitate manic episodes. Specific details about sleep–wake periods, including daytime naps, meal times, social activities, hobbies and other areas of interest, interpersonal attitudes, and ability to work and perform household tasks are helpful. Patients should be asked about a typical day.

Patients with mania or depression usually do not report characteristic psychological descriptors (e.g., elation, grandiosity, inflated self-esteem, racing thoughts, irritability, or agitation), so activities may provide diagnostic clues. For example, grandiose thinking may manifest as reckless gambling, spending sprees, or sexual promiscuity. Conversely, increased productivity, enhanced perceptual ability, altered view on interpersonal relationships, and fluctuating symptoms without substantial negative social or occupational consequences suggest hypomania.

Routine screening for depression is advised in primary-care settings, but attention should also be focused on screening for past episodes of hypomania or mania. The Mood Disorder Questionnaire (MDQ) is a validated screening tool for BD, which lessens the likelihood of underdiagnosis or a missed diagnosis. Use of the MDQ can identify 70% of persons with BD while eliminating the diagnosis for 90% of persons without it. More recently, there has been some question about whether or not the MDQ underdiagnoses BD II because of the requirement for moderate to severe impairment of functioning, as many patients feel that during a hypomanic episode they function better. Another instrument, the Bipolar Spectrum Diagnostic Scale, is better for ruling out the diagnosis of BD than for giving a positive diagnosis. If a patient scores positive for BD on this scale, further clinical evaluation is necessary to make the diagnosis.

Assessment for suicide risk is essential. Clinicians should inquire about suicide ideation and intentions, and about extent of plans or preparations for, prior attempts at, family history of, and recent exposure to suicide. This is essential both at presentation and during subsequent mood episodes because the lifetime risk for suicide in patients with BD is up to 15%. Most suicide attempts are associated with depressive episodes or during depressive features of mixed episodes.

MANAGEMENT

Pharmacological Management

The ideal treatment goals for patients with BD include complete remission of current symptoms, prevention of future affective episodes, and return to premorbid function. Mainstays of therapy are mood-stabilizing medications. Pharmacotherapy is used to achieve symptom remission and improve function in patients with BD. Mood stabilizers, second-generation antipsychotics, first-generation antipsychotics, and adjunctive anxiolytics and antidepressants are used to treat BD. Factors in determining which medication will most likely result in treatment remission depend on the diagnosis—BD I or BD II, manic versus depressed, acute or maintenance, rapid cycling versus non-rapid cycling, and whether psychotic symptoms exist. Attempts should be made to use the lowest possible dose to minimize side effects, particularly with first-generation agents.

Considerations before initiating therapy include the patient's age, because the elderly may be more sensitive to side effects of antipsychotic medications and anticonvulsants. It is essential to prescribe the lowest possible dose and monitor for side effects. The possibility of pregnancy should always be considered in women of childbearing age before initiating psychotropic medications. Knowledge of past treatment history, effectiveness, tolerability, failures, and side-effect profiles allows the practitioner to provide individualized, patient-centered care. It is likely there will be a need to change treatment modalities over time. Several weeks are required to assess the effects of a new treatment.

Collaboration with a psychiatrist will aid the clinician in selecting appropriate drug therapy to treat acute manic episodes in patients with BD. Treatment options for patients with BD I with hypomania, mania, or mixed episodes should begin with lithium, valproic acid (Depakote), or atypical antipsychotic agents. Carbamazepine (Tegretol) or oxcarbazepine (Trileptal) may also be used. If there is no response or a partial response, combination therapy such as lithium plus valproic acid, lithium plus an atypical antipsychotic, or an atypical antipsychotic plus valproic acid may be considered. If still not effective, clozapine (Clozaril) may be added or electroconvulsive therapy (ECT) may be introduced in treatment-resistant cases.

It is important that lithium be prescribed at a therapeutic dose. Valproic acid is usually preferred, however, due to its ease of administration. Carbamazepine, another anticonvulsant agent, is an alternative. Combinations of these agents may be used if patients do not respond to a single agent. If the patient does not respond fully, atypical antipsychotics may be added to one or more mood stabilizers. Lamotrigine is effective for patients who predominantly have had depressed episodes. Long-acting benzodiazepines, such as clonazepam and lorazepam, may be used for rapid treatment of manic symptoms and to calm and sedate patients until acute mania or hypomania has subsided and the mood stabilizer has taken effect. In the case of psychotic symptoms, antipsychotics may be added. ECT may be used for patients with severe BD with drug treatment–resistant mania or psychotic depression.

Episodes of depression pose particular challenges. There are fewer approved treatments for bipolar depression. Overall, antidepressant medications do not control depression as effectively in bipolar as in unipolar depression and may trigger mania. Mood stabilization is still the primary goal. If depression persists 2 to 4 weeks after optimization of the mood stabilizer, it is recommended that either lamotrigine (anticonvulsant, mood stabilizer) or an atypical antipsychotic be added. Antidepressants may be effective against depression but can precipitate mania and should not be given to a bipolar patient without a mood stabilizer, and even then they are reserved for extremely ill patients, after other options have failed. Bupropion is often the first antidepressant started because it is considered the least likely to induce mania. Any patient developing symptoms of hypomania while taking an antidepressant should stop taking it; in addition, patients should be slowly tapered off any antidepressants after a period of sustained remission. Patients with psychotic symptoms, such as delusions or hallucinations, will require treatment with antipsychotic medications.

Lithium remains the gold standard for treatment of BD and has been shown to be uniquely effective in decreasing suicidal behavior. Lithium appears to be most effective early in the course of the illness, for classic manic symptoms, in patients in whom depression immediately follows mania, and in patients with a strong family history of BD. However, lithium also has a number of potential adverse effects, including life-threatening neurotoxicity that can occur at serum levels higher than 2.0 mEq/L. Lithium levels should be obtained twice weekly until the patient's clinical status and levels are stable at which time they may be obtained every 1 to 3 months. Serum trough lithium levels are drawn 8 to 12 hours after the last dose.

Adverse drug interactions can occur when lithium is prescribed with thiazide diuretics, NSAIDs, angiotensin-converting enzyme inhibitors, and COX-2 inhibitors. Additional potential adverse effects include nausea, diarrhea, tremor, polyuria, polydipsia, and weight gain. Lithium may exacerbate psoriasis and acne, cause hypothyroidism (5%–35%), and in 20% of patients (usually after 15 or more years of treatment) lead to renal insufficiency. Lithium has also been associated with a rare birth defect called Ebstein's anomaly. This is a congenital heart defect in which the opening of the tricuspid valve is displaced toward the apex of the right ventricle of the heart. Lithium takes several weeks to become effective. Owing to potential adverse effects, lithium therapy should be preceded by an evaluation of renal, cardiac, and thyroid function, as well as a pregnancy test. Many patients do not stay on lithium. Some regret the loss of the exhilaration that occurs during a manic episode; some patients are concerned about weight gain or tremor. In one study, 50% of patients acknowledged some degree of medication nonadherence in the previous 2 years, and 32% reported only partial adherence in the preceding month.

Anticonvulsant medications are effective for the treatment and/or maintenance of mania and/or BD. These agents have become alternative treatments for patients who need a mood-stabilizing agent but who do not fare well with lithium; these medications also may be used in combination with lithium.

Divalproex/valproic acid is considered a first-line pharmacological treatment for acute mania, mixed episodes, rapid cycling, and maintenance treatment. There is some evidence of antidepressant effect as well. Divalproex appears to be most effective for rapid cycling and mixed episodes, in patients who have had more than three manic episodes, and in patients with comorbid alcohol abuse. Valproic acid is comparable to lithium in efficacy, and generally better tolerated. The most frequently observed side effects are nausea, vomiting, weight gain, tremor, dizziness, and sedation. Serious adverse effects include hepatotoxicity, pancreatitis, thrombocytopenia, and teratogenicity. Serum valproate levels, liver function tests, and CBCs should be monitored closely during treatment with valproic acid.

Valproic acid is a cytochrome 450 enzyme inhibitor and may engender metabolic interactions with other drugs. Valproic acid can induce menstrual irregularities and cause polycystic ovary syndrome (PCOS), affecting 2% to 7% of women in their reproductive years. PCOS is characterized by chronic anovulation and hyperandrogenism. VPA is teratogenic and can cause neural tube defects in 1% to 4% of neonates. VPA is also associated with congenital malformations, including spina bifida, atrial septal defect, cleft palate, hypospadias, polydactyly, and craniosynostosis. Troubling reports of lower IQ in children exposed in utero to valproate have been published. As a result, many authorities recommend avoiding VPA all together in women of child-bearing age.

Carbamazepine is approved for the treatment of bipolar mania and mixed episodes. Therapeutic serum levels for BD have not been established; usually concentrations used for seizure disorders (4–12 mcg/mL) are applied. Serum levels as well as CBC, platelets, and liver function must all be monitored as potential side effects which include agranulocytosis, aplastic anemia, hepatic failure, Stevens-Johnson syndrome, and pancreatitis. Carbamazepine reduces levels of other drugs, such as oral contraceptives and dihydropyridine calcium-channel blockers. Carbamazepine is contraindicated during pregnancy or lactation. It is associated with congenital malformations, including spina bifida, craniofacial defects, fingernail hypoplasia, and developmental delay.

Lamotrigine received approval as maintenance therapy for BD in 2003. This medication's antidepressant effects are stronger than its antimanic properties and it usually is not used as monotherapy for patients with BD I. The most significant adverse effect is rash (about 5% risk), which, in some cases can be Stevens-Johnson syndrome or toxic epidermal necrolysis, both of which can be fatal.

Typical antipsychotic agents such as haloperidol (Haldol) have been frequently used to treat acute bipolar mania. These agents work well in reducing symptoms such as paranoia, hallucinations, delusions, and thought disturbances. However, they are usually not used for the longer term or preventive management of BD and carry the risk of extrapyramidal symptoms (EPS), such as akathisia, dystonia (e.g. torticollis), parkinsonism, and tardive dyskinesia, as well as depression.

Newer second-generation, or atypical, antipsychotics have a lower propensity to induce EPS, but have been linked to weight gain and metabolic syndrome. Both classes of drugs block dopaminergic transmission, but the newer drugs also block serotonin receptors. These are standard agents for schizophrenia but most are now approved for use as monotherapy in mania, depression or for maintenance, with and without mood stabilizers. See Chapter 66 for further discussion of typical and atypical antipsychotics.

Maintenance drug therapy should be based on the patient's response to initial treatment and in conjunction with a psychiatrist. Patients at high risk for recurrence should consider lifelong therapy, generally with mood stabilizers. Lithium and valproic acid are first-line agents used in maintenance therapy, alone and in combination. Although there are some differences in side effects, the dropout rates are similar, and both agents demonstrate equal effectiveness. Carbamazepine may be used as an alternative.

Adjunctive drug therapy should be considered for comorbid disorders. For example, if a patient with BD is compliant with medication yet has a concurrent anxiety or substance use disorder, an antidepressant may be used with either a mood stabilizer or an antipsychotic. If a patient is persistently anxious, most psychiatrists will assess for a mixed state, occult substance abuse, or a medical condition. In summary, management options are based on the patients' primary symptoms of mania, depression, or mixed states (see Table 67.1).

Nonpharmacological Management

Patients living with BD may have difficulty discussing unusual events or thoughts and often have poor insight regarding symptoms or the need for treatment. They respond best to proactive, collaborative, and individualized treatment, as exemplified in the *Circle of Caring* model. Developing a therapeutic alliance is imperative, because BD is chronic and needs long-term management. Establishing a trusting relationship with a medical home will provide patients the opportunity to experience continuity of care, to attend to health maintenance and any chronic medical problems, and to maintain a collaborative connection with their behavioral health providers and supports.

Obtain a consultation with a psychiatrist if you suspect BD once you have excluded medical etiologies. Accurate diagnosis can be complicated because other psychiatric disorders may appear similar. Consultation will provide clinicians with a more accurate diagnosis as well as assistance with managing pharmacological regimens and acute crisis should it be necessary. Consider referral to an integrated treatment provider for dual-diagnosed patients with substance and/or alcohol dependence. Hospitalization is necessary for patients with BD who may be a danger to themselves or others or who are unable to care for their needs. Patients with mood disorders, particularly mania, are often unwilling to enter a hospital voluntarily and may require involuntary commitment.

A supportive primary-care provider can help in monitoring the patient's overall status, as well as encouraging adherence to the medication regimen. The clinician can also provide referral for specific psychosocial interventions for patients with BD. Along with a PMHNP or a psychiatrist, a behavioral health specialist may aid recovery by relieving depression, delaying episodes, and improving function and treatment adherence. Psychoeducation is aimed at providing information about BD and treatment and is an important resource for patients, families, and supports. The goals of psychoeducation are to increase knowledge and acceptance of the disorder and to address denial and nonadherence to the treatment plan. Meta-analysis has shown that patient education combined with drug treatment helps to improve adherence.

Psychotherapy, although not effective as monotherapy, can significantly enhance treatment response and prevent relapse. Interpersonal, family-focused, cognitive-behavioral, supportive, and psychoeducational approaches

TABLE 67.1 Management of Bipolar Disorder	
Symptomatology—Manic/Mixed	*Management Strategies*
First-line	Lithium plus an antipsychotic Valproate plus an antipsychotic (Second-generation antipsychotics are preferable) Carbamazepine Electroconvulsive therapy (may be used if preferred by the patient, patients with severe illness, or if patient is pregnant) For less ill patients, monotherapy with lithium, valproate, or an antipsychotic may be preferable
Adjunctive treatments	Benzodiazepine Gabapentin Topiramate
Nonresponse	Optimize the initial medication dose Add or change mood-stabilizing drug Add or change antipsychotic Add lamotrigine
Symptomatology—Depressed	*Management Strategies*
First-line	Lithium or lamotrigine Electroconvulsive therapy (for patients with life-threatening inanition, suicidality, or psychosis; severe depression/pregnancy)
Nonresponse	Optimize the initial medication dose Add another mood stabilizer Add an antipsychotic Add an antidepressant Electroconvulsive therapy

Sources: Adapted from American Psychiatric Association. *Diagnostic and statistical manual of mental disorders, fifth edition* (*DSM-5*). Arlington, VA; American Psychiatric Association; 2013; St. John D. Bipolar affective disorder. *Clin Rev.* 2013;15(6):47.

increase illness awareness, improve collaboration with health-care professionals and supportive family and friends, and may assist in lifestyle regulation. There is good evidence that cognitive behavioral therapy (CBT) protects against relapse, results in better treatment response, and helps support greater maintenance of treatment gains.

The onset of manic and depressive episodes is often associated with psychosocial stress. Patients should be encouraged to pace their activities at work and to maintain a regular schedule. A change in sleep patterns often heralds the onset of a manic or depressive episode. Insomnia may be a precipitant or a prodromal warning sign. Maintenance of regular sleep habits helps prevent escalation of mood symptoms into a full-blown episode. Educate BD patients and their families about the risks of stress, substance abuse, and irregular and inconsistent sleep patterns, meals, and other daily habits.

FOLLOW-UP AND REFERRAL

Education is a key component to effective adherence to therapy and to family support. Open discussion of all treatment options, side effects, and their management is critical and is a hallmark of patient-centered care. Monitoring and managing symptoms over time, including triggers and early warning signs, is essential. Self-monitoring and better symptom recognition are desirable goals. The prevalence of nonadherence with mood stabilizers ranges from 18% to 52%. Reasons include denial of diagnosis, unwillingness to take medication long term, perceived improvement in health, and adverse side effects of medications. Patient adherence to the medication regimen can make a difference in patient outcomes. In one 18-month study, 81% of partially adherent patients required hospitalization versus just 9% of adherent patients. Patients may ask if they will need to continue taking the same medication for life. The specific medications prescribed may change as new agents are introduced and as the individual's treatment needs are reassessed. What will remain constant is the need to monitor the patient with BD over their lifetime.

The practitioner can help the patient and family develop realistic treatment goals by actively listening and being responsive to patient needs and by regularly addressing mixed feelings about adherence to treatment. Patients with BD struggle with a variety of interpersonal and/or occupational issues. As stabilization management and supervision are lessened after an acute affective episode, patient attendance at follow-ups may decrease. During this postacute period, intensive collaboration with the patient and family can be invaluable for establishing the framework for long-term interactions that build on the therapeutic *Circle of Caring.*

Involvement of family and friends is critical to successful follow-up because progression of BD may be difficult to validate via self-report. Sensitivity to early warning signs of potential mood destabilization is important. Many patients do not try to achieve treatment goals. Symptoms of illness often preclude sound judgment, and patient unwillingness to tolerate medication side effects are some of the causes of apparent nonadherence.

Regularly reviewing with the patient "quality of life" versus "effects of treatment" and emphasizing the improved prognosis associated with maintenance therapy may improve medication compliance. CBT, family therapy, or interpersonal therapy should all target self-monitoring, treatment adherence, communication skills, and coping strategies to complement pharmacotherapy.

If a patient presents with early manifestations of relapse, promptly assess the clinical scenario and review the drug regimen. It is essential to investigate possible medication nonadherence, drug–drug interactions, and substance use and to obtain a drug level before initiating a change in the current regimen. If the cause of relapse is unclear or the symptoms fail to respond to standard treatment, a psychiatrist should be consulted. Periodically the patient should be reevaluated for known or new medical conditions or medication use that may complicate management; at every encounter, they should also be assessed for suicide risk.

Patient Education: Bipolar and Related Disorders

Educate the family and patient about the nature of bipolar illness and about the importance of medication compliance, regular visits for clinical and laboratory monitoring, and contacting their health-care provider before stopping or starting any medication (prescribed or over the counter). Patients should avoid complementary therapies such as St. John's wort, because they may interfere with some psychotropics or precipitate mania. Educating the patient and family about potential side effects of all medications is important, as is informing them of the many options available to minimize or eliminate side effects. Patients and their families need to understand the importance of maintaining adequate blood levels of medication in prevention of relapse and of contacting the health-care provider in the event of unpleasant side effects rather than stopping the medication.

At follow-up visits, the practitioner can counsel the patient and family about coping with stressors that may precipitate manic or depressive episodes, about maintaining a consistent lifestyle, about signs of relapse, and about medication adherence. Written patient instructions can reinforce the following recommendations:

- Limit "everyday" stimulants such as coffee, alcohol, and OTC medications that contain these substances because they can trigger mood episodes.
- Maintain regular sleep patterns.
- Avoid taking unnecessary or illegal drugs because they can trigger mood episodes; they can also prevent the benefits or increase the adverse side effects of necessary medications.

• Try to maintain a regular work schedule. If necessary, take time off rather than "tough it out" if mood symptoms hinder your ability to work.

As patients learn more about the stress of their illness on family members, it may help them reduce both their own stress and the disruption that it can cause. Patients may develop such insights by learning more about bipolar illness and by joining a bipolar support group or a mental health organization for lay people. Patients and families should be instructed to watch for early signs of relapse, including changes in sleep patterns, grooming habits, energy or sexual interest, concentration problems, mood instability, or changes in self-esteem. Most patients experience a change in sleep patterns early in the development of an episode of mania or depression. Even small amounts of stimulants may interfere with sleep patterns or mood and possibly trigger a relapse. Insomnia may be either a precipitant or a warning sign. Early recognition of these signals, promptly followed by contacting the primary-care provider, can help prevent relapse. Maintenance of regular sleep patterns, sometimes via judicious medication use, can prevent escalation of early symptoms into full episodes.

BD patients tend to minimize their limitations and vulnerabilities and may decide to discontinue treatment. There should be an individual action plan for coping and seeking assistance whenever the patient or family members suspect the patient is experiencing early manifestations of relapse. Knowing their assigned roles in the patient's action plan may be an important resource when the patient is tempted to stop therapy. They should feel free to contact their psychiatrist, counselor, or primary-care provider for advice whenever necessary, especially in light of self-destructive, aggressive behavior or any changes in daily routine that cause concern.

SUICIDE

Suicide is the result of wide-ranging disease states, disrupting biological, psychological, and social processes. In recent years, suicide has become an intensifying national public health crisis. In 2015, more than 44,000 Americans completed suicide, making it the tenth leading cause of death in the country. Since 2005, the suicide rate has increased every year. Suicide leaves a devastating legacy. Survivors are confronted with a myriad of distressing emotions and thoughts, which often continue to affect loved ones, family, children, friends, clinicians, and society long after the event.

Several terms are associated with suicidal behaviour. *Completed suicide* refers to self-inflicted death. *Attempted suicide* describes potentially lethal acts that did not result in death. *Aborted suicide* indicates potentially suicidal behaviour that was stopped before the action was completed. *Suicidal ideation* denotes thoughts of causing one's own demise. It can be accompanied by planning, intent, rehearsals, and obtaining the means to suicide.

Parasuicidal behavior describes patients who injure themselves in nonlethal, ocassionally attention-seeking gestures, such as superficial cuts on wrists, but who do not wish to die. The behavior is a risk factor for suicide.

Each person, and their life circumstances, who attempts suicide is unique. Unfortunately, there is no way to predict suicide. However, risk for suicide can be assessed, through analysis of risk factors, suicidal intent, and protective factors. If there is a shared personal characteristic, it is likely to be a profound sense of hopelessness, in the sense that the individual perceives there is no future or that the future they envision is somehow unattainable. Suicidal patients may be angry, sad, or confused. They may be quite honest about their suicidal plans or refuse to disclose their hidden thoughts and feelings.

Suicidal thoughts and feelings commonly are associated with mood disorders, principally major depressive disorder and bipolar disorder, although they also occur in other psychiatric disorders. Persons who are overwhelmed by severe psychosocial problems and/or medical illnesses may also experience suicidal thoughts.

Suicidal ideation can have acute onset, meaning that for a period of time, the person is at risk for acting on thoughts of suicide. Chronic suicidal thoughts are also not uncommon. In this case, the person never feels completely free of thoughts of taking their life. Impulsive suicidal behavior is the most difficult to assess because this type of behavior is likely to occur without warning. Patients who are troubled by thoughts of suicide but are clear about their determination not to act on their suicidal thoughts may be appropriate candidates for primary-care management. Any suggestion of impulsive behavior, chronic suicidal thoughts or evidence of acute suicidal ideation with intent, plan, and/or means is an indicator for emergent evaluation by a specialist.

In the month preceding a completed suicide, 45% of patients see their primary-care physician, only 20% see a mental health professional. Women and older patients are more likely to seek care before suicide compared to men and younger patients. Most antidepressant prescriptions (62%) in the United States are written by generalists, such as internists, pediatricians, and family physicians. Taken together, it is clear that primary-care clinicians provide the most depression treatment in the United States and are also the group most likely to see patients at risk of suicide in the month preceding their death. Therefore, they have the greatest opportunity to intervene (see The Patient's Voice 67.1.)

EPIDEMIOLOGY AND CAUSES

Suicide is the tenth leading cause of death in the United States and the second leading cause of death among adolescents and young adults, aged 15 to 24. Every 11.9 minutes another life is lost to suicide. Every day 121 Americans take their own lives, and more than 1,500

> ### The Patient's Voice 67.1
>
> The pain of the suicidal is private and inexpressible, leaving family members, friends, and colleagues to deal with an almost unfathomable kind of loss, as well as guilt. Suicide carries in its aftermath a level of confusion and devastation that is, for the most part, beyond description.
>
> *Kay Redfield Jamison*

attempt suicide. For every two victims of homicide in the United States, there are three deaths from suicide, and there are now twice as many deaths due to suicide than due to HIV/AIDS. More than half of all suicides occur in adult men aged 25 to 65. There are 3.3 male deaths by suicide for each female death by suicide, although there are 3 female attempts for each male attempt. Males are four times more likely to die from suicide than are females because they may use more lethal means, such as firearms. Sadly, many who make suicide attempts never seek professional care after the attempt. About 10% to 20% of all persons who attempt suicide eventually take their own lives.

Divorced, separated, single, and widowed persons of both sexes have a higher incidence of suicide. Adolescent (15–24 years) and geriatric (65 years and older) populations are at elevated risk, especially Native Americans and Caucasian males. Suicide is lowest in nonwhite females, including Hispanics and Asian/Pacific islanders.

In terms of methods, one study indicated that 91% of suicide acts involving firearms result in death, whereas drug overdoses lead to fatality only 2% of the time. Fatality rates associated with drowning were found to be 84%; hanging, 82%; and poisoning with gases, 64%. Firearm suicides account for 49.8% of suicide deaths. Suffocation/hanging is the second leading method of completed suicide at 26.8%.

Special at-risk occupations include physicians (especially female physicians and psychiatrists), musicians, dentists, law enforcement officers, firefighters, lawyers, and insurance agents. A number of CNS diseases increase the risk of suicide, specifically, epilepsy, multiple sclerosis, head injury, cardiovascular disease, Huntington's disease, and AIDS. All of these diseases are associated with mood disorders. Loss of mobility, disfigurement, and intractable pain are also associated with an increased risk of suicide. Certain drugs such as reserpine (Serpasil), corticosteroids, antihypertensive agents, and some antineoplastic agents can produce depression that may lead to suicide.

Suicide in Veterans

Among U.S. veterans, the rate of suicide is rising, too. An average of 20 veterans die by suicide each day. Veterans account for 18% of all suicide deaths but constitute only 8.5% of the adult population. Risk for suicide is 22% higher in veterans compared to civilians. Although women have lower rates of suicide compared with men in the general population, rates of suicide are increasing more among female veterans than males. In male veterans, suicide rates are highest in the younger and older years, whereas in female veterans, suicide rates are highest in the younger years.

Suicide in Elders

In 2015, the aged comprised 14.9% of the U.S. population, but accounted for 17.9% of suicide deaths. Suicide rates are highest among elderly white men, rising in this population to more than 45 suicides per 100,000 per year. This number is four times the nation's overall age-adjusted rate. Although elderly women (65 and older) account for 20% of suicide deaths among those 65 and older, this number is expected to rise as the population of older women increases.

Older age has been associated with more determined and planned self-destructive acts and with fewer warnings of suicidal intent. The most common mechanisms for suicide are firearms, hanging, self-poisoning, and falls from height. Among those who attempt suicide, elders are the most likely to die. In adolescence, the ratio of attempted to completed suicides is estimated to be 200:1, whereas the estimated risk for the general population is from 8:1 to 33:1. In contrast, there are approximately four attempts for each completed suicide in later life.

Several factors contribute to suicide in later life. Psychiatric illness is present in 71% to 97% of suicides, with depression the most closely associated with suicide. Poor physical health and functional impairment also contribute to elder suicide. Specific illnesses or conditions associated with suicide include congestive heart failure, chronic obstructive lung disease, seizure disorders, urinary incontinence, moderate to severe pain, visual impairment, neurological disorders, malignancy, and poor sleep quality. Serious physical illness in any organ category is an independent risk factor for geriatric suicide, and treatment for multiple illnesses is strongly related to higher risk of suicide. Serious physical illness and high overall burden of illness seem to be a stronger risk factor for suicide in men than in women. In addition to physical illness, the perception of poor health can contribute to suicidal behavior. Socially, disruption of ties, resulting in loneliness and loss of a confidant, are also significantly and independently associated with risk for suicide in later life.

PATHOPHYSIOLOGY

It is well documented that suicidal behavior, like other psychiatric disorders, tends to run in families. A family history of suicide increases the risk of attempted suicide and of completed suicide in most diagnostic groups. Twin studies suggest a genetic component in suicide. Over several studies, monozygotic twin pairs have had a significantly higher concordance for both attempted and completed suicide than dizygotic twins. Danish American adoption studies also have yielded strong evidence that adoptees who commit suicide have a strong family history of suicide in biological relatives, compared with no evidence of suicide in the adopting families. A further study of adoptees with mood disorders demonstrated that adoptee suicide completers with a situational crisis and/or impulsive behavior had more biological relatives who had committed suicide than controls. It was suggested that the genetic factors lowering the threshold for suicidal behavior may be decreased ability to control impulsive behavior. As such, environmental stress, in the presence of a psychiatric disorder, can be a potentiating mechanism that triggers impulsive behavior in the direction of suicide.

CLINICAL PRESENTATION

Clinicians must assess a patient's risk for suicide on the basis of the clinical examination. Suicidal behavior is multidimensional, with complex factors contributing to the overall risk of a future suicide attempt. Factors typically elicited include psychiatric symptoms such as depression, mania, psychosis, substance use, trauma, anxiety, personality pathology, sleep quality, and pain. When suicidal ideation is assessed, further detail should be obtained by asking about plan, intent, and availability of means, such as firearms or medications. Other factors contributing to suicidality include recent or severe psychological and social stressors. Asking about suicidal ideation does not trigger suicide or increase the risk of suicide but could save a life.

DIAGNOSTIC REASONING

Acute risk factors may include severe anxiety, rumination, insomnia, depression with psychotic features, and alcohol or other substance use. A prior suicide attempt is the most important risk factor for suicide. As such, suicide screening tools often focus on previous attempts or intent to commit suicide, with various supportive items such as demographic information, level of social support, and coexisting mental health disorders. Because the goal of a suicide scale is to prevent completion, the sensitivity of the scale must be high so as not to miss a potential suicide. This may result in an over-reliance on a history of suicide attempts when evaluating for risk of suicide. The Modified SAD PERSONAS Scale has an administration time of 1 to 2 minutes, and the authors suggest using this as a rapid screening tool for nonpsychiatrists to obtain the objective information necessary to make an initial assessment of suicidality. For adolescents and young adults aged 10 to 24, the Ask Suicide-Screening Questions (ASQ) Toolkit is a free resource for medical settings that can help clinicians identify youth at risk for suicide. The ASQ is a set of four screening questions that takes 20 seconds to administer.

Risk Factors: Acute Suicide Risk

The mnemonic "SAD PERSONS" may be used to evaluate a person's suicide risk. Consider risk factors within the context of the clinical presentation.

- S = Sex
- A = Age
- D = Depression
- P = Previous attempt
- E = Ethanol abuse
- R = Rational thinking loss
- S = Social support loss
- O = Organized plan
- N = No spouse
- S = Sickness

The score is calculated by giving one point for each "yes" answer:

- 0–4: Low risk of suicide
- 5–6: Medium risk of suicide
- 7–10: High risk of suicide

The following table presents a detailed description of acute suicide risk factors.

Sex	Male patients complete suicide (about one-half kill themselves using a gun) at a 3:1 ratio compared with females. Female patients are more likely to attempt suicide (usually by overdose) and act impulsively without warning than males.
Age	The risk of suicide increases with age, with persons aged 65 and older being more likely than younger persons to take their own lives (women peak at age 55; men at age 75). Older adults tend to use more lethal means and are less likely to voice their suicidal intent to others. Bereavement, social isolation, and deteriorating health status are thought to contribute to the high suicide rate in this group. Recent trends indicate that the suicide rate among young persons aged 25–34 years is increasing. Adolescents are a high-risk group, with suicide the second leading cause of death in this group. Gay adolescents who have been the victims of hate crimes or bullying, who fear social rejection, or who are socially isolated can be at increased risk for developing suicidal thoughts.
Race and Ethnicity	Caucasians are at the greatest risk for suicide; however, suicide is still one of the leading causes of premature death in minority groups (Drapeau & McIntosh, 2016).
Employment Status	Unemployed persons are at higher risk, although social class has not been shown to correlate strongly with increased risk for suicide.
Marital Status	Single, divorced, and widowed persons are at a significantly higher risk.
Immigration Status	Persons who migrate within the United States are at higher risk for suicide, as are those who immigrate to the United States. Social isolation appears to be a significant risk factor for immigrants.
Substance Abuse Problems	Persons with alcohol and drug problems are at extremely high risk for suicide, particularly when their substance abuse is complicated by other risk factors. More than one-third of persons who take their own lives are intoxicated at the time of their deaths. Alcoholism and substance abuse problems of a chronic nature account for 25% of all completed suicides.
Comorbidities	Major depression and bipolar disorders account for approximately 50% of all suicides. Schizophrenia and other psychotic disorders account for approximately 10% of completed suicides. Seventy percent of patients with borderline personality disorder will have at least one suicide attempt, with approximately 10% completing suicide.
Medical Conditions	Chronic, life-threatening, or painful physical illness is associated with increased risk for suicide. Specific high-risk illnesses include AIDS, Huntington's disease, cancer, peptic ulcer disease, spinal cord injury, head injury, renal disease requiring dialysis, chronic intractable pain, uncontrolled diabetes with amputation, and multiple sclerosis.
Medications	Certain medications increase suicidal risk: Steroids, antihypertensives (reserpine, methyldopa, clonidine), corticosteroids, opioids, antituberculosis drugs (isoniazid, ethionamide, cycloserine), anabolic steroid withdrawal, barbiturates, benzodiazepines, antidepressants, cocaine and amphetamine withdrawal. Of note, antidepressants carry a black-box warning for increased risk of suicidal thoughts or behavior (suicidality) in children, adolescents, and young adults up to and including age 24.
Other	Additional suicide risk factors include recent bereavement, legal and financial problems, recent arrest or impending court dates, and being a victim of abuse or sexual assault.

Adapted from Patterson, WM; Dohn, HH; Patterson, J; Patterson, GA (April 1983). "Evaluation of suicidal patients: the SAD PERSONS scale". *Psychosomatics*. 24 (4): 343–5, 348–9.

Hopelessness about the future, helplessness, and lack of future-orientation are "red flags" for possible suicidal intent, as well as suicidal thoughts, especially if accompanied by a plan and intent. Giving away personal possessions, quitting a job, and an appearance of peace may all signal that the person has made the decision to commit suicide.

Patients who are suicidal may state their intentions, but many will find it hard to volunteer this information. The impulsive patient will often appear to be so and will give information that shows a great deal of recent poor judgment. The determined patient may refuse to answer questions or may give information freely, thinking that his or her plan cannot be deterred. Confused patients are more likely to seem unable to protect themselves from harm. Confused patients include persons with auditory hallucinations instructing them to commit suicide and patients who are under the influence of drugs and alcohol. Suicidal patients may also express anger, rage, and have hidden thoughts or fantasies of homicide, as though taking their own life might be equivalent to taking the object of their anger's life.

MANAGEMENT

Suicide prevention is carried out at two levels—interpersonal and community. Interpersonal prevention includes risk assessment, intervention (e.g., medications, counseling, hospitalization), and referral to a specialist. Community prevention is based on the crisis model of 24-hour community hotline services and walk-in crisis counseling services. Crisis counseling services should include a crisis response team that is dispatched immediately to schools or locations where assistance may be needed. These response teams can intervene to reduce the risk of suicide pacts among peers or "copycat" suicides. One systematic review found that physician education and programs to reduce access to lethal means (especially firearms) were effective in reducing the risk of suicide.

In 2001, the Surgeon General organized the National Strategy of Suicide Prevention, under the auspices of the National Institutes of Health. Because suicide is such a serious public health problem, the *National Strategy* proposes public health methods to address it. The public health approach to suicide prevention represents a rational and organized way to marshal prevention efforts and ensure they are effective. Only within the past few decades has a public health approach to suicide prevention emerged with a better understanding of the biological and psychosocial factors, contributing to suicidal behaviors. Its five basic steps are as follows:

1. Clearly define the problem.
2. Identify risk and protective factors.
3. Develop and test interventions.
4. Implement interventions.
5. Evaluate effectiveness.

Careful assessment of suicide risk factors, consultation with other practitioners and specialists, and planning are the hallmarks of effective suicide risk management.

The assessment should cover the patient's personal history and pay special attention to recent stressful life events and changes in mental status. Reports of losses, humiliations, demoralizing experiences, substance use and abuse, and relationship problems should be explored. Persons who have been abusing drugs and/or alcohol can suddenly become highly motivated to end their lives due to various factors, including loss of control over their use, legal problems, financial issues, homelessness, and/or loss of social supports. Even a person who is recovering from substance abuse and has stopped using the substance can be at high risk for suicide when faced with the painful consequences of substance abuse, including withdrawal or severe drug cravings.

All suicidal statements should be considered *seriously.* One of the most valuable assessment tools for practitioners is the willingness to question a patient directly about his or her suicide risk. Two good general questions are:

- "How long can you go on the way you are?"
- "Are you feeling so bad that sometimes you wish you could go to bed and not wake up?"

Examples of more specific questions are:

- "Have you thought about hurting yourself or ending your life?"
- "Do you have a plan for suicide?"
- "Have you assembled what you need?"
- "Do you have a location picked out?"
- "What has stopped you so far?"

Suicide plans are assessed on their *specificity, availability,* and *lethality* (SAL): The more specific and detailed the plan and the more available and lethal the method, the higher the risk of suicide.

Once it is determined that the patient is suicidal, the level of risk will determine the direction of the intervention. A major decision to be made is whether the patient needs to be hospitalized. The absence of a strong social support system, history of impulsive behavior, an intention to die, a suicidal plan of action, hopelessness, helplessness, lack of future orientation, or the availability of means, such as weapons, are indications for hospitalization. If hospitalization is deemed necessary but the patient has no way of getting there, or if they refuse to go, it will be necessary to call 911 (or other local emergency services), to escort the patient, involuntarily, to the hospital. The primary goal of the intervention is to maintain the patient's safety. Therefore, the following considerations are important:

- Reduce or eliminate imminent danger.
- Never leave a patient alone who is actively suicidal.
- Involve family members or significant others who care so that they can stay with the patient until the crisis has passed.

The best predictor of suicide risk is a history of a previous suicide attempt. All persons with suicide gestures, attempts, and threats should be thoroughly screened for suicide risk factors and referred to a specialist for a full mental status exam, as well as psychiatric consultation and treatment. It is important to diagnose and treat any underlying psychiatric and/or substance abuse disorders. The clinician and the patient's family or significant others should ensure the patient's safety by the least restrictive method, starting with removing potentially lethal objects, such as firearms, and providing very close supervision. Some patients at acute high risk will require inpatient hospitalization for constant one-to-one supervision (including use of restraints, if indicated) and ongoing treatment. ECT may provide rapid, safe, and effective treatment for severely depressed, acutely suicidal patients.

Sometimes a no-suicide contract can be initiated. In the case of an angry or manipulative patient, this is usually not advisable. If a patient who is considered seriously suicidal cannot make the commitment to abide by a no-suicide contract, immediate hospitalization is necessary. A no-suicide contract is not a guarantee that a suicide will not happen, nor is it a substitute for clinical judgment. A mental health professional should be the person to implement a no-suicide contract. When it is appropriate to use them, no-suicide written contracts should include the following components:

- An agreement from the patient not to harm himself or herself
- An agreement that the patient will contact a mental health professional if the patient's suicidal impulses become unmanageable
- An agreement from the mental health-care provider to be available to the patient for a specified period of time, usually until the patient returns for a follow-up visit or another part of the intervention has taken place (e.g., when the patient has met with a psychotherapist for evaluation or therapy)
- Contact numbers for the mental health-care provider and emergency services

Both the patient and mental health-care provider sign the contract. A copy is given to the patient, and the original is kept in the agency records. However, it is important to bear in mind that research does not support the use of no-harm contracts as a method for preventing suicide, nor for protecting clinicians from malpractice litigation in the event of a patient suicide.

After this, it is essential to implement an ongoing program of help. This should involve the following:

- Treatment of the presenting symptoms
- Referral for individual or group therapy
- Referral for support groups
- Referral to a community program

If the patient is not hospitalized and until the treatment program is in effect, the clinician must continue to monitor the patient to ascertain their safety.

Appropriate documentation is critical. Follow the agency guidelines for documenting situations involving suicide risk. Records should include statements made by the patient; the decision-making process followed; potential ramifications of no treatment; what has been shared with the patient and the family; and the consultation process. To avoid malpractice litigation, practitioners need to perform and document a complete assessment addressing both the risk and the precautions taken and follow evidence-based guidelines. A standard of care exists for assessment of suicide risk but not for the prediction of suicide. Complete and accurate documentation is key (Box 67.4).

FOLLOW-UP AND REFERRAL

Safety plans for patients who are not acutely suicidal include a follow-up appointment within 24 hours of assessment and a follow-up telephone call for missed appointments. Patients and involved family and friends should be given the local 24-hour crisis telephone number and information regarding access to emergency services. Practitioners must take responsibility to ask patients about weapons and pill stashes, and then take steps to have these items located and

---

> **Box 67.4 Suicide Assessment and Management**
>
> **Suicide Assessment**
>
> 1. Psychiatric evaluation that includes the following:
>   - Specific psychiatric signs and symptoms
>   - Psychiatric history, including current treatment
>   - Past suicidal or other self-injurious behaviors (including intent of such acts)
>   - Family history of suicide, mental illness, and dysfunction
>   - Current psychosocial situation and nature of crisis
> 2. Inquire about suicidal thoughts, plans, behaviors (elicit presence of suicidal ideation, suicide plan, intent, and lethality of plan including access to weapons, pills)
> 3. Suicide risk estimation to include demographic factors, major psychiatric syndromes (primary and comorbid conditions), specific psychiatric symptoms, other aspects of psychiatric history and physical illness
>
> **Management**
>
> 1. Attend to patient's safety.
> 2. Establish and maintain a therapeutic alliance.
> 3. Determine a treatment setting (e.g., involuntary hospitalization, partial hospitalization, intensive outpatient programs, ambulatory settings).
> 4. Develop a plan of care.
> 5. Coordinate care and collaborate with other providers.
> 6. Promote adherence to treatment plan.
> 7. Provide education to the patient and the family.
> 8. Reassess safety and suicide risk (include suicide crisis and chronic suicidality).
> 9. Monitor psychiatric status and response to treatment.
> 10. Obtain consultation if needed.
>
> **Documentation and Risk Management**
>
> 1. Documentation issues specific to suicide
> 2. Be aware of own emotions and reactions, particularly when responding to those with severe or recurring suicidality or self-injurious behaviors—for difficult-to-treat patients, consultation and supervision from a colleague, as well as documentation of same, is recommended.
> 3. Suicide prevention contracts: limitations and clinical usefulness—not recommended in patients who are psychotic, agitated, impulsive, or using intoxicating substances.
> 4. Management of a suicide in one's practice.
> 5. Mental health intervention for surviving family and friends after suicide.

Source: Abstracted from American Psychiatric Association. Practice guideline for the assessment and treatment of patients with suicidal behaviors. https://psychiatryonline.org/pb/assets/raw/sitewide/practice_guidelines/guidelines/suicide.pdf. Published 2013.

removed for safekeeping. If medications are prescribed, the amount should not exceed a 1-week supply, with no refills. Patients who are at risk should be seen at least weekly, and social support systems must be mobilized. Be aware that caring for a patient contemplating suicide can be very challenging (see Box 67.5).

Box 67.5 Support for Health-Care Providers Caring for Patients at Risk for Suicide

- Be aware of your personal and professional limits and honor them.
- Know the legal standards about suicide, duty to report, confidentiality, and liability.
- Consult with others so that you are not the only decision-maker assessing the risk of the suicidal patient.

Patient Education: Suicide

Patient and family education includes providing suicide crisis hotline numbers to the patient and/or family members. Patients should be instructed to avoid alcohol. Encourage the patient to seek out adequate treatment for uncomfortable symptoms of physical illness, possibly including a prescription for analgesics to reduce pain. The patient should be informed that options often appear narrowed when a person is feeling depressed and suicidal. Alternative ways of thinking should be explored with the patient. Focus on building hope, especially for the future. Teach the patient to use specific, more constructive outlets for anger rather than self-destructive ones. Encourage patients to reach out for support and to reach out immediately when feeling the urge to harm themselves. Mobilize a social support system for the patient and educate significant others regarding suicidal risk and danger signs. Educate the patient and family that as the patient's mood "lifts" in response to antidepressant treatment, there can be an increased risk of suicide related to increased energy. At these times, patients must be monitored closely.

In the event that the patient does commit suicide, the clinician should prepare the family for a complex grief reaction that may follow. Suicide is particularly tragic because of the fallout that the death bequeaths to survivors. Edward Shneidman coined the term *postvention*, which refers to an intervention strategy that attempts to minimize the impact of patient suicide and to ensure that survivors of suicide have adequate services and support available to them. Postsuicide interventions by the clinician include the following:

- Educating family members about suicide
- Allowing family members to share their grief, including any burdens or other factors that family members may feel (e.g., guilt, shame, anger, inability to do anything, situation out of their control)
- Encouraging family members to attend support groups, such as Survivors of Suicide (SOS), which are available in most communities

The typical SOS group is sponsored by a mental health or social services agency and is facilitated by mental health professionals, survivor peers, or a combination of both.

Referrals to such groups following a completed suicide are essential. Clinicians may also require support after a patient suicide.

REFERENCES

Bipolar Disorder

Amann B, Gomar JJ, Ortiz-Gil J, et al. Executive dysfunction and memory impairment in schizoaffective disorder: A comparison with bipolar disorder, schizophrenia and healthy controls. *Psychol Med.* 2012;42:2127.

American Psychiatric Association. *Practice guidelines for the treatment of patients with bipolar disorder.* 2nd ed. https://psychiatryonline.org/pb/assets/raw/sitewide/practice_guidelines/guidelines/bipolar.pdf. Published 2002.

Baldessarini RJ, Tondo L, Visioli C. First-episode types in bipolar disorder: Predictive associations with later illness. *Acta Psychiatr Scand.* 2014;129:383.

Bellani M, Hatch JP, Nicoletti MA, et al. Does anxiety increase impulsivity in patients with bipolar disorder or major depressive disorder? *J Psychiatr Res.* 2012;46:616.

Bowden CL, et al. Bipolar disorder: Keys to diagnosis—strategies for effective management. *Consultant.* 2005;45:S2–S33.

Burton CZ, Ryan KA, Kamali M, et al. Psychosis in bipolar disorder: Does it represent a more "severe" illness? *Bipolar Disord.* 2018;20:18.

Calver L, Drinkwater V, Gupta R, et al. Droperidol v. haloperidol for sedation of aggressive behaviour in acute mental health: randomised controlled trial. *Br J Psychiatry.* 2015;206:223.

Castellani A, Girlanda F, Barbui C. *J Affect Disord.* 2015;174:45–50.

Chou YH, Lin CL, Wang SJ, et al. Aggression in bipolar II disorder and its relation to the serotonin transporter. *J Affect Disord.* 2013;147:59.

Craddock N, Sklar P. Genetics of bipolar disorder. *Lancet.* 2013;381:1654–1662.

Cusi AM, Macqueen GM, McKinnon MC. Patients with bipolar disorder show impaired performance on complex tests of social cognition. *Psychiatry Res.* 2012;200:258.

Dennehy EB, Marangell LB, Allen MH, et al. Suicide and suicide attempts in the Systematic Treatment Enhancement Program for Bipolar Disorder (STEP-BD). *J Affect Disord.* 2011;133:423.

Depp CA, Mausbach BT, Harmell AL, et al. Meta-analysis of the association between cognitive abilities and everyday functioning in bipolar disorder. *Bipolar Disord.* 2012;14:217.

Desmarais SL, Van Dorn RA, Johnson KL, et al. Community violence perpetration and victimization among adults with mental illnesses. *Am J Public Health.* 2014;104:2342.

Friborg O, Martinsen EW, Martinussen M, et al. Comorbidity of personality disorders in mood disorders: a meta-analytic review of 122 studies from 1988 to 2010. *J Affect Disord.* 2014;152–154:1–11.

Goodwin GM, Haddad PM, Ferrier IN, et al. Evidence-based guidelines for treating bipolar disorder: Revised third edition recommendations from the British Association for Psychopharmacology. *J Psychopharmacol.* 2016;30(6):495–553.

Gonzalez-Pinto A, Gonzalez C, Enjuto S, et al. Psychoeducation and cognitive-behavioral therapy in bipolar disorder: An update. *Acta Psychiatr Scand.* 2004;109(2):83–90.

Harford TC, Yi HY, Grant BF. Other- and self-directed forms of violence and their relationships to DSM-IV substance use and other psychiatric disorders in a national survey of adults. *Compr Psychiatry.* 2013;54:731.

Hirschfeld RM. Development and validation of a screening instrument for bipolar spectrum disorder: The Mood Disorder Questionnaire. *Am J Psychiatry.* 2000;157:1873.

Hirschfeld RM, et al. Screening for bipolar disorder in the community. *J Clin Psychiatry.* 2003;64:53–59.

Hirschfeld RM, et al. Screening for bipolar disorder in patients treated for depression in a family medicine clinic. *J Am Board Fam Pract.* 2005;18(4):233–239.

Jamison KR. *An unquiet mind.* New York, NY: Vintage Books; 1995.

Jentink J, Loane MA, Dolk H, et al. Valproic acid monotherapy in pregnancy and major congenital malformations. *N Engl J Med.* 2010;362:2185–2193.

Kahn D, et al. Treatment of bipolar disorders: A guide for patients and families. *Postgrad Med Rep.* 2004;209–116.

Kaye NS. Is your depressed patient bipolar? *J Am Board Fam Pract.* 2005;18(4):271–281.

Kendall T, Morriss R, Mayo-Wilson E, et al. Assessment and management of bipolar disorder: Summary of updated NICE guidance. *BMJ.* 2014; 349:g5673.

Lewandowski KE, Cohen BM, Ongur D. Evolution of neuropsychological dysfunction during the course of schizophrenia and bipolar disorder. *Psychol Med.* 2011;41:225.

Management of Bipolar Disorder Working Group. VA/DoD clinical practice guideline for management of bipolar disorder in adults. Washington, DC: Department of Veterans Affairs, Department of Defense; 2010. https://www.healthquality.va.gov/bipolar/bd_306_sum.pdf.

McCraw S, Parker G, Fletcher K, Friend P. Self-reported creativity in bipolar disorder: Prevalence, types and associated outcomes in mania versus hypomania. *J Affect Disord.* 2013;151:831.

McDermid J, Sareen J, El-Gabalawy R, et al. Co-morbidity of bipolar disorder and borderline personality disorder: Findings from the National Epidemiologic Survey on Alcohol and Related Conditions. *Compr Psychiatry.* 2015;58:18.

McIntyre RS, Soczynska JK, Cha DS, et al. The prevalence and illness characteristics of *DSM-5*-defined "mixed feature specifier" in adults with major depressive disorder and bipolar disorder: Results from the International Mood Disorders Collaborative Project. *J Affect Disord.* 2015;172:259.

Merikangas KR, Jin R, He JP, et al. Prevalence and correlates of bipolar spectrum disorder in the world mental health survey initiative. *Arch Gen Psychiatry.* 2011;68:241.

Miklowitz DJ, et al. A randomized study of family-focused psychoeducation and pharmacotherapy in the outpatient management of bipolar disorder. *Arch Gen Psychiatry.* 2003;60:904–912.

National Institute for Health and Care Excellence (NICE). Bipolar disorder: Assessment and management. http://www.nice.org.uk/guidance/CG185. Published September 2014. Accessed November 18, 2014.

National Institute for Health and Care Excellence (NICE). Antenatal and postnatal mental health: clinical management and service guidance (NICE clinical guideline 192). http://www.nice.org.uk/guidance/cg192. Published December 2014. Accessed May 16, 2016.

Ostergaard SD, Bertelsen A, Nielsen J, et al. The association between psychotic mania, psychotic depression and mixed affective episodes among 14,529 patients with bipolar disorder. *J Affect Disord.* 2013;147:44.

Reiger DA, et al. Comorbidity of mental disorders with alcohol and other drug abuse. Results from the Epidemiologic Catchment Area (ECA) Study. *JAMA.* 1990;264:2511–2518.

Sachs G. Approach to the patient with elevated, expansive, or irritable mood. In: Stern TA, Herman JB, Slavin PL, eds. *The MGH guide to psychiatry in primary care.* New York, NY: McGraw-Hill; 1998: 347.

Samamé C, Martino DJ, Strejilevich SA. Longitudinal course of cognitive deficits in bipolar disorder: a meta-analytic study. *J Affect Disord.* 2014;164:130.

Santos JL, Aparicio A, Bagney A, et al. A five-year follow-up study of neurocognitive functioning in bipolar disorder. *Bipolar Disord.* 2014;16:722.

Samamé C. Social cognition throughout the three phases of bipolar disorder: A state-of-the-art overview. *Psychiatry Res.* 2013;210:1275.

Subramaniam M, Abdin E, Vaingankar JA, Chong SA. Prevalence, correlates, comorbidity and severity of bipolar disorder: Results from the Singapore Mental Health Study. *J Affect Disord.* 2013;146:189.

Sylvia LG, Dupuy JM, Ostacher MJ, et al. Sleep disturbance in euthymic bipolar patients. *J Psychopharmacol.* 2012;26:1108.

Ten Have M, de Graaf R, van Weeghel J, van Dorsselaer S. The association between common mental disorders and violence: To what extent is it influenced by prior victimization, negative life events and low levels of social support? *Psychol Med.* 2014;44:1485.

Weissman MM, Bland RC, Canino GJ, et al. Cross-national epidemiology of major depression and bipolar disorder. *JAMA.* 1996;276:293.

Work Group on Psychiatric Evaluation, American Psychiatric Association Steering Committee on Practice Guidelines. Psychiatric evaluation of adults. Second edition. American Psychiatric Association. *Am J Psychiatry.* 2006;163:3.

Yatham LN, Kennedy SH, Parikh SV, et al. Canadian Network for Mood and Anxiety Treatments (CANMAT) and International Society for Bipolar Disorders (ISBD) collaborative update of CANMAT guidelines for the management of patients with bipolar disorder: update 2013. *Bipolar Disord.* 2013;15:1.

Yatham LN, Kennedy SH, Parikh SV, et al. Canadian Network for Mood and Anxiety Treatments (CANMAT) and International Society for Bipolar Disorders (ISBD) 2018 guidelines for the management of patients with bipolar disorder. *Bipolar Disord.* 2018;20(2):97–170.

Major Depressive Disorder

Ajinkya S, Jadhav PR, Srivastava NN. Depression during pregnancy: Prevalence and obstetric risk factors among pregnant women attending a tertiary care hospital in Navi Mumbai. *Ind Psychiatry J.* 2013;22(1):37–40.

Andrade L, Caraveo-Anduaga JJ, Berglund P, et al. The epidemiology of major depressive episodes: results from the International Consortium of Psychiatric Epidemiology (ICPE) Surveys. *Int J Methods Psychiatr Res.* 2003;12:3.

Austin M-P, Highet N; Guidelines Expert Advisory Committee. *Australian clinical practice guidelines for depression and related disorders—anxiety, bipolar disorder and puerperal psychosis—in the perinatal period. A guideline for primary health care professionals.* Melbourne, Australia: Beyond blue: The National Depression Initiative; 2011.

Baker R, Orton E, Kendrick D, Tata LJ. Maternal depression in the 5 years after childbirth among women with and without perinatal depression: a population-based cohort study. *Lancet.* 2015;386:S22.

Beck AT, et al. *Cognitive therapy of depression.* New York, NY: Guilford Press; 1979.

Blazer DG. The epidemiology of depressive disorders in late life. In: Roose SP, Sackeim HA, eds. *Late-life depression.* New York, NY: Oxford University Press; 2004:3.

Buchanan JL. Prevention of depression in the college student population: A review of the literature. *Arch Psychiatr Nurs.* 2012;26(1):21–42.

Byers AL, Yaffe K, Covinsky KE, et al. High occurrence of mood and anxiety disorders among older adults: The National Comorbidity Survey Replication. *Arch Gen Psychiatry.* 2010;67:489.

Center for Drug Evaluation and Research. *Drug safety and availability—FDA drug safety communication: Revised recommendations for Celexa (citalopram hydrobromide) related to a potential risk of abnormal heart rhythms with high doses.* https://www.fda.gov/Drugs/DrugSafety/ucm297391.htm. Published 2012.

Chaudron LH. Complex challenges in treating depression during pregnancy. *Am J Psychiatry.* 2013;170:12.

Cipriani A, et al. Comparative efficacy and acceptability of 12 new-generation antidepressants: A multiple-treatments meta-analysis. *Lancet.* 2009;373(9665):746–758.

Committee on Obstetric Practice. The American College of Obstetricians and Gynecologists Committee opinion no. 630. Screening for perinatal depression. *Obstet Gynecol.* 2015;125:1268.

Di Florio A, Forty L, Gordon-Smith K, et al. Perinatal episodes across the mood disorder spectrum. *JAMA Psychiatry.* 2013;70:168

Frasure-Smith N, et al. Elevated depression symptoms predict long-term cardiovascular mortality in patients with atrial fibrillation and heart failure. *Circulation.* 2009;120(2):134–140.

Gartlehner G, Gaynes BN, Amick HR, et al. *Nonpharmacological versus pharmacological treatments for adult patients with major depressive disorder.* Rockville, MD: Agency for Healthcare Research and Quality; December 2015. (Comparative effectiveness reviews no. 161). https://www.ncbi.nlm.nih.gov/books/NBK338245.

Gollan JK, Wisniewski SR, Luther JF, et al. Generating an efficient version of the Edinburgh Postnatal Depression Scale in an urban obstetrical population. *J Affect Disord.* 2017;208:615–620.

Greenberg PE, Fournier AA, Sisitsky T, et al. The economic burden of adults with major depressive disorder in the United States (2005 and 2010). *J Clin Psychiatry.* 2015;76:155.

Guille C, Newman R, Fryml LD, Lifton CK, Epperson CN. Management of postpartum depression. *J Midwifery Women Health.* 2013;58(6):632-642.

Gureje O, Kola L, Afolabi E. Epidemiology of major depressive disorder in elderly Nigerians in the Ibadan Study of Ageing: A community-based survey. *Lancet.* 2007;370:957.

Hazell P, et al. Tricyclic drugs for depression in children and adolescents. *Cochrane Database Syst Rev.* 2013; 6:CD002317.

Howard LM, Molyneaux E, Dennis CL, et al. Non-psychotic mental disorders in the perinatal period. *Lancet.* 2014;384:1775.

Katz IR. On the inseparability of mental and physical health in aged persons. Lessons from depression and medical comorbidity. *Am J Geriatr Psychiatry.* 1996;4:1.

Kendler KS, Gardner CO. Sex differences in the pathways to major depression: A study of opposite-sex twin pairs. *Am J Psychiatry.* 2014;171:426.

Kessler RC, Birnbaum H, Bromet E, et al. Age differences in major depression: Results from the National Comorbidity Survey Replication (NCS-R). *Psychol Med.* 2010;40:225.

Kessler RC, Ormel J, Petukhova M, et al. Development of lifetime comorbidity in the World Health Organization world mental health surveys. *Arch Gen Psychiatry.* 2011;68:90.

Kroenke K, et al. The PHQ-9: Validity of a brief depression severity measure. *J Gen Intern Med.* 2001;16:606–613.

Lin EH, et al. Depression and increased mortality in diabetes: Unexpected causes of death. *Ann Fam Med.* 2009;7(5):414–421.

Michigan Quality Improvement Consortium. *Primary care diagnosis and management of adults with depression.* https://www.phoenixhealthplan.com/Media/Default/Documents/Providers/Practice%20Guidelines/Depression.pdf. Updated January 2016.

Miklowitz DJ, et al. A randomized study of family-focused psychoeducation and pharmacotherapy in the outpatient management of bipolar disorder. *Arch Gen Psychiatry.* 2003;60:904–912.

Molyneaux E, Poston L, Ashurst-Williams S, Howard LM. Obesity and mental disorders during pregnancy and postpartum: A systematic review and meta-analysis. *Obstet Gynecol.* 2014; 123:857.

O'Connor E, Rossom RC, Henninger M, Groom HC, Burda BU. Primary care screening for and treatment of depression in pregnant and postpartum women: Evidence report and systematic review for the U.S. Preventive Services Task Force. *JAMA.* 2016;315(4):388–406.

Pedersen CB, Mors O, Bertelsen A, et al. A comprehensive nationwide study of the incidence rate and lifetime risk for treated mental disorders. *JAMA Psychiatry.* 2014;71:573.

Pop VM, Truijens SM, Spek V, Wijnen HA, van Son MM, Bergink V. A new concept of maternity blues: Is there a subgroup of women with rapid cycling mood symptoms? *J Affect Disord.* 2015;177:74–79.

Räisänen S, Lehto SM, Nielsen HS, et al. Risk factors for and perinatal outcomes of major depression during pregnancy: A population-based analysis during 2002–2010 in Finland. *BMJ Open.* 2014;4:e004883.

Richard LK, Daniel EF. Introduction: Chronic medical conditions and depression. The view from primary care. *Am J Med.* 2008;121(11):S1–S7.

Robert MC, Kenneth EF. Depression in patients with coronary heart disease. *Am J Med.* 2008;121(11):S20–S27.

Wayne JK. The comorbidity of diabetes mellitus and depression. *Am J Med.* 2008;21(11):S8–S15.

Yonkers K, Vigod S, Ross L, Yonkers KA, Vigod S, Ross LE. Diagnosis, pathophysiology, and management of mood disorders in pregnant and postpartum women. *Obstet Gynecol.* 2011;117(4):961–977.

Suicide Risk

Ballard ED, et al. Future disposition and suicidal ideation: Mediation by depressive symptom clusters. *J Affect Disord.* 2015;170:1–6.

Beck AT, et al. Hopelessness, depression, suicidal ideation and clinical diagnosis of depression. *Suicide Life Threat Behav.* 1993;23:139.

Campbell WH. Pearls: Revised "SAD PERSONS" helps assess suicide risk. *Curr Psychiatry.* 2004;13:3.

Conwell Y, et al. Age differences in behaviors leading to completed suicide. *Am J Geriatr Psychiatry.* 1998;6(2):122–126.

Conwell Y, et al. Risk factors for suicide in later life. *Biol Psychiatry.* 2002;52(3):193–204.

Conwell Y, et al. Suicide in Older Adults. *Psychiatr Clin North Am.* 2011;34(2):451–468.

Drapeau CW, McIntosh JL (for the American Association of Suicidology). *U.S.A. suicide 2015: Official final data.* Washington, DC: American Association of Suicidology; December 23, 2016. http://www.suicidology.org.

Eaton DK, et al. Youth risk behavior surveillance—United States, 2007. *MMWR Surveill Summ.* 2008;57:SS-4.

Gaynes BN, et al. Screening for suicide risk (Systemic evidence review no. 32). Rockville, MD: Agency for Healthcare Quality and Research; 2004. http://www.ahrq.gov/downloads/pub/prevent/pdfser/suicidser.pdf.

Holkup P. *Evidence-based protocol: Elderly suicide – Secondary prevention.* University of Iowa Gerontological Nursing Interventions Research Center; 2002. https://www.healio.com/nursing/journals/jgn/2003-6-29-6/%7Bdeca3678-aca1-4059-9ce0-8c179682dd48%7D/evidence-based-protocol-elderly-suicide—-secondary-prevention.

Juurlink DN, et al. Medical illness and the risk of suicide in the elderly. *Arch Intern Med.* 2004;164(11):1179–1184.

Lewis LM. No-harm contracts: A review of what we know. *Suicide Life Threat Behav.* 2007;37(1):50–57.

Mackenzie T, Popkin M. Medical illness and suicide. In: Blumenthal S, Kupfer D, eds. *Suicide over the life cycle: Risk factors, assessment, and treatment of suicidal patients.* Washington, DC: American Psychiatric Press; 1990:205.

McDowell AK, et al. Practical suicide-risk management for the busy primary care physician. *Mayo Clin Proc.* 2011;86(8):792–800.

Muzina DJ. Suicide intervention—how to recognize risk, focus on patient safety. *Curr Psychiatry.* 2007;6(9):30–46.

National Guideline Clearinghouse (NGC). Guideline summary: Final recommendation statement. Depression in adults: Screening. Rockville, MD: Agency for Healthcare Research and Quality; January 26, 2016. https://www.uspreventiveservicestaskforce.org/Page/Document/RecommendationStatementFinal/depression-in-adults-screening1. Accessed February 19, 2018.

Trangle M, Gursky J, Haight R. Adult depression in primary care. Institute for Clinical Systems Improvement. https://roar.nevadaprc.org/system/documents/4068/original/NPRC.3054.Depr-Interactive0512b.pdf?1471560355. Published 2016.

Turvey CL, et al. Risk factors for late-life suicide: A prospective, community-based study. *Am J Geriatr Psychiatry.* 2002;10(4):398–406.

U.S. Department Health and Human Services. National strategy for suicide prevention: Goals and objectives for action, 2012. https://www.surgeongeneral.gov/library/reports/national-strategy-suicide-prevention/index.html. Published 2012.

U.S. Preventive Services Task Force. Screening for suicide risk: Recommendation and rationale. *Am J Nurse Pract.* 2005;9(3):46.

Veterans Affairs Office of Suicide Prevention. Suicide among veterans and other Americans: 2001–2014. http://www.mentalhealth.va.gov/docs/2016suicidedatareport.pdf. Published August 3, 2016. Accessed February 12, 2018.

Waern M, et al. Burden of illness and suicide in elderly people: Case–control study. *Br Med J.* 2002;324:1355.

Web-Based Injury Statistics Query and Reporting System. Atlanta, GA: Centers for Disease Control and Prevention, National Center for Injury Prevention and Control; 2010. https://www.cdc.gov/injury/wisqars/index.html.

RESOURCES

Bipolar Disorder

Bipolar Disorder. Tell Me About Bipolar (Film). National Alliance on Mental Illness
https://www.nami.org/Learn-More/Mental-Health-Conditions/Bipolar-Disorder

Bipolar Disorder Across the Lifespan. Depression and Bipolar Support Alliance
http://www.dbsalliance.org/site/PageServer?pagename=education_bipolar_lifespan

Bipolar Disorder Among Adults Statistics. National Institute of Mental Health
https://www.nimh.nih.gov/health/statistics/prevalence/bipolar-disorder-among-adults.shtml

Bipolar Disorder Among Children. Statistics and Treatment. National Institute of Mental Health
https://www.nimh.nih.gov/health/statistics/prevalence/bipolar-disorder-among-children.shtml

Bipolar Disorder in Children and Teens brochure. National Institute of Mental Health
https://www.nimh.nih.gov/health/publications/bipolar-disorder-in-children-and-teens/qf-15-6380_152267.pdf

Bipolar Disorder Overview. Symptoms and Causes, Diagnosis and Treatment. Mayo Clinic.
https://www.mayoclinic.org/diseases-conditions/bipolar-disorder/symptoms-causes/syc-20355955

Bipolar Disorder Signs and Symptoms: Recognizing and Getting Help for Mania and Bipolar Depression. Help Guide and Harvard Health
https://www.helpguide.org/articles/bipolar-disorder/bipolar-disorder-signs-and-symptoms.htm

Bipolar Disorder: Overview, Signs and Symptoms, Risk Factors, Treatments and Therapies. National Institute of Mental Health
https://www.nimh.nih.gov/health/topics/bipolar-disorder/index.shtml

Do You Go Through Intense Moods? National Institute of Mental Health
https://www.nimh.nih.gov/health/publications/bipolar-disorder/index.shtml

Helping Someone With Bipolar: What Can You So To Support A Friend or Family Member. Harvard Health
https://www.helpguide.org/articles/bipolar-disorder/helping-someone-with-bipolar-disorder.htm

Living With Bipolar: Self Help Tips for Managing Your Symptoms and Staying Balanced. Harvard Health
https://www.helpguide.org/articles/bipolar-disorder/living-with-bipolar-disorder.htm

Systematic Treatment Enhancement Program for Bipolar Disorder (STEP-BD). National Institute of Mental Health
https://www.nimh.nih.gov/funding/clinical-research/practical/step-bd/index.shtml

Major Depressive Disorder

Depression. National Institute of Mental Health
https://www.nimh.nih.gov/health/topics/depression/index.shtml

Depression (Major Depressive Disorder). Mayo Clinic
https://www.mayoclinic.org/diseases-conditions/depression/symptoms-causes/syc-20356007

Depression and College Students: Answers To College Students' Frequently Asked Questions About Depression. National Institute of Mental Health
https://www.nimh.nih.gov/health/publications/depression-and-college-students/depression-college-students-pdf-new_151591.pdf

Depression in Older Adults. American Academy of Family Physicians
https://familydoctor.org/depression-in-older-adults/

Depression (Major Depressive Disorder) in Men. National Institute of Mental Health
https://www.nimh.nih.gov/health/publications/men-and-depression/mendepression-508_142046.pdf

Depression: What You Need to Know. National Institute of Mental Health
https://www.nimh.nih.gov/health/publications/depression-what-you-need-to-know/depression-what-you-need-to-know-pdf_151827_151827.pdf

Living with Depression: How to Keep Working. National Alliance of Mental Health
https://www.nami.org/Blogs/NAMI-Blog/April-2017/Living-with-Depression-How-to-Keep-Working

Major Depression. Cleveland Clinic
https://my.clevelandclinic.org/health/diseases/9290-depression-overview

The Geriatric Depression Scale (GDS). The Hartford Institute for Geriatric Nursing, New York University
https://consultgeri.org/try-this/general-assessment/issue-4.pdf

Types of Antidepressants. Handout. American Academy of Family Physicians
https://familydoctor.org/types-of-antidepressants/

Postpartum Depression

Action Plan for Depression and Anxiety Around Pregnancy. National Institute of Child Health & Human Development
https://www.nichd.nih.gov/ncmhep/initiatives/moms-mental-health-matters/moms/Documents/ActionPlan_DepressionAnxiety.pdf

Depression Among Women and Postpartum Depression. Centers for Disease Control and Prevention
https://www.cdc.gov/reproductivehealth/depression/

Depression During and After Pregnancy. Office of Women's Health
https://www.womenshealth.gov/a-z-topics/depression-during-and-after-pregnancy

Major Depression During Conception and Pregnancy: A Guide for Patients and Families. Women's Mental Health
https://womensmentalhealth.org/wp-content/uploads/2008/04/mdd_guide.pdf

Mom's Mental Health Matters: Depression and Anxiety Around Pregnancy. National Institute of Child Health & Human Development
https://www.nichd.nih.gov/ncmhep/initiatives/moms-mental-health-matters/moms/Pages/default.aspx

Postpartum Depression. American College of Obstetricians and Gynecologists Patient Education FAQ
https://www.acog.org/Patients/FAQs/Postpartum-Depression

Postpartum Depression: A Guide for Patients and Families
https://womensmentalhealth.org/wp-content/uploads/2008/04/postpartum_guide.pdf

Postpartum Support International
Support Helpline
http://www.postpartum.net

The Impacts of Depression During Pregnancy and Early Parenthood. National Alliance on Mental Illness. A Guide for Patients and Families. Women's Mental Health
https://www.nami.org/Blogs/NAMI-Blog/October-2016/The-Impacts-of-Depression-During-Pregnancy-and-Ear

Trying to Conceive, Pregnancy, and Mental Health. Office of Women's Health
https://www.womenshealth.gov/mental-health/pregnancy-conceive/#pregnancy

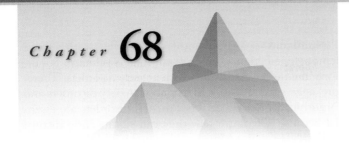

Chapter **68**

Anxiety, Stress, and Trauma-Related Disorders

Eugenia Millender, PhD, RN, MS, PMHNP-BC, CDE
Lynne M. Dunphy, PhD, APRN, FNP-BC, FAAN, FAANP

GENERALIZED ANXIETY DISORDER

Generalized anxiety disorder (GAD) is characterized by excessive worry (over 6 months) about multiple concerns that are difficult to control. Anxiety disorders are the most prevalent psychiatric syndrome in the United States population, and commonly present in primary-care settings. Persons with GAD experience a range of upsetting physical symptoms, along with hyperarousal and insomnia. A diagnosis of GAD requires evidence of disrupted or impaired occupational or social functioning. GAD is more disruptive than normal anxiety, which is characterized by apprehension and mild physical symptoms of upset such as headache. From 50% to 90% of patients with GAD have another comorbid mental disorder, most commonly depression.

EPIDEMIOLOGY AND CAUSES

Epidemiological studies indicate that, in general, the yearly prevalence of anxiety disorders in adults is approximately 17%. Women are diagnosed with anxiety disorders more often than men are (National Institute of Mental Health, 2016). Individuals with a history of trauma—recent, childhood, or adolescent—can be more vulnerable to anxiety disorders, including panic disorder and specific phobias, as well as depression. Exposure to childhood trauma and its effects in health and behavioral outcomes have been well documented in the Adverse Childhood Experience (ACE) Study. Onset of GAD often occurs during childhood or adolescence. Prevalence in the general population is 5% to 6%, but this proportion rises to approximately 25% in primary-care populations, is associated with an overall higher use of health services. GAD is common among patients with "medically unexplained" chronic pain and with chronic physical illness.

People with GAD have about a 60% or higher chance according to some studies of a comorbid psychiatric diagnosis, most often depression; this is associated with a poorer prognosis and greater functional impairment. A mixed anxiety and depressive disorder (MADD) has become common enough that a new disorder—mixed anxiety and depression—has been identified. According to ICD-10 criteria, MADD is characterized by co-occurring, subsyndromal symptoms of anxiety and depression, severe enough to justify a psychiatric diagnosis, but neither of which are clearly predominant. MADD appears to be very common, particularly in primary care, although prevalence estimates vary, often depending on the diagnostic criteria applied. There continues to be debate about the inclusion of this category in the *Diagnostic and Statistical Manual of Mental Disorders* (*DSM-5*) as of this writing.

There is solid evidence that at least some genetic component contributes to the development of anxiety disorders. For example, children of parents with an anxiety disorder have higher rates of anxiety disorders themselves. Data from twin registries support the hypothesis that anxiety disorders are at least partially genetically determined. No anxiety disorder, however, is likely to result from a simple Mendelian abnormality. Anxiety disorders commonly coexist with depression, substance abuse disorders, post-traumatic stress disorder (PTSD), and obsessive-compulsive disorder (OCD).

PATHOPHYSIOLOGY

It is well established that the autonomic nervous system of some patients with anxiety disorder, especially those with panic disorder, demonstrate increased sympathetic tone, adapt slowly to repeated stimuli, and respond excessively to moderate stimuli. The three major neurotransmitters associated with anxiety are norepinephrine, serotonin, and gamma-aminobutyric acid (GABA).

Functional brain-imaging studies, including positron emission tomography, single-photon emission computed tomography, and electroencephalography, of patients with anxiety disorders have variously reported abnormalities in the frontal cortex, the occipital and temporal areas, and, in one study of panic disorder, the parahippocampal gyrus.

CLINICAL PRESENTATION

The primary symptoms of GAD are anxiety, motor tension, autonomic hyperactivity, and cognitive vigilance. The anxiety is excessive and interferes with other aspects of the patient's life. Shakiness, restlessness, insomnia, and headaches are common manifestations of motor tension. Autonomic hyperactivity is commonly manifested by excessive sweating, various gastrointestinal symptoms (increased acidity, nausea, and epigastric pain), palpitations, concentration problems, tachycardia, headaches, and shortness of breath. Irritability and a quick-to-startle response are typical of cognitive vigilance. Often these patients seek help for their somatic symptoms. The distinction between GAD and normal anxiety is emphasized by the specification that the symptoms of GAD must cause significant impairment or distress.

It is important to screen for anxiety, and a variety of questionnaires are available. These include the Beck Anxiety Inventory, the Hamilton Anxiety Rating Scale, Generalized Anxiety Disorder 7-item (GAD-7) scale, the Anxiety Disorder Interview Schedule, Zung Self Rating Anxiety Scale and the Primary Care Evaluation of Mental Disorders (PRIME-MD) (see Advanced Assessment 68.1), which ask about somatic symptoms such as stomach, back, and chest pain; dizziness; and sweating; as well as mood-related symptoms such as depressed feelings and loss of interest in activities.

 Advanced Assessment 68.1: Screening and Diagnostic Tool

PRIME-MD

The PRIME-MD is a two-stage instrument that assesses common mood, anxiety, eating, alcohol, and somatoform disorders. It has a self-report *screening/case finding* component, the Patient Questionnaire (PQ), that is administered *before* the clinical encounter. It consists of 25 Yes/No questions about signs and symptoms present during the previous month and one question about the patient's overall health. The questions are divided into five groups corresponding to the five categories of mental disorders assessed by the PRIME-MD.

A current version of the PRIME-MD, the Patient Health Questionnaire (PHQ), increases the efficiency of PRIME-MD by making the entire screening and diagnostic process largely self-reported and taking only 3 minutes of the clinician's time. The PHQ is four pages long and contains questions similar to those in PRIME-MD-CEG (Clinical Evaluation Guide). However, the PHQ contains questions specific to women, with questions dealing with menstruation, pregnancy, and childbirth. The completed PHQ provides the clinician with most of the symptom-based information required to make the diagnoses at the beginning of the interview. This then allows more time for an assessment of the patient's life situation and personal history. This tool was designed for a low-health-literacy population, but the tool may still prove difficult for some patients to fill in by themselves. This is especially so for elderly patients, immigrants, refugees, and persons with low educational attainment. These populations are all at risk for mental disorders. Information from the PHQ can provide baseline data for some disorders and may prove useful in tracking the patient's response and progress over time with repeated administrations.

Numerous epidemiological and survey studies have demonstrated high rates of comorbid psychiatric conditions in children and adults with anxiety disorders. Therefore, aggressive measures to diagnose anxiety disorders and comorbid depression or other mental disorders are essential because, left untreated, they can significantly disrupt an individual's life. Moreover, because of familial correlations, consider screening children of parents with anxiety disorder, as well as parents with children who have been diagnosed with panic or other anxiety disorders.

DIAGNOSTIC REASONING

Symptoms

The *DSM-5* classifies anxiety disorders into the following categories:

- Generalized Anxiety Disorder
- Anxiety Disorder due to a general medical problem
- Substance-Induced Anxiety Disorder
- Anxiety Disorder Not Otherwise Specified
- Acute Stress Reaction/Disorder
- Posttraumatic Stress Disorder.

The main diagnostic criteria for GAD are excessive anxiety and worry predominating for at least 6 months. The intensity, duration, or frequency of the anxiety and worry are far out of proportion to the actual likelihood or impact of the feared event.

Many physiological symptoms that are included in the *DSM-5* criteria for GAD, such as palpitations, sweating, difficulty breathing, impaired concentration, impaired memory, and sleeping disturbance overlap with symptoms of some medical and substance use diagnosis that resembles anxiety. A detailed initial psychiatric assessment that includes a review of symptoms, medications, medical and drug use disorders including laboratory results must be completed to arrive at the correct mental disorder.

Differential Diagnosis

The differential diagnosis of GAD includes all medical disorders that may cause anxiety such as heart disease and hyperthyroidism (Box 68.1). Typically, a medical workup is necessary, including standard blood chemistry, electrocardiogram, and thyroid function tests specifically. Caffeine intoxication, stimulant abuse, and substance abuse, sedative, anxiolytic, and hypnotic withdrawal must all be ruled out. A complete list of all medications, both prescribed and over the counter including herbal and homeopathic agents, must be reviewed, including all herbal agents. An environmental/occupational assessment might also be called for as inhalation of volatile gases—such as gasoline, paint, insecticides, carbon monoxide, and carbon dioxide—may all cause symptoms of anxiety.

Box 68.1 Physiological Causes of Anxiety

- *Cancers:* carcinoid syndrome, pancreatic cancer, lung cancer, pheochromocytoma
- *Cardiac:* mitral valve prolapse, arrhythmia, congestive heart failure, ischemic heart disease
- *Pulmonary:* asthma, chronic obstructive pulmonary disease, sleep apnea, pulmonary embolism, hypercapnia, hypoxia
- *Neurological:* Ménière's disease, cerebrovascular accident (stroke), transient ischemic attack, multiple sclerosis, encephalopathy, subdural hematoma
- *Hematological:* anemia
- *Metabolic:* thyroid disease, hyperparathyroidism, Cushing's syndrome, Addison's disease, hypoglycemia, hyperglycemia, hyponatremia, hypokalemia
- *Nutritional:* Folate deficiency, vitamin B_{12} deficiency, iron deficiency

Medications and Medication Side Effects

Significant anxiety can develop as an adverse effect of prescribed or over-the-counter (OTC) medications. Medications commonly associated with drug-induced anxiety include:

- *Prescription drugs:* aminophylline, digitalis, dopamine, epinephrine, levodopa, lidocaine, neuroleptics, NSAIDs, steroids, SSRIs, theophylline, sympathomimetics, thyroid preparations
- *OTC drugs:* certain decongestants containing ephedrine and pseudoephedrine, caffeine, certain cough syrups, salicylates (in large doses), nicotine, monosodium glutamate, phenylpropanolamine
- *Herbal preparations:* ephedrine, ginseng, yohimbine
- *Illicit drugs:* amphetamines, marijuana, cocaine, ecstasy, methamphetamine, hallucinogenics
- *Others:* alcohol, caffeine, organic solvents

The history and mental status exam should explore the diagnostic possibility of panic disorder, phobias, and obsessive-compulsive disorder. Distinguishing GAD from major depressive disorder and dysthymic disorder is difficult because of the frequency of co-occurrence. In patients with comorbid depression and anxiety, the symptomatic profile may be balanced or either symptom can predominate. Patients may meet all the criteria for one disorder and only partially those for the other; they may meet the criteria for both disorders; or they may demonstrate symptoms of both disorders but may not meet the full diagnostic criteria for either.

Any patient who has symptoms of anxiety or depression should be evaluated for current symptoms of both disorders. Both GAD and social anxiety disorder are commonly comorbid with major depressive disorder. Identification and treatment of depression in this group of anxious patients can lead to improved outcomes and quicker recovery. The practitioner needs to perform a thorough suicide and/or homicide risk assessment in all patients who present with significant or alarming psychosocial issues.

MANAGEMENT

Education and Self-Care Management

Planning care for the patient with GAD begins with education. Often, the person with GAD lacks sufficient general information about GAD and has little understanding about his or her personal GAD symptoms. Patient education includes symptom recognition, effective interpretation of physical symptoms, different modalities of treatment, a decrease in the intake of stimulants such as caffeine and nicotine, and relaxation training. Patients should be aware that medication and counseling can be individually effective but yield better results as a combined treatment. Changes in coping should focus on developing more effective self-awareness and relaxation skills. Patients who develop routine methods of preventing acute anxiety and promoting relaxation are more successful than patients who attempt to cope with their GAD on an as-needed basis.

Areas of patient functioning that have been affected by anxiety should be well defined, and clear goals of improvement should be developed for each area. Some areas of functioning may be less affected by anxiety than others; however, improvement in major areas of functioning, such as being able to function at work or to maintain personal relationships, should be included.

Pharmacological Management

Selective serotonin reuptake inhibitors (SSRIs) are first-line medications for the treatment of GAD and are particularly helpful if the patient has a coexisting depression. Escitalopram (Lexapro), paroxetine (Paxil), and sertraline (Zoloft) have shown evidence of GAD symptoms remission and reduction. The serotonin-norepinephrine reuptake inhibitor (SNRI) venlafaxine (Effexor) is effective in the acute treatment of GAD as is the partial agonist buspirone (Buspar). Treatment up to 24 weeks is associated with greater response rates. When a sedating medication is needed, moderately sedating tricyclic antidepressants (TCAs; [imipramine]) can be considered. The goal of medication treatment for GAD should be to reduce or relieve symptoms sufficiently to enable effective self-care and to promote satisfactory levels of functioning (see Drugs Commonly Prescribed 68.1). Additional medications that have proven efficacy are the antipsychotic trifluoperazine (Stelazine), the antihistamine hydroxyzine (Vistaril), and the antiseizure medication pregabalin (Lyrica). If no response is noted with the first medication, consider maximizing dosage, changing to another SSRI or SNRI or adding another SSRI or SNRI. Response should be noted in 8 weeks.

Drugs Commonly Prescribed 68.1: Antianxiety Agents

DRUG	INDICATION	ADVERSE REACTIONS AND PRESCRIBING CONSIDERATIONS
Benzodiazepines: Half-Life <12 Hours		
Alprazolam	Anxiety, GAD, panic disorder	• Schedule IV controlled substance • All benzodiazepines are associated with potential anterograde amnesia, CNS depression, and paradoxical reactions • Sedation, memory deficits, ataxia, narrow-angle glaucoma; association with falls and injury in the elderly • Caution with depressed patients and substance abuse, impaired hepatic or renal function • Most contraindicated in obstructive sleep apnea • Metabolized by CYP450 3A4; check drug-gene interactions • Withdrawal symptoms with abrupt discontinuation • The onset of withdrawal symptoms is usually seen on the first day without drug and lasts 5–7 days—slow taper • Use lowest and shortest possible effective dose and time; risk of dependence for treatment longer than 12 weeks. • Avoid valerian, St. John's wort, kava kava, gotu kola • Potential severe allergic reactions (anaphylaxis, angioedema) and complex sleep-related behaviors, which may include sleep-driving, cooking, and eating food while asleep, and making phone calls while asleep
Oxazepam	Anxiety and alcohol withdrawal	See above
Temazepam	Insomnia, short-term	• See above • Administer 30 minutes before bedtime • Lack of active metabolites; excellent option for the elderly
Triazolam	Insomnia, short term	Not a drug of first choice for elderly because of the higher incidence of CNS adverse reactions in this population
Benzodiazepines: Intermediate Half-life (12–24 hours)		
Alprazolam XR	GAD, panic disorder, anxiety with depression	• Extended-release tablet: Should be taken once daily in the morning; do not crush, break, or chew. • Onset 1 hour and duration 12 hours
Estazolam	Insomnia short-term	No active metabolites
Lorazepam	Amnesia induction Anxiety sedation induction Status epilepticus	• Available in liquid and injectable formulation • Contraindicated if patient has angle-closure glaucoma
Benzodiazepines: Long Elimination Half-Life (>24 hours)		
Chlordiazepoxide	Anxiety, alcohol withdrawal	• The onset of withdrawal symptoms is usually seen after 5 days, with a duration of 10–14 days.
Clonazepam	Absence seizures Lennox-Gastaut syndrome Myoclonic seizures Panic disorder	• Less sedating than other anxiolytics; onset of full anxiolytic effect can take 3–6 weeks; less dependence. • Risk of suicidal ideation when used for seizures; monitor CBC, LFTs
Clorazepate	Anxiety, alcohol withdrawal, partial seizures (adjunctive)	• Increased risk of suicidal ideation when used for seizures • Long-acting metabolites; do not use in elderly • Monitor CBC, LFTs

Drugs Commonly Prescribed 68.1: Antianxiety Agents—cont'd

DRUG	INDICATION	ADVERSE REACTIONS AND PRESCRIBING CONSIDERATIONS
Diazepam	Amnesia induction, anxiety, drug-induced seizures, alcohol withdrawal, muscle spasms, partial seizures, sedation induction Status epilepticus, tetanus, tonic-clonic seizures	• Monitor CBC, LFTs • Only benzodiazepine with a rectal administration formulation
Flurazepam	Insomnia short-term	• Avoid in elderly and debilitated • Active metabolites with extended half-lives may lead to delayed accumulation and adverse effects
Quazepam	Hypnotic	• Long-acting; daytime sedation and fatigue, but this may prevent withdrawal symptoms when stopped
Nonbenzodiazepines		
Azapirones buspirone	Anxiety, GAD	• Low risk of cognitive or motor impairment, may cause dopamine-related movement disorders (restlessness) • Avoid St. John's wort, valerian, gotu kola, kava kava • May take 2–3 weeks to see full effect, little potential for abuse, needs continuous use, does not potentiate the effects of alcohol
Selective Serotonin Reuptake Inhibitors (SSRIs) escitalopram		See Drugs Commonly Prescribed 67.1
Selective Norepinephrine Reuptake Inhibitors (SNRIs) duloxetine venlafaxine		See Drugs Commonly Prescribed 67.1

Abbreviations: CBC, complete blood count; CNS, central nervous system; GAD, generalized anxiety disorder; LFTs, liver function tests.
Source: Clinical pharmacology [database online]. Tampa, FL: Gold Standard, Inc.; 2013. http://cp.gsm.com.

One helpful regimen for acute, severe, and debilitating GAD is to start the patient on both a benzodiazepine and an SSRI and then to taper the benzodiazepine as the SSRI reaches full effect. Some benzodiazepines (alprazolam and diazepam) can be helpful in the acute management of GAD, but it is important to remember that if the patient has comorbid depression, use of a benzodiazepine may exacerbate depressive symptoms. Dependence may also occur in those patients with predisposing factors and with long-term use. Nonetheless, unrelieved GAD symptoms can lead to additional new problems, such as substance abuse and severe social withdrawal. Psychopharmacogenetic testing may be considered in the pharmacologic treatment plan; this approach is becoming more common in the treatment of psychiatric disorders (see Box 68.2).

Nonpharmacological Management

In management of GAD, nonpharmacological management has similar efficacy to pharmacological therapy. Cognitive-behavioral therapy (CBT; see Box 68.3) has proven equally effective to SSRIs in dealing with GAD, as well as other disorders. Cognitive-behavioral treatment has a lower relapse rate in contrast to other forms of psychological modalities. Some have theorized that there are structural societal issues contributing to the current rates of anxiety and depression and suggest non-pharmacological approaches aimed at finding meaning, social connection, and mindfulness education.

FOLLOW-UP AND REFERRAL

Monthly follow-up appointments may be needed until the patient with GAD has established alternative resources for support and assistance. A clear follow-up plan decreases the problem of excessive or ineffective appointments. Ongoing assessment includes evaluation of the primary symptoms and the utilization of objective GAD tools, as well as assessment of the current risk of

---

Box 68.2   Psychopharmacogenetic Testing

"Precision medicine" or "personalized medicine" is a care approach that seeks to tailor treatment to the individual with the utilization of genetic testing as they relate to pharmacokinetics and pharmacodynamics for psychiatric medication to predict potential side effects and accelerate effective treatment (Brenan et al., 2015). Most drugs are prescribed in a "one-size-fits-all" fashion and are expected to work the same for all patients; however, genetics can affect medication efficacy. Pharmacogenomics uses information about a person's genetic makeup to help clinicians select the best drug and doses that will have the best efficacy for the person (Stahl, 2014). The same concept is used when addressing mental disorders, and it is referred to as *psychopharmacogentics*. This approach to care is extremely helpful because persons living with mental illness often undergo multiple trials of medications while experiencing negative side effects resulting in lower adherence to treatment before arriving at the right medication. Differences in each person's genes affect how their bodies respond to medications.

Understanding each individual's genetic uniqueness can help clinicians make more meaningful medication decisions. For example, a person's genes can affect blood levels of a drug (pharmacokinetic) by causing a medication to metabolize too slow, too fast, or normally, thus having an impact on how much drug reaches the brain to target a specific symptom. In this case, it may be as simple as increasing or decreasing the recommended medication dosage to reach the target outcome based on psychopharmacogenetic test results. On the other hand, if a patient is taking the correct dosage and reaches a therapeutic blood level, but symptoms have not improved, this may be due to the lack of receptor binding (pharmacodynamics). This gene–drug interaction problem can be solved by learning patient's specific phenotyping and selecting the best medication to target the correct sequence. Genetic test results can provide guidance on potential gene–drug interactions, side effects, and drug metabolization speeds and thus determine which medications may work best for the patient.

Some genetic tests are covered by health insurance, but most are not. Patients sign consent for this type of test and should pay attention of how this test results can be used, which may include clinical decision-making, billing and office operation, and quality improvement evaluation. Providers are reminded that test results are only part of the assessment. The use of psychopharmacogenetics has shown some early signs of clinical validity, as well as utilization and health cost savings, compared with patients receiving standard care (Benitez, J., Jablonski, M. R., Allen, J. D., & Winner, J. G. (2015).

Psychopharmocogenetics can be a powerful tool if used appropriately and in combination with a detailed clinical assessment, laboratory results, and patient education. Patients seem to appreciate that a test is available that can increase reliability and validate the provider's clinical decision. This may lead to greater patient optimism that medications will work, increasing adherence to the medication regimen and follow-up care. When patients and clinicians understand that pharmacogenetics is just one piece of the overall assessment, the additional information obtained from this type of testing may lead to faster symptom improvement.

Box 68.3   Cognitive-Behavioral Strategies

Assumptions

- Alterations in content of underlying cognitive processes alter affective states and behavioral problems (i.e., thinking alters feeling and doing).
- Correction of these faulty constructs ("stinking thinking") can lead to clinical improvement.
- A person's appraisal/perception of situations is reflected in his or her cognitions (both thoughts and visuals).
- Through therapy, patients become aware of these faulty constructs and learn to alter them.

Processes

- Identify and alter cognitive distortions that maintain symptoms
- Time-limited, usually 15–25 weeks, once weekly
- Collaborative empiricism
- Structured and directive
- Assigned readings
- Homework and behavioral techniques
- Desensitization in some patients
- Identification of irrational beliefs and automatic thoughts
- Identification of attitudes and assumptions underlying negative thoughts

Source: Saddock BJ, Saddock VA. *Kaplan & Sadock's synopsis of psychiatry.* 10th ed. Philadelphia, PA: Lippincott Williams & Wilkins; 2017.

---

suicide/homicide. Complete documentation of the evaluation and plan is essential. Practitioners may wish to make themselves available to anxious patients, and referrals to patient education and support groups may be helpful for some patients with GAD. The plan should include strict criteria for seeking emergency services. The goal is to protect the patient from unknowingly becoming overreactive to his or her GAD symptoms. Improvement can become more obtainable when a realistic understanding of the illness is maintained. Referral to a specialist should be considered if multiple comorbidities and co-occurring modalities exist or if no improvement is noted within 8 weeks from initiation of treatment.

Patient Education: Generalized Anxiety Disorder

Education about antianxiety medications should be reviewed with the patient and family members, including issues of overuse and dependency on medications, as well as potential adverse effects. The need to avoid combining antianxiety medications with alcohol should be stressed. The clinician should provide written instructions if the patient appears to have limited ability to concentrate. The practitioner should also discuss with the patient and family the causes and treatment of anxiety.

The provider may want to suggest to the patient and family complementary methods of anxiety management, such as relaxation techniques (see Complementary Therapies 68.1), guided imagery, music therapy, physical activity, yoga, and acupuncture. Physical exercise has consistently been shown to have good effect in control of anxiety. If appropriate, nutritional practices may need to be changed to include a healthier diet.

GAD cannot be managed with medication alone. Consistent and active patient self-care is required. At the same time, the highly symptomatic patient, no matter how motivated, is unlikely to be able to engage in self-care when his or her GAD symptoms are poorly controlled. GAD symptoms can increase the difficulty of learning new information, including learning new self-care skills. Many primary-care settings now have access to comprehensive patient education programs and team-based approaches in which the primary-care nurse practitioner can play a pivotal role. Giving patients enough time to practice newly adopted self-care skills, such as mindfulness-based stress reduction programs and meditation, may assist patients to cope with ongoing symptoms.

PANIC DISORDER

Panic disorder, which typically presents in young adulthood, is a disabling condition. It can impair an individual's social, family, and work lives. Panic disorder symptoms are recurrent, intense, short episodes of panic-level psychological and physical symptoms of anxiety. The initial panic episode must be spontaneous and unexpected, and it cannot occur when the person is the focus of others' attention, such as when speaking in front of an audience. A combination of sudden onset and severity of panic symptoms creates secondary symptoms of fear. These secondary fear symptoms essentially define this disorder. Fear compels the patient with panic disorder to seek emergency health-care services repeatedly. To the patient, panic symptoms are life-threatening and signal a serious health problem or an impending nervous breakdown. Patients endure an unshakable sense of doom and danger that they cannot define.

Patients who have lived with panic disorder for some time come to associate the onset of their symptoms with specific circumstances. They may or may not be accurate in their assessment, but they may nevertheless believe that a given situation or set of circumstances triggers their panic symptoms. When this is the case, the patient may develop methods of avoiding the trigger situations and circumstances. Panic symptoms can be triggered by a wide variety of stimuli such as substance use, a change in daily routine, or exposure to feared situations, such as being in crowds or closed-in spaces. Panic triggers may or may not be easy to avoid. An episode of panic typically lasts about 10 minutes or less; however, the secondary distress that follows a panic episode can last for hours.

Complementary Therapies 68.1: Relaxation Therapy Techniques

This breathing technique will help you relax, as well as provide increased energy, health, and concentration. Try using this technique for at least 15 minutes each day, on an empty stomach. Do not stand up suddenly after performing these exercises because they can lower blood pressure, making you dizzy.

Step 1: Sit in a comfortable chair and in a quiet location to minimize distractions.

Step 2: Close your eyes.

Step 3: Begin by taking a slow, deep breath in through your nose and breathe out through your mouth slowly and deeply, like blowing out a candle.

Step 4: Breathe in slowly for a count of four, hold for a count of seven, and breathe out for a count of eight. Repeat this several times.

Step 5: The following techniques may also help you to relax while doing the breathing exercise:

   a. Visualize a favorite, peaceful setting, such as a beach, forest, desert, or meadow.

   b. Play peaceful music in the background.

   c. Begin at your feet and repeat to yourself that your feet are warm and heavy. Once you have achieved that, move up to your legs, your torso, and then your arms and hands. The sensation of heaviness and warmth should spread throughout your entire body.

   d. Repeat a favorite phase, or mantra, with each breath.

   e. Tighten different muscles while inhaling and relax them while exhaling (start with your feet and move systematically up your body).

UTILIZATION OF TECHNOLOGY FOR MEDITATION

There are many free downloadable applications for phones and portable devices that walk a person step by step through how to meditate. Some of these are the following:

- Calm
- Headspace: Meditation
- Simple Habit: Meditation

The frequency and severity of panic episodes and the triggered emotional and behavioral responses to panic symptoms can vary from patient to patient. Individual patterns also may vary. Panic disorder differs from occasional panic attack, now defined in *DSM-5* as Panic Attack Specifier. The main distinction is that a diagnosis of panic disorder is based on a pattern of recurrent, unexpected panic attacks. At least one of these attacks must have been followed by 1 month or more of persistent worry and/or maladaptive changes in behavior. Persons with severe panic disorder become highly fearful of future panic episodes and may become preoccupied with searching for the "true meaning" of their panic symptoms. They are likely to make significant changes in their behavior and routines in the hope of avoiding future panic episodes. Without evidence of panic avoidance, it is difficult to confirm a diagnosis of panic disorder. Persons with panic disorder may become vigilant in their efforts to anticipate and thus avoid future panic episodes. Evidence of this anticipatory anxiety clarifies the diagnosis of panic disorder.

EPIDEMIOLOGY AND CAUSES

The prevalence of panic disorder is generally believed to be 1.5% to 3%, although perhaps 10% of the population has had at least one isolated panic attack. Panic disorder is more common also in persons with medical conditions. For example, in pulmonary clinics (where patients with asthma and other conditions that cause shortness of breath seek treatment), 10% to 20% of patients may be affected by panic disorder. Ten percent to 20% of patients who present to the emergency department with chest pain actually have a panic disorder.

Panic disorders typically appear in late adolescence or young adulthood, with a peak at 25 years of age. There is a second peak between 35 and 44 years. Panic disorder affects women approximately twice as often as men. Empiric research indicates that approximately 70% of patients with panic disorder have at least one major depressive episode during their lifetime. These patients also have social anxiety or social phobia; they may also be generally anxious, chronic worriers, with high rates of posttraumatic stress disorder (PTSD) and obsessive-compulsive disorder (OCD). Patients presenting with those disorders should always be tested first for an underlying anxiety and/or mood disorder.

Panic disorders appear to have a genetic component. Several studies have suggested that patients with panic disorder are at high risk for suicidal ideation and attempts. Comorbidity with major depression can increase the rate of attempted suicides. Further, panic disorder patients have a propensity to self-medicate with alcohol and drugs. These facts should alert the clinician to the serious nature of this disorder.

PATHOPHYSIOLOGY

Structural brain-imaging studies, such as magnetic resonance imaging, have demonstrated pathological involvement in the temporal lobes, particularly the hippocampus, in patients with panic disorder. Some studies use specific panic-inducing substances (such as caffeine, lactate, or yohimbine) to assess effects of panic on cerebral blood flow. Anxiety disorders and panic attacks are specifically associated with cerebral vasoconstriction. This in turn may cause central nervous system symptoms such as dizziness and peripheral nervous system symptoms such as hyperventilation and hypercapnia.

Genetic predisposition to panic disorders, especially in those with agoraphobia, has been established in a number of studies. The *DSM-5* now allows for panic disorder and agoraphobia to be diagnosed irrespective of each other, meaning that both diagnoses can be given to a patient if they meet criteria for each disorder.

First-degree relatives of those with panic disorder have a fourfold to eightfold higher risk for the development of the disorder than first-degree relatives of other psychiatric patients. Twin studies have demonstrated a higher concordance for panic disorder in monozygotic twins than in dizygotic twins. No data indicating association between a specific chromosomal location or mode of transmission and panic disorder exist at this time.

Studies have shown that patients with panic disorder typically experience greater distress about life events than control subjects, and that in the months before the onset of panic, they demonstrate a higher incidence of stressful life events. What was primarily a mild feeling of anxiety suddenly becomes an overwhelming feeling of apprehension and dread, replete with somatic symptoms.

The pathogenesis of the panic attacks may be related to neurophysiological factors triggered by psychological reactions that are likely precipitated by the unconscious meaning assigned to stressful events. When assessing a patient with panic disorder, the practitioner should conduct a complete assessment of possible triggers, including inquiry about current or past abuse, loss of significant others, and other stressful life events.

CLINICAL PRESENTATION

As with anxiety disorders, certain at-risk patients for panic disorder should be considered. Patients at risk include those patients with a family history of panic and/or anxiety disorders and patients who have a comorbid psychiatric disorder, such as major depression, bipolar disorder, or substance use disorders.

The patient should be asked to describe the panic/anxiety episodes in detail, noting frequency, duration, and precipitating events. Panic disorder is marked by recurrent and unpredictable panic attacks. The panic attacks come on unexpectedly, developing suddenly within 10 minutes and usually resolving within the hour. These attacks are distinct episodes of intense fear and discomfort associated with specific physical symptoms, such as sweating, shaking, rapid heart rate, a choking sensation, shortness of breath, nausea and/or GI distress, vertigo, feeling faint and light-headed, and/or shortness of breath. Frequency and severity of attacks vary from once a week to clusters of attacks separated by months of well-being. The first attack often occurs outside of the home.

Spontaneous panic attacks have no obvious stimuli, whereas situational panic attacks are in response to a phobic stimulus. Limited symptom attacks are spells manifesting one or two symptoms such as dizziness, tachycardia, or respiratory distress. Often limited symptom attacks occur early in the course of panic disorder or between panic attacks. Although panic disorder may occur without any obvious causative events, it can occur in early adult life after a loss, threat of a loss, physical illness, or an episode of drug abuse.

After having several panic attacks, as many as 80% of patients begin to fear the next attack. They also experience phobic avoidance of circumstances associated with attacks. This is called anticipatory anxiety, which may become more disabling than the panic attacks themselves. Patients may become agoraphobic, culminating in increasingly circumscribed lives; some patients eventually become completely homebound. Approximately 30% to 50% of individuals with agoraphobia are also diagnosed with panic disorder.

The risk factor with the best predictive power for panic disorder is a positive family history. Other types of mood and anxiety disorders often are comorbid in patients who experience panic disorder. It is important to look not only for panic disorders in the family history but also for the presence of other mental disorders.

DIAGNOSTIC REASONING

Symptoms

Panic disorder can be distinguished from other anxiety disorders based on the patient's history of repeated panic attacks. Patients with panic disorder exhibit persistent concern about the recurrence of panic attacks and may show behavioral changes as a result of this concern. The *DSM-5* provides complete diagnostic criteria for panic disorder.

Agoraphobia, which now has separate diagnostic criteria in the *DSM-5*, is characterized by overwhelming symptoms of anxiety when leaving home on at last two occasions. Symptoms include rapid heartbeat, chest pain, difficulty breathing, weakness, faintness, sweating, and a feeling of impending doom or fear of dying. Individuals with agoraphobia must also demonstrate avoidance behaviors, such as reluctance or refusal to leave home. See the *DSM-5* for complete diagnostic criteria for agoraphobia.

Differential Diagnosis

Diagnosis is generally clinical in nature. Tools that may provide a fairly accurate assessment in a relatively short time include the Mini-International Neuropsychiatric Interview (M.I.N.I.) and the PRIME-MD. Diagnosis will then structure appropriate treatment and follow-up. The array of medical, cultural, or other psychiatric conditions that may mimic symptoms/signs of panic disorder should be considered, especially with the onset of any anxiety disorder. Panic symptoms are common, for example, in patients with schizophrenia, bipolar

disorder, and depression. Clinicians also have to take into account cultural considerations and concepts of distress when assessing for panic disorder. The *DSM-5* has integrated cultural sensitivity tools to reflect cross-cultural presentations of mental disorders with person-centered assessments. Cultural expression of panic may include headache, tinnitus, and sobbing.

A comprehensive physical examination should be performed to rule out organic causes for the patient's symptoms. If the history suggests that significant organic disease is unlikely, the physical examination should be focused primarily on the organ system of most concern (e.g., the heart in a patient with chest pain). Laboratory tests to rule out physical causality should be considered.

Medical conditions that may accompany, contribute to, or cause panic symptomatology; these conditions include pheochromocytoma, hyperthyroidism, seizure disorder, and cardiac arrhythmias that may originate from an acute myocardial infarction. Consider that the use of or withdrawal from therapeutic or recreational drugs may cause panic attacks. Therapeutic drugs include theophylline and steroids. Recreational drugs include cocaine, amphetamines, and caffeine. Drug withdrawal symptoms are typically associated with drugs such as alcohol, barbiturates, and benzodiazepines. As described previously, the differential diagnosis of panic disorder is complicated by a high rate of comorbidity with other psychiatric conditions, especially abuse of alcohol and benzodiazepines, which patients may initially use in an attempt to self-medicate.

MANAGEMENT

Pharmacological Management

The pharmacological treatment of panic disorder is relatively straightforward and effective. The major recent advances in the treatment of panic disorder have been the advent of SSRIs and SNRIs and their recognition as powerful anti-panic drugs. Generally, they are recommended as first-line pharmacological therapy in panic disorder. Patients with panic disorder are often very sensitive to the pharmacological effects of various medications. When initiating pharmacological therapy, the practitioner may consider starting the drug at half of the recommended dose and gradually increasing the dose over several days. This strategy assists patients to slowly become acclimated to the effect of the medication. It is important to monitor and increase the dose until full therapeutic dosage is achieved. If the response to the initial SSRI is inadequate, the clinician may consider changing the drug, switching to another antidepressant, or adding a second medication. Additional medications shown to be effective include the tricyclic antidepressants (TCAs), benzodiazepines, valproic acid (Depakote), or gabapentin (Neurontin). One should avoid extensive use of the benzodiazepines, except in specific circumstances where the patient is unable to tolerate an SSRI/SNRI or TCA, and they should not be utilized in a depressed patient as monotherapy (American Psychiatric Association, n.d.). When they are used, a long-acting preparation is preferred, on an around-the-clock basis. When shorter-acting benzodiazepines are used "as needed," the risk is increased for greater tolerance and possible abuse or addiction. These particular anxiolytics can also exacerbate the depression that may coexist with panic disorder. After panic attacks have ceased, patients are maintained on medication for a minimum of 6 months. Pharmacological blockade of panic generally leads to a decrease in both anticipatory anxiety and phobic avoidance. A common approach is to use benzodiazepines for immediate relief. Other medications may be added, either concurrently or after symptoms are attenuated. Once these medications become effective, the benzodiazepine treatment may be tapered and discontinued.

Nonpharmacological Management

Cognitive behavioral therapy (CBT) (see Box 68.3) is the first-line treatment for panic disorder, and useful adjuncts are self-help CBT-based books and self-help programs. Patients who receive CBT have longer periods of remission and longer-term benefits. CBT is also useful to facilitate the gradual withdrawal from benzodiazepines, which are often used for immediate symptom relief in panic disorder. CBT is aimed at altering the unproductive and dysfunctional thinking that helps to generate and maintain anxiety. Patients with panic disorder learn to face their fear so that attacks are avoided. CBT is effective in treating maladaptive behaviors associated with anxiety, mainly by gradual exposure to more adaptive situations. CBT encompasses a range of treatments, each consisting of several elements, including breathing techniques, education, continuous panic monitoring, development of anxiety management skills, cognitive restructuring, and in vivo exposure. Some sources recommend brief, highly focused behavioral and cognitive psychotherapeutic techniques for panic. Hypnosis and alternative therapies (yoga, meditation) are sometimes useful as part of combined therapies but are not as effective as CBT. Some patients find relief in chiropractic treatment and acupuncture.

FOLLOW-UP AND REFERRAL

Patients with panic disorder can be managed in primary-care settings once a plan of care has been agreed to. Generally, pharmacological follow-up is scheduled every 1 to 2 weeks when initiating therapy, and then every 2 to 4 weeks until therapeutic dosage is achieved. Appointments can be spaced further apart as the dosage is stabilized and the symptoms reduced (see Box 68.4). As with any serious psychological condition, referral to specialist consultation or to hospital care should be made

---

Box 68.4   Advanced Practice Nursing Interventions for Panic Disorder

Management

Goal: full remission, elimination of panic attacks, anxiety, phobias, and disability; restoration of well-being.

Institute treatment with low-dose selective serotonin reuptake inhibitors (SSRIs); increase dose as tolerated to target dose.

Monitor closely for adverse effects.

Continue treatment for 12 to 24 months; phase out treatment slowly (over 4–6 months).

Refer to an anxiety disorder specialist if response is not satisfactory or if comorbid conditions are present.

Patient and Family Education

Teach the patient and family about panic disorder.

Advise patient not to abruptly stop medication.

Source: Adapted from American Psychiatric Association. *Practice guideline for the treatment of patients with panic disorder.* Retrieved from https://psychiatryonline.org/pb/assets/raw/sitewide/practice_guidelines/guidelines/panicdisorder.pdf. Updated January 2009.

---

as appropriate. This includes *mandatory* inquiry about suicidal history, ideation, or intent. Also, the practitioner should consider referring the patient to a psychiatrist if he or she fails to respond after 6 to 8 weeks of standard treatment. Similarly, patients should be referred to an appropriate medical specialist if an occult underlying organic disorder is suspected. The practitioner should assess the patient's response to treatment and symptom intensity and reinforce patient education at every visit, as well as review strategies to manage panic attacks. The ongoing therapeutic alliance with the primary-care clinician is crucial for long-term successful treatment.

Patient Education: Panic Disorder

For treatment to be effective, the patient and family must understand panic disorder and work together aggressively as active participants in the treatment plan. Moreover, the patient and family must be aware of the potential adverse effects of any drugs prescribed and work toward using relaxation techniques, deep breathing, and cognitive behavioral strategies to control panic.

Other approaches effective for GAD such as physical exercise, healthy nutrition, relaxation techniques and the like may also prove effective for panic disorder.

POST-TRAUMATIC STRESS DISORDER

PTSD is a syndrome that develops after a person witnesses, participates in, or experiences direct exposure to actual or threatened trauma, such as death, threatened death, serious injury, an event like sexual violence, and/or learning that a relative or close friend was exposed to a trauma. Additionally, indirect exposure to aversive details of the trauma, usually in the course of professional duties such as first responders, and medics, may also lead to the development of PTSD. This exposure can be repeated or onetime event. The reaction to this experience is typically fear and helplessness, reliving the event over and over, and trying to avoid being reminded of it. The traumatic event is persistently re-experienced in disabling ways such as recurrent nightmares, flashbacks, and intrusive thoughts and these symptoms must be severe enough to persist and/or develop more than thirty days after the initial exposure. Additionally, these manifestations must be disabling and significantly affect critical areas in the person's life such as interpersonal relationships and occupational roles. *Acute Stress Reaction/Disorder* is separated out from PTSD in the *DSM-5* and refers to the immediate aftermath of the exposure—typically, the first 30 days.

PTSD symptoms are responses to experiences that are overwhelming, for example, war, torture, natural disasters, terrorism, assault, rape, serious accidents, fires, and environmental and social experiences. Typically, persons continue to re-experience the trauma in their dreams and daily thoughts, and they try to evade anything that reminds them of the event. Patients can also undergo a "numbing" of responsiveness along with a physiological state of hyper-arousal. This is usually accompanied by depression, anxiety, cognitive difficulties, and often substance abuse. Comorbid disorders make persons more vulnerable to developing PTSD.

Nursing Situation: Post-traumatic Stress Disorder

Jennifer, a 45-year-old nurse and married woman with two children, presented to the Veteran's Administration Medical Center (VAMC). She lived in a rural community and served a total of 24 years in the military (13 years active duty in the U.S. Army and 11 years in the U.S. Army Reserves). She was deployed for 7 months during the Gulf War and for 19 months to Kuwait and Iraq. The deployment to Kuwait and Iraq was extended several times and her support system was also affected when various individuals of the medical team were reassigned to different locations. Jennifer denied any previous psychiatric history but reported a random sexual assault at age 20 for which she never received treatment.

During her Operation Iraqi Freedom deployment, she was at Abu Ghraib prison for 4 months and experienced mortar attacks, multiple casualties, prolonged working hours, and exposure to horrific injuries and death. She became adept at dissociating herself from these conditions until her fourteenth month of deployment. At that time, she lost interest in activities she normally enjoyed and became isolated from colleagues; her communication with family members also decreased. After redeployment, she began to have panic attacks, and she had

intrusive symptoms and nightmare. Sensory experiences such as hearing helicopters, seeing blood, or smelling seared meat would provoke intrusive symptoms. She became increasingly isolated and alienated.

Jennifer's recovery encompassed the three stages of PTSD recovery. Providing a safe environment is a prerequisite to begin the process. During empowerment, the survivor can choose to speak about the experience, to remember, and to mourn. Narrative reconstruction and reconnection allows the survivor to reprocess the traumatic events into a tolerable form. And third, reconnection allows the individual to confront the traumatic past, accept the personal changes, and to reengage with the world and actively recreate a future.

Jennifer sought treatment at a VAMC outpatient psychiatric clinic 3 months after redeployment with the initial diagnoses of major depression and panic attacks. Her initial treatment included an SSRI and trazodone for sleep. On her third appointment, after utilizing a validated tool for PTSD, she was diagnosed with mild-moderate PTSD. As her medications began to improve her symptoms, she began to verbalize the traumatic experiences she had witnessed and could then reframe those experiences. Unfortunately, after four sessions her psychiatrist retired, and Jennifer was referred to group therapy, which she was unable to do. She sought care at a community health provider for the next year and continued the medications. Jennifer continued to heal through family support, retiring from the military, and receiving new career training.

Many veterans receive treatment outside of the VA system, and it is important for APRNs to be aware of the evidence-based pharmacological and nonpharmacological treatments for PTSD.

Source: Adapted from Feczer D, Bjorklund, P. Forever changed: Posttraumatic stress disorder in female military veterans, a case report. *Perspect Pscyhiatr Care.* 2009;45(4):278–291.

EPIDEMIOLOGY AND CAUSES

The lifetime prevalence of PTSD in the general population is approximately 8% to 9%, and it is twice as common in women. Women in the military are most likely to have PTSD as a result of sexual assault or child sexual abuse. Men are more commonly affected by military combat or witnessing other forms of extreme violence (U.S. Department of Veterans Affairs, 2010). The prevalence of the disorder can therefore be higher among specific groups, such as war veterans, victims of terrorist attacks, or survivors of natural disasters. African American have a higher prevalence of PTSD diagnosis than white American, Hispanic American, or Asian American. Thus, the development of PTSD varies with the degree of exposure, the type of traumatic event, and the severity of the precipitating cause. For example, most studies of adult survivors of disaster have found a PTSD prevalence of 30% to 60% after a disaster.

Recent immigrants from areas of social and/or political instability can be highly susceptible to PTSD. However, for many reasons, immigrant patients may choose not to share their traumatic experiences with a practitioner. This reluctance may have to do with significant feelings of vulnerability that a recent immigrant may feel (U.S. Department of Veteran Affairs, 2015).

Other risk factors include female sex, age (the very young and the very old are especially susceptible), race, education, socioeconomic status, education, family history, reported abuse in childhood, reports of other adverse childhood factors or trauma, poor social and/or family support, and comorbidities. Comorbidities with PTSD include an increased association with anxiety, substance abuse, and mood disorders. There is at least one psychiatric disorder present in more than 70% of men and women diagnosed with PTSD and an increased incidence of depression and mania in patients with PTSD, compared with the general population.

Risk Factors: Post-traumatic Stress Disorder

- Physical or sexual childhood abuse
- Sexual or other life-threatening assault/accident
- Combat exposure
- Being involved in fire, flood, hurricane, or other natural disaster
- Witnessing someone being badly injured or killed
- History of mental health problems
- Refugee resettled in Western countries

(Fazel, Wheeler, & Danesh, 2005)

The prognosis for patients with PTSD is influenced by multiple factors, including whether the disorder is acute, chronic, or delayed; the presence or absence of previous mental disorders; the patient's premorbid personality; available support resources; compliance with treatment; and the patient's ability and desire to learn new coping mechanisms.

The adaptive person who develops acute PTSD after exposure to a traumatic event has a better chance for full recovery, especially if his or her family is supportive. Untreated, about 30% of patients recover completely, 40% continue to have mild symptoms, 20% continue to have moderate symptoms, and 10% remain unchanged or become worse.

PATHOPHYSIOLOGY

A number of biological variables have been implicated in PTSD. There is strong evidence, for example, for altered function in the noradrenergic system. Specifically, soldiers with PTSD-like symptoms may experience nervousness, high blood pressure, increased heart rate, palpitations, sweating, flushing, and tremors—all

symptoms associated with adrenergic drugs. Veterans with PTSD demonstrate increased epinephrine concentrations in 24-hour urine samples, and increased urine catecholamines have been found in 24-hour urine samples of sexually abused girls. Some studies have revealed cortisol hypersuppression in trauma-exposed patients who develop PTSD, compared with patients exposed to trauma who do not develop PTSD.

A personal predisposition may be necessary for symptoms to develop after a traumatic event, and individuals apt to develop PTSD may have a preexisting mood or anxiety disorder or a family history of anxiety or other psychiatric disorder. Patients with existing serious mental disorders are at risk for victimization and, at times, assault, and they may be more likely to develop PTSD. Symptoms must persist for more than 1 month, must cause significant distress and/or functional impairment, and these symptoms must not be due to other illness or substance use.

CLINICAL PRESENTATION

The principal clinical features of PTSD are painful reexperiencing of the event, a pattern of avoidance, and emotional numbing. These symptoms may never remit after the precipitating event or they may resolve within a few weeks, or even years, with a period of relative "normalcy," but then recurrent symptoms begin to creep in sometimes with major acceleration of distress. Typically, a combination of a trauma, the personal characteristics of the person experiencing the trauma, and a variety of post-traumatic factors all must coalesce for the person to develop PTSD. Patients should also be screened for suicide and comorbidities such as anxiety, depression, and substance use. A diagnosis of PTSD will rarely be made unless the patient exhibits at least one symptom from each symptom category.

- Reexperiencing the traumatic event or having intrusive thoughts, nightmares about the event, flashbacks about the event, emotional distress after exposure to traumatic reminders, and physical reactivity after exposure to traumatic reminders. This experience can manifest itself as a nightmare, a flashback, or simply sudden, vivid memories that are accompanied by painful emotions or images related to the trauma.
- Avoidance symptoms: The patient avoids any situation or activity that might revive memories of the trauma. This symptom can severely impair the patient's relationships with others because close emotional ties with family, friends, and colleagues may be included among the situations that the patient intentionally avoids. Patients with PTSD commonly complain that they cannot feel emotions, especially emotions toward those who are closest to them.
- Negative thoughts or feelings that began or worsened after the trauma and manifest in a variety of ways such

as a negative affect, exaggerated blame of self or others for causing the trauma, isolation.

- Hyperarousal symptoms: the third category includes hyperarousal symptoms. As a result of being hypersensitive or on edge, patients may experience episodes of unprovoked anger, jumpiness, and seem to be "on guard" most of the time. Patients may behave as though they are facing constant threats of danger or further trauma. They can become hyperreactive to unexpected sounds or encounters. Problems with concentrating or remembering current information are common, and terrifying nightmares can lead to severe insomnia.

In addition to hearing the patient's complaints, the practitioner needs to assess other pertinent factors to help establish goals for the patient as part of the planning process and to determine level of insight and functional status. A short diagnostic tool such as Primary Care PTSD Screen for *DSM-5* (PC-PTSD-5), the Short Post-Traumatic Stress Disorder Rating Interview, or Trauma Screening Questionnaire (TSQ) can help quickly assess whether the patient is experiencing PTSD and add an objective dimension to the clinical assessment that can track patient outcome over time.

DIAGNOSTIC REASONING

Symptoms

To meet the official *DSM-5* criteria for a diagnosis of PTSD, symptoms must have persisted for more than 1 month and must have caused clinically significant distress in social, occupational, or other areas of functioning. See the *DSM-5* for the complete diagnostic criteria for PTSD.

Differential Diagnosis

Diagnosis is generally clinical in nature. The patient must meet the criterion for exposure to death, threatened death, actual or real physical injury, or actual or threatened physical violence and requires direct exposure or direct witnessing of the trauma, learning that a relative or close friend was exposed to trauma, or indirect exposure to aversive details of the trauma, such as first-responders. Symptoms must persist for more than 1 month. A mental status exam should be done as well as a complete physical exam. A complete medication review should occur to rule out effect of substances as well as ruling out other comorbidities and substance use.

A comprehensive physical examination should be performed to rule out organic causes for the patient's symptoms. If the history suggests that significant organic disease is unlikely, the physical examination should be comprehensive to document ways that the disorder may physiologically affect the patient. Laboratory tests to rule out physical causality should be considered.

MANAGEMENT

Pharmacological Management

Various medications can improve symptoms. The SSRIs paroxetine (Paxil) and sertraline (Zoloft) are approved for use in PTSD, and they are at times effective in its acute treatment. They have been shown to improve all core PTSD clusters (numbing, intrusions, hyperarousal), and are effective in both genders, all trauma types, and in patients with comorbid disorders.

Prazosin is no longer recommended except for treatment of PTSD associated nightmares and improved the quality of sleep in in combat-related PTSD. For some patients, TCAs may be effective. Anxiolytic medications can be used for acute or short-term symptom management only. Buspirone (BuSpar) may reduce intrusive symptoms for some patients and is a relatively safe anxiolytic.

Nonpharmacological Management

Patients with PTSD will be presenting with new onset of symptoms of PTSD, history of trauma, positive screening, and/or be currently diagnosed with PTSD. There needs to be a safety assessment made, and the history needs to be established, including the trauma history and duration and current medications. In general, there is a lack of well-designed, randomized clinical trials to inform the pharmacological or nonpharmacological management of PTSD. There are gaps in the study of PTSD in subgroups, such as those individuals with traumatic brain injury, combat-related symptoms, or comorbid psychiatric disorders. There needs to be more rigorous research undertaken with veterans and an agreed-on "recovery" definition of the disorder. The Department of Veterans Affairs, Department of Defense Clinical Practice Guidelines for the Management of Post-traumatic Stress Disorder (2017) first-line treatment recommendation is to implement "trauma-focused psychotherapy," defined as therapy that uses cognitive, emotional, or behavioral techniques to facilitate processing a traumatic experience and in which the trauma focus is a central component of the therapeutic process. The trauma-focused psychotherapies with the strongest evidence from clinical trials are prolonged exposure (PE), cognitive processing therapy (CPT), and eye movement desensitization and reprocessing (EMDR). These treatments have been tested in numerous clinical trials, in patients with complex presentations and comorbidities, compared with active control conditions, have long-term follow-up, and have been validated by research teams other than the developers. PE is based in emotional processing theory, which posits that PTSD symptoms arise as a result of cognitive and behavioral avoidance of trauma-related thoughts, reminders, activities, and situations. PE helps the client interrupt and reverse this process by blocking cognitive and behavioral avoidance, introducing corrective information, and facilitating organization and processing of the trauma memory and associated thoughts and beliefs. PE was developed originally for women with sexual assault trauma and is an effective first-line treatment with sustained benefit over time. One technique of PE, called "imaginal exposure" has the patient imagine and describe the trauma and associated emotions. This has been proven effective in reducing PTSD symptom severity. In vivo exposure uses systematic desensitization to triggers of trauma. With desensitization, the patient is exposed to his or her trauma "trigger" in a controlled environment. Improvement is achieved by gradually increasing the time of exposure to the trigger until the patient no longer reacts with panic.

Other protocols that have sufficient evidence to recommend use are: specific cognitive behavioral therapies for PTSD, brief eclectic psychotherapy (BEP), narrative exposure therapy (NET), and written narrative exposure. There are other psychotherapies that meet the definition of trauma-focused treatment for which there is currently insufficient evidence to recommend for or against their use. Stress inoculation therapy (SIT) may be considered a "toolbox" for managing anxiety and focuses on correcting the patient's intrusive symptoms by teaching relaxation techniques, such as breathing exercises, that can be used to help self-manage intrusive symptoms when they occur. Present-centered therapy (PCT), and interpersonal psychotherapy (IRT) is a brief approach (three sessions) that was found to decrease chronic nightmares and improve sleep quality. All of these approaches are specialized forms of care, but practitioners in primary-care settings can refer patients to providers who can offer these services. Another intervention for PTSD is psychodynamic psychotherapy, although there is insufficient evidence to recommend for or against. This method focuses on helping the patient to examine personal values and how the experience of the traumatic event violated them. The goal is to resolve the conscious and unconscious mental conflicts that were created by the trauma. The patient works on strengthening his or her self-esteem as a way of increasing the ability to cope with the trauma.

Group therapy or peer-counseling groups are also effective interventions for PTSD. Health groups can encourage members to share similar traumas and symptoms safely. Through participation in these groups, individuals with PTSD can learn that they are worthy and that they are not somehow guilty for their trauma. Patients may find it easier to learn new coping techniques from other group members. Relaxation therapy and other forms of complementary therapies are also helpful for persons with PTSD. Massage, positive imagery, meditation, and yoga have all been shown to be beneficial.

Shared decision-making regarding goals, expectations, and treatment plan is a cornerstone of treatment.

FOLLOW-UP AND REFERRAL

If a patient is not fully recovering from a traumatic experience, is living with suicidality or comorbidities, he or she should be referred to a PMHNP or psychiatrist. The symptoms of PTSD can be very disturbing, and some patients will require more time and support than is available in primary-care settings. Pharmacological management may also require specialized management, especially if an SSRI has been tried and the patient proves refractory to treatment. Patients will most likely wish to continue with their primary-care practitioner for some aspects of their care. Recovery from trauma is a slow process; patients may stop and start treatment for years. When this is the case, their relationship with their primary-care practitioner becomes a stabilizing force.

Patient Education: Post-traumatic Stress Disorder

It is important that the patient with PTSD and his or her family have a good understanding of the disorder, the chronic nature of PTSD, and the potential adverse effects of any medications prescribed. For some patients, interventions of a holistic nature may prove beneficial. Regular physical activity, good nutritional practices, and other self-care interventions can help to control symptomatology. Disease progression could lead to suicidal ideation and/or violence. The patient and family should be counseled regarding danger signs and the need for close follow-up and possible intervention.

SEXUAL ASSAULT

Sexual assault (SA) is defined by the National Institute of Justice as any unwanted sexual behavior against the person's will or lack of consent due to age, disability, or being under the influence of alcohol or drugs (Breiding et al., 2014; National Institute of Justice, 2017). Sexual assault could be an actual event or threat of the following:

- Intentional touching of the victim's genitals, anus, groin, or breasts
- Voyeurism
- Exposure to exhibitionism
- Undesired exposure to pornography
- Public display of images that were taken in a private context or when the victim was unaware

Rape is a form of sexual assault, but not all sexual assault is rape. The term rape is often used as a legal definition, and as of 2013 specifically includes a definition of sexual penetration without consent. For its Uniform Crime Reports, the FBI (2013) defines rape as "penetration, no matter how slight, of the vagina or anus with any body part or object, or oral penetration by a sex organ of another person, without the consent of the victim."

This also includes incidents where penetration is from a foreign object, such as a bottle. Victims can be male or female, and the perpetrator may be the opposite sex or the same sex as the victim. Attempted rape includes verbal threats of rape. Rape and sexual assault are often combined into one victimization measure in some surveys, and incidence and prevalence rates for sexual assault are often inaccurate due to barriers in obtaining these data. Force does not need to be physical; perpetrators may use emotional coercion, psychological force, or manipulation to coerce a victim into nonconsensual sex. Some perpetrators will use threats to force a victim to comply, such as threatening to hurt the victim or his or her family or other intimidation tactics.

Sexual assault is a violent act, one of conquest and control. The offender's intent is to dominate, humiliate, and degrade the victim. Sexual assault is a highly traumatic event that can have long-term effects on the physiological and psychological well-being of the survivor. It is important to note that victims of sexual assault can be female or male (Bureau of Justice Statistics, 2017).

Sexual assault can be a life-threatening situation. Perpetrators may urinate or defecate on their victims, ejaculate into their faces and hair, force anal intercourse, insert foreign objects into the vagina and/or rectum, and cause other physical injury, including death. After the sexual assault, the victim may have an "acute stress reaction" to the trauma. They may experience shame, confusion, humiliation, fear, and rage. Victims may develop PTSD, depression, or alcohol and/or drug abuse and are more likely to contemplate suicide. Rape is the most underreported crime, with 63% of sexual assaults not reported to police. Only 12% of child sexual abuse is reported to the authorities.

The majority of perpetrators are someone known to the victim. Approximately seven out of 10 sexual assaults are committed by someone known to the victim, such as in the case of intimate partner sexual violence or acquaintance rape, or date rape. Acquaintance rape is far more common than rape by strangers. Research has suggested that more than 50% of the women who have had nonconsensual vaginal, oral, or anal intercourse against their will do not label these experiences as sexual assault or rape. Sexual assault also includes child sexual abuse, sexual hate crimes, incest, male sexual assault, sexual harassment, stalking, partner rape, and sexual exploitation by trusted professionals including health-care providers, therapists, teachers, priests, and police officers.

EPIDEMIOLOGY AND CAUSES

In 2016 in the United States, there were 321,500 victims (age 12 or older) of rape and sexual assault (Bureau of Justice Statistics National Crime Victimization Survey [NCVS]; Morgan & Kena, 2017). Young people aged 18 to 24 years account for 54% of this figure. Of those

incidents, 39.1% were committed by strangers, whereas 60.9% were committed by perpetrators known to the survivors. The U.S. study of sexual assault titled "Rape in America" estimates that only one in six sexual assaults is actually reported to law enforcement. According to the NCVS, women who are young, unmarried, and in a low-income group are the most frequent victims of sexual assault. Divorced and single women experience higher rates of sexual assault than married or widowed women, and women in low-income groups experience higher rates of assault than women in moderate or high-income groups. In addition, women of color report sexual assault twice as frequently as do white American women, with African American, American Indian/Alaskan women, and women of mixed race reporting the highest lifetime rates of rape or attempted rape. Sexual assault is more likely to occur in the survivor's home (43%) or in the home of a friend (15%). Most sexual assaults (65%) occur in the evening and during the summer months. Finally, most sexual assault survivors (78%) know their perpetrators. When the sexual assault is committed by a stranger, 31% of the time the sexual assault takes place in the home of the survivor or a friend's home. In some cases, sexual assault is part of the larger picture of intimate partner violence.

Men who commit rape, according to crime statistics, are typically between 25 and 44 years of age; 51% are white and tend to rape white victims; 47% are black and tend to rape black victims; the remainder are mixed. Thirty-four percent of all forcible rapes involve alcohol. The Violence Against Women Act of 2005 created the Sexual Assault Services Program, which is federally funded and dedicated to direct intervention and related assistance for survivors of sexual assault. State and local communities have responded as well to combat sexual assault. Annually, rape costs the United States more than any other crime ($127 billion), followed by assault ($93 billion), murder ($71 billion), and drunk driving ($61 billion). Health care is 16% higher for women who were sexually abused as children.

PATHOPHYSIOLOGY

Sexual assault is an act of violence and humiliation that is expressed through sexual means. Power and anger are expressed through rape or sexual assault and are often part of another crime. Perpetrators may threaten their victims with physical force or weapons and frequently inflict physiological injury.

CLINICAL PRESENTATION

Through their work with sexual assault survivors, experts have identified a set of immediate and long-term effects of sexual assault called the *sexual assault trauma syndrome*. Sexual assault trauma syndrome is considered a normal response to sexual assault. There are two identified phases of survivor responses—the *initial* or *acute phase,* characterized by a period of disorganization, and the *long-term phase,* characterized by a period of reorganization.

Initial or Acute Phase

During the initial or acute phase, many sexual assault survivors experience both physical symptoms and emotions such as fear, shock, and disbelief. Four major categories of physical symptoms have been identified:

- Physical trauma: symptoms include soreness and bruising from the physical attack on the hands, throat, neck, breasts, thighs, legs, arms, back, buttocks, head, and face.
- Skeletal muscle tension: symptoms include tension headaches, fatigue, and sleep disturbances.
- Gastrointestinal irritability: symptoms include stomach pains, nausea, and a decreased appetite.
- Genitourinary disturbance: symptoms include vaginal and/or anal bleeding and bladder and vaginal infections.

Several researchers have observed in their study of sexual assault survivors that survivors tended to have one of two emotional response patterns—expressed or controlled. The expressed style is the expression of fear, anger, and anxiety through behaviors such as crying, sobbing, paradoxical smiling, restlessness, and tenseness. The controlled style masks the psychological distress with a calm, composed, subdued affect. Research has indicated equal numbers of both expressed and controlled response styles among sexual assault survivors.

Long-Term Phase

In the long-term phase, psychological symptoms such as depression, anxiety, and fear are prominent. This phase has three components:

- Motor activity: sexual assault survivors often exhibit an increase in motor activity with a range of activities, such as changing their residence and telephone number and adopting a variety of personal safety and security measures. They may turn to family and friends for assistance with these activities. Survivors may make special trips home or to some location that symbolizes safety and social acceptance.
- Nightmares: nightmares after sexual assault are often upsetting, and violent dreams can occur for months after the sexual assault. The nightmares may contain images that are clearly connected to the sexual assault, but nightmare content may also fail to be obviously related to the sexual assault.
- Trauma-phobia: as the term implies, *trauma-phobia* is a phobic reaction to trauma in which the phobia develops as a psychological defense against the sexual

assault experience. The more common phobias are fear of being indoors, fear of being outdoors, fear of being alone, fear of being in crowds, fear of having people behind the individual, and sexual fears. Fear of sexually transmitted disease (STD), including HIV, is also a powerful source of psychological trauma. It has been estimated that 4% to 30% of sexual assault survivors are diagnosed with an STD as a result of the sexual assault.

- Some victims of sexual assault have what has been called a "silent rape reaction"; these survivors have not reported the assault to anyone. They experience psychological burdening and are not able to resolve their thoughts and feelings about the sexual assault. Consider unreported sexual assault as a basis for atypical psychological symptoms such as atypical anxiety; abdominal pain not otherwise specified; sexual relationship problems; significant changes in sexual behavior patterns; unexplained, sudden onset of phobias; and chronic low self-esteem.

DIAGNOSTIC REASONING

The diagnosis of sexual assault is made by patient complaint and confirmed by forensic evidence.

MANAGEMENT

During the initial or acute phase, sexual assault survivors may be seen in emergency departments, rape crisis centers, primary-care offices, or police stations. If the sexual assault has occurred within the last 72 hours, forensic physical evidence should be collected. If the survivor chooses to remain anonymous, a "Jane Doe Rape Kit" enables forensic evidence to be collected without revealing identifying information. Survivors are given a code number that can be used to identify themselves if they choose to report later. The Violence Against Women and Department of Justice Reauthorization Act of 2005 (and reauthorized in 2013) provides that states may not require those who have experienced sexual assault to participate in the criminal justice system or cooperate with law enforcement in order to be provided with a forensic medical exam. Under this provision, a state must ensure access to an exam free of charge even if the survivor chooses not to report to the police or otherwise cooperate with the criminal justice system (U.S. Department of Justice Office on Violence Against Women, 2013).

The use of a sexual assault nurse examiner (SANE), if one is available, is highly recommended. These nurses receive special training in collecting forensic evidence and providing crisis intervention and offer a number of advantages over emergency department practitioners. For example, the survivor is seen by one specialist rather than by several practitioners, which decreases the time a sexual assault survivor spends in the emergency department and ensures that she (or he) receives sensitive, nonjudgmental care by a practitioner who is a sexual assault specialist. Equally important, the nurse is skilled in the collection of forensic evidence, resulting in higher conviction rates of sexual assault. Law enforcement should be involved; however, patients may decline to discuss the assault with police. Conversely, in some cases, patients may choose to cooperate so that testing costs will be paid by law enforcement. Initial treatment for sexual assault survivors includes the sexual assault interview, physical exam for physical assessment and forensic evidence collection, and crisis intervention.

The Sexual Assault Interview

Before the interview, the capacity of the patient to consent to a forensic examination should be assessed. This can be done by evaluating understanding and appropriate responses when obtaining the diagnostic history. Drugs, alcohol, developmental disability, or young age may cause a delay in obtaining the patient's consent. In the case of severe head or critical injury, law enforcement may provide a court order to proceed with forensic evidence collection. Before doing a diagnostic physical exam, it is imperative to address psychological issues related to the examination itself. Patients presenting after sexual assault have undergone an experience that denied them the right to consent. There are important psychological and legal implications with obtaining forensic evidence, and the patient's consent and opportunity for a family member, friend, or patient advocate to be present should not be undervalued.

The sexual assault interview is performed in a room away from the waiting areas and exam rooms, while the survivor is still fully clothed, often with a police officer present. It should not be rushed and should be conducted with sensitivity. The sexual assault interview begins with general health information, including drug allergies, current medications including birth control, surgical history, tetanus, and hepatitis B immunization if relevant, major health problems, pregnancy status if known, first day of last menstrual period, gravidity, parity, history of STDs, and most recent consensual sexual contact.

Questions about the sexual assault follow the general health information questions. Although this history is difficult for the patient to report, it is important to obtain an accurate history for collection of forensic evidence in order for the examiner to locate all points of physical contact and penetration, as well as documenting the survivor's activity immediately after the sexual assault.

The sexual assault survivor is asked the date, time, and place of the sexual assault and all events surrounding the sexual assault. Inquire about the use of force or threats of force, including threats of future harm to the patient or acquaintance, presence of a weapon, or threats to expose a personal secret. Notation of the type of force; use of restraints; number of assailants; and type of assault, such as fondling, kissing, licking, penetration or attempted penetration of the mouth, vagina, or anus by finger, object, or penis need to be documented. "Drug-facilitated sexual abuse" associated with gamma-hydroxybutyrate (GHB) or alcohol may be suspected when the patient also reports lapses in consciousness, and GHB may be detected in urine up to 96 hours after consumption. Ask whether a condom was used. Ask about activities since the assault, such as bathing, urinating, defecating, douching, gargling, eating, brushing teeth, and washing or wiping self.

A complete physical exam should be performed, assessing for injury and potential evidence. All physical exam and forensic evidence collection procedures should be fully explained with ample opportunities for clarification if needed. The physical examination can be traumatic for survivors; thus, survivors should be allowed to control the exam as much as possible. This can be accomplished by letting survivors know they can refuse any part of the exam or stop the procedure at any time. Sexual assault survivors should also be encouraged to have a support person, such as a friend, spouse, or family member with them during the exam. In addition, a counselor or patient advocate from the local rape crisis center may also be available to support the sexual assault survivor during the exam. Although sexual assault survivors may decline such support, they should be offered and encouraged to accept it.

Physical Examination and Forensic Evidence Collection

The practitioner needs to be aware of state guidelines for evidence collection. The physical exam begins with the removal of all items of clothing. Each item of clothing worn at the time of the sexual assault is placed in a separate bag and then signed over to a law enforcement officer as forensic evidence. Physical forensic evidence that can be found on clothing includes hair, blood, semen, and saliva. Gloves should be worn throughout the physical exam to preserve evidence.

The sexual assault kit, available in most states, should contain all materials needed. Become familiar with the forms before doing the sexual assault exam. Document the general appearance of the patient and complete a head-to-toe assessment for signs of trauma, including an oral exam, skin exam for lacerations, swelling, broken fingernails, and foreign material such as leaves, grass, fibers, dried blood, and dried secretions anywhere on the body. Forensic evidence includes samples of the individual's hair (head and pubic) and saliva; oral, vaginal, and rectal swabs; and fingernail scrapings. It is important to label specimens accurately, noting the collection time and date and the signature of each person who provided and received them.

A detailed anogenital exam is performed to assess for injury. Pelvic, vaginal, and rectal exams are completed at the end of the exam. Colposcope and/or toluidine blue dye can be used to assess genital injury, providing permanent documentation of injuries that may heal very quickly and avoiding subjecting the patient to reexamination or potential loss of evidence. Toluidine blue dye is a nuclear stain that adheres to the areas of injury on subepithelial nucleated cells but not to intact epithelial cells;

therefore, it is not useful for mucosal surfaces, such as the vagina or anus. Almost half of genital exams done with a colposcope of women who have been raped will have a normal exam. Anoscopy is utilized to view the extent of rectal injuries. Genital injuries can also be detected when women participate in consensual intercourse. Although forensic evidence should be collected as soon as possible, exams performed several days after the sexual assault can still produce findings.

Laboratory testing for STDs is recommended only if treatment is deferred. STD testing at this time would detect only pre-assault infection. Consider testing in minors, because they are unable to give consent to engage in intercourse. However, serological testing for HIV, hepatitis B, and syphilis is recommended because the efficacy of prophylactic treatment is not complete. Seroconversion that is attributed to the assault may be covered by the Victims of Violent Crimes Fund. Further collection of blood, buccal, and urine specimens is recommended for crime lab testing for DNA, pregnancy testing for all women of childbearing age, and toxicology analysis if indicate. A 6-year, retrospective study of 1,421 sexual assault patients who presented to the emergency department found that 12% reported drug-facilitated sexual assault. This group had a longer delay in presentation to the emergency department, less often had police involvement, and had a decreased occurrence of genital and other injury. Hospitalization may be necessary to treat unstable medical conditions or to provide surgical intervention or psychiatric stabilization.

Nonpharmacological Treatment

Crisis intervention with sexual assault survivors includes encouraging them to talk about their feelings, validating these feelings, educating survivors about rape trauma syndrome, and identifying concerns related to the sexual assault. Psychological support is necessary to address the patient's needs and should be done before the sexual assault interview. These concerns include prevention of pregnancy and/or STDs, physical safety, and the need for specialized sexual assault psychotherapy and community support groups. Physical safety becomes a focus of concern for anyone who has just been assaulted. Sexual assault survivors can become preoccupied with the fear that their attacker will try to hurt them again. This is especially true when the survivor knows the identity of the attacker or the assault occurred in the survivor's home. Clinicians can help survivors start to problem-solve safety concerns and help to meet the survivor's immediate needs for safety. Some individuals may elect to live with friends or family until they begin to feel safe again.

A supportive approach and focusing on restoring the victim's sense of adequacy and control over his or her life are the best means for supporting the survivor provided there is no severe underlying pathology that might warrant a different treatment plan. Group therapy with homogeneous groups has been found to be effective for many. A rape victim fares best when he or she receives immediate support and can ventilate feelings of rage and fear to loving family members and to supportive clinicians and law enforcement officials. A longitudinal study of sexual assault survivors showed that negative social reactions and blame of the victim were associated with worsened PTSD symptoms.

Pharmacological Treatment

Medications to treat STDs and pregnancy should be offered. A tetanus booster is necessary if patients who experienced lacerations or abrasions have not been adequately immunized. HIV counseling, as well as testing and prophylaxis, should be offered to all survivors. Provider encouragement was shown to have an association with the patient's decision to start HIV prophylaxis treatment. Referral to an infectious disease specialist should be considered to guide antiretroviral therapy. Hepatitis B surface antibody testing with vaccination should be offered and hepatitis B immunoglobulin should be offered if there is a high risk of exposure by a known hepatitis B–positive assailant. Emergency contraception should be offered to female patients after penile-vaginal assault, especially to those patients who have not had a tubal ligation or do not have an intrauterine device (von Hertzen et al., 2002). Referral to an obstetrician/gynecologist and a urology specialist may be needed for treatment for specific traumatic injuries that require further care.

FOLLOW-UP AND REFERRAL

Sexual assault survivors should be encouraged to use the support services available from community rape counseling centers, such as individual therapy, group therapy, and self-defense training, as well as legal follow-up. The majority of rape counseling centers offer 24-hour crisis hotlines. Many individuals may not feel they need this support or that their family and friends are there for them. Survivors continue to be at risk for long-term problems, however, and to have grief and mourning needs long after the immediate crisis has passed and significant others have come to believe that the crisis is over. Rape counseling center personnel understand the long-term course of events of sexual assault. Some rape counseling centers are also able to provide advocates to support survivors as they deal with the legal and judicial systems. These services are often offered free of charge or at greatly reduced rates.

Medical follow-up after the initial visit includes reassessment of any traumatic injuries, review of laboratory results, post-HIV test counseling, and reassessment of psychological status and recovery. Retesting for pregnancy should be considered if the patient has not had the expected menstrual period. Repeat HIV, hepatitis B, and STD testing should be performed as indicated.

Patient Education: Sexual Assault

Education begins with the first patient encounter, allowing the survivor to regain control and become an active participant in her recovery, incorporating patient-centered care. Include education about the diagnostic work-up, management, psychological and medical recovery, and advice about community support services, as well as discussion of the long-term effects of sexual assault. Impress on the patient the need to engage with psychological evaluation early on. The most common long-term effect of sexual assault is the development of PTSD. Recent research has indicated that sexual assault survivors may be the largest single group of individuals with PTSD. PTSD was originally defined to explain the set of symptoms observed in survivors of natural disasters and military combat and includes symptoms such as anxiety, depression, nightmares, flashbacks, and sleep disturbances. Researchers have found that 94% of the women who had been sexually assaulted met the criteria for PTSD 12 days after the sexual assault and that 46% of these women still met the criteria 3 months later.

In addition to having higher rates of PTSD, sexual assault survivors report higher rates of drug and alcohol problems, depression, attempted suicide, anxiety, OCD, and medical care use. Sexual assault survivors were 13.4 times more likely to have had alcohol-related problems and 26 times more likely to have had problems with drug abuse, compared with women who were not sexually assaulted. Survivors were three times more likely to have had a major episode of depression, four times more likely to have had thoughts about suicide, and 13 times more likely to have attempted suicide compared with other women. Finally, survivors of sexual assault report more symptoms of illness across all body systems and perceive their health less favorably than do other women. Symptoms that are diagnosed at a much higher rate in sexual assault survivors include chronic pelvic pain, gastrointestinal disorders, headaches, general pain, and premenstrual symptoms. Every effort should be made to encourage the patient to initiate long-term support for dealing with the trauma of sexual assault. The health-care provider, practicing within a *Circle of Caring*, may be in the best position to maintain contact with the patient and facilitate growth and healing.

REFERENCES

Generalized Anxiety Disorder

Andrews G, Cuijpers P, Craske MG, McEvoy P, Titov N. Computer therapy for the anxiety and depressive disorders is effective, acceptable and practical health care: A meta-analysis. PLoS ONE 2010;5(10):e13196

Arch JJ, Ayers CR, Baker A, et al. Randomized clinical trial of adapted mindfulness-based stress reduction versus group cognitive behavioral therapy for heterogeneous anxiety disorders. *Behav Res Ther.* 2013;51:185.

Baker SL, et al. The Liebowitz Social Anxiety Scale as a self-report instrument: A preliminary psychometric analysis. *Behav Res Ther.* 2002;40:701–715.

Baldwin DS, et al. Evidence-based guidelines for the pharmacological treatment of anxiety disorders: Recommendations from the British Association for Psychopharmacology. *J Psychopharmacol.* 2005;19(6):57–59.

Benitez J, Jablonski MR, Allen JD, Winner JG. The clinical validity and utility of combinatorial pharmacogenomics: Enhancing patient outcomes. *Appl Transl Genom.* 2015;5:47–49.

Bereza BG, Machado M, Einarson TR. Systematic review and quality assessment of economic evaluations and quality-of-life studies related to generalized anxiety disorder. *Clin Ther.* 2009;31:1279–1308.

Bonadonna R. Meditation's impact on chronic illness. *Holist Nurs Pract.* 2003;17(6):309–319.

Brenes GA, Danhauer SC, Lyles MF, et al. Telephone-delivered cognitive behavioral therapy and telephone-delivered nondirective supportive therapy for rural older adults with generalized anxiety disorder: A randomized clinical trial. *JAMA Psychiatry.* 2015;72:1012–1020.

Brown TA, Barlow DH. Anxiety and Related Disorders Interview Schedule for *DSM-5* (ADIS-5), disorders interview schedule for *DSM-5*: Lifetime version (ADIS-5L), Clinician's manual. Oxford University Press; 2014

Christensen MC, Loft H, Florea I, McIntyre RS. Efficacy of vortioxetine in working patients with generalized anxiety disorder. *CNS Spectr.* 2017:1–9.

Craske M. *Cognitive behavior therapy.* Washington, DC: American Psychological Association; 2009.

Dear BF, Titov N, Sunderland M, et al. Psychometric comparison of the Generalized Anxiety Disorder Scale—7 and the Penn State Worry Questionnaire for measuring response during treatment of generalised anxiety disorder. *Cogn Behav Ther.* 2011;40:216–227.

Fava M, et al. Zolpidem extended-release improves sleep and next-day symptoms in comorbid insomnia and generalized anxiety disorder. *J Clin Psychopharmacol.* 2009;29(3):222–230.

Gommoll C, Durgam S, Mathews M, et al. A double-blind, randomized, placebo-controlled, fixed-dose phase III study of vilazodone in patients with generalized anxiety disorder. *Depress Anxiety.* 2015;32:451–459.

Hall J, Kellett S, Berrios R, et al. Efficacy of cognitive behavioral therapy for generalized anxiety disorder in older adults: systematic review, meta-analysis, and meta-regression. *Am J Geriatr Psychiatry.* 2016;24:1063–1073.

Hays P, Iwamasa G. Culturally responsive cognitive behavioral therapy: Assessment, practice, and supervision. Washington, DC: American Psychological Association; 2006.

Hofmann SG, Smits JA. Cognitive-behavioral therapy for adult anxiety disorders: A meta-analysis of randomized placebo-controlled trials. *J Clin Psychiatry.* 2008;69:621–632.

Huh J, Goebert D, Takeshita J, Lu BY, Kang M. Treatment of generalized anxiety disorder: A comprehensive review of the literature for psychopharmacologic alternatives to newer antidepressants and benzodiazepines. *Prim Care Companion CNS Disord.* 2011;13.

Katzman MA, Bleau P, Chokka P, et al.; Canadian Anxiety Guidelines Initiative Group on behalf of the Anxiety Disorders Association of Canada/Association Canadienne des troubles anxieux and McGill University. Canadian clinical practice guidelines for the management of anxiety, posttraumatic stress and obsessive-compulsive disorders. *BMC Psychiatry.* 2014;14(suppl 1):S1.

Kertz S, Bigda-Peyton J, Bjorgvinsson T. Validity of the generalized anxiety disorder—7 scale in an acute psychiatric sample. *Clin Psychol Psychother*. 2013;20:456–464.

Kishita N, Laidlaw K. Cognitive behaviour therapy for generalized anxiety disorder: Is CBT equally efficacious in adults of working age and older adults? *Clin Psychol Rev*. 2017;52:124–136.

Kreys TJ, Phan SV. A literature review of quetiapine for generalized anxiety disorder. *Pharmacotherapy*. 2015;35:175–188.

Locke, A, Kirst, N, Schultz, CG. Diagnosis and management of generalized anxiety disorder and panic disorder in adults. *Am Fam Physician*. 2015;91(9):617–624.

Miranda J, Bernal G, Lau A, et al. State of the science on psychosocial interventions for ethnic minorities. *Annu Rev Clin Psychol*. 2005;1:113–142.

Möller H-J, Bandelow B, Volz H-P, Barnikol UB, Seifritz E, Kasper S. The relevance of "mixed anxiety and depression" as a diagnostic category in clinical practice. *Eur Arch Psychiatry Clin Neurosci*. 2016;266(8):725–736.

National Institute of Mental Health. Women and mental health. https://www.nimh.nih.gov/health/topics/women-and-mental-health/index.shtml. Published 2016. Accessed September 3, 2018

Stahl S. *Essential psychopharmacology: The prescriber's guide*. 5th ed. New York, NY: Cambridge University/Stahl Press; 2014.

Stein MB, Sareen J. Clinical Practice. Generalized anxiety disorder. *N Engl J Med*. 2015;373(21):2059–2068.

Tully PJ, Cosh SM, Baune BT. A review of the affects of worry and generalized anxiety disorder upon cardiovascular health and coronary heart disease. *Psychol Health Med*. 2013;18:627–644.

Walkup J, Albano A, Piacentini J, et al. Cognitive behavioral therapy, sertraline, or a combination in childhood anxiety. *N Engl J Med*. 2008;359(26):2753–2766.

Weisberg RB. Overview of generalized anxiety disorder: Epidemiology, presentation, and course. *J Clin Psychiatry*. 2009;70(suppl 2):4–9.

Wetherell JL, Petkus AJ, White KS, et al. Antidepressant medication augmented with cognitive-behavioral therapy for generalized anxiety disorder in older adults. *Am J Psychiatry*. 2013;170:782–789.

Zhang X, Norton J, Carrière I. Risk factors for late-onset generalized anxiety disorder: results from a 12-year prospective cohort (the ESPRIT study). *Transl Psychiatry*. 2015;5:e536.

Zung WWK. A rating instrument for anxiety disorders. *Psychosomatics*. 1971;12:371–379.

Panic Disorder

Allen L, Barlow D. Treatment of panic disorder: outcomes and basic processes. In: Rothbaum B, ed. *Pathological anxiety: Emotional processing in etiology and treatment*. New York, NY: Guilford Press; 2006:166.

American Psychiatric Association. *Practice guideline for the treatment of patients with panic disorder*. 2nd ed. Washington, DC: American Psychiatric Association; 2009.

Antony MM, Ledley DR, Liss A, Swinson RP. Responses to symptom induction exercises in panic disorder. *Behav Res Ther*. 2006;44:85–98.

Arch JJ, Ayers CR, Baker A, et al. Randomized clinical trial of adapted mindfulness-based stress reduction versus group cognitive behavioral therapy for heterogeneous anxiety disorders. *Behav Res Ther*. 2013;51:185–196.

Cosci F, Knuts IJ, Abrams K, et al. Cigarette smoking and panic: A critical review of the literature. *J Clin Psychiatry*. 2010;71:606–615.

Cosci F, Schruers KR, Abrams K, Griez EJ. Alcohol use disorders and panic disorder: A review of the evidence of a direct relationship. *J Clin Psychiatry*. 2007;68:874–880.

Craske MG, Stein MB, Sullivan G, et al. Disorder-specific impact of coordinated anxiety learning and management treatment for anxiety disorders in primary care. *Arch Gen Psychiatry*. 2011;68:378–388.

Deacon B, Abramowitz J. A pilot study of two-day cognitive-behavioral therapy for panic disorder. *Behav Res Ther*. 2006;44:807–817.

Favreau H, Bacon SL, Labrecque M, Lavoie KL. Prospective impact of panic disorder and panic-anxiety on asthma control, health service use, and quality of life in adult patients with asthma over a 4-year follow-up. *Psychosom Med*. 2014;76:147–155.

Gloster AT, Sonntag R, Hoyer J, et al. Treating treatment-resistant patients with panic disorder and agoraphobia using psychotherapy: A randomized controlled switching trial. *Psychother Psychosom*. 2015;84:100–109.

Goodwin RD, Talley NJ, Hotopf M, et al. A link between physician-diagnosed ulcer and anxiety disorders among adults. *Ann Epidemiol*. 2013;23:189–192.

Grant BF, Goldstein RB, Saha TD, et al. Epidemiology of *DSM-5* alcohol use disorder: Results from the National Epidemiologic Survey on Alcohol and Related Conditions III. *JAMA Psychiatry*. 2015;72:757–766.

Hunt TKA, Slack KS, Berger LM. Adverse childhood experiences and behavioral problems in middle childhood. *Child Abuse Negl*. 2017;67:391–402.

Kabat-Zinn J, Massion AO, Kristeller J, et al. Effectiveness of a meditation-based stress reduction program in the treatment of anxiety disorders. *Am J Psychiatry*. 1992;149:936–943.

Kim S, Wollburg E, Roth WT. Opposing breathing therapies for panic disorder: A randomized controlled trial of lowering vs raising end-tidal $P(CO_2)$. *J Clin Psychiatry*. 2012;73:931–939.

Kimmel R, Roy-Byrne PP, Cowley DS. Pharmacological treatments for panic disorder, generalized anxiety disorder, specific phobia and social anxiety disorder. In: Nathan PE, Gorman JM, eds. *A guide to treatments that work*. 4th ed. New York, NY: Oxford University Press; 2015:337–353.

Klahn AL, Klinkenberg IA, Lueken U, et al. Commonalities and differences in the neural substrates of threat predictability in panic disorder and specific phobia. *Neuroimage Clin*. 2017;14:530–537.

Lessard MJ, Marchand A, Pelland MÈ, et al. Comparing two brief psychological interventions to usual care in panic disorder patients presenting to the emergency department with chest pain. *Behav Cogn Psychother*. 2012;40:129–147.

Metzler M, Merrick MT, Klevens J, et al. Adverse childhood experiences and life opportunities: Shifting the narrative. *Child Youth Serv Rev*. 2017;72:141–149.

Meuret AE, Rosenfield D, Seidel A, et al. Respiratory and cognitive mediators of treatment change in panic disorder: Evidence for intervention specificity. *J Consult Clin Psychol*. 2010;78:691–704.

Miller JJ, Fletcher K, Kabat-Zinn J. Three-year follow-up and clinical implications of a mindfulness meditation-based stress reduction intervention in the treatment of anxiety disorders. *Gen Hosp Psychiatry*. 1995;17:192–200.

Milrod BL, et al. Manual of panic-focused psychodynamic psychotherapy. Washington, DC: American Psychiatric Press; 1997.

Milrod B, Chambless DL, Gallop R, et al. Psychotherapies for panic disorder: A tale of two sites. *J Clin Psychiatry*. 2016;77(7):927–935.

Milrod B, Leon AC, Busch F, et al. A randomized controlled clinical trial of psychoanalytic psychotherapy for panic disorder. *Am J Psychiatry*. 2007;164:265–272.

Roy-Byrne P, Craske MG, Sullivan G, et al. Delivery of evidence-based treatment for multiple anxiety disorders in primary care: a randomized controlled trial. *JAMA*. 2010;303:1921–1928.

Sanderson W, Bruce T. Causes and management of treatment-resistant panic disorder and agoraphobia: A survey of expert therapists. *Cogn Behav Pract*. 2007;14:48–59.

Schneider AJ, Mataix-Cols D, Marks IM, Bachofen M. Internet-guided self-help with or without exposure therapy for phobic and panic disorders. *Psychother Psychosom.* 2005;74:154–164.

Smitherman TA, Kolivas ED, Bailey JR. Panic disorder and migraine: Comorbidity, mechanisms, and clinical implications. *Headache.* 2013;53:23–45.

Spek V, Cuijpers P, Nyklícek I, et al. Internet-based cognitive behaviour therapy for symptoms of depression and anxiety: A meta-analysis. *Psychol Med.* 2007;37:319–328.

Su VY, Chen YT, Lin WC, et al. Sleep apnea and risk of panic disorder. *Ann Fam Med.* 2015;13:325–330.

Stein DJ, Aguilar-Gaxiola S, Alonso J, et al. Associations between mental disorders and subsequent onset of hypertension. *Gen Hosp Psychiatry.* 2014;36:142–149.

Tully PJ, Turnbull DA, Beltrame J, et al. Panic disorder and incident coronary heart disease: A systematic review and meta-regression in 1131612 persons and 58111 cardiac events. *Psychol Med.* 2015;45:2909–2920.

Vos SP, Huibers MJ, Diels L, Arntz A. A randomized clinical trial of cognitive behavioral therapy and interpersonal psychotherapy for panic disorder with agoraphobia. *Psychol Med.* 2012;42:2661–2672.

White KS, Payne LA, Gorman JM, et al. Does maintenance CBT contribute to long-term treatment response of panic disorder with or without agoraphobia? A randomized controlled clinical trial. *J Consult Clin Psychol.* 2013;81:47–57.

Post-traumatic Stress Disorder

Ahmadpanah M, Sabzeiee P, Hosseini SM, et al. Comparing the effect of prazosin and hydroxyzine on sleep quality in patients suffering from posttraumatic stress disorder. *Neuropsychobiology.* 2014;69:235–242.

American Academy of Sleep Medicine. *International classification of sleep disorders.* 3rd ed. Darien, IL: American Academy of Sleep Medicine; 2014.

American Psychiatric Association. *Practice guidelines for the treatment of patients with acute stress disorder and posttraumatic stress disorder.* Arlington, VA: American Psychiatric Association; 2009. **https://psychiatryonline.org/pb/assets/raw/sitewide/practice_guidelines/guidelines/acutestressdisorderptsd-watch.pdf.** Reviewed 2018.

Anderson KN, Bradley AJ. Sleep disturbance in mental health problems and neurodegenerative disease. *Nat Sci Sleep.* 2013;5:61–75.

Blevins CA, Weathers FW, Davis MT, et al. The Posttraumatic Stress Disorder Checklist for *DSM-5* (PCL-5): Development and initial psychometric evaluation. *J Trauma Stress.* 2015;28:489–498.

Dedert EA, Calhoun PS, Watkins LL, et al. Posttraumatic stress disorder, cardiovascular, and metabolic disease: A review of the evidence. *Ann Behav Med.* 2010;39:61–78.

Department of Veterans Affairs, Department of Defense. Clinical practice guideline for management of post-traumatic stress, version 2.0. **http://www.healthquality.va.gov/guidelines/MH/ptsd.** Published October 2010. Accessed January 23, 2017.

Detweiler MB, Pagadala B, Candelario J, et al. Treatment of post-traumatic stress disorder nightmares at a Veterans Affairs Medical Center. *J Clin Med.* 2016;5(12).

De Venter M, Van Den Eede F, Pattyn T, et al. Impact of childhood trauma on course of panic disorder: Contribution of clinical and personality characteristics. *Acta Psychiatr Scand.* 2017;135:554.

Ehlers A, Clark DM, Hackmann A, et al. A randomized controlled trial of cognitive therapy, a self-help booklet, and repeated assessments as early interventions for posttraumatic stress disorder. *Arch Gen Psychiatry.* 2003;60(10):1024–1032.

Ehlers A, Grey N, Wild J, et al. Implementation of cognitive therapy for PTSD in routine clinical care: Effectiveness and moderators of outcome in a consecutive sample. *Behav Res Ther.* 2013;51(11):742–752.

Ehlers A, Hackmann A, Grey N, et al. A randomized controlled trial of 7-day intensive and standard weekly cognitive therapy for PTSD and emotion-focused supportive therapy. *Am J Psychiatry.* 2014;171(3):294–304.

Escamilla M, LaVoy M, Moore BA, Krakow B. Management of posttraumatic nightmares: A review of pharmacologic and nonpharmacologic treatments since 2010. *Curr Psychiatry Rep.* 2012;14:529–535.

Fazel M, Wheeler J, Danesh J. Prevalence of serious mental disorder in 7000 refugees resettled in Western countries: A systematic review. *Lancet.* 2005;365:1309–1314.

Feczer D, Bjorklund P. Forever changed: Posttraumatic stress disorder in female military veterans, a case report. *Perspect Psychiatr Care.* 2009;45(4):278–291.

Foa EB, Hembree EA, Cahill SP, et al. Randomized trial of prolonged exposure for posttraumatic stress disorder with and without cognitive restructuring: Outcome at academic and community clinics. *J Consult Clin Psychol.* 2005;73(5):953–964.

Forbes D, Phelps A, McHugh T. Treatment of combat-related nightmares using imagery rehearsal: A pilot study. *J Trauma Stress.* 2001;14:433–442.

Galea S, et al. The epidemiology of post-traumatic stress disorder after disasters. *Epidemiol Rev.* 2005;27(1):78–91.

Gauchat A, Séguin JR, Zadra A. Prevalence and correlates of disturbed dreaming in children. *Pathol Biol (Paris).* 2014;62:311–318.

George KC, Kebejian L, Ruth LJ, et al. Meta-analysis of the efficacy and safety of prazosin versus placebo for the treatment of nightmares and sleep disturbances in adults with posttraumatic stress disorder. *J Trauma Dissociation.* 2016;17:494–510.

Gradus JL, Farkas DK, Svensson E, et al. Posttraumatic stress disorder and cancer risk: A nationwide cohort study. *Eur J Epidemiol.* 2015;30:563–568.

Greenberg MS, Tanev K, Marin MF, Pitman RK. Stress, PTSD, and dementia. *Alzheimers Dement.* 2014;10:S155–S165.

Harb GC, Phelps AJ, Forbes D, et al. A critical review of the evidence base of imagery rehearsal for posttraumatic nightmares: Pointing the way for future research. *J Trauma Stress.* 2013;26:570–579.

Hartmann E. The underlying emotion and the dream relating dream imagery to the dreamer's underlying emotion can help elucidate the nature of dreaming. *Int Rev Neurobiol.* 2010;92:197–214.

Ho FY, Chan CS, Tang KN. Cognitive-behavioral therapy for sleep disturbances in treating posttraumatic stress disorder symptoms: A meta-analysis of randomized controlled trials. *Clin Psychol Rev.* 2016;43:90–102.

Husarewycz MN, El-Gabalawy R, Logsetty S, Sareen J. The association between number and type of traumatic life experiences and physical conditions in a nationally representative sample. *Gen Hosp Psychiatry.* 2014;36:26–32.

Jetly R, Heber A, Fraser G, Boisvert D. The efficacy of nabilone, a synthetic cannabinoid, in the treatment of PTSD-associated nightmares: A preliminary randomized, double-blind, placebo-controlled cross-over design study. *Psychoneuroendocrinology.* 2015;51:585–588.

Johannesson KB, Arinell H, Arnberg FK. Six years after the wave. Trajectories of posttraumatic stress following a natural disaster. *J Anxiety Disord.* 2015;36:15–24.

Khachatryan D, Groll D, Booij L, et al. Prazosin for treating sleep disturbances in adults with posttraumatic stress disorder: A systematic review and meta-analysis of randomized controlled trials. *Gen Hosp Psychiatry.* 2016;39:46–52.

Leeies M, Pagura J, Sareen J, Bolton JM. The use of alcohol and drugs to self-medicate symptoms of posttraumatic stress disorder. *Depress Anxiety.* 2010;27:731–761.

Levrier K, Marchand A, Belleville G, et al. Nightmare frequency, nightmare distress and the efficiency of trauma-focused cognitive behavioral therapy for post-traumatic stress disorder. *Arch Trauma Res.* 2016;5:e33051.

Lohr JB, Palmer BW, Eidt CA, et al. Is post-traumatic stress disorder associated with premature senescence? A review of the literature. *Am J Geriatr Psychiatry.* 2015;23:709–725.

Mason SM, Flint AJ, Roberts AL, et al. Posttraumatic stress disorder symptoms and food addiction in women by timing and type of trauma exposure. *JAMA Psychiatry.* 2014;71:1271–1278.

Monson CM, Fredman SJ, Macdonald A, et al. Effect of cognitive-behavioral couple therapy for PTSD: A randomized controlled trial. *JAMA.* 2012;308:700–709.

Nash WP, Boasso AM, Steenkamp MM, et al. Posttraumatic stress in deployed marines: Prospective trajectories of early adaptation. *J Abnorm Psychol.* 2015;124:155–171.

O'Donovan A, Cohen BE, Seal KH, et al. Elevated risk for autoimmune disorders in Iraq and Afghanistan veterans with posttraumatic stress disorder. *Biol Psychiatry.* 2015;77:365–374.

Pagura J, Stein MB, Bolton JM, et al. Comorbidity of borderline personality disorder and posttraumatic stress disorder in the U.S. population. *J Psychiatr Res.* 2010;44:1190–1198.

Paul F, Schredl M, Alpers GW. Nightmares affect the experience of sleep quality but not sleep architecture: an ambulatory polysomnographic study. *Borderline Personal Disord Emot Dysregul.* 2015;2:3.

Punamäki RL, Palosaari E, Diab M, et al. Trajectories of posttraumatic stress symptoms (PTSS) after major war among Palestinian children: Trauma, family- and child-related predictors. *J Affect Disord.* 2015;172:133–140.

Raskind MA, Peterson K, Williams T, et al. A trial of prazosin for combat trauma PTSD with nightmares in active-duty soldiers returned from Iraq and Afghanistan. *Am J Psychiatry.* 2013;170:1003–1010.

Roberts AL, Agnew-Blais JC, Spiegelman D, et al. Posttraumatic stress disorder and incidence of type 2 diabetes mellitus in a sample of women: A 22-year longitudinal study. *JAMA Psychiatry.* 2015;72:203–210.

Rosenberg L, Rosenberg M, Robert R, et al. Does acute stress disorder predict subsequent posttraumatic stress disorder in pediatric burn survivors? *J Clin Psychiatry.* 2015;76:1564–1568.

Schnurr PP. Focusing on trauma-focused psychotherapy for posttraumatic stress disorder. *Curr Opin Psychol.* 2017;14:56–60.

Schnurr PP, Hayes AF, Lunney CA, et al. Longitudinal analysis of the relationship between symptoms and quality of life in veterans treated for posttraumatic stress disorder. *J Consult Clin Psychol.* 2006;74:707–713.

Schredl M, Reinhard I. Gender differences in nightmare frequency: A meta-analysis. *Sleep Med Rev.* 2011;15:115–121.

Seda G, Sanchez-Ortuno MM, Welsh CH, et al. Comparative meta-analysis of prazosin and imagery rehearsal therapy for nightmare frequency, sleep quality, and posttraumatic stress. *J Clin Sleep Med.* 2015;11:11–22.

Shapiro F. Eye movement desensitization: A new treatment for post-traumatic stress disorder. *J Behav Ther Exp Psychiatry.* 1989;20(3):211–217.

Simor P, Horváth K, Gombos F, et al. Disturbed dreaming and sleep quality: Altered sleep architecture in subjects with frequent nightmares. *Eur Arch Psychiatry Clin Neurosci.* 2012;262:687–696.

Singh B, Hughes AJ, Mehta G, et al. Efficacy of prazosin in posttraumatic stress disorder: A systematic review and meta-analysis. *Prim Care Companion CNS Disord.* 2016;18(4).

Sjöström N, Waern M, Hetta J. Nightmares and sleep disturbances in relation to suicidality in suicide attempters. *Sleep.* 2007;30:91–95.

Spoont MR, Williams JW Jr, Kehle-Forbes S, et al. Does this patient have posttraumatic stress disorder?: Rational clinical examination systematic review. *JAMA.* 2015;314:501–510.

Taft CT, Watkins LE, Stafford J, et al. Posttraumatic stress disorder and intimate relationship problems: a meta-analysis. *J Consult Clin Psychol.* 2011;79:22–33.

Tribl GG, Wetter TC, Schredl M. Dreaming under antidepressants: a systematic review on evidence in depressive patients and healthy volunteers. *Sleep Med Rev.* 2013;17:133–142.

U.S. Department of Veterans Affairs. PTSD: National Center for PTSD. **https://www.ptsd.va.gov**. Accessed Sept. 4, 2018.

Villarreal G, Hamner MB, Cañive JM, et al. Efficacy of quetiapine monotherapy in posttraumatic stress disorder: A randomized, placebo-controlled trial. *Am J Psychiatry.* 2016;173:1205–1212.

Zhou P, Zhang Y, Wei C, et al. Acute stress disorder as a predictor of posttraumatic stress: A longitudinal study of Chinese children exposed to the Lushan earthquake. *Psych J.* 2016;5:206.

Sexual Assault

Abrahams N, Devries K, Watts C, et al. Worldwide prevalence of non-partner sexual violence: A systematic review. *Lancet.* 2014;383:1648–1654.

American Psychiatric Association. *Practice guidelines for the treatment of patients with acute stress disorder and posttraumatic stress disorder.* Arlington, VA: American Psychiatric Association; 2010.

Astrup BS, Ravn P, Thomsen JL, Lauritsen J. Patterned genital injury in cases of rape—a case-control study. *J Forensic Leg Med.* 2013;20:525–529.

Brawner BM, Sommers MS, Moore K, et al. Exploring genitoanal injury and HIV risk among women: Menstrual phase, hormonal birth control, and injury frequency and prevalence. *J Acquir Immune Defic Syndr.* 2016;71(2):207–212.

Breiding MJ, Smith SG, Basile KC, et al. Prevalence and characteristics of sexual violence, stalking, and intimate partner violence victimization—National Intimate Partner and Sexual Violence Survey, United States, 2011. *MMWR Surveill Summ.* 2014;63:1.

Bryant RA. Acute stress disorder as a predictor of posttraumatic stress disorder: A systematic review. *J Clin Psychiatry.* 2011;72:233–239.

Bryant RA, Friedman MJ, Spiegel D, et al. A review of acute stress disorder in *DSM-5. Depress Anxiety.* 2011;28:802–817.

Bryant RA, Nickerson A, Creamer M, et al. Trajectory of posttraumatic stress following traumatic injury: 6-year follow-up. *Br J Psychiatry.* 2015;206:417–423.

Bureau of Justice Statistics. Rape and sexual assault. **https://www.bjs.gov/index.cfm?ty=tp&tid=317**. Published 2017. **https://www.bjs.gov/index.cfm?ty=tp&tid=317**. Accessed September 4, 2018.

Bureau of Justice Statistics. Violence against women: Estimates from the redesigned survey. **https://www.bjs.gov/content/pub/pdf/FEMVIED.PDF**. Accessed February 23, 2018.

Bureau of Justice Statistics. Female victims of sexual violence, 1994–2010. **https://www.bjs.gov/content/pub/pdf/rsavcaf9513.pdf**. Revised May 31, 2016. Accessed February 23, 2018.

Campbell R, et al. Responding to sexual assault victims' medical and emotional needs: A national study of the services provided by SANE programs. *Res Nurs Health.* 2006;29:384–398.

Carey KB, Durney SE, Shepardson RL, Carey MP. Incapacitated and forcible rape of college women: Prevalence across the first year. *J Adolesc Health.* 2015;56:678.

Carr ME, Moettus AL. Developing a policy for sexual assault examinations on incapacitated patients and patients unable to consent. *J Law Med Ethics.* 2010;38:647–653.

Chivers-Wilson KA. Sexual assault and posttraumatic stress disorder: A review of the biological, psychological and sociological factors and treatments. *McGill J Med.* 2006;9(2):111–118.

Cowley R, Walsh E, Horrocks J. The role of the sexual assault nurse examiner in England: Nurse experiences and perspectives. *J Forensic Nurs.* 2014;10:77–83.

Crawford-Jakubiak JE, Alderman EM, Leventhal JM. Care of the adolescent after an acute sexual assault. *Pediatrics.* 2017;139.

Du Mont J, Macdonald S, White M, et al. Client satisfaction with nursing-led sexual assault and domestic violence services in Ontario. *J Forensic Nurs.* 2014;10:122–134.

Elklit A, Christiansen DM. ASD and PTSD in rape victims. *J Interpers Violence.* 2010;25:1470.

Ford N, Irvine C, Shubber Z, et al. Adherence to HIV postexposure prophylaxis: A systematic review and meta-analysis. *AIDS.* 2014;28:2721–2727.

Fantasia HC, Fontenot HB. The sexual safety of adolescents. *J Obstet Gynecol Neonatal Nurs.* 2011;40:217–224.

Hagemann CT, Nordbø SA, Myhre AK, et al. Sexually transmitted infections among women attending a Norwegian Sexual Assault Centre. *Sex Transm Infect.* 2014;90:283.

Kahn AS, et al. Calling it rape: Differences in experiences of women who do or do not label their sexual assault as rape. *Psychol Women Q.* 2004;27:233–242.

Larsen ML, Hilden M, Lidegaard Ø. Sexual assault: A descriptive study of 2500 female victims over a 10-year period. *BJOG.* 2015;122:577.

Linden JA. Clinical practice. Care of the adult patient after sexual assault. *N Engl J Med.* 2011;365:834–841.

Morgan RE, Kena G. Criminal victimization, 2016. Bureau of Justice Statistics National Crime Victimization Survey (NCVS), 2016. Department of Justice, Office of Justice Programs. https://www.bjs.gov/content/pub/pdf/cv16.pdf. Published 2017.

National Institute of Justice. Rape and sexual violence. https://www.nij.gov/topics/crime/rape-sexual-violence/Pages/welcome.aspx. Published 2017.

Nelson MS, et al. Validation of probe EFD52 (D17S26) for forensic DNA analysis. *J Forensic Sci.* 1996;41:557–568.

Peterson ZD, Voller EK, Polusny MA, Murdoch M. Prevalence and consequences of adult sexual assault of men: Review of empirical findings and state of the literature. *Clin Psychol Rev.* 2011;31:1–24.

Punamäki RL, Palosaari E, Diab M, et al. Trajectories of posttraumatic stress symptoms (PTSS) after major war among Palestinian children: Trauma, family- and child-related predictors. *J Affect Disord.* 2015;172:133–140.

Rothbaum BO, Astin MC, Marsteller F. Prolonged exposure versus eye movement desensitization and reprocessing (EMDR) for PTSD rape victims. *J Trauma Stress.* 2005;18(6):607–616.

Seña AC, Hsu KK, Kellogg N, et al. Sexual assault and sexually transmitted infections in adults, adolescents, and children. *Clin Infect Dis.* 2015;61(suppl 8):S856–S864.

Senn CY, Eliasziw M, Barata PC, et al. Sexual violence in the lives of first-year university women in Canada: no improvements in the 21st century. *BMC Women Health.* 2014;14:135.

Simpson Rowe L, Jouriles EN, McDonald R, et al. Enhancing women's resistance to sexual coercion: a randomized controlled trial of the DATE program. *J Am Coll Health.* 2012;60:211.

Straight JD, Heaton P. Emergency department care for victims of sexual offense. *Am J Health Syst Pharm.* 2007;64(17):1845–1850.

Sugar NF, et al. Physical injury after sexual assault: Findings of a large case series. *Am J Obstet Gynecol.* 2004;190:71–76.

Tiihonen Möller A, Bäckström T, Söndergaard HP, Helström L. Identifying risk factors for PTSD in women seeking medical help after rape. *PLoS One.* 2014;9:e111136.

Ullman SE, et al. The role of victim–offender relationship in women's sexual assault experience. *J Interpers Violence.* 2006;21:798–819.

U.S. Department of Justice Office on Violence Against Women. A national protocol for sexual assault medical forensic examinations. Adults/adolescents. 2nd ed. https://www.ncjrs.gov/pdffiles1/ovw/241903.pdf. Published April 2013. Accessed February 22, 2018.

U.S. Department of Justice, Office on Violence Against Women. *Frequently asked questions: Anonymous reporting and forensic examinations.* Updated September 2013.

Vrees RA. Evaluation and management of female victims of sexual assault. *Obstet Gynecol Surv.* 2017;72:39–53.

von Hertzen H, et al. Low dose mifepristone and two regimens of levonorgestrel for emergency contraception: A WHO multicentre randomised trial. *Lancet.* 2002;360:1803–1810.

Walters ML, Chen J, Breiding MJ. The National Intimate Partner and Sexual Violence Survey (NISVS): 2010 findings on victimization by sexual orientation. Retrieved from the Centers for Disease Control and Prevention, National Center for Injury Prevention and Control. http://www.cdc.gov/ViolencePrevention/pdf/NISVS_SOfindings.pdf. Published 2013. Accessed February 22, 2018.

WHO guidelines approved by the Guidelines Review Committee. Responding to intimate partner violence and sexual violence against women: WHO clinical and policy guidelines. Geneva, Switzerland: World Health Organization; 2013.

Young-Wolff KC, Sarovar V, Klebaner D, et al. Changes in psychiatric and medical conditions and health care utilization following a diagnosis of sexual assault: A retrospective cohort study. 2018;56:649–657.

RESOURCES

General

Anxiety Disorders: A Patient's Story. America Psychiatric Association
https://www.psychiatry.org/patients-families/anxiety-disorders/patient-story

Anxiety Disorders: Alprazolam (Xanax). National Alliance on Mental Illness
https://www.nami.org/Learn-More/Treatment/Mental-Health-Medications/Alprazolam-(Xanax)

Anxiety Disorders: Brief Overview of Signs' Symptoms, Risk Factors, Treatments and Therapies. National Institute of Mental Health
https://www.nimh.nih.gov/health/topics/anxiety-disorders/index.shtml

Anxiety Disorders: Bupropion (Wellbutrin). FDA Alerts
https://www.nami.org/Learn-More/Treatment/Mental-Health-Medications/Bupropion-(Wellbutrin)

Anxiety Disorders: Expert Q&A. American Psychiatric Association
https://www.psychiatry.org/patients-families/anxiety-disorders/expert-q-and-a

Anxiety Disorders: Mental Medications and Types of Medications. National Alliance on Mental Illness
https://www.nami.org/Learn-More/Treatment/Mental-Health-Medications

Anxiety Disorders: Overview, Symptoms, Types of Anxiety Disorders, Causes, Diagnosis, Treatment, and Related Conditions. National Alliance of Mental Illness
https://www.nami.org/Learn-More/Mental-Health-Conditions/Anxiety-Disorders

Anxiety Disorders: What Are Anxiety Disorders?
https://www.psychiatry.org/patients-families/anxiety-disorders/what-are-anxiety-disorders

Everyday Anxiety or Anxiety Disorder. Anxiety and Depression Association of America
https://adaa.org/understanding-anxiety#

Agoraphobia

Agoraphobia Among Adults. National Institute of Mental Health
https://www.nimh.nih.gov/health/statistics/prevalence/agora-phobia-among-adults.shtml
Agoraphobia Among Children. National Alliance on Mental Illness
https://www.nimh.nih.gov/health/statistics/prevalence/agora-phobia-among-children.shtml
Agoraphobia: Causes, Symptoms, Exams & Test, Treatments, and Support Groups. U.S. National Library of Congress. Medline Plus
https://medlineplus.gov/ency/article/000923.htm

Generalized Anxiety Disorder

Generalized Anxiety Disorder: A Brief Overview, Symptoms, Causes, Diagnosis, Treatment, Risk Factors, Complications, and Prevention. Mayo Clinic
https://www.mayoclinic.org/diseases-conditions/generalized-anxiety-disorder/symptoms-causes/syc-20360803
Generalized Anxiety Disorder: Causes and Treatments, Symptoms, and Everyday Life. American Academy of Families and Physicians
https://familydoctor.org/condition/generalized-anxiety-disorder/
Generalized Anxiety Disorder: When Worry Gets Out of Control. A Brochure. National Institute of Mental Health
https://www.nimh.nih.gov/health/publications/generalized-anxiety-disorder-gad/generalized-anxiety-disorder_124169.pdf
Generalized Disorder: Understanding GAD—The Symptoms and Treatment. Anxiety and Depression Association of America
https://adaa.org/understanding-anxiety/generalized-anxiety-disorder-gad

Panic Disorder

An Overview of Panic Disorder, Symptoms, Diagnosis, and Treatment. American Academy of Families and Physicians
https://familydoctor.org/condition/panic-disorder/?adfree=true
Panic Disorder: Understanding the Facts Anxiety and Depression Association of America
https://adaa.org/understanding-anxiety/panic-disorder#
Panic Disorder: When Fear Overwhelms Handout. National Institute of Mental Health
https://www.nimh.nih.gov/health/publications/panic-disorder-when-fear-overwhelms/index.shtml

Posttraumatic Stress Disorder

Post-Traumatic Stress Disorder (PTSD). American Academy of Families and Physicians
https://familydoctor.org/condition/post-traumatic-stress-disorder/?adfree=true
Post-Traumatic Stress Disorder Overview, Signs and Symptoms, Risk Factors, Treatments and Therapies, and Join a Study. National Institute of Mental Health
https://www.nimh.nih.gov/health/topics/post-traumatic-stress-disorder-ptsd/index.shtml
Posttraumatic Stress Disorder. American Psychiatric Association
https://www.psychiatry.org/patients-families/ptsd/what-is-ptsd

Post-Traumatic Stress Disorder. Substance Abuse and Mental Health Services Administration
https://www.samhsa.gov/treatment/mental-disorders/post-traumatic-stress-disorder
Posttraumatic Stress Disorder. University of Maryland Medical Center
http://www.umm.edu/health/medical/altmed/condition/post-traumatic-stress-disorder
Post-Traumatic Stress Disorder: Children's Mental Health. Signs, Causes, and Get Help for Treatment. Centers for Disease Control and Prevention
https://www.cdc.gov/childrensmentalhealth/ptsd.html
Posttraumatic Stress Disorder: Facts for Families. American Academy of Child and Adolescent Psychiatry
https://www.aacap.org/App_Themes/AACAP/docs/facts_for_families/70_posttraumatic_stress_disorder_ptsd.pdf
Posttraumatic Stress Disorder: Make The Connection. Information on Post-Traumatic Stress Disorder, Life Events and Experiences, Signs and Symptoms, Conditions, and Videos. U.S. National Department of Veteran Affairs
https://maketheconnection.net/conditions/ptsd
Post-Traumatic Stress Disorder: Symptoms, Causes, Diagnosis and Treatment. Mayo Clinic
https://www.mayoclinic.org/diseases-conditions/post-traumatic-stress-disorder/symptoms-causes/syc-20355967
Posttraumatic Stress Disorder: What You Can Do and Getting Help. American Psychological Association
http://www.apa.org/topics/ptsd/

Sexual Assault

Preventing Sexual Violence on College and University Campuses: A Summary of CDC Activities. Partnerships, Technical Assistance, and Research. Centers for Disease Control and Prevention
https://www.cdc.gov/violenceprevention/pdf/campusvsummary.pdf
PTSD: National Center for PTSD. Sexual Assault Against Females. U.S. Department of Veterans Affairs
https://www.ptsd.va.gov/public/PTSD-overview/women/sexual-assault-females.asp
Sexual Assault and Mental Health: What is Sexual Assault? Mental Health America
http://www.mentalhealthamerica.net/conditions/sexual-assault-and-mental-health
Sexual Assault: What is Sexual Assault? RAINN (RAPE, Abuse, Incest, National Network)
https://www.rainn.org/articles/sexual-assault
Sexual Violence Consequences: Physical, Psychological, Social and Health Risk Behaviors. Centers for Disease Control and Prevention
https://www.cdc.gov/violenceprevention/sexualviolence/consequences.html
Stop Sexual Violence: A Technical Package to Prevent Sexual Violence. Centers for Disease Control and Prevention
https://www.cdc.gov/violenceprevention/pdf/SV-Prevention-Technical-Package.pdf
Victims of Sexual Violence: Statistics. Rape, Abuse & Incest National Network
https://www.rainn.org/statistics/victims-sexual-violence

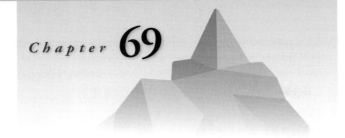

Chapter 69

Obsessive-Compulsive Disorders

Rehan Aziz, MD, FAPA

Denise Vanacore, PhD, DNP, APRN, ANP, PMHNP

Lynne M. Dunphy, PhD, APRN, FNP-BC, FAAN, FAANP

OBSESSIVE-COMPULSIVE DISORDER

Sigmund Freud called obsessive-compulsive disorder (OCD) the most fascinating of all mental illnesses. He published 14 major papers on it. He reasoned that the symptoms arose from unconscious psychological conflicts stemming from earlier stages of development. However, his account was not altogether satisfactory, and others before and after him have continued to grapple with explaining and treating the seemingly senseless rituals and tormenting thoughts associated with the condition.

OCD is characterized by the presence of obsessions, compulsions, or both. Only one category of symptoms is required for diagnosis. Obsessions are recurrent and persistent thoughts, urges, or images that are experienced as intrusive and unwanted. Compulsions are repetitive behaviors or mental acts that an individual feels forced to perform due to either an obsession or strict rules of conduct. Compulsions help to temporarily decrease anxiety from obsessions and thus, over time become reinforced.

OCD is grouped diagnostically with several related disorders, including body dysmorphic disorder (BDD), hoarding disorder (HD), trichotillomania (hair-pulling disorder), excoriation (skin-picking) disorder, and substance, medication, or another medical condition-induced obsessive-compulsive disorders. The linking feature of these ailments is repetitive behaviors, though otherwise, they have differing presentations, heritability, and treatments.

Due to shame, especially resulting from aggressive or sexual thoughts, patients often delay seeking help for OCD, and instead present to primary-care clinicians rather than psychiatrists. Only 40% of patients with OCD receive appropriate pharmacotherapy, and only 7.5% receive cognitive behavior therapy (CBT). According to the World Health Organization, OCD is the 10th most disabling condition worldwide due to lost income and decreased quality of life. As a result, it is imperative for primary-care providers to be able to screen for OCD and related disorders and, when they are suspected, begin treatment. Patients who have failed a course of CBT, pharmacotherapy, or both, along with those who have particularly disabling, complex, or high-risk symptoms, should be referred to specialists.

EPIDEMIOLOGY AND CAUSES

OCD occurs throughout the world, spanning all cultures and races. It is the fourth most common mental illness after depression, alcohol/substance use disorders, and social phobia. Lifetime prevalence is estimated at 2% to 3%. It is a chronic disorder, with a waxing–waning course. The disorder's onset is in childhood, late adolescence, or early adulthood, although it can present in older persons. There is a male preponderance in earlier-onset OCD, whereas females prevail when it is diagnosed at a later age. The sex ratio is equal. In many cases, onset of OCD is acute, typically after a significant stressful life event.

PATHOPHYIOLOGY

Obsessions are intrusive, recurrent, and persistent thoughts, urges, or images. They are experienced as alien and unwanted. Although unacceptable thoughts, such as an impulse to drive one's car off the road or jump onto the tracks before an approaching train, are not uncommon in the general population, in those with OCD, these thoughts are evaluated with an exaggerated, often horrifying, sense of personal responsibility for the thoughts themselves. The obsessions are emphasized further when the individual tries to avoid thinking about them. As a result, the person becomes preoccupied with the disturbing thoughts and attempts to control them. A brutal cycle then develops in which common unacceptable thoughts develop into pathological, tormenting obsessions. Compulsions follow from the obsessions. They are the patient's attempts to neutralize the irrational ideas, images, or urges for which they feel responsible. Compulsions help to lessen anxiety in the short term, but at the price of causing them to become needed tools for warding off obsessions. Accordingly, compulsions, adopting the form of behaviors or mental rituals, become ingrained and repetitive.

Individuals with OCD often have other psychopathology, requiring additional treatment. Many have a lifetime diagnosis of an anxiety disorder (76%) or a depressive/bipolar disorder (63%). Up to 60% to 80% of OCD patients will experience a depressive episode in their lifetime, and at least one-third of patients have concurrent major depressive disorder (MDD) at the time of evaluation. The commonality between OCD and depressive disorders is demonstrated by similarities in sleep electroencephalograph studies and neuroendocrine dexamethasone testing. Other psychiatric disorders found in patients with OCD include BDD, trichotillomania, excoriation disorder, schizophrenia, anorexia and bulimia nervosa, and Tourette's disorder.

With respect to childhood psychiatric disorders, the tic-related subtype of OCD occurs in individuals with a chronic tic disorder. It may account for as much as 10% to 40% of OCD cases diagnosed in childhood or adolescence. Early-onset cases with a personal history of tics show a male preponderance. Children with tic-related OCD typically have higher rates of disruptive behavior disorders, such as attention-deficit/hyperactivity disorder (ADHD) and oppositional defiant disorder, as well as trichotillomania and developmental disorders. OCD symptoms are also common in autism spectrum disorders. Such patients are likely to have repeating, hoarding, touching, tapping, and self-injurious behaviors, although fewer have somatic obsessions, obsessional thoughts, cleaning, and checking than patients with OCD only.

Genetic studies have demonstrated that both biological and environmental factors are important in the etiology of OCD. Family studies have indicated that OCD has a significant hereditable component, with relatives approximately fourfold more likely to develop OCD than the general population. Twin studies have found increased heritability estimates in child (45%–65%) compared with adult (27%–47%) OCD populations. Genes within the serotonin, dopamine, and glutamate pathways and those involved in white matter formation have been the focus of analyses. So far, the glutamate transporter gene, *SLC1A1*, is the only one that has been consistently associated with OCD.

Neurobiologically, there is evidence that the emergence of OCD is facilitated by hyperactivity in the orbitofrontal cortex, caudate nuclei, and anterior cingulate cortex, and/or by alterations to frontal corticostriatal thalamic circuitry. Any process affecting these circuits has the potential to cause OCD. Such conditions include gross neurological insults, such as strokes, brain tumors, Huntington's disease, Sydenham's chorea, frontotemporal dementia, or brain injury to the frontal lobe or basal skull. Subtler mechanisms, involving uncommon genes or environmental factors, can also be involved.

In childhood, a unique and rare presentation is pediatric autoimmune neuropsychiatric disorders associated with group A beta-hemolytic streptococcal infection (PANDAS). It is characterized by rapid onset and other neuropsychiatric symptoms, including tics, restricted eating, anxiety, and/or irritability. It is thought to be triggered by a throat infection or other illness, leading to the production of autoimmune antibodies against streptococci, which also cross-react with the basal ganglia. This cross-reaction is thought to result in neuropsychiatric symptoms, including OCD. A 2017 study looked at 1 million patients under age 18 years. Boys and girls

with a positive strep test had a significantly increased risk of OCD at 51% compared with individuals without a streptococcal test. However, PANDAS remains a diagnosis of exclusion and is not universally accepted.

CLINICAL PRESENTATION

In primary-care settings, patients with OCD may present with symptoms of either depression or anxiety because of distress or inability to function rather than state that they have OCD. These symptoms should prompt the clinician to maintain a high degree of suspicion for OCD. Patients with OCD often have good insight into their symptoms and can readily describe them, but occasionally they may have poor insight or even a delusional, fixed level of symptom intensity. Common obsessions, compulsions, and potential presentations seen in the primary care setting are in Table 69.1. The most common obsessions are fears of contamination, pathological self-doubt, intrusive thoughts, and symmetry. Patients with symmetry obsessions are concerned with exactness and feel distressed when items are misaligned or when something does not look "perfect." It is important to determine the frequency, intensity, duration, and severity of symptoms, as well as the symptom's impact on the patient's level of functioning. One should also ask about triggers, relieving factors, and avoidance of situations or things. Individuals will begin to avoid settings that trigger their obsessions or compulsions; for example, they may stop going to restaurants or using public restrooms. The patient may believe avoidance is better than the alternative (i.e., facing one's fears). In OCD, like other anxiety disorders, avoidance worsens the illness, leading to even greater loss of functioning and decreased quality of life.

DIAGNOSTIC REASONING

Screening questions for OCD only take a few moments to ask. If a patient responds positively to one of the following questions, a more formal diagnostic assessment and treatment plan may be in order.

- Are you ever bothered by frequent thoughts that are senseless but that you can't get out of your head? How do you deal with them?
- Do you spend a lot of time worrying about germs? Do you wash your hands a lot?
- Do you find yourself counting or repeating things over and over?
- Do you repeatedly check things like locks, plugs, or burners?
- Do you arrange things in a specific order? How do you feel if someone messes them up?
- How much time do you spend a day doing this?
- How does it affect your day-to-day life? Have you stopped going to certain places or doing certain things?

TABLE 69.1 Common OCD Symptoms and Presentations	
Type of Symptom	**Examples**
OBSESSIONS	
Aggressive impulses	Images of hurting a child or parent
Contamination	Becoming contaminated by shaking hands with another person
Need for order	Intense distress when objects are disordered or asymmetric
Religious	Blasphemous thoughts, concerns about unknowingly sinning
Repeated doubts	Wondering if a door was left unlocked
Sexual imagery	Recurrent pornographic images
COMPULSIONS	
Checking	Repeatedly checking locks, alarms, appliances
Cleaning	Hand washing
Hoarding	Saving trash or unnecessary items
Mental acts	Praying, counting, repeating words silently
Ordering	Reordering objects to achieve symmetry
Reassurance-seeking	Asking others for reassurance
Repetitive actions	Walking in and out of a doorway multiple times

Source: Fenske JN, Schwenk TL. Obsessive-compulsive disorder: Diagnosis and management. *Am Fam Physician*. 2009;80(3):239–245. Reproduced with permission from the American Academy of Family Physicians.

Rating scales for OCD severity include the 10-item Yale-Brown Obsessive-Compulsive Scale (Y-BOCS) and in children the Children's Yale-Brown Obsessive-Compulsive Scale (CY-BOCS). A seven-item self-report OCD screen (SOCS) has a high sensitivity (0.97) and specificity (0.88) for differentiating patients with OCD from healthy control subjects.

Symptoms

A diagnosis of OCD is established if distress is present, the acts are time-consuming (i.e., take more than one hour a day), or the illness significantly interferes with the individual's normal routine, occupation, or social activities. Please see the *Diagnostic and Statistical Manual of Mental Diseases*, 5th edition (*DSM-5*) for complete diagnostic criteria.

Differential Diagnosis

Differential diagnoses for OCD are presented in Differential Diagnosis 69.1.

MANAGEMENT

In general, due to shame and embarrassment from obsessions and compulsions, a strong therapeutic alliance and building of trust with patients are crucial for ongoing care. Families should be involved and given appropriate education and resources, such as information from the OCD Foundation Website.

Pharmacological Management

Selective serotonin reuptake inhibitors (SSRIs) are recommended as first-line pharmacological agents in the management of OCD in children and adults. Generally, higher dosages and trials of longer duration (up to 12 weeks) of SSRIs are required to treat OCD compared with depression or anxiety. All SSRIs are approved for OCD by the U.S. Food and Drug Administration (FDA) with the exception of escitalopram and citalopram. Although the use of SSRIs in children and adolescents carries a warning to be aware of a possible increase in suicidal ideation, studies have shown that in OCD, the benefits of treatment outweigh the risks. Clomipramine, a tricyclic antidepressant, can be used as a second-line therapy; however, the risks of seizures, weight gain, and cardiovascular events must be carefully considered. Other treatment strategies employed by specialists include adding lamotrigine, topiramate, acetylcysteine, or atypical antipsychotics, such as aripiprazole or risperidone. However, none of these strategies have been FDA approved for this indication.

Nonpharmacological Management

CBT is also regarded as a first-line management, either alone or in combination with an SSRI. CBT may be more effective than pharmacotherapy in OCD without other psychiatric comorbidities. CBT can be delivered

✖ Differential Diagnosis 69.1 Obsessive-Compulsive Disorder

Disorder	Clinical Features	Distinguishing Characteristics
Body dysmorphic disorder	Preoccupation with perceived defects or flaws in physical appearance, leading to repetitive behaviors or mental acts.	Obsessions and compulsions, such as checking, are limited to perceived physical defects. Patients often have poor insight.
Excoriation (skin-picking) disorder	Repeated skin picking results in skin lesions. The most common areas impacted are the face, arms, and hands.	The compulsive behavior is limited to skin-picking and is without the presence of obsessions
Hoarding disorder	Persistent difficulty discarding or parting with objects, regardless of their actual value or importance, due to a perceived need to save them and distress associated with discarding them.	In OCD, the behaviors are unwanted and bothersome. Excessive attainment of objects is usually not present, unless there is a specific obsession for it.
Trichotillomania (hair-pulling) disorder	Recurrent hair-pulling from any part of the body resulting in hair loss. There are repeated attempts to stop or decrease the hair pulling.	The compulsive behavior is limited to hair-pulling and is without the presence of obsessions.
Major depressive disorder	Depressed patients may have guilty or regretful ruminations, especially regarding the past. The ruminations are often mood-congruent. They may not be experienced as intrusive.	Depression does not involve obsessions or compulsions. In depression, the content of the ruminations is often varied and related to an overall depressed outlook. Obsessions in OCD are also usually linked to compulsions.
Generalized anxiety disorder (GAD)	GAD involves persistent worry about real-life issues. It is also accompanied by physical symptoms of anxiety, such as muscle tension or tachycardia.	OCD obsessions do not constitute real-life worries and normally include content that is odd, irrational, or of a magical nature. Obsessions in OCD are usually linked to compulsions.
Social anxiety disorder (social phobia)	In social anxiety disorder, the feared objects or situations are limited to social interactions. Avoidance is focused around reducing scrutiny by others.	Obsessions and corresponding compulsions are not present.
Illness anxiety disorder	There is a preoccupation with having or acquiring a serious illness, generally occurring in the absence of somatic symptoms. Patients have high anxiety about health. Patients also perform excessive health-related behaviors, such as checking their pulse.	In illness anxiety disorder, the fixations are consistent with one's sense of self and focused on having a disease. In OCD, the thoughts are intrusive, unwanted, and usually focused on fears of becoming diseased. Most patients with OCD will also have other obsessions and compulsions.
Pathological gambling/ substance use disorders/paraphilias	Gambling, substance use, and sexual behaviors can be performed repetitively by patients, not due to obsessions, but instead for pleasure. Typically, when the behaviors are given up, it is because of the consequences associated with them.	Compulsions are not pleasurable and are unwanted by the patient.
Obsessive-compulsive personality disorder (OCPD)	Despite the similarity in names, OCPD's defining feature is a pervasive pattern of preoccupation with orderliness, perfectionism, and a sense of control. OCPD begins by early adulthood and presents in a variety of contexts.	OCD differs from OCPD by the presence of obsessions and compulsions.
Autism spectrum disorder (ASD)	ASD patients exhibit deficits in social interactions and repetitive, restrictive ranges of interests or behaviors.	OCD symptoms are common in ASD, but OCD differs from ASD behaviors because obsessions and compulsions are unwanted by patients. OCD patients do not have social impairment.
Tics	Tics are sudden, painless, involuntary muscle contractions. They are preceded by localized uncomfortable sensations, rather than thoughts, which are relieved by the tic.	Tics can be mistaken for compulsions. The behavior is considered a compulsion rather than a tic if, for example, it is performed a certain number of times, in a certain order, in response to an obsession, is intended to reduce anxiety or prevent harm, and/or is voluntary.

individually, in group sessions, or with families. CBT with exposure and response prevention is one of the most effective treatments available for OCD. It is useful in both adult and pediatric populations. This technique involves repeatedly exposing patients to fear-producing stimuli in a hierarchical manner, beginning with less distressing situations and advancing to more feared encounters. During this time, patients are instructed to abstain from performing compulsive acts, thereby allowing for the fear response provoked by the obsessions to reduce via habituation over time. Patients also learn that feared stimuli are not as dangerous as imagined, that anxiety is not hazardous, and that anxiety can be tolerated.

Deep-brain stimulation (DBS) is FDA approved for OCD treatment as a last resort therapy on humanitarian grounds. The patient's OCD must be considered chronic, severe, and treatment-resistant. DBS is applied to the internal capsule and/or the adjacent ventral striatal region. Ablative surgery, such as anterior capsulotomy or anterior cingulotomy, has also been used for severe cases (Greenberg, Rauch, & Haber, 2010).

FOLLOW-UP AND REFERRAL

The primary-care practitioner should address medical concerns coexisting in the patient with OCD and be mindful of medication side effects or interactions. When a medication is started, the patient should be seen weekly for the first month, and a response should be seen between 4 and 12 weeks. Symptom severity can be assessed through the use of the aforementioned rating scales. OCD can be difficult to treat. Because each patient responds to treatment modalities quite differently, with improvement rates of 40% to 60%, it is recommended that care be provided in coordination with mental health specialists. Patients should be followed regularly, with attention paid to health maintenance issues. Referrals may be necessary for consequences of compulsive behaviors, such as referral to a dermatologist for trichotillomania, to a neurologist for co-occurring Tourette's syndrome, or for dental care due to excessive cleaning.

Patient Education: Obsessive-Compulsive Disorder

Education of the patient, family, and parents of the child with OCD is extremely important. Web sites provide information and links to support groups. Being educated and informed about the condition helps treatment compliance as well.

BODY DYSMORPHIC DISORDER

Body dysmorphic disorder (BDD) is among the obsessive-compulsive and related disorders. Its hallmark is a preoccupation with one or more perceived physical defects or flaws, often not visible or only slightly so to others. This is coupled with excessive repetitive behaviors, such as attempting to check, fix, conceal, or obtain reassurance about the perceived deformities. The course is often chronic. BDD causes significant distress and may result in decreased quality of life. It is associated with high rates of suicidality. Like OCD, it is often not recognized in clinical settings and may be misdiagnosed as OCD.

EPIDEMIOLOGY AND CAUSES

BDD is estimated to affect about 1% to 2% of the population and is about as common as OCD. BDD develops mostly in adolescence and is very unlikely to appear in adults past age 40. Men and women are affected equally. Many patients with BDD develop suicidal ideation. Rates of suicide attempts and completed suicide appear noticeably increased compared with the general population or to individuals with OCD.

In terms of psychiatric comorbidity, about 75% have a history of MDD, which is the most common comorbid disorder. BDD usually precedes MDD in onset. Approximately 40% of patients with BDD have a history of social anxiety disorder, and almost one-third have past or current OCD. Substance use disorders occur in 30% to 50%. Around 20% of men with muscle dysmorphia abuse anabolic steroids to increase muscle bulk.

PATHOPHYSIOLOGY

The pathophysiology of BDD is not clearly understood at this time. Results of twin studies in BDD indicate that genetic factors account for about 42% to 44% of the variance in symptoms, with the remaining difference accounted for by environmental influences. First-degree relatives of patients with BDD are thought to have a four times higher likelihood of developing BDD. BDD is also more common in first-degree relatives of patients with OCD. Data from visual processing studies suggest that patients with BDD actually perceive faces and objects differently than those without BDD. Patients may also have deficits with executive function (i.e., complex thinking). Neurotransmitter dysfunction, especially that of serotonin, may also play a role in BDD. Regarding the environment, a range of factors has been suggested that may influence the development of BDD, including childhood abuse, childhood neglect, bullying, peer teasing, and peer victimization.

CLINICAL PRESENTATION

Because patients feel ashamed about themselves and their bodies, they rarely report symptoms of BDD to primary-care providers. Instead, patients may present with symptoms of depression or anxiety and request referrals to dermatologists, plastic surgeons, orthodontists, or maxil-lofacial surgeons.

Regarding symptom profiles, women with BDD are more likely to be concerned about their weight, breasts, hips, legs, and body hair. They may frequently check mirrors, pick their skin, or camouflage their bodies to obscure disliked areas. Many women have comorbid eating disorders. Men may be consumed by having an "undersized" body, including muscle dysmorphia, thinning hair, or with their genital size. Men may have a comorbid substance use disorder.

DIAGNOSTIC REASONING

Helpful screening questions include the following:

- Do you think there is something wrong with the way you look? Does everybody notice?
- Do you think you look unattractive, ugly, or even hideous?
- How long do you spend looking in the mirror or on grooming?
- Have you stopped going out? Do you feel isolated?

The Yale-Brown Obsessive-Compulsive Scale modified for Body Dysmorphic Disorder (BDD-YBOCS) is both a reliable and valid tool to help identify BDD severity.

Symptoms

A diagnosis of BDD is made when an individual exhibits preoccupation with one or more imagined defects in appearance. Complete diagnostic criteria can be found in the *DSM-5*.

Differential Diagnosis

BDD deviates from normal concerns about appearance in several respects. In BDD, worries about appearance are excessive, and patients engage in time-consuming behaviors because of them. The symptoms also cause substantial distress and/or diminished functioning. Plainly visible physical defects, excluding lesions from skin picking, are not diagnosed as BDD. The preoccupations and repetitive behaviors of BDD differ from OCD obsessions and compulsions by centering only on appearance. Patients with OCD are typically aware of their illness, while those with BDD often lack insight. Many individuals with BDD even have delusional (i.e., false and fixed) beliefs about their appearance. This is diagnosed as BDD, not as a delusional disorder.

MANAGEMENT

Pharmacological Management

There are no FDA-approved treatments for BDD. However, high-dose SSRIs are considered the first-line pharmacological treatment for BDD. Agents prescribed have included fluoxetine, citalopram, escitalopram, fluvoxamine, and clomipramine. Trial duration is longer than for MDD, at 12 to 16 weeks.

Nonpharmacological Management

BDD-focused CBT has been shown to be effective for many patients. Techniques employed include cognitive restructuring, exposure and response prevention, and other specific approaches tailored to BDD, such as perceptual retraining.

FOLLOW-UP AND REFERRAL

Since poor or absent insight is common in BDD, it can be difficult to engage and retain patients in treatment. Phillips (2015) has suggested initially working on building a therapeutic alliance, by striving to build trust and rapport. Expressing empathy for the patient's plight while avoiding judgment is essential. Next, provide education regarding BDD. For patients considering or requesting referrals for cosmetic procedures, the clinician should discuss the likelihood that the results will be unsatisfying. Attempting to talk patients out of their appearance concerns is usually unsuccessful. Instead, the clinician can ask the patient to consider the possibility that they could be misperceiving their flaws. At this point, if the therapeutic alliance is well developed, the clinician should convey that psychiatric treatment is likely to be helpful and encourage the patient to consider it.

> ### Patient Education: Body Dysmorphic Disorder
>
> Patient and family education about BDD is vital to enhance diagnosis, increase support, and improve treatment compliance. The International OCD Foundation (IOCDF) provides information and links to other resources, including support groups, on its web site.

HOARDING DISORDER

In the past, hoarding was considered a subtype of OCD or a symptom of obsessive-compulsive personality disorder, but it is now recognized as a distinct diagnostic entity. Patients usually do not present complaining of hoarding but rather may be brought to clinical attention by a family member or friend, distressed by the individual's possessions and the state of their living environment.

EPIDEMIOLOGY AND CAUSES

HD is estimated to affect about 1.5% of the population. Men and women are affected equally. Its prevalence is greater in unmarried or divorced individuals. The majority of patients with HD have comorbid psychiatric illnesses such as post-traumatic stress disorder, generalized anxiety disorder, OCD, or MDD. In some individuals, symptoms of ADHD are present.

PATHOPHYSIOLOGY

The pathophysiology of HD is under active investigation. In some neuroimaging studies, the frontolimbic area of the brain has been implicated. There are also possible links between traumatic life events and its development.

CLINICAL PRESENTATION

The most prominent feature of HD is a cluttered home due to a patient's difficulty with discarding commonplace items such as magazines, plastic bags, empty containers, newspapers, or clothes. Some individuals collect animals. Patients often lack insight into their hoarding behaviors, as well as its impact on their level of functioning and home environment. They can also be resistant to change. HD can result in hazardous living conditions. Skin infections may arise owing to the environment. Due to clutter, patients, especially elders, are at risk for falls and possible fractures or trauma. Blocked windows and exits can make fires deadly.

DIAGNOSTIC REASONING

Symptoms

The essential features of hoarding disorder are a long-standing perceived need to save items and difficulty discarding or parting with possessions. The items may have little perceived value to others. Reasons given for this difficulty include the following:

- Perceived future utility of the items
- Perceived aesthetic value of the items
- A strong sentimental attachment to the possessions
- A sense of responsibility for the possessions
- A desire to avoid being wasteful
- Fearfulness of losing important information

Hoarding disorder is diagnosed when the behavior results in significant impairment in functioning, including the provision of a safe environment. Complete diagnostic criteria for hoarding disorder can be found in the *DSM-5*.

Assessment scales, such as the Structured Interview for Hoarding Disorder (SIHD) and the Hoarding Rating Scale, are available to help with the diagnosis of HD. Activities of Daily Living for Hoarding (ADL-H) and the Saving Inventory Revised are additional scales that can assist in determining the extent to which an individual is hoarding.

Differential Diagnosis

Hoarding disorder is not diagnosed if the symptoms are a consequence of obsessions or compulsions. In OCD, the excessive acquisition of objects is usually not present, unless the individual has a specific obsession for it, and then, it functions as a compulsion, as the individual does not have a genuine desire to possess the items. In OCD, the behavior is also generally undesirable and tormenting. The individual derives no pleasure from it.

MANAGEMENT

Nonpharmacological Management

CBT with exposure and response prevention, used in OCD, is generally not effective for HD. Instead, a specialized CBT approach for hoarding is employed. It involves office sessions and home visits, which are often the best way to begin the process of discarding possessions. Weekly meetings spanning 6 months or more may be needed depending on the extent of the hoarding and the severity of the patient's resistance to discarding objects. Follow-up home visits are conducted to ensure that the individual is following through with the cleaning and discarding process.

Pharmacological Management

Pharmacological studies of SSRIs have had mixed results. There is some research indicating that venlafaxine and paroxetine may have efficacy in treating hoarding disorder.

FOLLOW-UP AND REFERRAL

Due to the complex nature of the treatment for HD, most patients should be referred to specialists. However, primary-care practitioners should address medical concerns in patients, discuss home safety, and be mindful of medication side effects or interactions, if they are prescribed. Continued follow-up visits are vital to help prevent relapse.

Patient Education: Hoarding Disorder

Patient and family education about HD is critical to enhance diagnosis, increase support, improve home safety, and encourage treatment compliance. Two Web sites with information and links to other resources, including support groups and information for families are the following:

- https://hoarding.iocdf.org/
- https://www.psychiatry.org/patients-families/hoarding-disorder

The National Fire Protection Association also provides public education about hoarding and fire safety.

REFERENCES

Body Dysmorphic Disorder

American Psychiatric Association. Obsessive-Compulsive and Related Disorders. *Diagnostic and statistical manual of mental disorders.* 5th ed. Arlington, VA: American Psychiatric Association; 2013.

Bratiotis C, Steketee G. Hoarding disorder: Models, interventions, and efficacy. *Focus.* 2015;13(2):175–183.

Buhlmann U, Teachman BA, Naumann E, Fehlinger T, Rief W. The meaning of beauty: Implicit and explicit self-esteem and attractiveness beliefs in body dysmorphic disorder. *J Anxiety Disord.* 2009;23(5):694–702.

Deckersbach T, Savage CR, Phillips KA. Characteristics of memory dysfunction in body dysmorphic disorder. *J Int Neuropsychol Soc.* 2000;6(6):673–681.

Didie ER, Kuniega-Pietrzak T, Phillips KA. Body image in patients with body dysmorphic disorder: evaluations of and investment in appearance, health/illness, and fitness. *Body Image.* 2010;7(1): 66–69.

Feusner JD, Townsend J, Bystritsky A, et al. Visual information processing of faces in body dysmorphic disorder. *Arch Gen Psychiatry.* 2007;64:1417–1425

Feusner JD, Hembacher E, Moller H, et al. Abnormalities of object visual processing in body dysmorphic disorder. *Psychol Med.* 2011;41:2385–2397.

Greenberg BD, Rauch SL, Haber SN. Invasive circuitry-based neurotherapeutics: stereotactic ablation and deep brain stimulation for OCD. *Neuropsychopharmacology.* 2010 Jan;35(1): 317–336.

Greenberg JL, Mothi SS, Wilhelm S. Cognitive-behavioral therapy for adolescent body dysmorphic disorder: A pilot study. *Behav Ther.* 2016;47(2):213–224.

Krebs G, Fernández de la Cruz L, Mataix-Cols D. Recent advances in understanding and managing body dysmorphic disorder. *Evid Based Mental Health.* 2017;20:71–75.

Nordsletten AE, Fernández de la Cruz L, Pertusa A, et al. The Structured Interview for Hoarding Disorder (SIHD): Development, usage and further validation. *J Obsessive Compuls Relat Disord.* 2013;2:346–350.

Phillips KA. Body dysmorphic disorder: Clinical aspects and relationship to obsessive-compulsive disorder. *Focus.* 2015;13(2):162–174.

Wilhelm S, Greenberg JL, Rosenfield E, Kasarskis I, Blashill AJ. The Body Dysmorphic Disorder Symptom Scale: Development and preliminary validation of a self-report scale of symptom specific dysfunction. *Body Image.* 2016;17:82–87.

Wilhelm S, Phillips KA, Didie E, et al. Modular cognitive-behavioral therapy for body dysmorphic disorder: A randomized controlled trial. *Behav Ther.* 2014;45(3):314–327.

Hoarding Disorder

Brakoulias V, Eslick GD, Starcevic V. A meta-analysis of the response of pathological hoarding to pharmacotherapy. *Psychiatry Res.* 2015;229(1–2):272–276.

Mathews CA, Delucchi K, Cath DC, et al. Partitioning the etiology of hoarding and obsessive-compulsive symptoms. *Psychol Med.* 2014;44:2867–2876.

Nordsletten AE, Reichenberg A, Hatch SL, et al. Epidemiology of hoarding disorder. *Br J Psychiatry.* 2013;203:445–452.

Saxena S, Brody AL, Maidment KM, Baxter LR Jr. Paroxetine treatment of compulsive hoarding. *J Psychiatr Res.* 2007;41(6): 481–487.

Saxena S, Sumner J. Venlafaxine extended-release treatment of hoarding disorder. *Int Clin Psychopharmacol.* 2014;29(5):266–273.

Tolin DF, Meunier SA, Frost RO, Steketee G. Hoarding among patients seeking treatment for anxiety disorders. *J Anxiety Disord.* 2011;25:43–48.

Williams M, Viscusi JA. Hoarding disorder and a systematic review of treatment with cognitive behavioral therapy. *Cogn Behav Ther.* 2016;45(2):93–110.

Obsessive-Compulsive and Related Disorders

Alonso P, Cuadras D, Gabriëls L. Deep brain stimulation for obsessive-compulsive disorder: A meta-analysis of treatment outcome and predictors of response. *PLoS One.* 2015;10(7):e0133591.

American Psychiatric Association. *Diagnostic and statistical manual of mental disorders.* 5th ed. Arlington, VA: American Psychiatric Association; 2013.

American Psychiatric Association. *Practice guideline for obsessive compulsive disorder.* http://www.guideline.gov/search/search.aspx?term=obsessive+compulsive. Published November 2007 (reaffirmed 2012).

Blanco C, Olfson M, Stein DJ, Simpson HB, Gameroff MJ, Narrow WH. Treatment of obsessive-compulsive disorder by U.S. psychiatrists. *J Clin Psychiatry.* 2006;67:946–951.

Gilbert AR, Malouf FT. Pediatric obsessive-compulsive disorder: Management in primary care. *Curr Opin Pediatr.* 2008;20:544–550.

Grant JE. Obsessive–compulsive disorder. *N. Engl J Med.* 2014; 371:646–653.

Greenberg BD, Malone DA, Friehs GM, et al. Three-year outcomes in deep brain stimulation for highly resistant obsessive–compulsive disorder. *Neuropsychopharmacology.* 2006;31:2384–2393.

Guglielmi V, Vulink NC, Denys D, Wang Y, Samuels JF, Nestadt G. Obsessive-compulsive disorder and female reproductive cycle events: Results from the OCD and reproduction collaborative study. *Depress Anxiety.* 2014;31(12):979–987.

Kim SW, Dysken MW, Kuskowski M. The Yale-Brown Obsessive—Compulsive Scale: A reliability and validity study. *Psychiatry Res.* 1990;34:99–106.

Kim SW, Dysken MW, Kuskowski M. The Symptom Checklist—90: Obsessive-compulsive subscale: A reliability and validity study. *Psychiatry Res.* 1992;41:37–44.

Leckman JF, Denys D, Simpson HB et al. Obsessive-compulsive disorder: A review of the diagnostic criteria and possible subtypes and dimensional specifiers for *DSM-V. Depress Anxiety.* 2010;27(6):507–527.

Murray CJ, Lopez AD. *The global burden of diseases: A comprehensive assessment of mortality and disability from diseases, injuries and risk factors in 1990 and projected to 2020.* Boston: Harvard School of Public Health, World Health Organization, and World Bank; 1996.

Orlovska S, Vestergaard CH, Bech BH, Nordentoft M, Vestergaard M, Benros ME. Association of streptococcal throat infection with mental disorders: Testing key aspects of the PANDAS hypothesis in a nationwide study. *JAMA Psychiatry.* 2017;74:740–746.

Osborn I. *Tormenting thoughts and secret rituals: The hidden epidemic of obsessive-compulsive disorder.* New York, NY: Dell; 1999.

Pallanti S, Grassi G, Sarrecchia ED, Cantisani A, Pellegrini M. Obsessive-compulsive disorder comorbidity: Clinical assessment and therapeutic implications. *Front Psychiatry.* 2011;2:70.

Rapoport JL. The neurobiology of obsessive-compulsive disorder. *JAMA.* 1988;260(19):2888–2890.

Russell AJ, Mataix-Cols D, Anson M, Murphy DG. Obsessions and compulsions in Asperger syndrome and high-functioning autism. *Br J Psychiatry.* 2005;186:525–528.

Stewart SE, Pauls DL. The genetics of obsessive-compulsive disorder. *Focus.* 2010;8(3):350–357.

Shavitt RG, de Mathis MA, Oki F, et al. Phenomenology of OCD: Lessons from a large multicenter study and implications for ICD-11. *J Psychiatr Res.* 2014;57:141–148.

Veale D, Roberts A. Obsessive-compulsive disorder. *BMJ.* 2014; 348:g2183.

Veale D, Miles S, Smallcombe N, Ghezai H, Goldacre B, Hodsoll J. Atypical antipsychotic augmentation in SSRI treatment refractory obsessive-compulsive disorder: A systematic review and meta-analysis. *BMC Psychiatry.* 2014;14:317.

RESOURCES

Body Dysmorphic Disorder

Body Dysmorphic Disorder: A Brief Overview, Symptoms, Causes, Risk Factors, Complications, and Prevention. Mayo Clinic
https://www.mayoclinic.org/diseases-conditions/body-dysmorphic-disorder/symptoms-causes/syc-20353938

Body Dysmorphic Disorder: An Overview of Causes, Symptoms, Diagnosis, Treatment, Management and Prevention. Cleveland Clinic
https://my.clevelandclinic.org/health/diseases/9888-body-dysmorphic-disorder

Body Dysmorphic Disorder: Definition and Classification of BBD, Epidemiology, Demographic characteristics, Case Description, Insight Regarding Perceived Appearance Defects, Compulsions, Safety Behaviors, and Avoidance, Course of illness, Risk behaviors: suicidality, substance abuse, and violence. U.S. National Library of Medicine National Institute of Health
https://www.ncbi.nlm.nih.gov/pmc/articles/PMC3181960/

Body Dysmorphic Disorder (BDD): Characteristics of BBD, Symptoms, BBD and Other Mental Health Disorders, Diagnosis and Treatment. American and Depression Association of America
https://adaa.org/understanding-anxiety/related-illnesses/other-related-conditions/body-dysmorphic-disorder-bdd#

Body Dysmorphic Disorder: Description of the Research Program. Massachusetts General Hospital Research Institute
http://www.massgeneral.org/research/researchlab.aspx?id=1399

Body Dysmorphic Disorder: Recognizing and Treating Imagined Ugliness. World Psychiatry
https://www.ncbi.nlm.nih.gov/pmc/articles/PMC1414653/

Body Dysmorphic Disorder. John Hopkins Medicine
https://www.hopkinsmedicine.org/healthlibrary/conditions/mental_health_disorders/body_dysmorphic_disorder_134,216

The Mirror Lies of Body Dysmorphic Disorder: Demographics, Case Study, Etiology, Diagnosis, and Treatment. American Family Physician
https://www.aafp.org/afp/2008/0715/p217.html

The UCLA Eating Disorders and Body Dysmorphic Disorder Research Program: Symptoms, Research, and Treatment. Semel Institute for Neuroscience and Human Behavior
http://www2.semel.ucla.edu/edbdd

What Is BDD? Body Dysmorphic Disorder Foundation
http://bddfoundation.org/

Hoarding Disorder

A Patient's Story: Hoarding Disorder. American Psychiatric Association
https://www.psychiatry.org/patients-families/hoarding-disorder/patient-story

Hoarding Disorder. American Psychiatry Association
https://www.psychiatry.org/patients-families/hoarding-disorder/what-is-hoarding-disorder

Hoarding: Expert Q & A: Hoarding Disorder. American Psychiatric Association
https://www.psychiatry.org/patients-families/hoarding-disorder/expert-qa

Obsessive Compulsive Disorder (OCD)

Anxiety and Depression Association of America
https://adaa.org/understanding-anxiety/obsessive-compulsive-disorder-ocd

Obsessive Compulsive Disorder
https://www.mayoclinic.org/diseases-conditions/obsessive-compulsive-disorder/symptoms-causes/syc-20354432

Obsessive Compulsive Disorder: A Brief Overview, Symptoms, Causes, Diagnosis, and Treatment. National Alliance on Mental Illness
https://www.nami.org/Learn-More/Mental-Health-Conditions/Obsessive-Compulsive-Disorder

Obsessive Compulsive Disorder: A Brief Overview of Signs, Symptoms, Risk Factors, Treatments and Therapies. National Institute of Mental Health
https://www.nimh.nih.gov/health/topics/obsessive-compulsive-disorder-ocd/index.shtml

Obsessive Compulsive Disorder: When Unwanted Thoughts or Irresistible Actions Take Over. Brochure. National Institute of Mental Health
https://www.nimh.nih.gov/health/publications/obsessive-compulsive-disorder-when-unwanted-thoughts-take-over/508-ocd-qf-16-4676-12142016_150041.pdf

Obsessive Compulsive Disorder. American Academy of Families and Physicians
https://familydoctor.org/condition/obsessive-compulsive-disorder/

Obsessive Compulsive Disorder. Substance Abuse and Mental Health Services Administration
https://www.samhsa.gov/treatment/mental-disorders/posttraumatic-stress-disorder

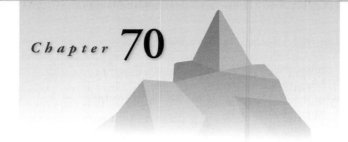

Chapter 70

Behavioral Disorders Related to Physical/Physiological Disturbances

Jason V. Lambrese, MD

Denise Vanacore, PhD, APRN, ANP-BC, FNP, PMHNP-BC

Lynne M. Dunphy, PhD, APRN, FNP-BC, FAAN, FAANP

EATING DISORDERS: ANOREXIA NERVOSA, BULIMIA NERVOSA, AND BINGE-EATING DISORDER

Eating disorders, which include anorexia nervosa (AN), bulimia nervosa (BN), and binge-eating disorder (BED), are not routinely assessed in primary care, although they can be a significant health problem. Eating disorders occur on a continuum; the number of individuals with subclinical symptoms exceeds those with full disorder symptomatology. Risk factors for developing an eating disorder include female sex, a family history of an eating disorder, perfectionism, obsessive personality traits, and susceptibility to societal pressures for thinness. At present, the incidence of eating disorders among males is low, but there is evidence of persistent increases over time, particularly in sexual minority males. *The Diagnostic and Statistical Manual of Mental Disorders* (5th edition; *DSM-5*) characterizes feeding and eating disorders as persistent disturbances from altered consumption or restriction of food intake, resulting in significant functional impairment. Included in the *DSM-5* classification are rumination disorder, avoidant/restrictive food intake disorder, anorexia nervosa, bulimia nervosa, and binge-eating disorder.

Anorexia Nervosa

AN is characterized by a refusal to maintain a minimally normal body weight and an intense fear of gaining weight due to a body image disturbance. In early adolescence, the patient may also fail to achieve expected weight and height gains. There are two types of AN—restricting and binge-eating/purging AN. With restricting AN, weight loss is usually accomplished by reducing or restricting all food intake or restricting dietary fat. With binge-eating/purging AN, there is binge eating followed by self-induced vomiting or chronic and excessive use of laxatives or diuretics. Providers can expect patients to resist changes in their diet or weight. AN can be accompanied by serious physiological consequences, including amenorrhea, signs and symptoms of starvation, and electrolyte abnormalities.

One in 10 patients with AN die suddenly from starvation, cardiac arrest, or suicide. AN is associated with depression in 65% of cases, social phobia in 34%, and obsessive-compulsive disorder in 26% of cases. AN is a serious medical disorder, with estimates of mortality ranging up to 20%. Patients with AN rarely self-identify and often demonstrate poor insight into their condition. Clinicians therefore have a responsibility to help patients recognize their diagnosis and work with them to assess their readiness to change and their integration with additional elements of care.

Bulimia Nervosa

Recurrent episodes of binge eating, followed by compensatory methods to prevent weight gain, and self-evaluation unduly influenced by body shape are the three essential features of BN. Binge eating is characterized by eating an excessive amount of food within a 2-hour period. Persons with BN undergo feelings of loss of control during bingeing episodes, and their self-esteem is excessively influenced by their body shape and weight.

Compensatory behaviors can include purging behaviors (self-induced vomiting and/or misuse of diuretics, laxatives, or enemas) or nonpurging behaviors (excessive exercise or fasting). In extreme cases, individuals may abuse thyroid hormone replacement medication or try other types of stimulant medication. The individual may feel an intense sense of shame about this behavior and may go to great lengths to keep it secret from others, including health-care providers.

Persons with BN who cycle between binging and extreme food restriction have a poorer prognosis than those who purge. The daily number of times the person with BN purges tends to increase over time and can lead to serious medical complications. In the primary-care setting, it is not unusual for persons with BN to refuse to disclose their symptoms.

Individuals with BN experience a sense of lack of control over eating during a binge episode and tend to misperceive themselves on the basis of their body weight and shape. Most patients with BN are not underweight; rather, they are of normal weight or overweight, distinguishing this from AN. Comorbidity with other psychological disorders is common, especially depression, anxiety, and substance abuse.

Binge-Eating Disorder

BED was first identified in 1959 by Stunkard and is characterized by the presence of recurrent episodes of binge eating without the compensatory use of vomiting, laxatives, emetics, or diuretics. BED was added to the *DSM-5* due to research supporting the clinical diagnosis. Binges are usually triggered by emotional responses to work, school-related stress, or fear of abandonment or loss. After the binge-eating episode, individuals are usually embarrassed by the amount of food that they consumed. BED is thought to be associated with a family history of BED or obesity. Similar to BN, patients with BED are often of normal weight or overweight.

EPIDEMIOLOGY AND CAUSES

The lifetime prevalence estimate for AN is 0.6%, for BN, 1.0%, and for BED, 5.5%. For each disorder, the risk is up to 10 times higher in women than in men, with a median age of onset between 18 and 21 years. An exact cause of eating disorders is not known but is likely due to a multifactorial combination of genetic, neurochemical, and sociocultural factors. Recent work indicates that childhood obesity may be a risk factor for BN, and there is evidence that familial transmission may occur. The state of starvation itself initiates dramatic physiological changes in a variety of body systems leading to a cascade-like cycle that makes it difficult to discern which biological change may have precipitated the process; nonetheless, it becomes self-perpetuating.

PATHOPHYSIOLOGY

Recent studies point to some genetic differences between AN, BED, and BN. When families of individuals with a high incidence of BN are examined, family members with an increased risk for obesity are found; however, in families of individuals with the restricting subtype of AN, there is no increased risk for obesity. Although these are two genetically related disorders, there clearly may be important differences between them. There is an increased frequency of BN in first-degree relatives of patients with this disorder. Some evidence points to higher concordance rates in monozygotic twins than in dizygotic. Sisters of patients with AN are more likely to be affected, but the causality involved may be more social than genetic. Cultural factors may be difficult to ascertain because few studies have looked at eating disorders and their occurrence in different countries, and populations without appropriate access to care may therefore not be accurately diagnosed.

CLINICAL PRESENTATION

Eating disorders are characterized by intense feelings of shame, guilt, and embarrassment. It is important to know key warning signs of eating disorders to provide care early in the disease process; early intervention has a better prognosis.

Focus on History: Anorexia Nervosa, Bulimia Nervosa, and Binge-Eating Disorder

Anorexia Nervosa

Warning signs: To assess for warning signs of anorexia, it is important to obtain answers to the following questions:

- Has the patient had any *substantial weight loss*?
- Does the patient have signs or symptoms of *depression or mood swings*?
- Does the patient have a *preoccupation with weight, calories, and food*?
- Does the patient *wear baggy clothes*?
- Does the patient have a history of *excessive exercise*?

Signs
- Physical exam: Emaciation/cachexia, dry skin, lanugo hair, peripheral edema, enlarged parotid glands (if purging)
- Vital signs: Hypotension, hypothermia, bradycardia, orthostasis
- Laboratory studies: Leukopenia, anemia, evidence of dehydration (elevated blood urea nitrogen, elevated urine specific gravity), elevated liver function tests, hypomagnesemia, hypophosphatemia, elevated thyroid-stimulating hormone, low bone mineral density

Symptoms
- Amenorrhea
- Constipation
- Abdominal pain
- Hypothermia
- Lethargy or fatigue
- Anxious energy
- Headaches

Bulimia Nervosa

Warning signs: To assess for warning signs of bulimia nervosa, it is important to obtain answers to the following questions:

- Has the patient had any significant *weight loss or gain*?
- Does the patient have signs or symptoms of *depression*?
- Does the patient have a *great concern for weight*?
- Does the patient *visit the bathroom after meals*?
- Has the patient alluded to *strict dieting/bingeing cycles*?
- Does the patient have *marked criticism of his or her body*?

Signs
- Physical examination: normal weight or overweight, tooth enamel erosion, enlarged parotid glands, periodontal disease, scars/calluses on dorsum of hand from self-induced vomiting (Russell's sign), esophageal bleeding/tears
- Laboratory studies: hypokalemia, hypochloremia, hyponatremia, elevated bicarbonate, metabolic alkalosis (due to vomiting) or metabolic acidosis (due to diarrhea from laxative abuse), elevated amylase

Symptoms
- Irregular menses
- Abdominal pain
- Fatigue or lethargy
- Peripheral edema
- Bloating
- Depression
- Acid reflux
- Sore throat

Binge-Eating Disorder

Warning signs: To assess for warning signs of binge-eating disorder, it is important to obtain answers to the following questions:

- Has the patient had any significant *weight gain*?
- Does the patient have a *negative body image*?
- Does the patient *eat rapidly until uncomfortably full*?
- Does the patient often eat large amounts of food *in isolation*?
- Does the patient have signs or symptoms of *depression*?

Signs
- Obesity
- Depression

Symptoms
- Abdominal pain
- Constipation
- Acid reflux

Individuals with eating disorders can present with that as a key symptom or problem, or with other somatic complaints. Therefore, the clinician must be alert to screen for these disorders among adolescents and young adults, particularly those thought to be at high risk. Assessment should be comprehensive and include physical, psychological, and social needs and a comprehensive assessment of risk to self. The primary-care provider should take responsibility for initial assessment and the initial coordination of care, including the determination of the need for emergency medical or psychiatric assessment (see Box 70.3). Where management is shared between primary and secondary care (e.g., pediatrics, adolescent/internal medicine, psychiatry), there should be a clear agreement in writing as to who should be monitoring the patient on a regular

basis. It should be shared with patient and family members so all lines of responsibility are clear.

Screening for eating disorders may use brief screening methods such as questionnaires and clinical interview. Assessment components are included in Box 70.1, and available screening instruments are listed in Box 70.2. The SCOFF consists of five questions designed to assess the core features of AN and BN. It is a mnemonic, with each letter based on a keyword in each question of the screening tool: **S**ick, **C**ontrol, **O**ne, **F**at, and **F**ood. It was designed to be brief, administered in primary care, and answered with yes-and-no responses. The EAT-26 is better validated but takes longer to administer and score. The EDI-2 is a standardized measure of symptoms associated with AN, BN, and other eating disorders. Although reliable and valid with good psychometrics, it does not yield a specific diagnosis but has utility as a screening instrument.

Assessment of body mass index (BMI), height, weight, and centile charts for age should be done on all patients. When AN or BN is suspected, a complete physical examination is needed to rule out other diseases or disorders that could produce severe weight loss.

Box 70.1   Assessment Components for Suspected Eating Disorder

- Complete history (highest and lowest weight, goal weight, dieting history, daily caloric intake, frequency of compensatory behaviors)
- Complete physical examination
- Height, weight, body mass index, and growth charts
- Vital signs (temperature, pulse, blood pressure)
- Laboratory studies (complete blood count, electrolytes, blood urea nitrogen, creatinine, liver function tests, thyroid function tests, glucose)
- Urinalysis
- Electrocardiogram

Sources: Lock J, La Via MC, American Academy of Child and Adolescent Psychiatry. Practice parameter for the assessment and treatment of children & adolescents with eating disorders. *J Am Acad Child Adolesc Psychiatry.* 2015;54(5):412–425; American Psychiatric Association. *Diagnostic and statistical manual of mental disorders.* 5th ed. Arlington, VA: American Psychiatric Association, 2013; Campbell K, Peebles R. eating disorders in children and adolescents: State of the art review. *Pediatrics.* 2014;134:582–592.

Box 70.2   Eating Disorder Screening Instruments

- SCOFF Questionnaire
- Eating Disorder Screen for Primary Care (ESP)
- Eating Attitudes Test (EAT-26)
- Eating Disorders Inventory-Second Edition (EDI-2)

Other physical assessments such as pulse, blood pressure, core temperature, cardiovascular and peripheral examination, and sit-ups/squat test for muscle power should be done on all patients. Laboratory investigations include complete blood count, endocrine testing, erythrocyte sedimentation rate, blood urea nitrogen (BUN) and electrolytes, creatinine, liver function tests (LFTs), random blood glucose, urinalysis, and electrocardiogram.

Excessive weight loss is often the most obvious sign of AN, but individuals with AN rarely complain of weight loss. Persons with AN are likely to deny that a problem exists although as they lose more weight, their fear of becoming fat intensifies. Severe weight loss eventually results in electrolyte imbalance and dehydration, with significant risks of serious medical complications such as cardiac arrhythmias. Long-standing amenorrhea can leave females at risk for developing osteopenia and osteoporosis.

Persons with BN vary in their weight and appearance, but most have a normal BMI. Many persons with BN have an extensive history of dieting. Assessment of dieting history, including both weight gain and loss, is important.

DIAGNOSTIC REASONING

Symptoms

The diagnosis of eating disorders is based on *DSM-5* criteria; please refer to the *DSM-5* for complete diagnostic criteria. Common symptoms include the following:

Anorexia Nervosa

- Self-imposed starvation (i.e., food restriction, compulsive exercising, or purging)
- Significant weight loss or emaciation and refusal to maintain body weight
- Fear of becoming obese, which can persist despite weight loss
- Body image disturbance, such as feeling fat even when emaciated

Bulimia Nervosa

- Recurrent episodes of binge eating
- Behaviors to reverse the effects of binging (e.g., self-induced vomiting or diarrhea, use of laxatives, excessive exercise, or fasting)
- Exaggerated concern about body shape and weight

Binge-Eating Disorder

- Frequent binge eating, including eating too quickly, until uncomfortable, or despite lack of hunger
- Negative feelings arise or persist from binge eating
- Not associated with compensatory behaviors (this would warrant a diagnosis of bulimia nervosa instead)

Differential Diagnosis

The differential diagnosis of eating disorders includes both primary medical conditions as well as psychiatric illnesses. A medical assessment, as described in Box 70.1, is an essential first step in the assessment of a suspected eating disorder. Medical conditions that can mimic AN include conditions that cause significant weight loss, including gastrointestinal disease, hyperthyroidism, malignancy, or HIV/AIDS; individuals with these conditions often do not manifest the fear of gaining weight or the body image disturbance that is present in AN and required for its diagnosis. The Kleine-Levin and Kluver-Bucy syndromes lead to excess eating but do not include the concern with body shape and weight that is often present in BN or BED.

Many psychiatric conditions can also mimic eating disorders. Individuals with major depressive disorder often have an appetite disturbance that can lead to weight loss or excess eating, although they do not have the body image disturbance present in eating disorders. Patients with social anxiety disorder may avoid eating in public due to embarrassment, and those with obsessive-compulsive disorder may have elaborate rituals involving eating or obsessions related to food (although they will also have other non–food-related obsessions or compulsions). Preoccupation with body shape without changes in food intake suggests body dysmorphic disorder. Impulsive behaviors, in the form of eating, can occur in the context of borderline personality disorder.

It is also important to distinguish between the different eating disorders based on the history and physical examination, as binging and purging are behaviors that cross diagnostic boundaries. An additional eating disorder, avoidant/restrictive food intake disorder (ARFID), manifests when patients have inadequate caloric intake that results in medical compromise, but there is no body image disturbance. Patients may have had a prior negative experience with food (e.g., choking, intense abdominal pain) that has led to decreased food intake, and the restriction is due to the anxiety of the negative experience happening again rather than a desire for thinness.

MANAGEMENT

The therapeutic relationship is central to management of the person with an eating disorder. Using the readiness to change model can help the patient and her or his family set realistic and safe goals. Factors that suggest the need for hospitalization are listed in Box 70.3. If the patient's condition does not require hospitalization, outpatient treatment of eating disorders can be effective. A multidisciplinary team, including the primary-care practitioner, nutritionist, and a psychiatric nurse specialist, is needed. Good communication between team members is essential because even motivated patients will have strong urges to resist treatment.

Box 70.3 Clinical Factors Suggesting Need for Hospitalization

- The presence of orthostatic hypotension
- Significant bradycardia
- Syncopal episodes
- Electrocardiogram abnormalities
- Abnormal electrolytes
- Acute food refusal for 24 hours
- Ideal body weight less than 85%
- Lack of response to outpatient treatment
- Active suicidal ideation
- Evidence of psychotic thinking (disorganized thought process, hallucinations, fixed false beliefs)
- Active substance abuse/withdrawal

Source: Yager J, Devlin MJ, Halmi KA, et al. *Guideline watch: Practice guideline for the treatment of patients with eating disorders.* 3rd ed. https://psychiatryonline.org/pb/assets/raw/sitewide/practice_guidelines/guidelines/eatingdisorders-watch.pdf. Published August 2012.

Inpatient Management

Goals for the patient who is hospitalized are fairly specific and include those listed in Box 70.4. The patient's psychological and nutritional status should be continuously assessed. A supportive, structured environment and programs should be provided, preferably in a specialized treatment center, or the patient should be admitted to a specialized eating disorder unit. If purging is involved,

Box 70.4 Goals of Inpatient Hospitalization of Eating Disorders

- Bedrest with supervised meals until the person has obtained a weight greater than 80% to 85% of his/her ideal body weight.
- Three hundred calorie stepwise, gradual increase in calories consumed.
- Stepwise increase in activity as weight increases.
- Establish the target weight.
- Weigh daily at first; as the weight gain progresses, this may be reduced to three times per week.
- Offer medication for symptom relief.
- Meals should be supervised.
- For the patient with anorexia, the goal is to achieve a weight gain of 1 to 2 pounds (0.45–0.91 kg) per week.
- Utilize nasogastric tube feedings as last resort if food refusal continues.
- For the patient with BN, restrict access to the bathroom for 2 hours after eating.

Sources: Lock J, La Via MC, American Academy of Child and Adolescent Psychiatry. Practice parameter for the assessment and treatment of children & adolescents with eating disorders. *J Am Acad Child Adolesc Psychiatry.* 2015;54(5):412–425; American Psychiatric Association. *Diagnostic and statistical manual of mental disorders.* 5th ed. Arlington, VA: American Psychiatric Association; 2013.

the clinician should identify the triggers and precipitants and help the patient work to establish alternative behaviors. Focused individual, group, and family therapies are also indicated.

Outpatient Management

On an outpatient basis, therapy involves building trust and a therapeutic alliance. The practitioner should involve the person with AN or BN in setting the target weight. The weight gain can be achieved gradually unless any danger signals surface.

The clinician should weigh the patient weekly at first, and later monthly if progress is being made. The focus should be on overall indices of health, not just on weight. The practitioner should prescribe medication if necessary for symptom relief and challenge any fear of uncontrollable weight gain. If purging is involved, precipitants should be identified, and alternative behaviors should be established. A cognitive-behavioral approach combined with education is often effective. Interpersonal therapy (IPT) or cognitive behavior therapy (CBT) should be offered to patients with BN and binge-eating disorder (Williams et al., 2008), although self-help programs are helpful for some patients (Williams et al., 2008). Studies indicate effectiveness of IPT or CBT for binge-eating disorder.

Family therapy as well as individual therapy may be necessary; the person should be referred to specialists in these areas. These may be advanced practice registered nurses, social workers, psychologists, or psychiatrists who have expertise in these areas. Family-based therapy (FBT), also known as the Maudsley approach, has been shown to be an effective approach for managing AN, with recent evidence indicating effectiveness for BN as well. FBT is an outpatient family therapy that empowers parents to take control of meal planning and take charge of the weight restoration. However, the primary-care provider can continue to play an important role on the interdisciplinary team and should maintain contact with the person being treated for an eating disorder.

Pharmacological therapy has been found to be effective in some cases, slightly more so with patients with BN (Level II; Williams et al., 2008). Antidepressant medications (especially selective serotonin reuptake inhibitors) have become mainstays of treatment of eating disorders. Fluoxetine (Prozac) 10 to 60 mg daily is the only U.S. Food and Drug Administration (FDA)-approved drug for BN, and it is sometimes necessary to use higher than normal doses for effective treatment of BN. Atypical antipsychotics can be useful to address rigid cognitions about body and weight and to assist with anxiety at mealtime, although acceptability is limited due to fear of weight gain. Lisdexamfetamine (Vyvanse) is approved for binge-eating disorder in adults, with typical dose range of 30 to 70 mg/day.

FOLLOW-UP AND REFERRAL

Treatment of eating disorders requires specialized care. Providers play the key role in helping patients accept referral to an eating disorders program. Making this decision is extremely difficult; patients may fail to follow through repeatedly before they accept treatment. Persons may appear to wish to have this decision made for them, but this is rarely the case, as involuntary treatment for an eating disorder is rarely effective. Persons who are dangerously malnourished and in need of emergency weight restoration must be hospitalized.

The course of illness with an eating disorder is long and highly variable. In a recent study of AN patients, about 50% achieved complete recovery, 21% had an intermediate outcome, and 26% had an outcome that was poor, with an overall mortality rate of 9.8%. Half of BN patients were reported to have recovered fully, 30% experienced occasional relapse, and almost 20% maintained the full criteria for BN. Relapse is common, especially during times of stress (e.g., marriage, childbearing). There is significant morbidity from severe malnutrition, cardiac arrest, and suicide. Poor prognosis is indicated by repeated hospitalizations, initial low weight, being married, and poor maturation. Depression is often a sequela of recovery. Eating disorders are best approached as chronic conditions marked by improvement and relapse. Recovered persons may continue to have complex feelings about food and their weight, but their self-care behaviors are more effective.

Patient Education: Eating Disorders

Information must be provided on the long-term effects of eating disorders. This may be especially important for the person with the disorder because she (or he) may simply be unaware of some of the long-term health consequences. See Box 70.5 for steps that the primary-care provider can take to provide support to patients and families.

SLEEP–WAKE DISORDERS

Description and classification of sleep–wake disorders have been expanded in *DSM-5* to reflect the important diagnostic overlay of medical conditions that affect normal sleep patterns. Of particular importance to primary care are insomnia disorder, obstructive sleep apnea hypopnea (OSAH) (see Chapter 29), substance/medication induced disorder (see Chapter 65), and restless legs syndrome (RLS). Insomnia disorder is presented in detail because it is an underpinning of each of these disorders. The criteria and important contributing factors for insomnia disorder and RLS are discussed.

Box 70.5 Education and Referral for Patients With Eating Disorders

- Provide information on eating disorder programs
- Review nutritional information and recommended dietary program and offer referral to a registered dietician
- Teach stress management and relaxation techniques for persons and families, to be used especially at mealtimes
- Provide education on health effects of laxatives and diuretics
- Reinforce the long-term nature of these disorders and the need for follow-up and treatment
- Point out that under stress, regressive behaviors can occur
- Involve the family in identifying symptoms to identify and report
- Encourage regular dental care for those who purge
- Teach strategies for managing self-destructive behaviors in ways that do not reinforce them
- Provide referral for individual or family therapy

Source: Vitousek KB, Orimoto L. Cognitive-behavioral models of anorexia nervosa, bulimia nervosa, and obesity. In: Kendall P, Dobson KS, eds. *Psychopathology and cognition.* San Diego, CA: Academic Press; 1993:191.

INSOMNIA DISORDER

Insomnia disorder, or difficulty sleeping, is an extremely common problem, yet it is one that is etiologically complex. It is defined as difficulty in falling or staying asleep, waking up too early in the morning, or any combination of these.

EPIDEMIOLOGY AND CAUSES

It is estimated that 10% to 15% of the primary-care population report daytime impairment because of insomnia, and that 6% to 10% meet criteria for the disorder. Women appear to be slightly more affected than men, and up to 50% of sufferers have a comorbid mental disorder. Difficulty maintaining sleep is the most common complaint.

Acute insomnia may be precipitated by physical or emotional discomfort. Examples include pain, acute illness, and environmental disturbances such as noise, light, and temperature. Sleeping at a time that is inconsistent with daily biological (circadian) rhythms because of plane travel across time zones (jet lag) or shift work may also precipitate acute insomnia. Pain may contribute to wakefulness; indeed, often the question "Does the pain awaken you at night?" is an important piece of information in determining the severity of pain.

PATHOPHYSIOLOGY

Normal sleep is a periodic state of rest accompanied by varying degrees of unconsciousness and relative inactivity. It is normally an easily reversible, regular, recurrent state. The functions of sleep are restorative and hemostatic, critical for normal thermoregulation and energy conservation. Sleep disturbance is often an early symptom of impending mental illness.

Two physiological states compose sleep: non–rapid eye movement (NREM) and rapid eye movement (REM) sleep. In NREM sleep, most physiological functions are markedly lower than in wakefulness, although there may be episodic, involuntary body movements during NREM sleep. In contrast, REM sleep is characterized by physiological activity levels similar to those in wakefulness and a high level of brain activity and is sometimes called paradoxical sleep. NREM sleep is composed of stages 1 through 4, with stages 3 and 4 being deep sleep. Typically, NREM sleep is punctuated with an REM cycle every 90 to 100 minutes during the night. The first REM period tends to be the shortest, lasting less than 10 minutes; later REM periods may last 15 to 40 minutes each. Most REM periods occur in the last third of the night; most stage 4 sleep occurs in the first third of the night.

These sleep patterns change over the course of a person's life. In young adulthood, REM comprises about 25% of sleep, and NREM approximately 75%. These figures remain fairly constant in normal sleep, although there is a reduction in both slow-wave sleep and REM sleep in older persons. NREM sleep increases after exercise and starvation and is thus thought to be associated with satisfying metabolic needs.

Daily variations in a variety of physiological functions affecting the endocrine, thermoregulatory, cardiac, pulmonary, renal, gastrointestinal, and neurobehavioral systems, as well as sleep–wake cycles, are governed by the 24-hour circadian rhythm in humans. The timing and internal architecture of sleep are coupled directly to the output of the endogenous circadian pacemaker. Misalignment of the output of the endogenous circadian pacemaker with the desired sleep–wake cycle can, therefore, induce insomnia, decrease alertness, and impair performance of shift workers, and accounts for the phenomenon of jet lag. Sleep deprivation for prolonged periods can lead to hallucinations, ego disorganization, and delusions, and REM-deprived patients may exhibit irritability and lethargy.

CLINICAL PRESENTATION

Insomnia may not be the chief reason for an office visit. It may be detected, however, by incorporating sleep-related questions into the general review of systems. Direct inquiry is important because patients with chronic insomnia often have never discussed their problem or have lived with it for so long that they think nothing can be done about it. The primary consequences of acute insomnia are sleepiness, negative mood, and impairment of performance, with severity related to the amount of sleep lost on one or more nights. Patients with chronic

insomnia frequently complain of fatigue, mood changes (e.g., depression, irritability), difficulty concentrating, and impaired daytime functioning.

The assessment should include questions about sleep, as well as questions about daytime functioning, where the full effects of altered sleep are manifested. The amount of sleep required for each individual to subjectively feel refreshed varies markedly. Although the ability to maintain sleep alters with age, the individual's need for sleep does not change significantly. The patient's medical history and comorbidities are other important parameters that should be documented. Many medical problems, such as gastroesophageal reflux disease, worsen at night because they may be aggravated by recumbency.

Focus on History: Insomnia Disorder

Questions to ask:

- How has the person been sleeping recently?
- How long has the person had difficulty sleeping?
- Does the person have any underlying psychiatric or medical conditions?
- Is the person's sleep environment conducive to sleep? For example, are there any problems that would make sleeping difficult, such as noise, temperature, light, or space?
- Does the person work shift work or odd hours?
- What does the person do in the evenings and to prepare to go to sleep?
- What time does the person usually go to sleep? Get up? Are these hours the same on the weekday as well as the weekend?
- Does the person travel frequently?
- Does the person use caffeine, alcohol, drugs, or tobacco? If so, how much, and what are the specifics concerning the patient's use?
- Does the person have difficulty staying awake or report dozing off during normal daily activities?
- Does the person report any daytime consequences of not sleeping?
- Does the person take daytime naps?
- Does the person (or his or her partner) report:
  - Loud snoring, gasping, or stop breathing at night? (suggests sleep apnea)
  - Legs or arms jerking during sleep? (suggests periodic limb movement)
  - Creeping, crawling, or uncomfortable feelings in the legs that are relieved by moving them? (suggests restless legs syndrome)

It may also be helpful for the patient to keep a sleep diary over 2 to 4 weeks. A sleep diary is a useful tool to track exactly when and under what conditions the patient sleeps, as well as diet, exercise, and drug habits that may help reveal the underlying problem. In addition, a record of all exercise and physical activity may prove helpful. The sleep diary also helps to further define the nature of the sleep problem, as patients should document what time they got into bed, what they did until they fell asleep, what time they recall falling asleep, any night-time awakenings (including ability to fall back asleep), and what time they awoke in the morning. Consider screening for insomnia as part of regular patient care (Schutte-Rodin et al., 2008).

DIAGNOSTIC REASONING

Symptoms

The diagnosis of insomnia disorder is made clinically using *DSM-5* criteria; please refer to the *DSM-5* for complete diagnostic criteria. Symptoms should occur frequently and for a significant duration of time. Common symptoms include:

- Poor quality of sleep (difficulty falling asleep, difficulty staying asleep, and/or early morning awakening)
- Trouble sleeping is not an effect of a medication or drug.

Collateral information from family or bed partners can be helpful to corroborate the diagnosis. Excessive daytime sleepiness can be assessed using the Epworth Sleepiness Scale. Polysomnography (sleep study) cannot distinguish those with insomnia from those without, and thus is only indicated if sleep apnea, periodic limb movements, or a REM sleep behavior disorder is suspected, or if usual treatment fail.

Differential Diagnosis

It is necessary to rule out all potential underlying causes of insomnia. Boxes 70.6 and 70.7 list medical and psychiatric causes of and contributors to insomnia. A thorough medication history must be taken, including all over-the-counter drugs, such as decongestants and cough syrups that contain decongestants, which act as stimulants. In addition, a complete history of all herbal remedies used, especially teas that may contain caffeine or ginseng and a variety of other central nervous system stimulants, should be obtained. When patients buy products in health food stores, they often do not think of them as "drugs." The patient also should be screened for any illicit drug and alcohol use.

MANAGEMENT

Nonpharmacological Management

Insomnia can be a chronic, lifelong illness, and given the chronic nature of this problem, long-term treatment is often advisable. Evidence supports the efficacy of CBT

Box 70.6 Medical Causes of and Contributors to Insomnia

- Painful conditions, such as arthritis and muscle cramps
- Fibromyalgia
- Delirium or dementia ("sundowning")
- Acid reflux, gastroesophageal reflux disease, or duodenal ulcers
- Conditions causing shortness of breath
- Thyroid disease
- Obesity (also associated with sleep apnea)
- Substance use, intoxication, or withdrawal
- Pregnancy or postpartum
- Nocturia
- Side effect of a medication

Source: Gutierrez C, Brady P. Obstructive sleep apnea: A diagnostic and treatment guide. *J Fam Pract.* 2013;62(10):565–572.

Box 70.7 Psychiatric Causes of and Contributors to Insomnia

- Major depressive disorder
- Generalized anxiety disorder
- Manic episode
- Psychotic illness, such as schizophrenia
- Traumatic events precipitating acute insomnia
- Post-traumatic stress disorder leading to hyperarousal
- Poor sleep hygiene
- Other sleep–wake disorders (OSAH, RLS)

Source: Roth T. Comorbid insomnia: Current directions and future challenges. *Am J Manag Care.* 2009;15:S6–S13.

---

for the first-line treatment of chronic insomnia (Schutte-Rodin et al., 2008). CBT can occur in an individual or group setting over 6 to 8 weeks. The clinician should review sleep hygiene strategies with the patient and identify any barriers to implementation (see Box 70.8). Any coexisting medical, psychiatric, or pain conditions should be adequately treated.

Reassurance and supportive counseling are essential; insomnia is not a complaint that should be taken lightly. Issues of caregiving for young children or older adults living in the home may be a part of the clinical picture. Again, diversionary lifestyle changes and situational support may be more effective than pharmacological measures for these patients. Sleep parameters can be reviewed and reemphasized several times during return visits before resorting to pharmacological measures (see Table 70.1).

Pharmacological Management

Evidence suggests that for some patients with persistent insomnia, adding a short course of a medication to CBT produces an additive benefit. Advantages of the

Box 70.8   Sleep Hygiene Strategies

- Maintain a regular sleep and wake schedule, 7 days a week
- Eat regular meals every day
- Develop a relaxing bedtime routine
- Limit amount of liquid consumed in the evening
- Limit amount of caffeine consumed later in the day
- Avoid tobacco and alcohol late in the day
- Avoid daytime naps
- Exercise regularly
- Limit exposure to bright lights in the evening; keep the bedroom as dark as possible; limit use of screens (phones, tablets, computers, TV) while in bed
- The bed should be used for sleeping and sex only; avoid doing other activities in bed that require wakefulness (e.g., reading) so that the bed is associated with sleepiness
- Turn any clocks to face away from the bed to avoid constant checking of the time
- If not asleep after 20 minutes, get out of bed and engage in a quiet activity, such as reading, outside of the bedroom before reattempting to fall asleep

Source: Sateia MJ, et al. Clinical practice guideline for the pharmacologic treatment of chronic insomnia in adults: An American Academy of Sleep Medicine Clinical Practice Guideline. *J Clin Sleep Med.* 2017;13(2):307–349.

sedative-hypnotics are that they hasten sleep onset, decrease the number of nighttime awakenings, increase total amount of sleep time (varies with medication duration of action), and make sleep more refreshing. Some of the disadvantages are that they may alter sleep architecture over time by decreasing slow-wave sleep and REM sleep and that they may cause residual sedation, psychomotor and cognitive impairment, psychological dependence in vulnerable individuals, and rebound insomnia.

Medications indicated for insomnia include five older benzodiazepines (estazolam, flurazepam, quazepam, temazepam, and triazolam) and three newer benzodiazepine-receptor agonist medications (eszopiclone, zaleplon, and zolpidem). The elimination half-lives and duration of action of the sedative-hypnotics (see Drugs Commonly Prescribed 70.1) vary tremendously. The advantages and disadvantages of a given duration of action must be assessed in light of each patient's individual needs. A limiting factor is that all agents in this class have some potential for abuse and are classified as Schedule IV by the Drug Enforcement Administration. In older adults, benzodiazepines should be avoided due to the risk of falls and rebound insomnia. Clinical trials have provided some evidence that sleep can improve to some degree without the use of any medication because patients receiving placebo often reported as much improvement during the

TABLE 70.1 Advanced Practice Nursing Interventions for Insomnia	
Behavioral Treatment	Relaxation therapy (progressive muscle relaxation therapy), autogenic training, electromyogram, biofeedback.
Sleep Restriction Therapy	Poor sleepers often increase their time in bed. Sleep restriction therapy curtails this time. For example, if a person reports sleeping only 5 hours per night, he or she should be counseled to stay in bed only 5 hours per night. As sleep improves, increase time in bed in 15- to 30-minute intervals. It works best to alter bedtime and keep rising time constant. Do not reduce sleep to less than 5 hours per night.
Stimulus Control Therapy	Functions on premise that insomnia is a conditioned response to temporal (bedtime) and environmental (bed/bedroom) cues. Objective is to reassociate the bed and bedroom with rapid sleep onset. Stimulus control therapy counsels: (1) Go to bed only when sleepy. (2) Use the bed only for sleep. (3) Get out of bed and go into another room when awake; go back into the bedroom only when sleepy. (4) Maintain a regular rise time, regardless of sleep deprivation during the night. (5) Avoid daytime napping.
Cognitive Therapy	Identify dysfunctional ideas about sleep and replace them with more functional approaches, e.g., 8 hours of sleep is not necessary for everyone; insomnia and less sleep does not have to destroy one's life. This approach helps minimize anticipatory anxiety around sleep.
Exercise	Regular physical activity will assist with sleep. Advise the patient not to exercise too close to bedtime.
Massage	Weekly massage may assist with relaxation.
Reassurance and Support	Active listening and patience; encourage expression of feelings, especially if stress is a component of the insomnia.

Drugs Commonly Prescribed 70.1: Sedatives and Hypnotics

DRUG	INDICATION	ADVERSE REACTIONS AND PRESCRIBING CONSIDERATIONS
Benzodiazepines		
		• Category IV controlled substance. • Risk of anterograde amnesia, CNS depression, paradoxical reactions, sedation, memory deficits, ataxia. • Use caution with narrow-angle glaucoma. • Association with falls and injury in the elderly. • Use caution with depressed patients and substance abuse, impaired hepatic or renal function. • Most contraindicated in obstructive sleep apnea. • Many drug–drug interactions (CYP pathways). • Withdrawal symptoms with abrupt discontinuation. The onset of withdrawal symptoms is usually seen on the first day without drug and lasts 5–7 days—slow taper. • Treatment longer than 4 months should be reevaluated to determine the patient's need for the drug. • Avoid valerian, St. John's wort, kava kava, gotu kola. • Potential severe allergic reactions (anaphylaxis, angioedema) • Risk of complex sleep-related behaviors, which may include sleep-driving, cooking and eating food while asleep, and making phone calls while asleep.
Estazolam (ProSom)	Insomnia, short-term	• Intermediate acting. • No active metabolites.
Flurazepam (Dalmane)	Insomnia, short-term	• Long acting. • Avoid in elderly and debilitated. • Active metabolites with extended half-lives may lead to delayed accumulation and adverse effects.
Temazepam (Restoril)	Insomnia, short-term	• Intermediate acting. • Administer 30 minutes before bedtime. • Lack of active metabolites—excellent option for the elderly.
Triazolam (Halcion)	Insomnia, short-term	• Short acting. • In elderly, higher incidence of CNS adverse reactions; not a drug of first choice.
Quazepam (Doral)	Insomnia	• Long-acting. • Risk of daytime sedation and fatigue. • May prevent withdrawal symptoms when stopped.
Benzodiazepine-Receptor Agonists ("Z-drugs")		
		• Category IV controlled substance. • Risk of daytime sedation, anterograde amnesia, rebound insomnia. • Less anxiolytic properties than the benzodiazepines. • All patients should be advised of residual morning effects and of complex sleep-related behaviors. This may include sleep-driving, cooking and eating food while asleep, and making phone calls while asleep. • All patients should be advised to get at least 4 hours of sleep after taking a short-acting agent and at least 7 hours of sleep with a long-acting agent.

Continued

Drugs Commonly Prescribed 70.1: Sedatives and Hypnotics—cont'd

DRUG	INDICATION		ADVERSE REACTIONS AND PRESCRIBING CONSIDERATIONS
Eszopiclone (Lunesta)	Insomnia, long-term		• Long half-life of 6 hours; good for sleep initiation and maintenance. • Advise to get 8 or more hours of sleep. • No hangover effect; may have metallic taste. • Risk of headache, dizziness, and somnolence. • Potentiates CNS depressants.
Zaleplon (Sonata)	Insomnia, short-term		• Short half-life, about 1 hour. • Good for patients that have difficulty falling asleep, not for sleep maintenance. • Advise to get at least 4 hours of sleep. • Dosage adjustment for hepatic impairment.
Zolpidem (Ambien)	Insomnia, short-term		• Half-life 1.4–2.4 hours. • Good for patients who have difficulty with falling asleep. • Risk of CNS depression, headache, dizziness, and somnolence. • Take with liquid—food can delay absorption. • No known rebound insomnia or hangover effect. • Reduced dosage in women and geriatric populations.
Zolpidem CR (Ambien CR [extended release])	Insomnia, long-term		• Half-life 1.4–2.4 hours, but released over a longer duration. • Risk of headache, dizziness, and somnolence. • Sleep may be impaired after discontinuation. • Abuse potential low. • Reduced dosage in women and geriatric populations. • Complex sleep-related behaviors, which may include sleep-driving, cooking and eating food while asleep, and making phone calls while asleep.
Melatonin Receptor Agonist			
Ramelteon (Rozerem)	Insomnia		• Indicated to promote sleep onset. • Peak concentrations within 1 hour if fasting, avoid high fat meal. • No withdrawal or rebound insomnia. • Does not affect REM sleep. • May affect testosterone and prolactin levels. • Risk of somnolence, dizziness, fatigue, nausea, and exacerbated insomnia. • Monitor liver transaminases.
Antihistamine			
Diphenhydramine (Benadryl)	Insomnia, short-term use less than 2 weeks		• Over the counter. • Many patients have used previously for other indications (suggests tolerance). • May have next-day sedation, dry mouth, decreased cognitive function. • Potentiates CNS depression. • Caution with asthma, other respiratory disorders; glaucoma; hyperthyroidism. • Can have a paradoxical effect in children and older adults.

Abbreviations: CNS, central nervous system; CYP, cytochrome P-450; REM, rapid eye movement.

study as those taking medication. In sleep studies, a placebo is not an "inactive" treatment in that all study participants must adhere to nonpharmacological regimens (such as going to bed and getting up at regular hours, not napping, avoiding caffeine and alcohol) that are recognized as effective remedies for insomnia.

Other agents often used to treat insomnia include antihistamines (diphenhydramine), antidepressants (trazodone, mirtazapine, doxepin), antipsychotics (quetiapine, olanzapine), melatonin, and the melatonin receptor agonist ramelteon. Of these, only doxepin and ramelteon are FDA approved for insomnia, with limited evidence for the others, despite their widespread use. Depression is the most common comorbid psychiatric diagnosis with chronic insomnia; however, antidepressants should be used most often in the setting of comorbid depression (Schutte-Rodin et al., 2008). Concurrent treatment of both insomnia and an underlying psychiatric comorbidity may result in greater improvements for the patient.

FOLLOW-UP AND REFERRAL

Transient insomnia may turn into chronic insomnia. For this reason, treatment is essential. Insomnia should resolve with patience, counseling, and treatment, and patients should be followed until the situation is resolved (Schutte-Rodin et al., 2008). A concern is daytime sleepiness (sleep apnea, for example, is highly correlated with car accidents). The patient may need to be referred for supportive counseling, especially if insomnia is related to a traumatic event.

Patient Education: Insomnia Disorder

The entire environmental situation of the patient and family should be assessed. Are there caregiver issues involved, and can external and additional support be provided or arranged for? Is there a need for diversionary activities, or a need to increase the individual's physical activity level? If sleep apnea is suspected, a polysomnogram should be ordered. In addition, all patients should be encouraged to maintain good sleep hygiene strategies, as outlined in Box 70.8.

RESTLESS LEGS SYNDROME

RLS is a neurological, sensorimotor condition that is typified by uncomfortable sensations in the lower extremities, such as burning, tingling, crawling, or itching, and an uncontrollable desire to move the legs, with associated sleep disturbance. Relief of symptoms is usually obtained once the individual moves his or her legs.

EPIDEMIOLOGY AND CAUSES

Prevalence rates of RLS vary from 2% to 7%, with women up to twice as likely as men to report symptoms. The prevalence of RLS increases with age, with onset typically occurring in the second or third decade of life. Those with familial RLS typically have an earlier age of onset and more progressive disease course. There is significant comorbidity with periodic limb movements of sleep, with up to 90% of individuals with RLS demonstrating periodic limb movements on polysomnogram.

PATHOPHYSIOLOGY

Dysfunction of dopaminergic systems is implicated in the pathophysiology of RLS, as evidenced by improvement of symptoms when dopaminergic drugs are administered. In addition, low iron levels can contribute to symptoms, so all patients should have iron studies completed, and appropriate supplementation should be implemented when necessary.

CLINICAL PRESENTATION

Symptoms occur when the patient is at rest and often worsen at night when attempting to initiate sleep. Patients often present complaining of an uncontrollable urge to move their legs that impairs their ability to initiate and maintain sleep. This leads to excessive daytime sleepiness and impaired functioning the next day. Bed partners may also notice the excessive movement during sleep. Many patients will report a family history of RLS.

DIAGNOSTIC REASONING

The diagnosis is based primarily on patient self-report, although a complete neurological examination and appropriate laboratory testing can help to rule out other possible diagnoses. In addition, patients should be referred for polysomnography.

Symptoms

Diagnosis is based on *DSM-5* criteria for RLS; please refer to the *DSM-5* for complete diagnostic criteria. Symptoms should occur frequently and for a significant duration of time. They include:

- An urge to move the legs
- An uncomfortable sensation in the legs
- The urge or discomfort begins or worsens when at rest, at night, or attempting to sleep
- The urge or discomfort is relieved by movement

Differential Diagnosis

RLS needs to be differentiated from leg cramps or positional discomfort. Important medical differential diagnoses are arthritis, peripheral neuropathy, peripheral vascular disease/ischemia, numbness, and radiculopathy, which may be associated with pain or discomfort in the extremities, but less often with the urge to move the extremities. Psychiatric comorbidity includes depressive disorders, anxiety disorders, panic disorder, and PTSD.

MANAGEMENT

The management of RLS includes reinforcing the sleep hygiene strategies listed in Box 70.8. Other interventions that can help include baths, whirlpool, massage, and exercise. The FDA has approved Relaxis, a vibrating pad that provides counter-stimulation to the legs. The American Academy of Sleep Medicine indicates that there is good evidence for use of the FDA-approved dopaminergic agents pramipexole (0.125–0.5 mg 2 to 3 hours before bedtime) and ropinirole (0.25–4.0 mg 1 to 3 hours before bedtime) in the treatment of RLS when there is moderate to severe impairment in sleep or daytime functioning.

FOLLOW-UP AND REFERRAL

All patients should be encouraged to maintain good sleep hygiene and keep a sleep diary. The primary-care provider should follow-up the response to the sleep hygiene strategies. Patients with suspected RLS should be referred for polysomnography. A trial of a dopaminergic agent is often warranted because a good response to these medications further supports the diagnosis of RLS. Patients who have complex sleep difficulties or are nonresponsive to first-line agents should be referred to a sleep specialist. In addition, patients with additional psychiatric comorbidity should be referred to a mental health provider for further assessment and management.

Patient Education: Restless Leg Syndrome

The patient and family members need to be reassured and counseled regarding the transient nature of RLS, including the lifestyle measures that can be instituted to assist with sleep. Appropriate sleep hygiene strategies should be emphasized. Care should be used with all pharmacological therapies because of the possible adverse effects and their potential for drug dependency, especially in elderly patients.

REFERENCES

Eating Disorders

American Psychiatric Association. *Diagnostic and statistical manual of mental disorders.* 5th ed. Arlington, VA: American Psychiatric Association; 2013.

Campbell K, Peebles R. Eating disorders in children and adolescents: State of the art review. *Pediatrics.* 2014;134:582–592.

Cotton MA, Ball C, Robinson P. our simple questions can help screen for eating disorders. *J Gen Intern Med.* 2003;18:53–56.

Crowther JH, Sherwood NE. Assessment. In: Garner DM, Garfinkel PE, eds. *Handbook of treatment for eating disorders.* 2nd ed. New York, NY: Guilford Press; 1997:34.

Davison GC, Neale JM. *Abnormal psychology.* 6th ed. New York, NY: John Wiley & Sons; 1994.

Jacobi C, et al. Coming to terms with risk factors for eating disorders: Application of risk terminology and suggestions for a general taxonomy. *Psychol Bull.* 2004;130(1):19–65.

Lock J, La Via MC; American Academy of Child and Adolescent Psychiatry. Practice Parameter for the assessment and treatment of children and adolescents with eating disorders. *J Am Acad Child Adolesc Psychiatry.* 2015;54(5):412–425.

Morgan JF, et al. The SCOFF questionnaire: Assessment of a new screening tool for eating disorders. *BMJ.* 1999;319:1467–1468.

National Collaborating Centre for Mental Health. *Eating disorders. Core interventions in the treatment and management of anorexia nervosa, bulimia nervosa and related eating disorders.* Leicester, United Kingdom: British Psychological Society; 2004. Retrieved from www.nice.org.uk/nicemedia/pdf/cg9fullguideline.pdf.

Rosen DS, and the Committee on Adolescence. Clinical Report—Identification and management of eating disorders in children and adolescents. *Pediatrics.* 2010;126:1240–1253.

Society of Adolescent Health and Medicine. Position Paper of the Society of Adolescent Health and Medicine: Medical management of restrictive eating disorders in adolescents and young adults. *J Adolesc Health.* 2015;56:121–125.

Striegel-Moore RH, Bulik CM. Risk factors for eating disorders. *Am Psychol.* 2007;62(3):181–198.

Vitousek KB, Orimoto L. Cognitive-behavioral models of anorexia nervosa, bulimia nervosa, and obesity. In: Kendall P, Dobson KS, eds. *Psychopathology and cognition.* San Diego, CA: Academic Press; 1993:191.

Walsh T, Garner DM. Diagnostic issues. In: Garner DM, Garfinkel PE, eds. *Handbook of treatment for eating disorders.* 2nd ed. New York, NY: Guilford Press; 1997:27.

Williams PM, et al. Treating eating disorders in primary care. *Am Fam Physician.* 2008;77(2):187–195.

Yager J, Devlin MJ, Halmi KA, et al. *Guideline Watch: Practice guideline for the treatment of patients with eating disorders.* 3rd ed. https://psychiatryonline.org/pb/assets/raw/sitewide/practice_guidelines/guidelines/eatingdisorders-watch.pdf. Published August 2012.

Insomnia

Allen RP, et al. Comparison of pregabalin with pramipexole for restless legs syndrome. *N Engl J Med.* 2014;370:621–631.

Aurora RN, et al. The treatment of restless legs syndrome and periodic limb movement disorder in adults—an update for 2012: Practice parameters with an evidence-based systematic review and meta-analyses. *Sleep.* 2012;35(8):1039–1062.

Bayard M, et al. Restless leg syndrome. *Am Fam Physician.* 2008;78(2):235–240.

Benca RM. Diagnosis and treatment of chronic insomnia: A review. *Psychiatr Serv.* 2005;56:332–343.

Buscemi N, et al. *Manifestations and management of chronic insomnia in adults.* Rockville, MD: Agency for Healthcare Research and Quality; 2005. http://www.ahrq.gov/clinic/tp/insomntp.htm.

Buysse DJ, et al. Clinical management of insomnia disorder. *JAMA.* 2017;318(20):1973–1974.

Earley CJ. Restless leg syndrome. *N Engl J Med.* 2003;348:2103–2109.

Gutierrez C, Brady P. Obstructive sleep apnea: A diagnostic and treatment guide. *J Fam Pract.* 2013;62(10):565–572.

National Institutes of Health. NIH State-of-the-Science Conference statement on manifestations and management of chronic insomnia in adults. https://consensus.nih.gov/2005/insomniastatement. pdf. Published 2005.

Palmer LJ, Redline S. Genomic approaches to understanding obstructive sleep apnea. *Respir Physiol Neurobiol.* 2003;135(2–3):187–205.

Roth T. Comorbid insomnia: Current directions and future challenges. *Am J Manag Care.* 2009;15:S6–S13.

Sateia MJ, et al. Clinical practice guideline for the pharmacologic treatment of chronic insomnia in adults: An American Academy of Sleep Medicine clinical practice guideline. *J Clin Sleep Med.* 2017;13(2):307–349.

Schutte-Rodin S, et al. Clinical guideline for the evaluation and management of chronic insomnia in adults. *J Clin Sleep Med.* 2008;4(5):487–504.

Winkelman JW. Insomnia disorder. *N Engl J Med.* 2015;373: 1437–1444.

RESOURCES

Anorexia Nervosa

Anorexia Nervosa. National Library of Medicine. PubMed Health
https://www.ncbi.nlm.nih.gov/pubmedhealth/PMHT0025745/

Anorexia Nervosa. Office on Women's Health
https://www.womenshealth.gov/files/documents/fact-sheet-anorexia.pdf

Anorexia Nervosa. Overview and Recommendations. Dynamed Plus
http://www.dynamed.com/topics/dmp~AN~T114614/Anorexia-nervosa

Anorexia: Overview and Statistics. National Eating Disorder Association
https://www.nationaleatingdisorders.org//anorexia-nervosa

Anorexia Nervosa: Signs, Symptoms, Causes, and Treatment. Harvard. Helpguide.org
https://www.helpguide.org/articles/eating-disorders/anorexia-nervosa.htm

Eating Disorder Support. National Alliance of Mental Illness
https://www.nami.org/Learn-More/Mental-Health-Conditions/Eating-Disorders/Support

Eating Disorder Types and Symptoms. National Association Anorexia Disorder
http://www.anad.org/get-information/about-eating-disorders/eating-disorder-types-and-symptoms/

Eating Disorders. Handout From the America Academy of Family Physicians
https://familydoctor.org/condition/eating-disorders/

How Is Anorexia Nervosa treated? Cleveland Clinic
https://my.clevelandclinic.org/health/diseases/9794-anorexia-nervosa/management-and-treatment

Let's Talk About It. Mental Health.Gov
https://www.mentalhealth.gov/what-to-look-for/eating-disorders/anorexia

Overview of Anorexia Nervosa. Mayo Clinic
https://www.mayoclinic.org/diseases-conditions/anorexia/symptoms-causes/syc-20353591

Women's Health.gov. Office of Women's Health, U.S. Department of Health and Human Services
https://www.womenshealth.gov/a-z-topics/anorexia-nervosa

Bulimia Nervosa

Bulimia Nervosa. Women's Health. Office of Women's Health
https://www.womenshealth.gov/a-z-topics/bulimia-nervosa

Bulimia Nervosa Overview and Statistics. National Eating Disorder Association
https://www.nationaleatingdisorders.org/bulimia-nervosa

Bulimia Nervosa Patient Information: Patient Plus Handout
http://m.patient.media/pdf/1894.pdf?v=636056672489531218

Bulimia Nervosa: Overview. Mayo Clinic
https://www.mayoclinic.org/diseases-conditions/bulimia/symptoms-causes/syc-20353615

Bulimia Nervosa: Overview and Recommendations. National Library of Medicine
http://www.dynamed.com/topics/dmp~AN~T114924/Bulimia-nervosa

Bulimia Nervosa: Signs, Symptoms, Treatment, and Self-Help. Help Guide. Harvard Health
https://www.helpguide.org/articles/eating-disorders/bulimia-nervosa.htm

Eating Disorder Treatment: Know Your Options. (Bulimia Nervosa). Mayo Clinic
https://www.mayoclinic.org/diseases-conditions/eating-disorders/in-depth/eating-disorder-treatment/art-20046234?p=1

Eating Disorders Among Adults-Bulimia Nervosa. National Institute of Mental Health
https://www.nimh.nih.gov/health/statistics/prevalence/eating-disorders-among-adults-bulimia-nervosa.shtml

Eating Disorders (Bulimia Nervosa) Teen's Health
http://kidshealth.org/en/teens/eat-disorder.html?view=ptr

Eating Disorders: About More Than Food. Booklet. National Institute of Mental Health
https://www.nimh.nih.gov/health/publications/eating-disorders/index.shtml

For Parents: Eating Disorders in Teens. American Academy of Family Physicians
https://familydoctor.org/for-parents-eating-disorders-in-teens/

Under Stress, Brains of Bulimics Respond Differently to Food. American Psychological Association
http://www.apa.org/news/press/releases/2017/07/stress-brains.aspx

Restless Leg Syndrome

A Guide to Living With Restless Legs Syndrome. Restless Legs Syndrome Foundation
https://www.rls.org/file/guide-to-living-with-rls.pdf

Restless Leg Syndrome. American Sleep Association
https://www.sleepassociation.org/patients-general-public/restless-legs-syndrome/

Restless Leg Syndrome. National Organization for Rare Disorders
https://rarediseases.org/rare-diseases/restless-legs-syndrome/

Restless Legs Syndrome: Brochure. National Institute of Neurological Disorders and Stroke
https://catalog.ninds.nih.gov/ninds/product/Restless-Legs-Syndrome/17-4847

Restless Leg Syndrome: Causes, Diagnosis, and Treatment for the Patient Living with Restless Legs Syndrome Brochure. Restless Legs Syndrome Foundation
https://www.rls.org/file/causes-092015.pdf

Restless Leg Syndrome: Overview, Facts, Causes, Symptoms, Self-Test, & Diagnosis, and Treatment. American Academy and Sleep Medicine
http://www.sleepeducation.org/essentials-in-sleep/healthy-sleep-habits

Restless Legs Syndrome: Overview, Outlook, Causes, Risk Factors, Treatment, and Living With National Heart, Lung, and Blood Institute
https://www.nhlbi.nih.gov/health-topics/restless-legs-syndrome

Restless Legs Syndrome: Treatment, Prognosis, Research, and Organizations. American Academy of Neurology
http://patients.aan.com/disorders/index.cfm?event=print&disorder_id=1053

Restless Leg Syndrome Fact Sheet: Patient and Caregiver Information. National Institute of Neurological Disorders and Stroke
https://www.ninds.nih.gov/Disorders/Patient-Caregiver-Education/Fact-Sheets/Restless-Legs-Syndrome-Fact-Sheet

Understanding Restless Leg: Watch the Basics of RLS. Restless Legs Syndrome Foundation
https://www.rls.org/understanding-rls

Sleep Disorders

Abnormal Sleep Behavior Disorders: REM Sleep Behavior Disorder. National Sleep Foundation
https://sleepfoundation.org/category/abnormal-sleep-behavior

About Narcolepsy: Epidemiology, Socioeconomic Impact, Symptoms, and Diagnosis. Stanford Medicine Center for Narcolepsy.
https://med.stanford.edu/narcolepsy/symptoms.html

Circadian Rhythm Sleep-Wake Disorders. American Academy and Sleep Medicine
http://www.sleepeducation.org/sleep-disorders-by-category/circadian-rhythm-disorders

Healthy Sleep Habits. American Academy and Sleep Medicine
http://www.sleepeducation.org/essentials-in-sleep/healthy-sleep-habits

Insomnia. American Academy of Family Physicians
https://familydoctor.org/condition/insomnia/?adfree=true

Insomnia Basics. National Library of Medicine
https://medlineplus.gov/insomnia.html

Insomnia Overview, Symptoms, Causes, Risk Factors, Complications, and Prevention. Mayo Clinic
https://www.mayoclinic.org/diseases-conditions/insomnia/symptoms-causes/syc-20355167?p=1

Insomnia: What is it? Causes, Signs and Symptoms, Diagnoses, Treatment, and Clinical Trials. National Heart, Lung, and Blood Institute
https://www.nhlbi.nih.gov/health-topics/insomnia

Narcolepsy Fact Sheet: National Institute of Neurological Disorders and Stroke
https://www.ninds.nih.gov/Disorders/Patient-Caregiver-Education/Fact-Sheets/Narcolepsy-Fact-Sheet

Narcolepsy—Overview and Facts, Symptoms, Self-Test, Diagnosis, and Treatment. American Academy and Sleep Medicine
http://www.sleepeducation.org/essentials-in-sleep/narcolepsy/overview-facts

Practice Standards/Practice Guidelines. American Academy of Sleep Medicine
https://aasm.org/clinical-resources/practice-standards/

Sleep Education. American Academy of Sleep Medicine
http://sleepeducation.org/

Understanding Sleep: Brain Basics Brochure. National Institute of Neurological Disorders and Stroke
https://catalog.ninds.nih.gov/ninds/product/Understanding-Sleep-Brain-Basics-/17-NS-3440-C

When Narcolepsy Lets Us Down, Understanding Lifts Us Up. Narcolepsy Network
https://narcolepsynetwork.org/

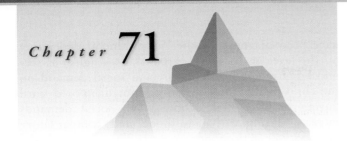

Chapter 71

Neurodevelopmental Disorders

Ronke Babalola, MD, MPH

Jason V. Lambrese, MD

Lynne M. Dunphy, PhD, APRN, FNP-BC, FAAN, FAANP

AUTISM SPECTRUM DISORDER

Autism spectrum disorder (ASD) is a neurodevelopmental disorder of childhood that, in the *Diagnostic and Statistical Manual of Mental Disorders* (5th edition; *DSM-5*), encompasses the following former diagnoses from the 4th edition of the *DSM*: pervasive developmental disorder not otherwise specified (PDD NOS), autistic disorder, Asperger syndrome, child disintegrative disorder, and Rett's syndrome. Core features for ASD include delays/deficits in social interaction and restricted or repetitive behaviors. ASD can present with or without intellectual disability or language impairment and may be associated with some genetic disorders.

EPIDEMIOLOGY AND CAUSES

The prevalence of ASD is thought to be approximately 1% of the population. Recent increases in the incidence of ASD may reflect a true increase in cases, increased awareness of the diagnosis, or the broadening of the criteria in *DSM-5*. ASD is more common in males than females (it is diagnosed four times more frequently in males), and females are more likely to experience intellectual disability. Severity of ASD is often increased with impairment in language or cognition, comorbid mental illness, or comorbid epilepsy.

The underlying etiology of ASD remains under investigation, though there is an apparent role for genetics given the elevated rate of diagnosis in siblings (up to 10 times higher than the general population) and the high concordance rate in monozygotic twins. Approximately 15% of cases of ASD are associated with a known genetic mutation. Repeated epidemiological studies have demonstrated no association between the MMR (measles, mumps, and rubella) vaccine and subsequent development of ASD, despite an initial faulty study that suggested otherwise. Environmental factors may contribute to ASD, including closer spacing of pregnancies, advanced parental age, premature birth, low birth weight, and fetal exposure to valproate.

PATHOPHYSIOLOGY

Symptoms of ASD usually appear during the second year of life but can be noted earlier or later depending on the severity of deficits. ASD is not a degenerative disorder, and the child will continue to develop throughout life, although at an altered pace compared with peers. Many patients with ASD will struggle socially throughout their lives, although those who are less impaired intellectually and behaviorally can lead independent lives. About 70% of individuals with ASD may have one comorbid mental disorder, and 40% may have two or more comorbid mental disorders. There is frequent co-occurring hyperactivity, anxiety, obsessive-compulsive symptoms, tics, and self-injury. In addition, up to 25% of individuals with ASD will have electroencephalogram (EEG) abnormalities or seizure activity. Intellectual disability is common, with only 20% of patients with ASD having an IQ in the normal range. Verbal skills are often more impaired than nonverbal skills.

CLINICAL PRESENTATION

Children with ASD can present with a variety of symptoms, but there are core features of ASD that can clue primary care providers in to the need for further assessment. A complete developmental history can provide context for the diagnosis.

Focus on History: Autism Spectrum Disorder

- Were there any difficulties with the pregnancy or in utero exposures?
- Were there any difficulties at delivery (e.g., preterm, low birth weight, need for emergent caesarian section)?
- Did the child experience any illness as in infant or toddler?
- At what age did the child reach developmental milestones (e.g., walking, talking, toileting)?
- Did the child develop normally, then experience a regression?
- How does the child interact with the caregiver? Does the child maintain eye contact, point at desired objects, seek out the parent?

- Does the child show empathy if the parent appears hurt?
- How does the child engage with other children?
- Does the child engage in pretend play?

Children on the autism spectrum (often referred to as "on the spectrum") have difficulty with imaginary play or sharing which would be appropriate to their age level. These children may present in primary care with the chief complaint of "sameness," such as self-restricted diet, and/or self-restricted activities such as lining up cars or watching the fan or toilet spin for hours at a time. Some may spin or twirl, and some may have repetitive movements such as hand flapping. They are inflexible about routine, become distressed over small changes, and parents might complain about their activities of daily living such as lack of or difficulty with showering, dressing, or eating. Although there are not exact percentages, most children on the spectrum have difficulty with sleeping and may function with less sleep. They sometimes demonstrate echolalia, which involves repeating words over and over, including those overheard from caretakers. People on the autism spectrum mostly self-talk, which can be misunderstood as a psychotic disorder. Self-talk in public is often due to a lack of social awareness.

Primary-care clinicians should pay attention to age-appropriate development. ASD children may also present with sensory issues and may be hyper- or hypo-reactive to pain, temperature, textures, certain smells, and specific sounds. Some nonverbal and severe ASD children have self-harming behavior such as banging their head on the wall, scratching or biting themselves, and/or displaying aggression toward others. The ASD population has been noted by parents and health-care workers to be stronger physically than their peers, especially during puberty. Physical exams, including providing immunizations and obtaining blood pressure or blood work, may prove difficult in some patients. Using clear, direct statements about what you are about to do will help to prepare children. It is also important to ask parents for self-soothing techniques that the child has found helpful that can be used during the examination.

DIAGNOSTIC REASONING

To diagnose a patient with ASD, there must be persistent deficits in social communication and interaction, and restrictive repetitive patterns in behavior, interests, and activities. When children or adults with ASD are evaluated, the clinician may observe a lack of emotional back-and-forth conversation, deficiencies in verbal and nonverbal communication, and deficiencies in understanding the interpersonal relationship. ASD may not

have been diagnosed earlier in childhood depending on the level of disability, verbal skills, English as second language, cultural beliefs, and social demand on the child. Mild ASD is at times not diagnosed until during or after high school when social demands increase during early adulthood and compensatory behaviors or actions no longer suffice. Although the diagnosis can be made later in life, the symptoms must have been present during the early developmental period on retrospect.

All young children should be screened for the presence of ASD features as part of routine developmental assessment. In addition, several tools are available that can be used to screen for ASD in primary care or mental health settings (see Box 71.1 for examples); some are rated by the clinician, others by the caregivers.

If there are significant concerns on screening, the child should undergo a comprehensive diagnostic evaluation, often accomplished through a referral to a developmental specialist (e.g., in developmental pediatrics or child and adolescent mental health). This assessment would ideally occur in a multidisciplinary team and include medical, developmental, psychological, and mental health assessments. A frequently used assessment tool is the ADOS (Autism Diagnostic Observation Schedule), which is administered by trained clinicians. Diagnoses should specify whether impairments in intellect or language are present. A comprehensive medical evaluation for organic causes of ASD should be completed (see Box 71.2).

Box 71.1	**Selected Screening Tools for Autism Spectrum Disorder**

- Autism Behavior Checklist (ABC)
- Childhood Autism Rating Scale (CARS)
- Checklist for Autism in Toddlers (M-CHAT)
- Autism Screening Questionnaire (ASQ)

Box 71.2	**Medical Evaluation of Suspected Autism Spectrum Disorder**

- Complete physical examination
- Hearing screen
- Wood's lamp examination for signs of tuberous sclerosis
- Genetic testing (karyotype, chromosomal microarray)
- Fragile X testing

Volkmar F, Wiesner L. Autism and related disorders. In: Carey WB, Crocker AC, Coleman WL, et al., eds. *Developmental-Behavioral Pediatrics*. 4th ed. Philadelphia, PA: Saunders Elsevier; 2009.

Differential Diagnosis

Differential diagnoses for ASD must be ruled out. Many medical conditions mimic or cause ASD (see Differential Diagnosis 71.1).

MANAGEMENT

ASD requires individualized treatment and referral, as no two ASD patients are alike. History obtained from parents and observation of the child is critical.

Differential Diagnosis 71.1: Autism Spectrum Disorder

- Deafness
- Tic or movement disorder
- Attention-deficit/hyperactivity disorder
- Selective mutism
- Social (pragmatic) communication disorder
- Language disorder
- Speech sound disorder
- Childhood-onset fluency disorder (stuttering)
- Stereotypic movement disorder
- Developmental coordination disorder or motor skills deficits
- Intellectual disability
- Schizophrenia
- Reactive attachment disorder
- Obsessive-compulsive disorder
- Fragile X syndrome
- Rett syndrome (when developmental regression is noted)
- Landau-Kleffner syndrome
- Tuberous sclerosis

Nonpharmacological Management

Educational and behavioral interventions have been shown to be effective for ASD and are first-line treatment options. Young children should be referred for Early Intervention Services. The most frequently used behavioral intervention is applied behavioral analysis (ABA), in which functional analyses are undertaken when maladaptive behaviors occur so that behavioral techniques can be identified to promote the desired behavior.

Assessment of the level and ability of the child's communication is critical. For children with minimal or absent verbal communication skills, forms of augmentative communication should be used, such as sign language, pictures, or communication boards. In addition, caregivers should be encouraged to speak with the school to discuss academic accommodations that may be beneficial, and they could consider requesting an evaluation for an Individualized Education Program (IEP). Because youth with ASD benefit most from structure and predictability, designing the school day to minimize disruptions can be beneficial. Consider the need to involve physical, occupational, and speech therapy. Finally, referral to a social skills program (some of which occur in schools) can help the patient develop and practice social pragmatic skills.

Pharmacological Management

Psychotropic medications should be considered when there is comorbid mental illness or if there are specific problematic target symptoms to address, such as severe irritability or aggression, sleep disturbances, or hyperactivity. Two agents have been approved by the Food and Drug Administration for the treatment of irritability (often manifesting as severe tantrums or aggression): risperidone and aripiprazole. Other medications have off-label uses for various target symptoms (see Drugs Commonly Prescribed 71.1).

Drugs Commonly Prescribed 71.1: Medications Used in the Treatment of Autism Spectrum Disorder

MEDICATION	INDICATION	ADVERSE REACTIONS AND PRESCRIBING CONSIDERATIONS
Second-Generation Antipsychotics (SGAs)		
Risperidone (Risperdal) (FDA approved)	Autism-associated irritability (including aggression, temper tantrums, self-injurious behavior, and quickly changing moods), bipolar disorder, disruptive behavior disorders, ADHD, Tourette's disorder, schizophrenia, delirium	• EPS (e.g., akathisia, dystonia etc.) • Drowsiness • Parkinsonian-like syndrome (common in children) • Increase in LFTs • Metabolic syndrome • Hyperprolactinemia, gynecomastia • Galactorrhea • Cardiovascular effect including prolongation of the QTc interval

Continued

Drugs Commonly Prescribed 71.1: Medications Used in the Treatment of Autism Spectrum Disorder—cont'd

MEDICATION	INDICATION	ADVERSE REACTIONS AND PRESCRIBING CONSIDERATIONS
Aripiprazole (Abilify) (FDA approved)	Autism-associated irritability (including aggression, temper tantrums, self-injurious behavior, and quickly changing moods), bipolar disorder, disruptive behavior disorders, ADHD, Tourette's disorder, schizophrenia, delirium	• EPS (particularly akathisia) • Drooling • Drowsiness • Parkinsonian-like syndrome (common in children) • Metabolic syndrome • Cardiovascular effect
Olanzapine (Zyprexa)	Bipolar disorder (including acute mania), schizophrenia, acute agitation, anorexia nervosa, Tourette's disorder	• EPS • Cardiovascular effect • Drowsiness • Weight gain • Metabolic Syndrome
Alpha-Agonists		
Clonidine (Catapres, Kapvay)	ADHD (particularly hyperactivity/impulsivity), disruptive behavior disorders, tic disorder, Tourette's disorder, hypertension, insomnia, anxiety	• Hypotension • Bradycardia • Drowsiness • Rebound hypertension • Epistaxis
Guanfacine (Tenex, Intuniv)	ADHD (particularly hyperactivity/impulsivity), tic disorder, Tourette's disorder, hypertension	• Hypotension • Bradycardia • Drowsiness • Increase in serum ALT • Skin rash
Melatonin		
Melatonin	Initial insomnia (difficulty falling asleep)	Rare, but headache, confusion, and fragmented sleep

Abbreviations: ADHD, attention-deficit/hyperactivity disorder; ALT, alanine aminotransferase; ASD, autism spectrum disorder; CNS, central nervous system; EPS, extrapyramidal symptoms; FDA, Food and Drug Administration; LFTs, liver function tests; NMS, neuroleptic malignant syndrome; ODD, oppositional defiant disorder; SGAs, second-generation antipsychotics.

Medications should be considered if behavioral interventions were ineffective or if symptoms are severe. Given the communication difficulties of some patients with ASD, response to medication may be judged by caregivers.

FOLLOW-UP AND REFERRAL

Because ASD is chronic and lifelong, the primary-care provider plays an important role in developing and maintaining a long-term relationship with the patient and family. Additionally, the needs of the patient and family will change over time and as the youngster develops. If the primary-care provider is a pediatric provider, plans around transition of care to an adult provider are

crucial. As these patients approach adulthood, planning around vocational training and the ability for independent living become highlighted. The primary-care provider should refer the patient to a multidisciplinary team for initial diagnostic assessment and support in management, and work in conjunction with this specialist team.

Patient Education: Autism Spectrum Disorders

Families should be encouraged to access local and national resources for ASD, engage in support groups, link with other families, access medical and mental health care, and maintain close lines of communication with the school system. Some schools are overwhelmed and underfunded such that some children are classified incorrectly and receive inappropriate interventions. Some caregivers are not aware of their rights when schools refuse special education evaluation, especially when the signs and symptoms of autism are not severe. Parents should request IEP assessments in writing, and by law the school needs to provide the assessment within a specified amount of time. There are laws and advocacy groups that can assist through this process, and parents and clinicians should become familiar with educational advocates in the area. Parents can be referred to the Autism Speaks Web site for further guidance around their rights.

INTELLECTUAL DISABILITY

Intellectual disability (ID), replacing the outdated term mental retardation, is present when there are deficits in cognition and adaptive functioning. Determining the presence of ID is important as it assists in the determination of the level of support that someone requires, particularly in school. ID onset must be during the development period with onset before age 18 years and has a range of severities. The most common conditions associated with ID are Down syndrome, fragile X syndrome, and fetal alcohol syndrome. Neuropsychological testing must be performed for the appropriate classification (mild, moderate, severe, and profound).

EPIDEMIOLOGY AND CAUSES

The prevalence of ID is estimated to be 1% to 3% of children, with a significant proportion being boys. People with ID are living longer than in the past and most are living in the community rather than in institutional settings. Patients with Down syndrome live, on average, twice as long as they did 25 years ago. Thus, the adult primary-care clinician will be providing health care for increasing numbers of patients with ID and cognitive impairment. Prevalence rates vary for the differing severity levels of ID, with the estimated prevalence of severe ID being 6 in 1,000. Challenging behaviors are present in up to 10% of individuals with ID. ID is a diagnosis in and of itself, although it can be associated with many underlying conditions that need to be assessed for and treated appropriately. Comorbidity with medical, mental, and neurodevelopmental conditions is common. The predominance of boys being diagnosed with ID is thought to be related to the many X-linked genetic disorders that can cause ID; of boys with an ID, 2% to 3% will have fragile

X syndrome. In addition to treatment of the underlying cause of the ID, supports often need to be put in place in school, home, and the community to address the differences in learning and adaptability that these children have.

PATHOPHYSIOLOGY

Intellectual disability describes a syndrome rather than a discrete diagnostic entity. As such, there is no unifying pathophysiological mechanism to explain the intellectual deficits observed in patients. ID can be the result of in utero insults (including genetic, toxic/metabolic, environmental, and structural malformations), perinatal/delivery complications, or postnatal illness (including ischemia, infection, traumatic brain injury, or toxic/metabolic exposures) which impede on normal neurological development, and subsequently, intellect. As ID can be associated with underlying medical causes, a comprehensive medical evaluation needs to be undertaken as part of the diagnostic process (see Box 71.3). Primary-care providers should consider referral to a medical geneticist and work closely with the geneticist in making the diagnosis.

CLINICAL PRESENTATION

Many patients with an intellectual disability will have delays in their developmental milestones; therefore, delays can first be identified within the first 2 years of life in severely affected children. Patients with ID will present with varying deficits in cognitive and adaptive

---

Box 71.3 **Evaluation for Medical Etiology of Intellectual Disability**

- Complete medical history, including a three-generation family history
- Complete physical examination, including assessment for dysmorphic features and a neurological examination
- Genetics referral for consideration of
  - Chromosomal microarray
  - Karyotype
  - Screening for inborn errors of metabolism
  - Testing for X-linked genetic disorders in boys, particularly fragile X syndrome
  - Testing for *MECP2* gene mutation in girls to rule out Rett syndrome
- Neuroimaging

Huang J, Zhu T, Qu Y, Mu D. Prenatal, perinatal and neonatal risk factors for intellectual disability: A systemic review and meta-analysis. *PLoS One.* 2016;11:e0153655.

functioning, depending on the severity of the disability. See Table 71.1 for clinical features in the conceptual, social, and practical domains that appear with increasing severity of ID.

DIAGNOSTIC REASONING

The diagnostic process includes diagnosing the ID and the underlying medical etiology, if one exists. The diagnosis of ID is based on meeting *DSM-5* criteria (see next section). Onset must be during the developmental period with deficits in conceptual, social, and practical domains. To assess for the criteria, neuropsychological testing of cognition (in the form of IQ) and adaptive functioning must be undertaken by a trained psychologist. Intellectual testing if often undertaken using standardized, structured assessments (e.g., Wechsler Intelligence Scale for Children) to assess intelligence quotient (IQ). The *DSM-5* stipulates that patients with ID should have intellectual functioning at least two standard deviations below the population mean; for IQ testing, this means an IQ of 70 or less. Adaptive functioning is also often assessed using standardized instruments, including the Vineland Adaptive Behavior Scale. Per *DSM-5* criteria, intellectual deficits can be in the domains of problem solving, planning, abstract thinking, judgment, academic learning, and learning from experience. Adaptive functioning deficits manifest in the activities of daily life, such as communication, school participation, and independent living.

Symptoms

The diagnosis of intellectual disability is based on *DSM-5* criteria; please refer to the *DSM-5* for complete diagnostic criteria. Though patients can present at any age, onset of symptoms must be during the developmental period. Common symptoms include:

- Cognitive deficits, such as low IQ, based on clinical assessment and testing.
- Deficits in adaptive functioning occurring across multiple environments that limit one's ability to successfully perform their activities of daily living.

Differential Diagnosis

In addition to diagnosis of the ID itself, a diagnostic assessment for underlying etiologies must be undertaken. Some children will present with characteristic physical features (e.g., Down syndrome) or behavioral features (e.g., Lesch-Nyhan syndrome) of the underlying cause. Discerning if children had a period of normal development prior to onset of symptoms will also help to narrow the differential diagnosis (see Differential Diagnosis 71.2). Assessment of comorbid mental illness should be undertaken as well (see Box 71.4).

MANAGEMENT

Pharmacological Management

There are no medications indicated for the treatment of ID. Treatment should be directed at any underlying

TABLE 71.1 Severity Levels for Intellectual Disability			
Severity	*Conceptual Domain*	*Social Domain*	*Practical Domain*
Mild	• Difficulties in learning academic skills • Impaired abstract thinking, executive functioning, or short-term memory	• Immature in social interactions and judgment • Concrete use of language and communication	• Functions well in personal care • Needs support in independent activities of daily living • Can excel in jobs that do not require conceptual skills
Moderate	• Language and academic skills markedly lag behind peers • Ongoing support needed into adulthood to manage day-to-day tasks	• Spoken language is simpler than peers • May misperceive social cues • Limited decision-making abilities	• With support, can manage ADLs and household tasks by adulthood • Considerable support required in employment
Severe	• Little understanding of written language or numbers • Limited attainment of conceptual skills	• Speech consists of single words or phrases • Understand simple language and gestures	• Support required for all ADLs • Cannot make responsible decisions regarding well-being

TABLE 71.1 Severity Levels for Intellectual Disability—cont'd

Severity	Conceptual Domain	Social Domain	Practical Domain
Profound	• Can use objects in a goal-directed way • Little understanding of conceptual processes • Motor or sensory impairments may be present	• Very limited understanding of symbolic communication • Uses nonverbal communication and gestures mostly	• Dependent on others for all aspects of daily care and recreational activities

Abbreviation: ADLs, activities of daily living.
Source: Volkmar F, Wiesner L. Autism and related disorders. In: Carey WB, Crocker AC, Coleman WL, et al., eds. *Developmental-behavioral pediatrics*. 4th ed. Philadelphia, PA: Saunders Elsevier; 2009.

 Differential Diagnosis 71.2: Intellectual Disability

- Down syndrome
- Fragile X syndrome
- Fetal alcohol syndrome
- Autism spectrum disorder
- Duchenne muscular dystrophy
- Lesch-Nyhan syndrome
- Rett syndrome
- Inborn errors of metabolism
- Structural brain malformations
- Maternal disease during the prenatal period
- Encephalopathy
- Hypoxic ischemic brain injury
- Traumatic brain injury
- Infections (e.g., meningitis, encephalitis)
- Seizure disorders
- Toxic metabolic syndromes
- Cerebral palsy

Box 71.4   Common Comorbid Mental Illnesses With Intellectual Disability

- Attention-deficit/hyperactivity disorder
- Depressive disorders
- Bipolar disorder
- Anxiety disorders
- Autism spectrum disorder
- Stereotypic movement disorder
- Impulse control disorders
- Major neurocognitive disorder

---

or comorbid medical or psychiatric condition. Challenging or dangerous behavior that is not responsive to behavioral or psychosocial interventions can be managed in a way similar to that described earlier for ASD. Off-label use of alpha-agonists (such as guanfacine and clonidine) or atypical antipsychotics (such as risperidone and aripiprazole) can be useful in managing challenging behaviors but should often be reserved for use only if there is a comorbid mental illness that would indicate use of these agents given the risk of side effects.

Nonpharmacological Management

Management of patients with ID should be focused on the underlying deficits of the individual. Specific adaptive deficits, such as those related to feeding, toileting, dressing, and recreational activities, should be managed with supports and coaching. Communication deficits may require augmentative communication, such as picture boards or use of apps on tablets. The environment may need to be changed to suit the needs and safety of the individual. Challenging behaviors may respond to behavioral interventions, such as functional behavior analysis, conducted by trained behavioral specialists. Educational needs should be addressed through the educational system, often through the use of an IEP or 504 Plan. Some individuals may benefit from schooling past 18 years old, depending on their developmental age. Many adults will benefit from consistent day structure, which can be provided through day programs or adult day cares.

FOLLOW-UP AND REFERRAL

In the initial assessment of a patient with suspected ID, referral for further diagnostic assessment is crucial. Patients should be referred to a genetic specialist for assessment of underlying medical causes, as well as a trained psychologist for structured diagnostic testing to determine the presence and severity of the ID. Patients with co-occurring psychiatric symptoms (e.g., depressed mood, irritability, aggression) should be referred for mental health assessment. The primary care provider should work in conjunction with the multidisciplinary team. In addition, as part of the ongoing management of the patient with ID, families should be referred for early intervention if they are of the appropriate age.

Patient Education: Intellectual Disability

Families should request an educational assessment for qualification for special education services through the implementation of an IEP. By law, schools are required to conduct an assessment free of charge within a specified amount of time and provide requisite supports and services if children qualify. Economic support for these programs varies state by state.

TIC DISORDERS

A tic is an involuntary muscular contraction or vocalization. Individuals can present with motor or vocal tics, or a combination of the two. Tic disorders often present during childhood, occasionally warrant treatment, and frequently self-resolve. The most common tic disorder is Tourette's disorder, characterized by the presence of motor and vocal tics. Behavioral and/or pharmacological treatment is warranted when tics interfere with activities or cause undue distress.

EPIDEMIOLOGY AND CAUSES

The prevalence of tic disorders is 0.5% to 3%, with approximately 7% of school-age children having tics in the previous year. Many youngsters will experience transient tic behaviors that do not rise to the level of a tic disorder. The average age of onset of tic disorders is 7 years old, although it can be much earlier. The severity often peaks by 12 years of age, and by adulthood, many individuals will find that their tics have resolved. Many patients struggle socially and have been shown to have greater psychological distress than their peers, and comorbidity with mental illness is common.

PATHOPHYSIOLOGY

Neuroimaging studies have pointed to deficits in motor areas of the brain in patients with tic disorders. Relatives of patients with tic disorders are more likely to have tics themselves, with at least a 10-fold increase risk of tics in first-degree relatives of individuals with tic disorders compared to the general population. In addition, there is significant concordance in monozygotic twins, pointing to a genetic basis. There are many conditions that can cause involuntary movements. See Table 71.2 for other involuntary movements that should be assessed for in the evaluation for tic disorder.

TABLE 71.2 Repetitive Movements of Childhood

Involuntary Movement	Description
Tics	Sudden rapid nonrhythmic movements
Dystonia	Muscle contractions that cause twisting or abnormal postures
Chorea	Random quick jerking movements that flow from joint to joint
Stereotypies	Rhythmic repetitive movements
Compulsions	Excessive meaningless activity used to avoid distress or worry
Myoclonus	Shock-like involuntary muscle jerk

CLINICAL PRESENTATION

Tics can present as simple (a rapid, meaningless movement) or complex (a purposeful or elaborate movement). See Box 71.5 for examples of common tics. The presence and severity of tics can wax and wane over time, with tics more prominent during times of stress, anxiety, fatigue, illness, or excitement. Tics are often preceded by a premonitory urge to tic, but it can be quite difficult to suppress the tic once the urge arises. There can be severe tension, itching, or a burning sensation if the person does not act on the urge.

DIAGNOSTIC REASONING

Tics are diagnosed when other causes of abnormal movements are ruled out, and when patients show the characteristic movements or vocalizations. Assessment should include gathering information on the types, frequency, and alleviating/aggravating factors of the tics. Family history should be ascertained. Rating scales can be used, such as the Yale Global Tic Severity Scale. Once medical causes of tics are ruled out, *DSM-5* criteria are used to diagnose a primary tic disorder (see next section). Laboratory testing should be undertaken (see Box 71.6). If focal neurological deficits are noted, neuroimaging should be performed to rule out structural lesion. Given the frequent comorbidity of psychiatric disorders, complete psychiatric assessment is warranted (see Box 71.7).

Symptoms

The diagnosis of a tic disorder is based on *DSM-5* criteria; please refer to the *DSM-5* for complete diagnostic criteria. Patients with a tic disorder will have symptoms onset at less than 18 years of age. Tics can be intermittent and vary in severity over time, though

Box 71.5   Common Tics

Common Motor Tics

- Simple tics
  - Eye blinks
  - Shoulder shrugs
  - Head jerks
  - Facial grimaces
  - Extension of extremities
- Complex tics
  - Tapping bottom of foot
  - Raising of finger
  - Simultaneous shoulder shrug and head turn

Common Vocal Tics

- Simple tics
  - Grunting
  - Sniffing
  - Snorting
  - Throat clearing
  - Humming
  - Coughing
  - Barking
  - Screaming
- Complex tics
  - Partial words/syllables
  - Words out of context
  - Repeated sentences
  - Coprolalia (swearing)
  - Echolalia (repeating)

van Egmond ME, Kuiper A, Eggink H, et al. Dystonia in children and adolescents: A systematic review and a new diagnostic algorithm. *J Neurol Neurosurg Psychiatry.* 2015;86:774; Scharf JM, Miller LL, Gauvin CA, et al. Population prevalence of Tourette syndrome: A systematic review and meta-analysis. *Mov Disord.* 2015;30:221.

Box 71.6   Laboratory Testing in Assessment of Tic Disorders

- Complete blood count
- Blood urea nitrogen, creatinine
- Liver function tests
- Thyroid panel
- Ferritin
- Urine drug screen

Sources: Singer HS, Mink JW, Gilbert DL, Jankovic J. *Movement disorders in childhood.* 2nd ed. Philadelphia, PA: Butterworth-Heinemann (Elsevier); 2015; Deng H, Gao K, Jankovic J. The genetics of Tourette syndrome. *Nat Rev Neurol.* 2012;8:203.

should last for at least one year. There are two tic disorders listed in the *DSM-5*, Tourette's disorder (in which both motor and vocal tics are present) and persistent tic disorder (in which either motor or vocal tics are present).

Box 71.7   Common Psychiatric Comorbidity With Tics

- Obsessive-compulsive disorder
- Attention-deficit/hyperactivity disorder
- Learning disabilities
- Autism spectrum disorder
- Anxiety disorders
- Major depressive disorder

Differential Diagnosis

Several medical and psychiatric conditions are associated with tics, which should be ruled out before a diagnosis of tic disorder (see Differential Diagnosis 71.3).

MANAGEMENT

Pharmacological Management

Because tics are often self-limited and transient, not every patient with tics or a tic disorder requires medication. When patients meet criteria for Tourette's disorder and tics are nonresponsive to behavioral interventions and cause significant impairment or distress, medications can be used. Alpha-agonists (guanfacine, clonidine) are often the initial choice of agent given their favorable side effect profile, with atypical antipsychotics (risperidone, aripiprazole) used if symptoms are nonresponsive or the patient cannot tolerate the alpha-agonists. Typical antipsychotics such as haloperidol are often saved for treatment-refractory cases. See Drugs Commonly Prescribed 71.2 for medication options. In addition, comorbid psychiatric conditions should be treated accordingly.

Differential Diagnosis 71.3: Tic Disorders

- Pediatric autoimmune neuropsychiatric disorder associated with streptococcus (PANDAS)
- Huntington's disease
- Postviral encephalitis
- Medication side effects (i.e., stimulants, bupropion, selective serotonin reuptake inhibitors, lamotrigine)
- Substance use (i.e., cocaine)
- Autism spectrum disorder (with stereotypies)
- Obsessive-compulsive disorder (with motor compulsions)
- Torticollis
- Central nervous system disease (tumor, trauma, anoxia)
- Wilson's disease

Drugs Commonly Prescribed 71.2: Medications for Tic Disorders

MEDICATION	INDICATION	ADVERSE REACTIONS AND PRESCRIBING CONSIDERATIONS
Clonidine (Catapres, Kapvay)	ADHD (particularly hyperactivity/impulsivity), disruptive behavior disorders tic disorder, Tourette's disorder, hypertension, insomnia, anxiety	• Hypotension • Bradycardia • Drowsiness • Rebound hypertension • Epistaxis
Guanfacine (Tenex, Intuniv)	ADHD (particularly hyperactivity/impulsivity), tic disorder, Tourette's disorder, hypertension	• Hypotension • Bradycardia • Drowsiness • Increase in serum ALT • Skin rash
Risperidone (Risperdal)	Autism-associated irritability (including aggression, temper, tantrums, self-injurious behavior, and quickly changing moods), bipolar disorder, disruptive behavior disorders, Tourette's disorder, schizophrenia, delirium	• EPS (e.g., akathisia, dystonia, etc.) • Drowsiness • Parkinsonian-like syndrome (common in children) • Increase in LFTs • Metabolic syndrome • Hyperprolactinemia • Gynecomastia • Galactorrhea • Cardiovascular effect
Aripiprazole (Abilify)	Autism-associated irritability (including aggression, temper tantrums, self-injurious behavior, and quickly changing moods), bipolar disorder, disruptive behavior disorders, Tourette's disorder, schizophrenia, delirium	• EPS (e.g., akathisia, dystonia; minimal compared with other SGAs) • Drooling • Drowsiness • Parkinsonian-like syndrome (common in children) • Metabolic syndrome • Cardiovascular effects
Haloperidol (Haldol)	Psychotic disorders, agitation, Tourette's disorder, delirium	• Prolongation of the QTc interval • EPS (more significant than with SGAs), • Oculogyric crisis • Neuroleptic malignant syndrome
Pimozide (FDA approved)	Tourette's disorder	• Cardiovascular • EPS (more significant than with SGAs) • Muscle rigidity • Myalgia • Stooped posture • Torticollis • Tremor

Abbreviations: ADHD, attention-deficit/hyperactivity disorder; ALT, alanine aminotransferase; ASD, autism spectrum disorder; EPS, extrapyramidal symptoms; FDA, Food and Drug Administration; LFTs, liver function tests; ODD, oppositional defiant disorder; SGAs, second-generation antipsychotics.

Nonpharmacological Management

Education about disease course and treatment options should be presented to the family. Classroom accommodations in the form of a 504 Plan or an IEP are sometimes necessary if the tic disorders are interfering with academic performance. For instance, teachers should be encouraged to ignore the tics.

Initial treatment options include habit reversal therapy, which involves awareness training, building a competing response, and social supports. As individuals feel the urge to have the tic, they do a competing behavior that prevents the tic from happening (e.g., if they feel an urge to jerk their shoulders, they are encouraged to sit on their hands with shoulders outstretched so that the jerking behavior does not happen). In addition, patients should be encouraged to develop coping strategies for managing the distress and anxiety that can accompany the tic behaviors.

FOLLOW-UP AND REFERRAL

Patients with abnormal movements should be referred to a neurologist for comprehensive neurological assessment. Patients with tic disorders can be managed in primary care, but complex or treatment refractory cases can be referred to neurology or psychiatry for further assessment and treatment.

Patient Education: Tic Disorder

Families should be aware that tics are often transient and self-limiting, and many children and adolescents experience them at some point in their lives. Determining the inciting triggers for tics can be useful for modifying the environment to reduce exposure to these triggers or developing a management plan for when exposure is inevitable, such as stressors.

ATTENTION-DEFICIT/ HYPERACTIVITY DISORDER

Attention-deficit/hyperactivity disorder (ADHD) is one of the most common neuropsychiatric disorders of childhood and adolescence and manifests with persistent patterns of hyperactivity, impulsivity, and/or inattention. These symptoms affect academic, behavioral, cognitive, emotional, and social functioning. Many children diagnosed with ADHD in childhood and adolescence continue to manifest significant impairment in occupational, academic, and social functioning into adulthood, continuing to meet the criteria for ADHD. Emotional dysregulation in adults with ADHD is common, and in some instances, the first diagnosis may not occur until in adulthood.

EPIDEMIOLOGY AND CAUSES

The reported prevalence of ADHD in children ranges from 2% to 18%; the prevalence in school-age children is reported to be 8% to 11%, which makes it one of the most common disorders of childhood. The prevalence increases in adolescents to approximately 14% and higher. In children, the male-to-female ratio is 2:1, and for adults the male-to-female ratio is 1.6:1. Although early onset is common (more than one-third of children are diagnosed before age 6), the overall prevalence for children and adolescents is 8% in the United States. Approximately 60% are estimated to be receiving treatment, and in as many as 30% to 60% the disorder persists into adulthood.

Current epidemiologic studies in adults aged 18 to 44 years estimate the prevalence of ADHD to be 4.4% in the United States and 3.4% internationally. Approximately 10% to 15% are receiving treatment. A 2012 study published in the *British Journal of Psychiatry*, the first epidemiologic study in older adults (aged 55–85), reports a prevalence of 4.2%, with men equal to woman (Michielsen et al., 2012).

In ADHD, comorbidities are the rule, not the exception. There appears to be a dose–response relationship between ADHD and comorbidity: the higher the number of ADHD symptoms, the greater the comorbidities (see Box 71.8). To date, no single etiology for ADHD has been identified. Data from biological, environmental, and psychosocial research suggest several *possible* risk factors or causes for the disorder. There is no strong scientific evidence that food additives, colorings, preservatives, or sugar contributes to ADHD, although some literature argues that certain subsets of populations, especially in children, may benefit from some forms of dietary controls.

Risk Factors: Attention-Deficit/Hyperactivity Disorder

Prenatal Factors
- Tobacco exposure
- Alcohol exposure
- Toxin exposure
- Zinc deficiency
- Genetic factors

Postnatal Factors
- Central nervous system infections
- Traumatic brain injury
- Cerebral palsy
- Lead exposure

Box 71.8 Psychiatric Comorbidities of Attention-Deficit/Hyperactivity Disorder (by Prevalence)

- Oppositional defiant disorder
- Social phobia
- Substance use disorders
- Bipolar disorder
- Major depressive disorder
- Persistent depressive disorder (dysthymia)
- Antisocial personality disorder
- Posttraumatic stress disorder
- Generalized anxiety disorder
- Obsessive-compulsive disorder

Data from Goldman LS, Genel M, Bezman RJ, Slanetz PJ. Diagnosis and treatment of attention-deficit/hyperactivity disorder in children and adolescents. Council on Scientific Affairs, American Medical Association. *JAMA*. 1998;279:1100.

There is a strong genetic component to this disorder. Children with parents or siblings with ADHD have two to eight times increased risk, with heritability estimated at 76% based on pooled data from twin studies. Results of behavioral genetic investigations using family, twin, and adoption studies converge with those of molecular genetic studies in showing that genes influence susceptibility to ADHD.

PATHOPHYSIOLOGY

Imbalances among the levels of norepinephrine, dopamine, and epinephrine all seem to be involved in the development of ADHD, suggesting a complex genetic mechanism through which the disorder is caused by the combined actions of several genes interacting with environmental risk factors. When examining the brains of children with and without ADHD with structural imaging, several differences emerge as well. There is literature indicating that those with ADHD demonstrate impaired executive functioning on neuropsychological testing and/or difficulties with response inhibition, confirming neuroimaging studies that demonstrate structural and functional abnormalities in prefrontal structures and basal ganglia. The noradrenergic system is involved in the modulation of higher cortical functions and animal models suggest that there is an imbalance in norepinephrine and dopamine systems in the prefrontal cortex that would account for the decrease in inhibitory dopamine activity and increase in norepinephrine activity.

CLINICAL PRESENTATION

Parents may be the first to note excessive motor activity (hyperactivity) during the toddler years. The disorder is not usually diagnosed during this time, however, because that is the normative developmental stage. By preschool, children with ADHD may have difficulty participating in sedentary activities, such as sitting still while listening to a story. Parents may describe the child as "always on the go," and the child may appear to constantly run, jump, and not sit still. There may also be excessive talking and interrupting of others.

ADHD is most often diagnosed during the childhood years (especially during elementary school) when the child's decreased attention span affects classroom work and academic performance. The school-aged child with ADHD will usually have difficulty remaining seated, be unable to complete assignments and turn them in, and talk out of turn. Hyperactive behaviors in these children may include constantly tapping their hands; shaking of their feet or legs; getting up during meals; and talking excessively while watching television, doing homework, or in other quiet activities.

In childhood and adolescence, the impulsive symptoms associated with ADHD may lead the individual to break rules. Disruptive behaviors and poor social skills can make bonding with peers difficult and may lead to association with deviant peer groups and substance and tobacco abuse. In adulthood, restlessness may lead to difficulty participating in sedentary activities, as well as to avoiding occupations, such as desk jobs, that provide limited opportunity for spontaneous movement. Adults with ADHD often complain of boredom and frustration with job and life routines.

Symptoms are often present and visible during the assessment of ADHD in the primary-care office, although inattention may be less obvious if the assessment is structured and the child answers questions appropriately. Children with ADHD may not be able to report their own symptoms accurately because of their age; therefore, information should be gathered from parents or guardians and supplemented by reports from teachers. It may be necessary to review early academic records or report cards for the presence of impulsivity, hyperactivity, and inattentive symptoms during the early school years. Additional questions related to family history of ADHD should be conducted. Adult patients may need to question their parents regarding ADHD behaviors that were evident from childhood. Key areas for questioning relate to complaints of boredom, disorganization or frustration in work, and a tendency for impulsive, impatient, and restless behavior.

Generally, diagnostic tests are not indicated, but a serum lead, ferritin, and/or thyroid level may be considered. EEG, diagnostic imaging, and genetic testing may be indicated for those patients who present with anomalies or soft neurological signs.

DIAGNOSTIC REASONING

Screening for psychosocial issues has become more common as providers become increasingly aware that many children exhibit emotional/behavioral problems. Utilizing a tool at regular well-child visits may help to identify this chronic condition, particularly in children with academic and behavioral issues. For adults, assessment should include prior history of ADHD, previous school performance, history of mental health diagnoses, substance abuse, and current or past medication use. When there are concerns for ADHD, various screening tools can be used (see Box 71.9).

Symptoms

The diagnosis of ADHD is based on *DSM-5* criteria; please refer to the *DSM-5* for complete diagnostic criteria.

Box 71.9   ADHD Rating Scales

Commonly used

- The National Institute for Children's Health Quality (NICHQ) Vanderbilt Assessment Scale (forms for teachers and parents)
- The Swanson, Nolan, and Pelham Questionnaire (SNAP IV)
- The Connors-3 (forms for teachers and parents)
- Adult ADHD self-reports scale (ASRS)

Others

- Strengths & Weaknesses of ADHD symptoms & Normal behavior (SWAN)
- Inattention/Overactivity With Aggression (IOWA)
- Achenbach Child Behavior Checklist (CBCL)

Computerized ADHD testing

- Testing of Variables of Attention (TOVA)
- Conner's Continuous Performance Test

Differential Diagnosis 71.4: Attention-Deficit/Hyperactivity Disorder

- Normal, age-appropriate behaviors
- Medical conditions
  - Thyroid disease
  - Lead toxicity
  - Iron deficiency
  - Fetal alcohol syndrome
- Genetic conditions
  - Fragile X syndrome
  - Turners syndrome
  - Neurofibromatosis type 1
  - Prader-Willi syndrome
  - Williams syndrome
- Psychiatric conditions
  - Learning disabilities
  - Autism spectrum disorder
  - Tic disorders
  - Conduct disorder
  - Oppositional defiant disorder
  - Major depressive disorder
  - Generalized anxiety disorder
  - Substance use disorder
- Drug-seeking behaviors

Symptoms must have been present for many months prior to age 12, though the diagnosis can be made anytime. Importantly, symptoms must be present across multiple settings (e.g.: home, school, work, social interactions), as symptoms in only one setting may indicate an environmental etiology and subsequent intervention. Categories of symptoms include:

- Inattention: difficulty focusing or sustaining attention, forgetfulness, or difficulty following instructions
- Hyperactivity: excessive motor activity and difficulty sitting still or in quiet activities
- Impulsivity: interrupting others, not thinking before acting or speaking

Differential Diagnosis

Various medical, psychological, and genetic conditions need to be assessed (see Differential Diagnosis 71.4). It is important for the clinician to be able to distinguish symptoms of ADHD from developmentally age-appropriate behaviors in active children. In addition, as many psychiatric conditions are associated with inattention, it is important to rule out other disorders.

MANAGEMENT

A comprehensive plan needs to address the chronic nature of the disorder, treatment options (pharmacological and nonpharmacological), and community and school resources. Reappraisal of the plan with medication reassessment needs to be done periodically and appropriate changes made.

Pharmacological Management

Pharmacotherapy in preschool-age children warrants precaution given their young age, and behavioral interventions are the first line of treatment. However, stimulants are approved for this age-group if the symptoms are severe or nonresponsive to behavioral treatment, and nonstimulants can be considered as well. For older children, adolescents, and adults, pharmacotherapy should be considered when symptoms cause clinically significant impairment at home, school, and/or work. There is strong evidence for the stimulant medications given their robust efficacy (with response rates of 75%–80%), and they are considered the first-line pharmacological treatment for ADHD.

The two stimulant classes are methylphenidate-based and amphetamine-based agents, with both immediate-release and sustained-release formulations available. The advantages for once-daily dosing include compliance, convenience, and confidentiality. Management includes beginning the stimulant at a low dose and titrating upward until symptoms are controlled (generally every 1–3 weeks) or side effects prohibit further titration. It is not necessary to begin with a short-acting agent before using a sustained-release agent, although this can be useful in dose titration, particularly with younger children. If the maximum dosage does not control the symptoms, switching to another stimulant is indicated. If the chosen stimulant does not provide adequate symptom control later in the day, addition of an afternoon "booster" can be useful, using either an immediate-release formulation of the same agent or an alpha-agonist (guanfacine or clonidine), with caution that dosing a stimulant too late in the day can lead to insomnia. If children cannot swallow pills, consider chewable or liquid options; in addition, some long-acting preparations come in capsules that can be opened and sprinkled. Medication diversion or abuse, especially to improve academic performance, is a consideration when prescribing for patients with ADHD. Stimulants may increase levels of seizure drugs, selective serotonin reuptake inhibitors, tricyclics, and warfarin (see Drugs Commonly Prescribed 71.3).

Common side effects of stimulants include weight loss, appetite suppression, abdominal pain, insomnia, and headache. The practitioner needs to be aware of the common side effects and have strategies to offset them,

including dose reduction, changing medication, and prescribing adjunctive medications. Tics are not an absolute contraindication to stimulant use, although for patients with medication-induced tics, reduction of dose or alternative medication may be necessary. Congenital heart disease including hypertrophic cardiomyopathy or significant cardiac-related symptoms should prompt cardiac evaluation, including electrocardiogram, before initiating pharmacological therapy.

Atomoxetine is a selective norepinephrine reuptake inhibitor (SNRI), which is used if stimulant drugs are not tolerated or contraindicated (active substance abuse, tics, comorbid anxiety, or mood lability). Atomoxetine has an effect both on ADHD and on comorbid anxiety. Atomoxetine affects weight and sleep less than the stimulants, and unlike stimulants (the effects of which are often seen soon after initiation), full clinical effect of atomoxetine may take up to 6 weeks. Although stimulants can be stopped

---

Drugs Commonly Prescribed 71.3: Attention-Deficit/Hyperactivity Disorder (ADHD) Medications

MEDICATION	INDICATION	ADVERSE REACTIONS AND PRESCRIBING CONSIDERATIONS
Methylphenidate (MPH) Derivatives†		
Ritalin Metadate Methylin Concerta‡ Daytrana Quillivant Aptensio Cotempla Focalin (dexmethylphenidate)‡	ADHD, narcolepsy	• Side effects: insomnia, weight loss, tics, tachycardia, elevated blood pressure, irritability • Age 6 years and older • Transdermal preparation (Daytrana) and OROS methylphenidate (Concerta) have less abuse potential
Amphetamine Derivatives†		
Mixed amphetamine salts (Adderall)‡ *d*-amphetamine sulfate (Dexedrine) Lisdexamfetamine dimesylate (Vyvanse)‡ Dyanavel Adzenys *d-&-l* amphetamine sulfate (Evekeo) *d*-amphetamine sulfate (Zenzedi) ProCentra	ADHD, narcolepsy	• Side effects: Insomnia, weight loss, tics, tachycardia, elevated BP, irritability • Stop slowly, not suddenly • Lisdexamfetamine: stimulant medication with less abuse potential • Age 3 years and older (mixed amphetamine salts) • Extended release: age 6 years and older
Selective Norepinephrine Reuptake Inhibitors		
Atomoxetine (Strattera)‡	ADHD: age 6 years and older; FDA approved for adults; ADHD plus enuresis; tic disorder; anxiety disorder	• Side effects: gastrointestinal upset; weight loss; mood swings, sedation, headaches • Once daily in a.m. (can split dose or give all at night if daytime sedation) • **Black-box warning:** suicide ideation

Drugs Commonly Prescribed 71.3: Attention-Deficit/Hyperactivity Disorder (ADHD) Medications—cont'd

MEDICATION	INDICATION	ADVERSE REACTIONS AND PRESCRIBING CONSIDERATIONS
Alpha-Agonists		
Clonidine (Catapres, Kapvay) Guanfacine (Tenex, Intuniv)	ADHD, Tourette's disorder	• More effective in treatment of impulsivity/hyperactivity than inattention • Must be tapered on discontinuation • Beneficial in comorbid Tourette's disorder and tics • Side effects: sedation, dizziness, hypotension • Helpful in treatment of stimulant-induced insomnia • Advantages of guanfacine over clonidine: less sedation and longer duration of action
Tricyclic Antidepressants*		
Imipramine (Tofranil)* Desipramine (Norpramin)*	ADHD, depression	• ECG recommended at baseline and with dose increases • Monitoring blood levels is useful in guiding dosing • **Black-box warning:** suicide ideation • Anticholinergic effect • Limited use due to risk of sudden death; use only if other agents not effective
Dopamine/Norepinephrine Reuptake Inhibitor		
Bupropion (Wellbutrin)*	ADHD, depression	• Side effects: insomnia, decreased appetite • Seizure risk
Antinarcoleptic		
Modafinil	ADHD, narcolepsy	• Insomnia • Headache • Decrease in appetite • Steven-Johnson's syndrome

Abbreviations: ECG, electroencephalogram; FDA, Food and Drug Administration.

*Off-label use.

†C-II controlled substance; available in short- and extended-release formulations; monitor growth parameters (height, weight), blood pressure, and pulse; do not use in severe cardiac disease or family history of sudden cardiac death at young age; caution in administration with history of drug or alcohol dependence; doses of stimulants should advance slowly every several days until appropriate response is obtained; stimulants may increase levels of seizure drugs, selective serotonin reuptake inhibitors, tricyclics, and warfarin.

‡Approved by the U.S. FDA for adults with ADHD. For a list of current FDA-approved medications for children with ADHD, see https://www.cms.gov/Medicare-Medicaid-Coordination/Fraud-Prevention/Medicaid-Integrity-Education/Pharmacy-Education-Materials/Downloads/stim-pediatric-factsheet11-14.pdf.

on weekends or school holidays if side effects warrant this and symptoms can be managed in the home, atomoxetine must be taken daily without "drug holidays."

Nonpharmacological Management

Behavioral interventions can be quite useful for all patients, particularly with younger children. Behavioral techniques include parental training, classroom management techniques, and peer interventions. Evidence-based group parent training programs and early educational programs are recommended as the initial step for preschool-age children, although these can be conducted in conjunction with medications in older patients. Referral for early intervention services or to a behavioral specialist may be useful. For adolescents and adults, study and organizational skills training including time management, study strategies, and empowerment to minimize distractions may increase functioning.

FOLLOW-UP AND REFERRAL

Follow-up for patients diagnosed with ADHD includes gathering information from the patient, parents, and teachers regarding symptom progression. The focus of follow-up visits includes physical parameters (height, weight, cardiac evaluation including blood pressure and pulse), assessment on behavioral progress (utilizing an ADHD scale helps to objectively identify and track behavioral changes from the parent and teacher), monitoring of medication compliance and side effects, and continued education and referral to support services if indicated. It is often useful to set specific parameters for tracking progress, such as grades, homework completion, or frequency of calls home from school. If appetite is so affected that the patient is falling on their growth chart, reevaluation of the treatment plan is necessary (including considering drug holidays, increasing caloric intake at the start and end of the day, or switching to a nonstimulant).

Children with ADHD are at increased risk for abuse, depression, and social isolation and should be monitored for these. Parents will need regular support and advice and may need referral for family therapy to cope with the added demands. Parents, teachers, and advisors should encourage career choices that allow autonomy and mobility. Adolescence offers new challenges, and the practitioner needs to address these issues both with the adolescent and the family. Increased independence, decision-making, and risk-taking behaviors need to be addressed. In addition, discussion about the continued need for and benefit of medication may ensue. In general, if the patient has been symptom free for longer than 1 year with no adjustment in medication dosage despite increases in weight and height, consideration about remission should occur. Summer vacation or prolonged vacation may be a good time to trial a drug holiday.

Monitoring for diversion of controlled substances is essential. If there are concerns regarding this, use of atomoxetine, extended-release guanfacine, or extended-release clonidine should be considered. In some situations, treatment with a stimulant agent that possesses a smaller risk for abuse could be used. College students are at high risk for nonmedical use of prescription stimulants as a study aid, particularly during exam time. Providers should be cautious when making a first-time diagnosis of ADHD in a college student, and retrospective history is extremely important, including speaking with previous providers and family, if possible.

Patient Education: Attention-Deficit/Hyperactivity Disorder

Adherence to the treatment plan is improved when the patient and family understand the chronic nature of ADHD and its potential impact on school, social life, and occupational functioning. Continued education about medications and management of side effects may improve adherence.

Utilization of various community support groups may also assist families and adults to deal with developmental challenges. There are many interventions that parents, family members, and teachers can do in addition to administering medication (Box 71.10). Parents should be educated regarding realistic expectations and should be made aware of support groups for themselves as well as child advocate groups.

Box 71.10   Patient Education: Attention-Deficit/Hyperactivity Disorder (ADHD)

Teach parents to do the following:

- Have the child do one task at a time.
- Use "time-out" periods for bad behavior.
- Make eye contact each time they are making a request.
- Reinforce good behavior or tasks the child does well with rewards and attention.
- Use behavior therapy, such as token systems.
- Stop unacceptable behavior before it escalates.
- Make use of parent support and advocacy groups.
- Deal with negative feelings and unrealistic expectations.
- Incorporate family therapy, anger-management training, and social training.
- Coordinate homework with teachers.
- Work closely with teachers for consistent behavioral plan.

Teach teachers to do the following:

- Make sure the child has a second set of books at home.
- Make work sessions short.
- Help the child deal constructively with negative feelings.
- Provide immediate consequences for bad behavior.
- Reinforce good behavior.
- Coordinate homework with parents.
- Work closely with parents for a consistent behavioral plan.

 For additional resources please visit
https://davisedge.fadavis.com/

REFERENCES

Attention-Deficit/Hyperactivity Disorder

American Academy of Pediatrics. Steering Committee on Quality Improvement and Management, Subcommittee on Attention-Deficit/Hyperactivity Disorder. Appendix to ADHD Clinical Practice Guideline: Implementing the key action statements—An algorithm and explanation for process of care for the evaluation, diagnosis, treatment, and monitoring of ADHD in children and adolescents. *Pediatrics* 2011;SI1–21.

Barkley RA. Theories of attention-deficit/hyperactivity disorder. In: Quay HC, Hogan AE, eds. *Handbook of disruptive behavior disorders.* New York: Kluwer Academic/Plenum; 1999:295.

Biederman J, Petty C, Fried R, et al. Impact of psychometrically defined deficits of executive functioning in adults with attention deficit hyperactivity disorder. *Am J Psychiatry.* 2006;163(10): 1730–1738.

Biederman J, Spencer T. Attention-deficit/hyperactivity disorder (ADHD) as a noradrenergic disorder. *Biol Psychiatry.* 1999;46:1234–1242.

Burgess-Champoux T, et al. Perceptions of children, parents, and teachers regarding whole-grain foods, and implications for a school-based intervention. *J Nutr Educ Behav.* 2006;38(4): 230–237.

Bush G, Frazier JA, Rauch SL, et al. Anterior cingulate cortex dysfunction in attention-deficit/hyperactivity disorder revealed by fMRI and the Counting Stroop. *Biol Psychiatry.* 1999;45:1542–1552.

Castellanos FX, Lee PP, Sharp W, et al. Developmental trajectories of brain volume abnormalities in children and adolescents with attention-deficit/hyperactivity disorder. *JAMA.* 2002;288:1740–1748

Daly BP, et al. Psychosocial treatments for children with attention deficit/hyperactivity disorder. *Neuropsychol Rev.* 2007;17(1):73–89.

Dickstein SG, Bannon K, Castellanos FX, Milham MP. The neural correlates of attention deficit hyperactivity disorder: an ALE meta-analysis. *J Child Psychol Psychiatry.* 2006;47:1051–1062.

Giedd JN, Blumenthal J, Molloy E, Castellanos FX. Brain imaging of attention deficit/hyperactivity disorder. *Ann N Y Acad Sci.* 2001;931:33 - 49.

Goodman D. Treatment and assessment of ADHD in adults. In: Biederman J, ed. *ADHD across the life span: From research to clinical practice—an evidence-based understanding.* Hasbrouck Heights, NJ: Veritas Institute for Medical Education; 2005.

Harrison AG, Nay S, Armstrong IT. Diagnostic accuracy of the Conners' adult ADHD Rating Scale in a postsecondary population. *J Atten Disord.* 2016. **https://doi.org/10.1177%2F1087054715625299.**

Hart H, Radua J, Nakao T, et al. Meta-analysis of functional magnetic resonance imaging studies of inhibition and attention in attention-deficit/hyperactivity disorder: Exploring taskspecific, stimulant medication, and age effects. *JAMA Psychiatry.* 2013;70:185–198.

Hauser TU, Iannaccone R, Ball J, et al. Role of the medial prefrontal cortex in impaired decision making in juvenile attention-deficit/hyperactivity disorder. *JAMA Psychiatry.* 2014;71:1165–1173.

Himelstein J, Newcorn JH, Halperin JM. The neurobiology of attention-deficit hyperactivity disorder. *Front Biosci.* 2000;5:D461–D478.

Makris N, Biederman J, Valera EM, et al. Cortical thinning of the attention and executive function networks in adults with attention-deficit/hyperactivity disorder. *Cereb Cortex.* 2007;17:1364–1375.

McCabe SE, et al. Medical use, illicit use and diversion of prescription stimulant medication. *J Psychoactive Drugs.* 2006;38(1):43–56.

McCarthy H, Skokauskas N, Frodl T. Identifying a consistent pattern of neural function in attention deficit hyperactivity disorder: A meta-analysis. *Psychol Med.* 2014;44:869–880.

McDonnell MA, Dougherty M. Righting a troubled course: Diagnosing and treating ADHD in adults. *Adv Nurse Pract.* 2005;8: 53–56.

Moriyama TS, Polanczyk GV, Terzi FS, et al. Psychopharmacology and psychotherapy for the treatment of adults with ADHD—a systematic review of available meta-analyses. *CNS Spectr.* 2013; 18:296–306.

MTA Cooperative Group. Moderators and mediators of treatment response for children with attention-deficit/hyperactivity disorder: The Multimodal Treatment Study of children with attention-deficit/hyperactivity disorder. *Arch Gen Psychiatry.* 1999;56(12):1088–1096. https://www.researchgate.net/publication/236585378_Moderators_and_mediators_of_treatment_response_for_children_with_Attention-Deficit_Hyperactivity_Disorder. Accessed February 19, 2018.

Pelham WE Jr, Fabiano GA. Evidence-based psychosocial treatments for attention-deficit/hyperactivity disorder. *J Clin Child Adolesc Psychol.* 2008;37(1):184–214.

Pennington BF, Ozonoff S. Executive functions and developmental psychopathology. *J Child Psychol Psychiatry.* 1996;37:51–87.

Rabiner DL, et al. The misuse and diversion of prescribed ADHD medications by college students. *J Atten Disord.* 2009;13(2):144–153.

Rigler T, Manor I, Kalansky A, et al. New *DSM-5* criteria for ADHD—Does it matter? *Compr Psychiatry.* 2016;68:56–59.

Ross MM, Arria AM, Brown JP, et al. College students' perceived benefit-to-risk tradeoffs for nonmedical use of prescription stimulants: Implications for intervention designs. *Addict Behav.* 2018;79:45–51

Rubia K, Overmeyer S, Taylor E, et al. Hypofrontality in attention deficit hyperactivity disorder during higher-order motor control: A study with functional MRI. *Am J Psychiatry.* 1999;156:891–896.

Rubia K, Smith AB, Brammer MJ, et al. Abnormal brain activation during inhibition and error detection in medication-naive adolescents with ADHD. *Am J Psychiatry.* 2005;162:1067–1074.

Russell V, Allie S, Wiggins T. Increased noradrenergic activity in prefrontal cortex slices of an animal model for attention-deficit hyperactivity disorder—the spontaneously hypertensive rat. *Behav Brain Res.* 2000;117:69–74.

Safren SA, et al. Cognitive-behavioral therapy for ADHD in medication-treated adults with continued symptoms. *Behav Res Ther.* 2005;43(7):831–842.

Seidman LJ, Valera EM, Makris N, et al. Dorsolateral prefrontal and anterior cingulate cortex volumetric abnormalities in adults with attention-deficit/hyperactivity disorder identified by magnetic resonance imaging. *Biol Psychiatry.* 2006;60:1071–1080.

Shaw P, Lerch J, Greenstein D, et al. Longitudinal mapping of cortical thickness and clinical outcome in children and adolescents with attention-deficit/hyperactivity disorder. *Arch Gen Psychiatry.* 2006;63:540–549.

Sowell ER, Thompson PM, Welcome SE, et al. Cortical abnormalities in children and adolescents with attention-deficit hyperactivity disorder. *Lancet.* 2003;362:1699–1707.

Spencer TJ, Brown A, Seidman LJ, et al. Effect of psychostimulants on brain structure and function in ADHD: A qualitative literature review of magnetic resonance imaging-based neuroimaging studies. *J Clin Psychiatry.* 2013;74:902–917.

Tannock R. Attention deficit hyperactivity disorder: Advances in cognitive, neurobiological, and genetic research. *J Child Psychol Psychiatry.* 1998;39:65–99.

Ustun B, Adler LA, Rudin C, et al. The World Health Organization adult attention-deficit/hyperactivity disorder self-report screening scale for *DSM-5. JAMA Psychiatry.* 2017;74:520–526.

Waite, R. Women and attention deficit disorders: A great burden overlooked. *J Am Acad Nurse Pract.* 2007;19:116–125.

Wolraich M, et al.; Subcommittee on Attention-Deficit/Hyperactivity Disorder; Steering Committee on Quality Improvement and Management. ADHD: Clinical practice guideline for the diagnosis, evaluation, and treatment of attention-deficit/hyperactivity disorder in children and adolescents. *Pediatrics.* 2011;128(5):1007–1022.

Zang YF, Jin Z, Weng XC, et al. Functional MRI in attention-deficit hyperactivity disorder: evidence for hypofrontality. *Brain Dev.* 2005;27:544–550.

Autism Spectrum Disorder

American Psychiatric Association. *Diagnostic and statistical manual of mental disorders.* 5th ed. Arlington, VA: American Psychiatric Association; 2013.

Antshel KM, Polacek C, McMahon M, et al. Comorbid ADHD and anxiety affect social skills group intervention treatment efficacy in children with autism spectrum disorders. *J Dev Behav Pediatr.* 2011;32:439–446.

Autism and Developmental Disabilities Monitoring Network Surveillance Year 2000 Principal Investigators; Centers for Disease Control and Prevention. Prevalence of autism spectrum disorders—autism and developmental disabilities monitoring network, six sites, United States, 2000. *MMWR Surveill Summ.* 2007;56:1–19.

Bearss K, Johnson C, Smith T, et al. Effect of parent training vs parent education on behavioral problems in children with autism spectrum disorder: A randomized clinical trial. *JAMA.* 2015;313:1524.

Chawarska K, Klin A, Paul R, Volkmar F. Autism spectrum disorder in the second year: stability and change in syndrome expression. *J Child Psychol Psychiatry.* 2007;48:128–138.

Ching H, Pringsheim T. Aripiprazole for autism spectrum disorders (ASD). *Cochrane Database Syst Rev.* 2012;(5):CD009043.

Estes A, Munson J, Rogers SJ, et al. Long-term outcomes of early intervention in 6-year-old children with autism spectrum disorder. *J Am Acad Child Adolesc Psychiatry.* 2015;54:580–587.

Farmer C, Thurm A, Grant P. Pharmacotherapy for the core symptoms in autistic disorder: current status of the research. *Drugs.* 2013;73:303–314.

Gringras P, Nir T, Breddy J, et al. Efficacy and safety of pediatric prolonged-release melatonin for insomnia in children with autism spectrum disorder. *J Am Acad Child Adolesc Psychiatry.* 2017;56:948–957.

Golan O, Baron-Cohen S. Systemizing empathy: teaching adults with Asperger syndrome or high-functioning autism to recognize complex emotions using interactive multimedia. *Dev Psychopathol.* 2006;18:591–616.

Goldstein H. Communication intervention for children with autism: A review of treatment efficacy. *J Autism Dev Disord.* 2002;32:373–396.

Guénolé F, Godbout R, Nicolas A, et al. Melatonin for disordered sleep in individuals with autism spectrum disorders: Systematic review and discussion. *Sleep Med Rev.* 2011;15:379–387.

Harfterkamp M, van de Loo-Neus G, Minderaa RB, et al. A randomized double-blind study of atomoxetine versus placebo for attention-deficit/hyperactivity disorder symptoms in children with autism spectrum disorder. *J Am Acad Child Adolesc Psychiatry.* 2012;51:733–741.

Hazlett HC, Gu H, Munsell BC, et al. Early brain development in infants at high risk for autism spectrum disorder. *Nature.* 2017;542:348–351.

Huffman LC, Sutcliffe TL, Tanner IS, Feldman HM. Management of symptoms in children with autism spectrum disorders: A comprehensive review of pharmacologic and complementary-alternative medicine treatments. *J Dev Behav Pediatr.* 2011;32:56–68.

Kasari C, Gulsrud AC, Wong C, et al. Randomized controlled caregiver mediated joint engagement intervention for toddlers with autism. *J Autism Dev Disord.* 2010;40:1045–1056.

Kasari C, Kaiser A, Goods K, et al. Communication interventions for minimally verbal children with autism: A sequential multiple assignment randomized trial. *J Am Acad Child Adolesc Psychiatry.* 2014;53:635–646.

Kasari C, Lawton K, Shih W, et al. Caregiver-mediated intervention for low-resourced preschoolers with autism: An RCT. *Pediatrics.* 2014;134:e72–e79.

Kasari C, Rotheram-Fuller E, Locke J, Gulsrud A. Making the connection: Randomized controlled trial of social skills at school for children with autism spectrum disorders. *J Child Psychol Psychiatry.* 2012;53:431–439.

Landa R, Garrett-Mayer E. Development in infants with autism spectrum disorders: A prospective study. *J Child Psychol Psychiatry.* 2006;47:629–38.

Landa RJ, Gross AL, Stuart EA, Faherty A. Developmental trajectories in children with and without autism spectrum disorders: The first 3 years. *Child Dev.* 2013;84:429–442.

Landa RJ, Holman KC, O'Neill AH, Stuart EA. Intervention targeting development of socially synchronous engagement in toddlers with autism spectrum disorder: A randomized controlled trial. *J Child Psychol Psychiatry.* 2011;52:13–21.

McConachie H, Le Couteur A, Honey E. Can a diagnosis of Asperger syndrome be made in very young children with suspected autism spectrum disorder? *J Autism Dev Disord.* 2005;35:167–176.

McElhanon BO, McCracken C, Karpen S, Sharp WG. Gastrointestinal symptoms in autism spectrum disorder: A meta-analysis. *Pediatrics.* 2014;133:872–883.

McGuire K, Fung LK, Hagopian L, et al. Irritability and problem behavior in autism spectrum disorder: A practice pathway for pediatric primary care. *Pediatrics.* 2016;137(suppl 2):S136–S148.

Miller M, Iosif AM, Hill M, et al. Response to name in infants developing autism spectrum disorder: A prospective study. *J Pediatr.* 2017;183:141–146.

Oono IP, Honey EJ, McConachie H. Parent-mediated early intervention for young children with autism spectrum disorders (ASD). *Cochrane Database Syst Rev.* 2013;(4):CD009774.

Ozonoff S, Iosif AM, Young GS, et al. Onset patterns in autism: Correspondence between home video and parent report. *J Am Acad Child Adolesc Psychiatry.* 2011;50:796–806.

Pearson DA, Santos CW, Aman MG, et al. Effects of extended release methylphenidate treatment on ratings of attention-deficit/hyperactivity disorder (ADHD) and associated behavior in children with autism spectrum disorders and ADHD symptoms. *J Child Adolesc Psychopharmacol.* 2013;23:337–351.

Pickles A, Le Couteur A, Leadbitter K, et al. Parent-mediated social communication therapy for young children with autism (PACT): Long-term follow-up of a randomised controlled trial. *Lancet.* 2016;388:2501–2509.

Reichow B, Steiner AM, Volkmar F. Social skills groups for people aged 6 to 21 with autism spectrum disorders (ASD). *Cochrane Database Syst Rev.* 2013;8(2):266–315.

Rogers SJ, Ozonoff S. Annotation: What do we know about sensory dysfunction in autism? A critical review of the empirical evidence. *J Child Psychol Psychiatry.* 2005;46:1255–1268.

Saint-Georges C, Mahdhaoui A, Chetouani M, et al. Do parents recognize autistic deviant behavior long before diagnosis? Taking into account interaction using computational methods. *PLoS One.* 2011;6(7):e22393.

Scahill L, McCracken JT, King BH, et al. Extended-release guanfacine for hyperactivity in children with autism spectrum disorder. *Am J Psychiatry.* 2015;172:1197–1206.

Scottish Intercollegiate Guidelines Network. Assessment, diagnosis and clinical interventions for children and young people with autism spectrum disorders. A national clinical guideline. Edinburgh: Scottish Intercollegiate Guidelines Network; 2007. http://www.sign.ac.uk/guidelines/fulltext/98/index.html. Accessed November 10, 2011.

Section on Complementary and Integrative Medicine; Council on Children With Disabilities; American Academy of Pediatrics, Zimmer M, Desch L. Sensory integration therapies for children with developmental and behavioral disorders. *Pediatrics.* 2012;129(6):1186–1189.

Solomon R, Van Egeren LA, Mahoney G, et al. PLAY Project Home Consultation intervention program for young children with autism spectrum disorders: A randomized controlled trial. *J Dev Behav Pediatr.* 2014;35:475–485.

Storebø OJ, Ramstad E, Krogh HB, et al. Methylphenidate for children and adolescents with attention deficit hyperactivity disorder (ADHD). *Cochrane Database Syst Rev.* 2015;(11): CD009885.

Teplin SW. Autism and related disorders. In: Levine MD, Carey WB, Crocker AC, eds. *Developmental-behavioral pediatrics.* 3rd ed. Philadelphia, PA: WB Saunders; 1999:589–605.

Thurm A, Manwaring SS, Luckenbaugh DA, et al. Patterns of skill attainment and loss in young children with autism. *Dev Psychopathol.* 2017;26:212–222.

Volkmar F, Siegel M, Woodbury-Smith M, et al. Practice parameter for the assessment and treatment of children and adolescents with autism spectrum disorder. *J Am Acad Child Adolesc Psychiatry.* 2014;53:237–257.

Volkmar F, Wiesner L. Autism and related disorders. In: Carey WB, Crocker AC, Coleman WL, et al., eds. *Developmental-behavioral pediatrics.* 4th ed. Philadelphia, PA: Saunders Elsevier; 2009:675.

Warren Z, Veenstra-VanderWeele J, Stone W, et al. Therapies for children with autism spectrum disorders (AHRQ Publication No.11-EHC029-EF). Rockville, MD: Agency for Healthcare Research and Quality; 2011.

Weitlauf AS, Sathe N, McPheeters ML, Warren ZE. Interventions targeting sensory challenges in autism spectrum disorder: A systematic review. *Pediatrics.* 2017;139.

World Health Organization. The ICD-10 classification of mental and behavioural disorders. Clinical descriptions and diagnostic guidelines. http://www.who.int/classifications/icd/en/bluebook.pdf. Accessed August 20, 2018.

Intellectual Disabilities

Battaglia A, Bianchini E, Carey JC. Diagnostic yield of the comprehensive assessment of developmental delay/mental retardation in an institute of child neuropsychiatry. *Am J Med Genet.* 1999;82: 60–66.

Baxter H, Lowe K, Houston H, et al. Previously unidentified morbidity in patients with intellectual disability. *Br J Gen Pract.* 2006; 56:93–98.

Bouhadiba Z, Dacher J, Monroc M, et al. MRI of the brain in the evaluation of children with developmental delay [in French]. *J Radiol.* 2000;81:867–880.

Bush A, Beail N. Risk factors for dementia in people with down syndrome: Issues in assessment and diagnosis. *Am J Ment Retard.* 2004;109:83–97.

Coppus AM, Evenhuis HM, Verberne GJ, et al. Survival in elderly persons with Down syndrome. *J Am Geriatr Soc.* 2008;56:2311–2316.

CDC response to Advisory Committee on Childhood Lead Poisoning Prevention Recommendations. Low level lead exposure harms children: A renewed call of primary prevention. http://www.cdc.gov/nceh/lead/ACCLPP/activities.htm. Accessed August 20, 2018.

Decobert F, Grabar S, Merzoug V, et al. Unexplained mental retardation: Is brain MRI useful? *Pediatr Radiol.* 2005;35: 587–596.

Fisher K, Kettl P. Aging with mental retardation: Increasing population of older adults with MR require health interventions and prevention strategies. *Geriatrics.* 2005;60:26–29.

Glover G, Bernard S, Branford D, et al. Use of medication for challenging behaviour in people with intellectual disability. *Br J Psychiatry.* 2014;205:6–7.

Hall SS, Lightbody AA, Reiss AL. Compulsive, self-injurious, and autistic behavior in children and adolescents with fragile X syndrome. *Am J Ment Retard.* 2008;113:44–53.

Hoffman-Zacharska D, Kmieć T, Poznański J, et al. Mutations in the PLP1 gene residue p. Gly198 as the molecular basis of Pelizeaus-Merzbacher phenotype. *Brain Dev.* 2013;35:877–885.

Hoffman-Zacharska D, Mierzewska H, Szczepanik E, et al. The spectrum of PLP1 gene mutations in patients with the classical form of the Pelizaeus-Merzbacher disease. *Med Wieku Rozwoj.* 2013;17:293–300.

Huang J, Zhu T, Qu Y, Mu D. Prenatal, perinatal and neonatal risk factors for intellectual disability: A systemic review and meta-analysis. *PLoS One.* 2016;11(4):e0153655.

Jarjour IT. Neurodevelopmental outcome after extreme prematurity: A review of the literature. *Pediatr Neurol.* 2015;52:143–152.

Jensen KM, Bulova PD. Managing the care of adults with Down's syndrome. *BMJ.* 2014;349:g5596.

McDonald L, Rennie A, Tolmie J, et al. Investigation of global developmental delay. *Arch Dis Child.* 2006;91:701–705.

Moeschler JB, Shevell M; Committee on Genetics. Comprehensive evaluation of the child with intellectual disability or global developmental delays. *Pediatrics.* 2014;134(3):e903–e918.

Moran JA, Rafii MS, Keller SM, et al. The National Task Group on Intellectual Disabilities and Dementia Practices consensus recommendations for the evaluation and management of dementia in adults with intellectual disabilities. *Mayo Clin Proc.* 2013;88:831–840.

Rice CE, Naarden Braun KV, Kogan MD, et al.; Centers for Disease Control and Prevention. Screening for developmental delays among young children—National Survey of Children's Health, United States, 2007. *MMWR Suppl.* 2014;63(2):27–35.

Scott Schwoerer J, Laffin J, Haun J, et al. MECP2 duplication: Possible cause of severe phenotype in females. *Am J Med Genet A.* 2014;164A:1029–1034.

Shevell M, Ashwal S, Donley D, et al. Practice parameter: Evaluation of the child with global developmental delay: Report of the Quality Standards Subcommittee of the American Academy of Neurology and the Practice Committee of the Child Neurology Society. *Neurology.* 2003;60:367–380.

Thomson A, Maltezos S, Paliokosta E, Xenitidis K. Risperidone for attention-deficit hyperactivity disorder in people with intellectual disabilities. *Cochrane Database Syst Rev.* 2009;(2): CD007011.

Tyrer P, Oliver-Africano PC, Ahmed Z, et al. Risperidone, haloperidol, and placebo in the treatment of aggressive challenging behaviour in patients with intellectual disability: A randomised controlled trial. *Lancet.* 2008;371:57–63.

U.S. Department of Health and Human Services. Closing the gap: A national blueprint to improve the health of persons with mental retardation. Rockville, MD: Office of the Surgeon General; 2002. http://www.nichd.nih.gov/publications/pubs/closingthegap/index.cfm. Accessed December 22, 2012.

van de Kamp JM, Betsalel OT, Mercimek-Mahmutoglu S, et al. Phenotype and genotype in 101 males with X-linked creatine transporter deficiency. *J Med Genet.* 2013;50:463–472.

van Schrojenstein Lantman-De Valk HM, Metsemakers JF, Haveman MJ, Crebolder HF. Health problems in people with intellectual disability in general practice: a comparative study. *Fam Pract.* 2000;17:405–7.

Tic Disorder

Albanese A, Bhatia K, Bressman SB, et al. Phenomenology and classification of dystonia: a consensus update. *Mov Disord.* 2013;28:863–873.

Albanese A, Jankovic J. Distingushing clinical features of hyperkinetic disorders. In: Albanese A, Jankovic J, eds. *Hyperkinetic movement disorders*. Oxford: Wiley-Blackwell; 2012:3.

Baizabal-Carvallo JF, Jankovic J. Movement disorders in autoimmune diseases. *Mov Disord.* 2012;27:935–946.

Baizabal-Carvallo JF, Stocco A, Muscal E, Jankovic J. The spectrum of movement disorders in children with anti-NMDA receptor encephalitis. *Mov Disord.* 2013;28:543–547.

Cuker A, State MW, King RA, et al. Candidate locus for Gilles de la Tourette syndrome/obsessive compulsive disorder/chronic tic disorder at 18q22. *Am J Med Genet A.* 2004;130A:37.

Deng H, Gao K, Jankovic J. The genetics of Tourette syndrome. *Nat Rev Neurol.* 2012;8:203–213.

Hacohen Y, Dlamini N, Hedderly T, et al. N-methyl-D-aspartate receptor antibody-associated movement disorder without encephalopathy. *Dev Med Child Neurol.* 2015;56:190.

Jankovic J. Medical treatment of dystonia. *Mov Disord.* 2013;28:1001–1012.

Leckman JF, Cohen DJ, Goetz CG, Jankovic J. Tourette syndrome: Pieces of the puzzle. *Adv Neurol.* 2001;85:369–390.

Mohammad SS, Fung VS, Grattan-Smith P, et al. Movement disorders in children with anti-NMDAR encephalitis and other autoimmune encephalopathies. *Mov Disord.* 2014;29:1539–1542.

Pauls DL, Fernandez TV, Mathews CA, et al. The inheritance of Tourette Disorder: A review. *J Obsessive Compuls Relat Disord.* 2014;3:380–385.

Singer HS, Mink JW, Gilbert DL, Jankovic J. *Movement disorders in childhood.* 2nd ed. Philadelphia, PA: Butterworth-Heinemann (Elsevier); 2015.

van Egmond ME, Kuiper A, Eggink H, et al. Dystonia in children and adolescents: A systematic review and a new diagnostic algorithm. *J Neurol Neurosurg Psychiatry.* 2015;86:774–781.

RESOURCES

Attention Deficit/Hyperactivity Disorder

ADHD for Parents and Caregivers: Comprehensive Assessment, How to Help Your Child Succeed at School, How to Make Life at Home Easier, and Parent Training. The National Resource on ADHD
  http://www.help4adhd.org/Understanding-ADHD/For-Parents-Caregivers.aspx

ADHD Tips and Resources. The National Resource on ADHD
  http://www.help4adhd.org/Support/Tips-and-Resources.aspx

ADHD: Attention Deficit Hyperactivity Disorder in Primary Care for School-Age Children and Adolescents. Agency for Healthcare Research and Quality
  https://www.icsi.org/guidelines__more/catalog_guidelines_and_more/catalog_guidelines/catalog_behavioral_health_guidelines/adhd/

Attention-Deficit Hyperactivity Disorder Guidelines for Adults. Agency for Healthcare Research and Quality
  https://www.guideline.gov/summaries/summary/46415?

Attention Deficit-Hyperactivity Disorder Information Page. National Institute of Neurological Disorders and Stroke
  https://www.ninds.nih.gov/Disorders/All-Disorders/Attention-Deficit-Hyperactivity-Disorder-Information-Page

Attention-Deficit Hyperactivity Disorder: Overview, Symptoms, Causes, Diagnosis, Treatment, and Resources. American Academy of Family Physicians
  https://familydoctor.org/condition/attention-deficit-hyperactivity-disorder-adhd/?adfree=true

Attention-Deficit/Hyperactivity Disorder (ADHD): The Basics. National Institute of Mental Health
  https://www.nimh.nih.gov/health/publications/attention-deficit-hyperactivity-disorder-adhd-the-basics/qf-16-3572_153275.pdf

Attention-Deficit/Hyperactivity Disorder. Symptoms and Diagnosis. Centers for Disease Control and Prevention
  https://www.cdc.gov/ncbddd/adhd/diagnosis.html

College Students with ADHD. American Academy of Child and Adolescent Psychiatry
  https://www.aacap.org/AACAP/Families_and_Youth/Facts_for_Families/FFF-Guide/College-Students-with-ADHD-111.aspx

Could I Have Attention-Deficit/Hyperactivity Disorder? Booklet. National Institute of Mental Health
  https://www.nimh.nih.gov/health/publications/could-i-have-adhd/qf-16-3572_153023.pdf

Focusing on ADHD. National Institutes of Health
  https://newsinhealth.nih.gov/2014/09/focusing-adhd

Helping Children and Youth with Attention-Deficit/Hyperactivity Disorder Systems of Care. Substance Abuse and Mental Health Services Administration
  https://store.samhsa.gov/shin/content//SMA05-4059/SMA05-4059.pdf

Autism Spectrum Disorder

Autism Initiatives. American Academy of Pediatrics
  https://www.aap.org/en-us/about-the-aap/Committees-Councils-Sections/Council-on-Children-with-Disabilities/Pages/Resources-for-Professionals-and-Families.aspx

Autism Resource Center. American Academy of Child and Adolescent Psychiatry
  http://www.aacap.org/AACAP/Families_and_Youth/Resource_Centers/Autism_Resource_Center/Home

Autism Society
  http://www.autism-society.org/

Autism Speaks
  http://www.AutismSpeaks.org

Autism. Healthy Children.org.
  https://www.healthychildren.org/English/health-issues/conditions/Autism/Pages/default.aspx

Intellectual Disability

A Summary of Evidence on Inclusive Education. National Association of Down Syndrome
  http://www.nads.org/wp-content/uploads/2017/06/A_Summary_of_the_evidence_on_inclusive_education.pdf

American Association on Intellectual and Developmental Disabilities
Center for Parent Information & Resources
Autism
    www.parentcenterhub.org/intellectual
Children with Intellectual Disabilities. American Academy of Pediatrics and Healthy Children.Org
    https://www.healthychildren.org/English/health-issues/conditions/developmental-disabilities/Pages/Intellectual-Disability.aspx
Fact Sheet on Intellectual Disability. Center for Parent Information & Resources
    http://www.parentcenterhub.org/intellectual/
Facts About Intellectual Disability for Parents. Centers for Disease Control and Prevention
    https://www.cdc.gov/ncbddd/actearly/pdf/parents_pdfs/IntellectualDisability.pdf
Individuals with Disabilities Education Act
    https://sites.ed.gov/idea/
Intellectual Disabilities. National Institute of Child Health and Human Development
    https://www.nichd.nih.gov/health/topics/idds/conditioninfo/Pages/default.aspx
Intellectual Disabilities: Definitions, Causes, and Treatment. American Psychiatric Association
    https://www.psychiatry.org/patients-families/intellectual-disability/what-is-intellectual-disability

Intellectual Disabilities: Facts for Families Guide. American Academy of Child & Adolescent Psychiatry
    https://www.aacap.org/AACAP/Families_and_Youth/Facts_for_Families/FFF-Guide/Children-with-an-Intellectual-Disability-023.aspx
Intellectual Disability Diagnosis, Treatment, and Policy. The Arc for People With Intellectual and Developmental Disabilities
    http://www.thearc.org/learn-about/intellectual-disability
Intellectual Disability: Causes, Symptoms, Exams, Treatment, Support Groups, and Prognosis. National Library of Medicine
    https://medlineplus.gov/ency/article/001523.htm
Intellectual Disability: Definition and Video Describing Intellectual Disability. American Association of Intellectual Disability
    http://aaidd.org/intellectual-disability/definition#.WkLuM9-nH4a

Tic Disorder

Tourette Association of America
    http://www.tourette.org

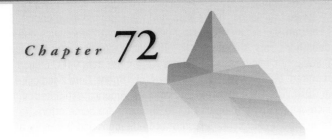

Chapter **72**

Common Urgent Care Complaints

Joe Holbrook, BS, BSN, MS, APRN

Jill E. Winland-Brown, EdD, APRN, FNP-BC

Brian Oscar Porter, MD, PhD, MPH, MBA

The definition of urgent care varies, but most experts agree that it is the provision of outpatient medical care for illness or injuries requiring immediate or prompt attention. Urgent care may be provided by a patient's primary-care provider in the office setting or by providers in at walk-in health-care clinics. These clinics are designed specifically to conveniently accommodate urgent care needs without the cost of an emergency department visit. The purpose of walk-in clinics is to provide convenient quality care at a fraction of the cost of an emergency department visit.

There are several types of walk-in clinics, allowing patients the convenience of unscheduled visits. These clinic models include walk-in primary care, on-site, retail, urgent care, freestanding emergency departments and traditional emergency departments. Box 72.1 explains the differences between these types of clinics.

Nurse practitioners (NPs) play an important role as clinicians in these clinics. Two-thirds of urgent care centers are staffed with nonphysician clinicians, and more than one-half do not have a physician on site. Many are staffed solely by NPs (Becker's Hospital Review, February 16, 2011). Urgent care NPs make about 5% more than the national average of all NPs.

The information presented in Figure 72.1 reflects data from an informal survey of an advanced practice registered nursing practice involving 155 visits at a suburban urgent care center in south Florida (Joe Holbrook, MSN, APRN, personal survey, 2017). This chapter also incorporates data from the National Urgent Care Chart Survey from the *Journal of Urgent Care Medicine* (2010). Discussion of these chief complaints includes epidemiology and triage information intended to help the practitioner decide which patients can be treated within an urgent care setting and which patients should be referred to other practitioners. If the disease, illness, or injury is also discussed in depth in another chapter, the reader is referred to that chapter.

PULMONARY COMPLAINTS

Pulmonary complaints comprise the highest percentage of chief complaints with almost 39% in the Urgent Care Survey (Braveheart Group, 2010) and almost 17% in the Florida study. Diagnoses include influenza, upper respiratory infection, bronchitis, and cough.

INFLUENZA

With an estimated annual attack rate of 5% to 10% in adults and 20% to 30% in children, patients with influenza present frequently to urgent care centers. In the Northern Hemisphere, the influenza season is from October through April; in the Southern Hemisphere, it is from May through September. In tropical regions, influenza may appear throughout the year. Persons at the highest risk for morbidity and mortality from influenza include children under age 5 years, older adults, immunocompromised persons, women who are pregnant during the flu season, and persons living in close quarters, such as long-term care facilities. Because morbidity and mortality may be reduced by widespread vaccination, an objective of *Healthy People 2020* is to "reduce, eliminate, or maintain elimination of cases of vaccine-preventable diseases."

TRIAGE

Common symptoms of influenza include high fever, chills, myalgias, and malaise. In the urgent care setting, the clinician must be alert to the development of complications that may further compromise the individual. Complications

---

Box 72.1   Types of Walk-In Clinics

Primary-Care Walk-in Clinics

When a clinic is labeled as a walk-in clinic, it may be one of several different health-care delivery models, including a primary-care office that allows patients to walk-in without an appointment. The scope of practice and on-site diagnostic testing is usually similar to other primary-care clinics.

On-Site Employee Clinics

Many employers are now offering on-site clinics for their employees. These clinics usually provide care for minor injuries, common illnesses, health education, and wellness exams.

Retail Clinics

There are more than 1,800 retail clinics in the United States, and the number is increasing. They are usually located at retail stores that have on-site pharmacies. The services they usually provide are care for minor injuries, common illness, and chronic conditions; vaccinations; health screenings for work or school; and physical exams. They usually maintain extended hours, including evening and weekends. They are most often staffed with a single nurse practitioner or physician assistant. The ability to access walk-in appointments, convenience, cost, and lack of a primary health provider are the three most common reasons patients cite for choosing retail clinics.

Urgent Care Clinics

Urgent care clinics provide urgent non–life-threatening treatment for illnesses and injuries. They are usually differentiated from other walk-in or retail clinics by the expanded services and diagnostics offered. These may include x-rays, lab tests such as electrolytes, complete blood counts, rapid flu tests, rapid strep tests, and computed tomography scans or ultrasounds. Many of the expanded services often include wound suturing, abscess incision and drainage, IV medications, IV fluids, basic fracture management, and sometimes on-site chiropractic treatment or physical therapy. Urgent care clinics are usually open 7 days a week and for longer hours than retail and primary-care clinics. There are no required certifications for urgent care clinics and definitions vary, therefore it is difficult to exactly quantify the number of clinics that exist. There were more than 9,000 clinics reported by the American Academy of Urgent Care Medicine in 2014. The Urgent Care Association of America estimated an increase by 23% from 2014 to 2016. There are some efforts to have urgent care centers require accreditation, and it is now a contractual requirement of some insurance companies.

Freestanding Emergency Departments

Freestanding emergency departments are open 24 hours a day, 7 days a week. They usually offer all the services of traditional emergency departments with the exception of hospital admissions and will transfer the patients who require admission to the appropriate hospital. They are designed to treat life-threatening injuries or serious illnesses. The average cost of care at these clinics is usually 9 to 15 times more than at an urgent care clinic. They are usually staffed with a physician and may also have nurse practitioners or physician assistants.

Traditional Emergency Departments

Traditional emergency departments are treated the same as freestanding emergency departments but are attached to a hospital where they may admit patients.

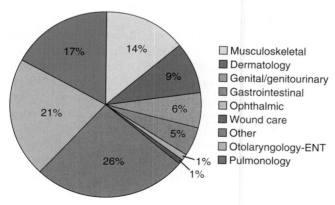

Figure 72.1. Distribution of patient visits at one suburban urgent care center based on 155 patient contacts. (Source: *Joe Holbrook, MSN, APRN, personal survey, 2017.*)

that may cause mortality and morbidity include primary influenza pneumonia; secondary bacterial pneumonia; myositis, myocarditis, and central nervous system (CNS) diseases such as seizure, encephalopathy, transverse myelitis, and Guillain-Barré syndrome. Myositis presents with myalgias, most often affecting the lower extremities, and is more common in children. Serum creatinine phosphokinase may be elevated, and myoglobinuria may be present. Myocarditis may present with electrocardiogram (ECG) or cardiac enzyme abnormalities, new-onset atrial or ventricular arrhythmias, complete heart block, or an acute myocardial infarction (MI)-like syndrome. For CNS diseases, seizure is the most common neurologic complication, and encephalopathy is the second most common. The clinician should be alert to an altered mental status, such as confusion, delirium, and behavioral changes.

UPPER RESPIRATORY INFECTION

The average adult has two to four colds per year, and the average school-age child has six to ten colds per year. Upper respiratory infection (URIs) are generally viral in origin. Cigarette smoking is associated with an increased risk of URIs.

TRIAGE

When assessing patients with URIs, clinicians should be alert for complications, which include otitis media, sinusitis, and an asthma exacerbation along with an exacerbation of any other pulmonary disease. URIs are covered in detail in Chapter 30.

BRONCHITIS

There were 563 deaths from chronic and unspecified bronchitis in 2014. Within the general category of chronic lower respiratory diseases, bronchitis is the third leading cause of death (Kochanek et al., 2016).

TRIAGE

Symptoms of acute bronchitis include cough (both productive or nonproductive), sputum, dyspnea on exertion, and wheezing, rhonchi, or other signs of obstruction. Purulent sputum occurs in approximately 50% of patients. There may be accompanying symptoms such as fever, sore throat, nasal congestion, or runny nose. Acute bronchitis is usually mild and does not cause complications. Diffuse wheezes and the use of accessory muscles are seen in more severe cases as well as a diffuse diminution of inspiration or stridor that may indicate bronchial or tracheal obstruction. Some of the symptoms of bronchitis may actually be those of heart failure. Symptoms of heart failure include dyspnea on exertion, fatigue and weight gain, cough, lower extremity edema, and shortness of breath when bending over. This differential diagnosis is critical. Heart failure is covered in Chapter 35.

Treatment of acute bronchitis is primarily supportive. Chronic bronchitis is covered in Chapter 31.

COUGH

In the 2010 National Urgent Care survey, a cough comprises almost 4% of all visits. Although a cough may be mild or intermittent, it is essential to properly diagnose the underlying condition, as the appropriate treatment should be started as early as possible.

TRIAGE

Diagnoses may include a chronic cough from smoking or lung cancer, or a new cough from allergies, a viral infection, sinusitis, postnasal drip, gastroesophageal reflux disease (GERD), or a relapse of bronchitis/chronic obstructive pulmonary disease. A cough may also be a factor in heart failure or pneumonia. Taking a history is the most important aspect in diagnosing a cough. A dry, irritating cough may indicate allergies, whereas a moist, heavy cough with sputum may be related to heart failure or pneumonia.

The patient's smoking history is vital. For a patient with a 40-pack-year history of smoking, a low-dose computed tomography (CT) scan of the lung should be ordered. A chest x-ray may rule out pneumonia or heart failure. Cough is covered in Chapter 28.

EYE/EAR/NOSE/THROAT (EENT) COMPLAINTS

Patients with eye/ear/nose/throat (EENT) complaints comprise the next highest percentage of chief complaints (28.7%) of urgent care visits according to the Urgent Care Survey. They comprise 22% of urgent care visits in the Florida study. Diagnoses in this category include conjunctivitis, sinusitis, rhinitis, sore throat, and ear pain.

CONJUNCTIVITIS

Conjunctivitis may be caused by allergic reactions or bacterial or viral infections. Acute conjunctivitis is the more commonly seen condition in urgent care settings, as these patients are more likely to seek immediate care for their symptoms than those with chronic conjunctivitis. Adenovirus is the most common cause of infectious conjunctivitis, which is more prevalent during summer and represents 20% to 62% of the cases. Risk factors include overcrowding or close quarters, an urban setting, and an exposure to infected persons.

The symptoms diagnostic of acute conjunctivitis can be ascertained during the physical exam. They include red conjunctiva; ocular discharge; eyelids that are "sticky" in the morning; and the feeling of itching, burning, or a foreign body sensation.

TRIAGE

A rapid in-office test (AdenoPlus) is sensitive and specific for detection of adenoviral conjunctivitis and may be used to rule out more serious conditions (Sambursky, 2013). Further examination with fluorescein staining may rule out a corneal abrasion. Ophthalmology consultation may be necessary, as eye pain may be the first sign of an ophthalmologic emergency such as acute angle-closure glaucoma, optic neuritis, orbital cellulitis, scleritis, infectious keratitis, and anterior uveitis. Red eye and conjunctivitis are covered in Chapter 19. Patients should be told not to wear contacts nor make-up until symptoms subside.

SINUSITIS

While most clinicians refer to the condition as sinusitis, the American Academy of Otolaryngology-Head and Neck Surgery Foundation refers to this symptomatic inflammatory condition as rhinosinusitis because other than the paranasal sinuses, the nasal cavity is almost always involved. Acute rhinosinusitis lasts less than 4 weeks. Chronic rhinosinusitis lasts longer than 12 weeks. In the National Urgent Care survey, sinusitis is the top diagnosis code of all the conditions at 10.6%.

Risk factors for sinusitis include smoking, a deviated septum, and asthma, among others. It is usually preceded by a viral URI. In one study involving 29 articles, viruses accounted for 67% of all sinus infections, while another study showed that *Streptococcus pneumonia* and *Haemophilus influenzae* resulted in up to 50% of all sinus infections. *Moraxella catarrhalis* is less frequent in adults, although more common in children (Smith et al, 2015).

TRIAGE

Sinusitis can be diagnosed by x-ray, although this is rarely performed. Diagnosis is usually made by signs and symptoms, including sinus tenderness, facial pain or headache, abnormal transillumination, history of colored nasal discharge, and a poor response to nasal sprays. See Chapter 24 for a thorough discussion and treatment of sinusitis.

RHINITIS

Millions of Americans are affected by rhinitis. The diagnoses of rhinitis may include vasomotor rhinitis, allergic or nonallergic rhinitis, or URI. Vasomotor rhinitis is not related to a specific allergen. A risk factor for vasomotor rhinitis is previous nasal trauma. Nonallergic rhinitis may also be an extraesophageal manifestation of GERD resulting in postnasal drip and/or a cough. Active and passive smoking are associated with an increased risk of allergic rhinitis (Saulyte et al., 2014).

TRIAGE

Rhinitis is not a medical emergency. There is no medication that is uniformly effective in controlling symptoms; however, a stepwise approach to symptom management may be tried. Rhinitis is covered in Chapter 24.

PHARYNGITIS/STREP THROAT

Annually, there are approximately 12 million ambulatory visits in the United States related to pharyngitis (Chow & Doron, 2017). Patients tend to present with pharyngitis to the urgent care setting after hours and on weekends.

Pharyngitis may be caused by viral or bacterial agents. Although most guidelines focus solely on group A β-hemolytic streptococcal infection, at least 10% of cases of bacterial pharyngitis are actually caused by

Fusobacterium necrophorum in older adolescents and individuals in their early 20s (Centor et al., 2015).

TRIAGE

Antibiotics are the recommended treatment for streptococcal pharyngitis, gonococcal pharyngitis, diphtheria, and *Haemophilus influenzae* type B. Symptoms suggestive of group A streptococcal pharyngitis include anterior cervical adenitis, persistent fever, and tonsillopharyngeal exudates. Triage may include using a rapid antigen detection test and/or culture to diagnose and treat (Harris, Hicks, & Qaseem, 2016). Pharyngitis is presented in Chapter 24.

EAR PAIN

Ear pain may indicate otitis externa, acute otitis media (AOM), otitis media with effusion (OME), acute mastoiditis, or a ruptured tympanic membrane (TM). Otitis externa most common affects children aged 7 to 12 years. Malignant otitis externa mainly affects elderly patients and those who are immunocompromised or have diabetes. One of the causes is a fungal infection of the external auditory canal more prevalent in this population (Abdelazeem, Gamea, Mubarak, & Elzawawy, 2015). Risk factors of otitis externa include water in the ear canal (especially water containing bacteria) from prolonged swimming, humidity and high ambient temperatures, and sweating. Items in the ear that disrupt the epithelium may also be a factor, such as hearing aids and ear plugs. Using cotton-tip applicators to clean ears is also a major risk factor for otitis externa. Patients should be warned against this practice.

Approximately one-half of all cases of AOM occur in children younger than age 5. A slight increase in cases also occurs in individuals older than age 75 years (Monasta et al., 2012). Viral causes of AOM include respiratory syncytial virus; rhinovirus, adenovirus, coronavirus, bocavirus, influenza virus; parainfluenza virus, enterovirus; and human metapneumovirus. The most common bacterial causes include *Streptococcus pneumoniae, Haemophilus influenza, Moraxella (Branhamella) catarrhalis* (Ngo, Massa, Thornton, & Cripps, 2016). Acute OME occurs predominantly in the first year of life with 90% of children affected by age 5 years. Risk factors include recent AOM or viral URI.

Acute mastoiditis is more common in children who have had AOM. The most dangerous complication of acute mastoiditis is an intracranial abscess. Signs and symptoms include headache, fever, otalgia, and otorrhea.

Ear pain with a ruptured tympanic membrane (TM) subsides quickly. There may also be clear, purulent, or bloody drainage from the ear, hearing loss, tinnitus, or vertigo, which may also include nausea or vomiting. The history and clinical presentation will diagnosis a ruptured TM. Causes may include otitis media, barotrauma, acoustic trauma from a loud sound, a foreign object in the ear, or severe head trauma.

TRIAGE

Diagnosis of these conditions is typically based on findings obtained during the physical exam. Mastoiditis is the most common serious complication of AOM in children. Other complications are rare and include meningitis, brain abscess, and facial nerve paralysis. If there is lack of improvement after treatment and/or focal neurological signs, which may indicate acute mastoiditis-related intracranial complications, a CT or magnetic resonance imaging (MRI) may be indicated. Ear pain is covered in Chapter 21, and otitis media is covered in Chapter 23.

MUSCULOSKELETAL COMPLAINTS

In the National Urgent Care study, nontraumatic and traumatic musculoskeletal pain account for almost 14.5% of chief complaints and 14% in the Florida study.

MUSCULOSKELETAL PAIN

NONTRAUMATIC MUSCULOSKELETAL PAIN

Low back pain (LBP) is probably the number one condition that clinicians manage each year. LBP may be due to occupational factors, poor body mechanics, or obesity. LBP is covered in Chapter 53.

Osteoarthritis (OA) or degenerative joint disease occurs in at least some joints in most persons older than age 40 years. According to the Arthritis Foundation, OA is the most common chronic condition of the joints, affecting approximately 27 million Americans. A person with OA will typically awaken with stiffness and a cracking sound in the joints; as the day progresses, the pain and stiffness will gradually lesson with movement. There may be mild swelling around the joint. Toward the end of the day, the pain may worsen. OA is the main reason for joint replacements. Arthritis is covered in Chapter 55.

TRAUMATIC MUSCULOSKELETAL PAIN

Sprains can occur during common activities or may occur due to falling, twisting, or being hit and forcing the body out of alignment. A sprain is caused by a stretched or torn ligament. A strain is a stretch or a tear in a muscle or tendon. Strains occur frequently in athletes and are more common in sports requiring repetitive motion, such as football, hockey, baseball, or tennis.

TRIAGE

Sprains and strains have similar symptoms of pain and inflammation with possible bruising at the affected area. Although pain is subjective, the clinician should use assessment techniques as described in Chapter 52 to make a diagnosis. These conditions are covered in Chapters 52 and 53.

FRACTURES

A bone fracture may either be caused by trauma (force or stress) or a disease such as osteoporosis or cancer (pathological). Acute musculoskeletal injury is covered in Chapter 52.

Fractures are prevalent until the early 20s, then level off until around age 60 when the incidence increases. Fractures related to violence are 10 times higher in African American (Pressley et al., 2011). The following section focuses on specific fractures.

Shoulder

Fractures of the humerus, clavicle, and acromion are common. A fracture of the clavicle typically occurs from a moderate fall (such as from a bicycle or down stairs) or from blows during a contact sport. Patients complain of sharp shoulder pain and are reluctant to move the upper extremity. It is important to verify that no neck pain or upper extremity paresthesias are present. These fractures usually best heal spontaneously after proper immobilization; they rarely require surgery.

Proximal Femoral (Hip) Fracture

Hip fractures are one of the most common of all adult fractures, accounting for at least one-half of all hospital days related to fracture care in the United States. There is a mortality rate of 50% 1 year after hip fracture surgery. The two primary types of hip fractures are femoral neck (intracapsular) and intertrochanteric, both of which occur most frequently in older adults who have sustained a fall at home or a similar low-energy trauma. The incidence of hip fractures doubles for each decade of life after age 50 years, with women affected twice as often as men.

Risks for hip fractures include increasing age, previous fracture, visual impairment, institutionalization, and osteoporosis. Pain in the hip area after trauma, such as a fall or motor vehicle collision, especially in patients older than age 50, should give rise to the suggestion of a fracture. However, neither a lack of trauma nor a long-standing history of hip pain rules out a fracture. In some cases, a fracture may occur as a pathological fracture secondary to an underlying neoplasm or chronic corticosteroid usage. The patient with a suspected hip fracture should be admitted to the hospital.

Patients with a suspected hip fracture should be asked if an injury occurred and if so, how the injury occurred and whether the fall was witnessed by anyone other than the patient. A loss of consciousness for any period of time necessitates a cardiac and neurological referral, as well as referral for orthopedic care. The clinician should determine the patient's mental status and try to obtain a realistic assessment of the preinjury functional status.

Physical exam typically reveals an externally rotated and shortened injured leg. Any motion to this extremity will produce severe pain center around the affected groin. The pelvic bony prominences should be examined for tenderness because pubis ramus fractures may also be present or may be confused with the hip injury. It is important to check for lower-extremity pulses and neurological function. The entire limb should be examined for fractures at sites such as the femur, tibia, or ankle. An anteroposterior view of the pelvis and "shoot-through" lateral views of the affected hip can provide definitive radiographic evidence to confirm the diagnosis. In most cases, surgical repair of the fracture is the treatment of choice.

Knee

A knee fracture is most likely to occur with direct trauma and result in acute onset of pain. Fractures of the knee and leg include those of the patella, tibial plateau, fibular head and shaft, and tibial pilon. Most, but not all, knee fractures are the result of significant trauma; fractures of the knee are often present in conjunction with injury to associated structures. Most fractures around the knee are associated with a large effusion. If the joint is tapped, the presence of hemarthrosis with fat globules is clinically indicative of a fracture. Swelling and significant pain on movement will be present. It is important to ensure that no neurovascular compromise is present in the lower leg. Radiography should be obtained, and immediate referral to an orthopedic surgeon is indicated. Patellar fractures are usually the result of a direct blow from a blunt object or can be attributed to a fall or motor vehicle collision (MVC). The patient with a patellar fracture is usually unable to flex the knee. Marked joint effusion is usually present.

Ankle

The patient with an ankle fracture will have pain, swelling, or inability to bear weight, decreased range of motion, and obvious bony disruption on x-ray film. Stress fractures of the ankle also may occur.

Stress Fractures

Stress fractures are common in patients who experience bone pain after initiating or increasing high-impact activity. Stress fractures are a result of repeated subtle bone trauma over a period of time that causes a gradual loss of bony substance. New bone is fragile until it calcifies. The cortex, temporarily weakened, is then susceptible to fracture. Common sites for stress fractures are the legs and feet.

Physical exam may reveal point tenderness over the bone. Ecchymosis and soft tissue swelling may be present. Often the patient has altered his or her gait to compensate for the pain and swelling, causing pain to the knee. Resistive motion of the joint is painless. Radiographs may reveal a periosteal reaction or a hairline radiolucency but are usually negative until 2 to 3 weeks after the injury has occurred. Bone scans or CT scans may be helpful.

TRIAGE

A fracture may be diagnosed on the clinical exam or may require an X-ray, CT, or MRI. Fractures require immobilization, which will range from casts or braces to surgery involving plates, screws, nails, or external fixators. Urgent care practitioners may apply a cast and/or braces depending on the level of swelling and refer patients requiring surgery to an orthopedic surgeon or the ED. Complications of fractures include malunion, osteomyelitis, and actual bone death or avascular necrosis. Other than a simple break, such as a greenstick fracture that may be treated with a cast in the urgent care setting, patients with a more involved bone fractures, just as a comminuted or impacted fracture, should be referred to acute care.

NEUROLOGICAL/ PSYCHOLOGICAL COMPLAINTS

In the Urgent Care study, there were 12.1% of visits categorized as neurological or psychological chief complaints. The most frequent diagnoses in this category are headache, anxiety, and depression.

HEADACHE

There are 150 diagnostic headache categories. The most common types of headaches are tension-type headache and migraines. Others include caffeine-withdrawal headaches, hunger headaches, or pathological headaches, such as those caused by an aneurysm, giant cell arteritis, or hypertension.

About 50% to 75% of the adult population globally has had a headache within the past year (World Health Organization, 2016). Primary headaches include tension, migraine, and cluster headaches. These types must be differentiated from secondary headaches that are caused by infection or vascular disease.

Primary headaches may be diagnosed by the patient's history. A tension-type headache produces bilateral mild to moderate pressure without other symptoms. A migraine headache may present with or without an aura. An aura may include visual, sensory, or speech symptoms that last less than 60 minutes and are reversible. A migraine usually occurs on one side of the head and lasts from 4 to 72 hours. Additional symptoms may include nausea, vomiting, photophobia, and/or phonophobia.

Cluster headaches are less common, but an estimated 500,000 Americans may experience a cluster headache at least once in their lifetime. Cluster headaches last from 15 to 180 minutes with severe head pain usually with associated symptoms of one-sided conjunctival redness, nasal congestion or rhinorrhea, eyelid edema, and forehead or facial swelling. The patient is usually restless or agitated.

TRIAGE

When taking a history of a patient with a headache, it is crucial to assess signs and symptoms that may indicate certain "red-flag" diagnoses that require immediate emergency care (see Box 72.2). If any of the signs and symptoms in the box are present, further evaluation should be done, including an erythrocyte sedimentation rate (ESR), lumbar puncture, and neuroimaging. Other than patients with suspected temporal arteritis, these patients should be sent to the ER for further diagnosis. Headaches are covered in detail in Chapter 9.

ANXIETY

There are many anxiety disorders, such as agoraphobia, generalized anxiety disorder, obsessive compulsive disorder, panic disorder; post-traumatic stress disorder (PTSD), and social anxiety disorder. Most of these disorders are chronic and long-standing. Patients with anxiety who typically seek urgent care are those experiencing a panic attack.

Box 72.2	Red Flags for Headache Diagnosis
Sign or Symptom	**Possible Diagnosis**
"The worst headache of my life"	CNS infection or intracranial hemorrhage
Headache triggered by coitus, a cough, or exertion	CNS lesion, subarachnoid hemorrhage
Change in mental status or LOC	CNS infection, intracerebral bleed, CNS lesion
Age greater than 50 years of age or	Temporal arteritis

Abbreviations: CNS, central nervous system; LOC, loss of consciousness.
(Adapted from Hainer & Matheson, 2013).

Panic disorder (PD) most commonly begins in early adulthood (age 20–29 years). The reported lifetime prevalence is just over 28% (Kessler et al., 2012). PD is most commonly associated with female sex, smoking, substance use disorders, stressful life events in childhood and adulthood, and a history of parental mental health disorders (Moreno-Peral, 2014).

TRIAGE

Patients with PD typically report an abrupt episode of fear or discomfort that usually peaks within minutes. Other symptoms include palpitations, sweating, trembling, shortness of breath, feelings of choking, chest discomfort, nausea, dizziness, and fear of losing control or dying (Lewis-Fernandez et al., 2010). A medication history should be obtained that may reveal possible triggers of the panic symptoms, such as sedatives, benzodiazepines, and pseudoephedrine. The patient should be asked about any illicit drug use as well as caffeine, nicotine, and alcohol use.

Proper diagnosis of panic disorder is essential because approximately 25% of persons who present to the ED or urgent care setting with chest pain are having a panic attack rather than a cardiac-related condition. To rule out a cardiac condition, a good history is essential, and an electrocardiogram (ECG) may be necessary. Once the patient has been diagnosed with PD, there are many treatment options, including lifestyle changes, nonmedical treatment such as cognitive behavior therapy, psychotherapy, and medications. For patients who are hyperventilating, some clinicians suggest breathing into a paper bag, while others encourage maximal exhalation and diaphragmatic breathing. See Chapters 64 and 68 for detailed information about anxiety disorders.

DEPRESSION

Depression is common and treatable, yet many Americans do not seek treatment. Nine percent of the U.S. population is currently depressed. Approximately 3.4% meet the criteria for major depression (Gonzalez & Berry, 2010).

Because depression often is not discussed, the U.S. Preventive Services Task Force recommends screening of all adults regardless of risk factors (AHRQ, 2016). Patients may be seen in urgent care settings because they know something is "wrong" and they may not have a primary-care provider. Depression is characterized by a persistent low mood with a lack of positive affect and anhedonia (loss of interest in pleasurable activities) that have been present for a period of at least 2 weeks. Depression is more common among persons with chronic health conditions and those with unhealthy lifestyles (smoking, drinking, lack of activity).

TRIAGE

Treatment of depression requires long-term therapy and/ or counseling. Although depression cannot be adequately treated in urgent care, it must be appropriately diagnosed and the patient referred. Suicide, a potential outcome of depression, was the 10th leading cause of death in 2015 (U.S. Department of Health and Human Services, 2017).

Signs and symptoms of depression include flat affect, self-reported changes in personal or workplace environments, weight gain or loss, irritable bowel syndrome, lack of energy, sleep disturbances, memory problems, difficulty concentrating, and increased stress. Many differential diagnoses should be considered, included bipolar disorder (the presence of mania or hypomania), postpartum depression, seasonal affective disorder, PTSD, an anxiety disorder, hypothyroidism, Cushing's disease, and bereavement or grief.

All patients who are depressed should be asked, "Have you thought about suicide?" If they say yes, the next question must be, "Do you have a plan?" See Chapter 68 for an in-depth discussion of acute suicide risk and depressive disorders.

GASTROINTESTINAL COMPLAINTS

In the National Urgent Care survey, gastrointestinal (GI) problems account for 10.6% and comprise 5.4% of chief complaints in the Florida study. Patients often present to urgent care with diarrhea, constipation, and heartburn. Patients presenting with heartburn may think that their chest pain is indicative of a heart attack.

DIARRHEA

Acute diarrhea is the passage of six or more stools daily without improvement for 3 or more days. Acute diarrhea may be caused by infections, noninfectious conditions, and medications.

Infections include bacterial, viral, parasitic, and other conditions such as foodborne illnesses, traveler's diarrhea, and infectious gastroenteritis. Most causes of acute diarrhea in adults are self-limiting and of infectious etiology.

Bacterial pathogens include *Vibrio cholerae* (which causes cholera), *Clostridium difficile*, *Escherichia coli*, *Legionella*, *Salmonella*, *Shigella*, and staphylococcal and streptococcal pathogens. Viral pathogens include dengue virus, HIV, norovirus, and rotavirus, among others. Parasitic infections include amebiasis, cryptosporidium, cryptosporidiosis, giardiasis, schistosomiasis, and strongyloidiasis.

In addition, there are noninfectious conditions that may cause acute diarrhea such as ulcerative colitis, Crohn's disease, irritable bowel syndrome, diverticulitis, and colorectal cancer.

Many medications may cause GI side effects, including antibiotics, laxatives, magnesium antacids, colchicine, and medications leading to immunocompromised conditions, such as long-term steroid use or chemotherapy (McCarthy, Lauwers, & Sheahan, 2015).

TRIAGE

A detailed history is essential to determine the cause of the diarrhea. Patients with a bacterial infection may have additional symptoms such as a fever, tenesmus, and/or bloody stools.

A person with a viral infection may present with nausea and/or vomiting with the onset 24 to 48 hours after possible exposure, whereas a foodborne illness usually experiences symptom onset 2 to 7 hours after possible exposure. If the diarrhea lasts more than 7 days, the clinician should suspect a parasitic infection. Testing may not be necessary, but guidelines are available for selection of the appropriate laboratory testing (Baron et al., 2013).

Treatment consists of rehydration and antimotility or antiperistaltic agents. They are contraindicated if the stool is bloody or fever or abdominal pain is present. See Chapter 38 for more information about diarrhea.

CONSTIPATION

Constipation is characterized by difficult stool passage, infrequent stools (fewer than three per week), or both. Primary constipation may be due to functional causes such as difficult or delayed evacuation, hard stools, and abdominal discomfort; slow or delayed transit; or outlet dysfunction such as anal stricture or cancer among others. Secondary constipation may be due to diet, lifestyle, pregnancy, older age, or medications.

Some medications that may cause constipation include calcium channel blockers, beta blockers, opioids, diuretics, and antidepressants. Chronic constipation is a symptom-based disorder and is more common in women. It can affect from 2% to 27% of the population. Constipation represents a major health problem as reflected by the millions of dollars spent yearly on laxatives (Pinto Sanchez & Bercik, 2011).

TRIAGE

It is important to assess the patient for fever, nausea and/or vomiting, unintentional weight loss of more than 10 pounds, anemia, hematochezia, or melena. A large or small intestinal obstruction or an ileus must be ruled out. If these etiologies are suspected, a fecal occult blood test may be performed; an x-ray may be ordered to rule out an obstruction; or the patient may be referred out for a colonoscopy. One of the most effective treatments for constipation is increased water intake. Patients should be drinking 2 L of water daily, which is just over eight glasses (which all persons would benefit from). Medications that may be causing the patients' constipation should be modified or stopped. A high fiber diet is recommended, along with psyllium supplements. Detailed information on constipation can be found in Chapter 38.

HEARTBURN

Heartburn, or functional dyspepsia, is most commonly caused by GERD which is caused by a relaxed lower esophageal sphincter (LES). GERD is common worldwide and has been increasing in prevalence. Fourteen percent of the global population reports frequent symptoms. In the United States, 10% of the population experience GERD symptoms daily, and more than 40% report symptoms every month.

TRIAGE

A history is crucial because some patients present to urgent care thinking that their pain is from a heart attack. The diagnosis of GERD is based on the history and physical examination and a trial of empiric therapy, if possible. An ECG and cardiac enzymes may be necessary if the patient is unclear about specific symptoms and a possible myocardial infarction (MI) is suspected.

Proton pump inhibitors or H_2 blockers may be ordered. Common triggers of GERD by affecting the LES include smoking, alcohol, citrus foods, spicy foods, caffeine, chocolate, and mints. Patients must be recommended to avoid all of these. A blood test for *Helicobacter pylori* to detect an ulcer may be performed if the empiric therapy does not improve the heartburn.

DERMATOLOGY COMPLAINTS AND WOUND CARE

In the National Urgent Care survey, dermatology and wound care issues comprise 14% of the chief complaints to clinics. In Joe Holbrook's Florida survey, they represent 9.4% of the chief complaints.

DERMATOLOGY

Patients sometimes present with a skin lesion and question whether it is cancer. It may be a common benign skin lesion, actinic keratosis, contact dermatitis, seborrheic keratosis, basal or squamous cell carcinoma, or a melanoma.

Some clinics will do a biopsy on site, but these patients may also be referred to a dermatologist.

TRIAGE

The clinician must rule out a melanoma. Patients should be taught the ABCDE's of skin cancer. A is for asymmetry; B is for border irregularity; C for color; D for diameter (greater than 6 mm); and E for evolving or elevation. All skin lesions are covered in Chapter 17.

WOUND CARE

Patients with lacerations frequently present to urgent care treatment. Suturing is the most common technique for closing the edges of a laceration. Staples are faster but are more likely to result in scarring if left in too long and should not be used on the face, neck, hands, or feet.

TRIAGE

Wound infection is a concern with laceration management, and the clinician should be especially alert for this complication in patients with diabetes, if there is any wound contamination, if the laceration is greater than 5 cm, or if the laceration is on a lower extremity. These conditions are risk factors for infection (Quinn, Polevoi, & Kohn, 2014). Laceration closure techniques and treatment are discussed in Chapter 73.

CARDIOVASCULAR COMPLAINTS

Patients present to urgent care with chest pain and symptoms related to hypertension. In the National Urgent Care survey, these complaints comprise 6.4% of the top diagnosis codes.

CHEST PAIN

Chest pain may occur in the chest or may radiate up to the jaw, neck, back, and one or both arms. Patients may describe it as stabbing, aching, or "an elephant sitting on my chest."

Chest pain may have a cardiac cause, or it can be caused by pulmonary, gastrointestinal, musculoskeletal, or psychological conditions. Life-threatening conditions may include a ST-elevation myocardial infarction, an acute coronary syndrome, thoracic aortic aneurysm and/or dissection, pulmonary embolism, esophageal rupture, or a tension pneumothorax.

TRIAGE

While an intrapericardial diaphragmatic hernia is rare, it may occur from blunt trauma such as a motor vehicle accident. Symptoms include chest pain, upper abdominal pain, dysphagia, and dyspnea. A chest CT is used to diagnosis this condition (Kuy et al., 2014). An ECG will diagnose a MI. GERD is a common condition found in patients presenting to urgent care centers suspecting they may have a heart attack. At that point, an ECG and cardiac enzymes would be done.

HYPERTENSION

The American Heart Association and the American College of Cardiologists issued new blood pressure guidelines in November 2017. For any individual with a 10% or greater risk factor of coronary disease, hypertension is defined as a blood pressure of 130/80 or higher. A calculator is available to determine a patient's coronary risk that takes into account the patient's age, cholesterol levels (total cholesterol as well as low-density lipoprotein and high-density lipoprotein), current blood pressure, and medical history (e.g., if being treated for HTN; history of stroke, angina, diabetes, peripheral artery disease, MI, or atherosclerotic cardiovascular disease) (Whelto et al., 2017).

The prevalence of hypertension is increasing, and many persons do not realize that they have it. Globally, the number of those diagnosed with HTN has increased from 594 million persons in 1975 to 1.13 billion in 2015 (NCD Risk Factor Collaboration, 2017).

More than 50% of persons aged 60 to 69 years and approximately 75% of persons older than age 70 years are affected by HTN. With the 2017 guidelines, the number of adults who are classified with HTN has increased by 14% in the United States.

TRIAGE

Patients may present with a severe headache or visual changes when in actuality it is due to HTN. To identify left ventricular hypertrophy, an echocardiograph is considered the gold standard. Some differential diagnoses for HTN that may need additional testing may include:

- Pheochromocytoma: plasma or urine metanephrines
- Sleep apnea: polysomnogram (sleep study)
- Thyroid disease: thyroid-stimulating hormone level and a thyroid panel
- Coarctation of aorta: computed tomography angiography, echocardiography, or MRI.

In the urgent care setting, a central alpha-agonist such as clonidine (Catapres) may be given initially and the patient should be instructed to sit quietly for 20 to 30 minutes to see if the blood pressure has decreased. Testing and home-care treatment can be initiated. See Chapter 35 for a complete discussion on HTN.

GENITOURINARY COMPLAINTS

Genitourinary complaints comprise 6.7% of the chief complains in the National Urgent Care survey.

URINARY TRACT INFECTION

A urinary tract infection (UTI) is a more frequent occurrence in women than men due to the shorter length of the female urethra. A UTI can usually be diagnosed on the history with complaints of frequency, urgency, and burning on urination. Patients may present to the urgent care setting when they do not want to wait for a doctor's appointment.

Risk factors in premenopausal women include being sexually active and having experienced a UTI previously (there is a 30%–44% risk of recurrent cystitis in women who have already experienced one episode). Risk factors in postmenopausal women include urinary incontinence and a history of a UTI prior to menopause. *E. coli* is the most common cause; others include *Klebsiella pneumonia, Enterococcus faecalis,* and *Proteus mirabilis.*

TRIAGE

The diagnosis can be confirmed with a urinalysis or urine culture that will identify the pathogen, which will then direct therapy. Women who have had prior UTIs may be able to make a self-diagnosis. Most clinics will empirically treat UTIs and stress the need for increased water intake. UTIs are covered in Chapter 44.

REFERENCES

General

American Academy of Urgent Care Medicine. What is urgent care? http://aaucm.org/about/urgentcare/default.aspx. Published 2017.

Braveheart Group. National Urgent Care Chart Surgery 2010. http://www.jucm.com/pdf/2010%20JUCM%20Urgent%20Care%20Chart%20Research-1.pdf.

More insurers are requiring urgent care center accreditation. *J Urgent Care Med.* Feb. 17, 2017. http://www.jucm.com/insurers-requiring-urgent-care-center-accreditation.

McNeeley S. Urgent care centers: An overview. *Am J Clin Med.* 2012;2(9):80–81.

Rappleye E. 7 key statistics on retail clinics. Integration and physician issues. *Becker's Hosp Rev.* April 23, 2015. https://www.beckershospitalreview.com/hospital-physician-relationships/7-key-statistics-on-retail-clinics.html.

10 Statistics on Urgent Care Centers. *Becker's Hosp Rev.* Feb. 16, 2011. https://www.beckershospitalreview.com/hospital-management-administration/10-statistics-on-urgent-care-centers.html. Accessed 10/23/18.

Urgent Care Association of America. Benchmarking report summary 2016. http://c.ymcdn.com/sites/www.ucaoa.org/resource/resmgr/benchmarking/2016BenchmarkReport.pdf. Accessed January 6, 2018.

Urgent Care Clinics. Industry FAQs. Urgent Care Association of America. http://www.ucaoa.org/general/custom.asp?page=IndustryFAQs. Accessed January 6, 2018.

Cardiovascular Complaints

Kuy S, Juern J, Weigelt JA. Laparoscopic repair of a traumatic intrapericardial diaphragmatic hernia. *JSLS*. 2014;18(2):333–337.

NCD Risk Factor Collaboration. Worldwide trends in blood pressure from 1975 to 2015: A pooled analysis of 1479 population-based measurement studies with 19·1 million participants. *Lancet*. 2017;389(10064):37–55.

Whelton PK, Carey RM, Aronow WS, et al. CC/AHA/AAPA/ABC/ACPM/AGS/APhA/ASH/ASPC/NMA/PCNA guideline for the prevention, detection, evaluation, and management of high blood pressure in adults. Journal of the American College of Cardiology (JACC). Published 2017. http://www.onlinejacc.org/content/early/2017/11/04/j.jacc.2017.11.006. Accessed 10/20/18.

Dermatology Complaints and Wound Care

Quinn, JV, Polevoi SK, Kohn MA. Traumatic lacerations: What are the risks for infection and has the "golden period" of laceration care disappeared? *Emerg Med J*. 2014;31(2):96–100.

Eye/Ear/Nose/Throat Complaints

Abdelazeem M, Gamea A, Mubarak H, Elzawawy N. Epidemiology, causative agents, and risk factors affecting human otomycosis infections. *Turk J Med Sci*. 2015;45(4):820–826.

Centers for Disease Control and Prevention. Adenovirus-associated epidemic keratoconjunctivitis outbreaks. *MMWR Morb Mort Wkly Rep*. 2013;62(32):637–641.

Chow A, Doron, S. Evaluation of acute pharyngitis in adults. UpToDate.com. http://www.uptodate.com/contents/evaluation-of-acute-pharyngitis-in-adults. Published 2017.

Ebell MH, Lundgren J, Youngpairoj S. *Ann Int Med*. 2013;11(1):5–13.

Harris AM, Hicks LA, Qaseem A; High Value Care Task Force of the American College of Physicians and for the Centers for Disease Control and Prevention. Appropriate antibiotic use for acute respiratory tract infection in adults: Advice for high-value care from the American College of Physicians and the Centers for Disease Control and Prevention. *Ann Intern Med*. 2016;164(6):425–434.

Marom R, Roth Y, Boaz M, et al. Acute mastoiditis in children: Necessity and timing of imaging. *Pediatr Infect Dis J*. 2016;35(1):30–34.

Monasta L, Ronfani L, Marchetti F, et al. Burden of disease caused by otitis media: Systematic review and global estimates. *PLoS One*. 2012;7(4):e36226.

Ngo CC, Massa HM, Thornton RB, Cripps AW. Predominant bacteria detected from the middle ear fluid of children experiencing otitis media: A systematic review. *PLoS One*. 2016;11(3):e0150949.

Sambursky, R, Trattler, W, Tauber, S, et al. Sensitivity and specificity of the AdenoPlus test for diagnosing adenoviral conjunctivitis. *JAMA Ophthalmol*. 2013;131(1):17–22.

Saulyte J, Regueira C, Montes-Martínez A, Khudyakov P, Takkouche B. Active or passive exposure to tobacco smoking and allergic rhinitis, allergic dermatitis, and food allergy in adults and children: A systematic review and meta-analysis. *PLoS Med*. 2014;11(3):e1001611.

Smith SS, Ference EH, Evans CT, et al. The prevalence of bacterial infection in acute rhinosinusitis: A systematic review and meta-analysis. *Laryngoscope*. 2015;125(1):57–69.

Gastrointestinal Complaints

Baron EJ, Miller JM, Weinstein MP, et al. A guide to utilization of the microbiology laboratory for diagnosis of infectious diseases: 2013 recommendations by the Infectious Diseases Society of America (IDSA) and the American Society for Microbiology (ASM)(a). *Clin Infect Dis*. 2013;57(4):e22–e121.

El-Serag HB, Sweet S, Winchester CC, et al. Update on the epidemiology of gastro-oesophageal reflux disease: A systematic review. *Gut*. 2014;63(6):871–880.

McCarthy AJ, Lauwers GY, Sheahan K. Iatrogenic pathology of the intestines. *Histopathology*. 2015;66:15–28.

Pinto Sanchez MI, Bercik P. Epidemiology and burden of chronic constipation. *Can J Gastroenterol*. 2011;25(Suppl B):11B–15B.

Genitourinary Complaints

Behzadi P, Behzadi E, Yazdanbod H, et al. A survey on urinary tract infections associated with the three most common uropathogenic bacteria. *Maedica (Buchar)*. 2010;5(2):111–115. https://www.ncbi.nlm.nih.gov/pmc/articles/PMC3150015/

Musculoskeletal Complaints

Pressley JC, Kendig TD, Frencher SK, et al. Epidemiology of bone fracture across the age span in blacks and whites. *J Trauma*. 2011;71(5 suppl 2):S541–548.

Neurological/Psychological Complaints

Gonzalez O, Berry JT. Current depression among adults—United States, 2006 and 2008. *Morb Mortal Wkly Rep*. 2010;59(38):1229–1235.

Hainer BL, Matheson EM. Approach to acute headache in adults. *Am Fam Physician*. 2013;87(10):682–687.

Kessler RC, Petukhova M, Sampson NA, et al. Twelve-month and lifetime prevalence and lifetime morbid risk of anxiety and mood disorders in the United States. *Int J Methods Psychiatr Res*. 2012;21(3):169–184.

Lewis-Fernandez R, Hinton DE, Laria AJ. Culture and the anxiety disorders: Recommendations for *DSM-V*. *Depress Anxiety*. 2010;27:212–229.

Moreno-Peral P, Conejo-Ceron S, Motrico E, et al. Risk factors for the onset of panic and generalised anxiety disorders in the general adult population: A systematic review of cohort studies. *J Affect Disord*. 2014;168:337–348.

National Guideline Clearinghouse. Guideline summary: Final recommendation statement: depression in adults: screening. In: National Guideline Clearinghouse. Rockville, MD: Agency for Healthcare Research and Quality; 2016. https://www.guideline.gov. Accessed November 12, 2017.

U.S. Department of Health and Human Services, Centers for Disease Control and Prevention, National Center for Health Statistics. *Chartbook on long-term trends in health*. May 2017. https://www.cdc.gov/nchs/hus/index.htm. Accessed 10/20/18.

World Health Organization. Headache disorders fact sheet. http://www.who.int/mediacentre/factsheets/fs277/en/. Updated 2016. Accessed November 9, 2017.

Pulmonary Complaints

Campigotto A, Mubareka S. Influenza-associated bacterial pneumonia: Managing and controlling infection on two fronts. *Expert Rev Anti Infect Ther*. 2015;13(1):55–68.

Centor RM, Atkinson TP, Ratliff AE, et al. The clinical presentation of Fusobacterium-positive and streptococcal-positive pharyngitis in a university health clinic: a cross-sectional study. *Ann Intern Med*. 2015;162(4):241–247.

Grohskopf LA, Sokolow LZ, Broder LR, et al. Prevention and control of seasonal influenza with vaccines: Recommendations of the advisory committee on immunization practices—United States, 2017–18 influenza season. *MMWR Recomm Rep*. 2017;66(2):1–20.

Kochanek KD, Sherry MA, Xu J, Tejada-Vera B. Deaths: final data for 2014. *Natl Vital Stat Rep*. June 2016;65(4). **https://www.cdc.gov/nchs/data/nvsr/nvsr65/nvsr65_04.pdf**. Accessed October 31, 2017.

Popescu CP, Florescu SA, Lupulescu E, et al. Neurologic complications of influenza B virus infection in adults, Romania. *Emerg Infect Dis*. 2017;23(4):574–581.

RESOURCE

Which Care Is Right? (Infographic)
  http://c.ymcdn.com/sites/www.ucaoa.org/resource/resmgr/infographics/UCAOA-OnDemandCare-Infograph.pdf

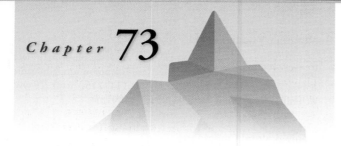

Chapter **73**

Common Injuries

Joe Holbrook, BS, BSN, MS, APRN

Jill E. Winland-Brown, EdD, APRN, FNP-BC

Mae De La Calzada-Jeanlouie, DO, MS

Brian Oscar Porter, MD, PhD, MPH, MBA

WOUNDS AND LACERATIONS

Wounds and lacerations result in a disruption of the continuity of skin commonly related to trauma. The mechanism and energy of the force causing the defect determine the type and severity of the wound. Wounds can range from trivial lacerations or abrasions, which occur daily in children on playgrounds, to more severe injuries such as stabbings or shootings that may require immediate surgical care. All wounds have the potential of becoming infected and should be evaluated for occult injury and retained foreign bodies. Proper evaluation and care will reduce the morbidity associated with wounds.

EPIDEMIOLOGY AND CAUSES

Statistics vary on the number of visits to urgent care and primary-care settings for wounds and lacerations. Because many clinicians do not suture in the office, most individuals seek out urgent care or emergency departments (EDs) where they know they can be treated. Thus, most clinicians will encounter these individuals at some point and need to be cognizant of their care. Adult wounds become infected about 5% of the time, whereas wounds in children become infected 1.2% of the time. Almost 75% of patients with wounds are men with an average age in the early 20s.

It is prudent in any case for the clinician to perform a thorough assessment and maintain complete documentation of wound care. Wound management accounts for a significant percentage of malpractice claims. Although culturing the wound can identify infectious complications and subsequently guide treatment, it is essential that the clinician visually appraise the wound initially for signs of infection to determine whether more invasive action is necessary and for proper antibiotic selection.

PATHOPHYSIOLOGY

The skin is made up of several layers, which are divided into the epidermis and dermis. The skin acts as a barrier to entry into the body, regulates body temperature, aids in the elimination of waste, and helps prevent dehydration. It also contains the cutaneous nerves, is a reservoir for nutritional stores and water, and is a source of vitamin D when exposed to sunlight. The ability of bacteria and other substances to penetrate the skin is related to the depth of the wound. Wounds that do not penetrate the stratum germinativum—the basement layer of the skin—do not leave scars.

The wound healing process involves many processes that occur simultaneously:

- *Injury phase.* This phase involves coagulation and platelet release. This process enhances the inflammatory response in the wound.
- *Inflammatory phase.* This phase is characterized by increased capillary permeability, which allows white

blood cells (WBCs) to migrate into the wound. Neutrophils and monocytes act as scavengers and rid the wound of debris and bacteria. In addition to providing wound defenses, inflammation stimulates other monocytes to promote fibroblast replication and neovascularization.

- *Epithelialization phase.* This phase begins within hours of tissue injury and involves the migration of cells at the wound edges from one side of the incision to the other. Within 24 to 48 hours, incisional wounds are epithelialized. Lacerations may heal by primary intention when the edges of the wound are approximated with sutures and allowed to heal by secondary intention from the inside out as granulation tissue fills in open lacerations whose edges are not approximated. Collagen synthesis in the healing wound peaks at day 7 posttrauma, and the tensile strength (which determines the ability of the wound to remain intact) increases rapidly at this stage. Typically, the wound will have only 15% to 20% of its normal tensile strength at 3 weeks and 60% by 4 months.

- *Remodeling phase.* In this final phase, the process involves wound contraction and tissue formation. This process begins on the third day after the injury and continues for up to 6 months. The appearance of the wound can change during this period; for this reason, plastic surgeons will usually wait 6 months before considering revising a scar.

CLINICAL PRESENTATION

Subjective

A thorough history of the injury must be obtained and documented. The mechanism of wounding is useful in determining the likelihood of deep structure injury, infection risk, extent of tissue damage, and likelihood of associated injuries. Questions regarding medical history should also be included. For example, a patient with diabetes or a history of vascular problems has a higher possibility of infection (see Focus on History: Wounds and Lacerations).

Focus on History: Wounds and Lacerations

History
- Mechanism of injury
- Potential for foreign body
- Potential for injury to underlying (deep) tissues
- Potential for infection
- Type of injury
- Age of wound
- Delayed or immediate presentation
- Tetanus immunization status
- Allergies
- Comorbidities (especially vascular problems)

Physical Examination
- Vital signs
- General examination
- Vascular injury
- Nerve involvement
- Located over joint
- Tendon damage
- Associated with fracture (open or closed)
- Range of motion
- Wound contamination
- Foreign body
- Avulsion injury
- Puncture

Objective

A description of any wound should include the length and depth (in centimeters) and the type of defect found. The depth of the wound is described as *partial thickness* if all layers of the skin have not been violated. If any subdermal tissue can be seen in the wound, it is considered a *full-thickness* defect. Wounds this deep may involve injuries to deeper structures, and further evaluation is necessary.

Different types of wounds are associated with specific types of associated injuries and special considerations. Refer to Advanced Assessment 73.1 for various types of wounds and special considerations associated with their assessment and treatment. See Therapeutic Procedure 73.1 for step-by step instructions for abscess drainage.

Any extremity that has sustained a wound injury should be evaluated for distal circulation and sensation. Circulation should be assessed by determining if the distal extremity has a strong pulse. For fingers or toes, the clinician should assess blanching and capillary refill time (normal is less than 2 seconds). Distal sensation should be checked to rule out nerve injury. A gross neurological screening examination comparing sensation on bilateral extremities should be done on all patients who present with wounds to the extremities.

All wounds must be explored to identify any deep structure injuries or foreign bodies and to help determine the type of closure required. After the wound is anesthetized, a bright light should be used to illuminate the wound. Wound edges should be retracted, but it is important not to cause trauma to the tissue that may impede normal healing. Blindly probing a wound can cause additional tissue destruction or nerve or vascular injury. Using an Adson forceps with teeth or tissue retractors, the clinician should hook the wound edge and retract it to expose deep structures. The clinician should probe the wound with gloved fingers only.

For large wounds, it is important to examine the full length of the wound because only a small section of the wound may be deep enough to cause deep structure injury. The defect should be examined for any tendon injury.

Advanced Assessment 73.1: Wounds and Lacerations

Type	Special Considerations
ABRASION	
A partial-thickness defect to the skin, usually associated with an abrasive force being applied to the skin.	• Ensure that the wound is thoroughly cleansed (this may require anesthesia). For cleansing larger areas of abrasion, consider using topical viscous lidocaine for analgesia. However, use caution with children because the amount of medication applied to large wounds may cause lidocaine toxicity. Allow 10–15 minutes after administration of lidocaine for sufficient absorption. • Remove all embedded dirt because it can lead to "tattooing" of the skin. Tattooing can occur when the skin has healed and the epidermis has grown over the embedded dirt, which is visible through the thin epidermis layer of skin. • Examine the entire area of the wound. Look for any deep lacerations, which may be hard to find because of the size of the wound. Any deep lacerations within an abrasion must be closed with sutures after thorough exploration, debridement, and irrigation. The goal of closure is to loosely approximate the edges. If the wound is deep, use a subcutaneous suture to allow the wound to heal without having to disturb the granulation tissue to remove the stitches later.
STELLATE OR FLAP LACERATION	
When the defect in the skin involves a flap or stellate defect; this usually occurs with a ripping mechanism or blunt trauma to a bony structure such as the skull.	• During exploration, fully retract the flap to allow for visualization to the base of the defect. Typically, this is the deepest part of the laceration. It is important to examine the area under the flap carefully for possible injuries to deeper structures. • Scalp lacerations should be explored for galea injury. The galea is a fibrous fascia that covers the skull. If the galea has a large defect (more than 3 cm), it should be closed with deep sutures. • If a flap laceration has a nonviable portion, it should be excised. When closing these types of defects, the first suture should bring all the sections of the flap or star together. Following the initial stitch, closure of the remaining defect can be accomplished using normal interrupted sutures.
LINEAR LACERATION	
Single linear or near-linear defect in the skin; usually caused by a sharp instrument.	• Thorough wound exploration is required to ascertain deep structure involvement. If tendons are involved, orthopedic consultation is recommended. • If muscular fascia is violated, such defects must be closed with deep sutures. If these wounds are not repaired, the possibility of muscular herniation is increased. • If a joint is violated, an orthopedic consultation is highly recommended. Depending on the mechanism of injury and how dirty or contaminated the wound is, surgical exploration and irrigation may be necessary. • Wounds in regions with low cosmetic significance, such as the scalp, can be closed using staples, which are faster and easier to place and remove than conventional sutures. Staples have a lower tissue inflammatory response and are well tolerated. Staples must be removed with special instruments, however, so follow-up must be considered when the decision regarding type of wound closure is made. • Wounds with low tension that do not cross a joint can be closed using tissue adhesive. This eliminates the need for suture removal and has been found to have similar or better cosmetic results than stitches. Using tissue adhesive to close wounds is much faster and decreases the amount of pain associated with wound closure. Before closing the wound, it is important to make sure that the wound has been thoroughly explored and cleaned. This may require infiltration with local anesthesia. Tissue adhesive can be used over wounds that have had subcutaneous sutures placed. Tissue adhesive can also be used to hold fingernails and toenails in place after nailbed repair. • Wounds under high tension must be closed with subcutaneous stitches or mattress sutures to reduce the tension on the skin edge. High-tension wounds will produce a larger scar and have a higher risk of dehiscence. To avoid this, sutures should remain in place longer in these types of wounds.

Advanced Assessment 73.1: Wounds and Lacerations—cont'd

Type	Special Considerations
BITE WOUNDS	
A defect caused by a high-pressure bite force, such as from a dog or human.	• These wounds have diminished vascularization related to tissue disruption and swelling. Debriding devitalized tissue is necessary to decrease bacterial load and eliminate that potential nidus of infection. • The clinician should consider whether delayed primary closure (tertiary intention) or allowing the wound to heal by secondary intention (filling of the defect by granulation tissue without approximation of the wound edges) is appropriate. • Given the source of the injury, antibiotic prophylaxis may be of benefit to the patient. • The need for tetanus vaccine (including booster shot) should be explored.
TENDON INJURY	
A force applied that is great enough to cause a disruption to a tendon; this could be from penetrating or blunt force trauma.	• All wounds near tendons must be explored for possible tendon injuries. If tendon damage is found, consultation with an orthopedist is recommended. • Extensor tendon injuries may be closed by the clinician. Early antibiotic prophylaxis is indicated. • Flexor tendon injuries usually require primary wound closure by an orthopedic specialist. There is a high morbidity associated with flexor tendon injuries. Early antibiotic prophylaxis is indicated.
JOINT VIOLATION	
A force, usually applied by a sharp, penetrating injury, that disrupts the joint capsule.	• All wounds near joints must be explored for potential violations of the joint capsule. If any such injury is found, consultation with an orthopedist is recommended. • If the wound is near a joint and a violation of the joint capsule cannot be ruled out, a saline-load test can be used to assess whether penetration of the capsule has occurred, although such tests may not have high sensitivity. In this test, sterile normal saline is injected directly into the joint space in a sufficient volume to assess for leakage, e.g., 150–200 mL for the knee joint. • If the metacarpophalangeal (MCP) joint is injured and any possibility of an injury from a bite (open mouth) exists, immediate follow-up by an orthopedist is needed. The area should be surgically irrigated to avoid joint morbidity.
CELLULITIS	
An infection of deeper tissue, usually caused by a defect in the integrity of the skin that was inoculated by bacteria. The infection usually involves *Staphylococcus aureus* and/ or *Streptococcus*.	• See Chapter 14 for more in-depth information. Mild cellulitis should be treated with an oral course of a first or second-generation cephalosporin. The patient should return for a wound check within 24–48 hours, depending on the extent of cellulitis, to determine if the antibiotic therapy is effective. The region of erythema should be outlined with a tissue marker on initial examination; this demarcation can be used to assess treatment effectiveness or failure if the erythema continues to increase. Wounds that exhibit fluctuance (palpable fluid under the skin) should be incised and drained to reduce the tension on the wound and decrease the bacterial load (see Therapeutic Procedure 73.1). • Patients with diabetes or other conditions that may involve vascular compromise need to be treated more aggressively. Treat the initial findings of cellulitis or wounds that appear dirty or contaminated with parenteral antibiotics and place the patient on oral antibiotics. Close follow-up is required, and these patients may need to be seen daily in the office, depending on the extent of cellulitis. • Patients who present with cellulitis should receive a thorough history and physical examination to determine the possible mechanism of injury. All hand and foot wounds that become infected should undergo x-ray to rule out foreign bodies. In addition, any wound that has a high potential of containing a foreign body should undergo x-ray. • Patients with wound infections involving angioedema or accompanied by fever or chills should receive parenteral antibiotics. Inpatient treatment should be considered for these patients.
ABSCESS	
A complication of a contaminated penetrating wound in which localized infection is walled-off, resulting in pus accumulation in a swollen and fluctuant pocket underneath the skin.	• Abscesses usually occur after the epithelium has been compromised. Patients with abscesses usually present with the complaint of a boil or spider bite. They often begin with superficial cellulitis, presenting with a localized area of erythematous, warm, tender, and fluctuant tissue. The most common pathogen is *Staphylococcus aureus*, especially methicillin resistant *S. aureus* (MRSA). Without proper pus evacuation via incision and drainage, the accumulated bacterial load can lead to disseminated or systemic infection and infection is unlikely to clear (see Therapeutic Procedure 73.1 Abscess Drainage).

Therapeutic Procedure 73.1: Abscess Drainage

1. **Protective Equipment**—Use gloves, gown, and face shield.
2. **Cleanse**—Clean with alcohol, betadine, or chlorhexidine.
3. **Analgesia and Anesthesia**—Before incision and drainage (I & D), the patient may be given by mouth or parental analgesics, and the site should be injected with a local anesthetic (e.g., lidocaine) in the roof of the abscess and around the circumference of the abscess. Injecting in the cavity may increase pain/pressure and is unlikely to anesthetize the surrounding tissue. Post I & D pain management with ibuprofen and acetaminophen is usually sufficient.
4. **Incision**—A linear incision should be made two-thirds to the full length of the area of fluctuance deep enough to enter the cavity. For small abscess, large-bore needle puncture and aspiration may be attempted. However, this is often not effective and requires repeat drainage if the infection exacerbates.
5. **Drainage**—After the initial spontaneous pus drainage, surrounding fluctuant areas may be compressed to produce additional fluid. Hemostats may be placed in the wound and opened at multiple directions within the cavity to break up all loculated compartments.
6. **Culture** of abscess fluid may be sent.
7. **Packing**—Some recent literature shows little or no utility with packing the wound. However, many clinicians continue to pack large open wounds. If packing is chosen, it should be done loosely with a continuous gauze strip, with approximately 2 cm of the packing extruding from the wound to prevent foreign body retention.
8. **Dressing**—The wound should be dressed with an appropriate dressing to cover the wound and absorb drainage.
9. **Antibiotics**—I & D alone is often sufficient intervention to facilitate healing and is required to overcome localized infection. Antibiotics are indicated for areas difficult to drain, poor response to I & D alone, septic phlebitis, extremes of age, immunosuppression, complicating co-existing conditions, rapid progression with cellulitis, fever, and severe or extensive disease (e.g., multiple sites, recurrences). Treatment should be directed toward treating MRSA infections with antibiotics such as trimethoprim-sulfamethoxazole (Bactrim), clindamycin (Cleocin), or doxycycline (see Evidence-Based Nursing Practice 73.1).
10. **Follow-up Care**—Patients should be instructed to change dressings daily or as needed due to saturation. The patient may apply warm compresses or soak the abscess in warm water to assist with drainage. A follow-up visit should be scheduled in 1 to 3 days for reassessment and removal or replacement of packing if indicated. The patient should be instructed to return to their primary-care practitioner or an ED if signs or symptoms of infection occur (e.g., erythema, pain, fever, swelling, myalgia, or vomiting).

Evidence-Based Nursing Practice 73.1

Daum RS, Miller LG, Immergluck L, et al. A placebo-controlled trial of antibiotics for smaller skin abscesses. *N Engl J Med.* 2017;376:2545–2555.

A multicenter, prospective, double-blind trial was conducted involving 786 participants with uncomplicated skin abscesses. *Staphylococcal aureus* was isolated from 527 participants and methicillin-resistant *Staphylococcal aureus* (MRSA) was isolated from 388 patients. Ten days after therapy with either clindamycin, trimethoprim-sulfamethoxazole (TMP-SMX) or placebo, the cure rate among patients in the clindamycin group was similar to that in the TMP-SMX group, and the cure rate in each active-treatment group was higher than that in the placebo group. Among the patients initially cured, new infections at 1 month of follow-up were less common in the clindamycin group than in the TMP-SMX group or placebo group, although more adverse events were in the clindamycin group. They concluded that when compared with incision and drainage alone, clindamycin or TMP-SMX in conjunction with incision and drainage improved short-term outcomes in patients with a simple abscess.

Exposed tendon will appear as a shiny white structure in the wound. The range of motion of the affected extremity or digit should be tested carefully against resistance in all planes in which the extremity can be moved. Pain during movement can indicate a partial tendon laceration.

Examination for injuries to underlying muscular fascia is required. If a large defect is found, the fascia must be closed to prevent herniation of the muscle in the future. If the wound is near a joint, violation of the joint capsule must be ruled out. The joint capsule is lined with a synovial membrane and contains synovial fluid, which lubricates the joint and also provides cushioning for the joint. If the synovial capsule is violated, the joint may become seeded (contaminated) with bacteria, in which case the possibility of developing a septic joint is likely.

The joint capsule is a shiny white structure; if it has been penetrated, bone ends are palpable and can be visualized. Again, the joint must be examined through the full range of motion to look for a defect. If a joint violation is suspected but cannot be confirmed by visualization, the clinician should order an x-ray of the joint, which may show air in the affected joint. Although specific for a penetrating joint injury, this is a rare finding and should not be relied on to rule out a joint violation.

A *saline-load test* can be performed to accurately determine if a joint violation has occurred. The practitioner should (using sterile technique) inject sterile saline in the joint, in a place away from the defect, and assess whether any saline escapes through the wound. The amount of saline to be injected is dictated by the size of the joint (e.g., 150–200 mL for the knee joint). Findings are considered negative when the saline injection causes distention of the joint without evidence of leakage or, in a conscious patient, distends the joint capsule to the point of discomfort.

DIAGNOSTIC REASONING

Diagnostic Tests

X-rays should be taken of wounds that may be associated with a bony abnormality or that raise suspicion of a retained foreign body. Wounds that may have a retained foreign body should be assessed before administration of anesthesia by palpating over the defect and margin of the wound to determine whether the patient can feel a foreign body in the wound. This sensation should be documented. X-ray studies can help to rule out foreign bodies, even fragments of glass of 1 mm in size. As an alternate imaging modality, the clinician may consider ultrasound to rule out radiopaque or radiolucent foreign bodies.

The presence of a fracture near the wound defect must be treated as an open fracture. Treatment requires consultation with an orthopedic surgeon and close follow-up. Depending on the type of wound and its size and location, surgical irrigation and closure may be necessary. Prompt antibiotic prophylaxis is indicated, within 2 to 3 hours of injury if possible, to prevent infection and osteomyelitis.

There is no indication for laboratory studies in the initial treatment of wounds and lacerations. One caveat is that if the patient is taking anticoagulants and the wound is bleeding profusely, the clinician should consider checking prothrombin time (PT) and international normalized ratio. A complete blood count (CBC) is indicated if the clinician suspects excessive blood loss. If the patient presents with cellulitis or if an abscess develops, a wound culture is indicated.

Differential Diagnosis

The aim of the differential diagnosis of otherwise clinically apparent wounds and lacerations is to determine the nature (type of wound, e.g., crush injury, trauma from a blunt or sharp object; presence of contamination or infection) and extent (e.g., depth, degree of damage to underlying structures) of the injury, as well as the underlying cause, which will inform short-term and long-term therapy. While the patient and individuals accompanying the patient to the care provider may readily provide a plausible history for the injury, the astute clinician must always consider other mechanisms of injury that may not be disclosed (e.g., domestic violence or other forms of physical or sexual abuse). Regardless of cause, however, the presentation of intentional or accidental injuries may provide an opportunity for patient education or other type of intervention that will minimize the risk of repeat injury in the future.

MANAGEMENT

A simple wound or laceration may be treated in the outpatient clinic. A patient with a large wound—especially one that needs major debridement or appears to be infected—should be referred to the ED. All patients with wounds should be asked about prior tetanus immunization. If more than 5 years have elapsed, a tetanus booster should be administered.

Wound Cleansing

After a thorough history and physical examination, all acute wounds must be cleansed. The most effective way to decrease the bacterial count in a wound is through irrigation with a high-pressure stream of solution aimed directly into the wound. Irrigation with a syringe and needle/catheter is more effective than bulb syringe irrigation for laceration cleansing and irrigation. Although traditionally most providers use normal saline, potable tap water is equivalent and may be superior to normal saline for laceration cleansing and irrigation. The amount of solution needed is dictated by the size and level of contamination of the wound. A good rule of thumb is to infuse 50 to 100 mL of solution per centimeter of wound length.

Saline irrigation or even soapy water is preferred to a dilute povidone-iodine (Betadine) solution, because povidone-iodine can be irritating and cytotoxic to lacerated tissue. The clinician should avoid hydrogen peroxide (H_2O_2), because it can be irritating to the wound. Scrubbing, if employed, needs to be done gently to ensure that the mechanical force applied does not cause additional tissue damage. Scrubbing with an ionic polymer solution such as Shur Cleanse may also be done, as it has been shown to loosen debris and remove superficial foreign bodies.

Wound Debridement

The wound needs to be debrided of devitalized tissue. Devitalized tissue is any tissue that is devascularized or extremely macerated. This type of tissue is a nidus for bacterial growth and disrupts tissue defenses. Debridement should be done using a sharp scalpel or scissors so that the debrided edge will be clean and sharp. Using a sharp instrument will cause less tissue trauma and vascular damage at the wound margin. It is important to remove only devitalized tissue. A wound with jagged edges should not be debrided unless the edges are devitalized tissue. Jagged wound margins give the clinician landmarks to use when closing the defect. The jagged edges also increase the surface area of the wound edge and decrease the amount of tension on the wound margin, which can decrease the size of the scar.

Wound Closure

Wound closure is done to reduce the size of scarring and decrease the risk of infection or other morbidity. The closure technique used is dictated by the type of wound. Depending on the size and location of the wound, the clinician should consider using sutures, staples, adhesive strips (Steri-Strips), or 2-octylcyanoacrylate tissue adhesives, such as Dermabond.

2-Octylcyanoacrylate tissue adhesives can be utilized for superficial lacerations less than 6 cm in length and in low-tension areas. They should not be used over a joint or on any grossly contaminated wounds. Caution should be exercised when repairing wounds near the eye because the adhesive is very fluid and can run into the eye, essentially gluing it shut. If this happens, the clinician must apply an antibiotic eye ointment to aid in slowly dissolving the adhesive. If it cannot be removed for an eye examination, the patient should see an ophthalmologist immediately.

For 2-octylcyanoacrylate tissue adhesive application, the skin must be clean and dry. The wound is approximated with sterile fingers or tissue forceps, taking care not to injure the tissue with the forceps. Once the wound is well approximated, with the fingers at least 1 cm away, the adhesive is applied in concentric circles, allowing 15 seconds in between applications. The patient should be advised not to scrub the adhesive and not to apply any antibiotic ointment to the wound, because this can dissolve the adhesive. Adhesive tape should also not be placed directly over the site.

Another application for cyanoacrylate tissue adhesive is in the repair of skin tears. Once the skin tear has been cleansed, the torn skin should be unfurled, which is teasing the curled-up pieces of skin back to their previous locations. Under no circumstances should the clinician cut the torn skin off because it can be used as an allograft. Then the cyanoacrylate adhesive can be applied with excellent results. This tissue adhesive also serves as a barrier against common bacterial microbes.

To decrease tension in high-tension areas, subcutaneous stitches will be helpful. To avoid obvious scars and poor cosmetic results, landmarks must be meticulously aligned and skin layers placed in the correct alignment, with the first suture being placed in the center of the wound. Suturing techniques are illustrated in Therapeutic Procedure 73.2. Scarring will be minimized if the following adage is followed: "approximate, don't strangulate."

Wound Dressings

The wound should be kept clean, dry, and covered. For sites that are difficult to keep bandaged, a thin layer of antibiotic ointment should be applied to protect the wound. Bandages should be changed daily or if they become wet or dirty. It is helpful to apply antibiotic ointment to the wound when the dressing is changed.

Antibiotic Therapy

Antibiotic prophylaxis for most wounds is not indicated. The risk of infection of a clean, recently injured wound in a well-vascularized area is low (only 3% to 5%). Grossly contaminated wounds or wounds that involve areas of diminished vascular supply, such as the fingers, toes, and ears, may benefit from prophylactic antibiotics. Wounds that have an increased risk of infection include the following:

- Crush injuries
- Dirty wounds
- Jagged wounds
- Wounds with devitalized tissue
- Wounds that are more than 12 to 19 hours old
- Bite wounds, especially from humans (particularly if they are meat eaters), cats, and dogs
- Wounds with retained foreign bodies
- Wounds closed with subcutaneous stitches

Patients with diabetes mellitus or who have a history of vascular compromise should be started on antibiotics prophylactically. Parenteral administration of ampicillin/sulbactam, cephalexin, or ceftriaxone is the initial treatment of choice. This should be followed by oral therapy with amoxicillin/clavulanate, cephalexin, or cefadroxil. If the patient has allergies to penicillin or cephalosporins, the clinician should consider prescribing doxycycline, with or without clindamycin, or ciprofloxacin.

When treating cellulitis or established infections, the clinician should consider initial parenteral therapy with ampicillin/sulbactam, cefoxitin, cephalexin, or ceftriaxone. The clinician should consider wound cultures before starting antibiotics for grossly infected wounds. If the patient has allergies to penicillin and cephalosporins, the clinician should consider using doxycycline, clindamycin, or ciprofloxacin. All parenteral therapy should be followed with oral antibiotic therapy for 7 to 10 days. Appropriate choices for oral therapy include cephalexin or cefadroxil for most infections. Wounds with a high risk of infection with anaerobic bacteria (i.e., wounds contaminated by mucus or feces) need to have broader antibiotic coverage with clindamycin or amoxicillin-clavulanate. See Evidence-Based Nursing Practice 73.1 for information about prescribing antibiotics for abscesses.

Severe infections require inpatient IV therapy. Outlining the area of erythema with a tissue marker during

Therapeutic Procedure 73.2: Suturing Techniques/Materials

SUTURE TECHNIQUE	ADVANTAGES	DISADVANTAGES
Buried suture	Allows good approximation of wound edges.	Minimal eversion occurs.
Running continuous suture	Quick, good for children; evenly distributed tension.	Entire suture must be removed.
Interrupted suture	Permits precise adjustments between sutures; allows selection of sutures.	Increased risk of uneven tension over the suture line; higher incidence of "railroad track" scarring.

Continued

Therapeutic Procedure 73.2: Suturing Techniques/Materials—cont'd

SUTURE TECHNIQUE	ADVANTAGES	DISADVANTAGES
Wound-closure strips	Minimal wound trauma; more resistant to wound infection.	Poor wound eversion; more difficult wound edge approximation.

SUTURE MATERIALS	CLINICAL CONSIDERATIONS
Nonabsorbable	
Silk	Not recommended due to frequent tissue reaction
Nylon	Most common
Polypropylene	Best for subcuticular and continuous suturing Easiest to remove
Absorbable (metabolized after ~3 weeks—used in inner tissues)	
Synthetic polymers	For deep layers Absorbed by hydrolysis (not used for skin)
Surgical catgut	Dissolves in an unpredictable time-frame Excites tissue reaction during its destruction
Tissue Adhesives	
	"Glue"-type adhesive of *n*-butyl 2-cyanoacrylate monomer is used in combination with or as an alternative to sutures for wound closure

SUTURE SIZE	USES
From smallest to largest size: 10/0—9/0—8/0—7/0—6/0—5/0—4/0—3/0—2/0—0—1—2—3—4—5—6—7—8—9—10 6/0 is thinner than a human hair; used for delicate suturing (e.g., eye surgery); family practice clinicians primarily use 3/0 and 4/0.	
Fine sizes	Plastic surgery Ophthalmic surgery Pediatric surgery Vascular surgery
Medium sizes	All other kinds of surgery
Heavy sizes	Retention Anchoring bone

Source: Colyar MR, Ehrhardt CR. *Ambulatory care procedures for the nurse practitioner*. Philadelphia, PA: FA Davis; 2004. Used with permission.

the initial visit will allow subsequent practitioners to assess treatment response more easily. Any extremity or digit that is infected should be immobilized to reduce the inflammatory response related to mechanical movement of the affected region. Close follow-up is important for the first 8 to 24 hours after therapy has been started. If the infection appears to be responding to therapy, the patient should continue oral therapy, with additional follow-up as indicated by the extent of the injury and infection.

FOLLOW-UP AND REFERRAL

Following the initiation of outpatient therapy, patients with high-risk wounds should be instructed to follow-up with the clinician who treated the wound or another provider in 1 to 2 days so that the wound can be evaluated for healing and signs of infection. Home health-care nursing is an effective mode of wound care follow-up in the outpatient setting.

Sutures must remain in place long enough to allow adequate tensile strength to develop during the healing process. The amount of time before suture removal varies with the location of the wound and the cosmetic importance of the wound site. Sutures that are left in too long can cause scarring, and the healing tissue can cover the sutures if left in too long; however, sutures over joints or areas of high skin tension must remain in place longer. If staples are used, follow-up will need to be with a clinician equipped with the appropriate staple removal equipment.

The following timeframes are recommended for the removal of sutures at various bodily sites:

- Face: 4 to 6 days; after suture removal, reinforce wound closure with adhesive strips (Steri-Strips)
- Scalp: 6 to 10 days
- Trunk: 7 to 10 days
- Arms: 10 to 14 days
- Legs: 10 to 14 days
- Joints: 14 days

Patient Education: Wounds and Lacerations

The patient may shower 12 to 24 hours after the initial wound repair. Wound healing processes form a protective barrier that will prevent bacterial invasion after as little as 8 hours. The wound should not be submerged in water, however, until after suture removal or scar formation. Aloe vera may provide mild pain relief, but it does not improve wound healing or reduce the risk of wound infection. Patients should be advised that taking ibuprofen (Motrin) or another NSAID will serve the same function.

Patients should monitor for signs of infection, including redness surrounding the wound area (cellulitis), red streaks extending from the wound (angioedema), and any purulent discharge from the wound (wound infection). Other secondary signs of infection include worsening pain, fever, and chills. Patients with high-risk wounds should understand the importance of follow-up in 1 to 2 days to evaluate for appropriate healing or signs of infection. Topical vitamin E preparations should be avoided because it is a weak steroid that can delay healing and cause dehiscence of high-tension wounds. Oral intake of vitamin E during the healing process is beneficial, however, although a well-balanced diet will provide a sufficient amount. Box 73.1 presents discharge instructions for patients with wounds and lacerations.

Box 73.1 Discharge Instructions: Wounds and Lacerations

- Keep the injured extremity elevated above the level of the heart if possible.
- Cleanse the wound daily with warm, soapy water. Gently remove debris and any scab that is present.
- Lacerations over joints should be immobilized until the sutures are removed to prevent further injury from mechanical irritation.
- For lower extremities, the patient should be advised to do isometric exercises to prevent a deep vein thrombosis while wearing a splint.
- Watch for signs of infection: redness, warmth, increased pain, swelling, fever, red streaks progressing up the extremity, any purulent discharge (pus) from the wound.
- Check wound as needed for any signs of infection—up every 24 hours for high-risk wounds.

ANIMAL AND HUMAN BITES

An animal bite is a bite wound to humans from dogs, cats, or other animals, including other humans. In most cases, bites result in puncture wounds, possible lacerations, and, in some cases, crush injuries. All bites, regardless of the source, are considered to be contaminated wounds and have a substantial risk for infection.

EPIDEMIOLOGY AND CAUSES

Millions of animal bites occur annually in the United States. Of these bites, 80% result in only minor injury, but 1% to 2% of these wounds result in hospitalization. Bite wounds occur in all age-groups but are most common in children. Animal bites cause more than 30 deaths annually in the United States and involve mostly infants and small children.

Dogs inflict 60% to 90% of mammalian bites, with an overall infection rate of 15% to 20%. Risks of infection from dog bites are greatest for puncture wounds, crush injuries, and bites to the hand. Dog bites in general have a 5% infection rate, but dog bites to the hand carry a 40% infection rate. The most common infectious organisms isolated from dog bites are *Staphylococcus aureus*, *Pasteurella multocida*, *Corynebacterium* species, and α-hemolytic *Streptococcus* species. One-half of all dog bite victims are children younger than 12 years of age. The majority of dog bite wounds are from a domestic pet known to the victim, with pit bulls being responsible for the most human deaths related to dog bites each year, followed by Rottweilers and Huskies.

Cats inflict 5% to 20% of mammalian bites. Their needle-like teeth result in puncture wounds with a high incidence of infection—around 50%. Specifically, cat bites are more common in women, although, in general, men receive more animal bite injuries than women. In more than 50% of cat bite wounds, *P. multocida* is isolated; this bacterium causes wound infections that develop within 24 hours of the bite, resulting in an intense inflammatory response and joint infection.

The third most common type of mammalian bites is those from other human beings. These bites account for 2% to 3% of all animal bites reported. Human bite injuries received during fistfights are common in teenagers and in alcohol-intoxicated men aged 30 to 35 years. Accidental human bites occur most commonly in children. Common infectious agents isolated from human bite wounds include *S. aureus, Streptococcus, Corynebacterium* species, *Bacteroides* species, and *Eikenella corrodens*.

Two percent of reported animal bites are from rodents. Some sick or injured wild animals—such as squirrels, skunks, and bats—will attack humans without provocation and may carry rabies caused by rhabdovirus. Clinicians should be familiar with state laws and regulations regarding bite wounds from mammals and rabies prophylaxis, especially in areas where rabies infection is endemic.

PATHOPHYSIOLOGY

The risk of bite wound infection depends on the wound location, tissue damage, patient characteristics, time elapsed before treatment, and the type of animal that inflicted the bite. Wounds should be classified as low risk or high risk to facilitate decision-making regarding antibiotic therapy and wound suturing. *Low-risk wounds* include lacerations involving the extremities, face, and body. Wounds at low risk for infection include bites on the face, ears, scalp, and mouth. Large, clean lacerations and bites by rodents are at low risk for infection. *High-risk wounds* include those in the distal extremities (hand, wrist, or foot), the scalp of an infant, a wound over a joint, or a penetrating wound of the cheek. Puncture wounds and nondebridable crush injuries are of high risk. Patients at high risk for infection are those older than age 50 years and individuals with prosthetic joints or heart valves, asplenia, chronic alcoholism, diabetes mellitus, altered immune status, or peripheral vascular disease, and patients who are on chronic corticosteroid therapy. Bites from domestic cats, large cats, primates, pigs, or humans (especially hand wounds) present the highest risk of infection.

Human bites in locations other than the hand have no greater risk of infection than a dog bite, if treated promptly. Most human bites are sustained in fights, but 15% to 20% of bites reported in one study were secondary to "love nips" (related to sexual activity). A closed-fist injury ("fight bite") occurs from a laceration over the metacarpophalangeal (MCP) joint caused by striking an opponent's tooth. When this occurs, infectious organisms

from the mouth are inoculated directly into the bone or joint, which can lead to septic arthritis or osteomyelitis. Also, when the fingers of the closed fist are extended, the injured extensor tendons retract proximally, sealing off the tissues. This sets the stage for a rapidly progressive infection of the tendon and adjacent tissue layers.

CLINICAL PRESENTATION

Subjective

The circumstances of the bite injury should be determined. These include the area(s) of the body injured, time elapsed since the injury, type of animal (including breed), current location of the animal, relationship of the animal to the victim, vaccination and health status of the animal, and whether the attack was provoked or unprovoked. The patient should be asked about his or her occupation, medical history and comorbid conditions, medication allergies, tetanus immunization status, any history of immunological compromise, and any specific musculoskeletal, neurological, or vascular complaints resulting from the bite. If the bite is on the patient's hand, the clinician should ask the patient which is the patient's dominant hand.

Objective

More than 70% of bite wounds are located on the extremities where the victim either handled or attempted to avoid the animal or another person. Injuries to the head and neck are the next most common bite wounds and are seen mostly in children. The clinician should inspect the skin and soft tissues, noting the presence or absence of lacerations, punctures, scratches, abrasions, swelling, crush injuries, and/or devitalized tissue. All puncture wounds should be examined carefully for injury to structures beneath the skin. A vascular examination should be performed, noting skin temperature, capillary refill time, and relevant pulses. The range of motion of all affected areas should be assessed, evaluating the functional status of potentially involved tendons. Motor and sensory nerve function should also be evaluated. To assess sensory function of the hand, the clinician should note sensation to light touch and two-point discrimination on the volar pads of the fingertips. The patient should be able to detect stimuli less than 5 mm apart in the axis of the digit, and the response should be compared with the uninjured side. The patient should be evaluated for skeletal injury and carefully assessed for neurovascular, joint, tendon, or osseous injury.

If the patient does not present with the bite wound until several hours to several days following the injury, the clinician should perform a careful search for evidence of local or systemic infection and regional adenopathy. Infection will be evidenced by increased pain, swelling, erythema, warmth, decreased range of motion at joints, or drainage from a puncture-wound site. A high index of suspicion should always be maintained for the possibility of a retained foreign body in the wound, especially when an infection develops at a puncture wound site.

DIAGNOSTIC REASONING

Diagnostic Tests

A radiograph of the affected area should be obtained if a fracture is suspected; a foreign body is present (e.g., tooth fragments, which are more common in bites from older animals); a bone, joint, or tendon has been penetrated; or a puncture wound has become infected. If the patient presents with a localized wound infection several hours or days after the bite, the clinician should obtain a site Gram stain and both aerobic and anaerobic cultures, after superficial decontamination of the wound but before debridement of devitalized tissues. Cultures of wounds are also indicated in cases in which an immunocompromised patient is infected, where there is sepsis, or when antibiotic therapy has failed. To obtain optimal wound cultures, the clinician should perform percutaneous or deep wound aspiration. If significant blood loss has occurred, it is important to obtain a CBC to assess for anemia.

If the patient is seriously ill with a bite wound infection, diagnostic tests should include a thorough laboratory evaluation (including a CBC with platelets, serum electrolyte panel, glucose level, blood urea nitrogen (BUN) and creatinine, and PT/partial thromboplastin time), at least two blood cultures, wound-site Gram stain and culture, and appropriate x-ray studies.

Differential Diagnosis

The diagnosis of animal bites is typically straightforward to determine by history, although the etiology of some bite wounds may be unclear in infants, young children, or incapacitated adults who cannot communicate the source of the bite. To properly direct management, it is critical that the animal source and extent (e.g., depth, affected structures) of the bite wound be characterized as thoroughly as possible.

MANAGEMENT

Analgesia

Pain management is commonly provided with analgesic agents such as NSAIDs and acetaminophen (Tylenol). If nonnarcotic oral agents are ineffective and the patient is in severe pain, ketorolac (Toradol) 30 to 60 mg may be effective.

Wound Cleansing

Bites and scratches should be cleansed with mild soap and water or 1% povidone-iodine (Betadine) solution to remove the animal's saliva from the wound, as well as any particulate matter. If the bite was caused by a potentially rabid wild animal (e.g., skunk, raccoon), the clinician, wearing protective gloves, should thoroughly irrigate the wound with 1% benzalkonium chloride, which has demonstrated effectiveness in inactivating the rabies virus.

Local Anesthesia

Using a 25-gauge or smaller needle, the clinician should infiltrate the wound edges with 1% lidocaine (without epinephrine) before closure if indicated. The maximum dose of lidocaine for local infiltration is 4 mg/kg (0.4 mL/kg of a 1% solution).

Wound Irrigation

The wound should be irrigated with 500 to 2,000 mL of normal saline. For wounds considered to be at high risk for infection, the clinician can use a 1% povidone-iodine (Betadine) solution. For irrigation, a 30 mL syringe with an 18- to 20-gauge plastic catheter should be used to achieve an irrigation pressure of 5 to 8 psi. This method of irrigation has been shown to reduce wound infection.

Wound Debridement

The clinician should remove foreign material, devitalized tissue, and eschar from the wound. The margins of puncture wounds should be debrided to approximately a 1- to 2-mm rim to allow for better drainage and improved cleaning.

Wound Closure

Approximately 10% of bite wounds require suturing and follow-up care. Fresh facial bites without signs of inflammation should be closed with sutures after thorough wound cleansing and preparation. Bite wounds of the hand should not be sutured. For bites to other areas in need of closure or bites greater than 24 hours old, delayed primary closure may be considered. A layer of fine-mesh gauze can be applied to the wound, which should be packed open, dressed, and followed closely. If there is no purulence or erythema of the wound margins at a 3- to 5-day clinic follow-up, wound closure may be performed.

Tetanus Immunization

Bite wounds are tetanus-prone injuries. If the patient has received a primary immunization series but not a booster within the past 5 years, a tetanus booster should be administered. For patients with absent or incomplete primary immunization, 250 units of tetanus immune globulin should be given in addition to the primary vaccination.

Antimicrobial Therapy

Patients should receive antibiotic prophylaxis for 3 to 5 days if the wound is a fresh bite wound; they were bitten by a cat; have a hand bite; have moderate to severe tissue damage; have a wound that may involve a tendon, bone, or joint; have one or more puncture wounds; or have a suppressed immune system. Patients with infected wounds should be given antibiotic therapy based on the results of aerobic and anaerobic cultures. Antimicrobial prophylaxis for cat bites, high-risk dog bites (e.g., bites to the hand or bites with considerable tissue damage), and human bites can be provided with amoxicillin/clavulanate for 3 to 5 days. An alternative that has fewer gastrointestinal (GI) side effects is cefuroxime, also for 3 to 5 days. Hospital admission and parenteral antibiotic therapy will be necessary for all significant human bites to the hand, especially closed-fist injuries and bites involving penetration of the bone or joint.

Positioning

The injured area should be elevated for several days after injury. For bites located over joints, the joint should be immobilized for 3 to 5 days in a proper position, depending on the bite location: 20 degrees wrist extension, 70 to 90 degrees flexion for metacarpophalangeal joints, and 10 degrees flexion for proximal interphalangeal and distal interphalangeal joints.

Rabies Prophylaxis

Rabies is caused by a rhabdovirus that can be found in the saliva of many mammals. The rabies virus is highly neurotoxic and can be fatal. The clinician should refer questions about postexposure prophylaxis to the local health department or an infectious disease specialist. If a dog or cat is healthy and available for 10 days of observation and shows no signs of rabies, no treatment of the exposed person is necessary. About 85% of all cases of animal rabies in the United States now occur in wildlife. Skunks, foxes, bats, raccoons, coyotes, bobcats, and other carnivores should be considered rabid unless proven negative by laboratory assessments. The risk of rabies in lagomorphs (rabbits) and rodents (e.g., mice, rats, chipmunks, and squirrels) is small.

If postexposure rabies is strongly suspected, both rabies immune globulin (RIG) and human diploid-cell rabies vaccine (HDCV) or rabies vaccine adsorbed (RVA) should be given as soon as possible before the completion of confirmatory laboratory testing. However, the vaccine course should be discontinued if fluorescent-antibody tests for rabies of the sacrificed animal's neural tissue are negative. Dosing is as follows:

- RIG: 20 IU/kg. If anatomically possible, one-half the dose should be infiltrated around the wound and the other half given intramuscularly (IM; in the gluteal muscle).

- HDCV: 1 mL IM in deltoid region on days 0, 3, 7, 14, and 28 if the patient has not been previously vaccinated.
- RVA: 1 mL IM in deltoid region on days 0, 3, 7, 14, and 28 if the patient has not been previously vaccinated.

Individuals who have been previously vaccinated with either HDCV or RA should not receive RIG; they should, however, receive 1-mL "booster" doses IM of either HDCV or RVA on days 0 and 3.

Hepatitis B and C Assessment

The clinician should also evaluate the potential for transmission of hepatitis B or C virus (HBV or HCV) in human bites. The type of intervention is dependent on prior receipt of the HBV vaccination series (no vaccination for HCV is currently available). If HBV prophylaxis is indicated (e.g., confirmed hepatitis B surface antigen positivity in the source of the animal bite), hepatitis B immune globulin, 0.06 mL/kg IM, should be administered immediately and repeated in 30 days. The primary HBV vaccine series should be completed, if not already done so, and a "booster" shot should be given if a protective post-vaccination titer has not been confirmed. If HCV-exposure is suspected, the patient should be assessed for HCV antibodies within 48 hours and, if positive, tested further for the presence of HCV RNA, which would be indicative of pre-existing disease. If negative, follow-up testing should occur after at least 3 weeks because positive results likely indicate new infection, which should then be referred for further treatment.

Post exposure HIV Prophylaxis

Although the risk of HIV transmission from a human bite is low, the clinician must also consider whether a human bite was from a known HIV-infected carrier, particularly if that individual had any bleeding in the mouth (such as from severe periodontal disease or from oral trauma during a fight). For example, health-care workers working with combative HIV-positive patients may be victims of human bite wounds or be exposed to needle stick injuries or have mucous membrane exposure to infectious fluids from their HIV-positive patients. The section on HIV infection in Chapter 63 discusses postexposure HIV prophylaxis in detail, which is considered an emergency problem that requires immediate intervention to minimize the risk of infection.

FOLLOW-UP AND REFERRAL

The patient should be discharged to home after thorough and meticulous wound management, with follow-up assessment within 48 hours. Infection, cellulitis, abscess, osteomyelitis, septicemia, tenosynovitis, septic joint (suppurative arthritis), rabies, and the loss of an injured body part are all potential complications of animal bites. Other systemic diseases that can occur as complications of animal bites are bubonic plague, cat-scratch disease, rat-bite fever, leptospirosis, tularemia, tetanus, and sporotrichosis.

Patients with severe cellulitis, systemic manifestations of infection, failure to respond to appropriate outpatient treatment within 48 hours, or bite-wound infections that involve a bone, joint, tendon, or nerve should be admitted to the hospital. The practitioner should obtain early consultation with an infectious disease specialist, if needed. Septic arthritis, osteomyelitis, and closed-fist injuries ("fight bites") require orthopedic consultation.

Patient Education: Animal Bites

If the bite was inflicted by a wild animal or occurred in an unprovoked attack by a domestic animal, the practitioner should ask the patient to have the animal that inflicted the bite evaluated for rabies, if possible. The patient or his or her family should contact the local health department and consult with an animal control officer about the patterns of rabies among animals in the local area. Individuals should be taught the importance of not petting or feeding unfamiliar or wild animals.

Patients should be reminded to elevate injured extremities to prevent swelling and to return for follow-up if signs of fever, redness, or swelling occur, given the subsequent risk of infection. The clinician should instruct patients to watch for red streaks, increased warmth at the wound site, increasing pain, foul odor, or increased drainage from the bite wound—all of which should trigger the patient to seek urgent assessment in the clinic or ED.

BURNS

According to the 2016 Fact Sheet of the American Burn Association, an average of 486,000 burn injuries receive medical treatment each year in the United States, with 3,275 fire-related and smoke inhalation deaths (2,745 from residential fires, 310 from vehicle crash fires, and 220 from other sources). The survival rate for a burn injury is 96.8%, with the majority of burn injuries being treated in the outpatient setting. Thus, it is important for clinicians to possess the knowledge and skills to treat burns.

EPIDEMIOLOGY AND CAUSES

The risk of all types of burns is highest in adults aged 18 to 35 years. The male-to-female ratio is 2:1 for both burn injuries and death. Burns are the second most common cause of accidental death in the United States. The death rate in patients older than 65 years of age is three times greater than that of the overall burn population. Approximately 73% of burns occur in the home, 8% at work, 5% on the street or highway, 5% from recreational or sport injures, and 9% at other locations. Mortality rates from burns have significantly decreased over the past 4 decades. This improvement in mortality rates is the result of a better understanding of the need for early resuscitation, metabolic support after the injury, early wound excision and closure, and control of infection.

About 40% of all reported occupationally related injuries concern the skin, and about 25% of these are caused by chemical burns. Common household chemical burns are caused by lye (found in drain cleaners and paint removers), sodium hypochlorite (found in disinfectants and bleaches), sulfuric acid (found in toilet-bowl cleaners), and phenols (found in deodorizers and sanitizers). The body sites most often burned by chemicals are the face, eyes, and extremities.

Burn-type injuries and other health problems can also result from overexposure to sunlight caused by ultraviolet (UV) radiation, which is commonly split into three bands: UVA, UVB, and UVC. UVB is particularly effective at damaging DNA, which contributes to melanoma and other types of skin cancer. UVC radiation is extremely dangerous but is absorbed by ozone and normal oxygen. Thus, overexposure to UV radiation not only results in painful sunburn but also causes malignant melanoma, basal cell carcinomas, squamous cell carcinomas, actinic keratoses, premature aging of the skin, cataracts, immune system suppression, sun poisoning (phototoxicity), and contact photodermatitis.

Sun poisoning (*phototoxicity*), also called *sun sensitivity,* is a systemic or allergic reaction to sun overexposure, usually occurring in conjunction with sunburn. The risk of sun poisoning is increased in persons who take medications that cause photosensitivity, such as oral contraceptives, tetracyclines, amoxicillin, sulfa drugs, and thiazide diuretics. Risk of sun poisoning also increases with metabolic disorders such as diabetes mellitus or thyroid disease and underlying infection. Patients who have had previous episodes of sun poisoning or who use immunosuppressive drugs are also at increased risk. Other contributing factors include medical disorders such as discoid lupus, systemic lupus erythematosus, or porphyria. Exposure to industrial light sources, such as welding arcs, also places people at greater risk for phototoxicity.

Contact photodermatitis is an acute or chronic inflammatory skin reaction resulting from the combined effects of a photosensitizing substance plus UV light, resulting in immunological delayed-type hypersensitivity. Agents that may photosensitize the skin include oral antidiabetic agents, NSAIDs, antibiotics, phenothiazines, sulfones/sulfonamides, chlorothiazides, and griseofulvin. PABA (*p*-aminobenzoic acid) in sunscreen lotion may also cause photosensitivity dermatitis.

PATHOPHYSIOLOGY

Local Response

Cellular injury from heat results in the release of cellular enzymes and pro-inflammatory vasoactive substances, such as histamine, kinins, serotonin, prostaglandins, leukotrienes, and interleukin-1. Complement is also activated. As a result, vascular permeability is altered, and significant hemodynamic, metabolic, and immunological effects occur locally and systemically. At the capillary level, there is a significant shift of protein molecules, fluid, and electrolytes from the intravascular space to the extravascular space. Lymph flow increases initially but subsequently decreases or ceases because the lymphatic vessels become blocked by serum proteins leaking through the walls of damaged capillaries.

In extensive burn injury (involving more than 25% total body surface area [TBSA]), edema forms in both burned and unburned areas because of a generalized increase in capillary permeability and hypoproteinemia. A decrease in cell transmembrane potential also occurs in extensive burns, causing a shift of extracellular sodium and water into the cell that results in cellular swelling. With adequate resuscitation, cell membrane potential is restored within 24 to 36 hours. However, edema may also result from the volume and oncotic pressure effects of large fluid resuscitation volumes during initial therapy. Maximum edema is typically seen 18 to 24 hours after a burn injury.

Systemic Response

The response of all organ systems to burn injury occurs in a biphasic pattern of hypofunction followed by hyperfunction. For example, even sunburn can alter the distribution and function of WBCs up to 24 hours after sun exposure. The degree of physiological change is proportionate to the extent of the burn, with a maximum response reached in patients with burns over 50% total body surface area (TBSA).

The metabolic response is one of the most significant alterations after burn injury. Protein wasting and weight loss occur in response to a severe burn, and the extensive healing process requires a rapid metabolic rate to support tissue anabolism, which reaches its peak 6 to 10 days after a burn injury. Hypermetabolism begins as resuscitation is completed and is probably mediated by the secretion of catecholamines. When a burn wound is closed, oxygen consumption and metabolic rate slowly returns to normal.

Wound Healing

When a burn injury disrupts the integumentary system, the body automatically responds with a series of overlapping physiological changes to repair and restore epithelial continuity. The *inflammatory response* begins at the moment of injury and lasts from 3 to 4 days after injury. Localized edema, erythema, heat, and tenderness are characteristic signs of the inflammatory response. During the *fibroblastic phase,* which occurs approximately 4 to 20 days after the injury, cells needed for tissue repair and reconstruction proliferate. Fibroblasts at the wound site migrate over the new capillary network, laying down a bed of granulation tissue (collagen) to fill the wound space. During *wound contraction,* which occurs as granulation tissue forms, myofibroblasts cause the wound edges to pull toward the center.

Epithelial cells from the burn margins then migrate across the wound and eventually reproduce to form a protective barrier. This process is called *epithelialization.* Epithelial cells also migrate from the hair follicles and sweat glands, forming small islands of cells known as *epithelial buds.* Newly forming epithelial cells are easily damaged by mechanical trauma and desiccation. If allowed to dry, the wound will form *neo-eschar,* retarding the healing process. The epithelial cells must secrete enzymes to dissolve the eschar in their path. The *maturation phase* occurs when immature granulation tissue is highly organized and serves to restore tissue strength. This phase begins approximately 20 days after the burn injury and continues beyond 1 year. Contractures can occur if a burn wound heals with extensive scar tissue formation over a joint. A *contracture* is the fixation of a joint or area of skin into a flexed or fixed position. This is caused by atrophy and shortening of muscle fibers or by scar formation and the loss of the normal skin elasticity.

Under optimal conditions, a partial-thickness burn heals in 2 to 6 weeks. The persistence of eschar on a full-thickness burn may delay healing; if the area involved is large, this will cause the patient to remain in a hypermetabolic state. As bacteria proliferate beneath the eschar, there is a possibility of infection. Approximately 2 weeks after a burn injury, the eschar will begin to separate from the underlying tissue as a result of microbial and leukocytic action on subeschar collagen fibers. Separation generally occurs from the wound margins inward but may occur in patches. Eschar may be removed earlier by surgical excision to facilitate healing.

CLINICAL PRESENTATION

Sun poisoning may present with urticaria, an erythematous rash accompanied by edema, fever, fatigue, dizziness, GI symptoms, or malaise. Hematuria, casts, and proteinuria may occur. Contact photodermatitis results in pruritic papules with erythema and occasionally vesicles 24 hours or more after sun exposure. The skin rash will occur in the area where the chemical was applied and sun exposure occurred.

In the past, burn injuries were classified as first through third degree. Currently second- and third-degree burns are classified as either partial-thickness or full-thickness. Partial-thickness injuries can be further categorized as superficial or deep. The signs and symptoms of the various depths of burn are as follows:

- *Superficial (first-degree) burns.* These burns involve the epidermal layer only. The patient presents with pain, hyperemia, and erythema. The surface is dry, with no vesicles or blisters, and blanches with pressure. The wound heals in approximately 5 days, without scarring. The prototype of a first-degree burn is a mild sunburn. If this type of burn occurs over a large surface area, it can result in fever, weakness, chills, and vomiting.
- *Superficial partial-thickness (second-degree) burns.* These burns involve the epidermis along with the upper layer of dermis. Signs and symptoms include erythema, hyperemia, pain, moist skin, and hypersensitivity to touch. Vesicles and blisters appear several hours after the injury. The healing time is within 21 days, with minimal scarring.
- *Deep partial-thickness (second-degree) burns.* These burns produce destruction of the epidermis, along with most of the dermis. Epidermal cells lining hair follicles and sweat glands remain intact. This level of burn may convert to a full-thickness injury. The burn wound is typically pale, mottled, pearly white, mostly dry, often insensate, and difficult to differentiate from a full-thickness burn. The burn will heal by wound contraction and re-epithelialization within 3 to 6 weeks. Often excision and grafting are done to provide a better functional cosmetic result and to decrease the healing time.
- *Full-thickness (third-degree) burns.* These burns result in destruction of all layers of the skin, down to or past the subcutaneous fat layer, sometimes involving fascia, muscle, and bone. The nerves are also typically destroyed. Hair will pull easily out of the follicles, but in a painless manner. The clinical picture typically includes a thick, dry, leathery eschar, with a wound that is white, cherry red, or brown/black in color. The tissue is insensate, with thrombosed blood vessels. These wounds typically require skin grafting.

DIAGNOSTIC REASONING

Diagnostic Tests

Initial laboratory studies for a patient with a major burn include a CBC, serum electrolyte panel, BUN and creatinine, and serum glucose. Pulse oximetry and arterial blood gas determinations should be done, given the effects that significant burns have on the circulatory system and oxygenation. In addition, because smoke inhalation injury is associated with significant fire-related burns, a carboxyhemoglobin (COHb) level should be checked to determine the percentage of hemoglobin bound to carbon monoxide and unavailable for oxygen transport.

The following COHb levels correlate with typical clinical symptoms:

- Less than 10% COHb: no symptoms
- 20% COHb: headache, nausea, vomiting, loss of dexterity
- 30% COHb: confusion, lethargy, ST-segment depression on electrocardiogram
- 40 to 60% COHb: coma
- More than 60% COHb: death

If the COHb level is less than 40%, treatment should consist of 100% oxygen administered by high-humidity flow mask. A patient with a COHb level of 40% or higher should be considered for transfer to a hyperbaric chamber, given its life-threatening consequences.

Differential Diagnosis

Although thermal injury is the most common cause of burn wounds, several other etiologies of burns exist. For example, chemical burns occur in industrial, military, home, agricultural, school, and research laboratory settings. For clinicians affiliated with these settings, especially student health-care settings that include a chemistry laboratory, it is important to have knowledge of the initial care of chemical burn injuries. Various agents that can cause burn injuries are listed in Table 73.1

Photodermatitis should be differentiated from contact dermatitis that may develop from one of the many substances in suntan lotions and oils. Sensitivity to the sun's rays may also be part of a more serious condition such as erythropoietic protoporphyria, systemic lupus erythematosus, pellagra, or porphyria cutanea tarda.

MANAGEMENT

If a patient with a major burn presents to an outpatient setting, it is necessary to assess and stabilize the patient so that he or she can be safely transported by emergency medical services (EMS) to a hospital ED or preferably a burn center. Therefore, all practitioners should understand the fundamentals of the initial assessment and treatment of burn injuries. See Figure 73.1 to estimate the extent of a burn injury using the "Rule of Nines." When burns are scattered on the body, a rule of thumb is that the size of the patient's palm is equal to approximately 1% TBSA.

Major Burns

A patient with a major burn should be immediately transported to a burn center or ED. A *major burn* is defined as follows:

- Partial-thickness burn greater than 25% TBSA in a person 10 to 50 years of age *or* greater than 20% TBSA in a child younger than 10 years of age or an adult older than 50 years of age

- Full-thickness burn greater than 10% TBSA in any individual
- Serious burn involving the hand, face, foot, or perineum
- A burn complicated by smoke or chemical inhalation injury
- An electrical burn
- A burn in an infant, an immunocompromised patient, or an elderly patient

Initial management of a patient with a major burn injury should include maintaining the patient's airway, breathing, and circulation. If there is time before transportation to the ED or burn center, the patient's clothing

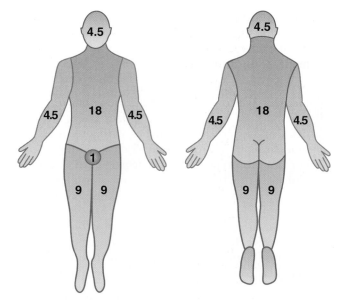

Figure 73.1 The Rule of Nines.

TABLE 73.1	**Burn Injuries**
Type of Injuries	*Characteristics*
Chemical	• *Damage:* Destruction of tissues from coagulation or desiccation of tissue protein; damage continues until agent is removed; skin penetration by many chemicals leads to systemic toxicity • *Effects:* Injury is generally deeper than it appears; small percentage of admissions to burn units
Cold liquids/gases	• *Damage:* Frostbite (freezing of tissue) results in ice crystal formation, which draws water out of the cells and into the extracellular space; crystals expand, causing mechanical destruction of cell membranes and organelles • *Effects:* Cellular destruction; serum electrolyte imbalances
Electrical	• *Damage:* Destruction of tissues from heat generated by electric current passing through tissues; arc burn or thermal injury • *Effects:* Injury is usually more extensive than it appears; cardiac conduction system may be affected, leading to sudden death or arrhythmias; severe muscle contraction can produce long bone or vertebral fractures; severe muscle destruction leads to release of myoglobin, which can affect kidney function
Radiation	• *Damage:* Occurs primarily by gamma or x-ray particles; affects the reproductive mechanisms of tissue cells, leading to cellular death • *Effects:* Proportional to the extent of injury and depth of tissue damage
Thermal heat	• *Damage:* Destruction of tissues from flames, scalding liquids, or steam • *Effects:* Proportional to extent of injury and depth; thermal burns account for highest percentage of admissions to burn units.

should be removed if further damage to the skin can be avoided. Jewelry should also be removed and secured in a safe place. The patient should be placed on and covered with a clean, warm sheet and clean blankets with overhead warmers if available. No other wound care is typically required until the patient reaches the ED or burn center.

For airway management, the clinician should assess the patency of the patient's airway while maintaining the head and neck in a neutral position. If a spinal cord injury is probable, the clinician should apply a cervical collar, sandbags, and backboard as appropriate.

For respiratory management, while the clinician is maintaining the patient's breathing, she or he should simultaneously observe the patient's skin color, monitor oxygen saturation via pulse oximetry (Spo_2), and auscultate the lungs to ensure effective bilateral ventilation. The clinician should be alert for signs of smoke inhalation and thermal airway injury if the patient was exposed to fire in an enclosed space. Signs and symptoms include facial burns, presence of soot around the mouth and nose and in the sputum, singed nasal hairs, coughing up of carbonaceous black sputum, difficulty swallowing, signs of hypoxemia including tachycardia, dysrhythmias, anxiety, or lethargy, increased or decreased respiratory rate, use of accessory muscles for breathing, intercostal or sternal retractions, inspiratory stridor, hoarseness, and expiratory stridor.

Once an airway injury has occurred, no measures can be taken to limit its progress, and complete airway obstruction can occur. If signs of airway injury are present, the patient will need to be intubated. After extensive swelling has occurred, intubation will be very difficult, so the decision to insert an artificial airway should be made early in the assessment of the patient with airway injury. In the non-intubated patient, humidified oxygen at 5 to 10 L/min should be administered by face mask along with a bronchodilator (albuterol 5 mg unit dose nebulized or 50 mcg/puff, four to eight puffs by metered-dose inhaler with a spacer, every 15 to 20 minutes as needed). If the patient has signs of carbon monoxide poisoning (e.g., headache, nausea, vomiting, dizziness, loss of manual dexterity, confusion, lethargy, unconsciousness, and cherry-red skin color), 100% oxygen should be administered via a nonrebreathing mask.

For circulatory management, if the patient presents in the outpatient setting with thermal injuries that involve more than 20% TBSA, the patient will need to be transported to a hospital ED or burn center. If there is evidence of burn-related shock and the patient can still take fluids orally, she or he should receive oral rehydration with balanced salt solutions. The patient should be encouraged to drink enough fluid to keep the urine clear and copious. If this is not possible, a large-bore (16- or 18-gauge) IV catheter should be inserted in an upper extremity vein, preferably through unburned skin. The clinician should infuse lactated Ringer's solution at an initial rate of 500 mL/hr.

Patients with major burns should receive tetanus prophylaxis. If the patient has not received a full primary vaccination series of at least three doses of tetanus toxoid, tetanus vaccine and tetanus immune globulin 250 U should be immediately administered, with the remaining vaccinations in the series administered according to age-appropriate guidelines. Fully vaccinated patients should receive a "booster" shot, if the last dose of vaccine was received within the past 5 years.

Minor Burns

A patient with minor burn injuries can usually be treated in an outpatient setting. Minor burn injuries include a burn of less than 15% TBSA in a patient 10 to 50 years of age or less than 10% TBSA in a child younger than 10 years of age or an adult older than 50 years of age.

Superficial (First-Degree) Burns

These burns should be cooled with wet compresses. Ice should not be placed directly on the skin. Aloe vera gel can be applied topically to the burn. Remedies (anesthetic sprays) with benzocaine or lidocaine may provide relief from pain, but these medications produce sensitivity reactions in some people. The patient can be given ibuprofen (Motrin) 800 mg every 8 hours, aspirin, or another NSAID, which work by blocking the production of prostaglandins that are mediators of pain in sunburned skin. If the sunburn is severe, the clinician should administer oral prednisone in a rapid taper: day 1, 80 mg; day 2, 60 mg; day 3, 40 mg; day 4, 20 mg; day 5, 10 mg. There are no benefits to prescribing topical corticosteroid ointments or creams.

Superficial Partial-Thickness and Deep Partial-Thickness (Second-Degree) Burns

These burns should be gently irrigated with cool water or saline solution to remove all loose dirt and skin. If the burn is chemical in nature, the caustic agent should be washed off with large amounts of water. Any necrotic skin should be peeled off or trimmed. Small, thick blisters should be left intact. Thin, fluid-filled blisters greater than 1 inch in diameter should be drained and the dead skin trimmed off using aseptic technique.

There are multiple methods for the outpatient management of superficial partial-thickness burns. One is to apply a topical antimicrobial preparation to the wound. Agents commonly used are presented in Drugs Commonly Prescribed 73.1. Silver sulfadiazine (Silvadene) is the most frequently used topical agent, although it cannot be used in patients with sulfa allergies or on the face because of silver staining. Alternative topical agents for facial burns include gentamicin ophthalmic ointment, Neosporin, or bacitracin. When these ointments are applied to the face, no overlying dressing should be used. If antibiotic creams are unavailable, aloe vera gel can be applied to the burn.

Burn wounds on areas other than the face should be covered with a dressing, which should be removed twice a day at home. The burn should be washed with mild antiseptic soap and water, then antibiotic ointment and a clean dressing should be re-applied. This regimen should continue for 7 to 10 days until the burn is healed. This particular method of therapy has some disadvantages in the outpatient setting. Some antimicrobial agents (such as Sulfamylon) encourage wound maceration and therefore cannot be used under a dressing. Also, most topical agents lose their potency in 6 to 24 hours after application, making frequent dressing changes necessary.

An alternative dressing for the superficial partial-thickness burn is to cover the burn with a fine-mesh gauze (e.g., Xeroform gauze) without a topical antibiotic. This gauze is covered with gauze pads, then a bulky absorbent dressing (e.g., Kerlix) is wrapped around the wound to provide protective bulk. The clinician should inspect the wounds and change the dressings the following day because the maximum amount of wound seepage occurs within the first 24 hours. The same type of dressing is reapplied, and the burn wound should also be assessed for infection, which should be aggressively treated.

The burn is then reevaluated after 4 days, and the bulky dressing removed. If a fluid collection has occurred beneath the fine-mesh gauze, the dressing will need to be removed, the wound cleansed, and new fine-mesh gauze applied. If the fine-mesh gauze is still in place without any apparent fluid collection, it should be left in place and the burn rewrapped. Another follow-up visit should be scheduled for reexamination in 5 days. At that time, the fine-mesh gauze, impregnated with the crust from the burn, should separate from the epithelium, revealing

Drugs Commonly Prescribed 73.1: Burns

TOPICAL	INDICATIONS	DOSAGE AND COMMENTS
Antimicrobial Agents		
Bacitracin ointment	Antimicrobial, especially for sensitive areas (e.g., lips, eyelids)	Apply to cleansed area 2–3 times daily. Does not penetrate eschar.
Clotrimazole cream (Lotrimin)	Fungal infections of burn wounds	Apply thin coat to wound; wait 20 minutes before applying dressing. Not for ophthalmic use. May cause skin irritation and blistering.
Mafenide acetate (Sulfamylon)	Active against most gram-positive and gram-negative organisms Drug of choice for electrical and ear burns	Apply 1–2 times daily using sterile gloves; do not use with dressings (may reduce effectiveness and cause skin maceration). Monitor for signs of acidosis, intake and output, and for signs of allergic skin reaction. Penetrates eschar better than other agents. Pain occurs on application to partial-thickness burns and for 30 minutes thereafter. Allergic maculopapular skin rash may occur. Use with caution in patients with impaired renal or pulmonary function. Hyperchloremic metabolic acidosis may occur. Superinfection with fungi possible.
Silver nitrate	Active against wide spectrum of bacterial pathogens and fungal infections Used for patients with sulfa allergy or toxic epidermal necrolysis syndrome	Apply 0.5% solution via wet dressings 2–3 times a day; ensure dressings remain moist. Preserve solution in a light-resistant container. Protect area with plastic to prevent staining from spills or splashes, as solution stains surfaces black (including unburned skin). Poor penetration of eschar. Electrolyte imbalances may occur. Methemoglobinemia may occur.
Silver sulfadiazine (Silvadene)	Active against wide spectrum of microbial pathogens Most frequently used agent for partial-thickness and full-thickness thermal injuries	Apply once or twice daily using sterile gloves; leave wounds exposed or apply gauze dressing over wound. Do not use if cream is dark in color. Transient neutropenia may occur after 2–3 days. Only moderate penetration of eschar. Bone marrow suppression may occur. Use with caution in patients with impaired hepatic or renal function.

healed epithelium underneath. Once the wound is left open, it must be kept clean and protected from extremes of temperature. The wound should epithelialize in approximately 3 weeks. Epithelialization, however, may not occur for 2 to 3 months if the wound is a deep partial-thickness burn in which the only skin remnants are the hair follicles or sweat glands.

Another method for outpatient burn wound management is to place a semisynthetic occlusive dressing (e.g., Biobrane), a xenograft, a moisture vapor-permeable dressing (e.g., Opsite), or a hydrocolloid dressing (e.g., DuoDerm) over the wound. These dressings are less readily available, however, and tend to be expensive. They are most useful for the immunocompromised patient because they minimize the risk of infection. They can be used on flat-surface superficial partial-thickness burns of the extremities and trunk. The goal is for the dressing

to adhere to the wound surface and for there to be no exudate or fluid between the dressing and the burn. The dressing is usually removed after 7 to 10 days because the wound is typically healed by then. If there is leaking or nonadherence at any time, the dressing must be changed. Superficial partial-thickness burn wounds heal faster using this method, and patients find this method easier to maintain with fewer dressing changes and more comfortable.

Oral antibiotics should be given only if the burn becomes infected, as prophylactic antibiotic therapy is not supported in acute burns. Any partial-thickness burn will convert to a full-thickness burn if it becomes infected, especially with *Streptococcus*. If infection occurs, the patient may have to be admitted for IV antibiotics. Signs of infection include pus, foul odor, cloudy blisters, increased swelling and redness in the normal skin around the burn, and fever greater than 101°F (38.3°C). Patients with infected minor burns should receive tetanus prophylaxis as described for major burns.

Chemical Burns

Consultation from clinicians at a burn center should be obtained for the treatment of chemical injuries. When a patient with a chemical burn is assessed, the clinician should don protective clothing and gloves. The first priority is to stop the burning process and arrange for rapid transportation to an ED or burn center. Any of the patient's garments that have become saturated with the chemical should be rapidly removed, and the patient should be rapidly transported to a shower irrigation area. All other garments should be removed from the patient before the irrigation is complete. If the agent is a powder-like material, such as lime, the clinician should brush off as much as possible from the patient before irrigating the burned area. The hair and the areas under the nails and between the toes should be checked for collections of the chemical. The patient may be more comfortable on a chair in a running shower, but any patient who is unstable should be kept in a horizontal position during the irrigation.

A chemical burn should be irrigated with water for no less than 30 minutes and preferably for 60 minutes. Irrigation may need to be continued for hours in the case of alkali burns. Irrigation decreases the concentration of the chemical agent and physically removes it from the wound; the rate and severity of reaction between the chemical and the tissue will thus be decreased. Following irrigation in the outpatient setting, the clinician should place wet towels over the patient and arrange for transportation to the hospital. Although wet towels help to relieve pain and continue to dilute the chemical, caution is needed to prevent hypothermia if the burned area is extensive. If possible, the patient should bring samples of the chemical agent with a product label to the ED. Use of pH-detection litmus paper may help determine the continued presence of alkali or acid in burn wounds. After irrigation and debridement of any remaining particles and devitalized tissue, antimicrobial agents should be used and tetanus prophylaxis updated as needed, as described for major burns.

For moderate to large burns caused by hot tar or asphalt, the wound should be rapidly cooled with a large volume of water. The tar can then be removed using a petrolatum-based product such as an antibiotic ointment (Neosporin). When a large body surface area is involved, a new (unopened) jar of mayonnaise will suffice. The wound can be dressed with a petrolatum-based dressing (e.g., Xeroform gauze). Tar can be removed from the cornea or conjunctiva with a polysorbate-containing neomycin sulfate preparation; consultation with an ophthalmologist is recommended.

Special consideration should be given to chemical or thermal burns that cause acute iritis (inflammation of the iris). Individuals will present with excess lacrimation, decreased vision, photophobia, and pain. Management should include consultation with an ophthalmologist and the use of a cycloplegic drug, as well as possibly topical corticosteroids.

Although not commonly considered a chemical burn, if a patient presents with skin that is adhered together with a fast-setting epoxy glue, the adhesive can be removed with acetone. If the glue is on the mucous membranes, the area can be swabbed with vegetable oil until the glue is removed. For glue in the eyes, the clinician should use an ophthalmic antibiotic ointment to facilitate removal. Referral to an ophthalmologist may be indicated, as care must be taken or else the drying glue can cause a corneal abrasion.

Some chemical exposures call for specialized agents as directed by an ED or burn center. If exposure to hydrofluoric acid (used in glass etching) or oxalic acid has caused a chemical burn, the affected area should be irrigated with water and then neutralized with subcutaneous injections of 10% calcium gluconate. However, this should be done only after consultation with clinicians at a burn center. If phenol (an acidic alcohol used in sanitizers and disinfectants) is the causative agent, the area should be irrigated with water only if a high-density shower is available. Phenol is more soluble in polyethylene glycol; therefore, a 50% solution of this agent should be used to irrigate the skin as soon as possible.

FOLLOW-UP AND REFERRAL

Although dressing changes for some types of burns may not be recommended until 5 to 7 days after the injury, all patients with a burn injury must still be reassessed in 24 hours to reevaluate the depth and extent of the burn. Infected burns must also be assessed within 1 to 2 days after starting antibiotic therapy to ensure improvement on the selected regimen.

Referral to an ED or specialized burn center is indicated for major burns, as well as minor burns that do not begin healing as expected. In addition, both thermal and chemical burns to highly sensitive parts of the body require rapid referral to appropriate specialty care (e.g., ophthalmology for eye injuries).

Patient Education: Burns

Patients should be advised to elevate the burned area, especially if it involves an extremity, and to return to the clinician's office or the ED if signs of an infection appear. Patients should also be given a prescription for analgesic medication. Given the risk of chemical burns from home-based cleaning products and other solvents, all parents should have the national Poison

Control Center Help Line (1-800-222-1222) readily available in the case of chemical injury.

Patients with sunburns should be informed that sunscreens with PABA may cause photosensitivity dermatitis. Photoplex broad-spectrum sunscreen lotion not only provides protection from UVB radiation but also offers absorbent protection from UVA rays and may be beneficial for patients who experience photosensitivity activated by UVA. Other useful substitutes are sunshades that contain titanium dioxide, zinc oxide, or talc. Patients should be informed about the sun protection factor (SPF) index—a system of evaluating the effectiveness of various formulations for protecting the skin from sun exposure. Protective agents are rated 1 to 50 by the U.S. Food and Drug Administration (FDA). An SPF of 15 means that the sunscreen provides 15 times the protection from sun as that of unprotected skin. A patient information sheet on sun exposure safety tips should be given to all patients, especially those who have sustained a sunburn severe enough to require treatment. Given the risk of infection to sun-damaged skin, the patient should also notify the health-care provider if pain and fever persist for more than 48 hours.

A patient information sheet on sun exposure safety tips should be given to all patients, especially those who have sustained a sunburn severe enough to require treatment (see Box 73.2).

HEAD TRAUMA

Types of head trauma that may be encountered in a primary-care setting include cerebral contusions, concussions, skull fracture, and epidural or subdural hematomas. In contrast, subarachnoid hemorrhage typically results from the spontaneous rupture of intracranial aneurysms (in greater than 80% of cases), rather than a traumatic etiology. The majority of head trauma patients will need to be transported to the nearest ED for emergent evaluation and care.

EPIDEMIOLOGY AND CAUSES

Head trauma is a leading cause of morbidity and mortality in the United States, resulting in about 30% of all injury deaths. Falls are the leading cause of head injury (disproportionately affecting the youngest and the oldest age groups, followed by being struck by or hitting an object, while motor vehicle accidents were the third leading cause [Centers for Disease Control and Prevention, 2017]). Although it is estimated that approximately 3.8 million concussions occur in the United States annually during competitive sports and recreational

---

Box 73.2   Patient Information: Sunburn

- Always wear sunscreen when outdoors on a sunny day. A sunscreen with a sun protection factor (SPF) of at least 15 will block most harmful UV radiation. For the average adult, the recommended dose is 1 ounce per application. Reapply every 2 hours after being in the water or after exercising and sweating.
- Use broad-spectrum sunscreens—those that contain active ingredients that absorb at least 85% of ultraviolet (UV) A and UVB rays of the sun.
- Protect sensitive areas such as the nose and rims of the ears. Use a lip balm containing a sunscreen. This can help keep some people from getting cold sores.
- Minimize exposure to the sun during the hours when the sun is directly overhead and exposure is most damaging, from 8 a.m. to 4 p.m. Sun (UV) exposure before 8 a.m. or after 4 p.m., when the sun is lower on the horizon, is typically only one-third that at midday. If your shadow is shorter than you are (around midday), you are being exposed to high levels of UV radiation.
- Wear sunglasses that block 99% to 100% of UV radiation. Babies and children should also be protected with sunglasses to prevent cataracts that may develop later in life.
- Wear a hat with a wide brim to provide protection to your eyes, ears, face, and the back of your neck.
- Wear tightly woven, loose-fitting clothes during prolonged periods in the sun.

- Avoid sunlamps and tanning parlors.
- Monitor the UV Index, as reported by the U.S. Environmental Protection Agency and consistent with World Health Organization guidelines:
  - UV Index 0–2 (minimal): precautions include wearing a hat.
  - UV Index 3–4 (low): precautions include wearing a hat and using a sunscreen with an SPF of at least 15.
  - UV Index 5–6 (moderate): precautions include wearing a hat, using a sunscreen with an SPF of at least 15, and staying in shady areas when outside.
  - UV Index 7–9 (high): precautions include wearing a hat, using a sunscreen with an SPF of at least 15, staying in shady areas when outside, and staying indoors between the hours of 10 a.m. and 4 p.m.
  - UV Index 10+ (very high): precautions include staying indoors as much as possible and taking other precautions when outdoors.
- Be aware that UV radiation increases 5% for every 1,000 feet of altitude. In North America, the sun is closest to the Earth on June 21, so spring skiing in the Rocky Mountains without adequate sun protection is dangerous. Snow and water can also reflect the sun's rays, making sun exposure more intense.

activities, half of those go unreported. In people older than 65 years of age, falls account for the majority of head injury deaths. Falls are the most common reason for an injury-related visit to an ED. Traumatic brain injury (TBI) may also be the result of drugs and alcohol, violence, and sports-related injuries.

PATHOPHYSIOLOGY

Mild head trauma is usually the result of a sudden deceleration injury or rotational force that causes shearing forces within the brain. These forces cause axonal and blood vessel damage. Injuries to small blood vessels can manifest themselves as petechial hemorrhages. If the bridging veins connecting the cortex to the venous sinuses are involved, acute subdural hematomas can occur that are potentially fatal. In contrast, subarachnoid hemorrhages, with their resultant meningeal findings including extreme headache and neck stiffness, result far more commonly from ruptured intracranial saccular (berry) aneurysms (in greater than 80% of cases), rather than from trauma.

The area of cerebral injury becomes ischemic and edematous. As edema increases, the autoregulatory control of intracranial vessels is lost. The blood–brain barrier breaks down, resulting in increased loss of fluid into the brain parenchyma, which in turn results in elevated intracranial pressure (ICP). As ICP increases, cerebral blood flow decreases, leading to tissue hypoxia, a decrease in the serum pH level, and an increase in carbon dioxide level. This process leads to cerebral vasodilation and edema, which further increases ICP (resulting in a vicious cycle). The increased ICP compromises cerebral perfusion and, if not treated and reversed, leads to increasing hypoxia and secondary brain injury. If left untreated, the brain herniates downward toward the brainstem, causing irreversible brain damage.

Cerebral Contusion

A *cerebral contusion* is a focal brain injury involving cortical bruising, and, at times, vessel lacerations. This is one of the most common cerebral injuries; it is associated with hemorrhage, edema, and brain swelling. Contusions are classified as *coup* (injury directly beneath the point of impact) or *contrecoup* (injury directly opposite the point of impact). Temporal and frontal lobes are the most common sites affected. Contusions are graded as mild or severe and superficial or deep. Superficial contusions usually involve the cortical and subcortical tissue, whereas deep contusions penetrate the white matter.

Concussion

A *concussion* involves diffuse brain injury. It is associated with a transient loss of consciousness (LOC) that occurs immediately following nonpenetrating blunt head trauma. Most patients with only a brief LOC (less than 5 minutes) are not admitted to the hospital if their subsequent neurological examination remains within normal limits. However, close observation by a responsible adult educated in the warning signs of neurological deterioration is critical for at least the next 24 hours.

A classic concussion, resulting in a LOC of less than 6 minutes, typically produces retrograde and posttraumatic amnesia and mild neurological impairment. The duration of amnesia can be a predictor of severity, as the longer the amnesia, the more severe the concussion. Multiple systems exist for the grading of concussions, as there are no universally agreed upon criteria to categorize severity. Some clinicians consider a mild concussion to be one with no LOC, but rather characterized by other neurologic manifestations, such as confusion, disorientation, and, at times, retrograde amnesia (i.e., an inability to recall events surrounding the injury) or post-traumatic amnesia. However, other experts feel that, by definition, concussions must involve LOC. Even with mild concussions, while confusion and disorientation immediately after the injury may last only minutes, recurrent dizziness, headache, and difficulty concentrating may last for months. More severe concussions with a greater LOC usually still present with a normal computed tomography (CT) scan of the head. Nonetheless, these patients should be admitted to the hospital for close observation, given the risk of significant neurologic sequelae.

Post-concussion syndrome is usually associated with mild head trauma and may follow any type of concussion. LOC does not have to occur for postconcussion syndrome to develop, and it is estimated that up to 50% of patients who suffer mild head trauma will experience this syndrome. The syndrome consists of the following signs and symptoms, which can start as early as 24 hours posttrauma and persist for up to 6 months after the injury:

- Headaches
- Dizziness
- Fatigue
- Irritability
- Insomnia
- Anxiety
- Impaired concentration
- Loss of memory

Skull Fracture

A *skull fracture* may occur with a severe blow to the head. A skull fracture increases the risk of an underlying epidural or subdural hematoma. In addition, patients with suspected or confirmed skull fractures require careful examination of the cranial nerves (CNs), particularly those that are most likely to be injured: olfactory nerve (CN I), optic nerve (CN II), oculomotor nerve (CN III), trochlear nerve (CN IV), trigeminal nerve (CN V), abducens nerve (CN VI), facial nerve (CN VII), and acoustic nerve (CN VIII).

A basilar skull fracture (i.e., a fracture of the base of the skull) can occur as an extension of a fracture in another area of the skull. Basilar skull fractures can cause leakage of cerebrospinal fluid (CSF), an entry point for bacteria leading to meningitis, and/or pneumocephalus (i.e., air entry into the CSF-filled spaces within the head). Several clinical manifestations can be associated with basilar skull fracture, including CSF leak through the cribriform plate of the skull causing nasal CSF rhinorrhea, hemotympanum (i.e., blood behind the tympanic membrane), ecchymosis over the mastoid process ("Battle's sign"), or periorbital ecchymosis ("raccoon eyes"). Routine x-rays may not reveal a skull fracture; therefore, radiographs are usually nondiagnostic and can cost precious minutes of critical care time. Thus, the clinician should be aware that basilar skull fracture is a clinical diagnosis and proceed immediately to EMS transport to the ED, if suspected.

Epidural Hematoma

Severe head trauma can cause intracranial bleeding that can put pressure on the brain tissue. The brain is surrounded by the *meninges,* three layers of protective membranes. The layers from the cranial bone going interiorly consist of the dura mater, arachnoid membrane, and pia mater (see Fig. 73.2). Between each membrane is a compartment or space where blood from ruptured vessels can collect. Between the cranial bone and dura mater is the epidural space. The middle meningeal artery courses through this space and can rupture when the cranium is fractured.

The middle meningeal artery runs tightly along the wall of the cranial bone, forming grooves in the bone. With a skull fracture, this artery is easily ruptured and bleeds rapidly within the epidural space, resulting in an *epidural hematoma.* The volume of blood may be large enough to displace the brain, causing neurological deficits and coma within hours after skull injury. Skull x-rays will reveal a fracture line that passes through a groove in the cranium, while a head CT scan can visualize the region of the bleed. Brain dysfunction is due primarily to parenchymal compression, which can be relieved with evacuation of blood from the epidural space.

A head CT to evaluate for bleeding should be considered for a head injury patient who meets any of the following criteria:

- Is on anticoagulants or has a history of bleeding dyscrasias
- Has sustained LOC
- Has altered mental status
- Is suspected of alcohol or drug ingestion
- Has vomited repeatedly
- Has a Glasgow Coma Scale (GCS) score below 15
- Is older than 60 years of age
- Has Battle's sign or raccoon eyes
- Is an infant with suspected shaken baby syndrome

Subdural Hematoma

Head trauma can also cause a *subdural hematoma,* which is a venous bleed within the subdural space—the compartment between the dura mater and the arachnoid membrane. Acute subdural hematomas commonly result from traumatic rupture of the bridging veins that span the cortex and the dural venous sinuses. If such acute bleeds require surgical intervention but are not rapidly treated within several hours after the injury, mortality rates are strikingly high (up to 90%). However, a subdural hematoma may can also be due to relatively mild head trauma or even spontaneous venous rupture and can develop slowly over days to weeks. Thus, in relation to the time postinjury, subdural hematomas can be acute (less than 72 hours old), subacute (between 3 and 20 days old), or chronic (greater than 20 days old).

Chronic subdural hematomas pose less of a mortality threat than acute subdural hematomas. The majority originate from subdural hygromas, which are potential spaces formed between the dura mater and the brain surface following separation of the dura–arachnoid interface due to ischemic or traumatic brain injury or atrophy resulting in a loss of brain parenchyma. These spaces

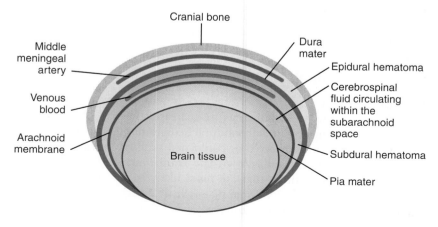

Figure 73.2 The layers of the meninges, cranial circulation, and location of hematomas.

become filled with CSF, and a neomembrane eventually forms that lines the space, becoming a site of neovascularization by fragile intracranial veins that are prone to rupture, with subsequent formation of a chronic subdural hematoma.

Neurological deficits may not be noted until a large volume of accumulated blood is present. Brain dysfunction is due primarily to parenchymal compression, which can be relieved with evacuation of blood from the subdural space. CT scans and x-ray studies may not clearly reveal a subdural hematoma, making it difficult to diagnose. Magnetic resonance imaging (MRI) can show displaced brain tissue away from the skull, which is a key finding of a subdural hematoma. Patients on anticoagulants, with coagulation deficiencies, or with liver impairment are particularly susceptible to subdural hematomas. Alcohol abusers are also susceptible to subdural hematomas, which may be acute or subacute, as a more slowly evolving source of increased ICP.

CLINICAL PRESENTATION

Subjective

A full history of the event causing the head injury is needed. This should include the mechanism of injury, an approximation of the amount of force involved with the trauma (if the event was witnessed), and whether the patient experienced LOC. Epidural hematomas are typically characterized by the patient losing consciousness briefly, followed by a brief lucid moment when the patient may be awake and talking, and then a return to a period of altered consciousness as the size of the epidural hematoma increases, becoming increasingly symptomatic and possibly progressing to coma.

Clinical presentation depends on the structures involved. General symptoms include behavior, motor, and speech deficits. If a family member or friend is with the patient, the clinician should ask that person if the patient appears normal; a person close to the patient can identify subtle behavioral changes that the clinician may not recognize. Patients may complain of headaches and confusion. When a patient complains of "the worst headache of my life," the clinician should suspect a subarachnoid hemorrhage.

Intoxicated patients present clinical challenges. Signs and symptoms of cerebral injury can be masked by alcohol intoxication. These patients require a head CT scan and transfer to an ED for close monitoring and serial neurological examinations until they are sober because their history and initial physical examination will be unreliable.

Objective

A patient presenting with a head injury should receive a rapid neurological examination to rule out significant cerebral injury. This examination should include checking mental status, cranial nerves, extremity strength, deep tendon reflexes, and cerebellar function. Hypoactive reflexes may result from damage to the spinal cord.

The GCS may also be used to rapidly evaluate the level of consciousness (see Advanced Assessment 73.2 for a description of a rapid neurologic assessment). The GCS establishes baseline neurologic status in each of three areas: eye opening (rated 1 to 4), motor response (rated 1 to 6), and verbal response (rated 1 to 5). Function in each of the three areas is rated on a progressive scale as noted, with a maximum score of 15 representing normal neurological function. A score of 7 usually indicates an unconscious patient, and a score of 3 represents a deep coma state. With any head trauma, the GCS should be done at least every 2 hours to assess for any change.

The clinician may note bradycardia, hypotension, somnolence, seizures, and focal deficits. With a cerebral hemorrhage, these clinical features generally develop immediately after the trauma. These symptoms develop several hours after the injury with an acute epidural hemorrhage. A subacute subdural hemorrhage may occur in the days to weeks (up to 21 days) following the head trauma, whereas a chronic subdural hemorrhage occurs from 3 weeks to months following the initial injury.

All patients should be monitored for signs of increased ICP. The early signs of increased ICP include headache, nausea and vomiting, amnesia, altered level of consciousness, changes in speech, drowsiness, agitation, restlessness, and/or loss of judgment. Any of these signs should prompt the caretaker to take the patient to the ED immediately.

Late signs of increased ICP are dilated, nonreactive pupils (from pressure on the oculomotor nerve), unresponsiveness to verbal or painful stimuli, abnormal posturing patterns (e.g., flexion, extension, or flaccidity), increased systolic blood pressure resulting in a widening pulse pressure, decreased pulse rate, and changes in respiratory rate and pattern. The last three are known as the *Cushing response or reflex*. These late signs are usually observed in patients who are hospitalized and being monitored.

In addition, a patient with a basilar skull fracture should be assessed for the following:

- Hemotympanum—blood behind the tympanic membrane
- Battle's sign—ecchymosis over the mastoid process
- Raccoon eyes—periorbital ecchymosis
- Rhinorrhea with CSF or otorrhea (ear drainage) with CSF

Typical alterations in cranial nerve function include the following:

- CN I: olfactory nerve—anosmia, may experience loss of smell or hyposmia
- CN II: optic nerve—blindness, visual field cuts, unreactive pupil to light

❖ Advanced Assessment 73.2: Rapid Neurological Examination

LEVEL OF CONSCIOUSNESS: GLASGOW COMA SCALE

Motor response	6		Follows commands
	5		Localizes pain on stimulus
	4		Withdraws from painful stimulus
	3		Shows abnormal flexion in response to pain
	2		Shows abnormal extension in response to pain
	1		No response
Verbal response	5		Oriented
	4		Confused
	3		Inappropriate words
	2		Unintelligible sounds
	1		No responses
Eye opening	4		Spontaneous
	3		Opens eyes on verbal command
	2		Opens eyes on painful stimulus
	1		No response
Score: 15 = normal; <7 = coma.			

MENTAL STATUS: FOGS

Family story
Orientation
General information
Spelling

CALCULATIONS

Count backward from 100 by sevens or repeat a three-digit number.

RECALL

Recall two objects.

CRANIAL NERVES

CN I	Olfactory	Smell (not usually assessed during acute examination)
CN II	Optic	Visual acuity, gross visual fields, funduscopic exam
CN III	Oculomotor	Pupillary response, eye movement (upward and medial gaze)
CN IV	Trochlear	Eye movement (downward and medial gaze)
CN V	Trigeminal	Teeth clenching, corneal reflex
CN VI	Abducens	Eye movement (lateral)
CN VII	Facial	Frown, smile, and puff cheeks; assess symmetry
CN VIII	Acoustic	Hearing
CN IX	Glossopharyngeal	Gag reflex
CN X	Vagus	Swallowing, gag reflex
CN XI	Spinal accessory	Shrug shoulders and turn head; assess strength and symmetry
CN XII	Hypoglossal	Articulation and tongue movement

GROSS MOTOR STRENGTH AND SYMMETRY

Upper and lower extremities	Look for symmetry and strength.

▓ Advanced Assessment 73.2 Rapid Neurological Examination—cont'd

CEREBELLAR FUNCTION

Romberg Test	Look for stability and pronator drift.
Coordination	Finger to nose and heel to shin
Reflexes	Biceps, triceps, patellar, Achilles, Babinski

- CN III: oculomotor nerve—problems indicative of increased ICP, loss of eye movements, diplopia, ptosis, dilated or unreactive pupil to light
- CN IV: trochlear nerve—impaired downward gaze, diplopia
- CN V: facial nerve—loss of sensation, absent blink/corneal reflex, muscle atrophy
- CN VI: abducens nerve—eye fails to abduct, diplopia
- CN VII: facial nerve—if lower motor neuron affected, ipsilateral (same side) weakness of entire side of face, loss of corneal reflex; if upper motor neuron affected, contralateral (opposite side) weakness of lower half of face; also, lost, delayed, or metallic taste
- CN VIII: acoustic nerve—dizziness, hearing loss

DIAGNOSTIC REASONING

Diagnostic Tests

For mild head injuries, if the patient did not have LOC, did not exhibit focal neurological signs, or have a history of a clinically significant mechanism of injury, close monitoring by a responsible adult is appropriate. Otherwise, patients with a history of LOC, significant mechanism of injury (which includes a fall that is equal to their height), a GCS score of 14 or less, impaired alertness or memory, positive findings on a rapid neurological examination, signs of increased ICP, a palpable depressed skull fracture, or an otherwise documented skull fracture (e.g., on x-ray) should undergo a head CT scan without contrast, which will also assess for intracranial bleeding (a CT with contrast is not indicated for minor head trauma).

If a cerebral hemorrhage is found, emergent surgery is indicated. Transportation to a hospital facility for electroencephalography may be helpful when a posttraumatic seizure disorder is suspected. A lumbar puncture may be done for support in diagnosing subarachnoid hemorrhage as indicated by the presence of red blood cells, elevated proteins, and a moderate reduction in glucose in the CSF. However, a lumbar puncture is contraindicated in the setting of intracerebral hemorrhage because it may precipitate a herniation syndrome in patients with a large hematoma. MRI can show displaced brain tissue away from the skull, a key finding with a subdural hematoma.

Differential Diagnosis

Typically, a patient with a head trauma will present following an injury, making the diagnosis obvious. However, a subdural hemorrhage may also be suspected in the absence of documented head trauma, as such bleeds may result from spontaneous rupture of bridging veins that cross the subdural space. Moreover, in a comatose patient with a closed-head injury, other conditions that can result in coma must be ruled out, such as drug overdose, cerebrovascular accident, diabetic ketoacidosis, and neuromuscular disorders. However, this type of assessment would typically be hospital-based, given the need for advanced intervention in a comatose patient.

MANAGEMENT

A thorough history and physical examination are necessary for any patient who presents with a head injury. Immobilization should be maintained until the patient is fully awake and CT findings are negative. It cannot be stressed enough that a head CT needs to be ordered on any head injury patient who is on anticoagulant medication such as warfarin or clopidogrel. If this diagnostic testing is not immediately available at the facility to which the patient presents, the patient should be transported to the nearest ED.

If serious complications of head injury have been ruled out and an adequate support network is evident, a patient with minor head injury may be sent home with a competent caregiver who is able to follow the instructions listed under Patient Education. However, patients with temporal cerebral injuries can be problematic because structures in this area are close to the tentorium and midbrain. Progressive edema can lead to elevated ICP and herniation. Thus, it is critical that these patients be transferred to the nearest hospital, so the clinician can monitor neurological assessments that represent the first signs of increased ICP because the earlier these signs are identified and treatment is begun, the better the prognosis for the patient.

FOLLOW-UP AND REFERRAL

A patient with a mild head injury who is sent home with a competent caregiver may not need any follow-up unless complications develop. The patient and caregiver must be alert to the signs and symptoms of increased ICP, which require immediate referral to emergency care. Very small bleeds may not be seen on the initial head CT and can bleed insidiously. Patients and family members should verbalize understanding of discharge instructions and return accordingly (see Patient Education).

Research has shown that the prevalence of any psychiatric illness in the first year after moderate to severe TBI approached 49%, and it approached 34% after mild TBI. Moreover, persons with a mild TBI with prior psychiatric illness had evidence of persisting psychiatric illness. Patients with any TBI should be followed closely and monitored for any affective disorders to determine the need for early postinjury psychiatric intervention.

Patient Education: Head Trauma

The patient with a mild head injury should remain with a responsible adult for the first 24 hours after injury. Decreased activity and a light diet are recommended for the first 24 hours. The patient should be awakened every 2 to 4 hours during the first 24 hours for repeated neurological evaluation to assess for changes. Moreover, it is critical for the patient and caregiver to report if the patient develops vomiting, an inability to move his or her arms or legs equally well, a temperature of 100°F (37.7°C), a stiff neck, pupils of unequal size or shape, convulsions, severe headache that does not improve with acetaminophen or ibuprofen, confusion, disorientation, or a change in personality or behavior. These signs and symptoms are indicative of increased ICP and demand immediate ED evaluation and intervention.

MUSCULOSKELETAL TRAUMA

Musculoskeletal trauma refers to injuries involving the musculoskeletal system. These injuries may present as minor innocuous wounds or with obvious deformities. The clinician needs to resist the urge to treat the obvious deformity or fracture while neglecting to look for occult injuries. Musculoskeletal sequelae can be associated with or caused by problems in other systems—neurological, endocrine, nutritional, or psychological. A thorough history and physical examination are required to rule out other bodily system involvement. This section discusses the musculoskeletal trauma of sprains, strains, and fractures.

EPIDEMIOLOGY AND CAUSES

Musculoskeletal injuries are one of the most common injuries seen in the office and emergency/urgent care setting. Patients of all ages are susceptible to injury. The annual cost of caring for people with musculoskeletal system injuries is in the billions of dollars. The loss of productivity to industry is staggering. Musculoskeletal disorders as a frequent cause of work disability account for productivity losses equivalent to 1.3% of the gross national product. There is an increase in the incidence of injuries among the younger population that can be attributed to higher participation in sports and riskier recreational activities such as in-line skating (rollerblading) and skiing.

Fitness classes and field sports are the most common culprits associated with musculoskeletal injuries in the younger population. Racket sports, walking, and low-intensity sports are associated with injuries in older adults. Usually the lower extremities are involved, especially the knees and ankles. Older patients tend to have more overuse injuries, such as metatarsalgia, plantar fasciitis, and meniscal knee injuries. Younger patients tend to have more patellofemoral syndromes and stress fractures. Knees and ankles are the most common sites injured in high school athletes. Sprains and strains are by far the most common types of injuries.

Occupational strains occur more often in the morning hours and in the first 4 hours of the work shift. Days earlier in the week, especially Monday, have a higher incidence of injury. Married workers 30 to 50 years of age are injured more frequently than other individuals. The occupations associated with a higher than average risk of musculoskeletal injuries include nurses and truck drivers.

Americans have a fracture rate of approximately 21.1/1,000 per year (23.5 per year per 1,000 males and 18.8 per year per 1,000 females), which is very similar to the rate in other industrialized countries. Males 15 to 49 years of age are almost three times more likely to sustain a fracture than females of the same age. There are three main peaks of fracture distribution—first among young adult males, second among older adults (affecting elderly men and women equally), and third, an increase in fractures, especially of the wrist, in women older than 40 years of age. Of note, 1.5 million fractures every year are caused by osteoporosis.

PATHOPHYSIOLOGY

Strains and Sprains

A *strain* involves microscopic and macroscopic stretching or tearing of muscle fibers. These injuries require more than just muscle contraction to occur; excessive stretching or stretching while the muscle is being activated is required for strain injuries. The injury usually occurs within the muscle's normal range of motion. The portion of the muscle that is typically injured is at the muscle–tendon junction. Research has shown that muscles that cross multiple joints or have a complex architecture are more susceptible to strains. Muscles most frequently injured include the hamstring, rectus femoris, gastrocnemius, and adductor longus muscles. A severe strain to the rectus femoris, hamstring, or abdominal wall muscles has been shown to have a poor prognosis for rehabilitation and may benefit from surgical repair.

A *sprain* is caused by stretching or twisting beyond the normal range of motion of a joint or musculoligamentous unit. A sprain can be impossible to differentiate from a strain during physical examination. Injuries involving joints are usually sprains because ligaments are more prominent around joint capsules. A history of overuse and/or excessive force, as opposed to a fall, hyperextension, or twisting of a joint, is more likely related to a strain. If bony tenderness at the injury site is found during the physical examination, x-rays are required to rule out fractures.

A high suspicion of fracture is required, especially in the young and in older adults. Infants and children are unable to provide an accurate history and fully cooperate during a physical examination. Many minor fractures (such as a torus fracture) are missed because the child does not complain and the parents or guardians are unaware of an injury. Older adults can have blunted pain perception, especially in the extremities, secondary to neuropathy. The clinician should be aware of this when considering obtaining x-rays on these patients.

Fractures

A *fracture* is a break in the continuity of a bone. Fractures are usually associated with a blunt force. Fractures are classified as *open* or *closed,* depending on whether they communicate with the external environment (i.e., through broken skin). Open fractures have an increased incidence of infection and must be aggressively treated. Many need to be surgically irrigated. Fractures can also be partial or complete. A *partial fracture* involves disruption of only a portion of the cortex, whereas a *complete fracture* involves circumferential disruption of the cortex. Complete fractures are unstable, and inappropriate initial stabilization can lead to additional injuries to the muscles or neurovascular structures.

When assessing the patient, the clinician should ask about the mechanism of injury. Fractures can occur at locations other than the obvious site of injury. The force can be transmitted to other areas of the body, causing fractures at distant sites. A person who fell off a roof and landed on his or her feet may have an obvious calcaneus (heel bone) fracture, but in addition, fractures of the hips, pelvis, and back must also be ruled out.

The goal of fracture management is to align the bones in a near-normal plane in order to allow the fragmented ends to heal together and return to normal function. The initial phase of healing starts with hematoma formation. This bridges the fractured fragments. The inflammatory phase follows, and granulation tissue forms on the fracture surfaces. During this process, the hematoma is reabsorbed, which provides the first continuity between the fragments. This occurs approximately 10 to 14 days after the injury. During this time, the bone surrounding the fracture line becomes less dense. This makes the fracture line easier to identify.

Callus is then formed on both the periosteal and endosteal surfaces of the bone, which acts as a biological splint. The calcification of the bone then begins. First, calcium phosphate is deposited, and then the bone undergoes osseous metaplasia. It takes approximately 2 to 3 weeks for the callus to be visible on x-rays. The callus is then slowly reabsorbed, and the fracture surfaces develop a firm bony union. During this phase, the calcified region undergoes organization, and the peripheral margins begin to smoothen. The process ends with remodeling and then consolidation. In a healthy adult, the whole process takes approximately 2 months for smaller long bones (such as the humerus) and up to 4 months for large bones (such as the femur).

CLINICAL PRESENTATION

Subjective

The predominant symptoms of a musculoskeletal injury are pain and disability. The history and mechanism of injury will help guide further assessment, including physical examination. The clinical presentation of the injury will help to focus on both obvious and occult areas of injury.

Objective

The importance of performing a thorough and complete physical examination for musculoskeletal injuries cannot be overemphasized. The signs of a musculoskeletal injury may include one or more of the following: tenderness, swelling, deformity, and abnormal range of motion (see Chapter 52). Life-threatening and occult injuries must be identified quickly. This is facilitated by completing a rapid initial survey, which can be accomplished in 90 seconds by an experienced practitioner. Following this primary survey, a more thorough secondary survey can be performed, during which fractures are typically identified.

DIAGNOSTIC REASONING

Diagnostic Tests

Suspected sites of musculoskeletal trauma must be radiographed to rule out fractures. Radiographic (x-ray) studies are the mainstay of orthopedic care, and it is critical that the clinician order the correct x-ray for the injury suspected. There are evidence-based guidelines to help clinicians choose the most appropriate imaging examination for patients' clinical condition. The latest version of the American College of Radiology (ACR) Appropriateness Criteria may be found on their website. Many x-ray studies include views of several joints and bones, but given the specialized nature of individual x-ray views, the clinician should focus on the area the specific x-ray examination is intended to visualize. Each x-ray examination uses a specific technique to ensure the correct joint angles, bony structures, and other information are included to allow the practitioner to rule out pathology to a specific region. If a patient has pain in the foot and the ankle, an ankle x-ray may miss foot pathology, and a foot x-ray may miss ankle pathology. Advanced Assessment 73.3 presents guidelines on reading an extremity x-ray film.

Many clinicians order routine comparison views of the uninjured extremity, especially in children with open growth plates. This may be helpful on rare occasions; however, this practice should not be condoned, because it exposes a growing child to unnecessary radiation, when a thorough examination usually pinpoints the location of the injury. When examining an infant or a child who will not move or bear weight on an extremity, the clinician should palpate the entire extremity while observing the patient's facial expressions. When the injury is palpated, the patient's face will reveal discomfort, which will assist the clinician in localizing the injured site before ordering the appropriate radiographic studies. Joint and soft tissue injuries are typically best visualized on MRI, which requires expert interpretation.

Differential Diagnosis

The goal of differential diagnosis in musculoskeletal trauma is to distinguish more serious bony fractures from strains and sprains, because these injuries are treated differently. As joint swelling and tenderness is a common presentation of such injuries, it is critical to consider a variety of rheumatological and infectious disorders, such as a septic joint, rheumatoid arthritis, or osteoarthritis. An appropriate history that seeks to characterize any preceding musculoskeletal trauma will typically differentiate these conditions.

The differential diagnosis for fractures also includes *reflex sympathetic dystrophy.* Also known as Sudeck atrophy and causalgia, this post-traumatic syndrome has three clinical stages—*early, dystrophic,* and *atrophic.* Early in the condition, a constant aching or burning occurs in the affected limb. Motion or external stimulation increases the symptoms, usually out of proportion to the original injury. In the dystrophic stage that follows, the skin of the affected extremity becomes glossy and cold and range of motion is limited. Finally, the atrophic stage is marked by skin atrophy and contracture. No correlation exists between incidence or symptom severity and the extent or type of the original musculoskeletal injury. Thus, early diagnosis of this syndrome is difficult, especially after an apparently trivial injury. Early diagnosis is extremely important, however, because the earlier treatment is initiated, the better the response, which is aimed at restoration of limb function through physical therapy. Antidepressant therapy and prednisone may also be beneficial.

MANAGEMENT

Management of the patient with musculoskeletal trauma initially consists of PRICE therapy, as described later in this section. However, confirmation of the appropriately of this therapy may require diagnostic x-ray imaging to identify damage to the joints or bony structures. If the patient can be seen immediately in an outpatient setting with radiographic capabilities, the patient may choose to see his or her primary-care practitioner or to go to an urgent care center. Otherwise, the patient should proceed directly to the ED for diagnostic studies (i.e., radiography) and further intervention as needed.

General Management: Strains and Sprains

After appropriate stabilization and 2 to 3 days of rest and elevation of the affected body part, the injury site can be examined more easily. The pain and swelling typically will be reduced, which will facilitate a better physical examination. Injuries that had negative x-rays initially but were extremely painful or suspicious for fracture can be re-radiographed in 10 to 12 days and read with an appropriate technique to maximize the chances of observing a fracture (see Advanced Assessment 73.3). Because of the healing process, the fracture line can be more easily visualized at that time.

⚬ Advanced Assessment 73.3: Reading an Extremity X-Ray

- Conduct a thorough history and determine the mechanism of injury, prior to ordering radiographic studies. This will help to determine the location and type of injury to expect. The area of injury should be examined, as these procedures will focus attention to the area of suspicion on the film. Always review the x-ray film after an examination, even if it was originally viewed before examining the patient.

- Using a well-lighted viewing box, follow the bony cortex of the injured area, looking for any defects. The cortex should be smooth and crisp; any area of haziness or any defect needs to be scrutinized using a bright (hot) light.

- Look at the soft tissue surrounding the area of concern. Injuries will cause soft tissue swelling. This may help focus your attention on the injured area. Scrutinize this region with a bright (hot) light.

- Several regions of the body, especially joints, have certain signs to look for that may reflect an occult injury. Confer with the collaborating physician or refer the patient to an orthopedic physician if occult injury is suspected.

PRICE Therapy

Protection, rest, ice, compression, and elevation (PRICE) are the mainstay of treatment for musculoskeletal strains and sprains:

- Protection of the injury involves both prevention and protection. Protection may refer to preventing the injury from occuring or making it less severe by wearing protective gear, such as helmets, wrist pads, and kneepads.
- *Rest* means no use of the affected limb or joint for minor injuries or sprains for 1 to 2 days, followed by slowly increasing use of the limb as tolerated by the patient. If the patient's activity being performed causes pain to the injury site, the level of activity needs to be reduced to levels that do not cause pain. However, mild discomfort after activity is considered normal during the rehabilitation phase. Generally speaking, the amount of limb rest needed depends on the severity of the injury.
- *Ice,* a potent anti-inflammatory, should be applied in repeated cycles of 30 minutes on and 30 minutes off, three to five times per day, to the injured site. Ice should not be applied directly to the skin, but rather over fabric or other material that transmits cold but minimizes the risk of thermal damage to the skin. The time of application "on" the injured site should be reduced in elderly patients, while "off" periods are critical for all patients to prevent frostbite. Ice therapy for 24 to 48 hours after the injury is recommended, as well as during the rehabilitation phase if mild pain after activity occurs. After that period, warm and moist heat to the region is advocated to increase circulation to the area, which promotes reabsorption of blood and edema that has collected at the injury site.
- *Compression* by elastic wrap or other splinting material is used to provide counterpressure at the site of injury to help tamponade bleeding to the region. This will help decrease the amount of swelling and blood collection at the injury site. The influx of blood causes localized inflammation, which leads to leaking of plasma and other substances into the injured area. The compression wrap must always include the distal portion of the extremity (i.e., the foot or hand) in order to prevent a tourniquet effect.
- *Elevating* the affected limb above the level of the heart will decrease bleeding into the tissue surrounding the injury and help to reduce pain. After the first 48 hours, when bleeding into the area has stopped, elevation of the affected body part will facilitate reabsorption of blood and tissue fluid at the injury site.

Pain Management

The use of NSAIDs for pain management is also recommended in conjunction with PRICE therapy. Muscle relaxants such as cyclobenzaprine (Flexeril) may be indicated for the management of acute painful musculoskeletal conditions associated with muscle spasm. They reduce tonic somatic muscle activity at the level of the brainstem.

General Management: Fractures

Initial fracture care involves stabilization of the bone ends to avoid further injury or damage to neurovascular structures. Immediate temporary splinting should be instituted. Patients with severely angulated long bone fractures should be transferred to an ED for sedation and straightened before they are splinted. Splints should be applied in such a way as to immobilize the joints above and below the fracture site to avoid motion of the bone ends involved. Commercially available metal and plastic splints are used for this purpose.

After radiographic assessment and confirmation of a non-displaced fracture, a more permanent splint should be applied. During immobilization, the clinician must consider the fact that fracture sites will continue to swell in the first 24 to 48 hours. In turn, placing a rigid circumferential cast on the patient in the first 24 to 48 hours can lead to vascular compromise and limb-threatening compartment syndrome. To avoid this, a plaster splint is placed on only half of the limb and can be adjusted or molded to allow optimal stabilization of certain fractures. The skin should be padded to avoid local necrosis, and the splint should be secured by an elastic bandage. This type of splint allows the extremity to swell without affecting distal circulation.

Even with the proper x-ray technique, some fractures are not visible initially and will not appear until 7 to 10 days after the injury. At that time, the margins of the fracture absorb and will widen the radiolucent line at the fracture site. New bone will also be produced beneath the periosteum at the margins of the fracture, which will accentuate the fracture line. This will allow fractures that were not identified initially to be visualized. If a fracture is suspected but not visible at the initial visit, the injury should be treated as a fracture and reexamined clinically and radiographically in 7 to 10 days. The patient should be informed of the rationale for this treatment. It is good practice to always add this to the patient's discharge instructions in writing and have the patient sign his or her understanding.

Oblique fractures typically heal more quickly than transverse ones. Children tend to heal more quickly than adults and older patients more slowly. Radiologic evidence of abundant organized callus formation at the fracture site, with bone ends that have remained stable on serial films, suggests stabilization of the fracture. Limited physical and weight-bearing activity for the affected limb is recommended until full strength is returned.

FOLLOW-UP AND REFERRAL

The patient should be reexamined by an orthopedic surgeon in 3 to 4 days after application of a cast or splint to evaluate his or her neuromuscular status. In addition, the patient should be instructed to report any of the following signs and symptoms, which may reflect compartment syndrome—intense pain, hypoesthesia (a dulled sensitivity to touch), paresthesia (numbness, prickling, or tickling), muscular weakness, swelling and color change of the digits (fingers or toes), or paralysis. The patient with these signs should be referred to an orthopedic surgeon immediately. In 6 weeks to 2 months after cast placement, a follow-up visit with an orthopedic surgeon and an x-ray of the injured area will determine whether bone consolidation has occurred and if the cast can be removed.

Patient Education: Musculoskeletal Trauma

Any site of a previous bony fracture will be weakened no matter how long after healing, and this site will always be more prone to a second fracture. Patients should always take this into account when deciding on what type of exercise or musculoskeletal activity in which to engage. In the future, it may be possible to predict which patients are at higher risk for fractures. Single bone mineral density measurements may be able to predict the risk of fragility fractures (e.g., distal radius, proximal humerus, hip, and vertebra) in women. This would help identify patients who would benefit from teaching and prevention strategies.

To avoid musculoskeletal injury, good physical conditioning is important. Consistent activity and exercise will strengthen muscles and reduce the chance of injury.

PNEUMOTHORAX AND HEMOTHORAX

Pneumothorax refers to the abnormal presence of air in the potential space between the parietal and visceral pleura in the thorax. *Hemothorax* refers to the abnormal presence of blood in the same region. For this potential space to become occupied by air or blood, there must be an injury to one of the pleurae. A pneumothorax is described as *closed* if the chest wall is intact or *open* if the chest is violated and communicates with the atmosphere.

EPIDEMIOLOGY AND CAUSES

Pneumothorax and hemothorax are usually the result of a trauma that penetrates the chest wall and violates the parietal pleura or of a blunt force trauma that fractures ribs, which violate the parietal or visceral pleura. These conditions can also be complications of in-hospital or emergency instrumentation in the chest, such as placement of a central venous line or arterial catheter that accidentally punctures the lung. In turn, these patients rarely seek care in outpatient settings.

Most patients (60%) who have suffered a penetrating or high-energy blunt trauma to the chest will develop a hemothorax and/or pneumothorax. A pneumothorax

(in 25% of patients) or other extrathoracic injuries (in 13%) will usually accompany a hemothorax. The etiology of pneumothorax can be traumatic (e.g., ribs piercing the pleura as a result of a motor vehicle accident), iatrogenic (e.g., a complication of central line insertion), idiopathic (spontaneous), or related to an underlying disease process (e.g., a ruptured emphysematous bleb in the lung apices in a patient with chronic obstructive pulmonary disease [COPD]). With the increased incidence of COPD, pneumothorax is becoming more common in the primary-care setting.

Spontaneous pneumothorax, which accounts for two-thirds of all pneumothoraxes, occurs most commonly and is more prevalent in tall, slender young men. It is usually the result of a rupture of a superficial bleb, which is an outpouching defect on the lung surface. Such defects may be inherited or related to forces placed on the lung during growth, development, and remodeling of inflammatory lung tissue. Cigarette smoking clearly predisposes an individual to bleb formation and spontaneous pneumothorax with a clear dose–response relationship, likely due to repeated inflammatory insults to the lung parenchyma.

Patients with connective tissue disorders, such as Marfan syndrome or homocystinuria, are also susceptible to spontaneous pneumothorax. In addition, women with thoracic endometriosis may suffer from recurrent catamenial pneumothorax or hemothorax, which are related to their menstrual cycles and bleeding from extrauterine endometrial implants. Catamenial pneumothorax occurs within 72 hours before or after the menstrual cycle. Thirty percent to 50% of patients with a history of spontaneous pneumothorax will have a recurrence of this condition.

Secondary pneumothorax is most often due to underlying emphysematous COPD or HIV-associated *Pneumocystis jiroveci* (formerly known as *Pneumocystis carinii*) pneumonia. Other etiologies for the clinician to consider include asthma, neoplasms, as well as pulmonary infarction. Other common predisposing conditions include cystic fibrosis and other conditions that cause significant bronchiectasis, as well as any cavitary lung infection, such as tuberculosis, in which cavities may rupture through the parietal pleura, leading to gas escape into the pleural space. Hemothorax may similarly result when cavitary lung lesions invade both blood vessels and the parietal pleura. However, penetrating chest trauma remains the primary cause of hemothorax.

PATHOPHYSIOLOGY

Although the underlying etiology of pneumothorax and hemothorax varies widely as described in the preceding text, the collection of either gas or blood within the pleural space ultimately results from a similar pathophysiological mechanism. The thorax contains the lungs, heart, and major blood vessels. A visceral pleural layer surrounds the outer surface of the lungs, and the chest wall is lined with a parietal pleural layer. The pleural space is a potential space resulting from the apposition of the two pleural membranes. The pleural cells that line the lungs and chest wall continually absorb any gas or fluid that collects in the pleural space, which maintains a negative pressure of −10 to −12 mm Hg. This thoracic pressure differential allows the lungs to expand during inspiration. Any trauma or membrane rupture that results in violation of either pleural membrane can eliminate this negative pressure and allow fluid or air to collect in this space. In turn, this has a negative impact on the ability of the lungs to expand effectively.

CLINICAL PRESENTATION

Subjective

The most frequent presenting symptoms in patients with pneumothorax and hemothorax are dyspnea and chest pain. The severity of the symptoms depends on the size of the pneumothorax or hemothorax. Typically, these conditions are associated with other injuries, which may mask the dyspnea or chest pain. For example, a patient who has a head injury or is unconscious may have altered breathing patterns related to a cerebral event. If the clinician is not alert to the possibility of chest pathology, a pneumothorax or hemothorax may be missed. Fractured ribs may mimic the type of pain encountered with a pneumothorax or hemothorax.

Objective

Because of decreased lung volume, patients with pneumothorax or hemothorax will usually have a lower than normal oxygen saturation and may present with cyanosis and varying levels of tachypnea and tachycardia. Lung sounds can be used to help determine the presence of a pneumothorax or hemothorax. Absent breath sounds on the affected side of the chest have a high positive predictive value for these conditions, but normal auscultation does not rule out the presence of pneumothorax or hemothorax. A patient with a large hemothorax can present with frank hypovolemic shock (low blood pressure).

DIAGNOSTIC REASONING

Diagnostic Tests

A high index of suspicion is needed when considering a pneumothorax or hemothorax. Any patient who has sustained blunt and/or penetrating chest trauma must have upright posterior-anterior and lateral chest x-rays to rule out pneumothorax or hemothorax. A supine chest x-ray can miss many significant thoracic injuries and should not be relied on to rule out these conditions. If rib x-rays are the only type of film ordered, the proper technique for this type of x-ray study may actually obscure the subtle radiographic findings of a pneumothorax.

When a pneumothorax is present, a subtle light line will be noted—this is the edge of the lung tissue. Beyond that point, the pleural cavity will have absent lung markings. It is helpful to use a bright viewing box, position the x-ray horizontally, and focus on the lateral and lateral-superior aspects of the pleural cavity, where the most pathology is found. If a pneumothorax is suspected but not found on an inspiratory chest film, the clinician should request an expiratory chest x-ray. During the expiratory phase, the thoracic volume is decreased, and the relative size of the pneumothorax is increased and, thus, may be more easily visualized. A pneumothorax is measured as a percentage of thoracic volume. A mild pneumothorax is less than 15%, a moderate one is 15 to 60%, and a severe one is more than 60% of thoracic volume.

If a hemothorax is suspected, the clinician should order a lateral decubitus view, which will reveal the shifting of blood to the lowest part of the pleural cavity. If doubt still exists or a more accurate determination of size of the defect is required, a chest CT scan is the definitive test.

Differential Diagnosis

The differential diagnoses for pneumothorax and/or hemothorax include pneumonia, pulmonary embolism, myocardial infarction, angina, and intercostal muscle strain. As the physical manifestations of these conditions may be similar, it is important to order the correct diagnostic tests, as well as to determine the cause of any confirmed pneumothorax or hemothorax.

MANAGEMENT

Most cases of pneumothorax can be treated in a non-urgent manner, although patients with significant respiratory distress will respond quickly to insertion of a chest tube. The patient with a pneumothorax or hemothorax is usually cared for and managed in the ED, where a chest tube is typically placed to facilitate drainage of air and blood. Thus, if a primary-care practitioner suspects that a patient presenting to a primary-care setting has a pneumothorax and/or hemothorax, EMS should be activated, the patient's respiratory and cardiovascular status should be evaluated and supported as needed, and the patient should be transported to the ED immediately. Patients should be placed on supplemental oxygen (up to 100% for a significant pneumothorax), even if the O_2 saturation is normal on room air, as this helps resorption of the pneumothorax. Patients with a tension pneumothorax require immediate stabilizing treatment (Box 73.3).

FOLLOW-UP AND REFERRAL

After a period of observation, patients with a mild pneumothorax who do not require a chest tube can be discharged with continued follow-up in 1 to 2 days. Patients with a large pneumothorax, a tension pneumothorax, or a hemothorax requiring a chest tube should not be discharged until the pleura has been drained of blood, and the lung has been reexpanded for at least 24 hours. Strenuous exercise should be limited until the patient has fully recovered because it is possible to reopen and aggravate the pleural defect if it has not yet fully healed. The patient should be advised to follow-up with a primary-care practitioner in 1 week for a repeat chest radiograph to evaluate for re-expansion of the lung volumes. If the pneumothorax is not fully resolved at this time, the patient should be referred to a cardiothoracic surgeon.

Box 73.3 Tension Pneumothorax

Patients with a tension pneumothorax usually have penetrating chest trauma, such as a gunshot or knife wound. A *tension pneumothorax* develops when air in the potential space between the parietal and visceral pleura is under pressure. The defect in the pleura allows air to enter the potential space during inspiration, but because of a flap mechanism (which functions like a one-way valve), air does not escape. This mechanism increases the pressure on the affected lung and, if not corrected, will lead to a complete collapse of that lung. If the defect is left untreated, the pressure will continue to increase and force the mediastinum to the unaffected side. This will cause the major blood vessels to kink and restrict normal blood flow to and from the heart, which can cause death within minutes.

A tension pneumothorax is a medical emergency and must be treated immediately. There is no time for x-ray evaluation to diagnose this condition. The emergent stabilizing treatment involves performing a needle thoracostomy. This is accomplished by inserting a large-bore (18-gauge or larger) needle into the chest. The needle should be inserted between the second and third ribs in the intercostal space at the midclavicular line. The needle should be inserted just over the third rib to avoid penetrating the neurovascular bundle that runs parallel to each rib along the inferior border.

Patient Education: Pneumothorax and Hemothorax

Patients who have been diagnosed with a spontaneous pneumothorax should be counseled that 23% to 30% of patients will have a recurrence at some point. An explanation of the signs and symptoms to watch for—dyspnea, persistent cough, and chest pain—should be given to all patients, regardless of the type of pneumothorax. The clinician should consider consulting a respiratory therapist before discharge to initiate incentive spirometry teaching for home use, as an aid in recurrence prevention.

FOREIGN BODY OBSTRUCTIONS

This section discusses ear, nose, throat, vaginal, and rectal foreign body (FB) obstructions. As FB obstructions may be an emergency, patients may present at whichever clinic or ED is the closest.

EPIDEMIOLOGY AND CAUSES

Foreign body obstructions are a common complaint seen in both the primary-care and urgent care settings. Most of these problems involve children, although adults may also present with this problem, either due to accidental or intentional insertion of a foreign body into a bodily orifice.

PATHOPHYSIOLOGY

The pathophysiology of a foreign body obstruction depends on the orifice that is obstructed. Otic (ear canal) occlusion may contribute to otitis externa or otitis media, especially if the tympanic membrane is ruptured. Nasal occlusion may predispose to rhinitis, sinusitis, malodorous discharge, or epistaxis (nosebleed). Moreover, nasal, pharyngeal, tracheal, or even esophageal occlusion may all result in varying degrees of respiratory compromise, if the respiratory tract is at all obstructed either internally or via external compression on the airway.

A vaginal occlusion, if unattended, can lead to toxic shock syndrome (mediated by infection with *Staphylococcus aureus* or *Streptococcus pyogenes*) or pelvic inflammatory disease. A bowel obstruction may result from a foreign body occluding the rectum if the object inserted is high enough in the GI tract. Early diagnosis and intervention will best protect against adverse effects from prolonged obstruction.

CLINICAL PRESENTATION

Subjective

The patient or caregiver (e.g., a parent, in the case of pediatric patients) will present with a complaint of a lodged foreign body, with signs and symptoms specific to the bodily orifice involved. However, if the individual is unaware of the presence of a foreign body, such as in the case of a forgotten tampon left in place, the patient may complain of a foul-smelling discharge from the affected orifice (such as the vagina). Thus, prolonged obstruction by a foreign body may lead to localized infection within the bodily orifice or even systemic symptoms, such as in toxic shock syndrome. In addition, a nasal or otic occlusion may lead to a feeling of head fullness or headache. Of note, many of these affected patients are children who may or may not be able to fully express their discomfort or pain verbally.

Objective

Based on the patient's signs and symptoms and the orifice involved, clinical signs of foreign body obstruction will vary:

- Ear: Foreign bodies in the auditory canal are common problems, especially in children. Foreign bodies can be vegetative, inanimate, or animate objects. Foreign bodies in the ear are usually asymptomatic unless they are left in the ear for a prolonged period of time and an infection develops. An insect or piece of cotton caught in the ear may cause equilibrium problems, dizziness, tinnitus, and diminished hearing on the affected side. The clinician should obtain a complete history to elicit whether there is a possibility of multiple foreign bodies. The practitioner should assess both ears to obtain a comparison view. It is important to try to ensure that there is no perforation of the tympanic membrane before trying to remove the foreign body. Some patients (especially children) can have a foreign body in the ear for such a long period that cerumen will eventually mask the foreign body.
- Nose: Nasal foreign bodies are most commonly seen in children. A foreign body in the nose of an adult is rare, unless the patient is significantly physically debilitated or has severe dementia, as insects have been known to lodge in the nose or ear of such patients. A foreign body obstruction may cause purulent discharge from the nares. The patient history is important, but children are usually reluctant to admit to what or how many objects they have placed into their nose. The diagnosis is made by direct visualization.
- Throat: Swallowed objects that become lodged in the throat are commonly seen by the primary-care practitioner. Usually, they are not life-threatening, but any object that becomes lodged in a position where it can obstruct the airway is a true emergency. If the object becomes lodged in the esophagus, the adult patient may present with the feeling of an object in the throat, pain, and the inability to swallow secretions and food. Pediatric patients may present with vomiting, gagging, choking, stridor, an inability to swallow, increased salivation, and a sensation of a foreign body in the chest.
- Vagina: Vaginal foreign bodies can be the result of children exploring their sexuality or an incident of child abuse. In adults, the foreign body may be a forgotten tampon, diaphragm, or cervical cap; however, the insertion of other objects into the vagina should also raise the suspicion of domestic violence in adults. A vaginal occlusion may result in a foul-smelling vaginal discharge. Emotional support and reassurance is important to patients (and parents).
- Rectum: A variety of objects have been inserted into the rectum, either accidentally or intentionally. A rectal occlusion may cause abdominal cramping, an increase in bowel sounds, and abdominal distention. As with objects inserted into the genitourinary tract, foreign body obstructions in the rectum should raise the suspicion of domestic violence or abuse, requiring an appropriate assessment and referrals, as needed.

DIAGNOSTIC REASONING

Diagnostic Tests

Diagnostic tests are usually not indicated, but radiological studies may be appropriate if physical examination is insufficient to fully characterize the obstructing object. However, because the majority of foreign bodies are not radiopaque, x-ray findings may be quite subtle, requiring formal interpretation by a radiologist. In some cases, direct endoscopy of the nasopharyngeal, respiratory, or GI tracts by properly trained professionals may be required to identify and remove the obstructing object.

Differential Diagnosis

The diagnosis is usually obvious from the patient's complaints and physical examination.

MANAGEMENT

Emergency Management

The clinician may attempt to remove the foreign body in the office, if the appropriate equipment is available.

This is typically limited to obstructions of the otic and nasal canals, if the foreign object is not inserted deeply. If the attempt is unsuccessful, the patient should be sent to an ED. In addition, obstructions in the rectum or vagina may be more complex to remove if inserted deeply or tightly, given the risk of tearing to the mucosa and bleeding. In addition, a more thorough evaluation than is capable in a primary-care or urgent care setting may be needed to ensure all foreign material is removed from the GI or genitourinary tracts, given the risk of severe systemic infection associated with retained foreign material.

General Management

The general management of ear, nose, throat, vaginal, and rectal foreign body obstructions is as follows.

Ears

Removal of inanimate objects is not always straightforward. If the patient is uncooperative or if the foreign body is difficult to grasp, ear, nose, and throat (ENT) consultation is suggested. If the object becomes lodged too deeply, it will be difficult to remove, and the patient may need general anesthesia for successful removal. If the object is small, irrigation is an option. If the object is appropriately shaped and accessible, alligator or bayonet forceps may be used to grasp and remove it. Suctioning may also assist in the removal of an object. A Yankauer suction catheter has a small orifice and a firm catheter tip that may facilitate foreign body removal.

A live insect trapped in the ear canal usually causes great distress. The patient will present with agitation, nausea, and tearing. The initial therapy is to immobilize the insect. This can be done by placing 2% lidocaine in the external ear canal, which will terminate the movement of the insect. The insect can then be removed using forceps.

After successful removal of the object, the ear canal needs to be checked for infections, superficial scratches, and tympanic membrane perforation. If there is no evidence of infection, the patient may be discharged home. If an infection is present, it should be treated as an otitis with appropriate antibiotics.

Nose

If the patient is uncooperative, a restraining device or sedation may be needed. If the patient is cooperative, the following steps may be used to remove the foreign body:

- Help the patient to blow his or her nose to see if the foreign object will be expelled.

- If the mucosa appears swollen, soak a pledget in a liquid decongestant such as phenylephrine (Neo-Synephrine) nasal spray and insert it into the affected nare to reduce swelling; care should be taken not to push the foreign body further into the nose.

- Using a nasal speculum and alligator or bayonet forceps, visualize the foreign body and gently remove it. Other methods include using an ear curette, single skin hook, or right-angle ear hook. Another method that has been used is to pass a small urinary catheter superior to (beyond) the object, inflate the balloon, and pull the object out, although this method should only be attempted by a properly trained clinician.

- All of these methods can be successful if the patient is cooperative. Care must be taken not to push the foreign body down the back of the patient's throat, where it may be aspirated into the trachea.

After successfully removing the object, the clinician should inspect the nares for other foreign bodies. No further treatment is necessary unless local infection is apparent, in which case appropriate antibiotic therapy is indicated. If removal is unsuccessful, however, referral to an ENT specialist may be necessary.

Throat

Although most swallowed objects will pass spontaneously, up to 10% to 20% require some type of intervention. There are several physiological narrow spaces in the esophageal-gastrointestinal tract that may restrict the movement of objects. In the pediatric population, the cricopharyngeal area is the most common site for obstruction, followed by (in order of frequency) the thoracic inlet, aortic arch, tracheal bifurcation, and hiatal narrowing. The majority of obstructions in adults occur at the distal end of the esophagus. Usually once the object has passed through the pylorus, it will pass through the rest of the GI tract without difficulty. If the object has sharp edges, however, it can injure the intestines and/or become lodged anywhere in the gastrointestinal tract. Ingested foreign bodies can also cause airway obstruction or perforation.

If there is a possible foreign body ingestion, a chest x-ray should be ordered to see if the object is lodged in the esophagus, although foreign bodies will only be visualized if they are radiopaque. If the object is in the stomach, the patient should be monitored for passage of the object through the GI tract. The stool will need to be examined. If the object is not found, an abdominal flat-plate x-ray can be used to determine the location of the object. Objects that fail to be expelled may have to be removed by invasive procedures such as colonoscopy or surgery.

The treatment for ingestion of a sharp object is controversial. Most practitioners recommend that sharp objects be removed so that they do not cause a perforation before they pass into the intestine.

A food bolus is usually the cause of ingested foreign bodies in the adult population. Typically, inadequately chewed meat is the main culprit. If the patient is unable to swallow salivary secretions, a chest x-ray should be obtained. Glucagon, a smooth-muscle relaxant, may be administered intravenously to relax the esophagus: a 1-mg dose is given IV and may be repeated after 20 minutes, if the object has not passed. The patient will usually vomit, which causes the foreign body to be expelled; it is important to ensure that the patient does not aspirate the vomitus. If glucagon has not produced the desired outcome, a GI consultation should be obtained. Some references recommend a barium swallow to visualize where the obstruction is located; however, most GI specialists prefer that no barium be given because it can obstruct the view of the bolus during endoscopy.

If a coin becomes lodged in the esophagus, it should be removed by endoscopy. Two other methods that may be tried by properly trained clinicians include passing an indwelling urinary catheter behind the object, inflating it, and pulling the object out. Smaller objects that become lodged in the esophagus can also be safely pushed into the stomach by a small urinary catheter.

In contrast, ingestion of button batteries is a true emergency situation. The batteries can cause burns to the gastrointestinal mucosa and must be removed quickly, as mucosal perforations may prove fatal.

Vagina

Typically, the only medical treatment necessary is removal of the foreign body, as most of the discharge and foul odor will disappear after the foreign body is removed. Privacy must be maintained to avoid undue embarrassment. If the foreign body is lodged in the side wall of the vagina, the clinician should irrigate the area with normal saline to gently remove the object from the wall. If a foreign body is suspected in a small child, referral to an ED or hospital setting for general anesthesia for exploration should be considered, if the object is not visible and cannot be removed by gently pulling on the labia.

Systemic signs of infection require an immediate referral to a more advanced clinical setting, given the risk of toxic shock syndrome from retained foreign material in the vagina. Antibiotic therapy is indicated, and a more thorough evaluation may be needed to ensure all foreign material has been successfully removed from the vagina.

Rectum

Foreign objects are usually found in the rectal ampulla and are palpable with digital examination. All patients presenting with the chief complaint of a foreign body in the rectum need x-ray examinations of the abdomen to reveal the position, shape, and number of foreign bodies in the rectum. A lateral decubitus abdominal film will also show if free air is present in the abdomen. This is indicative of a perforation of the bowel, which is the most serious potential complication and required immediate ED referral.

Removal of a foreign body from the rectum requires that the rectal sphincter be relaxed. If a brief attempt at removing the foreign body is unsuccessful, the practitioner should refer the patient to an ED for possible conscious sedation to relax the sphincter muscle. Conscious sedation requires close monitoring and is best carried out in an inpatient or emergency care setting. If there is any possibility of perforation, an emergent GI consultation is needed.

FOLLOW-UP AND REFERRAL

Follow-up is usually not indicated once the foreign body is removed. However, the patient should be alerted to signs and symptoms of an infection should one occur after removal, given the risk of severe systemic infection associated with retained foreign material in the genitourinary tract, in particular. If a rectal perforation has occurred as a result of a foreign body insertion or during its removal, an emergency gastroenterology referral is indicated.

Patient Education: Foreign Body Obstruction

Because children are usually involved in foreign body incidents, prevention is essential. Parents should be encouraged to buy age-appropriate toys and to keep small objects out of the reach of children. Also, children should be taught not to put objects in the various orifices of their bodies.

It should also not be assumed that foreign body obstructions in adults always occur accidentally, and an open and frank discussion of the risks of certain sexual practices or self-care (hygiene) behaviors may be needed, if it becomes apparent that the insertion of foreign bodies into the vagina or rectum was voluntary. Moreover, a domestic violence assessment with appropriate social service and police referrals should be completed on any patient presenting with a genitourinary or gastrointestinal foreign body obstruction, as a nonaccidental insertion may nonetheless be involuntary for the patient.

REFERENCES

General

Resnick LA, Shufeldt J. *The textbook of urgent care medicine*. Scottsdale, AZ: UrgentCare Textbooks; 2014.

Animal and Human Bites

Endom EE. Initial management of animal and human bites. http://www.uptodate.com/contents/initial-management-of-animal-and-human-bites. Published October 25, 2012.

Rivera J. Animal bite accident statistics. LegalMatch. http://www.legalmatch.com/law-library/article/animal-bite-accident-statistics.html. Published 2014. Accessed July 10, 2017.

Burns

American Burn Association. Burn incidence fact sheet. Burn incidence and treatment in the United States: 2016. http://ameriburn.org/who-we-are/media/burn-incidence-fact-sheet/. Accessed July 10, 2017.

Lee F, et al. Evidence behind the WHO guidelines: Hospital care for children: What is the role of prophylactic antibiotics in the management of burns? *J Trop Pediatr*. 2009;55:73–77.

Wasiak J, Cleland H. Burns: dressings. Systematic review 1903. *BMJ Clin Evid*. 2015;2015.

Foreign Body Obstructions

Colyar MR. *Advanced practice nursing procedures*. Philadelphia, PA: FA Davis; 2015.

Head Trauma

Centers for Disease Control and Prevention, National Center for Injury Prevention and Control, Division of Unintentional Injury Prevention. Traumatic brain injury & concussion. https://www.cdc.gov/traumaticbraininjury/get_the_facts.html. Published 2017.

Harmon KG, Drezner JA, Gammons M, et al. American Medical Society for Sports Medicine position statement: Concussion in sport. *Clin J Sport Med*. 2013;23(1):1–18.

Musculoskeletal Trauma

ACR Appropriateness Criteria. 2017 ACR appropriateness criteria. https://www.acr.org/Quality-Safety/Appropriateness-Criteria. Accessed July 10, 2017.

Statistics on Fractures. (2015). Statistics about fractures. Right Diagnosis. http://www.rightdiagnosis.com/f/fractures/stats.htm#medical_stats. Published 2015. Accessed July 10, 2017.

Pneumothorax and Hemothorax

Bintcliffe O, Maskell N. Spontaneous pneumothorax. *BMJ*. 2014;348:g2928.

Broderick SR. Hemothorax: Etiology, diagnosis, and management. *Thorac Surg Clin*. 2013;23(1):89–96, vi–vii.

Wounds and Lacerations

Daum RS, Miller LG, Immergluck L, Fritz S, et al. A placebo-controlled trial of antibiotics for smaller skin abscesses. *N Engl J Med*. 2017;376:2545–2555.

Ludtke H. Abscess incision and drainage. Society for Academic Emergency Medicine. https://www.saem.org/cdem/education/online-education/m3-curriculum/group-emergency-department-procedures/abscess-incision-and-drainage. Accessed July 5, 2017.

Storer A, Lindauer C, Proehl J, et al. Emergency nursing resource: Wound preparation. *J Emerg Nurs*. 2012;38(5):443–446.

RESOURCES

Burns

America Burn Association
   www.ameriburn.org
The Burn Resource Center
   www.burnsurvivor.com
UV Index. United States Environmental Protection Agency
   https://www.epa.gov/sunsafety/uv-index-scale-1

Head Trauma

American Association of Neurological Surgeons/Congress of Neurological Surgeons (AANS)
   www.aans.org
MedlinePlus: Traumatic Brain Injuries
   http://nlm.nih.gov/medlineplus/headandbraininjuries.html

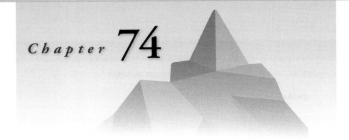

Chapter **74**

Toxic Exposures

Mae De La Calzada-Jeanlouie, DO, MS

Jill E. Winland-Brown, EdD, APRN, FNP-BC

Brian Oscar Porter, MD, PhD, MPH, MBA

POISONING

Poisons encompass a wide variety of toxic compounds, including pesticides, drug overdoses, carbon monoxide, as well as other toxins such as household chemicals and venom from biting or stinging organisms such as spiders, snakes, and scorpions.

EPIDEMIOLOGY AND CAUSES

According to 2015 data compiled by the U.S. Centers for Disease Control and Prevention, poisoning is the leading cause of injury-related death in the United States. In children younger than 5 years of age, poisonings are most often due to accidental ingestion. In the adolescent population, trauma and intentional self-harm are the first and second leading causes of death, and most adolescent and adult poisonings are self-inflicted and secondary to intentional ingestion.

It has been estimated that approximately 2.2 million poisoning accidents occur each year. The majority of these (46%) involve children, and more than 90% of all poisonings occur in the home. Adult toxicity events account for 80% to 90% of all hospital admissions due to poisonings. Most adult poisonings involve intentional ingestions, such as recreational drug exposures or suicidal gestures/attempts by overdose. The American Association of Poison Control Centers maintains a Toxic Exposure Surveillance System, which is a database of detailed toxicological information on more than 24 million poison exposures reported to U.S. poison control centers.

PATHOPHYSIOLOGY

The pathophysiology of poisonings varies widely, depending on the substance that the individual is exposed to and whether it is inhaled, topical, or ingested. Most

poisonings are dose-dependent. The diagnosis is usually made clinically and then supported by key laboratory evaluations.

For example, inhalation of motor vehicle exhaust leads to the chemical binding of carbon monoxide (CO) to hemoglobin in blood, thereby resulting in the formation of carboxyhemoglobin (COHb). COHb prevents the binding of oxygen to hemoglobin and the subsequent transport of oxygen to bodily tissues. While increasing COHb levels in the blood correlate to more severe clinical presentations, carbon monoxide poisoning may initially present in a clinically benign or ambiguous manner, such as with only a headache.

In contrast, a tricyclic antidepressant overdose (e.g., amitriptyline, nortriptyline, imipramine) can result in toxic cardiovascular and central nervous system (CNS) effects. These symptoms are secondary to the anticholinergic effects of the medication and alterations in cardiac cells. This leads to conduction disturbances such as QTc prolongation. Toxicology screening can confirm exposure through qualitative testing of urine or blood samples.

With a barbiturate overdose (e.g., phenobarbital), there is decreased neuronal activity, depressed central sympathetic tone, and inhibition of cardiac contractility. Barbiturates act directly on inhibitory gamma-aminobutyric acid (GABA) receptors by increasing the affinity of the GABA ligand to its cognate receptor, resulting in an increase in the average opening time of chloride ion channels. Benzodiazepines such as lorazepam (Ativan), alprazolam (Xanax), and diazepam (Valium) are also CNS depressants that enhance GABA receptor activity but at a molecularly distinct portion of the receptor. Benzodiazepines increase ligand affinity and the frequency of ion channel opening, but not the duration of time that the channel remains open. Given this mechanistic difference, benzodiazepines have less potential for toxicity than barbiturates, due to their saturable effects. Qualitative testing will confirm exposure to either barbiturates or benzodiazepines.

CLINICAL PRESENTATION

The primary-care practitioner should consider the clinical presentation of the specific type of poisoning suspected and confirm exposure with blood and urine toxicology screens when clinically warranted. Signs and symptoms of various types of poisonings are listed in Table 74.1.

Subjective

When evaluating an individual for a potential toxic exposure, the history is equally important to the physical examination of the encounter. The interview process can give the primary-care practitioner an opportunity to recognize possible exposures and understand the timeline of events. The clinician should consider obtaining

TABLE 74.1 Common Poisonings

Name/Type	Signs and Symptoms	Diagnosis	Management
Drugs			

Acetaminophen (Tylenol)	Varies; may be asymptomatic
	Nausea
	Vomiting
	24–48 hours postingestion:
	  Hepatic necrosis with jaundice
	  Hepatic encephalopathy
	  Renal failure
	  Possible death
		Acetaminophen level	Activated charcoal
			N-acetylcysteine IV (Acetadote) for 21 hours after ingestion

Barbiturates: Phenobarbital (Phenobarb) Pentobarbital sodium (Nembutal)	Decreased level of consciousness Drowsiness Confusion Ataxia Vertigo Slurred speech Shallow respirations Bradycardia Headache Cyanosis Hypothermia Cardiovascular collapse	Toxicology screen (urine or blood)	Gastric lavage with activated charcoal and cathartic agent Airway maintenance Ventilatory assistance Cardiovascular support
Benzodiazepines: Clorazepate dipotassium (Tranxene) Diazepam (Valium) Alprazolam (Xanax)	Central nervous system (CNS) depression Drowsiness Dizziness Headache Ataxia Hypotension Memory impairment	Toxicology screen (urine or blood)	Gastric lavage Symptomatic treatment Airway maintenance Ventilatory assistance Cardiovascular support
CNS stimulants: Methylphenidate (Ritalin, Concerta), amphetamine mixture (Adderall)	Vomiting Emotional lability Nervousness Fever Dizziness Hypertension Tachycardia Psychosis Dyskinesias Tourette's syndrome Seizures	Toxicology screen (urine or blood)	Supportive care
Cocaine	Nervous system stimulation Restlessness Hallucinations Tachycardia Dilated pupils Chills Fever Abdominal pain Vomiting Muscle spasms Irregular respirations, progressing to death	History of cocaine use Toxicology screen (urine or blood)	Diazepam (Valium) IV Emetic Gastric lavage Oxygen Symptomatic treatment

TABLE 74.1 Common Poisonings—cont'd

Name/Type	Signs and Symptoms	Diagnosis	Management
Heroin	Euphoria Flushing Pruritus Miosis Decreased level of consciousness Bradycardia Shallow, slow respirations Hypotension Hypothermia	History of heroin use Toxicology screen (urine or blood)	Maintain patent airway Oxygen Symptomatic treatment naloxone (Narcan) 2 mg IV
Lithium (Lithobid, Lithotabs, Duralith)	Vomiting Diarrhea Slurred speech Decreased coordination Drowsiness Muscle weakness or twitching	Cerebrospinal fluid lithium level Toxicology screen (urine or blood)	Gastric lavage Osmotic and saline diuresis (if renal function is normal) Urine alkalization Hemodialysis
Salicylates (aspirin, methylsalicylate)	Nausea Vomiting Gastritis Hyperpnea Tachypnea Tinnitus Agitation Confusion Coma Seizures Cardiovascular collapse Pulmonary edema Hyperthermia Possible death	Elevated prothrombin time Toxicology screen (blood) with a level >100 mg/dL Arterial blood gases reveal respiratory alkalosis (early) with underlying metabolic acidosis	Activated charcoal Gastric lavage Sodium bicarbonate IV Possible hemodialysis
Tricyclic antidepressants: Amitriptyline (Elavil), imipramine (Tofranil), nortriptyline (Pamelor) *Selective serotonin reuptake inhibitors (SSRIs) are relatively safe, even in overdose	Confusion Dizziness Decreased level of consciousness Hypotension Tachycardia Hyperthermia Mydriasis Dry mucous membranes Cardiac dysrhythmias Seizures	Toxicology screen (urine or blood)	Gastric decontamination with activated charcoal and cathartic agent Symptomatic treatment
Foods			
General food poisoning (foods consumed with toxins present)	Vomiting Abdominal cramping Afebrile	Toxins can be detected in food or stool specimens: *Staphylococcus aureus* *Bacillus cereus* *Clostridium perfringens* *Shigella* *Salmonella*	Fluids and electrolyte replacement Ciprofloxacin (use with caution, given adverse effect profile) Disease usually self-limited Anti-motility drugs
Poisonous fish	Abdominal cramps Nausea Vomiting Diarrhea Paresthesia Hypotension Respiratory paralysis	History of ingesting fish	Supportive treatment for symptoms

Continued

TABLE 74.1 Common Poisonings—cont'd

Name/Type	Signs and Symptoms	Diagnosis	Management
Scombroid fish poisoning (scombrotoxin-producing bacteria)	30 minutes to 2 hours after ingestion: Peppery sensation on the tongue Urticarial pruritic rash Headache Dizziness Periorbital edema Nausea Vomiting	History of ingesting fish	Gastric lavage Antihistamines Symptomatic treatment
Other Substances			
Arsenic	Metallic taste Garlic odor to breath Burning pain throughout Gastrointestinal (GI) tract Vomiting Dehydration Shock Seizures	Toxicology screen and/or attempt to discover type of material ingested by investigating all suspect containers	Gastric lavage Fluid and electrolyte management Treat shock and pulmonary edema Possible blood transfusions
Carbon monoxide	Deep respirations Pink (cherry red) tissues and skin (with carboxyhemoglobin [COHb]↑ 30%) Initial bradycardia, progressing to tachycardia Pounding pulse Dizziness Paresis Tinnitus Headache Faintness Nausea Dilated pupils	Carboxyhemoglobin (COHb) ↑	Supplemental oxygen via non-rebreather mask 100% oxygen under hyperbaric pressure (moderate to severe) Symptomatic treatment
Corrosive materials: Lysol, tincture of iodine, carbolic acid (phenol)	Burned tissues along gastrointestinal tract Brownish stains on lips and tongue Stridor from laryngeal swelling Nausea Vomiting Abdominal cramps Hematemesis Watery, mucoid, or bloody stools Violet or black mucous membranes Carbolic acid—white or gray mucous membranes Hydrochloric acid—grayish mucous membranes Nitric acid—yellowish mucous membranes Sulfuric acid—tan or dark-stained mucous membranes	Order toxicology screen and/or attempt to discover type of material ingested by investigating all suspect containers	Opiates for pain Possible tracheostomy Aggressive fluid and electrolyte resuscitation Antibiotics Corticosteroids

TABLE 74.1 Common Poisonings—cont'd

Name/Type	Signs and Symptoms	Diagnosis	Management
Iodine	Brown stains on lips and mouth Burning pain in mouth and throat Yellow emesis (blue if starch is present)	Diagnosis based on symptoms and open or empty container found at scene	Cornstarch or flour solution: 15 g in 2 cups of water given orally if patient is conscious or via gastric lavage if patient is comatose Morphine sulfate for pain
Lead: lead-based paints, lead-contaminated dust, hobbies (e.g., stained-glass windows)	Colicky abdominal pain Constipation Headache Irritability Coma Convulsions Chronic poisoning—learning disorders in children Motor neuropathy (wrist drop)	Blood levels: 10–50 mcg/dL—mild toxicity 50–70 mcg/dL—moderate toxicity 70–100 mcg/dL—severe toxicity Microcytic anemia	*Up to moderate toxicity:* Edetate calcium disodium (EDTA) Oral chelator—succimer (dimercaptosuccinic acid [DMSA]) *Severe toxicity:* EDTA IV (continuous infusion) dimercaprol (British Anti-Lewisite or BAL) IM
Strychnine	Sense of suffocation Cyanosis Dyspnea Hypoventilation Tachycardia Muscle rigidity Contractions Seizures	Lactic acidosis Metabolic acidosis	Gastric lavage Oxygen Sedatives Supportive care

additional information from friends and family who may provide supplemental details. Additionally, the clinician must remain mindful that a lack of symptoms does not preclude the possibility of an ingestion or exposure.

Objective

A toxic syndrome, or toxidrome, is a constellation of signs and symptoms associated with a distinct group of xenobiotics. Early assessment and clinical recognition can assist the provider in identifying potential ingestions and anticipate complications of toxicity. The five most common toxidromes are classified as follows: sympathomimetic, anticholinergic, cholinergic, sedative hypnotic/ethanol, and opioid. Each syndrome is characterized by vital signs and end organ manifestations associated with several bodily systems, as summarized in Table 74.2.

Evaluation of the poisoned patient begins with the primary survey: airway, breathing, and circulation (ABC). Barring clinical decompensation, evaluation for signs of trauma and central nervous system involvement should subsequently commence. Furthermore, individuals with a reported toxic ingestion or overdose should undergo an ECG (electrocardiogram), as specific findings can suggest exposure to certain agents. Radiographic studies may identify radiopaque foreign bodies (e.g., coins, needles) or capture substantial ingestions (e.g., concretion of pills, illicit drug body packers).

DIAGNOSTIC REASONING

Diagnostic Tests

Diagnostic testing will vary depending on the potential toxin(s). Laboratory testing includes a basic metabolic panel, liver function test panel, coagulation profile (PT/PTT/INR), lactic acid level, acetaminophen level, acetylsalicylic acid level, and urinalysis. A urine toxicology screen can be obtained, although the presence of a toxin does not confirm poisoning, but rather only exposure. In the setting of a known ingestion, quantitative levels of the specific substance can be obtained. However, depending on available laboratory testing equipment, specimens may need to be sent to an outside reference laboratory for certain tests.

Differential Diagnosis

A variety of clinical conditions can mimic each of the toxidromes; therefore, the primary-care practitioner should maintain a broad differential diagnosis

TABLE 74.2 Common Toxidromes: Clinical Manifestations						
Toxidrome	*Vital Signs*	*Mental Status*	*Pupils*	*Gastrointestinal*	*Skin*	*Other*
Sympathomimetic	↑ BP ↑ HR ↑ T	Agitated	Mydriasis	Normal/ hypoactive bowel sounds	Flushed Diaphoresis	Tremors Seizures
Anticholinergic	↑ BP ↑ HR ↑ T	Delirium	Mydriasis	Hypoactive bowel sounds	Flushed Dry	Urinary retention Dry mucous membranes
Cholinergic	±BP ±HR ↓ T	Normal Confusion Weakness	Varies	Hyperactive bowel sounds	Diaphoresis	**SLUDGE** **S**alivation **L**acrimation **U**rination **D**iarrhea **G**astrointestinal distress **E**mesis
Sedative hypnotic/ ethanol	↓ BP ↓ HR ↓ RR ↓ T	Depressed Confusion Coma	Varies	Hypoactive bowel sounds	Normal	Hyporeflexia
Opioids	↓ BP ↓ HR ↓ RR ↓ T	Depressed Confusion Coma	Miosis	Hypoactive bowel sounds	Normal	Hypoventilation Hyporeflexia

Abbreviations: BP, blood pressure; HR, heart rate; RR, respiratory rate; T, temperature; ↑, increased; ↓, decreased; ±, variable.

for suspected poisonings, eliminating possible diagnoses systematically. The list of differential diagnoses for toxidrome presentations is extensive and can vary from psychiatric disorders and sepsis to stroke-related symptoms. In the patient presenting with altered mental status, the primary-care practitioner should always consider head injury and other organic etiologies. Numerous xenobiotics produce gastrointestinal (GI), symptoms; thus, GI tract disorders should also be ruled out.

MANAGEMENT

In suspected poisonings, the priority of the primary-care practitioner is to treat the immediate medical condition. Although psychiatric evaluation becomes secondary to emergent treatment, a mental health evaluation and treatment is nonetheless an important and necessary component when treating the poisoned patient, given the strong association of poisonings with intentional ingestion, self-harm, depression, and suicidality. The American Association of Poison Control Centers has 55 poison information centers in the United States to help prevent and treat poison exposures. These centers are open 24 hours a day and 7 days per week; they can be reached at any time through the Poison Help Line at 1-800-222-1222.

Emergency Management

Utilizing the primary survey, the patient's ABCs are assessed. Emergency medical services should be immediately mobilized to transfer the patient to the nearest emergency department, while concomitantly monitoring the individual's respiratory and cardiovascular status. The patient is placed on a continuous cardiac monitor and treated conservatively with intravenous fluids and antiemetics. The local poison control center is then contacted for additional treatment recommendations.

General Management

A xenobiotic is a pharmacologically, endocrinologically, or toxicologically active substance not endogenously produced and, therefore, foreign to the patient. Toxicity occurs when a substance reaches its target end organ and overwhelms natural protective mechanisms against damaging biochemical processes. By limiting the amount of a substance that reaches target tissues, these effects can be mitigated. For management principles of common poisonings, see Table 74.1.

In the setting of a toxic ingestion, the xenobiotic must first dissolve in the GI tract before it can be absorbed and enter the systemic circulation. Therefore, GI decontamination aims at restricting the amount of xenobiotic from reaching the systemic circulation. Accepted modalities include activated charcoal, gastric lavage, and whole bowel irrigation.

Historically, syrup of ipecac was used as a form of decontamination, and parents were advised to keep a bottle readily accessible for unintentional childhood ingestions of toxins or medications. Children who were given syrup of ipecac would experience induced vomiting and theoretically prevent potential toxins from gaining access to the systemic circulation. However, in 2003, the American Academy of Pediatrics released a policy statement that no longer recommended the use of ipecac for the treatment of poisoning because studies showed a discordance in efficacy between times of ingestion among individuals.

The most common form of GI decontamination is the use of activated charcoal. To treat poisonings, charcoal is processed into a slurry that is introduced into the stomach through ingestion or via an orogastric tube. The charcoal particles act as an adsorbent material binding xenobiotic molecules of a certain size, thus hindering the absorption of potential toxins across the GI lumen. This results in the fecal elimination of unwanted substances. Nonetheless, activated charcoal has limitations. Its utility is optimized when it is administered within 1 hour of an ingestion, and delayed administration reduces its efficacy. In addition, activated charcoal does not adsorb nor protect against heavy metals, alcohol, caustics, or cyanide.

The dose of activated charcoal for children is 1 to 2 g/kg (25–50 g/dose), and for adults, the dose is 1 g/kg (25–100 g/dose). Activated charcoal may be given with or without sorbitol; addition of this cathartic assists in charcoal elimination through the GI tract, especially with multidose regimens. Of note, sorbitol may produce dehydration that can lead to an electrolyte imbalance in young children; therefore, it should be used with caution. A poison control center should be consulted for guidance with dosing and administration.

Gastric lavage attempts to evacuate toxins from the stomach before they can be broken down, dissolved, and absorbed through the GI tract. This modality is accomplished with the insertion of a large-bore orogastric tube and instillation of a normal saline solution into the stomach, followed by aspiration of stomach contents. Gastric lavage should only be performed in a patient with a protected airway, either in a conscious individual or someone who is intubated. The process is repeated until the aspirate is clear of particulate matter. Gastric lavage is often followed by the administration of activated charcoal to adsorb any remaining xenobiotics.

Whole bowel irrigation incorporates the use of a polyethylene glycol-electrolyte solution (PEG-ELS) to flush the contents of the GI tract before toxins can be absorbed through the GI membrane. This method produces liquid stool that is generated through a large volume of PEG-ELS (2 L/hr in adults and 0.5 L/hr in children), which is maintained until the rectal effluent matches the appearance of the solution entering the body. Many patients are unable to sustain the recommended rate of ingestion; therefore, a nasogastric tube may need to be used to consistently administer the irrigation fluid.

Theoretical indications for whole bowel irrigation include the elimination of xenobiotics that may have delayed absorption or illicit drug "body stuffers" with the potential to become symptomatic (e.g., from ruptured swallowed drug packets). Body stuffers differ from body packers in relation to the vehicle that encases the swallowed illicit substance. Body packers, also known as "drug mules," carry tightly sealed packages within their GI tract for illegal transportation into a country and eventual expulsion for distribution. In contrast, body stuffers are usually averting law enforcement and ingest baggies of illicit substances urgently that can subsequently dissolve and release contents into the GI tract.

Forced diuresis and alteration of urine pH can be used to remove certain toxins that undergo renal elimination. Acidic toxins can be trapped in alkaline urine, and alkaline toxins can be trapped in acidic urine. Sodium bicarbonate administration is used to alkalinize urine to a pH of greater than 7.0. Additionally, toxins can be eliminated through extracorporeal removal means such as, dialysis, plasmapheresis, and exchange transfusion. However, elimination of toxins is limited to xenobiotics that are water soluble, unbound to protein, and have a low volume of distribution. Chelation therapy is used for the removal of heavy metals such as lead, and hyperbaric oxygen may be indicated in moderate to severe carbon monoxide poisoning.

Adults who present with an undifferentiated depressed mental state may require dextrose, thiamine, and naloxone. Hypoglycemia can masquerade as a coma or even stroke, therefore necessitating its immediate reversal with 50 to 100 mL of 50% dextrose as an IV bolus. In malnourished patients or patients with suspected alcohol abuse, the diagnosis of Wernicke encephalopathy should be considered, and treatment should be initiated with 100 mg of intravenous thiamine. Respiratory depression and mental status depression due to opioid (e.g., heroin) toxicity can be reversed with naloxone 0.4 to 2 mg IV. Depending on the type of xenobiotic the opioid is integrated with, higher doses of up to naloxone 5 to 10 mg may be required, as the goal of opioid reversal is to alleviate respiratory depression.

FOLLOW-UP AND REFERRAL

Follow-up and referral will depend on the nature of the poisoning or overdose and the patient's clinical condition. If the poisoning or overdose is a suicide attempt or a call for attention, a psychiatric referral is indicated, which should be coordinated with the primary-care practitioner. The patient with suicidal ideation or an attempt should never be discharged home without having a psychiatric evaluation clearly documented with appropriate follow-up care arranged.

In addition, for unintentional poisonings, although urgent care or emergent intervention typically occurs in the emergency department setting, follow-up care should be coordinated with the primary-care practitioner to provide critical patient education for risk management against future toxic exposures in the home or workplace.

Patient Education: Poisons

In teaching the patient and his or her family about poisonings, the primary-care clinician should advise friends and family to call the Poison Help Line (1-800-222-1222) of the American Association of Poison Control Centers.

General teaching points for the prevention of poisonings include the following:

- Keep all medications and hazardous products locked up and out of the reach of children.
- Keep all medications in child-resistant containers.
- Never refer to medication as "candy" when administering to children.
- Dispose carefully of all unused or expired medications.
- Do not leave medications on countertops or tables, especially if children are present.
- Never transfer hazardous material from one container into another; keep all medications or other toxins in their original containers with appropriate labeling.
- Do not mix chemicals unless you know what the resultant reaction may be.

ARTHROPOD BITES AND STINGS

Arthropods are members of Arthropoda, a large phylum of animal life characterized by an external body support structure known as an exoskeleton, which includes lobsters and crabs, as well as mites, ticks, spiders, and insects. Arthropod bites and stings involve penetration of the skin by some part of the animal accompanied by the release of venom that can cause local or systemic symptoms. Some arthropods, such as ticks, can also transmit disease via infectious microorganisms. The majority of disorders caused by bites and stings of arthropods are from spider bites; bee, wasp, and ant stings; caterpillar spine irritation; interactions with sucking bugs, beetles, flies, and other winged insects; bites from lice, fleas, mites, and ticks; and stings from scorpions.

EPIDEMIOLOGY AND CAUSES

Millions of people in the United States are injured by venoms produced by insects and other arthropods each year, with a notable number of deaths. In one 10-year period, 65 deaths were reported to be caused by spiders in the United States. Of these, 63 deaths were from black widow spider bites. Bee and wasp stings cause more deaths annually than any other venomous animal. There are 40 to 50 fatalities each year from *Hymenoptera* stings. These insect stings result in a rapid progression of toxic effects: 80% of the deaths result from anaphylactic shock less than 1 hour after the sting. Spider bites, however, have a longer time interval between bites and time of death, with 89% of deaths occurring more than 12 hours after being bitten.

Ninety-five percent of all venomous animal fatalities occur from April to October, when animals and potential victims are most active in outdoor settings, heightening the risk of exposure. The risk of insect bites further increases with lack of protective measures and in areas with heavy insect infestations. Previous exposure to venom can predispose the victim to anaphylaxis upon reexposure to the same arthropod via venom-specific immunoglobulin (Ig)E-mediated mechanisms.

Wasps

The yellow jacket is the major cause of *Hymenoptera* insect-sting reactions. The yellow jacket, hornet, and other wasps feed on sugary sources and are attracted to foods commonly found in garbage cans and at picnics. When a wasp stings, it injects a venomous fluid under the skin. Yellow jackets, wasps, and hornets nest under logs, in the ground, or in walls; care should be taken to avoid disturbing these insects during gardening and lawn mowing.

Fire Ants

The imported fire ant is a small, light reddish brown to dark brown, wingless stinging insect that is responsible for an increasing number of acute allergic reactions. This insect attaches itself to its victim by biting with its jaws and then pivoting its body around its head, stinging in multiple sites in a circular pattern with its stinger located on the end of its abdomen. The fire ant's venom causes hemolysis, depolarization of cellular membranes, activation of the alternate complement pathway, and general tissue destruction.

Fire ants inhabit loose dirt and make nests that produce up to 200,000 ants during a 3-year period. They swarm if provoked and may attack in great numbers. The two species of imported fire ants (originally from Brazil) are found predominantly in nine southern states, particularly along the Gulf Coast. However, these colonies are gradually spreading westward and northward, accounting for increased exposure each year.

Brown Recluse Spiders

The natural habitat of the brown recluse spider (*Loxosceles reclusa*) is along the Mississippi River Valley, especially in northwestern Arkansas and southern Missouri. Because this spider can live in old boxes and furniture, it is easily transported to other states. The brown recluse spider prefers warm, dry locations such as woodpiles, cellars, and abandoned buildings; it is generally nocturnal in activity. The "fiddleback" spider has a characteristic violin-shaped marking on the dorsum of its cephalothorax (head and body section). The spider's venom contains sphingomyelinase D; it is chiefly cytotoxic, causing local tissue destruction. The necrosis is caused by an aggregation of leukocytes and platelets that forms a hemostatic plug in venules and arterioles.

Black Widow Spiders

Black widow spiders (*Lactrodectus mactans*) are relatively aggressive. They are found throughout the United States, predominantly in the South. Around houses, the black widow spider is found in protected places such as garages, storage sheds, crawl spaces under buildings, and rainspouts. Female spiders of the genus *Lactrodectus* carry the characteristic orange-red hourglass-shaped marking on the ventral abdomen. The *Lactrodectus* venom is a neurotoxin that acts on the myoneural junction and exerts its damage by releasing acetylcholine and norepinephrine. Black widow spiders are the most feared of all spiders because they injure their victims by injecting one of the most potent venoms secreted by any animal.

Scorpions

Found throughout the world, scorpions are nocturnal and spend the day under rocks, logs, and floors. The only species that is particularly dangerous, *Centruroides exilicauda* (the bark scorpion), is found mostly in the southwestern United States. This small Mexican scorpion is usually less than 2 inches long, yellow to brown, and possibly striped. The last segment of the scorpion's tail-like structure contains the venom glands and stingers. Most scorpions are relatively harmless, producing only local reactions, but the venom of *Centruroides exilicauda* has effects similar to those of black widow spider venom, producing severe systemic toxicity. The venom is predominantly a neurotoxin that causes repetitive firing of axons by the activation of sodium channels.

Ticks

Some of the more common ticks in the United States are the brown dog tick and the American dog tick. Ticks are frequently encountered by hikers and people who work outdoors. When feeding, ticks make a small hole in the skin, attach themselves with a modification of one of the mouthparts (which has teeth that curve backward), and insert barbed, piercing mouthparts to remove blood. The American dog tick (*Dermacentor variabilis*) may transmit Rocky Mountain spotted fever (caused by the intracellular bacteria *Rickettsia rickettsii*), tularemia (caused by the coccobacillus *Francisella tularensis*), and other diseases from animals to people. This tick has also been reported to cause paralysis if it attaches at the base of the skull or along the spinal column, due to a paralytic toxin secreted by the feeding tick.

Lyme disease (caused by the spirochete bacterium *Borrelia burgdorferi*) is also transmitted by ticks. Most disease transmission occurs in the New England states, where the primary vector is the deer tick/black-legged tick (*Ixodes scapularis*). Species that are close relatives to the deer tick, such as the western black-legged tick (*Ixodes pacificus*), are also capable of transmitting the disease.

Fleas

Fleas are wingless, blood-sucking insects, some species of which transmit arboviruses to humans by acting as a host or vector for the organism. Certain species of fleas transmit plague, murine typhus, and tularemia. Unfortunately, if a house has been previously occupied by pets that were infested with fleas, the abandoned hungry fleas may form a welcoming party for the newly arrived "human guests."

Chiggers

Chiggers or "red bugs" are the larvae of harvest mites. Infestations due to chiggers are caused by mite larvae that feed on the host skin cells. In other parts of the world such as India, Central and Southeast Asia, and Australia, chiggers may transmit scrub typhus (caused by the rickettsial bacteria *Orientia tsutsugamushi*). Chiggers become active in the spring, although in southern states such as Florida, they may be active all year. Chiggers attach themselves to the skin, hair follicles, or pores of humans or rodent hosts by inserting their piercing mouthparts. They prefer to attach themselves to parts of the human body where clothing fits tightly or where the flesh is thin, tender, or wrinkled; in rodents, they are often clustered on the inner skin of the ears.

During feeding, chiggers inject digestive enzymes into the skin, which dissolves tissue. Chiggers feed by sucking up the liquefied tissues; they do not burrow in the skin. After 3 days, when the larva is engorged, it drops off the human host. Chiggers are most often found in low, damp areas where vegetation is heavy, although some species prefer dry areas. They are most abundant in areas covered with shrubs and small trees, where rodents are numerous.

Biting Flies

The species of blood-sucking flies that can produce allergic reactions are deerflies, blackflies, horseflies, and sandflies. Fly bites can also result in cutaneous myiasis in which parasitism by fly larvae occurs. When a fly, such as the human botfly, deposits an egg on human skin, the egg hatches immediately, and the larva enters the skin through the bite or through another small break in the skin. The larvae grow to 15 to 20 mm under the skin, as a growing red, pruritic papule develops into a tender furuncle, with eventual emergence of the fly larvae.

Stinging Caterpillars

Stinging caterpillars include the puss caterpillar, saddleback caterpillar, and the hag moth caterpillar. These caterpillars are found primarily in the southeastern United States, especially in Texas and Florida. These caterpillars have spines that are hollow hairs containing poison sacs. When the spines break off, a toxin flows from the spines onto the victim's skin, causing a burning sensation.

Mosquitoes

Mosquitoes are blood-sucking arthropods attracted to hosts by moisture, carbon dioxide, estrogens, sweat, or warmth. They are vectors for many infectious diseases, and their bites also cause IgE-mediated immediate hypersensitivity reactions (erythematous urticarial lesions).

PATHOPHYSIOLOGY

The venoms produced by venomous insects and other arthropods can be classified according to their effects:

- Vesicating toxins (e.g., blister beetles, certain stinging caterpillars, and millipedes) produce blisters.
- Neurotoxins (e.g., black widow spiders, bark scorpions, certain ticks, wheel bugs, and *Hymenoptera* [honeybees, bumblebees, wasps, hornets, yellow jackets, and fire ants]) attack the CNS.
- Cytotoxic and hemolytic toxins (e.g., *Hymenoptera*, ground scorpions, mites, chiggers, wheel bugs, and the brown recluse spider) destroy tissue.
- Hemorrhagic toxins (e.g., lice, fleas, ticks, mites, true bugs [*Hemiptera*], and biting flies) prevent blood from clotting.

The normal or usual reaction following an insect sting is local erythema, pain, pruritus, and swelling. Insect stings almost always cause pain. This initial reaction should subside in 1 to 2 hours. The more significant reactions to insect bites can be categorized as large local reactions, toxic reactions, systemic or anaphylactic reactions, delayed reactions, and unusual reactions.

A *large local reaction* can spread more than 6 inches beyond the sting and is characterized by prolonged and marked edema at the site of the sting injury, peaking at 48 hours and lasting as long as 1 week. This reaction may be accompanied by nausea, vomiting, and fatigue.

A large local reaction can involve one or more neighboring joints and may even produce airway obstruction due to tissue swelling if the sting occurs in the mouth or throat. The history of a large local reaction is typically not associated with the risk of anaphylaxis upon future stings.

A *toxic reaction* occurs when there is a history of multiple stings, often more than 10 in number. Toxic reactions are caused by nonantigenic properties of *Hymenoptera* venom. They resemble systemic reactions but have a greater frequency of GI disturbances. Diarrhea, nausea, vomiting, light-headedness, and syncope are common signs. The patient may also have headache, drowsiness, fever, involuntary muscle spasms, edema without urticaria, and occasionally seizures. Urticaria and bronchospasm are not present, and symptoms usually subside within 48 hours.

Systemic or *anaphylactic reactions* may range from mild to fatal. The majority of such reactions occur within the first 15 minutes, and nearly all will occur within 6 hours after the insect sting, but some may not occur until 24 to 36 hours later. The shorter the interval between the sting and the onset of symptoms, the more severe the reaction. Fatalities that occur usually result from either hypotension or airway obstruction. The patient will present initially with generalized urticaria, pruritic eyes, a dry cough, and facial flushing. These symptoms may progress rapidly to chest or throat constriction, dyspnea, wheezing, laryngeal stridor, frothy sputum, cyanosis, diarrhea, abdominal cramps, nausea, vomiting, chills and fever, vertigo, shock, loss of consciousness, and involuntary loss of bowel and bladder function.

When an individual predisposed to *Hymenoptera* allergy is initially stung, there is an increase in the production of antigen-specific IgE antibodies. The antibodies become attached to mast cells and basophils, and the individual becomes sensitized to undergo an anaphylactic reaction after a subsequent sting. Anaphylaxis is a type I immediate hypersensitivity immune response to a triggering antigen/allergen found in insect venom. In this type of reaction, once introduced into the body, the circulating venom antigen binds to antigen-specific IgE molecules that are bound to mast cells and basophils. Binding of two or more cell membrane–bound IgE molecules to the same antigen (a process known as antibody cross-linking) leads to the degranulation of mast cell and basophil cytoplasmic contents and the release of preformed vasoactive mediators including histamine and tryptase. These substances are potent systemic vasodilators, accounting for the immediate flushing and life-threatening symptoms of hypotension, angioedema, and mucosal swelling with potential airway compromise.

Infusion of histamine into normal subjects causes the following effects and can be diminished by antagonists of specific histamine H_1 or H_2 receptors: flushing (H_1 plus H_2), hypotension (H_1 plus H_2), tachycardia (H_1), headache (H_1 plus H_2), pruritus (H_1), rhinorrhea (H_1), and bronchospasm (H$_1$). Honeybee venom contains histamine; wasp venom contains histamine and serotonin; hornet venom contains histamine, serotonin, and acetylcholine. The fact that histamine acts through both H$_1$ and H$_2$ receptors emphasizes the importance of administering both H$_1$- and H$_2$-blocking antihistamines during allergic reactions. However, the only reliable method of countering the life-threatening hypotension and mucosal edema associated with anaphylactic histamine release is with immediate administration of epinephrine, a potent vasoconstrictor.

Following this immediate response, through complex lymphocyte (e.g., T cell) and granulocyte interactions, other inflammatory vasoactive cytokines including prostaglandins, leukotrienes, and bradykinin begin to form several hours after exposure. These substances contribute to a second, later phase of anaphylaxis that typically occurs 6 to 12 hours after acute exposure to the triggering antigen. Leukotrienes and prostaglandins are responsible in part for vascular permeability, vasodilation, smooth-muscle contraction, and mucus secretion. Downregulation of the inflammatory response by these de novo–formed mediators is the goal of corticosteroid treatment in anaphylaxis.

Another type of *delayed reaction* to insect venom can appear 10 to 14 days after an insect bite or sting; this reaction is also antibody mediated, but by IgG or IgM, rather than by IgE. This type of reaction presents as a serum sickness–like illness, which is a type III antigen–antibody response in which immune complexes are deposited in the various tissues of the body. The patient's signs and symptoms include malaise, headache, fever, urticaria, lymphadenopathy, and polyarthritis.

Additional *unusual reactions* may be neurological or vascular in nature. They include nephrosis, vasculitis, serum sickness, encephalitis, and neuritis. The etiology of these reactions varies but may be due to an immunological pathogenesis.

CLINICAL PRESENTATION

Subjective

The primary-care practitioner should determine the history of the sting or bite, including the exact time of injury, and a precise description of the arthropod or species of insect, if possible. As the skin is inspected for signs of the insect or spider bite, the patient should first be evaluated for any anaphylactic symptoms or signs of a systemic reaction. The clinician should also determine if the patient has had previous allergies to insect bites, a history of allergies or asthma, or any known allergies to horses or horse serum, given the composition of certain antisera. A family history of anaphylaxis to bites or stings should also be elicited, as this increases the risk of anaphylaxis in the patient as well.

With stinging insects, the patient will usually remember the insult because the sting induces immediate pain. For biting insects, there may be some delay between the actual bite and the pruritus that follows. The patient's history should be carefully pursued to identify the probable source of exposure. For indoor exposure, fleas are common offenders although spider bites are also responsible for indoor bites. The primary-care practitioner should also inquire about whether pets have recently occupied the dwelling or if the patient has been to a home with pets.

Objective

Hymenoptera (bee and wasp) stings produce immediate pain and a red papule surrounded by a pale zone of edema, with varying amounts of local swelling. Large local reactions are common, spreading more than 6 inches (15.2 cm) beyond the sting, peaking at 48 hours, and lasting as long as 1 week. A mildly sensitive person will experience hives, malaise, wheezing, conjunctivitis, rhinitis, fever, and nausea. A severely sensitive person will suffer diffuse urticaria, facial swelling, laryngeal edema, bronchospasm, vomiting, cyanosis, abdominal pain, arrhythmias, and hypotension. Most fatalities occur within 1 hour of the sting.

Fire ant stings produce vesicles that become sterile pustules; these pustules subsequently become necrotic within several hours and may take up to 10 days to heal. If broken, the pustules may become infected. Systemic symptoms include nausea, vomiting, faintness, headache, fever, numbness, and muscle spasms.

Brown recluse spider bites are unusual in that persons bitten usually do not feel pain for 2 to 3 hours. A single necrotic lesion occurs, usually measuring 0.5 to 2 cm in size, self-limited in spread, and lacking adenopathy or sustained general toxicity. The typical bull's-eye lesion is created when the red blister is encircled by a pale, irregularly shaped and ischemic halo, which in turn is surrounded by extravasated blood. The pustule may gradually grow to form a crater-like lesion over 3 to 4 days, with associated lymphadenopathy and low-grade fever. Rarely, there is a generalized systemic reaction 24 to 48 hours after the spider bite, with fever, malaise, arthralgias, rash, and hemolysis.

Black widow spider bites create an initial puncture wound that disappears rapidly, leaving a local swelling where tiny red spots appear. Symptoms of envenomation occur within 10 to 60 minutes, including severe pain in the bitten extremity and muscle spasms of the abdomen and trunk. Diffuse paresthesias, ptosis, and hyperactive deep tendon reflexes may be noted. Victims experience agonizing pain and may develop hypertension, headache, muscular rigidity and spasm, hyperreflexia, vomiting, abdominal pain, agitation, or psychosis. Symptoms peak at 2 to 3 hours after the bite and may last up to 24 hours.

Scorpion stings are immediately intensely painful, with little or no erythema or swelling. Generalized reactions may occur within 1 hour and progress to maximum severity in 5 hours. The reactions can be graded as follows:

- Grade I: local pain and paresthesias at the site of envenomation
- Grade II: pain and paresthesias remote from the sting bite, along with local findings
- Grade III: either somatic skeletal or cranial nerve neuromuscular dysfunction, including blurred vision, wandering eye movements, hypersalivation, difficulty swallowing, upper airway obstruction, slurred speech, jerking of the upper extremities, restlessness, arching of the back, severe involuntary shaking, and jerking
- Grade IV: both cranial nerve and somatic skeletal neuromuscular dysfunction

Hypertension, nausea, vomiting, hyperthermia, tachycardia, and respiratory distress may also occur. Children younger than 10 years of age are more likely to have severe or prolonged reactions to scorpion stings. Older children and adults usually recover within 10 to 12 hours.

Tick bites can produce lesions that vary from small pruritic nodules to extensive ulceration, induration, and erythema. The lesions may be accompanied by malaise, fever, and chills. Tick-induced paralysis occurs more frequently during the spring and summer, when ticks are feeding. Symptoms occur 5 to 6 days after the adult female tick attaches and include irritability, restlessness, and paresthesias in the hands and feet. Over the next 24 to 48 hours, ascending, symmetric, and flaccid paralysis occurs, along with the loss of deep tendon reflexes. Within 1 to 2 days, severe generalized weakness may develop, accompanied by respiratory paralysis.

Flea bites produce lesions that are so similar to those of lice and scabies that diagnosis is often difficult. Flea bites produce itching papules, found in zigzag lines, especially on the legs and in the waist area. The lesions present as central hemorrhagic puncta surrounded by erythematous and urticarial patches. Pruritus is intense. Once the lesions clear, dull red spots may persist. Impetigo may develop as a complication. If the fleas remain in the environment, new lesions continue to appear.

Itching from *chigger bites* is usually noticed 4 to 8 hours after chiggers have attached or have been removed. Initially, a papule develops and ultimately enlarges over 24 to 48 hours to form a nodule. Pruritus peaks on the second day. The fluid injection causes nodules to appear, which may last for 2 weeks. Patients who exhibit an allergic reaction to the fluid (saliva) injected by the saliva will develop severe soft-tissue edema, pruritus, and fever. Chigger bites usually occur around the ankles, waistline, knees, or in the armpits. Mite infestations may be associated with an erythema multiforme–like rash and fever.

Biting flies can cause pain and subsequent pruritus when they pierce the skin, and allergic reactions can occur. If flies inject their eggs under the skin, the patient can also develop myiasis. As the fly larvae hatch and grow under the skin, the initial pruritic papule becomes a furuncle with a central opening that exudes serosanguineous fluid. The tip of the fly larva may even protrude from the central opening, or bubbles produced by its respiration may be seen.

The *puss caterpillar's sting* causes intense, immediate pain, often in spasms. This is followed by local edema, pruritus, and a rash of red blotches and ridges. The lesions consist of red or white papules and vesicles, often forming perfect gridlike markings where the caterpillar made contact. Ordinarily no systemic manifestations occur, and localized symptoms typically subside within 24 hours. In some patients, the intense pain can cause nausea and vomiting, as well as headache, fever, and lymphadenopathy. The papular or urticarial rash usually subsides within a few hours to 1 to 2 days after contact, and it can persist for up to 1 week.

An immediate skin reaction to *mosquito bites* includes erythema, wheal formation, and severe pruritus. A delayed reaction 12 to 24 hours later consists of more intense redness, edema, and a burning pruritus. Blistering and necrosis can also occur. The immediate reaction is of short duration, whereas the delayed reaction may persist for hours, days, and even weeks. Some individuals have a history of allergy to mosquito saliva, consistent with an increasing reaction to seasonal exposures accompanied by progressively more pronounced edema and pruritus. The allergic response can be accompanied by fever, generalized malaise, nausea, vomiting, and necrosis, with resultant scarring.

DIAGNOSTIC REASONING

Diagnostic Tests

In an arthropod bite or sting that results in systemic involvement, the clinician providing emergent care should order blood typing and crossmatch studies, coagulation tests, complete blood count, serum electrolytes, blood urea nitrogen, creatinine, and urinalysis. Serial arterial blood gases and pulse oximetry may also be necessary. For suspected tickborne diseases such as Rocky Mountain spotted fever and Lyme disease, further laboratory studies are in order. For example, spirochetes can be seen in the blood smear in 70% of cases of tickborne relapsing fever. Lyme disease, Rocky Mountain spotted fever, and tularemia, which all occur from tick bites, are diagnosed by specific antibody titers. However, results from these antibody titer assays are often not available for days to weeks, with empiric treatment often initiated before this. Thus, these tests are usually sent for confirmation only when a strong suspicion already exists for the infections and should not be sent indiscriminately. Acute infection is associated with elevated IgM titers, whereas past exposure (including from cleared infection) is characterized by elevated IgG levels.

Differential Diagnosis

Consultation with a regional poison control center may be indicated to correctly identify, diagnose, and/or treat arthropod bites and stings. It is helpful to know the specific arthropods that are indigenous to the local area, especially those that have caused recent infestations and injuries. Bites of fleas, lice, and scabies mites produce similar lesions that can complicate differentiation. Cercaria (i.e., larval schistosomes that develop in nonhuman hosts) cause similar lesions that appear after a patient has been exposed to infected water. Scabies have a more gradual onset but should also be considered in the differential diagnosis. The diagnosis of chigger infestations can usually be made on the basis of typical skin lesions in the setting of an outdoor exposure history. Patients who present with a "bull's-eye" rash following a suspected deer tick bite should be tested for Lyme disease.

When examining an urticarial reaction to an insect bite, other causes of urticaria should be considered, but if the hive (wheal) has a central punctum, its cause is likely an insect bite. Other foreign bodies can produce pruritic papules in the skin. Dermatitis herpetiformis should be included in the differential diagnosis, particularly when only excoriations are found. Eruptions associated with other viruses or with atopic dermatitis, allergic or irritant contact dermatitis, and drug sensitivity must also be considered. An uncommon idiopathic disorder, Mucha-Habermann disease, also presents with scattered necrotic papules and vesicles, but this type of rash is usually more generalized and symmetric. Some of the other skin conditions that may be confused with local or systemic reactions to arthropod stings and bites include streptococcal necrotizing fasciitis, focal cutaneous necrosis, various infections, local thromboses, punctures, trauma, drug reactions, vasculitis, purpura, Arthus (type III sensitivity or serum sickness) reactions, emboli to the skin, other bites that leave small puncture wounds, and artefacts.

Anaphylaxis from an insect sting may be confused with a vasovagal reaction, which is a disorder of central vasoregulation caused by increased parasympathetic tone mediated by the vagus nerve (cranial nerve X). A vasovagal reaction typically produces pallor, nausea, bradycardia, extreme diaphoresis, and hypotension that may result in syncope, whereas flushing, hypotension, tachycardia, and mucosal edema with severe bronchoconstriction are seen in anaphylaxis. Severe reactions to scorpion stings may present with symptoms similar to those of insecticide poisoning, with direct CNS effects.

Confirmation of stinging insect allergy is made by the detection of venom-specific IgE. This can be performed through an immediate reaction skin prick test, which measures the cutaneous histaminic response to dilute doses of allergen after scratching the skin surface with an antigen-coated needle tip, allowing for binding of allergen to IgE on tissue mast cells with subsequent degranulation. Yellow jacket, honeybee, yellow hornet, bald-faced hornet, and wasp extracts are available for diagnosis and treatment of stinging insect allergies. A patient is considered sensitive if a skin reaction of 1+ or greater occurs at a venom concentration of 1 mg/mL or less, provided that the 1+ reaction is greater than that of a diluent control. This is the most sensitive test for detecting allergic states and is commonly used as an allergy screening tool. However, it lacks specificity and may thus overestimate allergic states. In turn, as with all skin prick test results, its utility lies mainly in its negative predictive value.

IgE antibodies reacting with venom also may be measured by a serum detection assay known as the radioallergosorbent test (RAST). In this test, a patient's serum is applied to a culture plate surface coated with the specific allergen of interest, allowing for specific antibody-binding to the plate. After excess serum is rinsed away, a second fluorescent-labeled antibody specific for the constant region of IgE is applied to the plate to reveal any of the patient's antigen-specific IgE that bound to the plate during the first step of the assay. Thus, the greater the amount of fluorescence, the higher the concentration of antigen-specific IgE in the patient's serum. The RAST is not as sensitive as the skin test, although it is more specific and is thus more effective in ruling out, rather than ruling in an allergic state.

MANAGEMENT

Emergency Management

Anaphylactic shock and respiratory distress are true emergencies. The clinician should focus on stabilizing the patient while arranging for immediate transport to the emergency department. It should be stressed that anaphylaxis may be triggered by etiologies other than bites and stings. Anaphylactic reactions are extreme emergencies and can be caused iatrogenically by medications, environmental exposures, or certain food allergies, which are quite common. The treatment for anaphylaxis is standard and should be familiar to all practitioners who provide primary care, urgent care, or emergency care.

The clinician should place a conscious patient in a comfortable position, ensuring unimpeded ventilation. Hypotensive patients should be placed supine or in a modified Trendelenburg position if respiratory status allows. The clinician must help the patient maintain an adequate upper airway and give supplemental oxygen by mask or nebulizer with inhaled racemic epinephrine (0.5 mL of 2.25% epinephrine in 2 mL of normal saline), not to exceed three treatments in 60 minutes. Racemic epinephrine should not be considered an adequate substitute for systemic epinephrine in the case of a life-threatening attack. In the case of impending upper airway compromise, inadequate oxygenation, or profound shock, the clinician must prepare for immediate administration of systemic epinephrine (as described subsequently) and endotracheal intubation if necessary to maintain an open airway. Cricothyrotomy by a trained professional would be needed if severe angioedema precludes intubation via the oral route.

Epinephrine maintains blood pressure through beta-adrenergic cardiovascular effects, causes bronchial dilation, and antagonizes the adverse actions of the mediators of anaphylaxis. It also reduces the subsequent release of anaphylactic mediators through its action on mast cells and basophils. In the case of airway edema, bronchospasm, and/or cardiovascular instability (with or without cutaneous manifestations of urticaria or angioedema), the clinician should immediately administer aqueous epinephrine 1: 1,000 IM into the upper outer thigh, which provides the most rapid entry into the systemic circulation. The dose is 0.3 to 0.5 mg every 10 to 20 minutes as indicated. Injection of 0.1 to 0.2 mg of the epinephrine dose can be made directly into the sting or bite, causing vasoconstriction and reduction of swelling. If the reaction is limited to urticaria and pruritus, there is no wheezing or facial swelling, and the victim is older than 45 years of age, epinephrine can be withheld unless the patient's condition worsens. In addition to the immediate administration of epinephrine, albuterol may be used to treat bronchospasm, administered via nebulizer every 20 minutes as needed.

Antihistamines may be included in the treatment regimen. With H_1-blocking antihistamines, the primary-care practitioner may administer diphenhydramine by mouth (PO) (in severe anaphylaxis, 100 mg may be administered IV initially) or hydroxyzine IM as needed. The newer generation H_1-blockers such as cetirizine, fexofenadine, and desloratadine are less sedating and may be as effective as first-generation agents and can be used if the patient can take oral medications. For H_2-blocking antihistamines, the clinician may administer cimetidine or ranitidine. If available, cimetidine is the preferred H_2-blocker because it has greater peripheral effects than does ranitidine, which is more specific for the GI tract.

Circulatory support should be provided as needed in hypotensive patients. The clinician may infuse 0.5 to 1 L of either normal saline or lactated Ringer's solution every 20 to 30 minutes as needed to support the blood pressure at a level above 90 mm Hg systolic. The need for further fluid resuscitation should be determined by monitoring blood pressure, cardiac rhythm, and urine output. Usually, a total of 3 L can be given rapidly to an otherwise healthy adult without adverse effects. However, caution is needed in patients with congestive heart failure or the elderly, given the risk of pulmonary edema. Hypotension refractory to IV colloids requires treatment with IV pressor agents (e.g., norepinephrine, phenylephrine,

dopamine) in a hospital setting. Glucagon may be needed in patients who are already on beta-blocking agents, given that it stimulates inotropic and chronotropic cardiac function independent of the beta blockade.

If the allergic reaction is prolonged or severe or if the patient is regularly medicated with corticosteroids, the clinician should administer hydrocortisone, methylprednisolone, or dexamethasone (parenterally), with a 10-day oral taper to follow. If the therapy is initiated orally, the clinician should administer prednisone 60 to 100 mg daily. Even in the case of reactions that do not appear to be prolonged, systemic corticosteroid therapy should be administered for 24 to 48 hours after the onset of the initial reaction to minimize the chance of late-phase anaphylactic reactions, which may manifest up to 24 hours after the initial reaction and may be as severe as early-phase reactions. Corticosteroids are not administered to treat the acute inflammatory response in anaphylaxis, since agents such as hydrocortisone and methylprednisolone exert their peak effects at 4 to 8 hours after administration and are ineffective against the immediate life-threatening anaphylactic response.

General Management

Normal reactions to arthropod bites and stings do not require treatment other than local applications of cold compresses (ice) and analgesics. NSAIDs such as ibuprofen PO are effective if given immediately because they block the prostaglandins that mediate these typical reactions. Secondary infections are common with pruritic bites or stings that lead to frequent scratching. A topical antimicrobial ointment such as mupirocin 2% (Bactroban) should be applied three times daily for 5 days to sites of secondary infection.

Large Local Reactions

Large local reactions to arthropod bites or stings are treated with antihistamines, such as diphenhydramine and cimetidine. Intramuscular administration of diphenhydramine is not usually done because of the pain involved and the fact that the drug is absorbed very rapidly when administered orally. A corticosteroid such as methylprednisolone tapered over 5 days will hasten resolution of a large local reaction to a bee or wasp sting. Tapering slowly prevents a rebound flare-up of symptoms. Some clinicians also administer calcium gluconate. Importantly, large local reactions are not associated with the risk of anaphylaxis on future stings by the same type of insect.

The treatment of painful cases of venomous stings or bites with large local reactions includes nerve block anesthesia using 2% lidocaine, which can be repeated up to three times at 30- to 60-minute intervals. The use of oral analgesics may also be useful. In moderate and severe cases, which occur mainly in children, antivenin (antivenom) serum is indicated.

Delayed Serum Sickness-Type Reactions

Delayed serum sickness-type reactions in response to multiple bee, wasp, or fire ant stings can be managed with a corticosteroid such as prednisone (Deltasone) 60 to 100 mg, tapered over 2 weeks. The pruritus caused by these reactions can be controlled by a variety of oral antihistamines. Hydroxyzine is commonly prescribed because its dosage is flexible, and it produces few anticholinergic adverse effects. If patients are driving or working during the day, they should reserve the hydroxyzine for nighttime use to help with sleep. Treatment of urticaria may also require an H_2-blocking antihistamine, such as cimetidine.

For arthropod bites, when topical corticosteroids are used, class I (e.g., betamethasone dipropionate) or class II (e.g., fluocinonide) topical preparations may be applied twice daily. Lesions may take weeks to resolve. Topical antipruritics include lotions with 0.25% menthol, 1% phenol, or both (Sarna lotion) and topical anesthetics such as pramoxine (Pramosone). Topical antihistamines and benzocaine are not recommended because of their potential for allergic sensitization. Topical doxepin (Zonalon) is now available and is effective. Infected insect bites can be treated with topical mupirocin 2% (Bactroban) or neomycin. Extensive impetigo will need treatment with oral antibiotics, such as dicloxacillin or erythromycin.

Hymenoptera Stings

When a patient is stung by a honey bee, the stinger should be removed by scraping it away from the skin with a dull object. The stinger should not be grasped and pulled because this contracts the venom sac, thus releasing more toxin into the wound. Wasps and other bees do not leave a stinger in the patient's skin and are capable of stinging many times. The site should be cleaned, and an antiseptic should be applied. Blisters from fire ant stings should not be broken open. Ice should be applied with a cold compress pack, with or without a paste of papain (unseasoned meat tenderizer), and the body part should be elevated.

There is no specific antivenin for *Hymenoptera* stings. If the reaction is extensive or if there is envenomation from multiple stings, more aggressive therapy may be indicated in a hospital setting. This includes administering calcium gluconate IV with an antihistamine such as diphenhydramine IV or PO. Oral prednisone 40 mg daily for 2 to 3 days can be helpful in reducing localized swelling. Tetanus prophylaxis should be completed. In severe envenomation, an IV corticosteroid such as hydrocortisone 2 mg/kg should be administered at the earliest opportunity (see the section on anaphylactic reactions).

Brown Recluse Spider Bites

The patient should apply cold compresses intermittently for the first 4 days after the bite, over a sterile dressing. An oral antibiotic such as dicloxacillin, cephalexin, or erythromycin for 10 days can be administered. Elevation of the affected body part may be beneficial. Drug treatment is controversial; many brown recluse spider bites are minor and heal without specific treatment other than tetanus prophylaxis. One treatment for a severe wound in patients who screen negative for glucose-6-phosphate dehydrogenase (G6PD) deficiency is dapsone (Avlosulfon) 50 mg orally twice daily for 10 days. If G6PD deficiency is ultimately documented in a patient who has started dapsone empirically, the patient should discontinue dapsone immediately to avoid hemolysis.

Black Widow Spider Bites

The natural course of the envenomation is to resolve completely after a few days, with pain persisting for one week or more. Ice should be applied judiciously to the bite wound. The patient may require a narcotic analgesic, such as morphine. Opioids have a histaminic agonist effect, however, so these medications should be avoided in cases with significant histaminic responses. Muscle relaxants such as diazepam (Valium) may also be given for spasms.

The patient should be monitored for hypertension and administered a centrally acting or vasodilating antihypertensive if necessary. Inpatients may be given calcium gluconate via slow IV infusion to alleviate muscle spasms. Antivenin is reserved for seriously ill infants or older patients and is administered in a hospital-based critical care setting only, given the risk of anaphylaxis. Because many antivenins are derived from horse serum, horse serum sensitivity testing is needed to screen for potential anaphylactic reactions. One vial of antivenin is sufficient for most patients.

Scorpion Bites

The patient should apply ice for 30 minutes each hour to relieve local pain. Intense cooling should be avoided, and the affected body part should be immobilized but without a tourniquet. Opiate analgesics should be avoided because they potentiate the toxicity of the venom and may lead to apnea. The clinician should administer diazepam or phenobarbital to control seizures, along with a sympathetic antihypertensive agent to control hypertension. Hyperthermia from uncontrolled muscular contractions can be managed with cooling. The administration of antivenom (antivenin) is controversial given the risk of anaphylaxis and the needed for inpatient dosing. Horse serum sensitivity testing is done to rule out potential anaphylaxis.

Tick Bites

The clinician should always remove ticks. The tick can be covered with alcohol, machine oil, mineral oil, salad oil, or gasoline applied with a tissue or gauze pad. This blocks the tick's breathing pores and causes it to withdraw from the skin. It may take 30 minutes for the tick to disengage its mouthparts. Ticks should not be removed ion at the site of the tick bite. Most victims of tick paralysis will show improvement within hours of tick removal and return to their baseline status in several days. Patients with Rocky Mountain spotted fever or Lyme disease will require further treatment, including antibiotics and follow-up monitoring for chronic health problems.

Flea Bites

The patient should clean the bite lesions well with soap and water and apply a topical antiseptic ointment. To relieve pruritus and discomfort, calamine lotion with phenol can be applied. A systemic antihistamine such as hydroxyzine (Atarax) can be administered to control pruritus.

Chigger Bites

Chiggers are easily removed from the skin by taking a hot bath or shower and lathering with soap several times. The bath will kill attached chiggers. For moderate to severe cases, topical corticosteroid creams and oral antihistamines may provide some relief. Systemic corticosteroids will also provide relief for severe pruritus. Topical antibiotic therapy is indicated for secondary infection.

Mosquito Bites

Immediately after the person is bitten, he or she should apply a cold (ice) pack. A topical corticosteroid ointment can be applied to the site. Oral corticosteroids such as prednisone should be used only when the reaction is prolonged and severe, given their potential adverse effects.

Fly Bites

Fly bites are treated the same as mosquito bites. In addition, if the patient presents with cutaneous myiasis, the clinician should exert pressure to extrude the fly larva. The larva may emerge if its breathing hole in the skin is occluded with heavy oil, nail polish, or bacon fat. Alternatively, the clinician can inject 2 mL of local anesthetic into the base of the lesion, thus extruding the larva by fluid pressure. Care should be taken not to rupture the larva because an inflammatory reaction may result.

Caterpillar Spine Irritation

Broken-off spines in the skin can be removed by applying adhesive tape, a commercial facial peel, or a thin layer of rubber cement over the affected area. Then an oral antihistamine and/or NSAID can be administered. If the dermatitis is persistent and severe, the clinician should prescribe oral prednisone 60 to 100 mg for adults, to be tapered over 10 days.

FOLLOW-UP AND REFERRAL

After a severe allergic reaction to an arthropod sting or bite, further delayed reactions with a severe recurrence of symptoms are possible, particularly as the effects of treating medications decrease. Thus, patients may benefit from repeated doses of antihistamines and glucocorticoids over the next several days. All patients with severe allergic reactions who are discharged home should have a follow-up visit in 24 to 48 hours, and all such patients should be referred to an allergy specialist.

Individuals who have experienced a serious anaphylactic reaction should be prescribed three devices for the rapid self-administration of epinephrine by injection (EpiPen) and instructed on their use. These patients should also keep oral diphenhydramine and cimetidine readily available with injectable epinephrine in a portable kit. One kit should be kept in a bag or purse that is carried with the individual at all times, a second kit in the school or work setting, and a third kit should be kept in the home. Many individuals also keep a kit in the glove compartment of a personal vehicle; however, it is important to explain to the patient that extremes of heat and cold can affect the stability of many medicines, including life-saving epinephrine. Thus, storing a kit in the glove compartment of a vehicle is not recommended.

Individuals with a history of an acute allergic reaction (including systemic cutaneous reactions) with positive venom skin tests or a serum sickness-type reaction after an insect sting are considered at risk for subsequent sting reactions. Venom immunotherapy to prevent IgE-mediated allergic reactions to various types of *Hymenoptera* may be recommended, and referral to an allergist is required for specialized assessment that includes allergy testing (venom skin testing and venom-specific serum IgE–RAST testing). Of note, venom immunotherapy will not prevent future type III immune complex-mediated serum sickness reactions because these do not involve the IgE-allergic antibody. In addition, patients with large local reactions are not considered candidates for venom immunotherapy and do not require venom skin tests, because these reactions are not associated with the risk of anaphylaxis from future stings. Patients who have been treated for anaphylaxis and who use beta-adrenergic blocking agents should be switched to alternative medications, given the inhibitory effects of beta blockers on epinephrine.

Patient Education: Arthropod Bites and Strings

Patient education information regarding arthropod bites and stings is provided in Box 74.1.

Box 74.1 Patient Education: Arthropod Bites and Stings

- Avoid mowing lawns or working with flowering ornamental plants when bees and wasps are collecting nectar.
- Stand still if a stinging insect is near you. If it attacks, brush it off (do not slap at it) to prevent a sting.
- Do not walk in the yard in bare feet.
- Wear gloves when gardening.
- Keep garbage cans covered outdoors. Sweet items like soft drinks, ripened fruits, and watermelons attract bees and wasps and should be covered or in a sealed container when brought outdoors for consumption.
- Avoid perfumes, hair sprays, and colognes.
- Pick fruit as it ripens and dispose of rotten fruit.
- If you are attacked by a swarm of bees, wasps, yellow jackets, or hornets, leave the area immediately, using your arms to protect your face.
- Control wasps by applying insecticides to the nest.
- Avoid areas where insect exposure is likely to occur and always wear shoes when outdoors.
- Avoid wearing perfumes, aftershave lotions, and brightly colored clothing outdoors because these attract insects.
- If you are severely allergic to bee or wasp stings or to any medication, wear medical identification jewelry indicating the anaphylaxis-causing substance or event.
- Check bathrobes and bed sheets for spiders if you use them after a long absence.
- When you enter an attic or storeroom to open cardboard boxes, give the brown recluse spiders a chance to vacate because they will avoid you if they can.
- Have someone try to capture the spider for identification; immediately seek health care, and contact the local poison control center.
- Treat pets for ticks by using dusts, dips, or sprays.
- When you enter tick-infested areas, keep clothing buttoned, shirts tucked inside trousers, and trousers tucked inside boots.
- Wear light-colored clothing because this makes it easier to spot ticks; lighter clothing is also less attractive to biting flies.
- Do not sit on the ground or on logs in brush-filled areas.
- Keep brush cleared or pruned along frequently traveled areas. Use repellents to protect exposed skin; however, be aware that ticks will crawl over treated skin to untreated parts of the body.
- For treatment of flea infestations, treat not only the pet, but also professionally fumigate the house.
- If you are going into areas suspected of being infested with chiggers, wear protective clothing and use repellents.
- Apply a repellent containing *N,N*-diethyl-3-methylbenzamide and wear permethrin-impregnated fabric.
- Apply repellents to legs, ankles, cuffs, waist, and sleeves, either to clothing or directly to the body as directed by the repellant's label.
- Avoid unnecessary use of lights at campsites, and camp in a site that is high, dry, open, and uncluttered.

REFERENCES

Arthropod Bites and Stings

Haddad Jr. V, Amorim PC, Haddad Junior WT, Cardoso JL. Venomous and poisonous arthropods: identification, clinical manifestations of envenomation, and treatments used in human injuries. *Rev Soc Bras Med Trop.* 2015;48(6):650–657.

Hahlbohm D. Stinging insect allergy. *Adv NPs PAs.* 2013;4(4):20–22.

Poisoning

American Academy of Pediatrics Policy Statement. Poison treatment in the home. *Pediatrics.* 2003;112:1182–1185.

Gummin DD, Mowry JB, Spyker DA, et al. 2016 Annual Report of the American Association of Poison Control Centers' National Poison Data System (NPDS): 34th Annual Report. *Clin Toxicol.* 2017;55(10):1072–1252.

Kramarow E, Chen L-H, Hedegaard H, et al. Deaths from unintentional injury among adults aged 65 and over: United States, 2000–2013.

NCHS Data Brief, no. 199; May 2015. https://www.cdc.gov/nchs/data/databriefs/db199.pdf. Accessed December 19, 2017.

RESOURCES

Arthropod Bites and Stings

University of Iowa Hardin Library for the Health Sciences http://www.lib.uiowa.edu/hardin/md/insectbites.html.

Poisoning

American Association of Poison Control Centers http://www.aapcc.org

National Toxic Substance Incidents Program (NTSIP) of the Agency for Toxic Substances and Disease Registry (ATSDR) https://www.atsdr.cdc.gov/ntsip/

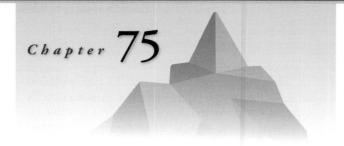

Chapter 75

Environmental Exposures

Joe Holbrook, BS, BSN, MS, APRN

Jill E. Winland-Brown, EdD, APRN, FNP-BC

Brian Oscar Porter, MD, PhD, MPH, MBA

Mae De La Calzada-Jeanlouie, DO, MS

HEAT-RELATED ILLNESSES

Heat-related illnesses include heat rash, heat cramps, heat syncope, heat exhaustion, and heat stroke. It is important to understand that heat-related illnesses are actually a continuum of conditions that range from mild to severe (see Table 75.1). Heat-related deaths are usually preventable.

Heat rash, also known as prickly heat or miliaria, is a group of skin conditions caused by environmental heat and excessive perspiration. The condition occurs when sweat is trapped under the skin due to closed pores. This forms an uncomfortable and often pruritic rash ranging from pinpoint to small, clear to red vesicles. The rash usually occurs on the face and neck. It is more common in the elderly, overweight persons, and infants.

Heat cramps are muscle spasms that usually occur in large muscle groups like the calves, abdomen, thighs and shoulders, during or shortly after exercising in the heat. The mechanism is thought to occur from either altered neuromuscular control of contraction caused by excessive muscle fatigue or electrolyte depletion from excessive perspiration or dilutional effects from excessive water consumption.

Risk factors for heat cramps include the following:

- a personal history of heat cramps
- an impaired ability to self-regulate body temperature, especially in the young and elderly
- alcohol use
- the use of certain medications, including anticholinergics, sympathomimetics, and diuretics

Heat syncope is a heat-related fainting episode. It may occur because of vasodilation and peripheral pooling of blood to release body heat, volume deficits, or sluggish vasomotor tone. Syncope occurs when the venous return of blood flow does not support the required cardiac output. Thus, heat syncope can result from inadequate cardiac output and postural hypotension. Typically, recovery is immediate once the patient lies flat.

Heat exhaustion occurs when the body overheats and is unable to maintain a normal core temperature. Symptoms may include thirst, heavy sweating, tachycardia, dizziness, nausea, vomiting, and weakness. Heat exhaustion is usually caused by strenuous work in hot and/or humid environments. Treatment includes rest, moving to a cooler environment, removal of clothing that prevents evaporative cooling, and hydration. Cold, electrolyte-balanced beverages ("sports drinks") are the best source of oral hydration. Intravenous 0.9% normal saline may also be given. Risk factors for heat exhaustion include the use of alcohol, dehydration, advanced age, and age younger than 5 years. The diagnosis is made by the presence of positive symptoms after heat exposure, with a body temperature of less than 104°F. Heat exhaustion can be prevented by proper hydration when exposed to heat, acclimatization to hot environments, proper cool down periods, avoiding alcohol, and wearing clothing that allows for evaporative cooling. Patients with heat exhaustion should be monitored for more severe symptoms of heat stroke until all symptoms have resolved and core body temperature has stabilized. The clinician may choose to perform diagnostic testing to confirm proper kidney function, electrolyte balance, and the absence of rhabdomyolysis.

Heat stroke or sunstroke is characterized by a core body temperature of 104°F (40°C) or higher, mental confusion, and more severe clinical manifestations that go beyond the symptoms of heat exhaustion. Heat stroke occurs when heat production is greater than heat loss. There may be damage to multiple organ systems and breakdown of muscle tissue (rhabdomyolysis), and mortality may be as high as 10%. The clinical presentation may include hot dry skin, a decreased level of consciousness, tachycardia, tachypnea, decreased urinary output, hypotension, seizures, nausea and vomiting, decerebrate posturing, diarrhea, and dilated, nonresponsive pupils. If the patient presenting to a primary-care setting has heat stroke, emergency medical services should be initiated while the patient's respiratory and cardiovascular status are evaluated and supported as indicated. The patient must then be transported to an emergency department (ED) immediately.

EPIDEMIOLOGY AND CAUSES

An average of 650 persons die each year of heat-related illnesses in the United States. Heat stroke is ranked third—behind head and neck trauma and cardiac disorders—as a cause of death among high school athletes in the United States. Factors associated with an increased risk of heat-related illnesses include age (both very young children

TABLE 75.1 Types of Heat-Related Illnesses

Type of Illness	Signs and Symptoms	Management
Heat rash	Pruritic rash of pinpoint to small, clear to red vesicles, usually on face and neck	Typically self-limited May use calamine lotion or topical corticosteroids for more severe cases
Heat cramps	Cramps, especially in the large muscle groups, such as shoulders, thighs, and abdominal wall muscles, following significant exercise in hot environment and profuse diaphoresis	Stop activity and rest; move to cool environment Muscle stretching Fluid and electrolyte replacement with oral electrolyte-balanced "sports drinks" or IV normal saline Monitor for progression to heat exhaustion and heat stroke Gradual acclimatization if exercising in hot or humid environments
Heat syncope	Orthostatic syncopal episode and dizziness due to vasodilation and peripheral pooling of blood, volume deficit, or sluggish vasomotor tone	Place the patient in a supine position Oral fluid replacement Cool environment and rest
Heat exhaustion	Prolonged fluid loss (e.g., from perspiration, diarrhea, or diuretic use) results in thirst, anxiety, anorexia, cramps in muscles, malaise, syncope, headache, dehydration, tachycardia, muscle weakness, orthostatic hypotension, nausea and vomiting, cutaneous flushing, and/or possible elevated temperature above 37.8°C	Remove the patient from hot environment into shady or cool place Elevate legs for postural hypotension Oral fluid replacement if no gastrointestinal symptoms and if alert and oriented; replace fluids and electrolytes at about 1 L/hr for several hour (recovery expected within 2–3 hours; otherwise, patient may need additional interventions)
Heat stroke	Medical emergency requiring rapid assessment at treatment, with core body temperature of at least 104°F (40.0°C), acute mental status changes, absent sweat, tachypnea, decreased urinary output, hypotension, seizures, nausea and vomiting, diarrhea, dilated nonresponsive pupils, decerebrate posturing	Rapid cooling (e.g., ice packs in groin and axilla) Monitor rectal temperature Supplemental oxygen, with intubation if necessary. IV fluids (usually 0.9% normal saline)

and older adults are at higher risk); a history of a chronic illness, such as cardiovascular, endocrine, neurological, or psychiatric disease; use of certain medications, such as antihistamines, beta blockers, and diuretics; fever or dehydration; a previous history of heat stroke; and heavy clothing that restricts evaporative heat loss.

Specifically, certain medications and medical conditions that impair the body's ability to self-regulate core temperature in the face of environmental heat extremes can contribute to the more severe forms of heat-related illness, such as heat exhaustion and heat stroke. Cholinergic blockade, beta-adrenergic blockade, and autonomic neuropathy are often unrecognized contributors to heat-related illnesses. Many drugs possess anticholinergic side effects that may result in an inability to perspire, while individuals on beta blockers may have a diminished ability to cope with heat. Monoamine oxidase inhibitors and sympathomimetics can cause a core temperature disturbance, leading to rapidly occurring muscle rigidity, extensive rhabdomyolysis, and electrolyte disorders that can prove fatal. Autonomic neuropathy associated with diabetes mellitus is an important risk factor for faulty heat dissipation and can also result in heat-related

illnesses. Certain living conditions, such as densely populated urban environments, living alone, and a lack of air conditioning during hot weather, are additional risk factors for heat-related illnesses. Exertion-related heat exhaustion and heat stroke may also be a complication of unconditioned amateur participants involved in strenuous athletic competitions.

PATHOPHYSIOLOGY

Heat loss is dependent on radiation, convection, conduction, and evaporation. Radiation and conduction result in direct transfer of heat from the body to the environment. When environmental temperatures reach 95°F (35°C), these mechanisms for heat transfer are no longer effective. Convection is heat loss related to air circulation, which is a process that relies on wind velocity. Evaporation of sweat is the only physiological mechanism for eliminating heat in an environment hotter than 95°F.

The body's ability to sweat is affected by skin conditions (e.g., sunburn), systemic diseases that affect the ability to sweat (e.g., cystic fibrosis), and drugs that inhibit sweating (e.g., phenothiazines). Increased core temperatures stimulate peripheral vasodilation and sweating. Venous return to the heart increases, resulting in increased cardiac output and heart rate. A concurrent sympathetic response is decreased blood flow to the kidneys, which can damage the kidneys if this process continues, with myoglobin produced as a byproduct. If this condition is not aggressively treated, it can lead to rhabdomyolysis. Respiratory function may be compromised by pulmonary edema. Hepatic function is often worsened because of the general decrease in perfusion. Clotting abnormalities with severe heat illness can range from thrombocytopenia to disseminated intravascular coagulation. As the metabolic rate rises, sweat production can increase to 1.5 L/hr, which may result in dehydration.

Acclimatization is a term that refers to the body's ability to adapt to heat stress. This adaptation primarily involves the sweating mechanism. In an unacclimatized person, each liter of sweat contains 30 to 50 mEq of sodium. This sodium level decreases to as little as 5 mEq/L in the fully acclimatized person, and the rate of sweating can be increased to 1.5 to 3 L/hr. This means that while the acclimatized person doubles sweat production, she or he loses only one-third to one-fifth of the total amount of sodium as the unacclimatized person.

Potassium wasting compensates for these sodium losses. Therefore, a fluid and electrolyte imbalance can develop quickly in an unacclimatized person. Cardiac output increases with acclimatization, as does aerobic muscle metabolism, which is more efficient metabolically. As the heart muscle responds, cutaneous circulation improves, and heat dissipation is augmented. The body develops a new, lower temperature set point at which sweating begins. Finally, increased secretion of aldosterone aids in sodium conservation by the kidneys and sweat glands. The additional sodium enhances extracellular fluid volume, which plays a part in the accelerated cutaneous blood flow and heat dissipation.

CLINICAL PRESENTATION

Subjective

For any heat-related illness, a complete history of the circumstances preceding the incident should be obtained. Any past history that may assist with the differential diagnosis is crucial. Medications that the patient is currently taking should be reviewed.

Objective

A complete physical examination, including monitoring the patient's cardiac status, vital signs, and core temperature, should be performed.

DIAGNOSTIC REASONING

Diagnostic Tests

Serum electrolytes should be assessed with more severe forms of heat-related illness (heat cramps, heat syncope, heat exhaustion, heat stroke) to assess for electrolyte imbalances or depletion, which may be corrected with IV saline infusion. With heat stroke in particular, hepatic and renal function tests should also be done to assess for end-organ dysfunction.

Differential Diagnosis

The differential diagnosis of heat stroke includes central nervous system infections, cerebrovascular accidents, and diabetic ketoacidosis. If the patient has recently traveled to countries in tropical or other endemic areas (e.g., certain countries in Africa and Asia), the primary-care practitioner should also consider malaria or typhoid fever. Additionally, with more severe presentations of heat exhaustion or heatstroke, the clinician should consider thyroid storm, meningitis, encephalitis, or brain abscess. Some toxicological issues to consider include salicylate, anticholinergic, phencyclidine (PCP), cocaine, or amphetamine toxicity.

MANAGEMENT

Treatment of heat-related illness is driven by the severity of presenting symptoms and the degree of electrolyte imbalance and end-organ damage. Treatment for milder forms such as heat rash is usually symptomatic because the condition is typically self-limited. Topical treatments include the use of calamine lotion applied directly to the rash and mild topical corticosteroids. Antibiotics may be prescribed if secondary infection develops. Heat rash can be prevented by minimizing exposure to heat and humidity, avoiding the use of tight fitting clothing, and by curtailing the use of creams and lotions. Heat cramps may be treated with muscle rest, but underlying causes must also be eliminated, such as dehydration and the use of contributing medications. Fluid-imbalances should also be addressed. Similarly, as patients suffering heat syncope often recover, as soon as they lie flat and postural hypotension is eliminated, treatment is focused on eliminating underlying aggravating factors.

For more severe forms of heat-related illness, such as heat exhaustion and heatstroke, general management focuses on cooling the patient. The safest and most practical method is to remove all clothing and spray warm water over the patient's entire body surface. Heat evaporation can be augmented with the use of fans, which should circulate air over as much body surface as possible. If ice packs are utilized, they should be placed in the axilla and groin, with the skin protected from local injury with a barrier between the skin and pack. Extremities should not be packed in ice, especially in older patients, because this treatment is poorly tolerated in older adults. Supplemental oxygen is also often administered.

Emergent referral to an ED is required for all patients with severe symptoms for further correction of fluid and electrolyte imbalances and directed therapy for any organ-specific damage (e.g., large-volume crystalloid infusions for rhabdomyolysis). The goal is to reduce the temperature to 102°F (38.8°C) within the first hour. To avoid hypothermia, further active cooling should cease when a core temperature of 101°F (38.3°C) is achieved. Antipyretics are ineffective in lowering the temperature in heat-related illnesses. IV fluids, such as normal saline or dextrose and half normal saline, are usually given. Chlorpromazine (Thorazine) 25 to 50 mg IV or diazepam (Valium) 5 to 10 mg IV may be given initially to control shivering and then every 4 hours. In addition, the patient's urinary output, rectal temperature, and cardiac status should be monitored.

FOLLOW-UP AND REFERRAL

As with other urgent care problems, follow-up assessments for heat-related illness depend on the severity and nature of symptoms and the risk of recurrence (e.g., due to persistent unavoidable environmental heat exposure). For example, while the immediate signs and symptoms of more severe forms of heat-related illness may be quickly corrected in the ED setting, outpatient follow-up by the primary-care practitioner is critical for patient teaching and to ensure contributing risk factors and underlying causes of heat-related illness have been eliminated to avoid repeated episodes.

Similarly, referral of patients with heat-related illness to an ED is driven by the severity of symptoms and the potential for subsequent sequelae. For example, some cases of heat exhaustion and heat syncope may require further evaluation in the ED setting, if these symptoms are felt to portend a more significant underlying disorder. Likewise, all cases of heat stroke require immediate ED evaluation and treatment to prevent permanent organ damage. In contrast, heat rash may be treated within the outpatient setting, and similarly, the primary-care practitioner can typically assess for contributing factors to heat cramps, in order to minimize recurrence, without the need for ED referral.

Patient Education: Heat-Related Illnesses

Heat-related illnesses, with their devastating effects, can be avoided or at least reduced in severity through simple preventive measures. These include the following:

- Pacing physical activity and becoming acclimatized to hot environments
- Avoiding alcohol consumption during exposure in hot, humid environments
- Wearing protective, light-colored clothing and a hat when outdoors in hot weather
- Ingesting adequate amounts of electrolyte-balanced liquids (e.g., Gatorade, "sports drinks") to maintain fluid and electrolyte balance, avoid dehydration, and maintain homeostasis

Patients should understand that if they have experienced a heat-related illness in the past, they are more prone to heat-related illnesses in the future. Patients should be taught to gradually build-up time spent in hotter conditions (acclimatization) and moderate physical activity until their bodies have adapted to the hot surroundings. It should be stressed that the higher the temperature and the greater humidity, the greater the risk for heat injury in certain settings. In turn, in these settings, fluids must be consumed even before there is an urge to drink, and prehydration is important if exercising. The ideal fluids are plain water or a low-sugar electrolyte drink.

Education about heat-related illnesses should also be a part of health maintenance, especially with regard to younger patients and the elderly. The primary-care practitioner should warn parents of the risks of leaving children in cars unattended. Older adults should be cautioned about the increased risk of heat-related illnesses, especially if they have medical conditions or are taking medications that increase the risk of heat-related illnesses. Athletes should drink more fluids and try to exercise during the coolest part of the day.

COLD-RELATED ILLNESSES

HYPOTHERMIA

Hypothermia is a medical emergency that can threaten life and limb and is defined by a core temperature of less than 95°F (35°C). If not treated promptly and accurately, the diagnosis carries a high mortality rate, with patient outcomes depending on underlying medical conditions and the duration of exposure to the elements.

EPIDEMIOLOGY AND CAUSES

The incidence and prevalence of hypothermia are difficult to quantify, because not all cases are reported. The hypothermic patient is more likely to be older (with a mean age of 45 years), to be uninsured, and to utilize more critical care than most other patients seen in the ED setting. Approximately 700 people die in the United States from accidental primary hypothermia (due to environmental temperatures) each year. The condition of hypothermia tends to affect economically disadvantaged patients due to unintentional environmental exposures to cold weather and is preventable with community engagement and social support for these patients. Problems with alcoholism, homelessness, and mental illness are common to patients in this category. The other category of affected individuals includes adventure-seekers, including hunters, skiers, climbers, boaters, and swimmers. Despite in-hospital treatment, 40% of patients with moderate to severe hypothermia die.

PATHOPHYSIOLOGY

The reduction in body core temperature starts with a cascade of events. First, there is a loss of heat from the body. This can involve evaporation, convection, conduction, respiration, and, most importantly, radiation through which 50% of body heat is lost rapidly. Common contributing factors to hypothermia include prolonged exposure to lower extremes of outdoor temperatures without protective clothing, alcohol and drug abuse, homelessness, and being elderly. The prognosis is highly dependent on the length of exposure, as well as the provider's recognition of the condition and rapid intervention. For example, progressive organ failure increases as core body temperature decreases; however, this situation is potentially reversible with adequate rewarming.

CLINICAL PRESENTATION

Subjective

The hypothermic patient may arrive with a core body temperature ranging from less than 82.4°F to 95°F (28°C–35°C). Depending on the core temperature, the patient may or may not be conscious enough to give a subjective history. If the patient is conscious, the primary complaint is coldness accompanied with a feeling of exhaustion.

Objective

In addition to an abnormally low body temperature, the physical signs of hypothermia depend on the degree of temperature decline.

Mild hypothermia is defined as a core temperature of 89.6°F to 95°F (32°C–35°C):

- The cardiopulmonary response includes vasoconstriction, hypertension, tachycardia, and tachypnea.
- The renal response is cold diuresis and defective distal tubular absorption of water and sodium.
- The neurological response involves shivering, ataxia, slowed mental processes, and an apathetic affect.

Moderate hypothermia is defined as a core temperature of 82.4°F to 89.6°F (28°C–32°C):

- The cardiopulmonary response is evidenced by hypotension, bradycardia, respiratory depression, and a J-wave on an electrocardiogram (ECG); atrial fibrillation and junctional bradycardia are both associated with a high mortality rate.

- The renal system clamps down (vasoconstricts), and urine output decreases.
- The neurological response leads to a diminished level of consciousness, dilated pupils, decreased reflexes (including the gag reflex), and an inability to mount a shivering reflex.

Severe hypothermia is defined as a core temperature of less than 82.4°F (28°C):

- The cardiopulmonary response may now reveal profound bradycardia with ventricular dysrhythmias or asystole, accompanied by pulmonary edema and/or apnea. Severe hypothermia can cause ventricular fibrillation and other malignant cardiac rhythms. Minimizing motion and jerking movements can help prevent these.
- Renal blood flow is greatly diminished, leading to oliguria.
- Neurologically, the patient loses consciousness, and coma rapidly ensues; the pupils are nonreactive.

DIAGNOSTIC REASONING

Diagnostic Tests

Given the emergent nature of the diagnosis, a laboratory work-up is initiated in the ED setting, following rapid transfer to a higher level of care. Initial laboratory tests consist of an arterial blood gas (ABG) to assess respiratory status and acid-base balance, complete blood count, basic metabolic panel with blood urea nitrogen and creatinine levels, alcohol and drug levels, coagulation studies including partial thromboplastin time, prothrombin time, and international normalized ratio, as well as a chest x-ray and an ECG. All tests may need to be repeated frequently during rewarming to assess for physiologic recovery.

Differential Diagnosis

The clinician should consider head injury, stroke, myocardial infarction, diabetic hypoglycemia or hyperglycemia, drug or alcohol intoxication, sepsis, and hypothyroidism. Typically, the patient's exposure history, as revealed by family or friends who accompany the patient, reveals the diagnosis. Unconscious hypothermic patients who present without accompanying persons to provide a reliable medical history require a comprehensive diagnostic assessment, while aggressively treating the underlying hypothermia.

MANAGEMENT

Hypothermia is a medical emergency and patients should be transported to the nearest hospital as quickly as possible. However, prehospital management should include prevention of heat loss, initiation of rewarming, and the avoidance of dysrhythmias. Wet clothing should be removed and replaced with warm blankets while drying the skin to avoid shivering, which depletes glycogen stores. Emergent management consists of assessing airway, affirming breathing, and monitoring circulation, with the initiation of basic life support measures as appropriate.

General management includes gradually rewarming the body by 1°C to 2°C (1.8°F–3.6°F) per hour via supportive care with warm IV fluids, cardiac monitoring, frequent vital signs, supplemental oxygen if needed, and repeating serum electrolytes, ABGs, and ECGs as needed. The clinician should be aware of the pathophysiological changes in acid–base balance upon initiating treatment. During rewarming, the pH remains constant until the core body temperature reaches 89.6°F (32°C). At this temperature, there is a decline in calcium (Ca^{2+}) and magnesium (Mg^{2+}), accompanied by an increase in pH. Serial ABGs and repeated serum electrolyte panels are essential to monitor acid–base balance.

FOLLOW-UP AND REFERRAL

Following discharge from ED or in-hospital care, the primary-care practitioner needs to consider the patient's age, psychological and medical status, and his or her living situation to plan appropriate follow-up care. If the patient is homeless, a wide social network must be engaged to prevent the recurrence of hypothermia, and a case manager should be consulted. The primary-care practitioner may have to discern if the patient has a home or a shelter in which to stay during the winter months and whether he or she has adequate clothing, including a winter coat, as well as adequate food availability.

Patient Education: Hypothermia

Each patient will have different educational needs, depending on the underlying risk factors for hypothermia. Basic education includes advice on dressing appropriately for cold weather and keeping the body dry and well covered when outdoors. The clinician should warn the patient to avoid alcohol and drug use, as well as overexertion during extremely cold temperatures.

FROSTBITE

Frostbite is freezing of an exposed area, usually the ears, cheeks, nose, fingers, or toes. If a previously frostbitten area becomes frostbitten again after it has healed, permanent tissue damage can occur, resulting in necrosis to that body part.

EPIDEMIOLOGY AND CAUSES

Because of the growing prevalence of homelessness and the increasing number of individuals participating in outdoor activities during cold weather, frostbite is a growing concern. The individuals at greatest risk for frostbite are adults aged 30 to 49 years. A cold environmental temperature is a universal risk factor for frostbite, but it is not the only factor. The duration of exposure to cold weather has a greater impact on frostbite severity and resultant tissue injury than the actual temperature itself.

In addition, ambient humidity, wind exposure, inadequate cold weather clothing, and preexisting medical conditions such as atherosclerosis, diabetes mellitus, and previous cold-related injuries predispose individuals to frostbite. In addition, alcohol consumption, tobacco smoking, poor self-care, immobility, drug abuse, and altered mental status all increase the risk of frostbite.

Although prolonged contact with a cold object can produce frostbite, it is cold humidity that contributes most to evaporative heat loss, as wet skin is more conducive to ice crystal formation. Wind exposure contributes to an increasing loss of heat at higher wind-chill factors. In addition to inadequate body coverage from clothing, overly constrictive clothing can also contribute to an increased incidence of frostbite, as constrictive clothing can reduce circulation to the extremities.

PATHOPHYSIOLOGY

The pathophysiology of frostbite occurs in several stages: tissue freezing, hypoxia, and the release of inflammatory mediators. As tissues cool, the circulation slows, allowing ice crystals to form, first extracellularly and then intracellularly, which damages the cell membrane. Crystals that form extracellularly exert osmotic force and pull fluid from the intracellular space into the extracellular space, resulting in cellular dehydration. As this process continues, the cell membrane is damaged. Intracellular crystals that subsequently form cause more damage to the cell as they expand within it.

Hypoxia results from cold-induced local vasoconstriction, which leads to acidosis and increased local blood viscosity, as well as hypoxia. Although the body has a natural defensive mechanism against the cold (called *cold-induced vasodilation* or the "hunting response," which prevents rapid freezing of the skin), prolonged exposure to the cold eventually causes this response to fail, and freezing occurs. As capillary blood flow ceases, arterioles and venules thrombose, leading to the release of inflammatory mediators. The release of prostaglandins and thromboxane promotes vasoconstriction, platelet aggregation, and blood vessel thrombosis, which worsen endothelial damage. If left unchecked, this process will lead to cell death and widespread tissue necrosis.

CLINICAL PRESENTATION

Subjective

Initially, the patient complains of a tingling sensation of the affected body part, followed by pain and eventual numbness.

Objective

The anatomical regions at greatest risk for injury are the hands and feet, which account for 90% of frostbite injuries. The ears, nose, cheeks, and penis are also prone to frostbite. Classically, the clinical presentation of frostbite has been categorized according to four degrees of injury. The classification should be applied after some rewarming has been initiated because most victims of frostbite initially present similarly, with tingling and redness followed by pallor and numbness.

- **First-degree frostbite (partial skin freezing):** Erythema, edema, hyperemia, no blisters or necrosis, occasional skin desquamation (5–10 days later), transient stinging and burning, and possible throbbing and aching; the patient may also have hyperhidrosis (excessive sweating).
- **Second-degree frostbite (full-thickness injury):** Erythema, substantial edema, vesicles with clear fluid, blisters that desquamate and form blackened eschar, numbness, and vasomotor disturbances in severe cases.
- **Third-degree frostbite (full-thickness injury and subcutaneous freezing):** Violaceous/hemorrhagic blisters, skin necrosis, and blue-gray discoloration; initially, no sensation (tissue feels like a block of wood), but shooting pains, burning, throbbing, and aching develop later.
- **Fourth-degree frostbite (full-thickness injury and subcutaneous tissue, muscle, tendon, and bone freezing):** Initially, skin is mottled, deep red, or cyanotic; later, skin becomes dry, black, and mummified. Minimal edema is present, with possible joint discomfort.

DIAGNOSTIC REASONING

Diagnostic Tests

There are no definitive diagnostic studies for frostbite, especially within the first week of injury. Doppler studies may be helpful to assess blood flow.

Differential Diagnosis

Differential diagnoses for frostbite include the following:

- Frostnip—a mild form of cold injury.
- Chilblain (erythema pernio)—tender red to red-blue itchy nodules on extremities triggered by cold weather and thought to result from chronic vasospasm; there is no actual freezing of the tissue.
- Immersion foot—hyperhidrosis (excessive perspiration) of the feet causing thickening, maceration, and tenderness of the skin due to prolonged submersion in water or cold (also called trench foot, because it affected soldiers camped for days in trenches during times of war).
- Hypothermia—see previous section for full description.

MANAGEMENT

Frostbite is a medical emergency because of the potential for extensive tissue necrosis and loss of limb. If the patient presenting to a primary-care setting has frostbite, the area should be rewarmed, and hot liquids such as coffee, tea, or broth should be administered. The basis of treatment for frostbite is to reverse the pathological effects of ice crystal formation, vasoconstriction, and the release of inflammatory mediators. Treatment should not be started if there is a possibility of refreezing. If it is suspected that the patient has second- to fourth-degree frostbite, hospitalization should be considered.

The first measure is to rewarm the affected area. Rewarming is accomplished by using warm water (104°F [40°C] to 108°F [42.2°C]). Care must be taken not to rub the affected area. If possible, the affected body part should be placed in water for 10 to 30 minutes until the tissue is pliable and red. This process can be very painful; therefore, narcotics should be administered and titrated for comfort.

Blister management in patients with frostbite is somewhat controversial. Blisters containing clear or milky fluid should be debrided and covered with aloe vera every 6 hours. Aloe vera is a potent antiprostaglandin agent. Hemorrhagic blisters should be left intact and covered with aloe vera. The affected area should be wrapped with a sterile dressing, splinted, and elevated. Topical Silvadene and bacitracin ointment have proven to be effective as antibacterials; however, use of these topical ointments may interfere with the effects of aloe vera.

It is unclear whether prophylactic antibiotic use is warranted for frostbite. The use of penicillin G 500,000 units IV every 6 hours for the first 72 hours has proven effective. Ibuprofen 400 mg PO every 4 to 6 hours should be administered for its antiprostaglandin activity. Ibuprofen is also a potential inhibitor of thromboxane and is more potent than other anti-inflammatory drugs. The patient's tetanus status should also be assessed, given the risk of infection through compromised skin. Patients who are being treated for frostbite should not be allowed to smoke, given the vasoconstrictive effects of tobacco smoke.

Patients may need daily hydrotherapy to debride devitalized tissue. In some instances, referral to a surgeon for a fasciotomy or escharotomy may be needed if there is limited range of motion in an extremity or if the possibility of "compartment syndrome" develops. Compartment syndrome occurs when any structure such as a nerve or tendon is being constricted in a closed space, such as an extremity. The sheath or tendon becomes enlarged because of the inflammation and is no longer able to move freely in the bodily compartment. This results in a restriction of circulation—a critical condition that may result in loss of a limb. Thus, compartment syndrome is an emergent situation that requires immediate referral to an ED.

FOLLOW-UP AND REFERRAL

The majority of patients with frostbite injuries should be admitted to the hospital for 2 to 4 days. If dressings are in place, the patient should be monitored every 2 to 3 days to assess healing. If debridement or grafting is necessary, the patient should be referred to a dermatologist or a vascular surgeon.

Patient Education: Frostbite

Patients should be taught to watch for signs of infection, to take all medications as prescribed, and to use extreme care regarding further exposure to cold. The following preventive measures should also be recommended:

- Do not go outdoors for prolonged periods of time.
- Wear a hat or earmuffs, mittens, and dress in layers.
- Keep dry and change out of wet clothing.
- Dress in natural materials such as cotton or wool.
- Avoid caffeine, tobacco, and alcohol when going outdoors in the cold, because these substances leave the skin more prone to thermal injury.
- Check the skin every 12 to 20 minutes for signs of frostbite when exposed to cold environments.

 For additional resources please visit
https://davisedge.fadavis.com/

REFERENCES

Frostbite

Fudge JR, Bennett BL, Simanis JP, Roberts WO. Medical evaluation for exposure extremes: Cold. *Wilderness Environ Med.* 2015; 26(Suppl 4):S63–S68.

Heat-Related Illnesses

Atha WF. Heat-related illness. *Emerg Med Clin North Am.* 2013;31(4):1097–1108.

Becker JA, Stewart LK. Heat-related illness. *Am Fam Physician.* 2011;83(11):1325–1330.

Fowler DR, Mitchell CS, Brown A, et al. Heat-related deaths after an extreme heat event. *MMWR Morb Mortal Wkly Rep.* 2013;62(22):433–436. https://www.cdc.gov/mmwr/preview/mmwrhtml/mm6222a1.htm. Accessed 10/23/18.

Gomez CR. Disorders of body temperature. *Handb Clin Neurol.* 2014;120:947–957.

Lipman GS, Eifling KP, Ellis MA, Gaudio FG, Otten EM, & Grissom CK. Wilderness Medical Society practice guidelines for the prevention and treatment of heat-related illness: 2014 Update. *Wilderness Environ Med.* 2014: 5(4); supplement S55–S65. https://www.wemjournal.org/article/S1080-6032(14)00270-1/abstract. Accessed 10/23/18.

Hypothermia

Brown DJ, Brugger H, Boyd J, Paal P. Accidental hypothermia. *N Engl J Med.* 2012;367:1930–1938.

Zafren K, Giesbrecht GG, Danzl DF, et al. Wilderness Medical Society practice guidelines for the out-of-hospital evaluation and treatment of accidental hypothermia: 2014 update. *Wilderness Environ Med.* 2014;25(4):425–445. https://ucdavis.pure.elsevier.com/en/publications/wilderness-medical-society-practice-guidelines-for-the-out-of-hos. Accessed 10/23/18.

RESOURCE

MEDDAC Preventive Medicine Climatic Injury Awareness and Prevention Site
http://www.alaska.amedd.army.mil/Preventive_Med/Preventive_Medicine.htm

Caring-Based Nursing:
The Practice

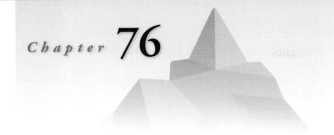

Chapter 76

Sports Physicals

Margaret Colyar, DSN, APRN, FNP-BC, PNP-BC

Lynne M. Dunphy, PhD, APRN, FNP-BC, FAAN,

FAANP

INTRODUCTION

The purpose of the sports physical, also known as the preparticipation physical, is to promote safe sports participation by identifying high-risk situations. Sometimes referred to as pre-participation physical evaluation (PPE), these exams are not meant to exclude athletes from participation. These exams are generally a formal requirement and are done annually before participation in junior high, high school, and college or professional. Objectives of the sports physical are listed in Box 76.1. A 2014 study documented that the requirements for PPE use and the content of the evaluations vary and are

determined by each state individually. To ensure comprehensive and consistent screenings, the authors conclude that there is a need for a nationwide standardized PPE form, preferably in an electronic format. Sudden cardiac death is the leading cause of death in young athletes during sports (Caswell, et al., 2015).

Sports are divided into five degrees of contact and intensity which the provider must consider when assessment an athlete for sports participation. A list of sports by level of contact and intensity is shown on Table 76.1.

EXAM FORMATS

The following are three types of exam formats for sports physicals:

1. **Office-based**—A single provider examines one athlete in the office setting. Office-based allows counseling at an important stage of life, establishes the importance of preventive care, provides privacy for open communication and provides continuity of care. However, it is usually more expensive.
2. **Assembly-line**—A single provider examines several athletes, one athlete after the other. This format is usually cheaper and quicker but lacks individual attention, causes possible communication problems, increases the risk that insufficient medical history is taken, and lacks continuity.
3. **Station**—Multiple examiners do different parts of the exam. This type saves time, is cost-efficient, and allows the use of providers with specialized expertise (cardiologist, optometrist, physical therapist, etc.). However, there is a tendency toward disorganization, as well as potential for inadequate integration of all findings. This format also is impersonal, lacks privacy, and may feel rushed to the athlete. It is best to use avoid the gymnasium setting due to privacy and noise issues.

Box 76.1 Objectives of the Sports Physical

Primary Objectives

- Determine the athlete is in general good health
- Assess the athlete's present fitness level
- Identify asymptomatic illness
- Identify athletes at risk for injury
- Evaluate any existing injuries of the athlete
- Detect conditions that may predispose the athlete to injury
- Detect congenital anomalies that increase the athlete's risk of injury
- Detect poor conditioning that may put the athlete at increased risk
- Detect conditions that may be life-threatening or disabling
- Find athletes at risk for sudden death
- Meet legal and insurance requirements

Secondary Objectives

- Determine general health
- Counsel on health-related issues
- Assess fitness level for specific sports

Source: Sanders B, Blackburn TA, Boucher B. Preparticipation screening—the sports physical therapy perspective. *Int J Sports Phys Ther.* 2013;8(2):180–193.

TABLE 76.1 Sports by Level of Contact

Contact	Collision	Noncontact
Field hockey	Soccer	Aerobics
Football	Wrestling	Track
Martial arts	Ice hockey	Fencing
Rodeo	Rugby	Swimming
Boxing	Baseball	Running
Lacrosse	Basketball	Weight lifting
		Archery
		Golf
		Tennis
		Crew
		Riflery

Source: Colyar MR. *Assessment of the school-age child and adolescent.* Philadelphia, PA: F.A. Davis; 2011.

COMPONENTS OF SPORTS PHYSICAL: HISTORY, PHYSICAL EXAMINATION, AND CLEARANCE

No matter what format is chosen, the sports physical can be divided into three main components: history, physical examination, and clearance.

History

The athlete's history gives the provider most of the information needed to make an informed decision about clearing or disqualifying an athlete. The athlete and parent should complete the history together prior to the examination. Specific items to screen for in the medical history, specific sports history, and family history are listed in Box 76.2.

The recommended baseline history includes the following areas:

- Medical conditions and diseases
- Surgeries
- Hospitalizations
- Medications (prescription, over the counter, supplements)
- Allergies (medications, insects, environmental)
- Immunization status
- Menstrual history
- Psychosocial history

Additional information that should elicited include the following pulmonary, neurologic, and musculoskeletal injuries or illnesses since the most recent exam:

- **Asthma**—Exercise-induced asthma is a common cause of exertional chest pain in young athletes and can be a sign of left ventricular outflow tract obstruction or coronary artery anomalies. If a new condition, the athlete should be referred to a pulmonologist.
- **Concussion**—Disqualification for athletes with a history of frequent or severe concussions is controversial. For athletes with a concussion history, the provider should determine the number of concussions the athlete has had, their duration, frequency, recovery time, and risk factors. Athletes with signs and symptoms of concussion (brief loss of consciousness after the injury, memory problems, confusion, drowsiness or feeling sluggish, dizziness, double vision or blurred vision, headache) or postconcussion syndrome (headaches, dizziness, fatigue, irritability, anxiety, insomnia, loss of concentration and memory, and noise and light sensitivity) should not be cleared for participation until all symptoms have resolved. Formal balance testing, such as the Balance Error Scoring System [BESS] (Table 76.2) and neuropsychologic testing, should be done before sports participation and when head injury occurs to determine when the athlete can return to play (Mirabelli, 2015).
- **Dyspnea on exertion**—Dyspnea on exertion and becoming easily fatigued may simply represent poor

Box 76.2 History Components of Sports Physical

Past Medical History

Allergies
Asthma
Birth defects
Burning/stinging pain caused by contact
Contagious diseases

- Chicken pox
- Hepatitis
- Measles
- Mononucleosis
- Pneumonia
- Rheumatic fever
- Tuberculosis

Diabetes
Disqualification from sports previously
Eating disorders
Glasses/contacts
Heart murmur
Heart problems
Heat problems
Hernia
High blood pressure
Immunization status
Kidney disease
Medications (prescription, over the counter, supplements)
Menstrual history
Mental disorders
Sickle cell disease
Seizures

Sports-Specific History

Chest pain with exercise
Dental trauma
Excessive shortness of breath
Excessive fatigue with exercise
Feeling faint or passed out with exercise
Orthopedic injuries

- Sprains
- Fractures
- Dislocations
- Surgeries
- Back or neck injuries

Family History

Diabetes
Heart disease
High blood pressure
Unexpected death before age 50

Source: American College of Sports Medicine. Pre-participation physical exams. https://www.acsm.org/docs/brochures/pre-participation-physical-examinations.pdf.

TABLE 76.2 Balance Error Scoring System Testing for Concussion

Test	Component	Timing
DOUBLE LEG STANCE		
• Stand with feet pelvic width apart • Hands on hips • Eyes closed	On firm surface	20 seconds
SINGLE LEG STANCE		
• Stand on the non-dominant leg with contralateral limb in approximately 20° of hip flexion, 45° of knee flexion • Hands on hips • Eyes closed	On firm surface	20 seconds
TANDEM STANCE		
• Dominant foot in front of the nondominant foot • Heel of the anterior foot touching the toe of the posterior foot • Hands on hips • Eyes closed	On firm surface	20 seconds
DOUBLE LEG STANCE		
• Stand with feet pelvis width apart • Hands on hips • Eyes closed	On foam surface	20 seconds
SINGLE LEG STANCE		
• Stand on the non-dominant leg with contralateral limb in approximately 20° of hip flexion, 45° of knee flexion • Hands on hips • Eyes closed	On foam surface	20 seconds
TANDEM STANCE		
• Dominant foot in front of the nondominant foot • Heel of the anterior foot touching the toe of the posterior foot • Hands on hips • Eyes closed	On foam surface	20 seconds

Note. No shoes should be worn.

Scoring: Count balance errors—opening the eyes, hands coming off hips, a step, stumble or fall, moving the hips more than 30 degrees, lifting the forefoot or heel, or remaining out of testing position for more than 5 seconds. Compare with pre–sports participation score.

Source: Bell DR, Guskiewicz KM, Clark MA, Padua DA. Systematic review of the Balance Error Scoring System. *Sports Health*. 2011;3(3):287–295.

conditioning. However, primary pulmonary hypertension, profound anemia, exercise-induced asthma, or an underlying cardiovascular disorder should be suspected. The athlete should be referred for a work-up before participation.

- **Eating disorders, psychiatric disorders, and abuse**—Athletes in weight-sensitive sports (boxing, wrestling) and aesthetic sports (diving, figure skating, dance, cheerleading) are at risk for eating disorders. Athletes with untreated mental illness should receive treatment and be stabilized before resuming athletic participation. Athletes with identified drug abuse should also receive treatment before returning to sports (Mirabelli, 2015).

- **Family history of premature sudden death**—A family history of premature sudden death is particularly relevant in identifying hypertrophic cardiomyopathy and is a major risk factor for long QT syndrome, arrhythmogenic right ventricular cardiomyopathy, Marfan syndrome, and coronary anomalies. Electrocardiography (ECG), echocardiography, exercise stress testing, and lipid panels should be used to evaluate for cardiovascular disease. A cardiology referral can be considered.

- **Hematologic disorders**—Athletes with bleeding disorders such as hemophilia and von Willebrand disease should be restricted from contact or collision sports. Athletes with sickle cell disease are limited to low-intensity activities. Those with sickle cell trait may participate in all activities; however, elevation, dehydration, and illness are risk factors that may cause exertional sickling.

- **Palpitations**—Palpitations may signify supraventricular tachycardia, sinus tachycardia, right ventricular cardiomyopathy, or long QT syndrome. Abruptness of onset, heart rate, and frequency of episodes should be evaluated. A sudden onset of a fast heart rate suggests supraventricular tachycardia, especially if it can be resolved with vagal maneuvers. A gradual onset and relief of palpitations on exertion suggests sinus tachycardia. The athlete should be asked about use of tobacco, caffeine, alcohol, over-the-counter medications, supplements, and illicit drugs. Sports participation should be restricted, and the athlete should be referred for a basic work-up (i.e., electrolyte testing, thyroid function testing, and careful ECG evaluation). If the etiology of palpitations is not clear, then further evaluation for malignant arrhythmia with Holter monitoring should be done.

- **Seizures**—Athletes with well-controlled seizures can participate in most sports, except those that could be fatal, such as skydiving, hang gliding, and scuba diving (Mirabelli, 2015).

- **Syncope and presyncope**—Athletes with exercise-related syncope or presyncope may have left ventricular outflow tract obstruction, arrhythmia, or congenital coronary anomalies and require further evaluation to rule out structural cardiovascular disease. They should not participate in sports until cleared by a cardiologist. A congenital coronary anomaly, most often a coronary artery that arises from the opposite aortic sinus, should also be suspected when an athlete presents with chest pain or syncope.

Physical Examination

The physical examination is a screening tool that emphasizes the areas of greatest concern in sports participation. Table 76.3 lists areas to focus on in each system.

Height and Weight

These measures evaluate growth and development and assess for problems with general fitness (obesity, anorexia) and pathology (eating disorders).

Head, Ears, Eyes, Nose Throat

Visual acuity is the focus of the eye exam. If the athlete's vision is greater than 20/40 in one or both eyes, they should be referred for an eye exam. Monocular vision and detached retina disqualify the athlete from contact sports. An otoscope examination of the ears, nose, and throat should be done, but abnormalities rarely indicate disqualification from sports participation.

TABLE 76.3   Physical Examination Focus Points

Area	Focus Points
Height/Weight	Anorexia athletica, morbid obesity
Head	Concussion
Eyes/ear/nose/throat	Visual acuity, monocular vision, detached retina
Pulses	Irregular rhythm
Blood pressure	Hypertension
Heart	Exertional syncope, dizziness, chest pain with activity, murmurs, palpitations, mitral valve prolapse
Lungs	Active tuberculosis, uncontrolled asthma, pulmonary insufficiency, and history of spontaneous pneumothorax
Abdomen	Hepatomegaly, splenomegaly
Genitourinary	Kidney problems, one kidney
Genitalia (boys)	Hernia–femoral or inguinal
Skin	Contagious diseases—tinea, boils, impetigo, herpes
Musculoskeletal	Fractures, sprains, torn tendons/ligaments, stiff joints, joint pain
Neurologic	Seizure disorder

Source: Colyar MR. *Assessment of the school-age child and adolescent.* Philadelphia, PA: F.A. Davis; 2011.

If the athlete reports burning pain, weakness, numbness, or tingling in all four or only the upper extremities, cervical spine impingement should be suspected. Other possible conditions are atlantoaxial instability, congenital fusions, and disk herniation (Kurowski & Chandran, 2000).

Cardiovascular System

All peripheral pulses should be assessed and all four valves of the heart auscultated. Any irregularity of heart rate should be checked by ECG as a prolonged QT interval can be the cause of sudden death. Serious arrhythmias are usually detectable when the athlete holds his or her breath. In addition, if any irregular heart sounds or murmur that has not been detected previously are found, the athlete should be referred for an echocardiogram.

Hypertension must be controlled before sports participation. Rough guidelines are a blood pressure of 125/80 mm Hg or less for those aged 10 to 15 years and 130/85 mm Hg for those aged 16 years and older (Chiolero, Bovet, & Paradis, 2013).

The most common cause of sudden cardiac death in athletes is hypertrophic cardiomyopathy. A systolic murmur heard along the left sternal border that increases with Valsalva maneuvers and standing and decreases with handgrip and squat maneuvers is the classic sign (Saglimbeni & Young, 2015). Symptoms usually occur during peak physical exertion or in volume-depleted states.

A consensus statement by the American College of Cardiology and the American Heart Association includes guidelines for eligibility for athletes who have previously been diagnosed with cardiac conditions based on the intensity of the sport. The guidelines allow athletes with known hypertrophic cardiomyopathy to participate in low-intensity activities, but recommend exclusion from most strenuous activities (Mirabelli, 2015).

Marfan syndrome is an inherited autosomal dominant disorder that affects connective tissue and commonly affects the heart, eyes, blood vessels, and skeleton. Signs an athlete has Marfan syndrome include long arms, legs and fingers, tall and thin body type, curved spine, chest sinks in or sticks out, flexible joints, flat feet, crowded teeth, and stretch marks on the skin that are not related to weight gain or loss. Because aortic root dilation is common with Marfan syndrome and can cause aortic dissection and sudden death, the American Heart Association recommends including examination for the physical signs of Marfan syndrome, auscultation of all four heart valves for heart murmurs, palpation of peripheral pulses, and brachial artery blood pressure taken in sitting position.

Evaluation including ECG, slit-lamp eye examination, and echocardiography to assess the aortic root is also recommended for males taller than 6 feet (1.83 m) and females taller than 5 feet 10 in (1.78 m) who have two or more physical manifestations of Marfan syndrome (Giese, O'Connor, Brennan, Depenbrock, & Oriscell, 2007).

Respiratory System

The respiratory rate should be measured and all lung fields auscultated, both anteriorly and posteriorly. Uncontrolled asthma and exercise-induced deoxygenation are reasons to restrict contact sports participation.

Musculoskeletal System

Flexibility, gait, muscle performance, joint laxity, and strength are key components for evaluation. Asymmetry of joints, muscles, range of motion, and strength should be assessed. The goal of this component of the sports physical is to identify risks of and prevent injury. Refer for evaluation of asymmetry of joints, muscles, range of motion, and unequal strength (Sanders, Blackburn TA, Boucher, 2013).

Neck/Cervical Spine. Range of motion of the neck should be evaluated. The athlete should be able to flex the cervical spine forward, backward, to the right and left sides and should be able to rotate the head from right to left.

Shoulders. Assessment includes trapezius muscle strength, deltoid muscle strength, and glenohumeral range of motion. The athlete should shrug and abduct their shoulders against resistance. External and internal rotation of the shoulders should be observed. Bilateral grip should be tested to evaluate upper extremity strength.

Elbows. Range of motion of the elbows should be assessed. The athlete should be able to extend and flex the elbows, pronate and supinate the forearm.

Wrist, Hands, and Fingers. Range of motion of the wrists with plantar flexion, dorsi flexion, internal and external rotation should be assessed. For the hands and fingers, the athlete should be instructed to make a fist and then spread the fingers.

Back. The spine should be assessed for scoliosis and range of motion, as well as hamstring flexibility. The athlete should be instructed to stand up straight and flex forward at the waist. Normal flexibility is 90 degrees. Scoliosis is seen when one scapula is higher than the other.

Legs. Strength, balance, and range of motion of hips, knees, and ankles are tested by instructing the athlete

squat down and duck-walk four steps. Calf strength, symmetry, and balance are assessment by instructing the athlete to walk on tip toes and walk on heels.

Gastrointestinal System

The abdomen should be palpated to check for pain or masses, and the liver and spleen size should be assessed because of the risk of rupture in contact sports. Any costal vertebral angle tenderness may indicate kidney problems.

Hernias

An inguinal hernia check should be done on all male athletes, and they should be taught how to do a testicular self-exam and what to look for. The need for a genital examination is an area of controversy among sports medicine physicians.

Skin

The athlete should be asked to show you any skin lesions. Tinea corporis, boils, impetigo, scabies, and herpes lesions will disqualify the athlete until corrected.

Clearance

Clearance can be divided into three categories:

1. Unrestricted clearance
2. Clearance after completion of further evaluation or rehabilitation
3. Disqualification or no clearance for certain types of sports or for all sports

Unrestricted clearance indicates the athlete is cleared for all sports and all levels of participation.

If the athlete has a health issue that needs evaluation or treatment or has suspicious signs or symptoms, further workup may be needed before sports participation. Clearance after completion of further evaluation or rehabilitation should be chosen.

Disqualification is the appropriate category when a known condition prohibits an athlete's participation in the given sport. Examples of conditions that can limit participation are shown in Table 76.4. The Committee on Sports Medicine has developed a list of recommendations for participation.

TABLE 76.4 Sports Participation Disqualification			
Problem	*Contact*	*Collision*	*Noncontact*
Acute infections			
Respiratory, genitourinary, mononucleosis, hepatitis, rheumatic fever, tuberculosis	X	X	X
Hemorrhagic disease—serious bleeding tendencies	X	X	X
Diabetes—inadequately controlled	X	X	X
—controlled	O	O	O
Eyes—single eye or detached retina	X	X	O
Corrected visual acuity <20/200	X	X	X
Glaucoma	X	X	O

Continued

TABLE 76.4 Sports Participation Disqualification—cont'd

Problem	Contact	Collision	Noncontact
Respiratory—*severe pulmonary insufficiency	X	X	X
Recurrent pneumothorax	X	X	O
Cardiovascular—*mitral/aortic valve stenosis/prolapse, aortic insufficiency, coarctation of aorta, cyanotic heart disease, recent carditis	X	X	X
Hypertension—uncontrolled	X	X	X
—controlled	O	O	O
Previous heart surgery	J	J	J
Liver—enlarged	X	X	O
Spleen—enlarged	X	X	O
Skin—boils, impetigo, herpes simplex	X	X	O
Hernia—inguinal or femoral	X	X	X
Musculoskeletal—inflammatory	X	X	X
Congenital or acquired problems that are incompatible with skills required	X	X	X
CNS—previous serious head injury	X	J	O
Seizure disorder—controlled	J	J	J
—uncontrolled	X	X	X
Previous head surgery	X	X	O
Kidneys—one kidney	X	X	O
Renal disease	X	X	X
Genitalia—one testicle	O	O	O
Undescended	O	O	O

Abbreviations: J, judge on individual basis with recommendations from cardiologist and/or surgeon; O, OK; X, exclusion.
*Refer and work-up.
Source: Colyar MR. *Assessment of The School-Age Child And Adolescent*. Philadelphia, PA: F.A. Davis; 2011.

For additional resources please visit
https://davisedge.fadavis.com/

REFERENCES

Bell DR, Guskiewicz KM, Clark MA, Padua DA. Systematic review of the Balance Error Scoring System. *Sports Health*. 2011;3(3):287–295.

Colyar MR. *Assessment of the school-age child and adolescent*. Philadelphia, PA: F.A. Davis; 2011.

Caswell, SV, Cortes, N, Chabolla, M et al. Pre-participation differences in school sports preparticipation physical evaluation policies. *Pediatrics* 2015;135. doi: 10.1542/peds.2014-1451. Originally published online Dec. 22, 2014.

Chiolero A, Bovet P, Paradis G. Screening for elevated blood pressure in children and adolescents: A critical appraisal. *JAMA Pediatr*. 2013;167(3):266–273. doi:10.1001/jamapediatrics.2013.438.

Giese EA, O'Connor FG, Brennan FH, Depenbrock PJ, Oriscell RG. The athletic preparticipation evaluation: Cardiovascular assessment. *Am Fam Physician*. 2007;75(7):1008–1014.

Kurowski KK, Chandran S. The preparticipation athletic evaluation. *Am Fam Physician*. 2000;61(9):2683–2690.

Mirabelli MH, Devine MJ, Singh J, Mendoza M, et al. The preparticipation sports evaluation. *Am Fam Physician*. 2015;92:371–376.

Saglimbeni AJ, Young CC. Sports physicals. *Medscape*. December 3, 2015. Updated Sep 04, 2018.

Sanders B, Blackburn TA, Boucher B. Preparticipation screening—the sports physical therapy perspective. *Int J Sports Phys Ther*. 2013;8(2):180–193.

RESOURCES

American College of Sports Medicine
www.acsm.org

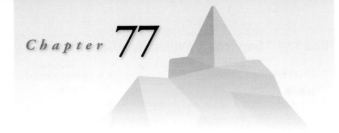

Chapter 77

Primary Care of Older Adults

Ruth McCaffrey, DNP, APRN, FNP-BC, GNP–BC, FAAN, FAANP

Lynne M. Dunphy, PhD, APRN, FNP-BC, FAAN, FAANP

Lori Martin-Plank, PhD, APRN, FNP-BC, GNP-BC, FAANP

Humberto Reinoso, PhD, FNP-BC, ENP-BC

"The impending crisis, which has been foreseen for decades, is now upon us. The nation needs to act now to prepare the health care workforce to meet the care needs of older adults."

(Institute of Medicine, 2008)

INTRODUCTION

The organic process of aging is called *senescence*, the medical study of the aging process is called *gerontology*, and the study of diseases that affect the elderly is called *geriatrics*. Aging presents unique challenges for older adults, their loved ones and families, their surrounding communities, as well as their health-care providers. The human life cycle—or "life expectancy"—varies from country to country. Old age is not a definite biological stage, as the chronological age denoted as "old age" varies culturally and historically. For purposes of this chapter, an older adult is one who is aged 65 or older because life expectancy in the United States exceeds that of many—but certainly not all—other countries.

Populations around the world are rapidly aging, with some of the fastest change occurring in low- and middle-income countries. Promoting healthy aging, emphasizing health prevention, and building systems to meet the needs of older adults are sound investments in a future where older people have the freedom to be and do what they value. The World Health Organization (WHO; 2016) has developed a global strategy and action plan on aging and health. The strategy (2016–2020) has two goals:

- Five years of evidence-based action to maximize functional ability that reaches every person
- By 2020, establish evidence and partnerships necessary to support a Decade of Healthy Ageing from 2020 to 2030

The strategy has five strategic objectives:

1. Commitment to action on Healthy Ageing in every country
2. Developing age-friendly environments
3. Aligning health systems to the needs of older populations
4. Developing sustainable and equitable systems for providing long-term care (home, communities, institutions)
5. Improving measurement, monitoring, and research on Healthy Ageing

Older adults often have limited regenerative abilities and are more susceptible to acute illnesses and complications, some of which can be complex, than younger adults. Additionally, older adults have a higher prevalence of chronic diseases that occur as the overall strength and resilience of the body declines. The elderly also face social issues around retirement, such as poverty, loneliness, and ageism.

With more Americans living longer and overall healthier lives, there is an increasing need to focus on health promotion in older adult populations and their specialized health-related needs. Health promotion and disease prevention in the older adult population requires close collaboration between health, social welfare, and community services (Pilotto et al., 2016; WHO, 2016). It has been suggested that health-care providers must rethink fundamental values related to the health care of older adults to include emotional, social, educational, and financial issues, as well as medical diagnosis and treatments (Osbourne, Moulds, Squires, & Doty, 2014; WHO, 2016). This is congruent with the *Circle of Caring* approach of this text, and reemphasizes the need for nursing-based approaches in this population including patient-centered care and teamwork.

Health systems have been traditionally designed to respond to episodic health needs than to the more complex and chronic health needs that tend to arise with increasing age. There is an urgent need to develop and implement comprehensive and coordinated primary health-care approaches that can prevent, slow, or reverse declines in intrinsic capacity, and, where these declines are unavoidable, help older people to compensate in ways that maximize their functional ability. Integrated-care approaches should be community-based, designed around the needs of the older person rather than the provider, and coordinated effectively with long-term care systems.

Services should be orientated around the needs of older people rather than the needs of the services themselves. Services should respond to a diversity of older people that ranges from those with high and stable levels of intrinsic capacity through those with declining capacity, to people whose capacity has deteriorated to the point of needing the care and support of others. According to the WHO (2016) Guidelines on Integrated Care for Older People (ICOPE), important elements of integrated care at the community level are as follows:

- A comprehensive assessment and care plan shared with all providers
- Common care and treatment goals across different providers
- Community outreach and home-based interventions
- Support for self-management
- Comprehensive referral and monitoring processes
- Community engagement and caregiver support (WHO, 2016)

Delivering ICOPE can support a transformation in the way health systems are designed and operate.

Not only do the numbers of older adult continue to increase but the cost of providing care to older adults escalates yearly (Segert, 2014). As the number of older adults continues to grow, providers and payers will need to find ways to provide needed care while holding costs to a sustainable level. *Healthy People 2020* lists the following emerging issues in the health of older adults:

- Person-centered care planning that includes caregivers and families
- Quality measures of care and monitoring of health conditions
- Fair pay and compensation standards for formal and informal caregivers
- Minimum levels of geriatric training for all health professionals
- Enhanced data on certain subpopulations of older adults, including the aging lesbian-gay-transgender-bisexual (LGBT) populations (Healthy People 2020, 2014)

Over 60% of older adults have two or more chronic diseases (National Council on Aging, 2016) that require a potentially complex plan of care centered around the wishes of the patient and family. Creating an effective care plan that functions across a continuum of settings, providers, and living conditions can improve the overall quality of life of older adults.

One of the most successful methods to assist older adults to improve their quality of life while meeting all their health-care needs is to use a team approach to care throughout care management. Geriatric care management assists older adults and their families find resources and manage stress. The care manager can be a medical office-based provider or a consultant who is available to older adults for a fee or insurance coverage (Box 77.1). In primary-care settings with many older adult patients, a list of local care managers might be useful to patients and families, especially when older adults do not live in the same vicinity as their family members.

Box 77.1   Services Provided by a Care Manager

- Assessment to determine what is needed to maximize elder's quality of life
- Complete evaluations and referral recommendations for where to turn and what to do for specific types of care
- Design, implement, and manage a comprehensive plan of care to relieve uncertainty, educate patient related to available services, and help older adults and their families understand the language and programs involved in eldercare.
- Family meetings to provide a safe space and a neutral party to listen to family concerns and help work toward resolving disagreements
- Coordination of services, appointments, and follow-up based on individual needs and decisions
- Assistance with living arrangement transitions
- Advocacy for elderly patients at doctor's visits and hospital stays and review of their care
- Assistance with screening, arranging, and monitoring services

---

DEMOGRAPHICS OF AGING

Why are the issues surrounding health promotion and chronic disease management in older adults so important? The population of the United States is aging, and the number of older adults in our society is growing as life expectancy lengthens. The Administration on Aging (2015) found that in 2014, 14.5% of the population, or one in seven people in the United States, were older than age 65. The U.S. Census Bureau speculates that this number will continue to rise until 17.8% of the U.S. population is older than age 65 by 2020 (Ortman, Welkoff, & Howard, 2014). It is estimated that each day, 10,000 baby boomers (those born in the years following World War II) retire and begin receiving Medicare and Social Security benefits (Insured Retirement Institute, 2016). These statistics can be compared to the population older than age 65 in 1900, which was only 4% of the population. This significant change also demonstrates the vitality of our current aging population. A child born in 2014 will live an average of 30 years longer than a child born in 1900. In 2015, 70% of men and 45% of women older than age 65 were married; 35% of women are widowed, and 20% either single never married or are divorced.

The U.S. Census Bureau uses the term "older population" to denote persons aged 65 and older. There are several subcategories within the older population group, including:

- Young-old = 65–74 years
- Old = 75–84
- Oldest-old = 85 and older

Baby boomers are defined as the population cohort born between mid-1946 and mid-1964. During these years, a sharp, unprecedented increase in the birthrate was observed. According to the Census Bureau, there were 76.4 million baby boomers living in the United States in 2012 (Ortman et al., 2014).

Population Projections

The older population (aged 65 and over) will nearly double in the next 4 decades, rising from 43.1 million in 2012 to 83.7 million in 2050. Most of this growth will occur between 2010 and 2030 as baby boomers reach age 65. The first of the baby boomers turned 65 in 2011; the last will turn 65 in 2029. In 2030, more than 1 in 5 (20.3%) U.S. residents will be counted among the older population—the largest proportion on record. Baby boomers will be better educated and more racially and ethnically diverse than previous generations of older adults.

The oldest-old (aged 85+) is the fastest-growing segment of the total population, doubling by 2036 and tripling by 2049. By 2050, 4.5% of the U.S. population will be aged 85 and older, up from 2.5% in 2030 (Segert, 2014). One of the goals of caring for older adults is to keep them independent and living at home. Currently, the overall percentage of older adults living in institutionalized settings such as nursing homes is 3.2% (U.S. Census Bureau, 2016). This percentage increases with lengthening life span; 10% of adults older than age 85 live in nursing homes. Among women older than age 75, 46% live alone. More than 500,000 older women live in a home with a grandchild and have the primary responsibility of caring for the grandchild who lives with them. In those living in homes or apartments, 81% were owners, and 19% were renters.

Ethnicity and Income

In 2014, 22% of older adults were members of an ethnic or racial minority. Hispanics represented 8% of this group, and African Americans represented 9% (U.S. Census Bureau, Population Division, 2016). The median income of older persons in 2014 was $31,169 for men and $17,375 for women. Among this group, 15% reported less than $10,000 in yearly income. In 2013, the major sources of income for older adults in the United States were Social Security (84% of older adults), income from assets (reported by 51% of older adults), earnings (reported by 28%), and private pensions (reported by 27%; U.S. Census Bureau, Current Population Survey, Economic Supplement FINC-01, 2016). More than 14% of older adults (more women than men) in the United States live below the poverty level.

Health and Health-Care Statistics Among Older Adults

In 2014, among noninstitutionalized older adults, 44% assessed their own health as excellent or very good (National Council on Aging, 2016). The most common chronic conditions were arthritis (49%), heart disease of all types (30%), cancer (24%), diabetes (21%), and hypertension (71%). Eight percent reported that they smoked, and 7% reported excessive alcohol consumption. Less than 3% reported that they experienced psychological distress. Only 2% of older adults said that they were unable to obtain needed medical care due to a financial barrier; however, the average out-of-pocket expense per year for older adults was $5,849, a 50% increase since 2004, with projected continued increases in out-of-pocket expenses. About 36% of older adults have one or more functional disabilities, defined as deficits in the areas of ambulation (23%), hearing (15%), independent living (15%), and cognition (9%) (Ortman et al., 2014).

THE AGING PROCESS

Aging is the natural process of wear and tear that continuously affects the body. Although there are several theories of why aging occurs, the normal aging process has been well studied and understanding what is normal allows the healthcare provider to prevent debilitation from normal aging processes and to assess for diseases that are not a part of normal aging.

There are many theories about the aging process that may work singly or together. Some of these theories include the following (Höhn et al., 2017):

- *Replicative senescence* is theory states that cells can replicate or divide a specific number of times. This ability tends to decrease with age. Although this safety mechanism protects against cancer risk in early life, it causes age-related conditions as cells stop replicating and replenishing themselves.
- *Oxidative damage* is the cumulative result of the aerobic metabolism, which generates chemicals called free radicals. Free radicals may interact with other chemicals in the body and cause damage to cells. Oxidative damage has been linked to several disease process, including cancer and Alzheimer's disease.
- *Telomere shortening* is a theory that links aging to a reduction in cell division. A telomere is a sequence of repetitive nucleotides at the end of each DNA strand that protects chromosomes from damage during replication. As we age, these telomeres shorten, reducing the ability of DNA to replicate and slowing down the cells' natural renewal processes.
- *Weakening of the immune response* leaves older adults more vulnerable to infection and debilitating diseases.

The normal aging process is accompanied by numerous physiological changes within different body systems. Even in the absence of disease, these physiological changes increase the older adults' vulnerability to morbidity and mortality. Many of these alterations involve decline in functional reserves with a reduced physiological response to stressors. For example, when older adults experience a physical stressor such as infection, their immune response is slower and less effective than that of a younger person. Normal age-related changes can adversely affect health and functionality and require corrective strategies to adapt to the changes. Too often the older adult or family members incorrectly accept the individual's decline in functionality as inevitable. Many of the physiological changes associated with aging are listed in Table 77.1, and changes in the laboratory values for older adults are listed in Table 77.2.

Normal changes of aging can create an altered or atypical presentation of common conditions response to treatment, and outcomes. For example, when a younger adult experiences a myocardial infarction, it is usually accompanied by crushing chest pain and diaphoresis. In the older adult, myocardial infarction often causes less obvious signs, such as nausea, confusion, and generalized weakness.

THE CHANGING FACE OF AGING IN THE UNITED STATES

Primary-care nurse practitioners (NP) are in a unique and pivotal position to guide and encourage health-promotion programs and individual efforts. From our nursing background, we bring a holistic orientation to health and wellness as well as knowledge of developmental tasks and the wellness-illness continuum.

TABLE 77.1   Physiological Influences of the Aging Process

Age-Related Change	Appearance or Functional Change	Implication
INTEGUMENTARY SYSTEM		
Loss of dermal and epidermal thickness	Loss of subcutaneous tissue and thin epidermis.	Prone to skin breakdown and injury
Decreased vascularity	• Atrophy of sweat glands resulting in decreased sweat production • Decreased body odor • Decreased heat loss • Dryness	• Alteration in thermoregulatory response • Fluid requirements may change seasonally • Loss of skin water • Increased risk of heat stroke
RESPIRATORY SYSTEM		
Decreased lung tissue elasticity	Decreased vital capacity	Reduced overall efficiency of ventilatory exchange
Cilia atrophy	Change in mucociliary transport	Increased susceptibility to infection
Decreased respiratory muscle strength	• Reduced ability to handle secretions and reduced effectiveness against noxious foreign particles • Partial inflation of lungs at rest	Increased risk of atelectasis
CARDIOVASCULAR SYSTEM		
Heart valves thicken and become fibrotic	Reduced stroke volume, cardiac output; may be altered	Decreased responsiveness to stress
Fibroelastic thickening of the sinoatrial node; decreased number of pacemaker cells	Slower heart rate	Increased prevalence of arrhythmias
Decreased baroreceptor sensitivity (stretch receptors)	Decreased sensitivity to changes in blood pressure	Prone to loss of balance, which increases the risk for falls
GASTROINTESTINAL SYSTEM		
Liver becomes smaller	Decreased storage capacity	
Decreased muscle tone	Altered motility	Increases risk of constipation, functional bowel syndrome, esophageal spasm, diverticular disease
Decreased basal metabolic rate (rate at which fuel is converted into energy)		May need fewer calories

Adapted from Kennedy-Malone L, et al. *Advanced practice nursing in the care of older adults.* Philadelphia, PA: FA Davis; 2014:643–650.

TABLE 77.2 Changes in Laboratory Values for Older Adults

Laboratory Test	Normal Values	Changes With Age	Comments
URINALYSIS			
Protein	0–5 mg/100 mL	Rises slightly	May be due to kidney changes with age, urinary tract infection, renal pathology
Specific gravity	1.005–1.020	Lower maximum in elderly 1.016–1.022	Decline in nephrons impairs ability to concentrate urine
HEMATOLOGY			
Erythrocyte sedimentation rate	Men: 0–20 Women: 0–30	Significant increase	Neither sensitive nor specific in aged
Iron binding	50–160 mcg/dL 230–410 mcg/dL	Slight decrease Decrease	
Hemoglobin	Men: 13–18 g/100 mL	Men: 10–17 g/mL	Anemia common in the elderly
	Women: 12–16 g/100 mL	Women: none noted	
Hematocrit	Men: 45%–52% Women: 37%–48%	Slight decrease speculated	Decline in hematopoiesis
Leukocytes	4,300–10,800/mm^3	Drop to 3,100–9,000/mm^3	Decrease may be due to drugs or sepsis and should not be attributed immediately to age
Lymphocytes	500–2,400 T cells/mm^3 50–200 B cells/mm^3	T-cell and B-cell levels fall	Infection risk higher; immunization encouraged
Platelets	150,000–350,000/mm^3	No change in number	
BLOOD CHEMISTRY			
Albumin	3.5–5.0/100 mL	Decline	Related to decrease in liver size and enzymes; protein-energy malnutrition common
Globulin	2.3–3.5 g/100 mL	Slight increase	
Total serum protein	6.0–8.4 g/100 mL	No change	Decreases may indicate malnutrition, infection, liver disease
Blood urea nitrogen	Men: 10–25 mg/100 mL Women: 8–20 mg/100 mL	Increases significantly up to 69 mg/100 mL	Decline in glomerular filtration rate; decreased cardiac output
Creatinine	0.6–1.5 mg/100 mL	Increases to 1.9 mg/100 mL seen	Related to lean body mass decrease
Creatinine clearance	104–124 mL/min	Decreases 10%/decade after age 40 years	Used for prescribing medications for drugs excreted by kidney
Glucose tolerance	62–110 mg/dL after fasting; <120 mg/dL after 2 hours postprandial	Slight increase of 10 mg/dL/decade after 30 years of age	Diabetes increasingly prevalent; drugs may cause glucose intolerance
Alkaline phosphatase	13–39 IU/L	Increase by 8–10 IU/L	Elevations >20% usually due to disease; elevations may be found with bone abnormalities, drugs (e.g., narcotics), and eating a fatty meal

Adapted from Kennedy-Malone L, et al. *Advanced practice nursing in the care of older adults.* Philadelphia, PA: FA Davis; 2014:643–650.

Our advanced practice education helps us to diagnose and treat patients in a way that supports their return to optimal level of function and/or maximizes their coping abilities within the limits of their existing function. This particular blend of NP competencies is especially valuable in working with older patients. Heterogeneity increases with aging, presenting the NP with the challenge of individualizing health-promotion recommendations for each patient. Most of the literature on older adult health is devoted to treatment of frail older adults, those with geriatric syndromes and dementia. There is a need to develop programs and measure outcomes in promoting health in older adults.

Images of older adults and old age are changing. Older adults have only recently begun to be more actively included in studies on health promotion (Bleijenberg et al., 2017). Single-focused interventions for health promotion often do not "fit" with the interrelatedness of older adult health-promotion challenges, and thus, clear age-specific preventive health guidelines for the older population are only recently becoming available. Many disorders in older adults encompass multiple risk factors that involve several systems and interventions to achieve outcomes; this presents a challenge when measuring and synthesizing evidence and reporting outcomes (American Gerontological Society [AGS] Guide to Multimorbidity, 2012). Medicare will only pay for A and B level recommendations that meet the U.S. Preventive Services Task Force (USPSTF) stringent evidence guidelines, leaving other beneficial interventions without coverage. Another confounding factor is the way that outcomes for screening are measured in terms of years of life saved; for older adults, quality of life or functional life is a more realistic goal (Friedman, Shah, & Hall, 2015).

The *Healthy People 2020* program has also set specific objectives for prevention in older adults; these include increased use of the Welcome to Medicare visit, an increased percentage of older adults who are up to date on all preventive services, and decreased use of the emergency department for falls by older adults, among others. Because of the focus on chronic disease management and the complexities of multiple comorbidities in older adults, many primary health-care providers are not oriented toward the potential of healthy aging and discount the importance of health promotion in this age-group (Friedman et al., 2015).

Current life expectancy is 78.8 years (CDC, 2015) with many people living to 100 years and beyond. It behooves us to focus on prevention and health promotion in our older patients to maximize the quality of these years. A collaborative plan should include consideration of the patient's health beliefs and goals, present and anticipated levels of function, risks and benefits of proposed interventions, and effectiveness of specific preventive interventions for older adults. The Welcome to Medicare visit provides a good opportunity to focus solely on preventive services and health promotion; this is followed by the Medicare-supported annual prevention visit. Health-promotion activities should be incorporated into every patient encounter, as opposed to being addressed selectively, and should be individualized to the patient. Recent efforts are being focused on partnering population-based, community-centered programs with personal health initiatives in older adults to make interventions more available and more economical and to increase socialization opportunities and harness the power of group support.

HEALTHY LIFESTYLE COUNSELING

The Welcome to Medicare visit provides an ideal opportunity for healthy lifestyle counseling. In addition to a thorough history (including some risk assessment, physical activity, diet, and tobacco and alcohol use), home safety and depression assessment are included. The Medicare MedLearn network has a link to guide providers covering all areas. Healthy lifestyle counseling should be addressed at each visit, using brief motivational interviewing (Lee, Choi, Yum, Yu, & Chair, 2016; Purath, Keck, & Fitzgerald, 2014).

Physical Activity

Older adults are the least active age group, although recent trends show an increase in physical activity in older adults. The American College of Sports Medicine and the American Heart Association issued updated recommendations for physical activity in all adults, with additional recommendations tailored to adults over age 65 and adults ages 50 to 64 with chronic conditions that are clinically significant or result in functional limitations. Counseling on physical activity should include any type of activity that the patient is able and willing to do. The health benefits of regular physical activity are well documented and include flexibility, increased muscle mass, maintenance of desirable weight, decreased insulin resistance, decreased peripheral vascular resistance, lower blood pressure, and a sense of well-being. Whenever possible, the components of aerobic activity (low to moderate), flexibility, balance, and strengthening (weight training) should be included, and the physical activity prescription should be individualized to the patient. Active hobbies, such as gardening, golfing, tennis, dancing, bowling, hiking, and swimming, are beneficial. Tai chi and yoga are helpful for stretching and balance. Frail elderly or older adults with impaired mobility can benefit from armchair exercises and modified ambulation; a recent study showed a decrease in risk of death in older adults with multiple morbidities who engaged in regular physical activity (Martinez-Gomez, Guallar-Castillon, Garcia-Esquinas, Bandinelli, & Rodriguez-Artalejo, 2017). Patients need to be reassured that expensive equipment or fitness memberships are not necessary to increase physical activity; motivation is the key. There are also many community exercise programs targeted to older adults as well as Web sites that can be shared if the patient has access to the Internet; these include Exercise is Medicine, the American Association of Retired Persons, the National Council on Aging, and the National Institute on Aging. Many programs are now targeting exercise and brain health to prevent cognitive decline. Several government and community group programs have handouts for patients. Before embarking on an exercise program, all patients should have an evaluation of health history, including medications, present physical activity and functional level, potential barriers to exercise, and a physical examination. Older adults with known or suspected cardiac risk factors should have a stress test before engaging in vigorous exercise. All participants should be reminded of the need for adequate hydration and use of caution during extreme weather conditions.

Nutrition

The heterogeneity of older adults is evident in the wide range of nutritional issues affecting them. Before initiating counseling on diet, obtain baseline information on current dietary intake and activity pattern and combine this with height and weight data and other health status information. For patients in the long-term care setting, this information is obtained easily from chart documentation. For community-dwelling older adults, a brief nutrition screening tool such as the Mini Nutritional Assessment (MNA) can be helpful. The abbreviated MNA consists of six questions, and there is a patient self-questionnaire that can be downloaded or mailed in advance of the visit. The MNA Web site contains a section on tools for clinicians, including a user guide and streaming video. It is available in multiple languages as well.

The importance of a healthy, balanced diet to the overall health of older adults cannot be overemphasized. Chronic illness and disability can interfere with the activities of daily living such as shopping or preparing meals. Financial hardship can limit food choices. Prescribed medications can affect absorption of nutrients, sense of taste, or appetite. Depression or social isolation can contribute to poor nutrition. Another problem commonly seen in community-dwelling older adults is obesity. Close to one-half of U.S. older adults are overweight or obese (Batsis & Zagaria, 2018). A recent systematic review of interventions targeting obesity in older adults found that programs combining physical activity and diet had better outcomes, although the findings were of low to moderate quality (Batsis & Zagaria, 2018). There is a need for further research to guide clinical interventions to decrease obesity. Overweight and obesity are associated with heart disease, certain types of cancer, type 2 diabetes, breathing difficulties, stroke, arthritis, and psychological problems. Although there is a decline in the prevalence of overweight and obesity after age 60 years, it remains a problem for many older adults. It is a major risk factor for decreased mobility and functional impairment as well as a cardiovascular risk. General guidelines for dietary counseling include the following.

- Limit fat and cholesterol.
- Maintain a balanced caloric intake.
- Emphasize the inclusion of grains, fruits, and vegetables daily.
- Ensure an adequate dietary calcium intake, especially for women.
- Limit alcohol, if used, to one drink daily for women and two drinks daily for men: one drink = 12 oz beer, 5 oz wine, or 1.5 oz of 80-proof distilled spirits.

Safety

Prevention of injury in the older adult is of paramount importance to continuing functionality and quality of life. Part of this counseling involves reinforcement of extant recommendations, including wearing lap and shoulder seat belts in a motor vehicle, avoiding drinking and driving, having working smoke detectors in the residence, and keeping hot water set below 120°F. For older adults who drive a motor vehicle, periodic assessment of their ongoing ability to drive safely is vital to the older adult and the public at large. Most motor vehicle accidents involve young drivers and old drivers.

Two recommendations are especially important for ensuring the safety of the older adult. The first involves the safe storage and removal of firearms. Possession of a firearm combined with depression, caregiver stress, irreversible illness, or decline in functional abilities can invite self-inflicted injury, suicide pacts, or other acts of violence. Counsel patients to avoid firearms in the home and to use alternative means for self-protection, such as alarm systems and pepper mace spray. The second recommendation involves the prevention of falls, the leading cause of nonfatal injuries and unintentional death from injury in older persons. Certain combinations of physiological and environmental factors place some patients at increased risk. About 85% of falls occur at home, in the later part of the day. Office-based providers can assess for falls by asking if there is a history of falling and by performing the Get Up and Go test in the office. If indicated, evaluation of risk factors and a home safety assessment by a home health nurse or a geriatric assessment team can provide direction for preventive intervention and education. Potential recommendations include exercise programs to build strength, modification of environmental hazards, monitoring and adjusting of medications, external protection against falling on hard surfaces, and measures to increase bone density. If urinary incontinence is a contributing factor, a urological work-up may be indicated. Falls are often alarming to patients and families; in some cases, family members may desire nursing home placement for the patient because of a fall. In other cases, patients may be fearful of ambulation as a result of a fall. Falls also pose a challenge in the long-term care environment. Education and counseling combined with an assessment of the patient's environment are helpful. Keeping water, call bell, telephone, and other necessities available and toileting regularly can minimize the potential for falling. Several home safety checklists are available on the Internet and can be given to patients for self-assessment.

Aging in Place

In the past few years technology such as SMART HOMES and sensors have been introduced to facilitate aging in place. Most these technologies are still in their infancy but offer hope in delaying institutionalization and promoting healthy functioning at home. Other programs, primarily in European countries, are targeting at risk "oldest old" and have designed comprehensive interventions to maintain them at home (Dahlin-Ivanoff et al., 2016). It is anticipated that more technological interventions will be implemented to promote healthy aging in place in the near future.

Sexual Behavior

Assumptions regarding lack of sexual expression in the healthy older adult are unfounded. With the possibility of pregnancy eliminated, many mature adults feel less restraint. As a result of divorce or widowhood, they may seek satisfaction with new partners yet lack the knowledge to protect themselves from sexually transmitted diseases, especially HIV. More than 42% of those living with HIV in the United States in 2013 were in people more than 50 years old (Centers for Disease Control and Prevention [CDC], 2017); 39% of deaths from HIV in 2014 were in adults older than 55 years (CDC, 2017). Older adults need to be taught methods for safe sex with use of a barrier to avoid sexually transmitted diseases, including HIV and hepatitis B. Using the patient's sexual history, explore patient needs, preferences, and medical or psychological obstacles to sexual expression. This exploration facilitates counseling and interventions to promote healthy sexual behavior.

Dental Health

Counseling regarding dental health in the older adult includes the need for regular visits to the dental-care provider, daily flossing, and brushing with fluoride toothpaste. Many elders have dentures or dental implants and assume that dental checkups are no longer necessary. Oral screening for cancer is still indicated, as is periodic assessment of denture fit and functionality. Another concern is for the condition of the remaining teeth of some older adults. Periodontal disease, erosion of dentin, or other problems may render the teeth nonfunctional for chewing and a potential source for infection. Dependence on others for transportation or lack of available dental resources for patients in long-term care settings further complicates the problem. Caregivers simply may overlook this aspect of preventive health, or financial considerations may preclude treatment. Patient and family education regarding dental health is essential.

Substance Use

Counseling about substance use (tobacco, alcohol, and drugs) and injury prevention can be combined naturally within the issue of safety. Smoking is the leading preventable cause of death in the United States. Smoking cessation yields many benefits to former smokers in terms of reduction of risk for several chronic illnesses and stabilization of pulmonary status. Clear and specific guidelines are available to help health-care providers advise tobacco users to quit and to provide them with follow-up encouragement and relapse prevention management. Quitting smoking may not be a choice for the institutionalized older adult but rather dictated by the policy of the institution. Health-care providers can offer support and encouragement, emphasizing the positive health changes that will result.

Counseling regarding alcohol or other drug use can be preventive or interventional, depending on the initial assessment. The Michigan Alcohol Screening Test (MAST), the CAGE questionnaire, or the Alcohol Use Disorders Identification Test (AUDIT) can be used to assess risk. The dangers of drinking and driving and the increased risk of falling while under the influence of alcohol or any drug that acts on the central nervous system should be emphasized. Patients should be informed about the coincidental interactions between alcohol and many prescription drugs, over-the-counter preparations such as acetaminophen, and herbal remedies. The contribution of alcohol abuse to problems, such as insomnia, depression, aggressive behaviors, and deteriorating social relationships, should be addressed. Likewise, the problem of dependence on prescription drugs, such as analgesics, hypnotics, tranquilizers, and anxiolytics, should be assessed and addressed. Counseling in the form of individual follow-up sessions, group support, or outpatient or inpatient rehabilitation may be indicated. In a group-living situation, the governing body (i.e., resident council) may become involved if the patient's behavior threatens the safety or well-being of the other group members.

IMMUNIZATIONS

Influenza vaccine is now recommended annually for all adults over 50 years old, unless contraindicated (Table 77.3). Residents of long-term care facilities that house persons with chronic medical conditions are at especially high risk for developing the disease. Healthcare workers also should receive the vaccine. Patients with a severe egg allergy or severe reaction to the influenza vaccine in the past and patients with a prior history of Guillain-Barré syndrome should talk with their health-care provider before getting the vaccine.

- *Tetanus-diphtheria toxoids with acellular pertussis vaccine (Tdap) vaccine* is administered as a once-in-a-lifetime booster to every adult. Following this, a tetanus-diphtheria *(Td)* booster is recommended every 10 years.

TABLE 77.3 Screening Guidelines for Older Adults		
Clinical Recommendation	*Evidence Rating*	*Reference*
The USPSTF concludes that the current evidence is insufficient to assess the balance of benefits and harms of screening for hearing loss in asymptomatic adults aged 50 years or older.	I	Moyer for USPSTF, 2012
The USPSTF recommends that clinicians screen for HIV infection in adolescents and adults aged 15 to 65 years. Younger adolescents and older adults who are at increased risk should also be screened.	A	Moyer et al. for USPSTF, 2013
The USPSTF recommends that clinicians screen adults aged 18 years or older for alcohol misuse and provide persons engaged in risky or hazardous drinking with brief behavioral counseling interventions to reduce alcohol misuse.	B	Currently under revision, 2017
The USPSTF recommends that clinicians ask all adults about tobacco use, advise them to stop using tobacco, and provide behavioral interventions and U.S. Food and Drug Administration (FDA)–approved pharmacotherapy for cessation to adults who use tobacco.	A	Siu et al. for USPSTF, 2015a
The USPSTF recommends screening for depression in the general adult population, including pregnant and postpartum women. Screening should be implemented with adequate systems in place to ensure accurate diagnosis, effective treatment, and appropriate follow-up.	B	Siu et al. for USPSTF, 2016a
The USPSTF recommends screening for high blood pressure in adults aged 18 years or older. The USPSTF recommends obtaining measurements outside of the clinical setting for diagnostic confirmation before starting treatment.	A	Siu et al. for the USPSTF, 2015b
The USPSTF recommends screening for abnormal blood glucose as part of cardiovascular risk assessment in adults aged 40–70 years who are overweight or obese. Clinicians should offer or refer patients with abnormal blood glucose to intensive behavioral counseling interventions to promote a healthful diet and physical activity.	B	U.S. Preventive Services Task Force (2016)
The USPSTF recommends that adults without a history of cardiovascular disease (CVD) (i.e., symptomatic coronary artery disease or ischemic stroke) use a low- to moderate-dose statin for the prevention of CVD events and mortality when all of the following criteria are met: (1) they are aged 40 to 75 years; (2) they have 1 or more CVD risk factors (ie, dyslipidemia, diabetes, hypertension, or smoking); and (3) they have a calculated 10-year risk of a cardiovascular event of 10% or greater. Identification of dyslipidemia and calculation of 10-year CVD event risk requires universal lipids screening in adults aged 40–75 years. See the "Clinical Considerations" section for more information on lipids screening and the assessment of cardiovascular risk.	B	Bibbins-Domingo et al. for USPSTF, 2016d
The USPSTF recommends one-time screening for abdominal aortic aneurysm by ultrasonography in men ages 65–75 who have ever smoked.		Topic under revision, June 2017
The USPSTF recommends screening all adults for obesity. Clinicians should offer or refer patients with a body mass index of 30 kg/m² or higher to intensive, multicomponent behavioral interventions.		Topic under revision, 2017
The USPSTF recommends biennial screening mammography for women aged 50–74 years.	B	Siu et al. for USPSTF, 2016b
The USPSTF concludes that the current evidence is insufficient to assess the balance of benefits and harms of screening mammography in women aged 75 years or older.	I	Siu et al. for USPSTF, 2016b
The USPSTF concludes that the current evidence is insufficient to assess the balance of benefits and harms of screening for impaired visual acuity in older adults.	I	Chou et al. for USPSTF, 2016
The USPSTF recommends screening for osteoporosis in women aged 65 years and older and in younger women whose fracture risk is equal to or greater than that of a 65-year-old white woman who has no additional risk factors.	B	USPSTF, 2011
Prostate cancer is common in older men.		USPSTF update in progress, 2017

Continued

TABLE 77.3 Screening Guidelines for Older Adults—cont'd

Clinical Recommendation	Evidence Rating	Reference
Screening for cognitive impairment in older adults		USPSTF update in progress, 2017
The USPSTF recommends screening for colorectal cancer starting at age 50 years and continuing until age 75 years (A recommendation).	A	Bibbins-Domingo et al. for USPSTF, 2016a
The decision to screen for colorectal cancer in adults aged 76–85 years should be an individual one, taking into account the patient's overall health and prior screening history (C recommendation).	C	Bibbins-Domingo et al. for USPSTF, 2016a
The decision to initiate low-dose aspirin use for the primary prevention of CVD and CRC in adults aged 60 to 69 years who have a 10% or greater 10-year CVD risk should be an individual one. Persons who are not at increased risk for bleeding, have a life expectancy of at least 10 years, and are willing to take low-dose aspirin daily for at least 10 years are more likely to benefit. Persons who place a higher value on the potential benefits than the potential harms may choose to initiate low-dose aspirin.	C	Bibbins-Domingo et al. for USPSTF, 2016b
The current evidence is insufficient to assess the balance of benefits and harms of initiating aspirin use for the primary prevention of CVD and CRC in adults aged 70 years or older.	I	Bibbins-Domingo et al. for USPSTF, 2016b

Abbreviations: CVD, cardivascular disease; USPSTF, U.S. Preventive Services Task Force.
Evidence ratings: A, consistent, good-quality, patient-oriented evidence; B, inconsistent or limited-quality, patient-oriented evidence; C, consensus, disease-oriented evidence, usual practice, expert opinion, or case series.

- *Pneumococcal vaccine* should be administered as a 1-time dose to PCV13-naïve adults at age 65 years, followed by a dose of PPSV23 12 months later.
- *Hepatitis B vaccine* is recommended for high-risk persons such as IV drug users, persons who are sexually active with multiple partners, those living with someone with chronic hepatitis B, patients <60 years with diabetes, and all desiring protection from Hepatitis B. The initial dose is given, followed 1 month later by the second dose, then the third dose is given 4 to 6 months after the second dose.
- *Zostavax* is recommended for all persons over age 60 as a single dose. Persons who have had a prior episode of zoster should be vaccinated (Advisory Committee on Immunization Practices, 2018).

GERIATRIC SYNDROMES

Older adults are living longer, healthier, and independent lives. Nonetheless, they may start to experience common geriatric syndromes that are not related to one specific disease, such as bladder control problems, sleep problems, delirium, dementia, falls, gait and balance, depression, visual acuity, and weight loss. Some of these conditions result from a combination of several diseases and may require detailed assessment, diagnosis, and treatment. These are called *geriatric syndromes.* A tool called "SPICES," developed in 2003, lists markers of early geriatric syndromes (Wallace & Fulmer, 2003; Box 77.2).

Box 77.2 SPICES Geriatric Syndrome Markers

- **S**leep Disturbances
- **P**roblems with eating or feeding
- **I**ncontinence
- **C**onfusion
- **E**vidence of falls
- **S**kin breakdown

Geriatric syndromes are not inevitable among older adults, and early implementation of preventive therapies and safety measures are important. Prevention is best provided using an interdisciplinary team approach with health-care providers who geriatric centered in their education and approach. The failure of health-care providers to identify, diagnose, and treat the underlying causes of geriatric syndromes can adversely affect the health of older adults. Early detection and correction of problems such as sensory deficits, confusion, and gait and balance issues can increase independence and longevity among this group. The focus of all health-care should be on maintaining function, dignity, and individual control to promote health and quality of life.

Geriatric syndromes are associated with substantial morbidity and poor outcomes (Hartford Institute for Geriatric Nursing, 2015; Inouye, Studenski, Tinetti, & Kuchel, 2008). Geriatric syndromes are multifactorial and although each is distinct, they share several risk factors. For example, older age, cognitive impairment, functional impairment, and mobility impairment are risk factors for falls, functional decline, delirium, and pressure ulcers. Therefore, identification of these risk factors must prompt an evaluation for multiple conditions. The following discussion focuses on geriatric syndromes and emphasizes their overlapping risk factors as well as overlapping symptoms.

Confusion

Confusion is defined as a state of bewildered or unclear thinking. In older adults, confusion is often caused by two problems: delirium and dementia.

Delirium describes a state of mental confusion that develops suddenly and can fluctuate over time. Symptoms of delirium include hallucinations, delusions, and a dreamlike state of incoherence and mental confusion. One in 10 hospitalized elderly patients has episodes of delirium, and these patients often have poor outcomes.

Common causes of delirium include infection (often urinary tract infection) anticholinergic medications, sedatives, antidepressant drugs, steroids, dehydration and electrolyte imbalance, metabolic encephalopathy, vitamin deficiencies, or diabetes and thyroid disease. An easy way to remember the causes of delirium in the older adult is the mnemonic DELIRIUM:

- D: Drugs
- E: Electrolyte imbalance
- L: Lack of drugs (withdrawal, uncontrolled pain)
- I: Infection
- R: Reduced sensory input (vision or hearing loss)
- I: Intracranial (e.g., cerebral vascular accident or subdural hematoma)
- U: Urinary retention or fecal impaction
- M: Myocardial/pulmonary

Prevention of delirium is best accomplished by treating or avoiding possible underlying causes. Unlike dementia, delirium has an underlying cause that if corrected can reduce or eradicate the delirium. Therefore, treatment of delirium begins with recognizing and treating the underlying cause, maintaining a quiet environment, and using simple communication methods and reassurance. In severe cases, antipsychotic drugs can reduce anxiety, hallucinations, aggressive behaviors, and delusion. However, use of drugs should not replace identification and treatment of the underlying cause of the delirium.

Dementia is another cause of confusion in older adults and differs significantly from delirium. Dementia has a gradual onset over months or even years. Dementia is defined as a chronic organic disorder of mental processes with symptoms of memory loss, personality changes, and impaired reasoning (Gandesha, Souza, Chaplin, & Hood, 2012). Over time these symptoms become severe enough to impair the patient's ability to complete activities of daily living. The most common type of dementia is Alzheimer's disease, followed by vascular dementia as a result of stroke. Dementia can be difficult to diagnose, but a standard diagnosis requires two of the following impairments to be present:

- Memory impairment
- Communication and language impairment
- Inability to focus or pay attention
- Reasoning and judgment impairment
- Visual perception impairment

Certain preventative measures have been shown to reduce the risk of dementia. These include monitoring the cardiovascular system for good blood flow to the brain and taking appropriate steps if the blood flow decreases. There is also evidence that regular physical exercise reduces the risk of dementia. A diet rich in grains, fruits and vegetables, fish, nuts, and healthy fats has also been shown to decrease the risk for dementia (Alzheimer's Organization, 2013).

Several types of medications may be used in the management of dementia. Cholinesterase inhibitors, such as donepezil, rivastigmine, or galantamine, reduce the breakdown of acetylcholine, which sustains the level of this neurotransmitter in the brain longer to promote brain function. Memantine regulates glutamate, a chemical messenger. Alternative therapies include modifying the environment to reduce clutter and noise to help focus attention and therapies that use modalities such as animals, art, music, aromas, and massage reduce agitation and aggressive behaviors that often accompany late-stage dementia. Vitamin E and omega -3 fatty acids show some evidence of improved attention in dementia patients. There are nontraditional therapies that assist patients Alzheimer's disease symptoms such as memory loss, agitation, and depression. Pet therapy, providing the patient with a pet to interact with and stroke, has been shown to decrease depression and anxiety. Pet therapy encourages communication and improves mood. Alzheimer's patients are usually comfortable with nonverbal communication (Hall, 2017). Music therapy has also been found to be a powerful memory stimulator and listening to familiar music can be comforting (Gallego & Garcia, 2017). Art therapy, such as walking through a gallery or museum or painting and drawing, can improve motor skills and help the Alzheimer's patient to express feelings (Chancellor, Duncan, & Chatterjee, 2014). Reminiscence and storytelling are methods for exercising long-term memory especially in the early stages of this disease (Asiret & Kapucu, 2016).

Dementia not only affects the patient but also the entire family and caregiver. For this reason, it is often called a family disease. Nearly 15 million caregivers provide unpaid care to persons living with Alzheimer's disease (Family Caregiver Alliance, 2014). As a healthcare provider, it is important to assess not only the patient but the caregivers as well. Providing resources for caregivers to obtain the assistance they need is an important part of providing health care to patients and families dealing with dementia. Team-based care with a social worker and access to a geriatric care manager is essential. Local and regional resources that offer education about the disease, emotional support, and finance and legal advice are important for families who care for someone with dementia (see Resources). Learning to manage challenging behaviors, feelings of grief and loss, a need for respite care (a break from caregiving duties), safety, medical care, stress relief, and planning for the future are all important issues that should be addressed with dementia caregivers. In the end stages of dementia, placement in a care facility and hospice services is often required for these patients.

Falls

As early as 2000, falls were identified as the leading cause of older adult injury-related visits to emergency departments in the United States (Fuller, 2000). Each year 2.8 million older adults are treated in the emergency room because of a fall; that is one person every 11 seconds (National Council on Aging, 2016). However, less than half of those who fall tell their health-care providers.

Risk factors for falls include previous falls, increasing age, medications, and cognitive deficits (CDC, 2015). Falls in older adults are the most common cause of traumatic injury and adjusted for inflation, resulting in direct medical costs $31 billion annually. Each year 800,000 older adults, one in five, are hospitalized because of a fall, most often because of a hip or head fracture. Older adults who have fallen or who feel they might fall should be evaluated for fall risk. Fall risk assessment can reduce the risks of falls, decrease the morbidity and mortality associated with falls in older adults, and improve the quality of life for both the elder and their family.

The Centers for Disease Control and Prevention has created Stopping Elderly Accidents, Deaths, and Injury (STEADI), a free falls risk assessment and prevention program for health-care professionals (CDC, 2016). This program includes physical assessment tools to assess for fall risk; instructions about how to identify patients at low, moderate, high risk for falls; and forms to track older adult falls. Provider guidelines for fall prevention are summarized using the memory device RITUAL:

* Review self-assessment from older adults
* Identify risk factors (e.g., scatter rugs in the home, lack of grab bars in bathrooms, stairs, and poor home lighting or poor vision)
* Test gait and balance (recommendation of programs such as yoga, tai chi, zumba, and other programs for older adults to improve strength, gait, and balance)
* Undertake multifactorial assessment
* Apply interventions (e.g., order appropriate fall prevention devices such as canes, walkers, and bathroom grab bars)
* Later follow up

Three questions are used to identify older adults who are at risk for falls:

1. Have you fallen in the past year?
2. Do you feel unsteady when standing or walking?
3. Do you worry about falling?

These questions are easily asked in the health-care provider's office. If the answer to any of these questions is yes, the STEADI program provides step-by-step instruction for further assessment, intervention, and treatments. Once fall risk is identified, the health-care provider is prompted to identify modifiable risk factors and offer effective interventions to prevent falls.

Fall risk is best reduced when a team effort is applied to the problem, including pharmacy, physical therapy, nursing, and medicine. Key interventions to reduce falls include patient education, enhancing strength and balance, modification of medications, management of hypotension, vitamin D and calcium supplementation, addressing foot and footwear issues, assessment of vision, and implementing home safety precautions.

MEDICATIONS IN THE OLDER ADULT

Polypharmacy can cause great harm in older adults and unfortunately is common because older adults often have multiple chronic diseases that require multiple medications (Guharoy, 2017; Jirón, Pate, Hanson, et al., 2016). Polypharmacy is defined as the practice of administering many different medications concurrently for a single disease or to treat coexisting conditions, a practice that increases the risk of adverse drug reactions (Rambhade, Chakarborty, Shrivastava, Patil, & Rambhade, 2012). Many older adults see numerous health-care providers; each provider may prescribe medications for the condition that he or she is treating. Many studies in ambulatory care define polypharmacy as a medication count of five or more medications. However, current medical practice guidelines often require multiple medications to treat each chronic disease state for optimal clinical benefit. Therefore, an elderly patient with at least two disease states, such as heart failure and chronic obstructive pulmonary disease, will usually exceed this arbitrary threshold of more than five medications (Boyd, Darer, Boult, et al., 2005). The concurrent use of multiple medications by a patient to treat frequently coexisting conditions may result in adverse drug interactions.

Health-care providers are not always aware of other medications taken by the older adult, whether prescribed by another provider or in the form of over-the-counter products that the older adult chooses to use. Additionally, the older adult population is at greater risk of adverse drug reactions from medications due to age-related changes in the absorption, distribution, metabolism, and elimination of medications (Breton, Froissart, Janus, et al., 2011; Garg, Papaioannou, & Ferko, et al., 2004).

Risks of Polypharmacy

Management of both prescribed and over-the-counter medications, including herbal substances, presents a special and significant challenge for older adults. Older patients may become confused about how to correctly take medications, especially when multiple medications are prescribed to be taken several times daily. Additionally, changes in how medications look—changes in shape and color of the pill itself related to various compounding processes among different pharmaceutical suppliers—have been demonstrated to also interfere with correct medication adherence and to be confusing to the consumer in general. The costs of medications, as well as side effects, may also lead to noncompliance. Enhanced drug coverage for older adults has been shown to be a powerful incentive to improve the use of beneficial therapies. A comparison of two groups of Medicare patients, as an example, found that statin use was 4.1% in patients without drug coverage and 27% in those with drug benefits (Federman et al., 2001). Significant utilization differences between insured and uninsured patients were seen even for the use of inexpensive medications such as beta-blockers and nitrates.

Unfortunately, polypharmacy has been linked to an increase in adverse events, including falls, confusion, extrapyramidal symptoms, and syncope (Fried, O'Leary, Towle, 2014; Lu, Wen, Chen, Hsiao, 2014). The risk of falling, for example, is directly correlated with the number of health conditions an elderly person has (Fernando et al., 2017; George & Verghese, 2017). Further, not to be underestimated is underutilization of prescribed drugs, not just overutilization (Lee, Pang, & Hui, 2013). Some sources say that in general less than 50% of people take medications as ordered and that this increases with age (Lee et al., 2013).

Factors leading to unintended underutilization include clinicians not recognizing medication benefit in the older population, affordability, and dose availability (Blanco-Reina et al., 2015).

Management of Polypharmacy

One strategy that may reduce the risks of polypharmacy is medication reconciliation. Medication reconciliation is the process of obtaining a list of all medications that a person is taking including dose and frequency and comparing that list to what has been ordered. This can provide valuable information on duplicate or overlapping drug regimens (Aronson, 2017). Asking older patients to bring all their medications in the original containers to each office visit can facilitate accurate medication reconciliation. The need for adoption of this strategy has grown, as older adults often see numerous health-care providers and are treated in different settings including hospitals, clinics, and physician offices (Greenleaf Brown, 2016). Patients' medications can change rapidly, which may result in confusion or inappropriate medication

administration, and periodic assessment of the benefits of individual medications in comparison to their risks is essential (Kuhn-Thiel, Weib, & Wehling, 2014).

Outpatient medication reconciliation, including patient and provider educational interventions, has shown promise for reducing medication discrepancies in medical records.

Another strategy to reduce polypharmacy risks is to be aware of which drugs frequently cause problems in this age-group (Kovačević et al., 2017). The AGS Beers Criteria (American Geriatrics Society, 2015) is a valuable resource for providers when prescribing medications. The AGS Beers Criteria identifies medications in which the risks may be greater than the benefits for individuals aged 65 and older. It includes the following classifications:

- Medications that are potentially inappropriate for use in older adults
- Medications that are potentially inappropriate for use in older adults due to drug–disease interactions or drug–syndrome interactions
- Medications that should be used with caution in older adults

Health-care providers should use the Beers Criteria as a guide for prescribing in all settings except for palliative care and hospice care (Terrery & Nicoteri, 2016).

END-OF-LIFE DECISION MAKING

Older adults should be asked about their end-of-life (EOL) preparations at annual office visits, when entering the hospital, or when undergoing an outpatient procedure. People differ in what they consider important, especially when thinking about the end of life. Patient preferences should be accommodated as much as possible when care is planned at the end of life. For this reason, elderly people, even those who are healthy, should be encouraged to document their wishes for EOL care and to discuss these instructions with their physicians.

Health-care providers should know state and federal laws and institutional policies regarding living wills, durable power of attorney, and procedures for refusal of extraordinary measures, such as resuscitation and initiation of life support. Such knowledge helps ensure that patients' wishes are followed when patients are no longer able to direct their own care. Patients, while they are still able, should be encouraged to document their wishes for EOL care and to discuss these instructions with their providers and family members (Box 77.3). Effective care for dying patients usually involves a team of caregivers because the skills and perspectives of several disciplines are needed (see Chapter 79).

Helping patients and their family members and friends find comfort in the experience of dying is often more important than adhering to medical routines or correcting symptomless physiologic abnormalities. However, distressing symptoms should be prevented or relieved as

---

Box 77.3   End-of-Life Medical Documents

- Living Will—A directive to health-care providers that communicates wishes for EOL medical care in case a person becomes unable to communicate them. Without documentation expressing those wishes, family members and health-care providers are left to guess what the patient would prefer, which can often lead to family disputes. Each state has regulations and laws regarding living wills; health-care providers should know what the requirements are in the state they practice in.
- Durable Power of Attorney—This document enables older adults to appoint an agent, such as a trusted friend or relative, to handle health decision making. If the patient is no longer able to make decisions for themselves, such as in advanced Alzheimer's disease or stroke or when a patient is comatose, the person listed as having durable power of attorney is someone who knows and understands the patients' health and EOL wishes and is authorized to speak for the patient.

 For additional resources please visit **https://davisedge.fadavis.com/**

effectively as possible. Preventing suffering is also important. Suffering is a global perception of distress caused by factors that together undermine quality of life; these factors include pain; dyspnea; delirium; asthenia; physical impairment; psychologic disturbances; and financial, social, family, and spiritual concerns.

Dying patients often have spiritual needs that should be recognized, acknowledged, and addressed. Patients who are dying often ask what their life means, who they really are, why illness has affected them, and what will happen to them when they die. Patients may question God's existence and love or may feel abandoned by God or a higher power. Some feel guilty or worry that their behavior is what caused their illness. Thus, dying can precipitate a spiritual crisis. Unresolved spiritual distress can lead to despair and hopelessness, which in turn can lead to anxiety, depression, and, for some, a desire to die or to commit suicide. Patients need help working through this distress so that despair can be transformed into hope and serenity.

CONCLUSION

The numbers of older adults in the U.S. population and around the world continue to grow and represent a larger segment of society. Caring for the health of older adults and acting as a primary-care provider for this group presents unique challenges and requires special knowledge and expertise. Although people are living longer, they often struggle with multiple chronic diseases and geriatric syndromes that diminish quality of life for both themselves and their families. Creating care plans specific to older adults enables the primary-care provider to improve the quality of life and longevity of older adults and aids families caring for their elderly loved ones.

REFERENCES

Administration on Aging, Agency for Healthcare Research and Quality and Centers for Medicare and Medicaid Services, Centers for Disease Control and Prevention. *Enhancing use of clinical preventive services among older adults.* Washington, DC: American Association of Retired Persons; 2011.

Advisory Committee on Immunization Practices. Immunization schedule for adults (19 years and older). **https://www.cdc.gov/vaccines/schedules/index.html.** Published 2018.

Alldred DP, Kennedy MC, Hughes C, et al. Interventions to optimise prescribing for older people in care homes. *Cochrane Database Syst Rev.* 2016;2:CD009095.

American Geriatrics Society. Updated Beers criteria for potentially inappropriate medication use in older adults. *J Am Geriatr Soc.* 2015;63(11):2227–2246.

American Geriatrics Society Expert Panel on the Care of Older Adults With Multimorbidity. Guiding principles for the care of older adults with multimorbidity: An approach for clinicians. *J Am Geriatr Soc.* 2012;60(10):E1–E25.

Aronson J. Medication reconciliation. *Br Med J.* 2017;356:i5336.

Batsis JA, Zagaria AB. Addressing obesity in aging patients. *Med Clin North Am.* 2018;102(1):65–85.

Bell HT, Steinsbekk A, Granas AG. Elderly users of fall-risk-increasing drug perceptions of fall risk and the relation to their drug use—a qualitative study. *Scand J Prim Health Care.* 2017;35(3):247–255.

Bibbins-Domingo K, Grossman DC, Curry SJ, et al. Screening for colorectal cancer: US Preventive Services Task Force recommendation statement. *JAMA.* 2016;315(23):2564–2575.

Bibbins-Domingo; U.S. Preventive Services Task Force. Statin use for the primary prevention of cardiovascular disease in adults: US preventive services task force recommendation statement. *JAMA.* 2016a;316(19):1997–2007.

Bibbins-Domingo; U.S. Preventive Services Task Force. Aspirin use for the primary prevention of cardiovascular disease and colorectal cancer: U.S. Preventive Services Task Force recommendation statement. *Ann Intern Med.* 2016b;164:836–845.

Bibbins-Domingo; U.S. Preventive Services Task Force. Aspirin use for the primary prevention of cardiovascular disease and colorectal cancer: U.S. Preventive Services Task Force recommendation statement. *Ann Intern Med.* 2016c;164:836–845.

Blanco-Reina E, Ariza-Zafra G, Ocaña-Riola R, León-Ortíz M, Bellido-Estévez I. Optimizing elderly pharmacotherapy: Polypharmacy vs. undertreatment. Are these two concepts related? *Eur J Clin Pharmacol.* 2015;71(2):199–207.

Bleijenberg N, Imhof L, Mahrer-Imhof R, et al. Patient characteristics associated with a successful response to nurse-led care programs targeting the oldest-old: A comparison of two RCTs. *Worldviews Evid Based Nurs.* 2017;14(3):210–222.

Bibbins-Domingo; U.S. Preventive Services Task Force. Statin use for the primary prevention of cardiovascular disease in adults: US preventive services task force recommendation statement. *JAMA.* 2016d;316(19):1997–2007.

Boulos C, Salameh P, Gateau P. Social isolation and risk for malnutrition among older people. *Geriatr Gerontol Int.* 2016;17:286–294.

Boyd CM, Darer J, Boult C, et al. Clinical practice guidelines and quality of care for older patients with multiple comorbid diseases: Implications for pay for performance. *JAMA.* 2005;294:716–724.

Breton G, Froissart M, Janus N, et al. Inappropriate drug use and mortality in community-dwelling elderly with impaired kidney function—the Three-City population-based study. *Nephrol Dial Transplant.* 2011;26:2852–2859.

Brown JD, Hutchison LC, Li C, Painter JT, Martin BC. Predictive validity of the Beers and Screening Tool of Older Persons' Potentially Inappropriate Prescriptions (STOPP) criteria to detect adverse drug events, hospitalizations, and emergency department visits in the United States. *J Am Geriatr Soc.* 2016;64(1):22–30.

Cadogan C, Ryan CA, Patton D, Hughes C. Theory-based interventions to improve medication adherence in older adults prescribed polypharmacy: A systematic review. *Drugs Aging.* 2017;34(2):97–113.

Centers for Disease Control and Prevention. Healthy aging & the built environment. **http://www.cdc.gov/healthyplaces/healthtopics/healthyaging.htm.** Published 2015.

Centers for Disease Control and Prevention. STEADI—older adult fall prevention. **https://www.cdc.gov/steadi/.** Published 2016.

Centers for Medicare and Medicaid Services. Frequently asked questions about billing the physician fee schedule for advance care planning services. **https://www.cms.gov/Medicare/Medicare-Fee-for-Service-Payment/PhysicianFeeSched/Downloads/FAQ-Advance-Care-Planning.pdf.** Published 2016.

Chancellor B, Duncan A, Chatterjee, A. Art therapy for Alzheimer's disease and other dementias. *J Alzheimer Dis.* 2014;39(1):1–11.

Chou R, Dana T, Bougatsos C, Grusing S, Blazina I. Screening for impaired visual acuity in older adults. Updated evidence report and systematic review for the US Preventive Services Task Force. *JAMA.* 2016;315(9):915–933.

Cigolle CT, Langa KM, Kabeto MU, et al. Geriatric conditions and disability: the Health and Retirement Study. *Ann Intern Med.* 2007;147:156–164.

Dahlin-Ivanoff S, Eklund K, Wilhelmson K, et al. For whom is a health-promoting intervention effective? Predictive factors for performing activities of daily living independently. *BMC Geriatr.* 2016;6:271.

Davidoff AJ, Miller GE, Sarpong EM, et al. Prevalence of potentially inappropriate medication use in older adults using the 2012 Beers criteria. *J Am Geriatr Soc.* 2015;63:486.

Duru Aşiret G, Kapucu S. The effect of reminiscence therapy on cognition, depression, and activities of daily living for patients with Alzheimer disease. *J Geriatr Psychiatry Neurol.* 2016;29(1):31–37.

Ekerstad N, Dahlin-Ivanoff S, Landahl S, et al. Acute care of severely frail elderly patients in a CGA-unit is associated with less functional decline than conventional acute care. *Clin Interv Aging.* 2017;12:1239–1249.

Family Caregiver Alliance. Alzheimer's disease and caregiving. **https://www.caregiver.org/alzheimers-disease-caregiving.** Published 2014.

Federman AD, Adams AS, Ross-Degnan D, et al. Supplemental insurance and use of effective cardiovascular drugs among elderly medicare beneficiaries with coronary heart disease. *JAMA.* 2001;286:1732

Fernando E, Fraser M, Hendriksen J. Risk factors associated with falls in older adults with dementia: A systematic review. *Physiother Can.* 2017;69(2):161–173.

Fried TR, O'Leary J, Towle V, et al. Health outcomes associated with polypharmacy in community-dwelling older adults: A systematic review. *J Am Geriatr Soc.* 2014;62:2261.

Fuller G. Falls in the elderly. *Am Fam Physician.* 2000;1(61):2159–2168.

Gallego M, Garcia J. Music therapy and Alzheimer's disease: Cognitive, psychological and behavioural effects. *Neurologia.* 2017;32(5):300–308.

Garg AX, Papaioannou A, Ferko N, et al. Estimating the prevalence of renal insufficiency in seniors requiring long-term care. *Kidney Int.* 2004;65:649.

George C, Verghese J. Polypharmacy and gait performance in community-dwelling older adults. *J Am Geriatr Soc.* 2017;65(9):2082–2087.

Gnanadesigan N, Fung CH. Quality indicators for screening and prevention in vulnerable elders. *J Am Geriatr Soc.* 2007;55(suppl 2):S417.

Gandesha, A, Souza, R, Chaplin, R, Hood, C, Adequacy of training in dementia care for acute hospital staff. Nurs Older People. 2012 May;24(4):26-31.

Greenleaf Brown L. Untangling polypharmacy in older adults. *Medsurg Nurs.* 2016;25(6):408–411.

Guharoy R. Polypharmacy: America's other drug problem. *Am J Health Syst Pharm.* 2017;74(17):1305–1306.

Hall K. Pet therapy for Alzheimer's disease. *Qual Health.* 2017;43(2):111–115.

Hazzard WR, Blass JP, Halter JB, Ouslander JG, Tinetti ME. *Principles of geriatric medicine and gerontology.* 6th ed. New York, NY: McGraw-Hill; 2016.

Höhn A, Weber D, Jung T, et al. Happily (n)ever after: Aging in the context of oxidative stress, proteostasis loss and cellular senescence. *Redox Biol.* 2017;11:482–501.

Hong SY, Park H. A meta-analysis of the risk factors related to falls among elderly patients with dementia. *Kor J Adult Nurs.* 2017;29(1):51-62. doi:10.7475/kjan.2017.29.1.51

Inouye S, Studenski S, Tinettin M, Kuchel G. Geriatric syndromes: Clinical research and policy of a core geriatric concept. *J Am Geriatr Soc.* 2008;55(5):780–791.

Insured Retirement Institute. Sixth annual update on the retirement preparedness of the boomer generation. **https://www.myirionline.org/docs/default-source/research/boomer-expectations-for-retirement-2016.pdf.** Published 2016.

Jirón M, Pate V, Hanson LC, et al. Trends in prevalence and determinants of potentially inappropriate prescribing in the United States: 2007 to 2012. *J Am Geriatr Soc.* 2016;64:788.

Kalsait AS, Lakshmiprabha R, Iyyar S, Mehta A. Correlation of cognitive impairment with functional mobility & risk of fall in elderly individuals. *Indian J Physiother Occup Ther.* 2017;11(2):7–11.

Kennedy-Malone L, Ryan KF, Martin-Plank L, et al. *Advanced practice nursing in the care of older adults.* Philadelphia, PA: FA Davis; 2014:643–650.

Kovačević SV, Miljković B, Ćulafić M, et al. Evaluation of drug-related problems in older polypharmacy primary care patients. *J Eval Clin Pract.* 2017;23(4):860–865.

Kuhn-Thiel AM, Weib C, Wehling M; FORTA authors/expert panel members. Consensus validation of the FORTA (Fit fOR The Aged) List: a clinical tool for increasing the appropriateness of pharmacotherapy in the elderly. *Drugs Aging.* 2014;31:131.

Lansdorp-Vogelaar I, Gulati R, Mariotto AB, et al. Personalizing age of cancer screening cessation based on comorbid conditions: model estimates of harms and benefits. *Ann Intern Med.* 2014;161:104.

Lee VW, Pang KK, Hui KC, et al. Medication adherence: Is it a hidden drug-related problem in hidden elderly? *Geriatr Gerontol Int.* 2013;13(4):978–985.

Lee WW, Choi KC, Yum RW, Yu DS, Chair SY. Effectiveness of motivational interviewing on lifestyle modification and health outcomes of clients at risk or diagnosed with cardiovascular diseases: A systematic review. *Int J Nurs Stud.* 2016;53:331–341.

Leipzig RM, Whitlock EP, Wolff TA, et al. Reconsidering the approach to prevention recommendations for older adults. *Ann Int Med.* 2010;153(12):809–814.

Lin FR, Yaffe K, Xia J, et al. Hearing loss and cognitive decline in older adults. *JAMA Intern Med.* 2013;173:293.

Lipitz-Snyderman A, Bach PB. Overuse of health care services: when less is more ... more or less. *JAMA Intern Med.* 2013;173(14):1277–1278.

Lomas-Vega R, Obrero-Gaitán E, Molina-Ortega FJ, Del-Pino-Casado R. Tai chi for risk of falls. A meta-analysis. *J Am Geriatr Soc.* 2017;65(9):2037–2043. doi:10.1111/jgs.15008

Lu WH, Wen YW, Chen LK, Hsiao FY. Effect of polypharmacy, potentially inappropriate medications and anticholinergic burden on clinical outcomes: A retrospective cohort study. *CMAJ.* 2015;187:E130.

Martinez-Gomez D, Guallar-Castillon P, Garcia-Esquinas E, et al. Physical activity and the effect of multimorbidity on all-cause mortality in older adults. *Mayo Clin Proc.* 2017;92(3):376–382.

Moyer VA on behalf of the U.S. Preventive Services Task Force. Screening for hearing loss in older adults: U.S. Preventive Services Task Force recommendation statement. *Ann Intern Med.* 2012;157:655–661.

Moyer VA on behalf of the U.S. Preventive Services Task Force. Screening for HIV: U.S. Preventive Services Task Force recommendation statement. *Ann Intern Med.* 2013;159:51–60.

Nagi S. A study in the evaluation of disability and rehabilitation concepts, methods and procedures. *Am J Pub Health.* 1965;54:1568–1579.

Nagi S. *Disability concepts revisited: Implications for prevention. Institute of Medicine, disability in America: Toward a national agenda for prevention.* Washington, DC: National Academy Press; 1991.

National Council on Aging. Chronic disease management. https://www.ncoa.org/healthy-aging/chronic-disease. Published 2016.

National Council on Aging. Falls prevention facts. https://www.ncoa.org/news/resources-for-reporters/get-the-facts/falls-prevention-facts. Published 2017.

National Institute on Alcohol Abuse and Alcoholism Helping patients who drink too much: A clinician's guide. http://www.niaaa.nih.gov/guide. Published 2005.

Nicholas JA, Hall WJ. Screening and preventive services for older adults. *Mount Sinai J Med.* 2011;78(4):498–508.

Niikawa H, Okamura T, Ito K, et al. Association between polypharmacy and cognitive impairment in an elderly Japanese population residing in an urban community. *Geriatr Gerontol Int.* 2017;17(9):1286–1293.

O'Connor MN, O'Sullivan D, Gallagher PF, et al. Prevention of hospital-acquired adverse drug reactions in older people using screening tool of older persons' prescriptions and screening tool to alert to right treatment criteria: A cluster randomized controlled trial. *J Am Geriatr Soc.* 2016;64:1558.

Office of Disease Prevention and Health Promotion. *Healthy People 2020.* https://www.healthypeople.gov/2020/topics-objectives. Published 2014.

Ortman J, Velkoff V. Hogan H. An aging nation: The older population in the United States population estimates and projections. U.S. Census Bureau. https://www.census.gov/prod/2014pubs/p25-1140.pdf. Published 2014.

Osborn R, Moulds D, Squires D, Doty MM. International survey of older adults finds shortcomings in access, coordination, and patient centered care. *Health Affairs.* 2014;33(12):2247–2255

Paliwal Y, Slattum PW, Ratliff SM. Chronic health conditions as a risk factor for falls among the community-dwelling US older adults: A zero-inflated regression modeling approach. *Biomed Res Int.* 2017;2017:5146378.

Paul KJ, Walker RL, Dublin S. Anticholinergic medications and risk of community-acquired pneumonia in elderly adults: a population-based case-control study. *J Am Geriatr Soc.* 2015;63:476.

Pilotto A, Cella A, Pilotto A, et al. Three decades of comprehensive geriatric assessment: Evidence coming from different healthcare settings and specific clinical conditions. *J Am Med Directors Assoc.* 2016;18(2):192e1–192e11.

Purath J, Keck A, Fitzgerald CE. Motivational interviewing for older adults in primary care: A systematic review. *Geriatr Nurs.* 2014;35(3):219–224.

Qato DM, Wilder J, Schumm LP, et al. Changes in prescription and over-the-counter medication and dietary supplement use among older adults in the United States, 2005 vs 2011. *JAMA Intern Med.* 2016;176:473.

Rambhade S, Chakarborty A, Shrivastava A, Patil UK, Rambhade A. A survey on polypharmacy and use of inappropriate medications. *Toxicol Int.* 2012;19(1):68–73.

Rasu R, Agbor-Bawa W, Rianon N. Impact of polypharmacy on seniors' self-perceived health status. *Southern Med J.* 2017;110(8):540–545.

Salahudeen MS, Hilmer SN, Nishtala PS. Comparison of anticholinergic risk scales and associations with adverse health outcomes in older people. *J Am Geriatr Soc.* 2015;63:85.

Saraf AA, Petersen AW, Simmons SF, et al. Medications associated with geriatric syndromes and their prevalence in older hospitalized adults discharged to skilled nursing facilities. *J Hosp Med.* 2016;11:694.

Schoenberg NE, Tarasenko YN, Bardach SH, Fleming ST. Patient and provider perspectives on the relationship between multiple morbidity management and disease prevention. *J Appl Gerontol.* 2015;34(3):359–376. http://doi.org/10.1177/0733464813499641

Segert L. New NIA report highlights health, aging trends. Association of Health Care Journalists. http://healthjournalism.org/blog/2014/07/new-nia-report-highlights-health-aging-trends. Published July 2014. Accessed February 10, 2018.

Shimizu, R, Bouchard, M, Mavriplis C. Update on age-appropriate preventive measures and screening for Canadian primary care providers. *Can Fam Physician.* 2016;62(2):131–138.

Singh DK, Pillai SG, Tan ST, Tai CC, Shahar S. Association between physiological falls risk and physical performance tests among community-dwelling older adults. *Clin Interv Aging.* 2015;10:1319–1326.

Siu AL; U.S. Preventive Services Task Force (2015). Behavioral and pharmacotherapy interventions for tobacco smoking cessation in adults, including pregnant women: U.S. Preventive Services Task Force recommendation statement. *Ann Intern Med.* 2015a;163:622–634.

Siu AL; U.S. Preventive Services Task Force. Screening for high blood pressure in adults: U.S. Preventive Services Task Force recommendation statement. *Ann Intern Med.* 2015b;163:778–786.

Siu AL and the U.S. Preventive Services Task Force. Screening for depression in adults. US Preventive Services Task Force Recommendation Statement. *JAMA*. 2016a;315(4):380–387.

Siu AL on behalf of the U.S. Preventive Services Task Force. Screening for breast cancer: U.S. preventive services task force recommendation statement. *Ann Intern Med*. 2016b;164:279–296.

Siu HY-H, White J, Sergeant M, Moore AE, Patterson C. Development of a periodic health examination form for the frail elderly in long-term care. *Can Fam Physician*. 2016;62(2):147–155.

Snyder AH, Magnuson A, Westcott AM. Cancer screening in older adults. *Med Clin North Am*. 2016;100:1101.

Tan JL, Eastment JG, Poudel A, Hubbard RE. Age-related changes in hepatic function: An update on implications for drug therapy. *Drugs Aging*. 2015;32:999.

Terrery JL, Nicoteri JL. The 2015 American Geriatric Society Beers Criteria: Implications for nurse practitioners. *J Nurse Pract*. 2016;12(3):192–200.

Tinetti ME. Making prevention recommendations relevant for an aging population. American College of Physicians Comment. *Ann Intern Med*. 2010;153(12):809–814.

Tommelein E, Mehuys E, Van Tongelen I, et al. Community pharmacists' evaluation of potentially inappropriate prescribing in older community-dwelling patients with polypharmacy: observational research based on the GheOP³S tool. *J Pub Health*. 2017;39(3):583–592.

United Nations, Department of Economic and Social Affairs, Population Division. World population ageing 2013. http://www.un.org/en/development/desa/population/publications/pdf/ageing/WorldPopulationAgeing2013.pdf. Published 2013.

U.S. Census Bureau. Selected characteristics of families by total money income. https://www.census.gov/data/tables/time-series/demo/income-poverty/cps-finc/finc-01.html. Published 2016.

U.S. Preventive Services Task Force. Aspirin for the prevention of cardiovascular disease: Preventive medication. http://www.uspreventiveservicestaskforce.org/Page/Topic/recommendation-summary/aspirin-for-the-prevention-of-cardiovascular-disease-preventive-medication. Published: March 2009. Accessed on October 6, 2014.

U.S. Preventive Services Task Force. Final update summary: Osteoporosis: screening. https://www.uspreventiveservicestaskforce.org/Page/Document/UpdateSummaryFinal/osteoporosis-screening. Published July 2015.

US Preventive Services Task Force, Bibbins-Domingo K, Grossman DC. Screening for colorectal cancer: US Preventive Services Task Force Recommendation Statement. *JAMA*. 2016;315(23):2564–2575

U.S. Preventive Services Task Force. Final recommendation statement: Abnormal blood glucose and type 2 diabetes mellitus: Screening. https://www.uspreventiveservicestaskforce.org/Page/Document/RecommendationStatementFinal/screening-for-abnormal-blood-glucose-and-type-2-diabetes. Published November 2016.

Veronese N, Stubbs B, Noale M, et al. Polypharmacy is associated with higher frailty risk in older people: An 8-year longitudinal cohort study. *J Am Med Directors Assoc*. 2017;18(7):624–628.

Wallace M, Fulmer T. Fulmer SPICES: An overall assessment tool of older adults. *Ala Nurse*. 2003;30(3):26.

Weng MC, Tsai CF, Sheu KL, et al. The impact of number of drugs prescribed on the risk of potentially inappropriate medication among outpatient older adults with chronic diseases. *QJM*. 2013;106:1009.

Whitcomb EL, Horgan S, Donohue MC, Lukacz ES. Impact of surgically induced weight loss on pelvic floor disorders. *Int Urogynecol J*. 2012;23:1111.

Wilson SR, Knowles SB, Huang Q, Fink A. The prevalence of harmful and hazardous alcohol consumption in older U.S. adults: Data from the 2005–2008 National Health and Nutrition Examination Survey (NHANES). *J Gen Intern Med*. 2014;29:312.

Wimmer BC, Cross AJ, Jokanovic N, et al. Clinical outcomes associated with medication regimen complexity in older people: A systematic review. *J Am Geriatr Soc*. 2017;65:747.

World Health Organization. The global strategy and action plan on ageing and health, 2016–2000. Retrieved from http://www.who.int/ageing/global-strategy/en/. Published 2016

World Health Organization. WHO guidelines on Integrated Care for Older People (ICOPE). http://www.who.int/ageing/publications/guidelines-icope/en/. Published 2017.

Zayas CE, He Z, Yuan J, et al. Examining healthcare utilization patterns of elderly middle-aged adults in the united states. Proceedings of the International Florida AI Research Society Conference. Florida AI Research Symposium. 2016:361–366.

Zia A, Kamaruzzaman SB, Tan MP. The consumption of two or more fall risk-increasing drugs rather than polypharmacy is associated with falls. *Geriatr Gerontol Int*. 2017;17(3):463–470.

RESOURCES

Ageing and Life Course. World Health Organization
   http://www.who.int/ageing/en/

Ageing: Levels and Trends in Population Ageing, Demographic Drivers of Population Ageing, Key Conferences on Ageing. United Nations
   http://www.un.org/en/sections/issues-depth/ageing/

Alzheimer's Foundation of America
   https://alzfdn.org/

American Geriatric Society (AGS)
   http://www.americangeriatrics.org/

Centers for Medicare and Medicaid Services
   https://www.cms.gov/Medicare/Medicare.html

End-of-Life Issues and Care. American Psychological Association
   http://www.apa.org/topics/death/end-of-life.aspx

Fact Sheet: Aging in the United States. Population Reference Bureau
   http://www.prb.org/Publications/Media-Guides/2016/aging-unitedstates-fact-sheet.aspx

Gerontological Advanced Practice Nurses Association (GAPNA)
   https://www.gapna.org/

Gerontological Society of America
   https://www.geron.org/

Health Information for Older Adults. Centers for Disease Control and Prevention: Healthy Aging
   https://www.cdc.gov/aging/aginginfo/index.htm

Health Systems That Meet the Needs of Older People. World Health Organization
   http://www.who.int/ageing/health-systems/en/

Healthy Aging: Empowering Older Adults to Live Healthier. National Council on Aging (NCOA)
   https://www.ncoa.org/healthy-aging/

Long-Term-Care Systems. World Health Organization
   http://www.who.int/ageing/long-term-care/en/

Making End-of-Life Decisions: What Are Your Important Papers? Family Caregiver Alliance: National Center on Caregiving
   Obtained from https://www.caregiver.org/making-end-life-decisions-what-are-your-important-papers

Measuring the Age-Friendliness of Cities: A Guide to Using Core Indicators. World Health Organization: Center for Health Development
   http://www.who.int/kobe_centre/publications/AFC_guide/en/

Medications & Older Adults: The 2015 American Geriatrics Society Updated Beers Criteria: Medications That Older Adults Should Avoid or Use With Caution.
http://www.healthinaging.org/medications-older-adults/

Medicines and You: A Guide for Older Adults. U.S. Department of Health and Human Services: U.S. Food & Drug administration
https://www.fda.gov/Drugs/ResourcesForYou/ucm163959.htm

Older Adult Falls. Centers for Disease Control and Prevention: Home and Recreation Safety
https://www.cdc.gov/homeandrecreationalsafety/falls/index.html

Older Adults: Behavioral Health Identification and Treatment, Screening and Assessment Tools, Evidence-Based Practices, Workforce, Financing, Resources for Individual and Families, and Federal and National Entities for Older Adults' Health. SAMHSA-HRSA Center for Integrated Health Solutions
https://www.integration.samhsa.gov/integrated-care-models/older-adults#Resources_for_Individuals&Families

The Demographics of Aging. Transgenerational Design Matters
http://transgenerational.org/aging/demographics.htm

The Growth of the U.S. Aging Population. SeniorCare.com
https://www.seniorcare.com/featured/aging-america/

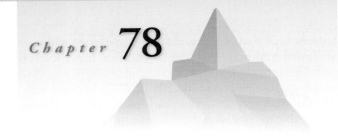

Chapter 78

Palliative Care and Pain Management

Ruth McCaffrey, DNP, APRN, FNP-BC, GNP –BC, FAAN, FAANP

Lynne M. Dunphy, PhD, APRN, FNP-BC, FAAN, FAANP

Palliative care provides physical, psychosocial, and spiritual care through thorough assessment and the development of a comprehensive treatment plan. "Palliative" is defined as relieving pain without dealing with the cause of the condition. This definition echoes the World Health Organization (WHO)'s definition of palliative care as a patient-centered approach that improves the quality of life of patients and families when they are experiencing life-threatening illnesses (WHO, 2015).

PRINCIPLES OF PALLIATIVE CARE

Palliative care focuses primarily on anticipating, preventing, diagnosing, and treating symptoms experienced by patients with a serious or life-threatening illness and helping patients and their families make medically important decisions. Helping patients and their families understand the nature of illness and prognosis is a crucial aspect of palliative care near the end of life. Receiving a diagnosis of life-threatening disease can be a frightening experience for the patient and family. Fear of potential suffering and pain, as well as fear of loss of control, relationships, and existence itself are some of the issues that confront the patient. Psychosocial distress may significantly influence treatment decisions, quality of life, and disease progression. All care providers and clinicians can improve the recognition and management of the distress related to a terminal diagnosis.

According to the National Consensus Project for Quality Palliative Care (NCP, 2013) on palliative care, the goal of palliative care is "to prevent and relieve suffering and to support the best possible quality of life for patients and their families, regardless of the stage of the disease or the need for other therapies. It can be delivered concurrently with life-prolonging therapies or as the main focus of care. Leadership, collaboration, coordination, and communication are key elements for effective integration of these disciplines and services" (NCP, 2013). Suffering is an experience of the whole person and is highly personal and subjective. The assessment of the level of a person's suffering requires the ability to consider complexity, multidimensionality, and subjectivity of symptoms and experiences beyond the outward symptoms of the disease.

The National Consensus Project for Quality Palliative Care (2013) has provided recommendations for care domains in palliative care. These recommendations are divided into eight domains of care (Table 78.1). In addition, the Institute of Medicine (2014) lists five areas that lead to quality palliative care:

1. Delivery of person-centered and family-focused care
2. Clinician–patient communication and advanced care planning
3. Professional education and development
4. Policies and payment system to support palliative care across all settings
5. Public education and engagement

TABLE 78.1 Domains of Palliative Care

Domain	Key Recommendation
1. Structure and process of care	Interdisciplinary team, comprehensive interdisciplinary assessment, education and training, relationship with hospice programs
2. Physical aspects of care	Pain and other symptoms are managed with the use of best practices.
3. Psychological and psychiatric aspects of care	Psychological and psychiatric issues are assessed and managed: grief and bereavement program is available for patients and families.
4. Social aspects of care	Interdisciplinary social assessments with appropriate care plan; referral to appropriate services.
5. Spiritual, religious, and existential aspects of care	Spiritual concerns are assessed and addressed linkages to community and spiritual or religious resources are provided as appropriate.
6. Cultural aspects of care	Culture-specific needs of patients and families are assessed and addressed; recruitment and hiring practices reflect the cultural diversity of the community.
7. Care of the imminently dying patients	Signs and symptoms of impending death are recognized and communicated; hospice referral is recommended when patient is eligible.
8. Ethical and legal aspects of care	Patient's goals, preferences, and choices form basis for plan of care; the team is knowledgeable about relevant federal and state statues and regulation.

Adapted from the National Project for Quality Palliative Care (2013).

PALLIATIVE CARE AND HOSPICE CARE

Hospice and *palliative care* are terms that are often used interchangeably. Both provide supportive medical, social, emotional, and spiritual services to patients and their caregivers. Both services rely on the combined knowledge and skill of interdisciplinary teams of professionals. Hospice care provides care to patients at the end of life. Palliative care provides comfort care and a support system to both the family and patient, integrating the psychological and spiritual aspects of patient care, throughout the trajectory of illness, from the time of diagnosis until death, and encompasses end-of-life care. Both palliative care and hospice care provide supportive medical, social, emotional, and spiritual services to patients and their caregivers. Both services rely on the combined knowledge and skill of interdisciplinary teams of professionals. Nevertheless, there are some key differences between the two types of care.

Primary practitioners who provide care to chronically ill patients with terminal conditions are expected to incorporate the basic elements of palliative care into their practice, regardless of setting. Palliative care is patient-centered care that provides comfort and support to both the family and patient by integrating the psychological and spiritual aspects of patient care. Care is provided throughout the entire span of illness, from the time of diagnosis until death. Because it also encompasses end-of-life care, palliative care may include offering help to bereaved family members after the death of a loved one. Additionally, palliative care provides care using a team of doctors, nurses, and other professional care givers and is most commonly administered through a hospital or medical provider. Costs are typically covered by insurance.

Hospice care *includes* palliative care; however, a referral from a physician is required to initiate hospice care. Hospice care is overseen by a team of hospice professionals in the home and occasionally in the hospital. A patient receiving hospice care must be considered terminally ill or within 6 months of death. Palliative care has no such restrictions, and patients can receive palliative care at any stage of their disease. Most hospice costs are covered through insurance providers, such as Medicare and supplemental insurance; however, it is important to check with each hospice program, as some can vary in costs and reimbursement. Some hospice programs offer subsidized care for the economically disadvantaged.

NEED FOR PALLIATIVE CARE

The need for palliative care providers has grown rapidly, especially since palliative care treatments have been shown to improve quality of life, reduce overall costs, enhance the ability to die at home, and actually increase longevity (Quill & Abernethy, 2013). From 2000 to 2012, hospital-based palliative care teams increased from 658 to 1,734, an increase of 164%. Benefits from palliative care practice include increased patient and family satisfaction with care, increased healthcare provider satisfaction, lower levels of stress for providers, and an increase in cost-effective models of care (Hughes & Smith, 2014). When patients with a life-threatening illness receive early palliative care, they are better able to cope with their disease and situation (Greer, 2016). Additionally, they have an overall better quality of life and improved mood.

Although palliative care has traditionally focused on treating people with cancer, there is a growing body of research to suggest that expanding palliative care services for other seriously ill populations, including patients with heart failure, chronic lung disease, end-stage renal disease, Alzheimer's disease, and others would be beneficial. As palliative care expands as an option for an aging population, more education will be needed to train health-care providers in palliative care standards, skills, and services. Nurse practitioners are well positioned to provide palliative care with their holistic understanding of human beings and their focus on caring and comforting, as well as healing.

Palliative care is ideally delivered by an interdisciplinary team that focuses on the needs of both the patient and family. The team often includes healthcare providers, nurses, social workers, chaplains, and other specialist providers that are required to assist individual patients. The focus of the team is to improve quality for those with serious illnesses and their families. Team goals include treatment of pain and other symptoms, addressing spiritual distress, communicating goals to the patient and family members, and coordination of care that supports patients, families, and loved ones (Box 78.1).

Box 78.1　Roles of the Palliative Care Team

- Treatment for the relief from pain and other distressing symptoms
- Coordination of care from all doctors and health-care providers
- Affirmation of life that regards dying as a normal process
- Provision of care that neither hastens nor postpones death
- Clarification of patient and family goals and options and assistance with medical decision making
- Integration of the psychological and spiritual aspects of patient care
- Provision of support to help patients live as actively as possible until death
- Assistance to help family members cope during the patient's illness and their own bereavement
- Enhancement of quality of life that may also positively influence the course of illness
- Treatments that are applicable early in the course of illness, in conjunction with other therapies that are intended to prolong life, such as chemotherapy or radiation therapy, and includes those investigations needed to better understand and manage distressing clinical complications

PALLIATIVE CARE AS PART OF PRIMARY-CARE PRACTICE

It is clear that palliative care is a specialty that needs to be integrated into primary-care practice. Ideally, primary-care providers come to know the patient and family, individualize care for the patient based on a long understanding of who they are and what their life has entailed, develop a full understanding of the needs and challenges faced by people with life-threatening illnesses, and can develop a plan to reduce suffering and pain. The requirement for palliative care does not always come at a specific time, and the primary-care provider can prevent gaps in the continuum of care by recognizing early signs of life limiting illnesses that may eventually require palliative care and begin a discussion with the patient and family. Integrating palliative care into a primary-care practice begins with a dialogue between all providers and staff within the practice. This dialogue should include definitions of palliative care, commitment to assisting those at the end of life or with life-threatening illnesses and what may already be happening within the primary-care practice that is really palliative care.

Second, the primary-care practice must compile and create connections with the needed professional and ancillary to provide adequate palliative care. These may include clergy, home health providers, councilors, medical equipment providers, and pharmacists. Staff training will be required to learn more about palliative care, what services should be provided, how care teams can be established, what resources and referrals might be required, what barriers may exist, and what infrastructure in need in billing and documentation.

The growing need for palliative care grows has led to a recognized need to advance and pay for palliative care in the community and provide a team approach to palliation before hospitalization. The California Healthcare Foundation is advocating for creating palliative care provision in community health centers and primary care.

The foundation lists the following challenges and opportunities for accomplishing this mission:

Challenges

- Not enough time to work with patients and families on goals of care and advance directives
- Added responsibility in a busy primary-care practice
- No real viable payment mechanism for reimbursement
- Differing resources required by different patients
- Lack of primary-care provider understanding of palliative care

Opportunities

- Providing an important service to the community
- Working with long-term patients whose history, family, and personal wishes are already known and understood
- Being on the cutting edge of an expanding concept for helping patients with long-term illnesses

The need for palliative care will continue to grow as the U.S. population ages.

Providing palliative care in the primary-care setting by creating teams led by nurse practitioners (NPs) seems the ideal method to promote end-of-life care, reduce the costs of unnecessary aggressive care, improve the quality of life of adults experiencing life-threatening illnesses and provide comfort, compassion and caring for patients and families at this difficult time.

PALLIATIVE CARE STANDARDS FOR PALLIATIVE CARE

In 2015, the Joint Commission revised standards for the provision of palliative care and the certification of providers of palliative care (Table 78.2). Managing palliative care programs requires the identification and minimization of risk to patients and families. All interdisciplinary team members should be provided with a comprehensive orientation to the program including a review of the domains of palliative care,

TABLE 78.2	Palliative Care Standards
Standard 1	Patients and families know how to access and use the program's care, treatments and services.
Standard 2	The palliative care program communicates with patients and families and involves them in decision making.
Standard 3	The program tailors care, treatments, and services to meet the lifestyle, needs, and values of the patient and family.
Standard 4	The interdisciplinary team assesses and reassess the patient's needs; these interdisciplinary teams can include volunteers and professionals.
Standard 5	The program provides care, treatment, and serves according to a plan of care. This plan of care addresses anorexia, confusion, constipation, dyspnea, fatigue, insomnia, nausea, pain, and restlessness, as well as psychological symptoms such as anxiety, stress, and grief. Referrals for these treatments are made as required.
Standard 6	The patient's care is coordinated using an interdisciplinary approach and the resolution of ethical issues discussed with all involved.

Source: © Joint Commission Resources. *Palliative care certification manual* (PCPC-2), effective January 1, 2018. Oakbrook Terrace, IL: Joint Commission on Accreditation of Healthcare Organizations; 2018. Reprinted with permission.

assessment and management of psychological symptoms and physical symptoms, communication skills, cross-cultural knowledge and skills, grief and bereavement, ethical principles that guide palliative care, and community resources for patients and families. The program should also provide a process for patients and families to address concerns.

INITIATING PALLIATIVE CARE

Although the steps to providing palliative care are important (Box 78.2), one of the most important aspects of working with patients in primary care is the initial discussion related to end-of-life decisions in general (Lo, Quill, & Tulsky, 2011). Building a trusting relationship with all patients is an essential aspect of advanced practice nursing; however, at the end of life, this trust becomes more essential to elicit the patient and families' concerns, goals, and values. Open communication and the building of trust will allow the patient and family to discuss and explore emotional, psychosocial, and existential concerns and spiritual suffering. The NP should use active listening skills and empathy for patients who are struggling to find closure in their lives. This type of caring can have a therapeutic value in and of itself.

The most important aspect of communication at this time is to let patients know that they are being heard and that their perspective is important. Open-ended questions can be asked to explore the need for palliative care, such as the following:

- What is your understanding of where things stand now with your illness?

- As you think about your illness, what is the best and the worst that might happen?
- What has been most difficult about this illness for you?
- What are your hopes, expectations, and fears for the future?
- As you think about the future, what is most important to you—what matters most to you?
- Do you have a strong religious or spiritual belief? If so, whom do talk to about spiritual matters? Would you like this person to be involved in your decision making at this time?
- Do you have any additional concerns?

Specific questions related to spiritual and existential issues include the following:

- What do you still want to accomplish during your life?
- What thoughts have you had about why you got this illness at this time?
- What might be left undone if you were to die today?
- What is your understanding about what happens after you die?
- Given that your time is limited, what legacy do you want to leave your family?
- What do you want your children and grandchildren or friends to remember about you?

In *Being Mortal*, Atul Gawande makes the point that answers to these questions may change as the patient and family experience the trajectory of illness. What is important at the beginning of that journey frequently changes as illness and symptoms progress, and time

---

Box 78.2 Advanced Practice Nursing Intervention: Dimensions of a Palliative Care Plan

1. Assess the extent of disease documented by imaging studies, laboratory data.
2. Assess and provide interventions for physical signs and symptoms including pain, dyspnea, delirium.
3. Assess coping strategies and psychological symptoms including presence and absence of depression, suicidal ideology.
4. Determine level and quality of support provided by family and friends. Is additional assistance needed in the home and can it be put into place? Determine community resources and identify what kind of assistance is available.
5. Identify coping strategies and psychological symptoms in family members or caregivers.
6. Perform a religious and spiritual assessment including degree of comfort from beliefs.
7. Evaluate the impact of disease on functional status. What can the patient do, and what assistance is needed with bathing, dressing, ambulation, meal preparation?
8. Evaluate what advance care planning has been done. Have the patient's wishes and preferences for resuscitation, artificial feeding, and hydration been discussed? Has the patient identified a surrogate decision-maker who knows the patient's

wishes? Is there documentation on advance directives in the medical record?
9. Evaluate overall quality of life and well-being. Does the patient feel secure that all that can be done is being done? Does the patient feel that physical and psychological symptoms are being satisfactorily addressed? Does the patient feel there is meaning to his or her life?
10. Identify the family burden of caring for the patient. Is attention being paid to support the caregiver so that burnout does not occur? What is the financial burden to the caregiver, and can he or she manage bill paying and reimbursement issues?
11. Determine the level of care needed in the home and provision for that care. What reimbursement issues affect obtaining the level of home care needed?
12. Is there a system in place for ongoing support and assistance to family members and caregivers after the death of the patient?
13. Has the patient identified his or her desire for their place of death? Has he or she communicated these wishes to the family, partner, caregiver?
14. Provide for bereavement counseling and support for the family beyond the life of the patient.

begins to seem short. Thus, these questions may need to be revisited and/or reaffirmed over time.

ASPECTS OF PALLIATIVE CARE

Total pain, is defined as the sum of the patient's physical, psychological, social, and spiritual pain, is a central concept to palliative care (Rome, Luminais, Bourgeois, & Blais, 2011). Optimal physical pain relief is not possible unless all elements of total pain are addressed. Managing total pain requires a team approach to determine the meaning of the pain to the patient, the extent of the physical pain, and the fear elicited by the physical pain. Increases in physical pain are often associated with dying by the patient and family, and can increase depression, distress, and muscular tension in the body. Until all of these issues are addressed, the patient's total pain may remain uncontrolled. Lack of adequate pain management by health-care providers increases anxiety and suffering in both the patient and family. The use of pain medications in palliative care, including opioids and barbiturates, is acceptable and necessary in order to promote comfort and optimal quality of life. The Centers for Disease Control and Prevention (CDC) guidelines for pain management and opioid use specifically state that the use of these drugs is necessary in end-of-life care.

Spiritual Care

Leleszi and Lewandowski (2016) have identified aspects of spiritual care that should be included in total pain evaluation. Spiritual suffering is an aspect of spiritual care that occurs with unresolved interpersonal or intrapsychic issues. This type of suffering is a longing for explanations and assurances spiritual belief that is struggling in the face of great challenges.

Another aspect of spiritual pain is inner resource deficiency. Resource deficiency often exists because of patients or family's diminished spiritual capacity, often exhibited by statements of unbelief or why they have been abandoned in spiritual guidance. One positive spiritual aspect identified at the end of life occurs when specific spiritually based requests are made to assist them in obtaining a sense of spiritual well-being. By attending to these spiritual and emotional needs as well as the physical needs for pain relief, the health-care provider is able to create palliative care that is individualized to each situation.

Physical Care

Managing common physical symptoms optimizes the quality of life throughout the palliative care process. Palliative care includes management of both end-of-life symptoms and therapies directed at the disease, such as chemotherapy and dialysis for people with life-limiting illnesses (Wilke & Ezenwa, 2012). In addition to management of physical symptoms such as pain, palliative care

also includes reducing prolongation of the dying process, giving the patient a sense of self-control, and relieving the care burden on families and loved ones while helping to strengthen these relationships.

Pain can be one of the most prevalent symptoms near the end of life and a frequent companion of those receiving palliative care. Pain is a multidimensional experience and requires careful and continuous assessment and evaluation of the effectiveness of treatment options. As a provider of palliative care to patients and families, it is essential to become competent in pain management. Opioid analgesics are the standard treatment for moderate to severe pain for patients with advanced illnesses. The unfounded fear that opioids induce respiratory depression and hasten death can be a barrier to providing adequate care. When opioids are given at appropriate doses, they are safe and provide comfort and relief from severe pain. Pain management is discussed in more detailed in the section "Pain Management."

Several studies have demonstrated that the most difficult end-of-life symptoms to manage are pain, respiratory distress, and confusional states. In a retrospective review of 100 patients in an inpatient palliative care unit, Fainsinger et al. (1991) identified 16% of the patients required sedation to control pain and delirium. In another evaluation of patients during the last week of life, Conill and colleagues (1997) assessed patients at two intervals—their initial consultation and then during the last 7 days of life. Asthenia, anorexia, and dry mouth were the three most common symptoms in both periods, but the incidence of confusional states doubled during the last week of life (30.1% and 68.2%, respectively). Potter et al. (2003) assessed 400 patients referred to palliative care services and found the most prevalent symptoms in the cancer population were pain (64%), anorexia (34%), constipation (32%), weakness (32%), and dyspnea (31%).

An important physical symptom that should be assessed and treated at the end of life is dyspnea. Dyspnea occurs in about 75% of heart failure patients and in patients with cancer or respiratory problems at a rate up to 90%. Oxygen, opioids, and benzodiazepines are the most widely prescribed medications for this problem. Oxygen, which must be medically ordered, is often the first treatment for dyspnea in end-of-life care. Decreased oxygen levels can cause confusion and anxiety in patients. However, not all dyspnea patients find oxygen therapy helpful as it may cause breathing to slow. The best practice is to ask the patient if the oxygen makes them feel better and if not, to remove the oxygen (Hanlon, 2015). Opioids and benzodiazepines relieve feelings of breathlessness and the inability to take in enough air, which can cause anxiety and distress; their effectiveness must be assessed frequently.

Terminal restlessness is an unsettling behavior that can occur at the end of life. Restlessness often is upsetting to family members as they believe this symptom is caused by discomfort. Restlessness can be characterized as anguish, anxiety, agitation, or cognitive failure. Signs of restlessness include fidgeting, purposeless yet coordinated movements, moans, groans, or grimaces. Causes for terminal restlessness include failing body organs, opioid toxicity, pain, drug interactions, and hypercalcemia. Medications to treat terminal restlessness include opioids, anxiolytics, antidepressants, antipsychotics, antiepileptic, steroids, and NSAIDS. Nonpharmacological solutions for restlessness include a quiet and calm environment, frequent reorientation of the patient to place and person, gentle touch, quiet voice, and soothing music.

Weakness and fatigue are often associated with end of life. Up to 99% of cancer patients experience fatigue, often beginning early in the disease process. Fatigue can be a protective mechanism at end of life and provide the patient with a coping mechanism for suffering. It is important to provide care that allows patients to decide how active they want to be.

Restlessness and agitation can be caused by delirium, which is defined as a sudden onset of a disturbed state of mind characterized by extreme restlessness, illusions, and incoherence of thought and speech (Darcy, 2012). Delirium is best treated by identification and elimination of the cause. The cause of delirium at end of life could be pain, hypoxia, decreased sensory stimulation, dehydration, infections, renal failure, or endocrine abnormalities. Haloperidol is the most effective medication for treating the agitation from delirium; however, removal of the cause of the dementia is the best overall treatment.

Constipation, nausea, and vomiting are also distressing symptoms at the end of life. Constipation can occur when the patient is receiving opioid pain relievers, and patients should always be prescribed a stool softener when receiving opioids to allow for easier passage of stool. Poor oral and fluid intake can also contribute to constipation. Polyethylene glycol laxatives such as MiraLAX increase the amount of water in the intestinal tract and stimulate bowel movements. Laxatives of any type should not be used if the patient has a suspected bowel obstruction. For nausea and vomiting, antiemetic medication, such as ondansetron, can be given around the clock.

Poor secretion control may cause the patient to have noisy rattling breathing and increase the patient's discomfort. Placing a scopolamine patch behind the patient's ear can decrease these sections and stop the rattling breath. At the end of life, nutrition and fluid intake can be problematic, although hunger during this time is usually suppressed. Family members may become concerned about lack of oral intake. However, the placement of a gastric tube is not recommended at the end of life because it only creates difficulty for caregivers and results in edema and painful swelling for the patient.

PAIN MANAGEMENT

Pain is a complex problem, and the management of chronic pain requires an ongoing round of assessments, adjustments, and treatments. There are many definitions of pain. The International Association for the Study of Pain (2012) defines pain as an "unpleasant sensory and emotional experience" and states that pain is always subjective and can have a psychological or emotional foundation. A person's experience of pain is not always supported by evidence of tissue damage.

Each person has a distinct level of pain tolerance or a distinct level of intensity of pain that is tolerable. The pain threshold is the lowest tolerable level in each individual, in which a stimulus can cause pain. Nociceptive pain represents a normal response to injury of tissue. This type of pain is divided into two categories: (1) somatic pain, which is pain arising from muscles joints, and cutaneous tissue; and (2) visceral pain, which is pain arising from organs and smooth muscle. Neuropathic pain is caused by somatosensory impulses in the nervous system. Diabetic neuropathy, postherpetic neuralgia, postamputation pain, and poststroke pain are all examples of neuropathic pain. Differentiating between nociceptive and neuropathic pain is important because these two types of pain require different treatments. Neuropathic pain responds poorly to both opioid analgesics and NSAID agents but often responds well to antiepileptic drugs, antidepressants, and local anesthetics.

Common Medications Used for Pain

Non-narcotic pain medications include aspirin; nonsteroidal antiinflammatory drugs (NSAIDs), such as ibuprofen (Motrin) and naproxen sodium (Aleve); acetaminophen (Tylenol); and tramadol (Ultram), a narcotic-like medication for moderate to severe pain (see Drugs Commonly Prescribed 78.1). All of these medications are available over-the-counter medications except for tramadol, which is a schedule "C" medication requiring a prescription and Drug Enforcement Administration (DEA) number. Aspirin is used for fever and pain relief and is also an anticoagulant because it reduces platelet aggregation. Aspirin should never be given to children younger than 8 years because it can cause Reye's syndrome, which can be fatal. NSAIDs can cause gastrointestinal problems, including bleeding and ulcers, as well as renal failure. Acetaminophen can cause hepatic failure, especially if it is taken with alcohol or other hepato-toxic drugs. Because acetaminophen is found in many over-the-counter cold medications, sleeping medications, and pain medications, overdose may occur when acetaminophen is combined with one of these medications. This is especially true with children.

Non-narcotic prescription pain relievers that are effective for neuropathic pain, such as sciatica, shingles, or diabetic neuropathy, include gabapentin and amitriptyline. Gabapentin is an antiepileptic medication that is effective for nerve pain. Amitriptyline is a tricyclic antidepressant that is effective for neuropathic pain as well.

Opioid pain medications require both a prescription and a DEA number. Morphine is considered the most

Drugs Commonly Prescribed 78.1: Pain Medications

DRUG	INDICATION	ADVERSE REACTIONS AND PRESCRIBING CONSIDERATIONS
Salicylates (OTC)	Chronic inflammatory pain	• Stomach pain, increased bleeding risk • Contraindicated in children due to Reye's syndrome
Acetaminophen (OTC) (Tylenol)	Chronic inflammatory pain, such as arthritis	• Half-life: 2–7 hours • Maximum dose per day 4,000 mg, less in older adults • Can cause liver enzyme elevation or liver failure if maximum dosage is exceeded
Gabapentin	Neuropathic pain	• Start at a low dose (100 mg daily) and increase up to 300 mg three times daily to reduce neuropathic pain.
NSAIDS (OTC and prescription)	Chronic inflammatory pain	• Many types; if one type is not effective others may be effective. • Can increase risk for renal failure and stomach ulcers.
Codeine	Opioid pain medication for mild to moderately severe pain	• Onset: 15 minutes. • Half-life: 4–6 hours. • Should not be used in children younger than 12 years or anyone who has had recent surgery to remove tonsils or adenoids. • High potential for allergic reaction. • Also available in cough syrups to relieve night time severe cough. • Common side effects include nausea, vomiting, stomach pain, constipation, sweating, and rash.
Hydrocodone (Vicodin, Lortab, Lorcet, Narco)	Moderate to severe pain	• Onset: 15 minutes. • Half-life: 3.5–4 hours. • Morphine is the opioid of choice unless contraindications exist. • Immediate-release and sustained-release forms available. • One relative contraindication is renal failure. • Can be constipating. • Usual starting dosage is 1 tablet (5 mg) every 4 hours. • A long-acting formulation has been approved.
Oxycodone (Percocet, Perco)	Moderate to severe pain	• Onset: 15–60 minutes. • Half-life: 2–3 hours. • See hydrocodone for adverse effects.
Fentanyl (Duragesic, Actiq, Fentora [transmucosal])	Very severe intractable pain use when opioids have failed or in combination	• Half-life: 72 hours for patch; 17 hours for oral forms. • Indicated for very severe intractable pain. • Onset of action: 12–16 hours after application; full effect takes 72 hours. • Transdermal patch is contraindicated for acute pain or opioid-naive patients. • Absorption affects effectiveness, application of external heat sources affects release. • Titration of the patch should not occur before three days after initial dose.
Methadone (Dolophine)	Severe long-term pain; use when opioids have failed	• Duration shorter than half-life—careful titration needed. • Steady state reached in 7 days. • This drug should only be administered by pain management specialist.
Hydromorphone (Dilaudid)	Severe pain or allergy to other opioids	• Five times the potency of morphine.

Continued

Drugs Commonly Prescribed 78.1: Pain Medications—cont'd

DRUG	INDICATION	ADVERSE REACTIONS AND PRESCRIBING CONSIDERATIONS
Tramadol (Ultram, Ultracet [tramadol plus acetaminophen])	Moderate to severe pain	• Narcotic-like pain reliever. • Comes in an extended-release form for round-the-clock pain management. • Should not be used in children under 18. • Seizures have occurred in patients taking tramadol. • Can be addictive. • Side effects include headache, dizziness, drowsiness, constipation, diarrhea, nausea, vomiting, itching, sweating.
Combination pain medications (Lorcet 10/650. Vicodin HP, Tylox, Percocet)	First-line opioid treatment of pain because the acetaminophen increases the pain-relieving action	• Most are combined with acetaminophen; use caution when prescribing with other medications containing acetaminophen.

Abbreviation: OTC, over the counter.

effective medication for pain in terminally ill patients because it has fewer side effects, can be given orally or intravenously, and has a simple route of metabolism. Hydrocodone and oxycodone are considered mild opioids and have actions similar to that of morphine. These drugs are often combined with acetaminophen or aspirin. Codeine is the most constipating opioid and is less effective than others when give alone. Hydromorphone is a major opioid and is similar to morphine in administration and side effects. Fentanyl is commonly used in transdermal preparations for severe chronic cancer pain. Methadone is also used for severe pain and may be effective for neuropathic pain. Methadone has a slow onset and long duration of action and half-life. It is best prescribed by pain management experts or by licensed providers certified by the Substance Abuse and Mental Health Services Administration in its administration (Hawley, 2012).

Acute Pain

Acute pain is a normal, predictable, physiological response to pain that lasts a short time. It is caused by an infection injury, such as a broken bone, cut, contusion, or a surgical incision. This type of pain is not as difficult to manage as chronic pain because it is short term, and once the injury heals, the pain goes away. However, acute pain that is inadequately managed is thought to lead to chronic pain. The continuum from acute to chronic pain is influenced by the initial pain experience and individual biopsychosocial factors (Blondell, Azadfard, & Wisniewski, 2013). According to the American Pain Society for the first-line therapy for mild to moderate acute pain, acetaminophen or NSAIDs are recommended first-line therapies (Blondell, Azadfard, & Wisniewski,

2013). If short-term opioids are necessary as with postoperative pain or a broken bone, combining the opioid with either acetaminophen or an NSAID provides better pain relief then an opioid alone (Gaskell, Derry, Moore, & McQuay, 2009). If opioid pain relievers are required for severe acute pain, prescribing a short course of a lower-dose, short-acting opioid is preferable. If the patient continues to experience acute pain, careful management of opioid use is recommended, and reassessment of the pain at least every week is recommended (Dowell, Haegerich, & Chou, 2016).

Chronic Pain

Chronic pain lasts longer than 12 weeks and often persists long after the cause of the pain is healed. Chronic pain may also begin with no clear cause. There are many symptoms that may accompany chronic pain including fatigue, movement limitations, sleep disturbance, and decreased appetite. In chronic pain management, the goal of treatment is to reduce pain and improve function so that the patient can complete day-to-day activities. Often, chronic pain cannot be cured, but it can be managed. Chronic pain can limit activities, decrease productivity, and reduce quality of life for patients. In order to affectively assess and treat this type of pain, compassionate patient care and careful consideration of the benefits and risks of treatment options is required (Medical Board of California, 2013).

Assessment

Unfortunately, there are no objective tests that can measure or locate pain empirically. Pain assessment is part of the patient history and because pain is a personal and subjective experience, the patient's own description of the pain is the only information the healthcare provider can obtain. While evaluating pain, it is important to identify and obtain a description of the pain (sharp, dull, cramping, achy), the timing of the pain (it happens after eating or prior to bowel movements), location of the pain, what makes it better, what makes it worse, and finally how long the pain has been present.

Chronic Pain Treatment Risks: The Opioid Epidemic

Opioid use disorder (OUD) is a diagnosis made when patients have a problematic pattern of opioid use that can lead to physical and mental impairment (see Box 78.3). OUD occurs when opioids are taken even when the pain is gone or when there have been unsuccessful efforts to reduce opioid use. In the National Survey on Drug Use and Health (2015), it was estimated that 91 million (37.8%) Americans used prescription opioids and that 11.5 (4.7%) misused them. Researchers estimate that 1.9 million Americans have opioid use disorder (Han, Wilson, Compton, Blanco, Crand, Lee, & Jones, 2017). The most common reason for opioid use is to relieve pain. The diagnosis of OUD is usually made when the patient exhibits problems at work school or home and in social relationships related to opioid use. Instances of opioid intoxication, opioid withdrawal, and opioid-induced mental disorder may be present for people who have OUD. When patients have been prescribed opioids for severe pain, such as cancer pain or end-of-life pain, it is not considered to be OUD but rather a method for achieve appropriate pain relief.

The diversion and abuse of prescription opioid medications has been growing over the last three decades (Maxwell, 2015). Since 2000, over 500,000 Americans have died from drug overdose, and the number of deaths attributed to overdose opioid has increased in parallel with the number of opioid descriptions written (CDC, 2016). Not only is this a sad statistic, but it is detrimental to all of society through increase crime rates, increased medical costs, and lost productivity. As new drug and drug combinations are created (such as mixing fentanyl with heroin), it is evident that law enforcement alone is inadequate in combatting this epidemic. Efforts to control the pace of the epidemic are focused on three areas: (1) monitoring patient need, (2) shortening the amount of time medication is prescribed, and (3) reducing the overall number of opioid prescriptions in medical practice. Another important effort is subsidized access to evidence-based, medication-assisted treatment for opioid use disorder (Kertesz, 2016).

Special populations present concerns about opioid medications. Several investigations have found that up to 50% of adolescents who present to primary care for headaches or sports injuries received an opioid medication (DeVries, Kock. Wall, Getchius, Chi & Rosenberg, 2014; Veils, Epstein-Ngo, Meier, Ross-Darrow, McCabe & Boyd, 2014). Another study found that 20% of adolescents with currently prescribed opioid medications reported using them intentionally to get high or increase the effects of alcohol or other drugs (McCabe, West, & Boyd, 2013). Misuse of opioid medications prior to high school graduation is associated with a 33% increase in the risk of later opioid misuse. Opioid misuse in adolescents is strongly associated with later onset heroin use (Miech, Johnston, O'Malley, Keyes, & Heard, 2015).

Health-care providers are often faced with balancing the risk of opioid addiction with treatment of chronic pain syndromes. Most health-care providers have not been educated to treat addiction issues in routine clinical practice, and there is a shortage of health-care providers who have expertise in this area. There are also conflicting societal pressures on health-care providers working with opioid addicted patients. For example, providing an opioid user with naloxone to prevent overdose and death is seen by some as supporting the opioid use rather than working with the patient. More research is needed to provide evidence-based recommendations about how to diagnose and treat opioid addiction in the health-care setting.

Box 78.3   Definitions of Tolerance, Dependence, and Addiction

(See Chapter 65 for more information about substance use disorders.)

Tolerance: The diminished response to a drug when a person uses a drug for a long time. For example, if a prescribed pain medication has been used for several months, the patient may begin to complain about the drug no longer being effective. This is often the case in cancer pain or long-term end-of-life pain and escalating doses of opioids are required to maintain pain relief.

Dependence: Changes in the body as a result of drug use. With prednisone, for example, the body adapts to repeated doses of the drug by decreasing its own cortisol production. For this reason, prednisone is not stopped suddenly after continued use because it takes time for the body's natural cortisol production to resume to normal levels. The same is true with opioids. The drug must be tapered slowly so that the body can readjust and withdrawal symptoms such as nausea, shaking, depression, and anxiety can be avoided.

Addiction: A disease characterized by compulsive drug-seeking and use, despite harmful consequences. Addiction is an uncontrollable or overwhelming need to use the drug that is long lasting and can return unexpectedly after a period of improvement. Addiction is the result of a complex interplay of social, biologic, and psychosocial factors such as genetics, economic status, family environment, and drug accessibility. Treating addiction is also complex and requires a team approach of medical, psychological, and behavioral counseling, as well as support of those around the patient.

Binswanger and Gordon (2016) suggest the following in helping health-care professionals understand the opioid epidemic and assists patients dealing with addiction:

- Blaming those who require opioids for pain management as weak or lazy is unlikely to be effective in resolving this complex problem. Creating a public dialogue about the complex issues in pain management and providing a venue for honest discourse founded on compassion and understanding could improve outcomes of pain management and avoid opioid overuse.
- The use of criminal sanctions against patients who use opioids and their providers is not helpful to stem the tide of the epidemic. OUD is a complex condition with medical, socioeconomic, and legal implications. Often the criminalization of opioid use alienates, disempowers, and abandons the patient at the time of need. The stigma of opioid overuse disorder is strengthened by pejorative language and attitudes that actually increase the risks and problems associated with disorder.
- Opioid overuse occurs in all types of people— young, old, homeless, wealthy, isolated, and living with loving families. This diversity makes assessment, diagnosis, and treatment difficult.
- Effective pharmacologic treatment of opioid disorder requires assistive medications and medication management that may not be supported by families and partners. Evidence-based recommendations for the treatment of the opioid disuse problem are lacking. Although health-care providers are anxious to avoid more deaths and create an effective treatment plan for people with opioid disorder, observational data alone are not sufficient to overcome this epidemic.

How should health-care providers approach opioid prescribing and identifying patients who may be at risk for opioid misuse syndrome? One example of an evidence-based program for opioid overuse comes from The Johns Hopkins Bloomberg School of Public Health (Johns Hopkins, 2015). This program is designed to inform action with evidence and intervene comprehensively to promote appropriate and safe use of prescription opioids. This program was presented at a conference hosted by the Bloomberg school of Public Health and the Clinton Health Matters Initiative. The steps in this program include the following:

- Increase education for providers and strengthen prescribing guidelines for opioid prescriptions.
- Mandate prescriber prescription drug monitoring programs and allowing third-party payers to use these data.
- Increase education related to overdose and naloxone use.
- Provide education and information on addiction treatment including expanded access to buprenorphine (Suboxone) and methadone.
- Develop patient-centered treatment for opioid overuse and study the outcomes and effectiveness of these programs.

Treatment of Chronic Pain

The need for pain management using opioids is still an important part of health care. In order to use opioids safety and avoid the risk of overdose or overuse, the CDC (Dowell, Haegerich, & Chou, 2016) created guidelines for primary-care clinicians who prescribe opioids for patients with chronic pain outside of active cancer treatment, palliative care, and end-of-life care (Dowell et al., 2016). When developing these guidelines, investigators found that opioid prescriptions per capita increased almost 8% from 2007 to 2012 with the largest increase in prescribing rates found among primary-care and internal medicine practices. They also found that rates vary across states that do not correlate with the underlying health status of the populations, which demonstrates a lack of consensus among clinicians. These guidelines are now a national standard of care for opioid prescribing and chronic pain management and will help to ensure that patients have access to safer, more effective chronic pain management as well as reducing the number of patients who misuse, abuse, or overdose on these drugs. The full guidelines can be accessed at the CDC website. The CDC also provides patient education information, facts sheets, and additional guidelines for providers as well as resources for overdose prevention.

In its review of the evidence, the CDC found that no benefits of opioid treatment for chronic pain 1 year after opioid therapy began. In addition, long-term opioid use is associated with possible harms, including overdose and motor vehicle injury. Finally, nonpharmacological and nonopioid treatments have benefits for patients with chronic pain. The CDC recommendations for opioid use in patients without active cancer or who are not receiving palliative and hospice care and those at the end of life are summarized as follows:

1. Nonpharmacologic therapy and nonopioid therapy should not be considered first-line or routine therapy for treating chronic pain. Opioid therapy should only be considered when the benefits of opioid use outweigh the risks.
2. Before starting opioid therapy for chronic pain, clinicians should establish treatment objectives and goals with both patients and families. These goals should include goals for function and how to discontinue opioids if benefits do not outweigh the risks. Opioids should be continued only if meaningful improvement in pain and function can be documented. Other nonopioid therapies should be used in conjunction with opioids to shorten the length of opioid use and improve function.
3. Before starting opioid therapy and each time a renewal of opioid medication is needed, the health-care provider should discuss the risks and benefits of therapy with the patient. The health-care provider should also discuss the plan for the patient's opioid treatment.

4. When initiating opioid use for patients with chronic pain, immediate-release preparations should be used instead of long-acting opioids. There is no clinical evidence that long-acting opioids are better at relieving chronic pain, and using these preparations increases the patient's risk for overdose, misuse, and addiction.

5. When opioids are necessary for chronic pain treatment, the clinician should prescribe the lowest effective dose and escalate dosage very slowly. If the dose must be adjusted upward or a stronger opioid used, the clinician should carefully document the reasons and the plan to monitor, reassess, and eventually lower the dose of opioids used.

6. Because opioid use often begins with treatment of acute pain, the lowest effective dose of immediate-release opioids should be prescribed, and no greater quantity should be dispensed than the expected duration of pain severe enough to warrant opioid use. To reduce acute pain, treatment for 3 days or fewer may be sufficient, and more than 7 days of opioid pain treatment is rarely necessary. If treatment for more than 7 days is required, reassessment of pain should be carefully documented.

7. Clinicians should document a reassessment of chronic pain every 4 weeks for patients on chronic opioids.

8. Before prescribing and at each patient visit, the clinician should evaluate and document risk factors for opioid-related harms, such as a history of substance abuse and use of benzodiazepines along with opioids. From this evaluation, the clinician should create a mitigation risk plan to reduce the risk of opioid-related problems, which may include providing naloxone to the patient to use in the case of opioid overdose. Prescribers should avoid prescribing opioids to patients with moderate to severe sleep-disordered breathing whenever possible.

9. Clinicians should review a patient's history of controlled substance use through state prescription drug monitoring programs (PDMP) data. There is a great deal of variation among states related to opioid prescription monitoring. Local pharmacies may have a database of patients and medication usage and can provide information related to opioid use. Clinicians should discuss the information found related to a patient's past opioid use with the patient. Occasionally, information is incorrect, many names are the same, or another person has used the patient's identity. If patients are found to have a history of taking high opioid dosages, dangerous combinations of medications, or multiple controlled substance prescriptions written by multiple providers, the clinician should discuss safety concerns such as respiratory depression and the risk of overdose and death with patients, especially when opioids are combined with benzodiazepines.

10. Avoid prescribing opioids and benzodiazepines concurrently.

11. If selling or sharing opioids is suspected, urine testing should be initiated. A negative urine test result may indicate that the patient is diverting opioids to others.

12. Consider the possibility of substance use disorder and discuss possible treatments with the patient. Also consider offering naloxone.

The CDC guidelines are aimed at changing clinical practice in primary care and to promote and improve communication between providers and patients. When patients and health-care providers work together, more effective and less dangerous pain management can be achieved.

Nonpharmacologic Treatments for Pain

Pain is a sensation that is evaluated by the brain that responds to the noxious stimuli based on past experience, pain tolerance, and ideas about pain. Several nonpharmacologic therapies have shown promise in the area of pain relief, either alone or in combination with pain medication (Abdulla et al., 2013). Acupuncture and dry needle therapy have shown promise for many types of pain including joint pain, muscle pain, and connective tissue disease. Transcutaneous electrical nerve stimulation (TENS) and massage have also been found to have efficacy in muscle and joint pain including lower back pain. TENs units are now sold over the counter and are reasonably priced. Some psychological approaches have been found to relieve pain, such as guided imagery, biofeedback, and relaxation. Gentle exercise programs such as yoga, tai chi, or stretching have been successful in reducing osteoarthritis pain and muscle pain.

Distraction from pain can also be effective in minimizing the need for pain medication. Those who are lonely and left to focus on their pain often require higher doses of pain medication than those who are surrounded by distracting conversation, music, or even television. Supportive interactions with family, friends, and communities such as churches who spend time with those in pain, such as during the postoperative period, can reduce pain as long as they are mindful of the patient's strength and tolerance for conversation. Mindful therapies such as prayer, chanting, or music therapy have been shown to decrease pain through distraction and focusing at a different psychological level.

CONCLUSION

Palliative and end-of-life care are elements of quality health care and well-being in our society. Assisting all patients no matter what stage of their illness with pain management can be challenging. As an NP, it is particularly important to pay attention to the state and national regulations for NP practice and stay within the confines of the NP scope of practice in the area of pain management.

When caring for patients with pain, use of a caring approach and gaining the patient's trust can help guide them toward appropriate therapies without putting them in danger of overuse. In end-of-life care either with hospice or palliative care, overuse is not as problematic and pain relief is essential. WHO has provided a three-step analgesic ladder for cancer pain that should be used in treating end-of-life pain. Addiction and dependence are acceptable for this group to ease pain and suffering. In others with pain, safe prescribing of pain medications using the CDC guidelines and, where appropriate, recommended alternative nonpharmacological pain relief methods can help patients manage pain and assist in healing.

In patients who are currently overusing opioids, it is important to provide them with information related to the risks associated with overuse. Patients may not be ready hear this information and be more likely to rely on the opioid response. In these cases, it is incumbent on the practitioner to continue to provide care by referring patients to an addiction specialist to have their situation assessed and handled appropriately.

For additional resources please visit
https://davisedge.fadavis.com/

REFERENCES

Abdulla A, Adams N, Bone M, et al. Guidance on the management of pain in older people. *Age Aging.* 2013;42(Suppl 1):1–57.

Binswanger I, Gordon A. From risk reduction to implementation: Addressing the opioid epidemic and continued challenges to our field. *Subst Abuse.* 2016;37(1):1–3.

Blondell R, Azadfard M, Wisniewski A. Pharmacologic therapy for acute pain. *Am Fam Physician.* 2013;1:87(11):766–772.

Conill C, Verger E, Herniquez I, et al. Symptom prevalence in the last week of life. *J Pain Sympt Manage.* 1997;14(6):328–331.

Darcy Y. Managing end-of-life symptoms. *Am Nurse Today.* 2012;7(7):23–31.

DeVries A, Koch T, Wall E, et al. A. Opioid use among adolescent patients treated for headache. *J Adolesc Health.* 2014;55:128–133.

Dowell D, Haegerich TM, Chou R. CDC Guideline for prescribing opioids for chronic pain—United States, 2016. *MMWR Recomm Rep.* 2016;65(No. RR-1):1–49. **https://www.cdc.gov/mmwr/volumes/65/rr/rr6501e1.htm.**

Fainsinger R, Young C. Cognitive failure in a terminally ill patient. *J Pain Sympt Manage.* 1991;6(8):492–494.

Gaskell H, Derry S, Moore RA, McQuay HJ. Single dose oral oxycodone and oxycodone plus paracetamol (acetaminophen) for acute postoperative pain in adults. *Cochrane Database Syst Rev.* 2009;(3):CD002763.

Gawande A. *Being mortal: Medicine and what matters in the end.* New York, NY: Metropolitan Books, Henry Holt and Company; 2014.

Greer J. Study confirms benefits of early palliative care for advanced cancer. **https://www.cancer.gov/news-events/cancer-currents-blog/2016/palliative-care-quality.** Published 2016.

Han B, Compton W, Blanco C, Crane E, Lee J, Jones C. Prescription opioid use, misuse, and use disorders in U.S. adults: 2015 National Survey on Drug Use and Health. *Ann Int Med.* 2017;167(5):293–301.

Hanlon P. The role of oxygen in palliative care. **http://www.rtmagazine.com/2015/06/role-oxygen-palliative-care.** Published 2015.

Hawley P. Methadone for pain in palliative care. *Br Med J.* 2012; 54(6):290–304.

Hughes MT, Smith TJ. The growth of palliative care in the United States. *Annu Rev Pub Health.* 2014;4(34):459–475.

Institute of Medicine. Dying in America: Improving quality and honoring individual preferences near the end of life. **http://www.nationalacademies.org/hmd/~/media/Files/Report%20Files/2014/EOL/Report%20Brief.pdf.** Published 2014.

International Association for the Study of Pain. IASP taxonomy. **http://www.iasp-pain.org/Taxonomy#Pain.** Published 2012.

Johns Hopkins Bloomberg School of Public Health. The prescription opioid epidemic: An evidence-based approach. **http://www.jhsph.edu/research/centers-and-institutes/center-for-drug-safety-and-effectiveness/opioid-epidemic-town-hall-2015/2015-prescription-opioid-epidemic-report.pdf.** Published 2015.

Kertesz S. Turning the tide or riptide? The changing opioid epidemic. *Subst Abuse.* 2016;38(1):194–201.

Leleszi J, Lewandowski J. Pain management in end-of-life care. *J Am Osteopath Assoc.* 2016;105(3 Suppl):S6–11.

Lo B, Quill T, Tulsky J. Discussing palliative care with patients. *Ann Intern Med.* 2011;156:744–749.

Maxwell JC. The pain reliever and heroin epidemic in the United States: Shifting winds in a perfect storm. *J Addict Dis.* 2015;34(2–3):127–140.

McCabe SE, West BT, Boyd CJ. Medical use, medical misuse and nonmedical use pr prescription opioids: Results from a longitudinal study. *Pain.* 2013;154 (5):708–713.

Medical Board of California. *Guidelines for prescribing controlled substances for pain.* **http://www.mbc.ca.gov/licensees/prescribing/pain_guidelines.pdf.** Published 2013.

Miech R, Johnston L, O'Malley PM, Keyes KM, Heard K. Prescription opioids in adolescence and future opioid misuse. *Pediatrics.* 2015;136:e1169–1177.

National Consensus Project for Quality Palliative Care. *Clinical practice guidelines for quality palliative care,* 3rd ed. Pittsburgh, PA: National Consensus Project for Quality Palliative Care; 2013.

Potter J, Hami F, Brya T. Symptoms in 400 patients referred to palliative care services: Prevalence and patters. *Palliat Med.* 2003;17(4):1231–1236.

Quill TE, Abernethy A. Generalist plus specialist palliative care—creating a more sustainable model. *N Engl J Med.* 2013;368:1173–1175.

Rome R, Luminais H, Bourgeois D, Blais C. The role of palliative care at the end of life. *Ochsner J.* 2011;11(4):348–352.

Veliz P, Epstein-Ngo QM, Meier E, et al. Painfully obvious: A longitudinal examination of medical use and misuse of opioid medication among adolescent sports participants. *J Adolesc Health.* 2014;54:333–340.

Wilkie DJ, Ezenwa MO. Pain and symptom management in palliative care and at end of life. *Nurs Outlook.* 2012;60(6):357–384

World Health Organization. Definition of palliative care. **http://www.who.int/cancer/palliative/definition/en/.** Published 2015. Accessed March 31, 2017.

RESOURCES

American Cancer Society
   https://www.cancer.org
National Hospice and Palliative Care Organization
   https://www.nhpco.org
Palliative Dementia Care Resources
   http://www.pdcronline.org
Veterans Guide to Palliative Care
   https://www.va.gov/GERIATRICS/Guide/LongTermCare/Palliative_Care.asp

Chapter 79

Ethical and Legal Issues of a Caring-Based Practice

Jill E. Winland-Brown, EdD, APRN, FNP-BC

Josie Weiss, PhD, FNP-BC, PNP-BC, FAANP

ETHICAL ISSUES

The American Nurses Association (ANA) designated 2015 as the Year of Ethics, 2016 as the Culture of Safety, and 2017 as the Year of the Healthy Nurse. For the past 15 years, Gallup Poll results have cited nursing as first on the list of professions with the highest ethical standards in their annual survey on honesty and ethics.

With economic, social, and legal constraints present in our everyday practice, it is no wonder that health-care providers face ethical dilemmas daily. This chapter begins with an overview of what ethics is, what constitutes an ethical dilemma, different theoretical approaches to analyzing dilemmas, and a description of ethical principles. Each of us lives by a moral code, whether or not we have taken the time to reflect on what this means. Some people live by the simple code of "an eye for an eye"; others use the "Golden Rule" that forms the core of some major religions (Table 79.1).

TABLE 79.1 Golden Rules	
Whatsoever ye would that men should do to you, do ye even so to them.	*Christianity (Jesus)*
What is hateful to yourself, don't do to your fellow man.	*Judaism (Rabbi Hillel)*
What you don't want done to yourself, don't do to others.	*Confucius*
Hurt not other with that which pains thyself.	*Buddhism*
May I do to others as I would that they should do unto me.	*Plato*
Do naught to others which if done to thee would cause thee pain.	*Hinduism (Mahabharata)*
Hurt no one so that no one may hurt you.	*Islam (Muhammad)*

It is becoming more difficult to practice ethically in health care today for many reasons, including dehumanizing procedures, technological advances that affect the quality of life, and the potential for unauthorized sharing of confidential information and violations of privacy because of easy access to data banks. Patients and providers must contend with these and many other problems. Historically, the "virtuous" man or woman who faithfully followed rules that were largely etiquette could be termed *ethical*. Even the ANA's first Code for Nurses in 1950 dealt with issues of etiquette as being synonymous with ethics. Today, in view of the questions posed by modern health-care practices, those rules seem simplistic.

Ethics

Ethics is a branch of philosophy that considers what is right and what one ought to do when confronted with moral choices. It is termed *bioethics* when those moral choices involve health care. Personal and professional values influence our daily professional lives. Many of these values are known and explicit; others are hidden and unknown. When involved in a professional practice, providers cannot escape the need to clarify their own values. Many excellent books on values clarification (see Resources) are available that can assist health-care providers in exploring their own values and in deciding what is meaningful or valued to them to facilitate self-understanding.

Ethics is integrally related to nursing because nursing is a practice with an inherent moral sense. Nursing ethics attempts to articulate that moral sense, to assess its fulfilment, to explore new possibilities for its fulfilment, and to appraise its adequacy. A classic saying is, "A patient doesn't care what a nurse knows until he knows a nurse cares." This could not be truer than in any situation with a health-care provider and a patient involving life and death choices. The patient wants to know that the provider is an advocate, a friend, and a trusted expert, not someone who is consumed with billing practices or always watching the clock. In addition, professional nursing is both valued within U.S. society as documented by the Gallup Poll and is uniquely accountable to that society.

The Skill of Ethical Action

Ethics is the standards or principles governing one's actions in professional practice. It is what the professional "ought" to do. Ethical behavior serves to protect the rights of human beings; a code of ethics is characteristic of all professions. To apply ethics, there are three basic philosophical skills that clinicians need to foster or acquire. First, the clinician must develop an ability for in-depth questioning, not just taking information at face value. Next, the clinician must develop the ability to understand different points of view and make a reasonable, empathetic effort to understand another person's opposing viewpoint. Finally, the clinician must not be afraid to argue a point logically.

A dialectic exchange occurs when both parties learn something; it is a win–win situation. It is similar to a formal debate in that those who do not know their opponents' arguments do not completely understand their own.

Professional Codes

The ANA has a Code of Ethics for Nurses; the American Medical Association has a code of ethics entitled the Principles of Medical Ethics; and the American Hospital Association has a Patient's Bill of Rights, which delineates the hospital's code of conduct owed to patients. There is also a Code of the International Council of Nurses. The ANA's Code of Ethics for Nurses (the Code) was first formally adopted in 1950, although the origins of the Code go back to the late 1800s when the ANA was founded (ANA, 2015). The Code of Ethics helped to legitimize nursing as a profession—one of the components of a profession is having a code of conduct that governs its actions. The Code was formulated by nurses, for nurses, and was voted on at a national ANA convention that had delegates representing all ANA members.

The Code serves as a contract between society and the nursing profession: It explicitly sets forth the values and ethical principles that guide the clinical decisions of all practicing nurses. The Code provides a framework within which nurses and advanced practice registered nurses (APRNs) can make ethical decisions and be held accountable to the public for those decisions. It also provides guidance for carrying out the professional role and aids in justifying differences between personal and professional values.

The primary purpose of the Code of Ethics is promotion of high-quality nursing care and protection of the public from incompetent or unethical nursing practice. The 2015 Code, the latest revision, continues to indicate that the recipient of care is the primary consideration in any conflict of interest. The Code sets the ethical standards for nursing, whereas the Nursing Practice Act of each state establishes the legal standards. The requirements of the Code may often exceed, but are never less than, those of the law. The interpretive statements add greater specificity for practice.

One of the provisions of the Code states that part of being an ethical professional is to advance the profession by being a member of the association that represents the professionals. For nurses, this is the ANA. Although there are many specialty nursing organizations, the ANA is the umbrella organization that speaks for all nurses. Yet only about 10% of nurses belong to the organization. Increasing membership, particularly among APRNs, is one of the challenges facing nurses who need to become active to effect legislative change. Involvement in the ANA is essential to assist nurses in participating in setting and monitoring national health objectives as in *Healthy People 2020,* including health literacy (Box 79.1).

Box 79.1   Healthy People 2020

Since 1979, *Healthy People* has set and monitored national health objectives that meet a broad range of health needs, encourage collaboration across geographic locations, guide individuals toward choosing informed healthy decisions, and measure the impact of preventive actions. *Healthy People 2010* led the way to achieve increased quality and years of healthy life and the elimination of health disparities.

Every 10 years, the U.S. Department of Health and Human Services uses scientific insights and lessons learned from the past decade, along with new knowledge of current data, trends, and innovations, to develop new guidelines. *Healthy People 2020* reflects assessments of major risks to health and wellness, changing public health priorities, and emerging issues related to the nation's health preparedness and prevention.

Regional public comment meetings across the nation were held to draft objectives and develop the framework for selecting the vision, mission, goals, focus areas, and criteria for prioritizing the objectives for the guidelines.

Ethical Dilemmas

Ethical dilemmas may stem from conflicts regarding what is "right" and other duties and obligations. These conflicts may be between two ethical principles one holds, between two possible actions that both seem right in some way, between the demand for action and the need for reflection, and between two unsatisfactory alternatives. Socrates said that we "must let reason determine our ethical decisions rather than emotion." This is why nursing students are taught to use ethical dilemma resolution guidelines to assist them in the process. Before we can resolve a dilemma, however, we must explore different theoretical approaches and discuss ethical principles.

Ethical Issues for Health-Care Providers

Although there are many ethical issues that confront providers in the health-care arena, some of the most common include the following:

- End-of-life issues: do-not-resuscitate (DNR) orders, allow natural death (AND) orders, advance directives, artificial nutrition, and hydration
- Health-care reform issues
- Cost-containment issues
- Breaches of patient confidentiality
- Incompetent and/or unethical conduct of other health-care professionals
- Pain management and palliative care
- Informed consent
- Access to care
- Health literacy

- HIV and AIDS issues
- Issues surrounding genetics/genomics

Theoretical Approaches

There are many ethical theories, from the developmental approach of Kohlberg with an ethic of justice, to the feminist perspective of Gilligan with her ethic of caring. Many studies have examined the ethical reasoning of males and females. At least one study comparing decision-making regarding dilemmas between medical students (mostly male) and nursing students (mostly female) found no difference in reasoning abilities. We all face dilemmas with different value systems. Because each individual may use different ethical theories as a basis for his or her decision-making, it is necessary to understand where someone else is coming from. These ethical theories suggest how to think and what to think about in dealing with conflicts that require choices. They do not solve dilemmas but rather suggest ways of structuring and clarifying the process.

Two of the most common approaches to analyzing ethical dilemmas are *deontology* and *teleology.*

Deontology

The term *deontology* literally means "from being." The concept involves the notion that there are specific duties we have as rational beings that cannot be broached without incurring moral evil. Immanuel Kant championed this moral perspective in his work. Some of the primary principles of the deontologic approach to ethics include the following:

- Act the same in similar situations (principle of universalizability).
- Consider the nature of the act itself and the principles or rules involved.
- "Duties" are based on "rights."
- The means justify the ends.
- "Do unto others as you would have others do unto you."

Teleology

The term *teleology* literally means "the study of goals or ends." The concept here is that there are specific goals or ends that human life is intended to achieve, and the role of living well is to enable a person to achieve those goals or ends. Typically, a teleological approach will claim that a human being ought to achieve happiness. Happiness is defined in different ways. The ethicist then provides principles or rules of attaining that end. There are many different forms of teleological ethical positions. The most well-known are Virtue ethics (Aristotle), Divine Command theory (Aquinas), and Utilitarianism (John Stuart Mill). The main principles of the teleological approach include the following:

- The greatest amount of happiness or the least amount of harm for the greatest number (utilitarianism).

- Consequences are considered; benefits are calculated. Theories focus on goals or ends.
- Ends justify the means.
- This approach is community-oriented and also considers future generations.

These two approaches to analyzing dilemmas may be further explained by comparing the ways both could be applied in several situations. In some situations, the same outcome may occur even though two different approaches are taken. Consider the patient who has just found out he is HIV-positive and does not want his partner to be told. A clinician using the deontological approach would act the same in any similar situation and would never tell a lie: The clinician would tell the partner that the patient was HIV-positive. A clinician using the teleological approach would focus on the ends justifying the means: The clinician would feel that the partner has a right to know because he could become infected. The clinician also would calculate the consequences of telling or not telling and would feel that it is best for everyone involved in this situation to know the truth about the patient's condition. In this situation, both the deontologist and the teleologist came to the same decision.

Another example of a situation in which these two approaches are used, but with different outcomes, is a situation involving a terminally ill patient who is on life support. The deontologist would consider the nature of the act itself (the sanctity of life), the uniqueness of each individual, and the high sense of duty, and would keep the patient on the ventilator. The teleologist, on the other hand, would consider the consequences of maintaining the dying patient on life support, would recognize and consider the suffering of the patient and family, both now and after long-term ventilator treatment, and would support the family in withdrawing life support. It is imperative that health-care providers look at both sides of ethical dilemmas and at both approaches to analyzing dilemmas so that they may effectively communicate with someone who is approaching the situation from a different viewpoint. If the clinician is unable to "speak the language" of others involved in the dilemma, there is no communicating, and the dilemma may remain unsolved. Communication among all parties is essential.

Ethical Principles

Just as we use principles of physics, biochemistry, psychology, and body mechanics in our everyday functioning as clinicians, we must incorporate principles of ethics in our everyday reasoning (Box 79.2). However, it is important to recognize that the nature of the principles of physics govern the motion or properties of physical reality in such a way that explains why some object acts as it does. Conversely, the principles in ethics usually contain or imply the moral term *ought.* This distinction is important, because unlike the principles of physics, the

---

Box 79.2   Ethical Principles

- Autonomy
- Beneficence
- Nonmaleficence
- Veracity
- Confidentiality
- Fidelity
- Justice

---

principles in ethics can be broken. We cannot violate the principle of gravity, but we can violate the principle of autonomy. In other words, when one thinks about the principles of ethics, these principles not only set a standard of behavior but also identify and explain why some actions fail to uphold the principle. These bioethical principles (relating to health care) help us respond to specific dilemmas despite the diversity of the moral traditions from which they are derived. Each ethical conflict that a clinician faces may call for the application of different principles. A dilemma may occur that requires one principle to be sacrificed in favor of another, depending on the situation. Just because the clinician may be clinically competent does not necessarily mean that he or she has expertise in dealing with ethical dilemmas. Reasoning at a principled level is a skill that each individual must practice to become morally competent.

Autonomy

The first ethical principle is *autonomy,* which deals with personal liberty of action and self-determination, along with respect for all persons as individuals. It is one of the most frequently mentioned moral principles in contemporary biomedical ethics. Autonomy, sometimes defined as "free will," is a principle deeply rooted in the liberal Western tradition emphasizing the importance of individual freedom and choice. *Autonomy* means "the ability to act or choose without outside interference." For example, if someone were persuaded to invest his or her life savings in a shady business venture, there is a real sense that that person acted freely. However, if you were asked to hold your hand over a button that, if pushed, would launch a terrible weapon, and your hand was then forced to push the button, it would not be reasonable to say that you acted freely. The main difference in these two examples is that someone interfered with your ability to choose and act by forcing your hand. Mayeroff (1971) suggested that autonomy is living the meaning of one's life. A truly autonomous person freely chooses actions that are authentic and in concert with basic values. Clinicians, as well as patients, are autonomous. Professional autonomy includes control over the terms of practice, content of the discipline, and the regulation of standards.

This principle of autonomy in bioethical contexts is the basis for medical decisions and informed consent, along with access to health care. The principle of autonomy involves giving patients options and allowing them to choose their own course of action, thereby nurturing the wholeness of the person. Informed consent addresses the strong advocacy component of the healthcare provider role and is a large component of autonomy (Box 79.3). Lack of informed consent accounts for about 10% of all lawsuits against providers.

Situations requiring informed consent include invasive procedures; treatment with significant risks, such as chemotherapy; clinical trials; and research. Situations that do not require informed consent include those involving therapeutic privilege, in which the provider anticipates harm from the knowledge that would be shared during the consent process, in an emergency situation, or with the therapeutic use of placebos. Informed consent at its best helps to ensure that the patient takes an active role in dealing with the medical uncertainties and potential problems associated with any procedure to be performed.

Certain behaviors in health care restrict patient autonomy. Health-care providers may assume that they know what's best for the patient and do what they deem to be appropriate, thus acting in a paternalistic manner toward patients, restricting their autonomy. The term for this behavior is *parentalism,* that is, acting as a parent would toward a child and assuming that one knows what is best. An example of parentalism is the clinician who orders a medication for a patient without obtaining his or her consent and says, "Take this; it's essential." Although the treatment may be the correct one, to respect the patient as a person, the clinician should involve the patient in the care decisions and obtain the patient's approval for treatment. By giving the patient a vested interest in the outcome of care, he or she may be more likely to adhere to the prescribed regimen.

Box 79.3   Elements of Informed Consent

Informed consent has two elements:

1. Informed: Information given to the patient about procedure or treatment
2. Consent: The patient's autonomous agreement

To be informed, the patient must receive, *in terms that he or she can understand,* all the information that would affect a reasonable person's decision to consent to or to refuse the procedure or treatment. The information should include all of the following:

1. Description of proposed procedure or treatment
2. Name and qualifications of person performing the procedure
3. Explanation of the potential for death or serious harm or for the discomforting side effects during or after the treatment
4. Alternative treatments available
5. The effects of not having treatment

Parentalism involves both paternalism and maternalism. *Paternalism* is the way a father would act toward a child, a sterner approach. A clinician who says, "Cigarettes will kill you. If you're not going to stop smoking, I can't care for you anymore," is using a paternalistic approach. *Maternalism* is the way a mother would react to a child. The end result is the same as paternalism, but it usually involves gentle coercion. A clinician addressing the same patient in a maternalistic manner might say, in effect, "Please don't smoke; it hurts my feelings when you don't follow my recommendations. I don't want to go to your funeral." The best way a clinician can respect a patient's autonomy is to give him or her all the facts and let the patient choose.

Parentalistic behavior, regardless of benevolent motives or the magnitude of the benefit to be secured or the harm to be avoided, overrides the right of each adult to be treated as a person. To respect another as a person and to maintain his or her autonomy is to take full account of the patient's values. To disregard these values and act paternalistic toward a patient shows contempt for the individual as a person. It regards the person as a mere object rather than one's equal as a person, even if the provider is trying to do something to benefit the patient or protect the patient from harm.

It is within this principle of autonomy that the patient's competence and capacity are considered when dealing with patients who exhibit mental status changes. *Competence* is a legal status; all adults older than age 18 years are assumed to be competent unless a judge specifically declares otherwise. *Capacity* is judged clinically and has to do with whether or not the patient is capable of understanding the options presented. *Substituted judgment* is a different approach to maintaining someone's autonomy because the patient's own value system is used in decision-making: one seeks to decide what the patient would have decided if the patient had been able to do so.

There are some instances in which the principle of autonomy may be overridden by the state. These situations include an emergency procedure that is necessary to protect a life, such as a blood transfusion for a child whose parents refuse treatment on religious grounds or an intervention when the potential for suicide exists. A provider can legally treat a patient without getting his or her consent if the patient needs immediate treatment to save his or her life; to prevent loss of an organ, limb, or function; if the patient is unconscious; or, in the case of a minor, if the family cannot be reached. In such situations, the law assumes that if a patient could decide, he or she would choose to receive treatment. This exception is limited. It does not apply if the provider knows the patient had previously said he or she would refuse such treatment if offered, or if the provider can wait for consent to be obtained. In only two instances is it legal to have a consent form signed by someone other than the patient: (1) in the instance of a minor and (2) when the patient has been declared legally incompetent.

Another exception to the need for informed consent is when a patient waives the requirement to be informed. A patient may not want to know the details. Nonetheless, the provider still has two responsibilities: (1) the provider must make sure the patient understands that risks and alternatives do exist, and (2) the provider must clearly document the patient's waiver of his or her right to receive information. Some facilities assume no responsibility for obtaining informed consent and supply no forms for doing so. Their premise is that even with detailed consent forms, it is impossible to provide all the relevant information and that completing the forms actually decreases the communication between the provider and the patient. The actual process of informed consent is what should be aimed for, rather than the completion of forms.

Beneficence

The second ethical principle is *beneficence*, which is mentioned in the Nightingale pledge. It is the provision of benefits and a balancing of harms and benefits and requires positive action. One must purposefully choose the right action, not merely by omission, and do what is in the best interest of the patient. Positive beneficence requires personal risk-taking. For example, clinicians who care for persons with AIDS are acting beneficently toward those patients by caring for them. Beneficence encompasses the principle of utility or proportionality when one weighs the probability of benefits and harms in order to produce the maximal net benefit (utility).

Nonmaleficence

The third ethical principle is *nonmaleficence*, the idea that a health-care provider should, above all, "do no harm," which is mentioned in the Hippocratic Oath. This principle, the foundation on which health care rests, forms the basis for most medical and nursing codes of ethics. It usually involves omissions and does not require taking positive action; the emphasis is on not taking the wrong action and doing something to harm the patient. Several moral rules, such as the prohibition of killing, are derived from nonmaleficence. It must be stressed, however, that it is almost always impossible to ensure someone's benefit without risking some harm. Consider the patient with cancer who is receiving chemotherapy. Chemotherapy may be considered a positive benefit, but the side effects are definitely deleterious. Paternalism is also deeply embedded within this principle because it is extremely difficult to respect a patient's autonomy while wanting to resolve the conflicts between beneficence and nonmaleficence. Most clinicians want the patient to choose the "right" decision. Consider the situation in which we know a patient would benefit from chemotherapy, yet the patient refuses because of a bad experience that a relative had with similar therapy. The patient's autonomy overrides our beneficent wish in this situation.

Veracity

The fourth principle is *veracity*, or truth-telling. Health-care providers may tell half-truths or may omit information because they feel that the patient cannot "handle" the news. Using the principle of autonomy, it is the right of the patient to know and to decide whether he or she wants any further information. As practitioners, we cannot make that decision for our patients. Veracity is important for obtaining informed consent. The critical issue here is that the patient understands or comprehends what the procedure will do or will cost. One must not only tell the truth but also tell it in a manner that is understandable by the listener.

Confidentiality

The fifth principle is *confidentiality*, which involves respecting privileged information. Maintaining a patient's confidentiality has become more difficult because computers can provide access to all kinds of personal information. Consider the situation several years ago of the patient who requested a breast cancer gene test to see if she was a candidate for prophylactic care, and an insurance company canceled her policy because she might develop breast cancer in the future. This practice is now illegal. Confidentiality, as well as veracity, are extremely important components of the provider–patient relationship.

Health-care providers need to be aware of the Health Insurance Portability and Accountability Act (HIPAA), which has been fully implemented since 2003. All health-care providers are responsible for maintaining secure electronic files and for ensuring confidentiality when sharing information between health-care providers and third-party organizations. Mandated development of electronic health records or electronic medical records increase both the potential ethical dilemmas and the positive aspects of efficiency/communication issues.

Fidelity

The sixth ethical principle is *fidelity*, or keeping promises. For example, a provider tells a patient that if treatment A does not work, he or she will try treatment B. When the time comes, however, the provider is unable to do so because a referral is not indicated, the treatment would make a negative impact on the audit that the insurance company will do shortly, or the insurance company will not pay for it. In another example, although providers try to do all they can to help a patient, when care is futile, the type of care must be changed to palliative rather than curative caring. Fidelity is critical because it avoids setting up false expectations. If a health-care provider claims that he or she will do something but fails to follow through, the patient may not request needed assistance later because the patient is expecting the promise-maker to once again fail to follow through. The result may be someone who does not receive a needed treatment.

Justice

The principle of justice or fairness involves weighing individual rights. Justice is the most complex and difficult principle to apply to health care. Health-care providers frequently use this principle to allocate scarce resources. The concept of justice in health care is what philosophers call *distributive justice*. This notion involves the idea of how to be fair to everyone involved while recognizing that some resources are scarce. For example, consider the following ways in which a tax refund could be distributed. If the government receives more revenue than needed, there are several ways to distribute the excess: (1) anyone who filed a tax form and overpaid could receive the same refund; (2) everyone who submitted a tax form and overpaid would receive back what that person overpaid; or (3) everyone who submitted a tax form and was born on a Sunday would receive the same share, but no one else would receive a share. All three of these possible distribution patterns of tax refunds are possible, but no one would think (unless that person was born on Sunday) that the third pattern was fair. The real debate is between the first and the second pattern of distribution. Typically, distribution patterns that are considered fair are ones in which proportionality of the scarce resource is balanced by the need or the immediacy of receiving the resource. There may be only four hearts available for transplant. Eight patients need a heart, but one patient may die within a few days without the transplant. The immediacy of the need is a major consideration into how these resources were distributed if the distribution were just. The decision must be based on principles rather than emotion; to be fair to patients, *like* cases should be treated *alike*. For example, if there are only so many patient-controlled analgesia pumps available and several candidates need one, who will get the last one? Who should get the liver transplant, and how many times should it be done before it is considered futile? Leaders in health care must continually address these questions. For example, one of the goals of *Healthy People 2010* was to eliminate health disparities. Some progress has been made and we will continue working to that end. In *Healthy People 2020,* one of the goals is to identify nationwide health-improvement priorities. With the 1,200 objectives in 42 topic areas in HP 2020, equitableness and fairness (the principle of justice) is the goal.

If these ethical principles are applied deliberately and consistently in practice, fewer mistakes will be made, less harm will be done to patients, autonomy will be respected, and decisions will be based on ethics. Changes in the health-care system are a challenge to health-care providers and themselves present ethical dilemmas. An *ethical dilemma* is a situation in which there is no satisfactory answer, and, although many options are available, one seems to conflict with another. The following Nursing Situation presents two ethical dilemmas.

Nursing Situation: Ethical Dilemmas

Situation 1

Shelly has been an APRN for several years and has been frustrated with the change in the health-care system and the resultant care that patients receive. When Joseph Harms, one of her patients, was cut back to part-time hours at work, he and his wife lost their health insurance. Mrs. Harms has been treated by Shelly for several years now for type 2 diabetes mellitus and has been very erratic in glycemic control. The Harmses cannot afford to come in as frequently as they did in the past and now must pay the office and pharmacy bills out of their own pockets. Shelly gives them free samples whenever possible and feels like she is not giving the best quality care when they insist they cannot afford any blood work—only the Accu-Chek in the office. Each office visit costs $60. Shelly has no control over billing.

1. What may happen if a fasting blood sugar, glycohemoglobin (Hb A1C), and urinalysis are not routinely ordered?
2. What may happen if Mrs. Harms cannot afford to see the ophthalmologist and podiatrist this year?

Situation 2

Jessica is 16 years old and is on birth control pills. Her relationship with her mother is precarious. Jessica's mom accompanies her to the nurse practitioner's (NP) office because of symptoms of bronchitis. Samantha, the NP, is not sure if Jessica's mom knows her daughter is taking birth control pills. Jessica's mom won't leave the room.

1. Jessica's mom already stated she would not leave Jessica alone in the room. Should Samantha insist?
2. Samantha doesn't want to let the opportunity pass and wants to talk about the fact that Jessica is on OCP with her mom. How far does the principle of confidentiality extend? Does the fact that Jessica is a minor play any part?

Resolution Guidelines

Although there is no blueprint for analyzing dilemmas, the mnemonic ETHICAL is a framework that can be used to provide a systematic method for acting consistently in ethical dilemmas, thus allowing reason rather than emotion to guide one's actions.

E Examine the data.
T Think about which person(s) should be making the decision.
H Humanize the options by constructing a decision tree.
I Incorporate the ethical principles, legal statutes, standards of care, and so on.
C Choose an option.
A Act.
L Look back and evaluate.

Consider the following situation and use **ETHICAL** as a framework to guide your actions:

Sylvia is a 76-year-old woman who presents with a massive suspicious breast lump and a new cough. She has not had a well-woman exam in years, nor has she done a monthly breast self-exam. The clinician explains that she wants Sylvia to get a mammogram. Sylvia refuses, stating that she does not want to know the results. What if the test is positive? Sylvia does not want surgery at her age. After a lengthy discussion, the clinician broaches the subject of advance directives. Sylvia states that, as a widow, she has nothing to live for, but she does not want to sign "a death sentence." She states, "When God wants me, he'll take me." This implies that she does not want extraordinary measures taken to keep her alive.

When applying the resolution guidelines in this situation, the first aspect to consider is **E**, examine the data. The clinician has detected a breast mass and recommends a mammogram as the next step in the diagnostic process. Sylvia has refused her clinician's recommendation to receive a mammogram. In this step of the resolution process, all of the information should be collected and the key participants identified. When interpreting the data, the conflicts presented in the situation should be identified. Are there conflicting rights and obligations? Is there a conflict between two unsatisfactory choices of action? The clinician should enter the world of the person involved and look at the situation from that perspective. The *Circle of Caring* model is definitely used in ethical dilemmas. The clinician should delineate the scope of responsibility and authority of each person. Factors should be identified that could limit each person's ability to participate in the decision-making, such as fear, coercion, and pain.

The second step, **T**, refers to thinking about and identifying the person(s) who should be making the decision. We do not know if other family members are involved in Sylvia's care, but because she is coming to the office by herself, the clinician assumes that she is independent, competent, and certainly capable of making her own decisions. Even if there were a son or daughter nearby, the decision would still be Sylvia's to make, although the clinician might ask Sylvia if he or she could discuss the situation with children and share their perspective. In most instances, there are other persons or ethical agents involved in the decision-making, such as the patient's family, physician, institution, clergy, social worker, and various therapists and consultants. The rights, duties, and responsibilities of each participant must be clarified and analyzed. In addition, because health-care ethics is a complex subject, there will always be difficult cases that will require consultation with people who have special training in relevant fields.

The third step, **H**, is to humanize the options by constructing a decision tree as shown in Figure 79.1. This allows all the options to be considered along with all the consequences of those options. Visualizing the results in this fashion can help narrow down acceptable options.

Resolution Guidelines: Constructing a Decision Tree

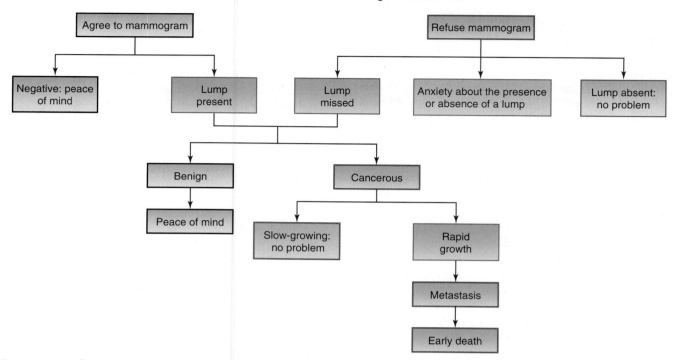

Figure 79.1 Resolution guidelines: constructing a decision tree. Each state defines the scope of practice within the state Nurse Practice Act. Every state has a Nurse Practice Act.

The fourth step, **I**, stands for incorporating all the extraneous data that must be considered when making ethical and/or legal choices. Certainly, the clinician is reflecting on his or her ethical principles. By allowing Sylvia the right to make her own choice, even though it conflicts with her own recommendation, the clinician is maintaining Sylvia's autonomy. If the clinician were to be beneficent in his or her actions, he or she might strongly urge (coerce) Sylvia to have the mammogram. But then what? Why pursue the mammogram if Sylvia has already stated that if it shows a problem, she will not consider any further action, for example, a biopsy, or more invasive surgery? Does Sylvia have the right to choose an option that might essentially be signing a "death warrant"? Yes, she does, as long as she is competent and has all the information presented to her. The decision tree allows Sylvia to see all the options and the resulting consequences. Although we cannot predict which branch of the tree this scenario will take, Sylvia has the right to consider all branches.

In this step in the ethical inquiry, all the basic principles should be considered. How does each ethical principle relate to the decision? The Code of Ethics for Nurses should help guide the action. Although codes by definition are brief and general, when used in combination with exploring the relationship of all the ethical principles to the proposed decision, the outcome will be ethical. This step usually points to the most ethical course of

action. The ultimate goal of laws is to protect individual rights without jeopardizing the welfare of the general population. Laws must be considered in directing action, seeking consultation, and requesting necessary assistance in selected patient-care situations.

The next step, **C**, involves choosing an action, and the following step **A** refers to actually acting on the decision. Sylvia has known all along what her choice would be—taking no action, which is actually choosing an action. The final step, **L**, stands for looking back or evaluating the situation, so that if the clinician were faced with a similar situation in the future, he or she might consider more choices and thus have more "branches" in the decision tree for consideration, or be aware of more legal precedence, and so forth. Especially when acting in the role of the primary moral agent, health-care providers need to keep abreast of the consequences of their own actions as well as those of others who are acting on behalf of the patient. Previous experience in similar situations can provide a frame of reference for comparisons and assist the clinician in making quality decisions. Although a decision tree is not meant to "lead" the patient to action, it does allow the patient and provider to consider more choices than may have been thought available. Brainstorming should be used; all choices proposed should be taken under consideration, even if they seem unrealistic at the time. Sometimes the first "irrational" choice ends up being the best choice for the patient and his or her family.

Institutional Ethics Committees

When health-care providers have difficult and unclear choices to make, the best course of action is to consult the local Institutional Ethics Committee (IEC). The Standards of The Joint Commission (TJC) state that an organization should have in place "a mechanism for the consideration of ethical issues arising in the care of patients and to provide education to caregivers and patients on ethical issues in health care." Although this mandate may be applied loosely and does not mean that the organization will have a standing ethics committee, assistance should be made available, such as a consulting with a parish nurse or a bioethicist. Some larger health-care institutions have ethics consultation services for ethical support for both patients/families and professional staff; the staff for these services may include ethicists who informally address nursing questions and concerns.

The purposes of IECs are to serve as a forum for health-care professionals' ethical concerns, as well as for conflict resolution between any of the parties involved. IECs provide advice, education, and consultation to the staff and patients and possibly to the community on actual and potential questions of ethics. They also provide recommendations for and help in developing institutional policies, procedures, and guidelines in areas of bioethical concern; assist in developing formal policies and procedures for identifying, reporting, and resolving ethical questions and in conducting retrospective reviews of decisions on ethical questions; and offer recommendations for improving policies and procedures used to resolve ethical issues.

IECs are usually multidisciplinary in nature because of the varied amount and types of health-care workers involved in any patient situation. They are composed of physicians, nurses, social workers, clergy, administrative personnel, legal counsel, a patient representative, and someone from the community. The patient representative must actively advocate for the patient, and in doing so, subordinate his or her own needs, opinions, and moral positions to those of the patient or family member. The patient representative works to focus and refocus the committee on the welfare and rights of patients. The ANA and the American Medical Association have developed position statements on specific topics such as referrals to the most appropriate provider and sexual harassment, to assist practitioners in drafting policies (see the ANA website for position statements). Health-care providers should not hesitate to use their professional organizations as resources (see Evidence-Based Nursing Practice 79.1).

Relationship Between Ethics and Law

Although clinicians strive to be ethical in all their actions, they must also think of legalities. Actions that are ethical are not always legal, whereas actions that are illegal are

 Evidence-Based Nursing Practice 79.1

Winland-Brown JE, Dobrin AL. A comparison of physicians' and nurses' responses to selected ethical dilemmas. Forum on Public Policy Online. http://forumonpublicpolicy.com/spring09papers/papers09spring.html. Published 2009.

The purpose of this study was to explore the similarities and differences between physicians' and nurses' responses to four ethical dilemmas. The dilemmas included surgical error, end-of-life care, possible physician or nurse drug use, and the medical repatriation of an illegal immigrant. Sixty-seven nurses and 26 physicians participated. This study found that physicians and nurses reason more alike than differently on ethical dilemmas. There was only one response to one dilemma for which physicians and nurses reasoned significantly differently. Similarly, an equal number of physicians and nurses had experienced moral distress in the past. The variables of religion, gender, education, and ethnicity were significant for some of the responses to the dilemmas. Strategies were suggested to enhance moral reasoning and possibly lessen some moral distress.

sometimes ethical (Table 79.2). APRNs should always strive to practice within the ANA Scope of Practice, their State Practice Act, and the Code of Ethics for Nurses, in addition to being cognizant of individual state laws on prescribing authority, signing death certificates, authorizing disabled parking permits, and other pertinent laws. The circumscribed actions and duties that are allowable in the profession are termed the *scope of nursing practice,* which are defined and guided by each state in the Nurse Practice Act and by common law. Common-law principles govern many interactions affecting nursing and are based on a traditional justice perspective. The state Nurse Practice Act, however, is the single most important piece of legislation for nursing because it is the Practice Act that affects all facets of nursing practice. The Nurse Practice Act cannot grant exceptions, waive the Act's provisions, or expand practice outside the Act's specific provisions.

TABLE 79.2	**Relationship Between Ethical and Legal Issues***	
	Legal	*Illegal*
Ethical	Assisting an older patient to complete an advance directive	Assisting in the death of a 99-year-old terminally ill patient
Unethical	Ordering emergency contraception in a Catholic Church–affiliated clinic	Billing for a treatment that was not done

*Although one may not agree with the choices of situations explaining ethical and legal issues, they are presented here for demonstration purposes—to explicate the intricacies of the ethical and legal relationship. Laws represent the minimum ethic governing behavior; compliance with them is mandated. Ethics operate at a higher level; they offer guidelines for resolving ethical dilemmas.

LEGAL ISSUES

Scope of Practice

The scope of practice defines the rules, regulations, and boundaries within which the APRN, with appropriate education and experience, can practice. The scope of APRN practice, which is regulated to ensure public safety, is evolving just as health care is evolving. As more supportive evidence for safe, effective APRN practice accumulates, the scope of practice is likely to broaden (National Council of State Boards of Nursing, 2012). In 2010, the Institute of Medicine (IOM) recommended scope of practice reform to allow APRNs to practice to the full extent of their education and training in all states. The importance of removing barriers to full practice authority was reinforced in 2017 in a report from the Robert Wood Johnson Foundation (2017).

The legislative agenda of major APRN organizations is to ensure full practice authority in all states to improve access to high quality care for all persons in the United States. Bringing uniformity to and removing barriers from state laws regarding scope of practice are two key goals of the National Council of State Boards of Nursing. Twenty-three states allow full practice authority as recommended by the IOM and national consensus statement. In 16 states, APRNs have reduced practice authority due to imposed barriers. In 12 states, even greater barriers are in place, including requirements for supervision, delegation, or team-management of practice. All states have prescriptive authority for controlled substances, with Florida the last state (in 2016) to gain that authority.

A model for future APRN practice was developed with the collaborative work of the APRN Consensus Work Group and the National Council of State Boards of Nursing APRN Committee (2008). This report established clear expectations for licensure, accreditation, certification, and education (known as LACE) for all APRNs, and ultimately these expectations will continue to shape future APRN practice.

Overview of Nurse Practitioners

There are more than 222,000 nurse practitioners (NPs) licensed in the United States today. Approximately 20,000 new NPs completed their graduate programs in 2015. With increased demand, the number is estimated to be 244,000 by 2025. According to a 2016 survey from the American Association of Nurse Practitioners (2017), the typical NP has the following characteristics:

- Has a graduate degree (96.2%)
- Is certified in an area of primary care (83.4%)
- Is 49 years old
- Has been in practice for 12 years as an NP
- Has an average full-time NP base annual income of $102,526
- Sees three or more patients per hour (60.7%)

- Prescribes medications (95.8%) and writes 23 prescriptions per day

Licensure and Certification

Many non-nursing individuals assume that licensing and credentialing are synonymous. It is the responsibility of the clinician to educate other providers and consumers regarding what he or she can and cannot do. Legal authority for all nursing practice, including advanced practice nursing, rests with the individual board that administers the legal statutes that define nursing practice in each state. Currently, for APRNs, this oversight varies. In some states, the Board of Nursing administers and defines advanced nursing practice; in others, it is the Board of Medicine; and in a few states, it is the Board of Pharmacy. The American Association of Nurse Practitioners recommends that only state boards of nursing regulate NP practice and prescriptive authority. Legal authority for professional practice was delegated to the states and territories by the U.S. Constitution and is not regulated by federal statutes.

An individual is permitted to practice basic or advanced practice nursing by licensure. *Licensure* protects the public from unsafe practitioners by ensuring a minimum standard of competency. Basic licensure as a registered nurse (RN) is a legal status granted by each state's Board of Nursing. Passing the National Council Licensure Exam (NCLEX-RN) is required for RN licensure, but does not ensure high nursing standards. The NCLEX is designed to assess minimum competency to practice safely. The curriculum of a nursing program, although providing a foundation of nursing knowledge that will graduate a safe and competent practitioner, is not specifically geared to the NCLEX exam. Nursing programs retain autonomy over their own curricula.

Similarly, the NP curriculum is under the control of the graduate faculty and is geared to advancing nursing-based knowledge. However, both undergraduate and graduate nursing programs must be accredited by national accrediting bodies such as the Commission on Collegiate Nursing Education for their graduates to take licensure and/or certification examinations. To bring more uniformity and rigor to nursing programs, curricular guidelines and competencies have been developed by leading educational organizations including the American Association of Colleges of Nursing and the National Organization of Nurse Practitioner Faculty. Upon completion of educational programs, each prospective APRN applies to the appropriate state board for an advanced nursing license. In some states, the graduate must pass a national certification exam to be eligible for this license. Although the licensing statutes may spell out prescriptive privileges for APRNs, they do not necessarily do that, nor is that the primary purpose of professional licensure. Some states mandate the filing of a protocol that documents physician oversight, but other states do not (Box 79.4 shows a

---

Box 79.4   Sample Advanced Practice Nursing Protocol

I. Requiring authority: Nurse Practice Act, Specific State—list Statutes, Chapters, Administrative Code. Administrative policies pertaining to certification of Advanced Practice Registered Nurses (APRN).

II. Advanced Practice Registered Nurse Certification: _____ (name, home address, phone number) is certified as an APRN #_____ by the (list State) Board of Nursing.
Supervising Professional: Name, address, license number, and DEA number of physician.

III. General Area of Practice: _____ may manage the health care for those patients for which he or she has been educated. His or her master's degree is in _____.
List practice address, including primary and satellite sites.

IV. Specific Management Areas:
  A. The following measures may be initiated by the APRN:
    1. Conduct a history and physical on patients.
    2. Take medication history, review medication profiles, and suggest necessary revisions.
    3. Order and interpret diagnostic tests necessary to treat, including, but not limited to, lab work, x-ray exams, pulmonary function tests, electrocardiograms.
    4. Diagnose and treat conditions within the scope of practice of a family nurse practitioner.
    5. Instruct patient and families in treatment and medications.
    6. Refer to other providers as appropriate.

  B. The following medications may be prescribed, initiated, monitored, altered, or ordered by the nurse practitioner in accordance with education: antibiotics, antihistamines, antihypertensives, anti-inflammatory agents, antigout agents, anticonvulsants, antimicrobial agents, antifungals, antiarrhythmics, antiparasitic agents, antianginals, antidepressants, antianxiety agents, antipsychotics, beta blockers, calcium-channel blockers, cathartics, laxatives, contraceptives, diuretics, expectorants, muscle relaxants, NSAIDs, optical agents, otic agents, over-the-counter agents, steroids, stimulants, vasodilators, vaccines.
Controlled substances may be initiated by the APRN only within the facility in which he or she practices, after appropriate federal and state guidelines have been followed by the supervising physician. (Will vary according to state.)

  C. Admit, initiate visits, and discharge patients in hospitals that have granted visiting privileges. Conduct histories and physicals, order diagnostic tests, treatments, and prescribe medications.

  D. Any other measures within the scope of preparation and experience of the APRN.

V. All of the above functions may be performed under the general supervision of the physician.

Signed: _____ APRN_____

Date: _____

Signed: _____ MD_____

Date: _____

---

sample protocol). Laws in most states do not mandate physician supervision of NPs. Protocols are similar to standing orders; they can be used as evidence to establish breach of the standard of care if they are not adhered to. Therefore, APRNs are often encouraged to make these protocols broad to accommodate changing practice environments.

Credentialing is a process used by certain health-care organizations to ensure that the NP meets certain criteria for practice. To become credentialed, an NP must demonstrate competency in certain areas such as licensure, education, and certification. Criteria for credentialing vary, depending on the credentialing body. A hospital, for example, may use credentialing to grant hospital privileges. Currently 49.9% of NPs hold hospital privileges, and 11.3% have long-term care privileges. This number is increasing daily. The granting of clinical privileges to practice in an institution is influenced by many factors. The primary factors governing the ability of an NP to obtain clinical privileges are the institutional policy, medical staff by-laws, state law, and TJC accreditation standards. Other factors include the approval of the medical staff including the collaborating physician (if required) and the NP's demonstration of competency, along with his or her eligibility for third-party reimbursement and prescriptive privileges.

Certification is a voluntary process with no legal authority. The primary purpose of certification is to validate the qualifications and knowledge of the APRN to practice. Although some states mandate that an NP pass a national certification exam before granting licensure to practice at an advanced level, not all states do. Currently 97% of all NPs hold national certification. National certification may be necessary to obtain third-party reimbursement; however, it is not the primary purpose of certification, nor is providing the public with information about the skills of the practitioners. Other than the specialty organizations, there are two predominate organizations that certify APRNs in adult/gerontology primary and/or acute care or family practice: the American Nurses Credentialing Center and the American Academy of Nurse Practitioners Certification Program. The certifying bodies also require recertification every 5 years, which includes educational credits in pharmacology. All national organizations guiding NP education and certification advocate that NPs obtain and maintain national certification.

Prescriptive Authority

Since the mid-1970s, APRNs have had some type of prescriptive authority. Prescriptive authority is an integral component of advanced nursing practice and is regulated differently from state to state. It is important for APRNs to know the extent of the prescriptive authority they have in the state in which they are practicing and what restrictions, if any, there may be. Restrictions may range from collaborative or supervisory requirements to a need for countersignatures, formulary restrictions, specific protocols, and/or site restrictions. All states grant statutory independent prescribing authority to APRNs. Some states require that APRNs have additional training to obtain prescriptive privileges. State-specific regulations affecting prescribing authority can severely limit the mobility of nurses who anticipate moving to another state. Both prescriptive authority and the mobility of the APRN's state license are legislative challenges facing APRNs today.

Unfortunately, the risk of medication errors accompanies prescriptive privileges. It is estimated that at least 44,000 and up to as many as 98,000 American deaths annually are due to preventable adverse events as a result of medication errors. Because many patients take three or more medications in a 24-hour period, drug–drug interactions are common. Of medical malpractice judgments against NPs, 16.5% are a result of medication-related problems. Malpractice rates for NPs remain low, however, with only 1.9% of NPs named as primary defendants. One policy approach to the problem of medication errors is to implement mandatory reporting of all medical errors. Employing educational strategies when errors occur, rather than punitive ones, can also be effective. In addition, prescribers must take steps to prevent medication errors, including asking each patient what medications he or she is taking before ordering a new one to avoid potential interactions. In addition, the healthcare provider must educate the patient about potential adverse effects of the medications, the signs and symptom of these effects, and when to notify the provider if a problem arises.

Reimbursement

Payment standards in the United States are driven by insurance companies, particularly those that administer Medicare and Medicaid. APRNs have made great strides in this area and now receive third-party reimbursement in most settings. Payment by private insurance companies is contract specific and varies with each state's insurance commission. Reimbursement has long been a controversial issue. In some areas, NPs are reimbursed at 85% of the physician rate, yet still provide the same services as physicians. Does this mean NPs only do 85% of the work of a physician or that they do only 85% of the work as well as a physician would have? If one asks the recipient of care, the patient will most likely state that the APRN gave the same level of care provided by or expected from a physician. In managed care contracts, a fixed, predetermined rate is given to all providers, whether APRN or physician. Reimbursement issues are another legislative challenge and barrier to full-practice authority facing APRNs. When reimbursement and scope of practice barriers are removed, APRNs will be able to achieve full practice authority, which is likely to improve access to care for all Americans.

Malpractice

The risk of malpractice is an important concern for APRNs. Three conditions must be present to establish malpractice:

1. The provider must have a duty to the patient.
2. The standard of care must be deviated from or breached.
3. Harm or damages must occur as a result of the duty and a breach of the standards of care.

A plaintiff must prove duty, breach of the duty, damages or injuries, and causation. *Duty* means that a relationship has been established between the defendant and the plaintiff. *Breach of the duty* is the failure to do what a reasonable and prudent person would have done in the same or similar circumstances. *Damages or injuries* include medical expenses; pain and suffering, both physical and mental; lost wages and lost earning capacity; loss of companionship, society, affection, and/or sexual relations; hedonic damages; and punitive or exemplary damages. *Causation* means that the plaintiff must prove a direct causal connection between the act of negligence and the alleged injuries.

The following example can be used to illustrate what malpractice is and what it is not: Sally is a clinician caring for Mr. B., who is suffering from congestive heart failure. Sally increases his diuretic but makes no note of his potassium level and orders no replacement potassium. When Mr. B. returns a week later for routine lab testing, his potassium level is found to be low. Sally orders a potassium supplement to begin immediately and a follow-up potassium-level measurement. Is Sally guilty of malpractice? No. Although Sally did have a duty to Mr. B. and she did deviate from the standard of care (which would have been to order a potassium supplement at the beginning), no harm came to Mr. B. Because all the components were not met, malpractice was not established. If patients were aware of this, many false claims would not be filed. If Mr. B. had died from a fatal arrhythmia due to his low potassium level, however, then Sally could be held liable.

In the outpatient office setting, the most common reason for a malpractice suit for both physicians and APRNs is the failure to make the correct diagnosis. Approximately one-third of the malpractice cases brought against general practitioners are due to failure to diagnose in a timely manner. These cases usually involve cancer, particularly cancer of the breast. Regarding NPs in particular, the most common reason for malpractice suits is related to failure to correctly diagnose or delay in diagnosis, with cancer and infections the leading conditions that are cited in liability suits.

APRNs must carry liability insurance to protect themselves and their assets against malpractice. Each APRN should have a lawyer who will represent him or her rather than the APRN's employment institution. However, nurses are often told that they should not carry their own insurance, and there are typically two reasons for this. The first is that a policy will encourage a lawsuit. There is no evidence to support this, and lack of coverage does not discourage a lawsuit, should there be a legitimate claim. The other reason is that nurses are told that their employer carries liability insurance that will also protect them. Although it is true that employers may provide insurance coverage for their employees, that coverage is subject to the provisions of the insurance agreement, and the employer is the client, not the nurse. Many physicians are "going bare," which means "opting out" of or not carrying malpractice insurance. They must post a sign in their office to that effect. Some hospitals, however, require physicians to provide a letter of credit guaranteeing payment in the case of a judgment against them. Some states, such as Florida, require NPs to carry malpractice insurance. In other states, some NPs are considering "going bare" as well. Before choosing to opt out of malpractice insurance, it is important to consider that a malpractice suit can destroy a life, both professionally and financially. As NPs would not consider being without health insurance, likewise, opting out of malpractice insurance should be considered very carefully.

Several types of malpractice insurance policies are available. One type, called the claims-made policy, covers only situations in which the incident occurred and the claim was made while the policy was in effect. With a claims-made policy, it is wise for practitioners to have a "tail policy" that covers claims made after the policy is terminated. An occurrence policy provides the most protection because it covers liability arising from all acts or omissions during the period the policy is in effect, no matter when the claim is brought. This is the ideal policy because a claim can be made several years after an incident occurs.

Professional liability policies may be expensive, so the practitioner may want to negotiate payment of the policy as part of the employment contract. Malpractice claims against NPs are on the rise, although slowly. The reasons can be attributed to three factors: changes in insurance markets due to fewer carriers, poor litigation laws that have arisen from current tort law practices, and the fact that the expanding scope of practice has made NPs more autonomous and therefore more vulnerable.

Excellent communication remains the best way that providers can avoid a costly judgment or settlement against them. Developing effective communication skills can significantly benefit NP practice. One study examined whether NPs used patient-centered communication styles or provider-centered communication styles in their patient encounters. Surprisingly, only a minority of NPs used patient-centered communication styles. As the rise in malpractice claims seems to be related to poor communication, NPs must be cognizant of the positive effects of patient-centered communication styles (see Evidence-Based Nursing Practice 79.2).

Collaboration

Collaboration between care providers from various professions, particularly NPs and physicians, can result in better health care at lower costs (Hain & Fleck, 2014). Collaboration implies collegiality, respect, and shared values that promote patient-centered care. Mutual understanding of and respect for each other's roles in this interdependent relationship can result in a constructive commitment to work toward the best interests of patients. Both the APRN and physician must respect the boundaries of their disciplines and value what the other has to offer and bring to the relationship.

Actualizing the IOM Report: The Future of Nursing, 2014 includes four critical messages:

1. Nurses should practice to the full extent of their education and training.
2. Nurses should achieve higher levels of education and training through an improved education system that promotes seamless academic progression.
3. Nurses should be full partners, with physicians and other health-care professionals, in redesigning health care in the United States.

 Evidence-Based Nursing Practice 79.2

Berry JA. Nurse practitioner–patient communication styles in clinical practice. *J Nurse Pract.* 2009;5(7):508–514.

Nurse practitioners (NPs) spend more than two-thirds of patient-encounter clinical time in intrapersonal communication. The NP literature has little on NP/patient communication styles. The purpose of this study was to examine and document the most common verbal communication style used by NPs in patient interactions. Content analysis was used to analyze 53 NPs/patient transcripts for communication style. On the basis of the transcript analysis, only a minority of NPs used a patient-centered communication style.

4. Effective workforce planning and policy-making require improved data collection and a developed information infrastructure.

While the report recommends that nurses should be full partners, collaboration with all providers involved is essential for optimal care of patients. The *Circle of Caring* model emphasizes the essential nature of collaboration between APRNs and all other health-care professionals, especially the physicians with whom they work.

APRN collaboration with physicians is also essential because many health-care needs are outside the scope of NP practice. Problems arise when the NP–physician relationship is one of supervision rather than collaboration. Different state boards of nursing delineate the NP's role in different ways. Some states require physician supervision or sponsorship of APRNs for licensure, which limits the nurse's scope of practice. Other states require a collaborative relationship. A major challenge for the APRN, especially in an environment that requires physician supervision, is to assert his or her autonomy and maintain a professional, collegial, and collaborative relationship with physicians.

In 1997, when the Oxford Health Plan allowed members to choose NPs as their primary-care providers and paid them the same rate as physicians for the same care, APRNs were finally recognized as independent practitioners who could provide quality care. In a situation such as this, collaboration is key because APRNs are the first to recognize that they are not expert in all areas.

Before being hired, it may be difficult to foresee whether a practice will be truly collaborative or not. Tools are available to assist a new NP in learning the skills of contract negotiation. One such comprehensive tool to aid in negotiating an employment or contractual arrangement is published by the American Association of Nurse Practitioners titled "Employment Negotiations."

Interprofessional Education

The IOM stresses the need for interprofessional education. Many university and community program leaders are creating opportunities for interprofessional learning activities to take place among nurses, physicians, social workers, and others (see Evidence-Based Nursing Practice 79.3).

Health-Care Reform

The United States is the only industrialized nation in the world without a national health insurance plan in place. The debate over health-care reform has centered on the following questions:

• Is there a fundamental right to health care for all?
• Who should have access to health care and under what circumstances?

 Evidence-Based Nursing Practice 79.3

Machin AI, Jones D. Interprofessional service improvement learning and patient safety: A content analysis of preregistration students' assessments. *Nurse Educ Today.* 2014;34(2):218–224.

A culture of continuous service improvement underpins safe, efficient, and cost-effective health and social care. This paper reports a qualitative research study of assessment material from one cohort of final year preregistration health and social care students' interprofessional service improvement learning experience. Initially introduced to the theory of service improvement, students were linked with an interprofessional buddy group and subsequently planned and implemented, if possible, a small-scale service improvement project within a practice placement setting. Assessment was by oral project presentation and written reflection on learning. Summative assessment materials from 150 students were subjected to content analysis to identify the following: service user triggers for service improvement, ideas to address the identified area for improvement, and perceptions of service improvement learning. Triggers for service improvements included service user disempowerment, poor communication, gaps in service provision, poor transitions, lack of information, lack of role clarity and role duplication, and difference between professions. Ideas for improvement included both the implementation of evidence-based best practice protocols in a local context and innovative approaches to problem solving. Students described both intrapersonal and interprofessional learning as a result of engaging with service improvement theory and practice. Service improvement learning in an interprofessional context has positive learning outcomes for health- and social-care students. Students can identify improvement opportunities that may otherwise go undetected. Engaging positively in interprofessional service improvement learning as a student is an important rehearsal for life as a qualified practitioner. It can help students to develop an ability to challenge unsafe practice elegantly, thereby acting as advocates for the people in their care. Universities can play a key support role by working collaboratively with service organizations, role modeling for effective interprofessional working, and supporting research to measure the impact of education on practice.

• What quality is achieved for the high prices currently being spent?
• Who will be responsible for the cost of a national health insurance plan?
• What services should be provided and within what timeframe?

The Patient Protection and Affordable Care Act of 2010

The Affordable Care Act (ACA) was signed into law on March 23, 2010 to reform health care in the United States. The health-care law includes reforms to health insurance and the way the health-care industry was run in the United States. The ACA aimed to greatly increase the number of Americans who have access to affordable health insurance. The ACA made the following changes:

- Expand Medicaid to America's poorest citizens
- Provide tax credits to employers who covered their employees
- Provide tax credits to individuals who need help paying for insurance
- Reform the health-care industry to rein in excess spending
- Tax higher earners and the health-care industry
- Create state-based, competitive, regulated, online health insurance exchanges (Marketplace) where individuals could buy insurance and receive cost assistance.

The goal of the ACA was to make health insurance coverage more secure and reliable for Americans who have it, make coverage more affordable for families and small business owners, and bring down skyrocketing health-care costs that have put a strain on individuals, families, employers, and the federal budget. The ACA required that all Americans have access to affordable health care (or pay a tax if they choose to opt out). *Affordable health care* is defined as costing 8% or less of annual income. The ACA also aimed to reform Medicare and Medicaid, as well as the other aspects of the health-care system, including the rates that insurance companies and private health-care facilities receive and patients' rights to health care.

At the time the ACA was established, the Congressional Budget Office determined that the ACA would be fully paid for and would provide coverage to more than 94% of Americans while staying under the established $900 billion limit. The ACA was designed to reduce the health-care deficit over the next 10 years and beyond. The ACA contains nine titles, each addressing an essential component of reform:

1. Quality, affordable health care for all Americans
2. The role of public programs
3. Improving the quality and efficiency of health care
4. Prevention of chronic disease and improving public health
5. Health-care workforce
6. Transparency and program integrity
7. Improving access to innovative medical therapies
8. Community living assistance services and supports
9. Revenue provisions

Unfortunately, there have been some concerns with the ACA. The predicted cost savings have not been as significant as originally projected. Although 32 states accepted Medicaid expansion, 19 did not for a variety of reasons, including increased state costs. As a result, Medicaid coverage was decreased rather than expanded in states that did not accept this expansion. With more

persons seeking insurance under the ACA, costs to insurance companies increased, resulting in many companies choosing to leave the ACA Marketplace. Patients felt this financial strain as their premiums and deductibles increased. With the decline in insurance companies and reduced revenues, fewer health-care providers were available to meet patient needs. In states where their practice is restricted, NPs could not help meet these increasing health-care needs. Patients had to travel further distances to see their primary-care and specialty-care providers, often a hardship for persons with low incomes.

The leading cause of personal bankruptcy in the United States is medical debt. Since 2010, the rate of bankruptcy has steadily declined and the ACA, along with changing bankruptcy laws, is an important contributing factor. The decline in devastating personal medical expenses is due not only to increased coverage but also to important provisions in the ACA that mandates coverage for preexisting conditions and ends annual and lifetime coverage caps (St. John, 2017).

Many organizations, including the ANA, have examined the potential outcomes of the ACA. Oregon, as an example, is one state with a successful unified health-care program. They accomplished this by rank ordering the community values of persons in the state. Their number-one value is prevention, followed by quality of life. Because nurses are advocates for patients and persons, their role is to continue to be involved in the development of public policy that will effect change in all aspects of health care (see Evidence-Based Nursing Practice 79.4).

With each new political administration, health care is always a major concern. The need for affordable health care is evident in the United States and the shift from

---

 Evidence-Based Nursing Practice 79.4

Winland-Brown JE, Dobrin AL. Medical repatriation: Physicians' and nurses' responses to a dilemma. *Southern Online J Nurs Res.* 2009;9(4).

Medical repatriation is an institutional dilemma that affects physicians and nurses. This study analyzed the responses of physicians and nurses to a hypothetical case study involving a young illegal immigrant involved in a truck accident who was deported back to Honduras for lack of medical resources. The only variable that was significant when considering deportation was ethnicity. There was no significant difference between the responses of either physicians or nurses whether the patient should be medically repatriated. When asked about solutions, respondents suggested involving the Hospital Ethics Committee, searching for additional resources to allow this patient to remain in the United States to receive rehabilitation services, and providing ethics training for physicians and nurses to enable them to resolve ethical dilemmas using principled thinking and to (it was hoped) decrease moral distress.

illness management, fee-for-service care to prevention and wellness with reimbursement based on patient outcomes is taking place. With the focus of health care on increased coverage, illness prevention, and cost-saving measures, APRNs are in an ideal position to help address these needs. Expansion of APRN scope of practice, allowing full practice authority for NPs to meet the health-care needs of all persons in all states, has never been more important. As health care evolves, the concepts of the Medical Home and expansion in both the number and practice authority of APRNs are essential.

All health-care providers have an ethical duty to actively engage in legislative efforts that will ensure the best possible conditions to optimize the health of the nation. As advocates, providers need to know their state legislators and governors. The ANA strongly believes that APRNs are one of the keys to solving America's health-care crisis. Their current efforts address the important role that APRNs must play in a reformed health-care system.

 For additional resources please visit **https://davisedge.fadavis.com/**

REFERENCES

American Association of Nurse Practitioners. NP fact sheet. https://www.aanp.org/all-about-nps/np-fact-sheet. Published 2017. Accessed April 1, 2017.

American Association of Nurse Practitioners. Employment negotiations. https://www.aanp.org/practice/business-management/68-articles/579-np-tips-for-contracting. Accessed July 18, 2017.

American Nurses Association. Code of ethics for nurses with interpretive statements. Silver Spring, MD: American Nurses Association; 2015.

APRN Consensus Work Group & the National Council of State Boards of Nursing APRN Advisory Committee. Consensus model for APRN regulation: Licensure, accreditation, certification & education. http://www.aacn.nche.edu/education-resources/APRNReport.pdf. Published 2008.

Buck JA. The looming expansion and transformation of public substance abuse treatment under the Affordable Care Act. *Health Aff.* 2011;30(8):1402–1410.

Centers for Medicare and Medicaid Services. Affordable Care Act in action at CMS. CMS.gov. http://www.cms.gov/about-cms/aca/affordable-care-act-in-action-at-cms.html. Accessed 10/23/18.

Davis K, Abrams M, Stremikis K. How the Affordable Care Act will strengthen the nation's primary care foundation. *J Gen Intern Med.* 2011;26(10):1201–1203. https://www.ncbi.nlm.nih.gov/pmc/articles/PMC3181291/. Accessed 10/23/18.

Green LV, Savin S. Primary care physician shortages could be eliminated through use of teams, nonphysicians, and electronic communication. *Health Aff.* 2013;32(1):11–19.

Hahn JA, Sheingold BH, Ott KM. Demystifying state health insurance marketplaces. *Nurs Econ.* 2013;31(3):119–143. https://www.researchgate.net/publication/255695674_Demystifying_State_Health_Insurance_Marketplaces. Accessed 10/23/18.

Hain D, Fleck LM. Barriers to NP practice that impact healthcare redesign. *OJIN Online J Issues Nurs.* 2014;19(2):2.

Henry J Kaiser Family Foundation. Summary of the Affordable Care Act. http://www.kff.org/health-reform/fact-sheet/summary-of-the-affordable-care-act/. Published 2017. Accessed July 18, 2017.

Institute of Medicine. The future of nursing: Leading change, advancing health. http://www.iom.edu/Reports/2010/The-Future-of-Nursing-Leading-Change-Advancing-Health.aspx. Published 2010.

Johnson SR. Controlling costs. Some follow Oregon's lead on Medicaid reform. *Mod Healthc.* 2013;43(36):7,12.

Kohlberg, L. *Philosophy of moral development.* San Francisco, CA: Harper & Row; 1981.

Mayeroff M. *On caring.* New York, NY: Harper & Row; 1971.

National Council of State Boards of Nursing. Changes in healthcare professions' scope of practice: Legislative considerations. https://www.ncsbn.org/Scope_of_Practice_2012.pdf. Published 2012.

Robert Wood Johnson Foundation. Charting nursing's future. http://www.rwjf.org/content/dam/farm/reports/issue_briefs/2017/rwjf435543. Published 2017. Accessed July 18, 2017.

St. John A. How the Affordable Care Act drove down personal bankruptcy. Consumer Reports. http://www.consumerreports.org/personal-bankruptcy/how-the-aca-drove-down-personal-bankruptcy. Published 2017. Accessed June 23, 2017.

Wyckoff M, Solano J, Ellingson S. Actualizing the IOM report: The future of nursing, 2014: A professional nursing practice providing consistent care from delivery to discharge. http://canpweb.org/canp/assets/File/2014%20Conference%20Presentations/IOM%20Report%20UC%20Davis%201.pdf. Accessed April 1, 2017.

Zamosky L. Obamacare's most vexing questions. Medical Economics. http://medicaleconomics.modernmedicine.com/medical-economics/news/obamacares-most-vexing-questions-physicians. Published 2013.

RESOURCES

American Academy of Nurse Practitioners
http://www.aanp.org

American College of Nurse Practitioners
http://www.acnpweb.org

American Nurses Association
http://www.nursingworld.org

End of Life Nursing Education Consortium Project (ELNEC)
http://www.aacn.nche.edu/elnec

Healthy People 2020
http://www.healthypeople.gov/hp2020/objectives/topicareas.aspx

National Alliance of NPs.
https://www.yelp.com/biz/national-alliance-of-nurse-practitioners-washington

National League for Nursing
http://www.nln.org

National Organization of Nurse Practitioner Faculties
http://www.nonpf.com

NP Central
http://www.npcentral.net

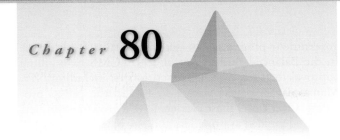

Chapter **80**

The Business of Advanced Practice Nursing

Marcella M. Rutherford, PhD, MSN, MBA, RN

INTRODUCTION

The Patient Protection and Affordable Care Act (ACA) was signed into law on March 23, 2010 to offer quality health care to more citizens. This legislation addressed controlling health-care spending by implementing a value-based payment system and improving health delivery outcomes. Those involved with drafting this legislation realized that the plan would need improvements. Transforming a fee-for-service payment model into a value-based care model was akin to turning around the Titanic before it hit a fast-approaching iceberg. But to manage continually rising health-care costs and declining quality, new approaches were worth trying.

Although there is a great deal of discussion about the state of the U.S. health-care system, one thing that everyone agrees on is the need for reform. Even with the ACA in place, many people are still not getting the health care they need—both in quantity and quality. In today's health-care market, prices for similar services vary by state, sometimes significantly (Dallas, 2015). Linking cost trends related to health-care delivery to the impact from improved care coordination (lowering costs and improving quality) are well documented.

Political opposition to this legislation has continued since the enactment of the ACA. On June 28, 2012, the Supreme Court found that the ACA Medicaid exchange was coercive to the states who were not prepared, ruling that the Department of Health and Human Services (HHS) had no enforcement authority over Medicaid expansion. States could opt not to accept Medicaid expansion funds, which reduced health-care services for Medicaid patient populations. However, this ruling left the expansion and other provisions of the ACA intact (Henry J. Kaiser Family Foundation, 2012a).

Polls confirmed that the monthly premiums for insurance coverage were increasing yearly, with citizens having difficulty paying copays, deductibles, and prescription drug costs (Henry J. Kaiser Family Foundation, 2012b). Policy experts attribute a significant portion of these rising health-care costs to overuse of medical technology and pharmaceuticals. Although growth rates in health-care spending have reached a 5-year record low, which could be the result of structural changes in the health-care delivery model, some analysts attributed much of the cost reduction to the 2008 recession (Roehrig, 2015). Less disposable income and low employment rates resulted in postponed health services. It is predicted, however, that health-care costs in 2015–2023 will rebound to prerecession levels with increases that will be higher than inflation (Leonard, 2014).

Although "repeal and replacement" of the ACA has been discussed for several years, it appears that, at least for now, the ACA remains in place. The main issues that stimulate the calls for replacement of the ACA are the high deductibles associated with the exchange plan offerings and the limited insurance plan options offered by some state exchange markets. In addition, the young and healthy have not signed up for the ACA in the numbers that were hoped for; this population is needed to mitigate the risk pool.

Advanced practice registered nurses (APRNs) are ideally positioned and have a unique opportunity to be part of the restructuring of the U.S. health-care system. In a system that is evaluating cost and quality, APRNs are integral to achieving these goals. The cost of care provided by an APRN is approximately one-half of that of an internal medicine physician and a quarter of that of a specialty physician (Porter & Lee, 2013). APRNs educational model focuses on a comprehensive care model that collaborates with all provider team members and places the patient and their family first when initiating a plan of care.

To be effective leaders in health care, APRNs also need to be knowledgeable in the business aspects that impact the health-care system. APRNs need the ability to document and communicate to other members of the health-care team, to the payers, and to consumers why their unique role offers a value to the community. Health care is moving away from fee-for-service and toward a reimbursement model that is based on performance, value, and risk. In this change-driven environment, providers will need a value agenda that focuses on maximizing the health of their patients.

Nurse practitioners (NPs) work in both rural and urban areas and are trained to provide care in various settings. This includes acute care facilities, community health centers, public health departments, hospitals and hospital clinics, school/college student health clinics, employee health settings, physician offices, independent medical offices, insurance organizations, rehabilitation and skilled nursing facilities, hospices, home health agencies, the armed forces, Veterans Administration facilities, and schools of nursing. Health-care change has shifted health-care services away from the acute patient care delivery model toward an outpatient setting whenever possible. Its focus is also shifting—from one that emphasizes care for the sick to a wellness care system. This shift fits well with the holistic, social-justice focus that is at the heart of all four APRN roles—nurse anesthetists, clinical nurse specialist, nurse midwife, and NP. This chapter will primarily focus on the NP role.

Today's growing older patient population has chronic health needs and is seeking health-care access in a system that has a limited number of care providers. The ACA has increased the role NPs play in accountable care organizations and patient-centered medical homes, with the position of team leader determined by the health-care provider best suited to lead. With the growing shortage of primary-care physicians, the rising number of insured individuals, and decreasing numbers of the uninsured (11.9% of population in the first quarter of 2015 were uninsured), there will be a need for more practitioners of all types. Practitioners are needed particularly in primary care, pediatrics, and obstetrics but resources have not yet been fully deployed or financially allocated. Primary-care providers who are equipped to treat an older, sicker population, who often have financial concerns, multiple chronic conditions, behavioral health issues, and substance abuse problems will be especially needed (Levy, 2015; Porter, 2015).

This chapter offers an overview of the current U.S. health-care environment, a review of third-party payer roles, the basics of the ACA, essentials of business practices, current reimbursement rules, tips for measuring and communicating value, and information for managing a health-care practice. In addition, NP business skills, NP professional choices, and the need for strategic and business planning are covered. Each section provides key elements that affect the ability of a practitioner to thrive and achieve professional goals.

THIRD-PARTY PAYER RULES

Whether NPs are employed by a hospital, a medical practice, a community health center (such as Federally Qualified Health Centers [FQHCs]) or are self-employed, a third-party payer most often determines reimbursement policies. Third-party payers fall into seven general categories:

1. Medicare
2. Medicaid
3. Indemnity insurance companies
4. Managed care organizations (MCOs)
5. Workers' compensation (WC)
6. Veterans Administration
7. Auto liability

In addition to these third-party payers, there are a limited number of patients without health insurance who pay out of pocket and who are considered private payers.

Each payer source has its own policies and fee schedules. All use guidelines provided by the CMS, the federal agency that runs the Medicare program. In addition, CMS works with the states to run the Medicaid program. CMS works to make sure that the beneficiaries in these government programs can get high-quality health care. In the Balanced Budget Act of 1997, CMS gave billing approval for nonphysician practitioners, including NPs. Managed care payers were slow to add the NP as providers. Over time, these carriers have a growing numbers NPs credentialed as providers and pay based on the CMS billing rules (85% of the fee schedule rate) or instruct NPs to bill under the physician's provider number.

Medicare

Health-care providers wishing to bill Medicare can join the program by submitting an application online at the Provider Enrollment Chain and Ownership System (PECOS) or by a using the traditional paper form (CMS-855I). Each Medicare provider is assigned a National Provider Identifier (NPI) for billing that must be used in Health Insurance Portability and Accountability Act (HIPAA) transactions. As a Medicare provider, the NP agrees to perform services for payment according to the current Medicare physician fee and guidelines. The NP's scope of practice, prescriptive authority, and requirement of physician collaboration are designated by state legislation. Each state gives authority for the nurse licensing board to regulate APRNs.

CMS payment policy is based on the annual *physician and nonphysician provider fee schedule* (Medicare Physician Fee Schedule [PFS]) (CMS, 2017a). For physicians, CMS identifies which services will be reimbursed (100% of the physician PFS) and then stipulates that 80% of the allowed rate will be paid by CMS and 20% is the responsibility of the patient. NPs are reimbursed by CMS at 85% of the physician's fee, with the patient still paying a 20% share (NP fees are typically 15% lower than that of physicians; Frakes, 2006). Most patients on the traditional Medicare plan acquire a secondary insurance plan to cover the 20% patient out-of-pocket expense. In addition to the 20% patient responsibility, Medicare has a yearly deductible. In 2017, the Medicare Part A (hospital services) deductible was $1,316. Out-of-pocket hospital fees are charged as follows:

- Hospital stays of 1 to 60 days: no additional payment in each benefit period
- Days 61–90: $329 per day coinsurance
- Days 91 days and beyond: $658 coinsurance per "lifetime reserved day" used—after 90 days for each benefit period the beneficiary can use up to 60 days over their lifetime.
- Beyond lifetime reserve days: all costs

The Medicare B (physician/provider and outpatient services) deductible is $183 per year. Once paid, the patient is charged 20% of the approved Medicare rate for physician office visits and some diagnostic tests. Information about Medicare beneficiary out-of-pocket expenses can be found at the official U.S. Government Site for Medicare, (CMS, 2017b).

Patient responsibility payments (copays and deductibles) should be collected before rendering services. This is especially important at the beginning of the calendar year when most Medicare beneficiaries have not yet met their deductible. Patient out-of-pocket payment responsibility should be verified at each medical treatment episode. If these fees are not collected before the services are rendered, they remain the patient's payment responsibility and will require direct patient billing. Patient billing increases the expense to the practice because of the cost and time involved in collecting funds. CMS providers are required to attempt to collect the co-payments and deductible patient payments and best practice recommends providers do so prior to rendering services.

Medicare Access and CHIP Reauthorization Act

The Medicare Access and CHIP Reauthorization Act (MACRA) final rule was released on October 15, 2016. This historic legislation repealed the Sustainable Growth Rate formula, creating a Quality Payment Program, and established a way for providers to be rewarded for quality outcomes by instituting a pay-for-performance system and combining existing CMS quality reporting into one program (American Medical Association [AMA], 2017). MACRA has resulted in several changes for Medicare providers and ultimately for beneficiaries (Haycock, Edwards, & Stanley, 2016). It offers two payment and reporting models for the provider to select from the following:

1. The Merit-Based Incentive System (MIPS) has three quality reporting categories: (1) a physician quality reporting system, (2) a value-based payment modifier, and (3) meaningful use. In addition, MIPS has four performance categories that are weighted by percentage of reporting in year 1: quality (50%), resource utilization and cost (10%), advancing care information (25%), and clinical practice improvement (15%).
2. The Advanced Alternate Payment Model (APM) includes specific requirements for participation. Participants must demonstrate an earning potential of 5% of the Medicare part B incentive payment. It also requires risk bearing (at risk for paying the lower of either losing 8% of its own revenues when Medicare expenditures are higher than expected or at risk of repaying CMS up to 3% of total Medicare expenditures) for monetary loss, use of an electronic medical record system for 50% of providers in the first year and 75% the second year, and a stated base payment on quality measures, similar to MIPS (AMA, 2016).

MACRA will affect all providers, including NPs who bill services to Medicare, starting with the first performance year CY 2017. All providers must choose either the APM or MIPS track, and those that do not will be automatically placed in MIPS. Providers seeking to use the APM track are realigning their practices into accountable care organizations (ACOs), clinically integrated networks (CINs), or integrated delivery networks (IDNs). Due to the risk of managing loss, all APMs must be able to analyze clinical claims data on population health, care pathways, or care models that focus on episodes of care and chronic condition management.

The focus of MACRA is value, including quality and resource utilization (cost). Providers under MIPS will face a potential 4% reduction in part B payments starting in year 1 (2019), increasing to a 9% reduction in subsequent years. MIPS providers may receive, however, payment increases of 4% in year 1 based on demonstration of high-quality care outcomes at a lower cost. APM providers are required to manage risk but may benefit from a team-based care approach. The decision is often not an easy one and both will require some system investment and an ability to capture quality data. Collection of performance measures in 2017 will drive reimbursement in 2019. Providers need to prepare for this change.

Medicare Advantage Plans

Medicare Advantage plans are Medicare MCOs. These plans must be approved by CMS as an alternative carrier for Medicare beneficiaries. They offer all of the benefits of Medicare and usually offer additional benefits and lower co-payments. Medicare Advantage carriers are paid subsidies per member by CMS for services rendered by their plan. These carriers offer traditional CMS services in addition to other health services at a lower cost. They are able to lower costs mainly due to economic efficiencies realized by their volume of commercial business relationships. However, problems have been noted with these plans. Because of the high medical utilization of and greater health-care costs incurred by their beneficiaries, many Medicare Advantage plans have found this market to be less financially viable. If a plan's pay-out exceeds the fixed CMS payment, the plan incurs a loss, causing many of these carriers to leave this market.

"Opting Out" of Medicare and "Going Bare"

As of 1998, all providers may choose to be a "nonparticipating" provider or to "opt out" of the Medicare program. To initiate this option, an affidavit must be filed with the CMS program. The opt-out period lasts for two years with no early-out clause. The physician practitioner and beneficiary must sign a contract explaining that neither the physician or patient can bill CMS for the balance of funds warranted to plan providers. As of 2015, these affidavits can be renewed automatically, and a 90-day notice must be submitted to change the opt-out status.

Nonparticipating practitioners can set his or her charge rate at 115% of the Medicare rate but can collect only 95% of the Medicare fee (CMS, 2017c). The Medicare program will pay 75% of the PFS, and the patient must pay the remaining 20% of the allowed (fee) amount, resulting in a 95% payment of the standard CMS fee to the opting-out provider. These physicians, however, are not subject to the billing restrictions set by CMS. In addition, these providers reduce their malpractice liability threshold. The physician can elect to be in the Medicare program only one time per year and must provide notice to patients and other referring physicians if he or she elects to become nonparticipating.

"Opting out" of the Medicare program limits the ability of participating physicians to use referral services. No participating Medicare physicians can refer patients to physicians who have opted out of the Medicare program. The "opting-out" physician must keep malpractice coverage or maintain a minimum of $250,000 available to cover any malpractice claims that may arise from health services. An NP working for an "opting-out" physician will not be able to bill as a Medicare participating physician for NP services. NPs that are employed by or leased by an "opting-out" physician are at a higher risk for being named in a malpractice case (CMS, 2017c).

Malpractice requirements and coverage can vary by state. In some high-risk states and practice specialties, physicians are choosing to practice without the security of malpractice insurance due to the rising costs of their malpractice premium coverage. State requirements generally require the physician to maintain a minimum escrow account (e.g., $250,000) to cover claims, post bond, obtain an irrevocable letter of credit, and notify all patients (prominently posted) that they do not carry insurance for malpractice. In addition, more recently insurance carriers have added policy options to allow physicians to settle the claim outside of court (Arthur G. Gallagher & Co.). It is prudent to review the status of any employer as to malpractice insurance of self-insurance practices and investigate what this means to your individual practice and actions that occur within and outside of the practice walls.

Medicaid

Medicaid offers medical assistance to individuals and families with low incomes and limited resources. Unlike Medicare, it was designed to be jointly funded by both federal and state governments. The federal government assists states in providing medical care to people who meet the program's financial eligibility criteria. Medicaid payments are made directly to the participating providers, who in turn must accept the Medicaid (lower) payment as payment-in-full. Two exceptions are (1) disproportionate-share hospital payments (hospitals that care for a disproportionate share of Medicaid-eligible patients) and (2) hospice care. Although lawmakers have discussed changing the Medicaid system, with an overarching focus of putting more control in the hands of the each state, currently no changes have been implemented.

Under Medicaid, states may impose nominal coinsurance and deductible rates. Emergency and family planning services must be exempt from the co-payment responsibility. Currently, the federal contribution matches the individual states' contribution as mandated by law. Reimbursement rates must remain sufficient to enlist enough providers willing to perform services and ensure that medical care is available to the general population in the region.

Guidelines for the Medicaid plan are available at the Medicaid Web site by state. Benefits for Medicaid were expanded and enhanced by ACA and are also outlined on the Medicaid website and updated at intervals (Affordable Care Act, 2015 (b); CMS 2013a). There are limitations and criteria for APRN reimbursable services outlined in each state's guidelines that can be located by selecting each state on the Web site.

Other Insurance Plans—Auto Liability; Workers' Compensation; ChampVA

Auto liability, workers' compensation, and CHAMPVA are additional health plans that guarantee that these population of patients, health-related services are covered under these specific carriers when indicated (e.g., auto accident injury, injury sustained while on the job, services provided to a veteran, etc.). ChampVA and the Tricare or Champus health services are often misunderstood. These plans have different provisions, billing criteria, and reporting criteria. For auto liability, it is important to identify when the auto insurance or medical insurance should be billed as the primary insurer. For example, when a Medicare patient receives care that should be paid by his or her auto liability plan, payment will be denied for medical services billed to Medicare. WC claims require notification to the person's employer, use of WC-contracted providers for care, and specific documentation for coverage that must be submitted to the plan. Traditionally, these plans limit the use of NPs for care delivery, but this should not deter a practitioner from seeking provider status.

Cash/Private Pay

Even with the ACA's progress in offering health insurance options, approximately 13% of Americans (30 million people) remain uninsured (Jester & Casselman, 2015). Many of these individuals are poor and live in underserved or rural areas. They may delay seeking health care, often entering the health-care system in acute need of care and requiring higher-cost treatment. The U.S. invests more than twice the resources in health care as other industrialized nations, yet it still ranks 37th based on health-care outcomes (infant mortality, maternal mortality, life expectancy, etc.) compared with other nations (Murray, Phil, & Frenk, 2010). The nation's poor return on investment for health care should spur economists and policy makers to look for alternative strategies to offer easier access, quality care, and lowest costs.

Affordable Care Act

In 2010, the ACA was signed into law and guaranteed certain health-care provisions including coverage for pre-existing conditions, removal of the lifetime cap on coverage, and continued coverage for children up to 26 years of age under their parent's plans. Also included in the ACA are less well-known provisions, which include the following:

- New federal insurance market rules that establish essential standard benefit packages included in all plans
- Limits on how much insurance companies can charge for administration and profits (with rebates to consumers if they charge too much) and state review of rates proposed by insurance companies (Altman, 2013).
- New health insurance exchanges that lower administrative costs, pool risk, and offer individuals and small businesses a choice of affordable plans
- A shared responsibility for health care by preserving employer-sponsored insurance and offering tax credits to small businesses
- Improvement of Medicare prescription drug benefits by slowly eliminating the "donut-hole" gap by 2020
- A long-term financing program to support the disabled
- Investment in a stronger primary-care foundation by increasing CMS payments for primary care, encouraging patient-centered medical homes, investing in primary-care training, and expanding community health centers
- An innovation center within CMS using payment methods to reward for quality versus volume of services; this innovation also encourages payment based on patient outcomes and provides incentives for productivity
- Creation of an Independent Payment Advisory Board that makes recommendations to reduce cost growth and improve quality
- Investment in infrastructure that offers publicly reported information on the quality, costs, and performance of providers; use of information technology in medical care and health insurance carriers; and policies on disease prevention, public health, quality, safety, and the health-care workforce (CMS, 2015a; Goldsteen & Goldsteen, 2013)

ACA provisions are detailed at the federal Web site managed by the U.S. Department of Health and Human Services.

At the core of the ACA are provisions to enhance the outcomes and value of the U.S. health-care system. ACA legislation is changing the way clinicians are organized and how health-care services are delivered; it is also focusing providers on reducing cost while improving quality of care outcomes. Since the ACA became law, more than 70% of the uninsured gained access to health care.

Physician and public support for this legislation remains mixed, with about 50% of the public questioning the benefits of the system. ACA, however, did generate discussion about the need for a comprehensive health-care system and a surge in demand for access and the need for providers to deliver health care.

The Nurse Practitioner's Role in the ACA

Finding a practitioner, particularly in rural and underserved areas, is challenging. The limited number of primary-care providers has caused many states to re-examine the scope of practice laws for NPs. NPs are educated to provide primary-care services in addition to geriatric, acute care, obstetrics, and psychology care, but the AMA has supported laws that limit the NP's scope-of-practice, citing concerns for patient safety (Iglehart, 2013). Currently, NPs provide essential primary care and disease management; enhance coordination of care and increasing patient care access; and offer high-quality oversight of health care at lower costs. Not only is the PFS payment for NPs 15% lower than the medical physician's payment, but (as of 2011) the family practitioner's yearly income was approximately $100,000 higher than the average family NP's annual salary (Medical Group Management Association, 2012).

Nurse practitioners represent the largest group of APRNs and function under various degrees of physician supervision, depending on the licensing state. Research demonstrates that NPs' primary-care outcomes are equal to or better than physicians' and that NPs rate equally or higher on patient satisfaction ratings compared with physicians (National Governors Association, 2012; Newhouse et al., 2012). The various House and Senate committees involved in implementing the ACA have included NPs as primary providers and acknowledge the shortage of primary-care physicians. In many rural communities and for hospice patients, NPs offer the only access to health care and are critical for reducing health-care costs and meeting the needs of the underserved citizens. In addition, the Institute of Medicine (IOM) has recommended that nurses be allowed to function to the full scope of their practice. Congress is set to address this issue, but patient demand is prompting each state to examine this issue as well. Only a few states have fully adopted the APRN Consensus Model, a uniform model supported by the American Nurses Credentialing Center to align licensure, accreditation, and certification in practice. This model must be adopted by all state boards of nursing for implementation. Fewer than 20 states allow NPs to practice independently of a physician based on their training (National Governors Association, 2012).

Insuring the Uninsured

The ACA was designed to allow the greatest number of U.S. citizens younger than age 65 years with employer insurance plans to continue to receive insurance coverage as part of their employer benefit package. Employers of more than 50 full-time (working 30 hours or more per week) employees are required to offer standard MCO plans. For small businesses (fewer than 50 employees), employees who work less than 30 hours weekly, and people who are not on employer plans, individual plans are available for purchase through state exchanges. The exchange allows citizens to select a plan that meets their financial and health needs. Tax incentives and penalties are used to encourage enrollment. Medicaid eligibility has also been expanded through the Medicaid plan.

The ACA's goal was to eventually enroll all uninsured U.S. citizens currently without health-care coverage. In 2017, ACA continues to reduce the number of uninsured. ACA legislation eliminates the high-deductible, low co-insurance, limited hospital coverage plans of the past and reduces pharmaceutical costs for all. This legislation has changed the health-care landscape because it requires all MCOs to offer preventive services with no additional cost to beneficiaries. All health plans must now offer the designated minimal benefits, and the beneficiaries can select from a variety of approved plans. Metrics are now provided online, allowing individuals to select the highest quality and lowest cost plans. It is hoped that competition for lower-cost and higher-quality providers and plans will shape health-care reform.

Technologies and Infrastructure

ACA efforts include supporting the use of telemedicine and other strategies that will offer a competitive advantage for providers. Hospitals and providers are joining ACOs and developing communication networks that expand their abilities to create efficient teams to treat the full range of patients' health needs. These efficient and effective ACOs support bundled payments and gain higher reimbursements, stimulating carrier and patient demand. Providers who are early adopters will seek out the most talented colleagues to join their ACOs. As a team, providers can focus on offering high-quality, low-cost health care, and the group will financially benefit from this effort. Data reporting and transparency of outcomes will drive health service choices, and those providers who consistently produce desired outcomes at competitive costs will be rewarded.

The use of technology also offers providers a competitive advantage. Electronic medical records (EMRs) and electronic health records (EHR) are now required and enhance business practices and reporting. EMR utilization facilitates improved care communication and care coordination between providers, aligning care offered to patients across the inpatient and outpatient spectrum.

BUSINESS ESSENTIALS

Without adequate funding, providers will need to reduce the services and resources that they can offer to their patients. NPs should understand the importance of maintaining adequate cash flow, obtaining payment for services, overseeing outstanding accounts receivables, implementing a collection policy, controlling overhead costs, utilizing the financial statements, and planning for success by creating and using a realistic operating budget.

Maintaining Cash Flow

Maintaining optimum cash flow is a fundamental goal in all businesses. Without adequate liquid capital, a business cannot grow or survive. Today, most health-related services are paid according to a fee schedule determined by a carrier contract. Providers are required to follow the carrier's billing guidelines. Continuous flow of funds from successful billing is needed to pay for expenses. In 2019, MACRA will change these rules.

In today's health-care industry, payment disbursement interruptions challenge providers; carrier and patient payments are not guaranteed solely because the service was delivered. Services can be medically indicated and result in healthy outcomes, but without supportive documentation matching medical coding, payment may be denied. The number of claims that result in slow payment (greater than 30–45 days) can range between 30% and 50%, and this delay negatively affects provider cash flow.

The profit margin in health care today is very slim. Medicare payments are designed to cover provider costs, and Medicaid payments range 15% to 20% lower than Medicare payments. Net profits for most providers are achieved from their MCO contracts and beneficiaries.

As with any major change in business, the ACA created a concern for providers. Physicians struggle to understand how health-care reform's bundled payment (payment to all providers involved in the complete episode of care) will affect individual provider cash flow. Bundled payment is designed to reimburse for the services of independent provider units, covering "the full care cycle for acute medical conditions, the overall care for chronic conditions for a defined period of time (usually a year), or primary and preventative care for a defined patient population (healthy children for instance)" (Porter & Lee, 2013, p. 60). Unlike fee-for-service or global capitation, this method aligns payment to care outcomes delivered by the team.

Health-care reform is aimed at bending the cost curve downward; therefore, further cost cutting is predicted and causes concern. Efficiency and quality outcomes will be rewarded in higher reimbursements. Payment models need to include severity adjustments, regional demographic differences, and unavoidable patient complications based on frailty, as well as provisions for unforeseeable high-cost medical events.

Obtaining Payment for Services

All third-party payments are based on the PFS, referred to as the carriers' "allowed amount" or plan fee schedule. As health-care costs continued to rise, all health-care plans looked for ways to keep insurance payment fees from increasing. Insurance plans have implemented higher patient out-of-pocket responsibilities by increasing the deductible and co-payment amounts. Patient out-of-pocket expenses became a larger portion, reducing the percent of the medical bill paid by insurance. ACA eliminated the pre-legislative high-deductible, high co-payment plans and stipulated a ceiling of profit that MCOs can realize from unspent premiums. In 2013, overpayments were refunded annually back to their beneficiaries. Without the healthy, young population in the risk pool electing for ACA plans, however, costs have risen, increasing deductibles and co-pays. The patient's out-of-pocket responsibility is deducted from the insurance plan's contracted service rate and is reflected on both the insurance plan's statement and the provider's billing; both are provided to the patient beneficiary. For the provider, collecting the patient responsibility for services is a significant portion of accounts receivable.

Provider profit margins have also decreased over the last 10 years. A provider's billing process starts when the patient's demographics are first collected (preadmission or at the time of admission) and continues until the bill is collected. Patients' benefit packages change yearly, and the change in the level of patient responsibility needs to be adjusted and verified. Because employers change carriers frequently, it is essential that the provider require proof of insurance eligibility at each patient visit. Collecting from the patient their portion of the service fee is a burden for the provider. If payments are not collected in a timely manner, cash resources to cover payables will become a problem. Slow collection of cash/payment also results in less money to support practice enhancements and resources needed for services. Billing oversight in claims processing can affect cash flow and include the following:

- "Unclean" claims, i.e., claims with missing patient demographics, medical coding, and required data elements
- Slow processing of billing records or posting of carrier payment
- Delay or failure to address bill denials and carriers' requests for additional documentation
- Failure to identify underpayments from plan carrier
- Changes in software data fields and software interfaces implemented by providers and/or carriers
- Failure to collect patients' responsibility before services

Overseeing Outstanding Accounts Receivable

Accounts receivable (AR) represents the money billed for services rendered to patients that remain unpaid. It is critical that a company's AR is monitored by its financial managers, ensuring that outstanding bills are collected or that changes in payment resulting from new billing requirements and regulations are identified in a timely manner. The longer money goes uncollected, the less likely it will be collected. When money goes uncollected beyond 120 days, it is very difficult to obtain payment. Uncollected expected payments (10% of the expected amount is often never collected in well managed practices) should be kept at the lowest percentage possible.

Accounts more than 30 days old should be reviewed to identify why the payment has not been received. Current and compatible claims software for claim tracking is required, but it is important to select software that enhances provider processes. Hiring knowledgeable coders and offering continuous education to medical billers will be supported by a lower AR.

Loss of experienced billing employees is a common reason for unanticipated cash-flow delays. Providers need to have a basic understanding of claims-management processes to be able to assist and troubleshoot cash-flow issues and to oversee the training of new billing managers.

Collection Policy

All patients require education about their payment responsibilities when accessing health-care services. Many patients do not understand their insurance policy benefits and payment responsibility. Patients often feel that they already pay substantial money for monthly health premiums and that this should entitle full coverage for needed health services. Co-payments and deductibles are perceived as excessive. Explanations of benefits that come after rendered service can cause the patient to become distrustful. In addition, many patients in today's economy are unable to pay the co-payment or deductible portion. Dedicating employee time to verify and explain eligibility and carrier benefits before treatment is worth the expense. Ensuring patient understanding of payment before services protects the patient–provider relationship.

Controlling Overhead Costs

Increasing practice efficiencies and controlling day-to-day costs enhance a practice's profitability. Implementing cost reduction measures, however, requires careful economic analysis of the impact on the quality of care and on the medical outcomes for patients. If the outcome choices are considered equal, the least costly service should be chosen. Health-care outcomes, however, are often difficult to measure, and, until recently, little emphasis was placed on measuring the cost-effectiveness of care outcomes. Economic analysis should evaluate both the cost benefits and cost-effectiveness of services.

Cost analysis involves understanding the resources and costs needed to provide a service. Direct costs—labor time, supplies, and minor equipment—are easy to identify and should always be evaluated before adding a new service. Indirect costs—administrative costs, cleaning, electricity, human resources costs, and the like—may be harder to allocate to each service but should be included in the analysis for a valid assessment. In addition, some costs are fixed whereas others are variable—fluctuating with the volume of activity. The office rent or mortgage payment, for example, is a fixed cost; supply expenses (printer paper, record documents, etc.) are variable. To make a profit, payment dollars must cover both direct and indirect expenses related to the services while covering associated variable costs and contributing to fixed expenses.

To maximize financial gain, practitioners and office managers tend to feel that cost shortfalls can be made up with increasing the volume of patients treated. The normal established-patient visit is commonly scheduled as a 15-minute block of time. New patients, however, require more time to gather the patient's history. Established-patient visits are more predictable. Managing patient visit scheduling offers efficiencies to the office and strategies that mingle established-patient visits with new-patient visits prevent patient bottlenecks. An appropriate mix of new and established patients is important to ensure a profitable office day.

A nurse practitioner's fee, according to Medicare, is set at 85% of the PFS. Physician overhead costs commonly hover around 50% of net revenue (Weiss, 2003). An NP's *value* can be linked to the resulting revenue (billed charges) and net revenue (collected payment less expenses associated with the services) generated by the NP. Table 80.1 and Box 80.1 provide examples of how to calculate the break-even analysis. Table 80.1 demonstrates a volume of patients across one year and Box 80.1 demonstrates the NP's financial impact/contribution to practice revenue. Hospital visits, procedures, and other services also need to be added to a complete estimate if warranted. Factors such as the number of new patients, the number of MCO patients (contracted fee rate ranges from 70%–120% of Medicare fees), the length of the visit, the number of private-pay patients, and other factors can affect the profitability of a provider's services. NPs should evaluate their individual patient care practice habits and the impact of these on the overall financial health of the practice.

Utilizing Financial Statements

Financial statements offer a business the ability to monitor the impact of monthly transactions taking place in the practice. The performance of a business can be reviewed using the following accounting reports:

- *Balance Sheet*—Quantifies the net worth of the business at a set time (monthly, quarterly, or yearly).
- *Operating or Income Statement*—Compares revenue to expenses in a period of time.
- *Cash-Flow Statement*—Details the movement of cash in and out of the business.
- *Net Income Statement*—Demonstrates whether assets grew as a result of the year's business activities.

An NP should review these documents to monitor the health of the company. These financial statements

TABLE 80.1   Profit/Loss Estimation for Patient Visits for Practice

CPT Code	Vol (# Pts)	% of visits	Fee	85%	Over-head (50% of fee)	Accounts Receive	Collections
99201	69	5%	$43.89	$37.31	$21.95	$1,514.21	$1,362.78
99202	345	25%	$74.51	$63.33	$37.26	$12,852.98	$11,567.68
99203	703.8	51%	$108.91	$92.57	$54.46	$38,325.43	$34,492.89
99204	220.8	16%	$164.67	$139.97	$82.34	$18,179.57	$16,361.61
99205	41.4	3%	$203.80	$173.23	$101.90	$4,218.66	$3,796.79
Total	1,380					$75,090.84	$67,581.75
99211	0	0%	$20.41	$17.35	$10.21	$—	$—
99212	745.2	18%	$43.89	$37.31	$21.95	$16,353.41	$14,718.07
99213	2484	60%	$72.81	$61.89	$36.41	$90,430.02	$81,387.02
99214	828	20%	$106.83	$90.81	$53.42	$44,227.62	$39,804.86
99215	82.8	2%	$142.90	$121.47	$71.45	$5,916.06	$5,324.45
Total	4,140					$156,927.11	$141,234.40
Net Revenue/ Year						$208,816.16	

Box 80.1 NP Valuation in the Practice Setting		
NP Cost		
Salary	$95,000	
Benefits	0.27	
Incidental	$1,5000.00	
Total	$122,150.00	$(122,150.00)
Practice value (net revenue)		$86,666.16 [208,816.16–122,150]
Assumptions		
Patient visits/day	30	
Productive hours	1,950	
Productive week/year	46	
Overhead estimate	50%	
Days/week	4	
Collection %	90%	

provide an overview of the company assets, as well as the corresponding liability or debt.

Planning for Success: Using the Operating Budget

Success in business does not just happen; it is a result of research, planning, financial knowledge, and hard work. The rate of rise in health-care costs can be controlled by "developing cost-effective technologies, delivering care in the most cost-effective settings, and using the most cost-effective practice available" (Emanuel, 2008). The APRN role fits well into this prescription for tomorrow's health-care system.

All businesses need direction and boundaries within which sound financial decisions can be made. Budgeting has several very important purposes for those managing a business. Budgets help planning, improve communication, facilitate coordination, improve motivation, help control expenses, and contribute to assessing performance. Budget preparation should involve all members of the business. Gathering all of the anticipated practice needs (expenses) for an upcoming year from all stakeholders will minimize variances to the budget. A successful practitioner sets goals and plans resource needs. The budget projects an estimate of the upcoming year's anticipated revenue and expenses based on obtaining the best information available from all care providers.

REIMBURSEMENT RULES

The provider plays an important role in ensuring the success of the business by clearly identifying the diagnosis and service codes that are appropriate for each patient's

visit. As a strong business partner, each practitioner who possesses reimbursement knowledge can optimize the billing payment. Specific documentation of key components of care can make a significant difference in the allowed reimbursement.

Current Procedural Terminology Coding

Current procedural terminology (CPT) offers the official procedural coding rules and guidelines required when reporting medical services and procedures performed by physicians and nonphysician practitioners (AMA, 2016). This reference text should be purchased yearly and should be readily available to each practicing provider. CPT coding lists and guides are also available electronically and can assist in the coding process with algorithms that assist those coding.

In 1977, the Health Care Financing Administration (HCFA) was developed within the HHS to control the spiraling costs of health care related to the Medicare program. Originally in 1965, Medicare was the responsibility of the Social Security Administration (SSA). Federal assistance to the Medicaid program was administered by the Social and Rehabilitation Service (SRS). The Department of Health, Education, and Welfare oversaw the SSA and SRS. HCFA was created to coordinate Medicare and Medicaid. HCFA was challenged with controlling costs, monitoring services, and updating code references used to uniformly document current care. These codes allowed assignment of descriptors to services as well as assigning reimbursement rates for each service code. HCFA (later to be overseen by CMS) selected CPT codes developed by the Editorial Board of the American Medical Association. Medicare used these codes at an increasing rate in the 1980s. By the early 1990s, commercial insurance carriers (MCOs) were using these codes in their contracts and billing records as well. The Resource-Based Relative-Value Scale (RBRVS) was authorized by Congress to be used to set reimbursement rates (Hsiao, 1987). The RBRVS scale is discussed later in the chapter.

CPT Coding Rules

Beginning in the 1990s, physicians were paid for office or surgical procedures based on calculated resource costs, which were designed to reflect the costs needed to provide services. These costs were calculated based on three components:

1. The physician's work or medical expertise, which accounts for approximately 54% of relative value unit (RVU)
2. The practice overhead expenses, which account for approximately 41% of the RVU
3. Professional liability and malpractice expenses, which are derived from a formula

The RVU is multiplied by a conversion factor, which is a monetary value determined yearly by HCFA/CMS and is adjusted for the cost of living and market-based rates in the geographical region. RVUs are assigned by CMS based on recommendations from the Relative-Value Update Committee of the AMA. Each specialty society in the AMA presents detail work and practice expenses to CMS when new CPT codes or fee rates are requested to be changed. These details are published in the Federal Register before finalization, allowing provider and user comments.

According to the AMA, the purpose of CPT is to provide a uniform language that describes medical, surgical, and diagnostic services, providing an effective means for reliable nationwide data collection and communications among all stakeholders. In 2000, the CPT Code Set was designated by the HHS as the national coding standard for physician and other health-care professional services and procedures under the HIPAA. Having a common nomenclature allows uniformity in management reporting, medical review, education, outcome measurement, and medical research. CPT is the accepted nomenclature utilized by all health-care facilities, providers, and vendors. Each service or procedure is represented by a five-digit code. CPT® code inclusion or exclusion does not indicate an endorsement by AMA of the procedure, nor does it guarantee payment.

As of 2005, all CMS billing is required to be sent electronically, unless certain exceptions were granted. The CPT code set was mandated for all billing records. To improve cash flow and minimize claim denials based on untimely submission, most providers benefit from electronic billing to insurance carriers.

The CPT manual and PFS offer three levels of CPT codes:

1. Category I—codes used in contemporary medical practice
2. Category II—tracking codes used for new or performance measurement
3. Category III—temporary coding used for new procedures, technology, and services

Yearly code updates are made available in October and implemented in January. Codes without an associated payment fee are commonly related to patient education and nursing services. Transition periods are often extended with reimbursement change.

The CPT manual Category I codes are presented in six sections:

1. Evaluation and Management (E&M)
2. Anesthesiology
3. Surgery
4. Radiology
5. Pathology
6. Medicine

CPT Unlisted Codes

Practitioners should select the code that provides the most specific and accurate match to the services performed. If no code exists that accurately identifies the provided services, an "unlisted" service code is provided in each of the six sections of CPT. Unlisted codes are discussed later in this chapter.

CPT Modifiers and Add-On Codes

Specific guidelines for CPT coding are presented at the beginning of each section in coding manual and should be reviewed before selecting a code. "Add-on codes" should accompany a primary procedure code. Examples of add-on codes for CPTs include "prolonged service" codes that indicate additional time spent with the patient. These codes should not be used alone and must be used with the appropriate primary or level of E&M code. A *modifier* provides a means to report that a service or procedure has been altered by the circumstances of its use. It is important that modifiers are appropriately used to obtain additional reimbursement. Modifiers are the only means for the practitioner to adjust standard payment rules. Box 80.2 provides an example of the use of a CPT modifier.

The CPT and payment fee values are applicable only to CMS services and are regulated and paid by the regional CMS carriers. MCOs can independently determine whether to use certain CPT code rules and/or the reimbursement values for the payment year.

New CPT Requests

It is important that practitioners participate in and provide CPT information directly or submit feedback through professional organizations. The CPT manual

---

Box 80.2   Case Example of Modifier Justifying Higher Payment for Level of Service

Significant, Separately Identifiable E&M Service on the Same Day as a Procedure or Other Service: Modifier 25

A previously treated patient is referred to a gynecological specialist's office following abnormal Pap test results. The patient's pathology is reviewed, and a vaginal exam is performed. From the examination, it is determined that a colposcopy procedure is warranted. The colposcopy procedure is performed on the same day as the evaluation and management (E&M) examination by the same physician. The practitioner will bill a 99213 for an established-patient visit of expanded focused complexity and add a −25 modifier to the CPT code in the billing record. The colposcopy is also billed on the same day of service and is ordered as a result of the E&M findings. Without the −25 modifier on the CPT code, the E&M visit would not be paid.

provides instructions on requesting updates to the CPT nomenclature. The effectiveness and accuracy of CPT relies on its ability to reflect actual practice; therefore, practitioners should communicate changes in practice and request coding changes that match provided services. As profit margins shrink, accurate coding becomes essential to maximizing the viability of the business. When requesting a new code, the practitioner should provide supportive information from research articles and medical journals, specific cost information related to the uniqueness of the code, and a specific recommendation concerning the new or existing codes. Suggestions should be submitted to the CPT Editorial Research and Development of the American Medical Association. Code changes can also be submitted online at the AMA/CPT Web site, and practitioners are encouraged to add, delete, or revise the CPT codes to ensure coding reflects changes in patient care practice.

"Incident To"

"Incident to a physician's professional service" is a billing phrase related to services furnished under the direct supervision of a physician. This does not mean that the physician needs to be in the room, but he or she must be in the same suite or office. The services are related to the course of treatment resulting from an initial visit with the physician and administered by a nonphysician. The nonphysician (often a registered nurse [RN] or NP) must be an employee of, leased by, or performing as an independent contractor of the physician. In this situation, services may be billed under the physician's provider number and reimbursement is made at 100% of the physician fee.

CMS provider rules offer guidance under "incident to" billing. NPs may bill and be reimbursed using their own NPI when a physician is not on site or in the office. These services, in comparison, are reimbursed at 85% of the PFS.

CPT Level II Codes

Each year, CMS releases its Healthcare Common Procedure Coding System (HCPCS) code set in the HCPCS Annual Update. HCPCS codes are established by CMS's Alpha-Numeric Editorial Panel and represent primarily items and supplies; physician services are not covered by CPT Level I coding. Drug administration, pharmaceuticals, and durable medical equipment supplies are located in this file. As stated in the previous section, new CPT codes are often assigned an HCPCS II code and are tracked for a year before a permanent CPT level code is identified. Demonstration codes used for data collection are also assigned an alphanumeric code. Payment may or may not be associated with these codes, but they are important for data tracking.

ICD-10-CM

The International Classification of Diseases (ICD) was developed to offer international comparability in the collection, classification, and review of health data, particularly mortality data. In October 2015, ICD-9-CM underwent an upgrade to ICD-10-CM. Changes in the upgraded version include the following:

- Larger and more specific listing of codes (three volumes vs. two volumes)
- Alpha-numeric format versus numeric only code categories
- Reorganization of certain conditions
- Minor changes related to mortality related events

The changes in diagnosis coding as a result of the ICD-10-CM implementation have required significant upgrades and education in EHR documentation for all practitioners.

Medicare Physician and Nonphysican Practitioner Fee Schedule

Each year CMS publishes the *Physician and Non-Physician Practitioner Fee Schedule* (CMS, 2017c). A Medicare Physician Fee Schedule (MPFS) search tool is available through the CMS website as well.

Electronic billing and automated electronic filing sets make timely transition to new PFS rates possible. This schedule provides a payment rate based on a state local base rate multiplied by the RBRVS (explained earlier in this chapter). The PFS is the payment rate for all Medicare services provided for that year. When procedures occur that have no CPT, the new code will be paid as a percentage of charge (managed care plans) or at a rate closest to a similar CPT code. Unlisted codes, provided in every CPT section, should be used as a last resort as payment for these nonspecific codes are delayed, requiring the provider to send medical documentation to detail the services provided. Manual billing, with the supporting documentation to substantiate services, delays payment beyond 45 to 60 days.

MCO plans negotiate contracts with providers based on payment at a percentage of charge or at a percentage of the Medicare fee. Carriers may pay some specialists higher than Medicare does but also can offer fees lower than Medicare rates. In many states, primary-care physicians and internists receive payments that are lower than Medicare's rates. General practitioners' and internists' practice volume, or payer mix, is composed of a high percentage of MCO-insured patients. To maintain their patient volume, internists are financially pressured to sign contracts at rates lower than the MPFS or risk losing a large number of clients. This atmosphere creates an environment where providers compete for healthy clients covered by better-paying carriers.

Accountable Care Organizations

Collusion—secretly and collectively sharing rates for the purpose of monopolizing or maintaining a higher payment rate—is prohibited by physician specialties. In addition, MCOs market their plans to employers and clients by demonstrating their large network availability. Periodic trends have surfaced with providers joining various ownership arrangements to facilitate fee negotiations. MCOs also may join to produce a larger number of providers with a substantial patient base. These large practice groups are often successful in negotiating higher commercial fee schedules. After ACA became law, this large provider group business model has been rejuvenated in the form of ACOs.

ACOs are groups of providers—providers, hospitals, outpatient-care facilities—that come together to coordinate the care of patients, seeking to offer a high quality of care at a lower cost. The concept was developed by CMS, and additional information can be found on their Web site (CMS, 2015b).

ACOs are an important part of ACA success, supporting CMS's goals to provide care for the chronically ill, eliminate duplication of services, and coordinate care. ACO members work together as a team, and all benefit from the efficiencies and quality of care they can collectively achieve. These low-cost, high-quality provider groups will receive higher bundled reimbursements shared by the ACO. ACO participation is optional for any provider. In a geographic area where provider networks are not robust, the MCO provider fee schedule may be adjusted to a higher payment rate to attract specialists in the region.

Evaluation and Management Documentation

EHR encounter tools are software programs that prompt clinicians to provide proper documentation that supports billing. In addition to billing support, coding also provides invaluable data, identifies patient trends, and allows providers to track future community needs. CPT E&M codes require providers to document the extent and complexity of the patient's history, physical exam, and medical decision-making. E&M codes relate to the recorded facts, findings, and provider observations and offer a consistent recorded care history.

The level of E&M coding, with 23 broad categories, such as office visits, hospital visits, observations, consultations, and case management, is based on the care setting. There are currently seven components that are used to define the levels of E&M services. The levels of E&M services are unique in its use and encompass a wide variety of skill, time, analysis, preventable care, and treatment. E&M components are as follows:

1. History
2. Examination
3. Medical decision-making
4. Counselling
5. Coordination of care
6. Time

The level of care needed in these various settings is provided in the documentation for these E&M codes. Documentation is often requested by the carrier to justify the level of care provided and billed. All practitioners should develop documentation forms and software records that contain the key elements of information for medical record documentation. Table 80.2 offers a chart audit tool that can be used to review the correct assignment of code levels.

Since 2013, CMS has expanded CPT codes and simplified CMS rules to include collaborative care management services. Additionally, CMS recognizes the increased work involved in the care of patients with behavioral health (mental health and substance use) care. In 2017, CMS issued a final rule that included a new code and fee to cover psychiatric services provided in a collaborative care model. The intent was to facilitate care payment so that behavioral health integration for psychiatric collaborative care would become part of care delivery when needed (Ross, 2017). Additional changes implemented in 2017 include coding used for conscious sedation provided in conjunction with a procedure; the code for moderate conscious sedation was removed. In 2017, CMS will also begin collecting data on the postoperative period for high-volume/high-cost procedures, new Medicare-G codes that can be used with telehealth services for dialysis and advanced care/critical care patients, revised methods to better calculate the differences in practice costs in certain regions, and new codes in primary care for interprofessional collaboration on resources needed to provide behavioral health services (Becker's Hospital CFO Report, 2017).

Electronic Medical Records

The American Recovery and Reinvestment Act legislation was designed to create a means to electronically capture and store patient medical records and make "meaningful use" of these data. This legislation mandated adoption of EMRs by 2014. Funding and incentives were made available for providers for several years before the 2014 deadline. EMRs are now required for all health-care providers; those who are not within compliance are subject to penalties (Athenahealth, 2012). MACRA legislation further impacts all providers reporting in 2017, requiring each to declare their track, APM or MIPS, which will centralize the quality outcome reporting outcome measures for each provider and direct reimbursements based on value in 2019.

The importance of all providers using EMRs is based on the principles of securing patient information and reducing administrative health-care costs. Standardizing EMRs and billing data will also improve provider cash

TABLE 80.2　E&M Chart Audit Tool—Reference Used to Justify CPT Coding

CPT	Focus	Elements		
New	**Visits**	**History**	**Exam**	**Medical Decision**
99201	New Patient, Level 1	HPI 1–3 Elements ROS: N/A PFSH: N/A	Single-system: 1–5 Multisystem: 1–5	Straightforward 10 minutes
99202	New Patient, Level 2	HPI: 1–3 Elements ROS: 1 PFSH: N/A	Single-system: 6+ Multisystem: 6+	Straightforward 20 minutes
99203	New Patient, Level 3	HPI: 4+ Elements ROS: 2–9 PFSH: 1	Single-system: 12 Multisystem: 12/2+ organ or 2 from 6 systems	Low complexity 30 minutes
99204	New Patient, Level 4	HPI: 4+ Elements ROS: 10 PFSH:—3	Single-system: all +1 from each system Multisystem: 2+ organs from 9 systems	Moderate complexity 45 minutes
99205	New Patient, Level 5	HPI: 4+ Elements ROS: 10 PFSH: 3	Single-system: all +1 from each system Multisystem: 2 from 9 systems	High complexity 60 minutes
Established Visits				
99211	Established Patient, Level 1	Minimal/RN visit	Minimal exam	None—may not require a provider 5 minutes
99212	Established Patient, Level 2	HPI: 1–3 Elements ROS: N/A PFSH: N/A	Single system: 1–5 Multisystem: 1–5	Straightforward 10 minutes
99213	Established Patient, Level 3	HPI: 1–3 Elements ROS: 1 PFSH: N/A	Single system: 6+ Multisystem: 6+	Low complexity 15 minutes
99214	Established Patient, Level 4	HPI: 4+ Elements ROS: 2–9 PFSH: 1	Single system: 12	Moderate complexity 25 minutes
99215	Established Patient, Level 5	HPI: 4+ Elements ROS: 10 PFSH: 3	Multisystem: 12/2+ organ or 2 from 9 systems Single system: all +1 from each system Multisystem: 2 elements from 9 systems	High complexity 40 minutes

New patients need all three criteria: History, Exam, and Medical Decision, whereas established patients require two out of three criteria (History, Exam, and Medical Decision). Counseling/coordination of care with other qualified professionals or agencies are provided consistent with nature of problem and patient and/or family needs.
Abbreviation: HPI, history of present illness; ROS, review of systems.

flow, allowing carriers to process claims more efficiently and reduce health-care costs.

Use of EMRs offers the following additional benefits:

1. Provides a longitudinal account of patient care
2. Allows tracking of care from the acute-care setting to nursing home, retirement home, or clients' private residences
3. Focuses on measurement of care quality across all settings rather than on episodes of care
4. Facilitates patient identification that allows providers to track the patient throughout the care delivery system and across the continuum of providers, offering information in a need-to-know environment
5. Provides practitioner alerts and reminders, communicates up-to-date resources, and links evidence-based bodies of knowledge used for clinical decision support
6. Presents real-time cost-effective options and enhances timely reimbursement through interconnectivity to

payers offering patient eligibility and authorization requirements

7. Matches patients to medications
8. Facilitates electronic transmission of payment to providers

VALUE MEASUREMENT

Practitioners should review common policies implemented to control and support practice decision making that fall under fraud and abuse/compliance plans, HIPAA, risk management, and performance improvement. In addition, all providers will benefit from data collection that allows them to demonstrate the value and quality of their performance. A plethora of data and quality indicators are now being generated from health-care delivery practices. Strategies related to information management, in which nurses are crucial participants, include integration of the EHR into all care settings; developing rapid online access to patient records, including information from other clinicians in alternate settings; participating in the creation of a repository of health information and nurse quality indicators; interacting with and utilizing online information services, including telemedicine; and use of various technology for health planning and scheduling.

Fraud and Abuse/Compliance Plans

As health care has evolved and become more sophisticated, the area of health-care ethics has grown. Ethical conflicts arise when providers balance competing pressures affected by professional values, changes in delivery systems, and financial regulations. An example is the investigations that the U.S. Department of Justice has pursued when dealing with Medicare fraud allegations. U.S. health-care fraud is persistent and costly and has caused the federal government to levy high fines and determine the need for whistleblower protection.

The health-care industry has not always been honest about its billing practices, and in response, Medicare requires audits of a certain percentage of charts or medical records to monitor practice coding and billing. As of 1996, to willfully and knowingly utilize deceptive billing is a legal violation. The False Claims Act was updated in 2006. Reckless disregard for the rules is auditable and subject to corrective audits and fines. Fines and damages can be levied up to three times the claim amount, with mandatory penalties of $5,000 to $10,000 per claim (CMS, 2009). Medicare Recovery Audit Contractors (RACs) and Medicaid as well as Medicaid Integrity Contractors (MICs) in addition to payment error rate measurement are means used to recover payment errors. Table 80.2 shows typical audit forms used to ensure correct CPT coding selection based on medical record documentation.

Compliance Plan

All health-care businesses should develop a compliance plan. A compliance officer identifies and assists in developing and maintaining a plan that includes practice safeguards to prevent episodes of fraud and abuse. Antikickback efforts, conflict of interest disclosure, and identification of questionable business practices are fostered. Adhering to a compliance plan is the responsibility of all employees to ensure that business practices discourage fraud and abuse.

Health Insurance Portability and Accountability Act

HIPAA can mean different policy concerns to different people. The act is separated into two parts, Title I and Title II:

- Title I of HIPAA protects health insurance coverage for workers and their families when they change or lose their jobs.
- Title II addresses administrative simplification and requires the U.S. Department of Health and Human Services to establish national standards for electronic health-care transactions and national identifiers for providers, health plans, and employers. It also addresses the security and privacy of health data. These standards were implemented to improve the efficiency and effectiveness of the nation's health-care system by encouraging the widespread use of electronic data interchange in health care (CMS, 2005).

HIPAA legislation is important to the daily management of the practitioner practice setting. This legislation focuses on password management, workstation security, e-mail and Internet use, and facility/physical security. Password protection ensures the privacy of patients' health-care information. With increased mandatory submission of electronic billing files and EMRs, a provider must take added precautions to protect the patient's electronic personal information.

Risk Management

Risk management is an extension of performance improvement. This program should be organization-wide, with a focus on identifying risks, controlling occurrences, preventing damage, and controlling legal liability. The goal of risk management is to prevent undesirable events and to minimize the impact of financial loss due to a malpractice claim. There are eight areas of responsibility for risk-management programs:

1. Risk identification
2. Loss prevention and reduction, including incident reports and investigations
3. Insurance claims management
4. Administration of workers' compensation and handling of medical/legal issues

5. Liability assessment of contracts
6. Risk management education
7. Handling product recall and Safe Medical Device Act issues
8. Ensuring compliance with accreditation standards and state and federal laws

Practitioners can be involved in any of these areas of risk management. With the rising number and cost of malpractice claims, risk management becomes a powerful tool to ensure appropriate health-care practices.

Health-Plan Employer Data and Information Set Reporting

Providers should be aware of performance reporting that is required by CMS. The Health-Plan Employer Data and Information Set (HEDIS) is a set of standardized performance measures identified as indicators for consumers so that they can evaluate the quality and cost aspects of health-care delivery. Indicators are selected based on current health issues such as cancer, diabetes, asthma, and heart disease. Examples include immunization age, screening mammography frequency, urinary tract infection occurrence, and cervical cancer screening frequency. HEDIS is supported and overseen by the National Committee of Quality Assurance.

Safety and Performance Improvement

Performance improvement initiatives should be part of the day-to-day routine of the medical practice. In some medical offices, the NP is the only professional nursing care giver and should therefore take the lead to encourage office personnel to undertake processes that focus on ongoing improvement. Data analysis of quality monitoring requires the ability to derive trends from statistical data. Once a negative trend is identified, a corrective action plan to address the trend is imperative, demonstrating and monitoring a successful turnaround and improvement.

Both medical and financial errors are common, occurring at a rate greater than acceptable to the public and medical community. According to the Institute of Medicine's (2000) study, *To Err Is Human: Building a Safer Health System,* a high number of medical errors were identified in the U.S. medical environment, but it took almost 7 years for comprehensive safety and quality outcome changes to be effected throughout the health-care system. Seventeen years later, health-care leaders are being challenged and reimbursement is being withheld for poor outcome performance. The task of reviewing existing medical practices processes using a systems approach is daunting; however, the benefits are worthwhile.

Other issues that affect the quality of a health-care practice involve patients' perceptions of their health-care experiences, including feeling depersonalized, shortened,

or rushed care delivery time, unwarranted denial of coverage, health-care choice restrictions, and overprescribing of unwarranted testing. Many health plans' policy regulations and benefit restrictions have been linked to an increase in malpractice liability claims. Maintaining and fostering a trusted relationship between the provider and the patient has a significant impact on patient participation in care, satisfaction with outcome, timely payment of bill responsibility, and limiting exposure to litigation.

APRNs play a valuable role in overseeing health-care outcome improvement efforts. Clinicians are highly valued for their ability to recognize familiar patterns and to use their gut instincts in times of complexity, identifying options for interventions (Kerfoot, 2004). A practitioner provides clinical problem solutions based on diagnostic testing, provides an economic impact of the care delivered in this clinical episode, and contributes to the practice's outcome metrics.

Value-Based Health Care

The Deficit Reduction Act of 2005, the programs Hospital-Acquired Conditions (HACs) Present on Admission Indicators Reporting and Hospital-Acquired Conditions Not Present on Admission instituted in 2007, and the 2012 Readmissions Reduction Program are aimed at lowering health-care costs and safeguarding the Medicare Trust Fund. There are 14 categories of HACs, with no new conditions added since 2014 (CMS, 2016).

Section 3025 of the Affordable Care Act added Section 1886(q) to the Social Security Act establishing the Hospital Readmissions Reduction Program, which requires CMS to reduce payments to Inpatient Prospective Payment System (IPPS) hospitals with excess readmissions, effective for discharges beginning on October 1, 2012 (CMS, 2013b). Currently, the policy does the following:

1. Defines *readmissions* as admissions within 30 days to the same or other hospital
2. Includes readmission diagnoses of acute myocardial infarction, heart failure, and pneumonia
3. Establishes a method to calculate the excessive readmission ratio for each condition and compares it to the ratio of the national hospital data set; this ratio is used to determine the adjustment to the reimbursement rate
4. Establishes a risk adjustment methodology for each diagnosis using National Quality Forum data, comparing each facility's readmission ratio to that of other similar facilities in the United States and adjusting the ratio for clinically relevant factors (demographics, patient frailty, etc.)

The final rule also included policies related to certain measures for FY 2017 through FY 2019, including performance periods and performance standards for those program years, as well as a new domain structure for FY 2017 based on the National Quality Strategy and its priorities of better patient outcomes, quality, safety, and lower cost for Medicare payments.

Provider Comparison Web sites

Many states have created Web sites for citizens to query data regarding many of these identified health outcomes, allowing citizens to compare individual providers and hospitals using common quality indicators. Transparency is desired by the consumer and creates a trusting provider relationship and providers and payers are being evaluated based on malpractice claims and health outcomes. Financial reward, therefore, is granted to medical providers with high-quality results. ACA's legislation includes initiatives to educate the public on both the costs and the quality of their health-care needs and choices, as well as embed a responsibility for making an informed consumer choices. Internet-available sources provide both quality and cost rankings and are designed to create competition and sway demand. Savvy providers may be able to showcase these sites as an opportunity to strengthen the trust of the community they serve.

MANAGING A HEALTH-CARE BUSINESS

NPs' strengths have always resided primarily in their clinical expertise and their holistic approach to patient care; as a patient advocate, an NP encourages patient independence, offers needed health-care diagnostic and treatment services, and teaches self-care. Today's practitioner is also challenged to assist patients as they navigate the Internet, coordinate care between networks of providers, and explain information retrieved from a variety of sources. More patients are using Internet resources for guidance when medical symptoms arise. NPs need to support patients who do not have access to a computer. The increased number of community members with insurance benefits creates a growing number of patients, as well as health-care access deficits. Health care is predicted to change more in the next decade than it has in the past 50 years, and many providers will struggle with the rules that reward health-care provider collaboration and information sharing. NPs will be seeking those practices that are poised to embrace the changes and to demonstrate their ability to offer high quality at a lower cost.

NP Business Choices

Selecting a business arrangement that offers a financially successful practice environment that embraces the NP role for its unique value to the practice is essential. To ensure success, communication and negotiation with practice providers will be essential. The business aspects and health of the organization as well as the clinical care role of the NP should be clearly communicated. Negotiations should include a frank discussion of salary, benefits,

hospital privileges, and on-call expectations. In addition, the NP should understand the inherent malpractice risks with the selected specialty and what arrangements are in place to mitigate these risks.

Negotiating Salaries and Benefits

Before signing an agreement with a practice site, the NP should draft a practice agreement as required by the state in which he or she wishes to practice. Each state board of nursing designates whether a collaborative agreement is needed and details the criteria that defines the level of collaboration required by an oversight physician. Prescriptive authority differs by state and should be discussed. Federal law defines the term *collaboration* to mean the following:

> A process in which a nurse practitioner works with a physician to deliver health-care services within the scope of the practitioner's professional expertise, with medical direction and appropriate supervision as provided for in jointly developed guidelines or other mechanisms as defined by the law of the State in which the services are performed. 42 U.S.C.S. § 1395x(aa)(6) [Buppert, 2018, p. 168].

The Balanced Budget Act of 1997 approved reimbursement to APRNs for Medicare patients, but it did not alter the language in the law. Some states do not require collaboration, whereas others do, and when the term *collaboration* is used, the definition above applies. Regulations vary by state, and collaboration requirements (no collaboration, collaborative relationship, or collaboration with a submitted written protocol) should be verified annually. With the advent of the ACA, states are being pressured to allow nurses to practice at their full scope of knowledge.

The practice specialty, colleague(s) personality, practice environment, patient population, and the current culture of the practice setting should be reviewed. Frank discussion of the degree of autonomy and role of the NP in the practice and the role of the other practitioners is essential. Topics to cover during a formal interview include the following:

- Are there any current or pending malpractice claims against the business?
- What is the practice's Medicare and Medicaid status?
- Will I have hospital privileges?
- What number and type of managed care contracts does the practice have? How do these carriers contract and reimburse NP services?
- What is the number of nurses (registered nurses [RNs] and licensed practical nurses [LPNs]/licensed vocational nurses [LVNs]) and support staff available to assist the NP?
- What expectations are there for a NP's net revenue generation?
- What is the expected number of patient visits per day?
- How will I be compensated for services?

There are four basic methods by which an NP can negotiate salary compensation:

1. Straight salary
2. Salary based on percentage of revenue payments
3. Salary plus a percentage (bonus) based on payments
4. Hourly rate

There are advantages and disadvantages with each method. The easiest payment method to calculate is a *straight salary*. The practitioner is paid a set amount weekly, biweekly, or monthly. If patent volume increases dramatically, affecting on-call time, rounds, discharge summaries, dictation, and so forth, there is no additional compensation.

A salary based on a *percentage of payments* is calculated from the percentage of payments collected during the prior month. Salaries calculated this way are based on an inconsistent salary dollar amount that fluctuates with care. The inconsistencies are due to the many factors that affect net payment, and the payments collected are often not within the practitioner's control. For example, the type of EHR system, number of billing staff, content of managed care contracts, and changes in referral sources can create dramatic changes in the cash flow. This payment method has the largest possibility for error and fluctuation.

The *salary plus percentage (bonus)* method allows the practitioner to profit from a higher volume of patients and longer work hours needed to provide services for patients seeking care. This method, however, must be set at a predetermined rate that is achievable. The practitioner should be paid a set amount weekly, biweekly, or monthly; when the payments generated by the practitioner reach a predetermined milestone, additional bonus payments are provided. The NP should make sure the base salary is adequate to meet the NP's financial commitments.

The last method of payment—*hourly payment*—is a well-understood payment method, and it is similar to how hospital employees and nurses have historically been paid. In this method, the practitioner provides time records with the hours worked for payroll payment. This method allows for fluctuations in patient flow and changes in time related to the needs of the job responsibilities. It also requires the nurse to essentially punch a time card or report hours worked, reducing the level of autonomy the practitioner has in the business.

Employment Benefits

When interviewing for a position, the practitioner should make a list of benefits that are necessary and then desired. The benefits that fall into the must-have category usually include health, dental, short-term disability, malpractice, life insurance, paid vacation time, a retirement plan or 401K plan, and paid sick time. On-call pay may be seen as a benefit if it allows NPs to enhance their salary base. Desirable benefits may include long-term disability

insurance, education allowance, car/parking allowance, investment options, and professional meetings reimbursement. Each practitioner should survey other NPs in their market to verify the standard benefits packages noted in the area. The NP should fully research all aspects of the practice and communicate needs and wants in writing. Negotiating requested salary and benefits can be supported by the revenue an NP can estimate generating for the practice.

Obtaining Hospital Privileges

All hospitals have credentialing approval processes that require the practitioner to submit and validate his or her educational preparation, licensing, certifications, and clinical competencies. Credentialing usually falls under the allied health validation process established by The Joint Commission and the medical staff hospital bylaws. Practitioners can obtain a copy of the hospital's rules and regulations and familiarize themselves with these regulations, ensuring all guidelines of the facility are achievable.

Practice Insurance

Insurance policies are critical for every business, allowing each business to meet the state's requirements for incorporation. The practitioner should be aware of the insurances needed for all businesses. Proof of insurance may be required to obtain the tax identification number (TIN or EIN), and these must be obtained to apply for a city, state, and county business license. Table 80.3 provides an overview of optional and mandatory insurance plans selected to protect businesses.

Practice liability insurance provides risk protection for an employer and practitioner against unforeseen events. As an owner, practitioner, or administrative employee of

TABLE 80.3 Corporation Insurance Plans

Type of Plan	Coverage
Workers' compensation	Medical expenses resulting from on-the-job injury, illness, and death
Unemployment insurance	State and federal coverage; provides payment for loss of employment
Liability insurance	Covers structure, furniture, equipment in the event of a disaster
Business interruption	Covers loss of payments/income in the event of a disaster
Employee fidelity bonds	Verifies employee honesty and deters theft
Life insurance	Many types and should be investigated; covers practitioners
Disability insurance	Risk of disability greater than death and creates financial hardship
Malpractice insurance	Protects practitioner in the event of lawsuit

the business, liability value of the practice (capital equipment and resources in the business) should be reviewed annually. As the practice grows and changes, these policies must remain current and reflect the worth of the current equipment and property owned by the practice. For example, significant growth in computers and software in the practice should be added to the practice liability policy, because these resources significantly increase the value of the practice.

A business expense that requires additional consideration includes WC insurance. WC insurance coverage has become very expensive over the past decade. With one or two employee claims in the fiscal year, WC coverage and available premiums may become limited and costly. High-risk businesses may be forced, based on the number of WC claims from employees, to seek plans through the Joint Underwriting Association at a high premium. WC premiums may be high enough to affect the financial health of a business. All practitioners should be aware of the practice policies and make sure employee screenings (protective measures against practice risk) are included in policy (e.g., drug screening, background verification, and employment screening). Yearly employee development education is essential and should include workplace safety processes. Employee actions that deviate from these processes should receive documented counseling to protect the practice from avoidable claims.

Malpractice insurance has become a much-discussed medical practice expense. Malpractice premiums have doubled and tripled for physicians and NPs over the past few years. The number of medical malpractice lawsuits is increasing, and practitioners are at risk. Practitioners work in a world that encourages patients to seek litigation when care outcomes are not as expected or to their liking. Certain physician specialties are more highly litigated, and these specialties have the alternative to "go bare." This option was discussed earlier in the chapter.

If the provider desires to carry insurance protection, he or she should purchase the highest amount of coverage affordable. The ideal coverage is an occurrence policy for $1 million per claim and $3 million in aggregate coverage. Because failure to have proper coverage can be catastrophic, or at least very expensive, it makes good sense to understand the product being purchased and the exposures that are not covered. Several states require that practitioners carry malpractice insurance or post a bond. When investigating choices in malpractice insurance plans, the practitioner should review and compare several different carriers for limits of coverage, whether the policy covers the business and employees, extent of coverage for legal costs, how long the insurance company has been in existence, and the differences between claims-made policies and occurrence policies. The rates can vary greatly. The stability of each carrier should be examined. It is important to calculate the price of tail coverage when shopping policies and understand the definition of disability for automatic tail provisions. *Tail coverage* is an insurance policy that insures the health-care providers for malpractice claims reported after a claims-made policy lapses. The status of the malpractice crisis for practitioners will affect how practitioners practice in the future.

Business and Strategic Plan

To compete in the business of health care, planning is essential. Developing both a strategic plan (with growth targets) and a business plan (showing the current progress on meeting targets) offers a practice a means of monitoring the success of a practice. Creating a business plan that fits the practice will guide, maintain, develop, and manage the company resources. This information should be used to meet strategic goals of retaining and attracting future patients.

A strategic and business plan helps the practice organize around a roadmap to success. This plan should span several years. The business plan will support the needs for funding and will allow lenders to assess the risk involved in investing. It is important that the practitioner review the practice's financial statements. Strategies for business success are detailed in the strategic plan that offers benchmarks and data sources that will allow collect and chronicle progress. Table 80.4 provides items to include in the business plan.

Marketing Plan

The ACA will affect the demand for NPs. Nurse practitioners tend to share their successes and inroads with those within the profession using nursing journals, conferences, and word-of-mouth communication between colleagues. Consumers, the media, and the public need to be included in the NP's ongoing marketing message.

NPs should identify marketing strategies and then measure the impact of these efforts. Some effective marketing strategies include the following:

- Practitioners can explore opportunities that inform patients and the public about the role and value of the NP. Print materials distributed to patients can offer clarification and explain differences in roles, as well as highlight educational and practice experiences.
- Media outreach to local news and broadcasting media that specialize in health can help publicize a practice. For example, practitioners can share data regarding care delivery outcomes, new offices, and public health issues via press releases. Practitioners can make themselves available to news media for commentary and interviews.
- All practitioners should be able to articulate the cost-savings their role uniquely brings to health care. With the health-care industry's increasing need to reduce the costs of health delivery, NPs have an opportunity to establish their role as leaders in the health-care team. Box 80.3 lists common policies and procedures that guide business managers and employees.

TABLE 80.4   Business Plan

Inclusions	Description
Company objectives	Summary of company key benchmarks
Executive summary	Company leadership and objectives
History of the company	Idea that started the company
Company goals	Short- and long-term goals, as well as identifying the customer • Strengths • Opportunities for growth
Management team	Background and responsibilities of the managers
Vision/mission statement	Unique aspects of your service
Capital and operating expenses	Costs of doing business
Value indicators	Quality measures
Marketing strategy	Convincing lenders and contributors of potential for the business • Analysis of competitors • Demand • Access • Advertisement and promotion
Research and practice evidence	Processes for submission, collection, and reporting
Financial projections	Balance sheet, income statements, cash flow, and units of service
Business risk	Risk management initiatives and monitoring
Change strategy	Benchmarks used to indicate success and failure

CONCLUSION

As the number of the U.S. citizens with health benefits grows, one question looms on the minds of all stakeholders: How will the nation cope with the surge of new patients and their demand for health services? There is already a shortage of primary-care physicians, creating a workforce issue. In addition, the population is growing, as is the percentage of individuals over 65 years of age. The NP workforce contributions in filling the gaps in caring for the growing number of insured and elderly Americans, the chronically illness will solve some of the pressures facing the health system. There remains an even larger issue in providing health access to the populations in underserved communities. The possibility of "repeal and replacement of ACA" is still looming, but minimal reform of ACA will be implemented over the next decade. These changes will create many challenges for practitioners. NPs have an opportunity to move past historical limitations of the APRN and to restructure their role in the new delivery system.

NPs who develop a professional vision, articulate their value to all stakeholders, demonstrate flexibility, and show an ability to adjust to health-care change offer a significate asset in today's and tomorrow's health-care system. Knowledge of the financial aspects of health care is essential to be able to adjust and participate in health-care policy decisions. Business knowledge enhances NP's emphasis on documenting data and share analysis chronicling the quality of their services. Data will be essential to highlight low-cost, high-quality care to maximize reimbursement. Clinical and economic expertise will enhance the value-drivers for the profession. The NP workforce offers unique solutions and enhances the ability of the health-care team to meet the new demands in the U.S. health-care system.

Box 80.3   Common Policies and Procedures

- Hours of practice
- Utilization of space and resources
- Forms and collection of patient information
- Collection of copayments and deductibles at the time of the visit
- Verification of eligibility and patient coverage before treatment on carrier Web site
- Implementation of frequent billing cycle (e.g., every 15 days)
- Acceptance of credit cards for copayments and deductible
- Establishment of payment plans for patients not able to pay in full
- Implementation of banking policies: collecting money, posting money, and depositing money should be handled by different employees; verification that billers make daily bank deposits and that receipts are matched daily to the posted payments of that day
- Protection of confidentiality and storage of patient records
- Hazardous waste disposal
- Credentialing of all providers
- Hiring and firing of employees is in accordance with state laws
- Risk management education
- Occupational Safety and Health Administration compliance and Health Insurance Portability and Accountability Act documentation
- External regulator reporting requirements
- Pharmaceuticals and resources needed for practice
- Quality assurance and effectiveness monitoring
- Compliance forms and yearly verification
- Emergency plans
- Employee education plan
- Equipment monitoring
- General liability for the practice
- Malpractice coverage for all providers
- Business and facility security
- Volunteer policy
- Advertisement and marketing

For additional resources please visit
https://davisedge.fadavis.com/

REFERENCES

Altman, D. Obamacare may be holding down costs. http://kff.org/health-reform perspective/how-obamacare-may-be-holding-down-costs. Published September 27, 2013.

American Medical Association. Current procedural terminology: CPT 2017 professional. Chicago, IL: CPT/DBP Intellectual Property Services.

American Medical Association. *Medicare Access and CHIP Reauthorization Act (MACRA) quality payment program final rule.* October 19, 2016.

American Medical Association. Understanding Medicare payment reform (MACRA). https://www.ama-assn.org/practice-management/understanding-medicare-payment-reform-macra.

Arthur J. Gallagher & Co. State regulations for medical malpractice. https://www.ajg.com/industries/healthcare/state-regulations-for-medical-malpractice.

Athenahealth. *Whitepaper: Making a smooth transition: Avoiding the top 5 risks of the ICD-10 conversion.* http://www.athenahealth.com/_doc/pdf/whitepapers/ICD-10_Preparing_Your_Practice.pdf. Published May 2012.

Becker's Hospital CFO Report. *8 changes to the Medicare physician fee schedule in 2017.* http://www.beckershospitalreview.com/finance/8-changes-to-the-medicare-physician-fee-schedule-in-2017.html. Published 2017.

Buppert C. *Nurse practitioner's business practice and legal guide.* 6th ed. Sudbury, MA: Jones & Bartlett Learning; 2018.

Centers for Disease Control and Prevention. International Classification of Diseases, Tenth Revision (ICD-10). https://www.cdc.gov/nchs/icd/icd10.htm. Published 2017.

Centers for Medicare and Medicaid Services. Accountable Care Organizations. http://www.cms.gov/Medciare/Medicare-Fee-for-Service-Payment/ACO/index.html. Published 2015a.

Centers for Medicare and Medicaid Services. Affordable Care Act. http://medicaid.gov/AffordableCareAct/Affordable-Care-Act.html. Published 2015b.

Centers for Medicare and Medicaid Services. False Claims Act. www.cms.hhs.gov/smdl/downloads/SMDO32207Att2.pdf. Published 2009.

Centers for Medicare and Medicaid Services. Health Insurance Portability and Accountability Act (HIPAA). http://www.cms.hhs.gov/hipaa. Published 2005.

Centers for Medicare and Medicaid Services. Hospital-acquired conditions (present on admission indicator). https://wwwww.coms.gov/Medicare/Medicare-Fee-for-Service-Payment/HospitalAcqCond/index.html. Published September 23, 2016.

Centers for Medicare and Medicaid Services. Hospital value-based purchasing. http://www.cms.gov/Medicare/Quality-Initiatives-Patient-Assessment-Instruments/hospital-value-based-purchasing/index.html. Published 2013(a).

Centers for Medicare and Medicaid Services. Medicare benefit policy manual. https://www.cms.gov/Medicare/Provider-Enrollment-and-Certification/MedicareProviderSupEnroll/OptOutAffidavits.html. Published 2017(c).

Centers for Medicare and Medicaid Services. Medicare.gov: Medicare costs at a glance 2017. https://www.medicare.gov/your-medicare-costs/costs-at-a-glance/costs-at-glance.html. Published 2017(b).

Centers for Medicare and Medicaid Services. Readmission reduction program. http://www.cms.gov/Medicare/Medicare-Fee-for-Service-Payment/AcuteInpatientPPS/Readmissions-Reduction-Program.htm. Published 2013b.

Centers for Medicare and Medicaid Services. Year 2017 Medicare Part B physician and non-physician practitioner fee schedule. https://www.cms.gov/Medicare/Medicare-Fee-for-Service-Payment/PhysicianFeeSched/PFS-Federal-Regulation-Notices-Items/CMS-1654-F.html. Published 2017c.

ChampusVA. Civilian health and medical program. https://nvf.org/champva-civilian-health-and-medical-program. Retrieved 03/01/17.

Dallas ME. Hospital prices vary widely across the United States. *US News and World Report.* http://www.lifelinescreening.com/community/health-facts.health-news.healthcare-rising-costs. Published December 26, 2015.

Emanuel E. *Healthcare guaranteed: A simple, secure solution for America.* Philadelphia, PA: Perseus Books; 2008.

Frakes MA. An overview of Medicare reimbursement regulations for advanced practice nurses. *Nurs Econ.* 2006;24(2):59–65.

Goldsteen RL, Goldsteen KR. *Jonas' introduction to the U.S. healthcare system.* 7th ed. New York, NY: Springer; 2013.

Haycock C, Edwards ML, Stanley CS. Unpacking MACRA: The proposed rule and its implication for payment and practice. *Nurs Admin Q.* 2016;40(4):349–355.

HCPCS Codes. HCPCS codes-level II: 2017 healthcare common procedure coding system. *2017.* https://hcpcs.codes. Retrieved February 28, 2017.

Henry J. Kaiser Family Foundation. Focus on health reform: A guide to the Supreme Court's decision on the ACA's Medicaid Expansion. https://kaiserfamilyfoundationfiles.wrdpress.com/2013/01/8347.pdf. Published August 2012a.

Henry J. Kaiser Family Foundation. Health care costs: A primer: Key information on health care costs and their impact. https://kaiserfamilyfoundation.files.wordpress.com/2013/01/7670-03.pdf. Published May 2012b.

Henry J. Kaiser Family Foundation. Polling data note: Beyond the ACA, the affordability of insurance has been deteriorating since 2015. http://kff.org/health-costs/press-release/polling-data-note-beyond-the-aca-the-affordability-of-insurance-has-been-deteriorating-since-2015/.ce. Published May 2, 2017.

Hsiao WC. The resource-based relative value scale: An option for physician payment. *Inquiry* 1987;24(4):360–361.

ICD10Data.com. *The web's free 2017 ICD-10-CM and ICD-10-PCS medical coding reference.* www.icd10data.com. Retrieved March 28, 2017.

Iglehart JK. Expanding the role of advanced nurse practitioners—Risks and rewards. *N Engl J Med.* 2013;368(20):1935–1941.

Institute of Medicine. To err is human: Building a safer health system. http://www.iom.edu/iom/iomhome.nsf. Published 2000.

Jester AM, Casselman B. 33 million Americans still don't have health insurance: Here's who they are. https://fivethirtyeight.com/features/33-million-americans-still-don't-have-health-insurance. Published September 28, 2015.

Kerfoot K. On leadership: Learning or intuition?—Less college and more kindergarten: The leader's challenge. *Nurs Econ.* 2004;21(5):253–255.

Leonard K. What's behind the slowdown in health care costs. *US News and World Report.* https://usnews.com/news/article/2014/09/26/whats-behind-the-slowdown-in-health-care-costs. Published September 26, 2014.

Levy J. In U.S., uninsured dips to 11.9% in first quarter 2015. http://www.gallup.com/poll/182348/uninsured-rate-dips-first-quarter.aspx. Published April 13, 2015.

Medicaid.gov. Keeping America health: Affordable Care Act. https://www.medicaid.gov/affordable-care-act/index.html. Published 2015.

Medical Group Management Association. *Physician compensation and production survey: 2012 report based on 2011 data.* Englewood, CO: Author; 2012.

Murray CJL, Phil D, Frenk J. Ranking 37th—Measuring the performed of the U.S. health care system. *N Engl J Med.* 2010;362:98–99.

National Governors Association. The role of nurse practitioners in meeting increasing demand for primary care. http://www.na.org/center. Published 2012.

Newhouse RP, et al. Policy implications for optimizing advanced practice registered nurse use nationally. *Policy Politics Nurs Pract.* 2012;13(2):81–89.

Porter ME, Lee TH. Providers must lead the way in making value the overarching goal. *Harv Business Rev.* http://www.acmha.org/content/summit/2014/Strategy_Fix_Healthcare.pdf. Published October 2013.

Porter S. Significant primary care, overall physician shortage predicted by 2025. http://www.aafp.org/news/practice-professional-issues/20150303aamcwkforce.html. Published March 3, 2015.

Physicians Practice. Physicians practice your: Your practice your way. Retrieved from http://www.physicianpractice.com/blog/medical-practice-guide-incident-billing. Published February 2, 2015.

Roehrig C. *What is behind the post-recession bend in the health care cost curve.* http://healthaffairs.org/blog/2015/03/23/what-is-behind-the-post-recession-bend-in-the-health-care-cost-curve/. Published March 23, 2015.

Ross M. PYA Healthcare Blog: Bridging business & healthcare: 2017 Medicare physician fee schedule proposed rule: Expanded payments for care management services. http://healthcareblog.pyapc.com/2016/08/articles/services/2017-medicare-physician-fee-schedule. Published August 5, 2017.

Weiss GG. *Exclusive survey: Practice expense.* http://medicaleconomics.modernmedicine.com/medical-economics/news/clinical/personal-finance/exclusive-survey-practice-expenses?page=full. Published November 7, 2003.

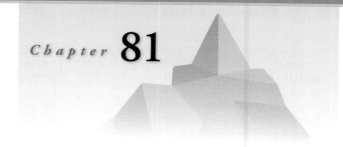

Chapter **81**

The 15-Minute Hour: Practical Approaches to Behavioral Health for Primary Care

Lynne M. Dunphy, PhD, APRN, FNP-BC, FAAN, FAANP

Brandi Cotton-Parker, PhD, APRN, PMHNP-BC

Contemporary advanced nursing practice presents many challenges, not the least of which is being on the frontlines of health management. Patients present for short office visits with complicated chief complaints, often seeking immediate relief from both physical and mental discomfort. In real-world clinical practice, the distinction between psychiatric and medical illness is often blurry, because mental and physical health interconnect. Specifically, psychological problems are often expressed as physical symptoms, and medical problems frequently precipitate psychological distress. Just as medical illness is usually best treated when detected in an early stage, early intervention is critical for psychological problems.

Additionally, the emphasis on behavioral health, self-care, prevention, and health promotion calls for the inclusion of a behavioral health specialist on primary-care teams. Changes in how health-care, including behavioral health care, is insured and funded continue to undergo changes. At the same time, the trend toward the integration of behavioral health care and primary care, prevention and health promotion interventions, the culture of well-being, and population health management will most likely remain constant.

The majority of psychiatric symptomatology is managed within the primary-care setting. In 1995, for example, a study by the World Health Organization sampled 1,500 patients around the world, in cities such as Ankara, Athens, Rio de Janeiro, Shanghai, Bangalore, Seattle, Berlin, and Manchester (Üstün & Sartorius, 1995) and found that 25% of patients met criteria for a psychiatric disorder. A more recent study by Smith et al. (2014) confirmed this finding, noting that 25% of patients in outpatient clinics met criteria for a *Diagnostic and Statistical Manual of Mental Disorders, Fifth Edition (DSM-5)*

diagnosis (more common than hypertension and diabetes combined). These authors argue for improved diagnostics and management of psychiatric symptomatology (Smith et al., 2014) and make the case for modification of educational curricula for medical students and residents with increased attention to psychiatric diagnoses and treatment.

Considering these statistics, it is unsurprising that patients present for primary-care visits reporting psychological concerns. Besieged by psychosocial stressors, patients seek relief for troubled relationships, stressful life events, recent losses, and economic strain. Although most providers agree that a thorough assessment of these contextual influences is important, the pressures of time-sensitive patient encounters create barriers to comprehensive and person-centered care. Given the significant impact of psychosocial factors on the prognosis of disease, building psychotherapeutic skills is critical for primary-care providers. Techniques such as reflective listening, validating emotions, and encouraging patient empowerment are easily used during short office visits. This chapter highlights the various modalities through which providers can assess and address acute stress and maladaptive responses that predict poorer prognosis of disease states; several therapeutic techniques are suggested for routine implementation during brief patient encounters.

STRESS

Stress is the physical and mental response that results from having to adapt to demands from the external and internal environments. When under stress, people generally cope less effectively than when they feel comfortable or pleasantly challenged. Distress is experienced when people's resources are overwhelmed by the constant challenges of life, leading to feelings of loss of control. Our understanding of the relationships among stress, coping, and health has been enhanced by the classic, long-term prospective studies of Vaillant (1979), whose findings suggest the following:

- Overwhelmed people regress functionally
- Poor adaptation is associated with ill health because risk of disease increases in those with anxiety, depression, and inadequate stress management
- Offering support to those under stress may facilitate their return to adaptive function and health

Given this understanding, health promotion and disease prevention require teaching constructive ways of coping with stress. When people become overwhelmed by the circumstances of their lives, whether due to a cataclysmic event, daily hassles, or even personality characteristics, they often become sick and may visit their primary-care provider. It is thus important to screen effectively for stressors and adopt techniques for providing support.

SOCIAL SUPPORT

Social support is a key element in stress management. When one's perception of control over life circumstances decreases, subjective feelings of stress increase dramatically. However, as social support increases, the stress level decreases. Not surprisingly, it has been shown that poor social support is deleterious to health. Health-care providers are in a position to convey essential social support by providing positive feedback to the patient or by suggesting strategies for handling a particular problem. When people are psychologically stressed or medically ill, they may be particularly vulnerable to negative feelings—namely, inadequacy and isolation. A key benefit of social support is that it augments a person's sense of competence and of connection. By reminding patients about their basic strengths, clinicians enhance patients' abilities to function in a healthy way.

THERAPEUTIC APPROACHES

By virtue of professional training and commitment to wellness, nurse practitioners are uniquely positioned to assist their patients in coping, regardless of the specific nature of the problem. Skillfully employed, the professional therapeutic persona of the clinician alone can decrease stress, feel less alone, and enable patients to cope more effectively. After discussions with a health-care provider about their concerns, patients often feel better and may even be able to solve formerly intractable problems. Many clinicians feel more comfortable calling this "counseling," but such interactions are essentially psychotherapy. Among the elements common to all major schools of psychotherapy noted by Goldfried and Padawer (1982) are (1) patient expectation of receiving help, (2) participation in a therapeutic relationship, (3) obtaining an external perspective, (4) encouraging corrective experience, and (5) repeated reality testing.

THERAPEUTIC TALK IN PRIMARY CARE: THE 15-MINUTE HOUR

Incorporating appropriate questions and responses regarding a patient's psychosocial situation is an acquired skill. The BATHE technique was developed by Marion Stuart, a psychologist, and Joseph Lieberman, a medical doctor, in their work with medical students and is elaborated in a full-length book by Stuart and Leiberman (2015) *The Fifteen Minute Hour: Therapeutic Talk in Primary Care*. The BATHE technique functions as both a quick screening test and an intervention for psychiatric problems, especially appropriate for new patients and those presenting with acute problems and mental distress. It has become an established method of identifying and addressing psychosocial aspects of patients' problems

during a brief office visit. It should be used early in the interview, usually after elicitation of the chief complaint (CC) and the history of the present illness (HPI). The acronym, intended to complement the "SOAP" method of medical documentation (see Chapter 4) stands for Background, Affect, Trouble, Handling, and Empathy.

Focus on History: BATHE

- **B**ackground. The simple question "What is going on in your life?" determines the context of the patient's visit.
- **A**ffect. Questions such as "How does that make you feel?" encourage patients to identify and report their emotional reactions to the circumstances described.
- **T**rouble. The question "What troubles you most about this?" helps both practitioner and patient focus on the situation's subjective meaning. Even when the patient's affect is positive, a modified version of this question should be asked: "Is there anything about it that troubles you?"
- **H**andling. The answer to "How are you handling that?" helps the practitioner assess the patient's level of functioning, helps the patient connect mind and behavior, and communicates the thought that the patient has indeed taken steps toward handling the situation.
- **E**mpathy. The statement "That must be very difficult" legitimizes the patient's reaction. Even when the patient is functioning suboptimally, it is important to reflect back the content of the circumstances and support the patient's attempts at resolution.

Although BATHE is not the only technique a clinician can employ, it brings order and efficiency to what may otherwise become a muddled and time-consuming attempt at psychosocial assessment. In the process, it helps tie the biomedical model to the psychosocial model in a way that is meaningful for both clinician and patient. By asking pointed, focused questions that lend themselves to brief but comprehensive answers, the clinician is able to incorporate this necessary form of assessment into a format that enhances rapport and also helps the patient express feelings, gain insight into the meaning of the situation, and become empowered. Most significantly, it satisfies all the aforementioned elements of psychotherapy: BATHE provides the expectation of help, a therapeutic relationship, an external perspective, the encouragement of new behavior, and the ongoing opportunity to test reality. The clinician must exercise discipline, however, and refrain from a lengthy exploration of the patient's life. BATHE's therapeutic effect derives simply from its focus on the patient's feelings, the subjective meaning of the situation, assessment of how things are being handled, and empathic demonstration of support.

Evidence for BATHE

The BATHE technique has empirical evidence to support its use in increasing patient satisfaction. In 2008,

Leiblum published a study exploring the use of the BATHE technique within the primary-care setting. Four experienced family medicine physicians working in a large urban outpatient office, who were trained in the BATHE technique, took part in a study that explored outcomes relating to patient satisfaction with this brief therapeutic intervention. Patients assessed with the BATHE technique were more likely satisfied with the information the physician provided and their perception of physician concern for them and were more likely to recommend their physician to others. In 2011, a study explored the use of the BATHE technique within the perioperative setting at Mount Sinai Medical Center in New York. One hundred surgical patients were randomly enrolled in the BATHE group or the control group. The use of the BATHE technique within this setting suggests that it is both clinically effective and practical: Findings suggest that use of the BATHE method increased patient satisfaction but did not increase the length of the physician evaluation (DeMaria et al., 2011).

Ownership

This technique helps the provider more fully assess the patient's situation and make therapeutic suggestions so the patient can deal with his or her problem more effectively. This is true whether the problem seems predominantly biomedical or psychosocial, because elements of each are invariably involved in the patient's overall situation. Nonetheless, it is crucial that the provider not assume responsibility for resolution of the patient's situation. The patient continues to "own" his or her problem; however, a more comprehensive understanding of the situation and its effect on the patient allows the provider to assist more effectively. Further, as the patient gains confidence that the provider is supportive and able to help, the element of trust in the therapeutic relationship is enhanced.

Applying the BATHE Technique

Practitioners may worry that application of the BATHE technique may uncover unanticipated issues that cannot be adequately addressed within the allotted time. However, BATHE's evaluative component is a *screening tool*, and the clinician must use judgment as to when and how extensively to explore what has surfaced. Sometimes it is important to say, "I am glad you brought this up. Let me examine you to see if there is some physical problem that we need to be concerned about, and afterward we can talk some more." In most cases, BATHEing the patient will take less than a minute and can help prevent the unexpected and time-consuming patient revelations sometimes held until the end of the visit. The essence of psychotherapy consists of making the patient feel competent and connected, and there are numerous additional and complementary techniques that can help accomplish this. The authors maintain that this can be accomplished

in a 15-minute visit. Many such strategies and examples can be found in Stuart and Lieberman's (2015) *The Fifteen Minute Hour*. In most cases, however, using the BATHE technique helps to clarify the situation. Once this is complete, patients should have their feelings validated and be supported in expressing those feelings. They should be provided brief information about the effects of stress along with specific suggestions for stress management and relevant problem-solving. If necessary, the patient should be invited to return and explore the situation further. As always, serious problems necessitate referral to a mental health professional, but the practitioner's role in uncovering important issues is invaluable; however, in many cases, a return 15-minute primary-care visit can provide continued support and, in some cases, resolution.

The Positive "BATHE"

The past decade has seen the emergence of a new mental health subfield called positive psychology. Researchers such as Martin Seligman, Edward Diener, and Christopher Peterson are encouraging psychologists to focus on human virtues, character strengths, and the benefits of happiness and personal growth, rather than the traditional exclusive concentration on the study and treatment of mental illness and disturbance. This approach is consistent with nursing's emphasis on health promotion and supporting patients' strengths. An impressive and growing body of literature links positive affect with health and longevity. Positive thought and emotion is believed to bolster the immune system and has even been associated with better health behaviors.

One specific area that has garnered attention is gratitude, a trait associated with a sense of well-being and positive feeling. In fact, investigators have shown empirically that related interventions, such as asking subjects to write gratitude letters or keep gratitude journals, lead to decreased physical and mental health symptoms (Peterson, 2006; Stuart & Lieberman, 2015).

Nearly 30 years after the first edition was published, *The Fifteen Minute Hour: Therapeutic Talk in Primary Care*, 5th edition (2015) continues to support primary-care practitioners in solving and often preventing many psychological and behavioural problems, while enhancing the therapeutic relationship with their patients. The simple and effective techniques are easily learned and designed to increase patient satisfaction without adding significantly to the length of a visit. Newer findings about brain plasticity, gene expression, and the epigenetic effects of constructively managing stress support this approach and also demonstrate the power of positive affirmation, mindfulness, and exercise on enhancing health.

In keeping with these themes, a new "Positive BATHE" intervention has been developed to help patients focus on autonomy and personal accomplishment, thankfulness, and general positive affect. Practically, learning this additional BATHE repertoire also allows the provider a second form of intervention, especially useful when interacting with the chronically ill or others who may return frequently for follow-up appointments. In this updated version, BATHE is an acronym for **B**est, **A**ccount, **T**hankfulness, **H**appen, and **E**mpowerment.

Focus on History: Positive BATHE

- **B**est. Asking patients "What's the best thing that has happened to you lately?" encourages recall of positive events, which likely leads to positive affect.
- **A**ccount. When patients reflect on the causes of positive events, they discover what they should do to promote recurrence of these events. Questions such as "How do you account for that?" advance this form of contemplation.
- **T**hankfulness. The question "What are you most thankful for?" is aimed at triggering gratitude related to the events mentioned and thereby positive feelings and good health.
- **H**appen. Asking "How can you make things like that happen again?" suggests that the patient be proactive in attaining positive experiences. It also challenges patients to put character strengths and adaptive traits to use in their day-to-day interactions.
- **E**mpowerment. Enthusiastic and empathic practitioner responses, such as "It sounds like you have a fantastic idea!" and "I am sure you can do it!" empower the patient to take the steps necessary for further success and achievement.

MOTIVATIONAL INTERVIEWING

Motivational interviewing (MI) is a therapeutic technique supported by a large volume of research. Employed within a wide array of clinical settings, MI is an empirically validated strategy for assisting patients with behavioral change. Developed by Robert Miller, PhD, as a target therapy for substance abuse, the tenets of MI extend to a wide range of clinical audiences.

MI asserts that ambivalence is a normal, nonpathological component of the change process. Clinicians assist patients in addressing ambivalence by exploring intrinsic motivation, values, and goals. The basic principles of MI promote respect for individual autonomy and belief that the patient is an expert on his or her own behavior. This is a consistent way of supporting the patient's self-care behaviors and taking responsibility for the patient's own health. MI involves empathetic listening and establishing a non-judgmental, non-confrontational patient approach. Collaboration and joint decision-making encourage "change talk." MI is a way of being with a client, not just a set of techniques for doing counseling (Miller & Rollnick, 1991). Techniques of MI include asking open-ended questions, offering affirmative and supportive statements, reflectively listening, and summarizing the patient's situation. MI also encourages clinicians to request permission before offering advice or interventions. Unsolicited advice is likely to promote resistance. If a patient is not yet ready to change a behavior (e.g., beginning a diet, monitoring glucose, adopting an exercise routine, decreasing substance use), it is unlikely that clinicians' advice will be well received (Miller & Rollnick, 2013).

The four principles of motivational interviewing use the acronym RULE (Rollnick et al., 2013):

- **R**esist the righting reflex.
- **U**nderstand your patient's motivation.
- **L**isten to your patient.
- **E**mpower your patient.

An important tenet of MI is the use of reflective listening, a key component in helping patients explore ambivalence and resistance to change. Reflective listening ranges from simple to complex: repeating, rephrasing, paraphrasing, and reflecting feeling. Dialogue is strategic; clinicians guide the conversation with reflective statements, not questions, accepting the patient regardless of her or his readiness for change (Rollnick et al., 2007). This is encapsulated in the approaches of open-ended responses, affirmations, reflective listening, and summarization. The acronym OARS highlights these four important components of MI (Miller & Rollnick, 2012):

1. **O**pen-ended response
2. **A**ffirming patient
3. **R**eflective listening
4. **S**ummarizing

The last part of MI is to ask the patient's permission to help him or her pursue a particular course of action. The accompanying Nursing Situations present examples of applying OARS to patient interviewing.

Nursing Situation: Motivational Interviewing: Alcohol Use

Martin is a 33-year-old man with a history of heavy alcohol use. He presents to his provider and reports a recent job loss due to excessive tardiness. He reports concern that his family faces eviction for failure to pay rent. Martin then discloses that much of his tardiness was a result of hangovers from heavy drinking. He has voiced concerns in the past, specifically reporting: "My wife nags me about spending too much time with my drinking buddies." He expresses concern that an intensive substance abuse program will be too time-consuming but reports several unsuccessful efforts to remain sober when using the 12-step program Alcoholics Anonymous (AA). Martin says, "I know I can really drink a lot after work. It relaxes me, you know. The job thing is tough—my wife has been pressuring me to get treatment or something. I tried AA, but it didn't work. A friend of mine did some intensive thing, but I don't have time for that. How am I supposed to spend 8 hours at some treatment facility when I need to be out looking for a job?"

Using the acronym OARS helps direct the patient interview:

O—Open-ended response:
- "What's this been like for you?"
- "What's most important to you at this point?"

A—Affirming patient:
- "It can be incredibly difficult to acknowledge these things. The fact that you are here today and talking with me about it shows a commitment to making things better."

R—Reflective listening:
- "So the drinking is causing strain. It's also a way for you to relax."
- "You want to find a program that is right for you."

S—Summarize:
- "From our last few visits, I know you've been thinking about cutting back on the drinking. It seems like today, after the job loss, you are more concerned than you were at our previous visits. You are thinking about treatment options, but it's really important to you to find a program that is going to fit your lifestyle."

ASK permission:
- "Do you want any information about alternative treatments in the area?"

Nursing Situation: Motivational Interviewing: Weight Loss

Anna is a 43-year-old woman with a body mass index of 35. She is the mother of two and works as a secretary. Anna is diagnosed with hypercholesterolemia and type 2 diabetes. She consumes a high-calorie diet and maintains a sedentary lifestyle. She states, "I know I need to lose weight. I keep planning on walking, but it's so cold now."

Using the acronym OARS helps direct the patient interview:

O—Open-ended response:
- "Tell me a little more about your goals in this area."

A—Affirming patient:
- "Implementing an exercise routine can be really difficult. The fact that you are considering how to make it work for you and your lifestyle is an important step."

R—Reflective listening:
- "Sounds like you want to exercise, but outdoor exercise isn't realistic in this weather."

S—Summarize:
- "You've been monitoring your weight over the past several months, and it seems like you're feeling discouraged with the results. Winter weather makes it even more challenging for you to meet your goals. You want a plan that's going to work for you."

ASK permission:
- "Several of my patients have had a lot of success with a new program—would you like to hear about it?"

MI is rooted in empathic listening and collaborative decision-making. Empirical data support these techniques as an effective strategy for increasing adherence to antivirals in HIV-positive patients, decreasing high-risk behaviors, promoting weight loss, treating eating disorders, increasing physical activity, and addressing domestic violence. The diverse application of MI principles suggests its promising role in promoting positive behavioral changes within a broad range of clinical settings (Miller & Rollnick, 2013).

SUMMARY

Patients' beliefs, values, perspectives, and health behaviors are situated within a broad social and environmental context. Understanding this context is essential to building and establishing rapport between patient and provider and providing holistic, person-centered care. Despite considerable time constraints, practitioners can use therapeutic tools to assist patients in changing maladaptive responses and unhealthful behaviors. Utilizing brief psychotherapeutic modalities, such as BATHE, Positive BATHE, and MI, can improve both patient satisfaction and health outcomes. Use of these techniques in the primary-care encounter also leads to positive and meaningful interactions.

 For additional resources please visit
https://davisedge.fadavis.com/

REFERENCES

Barnett E, Sussman S, Smith C, Rohrbach LA, et al. Motivational interviewing for adolescent substance use: A review of the literature. *Addict Behav.* 2012;37(12):1325–1334.

Bartrop RW, Luckhurst E, Lazarus L, Kiloh LG, Penny R. Depressed lymphocyte function after bereavement. *Lancet.* 1977;309:834–836.

Cobb S. Social support as a moderator of life stress. *Psychosom Med.* 1976;38:300–314.

Cohen S, Tyrrell DA, Smith AP. Psychological stress and susceptibility to the common cold. *N Engl J Med.* 1991;325:606–612.

DeMaria S, Jr, DeMaria AP, Silvay G, Flynn BC. Use of the BATHE method in the preanesthetic clinic visit. *Anesth Analg.* 2011;113(5):1020–1026.

Goldfried MR, Padawer W. Current status and future directions in psychotherapy. In Goldfried MR (Ed.), *Converging themes in psychotherapy: Trends in psychodynamic, humanistic, and behavioral practice.* New York: Springer; 1982:3–49.

Leiberman JA, Stuart, MA. Practicing biopsychosocial medicine. In: Rakel RE, ed. *Textbook of family practice,* 6th ed. Philadelphia, PA: Saunders; 2002:65–70.

Leiblum SR, Schnall E, Seehuus M, DeMaria A. To BATHE or not to BATHE: Patient satisfaction with visits to their family physician. *Fam Med* 2008;40:407–411.

Lindson-Hawley N, Thompson TP, Begh R. Motivational interviewing for smoking cessation. *Cohchrane Database Syst Rev.* 2015;(3):CD006936. doi: 10.1002/14651858.CD006936. pub3.

McCulloch J, Ramesar S, Peterson H. Psychotherapy in primary care: The BATHE technique. *Am Fam Physician.* 1998;57:2131–2134.

Miller WR, Rollnick S. *Motivational interviewing: Preparing people to change addictive behavior.* New York, NY: Guilford Press; 1991.

Miller WR, Rollnick S. *Motivational interviewing: Helping people change,* 3rd ed. New York, NY: Guilford Press; 2013.

Miller WR, Rose GS. Toward a theory of motivational interviewing. *Am Psychol.* 2009;64(6):527–537.

Motivational interviewing. Treatment Improvement Protocol (TIP) Series, No. 35. Rockville, MD: Center for Substance Abuse Treatment, Substance Abuse and Mental Health Services Administration; 1999.

Peterson C. *A primer in positive psychology.* New York, NY: Oxford University Press; 2006.

Rollnick S, Miller WR, Butler CC. *Motivational interviewing in health care: Helping patients change behavior (applications of motivational interviewing).* New York, NY: Guilford Press; 2008.

Rozanski A, Blumenthal JA, Kaplan J. Impact of psychological factors on the pathogenesis of cardiovascular disease and implications for therapy. *Circulation.* 1999;99:2192–2217.

Smith RC, Laird-Fick H, D'Mello D, et al. Addressing mental health issues in primary care: An initial curriculum for medical residents. *Patient Educ Counsel.* 2014;94(1):33–42.

Stuart MR, Lieberman JA III. *The fifteen minute hour: Therapeutic talk in primary care,* 5th ed. Radcliffe, UK: CRC Press Book; 2015.

Üstün TB, Sartorius N. *Mental illness in general health care: An international study.* New York, NY: Wiley; 1995.

Vaillant GE. Natural history of male psychologic health: Effects of mental health on physical health. *N Engl J Med.* 1979;301:1249–1254.

Vasilaki EI, Hosier SG, Cox WM. The efficacy of motivational interviewing as a brief intervention for excessive drinking: A meta-analytic review. *Alcohol Alcohol.* 2006;41(3):328–335.

RESOURCES

Center for Evidence Based Practices Motivational Interviewing
Case Western Reserve University
   https://www.centerforebp.case.edu/practices/mi
Motivational Interviewing Network of Trainers
   http://www.motivationalinterviewing.org/
Motivational Interviewing on YouTube:
   https://www.youtube.com/watch?v=67I6g1I7Zao
   https://www.youtube.com/watch?v=dm-rJJPCuTE
   https://www.youtube.com/watch?v=-zEpwxJlRQI
   https://www.youtube.com/watch?v=bTRRNWrwRCo

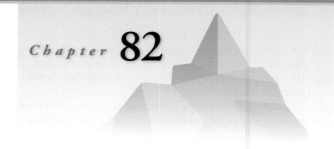

Chapter 82

Putting Caring Into Practice: Caring for Self

Mary Lavin, DNP, APRN, FNP-BC
Rebecca Carley, MS, DNP, APRN

The importance of self-care for the clinician cannot be overstated. As nurse practitioner (NP) students confront the demands of graduate school and, later, beginning practice, they realize the necessity of maintaining balance in their lives. Work and professional responsibilities, family and home life, coursework and clinical practicums all demand attention. Self-care and health promotion are major components of caring for patients; it is imperative that NPs care for themselves as well.

A review of the processes introduced in the *Circle of Caring* model provides a valuable starting point for the discussion of self-care of the APRN and indeed any health-care provider. Caring for others makes it incumbent for NPs to care for "self." The goal is to actualize the model by directing health-supporting activities toward oneself first, enabling the practitioner to experience and integrate the value gained from self-care, and to use this strength as a source of replenishment in helping others. This chapter provides an introduction to self-care definitions, explains some of the challenges to self-care, and suggests how to perform a self-assessment and apply practical healing strategies in advanced practice nursing and primary-care practice in general.

BACKGROUND: CARING AND SELF-CARE

Caring has long been considered the domain of nursing, although many other health-care providers care in their own ways. The *Circle of Caring* model presented in Chapter 1 and developed throughout this textbook helps us to deepen our conceptualization of the ways nursing contributes to the process of healing. This model provides for conceptualization instead of simply skills and techniques, and it expands the traditional medical model. The caring processes include patience, courage, advocacy, authentic presence, commitment, and knowing. Caring is central to the profession of nursing and is at the core of many, if not all, nursing theories.

Caring for others has been the traditional focus of nursing, but the need to retain nurses within the profession has fostered a new emphasis on self-care of the nurse. Defining *self-care* is difficult because there is no single definition that is broadly accepted in the literature. Godfrey et al. (2011) conducted an extensive evaluation of the concept of self-care by analyzing 139 self-care definitions that appeared in the literature between 1970 and 2009. Seven components of the definition of self-care were identified: health, illness and disability, general outcomes, performer of the self-care, action of the self-care, health-care professionals, and the health-care system. Self-care historically has been represented as a low-quality and ineffectual behavior, but the 2000s brought about a broadening of the term and a new appreciation of the importance of self-care.

Some commonly used definitions illuminate these components:

- The World Health Organization defines self-care as "a deliberate action that individuals, family members, and the community should engage in to maintain good health ... Self-care includes all health decisions people make for themselves and their family to become and remain physically and mentally fit such as eating healthy foods, exercising regularly, practicing good hygiene, and avoiding health hazards. People in good health, those who are ill or with disability can engage in self-care. ... Self-care is the ability of individuals, families, and communities to promote health, prevent disease, and maintain health and to cope with illness and disability with or without the support of a health-care provider" (cited in Godfrey et al., 2011, p. 16).
- Wilkinson and Whitehead (2009) define *self-care* as "not involving a health professional ... and the individual independently attains and preserves [his or her] desired level of health. Self-care could be understood as people being responsible for their own health and well-being through staying fit and healthy: physically, mentally, and where desired, spiritually" (p. 1,145).
- The American Holistic Nurses Association (AHNA) Standards of Holistic Practice requires the integration of self-care and personal development activities into one's life. Holistic nurses engage in self-assessment, self-care, and personal development and are aware of being instruments of healing. Holistic nurses value themselves and mobilize the necessary resources to care for themselves. They strive to achieve harmony and balance in their own lives and to assist others to do the same. The AHNA describes self-care practices as self-assessment, meditation, yoga, good nutrition, energy therapies, movement or dance, journaling, and creative expression (art, music).
- Orem defines self-care as comprising those activities performed independently by an individual to promote and maintain well-being throughout life (AHNA, 2014).

Regardless of the definition, many helping disciplines are beginning to focus on the issue of self-care for their members. A keyword search provides an abundance of literature that addresses this topic across many disciplines, including psychology, social work, medicine, education, and emergency medical services. The impact of stress and trauma on optimal functioning and retention of providers is of growing concern amid the changing health-care environment. Many professional associations have developed and incorporated self-care resources that are available on each association's website. For example, the American Nurses Association has recently implemented the Healthy Nurse initiative to address self-care issues among nursing professionals.

Nurse practitioners care for patients with a wide variety of lifestyles, health-care choices, acute-care illnesses, and chronic health-care conditions. To help their patients maintain optimal health, NPs frequently discuss and advocate for self-care programs with individuals and families. Modeling healthy lifestyle behaviors is an important aspect of patient support and teaching. By caring for himself or herself effectively, the NP will promote self-care in patients.

CHALLENGES TO SELF-CARE INHERENT IN ADVANCED PRACTICE NURSING

Self-care is an important strategy for NPs for many reasons. There is a great deal of stress inherent in the NP role in primary care. Recent changes in the U.S. health-care system are likely to profoundly change the roles and responsibilities of NPs. In addition, the introduction of new technologies, increased oversight from insurance providers, and societal and professional changes all have the potential to impact NPs both personally and professionally.

Changes in the Health-Care System

The Future of Nursing (Institute of Medicine [IOM], 2010) suggests that NPs will be called on to function to the full extent of their education and licensure, although state variations in scope of practice persist. Furthermore, the Affordable Care Act of 2010 increased patient access to care, and this has therefore increased the demand for primary-care practitioners. Many of these newly insured patients are sicker, with multiple comorbidities that are frequently co-joined to behavioral health and socioeconomic issues. This creates a challenging workplace, especially in safety-net settings such as community health centers where NPs often care for patients. The Quality and Safety Education for Nurses competencies also demand that NPs maintain patient safety standards, utilize evidence-based practice strategies, and implement continuous quality improvement.

Changes in Insurance and Technology

Additional challenges to NPs include compliance with insurance regulations, many of which constantly change maintenance of certifications and the introduction of new technologies, particularly in the areas of record keeping and billing. Insurance regulators have a major impact on time management   and reimbursement of NPs and other health-care professionals. Reimbursement rates for NP services are often less than the rates for physician providers who provide the same care (see Chapter 80, The Business of Advanced Practice Nursing). Primary-care practices provide many services not covered by insurance carriers, such as completion of prior authorizations for medications and diagnostic tests, as well as forms required for schools and camps.

The introduction and integration of the electronic health record (EHR) during the past decade has also created a challenge for all health-care providers to maintain effective communication with patients during office visits. Although the EHR has major benefits for documentation and continuity of care, there is also an increased time demand for documentation during patient visits. Increased time demands are also generated through the adoption of other technology, such as automated appointment scheduling, Web portals for accessing lab results, and texting patient reminders or encouragement for self-care. Although many of these technologies can enhance patient care, new systems must be implemented for the adoption of these practices. In addition, patients frequently search the Internet for answers to health-care questions. Sometimes this patient-conducted research allows for more informed questions for health-care providers, but it often also contributes to patients' anxiety regarding their symptoms.

Societal Changes

Social issues such as joblessness, poverty, immigration of undocumented persons, high costs for medications and other treatments, and the aging population all can adversely affect the health care and self-care of patients. Nurse practitioners in primary care are involved in the management of acutely ill and chronically ill patients whose care needs may be challenging and difficult to deal with emotionally. To further complicate matters, APRNs must also deal with confusion about professional boundaries, particularly considering the emerging doctorate of nursing practice (DNP) and changes in legislation and reimbursement.

Professional Changes

There has been an increasing demand by the IOM and other organizations for the development of interdisciplinary education and health-care teams. This is an overall positive initiative, but it does bring challenges. Roles may become blurred as different professionals attempt to remain viable and to expand their roles in health care. The roles and responsibilities of the NP are also changing to reflect these demands. Some of these transitions in scope of care will need legislative action or changes in rules and regulations within licensing and credentialing bodies.

The changing face of health care dictates the need for flexibility as we approach a new era in health care. APRNs have more opportunity to work independently, yet they experience increased risk of legal action. In addition, APRNs may feel squeezed between the conflicting values and roles of being both nurse and primary-care provider, constantly having to negotiate unique interprofessional relationships with other health-care providers. Nurses want to advocate for their patients in a system that does not always appreciate or, at times, even allow them to do their job appropriately and effectively.

COMPASSION FATIGUE AND BURNOUT

Providing excellent care day in and day out can lead to compassion fatigue and burnout for individual NPs. Several authors describe compassion fatigue and burnout as related but separate concepts (Lombardo & Eyre, 2011; Valent, 2002). *Compassion fatigue* occurs when a caregiver cannot rescue or save an individual from harm, leading to feelings of guilt and distress. Compassion fatigue appears suddenly and resolves quickly. *Burnout* occurs when a person cannot achieve his or her goals and results in "frustration, a sense of loss of control, increased willful efforts, and diminishing morale" (Valent, 2002, p. 27). Burnout arises and declines more slowly, but both burnout and compassion fatigue can have negative consequences for both the provider and the client (Sabo, 2006).

THE PRINCIPLES OF SELF-CARE MANAGEMENT

All nurses experience varying degrees of stress, compassion fatigue, or burnout at some point in their career. Nurse practitioners are easily able to identify problems within others but frequently avoid dealing with issues that might affect their own well-being. The most important strategy for NPs is to identify their stressors before they affect their well-being and that of their clients. Very often, an NP will know that something is wrong but will avoid taking the time needed to address the concerns in the middle of a highly packed day.

Focusing on personal and professional shortcomings does not lead to optimal health. Nurse practitioners are often able to understand and accept the deficiencies of others, yet they hold themselves to unattainable standards. Self-compassion is the ability to be compassionate

to oneself. Emotional intelligence is the ability of the person to recognize emotions, understand the meaning of the emotions, and realize how the emotions affect other people. Characteristics of emotional intelligence include self-awareness, self-regulation, motivation, empathy, and social skills. Heffernan et al. (2010) found a positive correlation between self-compassion and emotional intelligence among nurses. Two overarching principles of a self-care management plan are resilience and positive intentionality. These concepts are interrelated and can enhance the success of self-care practices.

Resilience

Resilience has been defined as the ability to keep functioning in the face of continued stress, difficult work conditions, or trauma. Resilience can be seen as a strategy for responding to difficult or adverse situations by positively adjusting to stressors. Resilience can be associated with hope, positivity, and self-efficacy (Sullivan et al., 2012). Some research suggests that resilience can be strengthened in nurses using different strategies. A review of the literature regarding resilience in health professionals by McCann et al. (2013) suggests that laughter/humor, self-reflection, beliefs/spirituality, and professional identity are all related to the characteristic of resilience. Developing positive relationships and encouraging positive attitudes and emotional insight will reinforce resilience.

Positive Intentionality

Positive intentionality is a form of focused consciousness and energy according to Jean Watson (2002). Holding thoughts of caring, loving, kindness, and open receptivity rather than having manipulative intent or seeking power over others leads to healing. Focusing on positive intentionality in thoughts and actions enhances caring energy, which leads to healing and improved health.

THE PROCESS OF SELF-CARE MANAGEMENT

Self-Assessment

Practicing nurses and experienced NPs are skilled at assessing a patient's readiness for change and developing plans to improve self-care, but these professionals may not take time to apply a similar process to themselves. The principles discussed in Chapter 3, "Health Promotion," and the alternative therapies discussed throughout this text can be applied to self-care of the nursing professional. Self-assessment of the provider's current status includes reflection on strengths and identification of areas that need support. This might include time for reflection and appropriate self-evaluation of performance. It might also include identification of strategies that are suggested and validated for stress management. A variety of self-assessment tools are available to assist in the identification of concerns with links to or suggestions for appropriate strategies to make changes. Many organizations have identified professional quality-of-life assessment tools, such as ProQOl (Stamm, 2008).

Self-care assessment can be used to examine the type of self-care strategies that the NP is using and identify other areas that might be important for self-care management. Some NPs will be able to identify stressors and concerns independently. Any method is acceptable if it leads to engagement in self-care behaviors.

Goal Setting

Each NP can identify individual areas to work on, setting goals depending on his or her perception of balance in life. Specific strategies such as increased exercise and adequate sleep may be important for one person, whereas another may need to focus on prayer or meditation. It is important for the NP to evaluate all aspects of the person—physical, psychological, spiritual, and professional and work domains—so that appropriate interventions are used to optimize well-being. The APRN engages in self-evaluation concerning clinical practice to monitor and ensure the quality of health-care practice. This is consistent with the National Organization of Nurse Practitioner Faculties (2017) core competency for NP practice.

Implementing Strategies

Strategies for self-care can be divided into categories for all components of well-being of the individual. These include physical aspects as well as psychosocial and spiritual components. It is important that each professional examine his or her practice to determine whether there are realistic expectations for performance in the clinical area. In addition, other life stressors such as family needs, chronic illnesses, holidays, vacations, and relationships can compound professional stressors.

Physical signs and symptoms of increased stressors such as insomnia, loss of appetite, overeating, and weight gain or loss can require interventions to ensure optimal well-being for the provider. Interventions suggested by personal health-care providers should be followed for optimal physical care. This might include weight loss programs, exercise programs, and strategies for sleep. Occasionally, a practitioner may benefit from some extra personal time for reflection and meditation. Access to and self-referral to treatment programs can be helpful in sustaining interventions.

Professionally, it seems important for NPs to develop their own "inner circle," a trusted peer group composed of people with similar beliefs, who can mentor them in individual needs. In the literature, the role is referred to as a "coaching" function for professionals (Marshall & Zolnierek, 2012). Discussion of stressors, alternative choices for managing stressors, and debriefing after difficult situations can help to promote self-confidence and self-efficacy. Peers can also be helpful during transition times. Positive, nurturing relationships are imperative for the development of resilience. The focus on positivity is an important strategy because positive feelings increase energy and help one feel more optimistic about challenging situations. Developing emotional insight and balance in life can also augment a person's resilience. The characteristic of resilience is associated with confidence and self-efficacy. These self-care strategies will help to prevent adverse effects of stress.

Many professionals are involved in various other self-care strategies. Because so many lay publications are devoted to self-care and self-help, there is a plethora of strategies that can be utilized for self-care. Many of these strategies are well researched and validated for effectiveness. But perhaps the most important consideration is that each professional must identify the most appropriate strategies for his or her own self-care. Many professionals participate in exercise programs, yoga, walking and running programs, or weight management programs; many use music, massage, and/or meditation to reduce stress.

Some newer modalities and older Eastern medicine modalities for self-care have also been researched and validated. The Centers for Disease Control and Prevention (CDC) provides ongoing research findings on alternative therapies and serves as an excellent resource of information. Two interesting modalities that are well researched are mindfulness-based stress reduction and energy field strategies:

- **Mindfulness-based stress reduction** is one strategy that has been shown to reduce stress, anxiety, and chronic depression and is recently being used for management of other lifestyle problems.
- **Energy field therapies**. *Therapeutic Touch* (TT) is a nursing strategy developed by Dora Kunz and Dolores Krieger. Krieger was a former student of Martha Rogers at New York University, who applied the principles of energy-field interactions to create a sequential process whereby nurses and caregivers direct their intentionality toward the patient's well-being. Research has shown that TT is useful in reducing pain, improving wound healing, aiding relaxation, and easing the dying process.
  Reiki is a form of complementary energy therapy that helps to rebalance the energy field around the person to help restore him or her to a balanced, positive state of energy flow. This therapy helps the individual to feel relaxed and peaceful and has been utilized in a variety of settings to manage stress (Cuneo et al., 2010; Natale, 2010).

Box 82.1   The Importance of Self Care

Jane R. has been a nurse practitioner for 10 years working in family primary care. Her current salaried position is in an urban community health center that provides care to a multicultural population. During an 8-hour workday, Jane will see 24 to 26 patients. She is the newest provider in the practice and is still building up her case load, so during most days she will see 4 to 6 new patients. Jane admits that most days she completes her EHR documentation at home, spending 2 to 3 hours most workdays and occasionally 1 day on the weekend reviewing and following up on labs and responding to patient e-mails or telephone calls. Jane is constantly worrying about what she is behind on or what she may have missed. Her children are grown and out of the house, but she finds little time to socialize or engage in activities she used to enjoy. She feels guilty that she is not spending more time with her husband. Her husband is concerned about her workload and the constraints work has put on her life.

Jane decides to discuss this issue with the NP who oriented her to this job. She was comforted to find out that her mentor was working as much as she was, but they both wondered if the other providers were having similar experiences. At the next monthly staff meeting, they raised the issue, and Jane was surprised to find that most of the providers were taking work home at night. The group decided to bring this issue to administration as an unacceptable situation. The issue is now being discussed and strategies for improving the situation are being considered. As a result of Jane's contemplation about work stressors, she realized that over time she has stopped exercising, eating well, or having restorative sleep. A colleague suggested that she make an appointment with a nurse who practices Therapeutic Touch. After undergoing several treatments, Jane notes that she is sleeping better, has energy to exercise, and feels less anxious.

Discussion

Jane R. experienced many of the work stressors discussed in this chapter. These stressors compromised her quality of life and her ability to participate in self-care. Reaching out to a colleague and eventually the other providers at her workplace helped Jane to realize that she was not alone. The cooperation and collaboration of her work group provided strength in approaching the administration of the health center. Through this process she realized that she has not been participating in self-care. She was able to seek support from colleagues and to improve her ability to function and participate in self-care.

CONCLUSION

In the role of health-care providers in primary care, NPs are exposed to many stressors and challenges that can lead to frustration and self-criticism, as well as compassion fatigue and burnout. Nurse practitioners are aware of the importance of self-care strategies and health promotion when caring for patients. It is imperative that NP students and practicing NPs internalize these same concepts of self-care, resilience, and positivity, as well as maintain their sense of intentionality, to attain and preserve well-being and professional excellence.

The NP must remain open to new strategies and modalities for self-care in the quest to balance personal and professional life. Many professional and other groups advertise conferences, lectures, and webinars on self-care strategies. These strategies can also be taught as self-care strategies for patients.

Nursing is the art and science of human caring. Self-care for practitioners and patients requires continual efforts and openness to new strategies and modalities for health promotion, health education, and patient advocacy. The resilience and positivity developed through self-care strategies will allow NPs to direct their skills and intentionality toward creating a peaceful, harmonious environment and to share and model excellent care for patients. Box 82.1 presents an example of how to initiate and implement some of these strategies.

 For additional resources please visit **https://davisedge.fadavis.com/**

REFERENCES

American Holistic Nurses Association. What is self-care? www.ahna.org. Published 2017. https://www.ahna.org/Portals/66/images/Resources/What's%20in%20Your%20Self-Care%20Toolkit_Aug%202017_p12.jpg?ver=2016-12-20-181700-607 accessed 10-25-18.

Cuneo CL, et al. The effect of Reiki on work-related stress of the registered nurse. *J Holist Nurs* 2010;29:33–41. Retrieved from http://dx.doi.org/10.1177/089801010377294

Godfrey CM, et al. Care of self—care by other—care of other: The meaning of self-care from research, practice, policy and industry perspectives. *Int J Evid Based Healthc.* 2011;9:3–24.

Heffernan M, et al. Self-compassion and emotional intelligence in nurses. *Int J Nurs Pract.* 2010;16:366–373.

Henry J, Henry L. *The soul of the caring nurse: Stories and strategies for revitalizing professional passion.* Silver Spring, MD: American Nurses Association; 2004.

Institute of Medicine. The future of nursing: Leading change, advancing health. http://iom.edu/Reports/2010/The-Future-of-Nursing-Leading-Change-Advancing-Health.aspx. Published 2010.

Kravits K, et al. Self-care strategies for nurses: A psycho-educational intervention for stress reduction and the prevention of burnout. *Appl Nurs Res.* 2010;23:130–138.

Lombardo B, Eyre C. Compassion fatigue: A nurse's primer. *Online J Issues Nurs.* 2011;16(1):3.

Lorenz JM. Making a self-care plan. http://www.nursing.advance-web.com/Continuing-Education/CE-Articles/Making-a-Self-Care-Plan.aspx. Published 2012.

Marshall J, Zolnierek C. Supporting nurses through critical practice incidents: The nurse advocate role. *Nurse Leader*. 2012;10(2): 34–44.

McCann CM, et al. Resilience in the health professions: A review of recent literature. *Int J Wellbeing*. 2013;3:60–81.

Moeini B, et al. The impact of cognitive-behavioral stress management training program on job stress in hospital nurses: Applying PRECEDE model. *J Res Health Sci*. 2011;11(2):114–120.

Natale G. Reconnecting to nursing through Reiki. *Creative Nurs*. 2010;16:171–176.

National Organization of Nurse Practitioner Faculties. Nurse practitioner core competencies content: A delineation of suggested content specific to the NP core competencies. file:///C:/Users/zrahemi2013/Downloads/2017_NPCoreComps_with_Curric%20(2).pdf. Published 2017.

Sabo BM. Compassion fatigue and nursing work: Can we accurately capture the consequences of caring work? *Int J Nurs Pract*. 2006;12:136–142.

Stamm BH. Professional quality of life: Compassion Satisfaction & Fatigue Scales, Rev. IV (ProQOL), 1997–2008. http://www.proqol.org.

Sullivan P, et al. Grace under fire: Surviving and thriving in nursing by cultivating resilience. *Am Nurse Today*. 2012;7(12).

Thrasher C. The primary care nurse practitioner: Advocate for self-care. *J Am Acad Nurse Pract* 2002;14(3):113–117

Valent P. Diagnosis and treatment of helper stresses, traumas and illness. In: Figley CR, ed. *Treating compassion fatigue*. Hove, UK: Brunner-Routledge; 2002:17–37.

Watson J. Intentionality and caring-healing consciousness: A practice of transpersonal nursing. *Holist Nurs Pract*. 2002;16(4):12–19.

Wilkinson A, Whitehead L. Evolution of the concept of self-care and implications for nurses: Literature review. *Int J Nurs Stud*. 2009;46:1143–1148.

Yoder EA. Compassion fatigue in nurses. *Appl Nurs Res*. 2010;23: 191–197.

RESOURCES

American Holistic Nurses Association
> http://www.ahna.org/Default.aspx?Tabname=Self-care

American Nurses Association Healthy Nurse Initiative
> http://www.ana.org

Centers for Disease Control and Prevention
> http://www.cdc.gov/feature/handlingstress
> http://www.cdc.gov/features/healthyliving.html

MindTools
> http://www.mindtools.com

Pumpkin Hollow Retreat Center—Therapeutic Touch
> http://www.pumpkinhollow.org
> www.therapeutictouch.org

The Happiness Project
> http://www.gretchenrubin.com

Index